CURRENT

Pediatric Diagnosis & Treatment

CURRENT

Pediatric Diagnosis & Treatment

Tenth Edition

Edited by

WILLIAM E. HATHAWAY, MD
Professor Emeritus, Department of Pediatrics
University of Colorado School of Medicine (Denver)

JESSIE R. GROOTHUIS, MD
Associate Professor of Pediatrics
University of Colorado School of Medicine (Denver)

WILLIAM W. HAY, JR., MD
Professor of Pediatrics and Head, Section of Neonatology
University of Colorado School of Medicine (Denver)

JOHN W. PAISLEY, MD
Consultant, Pediatric Infectious Disease
Emmanuel Children's Healthcare Center (Portland, OR)

and Associate Authors

The Department of Pediatrics at The University of Colorado School of Medicine is affiliated with The Children's Hospital of Denver, Colorado.

APPLETON & LANGE
Norwalk, Connecticut/San Mateo, California

Notice: Our knowledge in clinical sciences is constantly changing. As new information becomes available, changes in treatment and in the use of drugs become necessary. The authors and the publisher of this volume have taken care to make certain that the doses of drugs and schedules of treatment are correct and compatible with the standards generally accepted at the time of publication. The reader is advised to consult carefully the instruction and information material included in the package insert of each drug or therapeutic agent before administration. This advice is especially important when using new or infrequently used drugs.

Copyright © 1991 by Appleton & Lange
A Publishing Division of Prentice Hall
9th Edition copyright © 1987 by Appleton & Lange

91 92 93 94 95 / 10 9 8 7 6 5 4 3 2 1

Prentice Hall International (UK) Limited, *London*
Prentice Hall of Australia Pty. Limited, *Sydney*
Prentice Hall Canada, Inc., *Toronto*
Prentice Hall Hispanoamericana, S.A., *Mexico*
Prentice Hall of India Private Limited, *New Delhi*
Prentice Hall of Japan, Inc., *Tokyo*
Simon & Schuster Asia Pte. Ltd., *Singapore*
Editora Prentice Hall do Brasil Ltda., *Rio de Janeiro*
Prentice Hall, *Englewood Cliffs, New Jersey*

ISBN 0-8385-1429-4
ISSN 0093-8556

Production Editor: Christine Langan
Designer: Steven Byrum

PRINTED IN THE UNITED STATES OF AMERICA

Table of Contents

Contributors

Steven H. Abman, MD
Respiratory Tract & Mediastinum
Associate Professor of Pediatrics, Section of Pediatric Pulmonary and Critical Care Medicine, Department of Pediatrics, University of Colorado School of Medicine.

Frank J. Accurso, MD
Respiratory Tract & Mediastinum
Associate Professor of Pediatrics, Section of Pediatric Pulmonary and Critical Care Medicine, Department of Pediatrics, University of Colorado School of Medicine.

Roger M. Barkin, MD, MPH
Emergencies & Accidents
Chairman, Department of Pediatrics and Newborn Medicine, Rose Medical Center; Professor, Section of Emergency Medicine, Department of Surgery, University of Colorado School of Medicine.

Frederick C. Battaglia, MD
The Newborn Infant
Professor of Pediatrics, Section of Neonatology, Department of Pediatrics, University of Colorado School of Medicine.

Gary K. Belanger, DDS
Teeth and Periodontium
Associate Professor and Chairman, Division of Pediatric Dentistry, University of Colorado School of Dentistry.

Stephen Berman, MD
Ear, Nose, & Throat
Associate Professor of Pediatrics, Section of Ambulatory Pediatrics, Department of Pediatrics, University of Colorado School of Medicine.

John D. Burrington, MD
Emergencies & Accidents
Surgeon, Steamboat Springs, CO.

Bonnie W. Camp, MD, PhD
Developmental Disorders
Professor of Pediatrics and Psychiatry, Section of Developmental and Behavioral Pediatrics, University of Colorado School of Medicine; Director, John F. Kennedy Child Development Center, University of Colorado Health Sciences Center.

Paul S. Casamassimo, DDS, MS
Teeth and Periodontium
Professor of Pediatric Dentistry, The Ohio State University; Chief of Dentistry, Columbus Children's Hospital.

R. Barkley Clark, MD
Psychosocial Aspects of Pediatrics & Psychiatric Disorders
Assistant Clinical Professor, Division of Child Psychiatry, Department of Psychiatry, University of Colorado Health Sciences Center.

Carolyn R. Comer, MD
Allergic Disorders
Staff Physician, Department of Pediatrics, National Jewish Center for Immunology and Respiratory Medicine, Denver.

Anthony G. Durmowicz, MD
Diagnostic & Therapeutic Procedures
Senior Fellow, Section of Pediatric Pulmonary and Critical Care Medicine, Department of Pediatrics; Research Fellow, The Cardiovascular-Pulmonary Research Laboratory, University of Colorado School of Medicine.

Robert E. Eilert, MD
Orthopedics
Chairman, Department of Orthopedic Surgery, The Children's Hospital, Denver; Associate Clinical Professor of Orthopedic Surgery, University of Colorado School of Medicine.

Philip P. Ellis, MD
Eye
Professor and Chairman, Department of Ophthalmology, University of Colorado School of Medicine.

Leland L. Fan, MD
Respiratory Tract & Mediastinum
Associate Professor of Pediatrics, Section of Pediatric Pulmonary and Critical Care Medicine, Department of Pediatrics, University of Colorado School of Medicine.

Cynthia R. Gelman, BS Pharm
Drug Therapy
Consultant, Rocky Mountain Poison & Drug Center, Denver.

John H. Githens, MD
Hematologic Disorders
Professor Emeritus, Department of Pediatrics, University of Colorado School of Medicine.

Mary P. Glodé, MD
Infections: Bacterial & Spirochetal
Associate Professor of Pediatrics, Section of Pediatric Infectious Disease, Department of Pediatrics, University of Colorado School of Medicine; Associate Director of Infectious Disease, The Children's Hospital, Denver.

Stephen I. Goodman, MD
Inborn Errors of Metabolism
Professor of Pediatrics and Head, Section of Genetics, Metabolism and Birth Defects, Department of Pediatrics, University of Colorado School of Medicine.

Ronald W. Gotlin, MD
Endocrine Disorders: Diagnostic & Therapeutic Procedures
Professor of Pediatrics and Head, Section of Endocrinology, Department of Pediatrics, University of Colorado School of Medicine.

Carol L. Greene, MD
Inborn Errors of Metabolism
Assistant Professor of Pediatrics, Section of Genetics, Metabolism and Birth Defects, Department of Pediatrics, University of Colorado School of Medicine.

Randi Jenssen Hagerman, MD
Growth & Development
Associate Professor of Pediatrics and Head, Section of Developmental and Behavioral Pediatrics, Department of Pediatrics, University of Colorado School of Medicine.

K. Michael Hambidge, MD, ScD
Normal Childhood Nutrition & Its Disorders
Professor of Pediatrics, Section of Gastroenterology and Nutrition and Director, Pediatric Clinical Research Center, Department of Pediatrics, University of Colorado School of Medicine.

Keith B. Hammond, MS, FIMLS
Normal Biochemical & Hematologic Values
Senior Instructor of Pediatrics and Pathology, and Director of Pediatric Clinical Research Center Laboratory, University of Colorado School of Medicine.

William E. Hathaway, MD
Hematologic Disorders
Professor Emeritus, Department of Pediatrics, University of Colorado School of Medicine.

Anthony R. Hayward, MD, PhD
Immunodeficiency
Professor of Pediatrics and Medicine and Head, Section of Allergy and Immunology, University of Colorado School of Medicine.

J. Roger Hollister, MD
Rheumatic Diseases
Associate Professor of Pediatrics and Medicine, Section of Allergy and Immunology, University of Colorado School of Medicine; Senior Staff Physician, Department of Pediatrics, National Jewish Hospital and Research Center, Denver.

David W. Kaplan, MD, MPH
Adolescence
Associate Professor of Pediatrics and Head, Section of Adolescent Medicine, Department of Pediatrics, University of Colorado School of Medicine.

Georgeanna J. Klingensmith, MD
Endocrine Disorders
Associate Professor of Pediatrics, Section of Endocrinology, Department of Pediatrics, University of Colorado School of Medicine.

Nancy F. Krebs, MD, MS
Normal Childhood Nutrition & Its Disorders
Fellow, Section of Gastroenterology and Nutrition, Department of Pediatrics, University of Colorado School of Medicine.

Gary L. Larsen, MD
Respiratory Tract & Mediastinum
Associate Professor of Pediatrics and Head, Section of Pediatric Pulmonary and Critical Care Medicine, Department of Pediatrics, University of Colorado School of Medicine; Staff Member, Department of Pediatrics, National Jewish Center for Immunology and Respiratory Medicine, Denver.

Brian A. Lauer, MD
Infections: Bacterial & Spirochetal
Chief, Department of Pediatrics, and Co-Director, Clinical Virology Laboratory, Emanuel Children's Healthcare Center, Emanuel Hospital and Health Center; Adjunct Professor of Pediatrics, Oregon Health Sciences University, Portland.

Myron J. Levin, MD

Infections: Viral & Rickettsial

Professor of Pediatrics and Medicine and Head, Section of Infectious Disease, Department of Pediatrics, University of Colorado School of Medicine.

Gary M. Lum, MD

Kidney & Urinary Tract

Associate Professor of Pediatrics and Head, Section of Pediatric Renal Medicine, Department of Medicine, University of Colorado School of Medicine.

James V. Lustig, MD

History & Physical Examination; Fluid & Electrolyte Therapy

Associate Professor and Vice-Chairman, Department of Pediatrics, University of Colorado School of Medicine; Director, Medical Education, The Children's Hospital, Denver.

Kathleen A. Mammel, MD

Adolescence

Assistant Professor of Pediatrics, Section of Adolescent Medicine, Department of Pediatrics, University of Colorado School of Medicine.

David K. Manchester, MD

Genetics & Dysmorphology

Co-Director, Division of Genetic Services, The Children's Hospital, Denver; Associate Professor of Pediatrics and Pharmacology, Section of Genetics, Metabolism and Birth Defects, Department of Pediatrics, University of Colorado School of Medicine.

Paul G. Moe, MD

Neurologic & Muscular Disorders

Professor of Pediatrics and Neurology, Section of Child Neurology, Department of Pediatrics, University of Colorado School of Medicine.

John W. Ogle, MD

Infections: Bacterial & Spirochetal

Assistant Professor, Section of Pediatric Infectious Disease, Department of Pediatrics; Director, Child Health Associate Program, University of Colorado School of Medicine.

Malcolm Packer, MD

Critical Care

Critical Care Fellow, Section of Pediatric Pulmonary and Critical Care Medicine, Department of Pediatrics, University of Colorado School of Medicine.

John W. Paisley, MD

Infections: Viral & Rickettsial; Infections: Parasitic & Mycotic

Consultant, Pediatric Infectious Disease, Emanuel Children's Healthcare Center, Portland, OR.

David S. Pearlman, MD

Allergic Disorders

Clinical Professor of Pediatrics, University of Colorado School of Medicine; Senior Staff Physician, Pediatrics, National Jewish Center for Immunology and Respiratory Medicine, Denver.

Robert G. Peterson, MD PhD

Drug Therapy

Professor of Pediatrics and Pharmacology, University of Ottawa; Medical Director, Poison Information Centre, and Chief of Department of Pediatrics, Children's Hospital of Eastern Ontario, Canada.

Adam A. Rosenberg, MD

The Newborn Infant

Associate Professor of Pediatrics, Section of Neonatology, Department of Pediatrics, University of Colorado School of Medicine.

Barry H. Rumack, MD

Poisoning; Drug Therapy

Professor of Pediatrics and Head, Section of Clinical Pharmacology and Toxicology, University of Colorado School of Medicine; Director, Rocky Mountain Poison & Drug Center, Denver.

Barton D. Schmitt, MD

Ambulatory Pediatrics; Ear, Nose, & Throat

Professor of Pediatrics, Section of General Pediatrics, Department of Pediatrics, University of Colorado School of Medicine; Director of Consultative Services, The Children's Hospital, Denver.

Alan Seay, MD

Neurologic & Muscular Disorders

Associate Professor of Pediatrics and Neurology and Head, Section of Child Neurology, Department of Pediatrics, University of Colorado School of Medicine.

Arnold Silverman, MD

Gastrointestinal Tract; Liver & Pancreas

Professor of Pediatrics, Section of Gastroenterology and Nutrition, Department of Pediatrics, University of Colorado School of Medicine; Director of Pediatrics, Denver General Hospital.

Ronald J. Sokol, MD
Liver & Pancreas
Associate Professor of Pediatrics, Section of
Gastroenterology and Nutrition, Department of
Pediatrics, University of Colorado School of
Medicine.

Judith M. Sondheimer, MD
Gastrointestinal Tract
Associate Professor of Pediatrics and Head,
Section of Gastroenterology and Nutrition,
Department of Pediatrics, University of
Colorado School of Medicine.

David G. Spoerke, MS, RPh
Poisoning

Kurt R. Stenmark, MD
Critical Care
Associate Professor of Pediatrics, Section of
Pediatric Pulmonary and Critical Care
Medicine, Department of Pediatrics, and The
Cardiovascular-Pulmonary Research
Laboratory and Webb-Waring Lung Institute,
University of Colorado School of Medicine.

Janet Stewart, MD
Genetics & Dysmorphology
Associate Professor of Pediatrics, Section of
Genetics, Metabolism and Birth Defects,
Department of Pediatrics, University of
Colorado School of Medicine.

Eva Sujansky, MD
Genetics & Dysmorphology
Associate Professor of Pediatrics and
Biochemistry, Biophysics and Genetics,
Section of Genetics, Metabolism and Birth
Defects, Department of Pediatrics, University
of Colorado School of Medicine.

James K. Todd, MD
Antimicrobial Therapy of Pediatric Infections
Professor of Pediatrics and Microbiology/
Immunology, Section of Pediatric Infectious
Disease, Department of Pediatrics, University
of Colorado School of Medicine; Director of
Infectious Disease, The Children's Hospital,
Denver.

David G. Tubergen, MD
Neoplastic Diseases
Professor of Pediatrics, Section of
Hematology/Oncology, Department of
Pediatrics, University of Colorado School of
Medicine; Medical Director, The Children's
Hospital, Denver.

William L. Weston, MD
Skin
Professor of Dermatology and Pediatrics;
Chairman, Department of Dermatology,
University of Colorado School of Medicine.

Carl W. White, MD
Respiratory Tract & Mediastinum
Associate Professor of Pediatrics, Section of
Pediatric Pulmonary and Critical Care
Medicine, Department of Pediatrics,
University of Colorado School of Medicine;
Senior Staff Physician, National Jewish Center
for Immunology and Respiratory Medicine,
Denver.

Andrew M. Wiesenthal, MD
Immunization
Clinical Assistant Professor of Pediatrics,
Department of Pediatrics, University of
Colorado School of Medicine; Attending
Physician, Colorado Permanente Medical
Group, Denver.

James W. Wiggins, Jr., MD
Cardiovascular Diseases
Associate Professor of Pediatrics, Section
of Pediatric Cardiology, Department of
Pediatrics, University of Colorado School
of Medicine.

Robert R. Wolfe, MD
Cardiovascular Diseases
Professor of Pediatrics and Head, Section
of Pediatric Cardiology, Department of
Pediatrics, University of Colorado School
of Medicine.

Preface

The 10th edition of *Current Pediatric Diagnosis & Treatment* features practical, up-to-date, well-referenced information on the care of children from infancy through adolescence. *CPDT* emphasizes the clinical aspects of pediatric care while also covering the important underlying principles.

Intended Audience

Like all Lange medical books, *CPDT* provides a concise, yet comprehensive, source of current, clear, and correct information. Students will find *CPDT* an authoritative introduction to pediatrics and an excellent source for reference and review. Interns and residents will appreciate the concise descriptions of diseases and diagnostic procedures. Pediatricians, family practitioners, nurses, and other health care providers who work with infants and children will find *CPDT* a useful reference on all aspects of pediatric care.

Coverage

Thirty-nine chapters cover a wide range of topics, including growth and development of the healthy child, preventive medicine, and diagnosis and treatment of specific disorders. A wealth of tables and figures offer ready access to such important information as anti-infective agents, drug dosages, immunization schedules, differential diagnoses, and developmental screening tests. The final chapter serves as a handy guide to normal laboratory values.

New to this Edition

The 10th edition of *CPDT* is an up-to-date, comprehensive pediatric treatise and represents a significant revision and improvement of this classic book. The original intent of Drs Kempe, Silver, and O'Brien was kept in mind as the new team of editors and contributors substantially revised the book, providing recent medical advances, and increasing the book's emphasis on ambulatory care, cost effectiveness, and sensitivity and specificity of diagnostic tests. As editors and practicing pediatricians, we have tried to ensure that each chapter reflects the needs and realities of day-to-day practice. Sixteen of the 39 chapters are totally new; many others have been substantially revised. Every chapter has undergone revision, and 49 new figures and 155 new tables have been added.

The tenth edition of *Current Pediatric Diagnosis & Treatment* includes the following new chapters:

- The Newborn Infant
- Adolescence
- Critical Care
- Respiratory Tract & Mediastinum
- Neurologic & Muscular Disorders
- Psychosocial Aspects of Pediatrics and Psychiatric Disorders
- Infectious Diseases
- Inborn Errors of Metabolism
- Genetics & Dysmorphology
- Fluid & Electrolyte Therapy
- Antimicrobial Therapy of Pediatric Infections
- Immunization
- History & Physical Examination
- Growth & Development

Acknowledgements

We wish to thank Kate Palmer and the section of Pediatric Hematology-Oncology for organizational support.

William E. Hathaway, MD
Jessie R. Groothuis, MD
William Hay, MD
John Paisley, MD

October, 1990

History & Physical Examination

James V. Lustig, MD

PEDIATRIC HISTORY

The emphasis placed on anticipatory guidance and prevention of disease makes pediatrics unique among medical disciplines. To achieve disease prevention and provide anticipatory guidance, the pediatrician must have a comprehensive longitudinal data base depicting the child's progress to the present moment and pointing toward problems that the physician must anticipate. This emphasis results in certain unique aspects of the pediatric history. Addressing growth and development is a major goal in pediatrics, because children's ability to take their place in society is critical. The future of a child who fails to develop is clearly jeopardized. This must be recognized and treated early and effectively. Children's diets reflect much about their environment and growth. It is essential for the pediatrician to obtain data about the child's diet, especially the child's present diet.

Everyone is familiar with the importance of immunization, yet the number of children who have not received their full primary set of immunizations remains disappointingly high. This reflects not only the expense of immunization and the concerns of parents regarding the safety of immunizations but also our need to improve both our record keeping systems and our effectiveness in getting children into our offices to receive these important treatments.

The history must include information about the family's structure and the environment in which a child is reared. Children need a supportive, nurturing, and enabling environment. It is the physician's responsibility to help the family provide appropriate stimulation that simultaneously challenges children to develop and supports their success in development. An understanding of the social structure of a child's family is essential because it helps the physician interpret information elicited from the family of a child who presents with an acute problem.

Often, patients do not provide their own history. Usually one or both parents interpret the child's actions to the physician, who then reinterprets the parents' summary. The problem of not gaining the history directly from the patient is exacerbated by the vagueness of the complaints voiced by parents who bring children to the office. These vague complaints are often really statements of parents' concerns about the child's progress. Instead of hearing that Andy has had a "warm, red, tender, swollen knee for 2 days," the pediatrician is much more likely to hear that Andy has not played well this week or that he no longer wants to play on the soccer team. Many visits are precipitated by problems at school, such as poor grades or poor peer interaction. To separate organic from nonorganic illness, and to intervene appropriately without subjecting the child to inordinate testing, the physician must understand the family and its hopes and concerns for a given child. It is often necessary to ask specifically what it is a parent wishes to address and to discern what truly precipitated the visit by the patient and family. It is essential to elicit as much of the history as possible directly from the patient. Direct histories not only provide firsthand information but also reinforce the child's sense of self, give the child a degree of control over a potentially threatening situation, and may reveal family stress.

Ideally, a family's first trip to a pediatrician's office should be before the child is born. A prenatal visit goes a long way toward establishing rapport and helping the family to enjoy good, structured interaction with the physician. Families who know that a physician employs an extensive anticipatory guidance program are more confident that their concerns regarding growth, development, diet, and environment will be addressed. This also provides a natural framework for anticipating and preventing problems in these areas. Anticipating the information needed for each type of patient encounter helps the pediatrician structure inquiries, obtain data efficiently, and provide consistent patient care.

A child's medical record can be considered a longitudinal comprehensive data base. For this reason, different types of office visits need to be documented to provide comprehensive information, yet in a way that does not make data collection and maintenance of records burdensome to the physician or the office staff. The components of a comprehensive pediatric history are detailed in Table 1–1. Specific data elements are not included; rather, the goals of each component are listed.

Table 1–1. The pediatric historical data base.[1]

Demographic Data
Name, date of birth, sex, race, parents names (first and last), siblings' names, and the patient's nickname.

Problem List
The list of *all* of the child's problems, in a prominent place in the chart, including the date a problem became manifest, treatments employed, and the date of resolution.

Drug Allergies
Any drug allergies, prominently displayed in the data base, including the drug precipitating the reaction, the nature of the reaction, the treatment needed, and the date. (A medical alert bracelet should be obtained for all children with a significant reaction.)

Current Medications
The dose, vehicle, and frequency of medications currently employed by children who require chronic administration of medications.

Reasons for Visit
The patient's or parents' concerns, stated in their own words whenever possible, as a focus for the visit. A traditional "chief complaint" may be misleading.

Present Illness
A crisp, chronologic summary of the problems necessitating a visit, including the duration, progression, exacerbation, amelioration, and associations. The reactions of the historian, the patient, and the family to the problem are important in understanding the reason for the visit.

Past History

General State of Health
A statement regarding the child's functionality and general well-being, including a summary record of past significant illnesses, injuries, hospitalizations, and procedures, as well as decisions made about them, eg, the prophylactic use of penicillin due to the presence of rheumatic carditis.

Screening Procedures
The results of and actions taken in response to all screening procedures, maintained as a distinct part of the medical, including newborn screening, vision and hearing screening, any health screens, or screening labs. (Developmental screening results are maintained in the development section.)

Birth History
Mother: Health during pregnancy, including illnesses, medications, drugs used, complications of pregnancy; duration and ease of labor; form of delivery; analgesics/anesthetics used; need for monitoring; and labor complications.

Child: The birth weight, estimated gestational age, Apgar scores, and problems in the neonatal period. (These data often presage a child's subsequent development.)

Diet
Eating patterns, likes and dislikes, use of vitamins, parental assessment of eating, estimate of calories ingested, and relative amounts of carbohydrate, fat, and protein in the diet. (These data provide important insights not only into the nutritional adequacy of the diet but also familial interactions, attitudes, and concerns.)

Immunizations
The date of each immunization administered, the vaccine lot number, any reaction, and any contraindication to immunization, eg, immunodeficiency or evolving neurologic problem.

Family History
Should include, according to some authors, information about the illnesses of relatives (and the patient's relationship to those relatives) as well as a socioeconomic profile. (Maintaining these data in 2 distinct sections makes review of the history easier and more productive.)

Development
In 4 sections, (1) attainment of developmental milestones (including developmental testing results); (2) social habits and milestones (toilet habits, play, major activities, sleep patterns, discipline, development of relationships); (3) psychosocial data (family constellations, parents' education and occupation, religious preference, and stressors); and (4) school progress. (Maintaining date in distinct tables may be useful.)

Sexual History
Familial sexual attitudes, sex education, sexual development, sexual activity, sexually transmitted diseases, and birth control measures.

Reviews of Systems (ROS)
This area tends to be overlooked because of the work required to obtain a complete ROS and integrate data from the ROS into the patient's problems list and care plan. A focused ROS is essential if any problem is to be addressed adequately. For example, if a child is wheezing, it is important to know if the youngster required ventilatory support in the newborn period, had an antecedent or concurrent illness, has chronic diarrhea, or demonstrated failure to thrive. In such a case, it is also important for the examiner to determine whether (1) an atopic diathesis is present, (2) there is evidence of cardiac disease, (3) chronic or nighttime cough is present, and (4) symptoms are precipitated or exacerbated by exercise.

[1]The elements of this table should be included in a child's medical record. The medical record should be structured to allow easy review or updating of all data needed over time so that acute care visits are not disrupted.

TYPES OF VISITS

Prenatal Visits

A prenatal visit can greatly enhance a physician's relationship with a family. It enables the physician to learn about a family's desires, concerns, and fears regarding the anticipated birth of a child. Further, this visit fosters the development of trust in the pediatrician. If the child develops a neonatal problem, the physician who has not already met the family may have difficulty establishing rapport. Prenatal visits need not take a long time. They should be conducted in a relaxed atmosphere, with both parents present whenever possible. This is often a good time to elicit a family's medical history. The position (role) of the anticipated child in the family should be determined if possible. At this time, the physician should also elicit information about any problems that have occurred during the pregnancy.

If the family is new to a practice, the prenatal visit provides an easy way to acquaint them with the way that the practice is conducted. Parents want to know to whom they will speak when they call the office, when they may bring in children for acute care visits, and how their concerns regarding a child's developmental progress will be met. At the termination of the interview, the physician should have some understanding of the family's health care needs and should also be aware of the support systems available to aid the family through times of stress.

Although the prenatal visit is traditionally thought of in regard to new patients, it is often desirable to schedule a visit before all subsequent births in the family. This provides a relaxed forum in which the family can update and refocus their concerns and needs.

Acute Care Visits

Owing to the episodic nature of pediatric practice and the demands on a pediatrician's time, the acute care visit must be an efficient, structured part of the office routine. Office support personnel should have elicited the reason for the visit and provided the physician with a brief synopsis of the child's symptoms. Support personnel should list known drug allergies on the encounter form, which the physician should review in anticipation of the need to use medication. The historian should present the chronology of events related to the present problem and call attention to pertinent parts of the comprehensive record, such as immunization status, past illnesses, and related problems. The physical exam should be carefully detailed. The impression must be clearly shown. The record should include supporting laboratory data and should document treatments rendered and anticipatory guidance given, such as when to return to the office if the problem is not ameliorated.

Hospital Visits

Fortunately, hospital stays are not as frequent a part of pediatric care as they were in the past. When necessary, however, hospitalization is a time of stress for the patient and the patient's family. The physician must put aside time not only to answer questions about the immediate problem but also to give support and reassurance. Whenever possible, the patient must be included in discussions of anticipated treatment and progress. Because the history of a child's progress during hospitalization is often derived from nurses, technicians, house staff, and colleagues, the physician needs to interpret data not derived firsthand. Knowledge of the child's immunization status, history of past illnesses, allergy history, and problem list is important in the successful treatment of the hospitalized child with an acute problem.

Health Maintenance Visits

Because of the emphasis pediatricians place on prevention of disease and anticipatory guidance, the health maintenance visit has become a standard part

of practice. The goal of these visits is not only to provide anticipatory guidance but also to promote the health of the patient by ensuring that immunizations are up to date, no significant health problems have developed, growth continues to be normal, and development is progressing as expected.

The American Academy of Pediatrics, through its Committee on Practice and Ambulatory Management, has developed recommendations for preventive pediatric health care. These recommendations offer general guidelines for scheduling visits for children of different ages (Fig 1–1). Examples of specific issues to be addressed at different ages are presented in Table 1–2.

Preschool Visits

A trip to the physician's office before the child first starts school represents a special health maintenance visit. During the preschool visit, it is important for the physician to address development, elimination patterns, social behaviors, and diet. Examining development and social behavior helps the family anticipate problems the child may have at school and allows the family to ease the child's transition from home life to school. Control of bladder and bowel functions is important to the success of a child entering school. If there is a problem, it should be addressed before the child enters school, if possible. Traditionally, immunizations are given at the preschool visit. Screening of vision and hearing is also important at this time. Topics addressed during subsequent visits should include assessment of the past year's school performance, anticipated problems, and a critical review of both growth and development.

Sports Physicals

A physical examination is often needed before participation in organized sports programs. Time should be allotted not only to perform the physical exam but also to ask questions about the safety of the activities. What kind of protective equipment is provided? Are the supervisors and coaches trained to instruct children? What health care facilities are available? Will the patient require medication during competition (eg, beta agonists for the patient with exercise-induced asthma)? Will the patient be exposed to unnecessary hazards, such as a taking a turn at bat without a safety helmet or performing on the balance beam without a spotter? Does the program emphasize learning teamwork and skills, or is competition more important? Answering these questions can protect the child during an important experience of childhood.

COMPREHENSIVE PEDIATRIC HISTORY

Obtaining a comprehensive pediatric history is a major undertaking, given the time constraints of

RECOMMENDATIONS FOR PREVENTIVE PEDIATRIC HEALTH CARE
Committee on Practice and Ambulatory Medicine

Each child and family is unique; therefore these **Recommendations for Preventive Pediatric Health Care** are designed for the care of children who are receiving competent parenting, have no manifestations of any important health problems, and are growing and developing in satisfactory fashion. **Additional visits may become necessary** if circumstances suggest variations from normal. These guidelines represent a consensus by the Committee on Practice and Ambulatory Medicine in consultation with the membership of the American Academy of Pediatrics through the Chapter

Presidents. The Committee emphasizes the great importance of **continuity of care** in comprehensive health supervision and the need to avoid **fragmentation of care.**

A **prenatal visit** by the parents for anticipatory guidance and pertinent medical history is strongly recommended.

Health supervision should begin with medical care of the newborn in the hospital.

AGE[2]	INFANCY						EARLY CHILDHOOD					LATE CHILDHOOD					ADOLESCENCE[1]			
	By 1 mo.	2 mos.	4 mos.	6 mos.	9 mos.	12 mos.	15 mos.	18 mos.	24 mos.	3 yrs.	4 yrs.	5 yrs.	6 yrs.	8 yrs.	10 yrs.	12 yrs.	14 yrs.	16 yrs.	18 yrs.	20+ yrs.
HISTORY Initial/Interval	●	●	●	●	●	●	●	●	●	●	●	●	●	●	●	●	●	●	●	●
MEASUREMENTS Height and Weight	●	●	●	●	●	●	●	●	●	●	●	●	●	●	●	●	●	●	●	●
Head Circumference	●	●	●	●	●	●														
Blood Pressure										●	●	●	●	●	●	●	●	●	●	●
SENSORY SCREENING Vision	S	S	S	S	S	S	S	S	S	S	O	O	O	O	S	O	O	S	O	O
Hearing	S	S	S	S	S	S	S	S	S	S	O	●	S[3]	S[3]	S[3]	O	S	S	O	S
DEVEL./BEHAV.[4] ASSESSMENT	●	●	●	●	●	●	●	●	●	●	●	●	●	●	●	●	●	●	●	●
PHYSICAL EXAMINATION[5]	●	●	●	●	●	●	●	●	●	●	●	●	●	●	●	●	●	●	●	●
PROCEDURES[6] Hered./Metabolic[7] Screening	●																			
Immunization[8]		●	●	●			●	●		●		●					●			
Tuberculin Test[9]	←——————————————●						←————————●										←——————————————●			
Hematocrit or Hemoglobin[10]	←————————●						←————————●							●————→			←——————————————●			
Urinalysis[11]	←————————●						←————————●										←——————————————●			
ANTICIPATORY[12] GUIDANCE	●	●	●	●	●	●	●	●	●	●	●	●	●	●	●	●	●	●	●	●
INITIAL DENTAL[13] REFERRAL										●										

1. Adolescent related issues (e.g., psychosocial, emotional, substance usage, and reproductive health) may necessitate more frequent health supervision.
2. If a child comes under care for the first time at any point on the schedule, or if any items are not accomplished at the suggested age, the schedule should be brought up to date at the earliest possible time.
3. At these points, history may suffice: if problem suggested, a standard testing method should be employed.
4. By history and appropriate physical examination: if suspicious, by specific objective developmental testing.
5. At each visit, a complete physical examination is essential, with infant totally unclothed, older child undressed and suitably draped.
6. These may be modified, depending upon entry point into schedule and individual need.
7. Metabolic screening (e.g., thyroid, PKU, galactosemia) should be done according to state law.
8. Schedule(s) per Report of Committee on Infectious Disease, *1986 Red Book.*

9. For low risk groups, the Committee on Infectious Diseases recommends the following options: ① no routine testing or ② testing at three times—infancy, preschool, and adolescence. For high risk groups, annual TB skin testing is recommended.
10. Present medical evidence suggests the need for reevaluation of the frequency and timing of hemoglobin or hematocrit tests. One determination is therefore suggested during each time period. Performance of additional tests is left to the individual practice experience.
11. Present medical evidence suggests the need for reevaluation of the frequency and timing of urinalyses. One determination is therefore suggested during each time period. Performance of additional tests is left to the individual practice experience.
12. Appropriate discussion and counselling should be an integral part of each visit for care.
13. Subsequent examinations as prescribed by dentist.

N.B.: **Special chemical, immunologic, and endocrine testing** are usually carried out upon specific indications. Testing other than newborn (e.g., inborn errors of metabolism, sickle disease, lead) are discretionary with the physician.

Key: ● =to be performed: S=subjective, by history: O=objective, by a standard testing method.

September 1987

Figure 1–1. Recommendations for preventive pediatric health care. Reproduced, with permission, from the American Academy of Pediatrics Policy Statement, "Recommendations for Preventive Pediatric Health Care." *Pediatrics* (March) 1988;**81**:3. © 1988 American Academy of Pediatrics.

Table 1–2. Specific goals of selected health maintenance visits.

Initial Office Visit	2-Month Visit	5-Year Visit

History
1. Pregnancy, delivery, and neonatal history if not previously obtained.
2. Family history if not previously obtained.
3. How are the baby and family adjusting to home?
   A. Comfort level.
   B. Sleep and feeding patterns.
   C. Support Systems.
   D. Reactions of siblings.
   E. Elimination patterns.
   F. Is the child disruptive?
	Interval history (new problems).	1. Is the family ready for the child to go to school?
		2. Be careful to review bowel and bladder control.
		3. Does the child interact easily with others?
		4. Is separation from the parents a problem?

Diet 1. Frequency of feeding. 2. Duration. 3. Specifics of breast-feeding. 4. Formula preparation and amount consumed.	1. If mother is breast-feeding, is it beneficial to baby and family? 2. Familial pressure to introduce solid foods into diet. 3. Night feedings. 4. Check need for vitamin supplementation.	1. Review favorite foods. 2. Estimate caloric intake. 3. Will diet change for both mother and child due to child being in school?
Development 1. Regards face. 2. Smiles. 3. Moves all extremities. 4. Responds to noise. 5. Vocalizes. 6. Lifts head.	1. Smiles spontaneously. 2. Grasps rattle? 3. Follows object trajectory through 180 degrees. 4. Laughs. 5. Lifts head.	1. Copies a rectangle. 2. Draws a man with 6 identifiable parts. 3. Recognizes 6 colors. 4. Defines opposites. 5. Capable of backward heel-to-toe walk. 6. Knows letters of the alphabet. 7. Knows name, address, phone. 8. Dresses without supervision.
Screening 1. Subjective assessment of hearing and vision. 2. Response to noise, light.	1. Same as initial visit. 2. Informal vision screening.	1. Hearing. 2. Vision.
Physical 1. Complete exam. 2. BP, OFC, length, weight. 3. Growth chart. 4. Umbilical cord. 5. Congenital anomalies. 6. Birthmarks.	1. Monitor growth carefully. 2. Obtain blood pressure reading. 3. Check posture. 4. Check coordination.	Growth chart.
Procedures 1. Review newborn screening test. 2. Collect specimens for screening tests if there was early discharge from the nursery.	1. Hemoglobin. 2. Urinalysis.	
Immunizations	1. DPT. 2. OPV.	1. DPT. 2. OPV.
Anticipatory Guidance 1. Stress need for car seat if not obtained. 2. Review normal infant behavior patterns. 3. Anticipate adjustment of siblings to new baby if not already addressed. 4. Review symptoms of colic or food intolerance. 5. Give information about appropriate diet for age.	1. Immunization reactions. 2. Check family history for immunization prior to OPV. 3. Infant stimulation.	1. Review accident-prevention measures. 2. Anticipate school problems.

most pediatric offices. Many offices use questionnaires to facilitate the development of the comprehensive history. Such questionnaires, which are filled out prior to a patient's visit, enable the physician to anticipate problems and to learn about the patient before the visit takes place. They make office time more productive, allowing the physician to address problems in detail, while reviewing and dismissing areas that are not a problem. The longitudinally important elements of the comprehensive data base must be maintained in the medical records so that they are readily accessible as the child grows. In many practices, the front page of the medical record includes some minimal demographic data, a problem list, known drug allergies, current medication(s), and immunization status.

The Physical Exam

Detailed analysis of the pediatric examination is beyond the scope of this chapter. However, the approach to the exam and certain elements of the examination will be emphasized. Table 1–3 illustrates how the exam can be focused to provide information about key issues at different ages.

A. Approaching the Child: Adequate time must be allotted to allow the child to become familiar with

Table 1–3. Focusing the physical exam during health supervision visits.

Newborn
1. Congenital anomalies
2. Length, weight, head circumference
3. Fontanelles
4. Gestational age
5. Red reflex
6. Hip dislocation
7. Femoral and lower extremity pulses
8. Jaundice
9. Location of testes
10. Reaction to sound/light

6 months
1. Interaction with
   a. Parent
   b. Environment
2. Length, weight, head circumference
3. Vision and hearing
   a. Verbalization
   b. Strabismus
4. Developmental assessment
   a. Rolls over
   b. Sits up without support
   c. Vocalizes
   d. Laughs
5. Congenital anomalies

24 Months
1. Interaction
   a. Familial
   b. With examiner
   c. With environment
2. Length, weight, circumference
3. Hearing/vision
4. Developmental
   a. Climbs stairs while holding rail
   b. Vocabulary
     1. > 20 words
     2. 2-word phrases
   c. Response to commands
5. Sphincter tone

10 Years
1. Height, weight
2. Scoliosis
3. Tanner staging
4. Interaction

the examiner. Care must be taken to ensure that interactions with the child are appropriate for age and developmental level. A gentle approach, friendly manner, and a quiet voice help establish a setting that yields a productive physical exam and does not threaten the patient unduly. A physician who cannot establish rapport with the patient should perform the exam efficiently and systematically. In any pediatric exam, invasive or painful procedures, or those perceived as such by the child (eg, examining the ears of a toddler), should be done at the end of the examination.

Because the history is often incomplete, and since young children may perceive the examination as threatening and become fussy, inspection is very important. The examiner should make observations throughout the duration of the visit, paying special attention to how the child interacts with the environment. Observation also affords the examiner a chance to assess parent-child interactions.

Clothing should be removed slowly and gently to avoid chilling or threatening the child. Modesty, whenever a child exhibits it, should be respected, and drapes should be provided.

The sequence of the examination is important. Those areas in which the child's cooperation is needed should be addressed first. Painful or unpleasant procedures should be postponed until the end of the examination.

Examination tables are convenient, but a parent's lap is a safe haven for a toddler or young child. An adequate exam can be conducted on a "table" formed by parent's and examiner's legs as they sit facing each other.

B. The Growth Chart: After carefully measuring a child's height, weight, and, in children of 2 years of age or less, the head circumference, the examiner can compare a child's growth to normative values by plotting the data on a growth chart. Normal growth is one of the most reassuring pieces of information a physician can discern. Normal growth suggests the adequacy of genetic material, diet, and environment and at the same time implies the absence of major chronic disease. When a growth record is abnormal, the pattern of abnormality can help the physician establish a differential diagnosis. The approach to a child with failure to thrive can be established by an examination of the growth record. A pediatric evaluation simply is not complete if the growth chart is not plotted and reviewed.

Examination of the Newborn

The examination of the newborn is unique in that the examiner must rapidly assess the adequacy of transition from the womb to extrauterine life, discover and evaluate any congenital anomalies, and interact extensively with the family. This process is completed via a series of examinations starting in the delivery room and often culminating with a physical examination of the child in front of the child's parents to demonstrate the child's normalcy or explain any unusual findings. Although this is usually a joyous occasion, it is also a time of stress and anxiety as the parents grapple with their concerns about the normalcy of their child.

Screening & Developmental Testing

The incidence of hypertension in an open pediatric population is not high. The American Academy of Pediatrics Committee on School Health no longer suggests screening school-age children for hypertension because of the low yield of patients who ultimately require treatment. However, this recommendation is made in a setting in which blood pressure readings are routinely determined when a child is examined. This routine testing must continue, and physicians must routinely measure blood pressures in all infants and children for whom they provide care.

To assess development properly, the physician must know the level of the child's physiologic maturity. For this reason, the physician must pay careful attention to Tanner sexual staging (see Chapter 10). Similarly, in young children, physical development must be constantly monitored (eg, the time at which teeth appear).

Finally, the only way to assess a child's development is to do developmental testing. Time must be set aside for this testing, and both resources and personnel must be available at all times. The practicing pediatrician soon realizes how essential a part developmental assessment plays in the provision of care. Novices may be overwhelmed by the sophistication and meticulousness this assessment requires. Once practitioners become proficient, however, they realize they have mastered an essential set of techniques that are of great utility to both the physician and patients.

SELECTED REFERENCES

Barness LA: *Manual of Pediatric Physican Diagnosis,* 5th ed. Year Book, 1981.
Bates B: *A Guide to Physical Examination,* 4th ed. Lippincott, 1987.
DeGowin EL, DeGowin RL: *Bedside Diagnostic Examination,* 5th ed. Macmillan, 1987.
Frankenburg W et al: *Denver Developmental Screening Test Reference Manual,* rev ed. LADOCA Project & Publishing Foundation, 1975.

Green M. Richmond JB: *Pediatric Diagnosis,* 4th ed. Saunders, 1986.
Morgan WL, Engel GL: *The Clinical Approach to the Patient,* Saunders, 1969.
Zitelli BJ, Davis HW (editors): *Atlas of Pediatric Physical Diagnosis,* Mosby, 1987.

Growth & Development

Randi Jenssen Hagerman, MD

This chapter outlines the continuous and dynamic process of growth and development in children. It emphasizes the interative aspects of physical, cognitive, social, and emotional development so that the reader can appreciate the impact of each of these domains throughout the span of development.

Our understanding of development has undergone major shifts in this century as we have assimilated new information. Freud emphasizes how early emotional experiences determined by the environment shape personality and psychopathology. Piaget focuses on the predetermined unfolding of cognitive abilities over time in a specific progression that is innate to the child and relatively independent of the environment. In past decades, however, the influence of the environment has assumed an all-powerful role as people have appreciated how greatly the trauma of dysfunctional families and socioeconomic status affect optimal developmental outcomes. We have now reached a stage of regarding the environmental influences in a context that also takes into account the genetic components of temperament and cognitive abilities in a neurobiologic format. We can now understand development through the interaction of these forces so that the relative importance of any single factor is not inflated unless significant trauma or pathologic circumstances exist.

This chapter is divided into sections according to age so that the interactions of central nervous system maturation; physical, cognitive, and emotional growth; genetic variation; and environmental influences can be discussed at critical age levels. Major development theories are reviewed, and longitudinal changes are summarized in charts and tables to give readers an organizational framework by which to remember trends in development. Development occurs at a variable pace in each child. The developmental milestones cited refer to an average child or to group means, and the variability from child to child must be remembered.

THE NEWBORN

Normal newborns are endowed with a set of reflexes to facilitate survival, including rooting and sucking reflexes, and many sensory abilities. The newborn is no longer considered a blank slate—a totally unformed being who gradually gains abilities according to environmental influences. Instead, the newborn is seen as having genetic strengths and weaknesses in neurocognitive organization that are reflected in temperament, adaptability, responsiveness, and general interaction with the environment. These responses should in turn prompt reciprocal interactions from the parents, which further shape development. The Neonatal Behavioral Assessment scale by Brazelton was developed to measure many of the newborn's characteristics of temperament, including social behavior, orienting responses to stimuli, ability to deal with disturbing stimuli, state of arousal, and motor skills. When these abilities are described to the mother, this assessment can further sensitize her to the unique aspects of her child's behavior and responsiveness. This knowledge may in turn improve their interactions.

The newborn has significant sensory abilities, which have been better identified in the last decade. Hearing is well developed at birth, and speech sounds are preferred. The infant becomes alert and oriented to a female voice with high-pitched tones more readily than to a low-pitched male voice. The lower frequency tones of a male voice are more likely to soothe an infant. High-pitched crying is distressing not only to the newborn but also to adults. Infants can shut out loud or aversive stimuli and simply not respond. Within the first few weeks of life, they learn to recognize the mother's voice and differentiate it from other female voices.

Smell is well-developed at birth and plays a significant role in how infants orient themselves to the environment. Infants turn away from aversive smells and respond positively to pleasant ones. By 1 week of age, breast-fed infants recognize and discriminate the smell of their mother's breast pads. They recognize the smell of their mother, not the smell of milk alone. The infant has definite taste preferences at birth, preferring sweet tastes. Infants have more taste buds than adults do and avoid bitter or aversive tastes.

At birth, the retina is well-developed, but the lens is rather immobile. Fixation and tracking through the visual field are well-developed by 2 months of age. Infants prefer to gaze at a human face rather than geometric designs, and they also prefer curved lines, bright colors, and high contrast. The length of time that an infant fixates on a paired visual stimulus has been interpreted as visual preference and has also been correlated with later cognitive development. Visual fixation tasks are the basis of the "infant IQ" tests marketed recently. Although visual acuity is poor at birth (approximately 20/400), it improves rapidly in the first 6 months of life to 20/40. Strabismus is common after birth but usually resolves by 3 months of age. If it persists, referral to an ophthalmologist is appropriate at 6 months of age.

Brazelton TB: *Neonatal Behavioral Assessment Scale,* 2nd ed. Lippincott, 1984.

Brazelton TB, Yogman MW (editors): *Affective Development in Infancy.* Ablex, 1986.

Dixon SD, Stein MT: *Encounters with Children: Pediatric Behavior and Development.* Year Book, 1987. (An exceptional review of development with an emphasis on incorporating development issues into general pediatric care.)

Haith MM, Campos J: *Infancy and Developmental Psychobiology.* Vol 2 of: *Handbook of Child Psychology.* Mussen PH (editor). Wiley, 1983.

Kagan J: Canalization of early psychological development. *Pediatrics* 1982;**70:**474.

Yogman MW, Cook KV, Gersten M: Infant and toddler development: Active organization of the social world. *Curr Probl Pediatr* (May) 1988;**18:**259. (A detailed assessment of early cognitive and emotional development.)

THE FIRST YEAR

One of the most distressing features of infants is the amount of time they spend crying in the first few weeks of life. Crying gradually increases during the first 6 to 12 weeks of age because it is the main modality by which infants express responses to stimuli, both aversive and nonaversive. Crying can be a response to a variety of stimuli, including hunger, a wet diaper, fear, fatigue, and overstimulation. Crying gradually decreases after 12 weeks of age, as the infant develops other responses, such as smiling or reaching, or becomes more adept at self-soothing, such as by sucking the fingers or thumb. In the first weeks of life, however, crying can become a distressing problem for the parents, and crying associated with irritability is often labeled as colic. Particularly sensitive infants with a low tolerance for stimuli can be irritable and difficult to deal with at home. It is useful to help parents understand their infant's temperament and to teach them techniques for avoiding excessive stimuli (because parents often respond to excessive crying by creating excessive stimuli). Parents should be taught ways to calm the child, such as offering nonnutritive sucking, rocking the child, singing to the child, and walking while holding the child. Perhaps most important for the parents is an understanding of the developmental aspects of crying and the emergence of improved coping skills in the baby after 12 weeks of age.

Piaget describes the first 2 years of life as the sensorimotor period, during which infants learn with increasing sophistication how to link the sensory input from the environment with a motor response. Infants build on primitive reflex patterns of behavior (termed *schema;* sucking is an example) and constantly incorporate or assimilate new experiences to further elaborate their schema. The schema evolve over time as infants accommodate new experiences and as new levels of cognitive ability unfold in a rather orderly sequence. In the first year of life, infants' perception of reality revolves around themselves and what they can see or touch. They follow the trajectory of an object through the field of vision, but prior to 6 months, the object does not exist for them once it leaves the field of vision. At 9 to 12 months, infants gradually develop the concept of object permanence, or the understanding that objects exist even when they are not seen. They first apply the concept of object permanence to the image of the mother because of her emotional importance; this realization is a critical part of attachment behavior, discussed below. In the second year, children extend their ability to manipulate objects by using instruments, first by imitation and later by trial and error (Table 2–1).

Freud describes the first year of life as the oral stage because so many of the infant's needs are fulfilled by oral means. Nutrition is obtained through sucking on the breast or bottle, and self-soothing also occurs through sucking on fingers or a pacifier. As Mahler emphasizes, this is a stage of symbiosis with the mother, during which the boundaries between mother and infant are blurred. The baby's needs are totally met by the mother, and the mother has been described as manifesting "narcissistic possessiveness" of the infant. This is a very positive and critical interaction in the bidirectional attachment process known as bonding. The parents learn to be aware of and read their infant's cues, which reflect needs. However, a more sensitive emotional interaction process develops, which can be seen in the mirroring of facial expressions by mother and infant and in their mutual engagement in cycles of attention and inattention, which further develops into social play. A mother who is depressed or cannot respond to the baby's expressions and cues has a profound effect on the infant's future development and attachment. Erickson's terms of basic trust versus mistrust are another way of describing the reciprocal interaction that characterizes this stage (Table 2–1).

Turn-taking games, which occur between 3 and 6 months of age, are a pleasure for both the parents and the infant and are an extension of mirroring behavior. They also represent an early form of imitative behavior, which is important in later social and cognitive development. More sophisticated games, such as peek-a-boo, occur at approximately 9

Table 2–1. Perspectives of human behavior.[1]

	Theories of Development			Skill Areas		
Age	Freud	Erikson	Piaget	Language	Motor	Psychopathology
Birth–18 mo	Oral	Basic trust vs. mistrust	Sensorimotor	Body actions; crying; naming; pointing	Reflex sitting, reaching, grasping, walking	Autism; anaclitic depression, colic; disorders of attachment; feeding, sleeping problems
18 mo–3 yr	Anal	Autonomy v. shame, doubt	Symbolic (preoperational)	Sentences; telegraph jargon	Climbing, running	Separation issues; negativism; fearfulness; constipation; shyness, withdrawal
3–6 yr	Oedipal	Initiative vs. guilt	Intuition (preoperational)	Connective words; can be readily understood	Increased coordination; tricycle; jumping	Enuresis; encopresis; anxiety; aggressive acting out; phobias; nightmares
6–11 yr	Latency	Industry vs. inferiority	Concrete operational	Subordinate sentences; reading and writing; language reasoning	Increased skills; sports, recreational cooperative games	School phobias; obsessive reactions; conversion reactions; depressive equivalents
12–17 yr	Adolescence (genital)	Identity vs. role confusion	Formal operational	Reason abstract; using language; abstract manipulation	Refinement of skills	Delinquency; promiscuity; schizophrenia; anorexia nervosa; suicide
17–30 yr	Young adulthood	Intimacy vs. isolation	Formal operational	Reason abstract; using language; abstract manipulation	Refinement of skills	Schizophrenia; borderline personality; adjustment disorders; development of intimate relationship and difficulties with relationships
30–60 yr.	Adulthood	Generativity vs. stagnation	Formal operational	Reason abstract; using language; abstract manipulation	Refinement of skills	Depression; self-doubts; career development issues; family, social network; neuroses
60 yr and over	Old age	Ego integration vs. despair	Formal operational		Loss of functions (?)	Involutional depression; anxiety; anger; increased dependency

[1]Adapted and reproduced, with permission, from Dixon S: Setting the stage: Theories and concepts of child development. In *Encounters with Children.* Dixon S, Stein M [editors]. Yearbook, 1987.

months. The infant's thrill at the reappearance of the face that vanished momentarily demonstrates the emerging understanding of object permanence.

Eight to nine months is also a critical time in the attachment process because separation anxiety and stranger anxiety become marked. Kagan describes the infant at this stage as able to appreciate discrepant events that match previously known schema only partially. These new events cause uncertainty and subsequently fear and anxiety. Cognitively, the infant must be able to retrieve the memory of previous schema and integrate the new information to previous knowledge over an extended time. These abilities are developed by 8 months of age and lead to the fears that subsequently develop: stranger anxiety and separation anxiety. In stranger anxiety, the infant analyzes the face of a stranger, detects the mismatch with previous schema, and may subsequently respond with fear or anxiety, leading to crying. In separation anxiety, the child perceives the difference between the mother's presence and absence by remembering the schema of her presence. Perceiving the inconsistency, the child becomes uncertain and subsequently anxious and fearful. This begins at 8 months, reaches a peak at 15 months, and disappears

by the end of 2 years in a relatively orderly progression because central nervous system maturation facilitates the development of new skills. A parent can put the child's understanding of object permanence to good use by placing a picture of the mother near the child or by leaving an object where the child can see it during her absence. A visual substitute for her actual presence may comfort the child.

Brazelton TB, Yogman MW (editors): *Affective Development in Infancy.* Ablex, 1986.

Dixon SD, Stein MT: *Encounters with Children: Pediatric Behavior and Development.* Year Book, 1987.

Dworkin PH: The preschool child: Developmental themes and clinical issues. *Curr Prob Pediatr* (Feb) 1988; **18**:79.

Freud A: *Normality and Pathology in Childhood: Assessments of Development.* International Universities Press, 1965.

Ginsberg H, Opper S: *Piaget's Theory of Intellectual Development.* Prentice-Hall, 1969. (A readable review of Piaget's work.

Kagan J: Canalization of early psychological development. *Pediatrics* 1982;**70**:474.

Mahler MS, Pinme F, Bergman A: *The Psychological Birth of the Human Infant: Symbiosis and Individuation.* Basic Books, 1975.

Piaget J: *The Origins of Intelligence in Children.* Norton, 1952.

Piaget J, Inyhelder B: *The Psychology of the Child.* Basic Books, 1969.

Yogman MW, Cook KV, Gersten M: Infant and toddler development: active organization of the social world. *Curr Probl Pediatr,* (May) 1988;**18:**259.

GROWTH IN THE FIRST 3 YEARS

Fetal growth in length is most rapid at 4 to 6 months' gestation. However, adipose tissue begins to develop at 7 months, and weight gain accelerates, causing fetal weight to double during the last 2 months in utero. The rate of growth of males in late fetal development and during the first 6 months postnatally is more rapid than the growth rate of females because of a higher level of testosterone. The birth weight of the newborn correlates with the size, nutritional state, and general health of the mother and represents the influence of uterine constraints on ultimate size. Newborns may lose up to 10% of their birth weight in the first few days of life, but with normal nutrition birth weight is regained in approximately 10 days. The infant subsequently gains approximately 30 g per day for the first several months.

After the first 6 months of life, genetic factors influencing ultimate height begin to exert their effect. The growth percentile, therefore, may shift significantly in the first 4 to 18 months of life. This shift can be either up or down. An infant who is small for gestational age and has a genetic predisposition to larger stature usually experiences accelerated growth in the first 6 months, and by 18 months a relatively stable new growth percentile is established. The downward shift is seen in large infants who have a genetic predisposition to short stature. A falloff in their growth percentiles may often be misconstrued as failure to thrive, although a stable growth percentile should be achieved by 18 months of age.

By 1 year of age, infants weigh 3 times as much as they did at birth and are 1½ times as long. By 2 years of age, the growth velocity curve has stabilized into the rate for mid childhood, which is a weight gain of 2 to 3 kg/y and a height gain of 5 to 7.5 cm/y (Figs 2–1 through 2–9). At the second birthday, a child attains approximately one-half of adult height.

The energy requirement during growth also changes dramatically in the first few years of life. Approximately 110 kcal/kg/d is necessary in early infancy because up to 40% of this total energy requirement is used for growth. The percentage used for growth gradually decreases to 3% at 2 years of age and remains at this level even during adolescence. After 2 years of age, the overall energy requirement gradually decreases from 90 kcal/kg/d to 60 kcal/kg/d during middle childhood, and the ma-

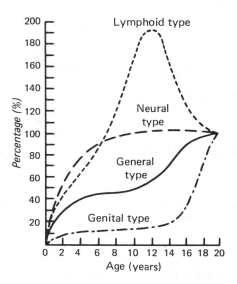

Figure 2–1. Graph showing major types of postnatal growth of various parts and organs of the body. *Lymphoid type:* thymus, lymph nodes, intestinal lymphoid masses. *Neural type:* brain and its parts, dura, spinal cord, optic apparatus, many head dimensions. *General type:* body as a whole, external dimensions (with exception of head and neck), respiratory and digestive organs, kidneys, aorta and pulmonary trunks, spleen, musculature as a whole, skeleton as a whole, blood volume. *Genital type:* testis, ovary, epididymis, uterine tube, prostate, prostatic urethra, seminal vesicles. (From RE Scammon. Redrawn and reproduced, with permission, from Holt LE Jr, McIntosh R, Barnett HL: *Pediatrics,* 13th ed. Appleton-Century-Crofts, 1962, as redrawn from Harris JA et al: *Measurement of Man.* University of Minnesota Press, 1930.)

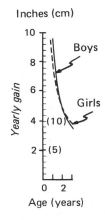

Figure 2–2. Growth rate from birth to age 3 (both sexes).

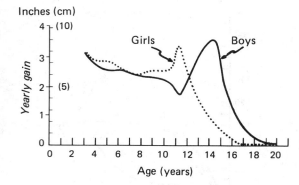

Figure 2–3. Growth rate from age 3 to 20 (both sexes).

Falkner F, Tanner JM (editors): *Developmental Biology: Prenatal Growth.* Vol 1 of: *Human Growth: A Comprehensive Treatise,* 2nd ed. Plenum Press, 1986.

Falkner F, Tanner JM (editors): *Postnatal Growth Neurobiology.* Vol 2 of: *Human Growth: A Comprehensive Treatise,* 2nd ed. Plenum Press, 1986. (A detailed analysis of current research in physical growth and brain development.)

Karlberg J, Engstrom I, Karlberg P, Fryer JG: Analysis of linear growth using a mathematical model. *Acta Paediatr Scand* 1987;**76:**478.

Lowrey GH: *Growth and Development of Children,* 8th ed. Year Book, 1986. (A detailed analysis of physical growth and development in children.)

Smith DW: *Growth and Its Disorders: Major Problems in Clinical Pediatrics,* Vol 25. Saunders, 1977. (A classic review of linear growth through childhood and adolescence.)

Tanner JM, Whitehouse RH, Takaishi M: Standards from birth to maturity for height, weight, height velocity; British children. *Arch Dis Child* 1965;**41:**454.

jority of the energy expenditure is accounted for by activity and basal metabolic rate of the tissues. The gradual decrease is secondary to a decline in the relative mass of organs, such as the brain and liver, that have a high requirement for energy compared to resting muscle. The relative energy expended during activity increases in adolescence, particularly for males. The percentage of body weight that is muscle increases from 22% at 3 months to 35% at 5 years and 40% at maturity in males. In contrast, organ weight is 17% of body weight in the infant, with 75% of organ weight accounted for by the brain. By maturity, only 5.1% of body weight is organ weight. Fat increases during the first year of life from 12% of body weight at birth. After the infant begins to walk and explore, however, the proportion of fat decreases and remains stable throughout childhood. In adolescence, the proportion of body weight that is fat increases with sexual maturation in girls but not in boys. For further information, see Chapter 5.

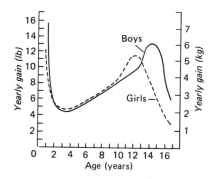

Figure 2–4. Yearly gain in weight. (Redrawn and reproduced, with permission, from Barnett HL: *Pediatrics,* 14th ed. Appleton-Century-Crofts, 1968.)

Brain Growth

Approximately 100 billion neurons are present in the fully developed brain, and replication of neurons is completed before birth. Most of this growth occurs in the first 3 months of gestation. Cell density subsequently decreases rapidly until birth. After birth, the decrease is slower, and ceases at 15 months. At birth, the head is three-fourths of its adult size and makes up one-fourth of the baby's length. This ratio changes dramatically in time so that by 25 years of age, the head measures one-eighth of the body length (Figs 2–9 through 2–11). Postnatally, the brain continues to grow rapidly, completing half of its lifetime growth by the end of the first year. The postnatal growth is due to an increase in white matter and a proliferation of synaptic connections. After 2 years of age, the head circumference increases only 2 cm/y during middle childhood. By 7 years of age, nine-tenths of brain growth is completed, and many 10-year-olds have the brain weight of an adult.

The cerebellum is the area of the gray matter that develops last. It begins its growth at 30 weeks of gestation and ends at approximately 1 year of age. It is, therefore, particularly vulnerable to trauma, which may occur in late gestation or at birth. The spinal cord extends through the length of the neural canal until the third month of gestation. After this time, the torso of the fetus grows faster than the spinal cord, which is fixed in position superiorly by the brain. The lower end of the spinal cord subsequently rests at a gradually higher vertebral level through later fetal life and, by birth, is located at the third lumbar vertebra. The spinal cord doubles its weight in the first year of life and has increased eightfold by adulthood.

Myelinization begins in the spinal cord by the fourth month of gestation and begins in the brain during the last trimester (Table 2–2). At birth, the

GIRLS: BIRTH TO 36 MONTHS
PHYSICAL GROWTH NCHS PERCENTILES*

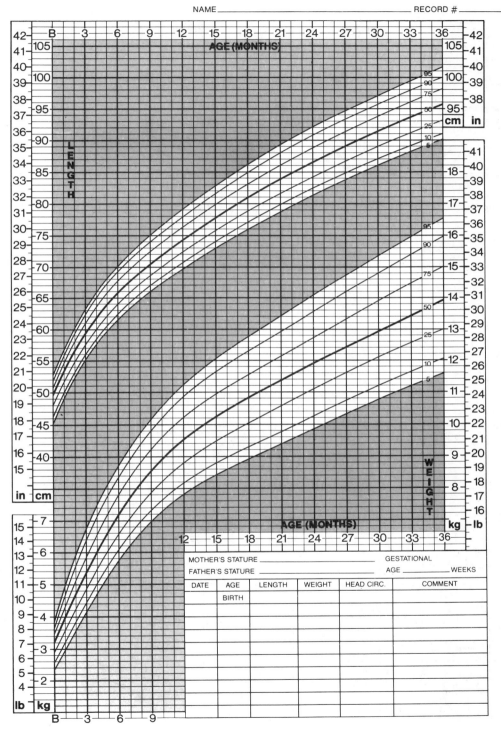

Figure 2–5. Percentile standards for weight and height in girls 0 to 3 years. (Reproduced, with permission, from Ross Laboratories, Columbus, OH. © 1982 Ross Laboratories.)

BOYS: BIRTH TO 36 MONTHS
PHYSICAL GROWTH NCHS PERCENTILES*

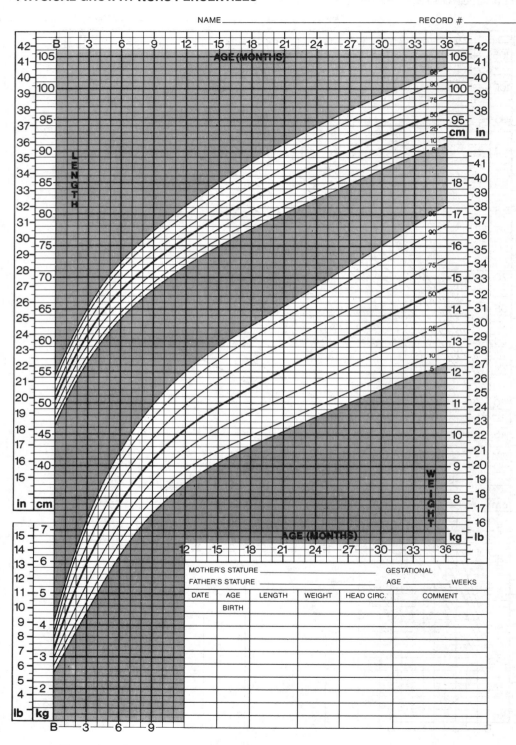

Figure 2–6. Percentile standards for weight and height in boys 0 to 3 years. (Reproduced, with permission, from Ross Laboratories, Columbus, OH. © 1982 Ross Laboratories.)

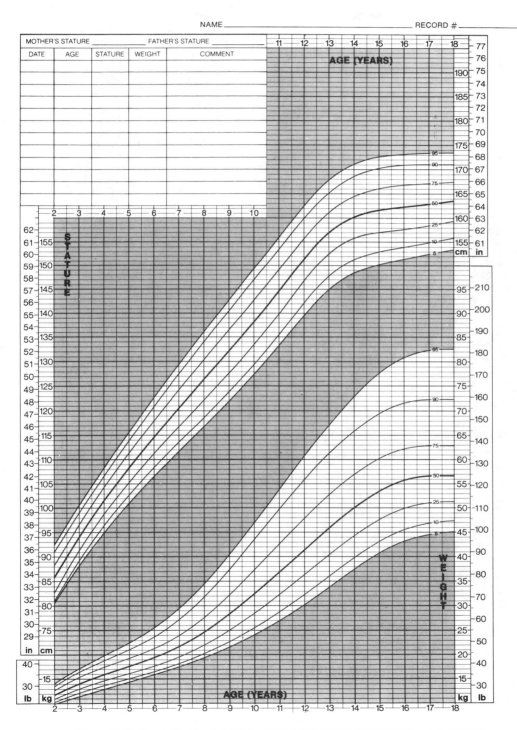

Figure 2–7. Percentile standards for weight and height in girls 2 to 18 years. (Reproduced, with permission, from Ross Laboratories, Columbus, OH. © 1982 Ross Laboratories.)

**BOYS: 2 TO 18 YEARS
PHYSICAL GROWTH
NCHS PERCENTILES***

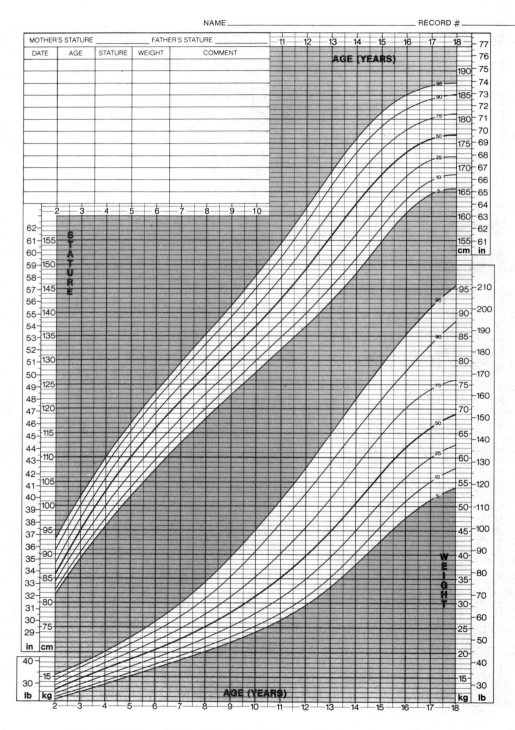

Figure 2–8. Percentile standards for weight and height in boys 2 to 18 years. (Reproduced, with permission, from Ross Laboratories, Columbus, OH. © 1982 Ross Laboratories.)

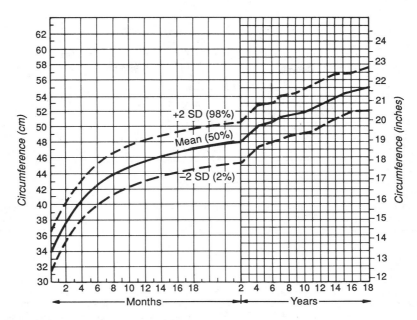

Figure 2–9. Head circumference of girls. (Modified and reproduced, with permission, from Nellhaus G: *Pediatrics* 1968;**41:**106.)

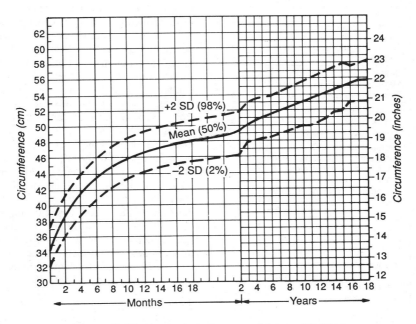

Figure 2–10. Head circumference of boys. (Modified and reproduced, with permission, from Nellhaus G: *Pediatrics* 1968;**41:**106.)

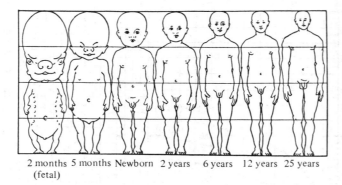

2 months 5 months Newborn 2 years 6 years 12 years 25 years
(fetal)

Figure 2–11. Relative proportions of head, trunk, and extremities at different ages. (From Stratz, modified by Robbins WJ et al: *Growth.* Yale Univ Press, 1928.)

Table 2–2. Human fetal development.[1]

		Fetal Age in Lunar Months
Integument	Three-layered epidermis	3
	Body hair begins	4
	Skin glands form, sweat and sebaceous	4
Mouth	Lip fusion complete	2
	Palate fused completely	3
	Enamel and dentin depositing	5
	Primordia of permanent teeth	6–8
Gastrointestinal	Bile secreted	3
	Rectum patent	3
	Pancreatic islands appear	3
	Fixation of duodenum and colon	4
Respiratory	Definitive shape of lungs	3
	Maxillary sinuses developing	4
	Elastic fibers appear in lung	4
Urogenital	Kidney able to secrete	2½
	Vagina regains lumen	5
	Testes descend into scrotum	7–9
Vascular	Definitive shape of heart	1½
	Heart becomes 4-chambered	3½
	Blood formation in marrow begins	3
	Spleen acquires typical structure	7
Nervous	Commissures of brain complete	5
	Myelinization of cord begins	5
	Typical layers of cortex	6
Special senses	Nasal septum complete	3
	Retinal layers complete, light-perceptive	7
	Vascular tunic of lens pronounced	7
	Eyelids open	7–8

[1]Reproduced, with permission, from Arey LB: *Developmental Anatomy: A Textbook and Laboratory Manual of Embryology,* 5th ed. Saunders, 1947.

autonomic system is matured and myelinated. The cranial nerves, except for the optic and olfactory nerves, are also myelinated. The cortex and most of its connection to the thalamus and basal ganglia are incompletely myelinated. It takes at least 2 years for myelinization of these areas and the spinal cord to be complete.

Newborn Reflexes

Reflex movement begins in fetal development as early as 9 weeks' gestation. However, most of the reflexes associated with the newborn develop between 20 and 38 weeks' gestation. Sucking, a basic reflex critical to survival, can first be seen in utero as early as 14 weeks' gestation. The rooting reflex begins by 28 weeks' gestation and is evidenced by the infant's pursing the lips and sucking after turning toward a touch to the cheek. The tonic neck reflex is elicited by forcibly turning the infant's head. In response, the infant extends the arm and leg on the side toward which the head is turned and flexes the opposite side (fencing position stance). This reflex disappears by 8 months of age unless myelinization or brain development is pathologic. The Moro embrace reflex (an embracing movement as a startle response), palmar grasp, and trunk incurving in response to a tactile stimulus to the side of the trunk all develop by 28 weeks' gestation but disappear by 3, 4, and 5 months of age, respectively. Babinski's reflex, which develops just prior to birth in a full-term infant, does not normally disappear until 12 to 16 months of age, when adequate myelinization has occurred.

EEG & Sleep

The brain also undergoes rapid maturation in the first 2 years of life. Prior to 26 weeks' gestation, the EEG is disorganized and without periodicity. By 8 months' gestation, however, low-amplitude fast waves occur at 16 to 18 cycles per second. At birth, the waking and sleeping cycles can be differentiated, and by 4 months, sleep spindles appear. During this period, the proportion of total sleep time occupied by active or rapid eye movement (REM) sleep decreases from 50 to 20%. The infant's sleep pattern at the onset of sleep also shifts from REM sleep to quiet sleep. The amount of quiet sleep also gradually increases to a maximum of 70 to 80% of total sleep time. These changes are a reflection of significant brain maturation, which has occurred by 4 months. Infantile reflexes, as previously mentioned, are disappearing, and the infant is becoming more alert and interactive with the environment. The infant is now reaching for and grasping objects, smiling and laughing out loud, anticipating food on sight, and sitting with support.

Motor Dexterity

The developmental progression of the grasp through the first year illustrates the gradual improvement in motor dexterity. The grasp begins as a raking motion involving mainly the ulnar aspect of the hand at 3 to 4 months. The thumb is used in the grasp just before 5 months, as the focus shifts to the radial side of the hand. The thumb opposes the finger for picking up a cube just before 7 months, but the neat pincer grasp used for smaller objects, such as a pellet, does not develop until approximately 9 months.

The changes in gross motor skills have a significant impact on the child's exploration of the environment. Sitting alone occurs at 6 months of age, but the onset of walking at 12 months (with a range of 9–17 months in the normal child) introduces the major theme of the second year of life, autonomy.

THE SECOND YEAR

Once children can walk independently, they can move away from the mother and explore the environment on their own. Although they use the mother as a home base and return to her frequently to reassure themselves that she is still there and available for them, they have definitely taken a quantum jump in independence and autonomy. These new themes are closely tied to the child's beginning sense of mastery over the environment and an emerging sense of self. These issues lead to the "terrible twos" and the frequent verbalizations "no" as children struggle to develop a better idea of what is under their control. This is a fragile time of ego development. Parents should not crush emerging autonomy but develop appropriate limits that foster independent exploration.

As children develop a sense of self, they begin to understand the feelings of others and develop empathy. They hug another who is in distress or become concerned when another is hurt. They begin to understand how another child feels when he or she is hit or hurt, and this realization helps them to inhibit their own aggressive behavior. They also begin to understand right and wrong and parental expectations. They realize when they have done something "bad" and may signify that awareness with "uh oh!" or distress. They also take pleasure in their accomplishments and become more aware of their bodies.

The development of these cognitive, emotional, and physical abilities is related to significant brain maturation, which occurs by 2 years of age. Myelinization is reaching its completion and, according to Rabinowicz, all the layers of the cortex reach a similar state of maturation between 15 and 24 months. Before this time, differences exist in the maturation level between cortical layers. These changes set the stage for toilet training after 18 months of age. Toddlers have developed the sensory abilities to be aware of a full rectum or bladder and are physically able to control their rectal sphincter. They also take great pleasure in their accomplishments, particularly in appropriate elimination, if it is positively reinforced. Children must be given some control over when elimination occurs. If severe restrictions are imposed, the accomplishment of this developmental milestone can become a battle between parent and child, and long-term struggles of control predisposing to encopresis may develop later. Freud terms this period the anal stage because the developmental issue of bowel control is the major task requiring mastery. It basically represents a more generalized theme of socialized behavior and overall body cleanliness, which is begun to be taught or imposed on the child at this age. The child is encouraged to control impulsive and aggressive behavior by acting in socially appropriate ways. Although Freud describes the by-products of anal regularity on personality development, including punctuality, reliability, cleanliness, and conscientiousness, these themes simply represent abilities emerging at the time that toilet is also being mastered. See Chapter 25.

Dixon SD, Stein MT: Encounters with Children: *Pediatric Behavior and Development*. Year Book, 1987.

Falkner F, Tanner JM (editors): *Postnatal Growth Neurobiology*. Vol 2 of: *Human Growth: A Comprehensive Treatise*, 2nd ed. Plenum Press, 1986.

Gesell A, Amatruda C: *Developmental Diagnosis*, 2nd ed. Harper & Row, 1965.

Kagan J: Canalization of early psychological development. *Pediatrics* 1982;**70:**474.

Lowrey GH: *Growth and Development of Children*, 8th ed. Year Book, 1986.

Rabinowicz T: The differential maturation of the cerebral cortex. In: *Postnatal Growth Neurobiology*, Vol 2 of: *Human Growth: A Comprehensive Treatise*, 2nd ed. Falkner F, Tanner JM (editors). Plenum Press, 1986.

Yogman MW, Cook KV, Gersten M: Infant and toddler development: Active organization of the social world. *Curr Probl Pediatr* (May) 1988;**18:**259.

LANGUAGE DEVELOPMENT: 1–4 YEARS

Communication is important from birth, particularly the nonverbal reciprocal interactions between the infant and caretaker, which have already been described. By 2 months of age, these interactions begin to include vocalizations that involve cooing and reciprocal vocal play between the mother and child. Babbling begins by 6 to 10 months of age, and the repetition of sounds, such as "da-da-da-da," is facilitated by increasing oral muscular control. Babbling reaches a peak at 12 months. The child then moves into a stage of having needs met by using individual words to represent objects or actions. It is common for children of this age to express wants and needs by pointing to objects. There is significant variability in the number of words acquired by 18 months, with an average of 20 to 50 words. The failure of parents or siblings to encourage vocalization and their overuse of nonverbal communication, such as pointing, slows the development of expressive vocabulary. Recurrent otitis media, which causes a fluctuating conductive hearing loss, may also have a significant impact on the achievement of early language milestones.

Receptive language usually develops more rapidly than expressive language. Word comprehension begins at 9 months; by 13 months, the receptive vocabulary may be as high as 20 to 100 words. After 18 months, there is a dramatic increase in expressive and receptive vocabulary, and by the end of the second year, a quantum leap occurs in language development. This leap represents a major change in cognitive development. The child begins to put words and phrases together and begins to use language to represent a new world, the symbolic world. Although the infant begins to use single words to represent objects or people in the latter part of the first year, it is not until the end of the second year that language ability begins to blossom. Children now begin to put verbs into their phrases and focus much of their language on describing their new abilities, often while they are doing them, eg, "I go out." They incorporate prepositions into speech and ask why and what questions more frequently. They also begin to appreciate time factors and to understand and use this concept in their speech (Table 2–3).

The Early Language Milestone Scale (ELM) (Fig 2–12) is a simple tool for assessing early language development in the pediatric office setting. It is scored in the same fashion as the Denver Developmental Screening Test–Revised (DDST-R) (Fig 2–13) but tests both receptive and expressive language areas in greater depth.

Piaget describes the 2- to 6-year-old stage as pre-

Table 2–3. Normal speech and language development.

Age	Speech	Language	Articulation[1]
1 month	Throaty sounds		Vowels: /ah/, /uh/, /ee/
2 months	Vowel sounds ("eh"), coos		
2½ months	Squeals		
3 months	Babbles, initial vowels		
4 months	Guttural sounds ("ah," "go")		Consonants: m, p, b
5 months			Vowels: /o/, /u/
7 months	Imitates speech sounds		
8 months			Syllables: da, ba, ka
10 months		"Dada" or "mama" nonspecifically	Approximates names: baba/bottle
12 months	Jargon begins (own language)	One word other than "mama" or "dada"	Understandable: 2–3 words
13 months		Three words	
16 months		Six words	Consonants; t, d, w, n, h
18–24 months		Two-word phrases	Understandable 2-word phrases
24–30 months		Three-word phrases	Understandable 3-word phrases
2 years	Vowels uttered correctly	Approximately 270 words; uses pronouns	Approximately 270 words; uses phrases
3 years	Some degree of hesitancy and uncertainty common	Approximately 900 words; intelligible 4-word phrases	Approximately 900 words; intelligible 4-word phrases
4 years		Approximately 1540 words; intelligible 5-word phrases or sentences	Approximately 1540 words; intelligible 5-word phrases
6 years		Approximately 2560 words; intelligible 6- or 7-word sentences	Approximately 2560 words; intelligible 6- or 7-word sentences
7–8 years	Adult proficiency		

[1]Data on articulation from Berry MF: *Language Disorders of Children.* Appleton-Century-Crofts, 1969; and from Bzoch K, League R: *Receptive-Expressive Emergent Language Scale.* University Park Press, 1970.

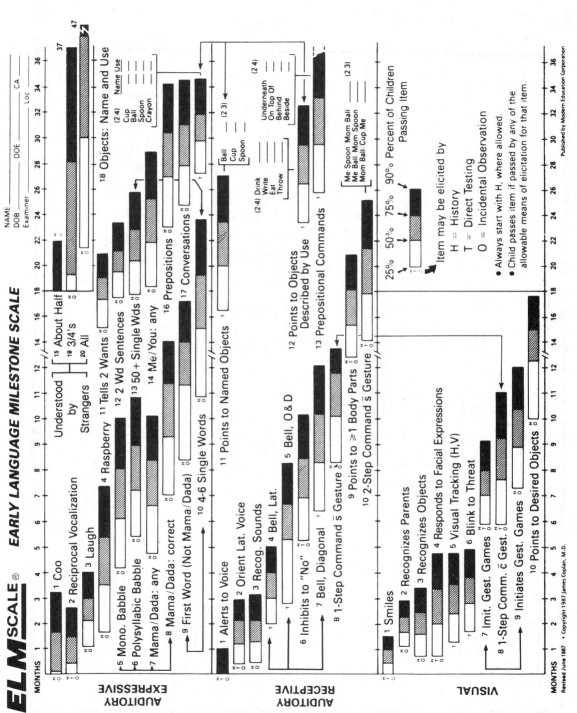

Figure 2–12. Early Language Milestone Scale. (Reproduced, with permission, from Coplan J: *Early Language Milestone Scale.* Pro Ed, Austin, TX. 1987.)

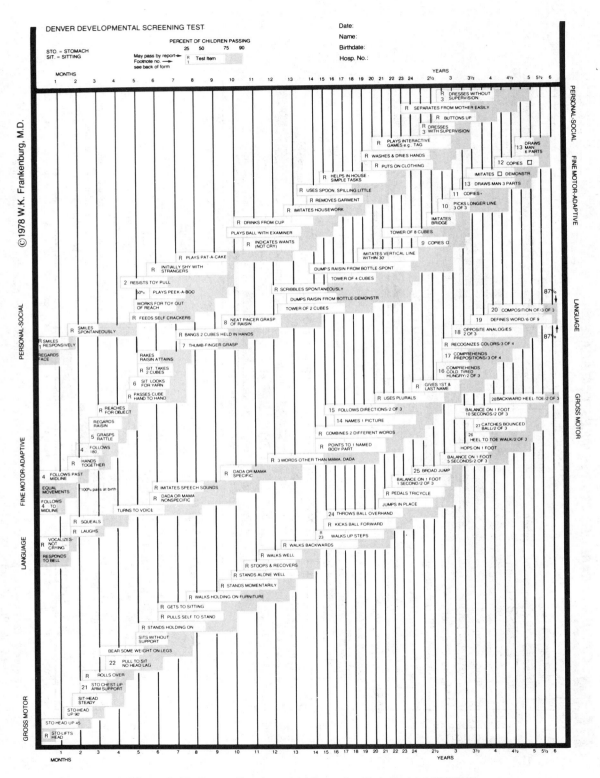

Figure 2–13. Denver Developmental Screening Test, Revised (DDST-R).

operational. This stage begins when language has facilitated the creation of mental images in the symbolic sense. The child begins to learn to manipulate the symbolic world. The child sorts out reality from fantasy imperfectly and may be terrified of dreams, wishes, and foolish threats. Most of the child's perception of the world is egocentric or interpreted in reference to wants, needs, or influence. Cause-and-effect relationships are confused with temporal relationships or interpreted egocentrically. For instance, children often focus their understanding of divorce on themselves; eg, "my father left because I was bad" or "my father left because he didn't love me." Illness and the need for medical care are also commonly misinterpreted at this age. The child may make a mental connection between a sibling's illness and a recent argument, a negative comment, or a wish that the sibling be ill. The child may experience significant guilt unless the parents are aware of these misperceptions and take time to sort them out.

At this age, children also endow inanimate objects with human feelings. They also assume that humans cause or create all natural events. For instance, when asked why the sun sets, they may respond that "the sun goes to his house" or "it is pushed down by someone else."

Magical thinking blossoms during the ages of 3 to 5 as symbolic thinking incorporates more elaborate fantasy. Fantasy facilitates development of role playing, sexual identity, and emotional growth. Children test new experiences in fantasy, both in their imagination and in play. In their play, children often create magical stories and novel situations that reflect issues they are dealing with, such as aggression, relationships, fears, and control issues. Children often invent imaginary friends at this time, and nightmares or fears of monsters are common. At this stage, other children become important in facilitating play, such as in a preschool group. Play gradually becomes more cooperative; shared fantasy leads to game playing. Freud describes the Oedipal phase between the ages of 3 and 6, when there is strong attachment to the parent of the opposite sex. The child's fantasies may focus on play acting the adult role with that parent, although by 6 years of age Oedipal issues are usually resolved, and attachment is redirected to the parent of the same sex.

Bayley N (editor): *Bayley Scales of Infant Development.* Psychological Corp, 1969.
Coplan J: *Early Language Milestone Scale,* Pro Ed, 1987.
Dixon SD, Stein MT: *Encounters with Children: Pediatric Behavior and Development.* Year Book, 1987.
Erikson EH: *Childhood and Society,* 2nd ed. Norton, 1963.
Fraiberg S: *The Magic Years.* Scribner, 1959.
Frankenberg WK, Dodds JB: The Denver Developmental Test. *J Pediatr* 1967;**71**:181.
Frankenberg WK et al: The newly abbreviated and revised Denver Developmental Screening Test. *J Pediatr* 1981; **99**:995.
Levine MD et al: *Developmental-Behavioral Pediatrics.* Saunders, 1983.
Lowrey GH: *Growth and Development of Children,* 8th ed. Year Book, 1986.
Piaget J, Inyhelder B: *The Psychology of the Child.* Basic Books, 1969.
Walker D, Gugenheim S, Downs MP, Northern JL: Early Language Milestone Scale and language screening of young children. *Pediatrics* (Feb) 1989;**83(2):**284.
Yogman MW, Cook KV, Gersten M: Infant and toddler development: Active organization of the social world. *Curr Probl Pediatr* (May) 1988;**18:**259.

THE EARLY SCHOOL YEARS: 5–7

Attendance in kindergarten at 5 years marks an acceleration in the separation/individuation theme initiated in the preschool years. The child is ready to relate to peers in a more interactive manner than demonstrated by previous parallel play. The brain has reached 90% of its adult weight. At approximately 6 years, a remodeling of the cortex occurs. The Betz cells decrease in length and increase in width. The cortex, in general, shows a decrease in total thickness, with an increase in the number of nerve cells in the different layers. Sensor-motor coordination abilities are maturing and facilitating pencil-and-paper tasks and sports, both part of the school experience.

Cognitive abilities are still at the preoperational stage, and children focus on one variable in a problem at a time. However, by 5½ years, most children have mastered conservation of length; by 6½ years, conservation of mass and weight; and by 8 years, conservation of volume.

By first grade, there is more pressure on the child to master academic tasks, including the recognition of numbers, letters, and words, and the ability to write. Piaget describes the stage of concrete operations beginning after age 6, when the child is able to perform mental operations concerning concrete objects that involve the manipulation of more than one variable. The child is able to order, number, and classify because these activities are related to concrete objects in the environment and because these activities are stressed in early schooling. Magical thinking diminishes greatly at this time, and the reality of cause-and-effect relationships is better understood. Fantasy and imagination are still strong and are reflected in the themes of play. Table 2–4 lists specific developmental abilities through middle childhood and adolescence.

MIDDLE CHILDHOOD YEARS: 7–11

Freud terms these the latency years, during which children are not bothered by significant aggressive or sexual drives but instead devote most of their energies to school and peer group interactions. In reality,

Table 2–4. Developmental charts.[1]

1–2 months

Activities to be observed:
Holds head erect and lifts head.
Turns from side to back.
Regards faces and follows objects through visual field.
Drops toys.
Becomes alert in response to voice.

Activities related by parent:
Recognizes parents.
Engages in vocalizations.
Smiles spontaneously.

3–5 months

Activities to be observed:
Grasps cube—first ulnar then later thumb opposition.
Reaches for and brings objects to mouth.
Makes "raspberry" sound.
Sits with support.

Activities related by parent:
Laughs.
Anticipates food on sight.
Turns from back to side.

6–8 months

Activities to be observed:
Sits alone for a short period.
Reaches with one hand.
First scoops up a pellet then grasps it using
    thumb opposition.
Imitates "bye-bye."
Passes object from hand to hand in midline.
Babbles.

Activities related by parent:
Rolls from back to stomach.
Is inhibited by the word *no*.

9–11 months

Activities to be observed:
Stands alone.
Imitates pat-a-cake and peek-a-boo.
Uses thumb and index finger to pick up pellet.

Activities related by parent:
Walks by supporting self on furniture.
Follows one-step verbal commands, eg,
    "Come here," "Give it to me."

1 year

Activities to be observed:
Walks independently.
Says "mama" and "dada" with meaning.
Can use neat pincer grasp to pick up a pellet.
Releases cube into cup after demonstration.
Gives toys on request.
Tries to build tower of 2 cubes.

Activities related by parent:
Points to desired objects.
Says one or two other words.

18 months

Activities to be observed:
Builds tower of 3 to 4 cubes.
Throws ball.
Scribbles spontaneously.
Seats self in chair.
Dumps pellet from bottle.

Activities related by parent:
Walks up and down stairs with help.
Says 4 to 20 words.
Understands a 2-step command.
Carries and hugs doll.
Feeds self.

24 months

Activities to be observed:
Speaks short phrases, 2 words or more.
Kicks ball on request.
Builds tower of 6 to 7 cubes.
Points to named objects or pictures.
Jumps off floor with both feet.
Stands on either foot alone.
Uses pronouns.

Activities related by parent:
Verbalizes toilet needs.
Pulls on simple garment.
Turns pages of book singly.
Plays with domestic mimicry.

30 months

Activities to be observed:
Walks backward.
Begins to hop on one foot.
Uses prepositions.
Copies a crude circle.
Points to objects described by use.
Refers to self as I.
Holds crayon in fist.

Activities related by parents:
Helps put things away.
Carries on a conversation.

3 years

Activities to be observed:
Holds crayon with fingers.
Builds tower of 9 to 10 cubes.
Imitates 3-cube bridge.
Copies circle.
Gives first and last name.

Activities related by parent:
Rides tricycle using pedals.
Dresses with supervision.

3–4 years

Activities to be observed:
Climbs stairs with alternating feet.
Begins to button and unbutton.
"What do you like to do that's fun?" (Answers using plurals,
    personal pronoun, and verbs.)
Responds to command to place toy *in, on,* or *under* table.
Draws a circle when asked to draw a man (girl, boy).
Knows own sex. ("Are you a boy or a girl?")
Gives full name.
Copies a circle already drawn. ("Can you make one
    like this?")

Activities related by parent:
Feeds self at mealtime.
Takes off shoes and jacket.

4–5 years

Activities to be observed:
Runs and turns without losing balance.
May stand on one leg for at least 10 seconds.

Table 2–4 (cont'd). Developmental charts.

Buttons clothes and laces shoes. (Does not tie.)
Counts to 4 by rote.
"Give me 2 sticks." (Able to do so from pile of 4 tongue depressors.)
Draws a man. (Head, 2 appendages, and possibly 2 eyes. No torso yet.)
Knows the days of the week. ("What day comes after Tuesday?")
Gives appropriate answers to: "What must you do if you are sleepy? Hungry? Cold?"
Copies + in imitation.

Activities related by parent:
Self care at toilet. (May need help with wiping.)
Plays outside for at least 30 minutes.
Dresses self except for tying.

5–6 years

Activities to be observed:
Can catch ball.
Skips smoothly.
Copies a + already drawn.
Tells age.
Concept of 10 (eg, counts 10 tongue depressors).
  May recite to higher number by rote.
Knows right and left hand.
Draws recognizable man with at least 8 details.
Can describe favorite television program in some detail.

Activities related by parent:
Does simple chores at home. (Taking out garbage, drying silverware, etc.)
Goes to school unattended or meets school bus.
Good motor ability but little awareness of dangers.

6–7 years

Activities to be observed:
Copies a $\triangle$.
Defines words by use. ("What is an orange?" "To eat.")
Knows if morning or afternoon.
Draws a man with 12 details.
Reads several one-syllable printed words. (My, dog, see, boy.)
Uses pencil for printing name.

7–8 Years

Activities to be observed:
Counts by 2s and 5s.
Ties shoes.
Copies a $\diamond$.
Knows what day of the week it is. (Not date or year.)
Reads paragraph # 1 Durrell:

Reading:
Muff is a little yellow kitten. She drinks milk. She sleeps on a chair. She does not like to get wet.

Corresponding arithmetic:

$$\begin{array}{cccc} 7 & 6 & 6 & 8 \\ +4 & +7 & -4 & -3 \end{array}$$

No evidence of sound substitution in speech (eg, *fr* for *thr*).
Adds and subtracts one-digit numbers.
Draws a man with 16 details.

8–9 years

Activities to be observed:
Defines words better than by use. ("What is an orange?" "A fruit.")
Can give an appropriate answer to the following:
"What is the thing for you to do if . . .

—you've broken something that belongs to someone else?"
—a playmate hits you without meaning to do so?"
Reads paragraph #2 Durrell:

Reading:
A little black dog ran away from home. He played with two big dogs. They ran away from him. It began to rain. He went under a tree. He wanted to go home, but he did not know the way. He saw a boy he knew. The boy took him home.

Corresponding arithmetic:

$$\begin{array}{cccc} & 45 & & \\ 67 & 16 & 14 & 84 \\ +4 & +27 & -8 & -36 \end{array}$$

Is learning borrowing and carrying processes in addition and subtraction.

9–10 years

Activities to be observed:
Knows the month, day, and year.
Names the months in order. (Fifteen seconds, one error.)
Makes a sentence with these 3 words in it: (One of 2. Can use words orally in proper context.)
  1. work . . . money . . . men
  2. boy . . . river . . . ball
Reads paragraph #3 Durrell:

Reading:
Six boys put up a tent by the side of a river. They took things to eat with them. When the sun went down, they went into the tent to sleep. In the night, a cow came and began to eat grass around the tent. The boys were afraid. They thought it was a bear.

Corresponding arithmetic:

$$\begin{array}{ccc} 5204 & 23 & 837 \\ -530 & \times 3 & \times 7 \end{array}$$

Should comprehend and answer question: "What was the cow doing?"
Learning simple multiplication.

10–12 years

Activities to be observed:
Should read and comprehend paragraph #5 Durrell:

Reading:
In 1807, Robert Fulton took the first long trip in a steamboat. He went one hundred and fifty miles up the Hudson River. The boat went five miles an hour. This was faster than a steamboat had ever gone before. Crowds gathered on both banks of the river to see this new kind of boat. They were afraid that its noise and splashing would drive away all the fish.

Corresponding arithmetic:

$$\begin{array}{ccc} 420 & & \\ \times 29 & 9\overline{)72} & 31\overline{)62} \end{array}$$

Answer: "What river was the trip made on?"
Ask to write the sentence: "The fishermen did not like the boat."
Should do multiplication and simple division.

12–15 years

Activities to be observed:
Reads paragraph #7 Durrell:

Table 2–4 (cont'd). Developmental charts.

Reading:
   Golf originated in Holland as a game played on ice. The game in its present form first apeared in Scotland. It became unusually popular and kings found it so enjoyable that it was known as "the royal game." James IV, however, thought that people neglected their work to indulge in this fascinating sport so that it was forbidden in 1457. James relented when he found how attractive the game was, and it immediately regained its former popularity. Golf spread gradually to other countries, being introduced in America in 1890. It has grown in favor until there is hardly a town that does not boast of a private or public course.

Corresponding arithmetic:

$$536 \overline{)\ 4762} \qquad \tfrac{1}{3} \qquad 7\tfrac{1}{6}$$
$$+ \tfrac{1}{3} \qquad - \tfrac{3}{4}$$

Reduce fractions to lowest forms.

Ask to write sentence: "Golf originated in Holland as a game played on ice."
Answers questions:
   "Why was golf forbidden by James IV?"
   "Why did he change his mind?"
Does long division, adds and subtracts fractions.

[1]Modified from Leavitt SR, Goodman H, Harvin D: *Pediatrics* 1963;**31**:499.

throughout this period there is a gradual increase in sexual drives, which is manifested by increasingly aggressive play and interactions with the opposite sex. Fantasy still has an active role in dealing with sexuality before adolescence, and fantasies often focus on movie stars and rock heroes. Organized sports, clubs, and other activities are other modalities that permit preadolescent children to display socially acceptable forms of aggression and sexual interest.

For the 7-year-old, the major developmental task focuses on achievement in school and acceptance by peers. Academic expectations have intensified and require the child to concentrate, attend, and process increasingly complex auditory and visual information. Children with significant learning disabilities or problems of attention may have difficulty in these tasks and subsequently may receive significant negative reinforcement from teachers and even parents. Such children may develop a poor self-image, which may be manifested as behavioral difficulties. The pediatrician must evaluate potential learning disabilities in any child who is not developing adequately at this stage or who presents with emotional or behavioral problems. Their abilities are not as easily documented as milestones in early development. In the school-age child, the quality of the response, the attentional abilities, and the child's emotional approach to the task can make a dramatic difference in how successful the child is at school. The clinician must consider all of these aspects to appropriately diagnose learning disabilities. See Chapter 3.

Hagerman RJ: Pediatric assessment of the learning disabled child. *J Develop Pediatr* 1984;**5**:274.
Levine MD et al (editors): *Developmental-Behavioral Pediatrics.* Saunders, 1983.
Piaget J, Inyhelder B: *The Psychology of the Child.* Basic Books, 1969.

PREPUBERTAL & PUBERTAL GROWTH

The pubertal growth spurt occurs at approximately 10 years in females and 12.5 years in males. The speed of growth increases, reaching a peak of approximately 9 cm/y in females and 10.3 cm/y in males. Different areas of the skeleton attain their peak growth at different times. This is seen most dramatically in the feet, which first experience a growth spurt. This is followed by a rapid increase in leg length and subsequently by trunk growth. Facial growth occurs after peak height velocity. The mandible changes most remarkably, demonstrating a 25% increase in height between 12 and 20 years of age, compared to only a 6–7% increase in the size of the cranial base.

Boys have just over 2 more years of preadolescent growth than girls do; during this time leg growth increases more dramatically than trunk growth. Girls have a greater spurt in hip width, related to stature, than boys do, although boys exceed girls in most other areas of bone growth.

The Hypothalamic-Pituitary-Gonadal Axis & Puberty

Gonadal development is initiated in the fetus by 10 weeks' gestation, and it is almost complete by age 3 months in the male. This process occurs without significant input from gonadotropins, although placental hCG plays a significant role in migration of germ cells and differentiation of Leydig's cells. By the 21st week of gestation, the hypothalamus secretes gonadotropin-releasing hormone (GnRH), and the anterior pituitary releases follicle-stimulating hormone (FSH) and luteinizing hormone (LH). Their levels reach a peak by the 23rd to 24th week of gestation, which coincides with oocyte maturation in utero, including the development of primary follicles.

In the newborn period, GnRH is secreted in a pulsatile fashion, causing episodic elevations of both FSH and LH. In females, FSH predominates, and in males LH predominates; they stimulate elevations in testosterone and estrogen in the first few months of life. After this period of significant neuroendocrine activity, a quiescent period, with almost undetectable levels of gonadotropins, sets in and lasts through childhood. Hypothalamic secretion of GnRH is suppressed until puberty.

The large fetal adrenal gland regresses significantly after birth until adrenarche at 6 to 9 years of age. Adrenarche refers to the regrowth of the zona reticularis and the activation of its enzyme systems to produce adrenal steroids such as dihydroepiandrosterone sulfate and 17-ketosteroids. These steroids are partially responsible for body odor, the development of pubic and axillary hair, and stimulation of linear growth. Adrenarche occurs before gonadarche and is probably under the control of ACTH.

Gonadarche is initiated by the pulsatile secretion of GnRH from the hypothalamus, which in turn stimulates the release of gonadotropins. In early puberty, FSH and LH are secreted during sleep, and there is an increasing amplitude in its pulses as puberty progresses. The efficacy of FSH and LH also changes in that biopotency of these hormones improves as puberty progresses.

In conjunction with adrenal steroids and growth hormone, testosterone, stimulated from Leydig's cells, promotes a relatively specific pattern of pubertal development. The testes increase in size before 10 years of age, and pubic hair subsequently develops at the base of the penis in the first stage of puberty. The scrotum becomes more pendulous, the penis increases in size, and a mild degree of gynecomastia develops in 70% of males in the second stage of puberty. In the third and fourth stages of puberty, the voice deepens because of laryngeal growth, and there is an increase in sebaceous and sweat gland activity, often accompanied by acne. Growth hormone potentiates the action of sex steroids in males and facilitates the pubertal growth spurt. Muscle mass increases; boys gain particularly in shoulder width.

Sex steroids have some effect on bone growth but a more dramatic effect on bone maturation (Fig 2–14). They promote the fusion of epiphyseal plates in a predictable order. For instance, the plate at the head of the femur fuses between 15 and 17 years in boys and between 14 and 16 years in girls. The distal epiphyses of the radius, ulna, tibia, fibula, and femur fuse at 18 to 20 years in boys and 17 to 19 years in girls. The stage of osseous development correlates better with sexual maturation than does chronologic age or any other growth parameter. Most females begin menarche when skeletal maturation is between 13 and 13.5 years.

In females, breast buds begin between 8 and 13 years, with an average onset at 11 years. Usually the growth spurt has already begun at 10 years, and pubic hair usually develops soon after 11 years. Within the next 3 to 4 years, the pubic hair increases, the breasts, areola, and nipples enlarge further, and the hip width increases. Growth in the breasts is initially due to elongation and thickening of the ducts secondary to estrogen stimulation. After ovulation, progesterone from the corpus luteum stimulates the distal ends of the ducts to form lobules and alveoli, further enlarging the breasts.

Menarche usually occurs approximately 2 years after the onset of breast development. However, approximately 50 to 90% of cycles are anovulatory during the first 2 years after menarche. Although the average age for menarche is 13 years, this age has decreased significantly over the last century. Malnutrition, a low socioeconomic level, and excessive exercise can all delay menarche. After menarche, the final stage of neuroendocrine regulation occurs, with a biphasic effect of estrogen on the hypothalamus. Estrogens initially suppress secretion of gonadotropins, but subsequently a positive feedback system develops. A critical concentration of estrogen causes a surge of FSH and LH secretion in mid cycle, which stimulates ovulation.

In late puberty and adulthood, the nighttime predominance of gonadotropin pulses ceases, and pulsatile secretion occurs throughout the day and night. After menarche, the average increase in height is 3 inches, with a range of 1 to 7 inches, in American girls. For further information on adolescent development, see Chapter 10.

Dixon SD, Stein MT: *Encounters with Children: Pediatric Behavior and Development.* Year Book, 1987.

Falkner F, Tanner JM (editors): *Postnatal Growth Neurobiology.* Vol 2 of: *Human Growth, a Comprehensive Treatise,* 2nd ed. Plenum Press, 1986.

Lowrey GH: *Growth and Development of Children,* 8th ed. Year Book, 1986.

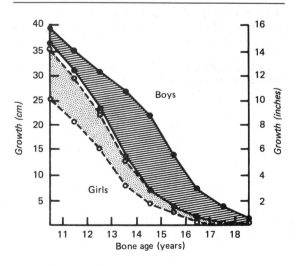

Figure 2–14. Growth expectancy at bone ages indicated. (Redrawn and reproduced, with permission, from Holt LE Jr, McIntosh R, Barnett HL: *Pediatrics,* 13th ed. Appleton-Century-Crofts, 1962, as redrawn from Harris JA et al: *Measurement of Man.* University of Minnesota Press, 1930.)

Orr DP, Ingersoll GM: Adolescent development: A biopsychosocial review. *Curr Probl Pediatr* (Aug) 1988; **18**:447.

Smith DW: *Growth and Its Disorders. Major Problems in Clinical Pediatrics,* vol 25. Saunders, 1977.

Tanner JM, Whitehouse RH, Takaishi M: Standards from birth to maturity for height, weight, height velocity: British children. *Arch Dis Child* 1965;**41**:454.

ADOLESCENT COGNITIVE & SOCIAL DEVELOPMENT

Adolescence is a difficult time because of the rehashing of earlier developmental issues, such as individuation and separation, but now in a context of a rapidly growing and maturing body and changing cognitive abilities. Piaget describes the development of formal operations in cognitive development at age 12. At this stage, abstract reasoning predominates in problem solving and understanding cause-and-effect relationships. Adolescents at this stage can better appreciate the relationship between current behavior and its long-term consequences. Egocentrism diminishes, and individuals are able to empathize and understand another's viewpoint.

The reality of the situation, however, is that very few young adolescents are in the stage of formal operations, and a substantial proportion of adolescents and adults never attain formal operational thinking. The thinking of early adolescents tends to be rigid and egocentric, with an overemphasis on concrete and physical aspects of social interaction. Some adolescents do not relate present actions to future consequences and cannot conceptualize. In an interview, they often give one-word answers and cannot discuss a concept at length. It is best to ask very concrete, specific questions to facilitate communication.

In mid adolescence, they begin to think abstractly, but the development of abstract thinking is a gradual process. It begins with introspection, which exacerbates the egocentrism of adolescence. Adolescents think about their own thinking and actions and develop pride in themselves, but often disdain for others, particularly adults, as they become critical of the thought processes of others. Their moral thinking advances, and they begin accepting the moral standards of the family and community rather than acting in certain ways for fear of punishment. Rules become more important, and dependence on and conformity to these rules dominate their lives, particularly at school. If they have difficulty succeeding in school, they may seek situations in which they can be successful, such as in a peer group that promotes antisocial behavior.

By mid to late adolescence, adult morality usually develops. It is marked by the development of moral principles that are autonomous and have validity apart from group rules. An individual is able to think abstractly about right and wrong and sort each problem out individually. Social cognitive growth, by late adolescence, is characterized by a lack of egocentrism and a true empathy for others. Rigidity is replaced by flexibility, and individuals become more accepting of those who are different from themselves. A lack of impulsiveness, an appropriate compliance, and an appreciation of long-term consequences facilitate the provision of health care at this stage. Some individuals do not reach this stage until adulthood, and some never achieve it. For further information, see Chapter 25.

Dixon SD, Stein MT: *Encounters with Children: Pediatric Behavior and Development*. Year Book, 1987.

Erikson EH: *Childhood and Society,* 2nd ed. Norton, 1963.

Ginsberg H, Opper S: *Piaget's Theory of Intellectual Development*. Prentice-Hall, 1969.

Orr DP, Ingersoll GM: Adolescent development: A biopsychosocial review. *Curr Probl Pediatr* (Aug) 1988; **18**:447.

Developmental Disorders

3

Bonnie W. Camp, MD, PhD

This chapter considers problems in development of cognitive and social competence. Competence is usually defined by comparing performance levels of an individual child with some norm derived from evaluating many children of the same age. Other standards of competence include comparison of the child's performance level with that of the adult norm and comparison of the child's present skills with skills needed to accomplish a given task or engage in a specific activity. Functional problems of mentally retarded children are discussed in this chapter; however, the main emphasis is on the larger group of children with learning and behavior problems that may or may not be associated with mental retardation.

Measurement of developmental competence is patterned on concepts of measuring intelligence. Although there is continued controversy over the extent to which heredity and environment determine intelligence, assessment of competence can be more usefully discussed independently of this issue. Assessment of competence hinges on the recognition that (1) children are able to perform increasingly more complex and difficult tasks as they get older; and (2) when tested at ages fairly close together, individual children tend to have a similar standing in relation to other children from one age to the next. By evaluating a child's performance on a variety of tasks requiring skills such as reasoning, abstract thinking, judgment, and planning and by determining how the child compares with other children of the same age, it is usually possible to predict school performance. Such assessments provide the basis for deriving an intelligence quotient and also may have implications for social behavior.

Measures of intelligence may be thought of as measures of general competence that attempt to determine what a child has learned in the process of exposure to an environment that provides unsystematic opportunities for learning that are grossly similar within a given culture. Anything that limits the breadth, variety, and depth of exposure or the ability of a child to profit from such exposure may place limits on the learning a given child will achieve in a given period. Anything that increases systematic exposure or increases breadth, variety, and depth of exposure potentially enhances learning.

Both biologic and psychosocial factors can increase or interfere with the growth-promoting effect of a child's general experience. Assessment of a child's general developmental or intellectual standing relative to other children sheds no light on the cause of the child's performance; consequently, it is important to determine whether an intelligence test gives a representative estimate of the child's usual functioning and whether other information might provide an explanation for low scores. Differences in experiential background often account for low scores of children from nondominant cultures given standard intelligence tests. Such explanations, however, do not necessarily alter the predictive value of scores from intelligence tests.

A variety of delays or deficiencies in the development of specific cognitive competence have also been identified and may or may not be associated with deficiencies in general competence. The most significant of these are associated with failure to acquire basic academic skills such as reading, writing, and arithmetic. Specific measures of competence are usually measures of achievement in areas where systematic instruction has been given (eg, music lessons, arithmetic lessons). Here again, both biologic and psychosocial factors (eg, "musical talent" or "math aptitude") may facilitate or interfere with development of competence in these specific areas. Measures of relative standing in specific areas of achievement correlate well with measures of intelligence. This correlation provides the basis for determining a child's expected level of achievement, whereas the discrepancy between expected and actual levels of achievement is a key factor for differential diagnosis in children with developmental problems.

Traditionally, social and emotional aspects of development have not been conceptualized as a dimension of competence. However, it is increasingly recognized that social competence is an important concept for assessing some aspects of social and emotional development. This is particularly true for aspects of behavior and social interaction such as empathy, distractibility, activity level, and aggression, which show strong, regular progression with age and which are associated with what has traditionally been termed cognitive development.

GENERAL PRINCIPLES IN EVALUATING COGNITIVE & SOCIAL COMPETENCE

Developmental evaluation should include (1) data that demonstrate a child's level of cognitive and social competence in both general and specific areas; (2) data that will assist in making an etiologic diagnosis; and (3) data relevant to management planning. An interdisciplinary team is often employed to develop the data base and a plan for management; this is the most thorough and effective approach. In addition to the pediatrician, the team usually includes a psychologist, social worker, educational specialist, and speech and language specialist. Assistance is also often needed from health care specialists in nursing, physical therapy, occupational therapy, ophthalmology, audiology, nutrition, and dentistry. Where an organized, functioning team is not available, the primary care physician can achieve similar results by requesting consultations from various professionals and obtaining information from other sources such as school personnel. It is also possible for the primary care physician to develop the minimal data base needed for initial assessment with only limited reliance on outside sources. The following discussion presents suggestions to assist the primary care physician in developing this data base through use of questionnaires and screening tests when assistance from other professionals is limited or unavailable.

History

A. Medical History: The medical history should focus on aspects of pregnancy, labor, and delivery that are likely to produce damage to the child's central nervous system (eg, use of drugs or x-rays during pregnancy; neonatal infections, asphyxia, and elevated bilirubin levels). Later evidence of central nervous system insults or injury, failure to thrive, chronic illnesses, hospitalizations, or abuse may also contribute significantly to a child's performance at school age. Neonatal records are often an important source of information, since they may reveal information forgotten by or unknown to parents. Recent studies have also focused on ways of combining psychosocial information about families from birth certificates to assess the risk for later problems in development.

B. Developmental History: The developmental history should include information about the age at which various milestones were passed, especially those pertaining to speech and language. Inability to use meaningful words other than "dada," "mama," "bye-bye," and "hello" by 18 months and inability to speak in short phrases by 24 months have been reported in association with specific learning disability as well as general slow learning and mental retardation. Development of motor skills is also important, particularly in assessing mental retardation, but deviance or delay in motor development may also be present in other conditions such as cerebral palsy and neuromuscular disorders. Information about sleep patterns, problems of temperament such as excessive crying or hyperactivity, and general problems may also be helpful.

C. Family History: Specific information regarding central nervous system disorders, mental retardation, epilepsy, or evidence of school problems or specific learning disabilities in other family members should be included. Details of the mother's pregnancy history, including stillbirths, deaths, and other problems, may also be helpful.

D. Educational and Learning History: In preschool children, considerable information can be obtained from a description of something the child has learned in an informal setting. If the child has been placed in a formal preschool setting, information should be obtained regarding the type of preschool and the child's relationships with other children and with teachers. Teachers can often give an excellent description of the child's performance and behavior in the classroom environment, and such assessments, even in the preschool period, are often as good as tests in predicting later problems.

Once a child has reached school age, the educational history should include details of grade placement, special educational evaluations and placement, repetition of grades, and other details of academic performance and participation in special programs. In the absence of a psychologist or educational specialist to provide this information, direct contact with school personnel is imperative for the primary care physician. Telephone conversations with the school nurse, teacher, social worker, or other professionals are very helpful in obtaining a clear picture of the child's performance and behavior in the school environment. Written reports from teachers using questionnaires that systematically address the most common types of learning problems can also be of great assistance.

E. Psychosocial History: Family problems and parental characteristics often interfere with development of both cognitive and social competence and foster deviant behavior in the child. Children of hostile, rejecting, highly authoritarian parents tend to be the most severely affected; these children often show advanced competence at 1 year of age but a progressive decline in competence beginning around 4 years of age. Children of nurturing parents with highly authoritarian parenting practices often do better; however, children of nurturing parents who are firm and verbal in providing guidance and setting standards without being rigidly authoritarian show advanced competence that increases with age. Parents who provide little nurturance or sense of belonging, who are too lax or too harsh in punishment, or who fail to supervise their children tend to have children who show early evidence of aggressive behavior problems that persist into adolescence and adulthood.

Because developmental and behavior problems in the child are often provoked by and associated with problems within the family or seem to be associated with a lack of family support for developing new skills, a good psychosocial history is an essential part of any developmental evaluation. Ideally, this should include assessment of the family's ability to promote cognitive and social development, which includes, as a minimum, information regarding the parents' linguistic and cultural background, quality of verbal interaction, disciplinary practices (use of positive reinforcement to shape behavior, reliance on physical punishment or limited use of reasoning or verbal explanations in discipline), ability to set standards, neglect, reliance on parenting practices that interfere with or inhibit development, family instability, marital discord, a hostile attitude toward the child, limitations in cognitive and social competence, depression, signs of maladjustment (eg, alcoholism, chronic unemployment, criminal or psychiatric problems), and general stress in the parents and chaos in the family that may contribute to and intensify developmental problems in the child.

In examining only the child, it is often difficult to distinguish behavior disorders associated with family problems from developmental disorders due to immaturity or alteration in development of the neurologic system. This difficulty has resulted in diagnosis by exclusion—ie, psychosocial assessment is used to determine whether there are social or emotional factors in the child's environment that can account for the observed learning or behavior problems. This is a practical approach in middle-class families, since it is often possible to ascertain that the family is reasonably stable and able to provide adequate support and stimulation to the child. Diagnosis by exclusion is, however, a very unsatisfactory approach for dealing with children from lower socioeconomic families, ie, the majority of children with behavior problems. The need for better assessment of these children is particularly acute, since they often have delays in both social and cognitive development and combinations of developmental delay and behavior problems. Ninety percent of the children who later show mental or emotional disorders are normal at birth and appear to be casualties of inadequate or pathologic environments.

At present, the most commonly used approach to family assessment is a global, clinical social history. Some of this information is usually included in the history obtained by the primary care physician. In most instances, however, a social worker will provide the most thorough and complete analysis. In preschool children, it is often helpful to supplement the usual clinical social history with the HOME (home observation for measurement of the environ-

ment) interview assessment of Bradley and Caldwell (see references, below). This is the most thoroughly studied approach to the systematic evaluation of the growth-promoting aspects of the child's environment. This interview, which requires a home visit, is used to identify economically disadvantaged families unlikely to support development in their children. It may be performed by any trained person but is usually done by a social worker or nurse. A shorter, questionnaire version of the HOME interview, the Home Screening Questionnaire (HSQ), provides most of the information obtained from the longer interview version and can be administered and scored by the pediatrician during a clinic or office visit. Although it has not yet been studied widely enough to determine its clinical usefulness, the HSQ appears to be a promising tool for use by the primary care physician. Neither scale is expected to be useful in evaluating children from middle or upper socioeconomic families.

Badger E, Burne D, Vietze P: Maternal risk factors as predictors of development outcome in early childhood. *Infant Ment Health J* 1981;**2**:33.

Bradley RH, Caldwell BM: Pediatric usefulness of home assessment. In: *Advances in Behavioral Pediatrics*. Vol 2. Camp BW (editor). JAI Press, 1981.

Coons CE et al: *The Home Screening Questionnaire Reference Manual*. LADOCA Publishing Foundation, 1981.

Physical & Neurologic Examination

It is essential that a thorough physical and neurologic examination be performed. A number of children will demonstrate neurologic "soft signs," eg, clumsiness, right-left confusion, disordered temporal orientation, overflow phenomena, choreiform movements, and finger agnosia. Although "soft signs" are commonly associated with school learning and behavior problems, the significance of these signs is controversial because they are also found in children who have no other problems and because most appear to represent delay in maturation rather than dysfunction. PANESS (physical and neurologic examination for soft signs), a standardized neurologic examination, has been studied and shows promising results for systematic evaluation of "soft signs."

In addition, recent studies linking minor physical anomalies with behavior disorders in childhood have prompted physicians to examine for the presence of dysmorphic features such as abnormal palmar creases, syndactyly, unruly hair, malformed ears, skin tags, and facial abnormalities. While these features are commonly seen in children with mental retardation, the implications of their presence in nonretarded children are not fully understood.

Holden EW, Tarnowski KJ, Prinz RJ: Reliability of neurobiological soft signs in children: Reevaluation of the PANESS. *J Abnorm Child Psychol* 1982;**10**:163.

Sensory Function

All children in whom developmental delay or mental retardation is suspected should be examined for visual and auditory problems. In infants and young children, sensory deficits may be mistaken for retardation. Retarded children often have sensory deficits in addition to their retardation, and this increases the complexity of their problem. In most nonretarded, school-aged children, vision and hearing can be satisfactorily evaluated by the usual screening methods and referral made to a specialist for further evaluation of children with abnormal screening results.

A variety of vision problems have been proposed as causes of reading problems, most without substantial research support. Learning to read can be accomplished quite satisfactorily with limited visual acuity. Although it is important that visual defects be corrected to improve the child's overall functioning, it is generally agreed that learning problems are seldom linked to refractive errors. Difficulty with convergence at near point, however, may interfere significantly with the process of reading and should receive careful evaluation.

Hearing loss has a significant impact on language development and may be associated with severe learning and behavior problems. Intermittent hearing loss, such as that due to otitis media, has been implicated in learning disabilities. In the past, deaf children have often been mistakenly labeled retarded. Losses in the high-frequency range may be associated with problems in discriminating speech sounds necessary for school learning. Others may have problems differentiating speech sounds despite normal hearing.

Emotional & Social Behavior

Although some information can be obtained directly from the child through interviews, play, and projective testing, typically one must rely on interviews with parents and reports from school personnel to obtain a picture of the child's social competence. Much of this information is obtained by social workers, psychologists, or psychiatrists. In evaluating reports of problem behavior at home and at school, it is helpful to assess the degree of deviance by comparing an individual child's behavior with children in general. Large studies of normal children indicate that most children show a few signs of deviant behavior. The truly deviant child, however, usually demonstrates this in a variety of ways. It is especially important to seek information about positive attributes, because these appear to be more powerful indicators of later mental health than negative attributes are of later maladjustment. Three of the most important positive attributes are school attendance (irrespective of performance), positive peer relations, and nondelinquency.

General adaptation and development of self-help are often included in developmental assessments of preschool children. Beginning around age 4 years (when abstract reasoning becomes the dominant factor in measures of cognitive development), it becomes increasingly important to include some assessment of general adaptation in the differential diagnosis of mental retardation. Children from minority cultures who perform poorly on IQ tests often appear less retarded when general adaptation is evaluated.

Rating scales of behavior, such as the ACTeRS scale (ADD-H: Comprehensive Teachers Rating Scale) (Table 3–1) for identifying children with attention deficit disorder, are important tools for assessing school behavior. The ACTeRS scale has been designed to identify clusters of problems in the areas of attention, hyperactivity, social skills, and oppositional behavior. Norms to assess the degree of deviance are available. The ACTeRS scale is readily acceptable to teachers and can be used by primary care physicians to assess the need for and response to stimulant medication.

A scale for obtaining teacher ratings of general behavior is also useful for identifying children with deviant behavior other than distractibility and hyperactivity and for assessing the degree and amount of prosocial (positive) behavior. Several such scales are available for assessing children as early as the preschool period, and some include rating scales to be completed by parents as well as the teacher.

Family & Social Resources

The type, extent, and cost of educational and counseling services available to the child and family, the family's ability to support and carry through with treatment plans, and other community resources should be assessed early in the evaluation. These factors often limit or modify the treatment plan developed for a child. Sixty percent of families presenting children for evaluation of learning problems have clear-cut social and emotional problems that need to be assessed and addressed as an integral part of treatment planning for the child. Social services are usually the principal sources of information in this area, and much of this information will be derived from the psychosocial history. In addition, however, the primary care physician should become familiar with resources in the community.

Intelligence

Measures of intelligence attempt to describe a child's general cognitive competence in relation to other children of the same age. The tests provide an increasingly difficult set of problems, and questions tend to tap general knowledge, reasoning, judgment, and organization of analytic skills that are expected to develop in the course of experiences encountered by most children in the process of growing up. Where children have grossly different experiences

A. Raw Scores

Table 3-1. ACTeRS scale. A: Raw Scores.

Child's Name: _____

Rater: _____

ID #: _____

Date: _____

NOTE:
Below are descriptions of behavior. Please read each item and compare the child's behavior with that of his or her classmates. Circle the number that most closely corresponds with your evaluation. Transfer the total raw score for each of the four sections to the profile sheet to determine normative percentile scores.

ATTENTION

	Almost Never				Almost Always
1. Works well independently	1	2	3	4	5
2. Persists with task for reasonable amount of time	1	2	3	4	5
3. Completes assigned task satisfactorily with little additional assistance	1	2	3	4	5
4. Follows simple directions accurately	1	2	3	4	5
5. Follows a sequence of instructions	1	2	3	4	5
6. Functions well in the classroom	1	2	3	4	5

Add items 1–6 and place total here_____

HYPERACTIVITY

	Almost Never				Almost Always
7. Extremely overactive (out of seat, "on the go")	1	2	3	4	5
8. Overreacts	1	2	3	4	5
9. Fidgety (hands always busy)	1	2	3	4	5
10. Impulsive (acts or talks without thinking)	1	2	3	4	5
11. Restless (squirms in seat)	1	2	3	4	5

Add items 7–11 and place total here_____

SOCIAL SKILLS

	Almost Never				Almost Always
12. Behaves positively with peers/classmates	1	2	3	4	5
13. Verbal communication clear and "connected"	1	2	3	4	5
14. Nonverbal communication accurate	1	2	3	4	5
15. Follows group norms and social rules	1	2	3	4	5
16. Cites general rule when criticizing ("We aren't supposed to do that")	1	2	3	4	5
17. Skillful at making new friends	1	2	3	4	5
18. Approaches situations confidently	1	2	3	4	5

Add items 12–18 and place total here_____

OPPOSITIONAL

	Almost Never				Almost Always
19. Tries to get others into trouble	1	2	3	4	5
20. Starts fights over nothing	1	2	3	4	5
21. Makes malicious fun of people	1	2	3	4	5
22. Defies authority	1	2	3	4	5
23. Picks on others	1	2	3	4	5
24. Mean and cruel to other children	1	2	3	4	5

Add items 19–24 and place total here_____

[1]Modified and reproduced, with permission, from Ullmann RK, Sleator EK, Sprague RL. ACTeRS Rating Form and Profile, copyright © 1986 by MetriTech, Inc., 111 North Market Street, Champaign, IL. (217) 398-4868.

34 / CHAPTER 3

Table 3–1 (cont'd). ACTeRS scale. *B:* Profile—girls' form.

B. Profile—Girls' Form

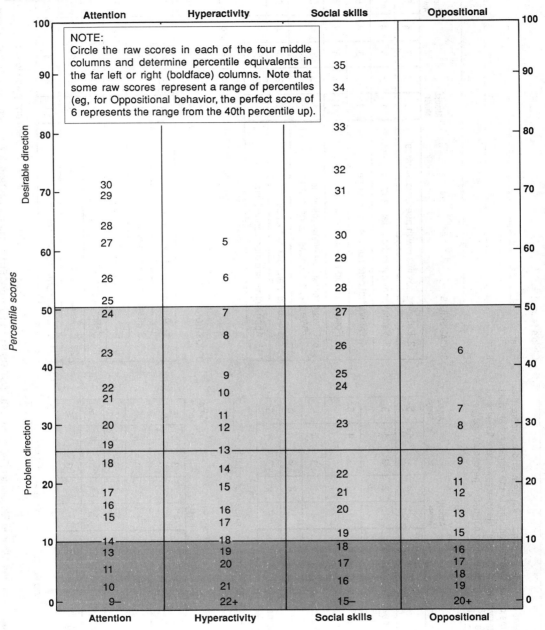

from those in the standard population, their scores may be expected to vary upward or downward. Originally, the IQ score obtained from such tests represented the percentage of expectancy a child had reached at a given age. This was derived by the formula (mental age ÷ chronologic age) × 100. Scores on most modern tests can still be reported in terms of MA/CA, but the most important tests yield IQ scores that represent a child's relative distance from the average child in standard score units.

In the preschool period, the principal diagnostic tests in general use are the Bayley Scales of Infant Development (for children under 30 months of age), the Stanford-Binet Intelligence Scale, the McCarthy Scales of Children's Abilities (for children 3 years of age and older), and the Kaufman Assessment Battery for Children (K-ABC). These are all individually administered tests, given by trained personnel. The screening tests used most commonly in the preschool period are the Revised Denver Developmental

Screening Test (Frankenberg); the Revised Developmental Screening Inventory (Knobloch et al); and, among older preschool children, the Early Screening Inventory (Meisels and Wiske). (See Table 3–2 for a summary of the screening tests discussed in this chapter.)

In recent years, several new assessment methods have been developed to capitalize on the caretaker's knowledge of the infant and preschool child. Procedures such as the Kent Infant Development Scale (KIDS) for children under 12 months of age and the Minnesota Child Development Inventory for children over 12 months of age use the caretaker's report to assess the child's general development, including cognitive, gross motor, fine motor, expressive language, self-help, and personal/social development. These procedures have several advantages: They provide for the inclusion of a large number of items at each age, are based on behavior readily observable at home, do not require extensive training for their administration, and can be used to plan and monitor appropriate intervention at home. Disadvantages include potential inaccuracy in the caretaker's reply and bias in reporting.

The Wechsler scales (Wechsler Adult Intelligence Scale [WAIS], Wechsler Intelligence Scale for Children, Revised [WISC-R], and Wechsler Preschool and Primary Scale of Intelligence [WPPSI] and the Stanford-Binet Intelligence Scale are the most widely used individual intelligence tests for school-age and older children. The Kaufman Assessment Battery for Children (K-ABC) is a relatively new test that is also gaining wide acceptance. The Stanford-Binet test is a highly verbal test with nonverbal items intermingled; results are reported as a single IQ score. The Wechsler scales are subdivided into 6 verbal and 6 nonverbal tests so that a verbal IQ and performance IQ can both be obtained as well as an IQ based on the full test (full-scale IQ). The Kaufman Battery is designed to assess differences in simultaneous and sequential processing of information as well as differences between aptitude and achievement. It is commonly thought that intelligence tests can reveal the potential for higher functioning, especially when scatter (the pattern of high and low scores) is examined carefully, and both the K-ABC and the Wechsler scales lend themselves particularly well to this task.

The standardized, individually administered tests of intelligence discussed above require extensive training for proper administration and are usually administered by trained psychologists. The Slosson Intelligence Test, however, is an abbreviated version of the Stanford-Binet test and is designed for use by nonprofessionals, including office assistants and primary care physicians. It is probably the most suitable screening test for estimating intelligence in children over 4½ years of age.

A number of briefer screening tests, such as the Peabody Picture Vocabulary Test and the Quick Test, are also suitable for use in office settings. These measure vocabulary skills alone, based on the fact that vocabulary has the best correlation with overall estimates of intelligence. A variety of other short screening tools are available, some of which rely on parent reporting or a combination of parent reporting and observation, but these often suffer from limited information regarding standardization data.

Achievement

Achievement usually refers to performance in specific school-related areas where a child has received instruction. In the preschool period, achievement is seldom distinguished from general development. By the time the child enters kindergarten, however, a variety of procedures are available for assessing readiness. In a child with a mental age of 6 years, 2 of the best predictors for readiness to enter the first grade are the ability to engage in sustained task-oriented behavior and the knowledge of letter names and sounds. A number of procedures are available to assess school readiness, and in recent years, testing programs have been specifically designed for early identification of children with learning disabilities. Although results of these programs appear to be about as accurate as teacher assessments of kindergarten performance, many feel that the programs represent an important advance. Most of the early identification testing programs are designed for use in schools or by psychologists. Several procedures are also available for use by primary care physicians in screening for school readiness at the time of well-child visits in the 4½- to 5½-year age range. These include the developmental screening tests described previously and the preschool portions of the Wide Range Achievement Test (WRAT; see below).

For school-age children, scores on a variety of achievement tests are often available through routine classroom testing done at school, and results of such testing should be included in the educational history. Where low scores are obtained on group testing of achievement, individual testing should be performed before accepting the results as representative of the child's ability. Many school systems with special education services can administer individual tests of achievement and give the test scores to the primary care physician. The Woodcock-Johnson Psych-Educational Battery is an individually administered battery of cognitive, achievement, and interest tests often used by educators to assess achievement and the discrepancy between aptitude and achievement.

Unfortunately, many children who are referred to a pediatrician for evaluation have no current achievement test scores in their school records. This is particularly true for children referred because of behavior problems. When an educational specialist or psychologist is unavailable to provide this information, the primary care physician may wish to make his or her own assessment through use of a screening test such as WRAT. WRAT is a rapid screening test for assessing achievement in reading, spelling, and arithmetic. It is suitable for testing children from kindergarten through college, and norms (available from the National Health Survey, as well as the publisher) are based on results in children from a representative sample of ethnic and economic groups throughout the country. The reading test covers only the accuracy of word reading and tends to yield higher scores than more thorough and comprehensive procedures do. However, WRAT is a simple and easy test to administer, and scores are reported in grade equivalents, percentiles, and standard scores that are comparable to many IQ test scores. In addition, the copying portions of the spelling test can be used to attain a rapid assessment of visual-motor coordination (discussed below).

Adaptive Behavior

Assessment of adaptive behavior is seldom addressed directly in children unless a child is suspected of being mentally retarded. Because poor performance on a cognitive test may result from many factors, it is essential that the accuracy of low scores be confirmed by assessment of functional level in everyday living. Scales such as the Vineland Adaptive Behavior Scales and the Scales of Independent Behavior are questionnaire/structured interview methods for assessing the child's developmental level in areas such as social interaction, communication, personal living, and community living.

Perceptual-Motor Function

In the early school years, a number of children with delays in copying and drawing skills will also demonstrate problems in learning to read. These problems have been variously termed visual-perceptual and visual-motor problems, and their presence in children beyond 7–9 years of age has often been thought to indicate the existence of central nervous system dysfunction, although this inference is controversial. There is a relationship between visual-perceptual problems and reading problems in the early school years; as children get older, however, reading achievement becomes more and more related to intelligence, even when the perceptual problems persist. Furthermore, perceptual problems are common among children from families in lower socioeconomic groups and even among children whose only history is confinement to bed for more than 2 months during the preschool years.

Because performance on tests of copying skills is highly correlated with intelligence, such tests are most useful when there is a discrepancy between the developmental level demonstrated on visual-perceptual tests and general intelligence. Methods for assessing the degree of this discrepancy are not

as well developed as for assessing the discrepancy between IQ and achievement. At a practical level, however, these problems may be severe enough to interfere with learning the skills of printing and writing. In this latter case, it is usually more helpful to analyze the child's writing, but several visual-perceptual tests, such as the Beery Test of Visual-Motor Integration, are commonly used to examine copying skills per se.

Speech & Language

Speech and language delays are common in mentally retarded children but may also occur in children with average or above-average intelligence. A number of children who appear to have specific learning problems will, on closer evaluation, show evidence of delay in language development or an articulation problem (or both). These problems can limit academic achievement in areas that depend on verbal skills (eg, reading). Speech and language delays in preschool children and methods for evaluating them have been discussed previously (see Chapter 2).

Most children should reach the adult proficiency level in language by 7–8 years of age, at which time evaluation of language skills typically becomes merged with evaluation of verbal intelligence. Scores on tests such as the Wechsler scale, the Stanford-Binet test, or the Slosson test will reflect language skills as well as intelligence. Specialized tests for assessing components of receptive and expressive language and language-processing skills are also available.

Motivation

Clinical assessment of motivation has received little attention despite mounting evidence that motivation is a key factor in determining how a child will use whatever time and help are provided for learning new skills. Studies of achievement motivation have suggested that 2 main motivational types can be identified, ie, those who are challenged by moderately difficult tasks and respond to success and those who are primarily motivated to avoid failure and will only attempt very easy tasks, where failure is unlikely, or very difficult ones, where failure carries no stigma. One of the major shifts that occurs in the age range of 5–7 years is from motivational dependence on social and external rewards to internal motivation for mastery of skills. Some children make this shift poorly or not at all and will fail to learn in the usual academic climate, which emphasizes mastery and competition. Often these are the children who seem primarily motivated to avoid failure and who need liberal support from external sources (praise, concrete incentives) just for trying. While motivational immaturity is seldom the principal problem, it is often a major determinant of how well a child will respond or progress in an educational program.

Table 3–2. Recommendations for use of assessment procedures.

Name	Type of Test	Age Range	Administered By
Wide Range Achievement Test	Achievement: reading, spelling, math, visual-perceptual	5 y–adult	Trained screener
Woodcock-Johnson Psych-Educational Battery	Aptitude and achievement	3 y–adult	Professional
Scales of Independent Behavior	Adaptive behavior	All ages	Professional
Vineland Adaptive Behavior Scales	Adaptive behavior	All ages	Professional
Bayley Scales of Infant Development	Development	3–30 mo	Professional
Revised Denver Developmental Screening Test (DDST)	Development	3 mo–6 y	Trained screener
Developmental Profile II (DPII)	Development	0–9 y	Trained screener
Early Screening Inventory	Development	4–6 y	Trained screener
Kent Infant Development Scale (KIDS)	Development	0–1 y	Caretaker response
Minnesota Child Development Inventory (MCDI)	Development	1–6 y	Caretaker response
Kaufmann Assessment Battery for Children (K-ABC)	Intelligence and achievement	2.5–12.5 y	Professional
McCarthy Scales of Children's Abilities	Intelligence	2.5–8.5 y	Professional
Slossen Intelligence Test	Intelligence	4.5 y–adult	Trained screener
Stanford-Binet Intelligence Scale	Intelligence	2 y–adult	Professional
Wechsler Intelligence Scale for Children-Revised (WISC-R)	Intelligence	6–16 y	Professional
Wechsler Preschool & Primary Scale of Intelligence (WPPSI)	Intelligence	4–6 y	Professional
Beery Test of Visual-Motor Integration	Visual-motor	2–15 y	Professional

Beery KE: *Revised Administration, Scoring, and Teaching Manual for the Developmental Test of Visual-Motor Integration.* Modern Curriculum Press, 1982.
Bruininks RH et al: *Scales of Independent Behavior.* DLM Teaching Resources, 1984.
Frankenburg WK: *Denver Developmental Screening Test Reference Manual (Revised).* LADOCA Foundation, 1975.
Jastak JF, Jastak S: *Wide Range Achievement Test.* Jastak Associates, 1984.
Knobloch H, Steven F, Malone AF: *Manual of Developmental Diagnosis.* Harper, 1980.
Meisels SJ, Wiske MS: *Early Screening Inventory.* Teachers College, 1983.
Slosson RL: *Slosson Intelligence Test for Children and Adults.* Slosson Educational Publications, 1985.
Sparrow SS et al: *Vineland Adaptive Behavior Scales: Interview Edition, Survey Form Manual.* American Guidance Service, 1984.

EVALUATING THE DISCREPANCY BETWEEN INTELLIGENCE & ACHIEVEMENT

The differential diagnosis of competence problems necessitates an evaluation of the significance of the discrepancy between expected achievement based on measures of general competence (intelligence) and actual achievement in specific areas of academic performance. The following material presents 2 methods of calculating the degree of discrepancy between IQ and achievement, based on grade equivalents and standard scores.

The United States Office of Education defines the discrepancy between achievement and IQ as significant when achievement is below 50% of expected grade level. The lowest level of achievement commensurate with age and intelligence is calculated by the following formula:

$$\text{Age } [(\text{IQ}/300) + 0.17] - 2.5 = \text{Lowest grade equivalent score which is commensurate with age and intelligence}$$

For an 8-year-old child with an IQ of 100, this formula indicates that a grade level of 1.5 is the lowest score that would be commensurate with age and intelligence. If this child's achievement test scores are below grade level 1.5, then there is a significant discrepancy. If they are at grade level 1.5 or higher, the discrepancy is not significant.

The following formula utilizes the direct correlation between intelligence test and achievement test scores to calculate the smallest difference between IQ and achievement test score needed to represent a significant discrepancy (D):

$$D = 1.96 \text{ SD } \sqrt{1 - r^2}$$ where SD = Standard deviation of scores on achievement test
r = correlation between IQ and achievement test scores

This formula can be used to compare an IQ obtained from a test such as the Slosson test with a standard score obtained from the WRAT. The Slosson test manual provides the information that the correlation coefficient with the WRAT is 0.72, and the WRAT manual provides the information that the standard deviation of scores on the WRAT is 15. According to this calculation, a difference of 20 points between IQ and achievement test score is needed before a difference between these 2 tests is significant at the $p = .05$ level of confidence or better.

Both of these approaches call attention to the fact that some difference between expected and actual achievement represents normal variation, while a significant discrepancy is defined in terms of an unusual degree of difference. Individual school districts are free to adopt their own criteria in determining the extent of this discrepancy that must exist for a child to qualify for special services.

TEMPERAMENTAL TRAITS & REACTIONS TO DEVELOPMENTAL CRISES

During the ages of 5–7 years and 10–13 years, major developmental changes occur in most children. In the 5- to 7-year period, children enter school, begin to develop operational thought, and shift from associative thinking to use of verbal mediation activity in learning and thinking. The 10- to 13-year period heralds the onset of puberty, entrance into junior high school, and development of formal operational thought. Inflections in the growth curve for intelligence occur during both periods, and there is a dramatic increase in a cluster of behavior problems that appear to be phase-specific reactions to the developmental changes occurring during these periods. These problems include restless sleep, disturbing dreams, physical timidity, irritability, overdependence, and jealousy. Emotional turbulence during one of these periods may or may not be associated with turbulence during the other period, and its occurrence in either does not seem to be indicative of serious long-term problems.

Often there is overlap between these phase-specific reactions and temperamental traits, which include characteristics such as shyness, oversensitiveness, somberness, and reserve. Both phase-specific reactions and temperamental traits may be a source of conflict between parents and children, but they do not in themselves indicate the presence of serious emotional disturbance. They usually resolve with support, and the child does not need treatment.

Kohlberg, L, LaCrosse J, Ricks D: The predictability of adult mental health from childhood behavior. In: *Manual of Child Psychopathology*. Wolman BB (editor). McGraw-Hill, 1972.

DISORDERS IN DEVELOPMENT OF COGNITIVE COMPETENCE (See Table 3–3.)

SPECIFIC LEARNING DISORDERS

Essentials of Diagnosis
■ Significant discrepancy between estimated intelligence (usually verbal) and achievement in one or more areas.
■ Achievement commensurate with intelligence in one or more academic areas.
■ No evidence of sensory deficits.
■ Either presence or absence (often absence) of behavior problems.

General Considerations
Specific problems may be experienced in any area of academic achievement, but the most common problems involve reading or spelling (dyslexia). Frequent but less common problems are specific to arithmetic (dyscalculia) or writing (dysgraphia). Intelligence is usually average or above average, but the key element in making the diagnosis is demonstrating a discrepancy between actual achievement and expected achievement in a specific area. (See previous section on discrepancy.)

Descriptive Classification
A. Reading and Spelling Disorders (Developmental Dyslexia): Dyslexia is the most common type of specific learning disorder. It occurs more frequently in boys than in girls (3:1), and in 34% of cases there is a strong family history, especially among the male relatives. Speech and language problems and problems in sequencing are the most common developmental problems associated with specific reading disorders. A variety of developmental problems such as clumsiness and incoordination, directional confusion, right-left confusion, disordered temporal orientation, and difficulties in naming colors and in recognizing the meaning of pictures have been reported in children with specific reading problems. These are of lesser importance than the speech and language problems and may be more related to intelligence than to reading disorder per se. A history of delays in speech and language development is present in at least one-third of cases. This involves delays such as failure to use meaningful words other than "mama," "dada," "hello," and "bye-bye" until after 18 months of age and failure to use 2-word phrases before 24 months of age. Although evidence of associated neurologic deficit or differential use of the right versus the left hemisphere can be demonstrated in some children, such results of neurologic investigations have generally contributed little to treatment or prognosis.

Traditionally, the definition of specific reading disorder (dyslexia) included failure to learn to read despite adequate sensory apparatus, conventional instruction, average intelligence, and sociocultural opportunity. Such diagnosis by exclusion was an attempt to distinguish between "unexpected" reading failure and reading failure that could be explained by a more general or pervasive factor, such as mental subnormality, cultural or educational deprivation, sensory defects, or emotional disturbance. With this

Table 3–3. Differential diagnosis of learning problems.

Type of Learning Problem	Characteristics	Treatment Issues
Disorders with IQ-achievement discrepancy		
Specific learning disorders:	Achievement is below IQ in an isolated area. The disorder is not due to sensory impairment. Other areas are at levels of expectancy.	Individualized instruction (often tutoring) in area of weakness should be provided. Normalized educational experiences in other areas is indicated.
Reading/spelling (dyslexia)	Achievement is below expectancy only in reading/spelling.	Specific instruction in reading/spelling/language arts is indicated. The child often exhibits generalized deficits in language processing. The child may have problems in math because of reading.
Arithmetic (dyscalculia)	Achievement is below expectancy only in arithmetic.	Specific instruction in math is indicated. Dyscalculia may be difficult to separate from a reading or writing disorder.
Writing (dysgraphia)	Achievement is below expectancy in written work.	Status of visual functioning must be clarified. Specific treatment for handwriting skill is indicated. Dysgraphia is often difficult to separate from dyslexia.
Hyperlexia	The child begins reading at a very early age (eg, 2 y). The child may appear autistic or show unusual discrepancies in abilities.	Comprehensive assessment and treatment in several areas of weakness is necessary. The prognosis for the autistic child is relatively good.
Nonspecific learning disorders:		
Underachievement	Achievement is below IQ in several areas. Underachievement may be due to environmental, behavioral (eg, ADHD), motivational, or situational problems, or to school absence.	The child often has emotional/behavior problems as well.
Generalized learning disability	Achievement is below IQ in several areas. The disability is not due to sensory impairment. The disability is often accompanied by evidence of visual/perceptual/motor difficulties. Associated environmental, emotional/behavioral, or motivational problems are often present.	Unusual combinations of discrepant functioning may be a reflection of abnormal brain functioning.
Disorders without IQ-achievement discrepancy		
Slow learner	IQ and achievement are commensurate but at low-normal to below normal levels.	Learning is slow but steady with appropriate programming.
Mental retardation	Both IQ and achievement are more than 2 SD below average.	
Educable	IQ is usually 50–70.	The child is capable of achieving rudiments of literacy.
Trainable	IQ is usually below 50.	The child is capable of acquiring preacademic and vocational skills.

approach, most children with reading problems tend to be excluded from the diagnosis of specific reading disorder—ie, their reading problems are attributed to the fact that they are slightly below average in intelligence, come from economically disadvantaged homes, or have emotional and behavior problems. Yet many in this large group show reading achievement below expectancy for their mental age; and in neurologic status, cognitive functioning, and other areas of achievement they are indistinguishable from the group defined in the traditional sense as having specific reading disorder. In addition, the presence of a significant discrepancy between actual and expected achievement is the only characteristic that is common to members of highly specific etiologic groups such as those with genetic dyslexia diagnosed on the basis of linkage studies.

Consequently, current thinking endorses the concept that subtypes of reading disability should first be described in terms of clear-cut characteristics irrespective of etiologic considerations. There have been 2 major approaches to this subtyping. One approach attempts to distinguish among different problems on the basis of analysis of reading and spelling errors; this has led to subtyping into 2 groups based on whether performance indicates heavier reliance on auditory-sequential-phonologic skills (auditory reader) or on visual-spatial-imagery (visual reader). The other approach uses associated disabilities such as those in language, perceptual-motor skills, and memory to distinguish the following probable subtypes: (1) a language disorder group with defects in understanding and expression of oral language; (2) a dyscoordination group with defects in speech articulation, copying skills, and understanding of oral language; (3) a visual-spatial-perceptual disorder group with visual, perceptual, and visual-constructive problems but intact oral language; and (4) a group with dysphonemic sequencing disorder.

B. Mathematics Disorders (Developmental Dyscalculia): Mathematics disorders have been studied primarily in relation to the developmental Gerstmann syndrome (dyscalculia, right-left disorientation, and finger agnosia) and often have been considered to be part of a reading disorder. However, limited studies of school children who demonstrate a significant discrepancy between actual and expected achievement in arithmetic suggest that a specific syndrome of mathematical disability does exist and affects approximately 6% of the population. Developmental disorder is distinguished from acquired disorder by the absence of clearly defined brain damage and neurologic findings in the former.

Several forms have been described and are characterized by difficulty in verbalizing, writing, reading, manipulating, or understanding mathematical operations. In individuals whose difficulties are confined to performance on numerical tests, signs of neurologic abnormalities tend to be few. In those who are unable to read or write numbers, the disorder may be associated with general disorders in reading and writing as well as mathematics, so that a learning disorder specific to mathematics may be difficult to demonstrate.

C. Writing Disorders (Developmental Dysgraphia): Children with reading problems often have illegible handwriting as well as spelling problems. In younger children, problems due to immature perceptual-motor development (eg, mirror writing, reversal of letters, and poor construction of letters) are common. Some children will have problems confined to illegible handwriting, inaccurate copying, or inability to transmit sequences of verbal information to paper. In some of these instances, illegibility is associated with mild cerebral palsy or general problems in fine motor coordination. Whether encountered alone or in combination with reading or math disability, specific training is often required to correct the penmanship problems.

A common syndrome seen in students during late elementary and junior high school involves not only elements of poor handwriting (slow, illegible, poor spatial organization) but also deficits in memory, expressive language, organization of ideas, and fluency. This has been termed "developmental output failure"; it is usually manifested by overall reduced productivity, with refusals to complete work, failure to submit assignments, and "forgetting" to do homework.

Left-handed children deserve special attention because they have frequently had poor instruction. In most instances, their problems in penmanship will improve with appropriate instruction. Despite common belief to the contrary, there is little evidence associating left-handedness with any kind of deficiency.

Etiologic Classification

Both psychobiologic and sociopsychologic factors appear to play a major causative role in specific learning disabilities. The group of children who fail to learn despite conventional instruction, adequate familial-cultural opportunity, and adequate intelligence have generally been thought to represent an idiopathic or genetically based syndrome. This group has been distinguished from children with emotionally, educationally, or culturally based limitations on the one hand and those with disorders secondary to sensory defects, brain damage, or mental retardation on the other.

In the idiopathic group, the term minimal brain dysfunction (MBD) has often been applied when neurologic "soft signs," poor motor coordination, and distractibility are present along with learning problems in children of average or above-average intelligence. The term has also been applied indiscriminately to children who show any one of these features alone, but the clinical picture of children with the full picture described above provides the most convincing evidence for attributing the problem to some type of neurologic handicap. However, because extensive research has failed to provide substantial evidence of dysfunction and because many of the characteristics are common in preschool children and tend to be present only in younger learning-disabled children, many have abandoned the concept of minimal brain damage altogether in favor of the view that the neurologic problem is one of immaturity.

Clinical Findings

A family history often reveals affected family members, especially among the males. Findings on physical examination are usually normal, and those on neurologic examination are normal except for the presence of "soft signs." Behavior problems may or may not be present. Intelligence test results often indicate average or above-average intelligence on nonverbal tests and may or may not show some decrease in verbal IQ. In contrast, achievement in the affected area of learning is significantly below nonverbal intelligence and sometimes below verbal intelligence. Achievement in nonaffected areas tends to progress normally. Vision and hearing are usually normal, although deficits in processing auditory sequential information are often noted on extensive testing.

Although reading disorders are common among brain-injured children (18–40%), a reading disorder is not necessarily associated with other evidence of altered cortical functioning. Furthermore, educational, language, and other psychometric tests are often of no help in distinguishing poor readers who are brain-injured from poor readers who are not brain-injured. Electroencephalography, CT scanning, and a variety of other procedures have been used in the past with little or no success.

Differential Diagnosis

The term "specific learning disability" is primarily a descriptive one that distinguishes between specific learning disorder, general learning disorder (slow learner), or mental retardation. Etiologic diagnosis is more difficult. The most important distinction is whether there is a strong family history, inadequate educational background, sociocultural disadvantage, or evidence of brain damage.

Treatment

The principal treatment for specific learning disorders is individualized instruction. Most of the children are best viewed as "hard to teach," and ultimate outcome will usually depend upon the child's access to individual instruction with an experienced and knowledgeable teacher and motivation to use the time and help provided. There have been many claims that instruction should be tailored to the sub-

type of reading disorder, but research has generally failed to support this claim. In part, this may result from the fact that discussions of reading instruction often deal only with questions of content. In this regard, there are basically 4 ways of altering the content of reading materials: (1) presentation of the whole word approach (look-say); (2) use of phonics (intrinsic or extrinsic); (3) use of a syllabary (or rebus); and (4) orthographic changes, eg, use of a modified alphabet such as the Initial Teaching Alphabet or use of words in color.

It is evident from considering the various structures of the reading programs and strategies used in teaching that the number of possible approaches to reading instruction is quite large. With the variety of approaches available, selection of the best approach for a particular child may require a series of learning trials. Most children will begin to demonstrate learning after 4–6 lessons. General principles for promoting progress, however, include introduction of some phonics or word attack skills at some level of teaching; mastery of early, less difficult material before proceeding to more difficult material; and continuation of instruction over a long enough period for results to be long-lasting. Approximately 40 lessons are required before most children will register a substantial and enduring gain in reading skills. More rapid increases are sometimes reported, but these can often be attributed to spuriously depressed initial scores.

A minority of children will fail to learn despite appropriate individual instruction. Special programs are needed to help these children profit from school attendance.

Several approaches to drug therapy for children with reading disability have been proposed, but none have yet received adequate study to warrant their recommendation. Furthermore, drug therapy prescribed for attention deficit disorder, if successful, may be expected to alter impulsive and distractible behavior but typically does not "cure" the learning problems if these are present. At best, the climate for learning is improved, but educational progress will still depend primarily on the quality and amount of instruction provided to the child.

Prognosis

With or without individual instruction, only a minority of children remain nonreaders into adulthood. There are, however, many adolescents and adults who read poorly. Ultimate level of skill usually depends on the child's intelligence, the type and amount of individual instruction provided, the severity of retardation, the age at which remediation is begun, motivation, and several other factors including the child's general emotional state. In some adults, poor spelling may be the only stigma of a childhood reading problem, whereas other adults may continue to show evidence of problems in reading and general language skills as well. Even with individual instruction, progress is often slow, sometimes slower than progress being made by children described as slow learners. In children with specific learning disorder, however, progress in nonaffected areas of achievement tends to proceed at a normal pace.

Kosc L: Developmental dyscalculia. *J Learning Disabilities* 1974;**7**:164.
Myklebust HR (editor): *Progress in Learning Disabilities.* Vols 1–5. Grune & Stratton, 1983.
Rutter M (editor): *Developmental Neuropsychiatry.* Guilford, 1983.
Schain RJ: *Neurology of Childhood Learning Disorders.* Williams & Wilkins, 1972.

SLOW LEARNER

Essentials of Diagnosis
- Achievement below average.
- No mental retardation but IQ often below average.
- No significant discrepancy between IQ and achievement.
- Performance usually poor in all subjects.
- School progress at a slower rate than average but nevertheless continuous.

General Considerations
The average IQ of children in this group tends to be in the 80s. Approximately 11% have definite evidence of neurologic dysfunction, 25% show questionable neurologic findings, and 60% have difficulty in copying forms. Clumsiness, motor impersistence, and right-left confusion are twice as common in this group as in children with specific learning disorders. Forty percent tend to have at least one sign of language delay (eg, first phrases after 24 months). The frequency of neurodevelopmental problems increases in children with lower IQs.

Clinical Findings
The most important characteristic is the lack of a significant discrepancy between intelligence and achievement. These children are often low-average to borderline in intelligence, and achievement is slow but commensurate with mental age. Usually the child is slow in all areas of achievement, but achievement in one area may be slower than in others. The lower the child's intelligence, the more one is likely to find evidence of neurodevelopmental problems and associated behavior problems. The history often reveals evidence of developmental delays, especially in the language area. A family history of school problems may or may not be present. In the absence of a positive family history, problems during the pregnancy, advanced maternal age, or difficulties in the newborn period are often cited as pos-

sible causes of early brain damage that might explain the appearance of such a child in a well-educated family. In many instances, however, the mother's educational and cognitive level will be consistent with that of the child whether signs of neurodevelopmental delay are present or not.

Treatment
Educational programming is the principal approach to this problem. Often, however, a major task is to help the family recognize and accept the fact that a child is a slow learner. This may require counseling or short-term psychotherapy to deal with the family's denial and their wish to find some explanation for the slowness that would relieve their feelings of guilt. Often the school has developed an appropriate educational plan for the child, and treatment needs to be directed toward helping the family accept the school's plan.

Prognosis
Given an appropriate educational opportunity to progress at their own rate, slow learners tend to make steady progress commensurate with their mental age. In many instances, long-term follow-up may show that these children actually make better progress in their areas of deficiency than do children with specific learning disorders.

NONSPECIFIC & EMOTIONALLY BASED LEARNING DISORDERS

Essentials of Diagnosis
- Usually, average or above-average intelligence.
- Significant discrepancy between intelligence and achievement, often in more than one academic area.
- Frequent association with emotional or behavior problems.
- Frequent incidence among children from culturally disadvantaged homes and large families.

General Considerations
Included in this group are the large numbers of children with learning disorders in association with psychiatric disorders and familial-cultural problems of motivation. A significant discrepancy between intelligence and achievement may exist in one or more areas, or the child may be generally slow. Family problems are usually apparent, and children frequently come from culturally disadvantaged homes and large families. These children have many of the same educational needs as children with more specific problems—and often more—but they have, unfortunately, been excluded from federal funding for education of the learning disabled.

This group also includes children with wide discrepancies in functioning that result from or appear to result from altered brain function, with or without attendant emotional or behavior problems. Reduced functioning in several areas without significant IQ impairment is frequently observed in children with documented neurologic disorders (eg, epilepsy, structural lesions, head injury).

Differential Diagnosis

Differentiation from specific learning disabilities is made primarily on the basis of motivational and emotional problems and a lack of specificity of learning problems in children with average or above-average intelligence. Slow learners or mentally retarded children with emotional problems may be indistinguishable. The most difficult differential diagnosis is between specific reading disabilities in an emotionally disturbed child and an emotionally based learning disability concentrated in the language area.

Children with documented head injury or brain damage may not present a diagnostic problem. Often, however, the pattern of performance on psychologic tests, particularly those that are sensitive to disturbance in cortical functioning, may be the only available evidence pointing to brain dysfunction. Neurologic tests such as EEGs or CT scans are seldom beneficial in making a diagnosis.

Treatment

Despite the problem in differential diagnosis, treatment for emotional and learning problems is indicated in all groups demonstrating both types of disturbance. Some schools provide special classrooms for children with emotional disturbances and behavior disorders. Often the severity of the emotional or behavior problem will be the final criterion for planning the child's educational program.

MENTAL RETARDATION

Essentials of Diagnosis

- Significantly limited intelligence ($\geq$ 2 SD below average [IQ below 70]).
- Adaptation significantly below age level.
- Possible presence of sensory defects not responsible for delay.
- Onset in the developmental period.

General Considerations

Mental retardation is a descriptive term defined as significantly subaverage intellectual functioning existing concurrently with deficits of adaptive behavior and manifested during the developmental period. Significantly subaverage intelligence is defined as 2 SD or more below average (IQ below 70 on the Wechsler scales or below 69 on the Stanford-Binet test) and by definition affects approximately 2–3% of the general population. An additional 6% are considered borderline in intelligence (IQ of 70–79). Adaptive deficiency is less easily evaluated.

About 10% of the retarded population are identified during infancy and early childhood. The majority fall in the moderate to profound retardation group (IQ below 50), and most of them have clear-cut evidence of brain damage, genetic disorder, or other pathologic conditions. Moderate to profound retardation is distributed equally among different socioeconomic groups but is more common in males than in females.

The remaining 90% of the retarded population tend to be mildly retarded (IQ of 50–69), and most are not identified before entering school, partly because limited efforts are made at earlier identification. The great majority of those with mild handicaps are diagnosed as cultural-familial retardates. They have no symptoms of central nervous system injury, and they come from families characterized by low intelligence and low socioeconomic status. Many who are mildly handicapped and identified primarily during the school years eventually blend into society and become at least marginally adequate citizens. There is a preponderance of males at all levels of retardation, except for those with organic disorders that are diagnosed after age 5 years.

Etiologic Considerations

Mental retardation is a descriptive diagnosis with a wide variety of causes. Many of the causative factors that can be identified are essentially untreatable. The basic data base will be helpful in deciding how far to pursue an etiologic diagnosis.

A. Genetic:

1. Inborn errors of metabolism—Aminoacidopathies, cerebral lipidoses, mucopolysaccharidoses, disorders of carbohydrate metabolism.

2. Chromosome disorders—Autosomal disorders, sex chromosome disorders such as fragile X syndrome.

B. Intrauterine: Congenital infections, placental-fetal malfunction, complications of pregnancy (maternal malnutrition, preeclampsia-eclampsia, use of drugs or radiation, intrauterine growth retardation).

C. Perinatal: Prematurity, postmaturity, metabolic disorders (hypoglycemia, hyperbilirubinemia).

D. Postnatal: Endocrinopathies, metabolic disorders, trauma, infections, poisoning, abuse.

E. Cultural-Familial: Low family intelligence, low socioeconomic status, environmental deprivation.

Clinical Findings

A. History: In infants and preschool children with developmental delays, there may be evidence of a genetic syndrome or factors in the prenatal or perinatal period that can account for delay. Often, however, there will also be evidence of maternal deprivation or neglect, particularly among children who are only mildly or moderately delayed. The older the child at the time of diagnosis, the more likely that retardation will be explained by deficiencies in early experience or by familial-cultural factors. Even when there are other family members with similar problems, a genetic basis for the retardation cannot be established unequivocally. Children who are not diagnosed until after entering school will often have a history of normal development in the first 2 years, and siblings may show a similar decline in relative competency as they get older. Children who come from nondominant cultural backgrounds will often show adequate functioning on measures of adaptation despite poor performance on standard intelligence tests. If behavior problems, especially disruptive and antisocial behavior, are absent, children who show relatively better adaptability than intelligence tend to blend into society after leaving school.

B. Symptoms and Signs: In mental retardation, the developmental or intellectual performance is at least 2 SD below the mean, and there is accompanying evidence of significant limitations in adaptability. In preschool children, developmental delay on screening tests may be the principal presenting finding. Sensory defects are also common, as are speech and language problems, motor handicaps, neurodevelopmental delays, seizure disorders, and behavior problems. Serious family problems are also common, and frequently the mentally retarded child merely appears to be enough slower than other members of the family to be identified as retarded rather than borderline or dull normal. If the child is examined adequately, signs of significant developmental delay including deficiencies in adaptation will often be evident by age 2 years.

Once the child reaches school age, general adaptation and achievement in all areas tend to be low but commensurate with mental age. Children with low IQs who are not retarded on measures of adaptation should not be diagnosed as mentally retarded. Occasionally, a mildly retarded or borderline child will show a significant discrepancy between actual and expected achievement in one academic area more than in others. This may technically represent a specific learning disability; however, if the child's overall intelligence is low enough (IQ below 70), special education will be indicated anyway. Idiot savants have been described as showing extraordinary ability in a circumscribed area while functioning on a mentally retarded level in all other ways. Neglect, abuse, and other family experiences damaging to growth may result in bizarre forms of behavior and emotional disturbance that are difficult to distinguish from autistic or psychotic behavior. Mentally retarded children are often transparent mirrors of disturbances going on within the family. The appearance of unusual behavior, sexual acting out, or bizarre activity in an otherwise stable retarded child is often an indication of a disturbance in the family.

C. Special Studies: General rules for ordering tests include (1) laboratory testing for treatable conditions when an etiologic diagnosis is unknown, eg, use of an amino acid or organic acid screen; and (2) ordering other tests such as electroencephalography, skull films, and chromosome studies only if clinical findings suggest specific syndromes or problems.

Differential Diagnosis

Once a descriptive diagnosis is made, the basic data base should provide enough information so that a decision can be made on how far to pursue an etiologic diagnosis. It is particularly important to distinguish the deaf, blind, and orthopedically handicapped from the mentally retarded. This is often difficult, since many retarded children also have sensory and orthopedic handicaps. It is also often difficult to differentiate between autism and retardation in very young children, particularly when family and social background indicates deprivation or neglect. Usually, however, the young retarded child shows delay in all areas of development, whereas the autistic child may be quite normal in motor development but show bizarre behavior and serious delays in language development.

Management

Mental retardation usually is diagnosed only after a significant period of developmental delay has been observed. The older the child at the time of diagnosis, the less the likelihood of reversing the signs of retardation even when a treatable cause can be identified. Prevention is therefore the only significant approach to treatment at present. A screening program for early detection of inborn errors of metabolism and institution of treatment before significant damage to the nervous system can occur represents the model approach to the problem of mental retardation. This same model has been used in developing preventive programs for children at risk for familial-cultural retardation. Controlled studies of stimulation programs for infants in sociocultural groups with high rates of mental retardation have shown significant long-range results after termination of the program when (1) parents have been involved in the program, (2) the infant participated in the program frequently (once every 2 weeks or more), and (3) the program continued for at least 2 years. Headstart has also been shown to decrease the number of children in special education classes and to increase the number of children from high-risk populations who remain in school.

In most instances, however, management of the retarded child does not involve treatment of the retardation per se but must be directed toward (1) assessing the impact on the family and providing support and psychotherapy, (2) providing protection for the child, (3) providing education and rehabilitation to maximize the child's potential, and (4) providing treatment of associated medical, emotional, and behavior problems.

A. Impact on the Family: The diagnosis of mental retardation is an event for which few families are prepared. Often parents can assess the mental age of their child within a few months but still refuse to accept the implications of this information. The tact and sensitivity with which the initial discussion of developmental delay is broached can determine how early the family will allow appropriate treatment, education, and rehabilitation to be started; thus, the primary care physician should be alert to parents' initial questions about developmental delay. A second opinion or repeated evaluation is almost mandatory when the impression of significant developmental delay arises unexpectedly from screening tests or school observations. Once the diagnosis is confirmed, the family will need continued assistance and support in adjusting to the diagnosis and in making contact with community resources.

Retarded children and adults can successfully remain within the family in most instances, but they usually require a host of family and community support services. These often include social services, infant education programs, and occupational and physical therapy programs and services for handicapped infants that begin as early as the newborn period. In school-age children, most services are organized through the public school systems, but the primary care physician may be called on to assist in difficult situations.

Once a severely handicapped child is "accepted" by the family, family resources may be totally consumed by care of the child, often to the detriment of normal siblings. Professionals involved with these families should provide help in developing priorities and alleviating parental guilt at being unable to do everything everyone suggests for the child. Less severely handicapped children are often less acceptable to the family, with resulting conflict and emotional disturbance as parents attempt to deny or seek more ego-syntonic diagnoses and explanations for the child's delays. Parental difficulty in accepting evidence of mild retardation often leads them to seek more than one evaluation as they pass through a mourning process and eventually develop more realistic expectations for the child. Parent support groups have been particularly helpful to families with retarded children.

B. Protection, Education, and Rehabilitation: Although they seldom alter the diagnosis, early intervention programs for developmentally delayed infants and young children are often associated with improved development of language, ambulation, and self-care. An emphasis on family life, whether within the biologic family, a foster family, or a group home, has been associated with a generally improved level of social competence and a decrease in the incidence of emotional and behavior problems. Current social and legislative trends are toward abolishment of institutions for individuals with developmental disabilities and emphasis on programs and services that promote productivity, independence, and community integration.

Mildly retarded children (IQ of 50–69) usually are considered educable and in many instances are able to blend into society with minimal or no protective custody. Moderately retarded children (IQ of 30–49) are considered trainable but require protective care (sheltered workshop, guardian, group home). More recently, the public schools have been required to provide services to members of this group who are ambulatory. Severely to profoundly retarded children (IQ below 30) usually require continuous care, and this group often includes the most severely deformed, nonambulatory, and minimally communicative individuals. Educational programs at all levels of disability stress providing an appropriate education in the least restricted, most normalized environment.

C. Treatment of Associated Medical, Emotional, and Behavior Problems: Sensory, motor, and orthopedic handicaps and other medical problems should be treated appropriately. The most controversial area of management concerns the use of psychotropic medication for treatment of emotional and behavior problems, especially in institutionalized retarded children. Although most of these medications are approved primarily for use in treatment of psychotic conditions, the phenothiazines in particular have been employed extensively in behavioral management of retarded persons.

Psychotropic medication practices have often resulted in too much being given for too long a time to too many institutionalized children. Frequently, several psychotropic drugs are given at the same time. Some children may be so heavily drugged that they are unable to respond maximally to educational and rehabilitative programs. These practices are often based on claims that the response to neuroleptic and psychotropic medications is altered in retarded children, but other evidence supports the interpretation that psychotropic medication often represents a "chemical straitjacket" that is used as a substitute for adequate personnel to provide more appropriate care. It is uncertain whether attention deficit disorder in mentally retarded children should be treated with stimulant medication. Some children appear to become worse with treatment (as do many psychotic children), whereas stimulant medication appears to be the treatment of choice for others. As children are withdrawn from heavy medication with phenothiazines and other major psychotropic drugs, symptoms such as dyskinesia may emerge, ie, withdrawal emergent symptoms, which require diagnosis and treatment in themselves. The most serious of these is tardive dyskinesia, which may also appear during treatment.

To avoid misuse of psychotropic medication in the mentally retarded, (1) a diagnosis of the emotional behavior problem should be made and an appropriate drug and dosage selected on the basis of the diagnosis; and (2) the patient's response to the medication should be carefully monitored by the physician through direct evaluation and observation as well as review of reports provided by caretakers.

MOTOR HANDICAPS

A variety of nonspecific problems in development of motor coordination has been observed in children with learning disorders and also as isolated problems. Mental retardation, cerebral palsy, or a neuromuscular disorder is also present in many cases. A larger group, estimated at about 6–7% of the population, shows clumsiness, awkwardness, choreiform movements, or generally poor coordination but no signs of systemic disease except for an increased incidence of other "soft signs" on neurologic examination. Many of the children in this group also show evidence of learning problems, and the motor problems have been cited as evidence of a neurologic basis for the learning problems. However, as with "soft signs" in general, this interpretation is controversial.

Clumsiness and awkwardness have also been reported in association with attention deficit disorder. In this instance, treatment with stimulant medications has frequently been accompanied by improvement in motor coordination. Occupational and physical therapy are often recommended for these children, though there are no adequately controlled studies with data to support the efficacy of these approaches for improving educational achievement. There is clear evidence that instruction in reading is better than perceptual-motor training in improving reading ability irrespective of the child's motor status. The whole area of mild motor disability has received so little formal scrutiny, however, that much is yet to be learned about ways of identifying and ameliorating developmental impairments in motor skills.

Connolly K: Motor development and motor disability. In: *Developmental Psychiatry.* Rutter M (editor). Heinemann, 1980.
Henderson A: Research in occupational therapy and physical therapy with children. In: *Advances in Behavioral Pediatrics.* Vol. 2. Camp BW (editor). JAI Press, 1981.

DEVELOPMENTAL-ADAPTATIONAL PROBLEMS

Developmental-adaptational problems are behavior problems that in normal children decline steadily with age either from infancy or from their appearance in the preschool years. Manifestations include fears, distractibility, hyperactivity, destructiveness, lying, negativism, temper tantrums, enuresis, and thumbsucking. Children with these manifestations often show no maladjustment later in life; absence of these manifestations does not rule out later maladjustment. The gradual decline in these behavior problems is associated with maturation of cognitive competence, including not only intelligence but moral maturity and ego development as well. When deficiencies in social character and cognitive adaptability persist in children beyond the early school years, they are more likely to have a poor prognosis.

ATTENTION DEFICIT HYPERACTIVITY DISORDER

Essentials of Diagnosis

- Distractibility, short attention span, hyperactivity, impulsivity.
- Duration of longer than 6 months.
- No association with psychosis.
- Association with aggressive behavior, sometimes but not always present.
- Onset before age 7 years.

General Considerations

Attention deficit hyperactivity disorder (ADHD) is characterized by heightened distractibility, short attention span, and impulsiveness. The rate of incidence is about 5%, and the disorder is more common in boys than in girls. Most of the children previously labeled hyperactive or said to have minimal brain dysfunction are children with attention deficit hyperactivity disorder. In normal children, attention span and ability to concentrate on cognitive tasks increase throughout childhood. Ability of preschool children to engage in sustained task-oriented behavior is one of the most reliable predictors of later school performance. Some evidence suggests that even in infants, attention span may be an early indication of later cognitive performance. In older children, attentiveness is one of the major characteristics of competent children with good peer relations.

The child who persists in immature forms of attentional behavior after age mates have matured is noticeably out of phase in cognitively stressful situations such as school. In these circumstances, children may appear driven to aimless, purposeless activity. Some children also show hyperactive behavior at home, on the playground, and in the physician's office, as well as in the classroom; others may only show problems under cognitive stress. Some children with attention deficit hyperactivity disorder have also been described as hypoactive rather than hyperactive.

In evaluating behavior problems, it is important to determine whether aggressive behavior problems or conduct disorders are also present. This mixture of behavior problems is common. It is not clear whether the presence of aggressive behavior alters the short-term response to treatment. However, long-term prognosis is poorer in those who have a mixed disorder than in those whose behavior problems are confined to distractibility, impulsiveness, and short attention span.

The causes of attention deficit hyperactivity disorder are not well understood, although there is evidence of a genetic or constitutional basis for the problem in many children. The diagnosis is largely descriptive, but it carries the implication that specific causes of distractibility and short attention span (eg, neurologic insult or injury, emotional trauma, psychosis, depression) have been eliminated. Immaturity in development of the central nervous system is one of the most likely underlying causes of the problem. However, children who show the functional disorder may or may not have evidence of "soft signs" on neurologic examination or abnormal findings on electroencephalography. The presence of neurodevelopmental signs has not been consistently related to treatment outcome.

Clinical Findings

A. History: The most important diagnostic information comes from a description of behavior in the classroom and teacher ratings on a scale such as the ACTeRS (Table 3–1). Ratings on this scale that fall below the 10th percentile on attention, hyperactivity, or both, regardless of ratings on the other scales, are usually indicative of attention deficit hyperactivity disorder. If problems with attention or hyperactivity are not evident at school, it is very unlikely that the child has attention deficit hyperactivity disorder. Physicians worried about teacher bias in completing the rating will often find that ratings obtained from several teachers will show similar results. However, ratings completed by parents may or may not show deviance. It is useful to review information about oppositional behavior and social skills and obtain information about intelligence and academic performance, because many children will also show other behavior or learning problems. The most common other behavior problem encountered among children with attention deficit disorder is aggressive behavior or conduct disorder. The family history is often positive for similar problems in childhood, particularly among male relatives. Children with attention deficit disorder are frequently described as active, colicky infants, and typically parents can recall many incidents indicating distractibility and hyperactivity in the preschool period. Attention deficit hyperactivity disorder is usually first recognized as a problem after a child enters school. The diagnosis can sometimes be made with great confidence in preschool children,

but many of these children are primarily in need of improved parental management.

B. Symptoms and Signs: The neurologic examination may or may not show signs of neurologic immaturity. There are usually no sensory impairments. A significant number of children also have learning problems that may be general or specific, usually depending on the child's level of intelligence. Attention deficit hyperactivity disorder occurs at all intellectual levels, but among children of average intelligence with behavior problems confined to the attention deficit hyperactivity disorder syndrome, achievement is often adequate despite teacher complaints that the child is "not learning." When a learning problem accompanies a behavior problem, the problems should be addressed separately.

Family problems may contribute to attention deficit hyperactivity disorder and increase the difficulty of treatment, especially in children who show aggressive behavior. Attention deficit disorder is excluded when a diagnosis of childhood psychotic disorder has been made, but the diagnosis may be made in mentally retarded children.

C. Special Studies: Tests measuring continuous performance or vigilance have been widely used in research on attention deficit hyperactivity disorder. These tests usually require that the child look for occurrences of one specified design among many, either on a page or sequentially flashing on a screen. One such system with norms is commercially available for electronic administration of a vigilance test; nevertheless, the clinical application of these procedures is incompletely worked out. No other special tests aid in diagnosis. If there is a question of seizure disorder or clear-cut evidence of neurologic disorder, investigation of these conditions is indicated.

Treatment

Two major effective forms of treatment are behavior modification programs in the classroom and stimulant drugs (methylphenidate [Ritalin], dextroamphetamine [Dexedrine; many others], and pemoline [Cylert]). Drug treatment, if effective, tends to have more dramatic results than behavior modification.

Approximately 50–80% of children with attention deficit hyperactivity disorder are responsive to stimulant drug therapy. Dose-response studies on methylphenidate suggest that a dose of 0.3 mg/kg produces optimal cognitive improvement (concentration) as well as significant improvement in social behavior. Greater improvement in social behavior can be achieved with higher doses, but this occurs at the expense of some loss in concentration. Peak action usually occurs 2 hours after ingestion, and most effects have dissipated after 6 hours. The usual regimen is to start with an early morning dose, followed by a dose at noon if needed. Morning activities often require the most concentration, and the noon dose may be unnecessary. If problems at home are also severe, a third dose may be given in the late afternoon. Medication on weekends and during school holidays should be tailored to the needs of the child and family. Dextroamphetamine and methylphenidate are quite similar in onset and duration of action, and most children who respond to one will respond to the other. Pemoline appears to be somewhat different in onset of action, and doses often require adjustment over a longer period of time.

Drug ''holidays'' are an important part of chronic drug therapy with psychotropic drugs. Medication should be withdrawn for at least 2 weeks of each year to determine whether therapy needs to be continued. Two convenient times for this are summer vacations and spring holidays. In the latter case, a week at home without medication can precede a week at school without medication.

Monitoring for side effects should be continuous. Weekly teacher reports (ACTeRS scale) during the first month are helpful for monitoring and evaluating treatment. The child should be reevaluated at 1 month to determine if the response is sufficient to justify continuing with medication.

Behavior modification programs are often tailored to an individual child's situation. Planning an individualized program usually involves the services of a psychologist or educational specialist. Think Aloud, a general cognitive behavior modification program for improving self-control in children 6–8 years of age, can be used in an office setting. Typically, it has been carried out by special teachers, psychologists, social workers, or other mental health workers but can be used by an intelligent parent or interested physician.

Prognosis

With or without treatment, the long-term outcome is better in the more intelligent children with stable families and uncomplicated attention deficit hyperactivity disorder. These children often require only short-term treatment (usually 2 years or less).

Camp BW, Bash MAS: *Think Aloud: Increasing Social and Cognitive Skills—A Problem Solving Program for Children.* Research Press, 1981.

Ingersoll B: *Your Hyperactive Child: A Parent's Guide to Coping With Attention Deficit Disorders.* Doubleday, 1988.

Wender PH: *The Hyperactive Child, Adolescent, and Adult.* Oxford Univ Press, 1987.

AGGRESSIVE ANTISOCIAL BEHAVIOR PROBLEMS

Essentials of Diagnosis

- Fighting and physically attacking other children or adults.

- Behavior often boisterous, disruptive, and argumentative, with a ''chip on the shoulder'' attitude.
- Probable evidence of family disturbance or disharmony.
- Frequent coexistence of poor achievement in children over 10 years of age.
- Incidence more common among less intelligent children.

General Considerations

Destructive, aggressive behavior is common in preschool children but declines significantly with the developmental shift at 5–7 years of age. Nevertheless, it is one of the most malignant behavior problems of childhood. It is more common in boys than in girls. By age 6–8, most normal children have shown a marked decrease in aggressive behavior. A significant number of those who continue to show aggressive behavior after 8 years of age will be aggressive in adolescence. Aggressive behavior is less likely to persist in children who identify with the values of one or both parents. Family disharmony and disturbance are the most important contemporaneous instigators of aggressive behavior problems at school.

Clinical Findings

A. History: Active destructive behavior is often seen at an early age and is frequently accompanied by risk-taking and other forms of behavior that make the child difficult to manage. The parents are often characterized as too strict or too lax, providing the child with little supervision or sense of belonging, and often openly rejecting the child. Aggressive behavior by the parents often complicates the diagnosis, since the child may be merely imitating the parents' behavior. Aggressive children of aggressive parents, however, often reject the parents' values even as they imitate the parents' behavior.

B. Symptoms and Signs: The most important information is from teacher, parent, and other reports of aggressive, antisocial, or disruptive behavior. Because some aggressive behavior is present in most children, only teacher and parent rating scales for general behavior that show increases of at least 1.5 SD above normal in amount of aggressive behavior should be considered significant. Neurologic examination usually shows normal results. Intelligence may be average or above average, but aggressive problems occur more frequently in children with lower IQs. Achievement may be average in the first few years of school but shows a steady decline after third grade, frequently accompanied by truancy. Learning delays in all areas are common in the aggressive delinquent adolescent, but 26% show evidence of specific learning disorders. (Most children with specific learning disability are not aggressive, however.) In early school years, the cognitive pattern of aggressive boys tends to show more impulsiveness and less verbal mediation activity than that of normal boys. By adolescence, the typical antisocial, aggressive boy shows a characteristic pattern of decreased verbal intelligence relative to nonverbal, impulsive stereotyped thinking and immaturity in ego development.

Treatment

Large-scale delinquency prevention programs for young aggressive boys have been unsuccessful even when they provided remedial reading instruction as well as counseling and family support. Small-scale behavior modification programs have had some success in normalizing cognitive and social behavior or slowing the increase in delinquent behavior. Psychotherapy and other methods of treatment have met with more modest success.

Behavior modification or other treatment programs are typically designed and monitored by psychologists or child psychiatrists. For younger children (6–8 years of age), the Think Aloud program has been used successfully by teachers, psychologists, social workers, and other mental health workers to help normalize both cognitive and social behavior at school.

When attention deficit disorder accompanies aggressive behavior problems, stimulant medication is sometimes helpful in decreasing general disruptive behavior as well as impulsiveness and distractibility, but the response may be quite variable.

Camp BW, Ray RS: Aggression. In: *Cognitive Behavior Therapy for Children.* Meyers A, Craighead LW (editors). Plenum Press, 1984.
Lefkowitz MM et al: *Growing Up to Be Violent.* Pergamon Press, 1977.

SELECTED REFERENCES

Levine MD et al: *Developmental and Behavioral Pediatrics.* Saunders, 1983.
Mussen PH (editor): *Carmichael's Manual of Child Psychology.* Vols 1–4. Wiley, 1983.
Reynolds CR, Mann L (editors): *Encyclopedia of Special Education.* Vols 1–3. Wiley, 1987.
Rubin IL, Crocker AC: *Developmental Disabilities: Delivery of Medical Care for Children and Adults.* Lea & Febiger, 1989.
Thompson RJ Jr, O'Quinn AN: *Developmental Disabilities: Etiologies, Manifestations, Diagnoses, and Treatments.* Oxford Univ Press, 1979.

4

The Newborn Infant

Adam A. Rosenberg, MD, & Frederick C. Battaglia, MD

Neonatology is a discipline that encompasses all care for newborn infants. By tradition, the first 28 days of life has been considered the newborn period. Practically, however, neonatal care includes all of the care provided until discharge from the nursery, ranging from a 24-hour stay for term, healthy infants to many months of care for sick, very immature infants. Follow-up care for most newborn infants is usually provided by family physicians and pediatricians. Neonatologists or other physicians skilled in developmental pediatrics, however, may provide special follow-up services for infants discharged from intensive care nurseries. Table 4–1 summarizes the levels of nursery care commonly encountered.

NEONATAL BIRTH WEIGHT & GESTATIONAL AGE DISTRIBUTION

The mortality rates have decreased steadily for infants in all birth weight-gestational age groups (see Fig 4–1, panels A and B). Since the collection of the data in Fig 4–1B, moreover, survival rates have continued to improve for infants of less than 28 weeks of gestation and 1000 grams. Eighty percent of infants survive at 28 weeks, 75% at 27 weeks, and 50% at 26 weeks. Mortality rates do remain very high for those infants born at less than 26 weeks of gestation. A few other points should be emphasized. There is no longer a difference between survival rates for term infants who are large for gestational age (LGA) and those who are appropriate for gestational age (AGA). This development is due in large part to better obstetric management of gestational and insulin-dependent diabetic patients. Furthermore, the use of ultrasound allows obstetricians to anticipate delivery of an LGA infant and, if necessary, perform cesarean section, avoiding much of the birth trauma associated with LGA infants in the past. However, the data in Fig 4–1B also indicate that the small-for-gestational-age (SGA) infant born prematurely is not doing very well; that is, mortality rates of these infants are comparable to those of premature babies of the same size. The same cannot be said, of course, for larger and more mature SGA infants, whose survival rate is much better than that of preterm infants of comparable size.

The birth weight and gestational age of all infants must be plotted on some appropriate standard. Birth weight-gestational age distributions vary from one population to the next. Table 4–2 lists some of the factors that affect these distributions. For these reasons, the standards should be prepared from data collected on the local population. When these are not available, any regional standard may be used: the birth weight-gestational age distribution of an infant is simply a screening tool that should always be supplemented by clinical data confirming a tentative diagnosis of intrauterine growth retardation or excessive fetal growth. These clinical data include not only the clinical features of the infant determined during the physical examination but also such factors as the size of each parent and the birth weight-gestational age distribution of infants previously born to the parents.

Table 4–1. Levels of nursery care.

Level 1 nurseries: These nurseries care for infants presumed healthy. In such units, screening and surveillance are primary responsibilities. "Rooming-in" units are encouraged, with emphasis on support of breast-feeding and assessment of parenting skills.

Level 2 nurseries: These nurseries care for infants > 30 weeks of gestation and ≥ 1200 gs who require special attention short of the need for circulatory or ventilator support and major surgical procedures. Because they address the greatest diversity of neonatal disorders, these nurseries present perhaps the greatest challenge to health care providers. A high percentage of the problems in such nurseries relates to obstetric complications (eg, birth trauma, fetal distress, obstetric anesthesia).

Level 3 nurseries: These nurseries are staffed and equipped to care for all newborn infants who are critically ill, regardless of the level of support required. They are regional institutions serving as referral centers for other nurseries and for this reason are often linked with transport services. Optimally, these nurseries should be part of a perinatal center.

Perinatal center: A perinatal center provides services both to high-risk mothers and to infants requiring level 3 nursery care. Ample data now clearly demonstrate a higher neonatal survival rate for high-risk pregnancies cared for in such centers. The transport of high-risk mothers to perinatal centers is preferred, therefore, to the transport of a critically ill infant following delivery.

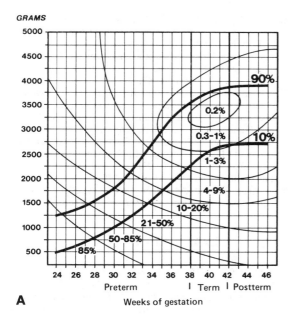

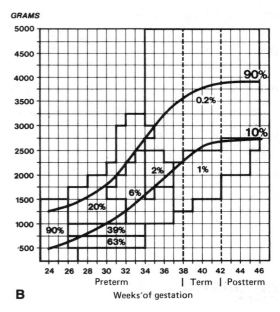

Figure 4–1. *A:* Neonatal mortality risk by birth weight and gestational age, 1958–1969, based on 14,436 live births at the University of Colorado Health Sciences Center. *B:* Neonatal mortality risk by birth weight and gestational age, 1974–1980, based on 14,413 live births at the University of Colorado Health Sciences Center. (Reproduced, with permission, from Koops BL, Morgan LJ, Battaglia FC: Neonatal mortality risk in relation to birth weight and gestational age: An update. *J Pediatr* 1982;**101**:969.

Table 4–3 lists causes of variations in neonatal size in relation to gestational age. A very important distinction to be made, particularly in SGA infants, is whether the growth disorder is symmetric (weight, height, and occipitofrontal circumference [OFC]; ≤ 10%) or asymmetric (sparing of growth in length and OFC). Asymmetric growth retardation implies a problem late in the pregnancy, such as pregnancy-induced hypertension or placental insufficiency of any cause. Symmetric growth retardation implies an event of early pregnancy: chromosomal abnormality, drug or alcohol use, congenital viral infections.

Knowledge of a baby's birth weight in relation to gestational age is also helpful in anticipating neonatal problems. LGA babies are at risk for birth trauma, hypoglycemia, polycythemia, congenital anomalies, cardiomyopathy, hyperbilirubinemia, and hypocalcemia. SGA babies are at risk for fetal distress during labor and delivery, polycythemia, hypoglycemia, and hypocalcemia.

Battaglia FC, Lubchenco LO: A practical classification of newborn infants by weight and gestational age. *J Pediatr* 1967;**71**:159.

Cnattingius S et al: Smoking, maternal age and fetal growth. *Obstet Gynecol* 1985;**66**:449.

Koops BL, Morgan LJ, Battaglia FC: Neonatal mortality risk in relation to birth weight and gestational age: Update. *J Pediatr* 1982;**101**:969.

Table 4–2. Factors affecting birth weight-gestational age distributions.

Socioeconomic factors that affect nutritional level and access to health care
Altitude
Incidence of environmental factors that affect birth weight, eg, smoking
Racial distribution

Table 4–3. Etiology of variations in neonatal size in relation to gestational age.

Infants large for gestational age
Infant of a diabetic mother
Infants small for gestational age
Asymmetric
Placental insufficiency due to pregnancy-induced hypertension or other maternal vascular diseases
Maternal age > 35
Poor weight gain during pregnancy
Multiple gestation
Symmetric
Maternal drug use
Narcotics
Cocaine
Alcohol
Chromosomal abnormalities
Intrauterine viral infection, eg, cytomegalovirus

Miller E et al: Elevated maternal hemoglobin A_{1c} in early pregnancy and major congenital anomalies in infants of diabetic mothers. *N Engl J Med* 1981;**304;**1331.

Mills JL et al: Lack of relation of increased malformation rates in infants of diabetic mothers to glycemic control during organogenesis. *N Engl J Med* 1988;**318:**671.

Molteni RA, Stys SJ, Battaglia FC: The relationship of fetal and placental weight in human beings: Fetal/placental weight ratios at various gestational ages and birthweight distributions. *J Reprod Med* 1978;**21:**327.

Sibai B, Anderson G: Pregnancy outcome of intensive therapy in severe hypertension in first trimester. *Obstet Gynecol* 1986;**67:**517.

Simmons M: Intrauterine growth retardation. *Semin Perinatol* 1984;**8:**73.

Warshaw J: Intrauterine growth retardation: Adaptation or pathology? *Pediatrics* 1985;**76:**998.

Briggs GG et al: *Drugs in Pregnancy and Lactation: A Reference Guide to Fetal and Neonatal Risk.* Williams & Wilkins, 1983.

Committee on Drugs, American Academy of Pediatrics: The transfer of drugs and other chemicals into human breast milk. *Pediatrics* 1983;**72:**375.

US Department of Health and Human Services: Cesarean childbirth: Report of a Consensus Development Conference sponsored by the National Institute of Child Health and Human Development in conjunction with the National Center for Health Care Technology and assisted by the Office for Medical Applications of Research, September 22–24, 1980. National Institutes of Health Publication No. (NIH) 82–2067, 1981.

Zuckerman BS et al: Adolescent pregnancy: Biobehavioral determinants of outcome. *J Pediatr* 1984;**105:**857.

EVALUATION OF THE NEWBORN INFANT

HISTORY

Taking the history in newborn medicine involves 3 key areas: (1) the medical history of the mother and father, including a relevant genetic history; (2) the previous obstetric history of the mother; and (3) the history of the current pregnancy.

Illnesses with genetic implications and all chronic illness in the mother known to effect intrauterine development are of particular importance. The past and current obstetric history must be as detailed as possible, including documentation of such procedures as ultrasound examinations, amniocentesis, screening tests, and biophysical profiles. The biophysical profile is the prenatal equivalent of an Apgar score, in which 5 or 6 indices of fetal well-being are assessed. If chorionic villus biopsy or cordocentesis (umbilical cord blood sampling) has been done, it should be documented together with the information obtained. An unusual dietary history, drug intake, smoking history, and potential exposure to infectious agents associated with congenital infection should be noted, as well as weight gain during pregnancy, the work place of the mother, and exercise level. The social history may assist the clinician in assessing parenting skills and the risks of child abuse. Acute problems in the mother, such as urinary tract infection, pregnancy-induced hypertension, bleeding, fetal distress, and meconium in the amniotic fluid should be noted. Knowledge of duration of ruptured membranes and chorioamnionitis should be obtained. In high-risk groups, the presence of HIV (human immunodeficiency virus) and HBsAg (hepatitis B surface antigen) must be determined.

PHYSICAL EXAMINATION

The extent of the physical examination of a newborn infant depends on the condition of the infant and the environment in which it is being performed. If the pediatrician is in attendance in the delivery room for a normal delivery, a physical examination is largely based upon observation coupled with auscultation of the chest and examination for congenital anomalies. Because the infant is recovering from "birth shock," the examination should not be extensive. The examination should include collecting sufficient information for an Apgar score (see Table 4–4) at 1 and 5 minutes of age. In the case of severely depressed infants, a 10-minute score should also be recorded. Serial Apgar scores provide a form of "bioassay" reflecting the severity of intrauterine distress or the quality of the resuscitative efforts made.

Table 4–4. Infant evaluation at birth (Apgar score).[1,2]

	Score		
	0	1	2
Heart rate	Absent	Slow (< 100)	> 100
Respiratory effort	Absent	Slow, irregular	Good, crying
Muscle tone	Limp	Some flexion	Active motion
Response to catheter in nostril (tested after oropharynx is clear)	No response	Grimace	Cough or sneeze
Color	Blue or pale	Body pink; extremities blue	Completely pink

[1]Reproduced, with permission, from Apgar V et al: Evaluation of the newborn infant—second report. *JAMA* 1958;**168:**1985. ©1958 American Medical Association.

[2]One minute and 5 minutes after complete birth of infant (disregarding cord and placenta), the following objective signs should be observed and recorded.

The color of the neonate's skin is a very useful indicator. Because there is normally a high blood flow to the skin, any stress that triggers a catecholamine response produces fairly dramatic changes in skin color secondary to changes in the distribution of cardiac output and perfusion of the skin. Cyanosis and pallor are 2 signs that are evaluated both as an index of oxygenation and as a reflection of changes in skin blood flow. In infants of very low birthweight, tissues are fragile and easily bruised. Thus, bruised areas should be considered an indication of deep tissue bleeding that may involve fairly extensive hemorrhage. The bruising not only produces problems with hyperbilirubinemia over the next few days but also can represent acute, significant blood loss that must be treated with volume expansion.

The skeletal examination immediately after delivery serves 2 purposes: (1) to detect any obvious congenital anomalies, and (2) to detect signs of birth trauma, particularly in LGA infants or infants in which there has been a prolonged second stage of labor.

The umbilical cord and the placenta should also be examined. The principal feature noted in the cord is the number of vessels. Normally, there are 2 arteries and one vein. In 1% of deliveries (5–6% of twin deliveries) the cord has only 2 vessels: an artery and a vein. The latter may be considered a vascular anomaly and, as is the case with other minor anomalies, carries with it a slightly increased risk of associated anomalies. The placenta is usually examined by the physician delivering it. Small placentas are always associated with small infants. The placental examination centers around the identification of membranes and vessels, particularly in multiple gestations. A single chorion always represents monozygotic twining, whereas a full set of double membranes, amnion and chorion, can be either mono- or dizygotic. The placenta is also examined for the frequency and severity of placental infarcts and for evidence of clot (placental abruption) on the maternal side.

General Examination

Heart rate should range from 120 to 160 (beats/min), and the respiratory rate is 30–60; blood pressure norms are a function of birth weight and gestational age (Fig 4–2). *Note:* an irregularly irregular heart rate, usually due to premature atrial contractions, is a common finding. This irregularity should resolve in the first days of life and is not of pathologic significance.

Plot length, weight, and head circumference on appropriate standards for percentiles.

Gestational Age Examination

Accurate maternal dates remain the best indicator of gestational age. Other obstetric observations, such as fundal height, auscultation of fetal heartbeat with a stethoscope, and early ultrasound examination, provide supporting information. A postnatal examination (Table 4–5) can also be used, because fetal physical characteristics and neurologic development progress in predictable fashion. Table 4–5 itemizes the physical and neurologic criteria to be examined. The upper panel is the neuromuscular examination assessing primarily muscle tone and strength. The lower panel catalogs a variety of physical characteristics.

Skin

Check for bruising, petechiae (common over presenting part), meconium staining, and jaundice. Peripheral cyanosis is commonly present when the extremities are cool or the infant is polycythemic. Generalized cyanosis merits immediate evaluation. Pallor may be due to acute or chronic blood loss. Plethora suggests polycythemia. Note vernix caseosa (a whitish, greasy material covering the body that decreases as term approaches) and lanugo (the fine hair covering the preterm infant's skin). Dry skin

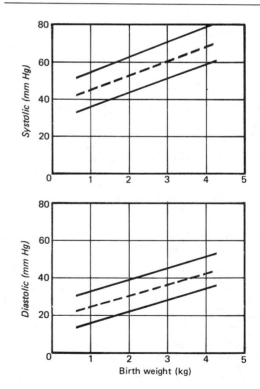

Figure 4–2. Aortic blood pressure during the first 12 hours of life in infants with birth weights of 610–4220 g. (Reproduced, with permission, from Versmold HT et al: Aortic blood pressure during the first 12 hours of life in infants with birth weight 610 to 4,220 g. *Pediatrics* 1981;**67**:607.

Table 4–5. A simplified score for assessment fetal maturation of newly born infants.[1,2,3]

	0	1	2	3	4	5
Neuromuscular maturity						
Posture						
Square window (wrist)	90°	60°	45°	30°	0°	
Arm recoil	180°		100°–180°	90°–100°	< 90°	
Popliteal angle	180°	160°	130°	110°	90°	< 90°
Scarf sign						
Heel to ear						
Physical maturity						
Skin	Gelatinous, red, transparent	Smooth, pink; visible veins	Superficial peeling, rash, or both; few veins	Cracking, pale area; rare veins	Parchment, deep cracking; no vessels	Leathery, cracked, wrinkled
Lanugo	None	Abundant	Thinning	Bald areas	Mostly bald	
Plantar creases	No crease	Faint red marks	Anterior transverse crease only	Creases anterior two-thirds	Creases cover entire sole	
Breast	Barely perceptible	Flat areola; no bud	Stippled areola; bud, 1–2 mm	Raised areola; bud, 3–4 mm	Full areola; bud, 5–10 mm	
Ear	Pinna flat; stays folded	Slightly curved pinna; soft; slow recoil	Well-curved pinna; soft; ready recoil	Formed and firm; instant recoil	Thick cartilage; ear stiff	
Genitalia (male)	Scrotum empty; no rugae		Testes descending; few rugae	Testes down; good rugae	Testes pendulous; deep rugae	
Genitalia (female)	Prominent clitoris and labia minora		Majora and minora equally prominent	Majora large; minora small	Clitoris and minora completely covered	

Score	5	10	15	20	25	30	35	40	45	50
Weeks	26	28	30	32	34	36	38	40	42	44

[1] Reproduced, with permission, from Ballard JL, Novak KK, Driver M: A simplified score for assessment of fetal maturation of newly born infants. *J Pediatr* 1979;**95**:769.
[2] Maturity rating.
[3] See text for a description of the clinical gestational age examination.

with cracking and peeling of the superficial layers is common in postterm infants. Edema may be generalized (hydrops) or localized (eg, on dorsum of the foot in Turner's syndrome). Check for birthmarks, eg, capillary hemangiomas (lower occiput, eyelids, forehead) and mongolian spot (bluish-black pigmentation over the back and buttocks). Milia (small white papules over the nose and face) are due to blocked ducts of sebaceous glands. Miliaria (pustules without a red base) are due to blocked ducts of sweat glands. Erythema toxicum is characterized by erythematous raised areas with pustules filled with eosinophils. Pustular melanosis is a pustular rash that shows pigment when the pustule ruptures. The pustules are noninfectious but contain neutrophils. Jaundice presenting in the first 24 hours of life should be considered abnormal.

Head

Check for cephalohematoma (within suture lines) and caput succedaneum (edema over presenting part that crosses suture lines). Subgaleal (beneath the scalp) hemorrhages are seen infrequently but are not limited by sutures, so that blood loss can be extensive. Skull fractures may be linear or depressed and may be associated with a cephalohematoma. Check size and presence of fontanelles. The anterior fontanelle varies from 1 to 4 cm in any direction, whereas the posterior fontanelle should be less than 1 cm. The third fontanelle is a bony defect along the sagittal suture in the parietal bones. Sutures should be freely mobile. Craniosynostosis is a prematurely fused suture.

Face

Odd facies may be associated with a specific syndrome. Bruising from birth trauma (especially with face presentation) and forceps marks should be identified. Facial nerve palsy is observed when the infant cries; the unaffected side of the mouth moves normally, giving a distorted facial grimace.

Eyes

Subconjunctival hemorrhages are seen frequently as a result of the birth process. Extraocular movements should be assessed. Occasional uncoordinated eye movements are common, but persistent irregular movements are abnormal. The iris should be inspected for abnormalities such as Brushfield's spots (trisomy 21) and colobomas. Examine for the red reflex of the retina. Leukocoria can be caused by glaucoma (cloudy cornea), cataract, or tumor (retinoblastoma). Infants at risk for chorioretinitis (congenital viral infection) should have the retina examined while the pupil is dilated.

Nose

Examine size and shape. In utero compression can cause deformities. Babies are obligate nose breathers; any nasal obstruction (eg, bilateral choanal atresia) can cause respiratory distress. Unilateral choanal atresia can be checked for by occluding each naris. Purulent nasal discharge suggests congenital syphilis.

Ears

Malformed or malpositioned (low-set or posteriorly rotated) ears are often associated with other congenital anomalies. The tympanic membranes should be visualized.

Mouth

Epithelial pearls are retention cysts along the gum margins and at the junction of hard and soft palates. Natal teeth may be present and need to be removed to avoid the risk of aspiration. Check integrity and shape of the palate; rule out cleft lip and palate. Small mandibles may be seen with Pierre Robin syndrome. This feature can result in respiratory difficulty as the tongue occludes the airway. A prominent tongue can be seen in trisomy 21 and Beckwith-Wiedemann syndrome. Excessive drooling suggests esophageal atresia.

Neck

Webbing is seen in Turner's syndrome. Sinus tracts may be seen as remnants of branchial clefts. Check for masses: midline (thyroid), anterior to the sternocleidomastoids (branchial cleft cysts), within the sternocleidomastoid (hematoma, torticollis), and posterior to the sternocleidomastoid (cystic hygroma).

Chest & Lungs

Check for fractured clavicles (crepitus, bruising). Increased anteroposterior diameter (barrel chest) can be seen with aspiration syndromes. Check air entry bilaterally. Diminished breath sounds suggest pneumothorax or a space-occupying lesion (eg, diaphragmatic hernia). Check the position of the mediastinum. A shift is seen with pneumothorax (tension) or with a space-occupying lesion. With pneumomediastinum, heart sounds are usually muffled. Expiratory grunting and decreased air entry are seen with hyaline membrane disease. Rales are not diagnostic of disease.

Heart

Examination of the heart is described in detail in Chapter 16. *Note:* murmurs are most often benign and are not necessarily present in serious congenital heart disease in the newborn. The 2 most common presentations of heart disease in the newborn are cyanosis and congestive heart failure with abnormalities of pulses. In hypoplastic left heart and critical aortic stenosis, pulses are diminished throughout. In coarctation, pulses are diminished in the lower extremities.

Abdomen

Check for softness, absence of distention, and good bowel sounds. Palpate for kidneys—most abdominal masses in the newborn are associated with the kidneys (multicystic-dysplastic, hydronephrosis, etc). When the abdomen is relaxed, normal-sized kidneys can be appreciated. A markedly scaphoid abdomen plus respiratory distress suggests diaphragmatic hernia. Absence of abdominal musculature (prune-belly) may occur in association with renal abnormalities. Check the size of the liver and spleen. The outline of a distended bladder may be seen and palpated above the symphysis pubica.

Genitalia & Anus

Male and female genitals show characteristics according to gestational age (Table 4–5). In the female, an imperforate hymen may be visible. During the first few days a whitish discharge with or without blood is normal. Rule out ambiguous genitals and abnormal anal openings or fissures. Check patency and location of anus.

Skeleton

Check for obvious anomalies, eg, absence of a bone, clubfoot, and fusion or webbing of digits. Check for extra digits. Examine for hip dislocation by attempting to dislocate the femur posteriorly and then abducting the legs to relocate the femur. Examine for extremity fractures and for palsies (especially brachial plexus injuries). Rule out myelomeningoceles and other spinal deformities (eg, scoliosis). Arthrogryposis (limited joint movement) is seen with in utero limitation of movement due to lack of amniotic fluid or from a congenital muscle disease.

Neurologic Examination

Observe resting tone (normal, term newborns should exhibit flexion of the upper and lower extremities) and spontaneous movements. Look for asymmetry of movements. Extension of extremities should result in spontaneous recoil to the flexed position. Assess character of cry; a high-pitched cry is indicative of disease of the central nervous system (eg, hemorrhage). Hypotonia and a weak cry are indicative of systemic disease or a congenital muscle disorder. Check for newborn reflexes:

(1) **Rooting reflex**—Head turns to the side of a facial stimulus.
(2) **Sucking reflex.**
(3) **Traction response**—Infant is pulled by the arms to sitting. Initially the head lags, then with active flexion comes to midline for a few seconds before falling forward.
(4) **Palmar grasp.**
(5) **Deep tendon reflexes.**
(6) **Placing**—Rub the dorsum of one foot on the underside of a surface. Then, the infant will flex the knee and bring the foot up.
(7) **Moro (startle) reflex**—Hold the infant, and support the head. Allow the head to drop 1–2 cm suddenly. The arms will abduct at the shoulder and extend at the elbow. Adduction will follow. The hands show a prominent spreading or extension of the fingers.
  Note: Several beats of ankle clonus and an upgoing Babinski reflex are normal.

American Academy of Pediatrics: *Guidelines for Perinatal Care.* American Academy of Pediatrics, 1988.

Brazelton TB: *Neonatal Behavioral Assessment Scale.* Spastics International Medical Publications. Heinemann, 1973.

Caputo AR et al: Dilation in neonates: A protocol. *Pediatrics* 1982;**69:**77.

Dubowitz LMS et al: Visual function in the newborn: Is it cortically mediated? *Lancet* 1986;**1:**1139.

Friedman S, Jacobs B, Werthmann M: Sensory processing in pre- and full-term infants in the neonatal. In: *Preterm Birth and Psychological Development.* Friedman S, Sigman M (editors). Academic Press, 1981.

Illingworth RS: *The Development of the Infant and Young Child: Normal and Abnormal,* 7th ed. Churchill Livingstone, 1982.

CARE OF THE NORMAL NEWBORN

CARE IMMEDIATELY AFTER DELIVERY

Gently suction the oropharynx. Obtain Apgar scores. Support body temperature by drying the skin, then swaddle or place the infant beneath a radiant heat source. If polyhydramnios is present at delivery or if excessive oral secretions are noted, pass a soft catheter into the stomach to rule out esophageal atresia. Routine eye prophylaxis must be done as defined by local health codes (eg, silver nitrate, 1%, or erythromycin ointment) to prevent gonorrheal conjunctivitis. Place identification-bands, and obtain footprint.

CORD BLOOD

Cord blood is used for blood typing, Coombs testing, and serology. Another tube is saved. Cord blood is also useful for other tests, eg, electrolytes, glucose, total protein, and toxicology screen. Blood from doubly clamped cord can also be used in testing for pH, base deficit, and lactate concentrations, if needed.

CARE IN TRANSITIONAL NURSERY

Check temperature stabilization. Give vitamin K, 1 mg intramuscularly, to prevent hemorrhagic disease of the newborn. Review pertinent history. Calculate birth weight and gestational age to assess risk for certain problems, eg, hypoglycemia. Indications that the baby is ready for feeding include the following: (1) alertness and vigor, (2) absence of abdominal distention, (3) good bowel sounds, and (4) normal hunger cry. All of these usually occur 2–6 hours after birth, but fetal distress or traumatic delivery may prolong this period. Check that all neonatal screening tests are completed.

CONTINUED CARE IN LEVEL 1

The primary responsibilities of the Level 1 nursery are care of the well infant, enhancing successful mother-infant bonding, feeding, and teaching the techniques of newborn care. However, surveillance is a key function of the staff; they must be alert for signs and symptoms of illness.

Admission

The prenatal history and immediate postnatal events should be reviewed so that as many problems as possible are anticipated. The determination of birth weight for gestational age is very helpful in this regard. The baby's initial physical examination should be performed within the first 12 hours of life.

Temperature Control

After delivery, body temperature may be labile until the infant has stabilized. Cooling should be avoided, because it can delay normal cardiovascular adjustments and predispose the infant to persistent pulmonary hypertension. Drying the skin is absolutely essential, and radiant heating devices are excellent adjuncts, allowing both heating of the infant and adequate observation.

Observation

The infant should be observed for signs of illness, including temperature instability, change in activity, refusal to feed, pallor, cyanosis, jaundice, tachypnea and respiratory distress, delayed (beyond 24 hours) passage of first stool or void, and bilious vomiting.

Screening Laboratory

Infants born to mothers with type O or Rh-negative blood should have a blood type and direct and indirect Coombs tests performed on cord blood. The indirect Coombs test is particularly important in the diagnosis of ABO incompatibility. Dextrostix or Chemstrip testing should be performed in the infants at risk for hypoglycemia. Values of less than 40 mg/dL should be confirmed with a blood glucose. He-

matocrit should be measured at 3–6 hours of age. Other tests include the serologic test for syphilis and state-sponsored screens for inborn errors of metabolism. These latter screens include tests for phenylketonuria, maple syrup urine disease, homocystinuria, galactosemia, sickle cell disease, hypothyroidism, and cystic fibrosis. In well newborns, these metabolic screens are performed just prior to discharge after the infant has received milk feedings. In hospitals with early discharge policies (ie, blood obtained at < 24 hours of age), a repeat screening at 1 week of age is required. In infants with prolonged hospital stays, the test should be performed at 1 week of age.

Duration of Stay

The trend over the last several years has been toward shorter hospital stays for well mothers and infants. Criteria for early discharge (< 24 hours) at the University of Colorado are presented in Table 4–6. These criteria have been adapted from those determined by the American Academy of Pediatrics (AAP). Early discharge has proved to be safe in indigent as well as middle-income populations provided that criteria such as those in Table 4–6 are met. Of considerable importance is the fact that most infants who manifest serious cardiorespiratory and infectious problems do so in the first 6 hours of life. Other problems, such as jaundice and difficulties in

Table 4–6. Criteria for early discharge.[1]

1. Delivery is vertex, single, sterile, and vaginal.
2. Apgar scores of > 7 at 1 and 5 minutes.
3. Gestational age of 38–42 weeks and weight of 2700–4000 g.
4. Minimum length of stay of 24 hours; a transition to normal thermoregulation in an open crib, completion of 2 successful feedings, evidence of stool and void, completion of neonatal screening for metabolic disease and blood type and Coombs' test (Rh-negative and O mothers) prior to discharge.
5. Vital signs within normal ranges at discharge:
   Axillary temperature   36.1–37.2 °C
   Heart rate   110–150 / min
   Respiratory rate   30–60 / min
6. A normal neonatal hospital course with no signs or symptoms that require continuous observation:
   Blood dextrose maintained > 45 mg/dL
   Hematocrit 45–65%
   ABO-incompatible infants must be held until 48 hours and released only if they do not require therapy for hemolysis.
7. Physical examination completed by the physician or a trained assistant.
8. Demonstration of mother's understanding and ability to provide adequate care for her newborn; infant care education provided on a one-to-one or classroom basis by the nursing staff prior to discharge.
9. Signed documentation by mother that states her obligation to participate in follow-up care.

[1]Reproduced, with permission, from Conrad PD, Wilkening RB, Rosenberg AA: Safety of newborn discharge in less than 36 hours in an indigent population. *Am J Dis Child* 1989;**143**:98. Copyright 1989, American Medical Association.

breast-feeding, typically occur later but can usually be handled on an outpatient basis provided that good follow-up has been arranged. The physician must order a more extended period of observation if there is any question about the hospital course and must realize that many infants will require a return appointment a few days after discharge rather than the customary 2 weeks.

Adapting Nursery Care to Meet the Needs of Mother

The life situation of the mother and family is important in their adaptation to the newly born infant. The caretaker needs to be aware of emotional support available to the mother (spouse or other family members), financial security, maturity of the mother, and past psychiatric, drug, or alcohol problems. To provide appropriate assistance, the nursery staff needs to get to know the family. The family should receive assistance with basic care skills such as feeding, bathing, and cord and circumcision care and information on common newborn problems. One-on-one teaching is the desired means of communication, supplemented on a busy service with videotapes and printed material. If the mother's condition permits, the baby should room-in with the mother as soon as possible. The mother and infant are then supervised by the nursery staff.

Circumcision

The American Academy of Pediatrics has published a statement to the effect that there is no longer any medical reason for neonatal circumcision. Undecided parents should be informed of the pros and cons of the procedure.

Discharge Preparation

1. Perform a physical examination.
2. Discuss cord and circumcision care.
3. Make sure the mother has mastered the essentials of newborn care.
4. Review signs and symptoms that cause concern:
   a. Increasing jaundice
   b. Poor feeding
   c. Lethargy: increased sleeping
   d. Vomiting
   e. Fever
5. Review feeding instructions.
6. Arrange follow-up.
7. Verify the identification of the infant and the person accepting the infant at discharge.
8. Check on all screening procedures.

American Academy of Pediatrics: *Guidelines for Perinatal Care.* American Academy of Pediatrics, 1988.

Britton HL, Britton JR: Efficacy of early newborn discharge in a middle-class population. *Am J Dis Child* 1984;**138:**1041.

Chowdhry P et al: Results of controlled double-blind study of thyroid replacement in very low-birth-weight premature infants with hypothyroxinemia. *Pediatrics* 1984; **73:**301.

Committee on Fetus and Newborn, American Academy of Pediatrics: Report of fetus and newborn: Report of the ad hoc task force on circumcision. *Pediatrics* 1975; **56:**610.

Conrad PD et al: Safety of newborn discharge in less than 36 hours in an indigent population. *Am J Dis Child* 1989;**143:**98.

Glorieux J et al: Follow-up at ages 5 and 7 years on mental development in children with hypothyroidism detected by Quebec Screening Program. *J Pediatr* 1985; **107:**913.

Grossman LK et al: Neonatal screening and genetic counseling for sickle cell trait. *Am J Dis Child* 1985; **139:**241.

Lane PA, Hathaway WE: Vitamin K in infancy. *J Pediatr* 1985;**106:**351.

Newborn screening for sickle cell disease and other hemoglobinopathies. *Pediatrics* 1989;**83(Suppl):**813.

New England Congenital Hypothyroidism Collaborative Study Group: Characteristics of infantile hypothyroidism discovered on neonatal screening. *J Pediatr* 1984;**104:**539.

New England Congenital Hypothyroidism Collaborative Study Group: Neonatal hypothyroidism screening: Status of patients at 6 years of age. *J Pediatr* 1985; **107:**915.

Nussbaum RL et al: Neonatal screening for sickling hemoglobinopathies. *Am J Dis Child* 1984;**138:**44.

Pittard WB III, Geddes K: Newborn hospitalization: A closer look. *J Pediatr* 1988;**112:**257.

Vichinsky E et al: Newborn screening for sickle cell disease: Effect on mortality. *Pediatrics* 1988;**81:**749.

Wiswell TE, Roscelli JD: Corroborative evidence for the decreased incidence of urinary tract infections in circumcised male infants. *Pediatrics* 1986;**78:**96.

PARENT-INFANT RELATIONSHIP

Interest in parent-infant bonding has grown in the last 20 years in part due to the observation of an excessive incidence of child abuse and nonorganic failure to thrive in infants who experienced a prolonged postdelivery separation from parents. This separation had its origin in the historical approach to neonatal care, which emphasized infant isolation for the prevention of infection. On the basis of this human experience and studies of mother-infant bonding in other species, the pendulum has now shifted to permit liberal nursery-visiting policies.

DEVELOPMENT OF PARENT-INFANT BONDING

The steps in maternal attachment can be outlined as follows: (1) planning the pregnancy, (2) confirming the pregnancy, (3) accepting the pregnancy, (4) feeling fetal movement, (5) accepting the fetus as an individual, (6) experiencing birth, (7) hearing and seeing the baby, (8) touching and holding the baby, and (9) caretaking. Numerous influences can affect this process. The actions and responses of the mother and father are a function of their own genetic endowment, interfamily relationships, cultural practices, past experiences with this or previous pregnancies, and, most important, the child-rearing practices of his or her own parents. Also critical is the in-hospital experience surrounding the birth—the behavior of doctors and nurses, separation from the baby, and hospital practices. It is particularly important for medical staff to recognize that many different parental approaches to the child are within the realm of good family interaction. Otherwise, needless and unfounded guilt and anxiety may be conveyed to the parents.

The first 1½ hours of life are an important time in the process of mother-infant bonding. The infant is alert and able to follow with the eyes, a response prompting meaningful interaction with mother. The infant's array of sensory and motor abilities evokes responses from the mother and initiates communication that may facilitate attachment and induction of reciprocal actions. Whether a critical time period for these initial interactions exists is not clear, but increased contact over the first 3 postpartum days is associated with improved parenting behavior. For these reasons, labor and delivery should pose as little anxiety to the mother as possible, and parents and baby should have time together immediately after delivery if the baby's medical condition permits. Prophylactic treatment of the eyes for gonococcal ophthalmitis should ideally be withheld until after the initial bonding has taken place. It can be performed safely within 1 hour of birth.

THE SICK INFANT

Mothers with high-risk pregnancies are at increased risk for subsequent parenting problems. The involvement of both obstetrician and pediatrician alike before the child's birth enables the family to prepare for anticipated aspects of the baby's care and provides reassurance that the odds are heavily in favor of a live baby who will ultimately be healthy. If the need for neonatal intensive care is anticipated before birth (known congenital anomaly, refractory premature labor), *maternal* transport to the proper facility should be planned. In this way, a mother can be with her baby during its most critical care. In addition, repeated studies have confirmed better survival rates for high-risk infants whose mothers were transported to perinatal centers for delivery compared to infants transported after birth to neonatal intensive care units. It is also very helpful to allow

the parents to tour before delivery the unit their baby will occupy. This practice greatly reduces parental anxiety after the birth.

The single basic principle in dealing with parents of a sick infant is to provide essential information clearly and accurately to both parents, preferably when they are together. Survival rates have improved, especially for premature babies; most do well. In most circumstances, one can be reasonably positive about the outcome. There is also no reason to emphasize problems that might occur in the future or to deal with individual worries of the physician. Questions, if asked, need to be answered honestly, but the tendency to overestimate the complications and handicaps should be avoided.

Before the parents' initial visit to the unit, a physician or nurse should describe what the baby and the equipment look like. When they arrive in the nursery, these details can again be reviewed. If the baby must be moved to another hospital, the mother should be given time to see and touch her infant before the transfer. The father should be encouraged to meet the baby at the receiving hospital so that he can become comfortable with the intensive care unit. He can serve as a link between baby and mother, providing information and photographs.

As a baby's course proceeds, the nursery staff can help the parents become comfortable with their infant. It is also important for the staff to discuss among themselves any problems that parents may be having and to keep a record of visits and telephone calls. This approach allows early intervention in dealing with potential problems.

CONGENITAL MALFORMATIONS

The birth of an infant with a congenital malformation is another situation in which staff support is essential. Parental reactions to the birth of a malformed infant follow a predictable course. For most parents, initial shock and denial are followed by a period of sadness and anger, gradual adaptation, and, finally, an increased satisfaction with and ability to care for the baby. The parents must be allowed to pass through these stages and, in effect, mourn the loss of the anticipated normal child. Again, information, including the prognosis for the particular problem, must be provided clearly and accurately to both parents.

DEATH OF AN INFANT

A stillbirth or the death of an infant is a highly stressful family event; there is a significant incidence of psychiatric disorders within 2 years of the death of a neonate. One of the major predispositions is a breakdown of communication between parents. The health care staff needs to encourage the parents to talk with each other, discuss their feelings, and display emotion. The staff should talk with the parents at the time of death and then several months later review the findings of the autopsy, answer questions, and see how the family is doing.

Committee on Bioethics, American Academy of Pediatrics: Treatment of critically ill newborns. *Pediatrics* 1983; **72:**565.

Hunter RS et al: Antecedents of child abuse and neglect in premature infants: A prospective study in a newborn intensive care unit. *Pediatrics* 1978;**61:**629.

Infant Bioethics Task Force and Consultants, American Academy of Pediatrics: Guidelines for infant bioethics committees. *Pediatrics* 1984;**74:**306.

Klaus M, Kennell J: *Parent-Infant Bonding.* Mosby, 1982.

Klaus MN, Kennell JH: Care of the parents. Page 147 in: *Care of the High Risk Neonate.* Klaus MN, Fanaroff AA (editors). Saunders, 1986.

Klein M et al: Low birth weight and the battered child syndrome. *Am J Dis Child* 1971;**122:**15.

Mahowald MB: Baby Doe committees: A critical evaluation. *Clin Perinatol* 1988;**15:**789.

Nance S: *Premature Babies: A Handbook for Parents.* Priam Books, 1982.

Schulman JL: Coping with major disease: Child, family, pediatrician. *J Pediatr* 1983;**102:**988.

Strain J: The American Academy of Pediatrics comments on the ''Baby Doe II'' regulations. *N Engl J Med* 1983;**309:**443.

FEEDING OF THE NEWBORN INFANT

WHAT, WHEN, & HOW MUCH TO FEED

The healthy, term infant should be allowed to feed every 2–5 hours on demand. The first feeding usually occurs at 2–6 hours of life. Breast-feeding can start as early as in the delivery room. Although there is a trend toward earlier institution of feedings, evidence that the infant is prepared for feedings should always be present—soft, nondistended abdomen, good bowel sounds, and a strong, rhythmic suck. Breast milk or formula (20 kcal/oz) can be given. Generally, the volume increases from 0.5–1 ounce per feeding initially up to above 1.5–2 ounces per feeding on day 3. By day 3, the average term newborn takes in about 100 mL/kg/d of milk.

METHODS OF FEEDING

Bottle Feeding

Most commercial bottles and nipples are satisfactory. The preterm infant usually requires a softer nipple with a larger hole.

Breast-Feeding

Although a wide range of infant formulas satisfy the nutritional needs of most neonates, breast milk is the standard on which formulas are based. The distribution of calories in human milk is 7% protein, 55% fat, and 38% carbohydrate. The ratio of whey to casein is 60:40. This allows ease of protein digestion, while fat digestion is aided by lipase. Despite low levels of several vitamins and minerals, bioavailability is high. Infants of mothers who are strict vegetarians should receive supplemental iron, folate, and vitamin B_{12}. Along with nutritional features, other advantages of breast milk include the following: (1) the presence of host resistance factors, including IgA and cellular components thought to decrease the incidence of upper respiratory and gastrointestinal infections in infancy; (2) the possibility that breast-feeding may decrease the frequency and severity of childhood eczema and asthma; and (3) promotion of mother-infant bonding.

The nursery staff must be cognizant of problems associated with breast-feeding and be able to provide help and support for mothers in the hospital. Feeding should be fairly frequent in early stages (every 2–3 hours) so that production of milk is stimulated. Initially, nursing time is limited to 5 minutes on each side, then increased to 10 minutes on each side. Care of the nipples should also be reviewed in hospital.

Gavage Feeding

Intermittent gavage feeding can be used for infants with a weak suck and swallow or for infants who tire easily, including preterm infants and those with medical conditions (eg, respiratory distress or congenital heart disease) precluding nipple feedings. An orogastric tube can be inserted for each feeding, or a soft, indwelling orogastric or nasogastric tube can be used. The position of the tube in the stomach should be checked prior to each feeding. The infant should be fed every 2–3 hours, depending on the age and size of patient. Generally, infants weighing less than 1500 grams require 2-hour feedings, whereas larger infants are fed at 3-hour intervals. Feedings are started at 10–25% of the child's nutritional needs and advanced to full requirements (100–120 kcal/kg/d) over 3–7 days. The more rapid advancement is used in infants weighing more than 1500 grams and the slowest in infants weighing less than 1000 grams.

Gastrostomy

Gastrostomy feedings are indicated for infants requiring indefinite tube feedings (eg, those with neurologic disease) and for those with certain surgical conditions (eg, some cases of esophageal atresia).

Parenteral Alimentation

Nutrition can effectively be provided with hyperalimentation solutions given either through peripheral or central venous lines. Table 4–7 illustrates the use of hyperalimentation in newborns. Parenteral nutrition is indicated for infants with gastrointestinal anomalies after surgical correction, for preterm infants with necrotizing enterocolitis and other forms of feeding intolerance, and for infants too sick for any reason to tolerate enteral feedings. Central hyperalimentation has now been facilitated by Silastic lines that can be placed in the nursery under local anesthesia percutaneously or through a basilic vein cutdown.

Anderson GH: Human milk feeding. *Pediatr Clin North Am* 1985;**32**:332.

Committee on Nutrition, American Academy of Pediatrics: Nutritional needs of low birthweight infants. *Pediatrics* 1985;**75**:976.

Dunn L et al: Beneficial effects of early hypocaloric enteral feeding on neonatal gastrointestinal function: Preliminary report of a randomized trial. *J Pediatr* 1988; **112**:622.

Farrell MK, Balistreri WF: Parenteral nutrition and hepatobiliary dysfunction. *Clin Perinatol* 1986;**13**:197.

Gilhooly J et al: Central venous silicone elastomer catheter placement by basilic vein cutdown in neonates. *Pediatrics* 1986;**78**:636.

Greene HL et al: Guidelines for the use of vitamins, trace elements, calcium, magnesium and phosphorus in infants and children receiving total parenteral nutrition. *Am J Clin Nutr* 1988;**48**:1324.

Kernan JA, Sunshine P: Parenteral alimentation. *Semin Perinatol* 1979;**3**:417.

Lawrence R: Breastfeeding. *Clin Perinatol* 1987;**14**:1.

Lemons JA et al: Nitrogen sources for parenteral nutrition in the newborn infant. *Clin Perinatol* 1986;**13**:91.

Oh W: Fluid and electrolyte therapy and parenteral nutrition in low birth weight infants. *Clin Perinatol* 1982; **9**:637.

Stahl G et al: Intravenous administration of lipid emulsions to premature infants. *Clin Perinatol* 1986;**13**:133.

Workshop on Current Issues in Feeding the Newborn Infant. *Pediatrics* 1985;**75(Suppl)**:135.

NEONATAL INTENSIVE CARE

GENERAL APPROACH

Neonatal intensive care should always have an anticipatory component; ie, obstetricians managing high-risk pregnancies should anticipate delivery as often as possible and discuss specific features of the pregnancy likely to affect the infant immediately after birth. In this way, the course of the labor and the condition of the infant during delivery are known to the baby's caregiver. A pediatrician or neonatologist should be in attendance at high-risk deliveries to provide prompt resuscitation of the infant, when needed. Furthermore, the pediatrician can request that blood tests be made on cord blood obtained at delivery, as appropriate.

TRANSPORTATION

Whenever possible, high-risk mothers should be delivered at perinatal centers so that transport of the infant after delivery can be avoided. In such circumstances, the infant is simply moved from the delivery room to the level 2 or 3 nursery. The transport

Table 4–7. Use of parenteral alimentation solutions.

	Volume (ml/kg/d)	Carbohydrate (g/100 mL)	Protein (g/kg)	Lipid (g/kg)	Calories (kcal/kg)
Peripheral: For short-term support (7–10 days)					
Starting solution	100–150	D10W	1	1	46–64
Target solution	150	D12.5W	2.5	3	102
Central: For long-term support (> 10 days)					
Starting solution	100–150	D10W	1	1	46–64
Target solution	130	D20W	3–3.5	3	123

Protein calories should be no more than 10% of total calories.
Advance dextrose in central hyperalimentation as tolerated by 2.5% per day as long as blood glucose remains normal.
Advance lipids by 0.5 g/kg every other day as long as triglycerides are normal.
Total water should be 100–150 mL/kg/d, depending on the child's fluid tolerance.
Monitoring
Chemstrips or blood glucose 2–3 times per day when changing dextrose concentration, then daily.
Electrolytes daily, then 2 times per week when the child is on a stable solution.
BUN, Cr, total protein, albumin, Ca, PO_4, Mg, direct bilirubin, alkaline phosphatase, and CBC with platelets weekly.
Zn, Cu monthly.

unit should be easily movable and be equipped to provide ventilatory assistance and oxygen therapy to the infant and to maintain body temperature. In transports from one hospital to another, equipment for intravenous infusions should be available, together with appropriate solutions to support circulating blood volume and extracellular fluid volume. Equipment should be on hand to monitor the infant (heart rate, respirations, blood pressure, oxygen saturation, and transcutaneous Po_2). All emergency equipment necessary to resuscitate an infant should be available. The infant should be stabilized prior to transport.

PERINATAL RESUSCITATION

Perinatal resuscitation involves the steps taken by the obstetrician during labor and delivery to support the infant, as well as the traditional resuscitative steps taken by the pediatrician after delivery of the infant. Intrapartum steps to support the infant include the following: maintaining maternal blood pressure with volume expanders if needed, administering maternal oxygen therapy, positioning the mother to improve placental perfusion, readjusting oxytocin infusions if appropriate, minimizing trauma to the infant (particularly important in infants of very low birth weight), suctioning the nasopharynx if meconium is present in amniotic fluid, obtaining all necessary cord blood samples, and completing an examination of the placenta.

Steps taken by the pediatrician or neonatologist center around support of the following physiologic areas: maintenance of perfusion, maintenance of effective ventilation, temperature support, and hydration and glucose regulation. These are generally accomplished as follows:

Resuscitation of the Newborn Infant

A number of conditions of pregnancy, labor, and delivery place the infant at risk for birth asphyxia: (1) maternal diseases such as diabetes, pregnancy-induced hypertension (PIH), heart and renal disease, and collagen-vascular disease; (2) fetal conditions such as prematurity, multiple births, growth retardation, and fetal anomalies; and (3) labor and delivery conditions, including fetal distress with or without meconium in the amniotic fluid and administration of anesthetics and narcotic analgesics.

Physiology of Birth Asphyxia

Birth asphyxia can be the result of several mechanisms: (1) acute interruption of umbilical blood flow (eg, prolapsed cord with cord compression), (2) premature placental separation, (3) maternal hypotension or hypoxia, (4) chronic placental insufficiency, and (5) failure to execute a proper newborn resuscitation.

The neonatal response to asphyxia follows a predictable pattern that has been demonstrated in a variety of species (Fig 4–3). The initial response to hypoxia is an increase in frequency of respiration and a rise in heart rate and blood pressure. Respirations then cease (primary apnea) as heart rate and blood pressure begin to fall. This initial period of apnea lasts 30–60 seconds. Gasping respirations (3–6/min) then begin, while heart rate and blood pressure continue to decline. Secondary or terminal apnea then ensues, with further decline in heart rate and blood pressure. The longer the duration of secondary apnea, the greater the risk for hypoxic organ injury. A cardinal feature of the defense against hypoxia is the sacrifice, ie, underperfusion, of certain tissue beds (eg, skin, muscle, and gastrointestinal tract), which allows the perfusion of core organs (ie, heart and brain) to be maintained.

The response to resuscitation also follows a predictable pattern. During the period of primary apnea, almost any physical or chemical stimulus causes the baby to initiate respirations. Infants in the stage of

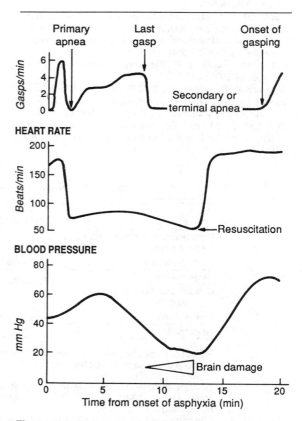

Figure 4–3. Schematic depiction of changes in rhesus monkeys during asphyxia and on resuscitation by positive pressure ventilation. (Adapted and reproduced, with permission, from Dawes GS: *Fetal and Neonatal Physiology.* Year Book, 1968.

secondary apnea require positive pressure ventilation. The first sign of recovery is an increase in heart rate, followed by an increase in blood pressure with improved perfusion. The time period required for rhythmic, spontaneous respirations to occur is related to the duration of the secondary apnea. As a rough rule, for each 1 minute past the last gasp, 2 minutes of positive pressure breathing are required before gasping begins, and 4 minutes are required to reach rhythmic breathing. However, these time periods can vary, depending on the degree and duration of intrauterine asphyxia. Not until sometime later do spinal and corneal reflexes return. Muscle tone gradually improves over the course of several hours.

Delivery Room Management

When asphyxia is anticipated, a resuscitation team of 2 persons, one to manage the airway and one to monitor heartbeat and provide assistance, should be present. The necessary equipment and drugs are listed in Table 4–8.

A. Steps in the Resuscitation: (Fig 4–4.)
1. Dry the infant well, and place the baby under the radiant heat source.
2. Gently apply suction to the oropharynx and nose.
3. Assess the infant's condition. The best criteria are the infant's respiratory effort (apneic, gasping, regular) and heart rate (> 100 or < 100). A depressed heart rate indicative of hypoxic myocardial depression is the single most reliable indicator of the need for resuscitation.

4. Generally, infants with heart rates over 100 beats/min (bpm) require no further intervention. Infants with heart rates less than 100 bpm and apnea or irregular respiratory efforts should be vigorously stimulated. The baby's back should be rubbed with a towel while oxygen is blown over the baby's face.
5. If the baby fails to respond to 15–20 seconds of stimulation, apply bag and mask ventilation, using a soft mask that seals well around the mouth and nose. For the initial inflations, pressures of 30–40 cm H_2O may be necessary to overcome surface-active forces in the lungs. An inspiratory time of 1–2 seconds may be helpful as well. In the premature infant, even higher pressures (40–60 cm H_2O) may be needed. Adequacy of ventilation is assessed by observing expansion of the infant's chest with bagging and a gradual improvement in color, perfusion, and heart rate. After the first few breaths, attempts should be made to lower the peak pressure. Rate of bagging should not exceed 40 breaths per minute.
6. Most neonates can be effectively resuscitated with a bag and mask. However, if the infant does not respond favorably in 30–40 seconds, the physician must proceed to intubation:
   a. Make sure that the head is stable with the nose in the sniffing position (pointing straight upward).
   b. Insert the laryngoscope blade, and sweep the tongue to the left.
   c. Advance the blade to the base of the tongue, and identify the epiglottis.
   d. Pick up the endotracheal tube with the right hand.
   e. Slide the laryngoscope anterior to the epiglottis, and gently lift along the angle of the handle of the laryngoscope.
   f. Identify the vocal cords.
   g. Insert the tube in the right side of the mouth, and visualize the tube passing through the vocal cords.
   h. Ventilate as described above.
   i. Failure to respond to intubation and ventilation can result from (1) mechanical difficulties (Table 4–9), (2) profound asphyxia with myocardial depression, and (3) inadequate circulating blood volume.
   j. Quickly rule out the mechanical causes in Table 4–9. Check to be sure the endotracheal tube passes through the vocal cords. Occlusion of the tube should be suspected when there is resistance to bagging and no chest wall movement. It is very unusual for a neonate to require either cardiac massage or drugs during

Table 4–8. Equipment for neonatal resuscitation.[1]

Clinical Needs	Equipment
Thermoregulation	Radiant heat source with platform, mattress covered with warm sterile blankets, servo control heating, temperature probe.
Airway management	*Suction:* bulb suction, DeLee suction apparatus, wall vacuum suction with sterile catheters. *Ventilation:* manual infant resuscitation bag connected to pressure manometer capable of delivering 100% oxygen, appropriate masks for term and preterm infants. *Intubation:* neonatal laryngoscope with No. 0 and No. 1 blades; endotracheal tubes—2.5, 3, 3.5 mm OD with Calgiswab stylet (nasopharyngeal calcium alginate applicator).
Gastric decompression	Nasogastric tubes—5 and 8 Fr.
Administration of drugs/volume	Sterile umbilical catheterization tray, umbilical catheters (3.5 and 5 Fr), volume expanders (Ringer's lactate, 5% albumin), drug box with appropriate neonatal vials and dilutions, sterile syringes, and needles.
Transport	Warmed transport isolette with oxygen source and manual resuscitator.

[1]Reproduced, with permission, from Rosenberg AA: Neonatal adaptation. In *Obstetrics Normal and Problem Pregnancies,* 1st ed. Gabbe SG, Niebyl JR, Simpson JL (editors). Churchill Livingstone, 1986.

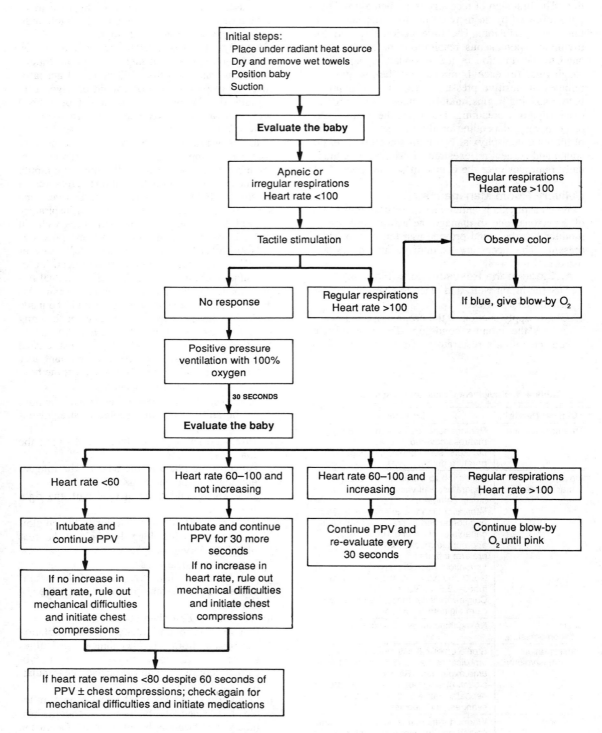

Figure 4–4. Delivery room management.

Table 4–9. Mechanical causes of failed resuscitation.

Etiology	Examples
Equipment failure	Malfunctioning bag; oxygen not connected or running
Endotracheal tube malposition	Esophagus, right mainstem bronchus
Occluded endotracheal tube	
Insufficient inflation pressure to expand lungs	
Space-occupying lesions in the thorax	Pneumothorax, pleural effusions, diaphragmatic hernia
Pulmonary hypoplasia	Extreme prematurity, oligohydramnios

Reproduced, with permission, from Rosenberg AA: Neonatal adaptation. In *Obstetrics Normal and Problem Pregnancies,* 1st ed. Gabbe SG, Niebyl JK, Simpson JL (editors). Churchill Livingstone, 1986.

resuscitation. Almost all newborns respond to ventilation with 100% oxygen.

k. If mechanical causes are ruled out, external cardiac massage should be performed for a heart rate persistently less than 100 bpm. Compression of 1–1.5 cm should be performed at a rate of 120 per minute. There is no need to pause for ventilation while doing cardiac massage.

l. If drugs are needed (rarely), the drug of choice is 0.1 mL/kg of epinephrine, 1:10,000 solution, through the endotracheal tube or an umbilical venous line. Sodium bicarbonate, 1–2 meq/kg of the neonatal dilution, can be used for an infant with *documented* metabolic acidosis. If volume loss is suspected, 10 mL/kg of a volume expander (5% albumin, Plasmanate) should be administered through an umbilical venous line.

The appropriateness of continued resuscitative efforts should always be reevaluated in an infant who fails to respond to all of the above efforts. Today, resuscitative efforts are made even in "apparent stillbirths," that is, infants whose Apgar scores at 1 minute are 0–1. However, efforts should not be sustained in the face of little or no improvement over a reasonable period (ie, 10–15 minutes).

B. Special Considerations:

1. In preterm infants, especially those weighing less than 1000 grams, proceed quickly to intubation.
2. In the case of narcotic administration to the mother during labor, perform the resuscitation as described above. When the baby is stable with good heart rate, color, and perfusion but still has poor respiratory effort, a trial of naloxone hydrochloride (0.1 mg/kg) is indicated.
3. Meconium-stained amniotic fluid:
   a. The obstetrician carefully suctions the oropharynx and nasopharynx after delivery of the head with a DeLee suction apparatus attached to wall suction.
   b. The delivery is then completed, and the baby is given to the resuscitator.
   c. If the baby is active and breathing, requiring no resuscitation, and if effective obstetric suctioning has been performed, the airway need not be inspected. Only further suctioning of the mouth and nasopharynx need be performed.
   d. The airway of any infant requiring ventilation must be checked (by passage of a tube below the vocal cords) before positive-pressure ventilation is instituted.

American Heart Association and American Academy of Pediatrics: *Textbook of Neonatal Resuscitation.* 1987.

Apgar V: A proposal for a new method of evaluation of the newborn infant. *Anesth Analg* 1953;**32:**260.

Brans YW: Equipment available for nurseries. *Clin Perinatol* 1983;**10:**263.

Carson BS et al: Combined obstetric and pediatric approach to prevent meconium aspiration syndrome. *Am J Obstet Gynecol* 1976;**126:**712.

Gregory GA et al: Meconium aspiration in infants: A prospective study. *J Pediatr* 1974;**85:**848.

Gupta JM et al: The sequence of events in neonatal apnea. *Lancet* 1967;**2:**55.

Linder L et al: Need for endotracheal intubation and suction in meconium stained neonates. *J Pediatr* 1988;**112:**613.

MacDonald HM et al: Neonatal asphyxia. 1. Relationship of obstetric and neonatal implications to neonatal mortality in 38,405 consecutive deliveries. *J Pediatr* 1980;**96:**898.

Main DM, Main EK, Maurer MM: Cesarean section versus vaginal delivery for the breech fetus weighing less than 1500 grams. *Am J Obstet Gynecol* 1983;**146:**580.

Phibbs RH: Delivery room management of the newborn. Page 212 in: *Neonatology: Pathophysiology and Management of the Newborn.* Avery GB (editor). Lippincott, 1987.

THE PRETERM INFANT

Premature infants account for the majority of high-risk newborns. The preterm infant faces a variety of physiologic handicaps:

(1) The ability to suck, swallow, and breathe in a coordinated fashion is not in place until 34–36 weeks of gestation. Therefore, enteral feedings must be provided by gavage. Furthermore, preterm infants frequently have gastroesophageal influx and an immature gag reflex, which increase the risk of aspiration of feedings.

(2) Decreased ability to maintain body temperature (see below).

(3) Pulmonary immaturity—both surfactant deficiency and structural immaturity in those infants of less than 26 weeks of gestation. Their condition is complicated by the combination of noncompliant lungs and a compliant chest wall.

(4) Immature control of respiration, leading to apnea and bradycardia.

(5) Persistent patency of the ductus arteriosus, leading to further compromise of pulmonary gas exchange due to left-to-right shunting.

(6) Immature cerebral vasculature, predisposing the infant to subependymal/intraventricular hemorrhage.

(7) Impaired substrate absorption by the gastrointestinal tract, compromising nutritional management.

(8) Immature renal function (including both filtration and tubular functions), complicating fluid and electrolyte management.

(9) Increased susceptibility to infection.

(10) Immaturity of metabolic processes, predisposing the infant to hypoglycemia and hypocalcemia.

CARE OF THE PRETERM INFANT

Delivery Room
See Perinatal Resuscitation.

Care in the Nursery
Some general principles, eg, thermoregulation, nutrition, and fluid and electrolyte management, are covered here. Other conditions unique to the preterm infant are discussed under specific headings in the chapter.

A. Thermoregulation: Maintaining a stable body temperature is a function of heat production and conservation balanced against heat loss. Heat is produced at the rate of 4.8 kcal/liter O_2 consumed. Heat production in response to cold stress can occur through voluntary muscle activity, involuntary muscle activity (shivering), and thermogenesis not due to shivering. Newborns produce heat mainly through the last of these three mechanisms. This metabolic heat production depends on the quantity of brown fat present, which is very limited in the preterm infant. Heat loss to the environment can occur through the following:

(1) Radiation—transfer of heat from a warmer to cooler object not in contact.

(2) Convection—transfer of heat to the surrounding gaseous environment. This is influenced by air movement and temperature.

(3) Conduction—transfer of heat to a cooler object in contact.

(4) Evaporation—cooling secondary to water loss through the skin.

Heat loss in the preterm newborn is accelerated because of a large ratio of surface area to body mass and reduced insulation of subcutaneous tissue. Furthermore, water loss through the skin is accelerated because of the immaturity of the skin (especially in infants < 27–28 weeks' gestation) and because of the limited ability of skin blood vessels to constrict in response to cold.

For these reasons, the thermal environment of the preterm neonate must be carefully regulated. The infant can be kept warm in an isolette in which the air is heated and convective heat loss minimized. Alternatively, the infant can be kept warm on an open bed with a radiant heat source. Although evaporative and convective heat losses are greater when the radiant warmer is used, this system allows easy access to a critically ill neonate. Ideally, the infant should be kept in a neutral thermal environment (Fig 4–5). The neutral thermal environment allows the infant to maintain a stable core body temperature with a minimum of metabolic heat production through oxygen consumption. In other words, heat losses have been minimized. This is a desirable goal in an infant that may be at risk for hypoxia due to cardiorespiratory disease. Furthermore, the infant is able to utilize calories for growth instead of heat production. The neutral thermal environment for a given infant depends on size, gestational age, and postnatal age. The optimal environment for infants (both dressed and undressed) in isolettes has been determined (Fig 4–6). Alternatively (for either isolette or radiant warmer care), the neutral thermal environment can be obtained by maintaining an abdominal skin temperature of 36.5 °C.

Temperature can be regulated in either isolettes or radiant warmers by manual or servo control adjustments. In manual control, skin temperature is regulated by manually adjusting the environmental temperature of an isolette or the heat output from a radiant warmer so that the infant maintains the desired skin temperature. In servo control, the heating equipment is adjusted automatically to maintain the desired skin temperature. The core temperature of the infant can be estimated from axillary temperatures. Although rectal temperatures provide a slightly better estimation of core temperature, they are discouraged because of the risk of rectal perforation. In infants weighing more than 1200 grams, skin temperature is less than core temperature; however, in infants of very low birth weight, core temperature is lower than skin temperature and invariably below normal in the first few hours of life. Generally, when infants reach 1800–2000 grams, they can maintain temperature while bundled in a bassinet.

B. Monitoring the High-Risk Infant: Care of the high-risk preterm infant requires sophisticated monitoring techniques. At a minimum, equipment to monitor heart rate, respirations, and blood pressure

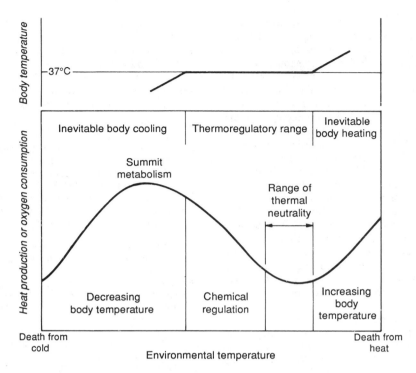

Figure 4–5. Effect of environmental temperature on oxygen consumption and body temperature. (Adapted and reproduced, with permission, from Klaus M, Fanaroff A, Martin RJ: The physical environment. Page 94 in: *Care of the High-Risk Neonate,* 3rd ed. Klaus MH, Fanaroff AA (editors). Saunders, 1986.

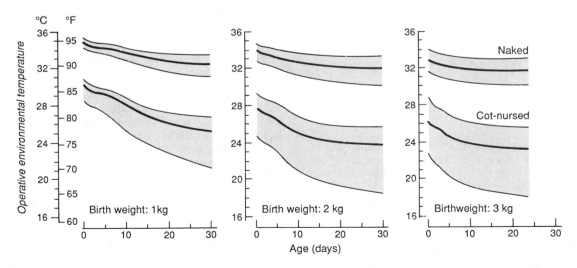

Figure 4–6. Range of environmental temperatures to maintain naked or dressed infants of 1, 2, or 3 kilograms in a neutral thermal environment. (Reproduced, with permission, from Hey E: The care of babies in incubators. Page 171 in: *Recent Advances in Paediatrics,* 4th ed. Gairdner D, Hull D (editors). Churchill, 1971.

should be available. The ideal monitor has memory capabilities to assess episodes of apnea and bradycardia. In the 1980s, the standard of care was to evaluate oxygenation using transcutaneous Po_2 monitors and pulse oximetry saturation. Although pulse oximetry is very simple and reliable, the measurement can be misinterpreted. In the sick newborn, knowledge of Pao_2 is also very important. For that reason, oxygen saturation (Sao_2) must be correlated with measures of Po_2 (eg, arterial blood gas or measure of $TcPo_2$). Finally, arterial blood gases, electrolytes, glucose, calcium, bilirubin, and other chemistries must be measured on small volumes of blood. Early in the care of a sick preterm infant, the most efficient way to sample blood for tests as well as provide fluids and monitor blood pressure is through an umbilical arterial line. Once the infant is stable and the need for frequent blood samples reduced (usually 4–7 days), the umbilical line should be removed. All indwelling lines are associated with morbidity from thrombosis/embolus, infection, and bleeding.

C. Fluid and Electrolyte Therapy: Fluid requirements in preterm infants are a function of (1) insensible losses (skin and respiratory), (2) urine output, (3) stool output (less than 5% of total), and (4) others, eg, nasogastric losses.

In most circumstances, the majority of the fluid requirement is determined by insensible losses and urine losses. The major contribution to insensible water loss is evaporative skin loss. The rate of water loss is a function of gestational age (body weight), environment (losses are greater under a radiant warmer than in an isolette), and the use of phototherapy. Respiratory losses are minimal when infants are breathing humidified oxygen. The renal contribution to water requirement is influenced by the decreased ability of the preterm neonate to concentrate the urine and conserve water.

Electrolyte requirements are minimal for the initial 24–48 hours until there is excretion in the urine. Basal requirements are as follows:

Sodium	3 meq/kg/d
Potassium	2 meq/kg/d
Chloride	2–3 meq/kg/d
Bicarbonate	2–3 meq/kg/d

In the infant of less than 30 weeks, sodium and bicarbonates losses in the urine are frequently excessive.

Initial fluid management after birth is determined by the infant's size. Infants weighing more than 1500 grams should start at 80–100 mL/kg/d of 10% dextrose in water (D10W), whereas those weighing less should start at 100–120 mL/kg/d of either D10W or 5% dextrose in water (D5W) (infants < 800 g and < 26 weeks often become hyperglycemic on D10W). The most critical issue in fluid management is monitoring. Measurements of body weight, urine

output, fluid and electrolyte intake, serum and urine electrolytes, and glucose (using Chemstrips) allow fairly precise determinations of the infant's water, glucose, and electrolyte needs. Once an infant has stabilized (usually by day 2–3), hyperalimentation solutions can be started to meet nutritional as well as water and electrolyte requirements.

Baumgart S: Reduction of oxygen consumption, insensible water loss, and radiant heat demand with use of a plastic blanket for low-birth-weight infants under radiant warmers. *Pediatrics* 1984;**74:**1022.

Hay WW et al: Neonatal pulse oximetry: Accuracy and reliability. *Pediatrics* 1989;**83:**717.

Hey E, Scopes JW: Thermoregulation in the newborn. Page 201 in: *Neonatology: Pathophysiology and Management of the Newborn.* Avery GB (editor). Lippincott, 1987.

Hey EN: The relation between environmental temperature and oxygen consumption in the newborn baby. *J Physiol (Lond)* 1969;**200:**589.

Hey EN, Katz G: The optimum thermal environment for naked babies. *Arch Dis Child* 1970;**45:**328.

Hey EN, O'Connell B: Oxygen consumption and heat balance in the cot-nursed baby. *Arch Dis Child* 1970;**45:**335.

Jennis MS, Peabody JL: Pulse oximetry: An alternative method for the assessment of oxygenation in newborn infants. *Pediatrics* 1987;**79:**524.

Mok JYQ et al: Effect of age and state of wakefulness on transcutaneous oxygen values in preterm infants: A longitudinal study. *J Pediatr* 1988;**113:**706.

Mok JYQ et al: Transcutaneous monitoring of oxygenation: What is normal? *J Pediatr* 1986;**108:**365.

Pasnick M, Lucey JF: Practical uses of continuous transcutaneous oxygen monitoring. *Pediatr Rev* 1983;**5:**5.

Ramanathan R et al: Pulse oximetry in very low birth weight infants with acute and chronic lung disease. *Pediatrics* 1987;**79:**612.

Scopes JW: Metabolic rate and temperature control in the human body. *Br Med Bull* 1966;**22:**88.

Wu PYK: Fluid balance in the newborn infant. *Clin Perinatol* 1982;**9:**3.

NUTRITION OF THE HIGH-RISK INFANT

This section addresses a nutritional approach to the very immature infant, for whom nutritional problems are most difficult. The end result of good nutrition is a steady weight gain. The daily weight of an infant should, therefore, be charted against one of the standard postnatal growth curves. It is helpful to include in this weight chart the total water intake (mL/kg/d) and total caloric intake (kcal/kg/d), as shown in Fig 4–7. This practice is particularly helpful in infants who have long nursery stays: it is relatively easy to distinguish infants who are not growing because of inadequate food intake from those not growing despite adequate caloric intake. Expected weight gain for the adequately nourished preterm infant is 10–30 grams per day or a minimum of 1% of the infant's weight.

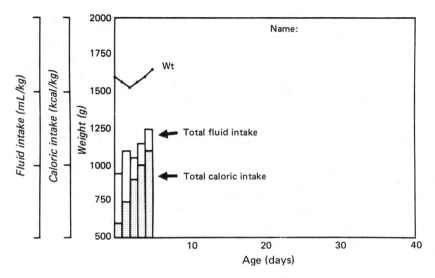

Figure 4–7. A convenient method of presenting a summary of hydration, nutrition, and body weight in newborn infants.

In general, the long-term nutritional support for infants of very low birth weight consists of either breast milk supplemented to increase protein and caloric density or infant formulas modified for preterm infants. In all of these formulas, protein concentrations (approximately 2 g per 100 mL) and caloric concentrations (approximately 24 kcal/oz) are relatively high. However, these feedings should not be started immediately. The infant should be gradually advanced to feedings of higher caloric density after the full volume of either breast milk or formula (20 kcal/oz) is tolerated.

Initial Feedings

Infants initially require intravenous glucose infusions to maintain blood glucose concentration in the range of 60–100 mg/dL. Infusions of 5–7 mg/kg/min (approximately 80–100 mL/kg/d of a 10% dextrose solution) are usually required. After stabilization, amino acids are added to the solution to provide nitrogen intakes of 1–2 g/kg/d. It is important to emphasize that the introduction of amino acids (as well as the introduction of intravenous lipids or milk feedings) is a decision predicated on the condition of the infant. The critically ill infant may receive only glucose and sodium salts until stabilization occurs.

The infant's first milk feedings ideally consist of colostrum, or early breast milk of the mother, unsupplemented. Alternatively, formulas for preterm infants at caloric concentrations of 20 kcal/oz can be used. Each of the first few feedings should be written as an order until it is clear that the infant is managing them without distention, respiratory difficulties, or other problems. Intermittent bolus feedings (if tolerated) are preferred, because these appear to stimulate the release of gut-related hormones and

may speed the maturation of the gastrointestinal tract. A suggested schedule for feedings is presented in Table 4–10.

Carbohydrates

Glucose is the only carbohydrate provided initially; once milk feedings are begun, however, the lactose in the milk provides galactose, an important carbohydrate for the newborn. It is important to measure blood glucose levels during the transition from intravenous to milk feedings (decreasing the reliance on intravenous glucose infusions), because infants fed only milk cannot sustain blood glucose concentrations unless gluconeogenesis is well-established.

Amino Acids

The amino acid composition of solutions available for intravenous use has been altered to provide a more readily usable form of nitrogen. Newer amino acid preparations (eg, Trophamin) produce amino

Table 4–10. Suggested feeding regimen for preterm infants.

	Initial			Time to Full
Weight (g)	Feeding (mL)	Frequency (hourly)	Advancement (mL/feeding)	Feedings (days)
500–800	1	2	1 every 12–24 h	6
800–1000	2	2	1 every 12 h	4–6
1000–1200	2–3	2	1 every 8–12 h	4
1200–1500	4	2	1 every 6–8 h	4
> 1500	5–10	3	1 every other feeding	3–4

acid profiles more similar to those seen in infants on breast milk. The same principle—breast milk as the gold standard—has been applied to the design of formulas for premature infants. The increase in protein concentration in these formulas can lead to nitrogen intakes of 3–3.5 gm/kg/d. These high intakes can be well utilized if caloric intake is also high.

Fats

Milk, whether breast milk or formula, constitutes a high-fat diet. A relatively high fat intake is important in establishing normal postnatal liver and gastrointestinal function. Deficiencies in essential fatty acids can develop quickly in the infant of very low birth weight, who has little body stores of essential fatty acids at the time of birth. Thus, it is important to make sure these babies receive an adequate amount of essential fatty acids, provided either intravenously or through milk feedings. Fatty acids are also required for oxidation, which in turn supports gluconeogenesis.

Vitamins

Vitamins are initially provided intravenously and later through milk feedings. It has been customary to supplement the vitamins provided in feedings with an oral multivitamin preparation because of the prolonged period before infants of very low birth weight consume enough milk to provide the necessary vitamins. However, fortified breast milk and the formulas for premature infants now provide adequate amounts of vitamins, with the exception of vitamin E. Vitamin E should therefore be supplied at a dose of 25 IU per day for several weeks after feedings are tolerated. This dose is adequate to prevent vitamin E deficiency hemolytic anemia. Vitamin K, 1 mg intramuscularly, is given once to all newborns immediately after delivery.

Minerals

Formulas for premature infants contain increased concentrations of calcium and phosphorus. Any premature infant receiving an adequate intake of either fortified breast milk or one of these formulas receives adequate amounts of calcium and phosphorus for bone mineralization. Osteopenia and occasionally rickets are still seen in infants receiving long-term parenteral nutrition or the calciuric diuretic furosemide. Iron supplementation (2mg/kg/d) is recommended for premature infants, beginning sometime in the first 2 months of life or at 36–39 weeks postconception. This can be provided by iron-supplemented formulas. Trace elements are discussed in Chapter 5.

DISCHARGE

Discharge policies are more flexible today. Term, healthy newborns may be discharged in 24 hours.

Very immature infants are usually discharged when they reach 2000–2500 g, but weight or postconceptual age alone no longer determines the time of discharge; a careful assessment of the infant's progress and the home environment also influences the decision. Factors such as the support for the mother at home and the stability of the family situation play a part in timing of discharge. The infant must at the very least be stable, eating well, and showing steady weight gain at the time of discharge. In addition, staff should observe the parents caring for the infant to confirm that the parents are capable of managing whatever special care the infant requires. Infants with special requirements, eg, oxygen therapy, may be discharged if the family clearly can manage to provide the additional support to the infant at home. The availability of a social worker or visiting nurse makes such discharge decisions easier.

FOLLOW-UP CARE

This term refers to follow-up visits to an ambulatory setting, for the purpose of tracking the achievement of behavioral and developmental landmarks in infants who have received neonatal intensive care. For infants discharged from level 2 nurseries, follow-up care can be provided by the pediatrician, with consultative visits at special care facilities as required. Infants discharged from level 3 nurseries require specialized follow-up care, because many families need help with physical or neurologic problems and management of home oxygen therapy. In addition, the family needs ongoing support during the first few years of the child's life. The frequency of repeated hospitalizations in many infants who have experienced complications (eg, chronic lung disease and the attendant growth disturbances) after neonatal intensive care underscores the need for such support.

Allen MC, Capute AJ: Neonatal neurodevelopmental examination as a predictor of neuromotor outcome in premature infants. *Pediatrics* 1989;**83:**498.

Amiel-Tison C, Grenier A: *Neurologic Examination of the Infant and Newborn.* Masson, 1983.

Ballard RA (editor): *Pediatric Care of the ICN Graduate.* Saunders, 1988.

Battaglia FC, Sparks JW: Perinatal nutrition and metabolism. Pages 145–171 in: *Perinatal Medicine.* Boyd RDH, Battaglia FC (editors). Butterworth, 1983.

Beaton GH: Nutritional needs during the first year of life. *Pediatr Clin North Am* 1985;**32:**275.

Committee on Nutrition, American Academy of Pediatrics: Nutritional needs of low birthweight infants. *Pediatrics* 1985;**75:**976.

Ellenberg JH, Nelson KB: Cluster of perinatal events identifying infants at high risk for death or disability. *J Pediatr* 1988;**113:**546.

Filer LJ (editor): Assessment of bone mineralization in infants. *J Pediatr* 1988;**113(Suppl):**165.

Franklin R, O'Grady C, Carpenter L: Neonatal thyroid function: Comparison between breast-fed and bottle-fed infants. *J Pediatr* 1985;**106:**124.

Georgieff MK et al: Effect of neonatal caloric deprivation on head growth and 1-year developmental status in preterm infants. *J Pediatr* 1987;**107:**581.

Hack M, Fanaroff AA: How small is too small? Consideration in evaluating the outcome of the tiny infant. *Clin Perinatol* 1988;**15:**773.

Hack M et al: Catch-up growth in very-low-birth-weight infants. *Am J Dis Child* 1984;**138:**370.

Hillman LS, Hoff N, Salmons S: Mineral homeostasis in very premature infants: Serial evaluation of serum 25-hydroxy vitamin D, serum minerals, and bone mineralization. *J Pediatr* 1985;**106:**970.

Kitchen W et al: Outcome in infants of birth weight 500–999 g: A continuing regional study of 5-year-old survivors. *J Pediatr* 1987;**111:**761.

Kitchen WH et al: Children of birthweight less than 1000 g: Changing outcome between ages 2 and 5 years. *J Pediatr* 1987;**110:**283.

Klein N et al: Preschool performance of children with normal intelligence who were very low-birth-weight infants. *Pediatrics* 1985;**75:**531.

Koops BL, Harmon RJ: Studies on long-term outcome in newborns with birth weights under 1500 grams. Pages 1–28 in: *Advances in Behavioral Pediatrics.* Vol 1. Camp BW (editor). JAI Press, 1980.

Kumar SP, Anday EK: Edema, hypoproteinemia, and zinc deficiency in low-birth-weight infants. *Pediatrics* 1984;**73:**327.

Laing IA, Glass EJ, Hendry GMA: Rickets of prematurity: Calcium and phosphorus supplements. *J Pediatr* 1985;**106:**265.

Nelson KB, Ellenberg JH: Antecedents of cerebral palsy. *N Engl J Med* 1986;**315:**81.

Oberkotter LV et al: Effect of breast-feeding vs. formula-feeding on circulating thyroxine levels in premature infants. *J Pediatr* 1985;**106:**822.

Sabio H: Anemia in the high-risk infant. *Clin Perinatol* 1984;**11:**59.

Sell EJ et al: Early identification of learning problems in neonatal intensive care graduates. *Am J Dis Child* 1985;**139:**460.

Stewart AL et al: Outcome for infants of very low birthweight: Survey of world literature. *Lancet* 1981;**1:**1038.

MULTIPLE BIRTHS

Multiple births represent an important area in perinatal medicine. Twinning occurs in 1 of 80 pregnancies. A clear distinction should be made between dizygotic (fraternal) and monozygotic (identical) twins. Race, maternal parity, and maternal age are associated only with the incidence of dizygotic twinning. Drugs that induce ovulation, such as clomiphene citrate or gonadotrophin therapy, increase the incidence of dizygotic twinning quite strikingly.

Examination of the placenta can help establish the type of twinning: 2 amnionic membranes and 2 chorionic membranes are found in all cases of dizygotic twins and in one-third of cases of monozygotic twins; 2 amnionic membranes and one chorionic membrane or one amnionic and one chorionic membrane always indicate monozygotic twins.

COMPLICATIONS OF MULTIPLE BIRTHS

Intrauterine Growth Retardation

There is some degree of intrauterine growth retardation in most multiple pregnancies of 36 or more weeks. If prenatal care is good, however, the growth retardation is rarely clinically significant. There are 2 exceptions; the first is the monozygotic twin pregnancy in which there is an arterial venous shunt from one twin's circulation to that of the other. The infant with the venous connection becomes plethoric and considerably larger than the other twin. Neonatal morbidity is more common in the larger of the 2 infants, in part due to the hypervolemia and hyperviscosity. Discordance in twins, that is, birth weights that are significantly different, can also occur when there are separate placentas; one placenta develops poorly, presumably because of a poor implantation site. In this instance there is no fetal exchange of blood, but there is a striking difference in the growth rate of the 2 infants.

Preterm Delivery

Gestation length tends to be inversely related to the number of fetuses. It is the prematurity that tends to increase the mortality or morbidity of twin pregnancies.

OBSTETRIC COMPLICATIONS

Obstetric complications, including polyhydramnios, pregnancy-induced hypertension, premature rupture of membranes, abnormal fetal presentations, and prolapsed umbilical cord, occur more frequently in women with multiple fetuses. In general, most of the complications can be avoided or minimized in terms of their impact on the infant by good obstetric management. Multiple pregnancy should always be identified prenatally with ultrasound examinations; doing so allows the obstetrician and pediatrician or neonatologist to plan their management jointly. The neonatal complications are usually related to prematurity. Prolongation of pregnancy, therefore, leads to a significant reduction in neonatal morbidity.

Follow-up studies of twin pregnancies have yielded conflicting results. In general, the studies do not suggest that twinning has a significant effect on the child's later development, especially if prematurity is excluded as a separate risk factor.

Berkowitz RL: Multiple gestations. Page 739 in: *Obstetrics: Normal and Problem Pregnancies*. Gabbe SG, Niebyl JR, Simpson, JL (editors). Churchill Livingstone, 1986.

Fukikura T, Froehlich LA: Mental and motor development in monozygotic co-twins with dissimilar birth weights. *Pediatrics* 1974;**53**:884.

Naeye RL, Tafari N: Twin gestations. Page 261 in: *Risk Factors in Pregnancy and Diseases of the Fetus and Newborn*. Naeye RL, Tafari N (editors). Williams & Wilkins, 1983.

Pettersson F, Smedby B, Lindmark G: Outcome of twin birth: Review of 1,636 children born in twin birth. *Acta Paediatr Scand* 1976;**65**:473.

Wilson RS: Twins: Measure of birth size at different gestational ages. *Ann Hum Biol* 1975;**1**:57.

SPECIFIC DISEASES OF THE NEWBORN INFANT

RESPIRATORY DISEASES

1. APNEA

Diagnosis

In preterm infants, recurrent apneic episodes are an important clinical problem. Significant apnea is defined as a respiratory pause lasting more than 20 seconds accompanied by cyanosis and bradycardia. Shorter respiratory pauses associated with cyanosis or bradycardia also qualify as significant apnea but must be differentiated from periodic breathing, which is common in term as well as preterm infants. Periodic breathing is defined as regularly recurring ventilatory cycles interrupted by short pauses not associated with bradycardia or color change. Apnea can be a response of the preterm infant's respiratory regulatory center to various peripheral stimuli. Causes for apnea in the preterm infant are listed in Table 4–11. The items listed in Table 4–11 require some comment. Both gastroesophageal reflux (GER) and apnea are common in preterm infants. The presence of GER, therefore, does not prove that GER is the cause of the apnea. The most precise diagnostic technique is to place an esophageal pH probe for 12 hours and correlate changes in esophageal pH with apneic episodes. Anemia is another difficult diagnostic entity. Recent work does suggest that frequency of periodic breathing and apnea can be decreased by giving the anemic child blood transfusions. This treatment for apnea, however, must always be weighed against the risk of transfusions.

Apnea of prematurity is the most frequent cause of apnea. Most apnea of prematurity is the so-called mixed apnea characterized by a centrally (brain

Table 4–11. Causes of apnea in the preterm infant.

Temperature instability—both cold and heat stress
Response to passage of a feeding tube
Gastroesophageal reflux
Hypoxemia
    Pulmonary parenchymal disease
    Patent ductus arteriosus
    ? Anemia
Infection
    Sepsis (viral or bacterial)
    Necrotizing enterocolitis
Metabolic causes
    Hypoglycemia
    Hyponatremia
Intracranial hemorrhage
Posthemorrhagic hydrocephalus
Seizures
Drugs, eg, morphine
Apnea of prematurity

stem) mediated respiratory pause preceded or followed by airway obstruction. Less common is pure central or obstructive apnea. Apnea of prematurity is due to immaturity of the central respiratory regulatory centers and of protective mechanisms that aid in maintaining airway patency. Onset, typically during the first 2 weeks of life, is gradual, with the frequency of spells increasing over time. Pathologic apnea can be suspected in an infant with a sudden onset of frequent apneic spells or a sudden onset of very severe spells. Apnea presenting from birth or on the first day of life is also very abnormal. This presentation suggests the presence of an acute (asphyxia or birth trauma) or chronic (congenital hypotonia, structural central nervous system lesion, etc) neuromuscular abnormality.

The workup is directed by the clinical presentation of the apnea. All infants, regardless of severity and frequency of apnea, require a minimum screening evaluation, including a general assessment of the infant's well-being (eg, tolerance of feedings, stable temperature, normal physical examination), a check of the association of spells to feeding, hematocrit, measurement of Pao_2 or SaO_2, glucose Chemstrip, and a review of drug history. Infants with sudden onset of severe apnea may require a more extensive evaluation, including a workup for infection. Other specific tests are dictated by signs in the infant, eg, evaluation for necrotizing enterocolitis in an infant with apnea and abdominal distention.

Treatment

The physician treating apnea should first address any underlying cause. If the apnea is due simply to prematurity, treatment is dictated by the frequency and severity of apneic spells. Simple measures include prophylactic cutaneous stimulation and use of a water bed. Apneic spells frequent enough to interfere with other aspects of care (eg, feeding) or severe enough to necessitate bag and mask ventilation to relieve cyanosis and bradycardia require more aggressive treatment. Intubation and ventilation can eliminate apneic spells but carry the attendant risks of long-term endotracheal intubation. Conclusive evidence that methylxanthines (theophylline and caffeine) are effective in the treatment of apnea have lead to their widespread use. Theophylline can be used, with a loading dose of 5 mg/kg and maintenance dose of 1–2 mg/kg every 6–12 hours. The loading dose of caffeine is 10 mg/kg (caffeine base) or 20 mg/kg (caffeine citrate); the maintenance dose is 2.5–5 mg/kg every 24 hours. These agents appear to work as central stimulants. Side effects include tachycardia, feeding intolerance, and (with overdosing) seizures. The minimum dose necessary to decrease the frequency of apnea and eliminate severe spells should be used. Desired drug levels are usually in the range of 5–10 μ/mL for both drugs.

Prognosis

In the majority of premature infants, apneic and bradycardic spells cease by 34–36 weeks postconception. Occasionally the episodes last longer, and outpatient therapy with methylxanthines may be indicated. Whether to provide home monitoring for such infants is controversial. Apneic and bradycardic episodes in the nursery are not precise predictors of later sudden infant death syndrome. However, home monitoring in infants still experiencing apnea and bradycardia at the time of hospital discharge is probably a prudent measure.

Aranda JV et al: Pharmacokinetic aspects of theophylline in premature newborns. *N Engl J Med* 1976;**295:**413.

Brazy JE et al: Central nervous system structural lesions causing apnea at birth. *J Pediatr* 1987;**111:**163.

Gerhardt T, Bancalari E: Apnea of prematurity. (2 parts.) *Pediatrics* 1984;**74:**58, 63.

Henderson-Smart DJ et al: Clinical apnea and brainstem muscle function in preterm infants. *N Engl J Med* 1983;**308:**353.

Joshi A et al: Blood transfusion effect on the respiratory pattern of preterm infants. *Pediatrics* 1987;**80:**79.

Kattwinkel J: Neonatal apnea: Pathogenesis and therapy. *J Pediatr* 1977;**90:**342.

Marchal F et al: Neonatal apnea and apneic syndromes. *Clin Perinatol* 1987;**14:**509.

Martin RJ et al: Pathogenesis of apnea in preterm infants. *J Pediatr* 1986;**109:**733.

NIH Consensus: Developmental Conference on Infantile Apnea and Home Monitoring. *Pediatrics* 1987;**79:**292.

2. RESPIRATORY DISTRESS IN THE NEWBORN

Diagnosis

Respiratory distress is among the most common symptom complexes seen in the newborn. Respiratory distress may be due to both noncardiopulmonary and cardiopulmonary causes (Table 4–12). The cardinal clinical features include a respiratory rate of more than 60 per minute with or without associated

Table 4–12. Respiratory distress in the newborn.[1]

Noncardio-pulmonary	Cardiovascular	Pulmonary
Hypothermia or hyperthermia	Left-sided outflow tract obstruction	Upper airway obstruction
Hypoglycemia	Hypoplastic left heart	Choanal atresia
Polycythemia	Aortic stenosis	Vocal cord paralysis
Metabolic acidosis	Coarctation of the aorta	Lingual thyroid
Drug intoxications; withdrawal	Cyanotic lesions	Meconium aspiration
Insult to the central nervous system	Transposition of the great vessels	Clear fluid aspiration
Asphyxia	Total anomalous pulmonary venous return	Transient tachypnea
Hemorrhage		Pneumonia
Neuromuscular disease	Tricuspid atresia	Pulmonary hypoplasia
Phrenic nerve injury	Right-sided outflow obstruction	Hyaline membrane disease
Skeletal abnormalities		Pneumothorax
Asphyxiating thoracic dystrophy		Pleural effusions
		Mass lesions
		Lobar emphysema
		Cystic adenomatoid malformation

[1]Reproduced, with permission, from Rosenberg AA: Neonatal adaptation. In *Obstetrics Normal and Problem Pregnancies,* 1st ed. Gebbe SG, Niebyl JR, Simpson JL (editors). Churchill Livingstone, 1986.

cyanosis, nasal flaring, intercostal and sternal retractions, and expiratory grunting. It is important to consider the noncardiopulmonary causes listed in Table 4–12, because the natural tendency is to focus on the heart and lungs. Most of the noncardiopulmonary causes can be ruled out by the history, physical examination, and a few simple laboratory tests. The evaluation of cardiovascular disorders is discussed in the next section.

The physician attempting diagnosis of pulmonary disorders must consider the following major concerns in the term infant: transient tachypnea, aspiration syndromes, and congenital pneumonia.

A. Transient Tachypnea: The syndrome of transient tachypnea (TTN) presents as respiratory distress in nonasphyxiated term infants (often delivered by cesarian section) or slightly preterm infants. The clinical features include tachypnea, cyanosis, grunting, flaring, and retractions presenting in the first hours of life. The chest x-ray film indicating prominent perihilar streaking and fluid in the interlobar fissures is the key to diagnosis. The symptoms generally abate within 12–24 hours, although they can persist longer. The cause of the disorder is thought to be delayed resorption of fetal lung fluid.

B. Clear Fluid Aspiration: At or before delivery, the infant can aspirate clear amniotic fluid or fluid mixed with blood. The clinical presentation is much like that of transient tachypnea, with the following differences: these infants usually require higher Fio_2 to be noncyanotic (30–60% versus 25–

40% in infants with transient tachypnea), and the course is more protracted (4–7 days). The chest x-ray film reveals hyperexpansion with a more patchy infiltrate pattern than that seen with transient tachypnea.

C. Meconium Aspiration Syndrome: The perinatal course in these infants is often marked by fetal distress, low Apgar scores, and meconium in the amniotic fluid. These infants exhibit tachypnea, retractions, cyanosis, an overdistended, barrel-shaped chest, and coarse breath sounds. The chest x-ray film reveals coarse, irregular infiltrates and hyperexpansion. There is a high incidence of air leaks and, in severe cases, a high rate of persistent pulmonary hypertension (see Cardiovascular Diseases).

D. Congenital Pneumonia: The lungs are the most common site of infection in the neonate. Both bacterial and viral infections can be acquired before, during, or after birth. Most commonly, infections ascend from the genital tract before or during labor. The rupture of membranes more than 24 hours prior to delivery is a major predisposing factor. The presence of chorioamnionitis in the mother further increases the risk. Infants with congenital pneumonia present with respiratory symptoms as early as in the delivery room, with the majority symptomatic by 6–12 hours of age. The chest x-ray is not helpful in distinguishing congenital pneumonia from other forms of neonatal lung disease. The presence of shock, poor perfusion, and absolute neutropenia on blood count provide corroborating evidence for pneumonia.

E. Spontaneous Pneumothorax: This entity occurs in 1% of all deliveries. Risk is increased by manipulations such as bagging in the delivery room. Clinically, the infants are tachypneic with a small oxygen requirement (25–40% Fio_2). Breath sounds may be asymmetric, and if the pneumothorax is under tension, the mediastinum may be shifted. The diagnosis can be confirmed on x-ray studies. There is a small increased risk of renal abnormalities associated with spontaneous pneumothorax. Therefore, a careful physical examination of the kidneys and observation of urine output are indicated.

F. Other Pulmonary Causes: Many of the other pulmonary causes of respiratory distress are fairly rare. Bilateral choanal atresia should be suspected if there is no air movement when the infant breathes through the nose. These infants present in the delivery room with good color and heart rate while crying. When they quiet down and resume normal breathing, they become cyanotic and bradycardic. Other causes of airway obstruction are usually characterized by some degree of stridor or poor air movement despite good respiratory effort. Pleural effusions can be suspected in hydropic infants (eg, those with erythroblastosis fetalis). Space-occupying lesions cause a shift of the mediastinum and asymmetric breath sounds.

G. Hyaline Membrane Disease: The most common cause of respiratory distress in the preterm infant is hyaline membrane disease (HMD). The incidence of this disorder increases from 5% at 35–36 weeks to 65% at 29–30 weeks of gestation. This condition is due to a deficiency of surfactant. Surfactant decreases surface tension in the alveolus during expiration, allowing the alveolus to maintain a functional residual capacity. The absence of surfactant results in poor lung compliance and atelectasis. The infant must expend a great deal of effort to expand the lungs with each breath, and respiratory failure ensues. Infants with hyaline membrane disease demonstrate all the clinical signs of respiratory distress. On auscultation, air movement is diminished despite vigorous respiratory effort. The chest x-ray film demonstrates diffuse bilateral atelectasis causing a "ground-glass" appearance. Major airways are highlighted by the atelectatic air sacs creating air bronchograms. In the unintubated child, there is doming of the diaphragms and hypoexpansion.

Treatment

The cornerstone of treatment of neonatal respiratory distress is the provision of adequate supplemental oxygen to maintain a Pao_2 of 60–70 mm Hg and an arterial saturation of 92–95%. Pao_2 levels less than 50 mm Hg are associated with pulmonary vascular vasoconstriction, and those greater than 100 mm Hg increase the risk of retinopathy of prematurity. Oxygen should be warmed, humidified, and given through an air blender. Concentration should be measured with a calibrated oxygen analyzer. An umbilical arterial line should be placed in any infant requiring more than 45% Fio_2 by 4–6 hours of life to allow frequent blood gas determinations. Noninvasive monitoring with a transcutaneous O_2 monitor (TCM) or pulse oximeter can provide continuous information.

Other supportive treatment includes intravenous provision of glucose and water if the infant is in too much distress to eat. Unless infection can be absolutely ruled out, blood cultures should be obtained and broad-spectrum antibiotics started. Colloid solutions (eg, 5% albumin) can be given in infusions of 10 mL/kg over 30 minutes for low blood pressure, poor perfusion, and metabolic acidosis. Sodium bicarbonate (1–2 meq/kg) is indicated for treatment of a documented metabolic acidosis that has not responded to oxygen, ventilation, and volume. While therapy is instituted, specific workup should be pursued as indicated by history and physical findings. In most cases, a chest x-ray study, blood gas, complete blood count, and glucose Chemstrip allow a diagnosis.

Intubation and ventilation should be undertaken for signs of respiratory failure ($Pao_2 < 60$ mm Hg in 70–80% Fio_2 or $Paco_2 > 50$ mm Hg). These guidelines, however, do not apply to infants with hyaline membrane disease. Indication for further respiratory support in these infants is a need for 50% Fio_2 to keep Pao_2 greater than 60 mm Hg. In infants greater than 30 weeks of gestation and 1500 grams, a trial of continuous positive airway pressure (4–8 cm H_2O) administered either nasally or by endotracheal tube can be attempted. If this fails to provide the desired result, the infant should be ventilated. Peak pressures should be adequate to produce chest wall expansion (usually 18–24 cm H_2O). Positive end-expiratory pressure (4–6 cm H_2O) should also be used. Ventilation rates of 20–50 are usually required. The goal is to maintain Pao_2 of 60–70 mm Hg and $Paco_2$ of 40–50 mm Hg.

Clinical trials evaluating the use of artificial surfactant in HMD are currently under way. Surfactant can be administered in the delivery room during resuscitation or in a ''rescue'' fashion after an infant has developed disease. Early results show that treated infants require lower ventilator settings and Fio_2 over the first 3 days of life.

Prognosis

Most of the conditions described in the term infant are acute and resolve in the first several days of life. Meconium aspiration syndrome and congenital pneumonia do have a significant rate of associated pulmonary morbidity (chronic lung disease) and mortality (approximately 25%). Mortality rates have decreased dramatically in infants with hyaline membrane disease through the use of continuous positive airway pressure and positive pressure ventilation. Mortality rates associated with hyaline membrane disease are less than 10% for infants of greater than 28 weeks' gestation. The major long-term sequela is the development of chronic lung disease (defined as the need for oxygen or ventilation after 1 month of age), which occurs in 20% of the survivors of hyaline membrane disease. The incidence is highest at lower gestational ages. The development of chronic lung disease is a function of lung immaturity at birth and exposure to high oxygen concentrations and ventilator barotrauma. Up to 10% of infants who develop chronic lung disease will die in the first 2 years of life because of respiratory failure, pulmonary infection, or sudden death. However, most infants with chronic lung disease do fairly well with good long-term recovery of pulmonary function. The use of artificial surfactants will likely decrease the incidence of severe chronic lung disease in the premature. Some infants with chronic lung disease require home oxygen therapy. This can be monitored with pulse oximetry, with Sao_2 kept at 92–95%. Systemic hypertension can be seen in these patients; frequent blood pressure determinations, therefore, are indicated, as are ECGs and echocardiograms to monitor for left and right ventricular hypertrophy.

Abman SH et al: Systemic hypertension in infants with bronchopulmonary dysplasia. *J Pediatr* 1984;**104**:929.

Avery ME, Mead J: Surface properties in relation to atelectasis and hyaline membrane disease. *Am J Dis Child* 1959;**97**:517.

Avery ME et al: Transient tachypnea of the newborn. *Am J Dis Child* 1966;**111**:380.

Dunn MS et al: Two-year follow-up of infants enrolled in a randomized trial of surfactant replacement therapy for prevention of neonatal respiratory distress syndrome. *Pediatrics* 1988;**82**:543.

Enhorning G et al: Prevention of neonatal respiratory distress syndrome by tracheal instillation of surfactant: A randomized clinical trial. *Pediatrics* 1985;**76**:145.

Gitlin JD et al: Randomized controlled trial of exogenous surfactant for the treatment of hyaline membrane disease. *Pediatrics* 1987;**79**:31.

Goldsmith JP, Karotkin EH (editors): *Assisted Ventilation of the Neonate.* Saunders, 1988.

Hallman M, Gluck L: Respiratory distress syndrome: Update 1982. *Pediatr Clin North Am* 1982;**29**:1057.

Hallman M et al: Exogenous human surfactant for treatment of severe respiratory distress syndrome: A randomized prospective clinical trial. *J Pediatr* 1985;**105**:963.

Horbar JD et al: A multicenter randomized, placebo-controlled trial of surfactant therapy for respiratory distress syndrome. *N Engl J Med* 1989;**320**:959.

Jobe A, Ikegami M: Surfactant for the treatment of respiratory distress syndrome. *Am Rev Respir Dis* 1987;**136**:1256.

Koops BL, Abman SH, Accurso FJ: Outpatient management and follow-up of bronchopulmonary dysplasia. *Clin Perinatol* 1984;**11**:101.

Merritt TA, Hallman M: Surfactant replacement. *Am J Dis Child* 1988;**142**:1333.

Northway WH Jr et al: Pulmonary disease following respirator therapy of hyaline membrane disease. *N Engl J Med* 1967;**276**:357.

Notter RH, Shapiro DL: Lung surfactants for replacement therapy: Biochemical, biophysical, and clinical aspects. *Clin Perinatol* 1987;**14**:433.

O'Brodovich HM, Mellins RB: Bronchopulmonary dysplasia: Unresolved neonatal acute lung injury. *Am Rev Respir Dis* 1985;**132**:694.

Saigal S, O'Brodovich H: Long-term outcome of preterm infants with respiratory disease. *Clin Perinatol* 1987; **14**:635.

Shapiro DL et al: A double-blind randomized trial of a calf lung surfactant extract administered at birth to very premature infants for prevention of the respiratory distress syndrome. *Pediatrics* 1985;**76**:593.

Surfactant Treatment of Lung Diseases: 96th Ross Conference on Pediatric Research. Ross, 1988.

CARDIOVASCULAR DISEASES

Diagnosis

Cardiovascular causes of respiratory distress in the neonatal period can be divided into 2 major groups—structural heart disease and a structurally normal heart with shunting through fetal pathways.

A. Structural Heart Disease: The central presenting features of symptomatic congenital heart disease in the first week of life include cyanosis and congestive heart failure. Cyanotic heart disease can be due to transposition of the great vessels, tricuspid atresia, certain types of truncus arteriosus, total anomalous pulmonary venous return, and right heart obstruction (eg, pulmonary and tricuspid atresia). Infants with these disorders present with early cyanosis. The hallmark of many of these lesions is cyanosis in an infant without associated respiratory distress. Although early cyanosis is the central feature in these disorders, tachypnea develops over time in many infants either because of increased pulmonary blood flow or secondary to metabolic acidosis from hypoxia. Infants with total anomalous venous return below the diaphragm present early with tachypnea, because the pulmonary venous return is obstructed and pulmonary edema develops. Diagnostic aids include comparing a blood gas obtained while the infant breathes 100% oxygen to one obtained while the child breathes room air. Failure of the Pao_2 to increase when 100% oxygen is breathed suggests cyanotic congenital heart disease. A chest x-ray film with decreased pulmonary markings is consistent with right heart obstruction, and an ECG with left-sided predominance suggests the hypoplastic right heart seen with tricuspid atresia. Diagnosis can be confirmed with echocardiography.

Infants with congestive heart failure generally have some form of left-sided outflow tract obstruction. Infants with left-to-right shunt lesions, such as ventricular septal defect, may have murmurs in the newborn period, but clinical symptoms do not occur until pulmonary vascular resistance drops enough to cause significant shunting and subsequent failure (usually 3–4 weeks of age). Infants with left-sided outflow obstruction generally do well the first day or two until the source of all or some of the systemic flow, the ductus arteriosus, closes. With ductal closure, tachypnea, tachycardia, congestive heart failure, and metabolic acidosis develop. On examination, all of these infants have abnormalities of the pulses. In aortic atresia and stenosis, pulses are all diminished, whereas in coarctation syndromes, differential pulses (diminished in the lower extremities) are evident. Chest x-ray films in these infants show a large heart and pulmonary edema. Arterial blood gases are remarkable for profound metabolic acidosis.

B. Shunting Through Fetal Pathways: The syndrome of persistent pulmonary hypertension (PPHN) occurs when the normal decrease in pulmonary vascular resistance after birth does not occur. Most infants with persistent pulmonary hypertension are full term or postterm and have experienced perinatal asphyxia. Other clinical associations include hypothermia, meconium aspiration syndrome, hyaline membrane disease, polycythemia, neonatal sepsis, chronic intrauterine hypoxia, and pulmonary hypoplasia.

There are 3 causes of persistent pulmonary hypertension: (1) acute vasoconstriction due to perinatal hypoxia, (2) prenatal increase in pulmonary vascular smooth muscle development, and (3) decreased cross-sectional area of the pulmonary vascular bed due to inadequate vessel number. In the first, an acute perinatal event leads to hypoxia and failure of the pulmonary vascular resistance to drop. In the second, abnormal muscularization of the pulmonary resistance vessels results in persistent hypertension after birth. Finally, the third includes infants with pulmonary hypoplasia (eg, diaphragmatic hernia).

Clinically, the syndrome is characterized by onset on the first day of life, usually from birth. Respiratory distress is prominent, and Pao_2 is usually poorly responsive to high concentrations of inspired oxygen. Many of the infants have associated myocardial depression with resulting systemic hypotension. Echocardiography reveals right-to-left shunting at the level of the ductus arteriosus or foramen ovale (or both).

C. Patent Ductus Arteriosus: Patent ductus arteriosus (PDA) is the most common cardiovascular disorder seen in the preterm infant. Clinically, significant patent ductus arteriosus usually presents on day 3–7 of life as the respiratory distress from hyaline membrane disease is improving. Presentation can be on day 1 or 2, especially in those infants of less than 28 weeks' gestation. The signs include a hyperdynamic precordium, increased peripheral pulses, and a widened pulse pressure, with or without a systolic heart murmur. These signs are often accompanied by an increase in respiratory support. The presence of significant patent ductus arteriosus can be confirmed by echocardiography. Before undertaking medical or surgical ligation, other structural heart disease must be ruled out.

Treatment

For congenital heart disease, early stabilization includes supportive therapy as needed (eg, intravenous glucose, oxygen, and ventilation for respiratory failure). Specific therapy includes infusions of prostaglandin E_1, O.1 μg/kg/min, to maintain ductal patency. In some cyanotic lesions (eg, pulmonary atresia), this improves pulmonary blood flow and Pao_2 by allowing shunting through the ductus to the pulmonary artery. In left-sided outflow tract obstruction, systemic blood flow is ductal dependent; prostaglandins improve systemic perfusion and resolve the baby's acidosis. Further specific management, including palliative surgical and cardiac catheterization procedures, are discussed in Chapter 16.

Therapy for persistent pulmonary hypertension involves supportive therapy for other postasphyxia problems (eg, anticonvulsants for seizures, careful fluid and electrolyte management for renal failure). Intravenous glucose should be provided to maintain normal blood sugar, and antibiotics should be administered for possible infection. Specific therapy is designed to get systemic pressure higher than pulmonary pressure to reverse the right-to-left shunting through fetal pathways. First-line therapy includes oxygen and ventilation (to lower pulmonary vascular resistance) and colloid infusions (10 mL/kg, up to 30 mL/kg) to improve systemic pressure. Ideally, systolic pressure should be greater than 60 mm Hg. With compromised cardiac function, systemic pressors can be used as second-line therapy (eg, dopamine 5–20 μg/kg/min or dobutamine 5–20 μg/kg/min, or both). If oxygenation is still not adequate (Pao_2 < 55 mm Hg), a trial of alkalosis by hyperventilation is indicated. Many babies improve as the pH rises above 7.55–7.6. Since alkalosis seems to be helpful, any base excess should be corrected with sodium bicarbonate to allow less vigorous hyperventilation. The final conventional therapies include use of vasodilators (isoproterenol, 0.1–1 μg/kg/min, tolazoline hydrochloride, 1–2 mg/kg intravenous push followed by an infusion of 0.2 mg/kg/h). The vasodilators produce very irregular results and, in fact, make some babies worse by causing systemic vasodilation. Therefore, they should be used with great caution and infused into superior vena cava drainage (right arm or head) to shunt them preferentially to the pulmonary circulation. Volume and increased systemic pressor infusions can counteract decreases in systemic pressure and may improve efficacy of the vasodilators.

Infants for whom conventional therapy is failing (poor oxygenation despite maximum support) may require extracorporeal membrane oxygenation (ECMO). The infants are placed on bypass with blood exiting the baby from the right atrium and returning to the aortic arch after passing through a membrane oxygenator. The lungs are essentially at rest during the procedure, and with resolution of the pulmonary hypertension, the infants are weaned from ECMO back to conventional ventilator therapy. This therapy can save infants who might otherwise die but has major side effects that must be considered prior to its institution.

The ductus arteriosus is managed by medical or surgical ligation. A clinically significant ductus causing compromise in the infant can be closed with indomethacin (0.2 mg/kg) given intravenously. The schedule of 3 doses is dependent on the infant's age. In about two-thirds of the cases, indomethacin is successful in closing the ductus. If the ductus reopens, a second course of drug may be utilized. If indomethacin fails to close the ductus or if a ductus reopens a second time, surgical ligation should be pursued. The major side effect of indomethacin is a transient oliguria, which can be treated by fluid restriction until urine output improves. Indomethacin does not increase the incidence and severity of intracranial hemorrhage. The drug should not be used if the infant is hyperkalemic, if the creatinine is greater than 2 mg/dL, or if the platelet count is less then 50,000/μl.

Prognosis

The prognosis for the congenital heart lesions, which depends on the type of lesion, is reviewed in Chapter 16. With persistent pulmonary hypertension, the mortality rate remains approximately 10–15%. Long-term neurologic morbidity occurs in approximately 10% of survivors. Recently, an increased incidence of hearing loss has been identified in this group of infants. The other major long-term morbidity is chronic lung disease secondary to the extensive ventilator support that many of these infants require.

Bartlett RH et al: Extracorporeal circulation in neonatal respiratory failure: A prospective randomized study. *Pediatrics* 1985;**76**:479.

Bhat R et al: Patent ductus arteriosus: Recent advances in diagnosis and management. *Pediatr Clin North Am* 1982;**29**:1117.

Clyman RI: Indomethacin therapy for patent ductus arteriosus: When is prophylaxis not prophylactic? *J Pediatr* 1987;**111**:718.

Cotton RB: The relationship of symptomatic patent ductus arteriosus to respiratory distress in premature newborn infants. *Clin Perinatol* 1987;**14**:621.

Fox WW, Duara S: Persistent pulmonary hypertension in the neonate: Diagnosis and management. *J Pediatr* 1983;**103**:505.

Gersony WM et al: Effects of indomethacin in premature infants with patent ductus arteriosus: Results of a national collaborative study. *J Pediatr* 1983;**102**:895.

Henricks-Munoz KD, Walton JP: Hearing loss in infants with persistent fetal circulation. *Pediatrics* 1988;**81**:650.

Kelley SR, Bohn DJ: The use of inotropic and afterload-reducing agents in neonates. *Clin Perinatol* 1988;**15**:467.

Murphy JD et al: The structural basis of persistent pulmonary hypertension of the newborn infant. *J Pediatr* 1981;**98**:962.

Rudolph AM: High pulmonary vascular resistance after birth. 1. Pathophysiologic consideration and etiologic classification. *Clin Pediatr (Phila)* 1980;**19**:585.

Short BL et al: Extracorporeal membrane oxygenation on the management of respiratory failure in the newborn. *Clin Perinatol* 1987;**14**:737.

Snider AR: Two-dimensional and Doppler echocardiographic evaluation of heart disease in the neonate and fetus. *Clin Perinatol* 1988;**15**:523.

Wung J-T et al: Management of infants with severe respiratory failure and persistence of the fetal circulation, without hyperventilation. *Pediatrics* 1985;**76**:488.

Yabek SM: Neonatal cyanosis: Reappraisal of response to 100% oxygen breathing. *Am J Dis Child* 1984;**138**:880.

JAUNDICE SECONDARY TO UNCONJUGATED HYPERBILIRUBINEMIA

General Considerations

Jaundice is a common neonatal problem, particularly in level 1 and 2 nurseries. Because many hospitals now implement early discharge policies, a proper approach is essential.

To understand neonatal jaundice, a brief description of the pathways of normal bilirubin metabolism is necessary. The normal destruction of circulating red cells accounts for about 75% of the newborn's daily bilirubin production. The remaining sources include ineffective erythropoiesis and tissue heme proteins. Heme is converted to bilirubin in the reticuloendothelial system. The lipid-soluble unconjugated bilirubin is transported bound to albumin, which enters the liver cells by dissociation from albumin in the hepatic sinusoids. Once in the liver cell, bilirubin is conjugated with glucuronic acid in a reaction catalyzed by glucuronyl transferase. The water-soluble conjugated bilirubin is secreted into the biliary tree for excretion via the gastrointestinal tract. The enzyme B-glucuronidase is present in the small bowel and hydrolyzes some of the conjugated bilirubin. This unconjugated bilirubin can then be reabsorbed into the circulation, adding to the total load of unconjugated bilirubin (enterohepatic circulation).

Diagnosis

Almost every newborn develops a serum unconjugated bilirubin of greater than 2 mg/dL (average of 5–7 mg/dL) during the first week of life. This transient hyperbilirubinemia has been called physiologic jaundice. Major predisposing factors are (1) increased bilirubin load due to increased red cell volume with decreased cell survival, increased ineffective erythropoiesis, and the enterohepatic circulation; and (2) Low levels of glucuronyl transferase leading to slower hepatic conjugation of bilirubin.

The clinical manifestations of physiologic jaundice are as follows: (1) jaundice does not present on day 1; (2) total bilirubin rises by less than 5 mg/dL/d, peaking at less than 12.9 mg/dL on days 3–4 (term infant) and 15 mg/dL on days 5–7 (preterm infant); (3) the conjugated fraction is less than 2 mg/dL; and (4) jaundice persists no longer than 1 week in the term infant and 2 weeks in the preterm infant. If criteria for a diagnosis of physiologic jaundice are not met, the cause of the jaundice needs to be investigated.

Etiology

A: Overproduction of Bilirubin:

1. Increased rate of hemolysis—All patients in this category have an increased unconjugated bilirubin concentration and an increased reticulocyte count.

a. Patients with a positive Coombs test.
   (1) Rh incompatibility.
   (2) ABO incompatibility.
   (3) Other blood group sensitizations.
b. Patients with a negative Coombs test.
   (1) Abnormal red cell shapes.
      (a) Spherocytosis.
      (b) Elliptocytosis.
      (c) Pyknocytosis.
      (d) Stomatocytosis.
   (2) Red cell enzyme abnormalities.
      (a) Glucose 6-phosphate dehydrogenase deficiency.
      (b) Pyruvate kinase deficiency.
      (c) Hexokinase deficiency.
      (d) Other metabolic defects.

2. Nonhemolytic causes of increased bilirubin load—Increased unconjugated bilirubin, normal reticulocyte count.

a. Extravascular hemorrhage.
   (1) Cephalohematoma.
   (2) Extensive bruising.
   (3) CNS hemorrhage.
b. Polycythemia.
c. Exaggerated enterohepatic circulation of bilirubin.
   (1) Gastrointestinal tract obstruction.
   (2) Functional ileus.

B. Decreased Rate of Conjugation: Unconjugated bilirubin elevated, reticulocyte count normal.

1. ''Physiologic'' jaundice.
2. Crigler-Najjar syndrome (type I glucuronyl transferase deficiency, autosomal recessive).
3. Type II glucuronyl transferase deficiency, autosomal dominant.
4. Breast milk jaundice.

C. Abnormalities of Excretion or Reabsorption: Conjugated and unconjugated bilirubin elevated, Coombs test negative, reticulocyte count normal. Conjugated hyperbilirubinemia is rare in the first week of life.

1. Hepatitis (viral, parasitic, bacterial, toxic).
2. Metabolic abnormalities (galactosemia, glycogen storage diseases, cystic fibrosis, hypothyroidism).
3. Biliary atresia.
4. Choledochal cyst.
5. Obstruction of ampulla hepatopancreatica (annular pancreas).
6. Sepsis.

Bilirubin Toxicity

Unconjugated bilirubin can enter nerve cells and produce cell death, causing a clinical syndrome of kernicterus. Kernicterus is the staining of certain areas of the brain (basal ganglia and hippocampus predominantly) by bilirubin. Severe kernicterus has a high mortality rate and in term infants is manifested by lethargy, refusal to feed, a high-pitched cry, hypertonicity, opisthotonos, seizures, and apnea. Survivors usually suffer sequelae, including athetoid cerebral palsy, high-frequency hearing loss, paralysis of upward gaze, and dental dysplasia. Fortunately, kernicterus is very rare with today's neonatal management. The risk of kernicterus in a given infant is not well defined. The only group in which a specific bilirubin level (20 mg/dL) has been associated with an increased risk of kernicterus is babies with Rh hemolytic disease. This observation has been extended to the management of other neonates with hemolytic disease, although no definitive data exist for these infants. The risk is likely negligible for term infants without hemolytic disease, even at levels greater than 20 mg/dL. Prematures of 32–38 weeks' gestation are probably safe up to levels of 20 mg/dL, but meaningful data for infants of less than 32 weeks of gestation are not available. Finally, auditory evoked potential studies have clearly identified a reversible entry of bilirubin into the central nervous system. The relevance of this finding to long-term outcome is unknown at this time.

Treatment

There are 2 modalities for treatment:

A. Phototherapy: Phototherapy is used most commonly, because it is relatively noninvasive and safe. Light at a wavelength absorbed by bilirubin (blue or white light) is used. The unconjugated bilirubin in the skin is converted to a water-soluble photoisomer excreted in bile, enhancing bilirubin excretion. Phototherapy is used in term and near term babies when bilirubin concentrations are still well below the level at which an exchange transfusion would be required (approximately 4 mg/dL below exchange level). In babies with hemolytic disease, phototherapy can be instituted earlier, at a level of 10 mg/dL on day 1 and 13 mg/dL on day 2. In very immature babies, many centers use phototherapy prophylactically. Alternatively, it may be begun at unconjugated bilirubin concentrations greater than 5 mg/dL. The use of phototherapy in this way has resulted in a decrease in the frequency of exchange transfusions for hyperbilirubinemia. When phototherapy is used, the infant's eyes should be shielded and extra water provided to compensate for increased evaporative losses. Other side effects of phototherapy include loose stools secondary to more rapid intestinal transit, skin rashes, and problems with thermoregulation. Finally, any baby placed under phototherapy requires a history, physical examination, and screening laboratory evaluation for pathologic hyperbilirubinemia (blood type, direct and indirect Coombs, complete blood count, reticulocytes, smear, fractionated bilirubin).

B. Exchange Transfusions: This procedure is used as the definitive treatment when bilirubin concentrations are approaching toxic levels. Table 4–13 lists guideline bilirubin levels for exchange transfusions according to the infant's weight. These are

Table 4–13. Serum levels of indirect bilirubin and exchange transfusion.[1,2]

Serum Bilirubin Level for Exchange Transfusion (mg/dL)		
Birth Weight (g)	Normal Infants[3]	Abnormal Infants[4]
< 1000	10	10[5]
1001–1250	13	10[5]
1251–1500	15	13
1501–2000	17	15
2001–2500	18	17
> 2500	20	18

[1]Reproduced, with permission, from American Academy of Pediatrics: Page 95 in: *Standards and Recommendations for Hospital Care of Newborn Infants,* 6th ed. American Academy of Pediatrics, 1977. Copyright American Academy of Pediatrics, 1977.
[2]These guidelines have not been validated.
[3]Normal infants are defined for this purpose as having none of the problems listed below.
[4]Abnormal infants have one or more of the following problems: perinatal asphyxia, prolonged hypoxemia, acidemia, persistent hypothermia, hypoalbuminemia, hemolysis, sepsis, hyperglycemia, elevated free fatty acids or presence of drugs that compete for bilirubin binding, signs of clinical or central nervous system deterioration.
[5]There have been case reports of basal ganglion staining at levels considerably lower than 10 mg.

only guidelines and, as noted above, are based in many cases on inadequate data. The indications have not been altered substantially over the last 8–10 years. When either fresh, whole blood or reconstituted citrate-phosphate-dextrose (CPD) blood is used, there is no need to attempt to correct the acidosis in the donor blood. Attempting to correct this may only cause problems; because the Pco_2 of stored CPD blood is greatly elevated, the pH quickly rises when the blood is introduced to the baby and equilibrates to the in vivo Pco_2 levels. Ionized calcium levels should be followed when CPD blood is used because of the binding of calcium by citrate. Two-volume exchanges should be done; a blood volume of 80% of body weight should be assumed. This procedure will replace more than 80% of the red cells and lower bilirubin concentrations substantially. The procedure is associated with significant mortality and morbidity rates, especially in the very immature infant. It should be carried out cautiously with full intensive care monitoring over a period of approximately 1–2 hours.

Exchange transfusions can be done in 2 other circumstances unrelated to the bilirubin level in the infant. The first is in the markedly hydropic erythroblastotic (Rh-sensitized) infant, in whom a partial exchange transfusion with packed red blood cells (approximately 35 mL/kg) may be carried out immediately after birth to correct anemia and adjust circulating blood volume and, thus, ease the high output failure. Fortunately, this indication is becoming rare because of better management of Rh-sensitized pregnancies, including direct intrauterine transfusion of severely sensitized infants.

The second indication for exchange transfusion not determined by bilirubin levels is in the severely sensitized erythroblasotic infant. A 2-volume exchange is carried out as shortly after delivery as possible after stabilization. The purpose of this exchange is to remove affected red cells and replace them with Rh-negative donor cells. This procedure is very effective in preventing a need for multiple exchange transfusions; sensitized red cells are removed prior to hemolysis and the potential bilirubin load for the infant is thus reduced. Again, good obstetric management has decreased the need for the procedure. Severely affected infants will have had in utero transfusions; consequently, when they are born, the majority of their red cells are donor Rh-negative cells. If more than 50% of cells are already donor cells, the exchange transfusion immediately after birth is not indicated.

1. BREAST MILK JAUNDICE

The key features of this disease are (1) jaundice that peaks late (within the first 3 weeks, usually between 6 and 14 days), (2) a well baby who is thriving, and (3) a peak bilirubin of 12–20. The jaundice is secondary to unconjugated hyperbilirubinemia. Breast milk jaundice can be distinguished from jaundice due to other causes by the prompt reduction in bilirubin concentration that occurs when formula is substituted for breast milk over a 2- or 3-day period. Thereafter, breast milk feedings can usually be resumed without difficulty. This entity is to be distinguished from jaundice in the breast-fed infant during the first week of life. Breast-fed infants have higher bilirubins than formula-fed infants. This phenomenon is due to decreased intake over the first several days of life. The treatment is not to stop breastfeeding but to increase the frequency of feedings.

2. ABO INCOMPATIBILITY

This incompatibility is most commonly seen in type O mothers with babies of type A or B. Naturally occurring IgG anti-A or anti-B in the mother crosses the placenta into the fetal circulation. The amount of these naturally occurring antibodies is variable; the disease picture is, therefore, also variable. This disease can be difficult to manage, because cord blood levels and early bilirubin levels provide no firm basis for predicting which infants will require therapy. These infants can have anemia with or without jaundice, jaundice with or without anemia, or neither. The peripheral smear (microspherocytes are indicative), a reticulocyte count, and a Coombs test (*Note:* direct Coombs may be negative, but indirect Coombs will be positive) identify

infants at risk, but management relies on phototherapy and serial bilirubin measurements to identify the occasional infant in whom an exchange transfusion is required. Phototherapy in term infants should be started if the bilirubin level is greater than 10 mg/dL on day 1; if it is greater than 13 mg/dL on day 2; and if it is 15 mg/dL or more on day 3 and beyond. An exchange transfusion is performed for a level at or greater than 20 mg/dL. Finally, after hospital discharge these infants should have serial hematocrits because of the possibility of late anemia.

3. ERYTHROBLASTOSIS

Isoimmunization to Rh antigens (D, C, E, d, c, or e), Kell, Duffy, Lutheran, and Kidd may cause erythroblastosis. Most commonly, it is due to sensitization from D. The involved red cell antigen is always absent from the mother's red cells. Therefore, if fetal red cells enter the maternal circulation (usually at delivery), the mother produces antibody to the foreign antigen. The antibody (IgG) enters the fetal circulation, causing hemolysis. The process is usually worse in successive at-risk pregnancies.

Obstetric Management of Erythroblastosis

(1) Serial antibody screening performed in Rh (D-negative) mothers is performed during pregnancy. Sensitization to other antigens can be detected by a single antibody screen (performed in all pregnant women). Significant sensitization to these other antigens is rare if the initial screen is negative. If the screen is positive, titers should be performed to assess significant sensitization.

(2) Amniocentesis to measure bilirubin (Δ 450) by absorbance is done to assess severity of sensitization. Further obstetric management (eg, fetal transfusions) is based on this determination.

Current obstetric practice aims at the prevention of this disease by passive immunization of pregnant women with high-titer $Rh_o(D)IgG$. This is given to nonsensitized women during pregnancy as well as immediately after delivery. The $Rh_o(D)IgG$ is also given for invasive procedures during the pregnancy, such as chorionic villus biopsy and amniocentesis.

Pediatric Management of Erythroblastosis

The key pediatric decisions relate to the following:

(1) The degree of cardiovascular and pulmonary compromise must be assessed. Where high output failure is severe, a partial exchange transfusion with packed red blood cells (35 mL/kg) for adjustment of blood volume and correction of anemia is used. Hydropic infants generally require ventilatory support, paracentesis of large volumes of ascitic fluid, and evacuation of pleural effusions, if present. Because

many of these infants are delivered early, their course is also complicated by hyaline membrane disease.

(2) Where intrauterine transfusions have not been done (either intra-abdominally or directly into the umbilical vein), the immediate poststabilization period is used for a 2-volume exchange transfusion to remove affected cells. Indications for this procedure are a cord blood hematocrit less than 40 or unconjugated bilirubin greater than 6 mg/dL (or both). This procedure is performed after initial cardiovascular and respiratory stabilization.

(3) Blood glucose concentration should be immediately supported (erythroblastotic infants have islet cell hyperplasia and are prone to hypoglycemia secondary to hyperinsulinemia), and water and electrolyte balance should be provided.

(4) The rate of rise of bilirubin concentrations should be graphically depicted to allow anticipation of the need for a 2-volume exchange transfusion prior to bilirubin concentrations listed in Table 4–13. An increase in serum bilirubin greater than 1.5 mg/dL per hour indicates the need for an exchange transfusion. This procedure is used in infants who did not have the initial early double volume exchange.

(5) Subsequent exchange transfusions are performed for bilirubins reaching a given infant's exchange level.

(6) Infants who have had repeated exchange transfusions should be followed closely for signs of coagulation disorders, severe anemia, or the development of a cholestatic syndrome.

4. EXTRAVASCULAR HEMORRHAGE

Bleeding within the body (eg, cephalhematoma, bruising, central nervous system hemorrhage) may result in unconjugated hyperbilirubinemia by creating an extra bilirubin load for the liver. Peak of jaundice tends to be at 3–4 days of age.

5. GASTROINTESTINAL TRACT OBSTRUCTION

Either functional or structural obstruction of the gastrointestinal tract can result in unconjugated hyperbilirubinemia due to enhanced enterohepatic circulation of bilirubin.

6. JAUNDICE SECONDARY TO CONJUGATED HYPERBILIRUBINEMIA

The category of jaundice secondary to conjugated hyperbilirubinemia includes a very long list of problems and, in most cases, involves both conjugated and unconjugated hyperbilirubinemia. The differential diagnosis of conjugated hyperbilirubinemia is covered in Chapter 21. However, a brief discussion of infectious causes is merited here. These are normally separated into 2 categories. In the first of these, hepatitis is a key feature of the infection. The infection can be caused by enteroviruses (coxsackie and echoviruses), hepatitis B, cytomegalovirus, toxoplasmosis, rubella, and herpes simplex. In such cases, the organism can be identified through culture and serologic techniques. Rarer causes include syphilis and tuberculous infections.

The second group includes infections that cause sepsis, which in turn produces a "toxic" effect upon the liver. No specific organism is associated with this form of jaundice, but almost all organisms known to cause sepsis in the newborn may be associated with jaundice secondary to a mixed hyperbilirubinemia. In some cases in which organisms produce hemolyzing toxins (eg, *Escherichia coli*), unconjugated hyperbilirubinemia can predominate.

7. PROLONGED UNCONJUGATED HYPERBILIRUBINEMIA

Causes of unconjugated hyperbilirubinemia after the first week of life are presented in Table 4–14.

Bowman JM: Neonatal management. Pages 200–239 in: *Modern Management of the Rh Problem.* Queenan JT (editor). Harper & Row, 1977.

Cashore WJ, Stern L: Neonatal hyperbilirubinemia. *Pediatr Clin North Am* 1982;**29:**1191.

Committee on Fetus and Newborn: Home phototherapy. *Pediatrics* 1985;**76:**136.

DeCarvalho M et al: Frequency of breast-feeding and serum bilirubin concentration. *Am J Dis Child* 1982; **136:**737.

Ennever JF et al: Phototherapy for neonatal jaundice: In vivo clearance of bilirubin products. *Pediatr Res* 1985; **19:**205.

Hovi L, Siimes MA: Exchange transfusion with fresh heparinized blood is a safe procedure: Experiences from 1069 newborns. *Acta Paediatr Scand* 1985;**74:**360.

Lascari AD: "Early" breast-feeding jaundice: Clinical significance. *J Pediatr* 1986;**108:**156.

Levine RL, Fredericks WR, Rapoport SI: Entry of bilirubin into the brain due to opening of the blood-brain barrier. *Pediatrics* 1982;**69:**255.

Levine RL, Maisels MJ (chairpersons): *Hyperbilirubinemia in the Newborn: Report of the Eighty-Fifth Ross Conference on Pediatric Research.* Ross Laboratories, 1983.

Maisals MJ: Light versus tin. *Pediatrics* 1988;**81:**882.

Table 4–14. Causes of prolonged unconjugat hyperbilirubinemia.

Hemolytic jaundice
Breast milk jaundice
Crigler-Najjar syndrome
Gastrointestinal tract obstruction
Hypothyroidism (can produce either un
   hyperbilirubinemia)

Maisals MJ: Neonatal jaundice. Page 534 in: *Neonatology: Pathophysiology and Management of the Newborn,* 3rd ed. Avery GB (editor). Lippincott, 1987.

McDonagh AF, Lightner DA: Bilirubin, jaundice and phototherapy. *Pediatrics* 1985;**75**:443.

National Institute of Child Health and Human Development: Randomized, controlled trial of phototherapy for neonatal hyperbilirubinemia. *Pediatrics* 1985;**75** (Suppl):381.

Osborn LM, Reiff MI, Bolus R: Jaundice in the full-term neonate. *Pediatrics* 1984;**73**:520.

Perlman M, Frank JW: Bilirubin beyond the blood-brain barrier. *Pediatrics* 1988;**81**:304.

Perlman M et al: Auditory nerve-brainstem evoked responses in hyperbilirubinemic neonates. *Pediatrics* 1983;**72**:658.

Poland RL: Breast-milk jaundice. *J Pediatr* 1981;**99**:86.

Ritter DA et al: A prospective study of free bilirubin and other risk factors in the development of kernicterus in premature infants. *Pediatrics* 1982;**69**:260.

Stevenson DK, Vremen HJ: S_N-protoporphyrin: A consideration of the first clinical trial in human neonates. *Pediatrics* 1988;**81**:880.

Watchko JF, Oski FA: Bilirubin 20 mg/dL = vigintiphobia. *Pediatrics* 1983;**71**:660.

INFECTION OF THE NEWBORN

GENERAL APPROACH

The fetus and newborn infant are very susceptible to infections. There are 3 major routes of perinatal infection:

(1) Blood-borne transplacental infection of the fetus (eg, cytomegalovirus, rubella, syphilis).

(2) Ascending infection with a disruption of the barrier provided by the amniotic membranes (eg, bacterial infections after ≥ 24 hours of ruptured membranes).

(3) Infection upon passage through an infected birth canal or exposure to infected blood at delivery (eg, herpes simplex, hepatitis B, bacterial infections).

The susceptibility of the newborn is related to immature both the cellular and humoral immune ...ature is particularly evident in ...ection against some ... IgG across the ... pregnancy. Pre- ...n at less than 30 ...the full amount of

obstetric histories are ...sis of neonatal infec- ...e of early onset (< 5

days) neonatal bacterial infection is 4–5:1000 live births. Rupture of membranes more than 24 hours prior to delivery is associated with an infection rate of 1:100, and rupture of membranes with chorioamnionitis with a rate of neonatal infection of 10:100. Irrespective of rupture of membranes, infection rates are 5 times higher in preterm infants. Other important historical points include immunization of the mother against rubella, a prior history of genital herpes, or viral illness around the time of delivery.

B. Symptoms and Signs: Early-onset bacterial infection is related to perinatal risk factors and presents most commonly on day 1 of life, with the majority of cases at less than 12 hours. Respiratory distress is the most common presenting sign. Other features include low Apgar scores without fetal distress, poor perfusion, and hypotension. Late-onset (presentation at > 5 days of age) bacterial infection presents in a more subtle manner, with poor feeding, lethargy, hypotonia, temperature instability, altered perfusion, new or increased oxygen requirement, and apnea. Signs suggestive of congenital viral infections include small size for gestational age, petechiae, jaundice, and hepatosplenomegaly.

C. Laboratory Findings: Low total white counts, absolute neutropenia (< 1000), and elevated ratios of immature to mature neutrophils are suggestive of neonatal bacterial infection. Thrombocytopenia is also a common feature. Other laboratory aids are hyperglycemia with no change in glucose administration and unexplained metabolic acidosis. In early-onset bacterial infection, pneumonia is invariably present; chest x-ray films show infiltrates, but these infiltrates cannot be distinguished from infiltrates due to other causes of neonatal lung disease. Antigen detection in urine or other body fluids has been helpful in the rapid identification of some bacteria (especially group B streptococcus). Definitive diagnosis is made by positive cultures from blood, cerebrospinal fluid, etc. Serologies and cultures are useful in the diagnosis of congenital viral infections.

Treatment

A high index of suspicion is important in the diagnosis and treatment of neonatal infection. Table 4–15 presents some guidelines for the evaluation and management of *term* infants with risk factors or clinical signs of infection. Because the risk of infection is greater in the preterm infant and because respiratory disease is a common sign of infection, any preterm infant with respiratory disease requires blood cultures and broad-spectrum therapy for 48–72 hours pending the results of cultures. An examination of cerebrospinal fluid should be performed in those infants in whom infection is highly suspected on a clinical basis (eg, associated hypotension, persistent metabolic acidosis, neutropenia). Other specific therapy includes the administration of intravenous gamma globulin (500 mg/kg) to infants with known

Table 4–15. Guidelines for evaluation of neonatal bacterial infection in the term infant.

Risk Factor	Clinical Signs[1]	Evaluation and Treatment
24 h rupture of membranes	None	Observation
> 24 h rupture of membranes, chorioamnninonitis	None	CBC, blood cultures, 48–72 h broad-spectrum antibiotics
> 24 h rupture of membranes, chorioamnionitis, maternal antibiotics	None	CBC, blood cultures, urine counterimmuno-electrophoresis (CIE), 48–72 h broad-spectrum antibiotics
None or present	Present	CBC, blood and cerebrospinal fluid (CSF) culture, ± urine culture, broad-spectrum antibiotics[2]

[1]If clinical signs consistent with infection are absent, close observation without treatment may be sufficient.

[2]Any infant, irrespective of age of presentation, who appears infected by clinical criteria should have a CSF examination. Urine culture is indicated in the evaluation of infants who were initially well but have developed symptoms after 2–3 days in the nursery.

infection or clinical signs very suggestive of true infection. Granulocyte transfusions have been used in neutropenic patients and exchange transfusions performed in sick infants unresponsive to other therapies. In sick infants, the essentials of good supportive therapy should be provided: intravenous glucose and water, colloid volume support, use of pressors as needed, and oxygen and ventilator support.

Prognosis

The prognosis for neonatal infection depends on the specific agent and type of infection. This issue is addressed in the discussion of specific infections.

SPECIFIC INFECTIONS

1. BACTERIAL SEPSIS

The most common organisms causing bacterial sepsis in the newborn are group B β-hemolytic streptococcus and gram-negative enterics (especially *E coli*). Other organisms to consider are *Staphylococcus aureus*, *Listeria monocytogenes*, enterococcus, and *Staphylococcus epidermidis* (most common in infants with indwelling central venous lines). Early-onset bacterial sepsis is usually acquired in vitro (ascending) or by passage through an infected birth canal. Late-onset bacterial sepsis is more often associated with infection of cerebrospinal fluid or other local infections (eg, osteomyelitis). Clinical signs, laboratory aids, and evaluation have been noted (see above and Table 4–15).

Antibiotic coverage should be directed initially towards suspected organisms. Early-onset sepsis is usually caused by group B streptococcus or gram-negative enterics; broad-spectrum coverage, therefore, should include ampicillin plus an aminoglycoside or third-generation cephalosporin. Specific doses and schedules are given in Chapter 38. Late-onset infections can also be caused by the same organisms, but coverage may need to be expanded to include staphylococci. In particular, the preterm infant with indwelling lines is at risk for *S epidermidis*, for which vancomycin hydrochloride is the drug of choice.

In the last several years, strategies for the prevention of bacterial infections in newborns have been developed. Intrapartum treatment with ampicillin or penicillin has proven effective in interrupting the transmission of group B streptococcal infections. In the nursery, administration of intravenous gamma globulin has been shown in some centers to decrease the incidence of late-onset sepsis in at-risk preterm infants.

2. FUNGAL SEPSIS

With more aggressive neonatal care associated with the survival of smaller infants, infection with *Candida albicans* has become more common. Infants of low birth weight with central lines who have had repeated exposures to broad-spectrum antibiotics are at highest risk. For infants less than 1500 g, colonization rates of 27% have been demonstrated, with many of these infants developing cutaneous lesions. A much smaller percentage develops systemic disease. Most infants with systemic candidiasis will have associated skin lesions. Other clinical features are indistinguishable from bacterial sepsis. Treatment is the antifungal amphotericin B.

3. MENINGITIS

Any newborn with bacterial sepsis is also at risk for meningitis. The incidence is low in infants with early-onset sepsis but is much higher in infants with late-onset infection. The workup for any infant with signs consistent with infection should include a spinal tap. Diagnosis is suggested by a protein greater than 250 mg/dL, glucose less than 30 mg/dL, more than 25 wbc/μL, and positive Gram stain. The diagnosis is confirmed by culture. Most common organisms are group B streptococcus and gram-negative enterics. While sepsis can be treated with 10–14 days of antibiotics, meningitis should be treated for 21 days with appropriate antibiotics. The mortality rate for neonatal meningitis is approximately 25%, with significant neurologic morbidity present in one-third of the survivors.

4. PNEUMONIA

The respiratory system can be infected in utero or upon passage through the birth canal. Early-onset neonatal infection is usually associated with pneumonia. Pneumonia should also be suspected in older neonates with a recent onset of tachypnea, retractions, and cyanosis. In infants already receiving respiratory support, an increase in oxygen requirement or ventilator settings may indicate pneumonia. Not only bacteria but also viruses (cytomegalovirus, respiratory syncytial virus, adenovirus, influenza, herpes simplex, parainfluenza), *Chlamydia,* and *Ureaplasma* can cause the disease. In infants with preexisting respiratory disease, intercurrent pulmonary infections may contribute to the ultimate severity of chronic lung disease.

5. URINARY TRACT INFECTION

Infection of the urine is uncommon with early-onset infection. Urinary tract infection (UTI) in the newborn is seen most commonly in association with genitourinary anomalies and is caused by gram-negative enterics. Urine should be evaluated as part of the workup for late-onset infection. Culture should be obtained either by suprapubic aspiration or bladder catheterization. Antibiotic therapy is continued for 10–14 days intravenously. Subsequently, evaluation for genitourinary anomalies, starting with an ultrasound, should be undertaken.

6. OSTEOMYELITIS

Osteomyelitis is an uncommon infection in the newborn. It is seen in association with late onset-septicemia, usually with *S aureus* or group B streptococcus. More detailed discussion of osteomyelitis can be found in Chapter 28.

7. OTITIS MEDIA

Otitis media may be present in a significant number of long-term nursery residents. It is particularly common in infants who have had prolonged endotracheal intubation. An evaluation for infection in such an infant is not complete without an ear examination. Gram-negative enterics are more common infecting agents in nursery residents than in outpatients.

8. OMPHALITIS

A normal umbilical cord stump will atrophy and separate at skin level. A small amount of purulent material at the base of the cord is common but can be minimized by keeping the cord open to air and cleaning the base with alcohol several times each day. The cord can become colonized with streptococci, staphylococci, or gram-negative organisms that can cause local infection. Infections are more common in cords manipulated for venous or arterial lines. Omphalitis is diagnosed when redness and edema are evident in the soft tissues around the stump. Local and systemic cultures should be obtained. Treatment is broad-spectrum intravenous antibiotics. Complications are determined by the degree of infection of the cord vessels and include septic thrombophlebitis, hepatic abscess, and portal vein thrombosis.

9. CONGENITAL VIRAL & PARASITIC INFECTIONS (See also Chapter 27)

Cytomegalovirus

Cytomegalovirus (CMV) is the most common virus known to be transmitted in utero. The incidence of congenital infection ranges from 0.2–2.2% among live births. Transmission of CMV can take place as a consequence of either primary or inactivated infection in the mother. The mother is usually asymptomatic from her illness, but CMV should be suspected in the face of a heterophile negative mononucleosis-like illness. Primary infection in pregnancy is more common in high than low socioeconomic groups. An important source of infection is children (especially those in daycare setting), who transmit the virus to parents. The incidence of primary infection in pregnancy is 1–4%, with a 40% transmission rate to the fetus. Of these infants, 85–90% are asymptomatic at birth, whereas 10–15% have clinically apparent disease—hepatosplenomegaly, petechiae, smallness for gestational age, direct hyperbilirubinemia, thrombocytopenia. The risk of neonatal disease is higher when the mother acquires the infection in the first half of pregnancy. The incidence of reactivated infection in pregnancy is less than 1%, with a 0–1% incidence of clinically apparent disease. Diagnosis in a suspected infant should be confirmed with culture of the virus (blood, cerebrospinal fluid, urine, throat, placenta, amniotic fluid). Pregnant caretakers should not take care of a child excreting CMV. Although experimental, ganciclovir has been used in some severely ill neonates.

The mortality rate in patients with symptomatic congenital CMV may be as high as 20%. Sequelae, including hearing loss, mental retardation, delayed motor development, chorioretinitis and optic atrophy, seizures, language delays, and learning disability, occur in 90% of symptomatic survivors. The incidence is 5–15% in asymptomatic infants; the most frequent finding is hearing loss.

Perinatal infection can also occur with acquisition of virus around the time of delivery. These infections are generally asymptomatic and without sequelae. Postnatal infection is usually asymptomatic but can cause hepatitis, pneumonitis, and neurologic illness in compromised seronegative prematures. The virus is usually acquired through transfusions, but the risk can be minimized by using frozen, washed red cells.

Rubella

Congenital rubella infection occurs as a result of rubella infection in the mother during pregnancy. The frequency of infection in the infant is as high as 80% in mothers infected during the first trimester. Infection rates then decline but increase again in the last month of pregnancy. A high incidence of defects can be attributed to infection acquired during the first trimester but declines with later infection. Clinical features of congenital rubella include adenopathy, bone radiolucencies, encephalitis, cardiac defects (pulmonary arterial hypoplasia and patent ductus arteriosus), cataracts, retinopathy, growth retardation, hepatosplenomegaly, thrombocytopenia, and purpura. The diagnosis should be suspected in cases of a characteristic clinical illness in the mother (rash, adenopathy, arthritis). Maternal illness can be confirmed with serologies. IgG titers in the infant can be compared to those in the mother, and specific IgM may be looked for in the baby. Diagnosis can be confirmed by culture of pharyngeal secretions.

There is no treatment for congenital rubella. Prevention, however, is possible with immunization. Nonimmune patients of childbearing age should be immunized prior to conception. Inadvertent immunization during pregnancy does not seem to carry a risk of causing significant illness in the fetus. Congenital rubella does cause significant, long-term sequelae, including mental retardation and hearing loss. Sequelae are most severe in infections acquired during the first trimester. Infants infected late in gestation do not suffer long-term sequelae.

Varicella

Congenital varicella is rare (5% after infection acquired during the first or second trimester) but does cause a recognizable constellation of findings, including limb hypoplasia, cutaneous scars, microcephaly, cortical atrophy, chorioretinitis, and cataracts. Perinatal exposure (5 days before to 2 days after delivery) can cause severe to fatal disseminated varicella. Diagnosis can be confirmed with a rise in maternal IgG titers, evidence of specific IgM in the neonate, or viral culture from vesicles. Prophylaxis and therapy are available for perinatal varicella. If maternal varicella develops within the perinatal risk period, 1.25 mL of varicella immune globulin should be given. If this has not been done, the illness can be treated with intravenous acyclovir. (see Chapter 27)

Toxoplasmosis

Toxoplasmosis is caused by the parasite *Toxoplasma gondii.* When infection occurs during pregnancy, up to 40% of the children become infected, of whom 15% have severe clinical damage. The means of acquisition include exposure to cat feces or ingestion of raw meat. Fetal damage is most likely to occur when the infection occurs in the second to sixth month of gestation. Clinical findings include growth retardation, chorioretinitis, seizures, jaundice, hydrocephalus, microcephaly, hepatosplenomegaly, adenopathy, cataracts, rash, thrombocytopenia, and pneumonia. The majority of affected infants are asymptomatic at birth but show evidence of damage (chorioretinitis, blindness, low IQ) at a later time. Serologies, first for IgG and then the specific IgM antibody, make the diagnosis.

10. PERINATALLY ACQUIRED VIRAL INFECTIONS (See also Chapter 27)

Herpes Simplex

Herpes simplex infection is most commonly acquired at the time of birth with passage through an infected birth canal. A mother can have either a primary or a reactivated secondary infection. Primary maternal infection, due to both high titer of organism and no maternal antibodies, poses the greatest risk to the infant. Most mothers with primary herpes at the time of delivery are asymptomatic. They tend to be young and to deliver prematurely. Time of presentation of localized or disseminated disease in the infant is usually 5–14 days of age. Central nervous system disease usually presents at 14–28 days of age. Up to 70% of infants present initially with local vesicles on the skin or oral mucosa. Progression of disease from localized skin or mucosal disease to CNS or disseminated disease occurs in a significant percentage of cases. The remainder present initially with CNS (lethargy, instability, seizures) or disseminated disease (pneumonia, shock, hepatitis). Preliminary diagnosis can be made by scraping the base of a vesicle and finding multinucleated giant cells. Viral culture, usually positive in 24–72 hours, makes the definitive diagnosis. Risk to the infant from secondary maternal infection is low (probably less than 1–2%).

Therapy for neonatal herpes is available with adenosine arabinoside or acyclovir. Acyclovir has fewer side effects and is the drug of choice. Both agents are effective in improving survival with CNS and disseminated disease and in preventing the spread of localized disease. Prevention is possible by not allowing delivery through an infected birth canal (eg, by cesarean section). However, antepartum cervical cultures are poor predictors of the presence of virus at the time of delivery. Furthermore, given the low incidence of infection in the newborn in secondary maternal infection, cesarean section is not indicated for these infants. If there is a history of recurrent herpes in the mother, both mother (cervix) and infant (eye, oropharynx, umbilicus, rectum) should be cultured. If the infant is colonized (positive cultures), treatment with acyclovir should be considered. In cases of documented primary infection at the time of delivery, the infant should be cultured and started on acyclovir pending the results of cultures. The major problem facing perinatologists is the high percentage of asymptomatic primary maternal infection. In those cases, infection in the neonate is currently not preventable. Therefore, any infant who presents at the right age with symptoms consistent with neonatal herpes should be cultured and started on acyclovir pending the results of those cultures.

Prognosis is good for localized skin and mucosal disease that does not progress. The mortality rate for both disseminated and CNS herpes is high, with significant rates of morbidity among survivors despite treatment.

Hepatitis B

Infants can be infected with hepatitis B at the time of birth. The presence of HBsAg should be determined in mothers at risk (eg, intravenous drug abusers, those of Far Eastern origin). If the result is positive, the infant should receive hepatitis B immunoglobulin (HBIG) as soon as possible after birth, followed by the hepatitis B vaccine in the first week of life with 2 subsequent doses. If an HBsAg has not been sent prior to birth in a mother at risk, the test should be sent after delivery and HBIG administered to the infant. Vaccination should be performed only if the maternal HBsAg is subsequently positive. Clinical illness is rare in the neonatal period, but exposed infants are at risk to become chronic HBsAg carriers and to develop chronic active hepatitis and are at increased risk for hepatic carcinoma.

Enteroviral Infection

Enteroviral infections occur with greatest frequency in the late summer and early fall. Infection is usually acquired in the perinatal period. There is often a history of a maternal illness (fever, diarrhea, rash) in the week prior to delivery. The illness presents in the infant in the first 2 weeks of life. Most commonly, the illness is characterized by fevers, lethargy, irritability, diarrhea, and rash but is not severe. Other symptom complexes include meningoencephalitis and myocarditis, as well as a severe disseminated illness with hepatitis, pneumonia, shock, and disseminated intravascular coagulation. Diagnosis can be confirmed by culture (rectum, cerebrospinal fluid, blood). There is no therapy of proved efficacy. Prognosis is good for all symptom complexes except severe disseminated disease, which carries a high mortality rate.

HIV Infection

Human immunodeficiency virus (HIV) can pass transplacentally, but infection is more likely at the time of birth. Transmission of virus occurs in about 30% of births. The longest documented incubation period prior to presentation of illness has been 7 years. However, the majority present within 2 years of birth. Diagnosis (discussed in detail in Chapter 27) is based upon clinical, immunologic, and serologic findings. Several drugs with activity against HIV have been developed (see Chapter 27).

Protection of health care workers is also an important issue to consider. Testing should be performed in the obstetric population at risk (intravenous drug abusers, those with multiple sexual partners). Because such testing will still fail to identify some infected patients, however, universal precautions should be used. Gloves should be worn during all procedures involving blood and blood-contaminated fluids, intubation, and any invasive procedures using needles. When a splash exposure is possible (eg, in the delivery room), a mask and eye covers should be used.

11. OTHER INFECTIONS

Congenital Syphilis

The infant is usually infected in utero by transplacental passage of the *Treponema pallidum*. Findings consistent with congenital syphilis include mucocutaneous lesions, lymphadenopathy, hepatitis, bony changes, and hydrops. However, in the newborn period, infants are most often asymptomatic, so that diagnosis is based on serologic testing. A definitive diagnosis can be made on those rare occasions when the organism is identified by darkfield or pathologic examination. See Chapter 28 for details of diagnosis and therapy.

Tuberculosis

Congenital tuberculosis is rare (seen only in the infant of a mother with hematogenously spread tuberculosis). Women with pulmonary tuberculosis are not likely to infect the fetus until after delivery. Management is based upon the mother's situation:

(1) Mother with a positive skin test and negative chest x-ray—the mother is treated with isoniazid, and the infant is followed with skin tests.

(2) Mother with active disease—the mother should be separated from the infant until adequate treatment has been administered to render the mother noncontagious. The infant should be followed with skin tests.

Conjunctivitis

Neisseria gonorrhoeae may colonize an infant during passage through an infected birth canal. Gonococcal ophthalmitis presents at 3–7 days with very purulent conjunctivitis. Diagnosis can be suspected when gram-negative intracellular diplococci are seen on Gram's strain and confirmed by culture (see Chapter 28 for treatment). Current therapy is aimed at prophylaxis with silver nitrate drops or erythromycin ointment at birth.

Chlamydia trachomatis is another important cause of conjunctivitis, presenting at 5 days to several weeks of age with congestion, edema, and minimal discharge. The organism is acquired at birth after passage through an infected birth canal. Acquisition occurs in 50% of infants born to infected women, with a 25–50% risk of conjunctivitis. Prevalence in pregnancy is over 10% in some populations. Diagnosis is by isolation of the organism or by rapid antigen detection tests. Treatment is oral erythromycin. Topical treatment alone will not eradicate nasopharyngeal carriage, leaving the infant at risk for the development of pneumonitis. Diagnosis in the infant requires therapy of the mother and her sexual partners.

INFECTION CONTROL

The single most important principal in nursery infection control is good hand washing. Hands should be washed with a germicidal soap for 3 minutes prior to entering the nursery to handle patients. This procedure should be repeated between patient visits. Personnel with upper respiratory tract infections should wear masks; those with gastrointestinal tract infections must be rigorous about hand washing. Wounds or herpetic lesions should be covered.

An infected infant with a communicable disease (eg, viral respiratory infection or necrotizing enterocolitis) should be isolated. Ideally, the infant should be placed in a separate room, but if one is not available, a remote site in the nursery and perhaps an isolette should be used. The number of staff caring for the infant and their exposure to other infants should be limited. Gown, gloves, and mask should be worn as indicated for type of infection, and exposed materials should be disposed of separately.

Nursery staff should also take precautions against acquiring HIV infection. Newborns should be handled with gloves prior to initial bathing to remove blood. Gloves should be worn when drawing blood and starting intravenous therapy. Aspiration of meconium from an infant's airway should be performed with wall suction.

Alkalay AL et al: Fetal varicella syndrome. *J Pediatr* 1987;**111**:320.

American Academy of Pediatrics: *Report of the Committee on Infectious Diseases.* American Academy of Pediatrics, 1988.

Arvin AM et al: Failure of antepartum maternal cultures to predict the infant's risk of exposure to herpes simplex virus at delivery. *N Engl J Med* 1986;**315**:796.

Baker CJ: Group B streptococcal infection in newborns. Prevention at test? *N Engl J Med* 1986;**314**:1702.

Baley JE: Neonatal sepsis: The potential for immunotherapy. *Clin Perinatol* 1988;**15**:755.

Baley JE, Silverman RA: Systemic candidiasis: Cutaneous manifestations in low birth weight infants. *Pediatrics* 1988;**82**:211.

Ballard RA et al: Acquired cytomegalovirus infection in preterm infants. *Am J Dis Child* 1979;**133**:782.

Berman SA, Balkany TJ, Simmons MA: Otitis media in the neonatal intensive care unit. *Pediatrics* 1978;**62**:198.

Boyer KM, Gotoff SP: Antimicrobial prophylaxis of neonatal group B streptococcal sepsis. *Clin Perinatol* 1988;**15**:831.

Boyer KM, Gotoff SP: Prevention of early-onset neonatal group B streptococcal disease with selective intrapartum prophylaxis. *N Engl J Med* 1986;**314**:1665.

Brown ZA et al: Effects on infants of a first episode of genital herpes during pregnancy. *N Engl J Med* 1987;**317**:1246.

Chin KC, Fitzhardinge PM: Sequelae of early-onset group B hemolytic streptococcal neonatal meningitis. *J Pediatr* 1985;**106**:819.

Chirico G et al: Intrauterine gamma globulin therapy for prophylaxis of infection in high risk neonates. *J Pediatr* 1987;**110**:437.

Christensen RD et al: Granulocyte transfusions in neonates with bacterial infection, neutropenia, and depletion of mature marrow neutrophils. *Pediatrics* 1982;**70**:1.

Conboy TJ et al: Early clinical manifestations and intellectual outcome in children with symptomatic congenital cytomegalovirus infection. *J Pediatr* 1987;**111**:343.

Conboy TJ et al: Intellectual development in school-aged children with cytomegalovirus infection. *Pediatrics* 1986;**77**:801.

Dashefsky B et al: Prevention of early-onset group B streptococcal sepsis. *J Pediatr* 1988;**112**:1039.

Dillon HC et al: Group B streptococcal carriage and disease: A 6 year prospective study. *J Pediatr* 1987;**110**:31.

Edwards MS et al: Long-term sequelae of group B streptococcal meningitis in infants. *J Pediatr* 1985;**106**:717.

Faix RG et al: Mucocutaneous and invasive candidiasis among very low birth weight (< 1500 grams) infants in intensive care nurseries. A prospective study. *Pediatrics* 1989;**83**:101.

Hinman AR: Prevention of congenital rubella infection: Symposium summary. *Pediatrics* 1985;**75**:1162.

Kumar ML et al: Congenital and postnatally acquired cytomegalovirus infections: Long-term follow-up. *J Pediatr* 1984;**104**:674.

Lake AM et al: Enterovirus infections in neonates. *J Pediatr* 1976;**89**:787.

Marion RW et al: Fetal AIDS syndrome score. *Am J Dis Child* 1987;**141**:429.

Miller E et al: Consequences of confirmed maternal rubella at successive stages of pregnancy. *Lancet* 1982;**2**:781.

Modlin JF et al: Risk of congenital abnormality after inadvertent rubella vaccination of pregnant women. *N Engl J Med* 1976;**294**:272.

Nicholas SW et al: Human immunodeficiency virus infection in childhood, adolescence, and pregnancy: A status report and national research agenda. *Pediatrics* 1989;**83**:293.

Paryani SG, Arvin AM: Intrauterine infection with varicella-zoster virus after maternal varicella. *N Engl J Med* 1986;**314**:1542.

Pass RF et al: Young children as a probable source of maternal and congenital cytomegalovirus infection. *N Engl J Med* 1987;**316**:1366.

Prober CG et al: Low risk of herpes simplex infections in neonates exposed to the virus at the time of vaginal delivery to mothers with recurrent genital herpes simplex virus infection. *N Engl J Med* 1987;**316**:240.

Prober CG et al: Use of routine viral cultures at delivery to identify neonates exposed to herpes simplex virus. *N Engl J Med* 1988;**318**:887.

Remington JS, Klein JO (editors): *Infectious Diseases of the Fetus and Newborn Infant*, 3rd ed. Saunders, 1989.

Sever JL et al: Toxoplasmosis: Maternal and pediatric findings in 23,000 pregnancies. *Pediatrics* 1988;**82**:181.

Stagno S, Whitley RJ: Herpesvirus infections of pregnancy. *N Engl J Med* 1985;**313**:1270.

Stagno S et al: Congenital cytomegalovirus infection: The relative importance of primary and recurrent maternal infection. *N Engl J Med* 1982;**306**:945.

St. Geme JW et al: Perinatal bacterial infection after prolonged rupture of amniotic membranes: An analysis of risk and management. *J Pediatr* 1984;**104**:608.

Task Force on Pediatric AIDS: Pediatric guidelines for infection control of human immunodeficiency virus (acquired immunodeficiency virus) in hospitals, medical offices, schools, and other settings. *Pediatrics* 1988;**82**:801.

Wald ER et al: Long-term outcome of group B streptococcal meningitis. *J Pediatr* 1986;**77**:217.

Weinstein RA, Boyer KM, Linn ES: Isolation guidelines for obstetric patients and newborn infants. *Am J Obstet Gynecol* 1983;**146**:353.

Whitley RJ: Neonatal herpes simplex virus infections. *Clin Perinatol* 1988;**15**:903.

Whitley RJ et al: The natural history of herpes simplex virus infection of mother and newborn. *Pediatrics* 1980;**66**:489.

GASTROINTESTINAL & ABDOMINAL SURGICAL CONDITIONS
(See also Chapter 20.)

CONGENITAL CONDITIONS

1. TRACHEOESOPHAGEAL FISTULA & ESOPHAGEAL ATRESIA

Diagnosis

These associated conditions are characterized by a blind esophageal pouch and a fistulous connection between either the proximal or distal esophagus and the airway. In 85% of infants with this condition, the fistula is between the distal esophagus and the airway. Polyhydramnios is common because of the high level of gastrointestinal obstruction. Infants present in the first hours of life with copious secretions, choking, cyanosis, and respiratory distress. Diagnosis can be confirmed with chest x-ray after careful placement of a nasogastric tube to the point at which resistance is met. On chest x-ray, the tube will be seen in the blind pouch. If a tracheoesophageal fistula is present to the distal esophagus, gas will be present in the abdomen.

Treatment

The tube in the proximal pouch should be placed on continuous suction to drain secretions and prevent aspiration. The head of the bed should be elevated to prevent reflux of gastric contents through the distal fistula into the lungs. Intravenous glucose and fluids should be provided and oxygen administered as needed. Definitive treatment is surgical and depends on the distance between the segments of esophagus. If the distance is not too great, the fistula can be ligated, gastrostomy (for feeding and decompression) performed, and the ends of the esophagus anastomosed. In instances where the end of the esophagus cannot be anastomosed, the initial surgery entails fistula ligation and a gastrostomy. Antibiotics are usually used postoperatively.

Prognosis

Prognosis is determined primarily by the presence or absence of associated anomalies. Vertebral, cardiac, renal, limb, and anal anomalies are also seen. Evaluation for other anomalies should be done early in the infant's course.

2. HIGH INTESTINAL OBSTRUCTION

Diagnosis

Infants with high intestinal obstruction present early with vomiting. A history of polyhydramnios is also common. In cases of duodenal atresia, vomitus does not contain bile; in cases of malrotation and midgut volvulus and high jejunal atresia, vomitus is bilious. Midgut volvulus is seen with malrotation and involves torsion of the intestine around the superior mesenteric artery that causes occlusion of the vascular supply of most of the small intestine. If not treated promptly, the infant can lose most of the small bowel to ischemic injury. Therefore, *bilious vomiting* in the neonate demands immediate attention and evaluation. Diagnosis of high intestinal obstruction can be confirmed with x-rays. Duodenal atresia is characterized by a double bubble sign (stomach and dilatated duodenum). In cases of midgut volvulus, the plain abdominal x-ray may not be definitive. Occasionally, air is present, stopping at the level of the ligament of Treitz (level of obstruction). However, air can also be present elsewhere, precluding accurate diagnosis on plain film. Diagnosis can be confirmed with a contrast enema indicating malposition of the cecum. If the results are equivocal and fail to confirm the diagnosis, an upper gastrointestinal series can be done to determine whether contrast material passes the ligament of Treitz.

Treatment

A nasogastric tube should be placed to suction for decompression, an intravenous needle should be placed for administering glucose and fluids, and supportive respiratory treatment should be given. The definitive treatment is surgery. Midgut volvulus is an indication for emergency surgery. Other conditions can be handled promptly but need not be done in an emergency fashion. Antibiotics are usually used for these conditions.

Prognosis

Duodenal atresia is associated with trisomy 21. Prognosis in that circumstance is related to other associated conditions (eg, cardiac). Infants with other high intestinal obstructions do well after surgical correction, except those with midgut volvulus who suffer loss of considerable amounts of ischemic small bowel.

3. DISTAL INTESTINAL OBSTRUCTION

Diagnosis

Low intestinal obstruction presents with an increasing intolerance of feedings (spitting progressing to vomiting), abdominal distention, and decreased or absent stooling. Imperforate anus can often be diagnosed on initial physical examination prior to onset of symptoms. In the case of a high rectal atresia, however, the obstruction can be missed on the initial examination. Other diagnostic clues to imperforate anus include the presence of perineal fistulas with meconium or the presence of meconium in the urine (rectovesical fistula). Other causes of distal intestinal obstruction include meconium ileus, Hirschsprung's disease, meconium plug syndrome, small left colon syndrome, ileal atresia, and colonic atresia. Plain film of the abdomen shows gaseous distention with air through a considerable portion of the bowel and air-fluid levels. Diagnosis of meconium ileus, meconium plug, and small left colon syndrome can be made by appearance on contrast enema. In cases of meconium plug syndrome, osmotic contrast material (eg, meglumine diatrizoate [Gastrografin]) has a therapeutic as well as a diagnostic use: it induces passage of the plug. Contrast enema and rectal biopsy showing absence of ganglion cells confirms the diagnosis of Hirschsprung's disease.

Treatment

Nasogastric suction to decompress the abdomen, intravenous glucose, fluid and electrotype replacement, and respiratory support as necessary should be instituted. Antibiotics are usually indicated. The definitive treatment for all these conditions (with the exception of meconium plug syndrome and small left colon syndrome) is surgery.

Prognosis

Up to 10% of infants with meconium plug syndrome are found to have cystic fibrosis (CF), whereas all infants with meconium ileus have CF. Small left colon syndrome is seen in infants of diabetic mothers. Once the child develops a normal stooling pattern, feedings will usually be tolerated and no further problems noted. Imperforate anus is associated (like tracheoesophageal fistula) with other anomalies—vertebral, renal, cardiac, limb. The other conditions usually carry an excellent prognosis after surgical repair.

4. ABDOMINAL WALL DEFECTS

Omphalocele

Omphaloceles are formed by the incomplete closure of the anterior abdominal wall after return of the midgut. The size of the defect is variable, but usually the omphalocele sac contains some intestine, stomach, liver, and spleen. The abdominal cavity is small and underdeveloped. The umbilical cord can be seen to insert onto the center of the omphalocele sac. There is a high incidence of associated anomalies, including cardiac, other gastrointestinal anomalies, and chromosomal syndromes (trisomy 13). Acute treatment involves covering the defect with sterile warm saline to prevent fluid loss, nasogastric tube decompression, intravenous fluids and glucose, and antibiotics. If the abdominal contents will fit, a primary surgical closure is done. If not, a staged closure is performed, with gradual reduction of the omphalocele into the abdominal cavity and a secondary closure. Postoperatively, third-space fluid losses may be extensive; fluid and electrolyte therapy, therefore, must be carefully monitored.

Gastroschisis

Gastroschisis is a defect in the anterior abdominal wall *lateral* to the umbilicus; there is no covering sac, and the herniated viscera is usually limited to intestine. Furthermore, the intestine has been exposed to amniotic fluid and has a thickened, beefy-red appearance. The herniation is thought to occur as a rupture through an ischemic portion of the abdominal wall. Other than intestinal atresia, associated anomalies are uncommon. Therapy is as described for omphalocoele; however, primary closures can be successfully performed more frequently.

Diaphragmatic Hernia

This congenital malformation consists of herniation of abdominal organs into the hemithorax (usually left) due to a posterolateral defect in the diaphragm. Infants usually present in the delivery room with respiratory distress, cyanosis, decreased breath sounds on the side of the hernia, and shift of the mediastinum to the side opposite the hernia. The infants are often difficult to resuscitate and require early intubation. The rapidity and severity of presentation with respiratory distress is dependent on the degree of pulmonary hypoplasia. The ipsilateral and, to some extent, the contralateral lung are compressed in utero due to the hernia. Treatment is to intubate and ventilate and to decompress the gastrointestinal tract with a nasogastric tube. An intravenous needle should be placed to administer fluids and glucose. A chest x-ray confirms the diagnosis. Emergency surgery is performed after the infant is stabilized to remove abdominal contents from the thorax and to close the diaphragmatic defect. The postoperative course is often complicated by pulmonary hypertension. The mortality rate for this condition is 50%, with survival dependent on the degree of pulmonary hypoplasia in the contralateral lung.

NECROTIZING ENTEROCOLITIS

Necrotizing enterocolitis (NEC) is the most common acquired gastrointestinal emergency in the newborn; it most often affects preterm infants. In term infants, NEC is seen in association with polycythemia, congenital heart disease, and birth asphyxia. The pathogenesis of the disease is multifactorial, related to previous intestinal ischemia, bacterial or viral infection, and immunologic immaturity of the gut. These 3 factors likely contribute to different degrees of disease severity in different infants. Many infants have well-defined risk factors for gut ischemia (eg, asphyxia, difficult respiratory course, presence of an umbilical arterial line). However, in up to 20% of patients, no risk factors for gut ischemia are present. The role of infection is supported by the epidemic nature of the disease.

Diagnosis
The most common presenting sign is abdominal distention. Other signs include vomiting or increased gastric residuals, heme-positive stools, abdominal tenderness, temperature instability, increased apnea and bradycardia, decreased urine output, and poor perfusion. The complete blood count may show increased white blood cell count with a bandemia or, as the disease progresses, an absolute neutropenia. Thrombocytopenia is often seen along with stress-induced hyperglycemia and metabolic acidosis. Diagnosis is confirmed by the presence of pneumatosis intestinalis (air in the bowel wall) on x-ray. There is a spectrum of disease, and milder cases may exhibit only distention of bowel loops with bowel wall edema.

Treatment
(1) Decompression of gut by nasogastric tube.
(2) Maintenance of oxygenation; ventilation if necessary.

(3) Intravenous fluids (colloid and normal saline) to replace third-space gastrointestinal losses. Enough fluid should be given to restore a good urine output.
(4) Broad-spectrum antibiotics.
(5) Close monitoring of vital signs, laboratory data (blood gases, white blood cell count, platelet count, and x-rays).

Indications for surgery are evidence of perforation (free air present on a left lateral decubitus film), a fixed dilatated loop of bowel on serial x-rays, abdominal wall cellulitis, and progressive deterioration despite maximal medical support. All these signs are indicative of necrotic bowel. In surgery, necrotic bowel is removed and ostomies are created. Reanastomosis is performed after the disease is resolved and the infant is bigger (usually > 2 kg). Infants managed either medically or surgically should not be refed until the disease is resolved—normal abdominal examination, resolution of pneumatosis on x-ray—usually a time period of 10–14 days. Nutritional support during this time should be provided by total parenteral nutrition.

Prognosis
Mortality from NEC occurs in 10% of cases. Surgery is needed in less than 25% of cases. Long-term prognosis is determined by the amount of intestine lost. Infants with short bowel require long-term support with intravenous nutrition and, therefore, have very long hospitalizations. Even for those infants, however, the outcome is favorable because of improved parenteral nutrition formulations. Late strictures can occur about 3–6 weeks after initial diagnosis. Some of these strictures are severe enough to require surgical intervention.

Prevention
Oral aminoglycosides and systemic antibiotics given prophylactically do not alter the incidence of NEC. Type of feedings and the method of advancing feedings also do not significantly alter the incidence of disease. The possibility that the administration of oral IgA may decrease the incidence of disease requires more detailed studies. Epidemics can be interrupted by careful measures to control infection.

Abbasi S et al: Long-term assessment of growth, nutritional status, and gastrointestinal function in survivors of necrotizing enterocolitis. *J Pediatr* 1984;**104**:550.

Book LS et al: Clustering of necrotizing enterocolitis. *N Engl J Med* 1977;**297**:984.

Brown EG, Sweet AY: Neonatal necrotizing enterocolitis. *Pediatr Clin North Am* 1982;**29**:1149.

Colombani PM, Cunningham MD: Perinatal aspects of omphalocele and gastroschisis. *Am J Dis Child* 1977;**131**: 1386.

Eibl MM et al: Prevention of necrotizing enterocolitis in low-birth-weight infants by IgA-IgG feeding. *N. Engl J Med* 1988;**319**:1.

Hendren WH, Lillahei CW: Pediatric surgery. *N Engl J Med* 1988;**319:**86.

Kliegman RM, Fanaroff AA: Necrotizing enterocolitis. *N Engl J Med* 1984;**310:**1093.

Kliegman RM, Fanaroff AA: Neonatal necrotizing entero-colitis: A nine year experiment. *Am J Dis Child* 1981; **135:**603.

Ostertag SG et al: Early enteral feeding does not affect the incidence of necrotizing enterocolitis. *Pediatrics* 1986; **77:**275.

Tejani A et al: Growth, health, and development after neo-natal gut surgery: A long term follow-up. *Pediatrics* 1978;**61:**685.

Vidyasagar D, Reyes H: Neonatal surgery. *Clin Perinatol* 1989;**16:**1.

HEMATOLOGIC DISORDERS
(See also Chapter 17.)

BLEEDING DISORDERS

Neonatal coagulation is discussed in detail else-where in the text. Bleeding in the newborn may re-sult from inherited clotting deficiencies (eg, factor VIII deficiency) or acquired disorders—hemorrhagic disease of the newborn (HDN), disseminated intra-vascular coagulation (DIC), liver failure, and throm-bocytopenia.

Hemorrhagic Disease of the Newborn

This disorder is due to the deficiency of the vita-min K-dependent clotting factors (II, VII, IX, X). Bleeding can occur on day 1 but usually occurs on day 2–3 in an otherwise well infant. Sites of bleed-ing include the gastrointestinal tract, umbilical cord, circumcision site, and nose. Bleeding from vitamin K deficiency is more likely to occur in infants of mothers taking anticonvulsants or sodium warfarin. Table 4–16 distinguishes clinical and laboratory fac-tors of HDN, DIC, and bleeding due to hepatic fail-ure. HDN is treated by administering 1 mg of vita-min K. DIC and liver failure are treated by addressing the underlying condition and replacing clotting factors.

Thrombocytopenia

Neonatal thrombocytopenia can be isolated or occur in association with a deficiency of clotting factors (see Table 4–16). The differential diagnosis for thrombocytopenia with distinguishing clinical features is presented in Table 4–17. Treatment of neonatal thrombocytopenia is transfusion of platelets (10 mL/kg of platelets increases the platelet count by approximately 70,000). Indication for transfusion in the term infant is clinical bleeding or a total count

Table 4–16. Features of infants bleeding from hemorrhagic disease of the newborn (HDN), disseminated intravascular coagulation (DIC), or liver failures.

	HDN	DIC	Liver Failure
Clinical	Well infant no prophy-lactic vitamin K	Sick infant; hypoxia, sep-sis, etc	Sick infant; hepatitis, inborn errors of metabo-lism, shock liver
Bleeding	Gastro-intestinal tract, umbili-cal cord, cir-cumcision, nose	Generalized	Generalized
Onset	2–3 d	Anytime	Anytime
Platelet count	Normal	Decreased	Normal or decreased
Prothrombin time (PT)	Prolonged	Prolonged	Prolonged
Partial throm-boplastin time (PTT)	Prolonged	Prolonged	Prolonged
Fibrinogen	Normal	Decreased	Decreased
Factor V	Normal	Decreased	Decreased

Table 4–17. Differential diagnosis of neonatal thrombocytopenia.

Disorder	Clinical Tips
Immune	
Passively acquired anti-body: idiopathic thrombocytopenic purpura, systemic lupus erythematosus, drug-induced	Proper history, maternal thrombocytopenia
Isoimmune sensitization to PLA-1 antigen	Positive antiplatelet antibod-ies in baby's serum, sus-tained rise in platelets by transfusion of mother's platelets
Infections	Sick infants with other signs consistent with infections
Bacterial	
Congenital viral infections	
Syndromes	Congenital anomalies, asso-ciated pancytopenia
Absent radii	
Fanconi's anemia	
Disseminated intravascular coagulation (DIC)	Sick infants, abnormalities of clotting factors
Giant hemangioma	
Thrombosis	Hyperviscous infants, vas-cular catheters
High risk infant with respira-tory distress syndrome, pulmonary hypertension, etc	Isolated decrease in plate-lets is not uncommon in sick infants even in the absence of DIC

less than 10,000–20,000/μL. In the preterm infant at risk for intraventricular hemorrhage, transfusion is indicated for counts less than 40,000–50,000/μL. Isoimmune thrombocytopenia requires transfusion of maternal platelets. In infants born to mothers with idiopathic thrombocytopenic purpura, corticosteroids have improved platelet counts.

Anemia

Anemia can be caused by hemorrhage, hemolysis, or failure to produce red cells. Anemia presenting in the first 24–48 hours of life is due to hemorrhage or hemolysis. Hemorrhage can occur in utero (fetoplacental, fetomaternal, or twin-to-twin), perinatally (cord rupture, placenta previa, incision through placenta at cesarean section) or internally (intracranial hemorrhage, cephalohematoma, ruptured liver or spleen). When the bleeding has been of a chronic nature in utero (eg, fetomaternal), infants are pale at birth but well-compensated, without signs of volume loss. The initial hematocrit is low. Acute bleeding presents with signs of hypovolemia (tachycardia, poor perfusion, hypotension). The hematocrit initially may be normal or decreased but after several hours of equilibration will be decreased. Hemolysis is caused by blood group incompatibilities, enzyme/membrane abnormalities, infection, and DIC. Initial evaluation should include a review of the perinatal history, a determination of the infant's volume status, and a complete physical examination. A Kleihaur Betke test for fetal cells in the mother's circulation should be done on maternal blood. A complete blood count, blood smear, reticulocyte count, and a direct and indirect Coombs should be performed. This simple evaluation should suggest a diagnosis in most infants.

ANEMIA IN THE PREMATURE INFANT

In the premature, the hemoglobin reaches its nadir at approximately 6 weeks and is 2–3 mg/dL lower than that in the term infant. The lower nadir in the premature appears to be the result of a decreased erythropoietin response to the low red cell mass. Symptoms of anemia include poor feeding, lethargy, increased heart rate, poor weight gain, and possibly apnea. The decision to transfuse is based on the presence of clinical symptoms. Transfusion is not indicated in an asymptomatic infant simply because of an arbitrary hematocrit number. Most infants become symptomatic as the hematocrit drops below 25%.

Premature infants are also at risk for a vitamin E deficiency hemolytic anemia. The syndrome presents at 4–6 weeks with a hemoglobin of 7–10 mg/dL, an increased relic count, thrombocytosis, and pedal edema. Infants at risk for this syndrome are those who have received a diet high in polyunsaturated fats, supplemental iron, and no supplemental vitamin E. Prevention is possible through the administration of 25 IU of vitamin E per day.

Supplemental iron should be started in preterm infants at 2–4 months after birth to prevent iron deficiency anemia.

POLYCYTHEMIA

Elevated hematocrits occur in 2–5% of live births. Although 50% of polycythemic infants are appropriate for gestational age, the proportion of polycythemic infants is greater in the SGA and LGA populations. Causes of increased hematocrit include (1) twin-twin transfusion, (2) maternal-fetal transfusion, (3) intrapartum transfusion from the placenta; associated with fetal distress, and (4) chronic intrauterine hypoxia (SGA infants, LGA infants of diabetic mothers).

The consequence of polycythemia is hyperviscosity since the major factor influencing blood viscosity in infants is red cell mass. Hyperviscosity decreases effective perfusion of the capillary beds of the microcirculation. Clinical symptomatology can be related to any organ system. (Table 4–18). Diagnostic screening can be done by measuring a capillary (heel stick) hematocrit. If the value is greater than 70%, a peripheral venous hematocrit should be measured. Values greater than 70% at less than 12 hours of age should be considered consistent with hyperviscosity. After 12 hours of age, values greater than 65% should be considered diagnostic.

Treatment for the acute symptoms is recommended for symptomatic infants. Treatment for asymptomatic infants based strictly on hematocrit is controversial. Definitive treatment is accomplished by an isovolemic partial exchange with 5% albumin. The amount to exchange is calculated using the following formula:

$$\frac{\text{Peripheral venous hematocrit} - \text{Desired hematocrit}}{\text{Peripheral venous hematocrit}} \times \text{Blood volume per kg} \times \text{Body weight}$$

Blood is withdrawn at a steady rate from an umbilical venous line while the replacement solution is infused at the same rate through a peripheral IV over 30–40 minutes. Desired hematocrit value is 50–55%; desired blood volume is 80 mL/kg.

Follow-up studies in infants with hyperviscosity show that at one and 2 years of age they demonstrate more motor problems, more abnormalities on neurologic examination, and more speech delays than do controls, with subtle deficits persisting through early school age. Partial exchange transfusions may slightly decrease the rate of neurologic sequelae, but the procedure does seem to increase the risk of necrotizing enterocolitis and other gastrointestinal symptoms acutely.

Table 4–18. Organ-related symptoms of hyperviscosity.

Central nervous system
  Irritability, jitteriness, seizures, lethargy
Cardiopulmonary
  Respiratory distress, secondary to congestive heart failure, or persistent pulmonary hypertension
Gastrointestinal
  Vomiting, heme-positive stools, distension, necrotizing enterocolitis
Renal
  Decreased urine output, renal vein thrombosis
Metabolic
  Hypoglycemia
Hematologic
  Hyperbilirubinemia, thrombocytopenia

Andrew M, Kelton J: Neonatal thrombocytopenia. *Clin Perinatol* 1984;**11**:359.

Barnard DR: Inherited bleeding disorders in the newborn infant. *Clin Perinatol* 1984;**11**:309.

Black VD, Lubchenco LO: Neonatal polycythemia and hyperviscosity. *Pediatr Clin North Am* 1982;**29**:1137.

Black VD et al: Developmental and neurologic sequelae of neonatal hyperviscosity syndrome. *Pediatrics* 1982; **69**:426.

Black VD et al: Gastrointestinal injury in polycythemic term infants. *Pediatrics* 1985;**76**:225.

Black VD et al: Neonatal hyperviscosity: Association with lower achievement and IQ scores at school age. *Pediatrics* 1989;**83**:662.

Black VD et al: Neonatal hyperviscosity: Randomized study of effect of partial plasma exchange transfusion on long-term outcome. *Pediatrics* 1985;**75**:1048.

Brown MS et al: Decreased response of plasma immunoreactive erythropoietin to available oxygen in anemia of prematurity. *J Pediatr* 1984;**105**:793.

Dallman PR: Erythropoietin and the anemia of prematurity. *J Pediatr* 1984;**105**:756.

Lane PA, Hathaway WE: Vitamin K in infancy. *J Pediatr* 1985;**106**:351.

O'Connor ME, Addiego JE: Use of oral vitamin K to prevent hemorrhagic disease of the newborn infant. *J Pediatr* 1986;**108**:616.

Oski FA, Naiman JL (editors): *Hematologic Problems in the Newborn.* Saunders, 1982.

Ramamurthy RS, Berlanga M: Postnatal alteration in hematocrit and viscosity in normal and polycythemic infants. *J Pediatr* 1987;**110**:929.

Schmidt B et al: Neonatal thrombotic disease: Prevention, diagnosis, and treatment. *J Pediatr* 1988;**113**:407.

Shannon KM et al: Circulating erythroid progenitors in the anemia of prematurity. *N Engl J Med* 1987;**317**:728.

Stockman JA et al: The anemia of prematurity. *N Engl J Med* 1977;**296**:647.

Stockman JA et al: Anemia of prematurity: Determinants of the erythropoietin response. *J Pediatr* 1984;**105**:786.

Wiswell TE et al: Neonatal polycythemia: Frequency of clinical manifestations and other associated findings. *Pediatrics* 1986;**78**:26.

Zipursky A et al: Oral vitamin E supplementation for the prevention of anemia in premature infants: A controlled trial. *Pediatrics* 1987;**79**:61.

METABOLIC DISORDERS

HYPOGLYCEMIA

The glucose concentration of the newborn infant at birth reflects maternal glucose concentration. The cord blood glucose concentration is approximately 15 mg/dL less than the maternal glucose concentration over a very wide range of maternal glucose concentrations. The cord blood glucose measurement is useful in all infants who are at risk of neonatal hypoglycemia: infants of diabetic mothers, SGA infants, erythroblastotic infants, and infants "stressed" by birth asphyxia, hypoxia, etc. The cord blood glucose allows a more precise interpretation of the first glucose concentration obtained in the nursery, because the clinician can then estimate the glucose clearance and arrive at a more precise estimate of the glucose intake required by the infant.

Glucose concentration normally decreases in all infants in the immediate postnatal period. Although a small number of term, normal newborns have glucose concentrations below 30–40 mg/dL, this phenomenon is quite rare; the range of 30–40 mg/dL is usually used for definition of hypoglycemia. By 3 hours of age, the glucose concentration in normal, term babies stabilizes between 50 and 80 mg/dL. After the first few hours of life, concentrations below 40 mg/dL should be considered abnormal.

The 2 most commonly encountered groups of newborn infants at high risk for neonatal hypoglycemia are infants of diabetic mothers (IDM) and infants with intrauterine growth retardation (IUGR).

Infant of a Diabetic Mother

The IDM baby represents an example of an infant with abundant carbon stores in the form of glycogen and fat who develops hypoglycemia because of an imbalance in insulin-glucagon secretion due to hyperinsulinemia from islet cell hyperplasia. In addition, there are other tissue sites that grow abnormally in utero, probably as a consequence of increased flow of nutrients (carbohydrates, amino acids, and fats) from the maternal circulation. The result is a macrosomic infant who is at increased risk for trauma (bruising, fractures, nerve root injuries, etc) during delivery. Other problems related to the in utero metabolic environment include a cardiomyopathy (asymmetric septal hypertrophy), which can present either as cardiac failure or as respiratory distress, and, more rarely, microcolon, which presents as a low intestinal obstruction. IDMs are also at increased risk for congenital anomalies likely related to first-trimester glucose control. Other neonatal problems include a hypercoagulable state and an increased risk for polycythemia, a combination that predisposes the infant to large venous thromboses. Finally, these infants are somewhat immature for their gestational age and are at increased risk for hyaline membrane disease, hypocalcemia, and hyperbilirubinemia.

Intrauterine Growth Retardation

The infant with intrauterine growth retardation (IUGR) has very little carbon stores in the form of glycogen and body fat and, therefore, is prone to hypoglycemia despite relatively appropriate endocrine adjustments to birth. In addition to problems with hypoglycemia (particularly in the very preterm SGA infant), marked hyperglycemia and a transient diabetes mellitus like syndrome occasionally may develop. These problems can usually be handled by adjusting glucose intake, although insulin is sometimes needed transiently.

Other Causes of Hypoglycemia

In addition, hypoglycemia can be found with other disorders associated with islet cell hyperplasia (Beckwith's syndrome [macroglossia, omphalocele, macrosomia], erythroblastosis fetalis, nesidioblastosis), inborn errors of metabolism (leucine sensitivity, glycogen storage disease, and galactosemia), and endocrine disorders (panhypopituitarism and other deficiencies of counterregulatory hormones). It may also occur as a complication of birth asphyxia, hypoxia secondary to cardiorespiratory disease, or other stresses, including bacterial and viral sepsis.

Diagnosis

Infants can present with a variety of clinical signs of neonatal hypoglycemia. Unfortunately, they are relatively nonspecific and are usually quite mild, including lethargy, irritability, poor feeding, and regurgitation. More severe symptoms are cardiorespiratory distress, apnea, and seizures. As the symptoms become more severe, one may find more signs associated with catecholamine release, including pallor, sweating, cool extremities, and an increased heart rate. Cardiac failure has been found when hypoglycemia has been severe, particularly in IDM babies with a cardiomyopathy. Infants with hyperinsulinemic states can also experience the onset of hypoglycemia very early (within the first 30–60 minutes of life).

Glucose concentration can be measured by one of the commercially available screening techniques that rely on a test strip method done on a drop of peripheral blood obtained by heel stick. All infants at risk should be screened, including IDMs who are not macrosomic and whose mothers have maintained good control of diabetes. In addition, all low or borderline values should be supplemented by direct measurement of blood glucose concentration determined with a glucose analyzer. There is far too great a variance in results obtained by the test strip meth-

ods to rely upon these alone in following the high-risk groups. It is important to continue surveillance of glucose concentration until the baby has been on full milk feedings for a 24-hour period. Relapse of hypoglycemia thereafter is very unlikely, but milk feedings constitute a low-glucose, high-fat intake; therefore, babies moving to full milk feedings are sustaining glucose concentration by a relatively high rate of gluconeogenesis. Because it is not certain that individual infants in the high-risk groups are capable of sustaining such a rate of gluconeogenesis, glucose surveillance must continue in this weaning period.

Infants with persistent hypoglycemia requiring intravenous glucose infusions for more than 5 days should be evaluated for less common causes of hypoglycemia. This workup should include evaluation for inborn errors of metabolism, hyperinsulinemic states, and deficiencies of counterregulatory hormones.

Treatment

Therapy is based on provision of glucose either enterally or intravenously. Suggested guidelines for treatment are presented in Table 4–19. It is also im-

Table 4–19. Hypoglycemia: suggested therapeutic regimens.

Screening Test	Presence of Symptoms	Action
Test strip 20–40 mg/dL	None	Confirm with blood glucose; if the infant is alert and vigorous, feed; follow frequent test strips. If the baby continues after 1 or 2 feeds to have test strips < 40 mg/dL, provide intravenous glucose at 6 mg/kg/min.
Test strip < 40 mg/dL	Present	Confirm with blood glucose; provide bolus[1] of 10% dextrose in water (D10W) followed by an infusion of 6 mg/kg/min.
Test strip < 20 mg/dL	+/–	Confirm with blood glucose; provide bolus[1] of D10W followed by an infusion of 6 mg/kg/min. If IV access cannot be obtained immediately, an umbilical venous line should be utilized.

In all cases, therapy should be instituted while confirmatory blood glucose results are awaited.
[1]Calculate bolus as follows:

10% glucose = 100 mg/mL
Assume glucose space of one-third of body weight
In 1000-g infant with blood sugar of 20:
Glucose space = $1000 \times 1/3 = 330$ mL
Desired glucose = 70
Less actual glucose = 20
Load = 50 mg/100 mL
$50 \times 3.3 = 165$ mg = 1.6 mL of 10% glucose.

portant to note that in hyperinsulinemic states rapid boluses of glucose are to be avoided. After initial correction with a bolus of D10W, 2 mL/kg, glucose infusion should be gradually increased as needed from a starting rate of 6 mg/kg/min. Finally, in both IDM and SGA babies, those with high hematocrits and hypoglycemia are most likely to show clinical signs of hypoglycemia. In such infants, both the hypoglycemia and polycythemia should be treated.

Prognosis

Prognosis of hypoglycemia is good if therapy is prompt. Central nervous system sequelae are seen in infants with neonatal seizures due to hypoglycemia.

Cowett RM, Stern L: Carbohydrate homeostasis in the fetus and newborn. Chap 30, in: *Neonatology,* 3rd ed. Avery GB (editor). Lippincott, 1987.

Fluge G: Neurological findings at follow-up in neonatal hypoglycemia. *Acta Paediatr Scand* 1975;**64:**629.

Hay WW Jr, Sparks JW: Placental fetal and neonatal carbohydrate metabolism. *Clin Obstet Gynecol* 1985;**28:** 473.

Lucas A et al: Adverse neurodevelopmental outcome of moderate neonatal hypogycemia. *Br Med J* 1988;**297:** 1304.

Pildes RS, Pyati S: Hypoglycemia and hyperglycemia in < 1000 gm infants. *Clin Perinatol* 1986;**13:**351.

Srinivasan G et al: Plasma glucose values in normal neonates: A new look. *J Pediatr* 1986;**109:**114.

HYPOCALCEMIA

Calcium concentration in the immediate newborn period decreases in all newborn infants. The concentration in fetal plasma is higher than that of the neonate or adult. Hypocalcemia is usually defined as a total serum concentration less than 7–8 mg/dL (equivalent to a calcium activity of 3–3.5 meq/L). In general, the higher range of 8 mg/dL is used as a cutoff for term infants and the lower of 7 mg/dL in preterm infants.

Diagnosis

The clinical signs of hypocalcemia and hypocalcemic tetany include a high-pitched cry, jitteriness, tremulousness (repetitive movement of the peripheral muscles), and seizures. ECG signs are primarily directed at recognition of an increased QT interval.

Hypocalcemia tends to occur at 2 different times in the neonatal period. The first peak occurs during the first 2 days of life, and the second toward the end of the first or second week of life. Early-onset hypocalcemia has been associated with infants of diabetic mothers, sepsis of the newborn, perinatal asphyxia, prematurity, and maternal hyperparathyroidism. Late-onset hypocalcemia has been reported in children receiving modified cow's milk, which has a high content of phosphorus. Mothers in third-world countries often suffer from vitamin D deficiency, which can also contribute to late-onset hypocalcemia.

Treatment

A. Oral Calcium Therapy: The oral administration of calcium salts is a preferred method of treatment because it avoids the potential complications of a slough from calcium solutions that infiltrate subcutaneously. In most infants with early-onset hypocalcemia who do not have frank tetany or seizures, oral administration can be successfully carried out. Calcium in the form of calcium gluconate can be given either as a dilute solution or added to formula feedings several times a day. A dose of 0.5–1 g/kg/d provides approximately 45–90 mg of elemental calcium per kilogram per day. If a 10% solution of calcium gluconate is used, the dose is 5–10 mL/kg/d given in divided doses every 4 or every 6 hours.

B. Intravenous Calcium Therapy: Intravenous calcium therapy is usually needed for infants with frank "tetany of the newborn" and certainly for infants with seizures associated with hypocalcemia. A number of precautions must be observed when calcium gluconate is given intravenously. The infusion must be given slowly, and it is helpful to dilute with an equal volume of 5% glucose. The infusion is administered slowly so that there is no sudden increase in calcium concentration in blood entering the right atrium, which would otherwise cause severe bradycardia and even cardiac arrest. Furthermore, the clinician must observe very carefully and terminate infusion if there is any infiltrate of the intravenous infusions: calcium in the soft tissues can cause a necrosis of the skin and underlying tissues. The intravenous administration of 10% calcium gluconate is usually given as a bolus of 2 mL/kg over approximately 10–20 minutes, followed by a continuous infusion (0.5–1 gm/kg/d) that is slowly tapered over a number of days. (*Note:* Calcium salts cannot be added to intravenous solutions that contain sodium bicarbonate because they precipitate as calcium carbonate.)

Prognosis

The prognosis is good for neonatal seizures entirely caused by hypocalcemia that is promptly treated.

Brown DR, Tsang RC, Chen I: Oral calcium supplementation in premature and asphyxiated neonates. *J Pediatr* 1976;**89:**973.

Shaw JC: Evidence for defective skeletal mineralization in low-birthweight infants: The absorption of calcium and fat. *Pediatrics* 1976;**57:**16.

Tsang RC, Donovan EF, Steichen JJ: Calcium physiology and pathology in the neonate. *Pediatr Clin North Am* 1976;**23:**611.

Venkataraman PS et al: Early neonatal hypocalcemia in very low birth weight infants: High incidence, early onset and refractoriness to supraphysiologic doses of 1,25-dihydroxyvitamin D$_3$. *Am J Dis Child* 1986;**140:**1004.

INFANTS OF MOTHERS WHO ABUSE DRUGS

The problem of newborn infants born to mothers abusing drugs is increasing in all parts of the country. The most common forms of abuse include smoking and its repercussions upon fetal growth and alcohol, marihuana, narcotic, and cocaine abuse. Because these mothers frequently abuse many drugs during pregnancy, it is often difficult to pinpoint which drug may be causing the morbidity seen in a newborn infant. The history of drug abuse is unreliable; because HIV screening is important in mothers who are using drugs intravenously, the physicians caring for the mother must be aware of the importance not only of the history but also of the physical examination of the mother.

NARCOTICS

Diagnosis

The withdrawal signs in infants born to mothers who are addicted to heroin or who have been on maintenance methadone programs are similar. Clinical manifestations begin early, usually within the first day or two of life. Symptoms are quite characteristic: irritability and hyperactivity, increased tremors, a high-pitched cry, excessive hunger and salivation, sweating, yawning, sneezing, nasal stuffiness, fist sucking, temperature instability, and regurgitation. More severely affected infants may have seizures, vomiting, and diarrhea, as well as respiratory distress in the form of tachypnea. The clinical picture characterized by excessive activity and irritability is typical enough to suggest a diagnosis even if the maternal history of drug abuse has not been obtained. The infants are often small for gestational age. Confirmation should be obtained by screening tests in the urine of the mother and infant. The clinical findings in infants born to methadone-maintained mothers seem to be, if anything, more severe and prolonged.

Treatment

Careful observation of the infant is a requirement. Supportive treatment includes swaddling the infant and providing a quiet, low-light environment. In general, specific treatment should be avoided unless the symptoms and morbidity in the infant warrant it. There is no single drug that has been uniformly effective, and the first choice varies among nurseries. The drugs that have been used include phenobarbital at an initial loading dose of 15–20 mg/kg intramuscularly, followed by a maintenance dose of 5 mg/kg/d in 2 divided doses usually given orally.

Paregoric and diazepam have also been used, although these authors prefer phenobarbital because of its safety and predictability of effect. Phenobarbital blood levels should be obtained in the more severely affected infants to ensure that the concentration of the drug remains within the therapeutic range. The treatment can then be tapered over some days, although some treatment may be necessary for weeks following delivery. Both handling and procedures in the nursery should be kept to a minimum. As an alternative, methadone has been used, particularly in the babies born to methadone-maintained mothers.

Prognosis

The prognosis is reasonably good in the immediate newborn period, although there is still a mortality rate in the more severe cases. Careful evaluation of the family situation must be made in each case. The long-term outcome in these children has not been encouraging, although it is not clear that the effects of the drug or drug withdrawal are directly responsible. Rather, the disorganized family and social situation in which drug abuse occurs is thought to play a greater role.

Infants of narcotic abusers have an increased risk of sudden infant death syndrome.

ALCOHOL

Diagnosis

Alcohol abuse, a common problem in the United States, unfortunately occurs in teenagers as well as in older women. The effects on the fetus and newborn are roughly proportionate to the degree of ethanol abuse. Fetal growth and development are adversely affected (intrauterine growth retardation and various dysmorphic features), and infants suffer withdrawal similar to that caused by narcotic abuse. The dysmorphic features include intrauterine growth retardation, short palpebral fissures, microcephaly, and a variety of anomalies, including cardiac anomalies and joint defects. The quoted congenital anomaly rate based on an alcohol intake equivalent to the consumption of 2 mixed drinks per day is 10%, rising to as high as 40% with much larger alcohol intakes per day.

Treatment

In addition to management of withdrawal, which should follow the treatment prescribed for narcotic withdrawal, it is imperative that the mother be encouraged to enter a program designed to cope with alcoholism. The infants themselves also commonly have the typical problems of infants who are small for gestational age, ie, hypoglycemia, polycythemia, and difficulty in maintaining body temperature.

Prognosis

The postnatal growth of infants with fetal alcohol

syndrome has been shown to be delayed. There is evidence of significant mental retardation in those most severely affected and hyperactivity, which contributes to school problems.

TOBACCO SMOKING

Smoking has been shown to have a significant impact on the growth rate of the fetus. The more the mother smokes, the greater the degree of intrauterine growth retardation. This is the only well-established complication of maternal smoking, and, of course, there is no treatment other than that prescribed for problems of IUGR infants in general. Prevention by education of expectant mothers is the key. Some studies have suggested an increase in obstetric complications such as abruptio placentae, placenta previa, and prematurity, although those issues remain controversial. It is important to recognize that multiple drug abuse applies to this category as well; that is, smokers tend to use alcohol and caffeine more than nonsmokers, and the potential interaction of these 3 factors on fetal growth and development must be considered.

COCAINE

Cocaine abuse is a growing problem in medicine. Its use has increased greatly; moreover, cocaine is often used in association with other drugs. Specific consequences of cocaine abuse are not yet well defined, but a number of associations have been noted. The most catastrophic effects include abruptio placentae in the mother and central nervous system infarcts in the baby. Other described complications include premature labor, intrauterine growth retardation, anomalies of the genitourinary system, and irritability of the central nervous system. In the presence of a maternal history of cocaine, a toxicology screen on the infant should be done, and the infant should be observed closely for drug effect and neurologic signs suggestive of an infarct (eg, seizures). As with the abuse of any drug, it is important to evaluate the social situation and the ability of parents to care for the child properly on discharge from the hospital.

OTHER DRUGS

There are 2 categories under which drugs and their effects on the newborn should be considered. In the first category are drugs to which the fetus is exposed because of exposure to the mother. Many times, these are drugs prescribed for therapy of maternal conditions. The human placenta is relatively permeable, particularly to lipophilic solutes. Thus, most drugs cross the placenta fairly rapidly. The effects on the fetus depend on the drug used. General anesthetics by and large cross the placenta rapidly, and if effective anesthesia is achieved in the mother, the baby will, in fact, be anesthetized and show these effects at birth. Generally, however, the anesthesia does not present much of a management problem if it is recognized. The babies are sleepy but recover quickly as the drug is excreted.

In the second category are drugs that the infant acquires from the mother during breast-feeding. Generally, most drugs taken by the mother either inadvertently or for therapy achieve appreciable concentrations in breast milk. In most instances, however, they do not present a problem to the infant. If the drug is one that could have adverse effects on the baby, timing breast-feeding to coincide with trough concentrations in the mother may be useful.

Berkowitz RL, Coustan DR, Mochizuki TK: *Handbook for Prescribing Medications During Pregnancy.* Little, Brown, 1981.

Briggs GG et al: *Drugs in Pregnancy and Lactation: A Reference Guide to Fetal and Neonatal Risk.* Williams & Wilkins, 1983.

Chasnoff IJ et al: Cocaine use in pregnancy. *N Engl J Med* 1985;**313:**666.

Chasnoff IJ et al: Perinatal cerebral infarction and maternal cocaine use. *J Pediatr* 1986;**108:**456.

Chasnoff IJ et al: Temporal patterns of cocaine use in pregnancy. *JAMA* 1989;**261:**1741.

Clarren SK, Smith DW: The fetal alcohol syndrome. *N Engl J Med* 1978;**298:**1063.

Committee on Drugs, American Academy of Pediatrics: Psychotropic drugs in pregnancy and lactation. *Pediatrics* 1982;**69:**241.

Davis PJM, Partridge JW, Storrs CN: Alcohol consumption in pregnancy: How much is safe? *Arch Dis Child* 1982;**57:**940.

Doberczak TM et al: Neonatal neurologic and electroencephalographic effects of intrauterine cocaine exposure. *J Pediatr* 1988;**113:**354.

Frank DA: Cocaine use during pregnancy: Prevalence and correlates. *Pediatrics* 1988;**82:**888.

Herlinger RA, Kandall SR, Vaughn NG: Neonatal seizures associated with narcotics withdrawal. *J Pediatr* 1977; **91:**638.

Lifshitz MH et al: Factors affecting head growth and intellectual function in children of drug addicts. *Pediatrics* 1985;**75:**269.

Meyer MB, Tonascia JA: Maternal smoking, pregnancy complications, and perinatal mortality. *Am J Obstet Gynecol* 1977;**128:**494.

Mills JL et al: Maternal alcohol consumption and birth weight: How much drinking during pregnancy is safe? *JAMA* 1984;**252:**1875.

Naeye RL: Abruptio placentae and placenta previa: Frequency, perinatal mortality, and cigarette smoking. *Obstet Gynecol* 1980;**55:**701.

Neumann LL, Cohen SN: The neonatal narcotic withdrawal syndrome: A therapeutic challenge. *Clin Perinatol* 1975;**2:**99.

Pedreira FA et al: Involuntary smoking and incidence of

respiratory illness during the first year of life. *Pediatrics* 1985;**75**:594.

Rantakallio P: The effect of maternal smoking on birth weight and the subsequent health of the child. *Early Hum Dev* 1978;**2**:371.

Rosett HL et al: Patterns of alcohol consumption and fetal development. *Obstet Gynecol* 1983;**61**:539.

Rothstein P, Gould JB: Born with a habit: Infants of drug-addicted mothers. *Pediatr Clin North Am* 1974;**21**:307.

Saxton DW: The behaviour of infants whose mothers smoke in pregnancy. *Early Hum Dev* 1978;**2**:363.

Streissguth AP, Herman CS, Smith DW: Intelligence, behavior, and dysmorphogenesis in the fetal alcohol syndrome: A report on 20 patients. *J Pediatr* 1978;**92**:363.

Tennes K, Blackard C: Maternal alcohol consumption, birth weight, and minor physical anomalies. *Am J Obstet Gynecol* 1980;**138**:774.

Wilson GS, Desmond MM, Wait RB: Follow up of methadone treated and untreated narcotic dependent women and their infants: Health, developmental and social implications. *J Pediatr* 1981;**98**:716.

Zuckerman B et al: Effects of maternal marijuana and cocaine use on fetal growth. *N Engl J Med* 1989;**320**:762.

RENAL DISORDERS

Renal function is dependent on postconceptual age. The glomerular filtration rate (GFR) is 20 mL/min/1.73 m^2 in term neonates and 10–13 mL/min/1.73 m^2 in infants 28–30 weeks of gestation. The velocity of maturation after birth is also dependent on postconceptual age. Creatinine can be used as a clinical marker of GFR. Values over the first month of life are shown in Table 4–20. The ability to concentrate urine and retain sodium is also dependent on gestational age. Infants less than 28–30 weeks of gestation are particularly compromised in this respect and, if not observed carefully, can become quite dehydrated and hyponatremic. Preterm infants also have an increased bicarbonate excretion and have a low tubular maximum for glucose (approximately 120 mg/dL).

RENAL FAILURE

Renal failure is most commonly seen in the setting of birth asphyxia, hypovolemic shock, and bacterial sepsis. The normal rate of urine flow is 1–3 mL/kg/hr. After a hypoxic or ischemic insult, acute tubular necrosis may ensue. Typically, there are 2–3 days of anuria or oliguria associated with hematuria, proteinuria, and a rise in serum creatinine. The period of anuria is followed by a period of polyuria and then gradual recovery. During the polyuric phase, excessive urine sodium and bicarbonate losses may be

Table 4–20. Normal values of serum creatinine (mg/dL).

Gestational Age at Birth (Weeks)	Postnatal Age	
	0–2 d	28 d
< 28	1.2	0.7
29–32	1.1	0.6
33–36	1.1	0.45
33–42	0.8	0.3

seen. The initial step in management is restoration of the infant's volume status with colloid as needed. Then, restriction of fluids to insensible water loss (40–60 mL/kg/d) without added electrolytes, plus milliliter-for-milliliter urine replacement, should be instituted. Serum and urine electrolytes and body weights should be followed frequently. These measures should be continued through the polyuric phase. After urine output has been reestablished, urine replacement should be decreased to a ratio of between three-fourths and one-half milliliter for each milliliter of urine output to see if the infant has regained normal function. If so, the infant can be returned to maintenance fluids. Finally, many of these infants do experience fluid overload and should be allowed to diurese back to birthweight. Hyperkalemia, which may lead to a dysrhythmia, may occur in this situation despite the lack of added intravenous potassium. When the serum potassium reaches 7–7.5, an infusion of insulin and glucose (1 unit of insulin for every 3 g of glucose administered) should be started. If an arrythmia occurs, calcium gluconate (100 mg/kg), followed by a glucose and insulin infusion, should be administered. Peritoneal dialysis is rarely, if ever, needed for the management of neonatal acute renal failure.

URINARY TRACT ANOMALIES

Abdominal masses in the newborn are most frequently due to renal enlargement. Most common is a multicystic/dysplastic kidney; congenital hydronephrosis is second in frequency. An ultrasound examination is the first step in diagnosis. In pregnancies with oligohydramnios, renal agenesis or obstruction due to posterior urethral values should be considered. Syndromes with multiple anomalies or chromosomal abnormalities frequently include renal abnormalities.

RENAL VEIN THROMBOSIS

Renal vein thrombosis (RVT) is seen most frequently in infants of diabetic mothers and in the context of dehydration and polycythemia. Of particular concern is the IDM infant, prone to hypercoagulability, who is also polycythemic. If fetal distress is superimposed on these problems, prompt reduction in blood viscosity is indicated. Thrombosis usually begins in intrarenal venules and can extend into larger veins. Clinically, there is evidence of a new renal mass, usually unilateral, and blood and protein in the urine. With bilateral RVT, anuria ensues. Diagnosis can be confirmed with an ultrasound examination of the kidneys. Treatment involves correcting the predisposing condition and systemic heparinization for the thrombosis. Prognosis is usually good with return of normal renal function. However, some infants will develop systemic hypertension.

Anand SK: Acute renal failure in the neonate. *Pediatr Clin North Am* 1982;**29**:791.
Aperia A, Zetterstrom R: Renal control of fluid homeostasis in the newborn infant. *Clin Perinatol* 1982;**9**:523.
Guignard J-P: Renal function in the newborn infant. *Pediatr Clin North Am* 1982;**29**:777.
Guignard J-P, John EG: Renal function in the tiny, premature infant. *Clin Perinatol* 1986;**13**:377.
Schmidt B et al: Neonatal thrombotic disease: Prevention, diagnosis, and treatment. *J Pediatr* 1988;**113**:407.

BRAIN AND NEUROLOGIC DISORDERS

HYPOXIC ISCHEMIA ENCEPHALOPATHY

Hypoxic ischemic brain injury is an important neurologic problem in the perinatal period for both term and preterm infants. In the premature, this encephalopathy is often associated with intraventricular hemorrhage; for this reason, it is difficult in many cases to determine whether neurologic morbidity is due to one or the other cause.

Diagnosis

Prenatal history, including abnormalities in antepartum testing, fetal distress with or without passage of meconium during labor, and low scalp pHs (< 7.2) are important in identifying infants at risk for hypoxic ischemic encephalopathy. Apgar scores, the response of the Apgar scores to resuscitation, the amount of resuscitation needed, and cord acid-base status are other important features to note. Clinical features of hypoxic ischemic encephalopathy progress over time:

(1) Birth–12 hours: decreased level of consciousness, poor tone, decreased spontaneous movement, periodic breathing or apnea, and possible seizures.

(2) 12–24 hours: more seizures, apneic spells, jitteriness and weakness.

(3) After 24 hours: decreased level of consciousness, further respiratory abnormalities (progressive apnea), onset of brain stem signs (oculomotor and pupillary disturbances), poor feeding, and hypotonia.

The severity of clinical signs and the length of time the signs persist correlate with the severity of the insult. Other evaluations helpful in assessing severity include EEG, technetium scan, CT scan, and evoked responses. As experience in the use of magnetic resonance imaging is gained, this technique may also prove useful. Markedly abnormal EEGs with voltage suppression and slowing evolving into a burst-suppression pattern are seen with severe clinical symptomatology. On technetium scans, ·increased uptake of the radionuclide on delayed (2–4 hours) images is suggestive of tissue injury. A CT scan early in the course may demonstrate diffuse hypodensity, whereas later scans may demonstrate brain atrophy and focal ischemic lesions. Visual and somatosensory evoked potentials provide information about function. In most instances, it is not necessary to use all these tests, but some are obtained to confirm an ominous prognosis.

Treatment

The critical management issue in infants with hypoxic-ischemic encephalopathy is to maintain adequate delivery of oxygen to the already injured brain by supporting a normal Pao_2 and blood pressure. Glucose should be administered to maintain a normal serum glucose. Modest fluid restriction should be maintained to avoid exacerbating cerebral edema, and seizures should be controlled with phenobarbital and other anticonvulsants as needed. No other specific therapy (eg, steroids or osmotic agents) has been shown to be helpful in improving the outcome in hypoxic ischemic encephalopathy.

Prognosis

Fetal heart rate tracings, cord pH, and 1- and 5-minute Apgar scores are not very precise predictors of long term outcome. Apgar scores of 0–3 at 5 minutes result in an 8% risk of death in the first year of life and a 1% risk of cerebral palsy among survivors. A 10-minute Apgar of 0–3 predicts death in the first year in 18% of cases and cerebral palsy among survivors in 5%; at 15 minutes, 48% and 9%, respectively; at 20 minutes, 59% and 57%, respectively. The single best predictor of outcome is the severity of clinical hypoxic, ischemic encephalopathy (severe symptomatology carries a 75% chance of death and 100% rate of neurologic sequelae among survivors). The major sequelae include cerebral palsy and mental retardation. Other prognostic features include prolonged seizures refractory to therapy, markedly abnormal EEGs, and CT scans with evidence of major ischemic injury.

INTRACRANIAL HEMORRHAGE

1. SUBDURAL HEMORRHAGE

Subdural hemorrhage is related to birth trauma; the bleeding is caused by tears in the veins that bridge the subdural space. Prospective studies relating incidence to specific obstetric complications are not available.

Three types of hemorrhage occur:

(1) Tentorial laceration with rupture of the straight sinus, vein of Galen, or lateral sinus. This results in an infratentorial bleed and lethal brain stem compression. The only treatment is immediate surgical drainage.

(2) Falx laceration with rupture of the inferior sinus. This hemorrhage is asymptomatic until the blood extends infratentorially, at which time immediate surgical drainage is the only treatment.

(3) The most common site is rupture of superficial cerebral veins with blood over the cerebral convexities. These hemorrhages can be asymptomatic or cause seizures with onset on day 2–3 of life, vomiting, irritability, and lethargy. Associated findings include retinal hemorrhages and a full fontanelle. Diagnosis is confirmed by CT scan. Specific treatment entailing needle drainage of the subdural space is rarely necessary.

The prognosis for the 2 rare types of bleeding is poor; the morbidity rate is high. In the third, more common type of bleeding, most infants survive, with 75% normal on follow-up. Fortunately, because of improved obstetric care, subdural hemorrhages in neonates have become rare altogether.

2. PRIMARY SUBARACHNOID HEMORRHAGE

Primary subarachnoid hemorrhage (SAH) is the most common type of neonatal intracranial hemorrhage. In the term infant, SAH can be related to trauma of delivery, whereas SAH in the preterm infant is seen in association with germinal matrix hemorrhage. Clinically, these hemorrhages can be asymptomatic or present with seizures and irritability on day 2 or, rarely, a massive hemorrhage with rapid downhill course. The seizures associated with SAH are very characteristic—usually brief, with a normal examination interictally. Diagnosis can be suspected on a spinal tap and confirmed with CT scan. Long term follow-up is uniformly good.

3. PERIVENTRICULAR-INTRAVENTRICULAR HEMORRHAGE

Periventricular-intraventricular hemorrhage is a lesion seen almost exclusively in premature infants. The incidence is 25–35% in infants of less than 31 weeks of gestation and 1500 g. Bleeding is most commonly seen in the subependymal germinal matrix (a region of developing glial cells). Bleeding can extend into the ventricular cavity and can also be seen in other areas of the cerebral hemispheres. In addition to prematurity, birth asphyxia, severe respiratory disease, and pneumothorax are also risk factors. The proposed pathogenesis of bleeding is presented in Fig 4–8. The critical event is likely ischemia/reperfusion injury to the capillaries in the germinal matrix or other brain regions.

Diagnosis

Up to 50% of hemorrhages occur at less than 24 hours of age, and virtually all occur by the fourth day. The clinical syndrome ranges from rapid deterioration (coma, hypoventilation, decerebrate posturing, fixed pupils, bulging fontanelle, hypotension, acidosis, acute drop in hematocrit) to a more gradual deterioration with more subtle neurologic changes to absence of any specific physiologic or neurologic signs.

Diagnosis can be confirmed by real-time ultrasound scan. This can be performed whenever bleeding is clinically suspected. If symptoms are absent, routine scanning should be done at 4–7 days in all infants of less than 31 weeks of gestation or in any "sick" infant of 31–35 weeks of gestation. Hemorrhages are graded as follows: (1) Grade I: germinal matrix hemorrhage only (60% of bleeds), (2) Grade II: intraventricular bleeding without ventricular enlargement, (3) Grade III: intraventricular bleeding with ventricular enlargement, and (4) Grade IV: any of the above plus intracerebral hemorrhage.

Follow-up ultrasounds, performed to follow for ventricular enlargement, should be done in infants with small bleeds on the initial scan at 2 weeks of age. In infants with grade III and IV hemorrhages, a follow-up scan should be done within a week of the initial scan. Further scans are dictated by the progression of ventricular enlargement. Scans should also be used in seeking evidence of another ischemic injury, periventricular leukomalacia (cystic changes in the periventricular white matter). This is usually evident by 17–21 days.

Treatment

During the acute hemorrhage, supportive treatment—restoration of volume and hematocrit, oxygenation, and ventilation—should be provided to avoid further cerebral ischemia. Progressive posthemorrhagic hydrocephalus (if it develops) can be controlled by decreasing the production of cerebrospinal fluid (furosemide 1 mg/kg/d, plus acetazolamide, increasing doses from 25–100 mg/kg/d) or by removal of cerebrospinal fluid (daily lumbar punctures). The process is usually self-limited and spontaneously resolves; the placement of a ventriculoperitoneal shunt is usually not needed.

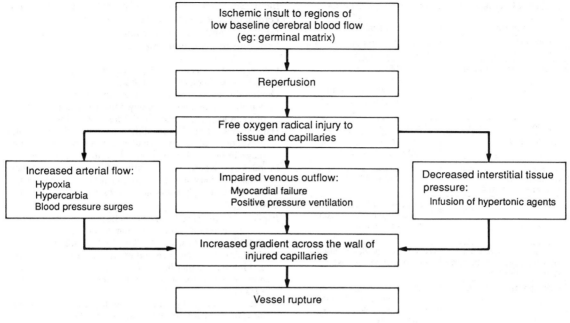

Figure 4–8. Pathogenesis of periventricular-intraventricular hemorrhage.

Interest in the last several years has focused on prevention of this complication of prematurity. Improved obstetric and neonatal care resulting in less asphyxia, improved fluid management, and improved ventilator therapy have decreased the incidence in infants of less than 31 weeks of gestation from 40–50% to 25–35%. The incidence of grade II–IV hemorrhages has also decreased; these formerly constituted 80% of all hemorrhages but now constitute only 40%. Other, less well proved treatments address the initial ischemia reperfusion injury. Agents that appear promising include postnatal vitamin E administration and antenatal phenobarbital.

Prognosis

There is no mortality due to grade I and II hemorrhages, whereas grade III and IV hemorrhages carry a mortality rate of 10–20%. Ventriculomegaly is rarely seen with grade I hemorrhages but is seen in 54–87% of grade II–IV hemorrhages. Very few of these infants will require a ventriculoperitoneal shunt. Long-term neurologic sequelae are seen no more frequently in infants with grade I and II hemorrhages than in preterm infants without bleeding. In infants with grade III and IV hemorrhages, severe sequelae occur in 20–25% of cases, mild sequelae in 35% of cases, and no sequelae in 40% of cases. The presence of severe periventricular leukomalacia and large parenchymal bleeds greatly increases the risk of neurologic sequelae.

SEIZURES

Newborns rarely have well-organized tonic-clonic seizures because of their incomplete cortical organization and a preponderance of inhibitory synapses. The most common type of seizure is characterized by a constellation of findings, including horizontal deviation of the eyes with or without jerking; eyelid blinking or fluttering; sucking, smacking, drooling, and other oral-buccal movements; swimming, rowing, or padding movements; and apneic spells. Strictly tonic or multifocal clonic episodes are also seen.

Diagnosis

Differential diagnosis of neonatal seizures is presented in Table 4–21. Information regarding antenatal drug use and the presence of birth asphyxia or trauma and family history (regarding inherited disorders) should be obtained. Physical examination focuses on neurologic features, other signs of drug withdrawal, concurrent signs of infection, dysmorphic features, and intrauterine growth. Screening workup should include blood glucose, calcium, and electrolytes in all cases. Further workup is dependent on diagnoses suggested by the history and physical examination. If there is any evidence of infection, a spinal tap should be done. Hemorrhages and structural disease of the central nervous system can be addressed with real-time ultrasound and CT scan.

Table 4–21. Differential diagnosis of neonatal seizures.

Diagnosis	Comment
Hypoxic-ischemic encephalopathy	Most common cause (60%); onset in first 24 h
Intracranial hemorrhage	Up to 15% of cases; periventricular-intraventricular hemorrhage, subdural or subarachnoid bleeding
Infection	12% of cases
Hypoglycemia	Small for gestational age, infant of a diabetic mother (IDM)
Hypocalcemia, hypomagnesemia	Infant of low birth weight, IDM
Hyponatremia	Rare, seen with syndrome of inappropriate secretion of antidiuretic hormone (SIADH)
Disorders of amino and organic acid metabolism, hyperammonemia	Associated acidosis, altered level of consciousness
Pyridoxine dependency	Seizures refractory to routine therapy; cessation of seizures after administration of pyridoxine
Developmental defects	Other anomalies, chromosomal syndromes
Drug withdrawal	
No cause found	10% of cases

Metabolic workup should be pursued when appropriate (see Chapter 24). EEG should be done; the presence of spike discharges must be noted and the background wave pattern evaluated.

Treatment

Adequate ventilation and perfusion should be ensured. Hypoglycemia should be treated immediately with a 2 mL/kg infusion of D10W, followed by 6 mg/kg/min of D10W (100 mL/kg/d). Other treatments, eg, calcium or magnesium infusion and antibiotics, are indicated to treat hypocalcemia, hypomagnesemia, and suspected infection. Electrolyte abnormalities should be corrected. Phenobarbital, 20 mg/kg intravenously, should be administered to stop seizures. Supplemental doses of 5 mg/kg can be used if seizures persist, up to a total of 40 mg/kg. In most cases, phenobarbital controls seizures. If seizures continue, therapy with phenytoin, sodium valproate lorazepam, or paraldehyde may be indicated. For refractory seizures, a trial of pyridoxine is indicated.

Prognosis

Outcome is related to the underlying cause of the seizure. The outcomes for hypoxic-ischemic encephalopathy and intracranial hemorrhage have been discussed. In these settings, seizures that are difficult to control carry a poor prognosis for normal development. Seizures due to hypoglycemia, infection of the central nervous system, some inborn errors of metabolism, and developmental defects also have a high rate of poor outcome.

Freeman JM, Nelson KB: Intrapartum asphyxia and cerebral palsy. *Pediatrics* 1988;**82**:240.

Guzzetta F et al: Periventricular intraparenchymal echodensities in the premature newborn: Critical determinant of neurologic outcome. *Pediatrics* 1986;**78**:995.

Hanigan WC et al: Administration of indomethacin for the prevention of periventricular-intraventricular hemorrhage in high-risk neonates. *J Pediatr* 1988;**112**:941.

Morales WJ, Koerter J: Prevention of intraventricular hemorrhage in very low birth weight infants by maternally administered phenobarbital. *Obstet Gynecol* 1986;**68**:295.

Papile LA, Munsick-Bruno G, Schaefer A: The relationship of cerebral intraventricular hemorrhage and early childhood handicaps. *J Pediatr* 1983;**103**:273.

Papile LA et al: Incidence and evolution of subependymal and intraventricular hemorrhage: A study of infants with birth weights less than 1500 grams. *J Pediatr* 1978;**92**:529.

Partridge JC et al: Optimal timing for diagnostic cranial ultrasound in low-birthweight infants: Detection of intracranial hemorrhage and ventricular dilation. *J Pediatr* 1983;**102**:281.

Rose AL, Lombroso CT: Neonatal seizure states: A study of clinical, pathological, and electroencephalographic features in 137 full-term babies with a long-term follow-up. *Pediatrics* 1970;**45**:404.

Sarnat HB, Sarnat MS: Neonatal encephalopathy following fetal distress: A clinical and electroencephalographic study. *Arch Neurol* 1976;**33**:696.

Scher MS, Painter MJ: Controversies concerning neonatal seizures. *Pediatr Clin North Am* 1989;**36**:281.

Shankaran S et al: Outcome after posthemorrhagic ventriculomegaly in comparison with mild hemorrhage without ventriculomegaly. *J Pediatr* 1989;**114**:109.

Shinnar S et al: Interventricular hemorrhage in the premature infant: A changing outlook. *N Engl J Med* 1982;**306**:1464.

Shinnar S et al: Management of hydrocephalus in infancy: Use of acetazolamide and furosemide to avoid cerebrospinal fluid shunts. *J Pediatr* 1985;**107**:31.

Sinha S et al: Vitamin E supplementation reduces frequency of periventricular hemorrhage in very preterm babies. *Lancet* 1987;**1**:466.

Volpe JJ: Intraventricular hemorrhage in the premature infant: Current concepts. *Ann Neurol* 1989;**25**:3,109.

Volpe JJ: Neonatal intraventricular hemorrhage. *N Engl J Med* 1981;**304**:886.

Volpe JJ: *Neurology of the Newborn.* Saunders, 1987.

Williamson WD et al: Survival of low-birth-weight infants with neonatal interventricular hemorrhage: Outcome in the preschool years. *Am J Dis Child* 1983;**137**:1181.

CONGENITAL ANOMALIES

Major congenital malformations are seen in 1.5% of live births and account for 22% of perinatal deaths, 18% of stillbirths, and 27% of neonatal deaths. This topic is discussed in detail in Chapter 34.

Inborn errors of metabolism. The individual errors of metabolism are rare, but collectively all inborn errors of metabolism create a significant clinical problem. These diseases are considered in detail in Chapter 33 but should be entertained in infants that present with sepsislike syndromes, recurrent hypoglycemia, neurologic syndromes (seizures, altered levels of consciousness), and unexplained acidosis.

Batshaw ML et al: New approaches to the diagnosis and treatment of inborn errors of urea synthesis. *Pediatrics* 1981;**68:**290.

Burton BK et al: Inborn errors of metabolism: The clinical diagnosis in early infancy. *Pediatrics* 1987;**79:**359.

Hudak ML et al: Differentiation of transient hyperammonemia of the newborn and urea cycle enzyme defects by clinical presentation. *J Pediatr* 1985;**107:**712.

Jones KL (editor): *Smith's Recognizable Patterns of Human Malformation,* 4th ed. Saunders, 1988.

Regemorter NV et al: Congenital malformations in 10,000 consecutive births in a university hospital: Need for genetic counseling and prenatal diagnosis. *J Pediatr* 1984; **104:**386.

SELECTED REFERENCES

American Academy of Pediatrics: *Guidelines for Perinatal Care,* 2nd ed. American Academy of Pediatrics, 1988.

Avery GB (editor): Neonatology: *Pathophysiology and Management of the Newborn,* 3rd ed. Lippincott, 1987.

Ballard RA (editor): *Pediatric Care of the ICN Graduate.* Saunders, 1988.

Battaglia FC, Meschia G: *An Introduction to Fetal Physiology.* Academic Press, 1988.

Fanaroff AA, Martin RJ (editors): *Neonatal-Perinatal Medicine, Diseases of the Fetus and Infant,* 4th Ed. Mosby, 1987.

Gabbe SG, Niebyl JR, Simpson JL (editors): *Obstetrics: Normal and Problem Pregnancies.* Churchill Livingstone, 1986.

Goldsmith JP, Karotkin EH (editors): *Assisted Ventilation of the Neonate,* 2nd ed. Saunders, 1988.

Hanshaw JB, Dudgeon JA (editors): *Viral Diseases of the Fetus and Newborn,* 2nd ed. Saunders, 1984.

Hastreiter AR (editor): Cardiovascular disease in the newborn. *Clin Perinatol* 1988;**15:**3.

Jones KL (editor): *Smith's Recognizable Patterns of Human Malformation,* 4th ed. Saunders, 1988.

Klaus MH, Fanaroff AA (editors): *Care of the High-Risk Neonate,* 3rd ed. Saunders, 1986.

Lubchenco LO: *The High Risk Infant.* Saunders, 1976.

Merritt TA, Northway WH, Boynton BR (editors): *Bronchopulmonary Dysplasia.* Blackwell, 1988.

Oski FA, Naiman JL (editors): *Hematologic Problems in the Newborn,* 3rd ed. Saunders, 1982.

Remington JS, Klein JO (editors): *Infectious Diseases of the Fetus and Newborn Infant,* 3rd ed. Saunders, 1989.

Stern L (editor): The respiratory system in the newborn. *Clin Perinatol* 1987;**14:**3.

Vidyasagar D (editor): The tiny baby. *Clin Perinatol* 1986;**13:**2.

Volpe JJ (editor): *Neurology of the Newborn,* 2nd ed. Saunders, 1987.

5

Normal Childhood Nutrition & Its Disorders

K. Michael Hambidge, MD, SCD & Nancy F. Krebs, MD, MS

NUTRITIONAL REQUIREMENTS

NUTRITION & GROWTH

The nutrient requirements of the child are influenced substantially by the rate of growth, body composition, and composition of new growth. These factors vary with the age of the subject and are especially important during early postnatal life. Growth rates are higher in early infancy than at any other stage of the life cycle, including the peak of the adolescent growth spurt (Table 5–1). These rates decline rapidly starting in the second month of postnatal life (proportionately later in the premature infant). Because of a more rapid rate of growth in early infancy, nutrient requirements for males are slightly higher than those for females.

Nutrient requirements also depend on body composition. In the adult, the brain, which accounts for only 2% of body weight, contributes 19% to the total basal energy expenditure. In contrast, in a term neonate, the brain accounts for 10% of body weight and for 44% of total energy needs under basal conditions. The liver accounts for a further 20% of basal energy expenditure. Thus, in the young infant basal energy expenditure is relatively high in relation to body weight, and the brain and liver account for a relatively high percentage of basal energy requirement.

Composition of new weight gain is a third factor that influences nutrient requirements and changes the nutrient requirements with age. For example, fat accounts for about 40% of weight gain between birth and 4 months but for only 3% between 24 and 36 months. The corresponding figures for protein are 11% and 21%; for water, 45% and 68%. The high physiologic rate of fat deposition in early infancy has implications not only for energy requirements but also for the optimal composition of infant feeds.

Because of the high nutrient requirements for growth, the body composition, and the relatively large size and continued growth of the brain of the young infant, undernutrition at this stage of life has profound implications. Slowed physical growth rate is an early and prominent sign of undernutrition in the young infant. The limited fat stores of the very young infant mean that energy reserves are unusually restricted. The relatively large size and continued growth of the brain render the central nervous system especially vulnerable to the effects of malnutrition in early postnatal life.

Beaton GH: Nutritional needs during the first year of life: Some concepts and perspectives. *Pediatr Clin North Am* 1985;**32**:275.

Table 5–1. Changes in growth rate, energy required for growth, and body composition in infants and young child.

Age (Mo)	Growth Rate (g/d)			Energy Requirements for Growth (kcal/kg/d)	Body Composition[1]		
	Male	Both	Female		Water	Protein	Fat
0–0.25		0 (See note 2.)			75	11.5	11
0.25–1	40		35	50			
1–2	35		30	25			
2–3	28		25	16			
3–6		20		10	60	11.5	26
6–9		15					
9–12		12					
12–18		8					
18–36		6		2	61	16	21

[1]Data from Fomon SJ (editor): *Infant Nutrition,* 2nd ed. Saunders, 1974.
[2]Birth weight is regained by 10 days. Weight loss of more than 10% of birth weight indicates dehydration or malnutrition.

ENERGY

The major determinants of energy expenditure are basal metabolism, metabolic response to food, physical activity, and growth. In addition, the efficiency of energy utilization may be a significant factor, and thermoregulation may contribute in extremes of ambient temperature if the body is inadequately clothed. Because adequate data on requirements for physical activity in infants and children are not available and individual growth requirements are quite variable, recommendations have been based on calculations of actual intakes by healthy subjects. The distinct recent trend toward lower figures for infants reflects a move away from hypercaloric and possibly inappropriate feeding practices that were in vogue between 1930 and 1970, when the growth data for the National Center for Health Statistics (NCHS) standards were collected. The lower figures approximate recent data for energy intake of healthy breastfed infants up to 6 months of age. After the first 4 years, energy requirements expressed on a body weight basis fall progressively to 40 kcal/kg/d by adolescence. Table 5–2 includes recent recommendations of the World Health Organization (1985), less the 5% added to estimated average intakes. Also included in Table 5–2 (in parentheses) are recent figures for energy requirements of infants and young

children based on actual measurements of energy expenditure together with a calculated increment for growth. Basal energy requirements for the premature infant are approximately 120 kcal/kg/d.

Approximate energy requirements can be calculated by adding 100 kcal/year to a base of 1000 kcal at 1 year of age. Appetite and growth are reliable indices of caloric needs of most healthy children, but intake also depends, to some extent, on the energy density of the formula. Individual energy requirements of normal infants and children vary considerably, and malnutrition and disease add enormously to this variation.

One method of calculating requirements for malnourished patients is to base these on the ideal body weight (IBW, ie, 50th percentile weight for patients length/height-age or 50th percentile weight-for-height) rather than actual weight. Alternatively, the extra requirement for ''catch-up'' growth can be calculated as:

$$\frac{5 \times weight\ (g)\ deficit\ below\ IBW\ kcal/day}{interval\ (days)\ for\ correction\ of\ deficit}$$

where 5 kcal is the energy cost of each gram of new tissue deposited.

These calculations should be adjusted on an ongoing basis according to the growth response.

Fomon SJ, Heird WC (editors): *Energy and Protein Needs During Infancy.* Academic Press, 1986.

Prentice AM et al: Are current dietary guidelines for young children a prescription for overfeeding? *Lancet* 1988; **2:**1066.

World Health Organization: *Report of a Joint FAO/WHO/UNU Expert Consultation: Energy and Protein Requirements.* WHO Tech Rep Ser No. 724, 1985.

PROTEIN

Only amino acids and ammonium compounds are usable as sources of nitrogen in human nutrition. Amino acids are provided by dietary protein. Dietary protein is hydrolyzed by pepsin in the stomach and by pancreatic trypsin digestion in the lumen of the small intestine. This is followed by peptidase digestion by pancreatic and intestinal peptidases. Nitrogen is absorbed from the gut lumen as amino acids and via short-peptide carrier systems. Absorption of nitrogen is more efficient from synthetic diets that contain peptides in addition to amino acids. Some intact proteins can be absorbed in early postnatal life and may result in allergies to these proteins. The liver plays a central role in amino acid metabolism, including regulation of the absorbed amino acids. Excess amino acids, including essential amino acids, are degraded in the liver, except for the branched-chain amino acids, which pass into the systemic circulation and are taken up primarily by muscle. Insulin stimulates this uptake and suppresses muscle

Table 5–2. Recommendations for energy and protein intake.[1]

Age	Energy (kcal/kg/d)		Protein (g/kg/d)
10 d–1 mo	120		(2.5) (See note 3.)
1–2 mo	115	(110) (See note 2.)	(2.25)
2–3 mo	105		
3–4 mo	95	(95)	(2)
4–6 mo	95		1.7
6–12 mo	90	(85)	1.5
1–2 y	105	(85)	1.2
2–3 y	100	(85)	1.1
3–5 y	95		1.1

	Male	Female	
5–7 y	90	85	1
7–10 y	78	67	1

	kcal/day		Male	Female
10–12 y	2200	1950	1	1
12–14 y	2400	2100	1	0.95
14–16 y	2650	2150	0.95	0.90
16–18 y	2850	2150	0.90	0.80

[1]Source: World Health Organization: *Report of a Joint FAO/WHO/UNU Expert Consultation: Energy and Protein Requirements.* WHO Tech Rep Ser No. 724, 1985.
[2]Figures in parentheses in this column are based on actual measurement of energy expenditure. (See Prentice AM et al: Are current dietary guidelines for young children a prescription for overfeeding? *Lancet* 1988;2:1066.)
[3]Recommendations in parentheses in this column are derived from extrapolation from intake of breast-fed infants and from factorial calculations (see reference in note 1, above).

protein catabolism. Protein turnover rates far exceed intake, indicating a marked reutilization of amino acids. However, some of these amino acids released from protein turnover are degraded. After removal of the amino group, the ketoacids are either utilized directly for energy or converted to carbohydrate and fat. Nitrogen is excreted primarily via the kidney as urea.

One hundred percent of body protein plays a role in body structure or function. Because there are no true stores of body protein, a continuous dietary supply is necessary, and any loss of protein decreases functional capacity. In infants and children, optimal growth depends on an adequate dietary protein supply. Relatively subtle effects of protein deficiency are now recognized, especially those affecting tissues with rapid protein turnover rates, such as the immune system and the gastrointestinal mucosa.

In relation to body weight, protein synthesis rates, protein turnover rates, and increments in body protein are exceptionally high in the infant, especially the premature infant. Eighty percent of the dietary protein requirement of the premature infant is required for growth, compared with only 20% in the 1-year-old child. Protein recommendations (Table 5–2) for infants and young children have undergone recent downward revisions. For comparison, calculated protein intakes of the fully breast-fed infant are (age in months in parentheses): 2.05 (0–1), 1.74 (1–2), 1.35 (2–3), 1.18 (3–4), and 1.03 (4–6) g/kg/d. The recommendations for premature infants weighing less than 1500 g is 3.0 g/kg/d or more. When this amount of nitrogen is administered to the infant of low birth weight, protein calories should not exceed 17% of total calories or 3 g protein/100 kcal.

Protein requirements increase in the presence of unusual cutaneous or enteral losses, burns, trauma, and severe sepsis. Requirements also increase during times of catch-up growth accompanying recovery from malnutrition (approximately 0.2 g protein per gram of new tissue deposited). In a young infant during rapid recovery, this could amount to as much as 1–2 g/kg/d of extra requirement. By 1 year of age, this is unlikely to be more than 0.5 g protein/kg/d. Circumstances in which the intake of protein may be deficient include significant low-protein supplementation (eg, fruit juices) in the breast-fed infant, protein malabsorption (cystic fibrosis), or the use of a low-protein weaning food (eg, cassava) as the dietary staple.

The quality of protein depends on its amino acid composition. Infants require 43% of protein as essential amino acids, and children require 36%. Eight essential amino acids cannot be synthesized by adults: isoleucine, leucine, lysine, methionine, phenylalanine, threonine, tryptophan, and valine. Histidine may be added to this list. Cysteine and tyrosine are considered partially essential because their rates of synthesis are limited and may be inadequate in certain circumstances. During early development, rates of synthesis of cysteine, tyrosine, and perhaps taurine do not provide sufficient amounts of these substances. Lack of an essential amino acid leads to weight loss within 1–2 weeks. Wheat and rice are deficient in lysine, and legumes are deficient in methionine. Appropriate mixtures of vegetable protein are therefore necessary to achieve high protein quality.

Because the mechanisms for removal of excess nitrogen are efficient, moderate excesses of protein are not harmful and may help to ensure an adequate supply of certain micronutrients. Adverse effects of excessive protein intakes may include increased calcium losses in urine and, over a life span, increased loss of renal mass. A gross excess of protein may cause elevated blood urea nitrogen, acidosis, hyperammonemia, and, in the premature infant, failure to thrive, lethargy, and fever.

Ashworth A, Millward DJ: Catch-up growth in children. *Nutr Rev* 1986;**44:**157.

LIPIDS

Fats are the main dietary energy source for infants and account for up to 50% of energy in human milk. Over 98% of these fats are in the form of triglycerides, which have an energy density of 9 calories per gram. Fats can be efficiently stored in adipose tissue with a minimal energy cost of storage. This is especially important in the young infant. Fats are required for the absorption of fat-soluble vitamins and for myelination of the central nervous system. Fat also provides essential fatty acids (EFA) necessary for brain development, for phospholipids in cell membranes, and for the synthesis of prostaglandins and leukotrienes. The EFA are polyunsaturated fatty acids derived from linoleic acid (18:2ω6, ie, 18 carbons and 2 double bonds from the methyl [omega] end) and linolenic acid (18:3ω3) by elongation and further desaturation. Among these are arachidonic acid (20:4ω6), which can be obtained from dietary linoleic acid and is present primarily in membrane phospholipids. Oxygenation of arachidonic acid through the lipoxygenase pathway yields leukotrienes and through the cyclooxygenase pathway yields prostaglandins. Important derivatives of linolenic acid are eicosapentaenoic acid (20:6ω3) and docosahexaenoic acid (22:6ω3), which is found in human milk and brain lipids. Visual acuity of formula-fed premature infants is improved with the addition of 20:6ω3, which is not derived readily from 18:3ω3.

Clinical features of EFA ω6 deficiency include growth failure, abnormal scaliness, erythematous skin lesions, decreased capillary resistance, increased fragility of erythrocytes, thrombocytopenia, poor wound healing, and increased susceptibility to infection. Clinical features of deficiency of ω3 fatty acids is less well defined, but dermatitis and neurologic abnormalities—including blurred vision, peripheral neuropathy, and weakness—have been reported. Fatty fish are the best dietary source of ω3 fatty acids. A high intake of fatty fish is associated with a decrease in platelet adhesiveness and decreased inflammatory response.

Up to 8–10% of fatty acids in human milk are polyunsaturated. The majority of these are ω6 series, but long-chain ω3 fatty acids are also present. Breast milk also contains about 40% of fatty acids as monounsaturates, primarily oleic acid (18:1) and up to 10% of total fatty acids as medium-chain triglycerides (MCT). In general, the percentage of calories derived from fat is a little lower in infant formulas than in human milk. Typically, these formulas contain a relatively high percentage of linoleic acid but very little long-chain ω3. The American Academy of Pediatrics recommends that infants receive a minimum of 30% of calories from fat, including a minimum of 1.7% of total calories from ω6 fatty acids and 0.5% of calories from ω3. Providing up to 40–50% of energy requirements as fats is desirable at this age. In contrast, children older than 2 years should derive a maximum of 30% of total calories from fat, and no more than 10% of calories either from saturated fats or polyunsaturated fats.

Triglycerides are hydrolyzed to monoglycerides, free fatty acids, and glycerol in the lumen of the gut. Substantial hydrolysis of triglycerides in milk formulas occurs in the stomach by the action of lingual and gastric lipases. Pancreatic lipases and bile salt levels are relatively low in early postnatal life, but breast milk contains a bile salt–stimulated lipase that is effective in the lumen of the duodenum. Bile salts promote the formation of the colipase-lipase complex, which adheres to the triglycerides prior to hydrolysis. Bile salts also have a major role in the emulsification of fatty acids, allowing their passage through the unstirred water layer to the surface of the mucosal cell. After passage into the enterocyte, long-chain ($\geq$ C12) fatty acids and monoglycerides are reesterified to triglycerides and are packaged with phospholipids, cholesterol, and protein into chylomicrons, which are transported in the lymphatics to the systemic circulation. At the capillary endothelial surfaces in adipose and muscle tissue, lipoprotein lipase (LPL) hydrolyzes triglycerides from chylomicrons, releasing free fatty acids and glycerol, which are taken up by the adjacent cells. LPL also hydrolyzes triglycerides synthesised in the liver and transported to peripheral tissues as very low density lipoproteins.

β-Oxidation of fatty acids takes place in the mitochondria of muscle and liver. Carnitine is necessary for the oxidation of the fatty acids, which must cross the mitochondrial membranes as acylcarnitine. Carnitine is synthesized in the human liver and kidney from lysine and methionine. Carnitine needs of infants are met by breast milk or formulas, and carnitine has recently been added to soy-based formulas but is not present in intravenous infusates. In the liver, substantial quantities of fatty acids are converted to ketone bodies, which are then released into the circulation and provide an important source of fuel for the brain in the young infant.

Medium-chain triglycerides (MCT C8 and C10, ie, energy density 7.6 kcal/g) are sufficiently soluble that micelle formation is not required for them to diffuse through the unstirred water layer. They are much more readily absorbed than long-chain triglycerides and are then transported directly to the liver via the portal circulation. MCTs are rapidly metabolized in the liver, undergoing β-oxidation or ketogenesis. They do not require carnitine to enter the mitochondria. Ketones are formed from MCT even when provided orally. MCTs are useful for patients with luminal phase defects (eg, cirrhosis), absorptive defects (eg, short-bowel syndrome) and chronic inflammatory bowel disease. The potential side effects of MCT administration include diarrhea when they are given in large quantities, high octanoic acid levels in patients with cirrhosis, and, if they are the only source of lipids, deficiency of essential fatty acids.

Roy CC, Levy E: Role of medium-chain triglycerides in infant nutrition. Pages 51–64 in: *Nutritional Requirements of the Low-Birth-Weight Neonate*. Roy CC (editor). Key Largo, 1987.

CARBOHYDRATES

The energy density of carbohydrate is 4 kcal/g. Approximately 40% of caloric intake in human milk is in the form of lactose, or "milk sugar." The percentage of energy from lactose in cow's milk is only 20%, but infant formulas generally provide a somewhat higher percentage of energy from carbohydrates than does human milk.

After the first 2 years of life, 60% or more of energy requirements should be derived from carbohydrates, including no more than 10% from simple sugars. These dietary guidelines are, unfortunately, not reflected in the diets of North American children, who typically derive 25% of energy from sucrose and less than 20% from complex carbohydrates. Diets high in complex carbohydrates are, however, typical for the majority of the world's population of children.

The rate at which lactase hydrolyzes lactose to glucose and galactose in the brush border determines how quickly milk carbohydrates are absorbed. Lactase levels are highest in young infants, declining by more than 50% later in the first year. Lactase levels decline further with age, especially in children who are not of Northern European descent. Many black and Hispanic children cannot consume large amounts of dairy products without some evidence of lactose intolerance, eg, flatulence and loose stools. Lactase is located predominantly at the tip of the intestinal villi, where it is especially vulnerable to the effects of gastroenteritis or malnutrition. Thus, it may be helpful to avoid giving lactose-containing foods to children recovering from gastroenteritis or malnutrition, though this is not universally necessary. Galactose is preferentially converted to glycogen in the liver, prior to conversion to glucose for subsequent oxidation. Infants with galactosemia, an inborn metabolic disease caused by deficient galactose-1-phosphate uridyltransferase, require a lactose-free diet starting in the neonatal period.

Starch is broken down in the lumen of the gut into disaccharides and oligosaccharides, which are hydrolyzed into glucose by maltase, isomaltase, and glucoamylase in the brush border. Glucoamylase, which hydrolyzes oligosaccharides of 4–9 glucose units, is located predominantly at the base of the villi, where it may be protected from partial villus atrophy. Glucose polymers of this length are used extensively in special infant formulas and for caloric supplementation. Advantages include a relatively low osmolal effect in the lumen of the intestine as well as relatively easy hydrolysis by the compromised mucosa. Glucose and galactose are absorbed actively with sodium. This provides the theoretical basis for the composition of oral rehydration solutions in the management of diarrhea. The glucose enhances the absorption of sodium (and thus of water) and also supplies some energy.

During and immediately following a meal, plasma glucose levels are maintained by glucose absorption. If less than 10% of dietary energy is provided by carbohydrate, ketosis results. Within 2–4 hours of a meal, maintenance of plasma glucose depends increasingly on utilization of hepatic glycogen stores. These provide only 100–150 g glucose in the adult and only 6 g in the neonate. Subsequently, until the next meal, there is progressive dependence on gluconeogenesis. Glucose is the principal fuel for the brain and is a necessary energy source for certain other tissues, including red and white blood cells.

Children and adolescents in North America consume large quantities of sucrose (table sugar) in such items as soda pop, candy, syrups, and sweetened breakfast cereals. Average consumption by adolescents is 210 lb per year. A high intake of sucrose predisposes the individual to obesity and is a major risk factor for dental caries. Sucrase hydrolyzes sucrose to glucose and fructose in the brush border of the small intestine. Fructose is absorbed more slowly than and independently of glucose by a facilitated diffusion process. This characteristic provides a distinct advantage. Neither fructose nor galactose stim-ulates insulin secretion. Fructose, however, is easily converted to hepatic triglycerides, which may be especially undesirable in malnourished subjects.

Dietary fiber can be classified into 2 major types: nondigested carbohydrate (β1-4 linkages) and noncarbohydrate (lignin). Insoluble fibers (cellulose, hemicellulose, and lignin) increase stool bulk and water content and decrease gut transit time. They may to some extent impair mineral absorption. Soluble fibers (pectins, mucilages, and oat bran) bind bile acids and reduce lipid and cholesterol absorption. Pectins also slow gastric emptying and the rate of nutrient absorption. Fiber intakes are exceptionally low in North America. Few data regarding the fiber needs of children are available.

MAJOR MINERALS
(See Table 5–3 for recommended intakes.)

Calcium

The major dietary sources of calcium are milk and other dairy products. Although some calcium is available from other sources, including fortified cereals, it is difficult to achieve an adequate intake of calcium if dairy products are excluded from the diet. In such cases, a calcium supplement may be desirable. Average calcium absorption, which depends on calcium status and intake, is 20–30%, but calcium absorption from human milk is 60%. Absorption is enhanced by lactose, glucose, and protein and is impaired by phytate, fiber, oxalate, and unabsorbed fat. Control of calcium absorption is exerted primarily by changes in levels of 1,25-dihydroxycholecalciferol, which are increased in response to an increase in circulating parathormone (PTH). PTH, which is secreted in response to a fall in plasma-ionized calcium, also increases the release of calcium from bone. The desirable ratio of dietary calcium:phosphorus is 1.5:1 or greater in the young infant and 1:1 or greater at all other ages. The low calcium:phosphorus ratio found in unmodified cow's milk can cause hypocalcemic tetany and convulsions in the neonate. Calcium is excreted primarily via the kidney. It is the most abundant mineral in the body, and more than 99% is in the skeleton. Many vital cellular processes depend on calcium, especially changes in cytosolic free calcium levels. Changes in these levels also occur in various pathologic states and can grossly disturb intracellular metabolism. A deficiency in dietary calcium can occur in premature infants and lactating adolescents as a result of a restricted milk intake and also in patients with steatorrhea. The effect is a decrease in bone density, possibly progressing to rickets.

Chan GM et al: Decreased bone mineral status in lactating adolescent mothers. *J Pediatr* 1982;**101:**767.

Kooh SW et al: Rickets due to calcium deficiency. *N Engl J Med* 1977;**297**:1264.

Marie PJ et al: Histological osteomalacia due to dietary calcium deficiency in children. *N Engl J Med* 1982; **307**:584.

Phosphorus

Phosphorus is abundant in meats, eggs, dairy products, grains, legumes, and nuts. Phosphorus levels are high in processed foods and very high in cola and soft drinks. Approximately 80% of dietary phosphorus is absorbed; the kidney is responsible for homeostatic control. PTH decreases tubular reabsorption of phosphorus. More than 85% of body phosphorus is in bone. Phosphorus is also a component of many organic compounds that have a vital role in metabolism, including adenosine triphosphate (ATP) and 2,3-diphosphoglycerate. Many of the clinical effects of phosphorus depletion are attributable to cellular energy depletion from lack of ATP or to cellular anoxia secondary to impaired release of oxygen from hemoglobin. Other key compounds containing phosphorus include cell membrane phospholipids and nucleotides.

Nutritional phosphorus deficiency is rare but has been documented in very premature infants fed human milk, in whom it can cause osteoporosis and rickets, and in patients undergoing rehabilitation from protein-energy malnutrition. Nonnutritional causes of phosphorus depletion include the ingestion of phosphorus-binding antacids. Severe hypophosphatemia results from a deficiency together with an acute extracellular to intracellular shift in phosphorus. This shift can be triggered by a glucose load, by insulin, or during nutritional rehabilitation of the malnourished patient. Phosphorus deficiency affects most organ systems, including muscle (weakness progressing to rhabdomyolysis), cellular components of blood (both physiologic and functional changes), the gastrointestinal system, the central nervous system, and bone (bone pain, osteomalacia, rickets). Respiratory insufficiency may result from weakness of the diaphragm. Phosphate depletion in the premature infant can cause hypercalcemia. Phosphorus depletion can be treated with phosphorus salts, cola, or skimmed milk. Phosphorus excess may cause neonatal tetany due to decreased calcium. Phosphorus retention in chronic renal disease leads to metabolic bone disease.

Knochel JP: The clinical status of hypophosphatemia. *N Engl J Med* 1985;**313**:447.

Miller RR, Menke JA, Mentser MI: Clinical and laboratory observations: Hypercalcemia associated with phosphate depletion in the neonate. *J Pediatr* 1984;**105**:814.

Sagy M et al: Phosphate-depletion syndrome in a premature infant fed human milk. *J Pediatr* 1980;**96**:683.

Magnesium

Two-thirds of dietary magnesium is derived from vegetables, cereals, and nuts. The kidney exerts very effective control of magnesium homeostasis. When intake is low, excretion is minimal, and intracellular levels are maintained very effectively. Magnesium is the second most abundant intracellular cation; 50% is in bone. Levels in the cell cytosol are 10 times those of the extracellular fluids and are especially high in mitochondria. Magnesium activates many enzymes, especially phosphorus-hydrolyzing and transferring enzymes involved in energy metabolism. Magnesium also plays major roles in nucleic acid metabolism.

Dietary magnesium deficiency is not recognized except as a component of protein-energy malnutrition, but magnesium depletion may occur secondary to renal disease or intestinal malabsorption. Clinical effects include increased neuromuscular excitability, muscle fasciculation and tremors, personality changes, neurologic abnormalities, and electrocardiographic changes (depression of ST and T). Disturbance of PTH metabolism can cause secondary hypocalcemia. Acute states of magnesium depletion can be treated with a 50% solution of $MgSO_4$ providing 0.3–0.5 meq of magnesium per kilogram (3–6 meq maximum) given intravenously over 3 hours and repeated over the remainder of a 24-hour period. Magnesium excess can cause respiratory depression, lethargy, and coma.

Zelikovic I et al: Severe renal osteodystrophy without elevated serum immunoreactive parathyroid hormone concentrations in hypomagnesemia due to renal magnesium wasting. *Pediatrics* 1987;**79**:403.

Sodium

In the USA and Western Europe, only 10% of sodium intake is derived directly from food. Fifteen percent is derived from cooking and 75% from processed foods. The 10% derived from unprocessed foods is more than adequate to meet the normal requirement. Current dietary recommendations include a reduction from the typical intakes of North Americans, in which the ratio of sodium to potassium is 2:1; this ratio is 0.25:1 in other societies and in other mammalian species. High sodium:potassium ratios have been implicated in the pathoetiologic origins of hypertension, especially if the intake of dietary calcium is low. Fifteen percent of the population may be susceptible to adverse effects from high sodium:potassium ratios. The sodium intake of breastfed infants, while adequate (4–6 mmol/d), is low in comparison to that of most formula-fed infants.

Excessive sweating or cystic fibrosis may increase sodium requirements. Sodium deficiency, which occurs most commonly as a result of diarrhea and vomiting, causes dehydration. Anorexia, vomiting, and mental apathy may result from chronic depletion of sodium chloride. Hyponatremic and hypernatremic dehydration are discussed in Chapter 36.

Severe malnutrition and severe stress/hypermetabolism can disturb the ionic gradient across cell membranes and lead to an excess in intracellular sodium, which can adversely affect cellular metabolism. Sodium should be administered only with great caution in these circumstances.

Chloride

The intake and homeostasis of dietary chloride are closely linked with those of sodium. However, chloride is itself important in the physiologic mechanisms of the kidney and of the gut. Active chloride transport in the ascending loop of Henle is necessary for the passive reabsorption of sodium. Thus, a deficiency of chloride leads to a decrease in the absorption of sodium in the ascending loop of Henle and an increase in the amount of sodium presented to the lumen of the distal tube. This sodium is exchanged for H+ and K+, which can result in hypokalemic alkalosis.

Infants fed formulas low in chloride have experienced a nutritional deficiency of chloride. Other causes of chloride deficiency include cystic fibrosis, pyloric stenosis and other causes of vomiting, familial chloride diarrhea, chronic diuretic (furosemide) therapy, and Bartter's syndrome. Chloride deficiency has been associated with failure to thrive and may especially affect head growth. Other clinical features may include anorexia, lethargy, muscle weakness, vomiting, dehydration, and hypovolemia. Laboratory features include hypochloremia, hypokalemia, metabolic alkalosis, and hyperreninemia. Urine chloride levels depend on the cause of the depletion.

Perlman JM et al: Is chloride depletion an important contributing cause of death in infants with bronchopulmonary dysplasia? *Pediatrics* 1986;**77**:212.

Soriano-Rodriguez J et al: Biochemical features of dietary chloride deficiency syndrome: A comparative study of 30 cases. *J Pediatr* 1983;**103**:209.

Potassium

Potassium is readily available in unprocessed foods, including nuts, whole grains, meats and fish, beans, bananas, and orange juice. Relatively high potassium intakes are encouraged except in the presence of renal failure. The kidneys control potassium homeostasis via the aldosterone-renin-angiotension endocrine system. Potassium is the principal intracellular cation. The amount of total body potassium, therefore, depends on lean body mass. Potassium deficiency occurs in protein-energy malnutrition and, if not aggressively treated during the acute management stage, can be a cause of sudden death from cardiac failure. Because of loss of lean body mass, excessive potassium is excreted in the urine in any catabolic state. Again, this requires aggressive replenishment during recovery. In acidosis, intracellular potassium is exchanged for H+. Potassium, thus shifted into the extracellular fluid, is subsequently lost in the urine, and total body potassium is depleted (eg, in diabetic ketoacidosis) despite normal or elevated levels of plasma potassium. Other prominent causes of potassium deficiency include diarrhea and the use of diuretics. The effects of potassium deficiency are muscle weakness, mental confusion, and sudden death from arrythmias. Electrocardiographic findings include depression of the ST seg-

Table 5–3. Suggested dietary intakes of minerals and trace elements[1]

Nutrient	Premature Infant[2]	Term Infant	Children > 1 Year
Sodium		50 mg/kg/d (2 mmol/kg/d)	250–500 (10–20 mmol/d)
Potassium		80 mg/kg/d (2 mmol/kg/d)	800 (20 mmol/d)
Chloride		70 mg/kg/d (2 mmol/kg/d)	700 (20 mmol/d)
Calcium	180	400 (200) (See note 3.)	800
Phosphorus	150	300 (100) (See note 3.)	600
Magnesium	15	40	100
Iron	2 (after first 1–2 mo)	1 mg/kg/d ($\leq$ 0.1) (See note 3.) (after 2 mo)	10 (18 in adolescence)
Zinc	1.5	4 → 2 (2 → 0.75)	2–10
Copper	0.12	0.2–0.4	0.5–2
Selenium	0.003	0.01–0.03	0.03–0.1
Iodine	0.01	0.05	0.07–0.15

[1]Amounts expressed in mg/d unless otherwise indicated.
[2]The figures in this column indicate mg/kg/d.
[3]Amounts in parentheses are for the fully breast-fed infant aged less than 4–6 months.

ment and low T waves. Hyperkalemia may result from renal insufficiency.

TRACE ELEMENTS

Trace elements that have a recognized role in human nutrition are iron, iodine, zinc, copper, selenium, manganese, molybdenum, chromium, cobalt (as a component of vitamin B_{12}), and fluoride. Dietary requirements of trace elements are summarized in Table 5–3. Iron deficiency is discussed in Chapter 17. In general, good dietary sources of trace elements include human milk, meats, shellfish, legumes, nuts, and whole-grain cereals. Fish are a good source of selenium. Absorption of iron, zinc, copper, and probably other trace elements from human milk is especially favorable; the breast-fed infant does not normally require other sources of trace elements, including iron, for the first 4–6 months. Factors affecting the absorption of trace elements include the quantity of that trace element in the diet; dietary factors that form insoluble complexes (phytate, fiber, phosphate, oxalate); factors affecting oxidation state (ascorbic acid increases iron absorption and decreases copper absorption); chemical form (heme versus nonheme iron); competitive inhibition at mucosal cell (interactions of iron, zinc, and copper); and host factors (including nutritional status, diarrhea, impaired mucosal function). The gastrointestinal tract is the major site of homeostatic control for iron and zinc, the liver for copper, the intestinal tract and liver for manganese, and the kidneys for selenium, chromium, and iodine.

Deficiencies of iron, zinc, and possibly copper occur in the free-living population; in certain geochemical areas, the same is true of iodine and selenium. Infants fed cow's milk are at risk for deficiencies in iron and copper. Excessive losses, factors impairing absorption, or iatrogenic factors can cause deficiencies of iron, zinc, or copper. Deficiencies in these elements, as well as selenium, chromium, manganese, and molybdenum, have been associated with the use of synthetic diets, especially intravenous feeding. Protein-energy malnutrition may be complicated by deficiencies in iron, zinc, copper, selenium, or chromium. Finally, deficiencies in zinc, copper, iron, and molybdenum occur as a result of specific inborn metabolic diseases affecting the metabolism of these elements.

Hambidge KM: Trace element requirements in premature infants. In: *Textbook of Gastroenterology and Nutrition in Early Childhood*, 2nd ed. Lebenthal M (editor). Raven Press, 1988.

Zinc

Zinc is a component of many enzymes, plays multiple roles in nucleic acid metabolism and protein synthesis, and is important for membrane structure and function. Causes of zinc deficiency include diets low in available zinc during periods of rapid growth in infancy and childhood, synthetic oral or intravenous diets lacking adequate zinc supplements, diseases associated with impaired absorption (eg, regional enteritis) or excessive losses (eg, chronic diarrhea) of zinc, and one or more inborn diseases of zinc metabolism. Zinc deficiency may be a factor of secondary importance in some cases of anorexia nervosa. Clinical effects of a mild deficiency include impaired growth and poor appetite. More severe cases are characterized by changes in mood, irritability, and lethargy. Impairment of the immune system, especially T cell function, has been linked to increased susceptibility to infection. The most severe cases are characterized by an acro-orificial skin rash, usually accompanied by diarrhea and alopecia. These features occur in patients with acrodermatitis enteropathica, an inborn error of zinc metabolism; in those undergoing intravenous feeding without adequate zinc supplements; and in some premature breast-fed infants whose mothers have a defect in the secretion of zinc by the mammary gland. Plasma zinc collected before breakfast is below 6 mmol/L (40 μg/dL) in cases of severe zinc deficiency and 6–9 mmol/L (40–60 μg/dL) in cases of moderate zinc deficiency. In cases of mild zinc deficiency, plasma zinc concentrations may be within the normal range (9–15 mmol/L). Moderate hypozincemia occurs in response to release of interleukin-1 and in pregnancy even when zinc intake is adequate. Suspected dietary zinc deficiency can be treated with 1 mg/kg/d of zinc for 3 months (eg, 4.5 mg $ZnSO_4 \cdot 7H_2O$ per kilogram per day), preferably administered separately from meals and from iron supplements. Sustained clinical remissions in acrodermatitis enteropathica are usually achieved with 30–50 mg Zn^{2+} per day, but larger quantities may be required.

Hambidge KM: Zinc deficiency in the premature infant. *Pediatr Rev* 1985;**6**:209.
Walravens PA, Koepfer DM, Hambidge KM: A double-blind, controlled study of zinc supplementation in infants with a nutritional pattern of failure to thrive. *Pediatrics* 1989;**83**:532.

Copper

Copper is a vital component of several oxidative enzymes, including cytochrome *c* oxidase, the terminal oxidase in the electron transport chain; cytosolic and mitochondrial superoxide dismutases, which have key roles in the body defense against free radicals; lysyl oxidase, which is necessary for the cross linking of elastin and collagen; and ferroxidases (including ceruloplasmin) necessary for the oxidation of ferrous storage iron to ferric iron prior to attachment to transferrin for transport to the red cell precursors in the bone marrow. Cu^{2+} is highly reactive and must be transported in the circulation tightly bound to ceruloplasmin so that its oxidative potential (when it is free or loosely bound) can be contained.

Copper deficiency may occur in the following circumstances: in premature infants fed milk preparations low in copper; in association with prolonged feeding with unmodified cow's milk; in association with more generalized malnutritional states; in patients maintained on prolonged total parenteral nutrition without copper supplementation; and secondary to intestinal malabsorption states or prolonged diarrhea.

Osteoporosis is an early finding. Later skeletal changes include enlargement of costochondral cartilages, cupping and flaring of long-bone metaphyses, and spontaneous fractures of the ribs. The radiologic findings must be distinguished from battering (not symmetric), rickets, and scurvy. Neutropenia and hypochromic anemia are other early manifestations. The anemia is unresponsive to iron therapy. Very severe central nervous system disease is present in Menkes' steely (kinky) hair syndrome, in which a profound copper deficiency state results from a specific X-linked inherited defect in cellular metabolism of copper.

A low plasma copper or ceruloplasmin level helps confirm the diagnosis of copper deficiency. However, these levels are normally very low in the young infant, especially the premature infant, and are higher than adult values in later infancy and early childhood. Hence, carefully age-matched normal data are necessary for comparison. Interleukin-1 grossly elevates ceruloplasmin and copper levels; these levels are also very high in pregnancy.

Copper deficiency can be treated with a 1% solution of copper sulfate (2 mg of the salt or 500 μg of elemental copper per day for infants).

Selenium

Selenium is an essential component of glutathione peroxidase, which catalyzes the reduction of hydrogen peroxide to water in the cell cytosol by the addition of reducing equivalents derived from glutathione. Hence, selenium plays an important role in the body's defenses against free radicals.

Selenium deficiency is now recognized as the major etiologic factor in Keshan disease, an often fatal cardiomyopathy affecting primarily infants, children, and young women in a large area of China where there is a severe geochemical deficiency of selenium. Similar cases have been identified in the USA in patients maintained on long-term total parenteral nutrition without adequate selenium supplements. Other patients on parenteral nutrition have manifested selenium deficiency with incapacitating skeletal muscle pain and tenderness. Macrocytosis and loss of hair pigment occur in milder states of selenium deficiency. Blood levels are especially low in premature infants with bronchopulmonary dysplasia. It appears that the selenium intake of infants,

especially premature infants, is suboptimal and is likely to be increased in the near future.

A plasma selenium level less than 0.5 mmol/L (less than 40 μg/L) is compatible with mild selenium deficiency; a level less than 0.12 mmol/L (less than 10 μg/dL) indicates a possible severe selenium deficiency.

Iodine

Endemic goiter due to iodine deficiency has been eradicated in North America by effective prophylactic measures but continues to be a major health problem in many developing countries. Goiter occurs when iodine intake or excretion in urine is less than 20 μg/d. Most goitrous persons are clinically euthyroid. Maternal iodine deficiency causes endemic cretinism in about 5–15% of neonates who develop endemic goiters.

"Neurologic" endemic cretinism, seen clinically in most regions, is characterized by severe mental retardation, deaf-mutism, spastic diplegia, and strabismus. Clinical evidence of hypothyroidism is usually absent, and it is thought that the neurologic damage may be due to a direct effect of fetal iodine deficiency or to an imbalance between T_4 (low) and T_3 (normal or elevated). "Myxedematous" endemic cretinism predominates in some central African countries. Signs of congenital hypothyroidism are seen in this type. Milder neurologic damage occurs in many other cases of endemic neonatal goiter.

In North American countries, the use of iodized salt has been highly effective in preventing goiter. In areas where endemic goiter occurs, intramuscular depot injections of iodized oil have also been used extensively for prevention.

Fluoride Supplementation

When fluoride is incorporated into the hydroxyapatite matrix of dentin, it affords an inexpensive and effective means of helping to prevent dental caries. Fluoride is most effectively administered in the drinking water, but in infancy and childhood, fluoride in vitamin preparations or tablets serves the same purpose. Ready-made formulas provide less than 0.3 ppm. A dosage schedule as recommended by the American Academy of Pediatrics is given in Table 5–4. Breast-fed infants should be given fluoride supplements after 6 months of age. Earlier sup-

Table 5–4. Supplemental fluoride requirements (mg/d).

Age	Concentration of Fluoride in Drinking Water		
	< 0.3 ppm	0.3–0.7 ppm	> 0.7 ppm
2 wk to 2 y	0.25	0	0
2–3 y	0.5	0.25	0
3–16 y	1	0.5	0

plementation for the breast-fed infant, although its value has not been demonstrated conclusively, has been recommended by the American Academy of Pediatrics Committee on Nutrition.

VITAMINS

1. FAT-SOLUBLE VITAMINS

Because they are insoluble in water, the fat-soluble vitamins require digestion and absorption of dietary fat and a carrier system for transport in the blood. Deficiencies in these vitamins develop more slowly than deficiencies in water-soluble vitamins because the body accumulates stores of fat-soluble vitamins. Excessive intakes carry a considerable potential for toxicity (Table 5–5).

Moran JR, Greene HL: Nutritional biochemistry of fat-soluble vitamins. Pages 69–86 in: *Pediatric Nutrition:*

Table 5–5. Effects of vitamin toxicity

Thiamin
(Very rare.) Anaphylaxis; respiratory depression.
Riboflavin
None.
Pyridoxine
(Very rare.) Sensory neuropathy.
Niacin
Histamine release → cutaneous vasodilation; cardiac arrythmias; cholestatic jaundice; gastrointestinal disturbance; hyperuricemia; glucose intolerance.
Pantothenic acid
Diarrhea.
Biotin
None.
Folate
None (except masking B_{12} deficiency).
Cobalamin
None.
Vitamin C
Interference with copper absorption; decreased tolerance to hypoxia; increased oxalic acid excretion.
Carnitine
None recognized.
Vitamin A
($>$ 20,000 IU/d): Vomiting; increased intracranial pressure (pseudotumor cerebri); irritability; headaches; insomnia; emotional lability; dry, desquamating skin; myalgia and arthralgia; abdominal pain; hepatosplenomegaly; cortical thickening of bones of hands and feet.
Vitamin D
($>$ 40,000 IU/d): Hypercalcemia; vomiting; constipation; nephrocalcinosis.
Vitamin E
? 25–100 mg/kg/d IV: Necrotizing enterocolitis and liver toxicity (but probably due to polysorbate 80 used as a solubilizer).
Vitamin K
Lipid-soluble vitamin K: very low order of toxicity; Water-soluble, synthetic vitamin K: vomiting, porphyrinuria, albuminuria, hemolytic anemia, hernoglobinuria, hyperbilirubinemia (do not give to neonates).

Theory and Practice. Grand RJ et al (editors). Butterworth, 1987.
Tsang RC (editor): *Vitamin and Mineral Requirements in Preterm Infants.* Dekker, 1985.

Vitamin A

Dietary sources of vitamin A include dairy products, fortified margarine, eggs, liver, meats, fish oils, and corn. The vitamin A precursor, β-carotene, occurs in abundance in yellow and green vegetables. Dietary retinyl palmitate requires hydrolysis by pancreatic and intestinal hydrolases. β-Carotene is cleaved in the intestinal mucosal cells by dioxygenase to yield 2 molecules of retinal (retinaldehyde), which is then reduced to retinol (vitamin A alcohol). Dioxygenase is stimulated by thyroxin; thus, individuals with hypothyroidism accumulate carotene because they cannot convert it to retinol. Carotene appears to have an important physiologic role in its own right as a powerful antioxidant. Data on the in vivo role of carotene in children are currently extremely limited.

Retinol is reesterified in the mucosal cells and transported in chylomicrons to the liver, where it is stored. From the liver, vitamin A is transported to the rest of the body attached to retinol-binding protein (RBP) complexed to prealbumin. RBP may be decreased in liver disease or in protein-energy malnutrition. Circulating RBP may be increased in chronic renal failure.

Vitamin A has a unique and specialized role in the photochemical basis of vision. The photosensitive pigment rhodopsin is formed from retinal and a protein called opsin. Vitamin A also modifies differentiation and proliferation of epithelial cells, especially in the respiratory tract. Vitamin A is necessary for glycoprotein synthesis and for the integrity of the immune system and may affect gene expression. Retinol can be irreversibly oxidized to retinoic acid, which is effective in glycoprotein synthesis but is ineffective for vision.

Vitamin A deficiency occurs in premature infants, in association with intravenous nutrition with inadequate vitamin A supplements, and in association with protein-energy malnutrition when the manifestations are frequently made more severe by measles. Other causes of vitamin A deficiency are cultural factors (failure to grow vegetables even when practical, eg, in Central America and the Philippines); fat malabsorption syndromes, including biliary atresia, giardiasis, and cystic fibrosis.

The classic features of vitamin A deficiency are primarily related to the eye and vision. Night blindness progresses to xerosis (dryness of cornea and conjunctiva), xerophthalmia (extreme dryness of conjunctiva), Bitot's spots, keratomalacia (clouding and softening of the cornea), ulceration and perforation of the cornea, prolapse of lens and iris, and eventually blindness. Vitamin A deficiency is the leading cause of irreversible blindness in children worldwide. Other features of vitamin A deficiency can include follicular hyperkeratosis (dry, thickened, rough skin) pruritus, growth retardation, increased susceptibility to infection, anemia, and hepatosplenomegaly. Vitamin A deficiency in the neonatal period may be an etiologic factor in the onset of bronchopulmonary dysplasia in premature infants.

Serum levels of retinol below 20 μg/dL are considered low; a level below 10 indicates deficiency. A ratio of retinol:RBP below 0.7 is also indicative of vitamin A deficiency.

Suggested intakes of vitamin A are summarized in Table 5–6. Therapy of xerophthalmia requires 50,000–100,000 units orally or intramuscularly. The standard maintenance dose in fat malabsorption syndromes is 2500–5000 international units (800–1600 μg). Doses as high as 25,000–50,000 IU/d may be needed, but monitoring to avoid toxicity is essential. Vitamin A can be provided in these circumstances as a water-soluble preparation, Aquasol A (1 mL = 50,000 IU). The effects of vitamin A toxicity are summarized in Table 5–5.

Carpenter TO et al: Severe hypervitaminosis A in siblings:

Evidence of variable tolerance to retinol intake. *J Pediatr* 1987;**111**:507.
Shenai JP et al: Clinical trial of vitamin A supplementation in infants susceptible to bronchopulmonary dysplasia. *J Pediatr* 1987;**111**:269.

Vitamin D

Vitamin D requirements are normally met primarily from ultraviolet radiation of dehydrocholesterol in the skin with the formation of cholecalciferol (vitamin D_3). Similarly, vitamin D_2, or ergocalciferol, is derived from radiation of ergosterol. Vitamin D is transported from the skin to the liver attached to a specific carrier protein. The primary dietary source is vitamin D-fortified milk and formulas. Egg yolk and fatty fish contain some vitamin D. Vitamin D absorption depends on normal fat absorption. Absorbed vitamin D is transported to the liver in chylomicrons. Vitamins D_2 and D_3 undergo 25-hydroxylation in the liver and then 1-α hydroxylation in kidney proximal tubules to yield 25-hydroxycholecalciferol and 1,25-dihydroxycholecalciferol, respectively. Parathormone activates the 1-α-hydroxylase enzyme in the kidney. Calcidiol (25-hydroxycholecalciferol) is the major circulating form of vitamin D. Calcitriol (1,25-dihydroxycholecalciferol) is the biologically active form of vitamin D. Calcitriol stimulates the intestinal absorption of calcium and phosphate, the renal reabsorption of filtered calcium, and the mobilization of calcium and phosphorus from bone.

Vitamin D deficiency results from lack of adequate sunlight coupled with a low dietary intake. An infant requires only half-hour total body exposure or 2-hour head exposure to the sun per week to maintain adequate vitamin D status. Even without exposure to sunlight, the breast-fed infant can acquire sufficient vitamin D from human milk if the mother's vitamin D status is optimal. Otherwise, a vitamin D supplement is required to avoid risk of rickets. In the United States, cow's milk and infant formulas are routinely supplemented with vitamin D. Nutritional rickets may occur in older infants and children who are not exposed to sun and who do not consume vitamin D-fortified milk. Vitamin D deficiency also occurs in fat malabsorption syndromes, including small intestinal disease, cholestasis, and lymphatic obstruction. Use of P450-stimulating drugs may decrease hydroxylated vitamin D, which can also be decreased by hepatic and renal disease and by inborn errors of metabolism. End-organ unresponsiveness to calcitriol may also occur. The clinical effects of vitamin D deficiency are osteomalacia (adults) or rickets (children), in which there is an accumulation in bone of osteoid (matrix) with reduced calcification. Cartilage fails to mature and calcify. The effects include craniotabes, rachitic rosary, pigeon breast, bowed legs, delayed eruption of teeth and enamel defects, Harrison's groove, scoliosis, kyphosis, dwarfism, painful bones, fractures, an-

Table 5–6. Suggested intakes of vitamins.

	Premature Infants[1] (per kg/d)	Term Infants[1] (per day)	Adults[2] (per day)
Thiamin (mg)	0.35	12	1.5
Riboflavin (mg)	0.2	0.5	1.7
Pyridoxine (mg)	0.2	0.6	2.0
Niacin (mg NE)[3]	7	17(NE)	19(NE)
Pantothenic acid (mg)	2	5	4–7
Biotin (μg)	6	20	30–100
Folic Acid (μg)	50	140	200
Cobalamin (μg)	0.3	1	2.0
Vitamin A (μg RE)[4]	500	700	1000
Vitamin C (mg)	25	80	60
Vitamin D (μg) (cholecalciferol)	4 (160IU)	10 (400 IU)	5
Vitamin E (mg) (α-tocopherol)	3 (See note 5)	7	10
Vitamin K (μg)	80	20	80

[1]Based on recent recommendations for intravenous vitamins. (Greene HL, Hambidge KM, Schanler R, Tsang RC: Guidelines for the use of vitamins, trace elements, calcium, magnesium, and phosphorus in infants and children receiving total parenteral nutrition: Report of the Subcommittee on Pediatric Parenteral Nutrient Requirements from the Committee on Clinical Practice Issues of The American Society for Clinical Nutrition. *Am J Clin Nutr* 1988;**48**:1324 © *Am J Clin Nutr*. American Society for Clinical Nutrition.)
[2]Based on *Recommended Dietary Allowances*, 10th ed. National Research Council, National Academy Press, 1989.
[3]NE Niacin equivalents.
[4]RE Retinol equivalents (1 μg retinol or 6 mg β-carotene = 1 RE; 1 IU = 0.3 μg retinol).
[5]Oral doses up to 25 mg/d are now frequently used with the expectation that this may help to combat oxidant stress.

orexia, and weakness. X-ray findings include cupping, fraying, and flaring of metaphyses; the loss of sharp definition of bone trabeculae accounts for the general decrease in skeletal radiodensity. The diagnosis is supported by characteristic radiologic abnormalities of the skeleton, low serum phosphorus levels, high serum alkaline phosphatase levels, and high parathormone levels. The diagnosis can be confirmed by a low level of serum 25-hydroxycholecalciferol.

Rickets is treated with 1600–5000 IU/d of vitamin D_3 (1 IU = 0.25 μg). If this is poorly absorbed, 25-hydroxycholecalciferol, 2 μg/kg/d, or 1,25-dihydroxycholecalciferol, 0.05–0.2 μg/kg/d, is given. Renal osteodystrophy is treated with 1,25-dihydroxycholecalciferol.

Suggested dietary intakes for vitamin D are summarized in Table 5–6, and toxic effects in Table 5–5.

Specker BL et al: Sunshine exposure and serum 25-hydroxyvitamin D concentrations in exclusively breastfed infants. *J Pediatr* 1985;**107:**372.

Vitamin D: New perspectives. (Editorial.) *Lancet* 1987; **1:**1122.

Vitamin E

Vegetable oils provide the main dietary source of vitamin E. Coconut and olive oils, however, are low in vitamin E. Some vitamin E is present in cereals, dairy products, and eggs. Activity may decrease with processing, storage, or heating. Vitamin E is a family of compounds, the tocopherols. There are 4 major forms: alpha, gamma, beta, and delta; α-tocopherol has the highest biologic activity. Vitamin E can donate an electron to a free radical molecule to stop oxidant reactions. Oxidized vitamin E is then reduced by ascorbic acid or glutathione. The reduced tocopherol is able to "scavenge" another free radical. The nutrients that participate in antioxidant defenses include β-carotene, vitamin C, selenium, copper, manganese, and zinc. Vitamin E is located at specific sites in the cell to protect polyunsaturated fatty acids in the membrane lipids from lipid peroxidation and to protect thiol groups and nucleic acids. Vitamin E also functions as a cell membrane stabilizer, may function in the electron transport chain, and may modulate chromosomal expression.

Vitamin E deficiency may occur in the following circumstances: in the premature infant; in cholestatic liver disease, pancreatic insufficiency (including cystic fibrosis), abetalipoproteinemia, and short bowel syndrome; as an isolated inborn error of vitamin E metabolism; and possibly as a result of increased utilization due to oxidant stress.

Vitamin E deficiency shortens red cell half-life and may cause a hemolytic anemia. Chronic vitamin E deficiency secondary to malabsorption results in a progressive neurologic disorder with loss of deep tendon reflexes, loss of coordination, loss of perception of vibration and position sensation, abnormalities in eye movements, weakness, scoliosis, and degeneration of the retina. In premature infants, vitamin E deficiency may contribute to oxidant injury of the lung, retina, and brain (brain hemorrhage). These putative adverse effects in the premature infant require confirmation.

Vitamin E nutritional status can be partially assessed with serum vitamin E (normal range for children is 3–15 μg/mL). The ratio of serum vitamin E:total serum lipid is normally more than 0.8 milligrams per 1 gram. Hydrogen peroxide-induced hemolysis is also used as a test of vitamin E status.

Suggested intakes are summarized in Table 5–6. Requirements increase if dietary polyunsaturated fatty acid (PUFA) increase (need 0.4–0.5 mg of vitamin E per gram of PUFA in the diet). One international unit = 1 mg of dl-α-tocopheryl acetate.

Large oral doses (up to 100 IU/kg/d) of vitamin E correct the deficiency resulting from most malabsorption syndromes. Intramuscular injections (5–7 mg/kg/week) may be necessary in some cases of cholestatic liver disease. For abetalipoproteinemia, 100–200 IU/kg/d of vitamin E are needed. Vitamin E therapy in ischemia-reperfusion injury and in the prevention of intracranial hemorrage in the preterm infant remains experimental. Toxic effects of vitamin E are summarized in Table 5–5.

Machlin LJ, Bendich A: Free radical tissue damage: Protective role of antioxidant nutrients. *FASEB J* 1987; **1:**441.

Sokol RJ: Vitamin E deficiency and neurologic disease. *Annu Rev Nutr* 1988;**8:**351.

Vitamin K

Vitamin K_1 (phylloquinone) is obtained from leafy vegetables, soybean oil, fruits, seeds, and cow's milk. Vitamin K_2 (menaquinone), which has 60% of the activity of K_1, is synthesized by intestinal bacteria. K_2 may be a major source of vitamin K in infants and young children, but less is produced in the intestine of the breast-fed infant.

Vitamin K is necessary for the posttranslational carboxylation of glutamic acid residues of the vitamin K-dependent coagulation proteins. Carboxylation allows these proteins to bind calcium, thus leading to activation of the clotting factors. Thus, vitamin K is necessary for the maintenance of normal plasma levels of coagulation factors II (prothrombin), VII, IX, and X and is also necessary for the maintenance of normal levels of the anticoagulation protein C. Vitamin K deficiency occurs in newborn, especially those who are breast-fed and who do not receive vitamin K prophylaxis at delivery. This deficiency results in hemorraghic disease of the newborn. Later, vitamin K deficiency may result from fat malabsorption syndromes and the use of nonabsorbed antibiotics and anticoagulant drugs (eg, Warfarin). Clinical features are hemorrhage into the skin (purpura), gastrointestinal tract, genital urinary tract, gingiva, lungs, joints, and central nervous system, which may be fatal. Vitamin K status can be assessed with plasma levels of protein-induced vitamin K absence (PIVKA) or by prothrombin time.

Vitamin K requirements are summarized in Table 5–6. Newborns require prophylactic intramuscular vitamin K (0.5–1 mg). For older children with acute bleeding, 3–10 mg of vitamin K is given intramuscularly or intravenously. For chronic malabsorption syndromes, 2.5 mg twice weekly to 5.0 mg/d is given orally. To reverse Warfarin effect, 50–100 mg of intravenous vitamin K is given. Toxic effects are summarized in Table 5–5.

Lane PA, Hathaway WE: Vitamin K in infancy. *J Pediatr* 1985;**106:**351.

2. WATER-SOLUBLE VITAMINS

Deficiencies of water-soluble vitamins are much less common in the USA because many foods are fortified, particularly with B vitamins. Most bread and wheat products are now routinely fortified with B vitamins.

The danger of toxicity from water-soluble vitamins is not as great because excesses can be excreted in the urine. However, deficiencies in these vitamins can also develop more quickly than deficiencies in fat-soluble vitamins because of the limited stores.

Additional salient details are summarized in Tables 5–6 through 5–11. Although dietary intake of the water-soluble vitamins on a daily basis is not necessary, these vitamins, with the exception of vitamin B_{12}, are not stored in the body.

Carnitine is synthesized in the liver and kidneys from lysine and methionine. In certain circumstances (Table 5–10), however, synthesis is inadequate, and carnitine can then be considered a vitamin. A dietary supply of other organic compounds, such as inositol, may also be required in certain circumstances.

Ek J, Magnus E: Plasma and red cell folate values and folate requirements in formula-fed term infants. *J Pediatr* 1982;**100:**738.

Hallman M, Arjomaa P, Hoppu K: Inositol supplementation in respiratory distress syndrome: Relationship between serum concentration, renal excretion, and lung effluent phospholipids. *J Pediatr* 1987;**110:**604.

Table 5–7. Summary of biologic roles of water-soluble vitamins.

B-vitamins involved in production of energy of metabolism
Thiamin (B_1)
 Thiamine pyrophosphate is coenzyme in oxidative decarboxylation (pyruvate dehydrogenase, alpha ketoglutarate dehydrogenase, and transketolase).
Riboflavin (B_2)
 Coenzyme of several flavoproteins (eg, flavin mononucleotide [FMN] and flavin adenine dinucleotide [FAD]) involved in oxidative/electron transfer enzyme systems.
Niacin
 Hydrogen-carrying coenzymes: nicotinamide-adenine dinucleotide (NAD), nicotinamide-adenine dinucleotide phosphate (NADP); decisive role in intermediary metabolism.
Pantothenic acid
 Major component of coenzyme A.
Biotin
 Component of several carboxylase enzymes involved in fat and carbohydrate metabolism.
Hematopoietic B vitamins
Folic acid
 Tetrahydrofolate has essential role in one-carbon transfers. Essential role in purine and pyramidine synthesis; deficiency → arrest of cell division (especially bone marrow and intestine).
Cobalamin (B_{12})
 Methyl cobalamin (cytoplasm): synthesis of methionine with simultaneous synthesis of tetrahydrofolate (reason for megaloblastic anemia in B_{12} deficiency). Adenosyl cobalamin (mitochondria) is coenzyme for mutases and dehydratases.
Other B vitamins
Pyridoxine (B_6)
 Prosthetic group of transaminases, etc involved in amino acid interconversions; prostaglandin and heme synthesis; central nervous system function; carbohydrate metabolism; immune development.
Other water-soluble vitamins
L-Ascorbic acid (C)
 Strong reducing agent—probably involved in all hydroxylations. Roles include collagen synthesis; phenylalanine → tyrosine; tryptophan → 5 OH tryptophan; dopamine → norepinephrine; Fe^{3+} → Fe^{2+}; folic acid → folinic acid; cholesterol → bile acids; leukocyte function; interferon production; carnitine synthesis. Copper metabolism; reduces oxidized vitamin E.
Carnitine
 Transfer of long-chain fatty acids from cytosol to mitochondria (necessary for β-oxidation).

Table 5–8. Major dietary sources of water-soluble vitamins.

Thiamin
 Whole grains, cereals (including fortification), lean pork, liver
Riboflavin
 Dairy products, meat, poultry, wheat germ, leafy vegetables
Pyridoxine
 All foods
Niacin
 Meats, poultry, fish, legumes, wheat, all foods except fats, synthesized in body from tryptophan
Panthothenic acid
 Ubiquitous
Biotin
 Yeast, liver, kidneys, legumes, nuts, egg yolks (synthesized by intestinal bacteria)
Folic acid
 Leafy vegetables (lost in cooking), whole grains, wheat germ, liver, yeast, eggs
Cobalamin
 Eggs, dairy products, liver, meats; none in plants
Vitamin C
 Fresh fruits and vegetables
Carnitine
 Meats, dairy products, none in plants

Table 5–9. Circumstances in which the possibility of vitamin deficiencies merit particular consideration.

Circumstance	Possible Deficiency
Prematurity	All vitamins
Protein-energy malnutrition	B_1, B_2, folate, A
Synthetic diets (including TPN)	All vitamins
Inherited disorders	Folate, B_{12}, D, carnitine
Vitamin-drug interactions	B_6, biotin, folate, B_{12}, carnitine, fat-soluble vitamins
Fat malabsorption syndrome	Fat-soluble vitamins
Breast-feeding	B_1,[1] Folate,[2] B_{12},[3] D,[4] K[5]

[1]Alcoholic or malnourished mother
[2]Folate-deficient mother
[3]Vegan mother
[4]Infant not exposed to sunlight and mother's vitamin D status suboptimal
[5]Maternal status poor; neonatal prophylaxis omitted

Table 5–10. Causes of deficiencies in water-soluble vitamins.

Thiamin
Infantile beriberi; seen in infants breast-fed by mothers with history of alcoholism or poor diet; has been described as complication of total parenteral nutrition (TPN); protein-energy malnutrition; prematurity.
Riboflavin
General undernutrition; prematurity; inactivation in TPN solutions exposed to light.
Pyridoxine
Prematurity (these infants may not convert pyridoxine → pyridoxal-5-P); B_6 dependency syndromes; drugs (isoniazid); heat-treated formulas (historical).
Niacin
Maize or millet diets (high leucine and low tryptophan intakes); prematurity.
Pantothenic acid
None.
Biotin
Suppressed intestinal flora and impaired intestinal absorption.
Folic acid
Prematurity; seen in term breast-fed infants whose mothers are folate deficient and in term infants fed unsupplemented processed cow's milk or goat's milk; kwashiorkor; chronic overcooking; malabsorption of folate due to a congenital defect; sprue; celiac disease; drugs (phenytoin).
Increased requirements: chronic hemolytic anemias, diarrhea, malignancies, hypermetabolic states, infections, extensive skin disease, cirrhosis.
Cobalamin
Rare; seen in breast-fed infants of mothers with latent pernicious anemia or who are on an unsupplemented strict vegetarian diet; absence of luminal proteases; congenital malabsorption of B_{12}.
Vitamin C
Prematurity; maternal megadoses during pregnancy → deficiency in infants; lack of fresh fruits or vegetables; seen in infants fed formula and pasteurized cow's milk (historical).
Carnitine
Seen in premature infants fed unsupplemented soy formula or fed intravenously; dialysis; inherited defects in carnitine synthesis; organic acidemias; valproic acid.

Table 5–11. Clinical features of deficiencies in water-soluble vitamins.

Thiamin
Infantile beriberi (cardiac; aphonic; pseudomeningitic).
Riboflavin
Cheilosis; angular stomatitis; glossitis; soreness and burning of lips and mouth; dermatitis of nasolabial fold and genitals; ± ocular signs (photophobia → indistinct vision).
Pyridoxine
Listlessness; irritability; seizures; gastrointestinal disturbance; anemia; cheilosis; glossitis.
Niacin
Pellagra (weakness; lassitude; dermatitis of exposed areas; diarrhea; dementia).
Pantothenic acid
Weakness; gastrointestinal disturbance; burning feet.
Biotin
Scaly dermatitis; alopecia; irritability; lethargy.
Folate
Megaloblastic anemia; neutropenia; thrombocytopenia; growth retardation; delayed maturation of central nervous system in infants; diarrhea (mucosal ulcerations); glossitis; jaundice; mild splenomegaly.
Cobalamin
Megaloblastic anemia; neurologic degeneration.
Vitamin C
Anorexia; irritability; apathy; pallor; fever; tachycardia; diarrhea; failure to thrive; increased susceptibility to infections; hemorrhages under skin, mucous membranes, into joints and under periosteum; long-bone tenderness; costochondral beading.
Carnitine
Increased serum triglycerides and free fatty acids; decreased ketones; fatty liver; hypoglycemia; genetic: progressive muscle weakness or cardiomyopathy or hypoglycemia.

Levine M: New concepts in the biology and biochemistry of ascorbic acid. *N Engl J Med* 1986;**314**:893.

Mock DM et al: Biotin deficiency complicating parenteral alimentation: Diagnosis, metabolic repercussions, and treatment. *J Pediatr* 1985;**106**:762.

Schmidt-Sommerfeld E, Penn D, Wolf H: Carnitine deficiency in premature infants receiving total parenteral nutrition: Effect of L-carnitine supplementation. *J Pediatr* 1983;**102**:931.

INFANT FEEDING

BREAST-FEEDING

Breast-feeding, one of the most important influences on children's health worldwide, provides optimal nutrition for the normal infant during the early months of life. Numerous immunoactive components of breast milk (including secretory IgA, lysozyme, lactoferrin, bifidus factor, and macrophages) help to provide protection against gastrointestinal and upper respiratory infections. In developing countries, lack of refrigeration and contaminated water supplies frequently make formula feeding especially hazardous. Allergic diseases are less common among infants who have been breast-fed. Although formulas have improved progressively and are made to resemble breast milk as closely as possible, it is impossible to mimic the nutritional or immune composition of human milk. Additional differences of physiologic importance continue to be identified; recently identified examples include the substantial quantities of taurine and docosahexaenoic acid found in human milk. Furthermore, the relationship developed through breast-feeding can be an important part of early maternal interactions with the infant and provides a source of security and comfort to the infant.

In the last decade, breast-feeding has been reestablished as the predominant mode of feeding the young infant in the United States. Unfortunately, breast-feeding rates remain low among several subpopulations of women, including low-income, minority, and young mothers; many mothers face obstacles in maintaining lactation once they return to work. Skilled use of the breast pump may help to maintain lactation in these circumstances.

Absolute contraindications to breast-feeding are rare. They include tuberculosis (in the mother) and galactosemia (in the infant). Although breast milk may serve as a vehicle for transmission of the human immunodeficiency virus (HIV), preliminary evidence suggests this is not a major route of transmission. Current recommendations are that HIV-infected mothers in developed countries refrain from breast-feeding because of the widely available, safe alternatives. In developing countries, the risk of HIV infection via breast-milk is generally considered less than the known benefits of breast-feeding, particularly when alternative feeding methods may be hazardous.

The premature infant under 1500 grams may benefit from the addition of a milk fortifier, particularly to increase the density of protein, energy, calcium, and phosphorus. Breast-fed infants with cystic fibrosis quite frequently need an energy and protein supplement.

Management of Breast-Feeding

Because today's grandmothers predominantly bottle-fed their children, the "art" of breast-feeding is no longer automatically passed from mother to daughter. Hence, the role of the health professional in supporting and promoting breast-feeding is of outstanding importance. Organizations such as the La Leche League have been very effective in promoting breast-feeding.

Perinatal hospital routines and follow-up pediatric care have a great impact on the successful initiation of breast-feeding. Breast-feeding is promoted by prenatal and postpartum education, frequent mother-baby contact after delivery, one-on-one advice about breast-feeding technique, demand feeding, rooming-in, avoidance of bottle supplements, early follow-up after delivery, maternal confidence, family support, adequate maternity leave, and accurate advice for common problems such as sore nipples. Breast-feeding is undermined by mother and baby separations, feeding babies in the nursery at night, routinely offering supplemental bottles, conflicting advice from staff, incorrect infant positioning and latch-on, scheduled feedings, lack of maternal confidence or support, delayed follow-up, early return to employment, and inaccurate advice for common breast-feeding difficulties.

It is important for the mother to know that very few women are unable to nurse their babies. The newborn is generally fed ad libitum every 2 to 3 hours, with longer intervals (4 to 5 hours) at night. Thus, a newborn nurses 8 to 10 times a day, so that a generous milk supply is stimulated. This frequency is not an indication of inadequate lactation. Mothers also frequently need to be reassured about stooling pattern. In early stages, a loose stool is often passed with each feeding; later, there may be several days between stools.

Expressing milk may be indicated if the mother returns to her job or if the infant is premature, cannot suck adequately, or is hospitalized. Modern electric breast pumps are very effective and can be borrowed or rented.

Technique of Breast-Feeding

Breast-feeding can begin after delivery as soon as both mother and baby are stable. Correct positioning and breast-feeding technique are necessary to ensure effective nipple stimulation and optimal breast emptying with minimal nipple discomfort.

If the mother wishes to nurse while sitting, the infant should be elevated to the height of the breast and turned completely to face the mother, so that their abdomens touch. The mother's arms supporting the infant should be held tight at her side, bringing the baby's head in line with her breast. The breast should be supported by the lower fingers of her free hand, with the nipple compressed between the thumb and index fingers to make it more protractile. The infant's initial licking and mouthing of the nipple helps make it more erect. When the infant opens his or her mouth, the mother should rapidly insert as much nipple and areola as possible.

Some breast-fed infants fail to thrive. The most common cause of early failure to thrive is poorly managed mammary engorgement, which rapidly decreases milk supply. Unrelieved engorgement can result from inappropriately long intervals between feeding, improper infant suckling, a nondemanding infant, sore nipples, maternal or infant illness, nursing from only one breast, and latching difficulties. The mother's ignorance of technique, inappropriate feeding routines, and inadequate amounts of fluid and rest for the mother can all be factors. Some infants are too sleepy to do well on an ad libitum regimen and, in particular, may need waking to feed at night. Primary lactation failure is rare but does occur. Some decline in weight for age percentiles after 3 months should not necessarily be interpreted as an indication of inadequate nutrition, because the commonly used percentile charts have been constructed primarily from data on infants who have been formula-fed.

Rigid time restrictions should not be imposed. The sensible guidelines are 5 minutes per breast each feeding the first day, 10 minutes on each side at each feeding the second day, and approximately 15 minutes per side thereafter. A vigorous infant can obtain most of the available milk in 5–7 minutes, but additional sucking time ensures breast emptying and ongoing milk production and satisfies the infant's sucking urge. The side on which feeding is commenced should be alternated. The mother may break suction gently after nursing by inserting her finger between the baby's gums.

Follow-Up

Individualized assessment should identify before discharge the mothers and infants needing additional support. All cases require early follow-up after discharge. The onset of copious milk secretion between the second and fourth postpartum day is a critical time in the establishment of lactation.

Common Problems

Mild nipple tenderness requires attention to proper positioning of the infant and correct latch-on. Ancillary measures include nursing for shorter periods, beginning feedings on the less sore side, air drying the nipples well after nursing and the application of lanolin cream. Severe nipple pain and cracking usually indicate improper infant attachment. Temporary pumping, which is well tolerated, may be needed.

Breast-feeding jaundice is exaggerated physiologic jaundice associated with inadequate intake of breast milk, infrequent stooling, and unsatisfactory weight gain. If possible, the jaundice should be managed by increasing the frequency of nursing and, if necessary, augmenting the infant's sucking with regular breast pumping. Supplemental feedings may be necessary, but care should be taken not to decrease breast milk production further.

In a small percentage of breast-fed infants, breast milk jaundice is caused by an unidentified property of the milk that inhibits conjugation of bilirubin. In severe cases, interruption of breast feeding for 24–36 hours may be necessary. The mother's breast should be emptied with an electric breast pump during this period.

Maternal mastitis should be suspected when a nursing mother complains of a ''flulike'' illness with local breast tenderness. Antibiotic therapy providing coverage against β-lactamase-producing organisms should be given for 10 days. Analgesics may be necessary, but breast-feeding should be continued. Breast pumping may be a helpful adjunctive therapy.

Maternal Drug Use

Many factors play a role in determining the effects of maternal drug therapy on the nursing infant, including the route of administration, dosage, molecular weight, pH, and protein binding. In general, any drug prescribed therapeutically to newborns can be consumed via breast milk without ill effect. Very few therapeutic drugs are absolutely contraindicated; these include radioactive compounds, antimetabolites, lithium, diazepam, chloramphenicol, and tetracycline. For up-to-date information, a regional drug center should be consulted.

Maternal use of illicit or recreational drugs is a contraindication to breast-feeding. If a woman is unable to discontinue drug use, she should not breast-feed. Expression of milk for a feeding or two after use of a drug is not an acceptable compromise. The breast-fed infants of mothers taking methadone as part of a treatment program (but no alcohol or other drugs) have generally not experienced ill effects when the daily maternal methadone dose is under 40 mg.

Nutrient Composition

The nutrient composition of human milk is summarized and compared with that of cow's milk and formulas in Table 5–12. Outstanding characteristics include (1) the relatively low protein content, which is, however, quite adequate for the normal infant; (2) a generous, but not excessive, quantity of essential fatty acids; (3) the presence of long-chain unsaturated fatty acids of the ω3 series, of which docosahexaenoic acid is thought to be especially important; (4) a relatively low sodium and solute load; and (5) very favorable absorption of calcium, iron, and zinc, which results in the provision of adequate quantities of these nutrients to the normal breast-fed infant for 4–6 months despite the relatively low intakes.

Weaning

Weaning can take place according to the needs and desires of both infant and mother. Gradual weaning, starting typically after 4–6 months, is preferred. Bottle feedings (or cup feedings) are increased progressively over a period of several weeks as breast feedings are omitted.

Bowes WA Jr: The effect of medications on the lactating mother and her infant. *Clin Obstet Gynecol* 1980; **23:**1073.

Committee on Nutrition, American Academy of Pediatrics and Canadian Paediatric Society Nutrition Committee: Breast-feeding. *Pediatrics* 1978;**62:**591.

Table 5–12. The composition of milk (per 100 kcal).

Nutrient (Unit)	Minimum Level Recommended[1]	Mature Human Milk	Typical Commercial Formula	Cow's Milk (Mean)
Protein (g)	1.8 (See note 2.)	1.3–1.6	2.3	5.1
Fat (g)	3.3 (See note 3.)	5	5.3	5.7
Carbohydrate (g)	. . .	10.3	10.8	7.3
Linoleic acid (mg)	300	560	2300	125
Vitamin A (IU)	250	250	300	216
Vitamin D (IU)	40	3	63	3
Vitamin E (IU)	0.3 FT 0.7 LBW 1 g linoleic	0.3	2	0.1
Vitamin K (μg)	4	2	9	5
Vitamin C (mg)	8	7.8	8.1	2.3
Thiamine (μg)	40	25	80	59
Riboflavin (μg)	60	60	100	252
Niacin (μg)	250	250	1200	131
Vitamin B_6 (μg)	15 μg/g protein	15	63	66
Folic acid (μg)	4	4	10	8
Pantothenic acid (μg)	300	300	450	489
Vitamin B_{12} (μg)	0.15	0.15	0.25	0.56
Biotin (μg)	1.5	1	2.5	3.1
Inositol (mg)	4	20	5.5	20
Choline (mg)	7	13	10	23
Calcium (mg)	5	50	75	186
Phosphorus (mg)	25	25	65	145
Magnesium (mg)	6	6	8	20
Iron (mg)	1	0.1	1.5 in fortified	0.08
Iodine (μg)	5	4–9	10	7
Copper (μg)	60	25–60	80	20
Zinc (mg)	0.5	0.1–0.5	0.65	0.6
Manganese (μg)	5	1.5	5–160	3
Sodium (meq)	0.9	1	1.7	3.3
Potassium (meq)	2.1	2.1	2.7	6
Chloride (meq)	1.6	1.6	2.3	4.6
Osmolarity (mosm)	. . .	11.3	16–18.4	40

[1]Committee on Nutrition, American Academy of Pediatrics.
[2]Protein of nutritional quality equal to casein.
[3]Includes 300 mg essential fatty acids.

Jelliffe DB, Jelliffe EFP: *Human Milk in the Modern World.* Oxford University Press, 1979.

Lawrence RA: *Breast-Feeding: A Guide for the Medical Profession.* Mosby, 1989.

Neifert MR: Returning to breast feeding. *Clin Obstet Gynecol* 1980;**23**:1061.

Neville MC, Neifert MR (editors): *Lactation: Physiology, Nutrition, and Breast-Feeding.* Plenum Press, 1983.

Oxtoby MJ: Human immunodeficiency virus and other viruses in human milk: Placing the issues in broader perspective. *Pediatr Infect Dis J* 1988;**7**:825.

Whitehead RG, Paul AA: Growth charts and the assessment of infant feeding practices in the Western world and in developing countries. *Early Hum Dev* 1984; **9**:187.

SPECIAL DIETARY PRODUCTS FOR INFANTS

Soy protein Formulas

The major indication for the use of soy protein formulas is lactose intolerance. For example, it is reasonable to recommend a soy protein formula during recovery from acute gastroenteritis for a period of 2–4 weeks. Soy protein formulas are also used frequently in cases of suspected intolerance to cow's milk protein. However, infants who have true cow's milk protein intolerance may also be intolerant of soy protein. Many infants in the United States are currently fed soy protein formulas without good reason.

Semielemental Formulas

These formulas include Pregestimil (Mead Johnson), Nutramigen (Mead Johnson), and Alimentum (Ross). The major nitrogen source of each of these products is casein hydrolysate, supplemented with selected amino acids. Each contains an abundance of EFA from vegetable oil; Pregestimil and Alimentum also provide substantial amounts of medium-chain triglycerides (MCT). Pregestimil contains corn syrup solids; Nutramigen contains sucrose, which also provides part of the carbohydrate content in Alimentum.

These formulas are invaluable in a wide variety of malabsorption syndromes, including short bowel syndromes, some cases of chronic diarrhea, and some cases of cystic fibrosis. They are also effective in feeding infants who cannot tolerate cow's milk and soy protein.

Formula Supplements

The most useful formula supplements are MCT oil and polycose, both of which may be used to increase the energy density of a formula. Often it is more appropriate, however, to increase the concentration of the parent formula and thus increase the density of all nutrients.

Special Formulas

These formulas include those in which one component, often an amino acid, is reduced in concentration or removed for the dietary management of specific inborn metabolic diseases. Also included under this heading is Amin-Aid (American McGaw).

Complete information regarding the composition of these special formulas, the standard infant formulas, and special formulas for premature infants can be found in standard reference texts such as the Harriet Lane handbook (*A Manual for Pediatric House Officers*) and in the manufacturer's literature.

PRUDENT DIET

A prudent diet should be encouraged for all children 2 years of age and older: children with high cholesterol levels tend to become adults with high cholesterol levels and are likely, therefore, to have an increased risk of coronary heart disease. Nutritional habits are formed early in life; dietary intervention may, therefore, be exceptionally effective when started in early childhood.

Salient features of a prudent diet include the following:

(1) Total fat should constitute less than 30% of caloric intake, with saturated fats and polyunsaturated fats providing less than 10% each. Thus, monounsaturated fats should provide 10% or more of caloric intake from fat.
(2) Cholesterol intake should be less than 300 mg/d.
(3) Carbohydrates should provide 60% or more of daily caloric intake, with 50% or more in the form of complex carbohydrates (ie, no more than 10% in the form of simple sugars). A high-fiber diet is also recommended.
(4) The diet should be nutritionally complete, include a variety of foods, and be adequate for optimal growth and activity.
(5) A low salt intake is also advised.

The consumption of lean cuts of meats and poultry should be encouraged. Fish should be broiled or baked. Skim milk, soft margarine, and vegetable oils (especially olive oil) should be used. Consumption of egg yolks should be limited to 2–3 times per week. Whole-grain bread and cereals and plentiful amounts of fruits and vegetables are recommended. The consumption of processed foods, soda pop, desserts, and candy should be limited.

A prudent diet should be only one component of counseling on life-styles for children. Other aspects are the maintenance of ideal body weight, a regular exercise program, avoidance of smoking, and screening for hypertension. All children beyond the age of 3 years should be screened for total cholesterol. If an abnormal result is obtained, the screen should be repeated before proceeding to a more complete evaluation.

INTRAVENOUS NUTRITION

INDICATIONS

Supplemental Peripheral Nutrition

Supplemental peripheral nutrition is indicated when complete enteral feeding is not possible or desirable (eg, in the premature infant of very low birth weight during the first few days of postnatal life or in the malnourished surgical patient during the early postoperative period). Short-term partial intravenous feeding is a preferred alternative to dextrose electrolyte solutions alone. A suitable central line, if already available, can be used, but supplemental short-term nutrition may also be administered via a peripheral vein. Because of the osmolality of the solutions required, it is usually impossible to achieve total parenteral nutrition via a peripheral vein.

Total Parenteral Nutrition

Total parenteral nutrition (TPN) should be provided only when clearly indicated. Apart from the expense, numerous risks are associated with this method of feeding (see below). In addition, the powerful homeostatic control mechanisms provided by the intestine and the liver are bypassed. Even when TPN is indicated, every effort should be made to provide at least a minimum of nutrients enterally to help preserve the integrity of the gastrointestinal mucosa and of gastrointestinal function. Such feeding helps, at least to some extent, to maintain the physiologic release of gut hormones, bile flow, and the integrity of the enterocyte.

The primary indication for TPN is the loss of function of the gastrointestinal tract that prohibits the provision of more than a small proportion of required nutrients by the enteral route. Important examples include short bowel syndrome and some congenital defects of the gastrointestinal tract.

CATHETER SELECTION & POSITION

The Broviac is the catheter of choice for long-term intravenous nutrition. For periods of up to 3–4 weeks, a percutaneous central venous catheter threaded into the superior vena cava (SVC) from a peripheral vein can be used. For the infusion of dextrose concentrations higher than 12.5%, the tip of the catheter should be located in the SVC or right atrium. After placement, a chest x-ray must be obtained to check this position. If the catheter is to be used for nutrition and medications, a double-line catheter should be inserted.

COMPLICATIONS

Mechanical Complications
A. Related to Catheter Insertion or to Erosion of Catheter Through Major Blood Vessel: There is an extensive list of complications involving trauma to adjacent tissues and organs, including damage to the brachial plexus, hydrothorax, pneumothorax, hemothorax, and cerebrospinal fluid penetration. The catheter may slip, especially if care is not taken at the time of dressing or tubing change. The patient may manipulate the line.

B. Clotting of the Catheter: Addition of heparin (1 unit/mL) to the solution is an effective means of preventing this complication. If a catheter does become occluded, urokinase can be administered for clot lysis.

C. Related to Composition of Infusate: Calcium phosphate precipitation is a major problem if excess amounts of calcium or phosphorus are administered. The quantities of calcium and phosphate that can be added to the infusate vary widely, depending upon the particular commercial amino acid source. Intravenous calcium boluses should not be administered through a Broviac catheter. Factors that increase the risk of calcium phosphate precipitation include increasing pH and decreasing concentrations of amino acids. Precipitation of medications incompatible with TPN or lipids can also cause clotting.

Septic Complications
Septic complications are the most common cause of nonelective catheter removal, but strict use of aseptic technique and once-daily entry into the catheter at tubing change can result in greatly reduced rates of line sepsis. *For this reason, strict adherence to the standardized nursing protocol (for nurses and physicians) is mandatory.*

Metabolic Complications
A wide variety of metabolic complications associated with total parenteral malnutrition has been documented. Many of these have been related to deficiencies or excesses of specific nutrients. The incidence of these complications has decreased as a result of improvements in amino acid solutions and lipid emulsions and a better understanding of how to achieve appropriate intakes of most nutrients. However, specific deficiencies still occur, especially in the premature infant. Avoidance of deficiencies and excesses and of metabolic disorders requires careful attention to the nutrient balance, electrolyte composition, and delivery rate of the infusate and careful monitoring, especially when the composition or delivery rate is changed.

Currently, the most challenging metabolic complication is cholestasis, particularly common in premature infants of very low birth weight. Amino acids competing for and blocking bile acid receptors at the hepatocyte appear to be one critical factor in the pathogenesis of this disorder. Complete lack of oral feeding, sepsis, free radical damage, or toxic factors present in TPN solutions may contribute to this problem. There are no amino acid solutions currently available that have been proved to decrease cholestasis. Maneuvers that *may* minimize cholestasis include administering some enteral feedings (even if very small) as soon as feasible, protecting the TPN solutions from light, and alternating relatively larger doses with lower doses of amino acids every other day (eg, 1 g/kg/d alternating with 3 g/kg/d rather than administering 2 g/kg/d daily).

NUTRIENT REQUIREMENT & DELIVERY

Energy
When patients are fed intravenously, no fat and carbohydrate intakes are unabsorbed, and no energy is used in nutrient absorption. These factors account for at least 7% of energy in the diet of the enterally fed subject. The intravenously fed patient also expends less energy in physical activity because of some impediment to mobility. Average energy requirements are, therefore, at least 7% lower in children fed intravenously, and the decrease in activity probably increases this figure to a total reduction of 10–15%. Caloric guidelines for the intravenous feeding of infants and young children are as follows:

Age (mo)	Requirements (kcal/kg/d)
0–2	100–110
2–4	90–100
4–36	75–80

These guidelines are averages; individuals vary considerably. Some older infants require 70 kcal/

kg/d or fewer and on higher intravenous intakes will become obese. A multitude of factors can significantly increase energy requirement, including exposure to a cold environment, fever, sepsis, burns, trauma, cardiac or pulmonary disease, and "catch-up" growth after malnutrition.

With few exceptions, eg, some cases of respiratory insufficiency, at least 60% of energy requirements is provided as glucose. Up to 40% of calories may be provided by intravenous fat emulsions.

Dextrose

The energy density of intravenous dextrose (monohydrate) is 3.4 kcal/g. Thus, a 10% solution of dextrose in water (D10W) provides 0.34 kilocalories per milliliter. Dextrose is the main exogenous energy source provided by total intravenous feeding. Intravenous dextrose suppresses gluconeogenesis and provides a substrate that can be oxidized directly, especially by the brain, red and white blood cells, and wounds. Because of the high osmolality of dextrose solutions (D10W yields 505 mosm/kg H_2O), concentrations greater than 10–12.5% cannot be delivered via a peripheral vein or improperly positioned central line.

It is customary to think only in terms of dextrose concentrations when ordering intravenous solutions. However, the amount of glucose supplied is determined by the rate of administration as well as the dextrose concentration. Consequently, it is important to calculate the desired glucose load in planning dextrose infusions. If fluid volume is restricted, a higher dextrose concentration can be used to deliver the same quantity of dextrose per unit of time into the superior vena cava. Conversely, if unusually rapid initial flow rates are being used, a correspondingly lower dextrose concentration is indicated.

The standard initial quantity of dextrose administered is 10 g/kg/d, which provides 34 kcal/kg/d. This is typically, but not necessarily, provided as 100 mL/kg/d of D10W. Tolerance to intravenous dextrose normally increases rapidly, primarily because hepatic production of endogenous glucose is suppressed. Dextrose can be increased by 2.5 g/kg/d. Standard final infusates for infants usually contain D20W, but if necessary (especially at low flow rates), concentrations up to D30W or greater may be used. Again, these high concentrations should be delivered only into the superior vena cava or right atrium. Tolerance to intravenous dextrose loads is markedly diminished in the premature neonate and in patients in hypermetabolic states.

Problems associated with intravenous dextrose administration include hyperglycemia, hyperosmolality, and glucosuria (with osmotic diuresis and dehydration). Possible causes of unexpected hyperglycemia include the following: (1) inadvertent infusion of higher glucose concentrations than ordered; (2) uneven flow rate; (3) sepsis; (4) a stress situation;

(5) pancreatitis. Intravenous insulin reduces hyperglycemia but does not increase glucose oxidation rates; it may also decrease the oxidation of fatty acids, resulting in less energy for metabolism. Hence, insulin should be used very cautiously. A standard intravenous dose is 1 unit per 4 grams of carbohydrate, but much smaller quantities may be adequate. Exogenous insulin is probably contraindicated in hypermetabolic states.

Hypoglycemia may occur after an abrupt decrease in or cessation of intravenous glucose. When cyclic intravenous nutrition is provided, the intravenous glucose load should be decreased steadily for 1–2 hours prior to discontinuing the infusate. If the central line must be removed, the intravenous dextrose should be gradually tapered over several hours.

Quantities of exogenous dextrose in excess of maximal glucose oxidation rates are used initially to replace depleted glycogen stores; hepatic lipogenesis occurs thereafter. Excess hepatic lipogenesis may lead to a fatty liver when hepatic secretion of very low density lipoproteins fails to keep pace with lipogenesis. Lipogenesis results in release of carbon dioxide, which when added to the amount of carbon dioxide produced by glucose oxidation (which is 40% greater than that produced by lipid oxidation) may elevate the $Paco_2$ and aggravate respiratory insufficiency or impede weaning from a respirator.

Lipids

Several commercial fat emulsions are now available for intravenous use. All consist of more than 50% linoleic acid and 4–9% linolenic acid. It is recognized that this high level of linoleic is far from ideal except when small quantities of lipid are being given to prevent a deficiency in essential fatty acids. Ultimately, improved emulsions are anticipated. The particle size is approximately that of chylomicrons (0.5 μm), but the particle contains no protein. Thus, the infused fat emulsion must acquire apolipoprotein C-II from HDL particles before it can be acted on by endothelium-bound lipoprotein lipase (LPL) or hepatic triglyceride lipase. The level of LPL activity is the rate-limiting factor in the metabolism and clearance of fat emulsions from the circulation. LPL activity is inhibited or decreased by malnutrition, leukotrienes, immaturity, growth hormone, hypercholesterolemia, hyperphospholipidemia, and theophylline. LPL activity is enhanced by glucose, insulin, lipid, catecholamines, and exercise. Heparin releases LPL from the endothelium into the circulation and enhances the rate of hydrolysis and clearance of triglycerides. In small premature infants, low-dose heparin infusions may increase tolerance to intravenous lipid emulsion. After hydrolysis of the triglycerides, the residual phospholipid forms a vesicle that acquires free cholesterol from peripheral cell membranes, forming an abnormal lipoprotein particle (LpX). This particle is metabolized only slowly by the liver and accounts for the hyperphospholipidemia and hypercholesterolemia that may occur during administration of intravenous fat emulsions. Because 10% and 20% lipid emulsions contain the same concentrations of phospholipids, a 10% solution delivers more phospholipid per gram of lipid than a 20% solution. Twenty percent lipid emulsions are preferred for all patients.

The advantages of using fat emulsions to provide up to 40% of caloric intake include the following:

(1) The energy density, which is 2 kcal/mL for 20% emulsions, allows more energy to be provided via a peripheral vein than with dextrose alone.
(2) The osmolality is low: 280 mosm/kg H_2O.
(3) Deficiencies in essential fatty acids can be prevented.
(4) The production of CO_2 is 40% lower per unit of energy, an important consideration in cases of pulmonary insufficiency.
(5) The energy cost of fat storage is negligible (energy does not have to be synthesized from dextrose).
(6) The risk of fatty liver is decreased because of decreased hepatic lipogenesis from dextrose.

Potential disadvantages of fat emulsions include the following:

(1) Impairment of function of lymphocytes, neutrophils, macrophages, and the reticuloendothelial system.
(2) Coagulation defects, including thrombocytopenia, elevated prothrombin time (PT) and partial thromboplastin time (PTT).
(3) Decrease in pulmonary oxygen diffusion.
(4) Competition with bilirubin and drugs for albumin-binding sites.
(5) Increase in LDL cholesterol.

In general, these adverse effects can be avoided by starting with modest quantities and advancing cautiously in light of results of triglyceride monitoring and clinical circumstances. In cases of severe sepsis, special caution is required to ensure that the lipid is effectively metabolized. Continuous monitoring with long-term use is also essential.

Start with 1 g/kg/d. Advance every 1–2 days by 0.5–1 g/kg/d up to 2.5 g/kg/d in an infant and 3.5 g/kg/d in a child. Check serum triglycerides before starting and before and after increasing dose. Request results the same day. As a general rule, do not increase dose if serum triglyceride is greater than 250 mg/dL during infusion (150 mg/dL in neonates and septic patients). Clearance 4 hours postinfusion should also be monitored.

Note: Linoleic acid must constitute 2–3% of caloric intake (300 mg linoleic acid per 100 kcal) so that a deficiency in essential fatty acids can be avoided. Linolenic acid (1%) is also needed and is adequately supplied when linoleic acid needs are met.

Nitrogen

One gram of nitrogen is yielded by 6.25 grams of protein (1 gram of protein contains 16% nitrogen). Caloric density of protein is equal to 4 kcal/g (but protein calories must *not* be included in calculations of daily caloric intake).

A. Protein Requirements: Protein requirements for intravenous feeding are the same as those for normal oral feeding (Table 5–2).

B. Protein-Energy Interactions: There are important interactions between protein and energy requirements. A positive nitrogen balance cannot be achieved on a hypocaloric diet, because protein will be catabolized for energy. When energy intakes are low, the administration of some amino acid does, however, improve the severity of the negative nitrogen balance. Conversely, when nitrogen intake is low, the provision of calories improves nitrogen balance to some extent. In infants, the energy necessary to minimize nitrogen loss associated with an amino acid-free diet is approximately 70 kcal/kg/d. At this level of energy intake, a positive nitrogen balance can be achieved to a degree that depends on the level of nitrogen intake and is independent of further increase in energy intake.

In infants receiving about 50 kcal/kg/d, increasing protein intake up to 3 g/kg/d improves the nitrogen balance. In these circumstances, therefore, a ratio of grams of nitrogen per kilocalorie as low as 1:100 can be advantageous. However, at higher levels of energy intake, ratios of 1:150–250 or more are optimal. Although these ratios provide a useful crude check, they are not usually the best means of determining protein requirements.

C. Intravenous Amino Acid Solutions: Nitrogen requirements are provided by one of the commerically available amino acid solutions. All of the standard preparations are equally good sources of amino acids. There is some preliminary evidence, however, that the use of Trophamine in premature infants is associated with superior nitrogen retention. The putative benefits of Trophamine are quite likely attributable in part to the cysteine that can be added to the solution immediately before use. Forty milligrams of cysteine is added for each gram of Trophamine. Thus, a liter of 2% solution requires an addition of 800 mg of cysteine. Cysteine provides a good source of taurine.

Normally, the final infusate contains 2–3% amino acids, depending on the rate of infusion. In the very low birth weight or severely malnourished infant, the initial amount should be 1 g/kg/d.

Because of the high osmolality of amino acid solutions, the concentration should not be advanced beyond 2% in peripheral vein infusates.

D. Monitoring: Monitoring for tolerance of the intravenous amino acid solutions should include routine blood urea nitrogen (BUN). Blood ammonia should be assayed if clinically indicated, but the incidence of hyperammonemia has decreased since the development of the newer intravenous nitrogen preparations. More important are assays (serum alkaline phosphatase, γ-glutamyltransferase) to detect the onset of cholestatic liver disease.

E. Special Amino Acid Preparations: Some solutions are designed to provide high concentrations of branched-chain amino acids (BCAA). These solutions are expensive and should not be ordered without a specific reason, which does not include their routine use in liver disease. They may be indicated in hepatic failure and are also undergoing experimental use in multisystem organ failure. In this circumstance, the BCAA are given as a source of metabolizable energy, providing up to 25% of energy intake. Solutions containing only essential amino acids have some application in the management of patients with renal failure.

F. Albumin: Albumin (0.5–1 g/kg/dose) can be added to the infusate when clinically indicated to restore blood volume. If the pathoetiologic origin of hypoalbuminemia is considered to be primarily nutritional, however, the hypoalbuminemia—even if severe—should be managed by careful nutritional rehabiliation rather than by intravenous administration of albumin. Albumin is deficient in isoleucine and tryptophan and has too long a half-life (15–20 days) to be considered a useful nutritional source of amino acids.

Minerals & Electrolytes

A. Calcium, Phosphorus, and Magnesium: The results of 2 recent studies have indicated that the intravenously fed premature and term infant should be given relatively high amounts of calcium and phosphorus. Although lower amounts of calcium are routinely provided in many centers, current recommendations are as follows: calcium, 500–600 mg/L; phosphorus, 400–450 mg/L; and magnesium, 50–70 mg/L. After the age of 1 year, the recommendations are as follows: calcium, 200–400 mg/L; phosphorus, 150–300 mg/L; and magnesium, 20–40 mg/L. The calcium:phosphorus ratio should be 1.3:1 by weight or 1:1 by molar ratio. These recommendations are deliberately presented on a per liter infusate basis to avoid inadvertent administration of concentrations of calcium and phosphorus that are high enough to precipitate in the tubing. During periods of fluid restriction, care must be taken not to inadvertently increase the concentration of calcium and phosphorus in the infusate. These recommendations assume an average fluid intake of 120–150 mL/kg/d and an infusate of 25 grams of amino acid per liter. With lower amino acid concentrations, the concentrations of calcium and phosphorus should be decreased.

B. Electrolytes: Standard recommendations are given in Fig 5–1. After chloride requirements are met, the remainder of the anion required to balance the cation should be given as acetate to avoid the possibility of acidosis resulting from excessive chloride. The required concentrations of electrolytes depend to some extent on the flow rate of the infusate and must be modified if flow rates are unusually low or high and if there are specific indications in individual patients. Intravenous sodium should be administered very sparingly in the severely malnourished patient because of impaired membrane function and high intracellular sodium levels. Conversely, generous quantities of potassium are indicated. Replacement electrolytes and fluids should be delivered via a separate infusate.

C. Trace Elements: Recommended intravenous intakes of trace elements are given in Fig 5–1.

When intravenous nutrition is only supplemental or limited to less than 2 weeks, only zinc need routinely be added.

Intravenous copper requirements are relatively low in the young infant because of the presence of hepatic copper stores. These are significant even in the 28-week fetus. Circulating levels of copper and manganese should be monitored in the presence of cholestatic liver disease. If monitoring is not feasible, temporary withdrawal of added copper and manganese is advisable. Copper and manganese are excreted primarily in the bile, but selenium, chromium, and molybdenum are excreted primarily in the urine. These trace elements, therefore, should be administered with caution in the presence of renal failure.

For patients on long-term parenteral nutrition, a dose of 1 μg/kg/d of iodine avoids any risk of iodine deficiency and does not increase the risk of toxicity from accidental absorption of topical iodine-containing preparations.

Although low doses of iron are routinely added in some centers to the intravenous infusate for infants and children, no official recommendation has been made because of the lack of adequate published data regarding compatibility. Iron added to the infusate should be in a diluted form of iron dextran in a concentration of 1 mg/L. After 2 months of age, maintenance intravenous iron requirements for the term infant are approximately 100 μg/kg/d intravenously. After the first month, the premature infant requires up to 200 μg/kg/d intravenously. Although overload is unlikely to occur during short-term parenteral nutrition, a surreptitious accumulation of extra iron could occur if parenteral nutrition is prolonged. This risk is enhanced if the patient has received blood transfusions. A second concern is that the potential for free iron is increased in malnourished infants with low transferrin levels. Excess iron is thought to enhance the risk of gram-negative septicemia. Iron has powerful oxidant properties and can enhance the

---

PEDIATRIC PARENTERAL NUTRITION (PN) ORDER FORM

Imprint Patient Plate

_____

Weight of patient _____ kg   Central line _____   Peripheral line _____

Rate _____

	Standard Order	Modifications To Standard Order	*Adjustments for Neonates and Premature Infants (Circle these when required and cross out corresponding items* under "standard order").
Protein (as amino acid)*	g%		*Use trophamine and cysteine for patients in level II and III nurseries who have a central line or are on day 6 of peripheral therapy.
Dextrose	g%		
Na	30 meq/L		
K	25 meq/L		
Cl	20 meq/L		
Acetate	45 meq/L		
Ca (as gluconate) (10 mM Ca/L)	20 meq/L		
Mg (as sulfate)	3 meq/L		
P	10 meq/L		
MVI Pediatric	*5.0 mL/d		*2 mL/kg/d for patients < 2.5 kg
Zinc	*1.0 mg/L		*Zn: 400 µg/kg/d < 2 kg body weight
Copper	200 µg/L		250 µg/kg/d others < 3 mo old
Manganese	5.0 µg/L		
Chromium	2.0 µg/L		
Selenium	20.0 µg/L		
Iodide	10 µg/L		
Heparin	1000 Units/L		
Cysteine (40 mg/g trophamine)*	._____ mg/L		*Use only with trophamine

Pharmacy will automatically account for electrolytes provided in amino acid preparation.
Changes in Na or K to be made as: Cl only __, or Acetate only __, or Cl: Acetate 1:1 __, or other Cl: Acetate ratio (specify _____).

Date: _____   Signature: _____ M.D.

Figure 5–1. Example of pediatric parenteral nutrition order. Standard recommendations for minerals and trace elements are indicated.

---

demand for antioxidants, especially vitamin E. None of these concerns appear to preclude the routine use of iron supplements during intravenous nutrition, but they do emphasize the need for a conservative attitude in determining dosage schedules.

Currently, intravenous infusates are contaminated with aluminum. In infants, aluminum accumulation in bone after 3 weeks of intravenous feeding can be marked. Aluminum intakes should be measured when possible, especially in the premature infant and in the infant or child with impaired renal function.

Vitamins

Recommendations for intravenous vitamin intakes are given in Table 5–6. MVI Pediatric (Armour) meets the guidelines for term infants. The recommended dose of MVI Pediatric for premature infants is 2 mL (40%) of a single-dose vial per kilogram per day. This formulation is not optimal (too little vitamin A, excessive amounts of water-soluble vitamins), but it is currently the best available.

Intravenous lipid preparations contain enough tocopherol to effect total blood tocopherol levels. The majority of tocopherol in soybean oil emulsion is γ-tocopherol, which has substantially less biologic activity than α-tocopherol, which is present in safflower oil emulsions. Premature infants may possibly be susceptible to liver damage from excessive intakes of vitamin E. The intravenous administration of 25–100 mg/d of α-tocopherol acetate for as little as one week has been associated with coagulopathy and progressive liver failure in several infants of very low birth weight. The toxicity may well have been due to the solubilizer, polysorbate 80, rather than to the α-tocopherol.

Recent data indicate that a dose of 40 IU/kg/d of vitamin D (maximum 400 IU/d) is adequate for both term and preterm infants. The higher dose of 160 IU/kg/d has not been associated with any complication and continues to be recommended.

Fluid Requirements

The initial fluid volume and subsequent increments in flow rate are determined by basic fluid requirements, the clinical status of the patient, and the extent to which additional fluid administration can be tolerated and may be required to achieve adequate nutrient intake. Calculation of initial fluid volumes to be administered should be based on standard pediatric practice. Tolerance of higher flow rates must be determined on an individual basis. If replacement fluids are required for ongoing abnormal losses, these should be administered via a separate line.

Ordering

An example of a parenteral nutrition order form for pediatrics is given in Fig 5–1. Orders should be reviewed daily when changes are made and when the patient is acutely ill.

Monitoring

Vital signs should be checked at each shift.

With central catheter in situ and fever more than 38 °C, peripheral and central line blood cultures, urine cultures, complete physical examination, and examination of intravenous entry point are required. Instability of vital signs, elevated white blood cell count with left shift, and glycosuria suggest sepsis. Appropriate antibiotic therapy should be instituted after cultures and blood cultures repeated every 24 hours until results are negative. Removal of the central venous catheter should be considered if patient is toxic or unresponsive to antibiotics (the patient must be weaned of dextrose prior to removal of the catheter).

A. Physical Examination: Monitor especially for hepatomegaly (differential diagnoses include fluid overload, congestive heart failure, steatosis, and hepatitis) and edema (differential diagnoses: fluid overload, congestive heart failure, hypoalbuminemia, thrombosis of superior vena cava).

B. Intake/Output Record: Calories and volume delivered should be calculated from previous day's intake and output sheets (that which was delivered rather than that which was ordered). The following should be recorded on flow sheets: intravenous, enteral, and total fluid (mL/kg/d); dextrose (g/kg/d); protein (g/kg/d); lipids (g, kcal/kg/d); energy (kcal/kg/d).

C. Growth, Urine, and Blood: Routine monitoring guidelines given in Table 5–13 are only a guide. These are minimum requirements, except in the very long term stable patients. Individual variables should be monitored more frequently as indicated, as should additional variables or clinical indications. For example, a blood ammonia should be ordered in an infant with lethargy, pallor, poor growth, acidosis, azotemia, and elevated liver enzymes.

Fomon SJ, Heird WC (editors): *Energy and Protein Needs During Infancy.* Academic Press, 1986.

Greene HL et al: Guidelines for the use of vitamins, trace elements, calcium, magnesium, and phosphorus in in-

Table 5–13. Routine monitoring summary.

Variables	Acute Stage	Long-Term
Growth		
Weight	Daily	Weekly
Length	Weekly	
Head circumference	Weekly	
Urine		
Glucose (dipstick)	Void	Twice weekly
Specific gravity	Void	
Volume	Daily	
Blood		
Glucose	4 h after changes,[1] then daily for 2 days, then twice weekly.	Twice weekly
Na, K, Cl, CO_2, BUN	Daily for 2 days after changes, then twice weekly.	Twice weekly
Ca, Mg, P	Initially, then twice weekly.	Weekly
Total protein, albumin bilirubin, AST, and alkaline phosphatase	Initially, then weekly.	Weekly
Zinc and copper	Initially, then weekly.	Monthly
Triglycerides	Initially, 1 day after changes, then weekly.	Monthly Weekly
CBC	Initially, then twice weekly; according to clinical indications (see text).	Twice weekly

[1]Changes include alterations in concentration or flow rate.

fants and children receiving total parenteral nutrition: Report of the Subcommittee on Pediatric Parenteral Nutrient Requirements from the Committee on Clinical Practice Issues of the American Society for Clinical Nutrition. *Am J Clin Nutr* 1988;**48:**1324.

Heird WC et al: Amino acid mixture designed to maintain normal plasma amino acid patterns in infants and children requiring parenteral nutrition. *Pediatrics* 1987; **80:**401.

Kerner JA (editor): *Manual of Pediatric Parenteral Nutrition.* Wiley, 1983.

INTENSIVE CARE NUTRITION

Intravenous Delivery of Nutrients

The availability of sufficient intravenous lines for nutrition in addition to other multiple needs for intravenous access is a perennial problem in the intensive care setting. In many instances, the position of these lines, frequently placed for other purposes under emergency conditions, also prevents their use for nutrition support. Double-lumen catheters, with tips located in the superior vena cava or right atrium, should be placed whenever possible so that these difficulties can be minimized. Sometimes, these catheters can be placed electively prior to major procedures.

The need for fluid restriction, combined with extensive administration of fluids for nonnutritional purposes, also limits opportunities to provide adequate nutrition. This problem can be mitigated to some extent by the immediate use of more concentrated solutions of dextrose, amino acids, vitamins, and trace elements. Provided that the catheter tip is placed in the superior vena cava, the most important factor is the quantity delivered and not the concentration in the line. The only exceptions to this principle are calcium and phosphorus.

Provision of Nutrients in Hypermetabolic States

The most important principle is to continue enteral feeding whenever possible. If enteral feeding must be discontinued, it should be reintroduced as soon as possible so that the integrity of the enterocytes can be maintained. The increase in energy requirements varies according to the severity of hypermetabolism and its cause. Requirements are highest in burn patients, but major trauma and severe sepsis increase energy expenditure by 20–50%.

The uncontrolled muscle proteolysis and negative nitrogen balance, which are among the most outstanding features of hypermetabolic states, cannot be counteracted totally by aggressive nutrition support or by other known therapeutic modalities. However, optimal nutrition support does help significantly in reversing the adverse effects of hypermetabolism. Negative nitrogen balance can be improved by providing 1.5–2 times the basal protein requirement for

that age. Larger quantities do not further improve nitrogen balance; furthermore, they require substantial energy expenditure for their oxidation and increase CO_2 production. Additional amounts of branched-chain amino acids, however, are currently being used experimentally as an energy source to provide up to 25% of caloric needs.

Another major metabolic aberration in hypermetabolic states, compared with the metabolic response to fasting, is persistent, uncontrolled hepatic gluconeogenesis. Elevated blood glucose concentrations are one of the early laboratory indicators of hypermetabolism. Gluconeogenesis is not switched off—as would normally be expected—by the administration of intravenous dextrose. Although some exogenous dextrose will be oxidized, the amount is likely to be quite limited. Dextrose administration tends to aggravate hyperglycemia and increase hepatic lipogenesis. The aim should be to provide at least 50% of energy requirements as dextrose, but in some patients (especially those who develop multisystem organ failure), only very modest quantities will be tolerated. If severe hyperglycemia and glycosuria occur, temporary insulin therapy is necessary. However, the putative effects of insulin in hypermetabolic states are complex and not well clarified. Hypermetabolism is characterized by insulin resistance. Insulin does not reverse the uncontrolled muscle catabolism and gluconeogenesis, nor does administration of insulin increase glucose oxidation. Theoretically, insulin administration could decrease lipolysis and thus deprive the hypermetabolic patient of some of the major sources of utilizable endogenous fuel.

Lipolysis is increased in hypermetabolic states; β-oxidation of fatty acids is also increased initially. Ketogenesis, although it occurs in starvation states, does not occur in hypermetabolic states. Utilization of exogenous lipids depends on the rate of release of endogenous fatty acids versus the rate of β-oxidation. Intravenous lipids can usually be utilized quite well in early stages, and up to 50% of energy may be provided as lipid. Metabolically, lipid is the preferred fuel in patients with severe sepsis. Lipid tolerance deteriorates in advanced multisystem organ failure. Carnitine deficiency may limit utilization in some cases.

The metabolic and nutritional advantages of lipid as a fuel must be balanced against potential adverse effects in the septic child. These may include some impairment of the function of lymphocytes, neutrophils, and macrophages and possible coagulation defects. It is important to monitor these factors closely (including triglyceride, PT, PTT, and platelets) and not to administer fat emulsion in excess of quantities that can be cleared effectively from the circulation.

In summary, nutritional management of hypermetabolic states includes the administration of only modest quantities of intravenous glucose; more liberal use of intravenous fat emulsions in some cases;

and the administration of 1.5–2 times the basal amino acid requirement. These intakes should be tailored to the tolerance of each individual patient and should be very closely monitored. On a research basis, additional amounts of branched-chain amino acids may be given as an energy source. Sodium intake should be strictly limited because of increased intracellular levels. Enteral feeding should be recommenced at the earliest possible moment.

Hypoalbuminemia may occur in hypermetabolic states because of the direct effect of interleukin-1 and as a response to sepsis. Hence, low serum albumin does not necessarily result from protein deficiency in these circumstances.

Filkins JP: Monokines and the metabolic pathophysiology of septic shock. *Fed Proc* 1985;**44**:300.
Nanni G et al: Plasma carnitine levels and urinary carnitine excretion during sepsis. *J Parenter Enter Nutr* 1985;**9**:483.
Shaw JHF, Wolfe RR: Energy and protein metabolism in sepsis and trauma. *Aust N Z J Surg* 1987;**57**:41.

6 Immunization

Andrew M. Wiesenthal, MD

The routine use of immunization has become an integral part of pediatric practice in the United States over the last 50 years. Despite the threats of complacency, increased cost, and litigation, immunizations continue to be a critical part of the well-child care provided by the practitioner. Experience with smallpox has shown that complete eradication of a disease is possible when mass coverage with an effective immunization is attained and maintained.

Every immunization is intended to prevent either the primary manifestations of infection by an organism or secondary phenomena resulting from that infection. To decide which children should routinely receive a particular product, public health officials pay careful attention to the likely benefits of the use of the product as well as the risks inherent in its use. This principle not only informs public health strategies for the mass use of immunizations but also guides the individual practitioner as each child presents for health maintenance.

An immunization confers a benefit to the extent that it eliminates the risk of a particular illness or its complications. Any calculation of benefit must take into account the likelihood that the illness will occur in a defined population or individual as well as the likelihood that the immunization will effectively prevent that illness. This measure of the risk of not using the product must be weighed against the risk to the individual child of using it. It is the obligation of the physician to present this information to parents and to document their consent to the use of an immunization in their child's medical record. Although there is no single right way for a physician to conduct such a discussion with parents (nor, indeed, is it required in most jurisdictions), the responsible physician must do so. See the section at the end of the chapter for a fuller discussion of the legal implications of childhood immunization.

The recommendations for use of immunizations outlined in this chapter are current as of this writing. However, as technology and epidemiology change, the recommendations are bound to change as well. The most useful sources for current information are the following:

(1) *Morbidity and Mortality Weekly Report*. Published weekly by the Centers for Disease Control (CDC), Atlanta, GA 30333. *MMWR* contains the recommendations of the US Public Health Service Advisory Committee on Immunization Practices (ACIP).

(2) *Report of the Committee on Infectious Diseases*. Published at 2-year intervals, the *Red Book* is available from the American Academy of Pediatrics, 141 Northwest Point Boulevard, PO Box 927, Elk Grove Village, IL 60009–0927. Updates are published in *Pediatrics* as needed.

SAFETY OF IMMUNIZATION

Vaccine Factors

All vaccines licensed for use in the United States are subjected to rigorous testing for purity and uniformity of content. The safety standards established by the Food and Drug Administration (FDA) require regular examination of manufacturing techniques as well as production lots of vaccine. As a result of these standards, no incidents of bacterial or viral contamination of vaccines have occurred at the factory level in the United States for decades.

Factors Related to Vaccine Administration

The use of disposable syringes and needles or a single-dose vaccine unit is preferred to minimize the opportunity for contamination. If reusable glass syringes are employed, they must be thoroughly cleaned and autoclaved after each use. The American Academy of Pediatrics recommends that the autoclave be set at 121 °C (249.8 °F) for 15 minutes at 15 lb pressure. If autoclaving is not possible, dry heat of 170 °C (338 °F) for 2 hours or boiling for 30 minutes are acceptable alternatives. A solution of 70% alcohol is appropriate for disinfecting the stopper of the vaccine container and the skin at the injection site.

Adherence to the manufacturer's recommendations for route and site of administration of injectable vaccines is critical to both the safety and efficacy of these preparations. In general, all vaccines that contain an adjuvant (eg, alum) must be administered intramuscularly to avoid significant pain or sterile abscesses. Such injections should be given in the anterolateral thigh (not intragluteally) in infants and may be given in the deltoid or triceps muscle in older children and adults. Aqueous vaccines may be administered intramuscularly or subcutaneously. Good injection technique, including aspiration prior to injection, must always be followed.

It is safe to administer many combinations of vaccines simultaneously without increasing the risk of adverse effects (see below under individual preparations for further discussion). If any doubt exists about either the safety or efficacy of simultaneous immunization, then at least 30 days should elapse between the administration of one vaccine and the next. If an immunoglobulin has been administered, live virus immunization should ordinarily be delayed by at least 90 days to avoid interference with the immune response. Exceptions to this include the simultaneous administration (same time, different sites) of several human hyperimmune globulins (tetanus, hepatitis, rabies) along with their associated vaccines under the appropriate clinical circumstances (see below under the specific preparations).

Host Factors

A. Healthy Children: Healthy children are ideal candidates for immunization. Minor, nonfebrile (temperature < 37.5 °C [99.5 °F]), acute illnesses are not contraindications to immunization because such illnesses are so common in early childhood and because there is no evidence that immunization under these conditions increases the rate of adverse effects or decreases efficacy. Fever greater than 37.5 °C (99.5 °F) may constitute a contraindication.

B. Children With Chronic Illnesses: Most chronic diseases are not of themselves contraindications to immunization. In fact, children with chronic diseases may be at greater risk than healthy children for complications from illnesses preventable by immunization, making immunization even more important for the former. Premature infants are a good example. It is clear that they should be immunized according to their chronologic, not gestational, age, especially in view of the many chronic debilities they often suffer. The one exception to this rule may be children with progressive central nervous system disorders. Immunization may be deferred or avoided entirely for them, whereas children with static central nervous system diseases are candidates for immunization.

C. Immunodeficient Children: Congenitally immunodeficient children should not be immunized with live viral or live bacterial vaccines. Depending on the nature of the immunodeficiency, other vaccines are safe and may be capable of evoking an immune response. Children with cancer and children being treated with corticosteroids or other immunosuppressive agents should not ordinarily be immunized with live viral or live bacterial vaccines. This contraindication does not apply if the malignant disorder is in remission and chemotherapy has not been administered for at least 90 days. In addition, the following children may all receive live vaccines safely: children being treated with low to moderate

doses of corticosteroids for less than 14 days, children on alternate-day steroid therapy, children on physiologic corticosteroid maintenance therapy without other immunodeficiency, and children using only topical or intra-articular corticosteroids. These guidelines apply as well to children with documented human immunodeficiency virus (HIV) infection, except that oral attenuated poliovirus vaccine is not recommended for these children, although live measles, mumps, and rubella immunizations are recommended. No distinction is made between children with asymptomatic HIV infection and those with symptomatic infection for the purpose of this recommendation. Siblings of a child who is immunodeficient should not receive oral poliovirus vaccine unless the immunodeficient child has been successfully immunized against poliomyelitis. If not, the siblings should receive inactivated poliovirus vaccine. Measles, mumps, and rubella vaccines are not contraindicated under these circumstances.

D. Allergic or Hypersensitive Children: Hypersensitivity reactions are rare following immunization. They are generally attributable to a trace component of the vaccine rather than to the antigen itself. Measles, mumps, and rubella vaccines now contain microgram quantities of neomycin. Children with known anaphylactic responses to this antibiotic should not be given these vaccines. Trace quantities of egg antigens may be present in influenza vaccines, which are grown in eggs, and in vaccines raised in fowl-derived tissue culture, including measles and mumps vaccines. Children who have had anaphylactic reactions to eggs should not be given these vaccines. Children with less serious reactions to eggs may generally be safely immunized with these products. If doubt exists about the nature of a child's egg sensitivity, a skin testing procedure is outlined in the *Report of the Committee on Infectious Diseases* ("Red Book").

Centers for Disease Control: Immunization of children infected with human immunodeficiency virus: Supplementary ACIP statement. *MMWR* 1988;**37:**181.

Centers for Disease Control: Immunization of children infected with human T-lymphotropic virus type III/lymphadenopathy associated virus. *MMWR* 1986;**35:**595.

COMPOSITION OF IMMUNIZING AGENTS

Active Immunization

Although each vaccine is unique in some fashion, it is helpful for the practitioner to be familiar with the general constituents of vaccines. The antigenic component, or immunogen, may be a single, well-defined entity, such as tetanus toxoid, or it may be a mixture of defined entities, such as the capsular polysaccharides of pneumococcal vaccine. The immunogen may be a live, attenuated organism, like that in bacille Calmetle-Guérin (BGG) or measles vaccine, or it may be whole, killed organisms, such as inactivated poliovaccine contains. The antigenic component may be a complex of killed, disrupted organisms and products, as in pertussis vaccine. All antigens are not equally capable of inducing an immune response in all hosts. The factors influencing host responses include genetic variability in the predisposition to respond to certain antigens, age at first exposure, and any prior experience with the antigen. A proportion of children receiving certain antigens simply do not mount a response that is capable of conferring protection against future infection. For this reason, every vaccine has a definable failure rate.

The immunogen is suspended or dissolved in a fluid, such as sterile water or saline solution. The fluid may also be more complex, such as tissue culture medium, and it may contain constituents from the biologic system used to produce the immunogen.

Most vaccines contain materials, particularly mercurials, to preserve or stabilize the immunogen. In addition, trace amounts of antibiotics, such as neomycin, may be present to prevent bacterial overgrowth.

Some vaccines contain adjuvants, eg, alum, aluminum hydroxide, and aluminum phosphate, which are nonspecific immune stimulants. They also help to retain the immunogen in a "depot" site for a prolonged time, thus increasing the antigenic response evoked by the primary immunogen.

Finally, despite rigorous testing and high standards of mechanical and biologic purity and stability, vaccines may contain unwanted and undetectable antigens and other materials. Although this eventuality is not likely, vaccine administration could, on rare occasions, have wholly unforeseen adverse consequences.

Passive Immunization

Immune globulin (IG) is derived from pooled donations of large numbers of individuals (more than 1000 per lot). IG is prepared by alcohol fractionation, is sterile, and is not known to transmit any infectious agents (including hepatitis B virus and HIV). It is a 16.5% solution consisting primarily of immunoglobulin G (IgG) with small amounts of IgA and IgM.

ROUTINE CHILDHOOD IMMUNIZATIONS

See Table 6–1 for a detailed schedule of the administration of routine childhood immunizations to normal infants and children. Even if the interval elapsed between doses in a series of immunizations is longer than recommended, that series can be resumed as if no interruption had taken place; it is not necessary to begin the series again. Table 6–2 sets forth recommended schedules for children whose immunization was not initiated at the recommended time during the first year of life. Variations from these schedules may be necessitated by epidemiologic or individual clinical circumstances. These variations are discussed in the sections on specific vaccines.

DIPHTHERIA

Diphtheria toxoid is prepared by the formaldehyde inactivation of diphtheria toxin. The toxoid content of the several available preparations varies and is measured in flocculating units (Lf). The protective efficacy of diphtheria toxoid has never been measured on a mass scale, but it is estimated to be greater than 85% and less than 100%.

Preparations Available

A. Diphtheria Toxoid: This preparation is used only when tetanus toxoid and pertussis vaccine are both contraindicated. It contains 10–12 Lf per immunizing dose.

B. Diphtheria-Tetanus (DT) (Pediatric): These toxoids are used when pertussis vaccine is contraindicated. DT contains 10–12 Lf per dose. Pediatric DT should not be used in adults because of potentially severe adverse reactions.

C. Tetanus-Diphtheria (Td) (Adult): This preparation contains 10% of the diphtheria antigen content of pediatric preparations ($\leq$ 2 Lf per dose) and is far less likely to produce local reactions while still eliciting a booster response. This is the preparation ordinarily used in individuals beyond the appropriate age for pertussis immunization.

D. Diphtheria-Tetanus-Pertussis (DTP): This is the standard immunizing agent for healthy children. It contains 10–20 Lf per dose. See the section on DTP below.

Dosage & Schedule

All the above preparations are administered intramuscularly in a dose of 0.5 mL. See Table 6–1 for the routine schedule and Table 6–2 for schedules for children not appropriately immunized during the first year of life.

Adverse Effects

No significant adverse reactions have been associated with diphtheria toxoid alone.

Antibody Preparations

Equine diphtheria antitoxin is available for use in the treatment of the disease. Dosage depends on the

Table 6–1. Recommended schedule for active immunization of normal infants and children.[1,2]

Recommended Age	Immunization(s)[3]	Comments
2 mo	DTP, OPV	Can be initiated as early as age 2 wk in areas of high endemicity or during epidemics.
4 mo	DTP, OPV	2-mo interval desired for OPV to avoid interference from previous dose.
6 mo	DTP	A third dose of OPV is not indicated in the USA but is desirable in geographic areas where polio is endemic.
15 mo	Measles, mumps, rubella (MMR),[4] DTP,[5] OPV, PRP-D	MMR preferred to individual vaccines; tuberculin testing may be done at the same visit. The ACIP now recommends that the fourth DTP and the third OPV and PRP-D be routinely given at 15 months along with MMR, rather than at 18 months.
4–6 yr	DTP[7] OPV	At or before school entry.
14–16 yr	Td	Repeat every 10 yr throughout life.

[1]Modified and reproduced, with permission, from *The 1988 Report of the Committee on Infectious Diseases*, 21st ed. © 1988 American Academy of Pediatrics.
[2]For all products used, consult manufacturer's package insert for instructions for storage, handling, dosage, and administration. Biologics prepared by different manufacturers may vary, and package inserts of the same manufacturer may change from time to time. Therefore, the physician should be aware of the contents of the current package insert.
[3]DTP = diphtheria and tetanus toxoids with pertussis vaccine; OPV = oral poliovirus vaccine containing attenuated poliovirus types 1, 2, and 3; MMR = live measles, mumps, and rubella viruses in a combined vaccine (see text for discussion of single vaccines versus combination); PRP-D = *Haemophilus* b diphtheria toxoid conjugate vaccine; Td = adult tetanus toxoid (full dose) and diphtheria toxoid (reduced dose) for adult use.
[4]In July 1989, in response to the national increase in reported measles cases in 1989 (despite high levels of immunization), the Red Book Committee of the American Academy of Pediatrics recommended that a second dose of MMR be given at the time a child enters junior high school. The official ACIP recommendation on a second dose of MMR was not available at the time of final editing of this chapter, but it is believed that it will be to give a second dose between the ages of 4 and 6 years at the time of primary school entry. If a child has already had two doses of MMR by the time he or she reaches junior high school, the Red Book Committee has said that an additional dose at the time is not necessary.
[5]Should be given 6 to 12 months after the third dose.
[6]*MMWR* 1989;**38**:205.
[7]Up to the seventh birthday.

size and location of the diphtheritic membrane and an estimation of the patient's level of intoxication. Before proceeding with the use of this preparation, the physician must determine the presence or absence of equine serum sensitivity. If it is present, desensitization must be undertaken. If it is absent, the following doses should be considered:

Site	Duration of Lesion	Toxic?	Dose
Pharyngeal or laryngeal	< 48 h	—	20,000–40,000 units
Nasopharyngeal	—	—	40,000–60,000 units
Extensive	> 72 h	Yes	80,000–100,000 units

The antitoxin should always be administered intravenously to neutralize circulating toxin as rapidly as possible.

TETANUS

Tetanus toxoid is also prepared by inactivating the toxin with formaldehyde. Its activity is measured in flocculating units (Lf) and is generally 4–10 Lf per immunizing dose for adsorbed products and 4–5 Lf per dose for the fluid product. The protective efficacy of tetanus toxoid has also never been measured in any large study, but it is believed to be high.

Preparations Available
A. Tetanus Toxoid (Fluid): This preparation is used rarely, only when rapid immunization is desirable.

B. Tetanus Toxoid and Aluminum Phosphate Adsorbed: This is the standard single antigen "booster" toxoid.

C. Tetanus-Diphtheria (Pediatric DT and Adult Td): See above.

D. Diphtheria-Tetanus-Pertussis (DTP): See the section on DTP below.

Dosage & Schedule
All the above preparations are administered intramuscularly in a dose of 0.5 mL. See Table 6–1 for the routine schedule and Table 6–2 for the schedule for children not appropriately immunized during the first year of life.

Table 6–2. Recommended immunization schedules for children not immunized in first year of life.[1]

Recommended Time	Immunization(s)	Comments
Less than 7 years old		
First visit	DTP, OPV, MMR	MMR if child ≥ 15 mo old; tuberculin testing may be done at same visit.
Interval after first visit: 1 mo	PRP-D	For children aged 15–60 mo; can be given concurrently with DTP (at separate sites) and other vaccines.[2]
2 mo	DTP, OPV	
4 mo	DTP	A third dose of OPV is not indicated in the USA but is desirable in geographic areas where polio is endemic.
10–16 mo.	DTP, OPV	OPV is not given if third dose was given earlier.
4–6 yr (at or before school entry)	DTP, OPV	DTP is not necessary if the fourth dose was given after the fourth birthday; OPV is not necessary if recommended OPV dose at 10–16 mo following first visit was given after the fourth birthday.
10 yr later	Td	Repeat every 10 yr throughout life.
7 Years Old and Older		
First visit	Td, OPV, MMR	
Interval after first visit: 2 mo	Td, OPV	
8–14 mo	Td, OPV	
10 yr later	Td	Repeat every 10 yr throughout life.

[1]Modified and reproduced, with permission, from *The 1988 Report of the Committee on Infectious Diseases*, 21st ed. © 1988 American Academy of Pediatrics.
[2]The initial 3 doses of DTP can be given at 1- to 2-month intervals; so, for the child in whom immunization is initiated at age 24 months or older, one visit could be eliminated by giving DTP, OPV, and MMR at the first visit; DTP and PRP-D at the second visit (1 month later); and DTP and OPV at the third visit (2 months after the first visit). Subsequent DTP and OPV 10 to 16 months after the first visit are still indicated. PRP-D, MMR, DTP, and OPV can be given simultaneously at separate sites if return of vaccine recipient for future immunizations is doubtful.

Adverse Effects

Significant reactions to tetanus toxoid, historically an extremely safe preparation, are very unusual. Some older individuals who have had repeated doses may experience severe local reactions.

Antibody Preparations

Tetanus immune globulin (TIG) is indicated in the management of tetanus-prone wounds occurring in individuals who have had an uncertain number or fewer than 3 tetanus immunizations. Fully immunized persons need not receive TIG regardless of the nature of their wound. The dose is 250–500 units (1–2 vials).

PERTUSSIS

Pertussis vaccine as currently used in the United States is a preparation of killed whole cells. Bacterial inactivation is carried out by a variety of means. The immunogenicity of the vaccine is standardized in an indirect but reproducible assay, the mouse protection test. The currently available preparations have a proved protective efficacy of 80–90%. Further epidemiologic evidence of the efficacy of pertussis vaccine is provided by the observation of a large increase in reported pertussis cases in Great Britain and Japan after those 2 countries reduced or discontinued the use of the vaccine.

Preparations Available

A. Pertussis Vaccine (Adsorbed): This is manufactured by the Michigan Department of Public Health for use in that state. It may be obtained for other use by consultation with the department.

B. Diphtheria-Tetanus-Pertussis (DTP): See the section on DTP, below.

Dosage & Schedule

Each of the available preparations is administered intramuscularly in a dose of 0.5 mL. See Table 6–1 for the routine schedule and Table 6–2 for the schedule for children not appropriately immunized during the first year of life.

Adverse Effects

A large number of adverse reactions have been attributed to pertussis vaccine. These can be divided into 3 categories: local, mild to moderate systemic, and severe systemic reactions. Local reactions include pain, swelling, and redness at the injection site. Typical mild to moderate reactions include a fever equal to or greater than 38 °C (100.4 °F) but less than or equal to 40.5 °C (104.9 °F), drowsiness, fretfulness, anorexia, and vomiting. Severe reactions include persistent crying, high-pitched cry, hypotonic-hyporesponsive episodes, convulsions, and fever equal to or greater than 40.5 °C (104.9 °F). The estimated rates of these reactions within the first 48 hours after immunization are shown in Table 6–3. Rarer systemic reactions include acute (onset within 7 days of immunization) encephalopathy, which is estimated to occur at a rate of 1:140,000 doses administered, and consequent permanent neurologic deficit, which is estimated to occur at a rate of 1:330,000 doses administered. All of the severe systemic reactions, including the rare ones, are considered absolute contraindications to the further use of pertussis vaccine, whether they occur after the administration of pertussis vaccine alone or of DTP. (High fever is considered a contraindication on the condition that no other and more plausible cause is apparent.) Caution must be exercised when causality is presumed on the basis of temporal proximity. For example, in some cases of encephalopathy or permanent neurologic deficit, it is possible that the vaccine is merely uncovering a neurologic abnormality that already existed and would have become manifest in any event. The fallacy of assuming causality by virtue of close temporal association became apparent when careful epidemiologic investigations demonstrated that infantile myoclonic seizures and sudden infant death syndrome were both clearly unrelated to pertussis vaccine use. The issue of causal association had been raised for both because their onset tends to be during the first 6 months of life, a time when pertussis immunization is also a common event.

Antibody Preparations

No antibody preparations are available. Pertussis immune globulin, available at one time, is ineffective in either the prophylaxis or treatment of pertussis.

Table 6–3. Adverse events occurring within 48 hours of pertussis immunization.[1,2]

Categories	Rate (%) per Dose
Redness at site > 2.4 cm	7.2
Swelling at site > 2.4 cm	8.9
Pain at site	51
Fever: temperature ≥ 38 °C	47
(100.4 °F)	
temperature ≥ 40.5 °C	0.3
(104.9 °F)	
Drowsiness	32
Fretfulness	53
Anorexia	21
Vomiting	6
Persistent crying (3 to 21 hr duration)	1
High-pitched, unusual cry	0.1
Convulsions	0.06
Collapse with shocklike state	0.06

[1]Modified and reproduced, with permission, from *The 1988 Report of the Committee on Infectious Diseases*, 21st ed. © 1988 American Academy of Pediatrics.
[2]These data are derived from 15,752 DTP immunizations (modified from: Cody CL, Baraff LJ, Cherry JD, Marcy SM, and Manclark CR: Nature and rates of adverse reactions associated with DTP and DT immunizations in infants and children. *Pediatrics* 1981;**68**:650.).

DIPHTHERIA-TETANUS-PERTUSSIS (DTP)

Diphtheria and tetanus toxoids and pertussis vaccine (DTP) is the recommended vehicle for the immunization of healthy infants against the 3 diseases. It has been in wide use in the United States for more than 40 years. It has the combined clinical efficacy of the 3 single preparations, and the efficacy of pertussis vaccine may even be enhanced by the adjuvant effect of the toxoids. It can be safely and effectively administered simultaneously along with both live attenuated poliovaccine or inactivated poliovaccine, measles-mumps-rubella vaccine, and *Haemophilus influenzae* type b conjugate vaccine.

Preparations Available

Combined diphtheria and tetanus toxoids and whole cell pertussis vaccine adsorbed with one of several adjuvants (alum, aluminum phosphate, or aluminum hydroxide, depending on the manufacturer).

Dosage & Schedule

DTP is administered intramuscularly in a dose of 0.5 mL. See Table 6–1 for the routine schedule and Table 6–2 for the schedule for children not appropriately immunized during the first year of life.

Adverse Effects

See above under the individual component vaccines.

Antibody Preparations

See above under the individual component vaccines.

Baraff LJ et al: Infants and children with convulsions and hypotonic-hyporesponsive episodes following diphtheria-tetanus-pertussis immunization: Follow-up evaluation. *Pediatrics* 1988;**81**:789.
Bernbaum JC et al: Response of preterm infants to diphtheria-tetanus-pertussis immunizations. *J Pediatr* 1985;**107**:184.
Centers for Disease Control: Diphtheria, tetanus, and pertussis: Guidelines for vaccine prophylaxis and other preventive measures. *MMWR* 1985;**34**:405.
Griffin MR et al: Risk of seizures and encephalopathy after immunization with the diphtheria-tetanus-pertussis vaccine. *JAMA* 1990;**263**:1641.
Stetler HC et al: History of convulsions and use of pertussis vaccine. *J Pediatr* 1985;**107**:175.

POLIOMYELITIS

Vaccines directed against poliovirus infections have largely eliminated naturally occurring disease in the developed world. In the United States, the annual number of reported cases of paralytic poliomyelitis has fallen from more than 18,000 in 1954 to less than 13 per year, on average, during the 1970s.

The provisional total reported for 1988 was 2. Despite—or perhaps because of—this extraordinary success, controversy continues over the appropriate poliovaccine for mass usage. Live attenuated poliovaccine (OPV) is prepared via passage in monkey kidney cells or human diploid cells, depending on the manufacturer. Inactivated poliovaccine (IPV) is currently grown in human diploid cells and then inactivated by formaldehyde. Until recently, IPV had been grown in monkey kidney cells. The newer preparation is more potent than the vaccine grown in monkey kidney cells, and field trials have demonstrated that fewer doses are required to attain comparable immunity to that conferred by OPV.

Because it is inactivated, IPV cannot cause poliomyelitis, whereas OPV can cause such cases rarely. The rate of these complications in the USA is estimated to be one case of paralytic disease in a healthy recipient per 12 million doses of OPV administered, one case in a healthy person having close contact with a vaccinee per 5 million doses, and one case in an immunodeficient person (either vaccinee or close contact) per 24 million doses administered. (These rates are calculated on the basis of total doses administered and not on the basis of specific denominators for each risk category, because these denominators are unknown. The risk of paralysis in the immunodeficient population may be as much as 10^4 times that in the healthy population.) IPV cannot multiply in the gut as OPV does—in theory not protecting against intestinal infection with wild virus as OPV can—and IPV cannot produce "secondary vaccination" among those in close contact with vaccinees. IPV has the practical advantage of not requiring freezing for storage as OPV does, whereas the mass administration of OPV requires no needles and syringes.

Weighing all the advantages and disadvantages of each vaccine, a special expert committee of the Institute of Medicine of the National Academy of Sciences and the Committee on Infectious Diseases of the American Academy of Pediatrics both continue to recommend the use of OPV under most circumstances in the USA. Exceptions include immunodeficient recipients, recipients with immunodeficient persons in their households, and unvaccinated adults, all of whom should receive IPV. In addition, anyone who is informed of the risks and benefits of OPV should be permitted to elect to receive IPV if they are prepared to commit to a full schedule of immunization with that preparation. This recommendation is regularly reexamined and could be changed if the epidemiology of poliomyelitis in the USA changes.

Preparations Available

A. Inactivated Poliovaccine (IPV): This vaccine contains types 1, 2, and 3 virus, all formaldehyde-inactivated.

B. Trivalent Live Attenuated Poliovaccine (OPV): This vaccine contains larger quantities of types 1 and 3 than of type 2 because multiplication of the last may inhibit that of the former two.

Dosage & Schedule

A. IPV: If the vaccine is of enhanced potency (grown in human diploid cells), the dose is 0.5 mL given intramuscularly. The dose of vaccine grown in monkey kidney cells is 1.0 mL given intramuscularly. See Table 6–1 for the routine schedule and Table 6–2 for the schedule for children not appropriately immunized during the first year of life.

B. OPV: A single thawed ampule is given orally for each dose. See Table 6–1 for the routine schedule and Table 6–2 for the schedule for children not appropriately immunized during the first year of life.

Adverse Reactions

IPV is associated with essentially no adverse reactions. OPV carries a risk (described above) of vaccine-associated paralytic disease, especially among immunodeficient recipients, immunodeficient people in contact with recipients, and unvaccinated healthy adults in contact with recipients. No other adverse reactions to OPV are known.

Antibody Preparations

No antibody preparations are available.

Centers for Disease Control: Poliomyelitis prevention. *MMWR* 1982;**31**:22.

Hinman AR et al: Live or inactivated poliomyelitis vaccine: An analysis of benefits and risks. *Am J Pub Health* 1988;**78**:291.

Robertson SE et al: Clinical efficacy of new, enhanced-potency, inactivated poliovirus vaccine. *Lancet* 1988;**1**:897.

MEASLES

Since the introduction of measles vaccine in 1963, the annual number of reported cases of this disease in the United States has decreased from well over 400,000 to 2933 in 1988. However, by the 35th reporting week of 1989, 9674 cases had been reported, as compared to 2174 cases during the same period in 1988. This dramatic increase prompted the Red Book Committee to recommend a second dose of MMR at junior high school entry (see notes, Table 6–1). Initially, an inactivated and a live attenuated vaccine (Edmonston B strain) were used, the former until 1967 and the latter until 1972. (The problem of atypical measles in inactivated vaccine recipients is, by virtue of their age, no longer an issue for pediatricians.) A further attenuated form of the Edmonston B strain (Schwarz strain) was licensed in 1965, and a similar preparation (Moraten strain) became available in 1968. The latter 2 strains are as effective as Edmonston B and have fewer adverse effects.

Given the efficacy rate of the current vaccine (> 95%), the elimination of indigenous measles from the United States is an attainable public health goal (currently, about 10% of all cases reported each year are either acquired outside the USA or result from exposure to such a case). Each year, about one-third of reported indigenous cases are judged to be potentially preventable. One-quarter occur in persons who would not have been immunized by virtue of age or exemption, and about 40% occur in persons with a history of adequate immunization. An aggressive campaign directed at ensuring that all eligible candidates are immunized at the appropriate age would certainly reduce the number of cases to a minimum and might eliminate indigenous transmission completely.

Preparations Available

A. The Moraten Strain: This is the only vaccine currently available in the United States. It is derived from the Edmonston B strain after multiple passages in chick embryo tissue culture.

B. Combined Vaccines: The Moraten strain is also available in combination with mumps vaccine (MM), rubella vaccine (MR), and mumps and rubella vaccines (MMR). It is equally effective alone and in each of these combinations.

Dosage & Schedule

Under ordinary circumstances, measles vaccine should be given routinely as MMR to 15-month-old children and again to children when they enter junior high school. A dose of 0.5 mL, whether alone or in combination, should be given subcutaneously. If the epidemiologic setting is unusual (an outbreak or increased local incidence, travel to an endemic area, etc), monovalent measles vaccine may be administered to a child as young as 6 months of age. The ACIP has recently recommended that, in counties "reporting more than five cases of measles among preschool-aged children during each of the previous 5 years," monovalent vaccine be given at 9 months of age or during the first visit thereafter and that these children be reimmunized with MMR at 15 months of age. If a 2-dose regimen is impractical, then MMR should be given at 12 months of age. Children immunized before their first birthday should be reimmunized at 15 months. Children with an unclear or unknown immunization history should be reimmunized with MMR. Measles immunization is contraindicated in pregnant women, women intending to become pregnant within the subsequent 90 days, immunocompromised persons (except those with HIV infection), persons with anaphylactic egg allergy, and persons with anaphylactic neomycin allergy. Children with minor acute illnesses (including febrile illnesses), nonanaphylactic egg allergy, or a history of tuberculosis should all be immunized.

Monovalent measles or MMR may be safely administered simultaneously with DTP and OPV.

Adverse Effects

Between 5% and 15% of vaccinees experience fever of up to 39 °C (103 °F) or higher approximately a week after immunization, and 5% may develop a transient morbilliform rash. Encephalitis and other central nervous system conditions are reported to occur at a rate of one per 3 million doses in the United States. This rate is lower than the rate in the general unvaccinated population, implying that the relationship between these conditions and measles immunization may not be causal.

Antibody Preparations

IG, given intramuscularly at a dose of 0.25 mL/kg (0.5 mL/kg in the immunocompromised) is effective in preventing or modifying measles after exposure if given within 6 days after exposure. If a child is seen within 72 hours after exposure, immunization is the preferred method of protection. If IG has been given for this or any other reason to an unimmunized child, immunization is indicated but must be deferred for at least 90 days.

Centers for Disease Control: Measles prevention. *MMWR* 1987;**36**:409.
Centers for Disease Control: Measles prevention: Supplementary statement. *MMWR* 1989;**38**:11.
Deforest A et al: Simultaneous administration of measles-mumps-rubella vaccine with booster doses of diphtheria-tetanus-pertussis and poliovirus vaccines. *Pediatrics* 1988;**81**:237.
McGraw TT: Reimmunization following early immunization with measles vaccine: A prospective study. *Pediatrics* 1986;**77**:45.
Simoes EA et al: Antibody response of children to measles vaccine mixed with diphtheria-pertussis-tetanus or diphtheria-pertussis-tetanus-poliomyelitis vaccine. *Am J Dis Child* 1988;**142**:309.

MUMPS

Although the reporting of mumps in the United States is incomplete, it is clear that the use of mumps vaccine has greatly reduced the incidence of this infection and the complications and mortality associated with it. In the last decade, fewer than 20 cases of mumps encephalitis and fewer than 2 deaths due to mumps have been reported annually. An inactivated mumps vaccine was first produced in 1950, but its efficacy was 80% or less, and the duration of immunity was less than one year. It was withdrawn from use in 1976. A live attenuated vaccine was first licensed in the United States in 1967. This vaccine, the Jeryl Lynn strain, was prepared from virus isolated from a child and subjected to passage in embryonated hens' eggs and in chick embryo tissue culture. The duration of protective immunity conferred by this vaccine is at least 19 years.

Preparations Available

A. The Jeryl Lynn Strain: This is the only preparation available in the United States as monovalent vaccine.

B. Combined Vaccines: The Jeryl Lynn vaccine is also available in combination with measles vaccine (MM), rubella vaccine, and measles and rubella vaccines (MMR).

Dosage & Schedule

Mumps vaccine is routinely given to children in the combination vaccine MMR at the age of 15 months and at junior high school entry. As monovalent vaccine, it is safe and effective if given after the first birthday. The dose of either is 0.5 mL given subcutaneously. The use of the monovalent vaccine is now limited to susceptible patients with proved immunity to the other constituents of MMR. Reimmunization with mumps vaccine or any of the vaccines in MMR is not harmful. Anyone with an unclear immunization history should therefore be immunized. The same contraindications apply to mumps vaccine as to measles vaccine (see above).

Adverse Effects

Illness reported after mumps vaccination is most unusual and is believed not to be causally related in virtually all circumstances.

Antibody Preparations

No antibody preparations are available.

Centers for Disease Control: Mumps vaccine. *MMWR* 1982;**31:**617.
Cochi SL, Preblud SR, Orenstein WA: Perspectives on the relative resurgence of mumps in the United States. *Am J Dis Child* 1988;**142:**499.
Kaplan KA et al: Mumps in the workplace. *JAMA* 1988; **260:**1434.

RUBELLA

Rubella vaccine is unlike the other immunization products discussed in this chapter because it is not intended to protect individuals from the consequences to themselves of rubella infection. Rather, it is intended to prevent congenital rubella syndrome. In the United States, the approach has been to immunize young children. The intent is to reduce transmission to women of childbearing age via a herd immunity effect and to confer protection lasting through childbearing age to girls. Other countries, notably the United Kingdom, take the approach that pubertal girls (ages 11–14) are candidates for immunization. The relative efficacies of these 2 strategies in the prevention of congenital rubella syndrome are not clear. Although the incidence of congenital rubella syndrome has fallen in the United States since the introduction of vaccine in 1970 (from 4 to 8 cases per 10,000 pregnancies to less than 0.01 per 10,000 pregnancies), and the incidence of postnatal rubella has declined similarly, many authorities have wondered whether a second dose of vaccine ought to be administered to adolescent girls. For this reason, the Red Book Committee advocated a change in the recommendations for rubella (as well as measles) in July 1989. The vaccine currently in use is the RA 27/3 strain, grown in human diploid cell tissue culture.

Preparations Available

A. The RA 27/3 Strain: This is the only vaccine available in the United States.

B. Combined Vaccines: The RA 27/3 strain is available in combined preparations with measles vaccine (MR), mumps vaccine, and measles and mumps vaccines (MMR).

Dosage & Schedule

Either the monovalent or combined form should be administered subcutaneously in a dose of 0.5 mL. Current practice is to use MMR vaccine at 15 months of age and again at entry to junior high school. Susceptible pubertal girls and postpubertal women identified by premarital or prenatal screening should also be immunized. All susceptible adults in certain institutional settings, including colleges, daycare centers, military settings, and hospital and health care settings, should also be immunized. Whenever rubella immunization is offered to a woman of childbearing age, the woman should be questioned about the possibility of pregnancy. If necessary, a test should be performed to rule out pregnancy, and an effective means of contraception should be advised to prevent conception during the 90 days following immunization. These precautions may be unnecessary, because current data suggest that the risk of fetal infection after the inadvertent immunization of a pregnant woman with RA 27/3 vaccine approaches zero. Otherwise, the contraindications to immunization are the same as for measles (see above).

Adverse Effects

In children, adverse effects from rubella immunization are very unusual. In adults, the most important complications are arthralgia or arthritis, occurring in 14% of vaccinees in one study. Rash occurs alone or as mild rubella in 1–4% of adults. Rare complications include peripheral neuritis and neuropathy, transverse myelitis, and diffuse myelitis.

Antibody Preparations

No antibody preparations are available.

Bart SW et al: Fetal risk associated with rubella vaccine: An update. *Rev Infect Dis* 1985;**7(Suppl):**103.

Centers for Disease Control: Rubella prevention. *MMWR* 1984;**33**:301.

Chu SY et al: Rubella antibody persistence after immunization: Sixteen-year follow-up in the Hawaiian Islands. *JAMA* 1988;**259**:3133.

HAEMOPHILUS INFLUENZAE TYPE B

A vaccine against *Haemophilus influenzae* type b is the most recent addition to the armamentarium of physicians providing routine childhood immunizations. The first vaccine licensed against the organism became available in the United States in 1985 for use in 2-year-olds, primarily on the basis of a large field trial conducted in Finland, along with much smaller safety and immunogenicity trials in the United States. That vaccine, composed of purified capsular polysaccharide (PRP), became controversial within 2 years after its licensure when studies in several states, notably Minnesota and Missouri, indicated that it might lack clinical efficacy. Furthermore, case reports and data from laboratory animal experiments supported the conclusion that in those children with small quantities of preexisting anticapsular antibody, immunization actually might increase the risk of disease during a brief period within the first week after vaccine administration.

In late 1987, a conjugate vaccine consisting of the same type b capsular polysaccharide covalently linked to diphtheria toxoid was licensed, also based on the results of a Finnish trial. This vaccine, approved for use in 15-month-olds, has completely supplanted the original vaccine. Whether the same problem of increased risk of infection during the first week after immunization exists for the conjugate vaccine is not yet clear, but results of the Finnish trial indicate no such risk. Studies of various conjugate vaccines are currently under way to see if they might be incorporated into the routine schedule at 2, 4, 6, and 15 months of age and afford good protective efficacy. Conjugate vaccines using diphtheria toxoid or toxin are not immunizing agents against diphtheria.

Preparations Available
A. Purified Capsular Polysaccharide Linked to Diphtheria Toxoid (PRP-D): PRP-D is an *H influenzae* type b capsular polysaccharide molecule covalently linked to diphtheria toxoid by a 6-carbon spacer molecule (Connaught Laboratories, licensed December 1988).

B. Vaccines Linked to Diphtheria Toxin: These are type b capsular oligosaccharides directly linked in a variety of ways to a mutant diphtheria toxin, CRM_{197} (Praxis Biologics, licensed January 1989). Although the 2 preparations are clearly different chemically, there are no established differences between them in terms of immunogenicity, safety, or efficacy.

Dosage & Schedule
Regardless of which preparation is used, 0.5 mL should be given intramuscularly as a single dose at 15 months of age. There is no current knowledge about the possible need for booster doses. Children immunized prior to 24 months of age with the PRP vaccine should be reimmunized with a conjugate vaccine. Children who have developed invasive *H influenzae* type b disease prior to 15 months should be immunized. Previously unimmunized children between the ages of 2 and 5 years may be immunized. Functionally or anatomically asplenic individuals as well as other immunosuppressed or immunocompromised individuals who have not been previously immunized should be immunized. These vaccines may be given simultaneously (at different sites) with DTP. Data are lacking on the simultaneous use of MMR or OPV, but these may be given simultaneously with DTP to children unlikely to return for further immunization.

Adverse Effects
These are the first vaccines for which a new FDA requirement for active surveillance of adverse reactions has been in effect after licensure. Accordingly, there are good early data reporting that fewer than 5% of those immunized develop any minor and local or systemic reaction (including fever) to the Connaught preparation. There have been no reports of more severe reactions.

Antibody Preparations
There is no commercially available antibody preparation. The Massachusetts Biologic Laboratory is investigating a bacterial polysaccharide immune globulin obtained from adult donors who have been immunized with PRP and with polyvalent pneumococcal and meningococcal vaccines. The routine use of IG or IVIG may prevent *H influenzae* type b infections in antibody-deficient children, such as those with agammaglobulinemia or HIV infection.

Black SB et al: Efficacy of *Haemophilus influenzae* type b capsular polysaccharide vaccine. *Pediatr Infect Dis J* 1988;**7**:149.

Centers for Disease Control: Update: Prevention of *Haemophilus influenzae* type b disease. *MMWR* 1988;**37**:13.

Lepow ML et al: Persistence of antibody to *Haemophilus influenzae* type b at 4 years of age in children previously immunized with polysaccharide antigen alone or conjugated with diphtheria toxoid. *J Pediatr* 1988;**112**:741.

IMMUNIZATIONS FOR SPECIAL SITUATIONS

INFLUENZA

Influenza occurs regularly each winter and early spring and equally regularly is associated with significant morbidity and mortality rates in certain high-risk individuals, including children with chronic cardiac, pulmonary, metabolic, renal, and neurologic disease. All physicians caring for children should be responsible for identifying such children in their practices and actively encouraging parents to seek influenza immunization for these children each fall. In pandemic years, it may be important to advocate immunization in all children, regardless of their usual state of health. Influenza immunization has been calculated to have a 65–80% efficacy in protecting against disease.

Each year, recommendations are formulated in the spring and summer regarding the constituents of influenza vaccine for the coming season. These recommendations are based on the results of surveillance in Asia and the southern hemisphere during the spring and summer. Each year, the vaccine typically contains antigens from one or more strains of influenza A and influenza B. Influenza vaccines are grown in hens' eggs and then formalin-inactivated. These whole-virus preparations may be further treated with a variety of detergents to produce split-virus or component virus vaccines.

Preparations Available

Several manufacturers produce vaccines each year, but they are all similar in nature. Whole-virus vaccines produce unacceptably high rates of adverse reactions in children and are therefore contraindicated. Only split-virus preparations should be used. These are also effective in adults, and so practitioners need not concern themselves with which vaccine to use in adolescents. Split-virus preparations should be the rule.

Dosage & Schedule

Children under 6 months of age cannot be immunized. For all others, what dose to give and whether the child will require one dose or 2 doses separated by 30 days depends on the strains circulating and the child's prior experience with vaccines. Public health authorities should be consulted annually for proper dosage information. Because this vaccine is inactivated, pregnancy is not an absolute contraindication to use.

Adverse Effects

A small proportion of children experience some systemic toxicity evidenced by fever, malaise, and myalgias. These symptoms generally begin 6–12 hours after immunization and may last 24–48 hours. Rarely, some children have anaphylactic reactions, presumably due to hypersensitivity to eggs. Guillain-Barré syndrome, although seen with some increased frequency following swine influenza immunization in 1976–1977, has not been noted to occur since, despite efforts at active surveillance for the syndrome. It is not currently felt to be a complication of most influenza immunizations.

Antibody Preparations

No antibody preparations are available.

Bernstein DI et al: Clinical reactions and serologic responses after vaccination with whole-virus or split-virus influenza vaccines in children aged 6 to 36 months. *Pediatrics* 1982;**69**:404.

Centers for Disease Control. Prevention and control of influenza. *MMWR* 1988;**37**:361.

Kilbourne ED: Inactivated influenza vaccines. In: *Vaccines,* Plotkin SA, Mortimer EA (editors). Saunders, 1988.

Murphy KR, Strunk RC: Safe administration of influenza vaccine in asthmatic children sensitive to egg proteins. *J Pediatr* 1985;**106**:931.

HEPATITIS B

The first vaccine to be prepared entirely from material derived exclusively from human donors, hepatitis B vaccine was first licensed for use in the United States in 1981. Although it was initially developed as a means of preventing infection via percutaneous and sexual exposure, subsequent studies have shown it to be more than 85% effective in preventing perinatally acquired infection and 95% effective in preventing most postnatally acquired infections.

In 1988, the American College of Obstetrics and Gynecology recommended that all pregnant women be screened for the presence of hepatitis B surface antigen (HBsAg) as a routine part of prenatal care. Positive women should be considered chronic carriers of hepatitis B virus, and children born to such women are highly likely to become chronic carriers themselves. In turn, they have the long-term increased risk of hepatocellular carcinoma that chronic carrier status implies. Female infants are highly likely to pass the infection perinatally to their own offspring once they attain childbearing age, thus perpetuating the cycle. The use of hepatitis B vaccine along with hepatitis B immune globulin (HBIG) has been established as an effective means of interrupting this cycle in all but the 2–3% of infants who acquire hepatitis B in utero. It is therefore imperative that pediatricians and obstetricians establish effective means of communicating the HBsAg status of every woman while she is in labor so that appropriate preventive measures can be instituted as soon as possible after delivery.

In addition to newborns at high risk, several other categories of persons at high risk of acquiring hepatitis B have been defined as target populations for immunization. Those that are relevant to physicians caring for children include clients and staff in institutions for the developmentally delayed, clients and staff of hemodialysis units, recipients of clotting factor concentrates, homosexually active males, users of illicit injectable drugs, household contacts of chronic hepatitis B carriers, and health care personnel (including pediatricians and family physicians and their office staff). In all cases except high-risk neonates, persons identified as being at high risk should be screened for markers of past infection and immunized only if they are proved susceptible. Because this vaccine consists of a purified, inactive subunit of the virus and is not infectious, its use is not contraindicated in immunosuppressed individuals or in pregnant women.

Preparations Available
A. Purified HBsAg Obtained from the Plasma of Positive Human Donors.

B. Recombinant Vaccine: Licensed in 1986, this vaccine is made by inserting into baker's yeast a plasmid containing the gene for one subtype of HBsAg and then harvesting the HBsAg by lysing the yeast cells. It is immunologically indistinguishable from the HBsAg found in chronic carriers.

Dosage & Schedule
A. Neonatal: Infants of HBsAg-positive mothers should be cleansed of the bloody products of conception in the delivery room. Both hepatitis B vaccine (dose 0.5 mL IM) and hepatitis B immune globulin (HBIG, dose 0.5 mL IM) should be administered simultaneously at different injection sites as soon as possible, preferably also in the delivery room. The vaccine dose should be repeated at 30 and 180 days after the initial immunization. At 9 months of age, every immunized infant should be tested for hepatitis B surface antibody. If the antibody test is positive, immunization has been effective. If it is negative, the infant should be screened for the antigen (HBsAg). If the antigen test is positive, immunization has failed, and the infant is a chronic carrier. If the infant is HBsAg-negative, a fourth dose of vaccine should be administered, and the same testing sequence should be repeated after another 30 days.

B. All Others: The dose of HBIG is 0.06 mL/kg (maximum 5 mL). In children less than 10 years of age, the vaccine dose and schedule are identical to those for the neonates. In children 10 years or older, the dose is 1.0 mL given intramuscularly according to the same schedule. Although vaccine and HBIG may be administered simultaneously, the vaccine may be delayed as much as 7 days after HBIG ad-

ministration and still be effective. It is recommended that renal dialysis patients and immunosuppressed persons being immunized receive twice the above doses of vaccine (not of HBIG) because of their poorer response. Currently, they should be given only the plasma-derived vaccine, because the aluminum hydroxide content of the recombinant vaccine would be excessive in the volume required.

Adverse Effects
The overall rate of adverse effects has been one per 10,000 doses. Such effects have all been minor, and they include arthralgia and pain at the injection site. There is no evidence for the transmission of HIV infection or any other blood-borne infection via the plasma-derived vaccine or via HBIG.

Antibody Preparations
The use of HBIG, prepared from donors with high titers of hepatitis B surface antibody, is described above.

Centers for Disease Control: Prevention of perinatal transmission of hepatitis B virus: Prenatal screening of all pregnant women for hepatitis B surface antigen. *MMWR* 1988;**37**:341.

Centers for Disease Control: Update on hepatitis B prevention. *MMWR* 1987;**36**:353.

Ghendon Y: Perinatal transmission of hepatitis B in high-incidence countries. *J Virol Methods* 1987;**17**:69.

Hsu-Mei H et al: Efficacy of a mass hepatitis B vaccination program in Taiwan. *JAMA* 1988;**260**:2231.

PNEUMOCOCCAL INFECTIONS

Infections with *Streptococcus pneumoniae* account for an important proportion of the morbidity and mortality in certain high-risk groups of children. Among these are children with anatomic and functional asplenia (including sickle cell disease), nephrotic syndrome, cerebrospinal fluid leaks, and immunosuppression (including those with HIV infection). The vaccine is ineffective in children less than 2 years of age and therefore should not be given to children in the above groups until their second birthday. It is not indicated for children having only recurrent upper respiratory tract infections, such as otitis media or sinusitis. The protective efficacy of the vaccine in high-risk children has not been well studied but is presumed to be roughly 60%, based on extrapolation from investigations in adults. The initial licensure of a 14-valent vaccine in the United States was in 1977. The currently used 23-valent vaccine was licensed in 1983.

Preparations Available
The standard dose of currently available vaccines contains 25 μg each of the purified capsular polysac-

charide antigen of 23 serotypes of *S pneumoniae*. These 23 serotypes cause 88% of the bacteremic pneumococcal disease in the United States. Cross-reactive antibody responses may protect against an additional 8% of bacteremic serotypes.

Dosage & Schedule

The dose is 0.5 mL given intramuscularly or subcutaneously, and the vaccine is generally given only once. If splenectomy or immunosuppression can be anticipated, the vaccine should be given at least 2 weeks previously. Routine revaccination is not indicated because of an increased risk of adverse reactions. However, some centers reimmunize children with sickle cell anemia 3–5 years after initial immunization because of their very high risk of pneumococcal infection. Children who received initial immunization during chemotherapy for Hodgkin's disease should be reimmunized 3–4 months after the cessation of chemotherapy. Immunization does not preclude consideration of antibiotic prophylaxis in certain high-risk children.

Adverse Effects

Half of all vaccine recipients develop pain and redness at the injection site. Less than 1% develop systemic side effects, such as fever and myalgia. Anaphylaxis occurs very rarely.

Antibody Preparations

A high-titer bacterial polysaccharide immune globulin, as described above under *H influenzae* type b, is under investigation. Some authorities recommend the routine use of IG or IVIG in agammaglobulinemic patients or patients with HIV infection, in part to prevent pneumococcal disease.

American Academy of Pediatrics Committee on Infectious Diseases: Recommendations for using pneumococcal vaccine in children. *Pediatrics* 1985;**75**:1153.

Centers for Disease Control: Pneumococcal polysaccharide vaccine. *MMWR* 1989;**38**:64.

Konradsen HB, Pedersen FK, Henrichsen J: Pneumococcal revaccination of splenectomized children. *Pediatr Infect Dis* 1990;**9**:258.

Paton JC et al: Antibody response to pneumococcal vaccine in children aged 5 to 15 years. *Am J Dis Child* 1986;**140**:135.

RABIES

Human rabies has been rare in the United States over the last several decades, but animal rabies persists in many domestic and feral animal species throughout the country. The risk of rabies transmission depends on the nature of the animal-to-human contact, the species of animal involved, and the locale of the incident. Local public health officials are well-versed in the epidemiology of animal rabies in their jurisdictions, and they should always be consulted before any postexposure rabies prophylaxis is undertaken. First, they can avert unnecessary immu-

nization. Second, they can assist in the proper handling of the involved animal, if either confinement or testing is appropriate. Third, they can supply needed biologics that may not be routinely stocked in hospitals, offices, or pharmacies. In some jurisdictions, these biologics are supplied at no expense to the recipient if the use is authorized by the appropriate public health official. To facilitate discussion, the physician should have the following information at hand: the species of animal, its availability for testing or confinement, the nature of the attack (provoked or unprovoked), and the nature of the exposure (bite, scratch, lick, aerosol of saliva, etc). Confinement and observation of the biting animal are appropriate *only* when that animal is either a dog or a cat and the animal appears well.

Preexposure prophylaxis is indicated for veterinarians, animal handlers, and all persons, including children, whose work or home environment potentially places them in close contact with animal species—eg, bats, skunks, raccoons, and foxes—in which rabies is endemic.

Preparations Available

Two vaccines are currently available in the United States. Both consist of virus grown in human diploid cell culture and then inactivated. The preparations differ only in the inactivation process and are otherwise equivalent. The vaccine is called human diploid cell vaccine or HDCV.

Dosage & Schedule

Each dose is 1.0 mL of vaccine given intramuscularly. Care must be taken to inject into good muscle mass, or the antibody response may be inadequate.

A. Preexposure Prophylaxis: This consists of a 3-dose regimen of the above dose on days 0, 7, and 28. Antibody levels should be measured every 2 years, and the decision to boost should be made on the basis of the results.

B. Postexposure Prophylaxis: The wound should be immediately and thoroughly cleaned with soap and water. As soon as possible after the exposure, administer 20 IU/kg of human rabies immune globulin (HRIG) intramuscularly (if possible, half the dose should be infiltrated at the wound and the other half given intramuscularly). At a different site—also as soon as possible after exposure—administer the first dose of HDCV. Four subsequent doses of HDCV should be given on days 3, 7, 14, and 28. The World Health Organization recommends an additional dose on day 90, but the ACIP does not.

Adverse Effects

HDCV is relatively free of side effects. Approximately 20% of adults experience pain at the injection site, 7% have headache, 5% have nausea, and 4% have fever. Children complain of side effects less frequently. Allergic reactions occur, primarily after booster doses. The rate of anaphylaxis in this setting is estimated to be one per 10,000 doses.

Antibody Preparations

HRIG is prepared from the plasma of human volunteers hyperimmunized with rabies vaccine. It is very safe and free of adverse effects. Usage is described above.

Centers for Disease Control: Rabies prevention: United States, 1984. *MMWR* 1984;**33**:393.

Wiktor T, Plotkin SA, Koprowski H: Rabies vaccine. In: *Vaccines,* Plotkin SA, Mortimer EA (editors). Saunders, 1988.

MENINGOCOCCAL DISEASE

A quadrivalent vaccine containing 50 μg each of purified bacterial polysaccharide antigen from capsular groups A, C, Y, and W135 is available in the United States. Because meningococcal infection is not endemic in the United States, routine use of this vaccine is unnecessary. However, functionally or anatomically asplenic children should be immunized, and immunization should be considered for children deficient in the terminal components of complement. In general, the vaccine should not be administered to such children before their second birthday. The dose is 0.5 mL given subcutaneously once. Adverse reactions are unusual, consisting of local pain and erythema at the injection site when they do occur.

Centers for Disease Control: Meningococcal vaccines. *MMWR* 1985;**34**:255.

CHOLERA

The currently available cholera vaccine is a phenol-killed whole bacterial cell preparation. Its use is limited because it has a maximum protective efficacy of only 50% with a duration of protection of only 3–6 months. Its primary importance is to satisfy the entrance requirements for travel to some countries. Immunization frequently results in redness and pain at the injection site, and fever, malaise, and myalgia occur in approximately 1% of people vaccinated. The vaccine may be administered subcutaneously or intramuscularly, and a primary series consists of 2 doses at least 1 week apart. Boosters may need to be given as frequently as every 6 months. For the quantity to administer, see below. Vaccine should not be given to children less than 6 months of age.

Age at Immunization

	6 mo–4 y	5–10 y	> 10 y
Dose	0.2 mL	0.3 mL	0.5 mL

Centers for Disease Control: Cholera vaccine. *MMWR* 1988;**37**:617.

PLAGUE

Plague vaccine is composed of inactivated whole bacteria (*Yersinia pestis*). It should be used in children who reside in or are traveling to endemic areas. It should be administered intramuscularly according to the following dosage schedule:

	Age (in Years)			
	< 1	**1–4**	**5–10**	**> 10**
Day 0 (dose 1)	0.1 mL	0.2 mL	0.3 mL	0.5 mL
Day 30 (dose 2)	0.1 mL	0.2 mL	0.3 mL	0.5 mL
Day 60–120 (dose 3)	0.04 mL	0.08 mL	0.12 mL	0.2 mL

Booster doses in the amount of the last dose above should then be given at 6-month intervals until a total of 5 doses has been given. Boosters should then be given at 1–2 year intervals as long as the child resides in the endemic area.

Centers for Disease Control: Plague vaccine. *MMWR* 1982;**31**:301.

TUBERCULOSIS

Bacille Calmette-Guérin (BCG) is a vaccine consisting of live attenuated *Mycobacterium bovis*. Several large clinical efficacy trials have been conducted, and the results are conflicting. BCG is not currently indicated for mass use in the United States, primarily because of doubts about its efficacy. It may be useful in tuberculin-negative infants or older children residing in households where untreated or poorly treated individuals with active infection also reside. It is given intracutaneously in a dose of 0.05 mL for newborns and 0.1 mL for all other children. Adverse effects in healthy individuals are rare. It may cause disseminated, fatal infection in immunocompromised individuals, including those with HIV infection, and is therefore contraindicated in them. BCG almost invariably causes its recipients to be tuberculin-positive. In a child with a history of BCG immunization who is being investigated for tuberculosis as a case contact, a positive PPD should be interpreted as indicating infection with *M tuberculosis*. The child should be evaluated and treated in that light; ie, the history of BCG vaccination is essentially ignored.

Centers for Disease Control: Use of BCG vaccines in the control of tuberculosis: A joint statement by the ACIP and the Advisory Committee for Elimination of Tuberculosis. *MMWR* 1988;**37**:663.

Eickhoff TC: Bacille Calmette-Guérin (BCG) vaccine. In: *Vaccines,* Plotkin SA, Mortimer EA (editors). Saunders, 1988.

TYPHOID FEVER

Typhoid vaccine also has shown variable efficacy in field trials. Protective efficacy is inversely related to inoculum size in laboratory-based volunteer studies, and this may be the reason why some field trials have had disappointing results. Two vaccines are available in the United States—a heat-phenol inactivated whole bacterial vaccine for parenteral use and a live attenuated vaccine for oral use (TY 21A). The oral vaccine is an enteric coated capsule; since stomach acid kills *Salmonella*, the capsule should be taken intact. Typhoid vaccine is indicated for use in children who reside in a household with a proved typhoid carrier or in children who are traveling to (and going to reside in) an endemic area. The parenteral vaccine is given subcutaneously in a series of 2 injections 3 weeks or more apart, with booster doses every 3 years if residence in an endemic area continues. The dose is 0.25 mL per injection in children aged 6 months to 9 years and 0.5 mL in those 10 years of age or older. Vaccination usually produces 1–2 days of discomfort at the injection site. Fever and other systemic reactions are much less common. The oral vaccination schedule is one capsule every other day for four days. Children under 6 years old should receive the parenteral vaccine. A liquid oral vaccine is being tested.

Levine MM, Taylor DN, Ferreccio C: Typhoid fever vaccines come of age. *Pediatr Infect Dis* 1989;**8:**374.

YELLOW FEVER

Immunization against this disease is indicated for children traveling to endemic areas or to countries that require it for entry. Public health authorities maintain updated information on these requirements and must be consulted. This live attenuated viral vaccine is contraindicated in infants less than 6 months of age, pregnant women, persons with anaphylactic egg allergy, and immunocompromised individuals. It can be administered only at licensed yellow fever vaccination sites (usually public health departments). The dose is standardized to 1000 mouse LD50 units by WHO. The package insert must therefore be consulted to determine the appropriate volume (generally 0.5 mL). It is administered subcutaneously. Adverse reactions are generally mild—fever, headache, and myalgia 5–10 days after immunization—and uncommon, occurring in 2–5% of vaccinees. Encephalitis occurs rarely within 30 days following immunization.

Centers for Disease Control: Yellow fever vaccine. *MMWR* 1984;**32:**679.

INVESTIGATIONAL VACCINES

Vaccines against many common childhood pathogens are currently under investigation. Among them are rotavirus vaccines, respiratory syncytial virus vaccines, hepatitis A vaccines, adenovirus vaccines, rhinovirus vaccines, and HIV vaccines. Two vaccines that are not yet licensed but are very close to licensure in the United States—acellular pertussis vaccine and varicella vaccine—bear further comment.

ACELLULAR PERTUSSIS VACCINE

The 2 main immunizing antigens of *Bordetella pertussis* are filamentous hemagglutinin (FHA) and pertussis toxin or lymphocyte-promoting factor (PT or LPF). A vaccine containing these 2 antigens in purified form has been produced in Japan and successfully field-tested there and in Sweden. Preliminary results indicate that this vaccine, when used in combination with standard diphtheria and tetanus toxoids, is less likely to produce adverse effects than standard DTP is and may have similar protective efficacy. Field trials are currently under way in the United States. One disturbing unanticipated result in the Swedish trial was an increase in the number of serious bacterial infections from unrelated bacteria in the experimental vaccine group. This result has not been noted in Japan, where the vaccine is currently in regular clinical use, and it is being looked for actively in the US trials.

Anderson EL, Belshe RB, Bartram J: Differences in reactogenicity and antigenicity of acellular and standard pertussis vaccines combined with diphtheria and tetanus in infants. *J Infect Dis* 1988;**157:**731.
Aoyama T et al: Efficacy of an acellular pertussis vaccine in Japan. *J Pediatr* 1985;**107:**180.

VARICELLA

A live attenuated varicella vaccine, the OKA strain, has been developed in Japan and thoroughly field-tested both there and in the United States. The initial population studied in both countries was susceptible leukemic children whose chemotherapy was temporarily interrupted for the purpose of immunizing them. The vaccine has also been extensively evaluated in normal children in both countries. It has been proved safe and effective in both healthy and leukemic children, and initial longer-term follow-up on the leukemic children immunized in the United States shows that the incidence of herpes zoster is less than expected in the absence of immunization.

The dose of vaccine virus that has shown efficacy is between 300 and 500 plaque-forming units (PFU) administered subcutaneously. Because the vaccine is not yet commercially available, it is not clear what volume of injection this will ultimately involve. Adverse effects in leukemic children included mild varicella rash in roughly 20% of recipients and fever in a smaller proportion. The incidence of these side effects is less than 5% in immunized healthy children.

Licensure by the FDA is thought to be imminent. It is not clear whether this vaccine will be licensed for use only in leukemic children or for routine use in the immunization of all children.

Until—and very likely after—the licensure of varicella vaccine, the only effective means of preventing or modifying varicella infection in exposed susceptible individuals will be varicella-zoster immune globulin (VZIG). The use of this preparation, obtained from pooled plasma donations from individuals known to have high titers of antivaricella antibody, is indicated in several categories of high-risk exposed and susceptible individuals. These include immunocompromised persons, healthy persons 15 years of age or older, newborns whose mothers develop varicella between 5 days before and 48 hours after delivery, premature infants ($\geq$ 28 weeks' gestation) whose mothers are susceptible, and premature infants less mature than that regardless of maternal status. Exposure is defined as household contact, playmate contact ($>$ 1 h/d), hospital contact (in the same contiguous room or ward), and newborn contact (as defined above). Susceptibility is defined as the absence of detectable antibody on the fluorescent antibody against membrane antigen (FAMA) test. To be effective, VZIG must be administered within 96 hours of exposure. Maximum effectiveness is achieved if VZIG is administered within 48 hours of exposure. Newborns should be given 125 units intramuscularly. The dose for all others is 125 units per 10 kg of body weight given intramuscularly to a maximum dose of 625 units. VZIG should be readministered if more than 3 weeks have elapsed since the last dose of VZIG and a susceptible, high-risk person is reexposed.

Brunell PA et al: Risk of herpes zoster in children with leukemia: Varicella vaccine compared with history of chickenpox. *Pediatrics* 1986;**77**:53.

Englund JA et al: Placebo-controlled trial of varicella vaccine given with or after measles-mumps-rubella vaccine. *J Pediatr* 1989;**114**:37.

Johnson CE et al: Live attenuated varicella vaccine in healthy 12- to 24-month-old children. *Pediatrics* 1988; **81**:512.

Lawrence R et al: The risk of zoster after varicella vaccination in children with leukemia. *N Engl J Med* 1988; **318**:543.

Weibel RE et al: Live attenuated varicella virus vaccine. Efficacy trial in healthy children. *N Engl J Med* 1984; **310**:1409.

IMMUNE GLOBULINS

Immune globulin (IG) is indicated as replacement therapy in patients with antibody deficiency disorders at a dose of 0.6 mL/kg/month. It may prevent or modify infection with hepatitis A virus if administered in a dose of 0.02 mL/kg within 14 days of exposure. Measles infection may be prevented or modified in a susceptible individual if IG is given in a dose of 0.25 mL/kg within 6 days of exposure. Special forms of IG include tetanus immune globulin (TIG), hepatitis B immune globulin (HBIG), rabies immune globulin (RIG), and varicella-zoster immune globulin (VZIG). These are obtained from donors known to have high titers of antibody against the organism in question. Their use has been described in the corresponding sections above. All of these forms of immune globulin are intended to be administered intramuscularly only. The dose varies according to the clinical indication. Adverse reactions include pain at the injection site, headache, chills, dyspnea, nausea, and anaphylaxis, though all but the first are rare.

There is also an intravenous immune globulin (IVIG), prepared in a similar fashion to IG. Its primary indications are for replacement therapy in antibody-deficient individuals, the treatment of Kawasaki disease, and the treatment of some patients with idiopathic thrombocytopenic purpura. It may also be beneficial in children with congenital HIV infection. It must be administered intravenously only. Adverse reactions include headache, flushing, diaphoresis, hypotension, fever, nausea, vomiting, and anaphylaxis.

Finally, some immune globulins of animal origin are available for use in certain situations. These include botulism antitoxins, diphtheria antitoxin, and snake and spider antivenins. A variety of adverse reactions, including acute febrile responses, anaphylaxis, and serum sickness, may develop as a result of the use of these products. Their use should therefore be restricted to clinical circumstances in which the need is clear. A schedule for hypersensitivity testing and desensitization for antisera of equine origin can be found in the *Report of the Committee on Infectious Diseases* (the *Red Book*).

LEGAL ISSUES IN IMMUNIZATION

The National Childhood Vaccine Injury Act of 1986 was funded on and effective as of October 1, 1988. It provides that liability claims against those who administer or manufacture vaccines must be adjudicated by a federal compensation board before a civil suit may be filed. Compensation may be sought for certain events following certain immunizations within specified time intervals (see Table 6–4). Parents must reject the judgment rendered by this compensation board before filing a civil suit in either state or federal court. The compensation system will be funded by a trust fund created by an initial grant of $80 million from Congress and a continuing sur-

charge levied against the manufacturers for each dose of the specified vaccines that is distributed.

The act requires strict record keeping and reporting of adverse reactions by physicians who administer vaccines. For each dose administered, the medical record of the vaccinee or some other permanent record maintained in the administrator's office must reflect the date of administration, the name of the manufacturer and lot number of the vaccine, and the

Table 6–4. Reportable events following vaccination.[1]

Vaccine/Toxoid	Event	Interval From Vaccination
DTP, P, DTP/Polio Combined	A. Anaphylaxis or anaphylactic shock	24 hours
	B. Encephalopathy (or encephalitis[2])	7 days
	C. Shock-collapse or hypotonic-hyporesponsive collapse[2]	7 days
	D. Residual seizure disorder[2]	(See Aids to Interpretation[2])
	E. Any acute complication or sequela (including death) of above events	No limit
	F. Events in vaccinees described in manufacturer's package insert as contraindications to additional doses of vaccine[3] (such as convulsions)	(See package insert)
Measles, Mumps, and Rubella; DT, Td, Tetanus Toxoid	A. Anaphylaxis or anaphylactic shock	24 hours
	B. Encephalopathy (or encephalitis)[2]	15 days for measles, mumps, and rubella vaccines; 7 days for DT, Td, and T toxoids
	C. Residual seizure disorder[2]	(See Aids to Interpretation[2])
	D. Any acute complication or sequela (including death) of above events	No limit
	E. Events in vaccinees described in manufacturer's package insert as contraindications to additional doses of vaccine[3]	(See package insert)
OPV	A. Paralytic poliomyelitis	
	—in a nonimmunodeficient recipient	30 days
	—in an immunodeficient recipient	6 months
	—in a vaccine-associated community case	No limit
	B. Any acute complication or sequela (including death) of above events	No limit
	C. Events in vaccinees described in manufacturer's package insert as contraindications to additional doses of vaccine[3]	(See package insert)
IPV	A. Anaphylaxis or anaphylactic shock	24 hours
	B. Any acute complication or sequela (including death) of above event	No limit
	C. Events in vaccinees described in manufacturer's package insert as contraindications to additional doses of vaccine[3]	(See package insert)

[1]Modified and reproduced, with permission, from U.S. Department of Health and Human Services Public Health Service: National childhood vaccine injury act: Requirements for permanent vaccination records and for reporting of selected events after vaccination. *Morbidity and Mortality Weekly Report;***37** (No. 13):197.

[2]**Aids to Interpretation:** Shock-collapse or hypotonic-hyporesponsive collapse may be evidenced by signs or symptoms such as decrease in or loss of muscle tone, paralysis (partial or complete), hemiplegia, hemiparesis, loss of color or turning pale white or blue, unresponsiveness to environmental stimuli, depression of or loss of consciousness, prolonged sleeping with difficulty arousing, or cardiovascular or respiratory arrest.

Residual seizure disorder may be considered to have occurred if no other seizure or convulsion unaccompanied by fever or accompanied by a fever of less than 38.9 °C (102 °F) occurred before the first seizure or convulsion after the administration of the vaccine involved.

AND, if in the case of measles-, mumps-, or rubella-containing vaccines, the first seizure or convulsion occurred within 15 days after vaccination OR in the case of any other vaccine, the first seizure or convulsion occurred within 3 days after vaccination.

AND, if 2 or more seizures or convulsions unaccompanied by fever or accompanied by a fever of less than 38.9 °C (102 °F) occurred within 1 year after vaccination.

The terms *seizure* and *convulsion* include grand mal, petit mal, absence, myoclonic, tonic-clonic, and focal motor seizures and signs. Encephalopathy means any significant acquired abnormality of, injury to, or impairment of function of the brain. Among the frequent manifestations of encephalopathy are focal and diffuse neurologic signs, increased intracranial pressure, or changes lasting at least 6 hours in level of consciousness, with or without convulsions. The neurologic signs and symptoms of encephalopathy may be temporary with complete recovery, or they may result in various degrees of permanent impairment. Signs and symptoms such as high-pitched and unusual screaming, persistent unconsolable crying, and bulging fontanelle are compatible with an encephalopathy, but in and of themselves are not conclusive evidence of encephalopathy. Encephalopathy usually can be documented by slow wave activity on an electroencephalogram.

[3]The health-care provider must refer to the CONTRAINDICATION section of the manufacturer's package insert for each vaccine.

name and work address of the person administering the vaccine. Physicians administering the specified vaccines are also obliged by the act to report any of the specified reactions (see Table 6–4) to a public health authority. If the vaccine was purchased with public funds, the reaction must be reported by the administrator to the local, county, or state health department, which in turn reports to the Centers for Disease Control. If the vaccine was purchased with private funds, the administrator must complete FDA form 1639 (available from the FDA and the *FDA Drug Bulletin*) and forward the form directly to the FDA in Rockville, Maryland. The act provides for no penalty for failure to report.

Because the act has only recently taken effect, it remains to be seen what effect, if any, it will have on the volume of malpractice litigation deriving from vaccine injury claims or on the size of individual court awards. For the present, it would seem prudent to comply with the record keeping and reporting requirements of the act.

Centers for Disease Control: National Childhood Vaccine Injury Act: Requirements for permanent vaccination records and for reporting of selected events after vaccination. *MMWR* (April 8) 1988;**37**(13):197.

Ambulatory Pediatrics

Barton D. Schmitt, MD

This chapter offers guidelines for the conduct of 4 specific types of pediatric visit: (1) health maintenance care, (2) acute illness care, (3) chronic disease follow-up, and (4) consultation. Each type of visit requires a specific service that is different in many ways from the others. If the pediatrician and the office staff can mentally classify the patients in this way and vary their approach accordingly, the delivery of pediatric care will become more logical and consistent.

This organization of ambulatory care has 3 general advantages: (1) The quality of care improves because the patient benefits from the comprehensiveness of care that only a systematic approach can ensure. (2) The practice of pediatrics becomes more enjoyable because the establishment of clear office guidelines and policies prevents many frustrations and much duplication of effort by the physician. (3) The cost of medical care is reduced by increasing the efficiency of health care delivery.

HEALTH MAINTENANCE VISITS

OBJECTIVES

Health maintenance or health supervision visits are the key to preventive pediatrics. These visits involve 3 people: the physician, the parent, and the child. Children should assume more active roles in their own health care with each passing year. The visit has multiple purposes: responding to the parent's or child's current concerns, presenting age-appropriate anticipatory guidance, assessing growth and development (see Chapter 2), performing a physical examination (Chapter 1), obtaining laboratory screening tests, and administering immunizations (Chapter 6). A natural outcome of these visits is a deepening of family-physician rapport.

PARENTAL CONCERNS

The first part of each well child visit should be directed toward dealing with the current concerns of the parent, usually the mother. Most expectant mothers have many questions that should be discussed with their pediatrician several weeks prior to delivery. The most frequent concerns include arguments for and against breast-feeding and circumcision, preparation of the breasts if breast-feeding is to be chosen, hospital policies about rooming-in and parent-infant contact in the delivery room, essential baby equipment, separation problems with other children during the mother's confinement, and ways of decreasing sibling jealousy. It has been traditional for the first newborn office visit to take place at 6 weeks, probably because 6 weeks is the traditional time for the mother's first postdelivery obstetric visit. However, most mothers—particularly primiparas—have many questions and concerns well before this traditional interval after birth. A 2-week postpartal office visit is much more logical.

A health maintenance visit without parental concerns is uncommon. Some mothers bring a list of questions, "How much should babies cry?" "How do I know he's getting enough to eat?" "Can I spoil her by picking her up too much?" "Is it all right to spank children?" "How old should Johnny be before I let him cross the street alone?" Many of the questions have no clear-cut answers. The seasoned pediatrician usually enjoys the challenge of these discussions and the satisfaction that comes with reassuring an anxious parent.

Anderson FP: Evaluation of the routine physical examination of infants in the first year of life. *Pediatrics* 1970;**45**:950.

Charney E: Counseling of parents around the birth of a baby. *Pediatr Rev* 1982;**4**:167.

Green M et al: The changing picture of well-child care. *Contemp Pediatr* 1988;**5(8)**:14.

Hoekelman RA: What constitutes adequate well-baby care? *Pediatrics* 1975;**55**:313.

ANTICIPATORY GUIDANCE

Anticipatory guidance usually includes nutritional counseling, accident prevention, behavioral counseling, suggestions for developmental stimulation, sex education, dental recommendations, medical information, etc. Special counseling is in order for adolescents (see Chapter 10). A list of suggested topics to be discussed at particular ages is found on the health maintenance forms presented at the end of the chapter. A blank space or line on these forms indicates that a comment is required following that item. All anticipatory guidance advice is followed by the optimal age for discussion in parentheses. A check mark in the box that follows each of these advice items indicates that this counseling was done. These topics can be covered in a variety of ways. Some physicians prefer to discuss all the items with the parents personally; others prefer to delegate the discussion of some of these issues to the office nurse, and still others use printed materials to expand upon what the physician covers personally.

ACCIDENT PREVENTION

Injuries kill more children than the 6 other leading causes of childhood deaths combined. Between ages 1 and 14, over 50% of deaths are due to injuries, and between ages 15 and 23, over 80% are due to injuries. Each year 100,000 children under 15 years of age are left with permanent disabilities due to injuries. During the first 3 years of life, children have little sense of danger or self-preservation. They are totally dependent on adult supervision for their safety.

Accident prevention advice should be an integral part of medical care provided for all infants and children. Several years ago, the American Academy of Pediatrics established the Injury Prevention Program (TIPP), which includes parent questionnaires for assessing risk and information sheets to aid parents in preventing accidents. The main thrust of the program is to advise parents of the following 5 preventive measures: (1) approved car restraints for children, (2) smoke detectors, (3) hot water heater set to less than 130 °F, (4) guards for windows and gates for stairways, and (5) syrup of ipecac.

The Injury Prevention Program (TIPP) materials can be obtained from the American Academy of Pediatrics, Publications Department, 141 Northwest Point Boulevard, PO Box 927, Elk Grove Village, IL 60007 (telephone 1-800-433-9016).

Motor Vehicle Accidents

The foremost killer and crippler of children in the United States is the motor vehicle accident. Proper use of car safety seats can reduce fatalities and hospitalizations by at least 70%. Laws have been passed in all 50 states requiring that children riding in cars be restrained in an approved safety seat. The child's weight determines the type of safety seat to be used. In general, the smaller seats are more protective and should be used as long as they are appropriate:

Less than 20 pounds: rear-facing infant seat
20–40 pounds: forward-facing toddler seat
40–60 pounds: booster seat with lap belt
Over 60 pounds: regular lap belt
Over 48 inches (4 feet): shoulder strap with lap belt.

Prevention of Burns

(1) Never drink anything hot while holding a baby.
(2) Keep hot substances away from the edge of a table or stove.
(3) Do not let a child turn the faucet handles in the bathtub.
(4) Set hot water heaters to less than 130 °F.
(5) Use flame-resistant sleepware.
(6) Install smoke detectors in the home.
(7) Keep cigarette lighters and matches away from children.
(8) Keep electric cords unplugged or out of the reach of children.

Prevention of Choking

(1) Do not give a child any foods that are commonly aspirated into the lungs (nuts of any kind, sunflower seeds, orange seeds, cherry pits, raw carrots, raw peas, raw celery) until the child is old enough to chew or spit out such foods (usually 4 years of age).
(2) Carefully chop up any foods that might block the windpipe, such as hot dogs, grapes, caramels.
(3) Warn babysitters and siblings not to share these foods with small children.
(4) Do not allow a child with food in the mouth to run or play.
(5) Avoid toys with small detachable parts that could enter the windpipe.
(6) Be especially careful when disposing of button batteries.

Prevention of Drowning

(1) Never leave a child under age 3 unattended in the bathtub or a wading pool.
(2) Never leave a child who cannot swim unattended near a swimming pool. (More children drown in backyard swimming pools than at beaches or in public pools.)
(3) Remember that infant water programs are for fun, not for learning how to swim. (Children cannot be made water safe before age 3.)
(4) Try to arrange swimming lessons for your child between ages 3 and 8.

Prevention of Head Trauma

(1) Never leave an infant of any age alone on a high place.
(2) Always keep the side rails on the crib up.
(3) Avoid bunk beds.

(4) Avoid baby walkers. (Over 35% of infants using them have an accident requiring emergency care. The most serious accidents occur when a child in a walker falls down a stairway. Keep a sturdy gate at the top of all stairways.)

(5) Teach children to cross the street safely at age 4 or 5.

(6) Do not teach a child to ride a bicycle until age 7 or 8.

(7) Forbid trampolines.

Prevention of Poisoning

(1) Remember to keep drugs and chemicals locked up and out of reach.

(2) Keep in mind that drain cleaners, furniture polish, and insecticides are the most dangerous of the common poisons (other than drugs).

(3) Keep the safety cap on all drug containers.

(4) Keep some syrup of ipecac handy.

(5) Know the telephone number of the nearest poison control center.

Greensher J: Recent advances in injury prevention. *Pediatr Rev* 1988;**10**:171.

Wilson M: Injury prevention: Protecting the under-6 set. *Contemp Pediatr* 1988;**5(5)**:19.

The Injury Prevention Program (TIPP) materials can be obtained from the American Academy of Pediatrics, Publications Department, 141 Northwest Point Boulevard, PO Box 927, Elk Grove Village, IL 60007 (telephone 1-800-433-9016).

PHYSICAL EXAMINATION

A complete physical examination should be performed during most health maintenance visits (see Chapter 1). Height, weight, and head circumference should be measured and plotted on growth curves (see Chapter 2). During childhood, most chronic diseases will affect growth. Although these examinations are usually normal, they serve as a point of reference in evaluating future illnesses. Therefore, the extent of the examination should be carefully recorded. To save time, the checklist shown in Table 7–1 can be used. Elaboration is required only for the abnormal findings.

Some physical findings are silent—ie, they are not noticeable to parents and cause few if any symptoms. Of greatest concern are disorders that are treatable if detected early but potentially serious when not detected. A routine examination will diagnose most such conditions (eg, congenital heart disease). A few conditions are detected only by a detailed examination (eg, retinoblastoma [red fundus reflection test], strabismus [corneal light reflection test], congenital hip dislocation [Ortolani maneuver, or restricted abduction], scoliosis, coarctation of the aorta [femoral pulses], hypertension, lower urinary tract obstruction [inquire about urine stream], imperforate hymen, and labial adhesions). Visual deficits (eg, refractive errors or color blindness) and hearing deficits can also be missed if appropriate testing is not included. Dental caries may be overlooked by physicians who assume, not always rightly, that their patients are receiving periodic dental examinations (see Chapter 13). Early cancer detection can be improved by teaching self-examination of the breasts or testes.

Strong WB, Linder CW: Preparticipation health evaluation for competitive sports. *Pediatr Rev* 1982;**4**:113.

Table 7–1. Checklist for physical examination.

	Normal	Abnormal
1. GENERAL APPEARANCE: well nourished, hydrated, alert		
2. SKIN: color, rash, swelling, hair, nails		
3. HEAD: shape, anterior fontanelle		
4. EYES: conjunctiva, cornea, pupils, extraocular movement		
5. EARS: pinnae, canals; tympanic membrane appearance, mobility		
6. NOSE: nares, turbinates		
7. MOUTH: tongue, teeth, oral mucosa, tonsils, pharynx		
8. NECK: thyroid, range of motion		
9. NODES: cervical, axillary, inguinal, other		
10. CHEST: symmetry, expansion, breasts		
11. LUNGS: rate, auscultation, percussion		
12. HEART: rate, rhythm, S_1, S_2, murmur, femoral pulses		
13. ABDOMEN: contour; palpation of liver, spleen, and kidney; mass; tenderness		
14. GENITALIA: ♀ external; ♂ penis, meatus, testes, hernia		
15. SPINE: curvature (scoliosis), sacral area		
16. EXTREMITIES: range of motion, tenderness, edema, clubbing		
17. NEUROLOGIC (SCREEN): cranial nerves 3, 4, 6, 7, and 12; gait; cerebellar function; motor system (strength, tone)		
18. NEUROLOGIC (COMPLETE): above plus other cranial nerves; sensory and motor systems (deep tendon reflexes, clonus)		

THE SCHOOL READINESS EXAMINATION

The preschool examination of the 4- or 5-year-old child should be designed to answer the basic question, "Is the child ready for school?" Auscultation of the heart and lungs at this time is probably far less important than noting any abnormalities of speech, hearing, or vision and determining if developmental age is commensurate with chronologic age, if attention span is adequate for learning, and if parents have adequately prepared the child for separation when entering school. These problems should also be investigated earlier, but they are of greatest significance at the preschool examination.

Vision

Five to 10% of preschool children have some kind of visual impairment. The illiterate E chart, Snellen chart, STYCAR test, or Allen picture cards can be used for checking visual acuity, and each eye should be tested separately. Testing should be attempted at age 3. The 5-year-old child should have a visual acuity of 20/30 (6/9) or better in both eyes, and there should be no more than a 1-line difference between the 2 eyes. Suppression amblyopia affects 2–5% of children and must be detected early before permanent loss of vision occurs. Amblyopia is often secondary to strabismus, which can be detected by noting the position where light is reflected off both corneas or by the cover test (see Fig 12–4). Alignment can be tested by 6 months of age.

Hearing

Hearing deficits occur in approximately 1% of young school children, and in 10% the loss is profound and bilateral. Most children with hearing loss have recurrent purulent otitis media or serous otitis media. Even children with a single episode of otitis media may have some degree of hearing impairment for 3–6 months after the acute episode. Although the losses are generally not too severe, if they occur at an inopportune time they may be sufficient to prevent an early school-age child from learning phonics; hence, the effect of the loss may be carried on and magnified throughout much of the school years (see Chapter 14). If such losses are detected before entry into school, some of the learning, behavior, and discipline problems that occur secondary to poor attention might be averted. Detection of such problems is as much a part of preventive pediatrics as is the immunization routine. Audiologic screening tests can be performed by nonprofessional technicians and should be a part of the preschool examination.

Speech

The child entering school should be able to speak distinctly and clearly without difficulty; should be able to answer questions; and, after a period of getting acquainted, should be able to carry on a conversation with the physician about recent events. Poor speech may impair performance in school. An easily administered screening articulation test (Early Language Milestones Scale) has been developed to identify children who should be referred to a speech pathologist for definitive evaluation (see Fig 2–12).

Emotional Development & Behavior

The assessment of emotional development and behavior is an important part of the preschool examination. In one study, 42 physicians were observed conducting 673 well-child clinic visits. On the average, they said fewer than 2 sentences per visit to the mother that were relevant to child behavior. Yet, when given the opportunity to respond to a questionnaire about behavior, 85% of mothers of preschool children (ages 1½–6 years) indicated one or more such concerns (mean of 3.5 concerns per child). A simple self-administered questionnaire is an effective and efficient device which not only indicates to the parent that the physician is interested in discussing behavioral problems and emotional growth but also helps the physician to concentrate on areas of guidance most relevant to the parent's concerns. The pediatric health maintenance forms (provided at the end of this chapter) stress anticipatory guidance and counseling for behavioral aspects of pediatrics.

Physical, emotional, and developmental maturation proceeds at different rates for different children. Some children are ready for school long before their fifth birthday; others are not nearly ready at that age. Some parents tend to push their children into experiences that are beyond their capacities at a given age. Children should begin their school experiences with successes; the child who starts with failure is often criticized and becomes discouraged and less interested in school, so that a pattern of failure may develop. The child may continue to lag behind and miss the early fundamentals of learning, which are the basis for further education. Many children develop behavioral disorders and truancy simply because they cannot read and so are unable to understand what is going on in the classroom. Part of the physician's role is to help parents recognize physical, emotional, and developmental lags early, so that corrective measures can be taken to prepare the child for school. A number of easily administered developmental tests are available. The Denver Developmental Screening Test (see Chapter 2) is extremely helpful in the younger age groups. If, despite intervention, the child is not ready for school, the physician must advise the parents appropriately.

Committee on Nutrition, American Academy of Pediatrics: Indications for cholesterol testing in children. *Pediatrics* 1989;**83**:141.

Committee on Practice and Ambulatory Medicine, American Academy of Pediatrics: Vision screening and eye examination in children. *Pediatrics* 1986;**77**:918.

Coplan J, Gleason JR: Unclear speech: Recognition and significance of unintelligible speech in preschool children. *Pediatrics* 1988;**82**:447.

Dworkin PH: Educational readiness. *Pediatrician* 1986; **13**:62.

Joint Committee on Infant Hearing, American Academy of Pediatrics: Position Statement of 1982. *Pediatrics* 1982; **70**:496.

Nozza R: Screening audiometry: A sound investment for your practice. *Contemp Pediatr* 1986;**3**(9):71.

Palfrey JS, Rappaport LA: School placement. *Pediatr Rev* 1987;**8**:261.

LABORATORY SCREENING TESTS

A health maintenance flow sheet (see example provided at the end of this chapter) is a helpful reminder to the nurse and physician that certain procedures, laboratory tests, developmental evaluations, and immunizations need to be done. All of these items can be initiated by the nurse or aide if the physician establishes the routine to be followed.

Blood

Iron deficiency anemia (see Chapter 17) is found more often in lower socioeconomic populations and has its highest incidence in infants between 9 and 24 months of age. A routine hemoglobin or hematocrit is recommended in this age group and is particularly important in the child whose diet is low in iron-containing foods.

Children with sickle cell disease (see Chapter 17) must be diagnosed before 6 months of age to prevent death due to sepsis or splenic sequestration (10–20% mortality rate). Do not wait for the routine hematocrit at age 9 months. Prophylactic antibiotics should be started by age 3 months. It is strongly recommended that all black newborns have hemoglobin electrophoresis performed on cord blood or in conjunction with heel-stick testing for phenylketonuria. If not, the test should be performed at the 2-month check up.

Screening for phenylketonuria (see Chapter 33) should be done by blood test in the hospital nursery prior to the infant's discharge, and in all states such a test is required by law. An infant with this disorder who failed to ingest sufficient milk protein may have a negative test in the first few days of life. Therefore, most centers recommend a repeat test at 10–14 days of age if the first test was performed before 48 hours of age. Screening newborns for other treatable causes of mental retardation, congenital hypothyroidism and galactosemia, is required in most states and should be performed even where not required by state law. A T_4 or TSH assay can be done using cord blood.

Screening for lead poisoning (see Chapter 30) is extremely important in areas where the child has access to lead-based paint or soil contaminated by lead. Children living in such neighborhoods should have a routine blood lead level performed at 18–24 months of age. This test should be repeated at 6-month intervals until age 3 years in children with pica or where there is an index case in their building.

Routine cholesterol testing of all children is controversial. For now, the American Academy of Pediatrics recommends elective testing of those children who have a family history of hyperlipidemia or early myocardial infarction (< 50 years of age in men and < 60 in women). Testing of these children should be performed at age 2–3 years.

Urine

Routine urinalysis has a low yield in the asymptomatic patient. In contrast to the adult population, it is unusual for a child to have asymptomatic diabetes, and proteinuria is a rare presenting sign for a renal abnormality in an asymptomatic child. Transient orthostatic proteinuria is common in adolescents but benign. Although many recommend that the urine dipstick test be performed only on symptomatic children, testing once at age 3 or 4 is not unreasonable.

In screening for asymptomatic urinary tract infection, microscopic examination of the urinary sediment is time-consuming and not reliable. Several inexpensive methods are available to screen a first morning specimen for bacteriuria (eg, nitrite or glucose detection strips), followed by a urine culture if the dipstick test is positive. Since untreated asymptomatic bacteriuria usually clears spontaneously and does not lead to renal damage, screening should be reserved for high-risk groups (eg, children with diabetes). However, the clinician must not hesitate to check a specimen for bacilluria in any child with unexplained fevers, unexplained abdominal pain, enuresis, foul-smelling urine, or other vague symptoms.

Teenage girls who are sexually active will benefit from annual gonococcal cultures and Papanicolaou smears. Birth control counseling and sexuality counseling can also be offered at this time.

Gutgesell M: Practicality of screening urinalyses in asymptomatic children in a primary care setting. *Pediatrics* 1978;**62**:103.

Hein K et al: The need for routine screening in the sexually active adolescent. *J Pediatr* 1977;**91**:123.

Holtzman C et al: Descriptive epidemiology of missed cases of phenylketonuria and congenital hypothyroidism. *Pediatrics* 1986;**78**:553.

IMMUNIZATIONS

A child's immunization status can be easily monitored on the health maintenance flow sheet (see example provided at the end of this chapter). A record of the child's immunizations should also be given to the parents and updated by the nurse as additional immunizations are given. The details of routine immunization of children are presented in Chapter 6.

GROUP WELL-CHILD CARE

The newest model for providing health supervision visits is seeing 4 or 5 patients of the same age group during a 1-hour block. This model has been pioneered by Dr Lucy Osborn. The first 45 minutes are spent on health education, using lectures, videotapes, and discussion. Children are present during this time. The last 15 minutes are used to perform physical examinations on the children and to give immunizations.

For the parents, the advantages of group visits include the following: (1) Parents can benefit from a complete curriculum of anticipatory guidance topics. (2) They hear the concerns of other parents. (3) They are able to observe other infants' behaviors, and (4) they acquire a social support group. For the physician, the main advantages include (1) more contact time per parent, (2) more time to address behavior problems, (3) fewer telephone calls at later times regarding these topics, (4) a higher percentage rate of kept appointments, (5) more referrals generated by the parents, and (6) more stimulating interaction. It should be noted that this process does not save physician time or increase the overall fees generated.

Dr Osborn suggests that the 2-week visit be an individual one and that this program begin with the 2-month visit. She prefers to schedule the first hour in the morning and the first hour in the afternoon for group care. Adequate space for meeting with 5 or more adults is required. Any sensitive issues that the parents need to address can be covered during the time of the physical examination. In summary, this new model was preferred by the majority of parents and physicians who followed it.

Osborn LM: The use of groups in well-child care. *Pediatrics* 1981;**67**:701.

ACUTE ILLNESS VISITS

The episodic office visit for the child with an acute illness places special demands on the physician.

OBJECTIVES

Diagnosis and treatment of the chief complaint is the first priority for the parents, patient, and physician. Extenuating circumstances (eg, a crowded waiting room) rarely justify an incomplete workup of an acute chief complaint. Detection of patients who have a chronic disease or an undiagnosed chronic complaint should lead to a follow-up visit of appropriate length.

COMMON TYPES OF ACUTE ILLNESSES

The following diagnoses or conditions are the acute illnesses most commonly seen in office practice, listed in approximate order of frequency. Any health care provider who sees children must master the evaluation and management of these disorders: common colds, acute otitis media, viral pharyngitis and tonsillitis, gastroenteritis, acute tracheitis and bronchitis, conjunctivitis, streptococcal pharyngitis, diaper rash, thrush, impetigo, chickenpox, viral maculopapular rashes, skin trauma, head trauma, facial trauma, sprains, urinary tract infection, pneumonia, croup, cellulitis and boils, and ingestions.

ASSESSING ACUTE ILLNESS

Optimal management of an acute illness mainly includes telephone triaging, office triaging, diagnosis, assessment of the need for hospitalization, home therapy, and a follow-up plan.

The detection of multiple health problems is best accomplished by using a brief screening questionnaire, which should be completed for any new patient. Some parents have only crisis care available to their families (eg, in rural areas). Other parents have access to comprehensive health care but use only crisis care. The screening questionnaire is unnecessary for patients already being followed for health maintenance care. The parent can complete the questionnaire while waiting to see the physician. If chronic physical, emotional, or school problems are detected, the doctor should strongly recommend a follow-up appointment for a complete evaluation.

Katcher AL: Efficient office practice. *Pediatrics* 1977;**59**:533.

1. TELEPHONE TRIAGING & ADVICE

Does the Patient Need to Be Seen?

The physician is the person best qualified to give medical advice, both in the office and over the phone. However, because talking with parents on the phone may take too much physician time, this function is usually delegated to another member of the office team. Most of the questions are routine ones that require only routine answers. An office nurse specifically trained for the role is probably the best person to take routine calls. Office policies about medical advice over the phone should be standardized. Routine instructions for handling minor infections, minor injuries, reactions to immunizations, infant feeding problems, newborn care, and prescription refills are easy to communicate to parents if they are written down in an office protocol book. The protocol book should also specify the point at which each problem requires an office visit. This decision depends on (1) the type of symptom, (2) the duration of the symptom, (3) the age of the patient, (4) whether or not the patient acts "very sick," (5) an assessment of the parents' anxiety, and (6) the presence of any underlying chronic disease. (For example, most patients under 1 year of age with diarrhea and vomiting need to be examined.) After telephone baseline data are gathered, the nurse must be able to decide whether the child needs an appointment or not; the nurse should err on the side of giving an appointment when in doubt. For patients not seen, any pertinent telephone data should be entered on a temporary log sheet. If an office visit later becomes necessary, the data should be transferred to the patient's chart.

It is helpful if parents understand 2 general telephone rules: (1) The nurse will screen all calls during office hours except emergency ones and (2) nighttime calls should be restricted to emergencies or urgent problems that cannot wait until morning. Many routine calls come from overanxious, insecure parents who need reassurance and acceptance, not brisk criticism and implied rejection. The conversation with the nurse should help to build up a young mother's confidence. The mother can be asked what she had considered doing, and that plan of action should be strongly endorsed if possible. If parents are helped to become more confident and independent in these matters, unnecessary visits will be less frequent, as will medical costs for society in general. However, the conversation should convey the message that telephone calls are an important aid in medical care and that the parent is free to call again.

The physician directly accepts some calls: (1) emergency calls from parents, (2) calls from physicians and other professionals, (3) calls regarding hospitalized patients, (4) long distance calls, (5) calls from a parent who "demands" to talk to the physician, and (6) calls where the nurse is unclear about what should be done. These exceptions to the rule are obvious. Parents reasonably expect that their child's personal physician or a designated substitute should be readily available for emergencies, even if the "emergency" exists only from their viewpoint. The physician must be conscientious about accepting calls after midnight, for they often relate to psychosocial crises or urgent medical problems that cannot be ignored even for a few hours.

There are 4 other possible methods of dealing with telephone calls, any of which may serve as an alternative to having an office nurse screen and give telephone advice: (1) The physician can accept calls continuously throughout the day. These interruptions are unacceptable to most physicians and parents. (2) The physician can have a telephone hour at the beginning, middle, and end of the day and accept only emergency calls at other times. The disadvantages of this approach are that some parents must then wait for answers to urgent questions, and the physician lengthens his or her day with many routine calls. (3) The physician may charge for telephone advice. This decreases the number of calls, but in the process it may discourage important calls and thus interfere with preventive pediatrics. High charges for nighttime calls may help control these calls; however, the cost of billing makes charges for calls during office hours impractical. (4) The physician can allow various nonmedical office personnel to accept telephone calls randomly themselves. This approach would result in inconsistent medical advice and could be dangerous. The physician is of course legally liable for any harm to a patient proximately caused by improper advice given over the phone by employees.

Fosarelli P, Schmitt B: Telephone dissatisfaction in pediatric practice: Denver and Baltimore. *Pediatrics* 1987; **80**:28.
Katz, HP: *Telephone Manual of Pediatric Care.* Wiley, 1982.
Perrin EC, Goodman HC: Telephone management of acute pediatric illness. *N Engl J Med* 1978;**298**:130.
Schmitt BD: *Pediatric Telephone Advice.* Little, Brown, 1980.

When Does the Patient Need to Be Seen?

Some patients must be seen immediately (eg, for a foreign body in the eye). Others can be seen later the same day (eg, for a cough that kept the patient awake much of the preceding night). Other patients can be scheduled 1–2 days later (eg, for recurrent epistaxis). The nurse can make these decisions.

Where Should the Patient Be Seen?

Most sick patients can be seen in the physician's office by appointment. The physician can keep the first and last hour of each day plus at least 15 minutes out of each hour reserved for acute problems. Most of the first-hour appointments will be given to parents who call the physician during the preceding evening.

Another facility where patients can be seen for medical care is the hospital emergency room. This routing applies to patients who are highly likely to be admitted (eg, for croup). Some physicians also send patients with poisonings, lacerations, or possible fractures to the nearest emergency room.

A third possibility is a house call. Most physicians consider this disadvantageous to themselves financially and to the patient medically, because laboratory services are not available. A rare indication for a house call might be a contagious disease that needs confirmation (eg, varicella). The physician could occasionally see such a patient in the office parking lot.

2. OFFICE TRIAGING & PROCEDURES

How Sick Is the Patient?

The nurse should screen all sick patients as soon as possible after they arrive at the office. They can be thought of in terms of 3 general groups: emergency, contagious, and minor illness. Most patients have a minor illness (eg, cold, accident, earache) and can be seen at their appointed time. Some patients are contagious until proved otherwise and should quickly be moved from the waiting room to an isolated examining room (eg, febrile illnesses with rashes, lice, jaundice, possible pertussis). An attempt should be made to keep children with bronchiolitis or croup away from infants. When an office emergency (eg, febrile seizures, respiratory distress) is recognized by the nurse, the physician should be notified immediately. The physician can take appropriate emergency action, stabilize the patient, and arrange for transfer to the hospital if necessary (eg, an acidotic, dehydrated infant). (See Chapter 8.)

Russo RM et al: Triage abilities of nurse practitioner vs pediatrician. *Am J Dis Child* 1975;**129**:673.

Preparation of the Patient for the Physician

The office aide can record the sick patient's temperature, height, and weight. The office nurse can record the chief complaint. Depending upon the symptom, the nurse can take vital signs and initiate the office's standing orders on laboratory procedures and symptomatic treatment listed below.

Initial Treatment & Laboratory Workup

Steps in initial management are listed below. Details of procedures are outlined elsewhere in the text.

A. Abdominal Pain: Take samples for urinalysis and urine culture; save stool specimen for occult blood testing.

B. Animal Bite: Wash out immediately with benzalkonium chloride for 10 minutes. Initiate the official reporting form, and call the county health department. Delay irrigation if the wound is infected and a culture is needed.

C. Cough: If present over 1 month, apply a tuberculin skin test.

D. Diarrhea: Take a sample for stool culture if the stool contains blood or mucus or if diarrhea has persisted for more than 1 week at any age. For children under age 2, give 180 mL (6 oz) of an oral electrolyte solution, and record the naked weight on each visit. If a child appears dehydrated, collect urine for specific gravity.

E. Earache: Give acetaminophen if in obvious pain. If there is a possibility of mumps, isolate the patient.

F. Eye Injury: Test visual acuity if child is over age 3. Place eye tray in the examining room.

G. Fever Over 39 °C (102.2 °F): Give acetaminophen at a dose of 15 mg/kg. Put the child in an examining room and assist with undressing. Give a sponge bath if temperature exceeds 40 °C (104 °F) despite drugs and if the child is uncomfortable. Provide a bag for urine if the child is not toilet trained, and save urine in refrigerator for analysis and culture. If unexplained fever has been present over 24 hours, order a white count and differential. If the infant is under 2 months of age, notify the physician immediately.

H. Fractures: Notify physician immediately, obtain equipment to immobilize the site, and fill out the x-ray request.

I. Head Injury: Record vital signs and level of consciousness, and check pupils for equal size and reaction to light.

J. Infectious Hepatitis Exposure: Record weights of persons who have had intimate contact with the patient, and anticipate giving immune globulin, 0.03 mL/kg intramuscularly.

K. Lacerations: Wash thoroughly (at least 10 minutes). Check date of last tetanus shot and record. (The physician must decide if tetanus booster or antitoxin is needed.) Shave around the wound edges if necessary (but never shave eyebrows). Have parents sign consent for suturing.

L. Nosebleed: Instruct the parent or child on how to compress the bleeding site for 10 minutes. Check blood pressure and perform fingerstick for hematocrit.

M. Painful Urination (Burning or Frequency): Take sample for urinalysis, urine culture, nitrite dipstick, and a gram-stained smear of unspun drop.

N. Pinworms: Record the approximate weights of all family members if the infection is a recurrent one (for calculation of dosage of medication, see Chapter 29).

O. Sore Throat: Take material for throat culture (contraindicated if the patient has croup).

P. Streptococcal Sore Throat (Culture Positive): Inquire about penicillin allergy and record. Arrange for symptomatic family contacts to have throat cultures taken.

Q. Vomiting: Record exact weight. Give patient emesis basin and sips of ice water while waiting. If patient appears dehydrated, collect urine for specific gravity.

3. THE WORKING DIAGNOSIS

The physician makes the final decision about the diagnosis and the severity of the disease. Emergency conditions (eg, shock or meningitis) may be noted and emergency intervention initiated. History taking can be modified to emphasize the chief complaint. A history of recent contact with persons with contagious diseases is often important. Severity can be partially assessed by inquiries about playfulness, energy, ability to sleep, and the parent's feelings about how sick the child is this time compared to other times. If a family of sick children is brought in, the physician should ask the mother which children she considers the sickest. The physical examination should be mainly directed toward the chief complaint. A patient with a dog bite does not require a complete examination, but a patient with an earache must be checked for mastoid swelling and meningeal signs in addition to otoscopic examination.

Utilizing the conventional techniques of history, physical examination, and laboratory tests, the physician will correctly diagnose most acute chief complaints. However, a vigilant clinical mind is necessary in order not to miss a diagnosis of septicemia. Septic children usually present with unexplained fever, but (unlike children with acute viral fevers) they often will not smile or play, even with their parents. They frequently are physically exhausted and too weak to resist the physical examination, constantly irritable and unable to sleep, and respond paradoxically to cuddling by the mother. Irritability usually stems from pain or hypoxia. A less common finding in the toxic child is constant lethargy or sleepiness. This is difficult to assess because most sick children sleep more than normally. A child with suspected septicemia requires an intensive workup and therapy in a hospital setting. These more complicated acute illness evaluations can be expedited if the physician has studied appropriate decision-making algorithms (see Chapter 14).

McCarthy PL et al: Predictive value of abnormal physical examination findings in ill-appearing and well-appearing febrile children. *Pediatrics* 1985;**76**:167.

Nelson KG: An index of severity for acute pediatric illness. *Am J Public Health* 1980;**70**:804.

4. INDICATIONS FOR HOSPITALIZATION

For every acute problem, the physician must decide whether to treat the child at home or in the hospital.

Patients whose problems fit into one of the following 3 groups of indications should be hospitalized:

Major Emergencies

Some examples of obvious life-threatening conditions are shock, severe dehydration, coma, meningitis (bacterial or of unknown cause), respiratory distress, congestive heart failure, symptomatic hypertension, acute renal failure, status epilepticus, and surgical emergencies.

Potentially Life-Threatening or Crippling Illnesses

Some patients are not in critical condition when first seen but require hospitalization because their problem may be rapidly progressive during treatment. If deterioration occurs in the hospital, emergency therapy can be rapidly instituted. Most of the entities in this group are caused by infection or trauma. Endogenous diseases rarely change this rapidly. Although absolute rules cannot be formulated for every situation, the following guidelines can be applied to most cases of acute illness. Obviously, these rules will have some exceptions such as when the emergency room has a 8-hour observation area. Also, the list is not complete (eg, chronic diseases are not listed).

These problems are listed according to body systems:

A. Skin:

1. Cellulitis if the patient is less than 2 months old; if there is buccal involvement or the cavernous sinus drainage area is involved; if underlying sinusitis or osteomyelitis is suspected; if cellulitis is secondary to a puncture wound in the foot; or if there is no response after 2 days of therapy.
2. Erysipelas, toxic epidermal necrolysis, or acute necrotizing fasciitis. Omphalitis if the patient is less than 2 months old.
3. Suspected thrombophlebitis.
4. Burns (second- or third-degree) involving more than 10% of surface area (> 15% if the patient is more than 1 year old); burns of perineal area, hand, or face if they might need grafting; all inhalation burns; and most electrical burns.
5. Pupura with fever, without fever but unexplained, or without fever but progressive.

B. Eyes:

1. Gonococcal conjunctivitis or bacterial keratitis.
2. Eye injury if visual acuity is decreased.
3. Papilledema.

C. Ears, Nose, and Throat:

1. Acute otitis media if the patient is less than 1 month old with fever, systemic symptoms, or no response after 2 days of therapy.
2. Mastoiditis.
3. Sinusitis if overlying redness or edema is present.
4. Nasal obstruction if the patient is less than 6 months old and an apneic episode has occurred.
5. Epistaxis if uncontrolled; if hypertension is present; if there is bleeding elsewhere; or if severe anemia is present.

6. Fluctuant tonsillar abscess.
7. Retropharyngeal abscess.
8. Diphtheria (any symptoms at any age).
9. Cervical adenitis if the patient is toxic, dehydrated, dysphagic, dyspneic, or less than 6 months old and needs treatment by incision and drainage.

D. Respiratory System:

1. Epiglottitis (all cases).
2. Viral laryngitis if there is stridor at rest, dyspnea, or drooling; if the child has repeatedly awakened from sleep with stridor; if the illness is currently progressive; if there is a history of a previous bout with rapid progression; if there are apneic or cyanotic episodes; or if the patient is less than 1 year old and the stridor is easily provoked (eg, occurs with any crying).
3. Pertussis if symptomatic and the patient is less than 1 year old; pertussis at any age if accompanied by apnea, respiratory distress, a whoop, or weight loss.
4. Bronchiolitis if the patient is dyspneic, has apneic or cyanotic episodes ($Po_2 < 50$), has poor fluid intake, or is unable to sleep.
5. Asthma if respiratory distress persists after 2 injections of epinephrine, one nebulized dose of a beta-agonist, or both.
6. Pneumonia if the patient is less than 1 month old; if bacterial pneumonia is suspected and the patient is less than 6 months old; if there is a history of apnea, cyanosis, or choking spells; if there is dyspnea (any age); if there is pleural effusion; if staphylococcal pneumonia is suspected (any age); if aspiration pneumonia is present; if fluid intake is poor; if there is underlying cystic fibrosis or congenital heart disease; or if there is no response after 2 days of therapy.
7. Suspected foreign body of the airway.
8. Hemoptysis if unexplained; if there is bleeding elsewhere; or if anemia is present.
9. Apnea in all cases except periodic breathing, breath-holding spells, or mild choking on food.

E. Cardiovascular System:

1. Suspected subacute bacterial endocarditis.
2. Any myocarditis or pericarditis.
3. Acute hypertension or shock.
4. Unexplained dysrhythmias.

F. Gastrointestinal System:

1. Vomiting with dehydration, delirium, or persistent abdominal pain.
2. Hematemesis if documented and not caused by swallowed blood.
3. Diarrhea if explosive in character; if accompanied by abdominal distention or associated Kussmaul respirations; if typhoid fever is suspected in a patient of any age; if acute *Shigella* infection is suspected in a patient less than 1 year old; or if

staphylococcal enterocolitis is suspected in a patient less than 1 year old who has moderate dehydration or mild dehydration with vomiting.
4. Melena or unexplained bright-red blood mixed in the stools.
5. Suspected appendicitis, peritonitis, or intussusception.
6. Abdominal trauma if penetrating injury has occurred or if damage to the spleen, liver, kidneys, pancreas, or intestines is suspected.
7. Toxic ileus.

G. Urinary System:

1. Pyelonephritis if the patient is less than 2 months old, toxic, or unimproved after 2 days of therapy; if gram-negative sepsis is suspected; if underlying renal disease is present; or if recurrences have been frequent.
2. Acute edema, oliguria, or azotemia.
3. Hematuria with symptoms listed in (2), renal colic, and unexplained or posttraumatic gross hematuria.
4. Acute urinary retention.

H. Genitalia:

1. Vaginitis if associated with salpingitis.
2. Vaginal injury with sharp object.
3. Suspected testicular torsion.
4. Priapism.

I. Skeletal System:

1. Suspected osteomyelitis.
2. Arthritis if possibly septic or acute rheumatic fever.
3. Wringer injury if above the elbow; if a hematoma or avulsed skin is present; if a fracture or nerve injury is present; or if the peripheral pulse is diminished.

J. Nervous System:

1. Aseptic meningitis if the level of consciousness is depressed or there is a motor deficit.
2. Suspected tetanus.
3. Suspected epidural spinal abscess or brain abscess.
4. Febrile or afebrile seizures if they continue more than 30 minutes; if there are persistent neurologic signs; if the level of consciousness is decreased; or if serious underlying disease cannot be ruled out.
5. Head injury if the patient has been unconscious longer than 5 minutes; if there are persistent neurologic signs; if the level of consciousness is decreased; if a seizure has occurred; if cerebrospinal fluid rhinorrhea or otorrhea is present; if there is significant swelling over the middle meningeal artery; if there are retinal hemorrhages or progressive headaches; or if abnormal or irregular vital signs are present.

6. Skull fractures that are depressed or compound (ie, into air sinuses or overlying scalp laceration), fractures across the middle meningeal artery or venous sinus, occipital fracture into the rim of the foramen magnum, or any fracture with an underlying bleeding disorder.
7. Suspected spinal cord trauma.
8. Acute muscle weakness.
9. Acute cognitive deterioration, including delirium that is unexplained or persists longer than 2 hours.
10. Suspected increased intracranial pressure.

K. General:

1. Fever if the patient is less than 2 months old; if toxicity is evident and serious underlying disease cannot be ruled out; or if fever is due to heat stroke.
2. Poisoning if the patient is symptomatic (eg, respirations slow or irregular, drowsiness, etc); the agent or dosage is unknown; or the dosage is a potentially fatal one.
3. Suspected lead poisoning.
4. Unexplained mass.
5. Failure to thrive if severe or unexplained or if serious neglect is suspected.
6. Unexplained hypoglycemia.
7. Suspected anaphylactic reaction with laryngeal reaction, bronchospasm, hypotension, or dysrhythmias.

Gururaj VJ: Short stay in an outpatient department. *Am J Dis Child* 1972;**123**:128.
Lovejoy FH et al: Unnecessary and preventable hospitalizations: Report on an internal audit. *J Pediatr* 1971; **79**:868.

Psychosocial Indications for Hospitalization

Patients with acute psychosocial problems now comprise a larger proportion of hospitalized children than was formerly the case. In many cities, a child can be placed in an emergency receiving home or an acute psychiatric ward. Sometimes the child can temporarily stay with a relative. Indications for hospitalization fall into 3 general groups: parent, child, and disease problems.

A. Parent Problems:

1. Child abuse (eg, battering, failure to thrive secondary to neglect, or incest).
2. Incipient battering (eg, the parent has made a homicidal threat against a child).
3. Absent parents (eg, abandonment, emancipated minors without caretakers, or the parents themselves are hospitalized).
4. Physically exhausted parents (eg, no sleep for 2 nights).
5. Severely overanxious parents (eg, if the parents remain immobilized and extremely anxious after a careful explanation of their child's illness).

6. Neglectful parents who seem uninterested in their child's illness or therapy (eg, neglected eczema). This is a rare situation compared to overly anxious parents.
7. Intellectually incompetent parents (eg, a mentally retarded mother who cannot reliably follow verbal or written instructions).
8. Emotionally disturbed parents who need psychiatric hospitalization and treatment for their own problems (eg, a floridly psychotic mother).
9. Parent who is alcoholic or drug abuser.

B. Child Problems:

1. Suicide attempt—a short hospital admission allows time for the mental health worker to make an evaluation and for the family to look seriously at their problems.
2. A destructive, dangerous child can be held on a pediatric ward pending placement. A dangerous adolescent will require a psychiatric care facility.
3. An incapacitating emotional symptom (eg, a severe conversion reaction such as paraplegia or blindness).

C. Disease Problems:

1. An incapacitating (but not life-threatening) physical disease (eg, severe Sydenham's chorea).
2. Initial diagnosis of a disease with a complex treatment regimen. The parents and patient deserve a careful, unhurried, and organized introduction to the complex home management of some chronic diseases (eg, diabetes mellitus).
3. Initial diagnosis of a fetal disease—This gives the family time to work through the impact phase (eg, leukemia).
4. Terminal care if the family does not want the child to die at home.
5. Chronic diseases that are exacerbated by family conflicts (eg, ulcerative colitis).
6. Hazardous home (eg, carbon monoxide or lead poisoning).

Unnecessary Hospitalization

In the USA, overhospitalization is currently a greater problem than underhospitalization. In recent studies, at least 20% of hospitalizations were judged to be unnecessary. Moreover, 25% of unnecessary patient days were due to delayed discharge because the patient was simply waiting for transportation home. Overhospitalization takes 3 general forms: (1) Hospitalization for an acute illness sometimes occurs because the primary physician is uncertain of the diagnosis and prognosis (eg, viral rashes). Reassurance in the face of such uncertainty can often be gained by immediate consultation with a colleague. (2) Hospitalization is sometimes arranged for a diagnostic evaluation and tests because the patient has no outpatient insurance (eg, urinary tract infection). Unless the parents are in serious financial difficulty, this custom is unethical. It is to be hoped that more realistic insurance coverage will make ambulatory studies equally reimbursable. (3) Periodic hospitalizations sometimes are ordered for routine reevaluations of a chronic disease (eg, chronic glomerulonephritis). Even if the patient travels a great distance, this reevaluation can be done on an ambulatory basis if it is carefully planned in advance. The combined costs of the special studies plus hotel accommodations will be far less than hospitalization charges. In cases of elective hospitalization, preadmission evaluations can reduce hospital stays by 2 or 3 days.

The indications for hospitalization are becoming more selective. The time has passed when every child with infectious mononucleosis, hepatitis, pneumonia, gross hematuria, or a urinary tract infection is automatically admitted. Fewer than 10% of patients with these acute disorders require hospitalization. In fact, in emergency rooms with special observation units, children with moderate dehydration, diabetic ketoacidosis, status asthmaticus, etc, are treated and released in 3–6 hours.

Unnecessary hospitalization carries 5 main problems or risks, the last one probably being the most serious: (1) Children under 3 years of age can experience separation problems. (2) The parents' confidence in caring for a sick child themselves is undermined. (3) There is a danger of cross-infection to the patient and others. (4) There is a risk of medical error, such as the wrong medication or wrong dosage. (5) Society sustains an endlessly rising cost for medical care.

An acutely ill child can be observed in the office for several hours if it is not clear whether or not hospitalization is necessary. This will allow time for any reassurance given to the mother to take effect, and it permits the physician to compare the patient at 2 points in time and determine whether the condition is improving or getting worse. This interval also helps one decide what to do when the mother's history and the physical examination are inconsistent (eg, "recurrent vomiting" without dehydration, "no urination" without bladder distention). If necessary, another physician can be called in for consultation during this time.

Goldbloom RB, Macleod MU: Impact of preadmission evaluations on elective hospitalization of children. *Pediatrics* 1984;**73**:656.

Kemper KJ: Medically inappropriate hospital use in a pediatric population. *N Engl J Med* 1988;**318**:1033.

5. TREATMENT OF THE NONHOSPITALIZED PATIENT

Words are as necessary as drugs in the treatment of a sick child. The parents expect to be told their child's diagnosis and its causes, prognosis, and treatment. They also need to have their special concerns acknowledged and clarified. If this communication does not take place, the parents will often be dissatisfied with the quality of care being given, and their compliance with regard to medications, advice, and follow-up will probably be less than optimal.

If the child has a mild acute illness (eg, viral nasopharyngitis), the parent would be reassured by the following general types of comment:

Diagnosis

"David has a cold." The diagnosis should be conveyed in plain English, not in medical jargon. If the physician does not specifically state the diagnosis, the parents may assume none has been arrived at. (See also Ambiguous Diagnosis, below.)

Etiology

"It's due to a virus." This means to most parents that the infection is not serious. Some parents need an added statement that there was nothing they could have done to prevent it—eg, "Everyone is coming down with this."

Parents' Concerns

Mothers often do not listen to their physician's instructions until their own main concerns have been discussed. These concerns are easily elicited by Korsch's 3 questions: (1) "Why did you bring David to the clinic today?" (2) "What worried you most about him?" (3) "Why did that worry you?" After these concerns are out in the open, the physician is in a position to clarify misconceptions. Reassurance can be specific—eg, "He doesn't have meningitis," or, "It won't turn into leukemia."

Treatment

In self-limited disease, the goal of medication is to keep the patient comfortable. A list of useful approaches to management (sometimes overlooked) is as follows: (1) An antipyretic is useful if the patient's fever causes discomfort. (2) Dextromethorphan can be used for acute cough that interferes with sleep. Teaching the parent how to suction the nose properly can turn a restless baby into a sleeping one. (3) Advice about diet, bed rest, isolation, and mood is also appreciated by the parent. The patient can usually be allowed to dictate the diet during periods of illness. (4) In most cases, the patient can also be allowed to decide whether to stay in bed, to be up in pajamas watching television, etc. (5) Isolation within the family structure is rarely indicated, because exposure has usually preceded the diagnosis. (6) Parents can be reassured about temporary emotional regression during an acute illness. A return to the previous level of maturity need not be encouraged until good health returns.

Prognosis

"David will probably feel better in 2 or 3 days.

This is not a serious infection. If his fever lasts over 3 days or he gets worse, give me a call.'' Nothing is gained by mentioning all the possible complications. Without promoting anxiety, the door to additional medical evaluation is quietly left open for any new problems that might arise.

Closing

''You're doing a fine job with David. Just hold the fort and he will be his old self in a few days.'' The visit should close on a positive note, even a compliment if possible. If David is older, an attempt can be made to boost his morale as well—eg, ''This won't keep *you* out of action for long.''

The Ambiguous Diagnosis

An unclear diagnosis presents special problems in communication with the parents. The physician must be honest about the inconclusive diagnosis and yet not unduly alarm the parents. ''David's illness is not far enough along to be diagnosed exactly. Another day or so will be needed to pinpoint the problem. I can tell you a few things for certain. He is not in any serious trouble. He doesn't have meningitis. I definitely want to see him tomorrow. Call me sooner if there are any new developments.''

Symptomatic therapy should also be prescribed.

Carey WB, Sibinga MS: Avoiding pediatric pathogenesis in the management of acute minor illness. *Pediatrics* 1972;**49:**553.

Korsch B et al: Practical implications of doctor-patient interaction analysis for pediatric practice. *Am J Dis Child* 1971;**121:**110.

Waller DA, Levitt EE: Concerns of mothers in a pediatric clinic. *Pediatrics* 1972;**50:**931.

6. FOLLOW-UP OF THE NONHOSPITALIZED PATIENT

Many children seen in an emergency room have conditions that require following (eg, asthma, bronchiolitis, croup, pneumonia, otitis media, burns, and seizures). If a child has an ambiguous diagnosis (eg, high fever of unknown origin) or an unpredictable course (eg, vomiting), daily follow-up is necessary. This protects both the patient and the physician. This follow-up can be accomplished by revisits, telephone calls, or a visiting nurse.

Revisits

Daily office visits are the best approach to the more serious problem. The weight of an infant with diarrhea and the degree of respiratory distress in a child with croup cannot be estimated over the phone. If a scheduled appointment is not kept, the office clerk should immediately notify the physician, and a phone call or home visit should be made on that same day. If transportation is a problem for the par-

ent, a community service agency can usually help. If the late results of laboratory tests indicate that an illness is quite serious (eg, stool culture growing *Salmonella* in a 2-month-old infant) and reasonable attempts to locate the parents fail, the police may be asked to find and bring the patient to the clinic or office.

Telephone Calls

A daily telephone call will suffice for milder problems when only historical follow-up data are needed (eg, vomiting or lethargy). Since these calls are essential to proper management, the physician or nurse should make them. A daily telephone list can be kept and the charts pulled prior to calling. If the follow-up is felt to be important, parents should not be depended upon to initiate these calls. Telephone calls become the realistic choice of follow-up when long distances are a factor.

Home Visits

The evaluation of children with allergies, obesity, failure to thrive, recurrent accidents, recurrent ingestions, or behavior problems is enhanced by a home visit. The follow-up of early-discharge newborns is simplified by home visits. Dressing changes of burns or wounds can readily be done in the home. Most of these house calls are made by the public health nurse, but the office nurse or physician can also become involved. Mothers of large families who have both a baby-sitter problem and a transportation problem appreciate this type of follow-up. Mothers who have several sick children or who are themselves in poor health also benefit from home visits.

Berger LR, Samet KP: Home visits: Extending the boundaries of comprehensive pediatric care. *Am J Dis Child* 1981;**135:**812.

DeAngelis C, Fosarelli P: Assignment of follow-up appointments from an emergency room by pediatric residents. *Am J Dis Child* 1985;**139:**341.

Weitzman M, Moomaw MS, Messenger KP: An after-hours pediatric walk-in clinic for an entire urban community. *Pediatrics* 1980;**65:**964.

MEDICOLEGAL PROBLEMS

The management of acute illness offers the greatest potential for malpractice litigation in pediatrics. Physicians are legally liable for damage proximately caused not only by their own mistakes but by the mistakes of their employees as well. Errors can be made in any of the areas previously discussed. An error in telephone triaging can result in a delay in diagnosis (eg, calling meningococcemia a viral exanthem, or arranging an appointment for the next day for scrotal pain that turns out to be testicular torsion). An error in underhospitalization can lead to death (eg, epiglottitis being treated on an outpatient basis). Errors in therapy may result in sciatic nerve palsy if an injection is given into an inappropriate quadrant of the buttocks or may result in acute rheumatic fever if penicillin is not given for a streptococcal sore throat because it was not cultured. Errors in follow-up can result in undiagnosed abdominal pain silently progressing to ruptured appendix.

The physician should obtain parent consent forms for all medical procedures (eg, lumbar puncture, suturing) unless an emergency exists. Consultation should be sought whenever a physician is uncertain about what is happening with an acutely and perhaps seriously ill patient.

The errors listed above are not difficult to prevent if the physician bases all medical decisions on what is best for the patient.

Markham BF: Legal issues for the practicing pediatrician. *Pediatr Clin North Am* 1981;**28**:617.

Robertson WO: Medical malpractice: 1984. *Pediatr Rev* 1985;**6**:229.

CHRONIC DISEASE FOLLOW-UP VISITS

At least 7.5% of children in the USA have one or more chronic illnesses; management of these patients is thus a major part of pediatric practice. Office visits for a child with known or potential chronic disease present special problems. There are 5 broad types of chronic disease, each being progressively more difficult to manage: (1) potential chronic disease (eg, the small premature infant, the newborn who has recovered from hypoglycemia, or the older child who has recovered from meningitis; (2) reversible chronic disease (eg, tuberculosis, eczema, or idiopathic thrombocytopenic purpura); (3) statis chronic disease (eg, cerebral palsy, deafness, or dwarfism); (4) progressive chronic disease (eg, diabetes mellitus or sickle cell anemia); and (5) fatal disease (eg, some cancers). Children with these problems usually receive excellent care when they are hospitalized. They should also receive the same thoughtful care when they do not occupy a hospital bed or have an interesting complication.

COMMON TYPES OF CHRONIC ILLNESSES

The following diagnoses or conditions are the chronic disorders most commonly seen in office practice: serous otitis media, hay fever, asthma, obesity, enuresis, recurrent abdominal pain, recurrent headaches, acne, developmental delays or mental retardation, seizures, learning disabilities, attention deficit disorder, menstrual problems, visual acuity defect, hearing defect, depression, child abuse, recurrent urinary tract infections, hypertension, congenital heart disease, failure to thrive, short stature, eczema, cerebral palsy, constipation or soiling, recurrent hematuria, scoliosis, chronic diarrhea, peptic ulcer, and diabetes mellitus.

OBJECTIVES

There are 2 primary objectives in the management of a chronic disease. The first is to counteract the effects of the disease to the extent possible. This requires the aggressive use of every available treatment measure that could be useful for the individual patient's problems. The second objective is to help the patient and parents make a suitable emotional adjustment to the treatment regimen and to the effects of the disease that cannot be controlled. Except for necessary restrictions imposed by the disease, the child should be reared just like other children. The goal of management is to enable the patient to live as normal a life as possible in all positive respects.

Chronic disease management is optimal when the following receive ongoing attention: continuity of care, frequent visits, problem-oriented records, chronic disease flow sheets, personal medical identification documents, a chronic disease patient registry kept in the office, and medical passport.

1. CONTINUITY OF CARE

The patient with a chronic disease may have multiple problems that are difficult to manage. If anyone deserves continuous medical care from one physician, this person does. Discontinuous care by several physicians (eg, in emergency rooms) often results in a confused and maladjusted patient. When the patient has a progressive or fatal disease, depression can occur. In such a situation, patients depend upon a single sustaining physician to help them maintain their tenuous hope for the child's survival. Fragmented medical care usually accentuates a poor psychologic adjustment. The physician who agrees to care for a patient with a chronic disease should be available by phone at all times, even when at home. If the physician cannot deal with a problem personally, arrangements can be made for the patient to be seen by another physician who has been fully briefed. If the physician must be away for any reason, a substitute physician who has been designated well in advance should be available.

Becker MH et al: Continuity of pediatrician: New support for an old shibboleth. *J Pediatr* 1974:**84**:599.

2. FREQUENT VISITS

The patient with a chronic disease should be contacted frequently. Monitoring the patient's disease and response to therapy is impossible without periodic visits or telephone communications. If the problem is stabilized, the patient should be seen personally at least every 6 months; 3-month intervals are better for progressive diseases. If the disease is in relapse, the patient may need to be seen daily.

3. PROBLEM-ORIENTED RECORDS

In addition to a personal physician, comprehensive care of the chronically ill patient depends upon good record keeping. No physician's memory is completely reliable, and in any case the patient must have accurate office records when the physician moves away from the city or dies. An excellent system of record keeping has been developed and refined in a practice setting (see references, below). It has 4 components: the initial data base, the active problem sheet, the plan for each problem, and the progress notes that contribute to the continually expanding data base and problem list.

Initial Data Base

The conventional present illness, review of systems, past medical history, family history, psychosocial history, physical examination, and laboratory screening tests comprise the data base. Information from all accessible sources is used. (See Chapter 1.)

Active Problem Sheet

The active problem list is the keystone of this system. It lists all of the patient's significant problems, including psychosocial ones. These problems are defined from the data base currently at hand. They can be expressed as an etiologic diagnosis (eg, rheumatic heart disease); a pathophysiologic state (eg, congestive heart failure), or a sign or symptom (eg, edema). When the therapy carries considerable risk, it should be defined as a problem (eg, corticosteroids or tracheostomy). An attempt is made to list the problems in order of priority. Each problem is then assigned a permanent number. Thereafter, this number should precede any entry in the chart concerning this problem. The active problem sheet should be kept in the front of the patient's chart as a table of contents. The dates should be date of onset or resolution. New problems are added as identified, and old problems are transferred to the "resolved or inactive" column when appropriate. Symptom problems should be reidentified as diagnosed problems when the data accumulated justify doing so. When a patient with multiple diseases is cared for by several physicians, the last column on the active problem list

can be used to list the responsible physician for each problem. This technique is especially helpful for improving continuity of care in a large medical center.

The active problem list can become somewhat standardized if "#1" is always used for "health maintenance care" (or well child care) and "#2" is always used for "minor acute illnesses" (or temporary problems). The latter category is a convenient place to bury self-limited minor illnesses that do not warrant being given individual permanent numbers. Examples are colds, coughs, gastroenteritis, conjunctivitis, mumps, viral exanthems, impetigo, diaper rash, insect bites, minor trauma, etc. Acute illnesses that can be serious (eg, pneumonia) or recurrent (eg, otitis media) obviously should be given different numbers.

Plan for Each Problem

Each problem as listed in the active problem sheet needs an individual diagnostic, therapeutic, and educational plan. If the plans for all the problems are combined, omissions are likely to occur.

Progress Notes

Progress notes contain newly collected data, an analysis of the data, and a reassessment of the plan. These notes should always pertain to one of the problems on the active problem sheet and be so labeled both by number and by title, eg, as follows:

Seizures, grand mal:
Subjective—Two seizures last week, lasting 1 minute and 5 minutes. Occurred at 7:00 AM and 10:00 AM. No precipitating events apparent. Last seizure 3 months ago. No headaches or vomiting. Not drowsy from medication.
Objective—Neurologic examination and fundi normal. No nystagmus.
Assessment—Seizures still in poor control.
Plan—Continue phenobarbital, 90 mg/d. Recheck blood level. Reviewed reasons for strict compliance.

Gordon IB: Office medical records. *Pediatr Clin North Am* 1981;**28**:565.

4. THE CHRONIC DISEASE FLOW SHEET

There are many variables in the management of a chronic disease. The variables can become lost in the substance of the chart and relatively unavailable for comparison and interpretation. For a patient with a chronic disease or multiple problems, critical data from the progress note should be recorded on a chronic disease flow sheet which tabulates variables so that trends and correlations can be accurately determined. The long axis of the flow sheet has time intervals. Inpatient flow sheets maintained for a critically ill child usually monitor vital signs, intake and output, blood gases, and numerous chemical determinations. Outpatient flow sheets often contain little of the above. Although a specific flow sheet is designed for each chronic disease, the following variables are commonly present in the ambulatory management of most chronic diseases. An example of how to use a flow sheet for a patient with diabetes mellitus is provided at the end of this chapter.

Disease Status

One must monitor the activity level of the disease to know whether therapy is being effective or not. Such activity can be evaluated through the history, physical findings, laboratory data, consultations, and hospitalizations. Variables so determined can be tabulated on the flow sheet.

A. Symptom Data: Frequency of attacks and duration of attacks are the main determinants of the success of asthma therapy. Migraine headaches, seizure episodes, and psychogenic recurrent abdominal pain must also be monitored largely by attack rates.

B. Physical Findings: Childhood nephrosis must be followed by weighing the patient and observing the presence or absence of edema. Splenomegaly is an important variable in leukemia. Motor milestones are important in cerebral palsy.

C. Laboratory Data: Chest films are important for following tuberculosis, liver enzyme levels for chronic active hepatitis, urine cultures for recurrent urinary tract infection, etc.

D. Data for Early Detection of Complications: Some chronic diseases have complications that are not preventable but respond much better to therapy if they are detected early. Warning signs of these complications should be listed on the flow sheet. Examples are (1) head circumference measurements to detect early subdural effusions or hydrocephalus after meningitis and (2) blood pressure measurements to detect early hypertension in chronic renal disease. Once hypertension is discovered, it is no longer an anticipated complication but an indicator of disease activity.

E. Consultations: One of the patient's problems may be managed by another specialist. The primary physician should record on the flow sheet, under the dates of these visits, the consultant's name and a brief note about that specialist's conclusions. The date will permit easy location of the consultation report in the chart when it is needed.

F. Hospitalizations: All hospitalizations should be recorded under the problem they were required for. They usually represent a marker of increased activity of the disease.

G. Emotional Status: Emotional maladjustments are a frequent and often unnecessary side effect of chronic diseases. The physician can prevent them in many instances by reviewing an emotional problem checklist on *every* visit. Some of the more common but unspoken maladjustments are necessary restrictions, overprotectiveness, favoritism, school phobia, underdiscipline, and teasing by peers. This subject is more fully discussed in Chapter 25.

Treatment Regimen

Therapy may or may not be responsible for improvements in clinical status. Examining the temporal relationship of one to the other allows the physician to decide if treatment has been effective. A chronic disease flow sheet should supply this information.

A. Medications: All medications and dosages should be listed with the dates when started, when discontinued, and when the dosage is changed. The dosage may be increased because the patient has outgrown it or because the problem is not under optimal control (eg, increasing the dosage of digoxin in persistent congestive heart failure). New drugs should be added when other drugs have been pushed to tolerance without adequate control (eg, adding metaproterenol to daily theophylline therapy in asthma). Any drug the patient is receiving should have at least one related variable listed under disease status that permits rapid assessment of the efficacy of the drug (eg, bowel movements per day recorded for the patient with ulcerative colitis who is taking sulfasalazine).

B. Toxicity: If drugs with side effects are being used, these problems should be anticipated. The bone marrow, kidney, or liver function tests that need monitoring should be recorded on the flow sheet, as well as the required frequency of testing. If the potential toxicity is high, the drug should also be recorded on the problem list. If suddenly discontinuing the drug could lead to a severe adverse reaction, this risk should be frequently discussed with the patient (eg, anticonvulsants).

C. Nondrug Therapy: Other methods of treatment besides drugs should be recorded on the flow sheet so that their effect on the course of the disease can be estimated. Examples are specific food avoidance in recurrent urticaria or bubble bath avoidance in recurrent urinary tract infection. In static diseases, compensatory devices (eg, braces in cerebral palsy or hearing aids in deafness) should be listed, as well as the recommended interval for routine checks of these devices. Reassurance and other forms of supportive psychotherapy will generally be given on every visit and need not be listed here.

D. Therapy for Prevention of Complications: Many chronic diseases have predictable complications that are preventable if therapy is instituted in advance. If these are listed in the flow sheet, the physician will be certain to remind the parent of them on each visit. Examples are performing daily range-of-motion exercises to prevent contractures in rheumatoid arthritis, requesting penicillin prophylaxis before dental procedures to prevent subacute bacterial endocarditis in congenital heart disease, avoidance of altitudes over 10,000 feet to prevent a crisis in sickle cell disease, and carrying an antihypoglycemic food in the pocket at all times in diabetes mellitus.

E. Compliance With Therapy: The best treatment regimen is useless unless the patient complies with it. A check on the patient's compliance can be performed by inquiring about the degree of satisfaction or dissatisfaction with the medical care received; by asking if the medications have been difficult to take; or in some cases by measuring blood or urine levels (eg, aspirin, penicillin).

F. Disease Education Reviews: Patients may not cooperate with a therapeutic plan until they are intellectually and emotionally committed to it. Unless the family fully understands what they are expected to do, they cannot do it. Unless they understand priorities, they may unknowingly discontinue some critical element in the treatment program when the program as a whole becomes frustrating. Optimal patient education is reached when patient and family know as much about the home treatment of the disease as the physician does and when they can make minor adjustments in treatment independently.

When facts regarding the disease and its treatment are reviewed, one should begin with basic information even though it has been covered many times before. After the first session, the subject is reviewed by asking the patient questions. In the early years, the facts are covered with the patient and both parents present. If the father does not share responsibility for medical care of the child, serious marital problems may develop. In the adolescent years, the review sessions should be done privately with the teenager. The patient's understanding of the problems should be explored approximately every 6 months. In the period immediately following diagnosis, it should be covered on every visit for a few months.

G. School Notification: Each fall the physician should notify the school nurse about any patient whose disease may become manifest or cause a problem of any sort at school. This notification will prevent emotional problems secondary to mishandling of the physical problem by the school. The patient with chronic heart or lung disease may need a gym excuse (no gym) or a modified gym status (eg, no gym on days of wheezing; no rope climbing). Both nurse and teacher need to know how to respond to a seizure or insulin reaction at school. The physician should have this listed on the flow sheet so it is never overlooked. The parents of the patient's closest friends should also have this information, as should the baby-sitters.

Paulson JA: Patient education. *Pediatr Clin North Am* 1981;**28:**627.

Schmitt BD: The chronic disease flow sheet in ambulatory pediatrics. *Pediatrics* 1973;**51:**722.

5. THE MEDICAL IDENTIFICATION CARD

The patient with a chronic disease should carry an identification card that sets forth the active problem list, medications being taken currently, the physician's telephone number, and the parents' telephone numbers at home and at work. If the disease can lead to sudden changes in consciousness (eg, insulin reaction in diabetes mellitus) or if an allergy is present that could be fatal if violated (eg, penicillin hypersensitivity), the patient should obtain a medical identification bracelet or necklace. These can be ordered from Medic Alert Foundation International, Turlock, CA 95380.

6. CHRONIC DISEASE PATIENT REGISTRY

Every effort should be made to keep certain patients from being "lost to follow-up." People with chronic diseases (eg, those with rheumatic heart disease receiving prophylactic penicillin) fall into this group. To prevent the disappearance of any of these patients, the physician should keep them listed in a chronic disease patient registry. Their charts should have a special mark placed on the corner of the cover to show that they are special high-risk patients. These patients should be sent a reminder card 1 week prior to appointments. If the parent cancels an appointment and promises to call back and make another one, the patient's name should be placed on a critical phone call list that automatically goes into effect if the appointment is not remade within 2 weeks. If the patient misses an appointment, the physician should be notified that same day and should call the patient. If the parent has no phone, a letter should be sent. If there is no response to the letter, a visiting nurse referral should be sent. This usually returns the patient to the physician or shows that the family has changed physicians. If the family does not wish further medical care from anyone and the patient's disease is life-threatening but treatable (eg, tuberculosis, chronic pyelonephritis), the physician should report the case to the local child protective services. Since this is an example of medical care neglect, a court order will be issued for treatment of the child. The physician should assume personal responsibility for following any high-risk patient until transfer of care occurs.

7. THE MEDICAL PASSPORT

Every year, 20% of North American families change residences. Some of them have children with chronic diseases. Nothing is more frustrating for a physician than to take a complicated new patient with no past records. Legally, the records belong to the physician; but morally, the records belong to the patient. The patient who moves should carry a copy of the active problem list, chronic disease flow sheet, health maintenance flow sheet, consultation reports, hospital discharge summaries, pertinent x-ray reports, and a covering letter. Original copies should never be sent, because they may be lost. The physician should also give the family the names of 2 or 3 pediatricians they might use in the city they are moving to. These may be personal acquaintances or selections made from the American Academy of Pediatrics *Fellowship Directory*.

CONSULTATIVE VISITS

The physician must know both how to serve as a consultant and how to seek consultation when it is called for. The practicing pediatrician is still the best consultant for most pediatric problems.

OBJECTIVES

The usual purpose of a consultation is the evaluation of an undiagnosed problem followed by therapeutic recommendations. Some referrals are for treatment advice only. A secondary goal of consultation is to provide the referring physician with a continuing medical educational experience.

THE PEDIATRICIAN IN THE ROLE OF CONSULTANT

Referring Source

A. Self-Referral: Although not technically a consultation, some problems require the same kind of intensive approach that is needed when consulting with a colleague. A problem requiring a careful diagnostic evaluation may be detected during a well-child visit or a sick child visit. These "big" problems are often not mentioned by the parent until the end of the visit or may be detected by a screening questionnaire. The physician should arrange to see such patients again. These diagnostic evaluations can keep practice stimulating. If the physician is unsure about the workup of a particular problem, it will be necessary to review the literature ahead of time.

B. Physician Referral: Family practitioners or other specialists occasionally refer patients to a pediatrician for consultation. Within the pediatric community, some pediatricians refer patients to other

physicians who have a subspecialty interest or expertise in a specific disease. This is more common within a group practice.

C. Nonphysician Referral: A physician who is well thought of receives referrals from dentists, school officials, psychologists, social workers, nurses, and other patients. Some of these referred patients will require a consultation type of visit.

Appointments

Consultations usually require 1-hour appointments. In some cases, 2 or more visits may be required to complete the evaluation. The average pediatrician will need to have 2–5 of these 1-hour appointments scheduled each week. The visit will be considerably more productive if a screening questionnaire is completed in advance (eg, using forms such as those presented at the end of this chapter). The questionnaire delineates the patient's physical, intellectual, and emotional problems and serves as an initial data base. The psychosocial portion is different for each of 4 age groups. The physician will then have a tentative problem list at hand when the patient is first seen.

These long appointments are easily arranged when the patient is referred by another professional, because a telephone call or letter usually precedes the patient. However, a patient with almost any problem requiring a careful evaluation can walk into a physician's office at any time. When the mother of a 10-year-old patient who is being seen for acute otitis media mentions that her child has experienced 4 years of encopresis or 6 months of "staring spells" at school, the busy physician may feel under some pressure to make a quick recommendation. The temptation may be strong to do a 5-minute workup and order some laboratory tests, or to hospitalize the patient for evaluation at greater leisure, or even to disregard the complaint or minimize its importance. Needless to say, these responses do not serve the patient's best interests. Long-standing diagnostic dilemmas require a comprehensive assessment that takes at least an hour. Most such evaluations can be done on an ambulatory basis. Shortcuts can lead to tentative conclusions, unconvinced parents, postponement of the indicated workup, "doctor shopping," secondary gain for the patient, and an unresolved problem.

The first visit can serve a useful purpose. One can tell the parents that the child's problem is complicated and demands a complete evaluation. A few screening laboratory tests such as a blood count and erythrocyte sedimentation rate may be ordered. The parent can fill out the screening data questionnaire. A release can be signed for hospital discharge summaries, prior consultation reports, laboratory test results (especially any tests that are dangerous, painful, or expensive), school reports, and growth information. These data will make the consultation visit more meaningful and avoid duplication of effort. In these consultations (unlike hospitalized consultations), an immediate appointment is rarely needed, and the patient can be rescheduled for the following week or later if more time is needed to accumulate data.

Extent of Services

When the patient is referred by the parents or a nonphysician, the request is usually for total care. When the patient is referred by a physician, there are 5 possible degrees of service the consulting physician can offer. If the referring physician does not specify precisely what is needed, the consulting physician may either ask for more specific details about what is wanted or may assume that this cannot be predicted in advance and must await the results of the evaluation.

A. Evaluation Only: The consultant can do a diagnostic evaluation on a patient and tell the parents nothing except that the findings will be discussed with their primary physician. Parents generally do not like this. They are paying for the consultation, and they want to hear something from the expert personally. Common courtesy suggests that they are right.

B. Evaluation and Interpretation: After the evaluation is completed, the consultant usually discusses the diagnosis and the causes of the problem with the family. Recommendations for therapy should be mentioned, if at all, only in very general terms and with the clear understanding that the referring physician will be coordinating the therapy. The patient should then be returned to the referring physician, who will make specific therapeutic recommendations to the family. A specific return appointment date with the referring physician should be given. This is the usual type of referral process for a patient with a chronic disease. The consultant may be called upon periodically to reassess the response to therapy and to offer revised recommendations.

C. Evaluation and Treatment of an Isolated Problem: Sometimes the referring physician wants the consultant to assume responsibility for management of the problem that is the subject of referral. This usually happens with treatable problems that will require only 3–6 visits (eg, recurrent headaches, breath-holding spells, ringworm, Sydenham's chorea). The consultant should clearly define and support the referring physician's role as the continuing provider of health supervision and acute illness care during this interval. When the problem is resolved, the patient should be returned to the referring physician for resumption of care.

D. Total Health Care: Occasionally, a physician refers a patient to a consultant for management of a specific problem plus all future medical care. This may occur when the family is moving to a new area or is unable for financial reasons to maintain the contact with a private physician. In the latter instance, referral should be to a community-based clinic rather than another private physician.

E. Evaluation and Referral for Additional Consultation: The patient's problem may require the expertise of a subspecialist (eg, pediatric hematologist). Before this step is taken, permission must be sought from the original physician for further consultation. The pediatrician's advice about where to seek further expert consultations will usually be heeded.

Communication With the Referring Source

Communication is the key to a satisfactory referral process. The consulting physician is mainly responsible for this aspect of consultation. The referring physician should not have to ask the consultant for the results. The following procedure serves as an appropriate format for completing the process diplomatically.

A. Acknowledge the Referral: As soon as a referral letter is received, the consulting physician should send the referral source a brief note acknowledging the referral. Additional information can also be requested at this time: "Thank you for your recent referral letter on David Jones. I have sent the parents a screening data questionnaire. As soon as it is returned, he will be scheduled for a full evaluation. I will be in contact with you regarding the results. Best regards."

B. Send a Consultation Report: This report should be sent promptly. The content of the final report depends on the referring source. School officials do not want to know medical details; they usually just want to know if the patient is physically healthy or, if not, what their responsibility is. A referring physician expects a full report that will be helpful in treating the patient. Recommendations should therefore be specific (drugs, dosages, other forms of therapy, duration of therapy, specific laboratory tests, the frequency of these tests, etc). A copy of or reference to a recent review article on the subject will also be appreciated.

This evaluation should be typed as a formal consultation report. It should not contain personal comments or resemble a letter. When written in this style, it can serve as an official evaluation report for anyone who might request a copy of it in the future. To make this communication to the referring physician more personal, it should be accompanied by a covering letter: "It was a pleasure to see David Jones today. A complete summary of his evaluation is included. The recommendations may need to be modified in the light of your previous experience with this family. As you know, the marital situation is very stormy. It would be a privilege to see David again if you feel the need arises."

C. Call the Referring Physician Selectively:

Most referring physicians prefer a consultation report to a phone call because the former can become a permanent part of the patient's record. Some cases require a brief telephone report in addition to the written consultation report. These cases include situations where the patient needs to return to the referring physician before a consultation report can be sent, where the patient needs to be referred to an additional specialist, or where a question exists about proper disposition.

D. Arrange a Return Appointment With the Referring Physician: At the end of the consultation, the consultant should tell the parents when the patient should see the primary physician—usually in 1–2 weeks. Positive comments about the referring physician's competence and judgment should be made. The parents must feel confident that the primary physician can provide the necessary follow-up care. If the referring physician had tentatively made the correct diagnosis prior to referral, the consultant's corroboration should be made clear to the parents and recorded in the consultation report.

Fees for Services Rendered

Many pediatricians are reluctant to charge adequately for their time. This seems illogical, since an ambulatory consultation can prevent the high cost of an unnecessary hospital workup. Even if ambulatory insurance does not cover the full cost of such an evaluation, the pediatrician should bill for these evaluations as "office consultations" and charge for the time allotted. An hour is worth the same whether it is spent with one consultation or several well or sick children.

THE PEDIATRICIAN IN THE ROLE OF REFERRING PHYSICIAN

Indications for Referral

There are generally 8 indications for seeking consultation. The last 2 are primarily to help the parents deal with reality.

A. Uncertain Diagnosis: Referral for a diagnostic evaluation is a time-honored indication. The ambulatory consultation is preferable to hospitalization.

B. Treatment Requires Special Expertise: *Examples:* Surgery, cancer chemotherapy.

C. Treatment is Nonmedical: *Examples:* Services of psychiatrists, psychologists, social workers, special teachers, speech therapists.

D. Treatment is Complex: The treatment of some diseases is so complex that the physician unfamiliar with it should refer those patients. *Examples:* Cystic fibrosis, muscular dystrophy, leukemia.

E. Conventional Treatment is not Effective: When the patient is not doing as well as expected, 2

heads are better than one. Even with diseases the physician has successfully treated many times, an atypical problem may arise that requires a fresh opinion (eg, recalcitrant seizures). Phone consultation with the appropriate subspecialist will sometimes solve the problem.

F. Medicolegal Problems: Parents bring in children with injuries for which they are suing a physician or other person. The pediatrician's main task is to decide if the alleged disability or defect is real. If the injury proves to be significant, the physician can help the family find an expert consultant whose testimony will be received in court (eg, an orthopedist in the case of a hand injury). If it seems that the parents are exaggerating the disability for financial gain, the physician should declare the child healthy and recommend return to full activity without confronting the family with such suspicions.

G. Parents Insist on Overtreatment: The pediatrician can help the family avoid uselessly aggressive intervention by recommending consultation with experts known to have conservative views. Even though there are honest differences of opinion about the indications for tonsillectomy, "corrective shoes," hyposensitization, etc, it is often in the patient's best interests not to have to undergo further painful or protracted procedures with little chance of substantial benefit.

H. Parents Are Thinking About a Consultation: When the parents have to ask for a consultation or obtain one without telling the physician, the pediatrician has waited too long. Such an attitude should be suspected when the parents seem angry or critical or uncertain about following advice. The parents' tendency to deny an unfavorable prognosis can be anticipated with certain diseases (eg, fatal diseases and mental retardation). This denial should be respected if it does not interfere with therapy.

A rare or fatal disease is not as such an indication for referral. Some physicians automatically seek "confirmation" of a diagnosis they are already sure of or "approval" of a treatment regimen they are already familiar with. This practice is wasteful of medical resources and may undermine the family's confidence in the doctor.

Method of Referral

A. Obtain Permission from the Family: The family will usually agree to a referral if the reason for it is made clear. Patients sometimes feel that a referral means they are being abandoned by their physician. The referring physician's continuing availability for primary medical care must be made clear. The family should also be told in advance that the consultation will cost more than a regular visit but that it will be worth more.

B. Help the Family Choose a Consultant: The physician should maintain a file listing the best consultants locally and at the nearest medical center.

The parents can be given the names of 2 or 3 competent physicians. If one is outstanding, the pediatrician should not be reluctant to state a preference. If the parents suggest someone they have heard of but who the physician feels is unqualified, the pediatrician should express doubts about that person's degree of expertise in this particular kind of case. It often happens that only one subspecialist is available in the community (eg, oncologist) and that no choice exists.

C. Make an Appointment for the Family: After the family has agreed to the referral, the physician's secretary should arrange an appointment. This increases compliance. If the case is particularly complicated, a long consultation visit should be requested.

D. Send a Referral Letter: A referral letter should be sent immediately so that it will arrive well in advance of the appointment with the consultant. All pertinent information, such as copies of previous evaluations, hospital discharge summaries, and laboratory results, should be included. If time is short, the consultant can be prepared for the visit by phone and pertinent data can be sent along with the patient.

E. Specify the Service Requested: The specific questions to be answered and the future role of the referring physician should be clarified if possible in the referral letter.

Stickler GB: The pediatrician as a consultant. *Am J Dis Child* 1989;**143**:73.
Survey: The pattern of pediatric referrals. *Contemp Pediatr* 1988;**5(12)**:20.

QUALITY CONTROL OF AMBULATORY PEDIATRIC CARE

The concept of peer review or medical audit can be implemented by any group of physicians for purposes of self-education as well as continuing improvement of quality. In a good hospital with an interested staff—especially where house staff are present—quality control is almost a built-in feature. Frequent reassessments of the inpatient's status by the physician, plus constant review by other medical and paramedical personnel, make "peer review" an ongoing process.

Care of ambulatory patients, on the other hand, usually is not reviewed systematically. The following is a suggestion for developing a program that will both improve the quality and cost-effectiveness of ambulatory practice and make it more challenging and satisfying. Physicians can attempt to schedule 1

hour a week for chart review. Several pediatricians should be present to make this a maximal learning experience. In group practice, the participants are already available. The pediatrician in solo practice can meet with the one or 2 pediatricians who share the responsibility for responding to night calls. The group can focus on random charts or on selected charts that cover a specific problem. The latter method requires an office data retrieval system.

CHART REVIEWS

Health Maintenance Chart Review

The delivery of comprehensive health maintenance care can be easily audited by reviewing the health maintenance flow sheet (see Table 7–2). Because the nursing staff is primarily responsible for filling out these flow sheets, this type of review is largely a check on their ability to comply with office protocol and need not be done very often. The office protocols themselves require periodic review and revision.

Acute Illness Chart Review

Acute illness charts can be audited for completeness in diagnosis and therapy of the chief complaint. The following questions can be asked: (1) Was the diagnosis valid? Validity is substantiated if the chart contains adequate historical, physical, or laboratory data to document the diagnosis. (2) Was the therapy optimal? (3) Was the follow-up plan optimal? Charts of patients with a specific acute illness (eg, acute lymphadenitis, streptococcal pharyngitis, or infectious hepatitis) can be pulled and audited to test the group consensus about therapy and follow-up.

Chronic Disease Chart Review

Examination of the chronic disease flow sheet is an easy way to audit chronic disease management. If no such flow sheet exists for the patient, the variables recommended above for monitoring chronic disease can be assessed as one reviews the entire chart. This process could then result in the formation of a chronic disease flow sheet for that patient. Chart review sessions can be more educational if only one chronic disease is considered each time and if an "expert" on that disease is present. The expert can be an actual subspecialist or a member of the group who has reviewed the literature or attended a workshop on this disease.

Diagnostic Problem Chart Review

An easy way to review consultations is to criticize the consultation report. The following questions can be asked: (1) Was the data base adequate? (2) Were all of the active problems identified? (3) Was the diagnostic plan for each problem optimal? (4) Were the final diagnoses valid? (5) Was the recommended

Table 7–2. Health Maintenance Flow Sheet.

Name: _____ Hosp. No.: _____ Date of Birth: _____

Directions: Record date only for all immunizations.
Record value for head circumference, height, weight, BP, and Hct.
Record N (normal) or ABN (abnormal) for all other items.

	NB	2 wk	2 mo	4 mo	6 mo	9 mo	12 mo	15 mo	18 mo	2 yr	3 yr	4 yr	5 yr	6 yr	8 yr	10 yr	12 yr	14 yr	16 yr	18 yr
Today's date																				
Head circumference																				
Height (cm)																				
Weight (kg)																				
BP																				
Dental caries screen																				
DTP (Td after 6 years)																				
OPV																				
Measles, mumps, rubella																				
Haemophilus influenzae type b conjugated vaccine																				
TB test[6]																				
PDQ or DDST = R[7]																				
Speech (ELM)																				
Hearing[1]																				
Vision[2]																				
Biochemical screen[3]																				
Hct																				
Sickle cell test for black patients[4]																				
Pap smear/GC[5]																				

LEGEND:

[1] High-risk inquiry (NB)
Listens to soft sounds (2m)
Turns to sound (6m)
Audiometrics (4y and thereafter)

[2] Red reflex (NB or 2w)
Regards smiling face (2m)
Follows past midline (4m)
Corneal light reflections test (6m)
Visual acuity (3y and thereafter)
Color vision once (6y)

[3] PKU, thyroid, galactosemia (newborn nursery)
PKU retest (2w) if first test done before 48 hours

[4] If not performed in newborn, perform at 2 months of age

[5] Sexually active patients

[6] High risk groups; TB test yearly

[7] Screen with PDQ if high school graduate. Screen with DDST=Revised if parent did not complete high school. If child fails PDQ or DDST=R, perform complete DDST.

therapy for each diagnosis optimal? (6) Was the role of the referring physician clarified and the patient reappointed to him or her? If these consultations are concerned with general pediatric problems, an outside consultant will usually not be required.

Berwick DM: Measuring health care quality. *Pediatr Rev* 1988;**10**:11–16.

Haggerty RJ: Quality assurance: The road to PSRO and beyond. *Pediatrics* 1974;**54**:90.

Starfield B et al: Private pediatric practice: Performance and problems. *Pediatrics* 1973;**52**:344.

MEDICAL CARE COMPLIANCE

Correct diagnoses and optimal therapeutic recommendations can be ensured by the voluntary type of peer review discussed above. An aspect of the quality of care not easy to assess by chart review but which needs to be borne in mind is patient compliance. Superb recommendations do not guarantee anything. Medical care does not become effective until the parent accepts the diagnosis and carries out the therapeutic recommendations. Compliance is improved by providing written instructions, including the parents in treatment planning, simplifying the treatment regimen, linking medication taking with daily routines, explaining the reason for each treatment, and clarifying misconceptions. Strong parent-physician rapport also enhances compliance. The physician must make an effort to find out why appointments are not kept, medications are not given, etc; otherwise, even the best-conceived therapeutic goals will often not be achieved.

Charney E: Patient-doctor communication: Implications for clinicians. *Pediatr Clin North Am* 1972;**19**:263.

Maiman LA et al: Improving pediatricians' compliance-enhancing practices. *Am J Dis Child* 1988;**142**:773.

PRACTICAL TIPS FOR AMBULATORY CARE

FOREIGN BODIES

Metallic Foreign Body in the Soft Tissues

Tape a straight pin with the point over the site where the metallic object entered the skin. Then obtain an x-ray of the area. An exact measurement can then be obtained to locate the foreign body in relation to the straight pin. Located in this manner, the foreign body can be removed with minimal exploration.

Splinters Under the Nails

With a single-edged razor blade or a sharp thin scalpel, gently shave the nail over the distal end of the splinter until the splinter is exposed. The sliver can then be easily pulled out with a pair of fine-pointed tweezers.

Embedded Fishhook

Fishhooks can be removed (eg, from a finger) without wire cutters by bringing them back through their point of entry. For shallow wounds, the skin overlying the metal can be cut and the fishhook lifted out. For deeper wounds, a technique that does not include yanking is preferred. An 18-gauge needle is inserted into the wound through the point of entry. After the needle bevel is locked firmly over the barb, the fishhook and needle can be slowly withdrawn through the original wound as a unit. Local anesthesia helps.

A technique that includes yanking is preferred by fishermen in remote areas. A piece of fishline is looped around the curve of the fishhook. The 2 ends of the fishline are wrapped tightly about the physician's forefinger about 1 foot from where it is looped around the hook. The patient's finger is held against a firm surface to stabilize it. The free shank of the fishhook is pressed against the patient's finger with the physician's free hand until the barb is disengaged and the barb's long axis is parallel to the line of intended expulsion. With the string in this same axis, a quick yank expels the hook immediately.

Friedenberg S: Removing an embedded fishhook. *Hosp Physician* (Aug) 1971;**7**:48.

Longmire WT: Another twist on a fishhook. *Emergency Med* (July) 1971;**3**:98.

Feasting Ticks

Grasp the tick as close to the skin surface as possible with tweezers. Pull straight upward with steady, even pressure. Do not twist or jerk the tick, as this may cause the mouth parts to break off. Wash the site of the bite and the hands thoroughly after removal. While traction is uniformly effective, covering the tick with petroleum jelly, fingernail polish, or rubbing alcohol is uniformly ineffective. Applying a hot match also fails to induce detachment.

Needham GR: Evaluation of five popular methods for tick removal. *Pediatrics* 1985;**75**:997.

The Zipper-Entrapped Foreskin

A young child in a hurry to urinate can inadvertently catch his foreskin in his zipper. A zipper is composed of 2 rows of zipper teeth plus a zipper fastener in the middle. The zipper fastener is composed of an upper and a lower plate. The plates are joined by a U-shaped median bar. This U-shaped bar should be cut with bone cutters or wire cutters. After this is done, the zipper fastener will come apart, and this will usually free the skin. If the skin remains attached to the zipper teeth, these can be separated by grasping them on both sides and using a circular motion, rotating the 2 sides away from each other. Use local anesthesia for initial pain.

Saraf P, Rabinowitz R: Zipper injury of the foreskin. *Am J Dis Child* 1982;**136**:557.

Ring on a Swollen Finger

In most cases, an attempt is made to save the ring. The key to removing the ring is reducing finger edema. At 5-minute intervals, the patient should alternate soaking the hand in ice water and holding it (fingers extended) high in the air. At 30 minutes (after the hand has been elevated for the third time), mineral oil or cooking oil can be applied to the finger. While the hand remains elevated, steady upward pressure can be applied until the ring slides off.

A string technique may work in some resistant cases. Pass a piece of string under the ring and then wind the distal end of the string in close loops tightly from the distal edge of the ring past the knuckle. Exert a slow, firm pull on the proximal end of the string. The edema passes underneath the ring, and the ring is slowly pulled distally as the cord unwinds.

As a last resort, the ring must be cut off. If there is a dentist's office nearby, have the dentist cut it off with a Carborundum disk attached to the drill. The flesh of the finger must be protected by an inserted strip (eg, a tongue blade segment). This method has the disadvantage of destroying the ring and possibly heating the ring enough to burn the finger.

Hair Wrapped Around a Digit

A piece of fine hair wrapped about an infant's digit and left unnoticed can cause severe edema or even amputation. Removal of the hair is usually difficult because it cannot be readily grasped. Application of a liquid hair remover (eg, Nair) will usually dissolve the hair within 15 minutes.

Douglas ED: (Correspondence.) *J Pediatr* 1977;**91**:162.

Gum in the Hair

An easy and nontraumatic way to remove gum from children's hair is by rubbing the gum with peanut butter until the hairs are freed from the gum. This technique is far superior to pulling or cutting the gum out of the hair.

Tar on the Skin

Tar can be removed by applying ice to it or soaking it in ice water for 1 or 2 minutes. The ice causes the tar to become hard and nonsticky, so that it can be easily peeled from the skin. Hydrocarbon solvents merely soften the tar and smear it around, and they are painful if a wound is present.

Fiberglass Spicules or Cactus Spines

The small glass spicules from fiberglass can be removed by applying a layer of wax depilatory (hair remover). Either let it air dry for 5 minutes or accelerate the process with a hair dryer. Then peel it off. White glue can also be tried, but it is less effective. This treatment is also helpful for some plant stickers (eg, cactus, stinging nettle). A corticosteroid cream applied twice daily for 1–2 days may be helpful after the treatment.

LACERATIONS

Wound Cleaning in a Resistant Child

The wound can be covered with gauze saturated with 1% lidocaine for 15 minutes. More recently, TAC (tetracaine, adrenaline, cocaine) liquid when applied topically has been shown to provide complete anesthesia in over 95% of minor lacerations. This will cause only momentary discomfort. The area will then be relatively anesthetized, and vigorous wound cleaning will be tolerated. The subcutaneous injection of additional lidocaine after the wound is cleaned will also be better tolerated.

Bonadio WA, Wagner V: Efficacy of TAC topical anesthetic for repair of pediatric lacerations. *Am J Dis Child* 1988;**142**:203.

Avoiding Unwanted Tattoos

Dirty abrasions of the knee, face, and elbow can result in permanent tattooing if all foreign particulate matter, especially carbon particles, is not meticulously removed. The area should be anesthetized as described above and then scrubbed gently with an antibacterial cleanser and a soft surgical nail brush. Tar can usually be removed by rubbing with petrolatum. Some contaminated pieces of skin may need debridement.

Laceration Closure in a Frightened Child

Wounds can often be closed without local anesthesia or sutures by using microporous adhesive tape (Steri-Strip). The skin adjacent to the laceration is made tacky with tincture of benzoin. The ⅛-inch strips of tape are applied in either a parallel or crisscross pattern. This microporous tape is a decided improvement over "butterfly" tape.

Suture Removal

There is a way to avoid having to dig embedded sutures out of the skin of a struggling child. At the time the laceration is closed, a straight needle threaded with silk can be passed under each suture used for skin closure. The ends of this silk suture can be tied together, leaving a loose loop. At the time of removal, picking up this loose loop will lift the sutures that have been used to close the wound. The scissors can then be easily slid underneath the sutures for snipping. A new, inexpensive sterile stitch cutter makes suture removal easy.

Traumatic Amputations

When a patient loses a significant piece of skin (eg, a fingertip) in an accident, the skin should be placed in cold normal saline solution and sent with the patient to a plastic surgeon. A watchful waiting approach in children less than 10 years of age will usually result in spontaneous regeneration of the distal digit.

Rosenthal LJ, Reiner MA, Bleicher MA: Nonoperative management of distal fingertip amputations in children. *Pediatrics* 1979;**64**:1.

BLUNT TRAUMA

Subungual Hematomas

The painful pressure secondary to a subungual hematoma can easily be relieved by applying a redhot paper clip or other thick wire to the nail surface. The paper clip is held by a clamp. A hole is quickly bored through the nail, and the blood is allowed to escape. This ''hot iron'' approach can be very frightening for a child. If there is a dentist's office nearby, it is preferable to have the dentist bore a hole quickly through the nail with a high-speed drill.

Traumatic Tooth Avulsion

Reimplantation of a tooth is possible only with the permanent teeth. The physician or parent should attempt to replace the avulsed tooth in its socket prior to going to the dentist. If this proves impossible, the tooth should be placed in cold normal saline solution and sent with the patient to the dentist. The deadline for successful replacement is 2 hours.

MISCELLANEOUS PROCEDURES

Genital Labial Adhesions

Labial adhesions can usually be separated by introducing a probe into any opening remaining in the introitus and then separating the adhesions. This method is only acceptable for thin adhesions. An ointment should be applied to the newly separated surfaces for several days to prevent them from resealing. A nontraumatic method for separating thicker labial adhesions is application of estrogen cream (eg, Premarin) twice daily to the medial line for 3 or 4 days.

Hiccup

One teaspoonful of ordinary white granulated sugar swallowed ''dry'' will result in immediate cessation of hiccup in most patients. If the hiccups recur, this method will again be effective. Recalcitrant hiccups may respond to stimulation of the nasopharynx with a rubber catheter.

Inadvertent Subcutaneous Injections

When intramuscular agents are given subcutaneously by mistake, complications can result. The location of the needle point can be rapidly assessed by trying to wiggle it prior to injection. If it is in a muscle mass, the needle point will be relatively fixed. If it is in the subcutaneous fatty tissues, it can be felt to move freely.

Painful Bee Stings or Other Insect Bites

A dash of meat tenderizer (papain powder) and a drop of water massaged into the sting site for 5 minutes will quickly relieve the pain. If these ingredients are not available, an ice cube often helps.

Paraphimosis

In this condition, the foreskin has become retracted and trapped behind the corona. Manual reduction can usually be achieved by placing the tips of the index and middle fingers of one hand behind the swollen foreskin, the thumb of the other hand over the urethral meatus, and applying gradual pressure. The foreskin will usually return to its normal position after this technique has been applied continuously for 4–5 minutes. If this approach fails, a urologist should be consulted for an emergency dorsal slit.

Plastibell Circumcision Ring Paraphimosis

Sometimes the Plastibell circumcision ring slips behind the glans onto the shaft of the penis and cannot be slipped forward. Local swelling can be reduced by applying cold compresses for 10 minutes. The plastic ring can then be cut with a pair of scissors. Mineral oil can be applied to allow the scissors blade to slip easily under the ring. If the operator is worried about cutting the skin, a piece of a small feeding tube can be threaded under the ring and used as a guide for the scissors. This problem can be prevented if parents are told to call their physician if the ring has not fallen off by day 12.

Postcircumcision Skin Tags

Parents occasionally bring their infant in during the first month of life because the foreskin has an irregular skin tag. A clamp can be applied along the desired line of cleavage for 1 minute. After the clamp is removed, an iris scissors can be used to cut along the crushed skin line without causing any significant bleeding.

SELECTED REFERENCES

Ambulatory Pediatrics Association: *Educational Guidelines for Training in General/Ambulatory Pediatrics.* Ambulatory Pediatrics Association, 1984.

American Academy of Pediatrics: *Guidelines for Health Supervision II.* American Academy of Pediatrics, 1988.

American Academy of Pediatrics: *Management of Pediatric Practice.* American Academy of Pediatrics, 1986.

Charney E: Well-Child Care. Ross Roundtable, 17th Report, Ross Laboratories, 1986.

Gordon IB, Paulson JA: Issues for the practicing pediatrician. *Pediatr Clin North Am* 1981;**28:**535. [Entire issue.]

Green M, Haggerty RJ (editors): *Ambulatory Pediatrics.* Vols 1, 2, and 3. Saunders, 1968, 1977, and 1984.

Hoekelman RA et al (editors): *Primary Pediatric Care.* Mosby, 1986.

Table 7-3. Pediatric Health Maintenance Charts.

PEDIATRIC HEALTH MAINTENANCE

Birth through 3 months

Patient's concerns

Newborn data base
Birth weight _____ Gestational age _____
Pregnancy or delivery problems _____ Neonatal problems _____

Growth (comment on growth curve)

Feeding advice
Formula _____ oz/24 hours
Breast feeding: Frequency _____ min/feeding
Vitamins _____ Iron
Solids _____ Fluoride drops
Feeding problems
Advice: Introduce bottle in breast fed (2w) □ Introduce fluids other than milk (2m) □

Developmental status
Stimulation advice: Hold baby (2w) □ Talk to baby (2w) □

Child rearing advice
Sleep pattern
Crying or colic
Mother-child interaction
Sibling rivalry (2w)
Advice: Paternal involvement, family planning (2w) □ Utilize sitter (2m) □

Family status

Accident prevention advice
Car seats, crib safety (2w) □ Rolling over (2m) □ Smoke detector □

Medical Advice
Demonstrate use of bulb syringe for nose (2w) □ Foreskin or circumcision care ♂ (2w) □
Temperature taking, Tylenol and fever handout (2m) □ Discuss when to call doctor (2m) □

Intercurrent illness

PEDIATRIC HEALTH MAINTENANCE

4 months through 14 months

Parent's concerns

Growth (comment on growth curve)

Feeding advice
Formula _____ oz/24 hours
Breast feeding: Frequency _____ min/feeding
Vitamins _____ Iron
Solids _____ Fluoride drops
Feeding problems
Advice: No bottles in bed; introduce solids, spoon, cup (4m) □
Confirm intake of iron-rich solids (6m) □ Introduce finger foods, confirm on 3 meals/day (9m) □
Entirely on table foods. Phase out bottle by 18m (12m) □

Developmental status
Stimulation advice: Toys for reaching (4m) □ Avoid confining baby equipment (6m) □
Repeat baby's sounds (9m) □ Name objects and pictures for baby (12m) □

Child rearing advice
Sleep pattern _____
Behavior problems _____
Advice: Sleeps through the night (4m) □ Normal separation anxiety (6m) □
Discipline: Use negative voice and eye contact rather than physical punishment (9m) □
Don't punish for normal exploratory behavior, discuss positive strokes for good behavior (12m) □

Family status

Accident prevention advice
Safe toys (4m) □ Stairs and gates, drowning in bathtub (9m) □
Electrical cords (6m) □ Ipecac and poison talk (12m) □

Medical advice
Teething myths (6m) □ Avoid expensive shoes (9m) □ Use of 911 (12m) □

Intercurrent illness

Table 7-3 (cont'd.). Pediatric Health Maintenance Charts.

PEDIATRIC HEALTH MAINTENANCE

4 years through 5 years

To be completed by parent

School readiness:		Check correct answer
1. Does your child pay attention when being read to?	Yes	No
2. Can your child play quietly alone for over ½ hour?	Yes	No
3. Does your child mind adults and follow instructions?	Yes	No
4. Does your child speak clearly enough for others to understand?	Yes	No
5. Does your child object to being with a sitter?	No	Yes
6. Can your child dress without help?	Yes	No
7. Does your child ever wet or soil him/herself during the day?	No	Yes

To be completed by physician or nurse

Parent's concerns

Growth (comment on growth curve)

Diet

School readiness
Problems detected by above questions _____ Weak category _____
Development: PDQ (4, 5) Score _____
DDST (if fails PDQ) Result _____
Articulation: DASE (4) Score _____ Percentile _____
Advice: Preschool if any problems (4) □

Accident prevention advice
Adult seat belts, petting dogs (4) □ Crossing street, trampoline (5) □

Dental advice
No daytime thumb-sucking (4) □ No nighttime thumb-sucking (5) □
Frequency of brushing _____ Type of toothpaste _____ Fluoride intake _____

Intercurrent illness

PEDIATRIC HEALTH MAINTENANCE

15 months through 3 years

Parent's concerns

Growth (comment on growth curve)

Diet
Milk _____ oz/24 hours
Eating problems _____
Advice: Entirely on table foods, off all bottles (18m) □
Normal decreased intake, iron intake (2y) □

Developmental status
Advice: Read to child (1½, 2) □ Listen to child (2) □ TV rules (3) □

Child rearing advice
Sleep problems _____
Behavior problems _____
Frequency of spanking _____
Advice: Don't punish for normal negativism, ignore temper tantrums (1½) □
Discuss toilet training and readiness (1½, 2, 3) □ Discuss positive "strokes" for good behavior (2) □
Emphasize consistency in discipline and use of time-out room (2, 3) □

Family status

Accident prevention advice
Scalds, aspiration foods (1½) □ Street/garage safety (2) □
Drowning in ditch and pools (3) □

Dental advice
Brushing frequency _____ Fluoride intake _____
Advice: Avoid snacks that cause cavities (1½) □ Benefits of fluoride toothpaste (2) □
Brushing techniques (3) □

Intercurrent illness

Table 7-3 (cont'd.). Pediatric Health Maintenance Charts.

PEDIATRIC HEALTH MAINTENANCE

6 years through 11 years

Parent's concerns

Diet

School
Name of school _____ Grade _____
Academic performance
Attendance
Behavior
Advice: Child's responsibility for schoolwork (6) □ Adult at home before and after school (6, 10) □

Behavior
Behavior problems
Chores
Friends
Advice: TV less than 2 h/d (6) □ Understanding of death (6) □
One sport or club (8, 10) □ Smoking (10) □

Family status

Sex education
Discuss puberty and menarche before junior high school (10) □
Menstrual status (10 ♀)

Accident prevention advice
Bicycle safety (6) □ Swimming lessons (8) □
Fires, matches (10) □

Dental advice
Frequency of brushing _____ Type of toothpaste _____ Fluoride intake _____
Dental referral (6) □

Intercurrent illness

PEDIATRIC HEALTH MAINTENANCE

12 years through 18 years

Parent's concerns

Adolescent's concerns

Growth (comment on growth curve)

Diet

School
Name of school _____ Grade _____
Academic performance
Attendance
Behavior
Career plans

Behavior
Free time/friends
Chores/job
Person to confide in
Predominant mood
Advice: Discuss values of babysitting (12) □ Discuss drugs and alcohol (12, 16) □
Discuss smoking (14) □

Family status
Advice: Discuss independence and parent's trust (16) □

Sex Education
Dating, masturbation (14) □ Marriage (18) □
Sexual activity, preventing pregnancy, venereal disease (14, 16, 18)

Accident prevention advice
Firearms (12) □ Cycling safety (14) □ Driving safety, water safety (16) □
Motorcycles, seat belts (18) □

Dental advice
Frequency of brushing _____ Type of toothpaste _____

Medical advice
Acne □ Personal hygiene (14) □ Teach self-examination of breasts (16♀) □

Intercurrent illness

Emergencies & Accidents

8

Roger M. Barkin, MD, MPH, & John D. Burrington, MD

CARDIOPULMONARY ARREST

Cardiopulmonary arrests in children are primarily respiratory in origin, resulting from obstruction or hypoxia. The precipitating causes are often preventable or identifiable prior to the arrest.

Resuscitation should be initiated when peripheral pulses are not palpable or severe bradycardia exists. Irreversible central nervous system damage occurs within 4 minutes if circulation is not restored.

Principles of Management

A. Verification of Unconsciousness: Establish unresponsiveness or respiratory difficulty. Gently shake the patient to determine consciousness. If resuscitation is required, position the patient for basic life support without subjecting the patient to further injury. Call for help.

B. Airway: Airway management must reflect the nature of precipitating causes of respiratory difficulty and the potential for cervical spine injury.

1. Clear the upper airway by one of the following methods:

a. Lift the occiput slightly off the bed or flat surface by placing a towel roll or hand under the occiput.

b. With one hand under the neck and the other on the forehead, lift the neck slightly and tip the head backward with gentle pressure on the forehead (head tilt and neck lift method; Fig 8–1A).

c. Extension of the neck can also be maintained by applying pressure on the forehead while using the tips of the fingers of the hand that had been under the neck to lift the bony part of the jaw (chin) forward (head tilt and chin lift method).

2. Maintain patency of the airway. Adjuncts to management include the following:

a. Suction and clear debris as necessary. Remove loose teeth.

b. An oropharyngeal or nasopharyngeal airway may be useful in maintaining patency. The oropharyngeal airway (Fig 8–2) is poorly tolerated by the conscious patient.

c. Endotracheal intubation provides a stable airway and is indicated if there is continued obstruction or if assisted ventilation will be required on a prolonged basis. The choice of oral or nasal route depends on the expertise of the clinician. The size of the tube to be used may be estimated by selecting a tube that approximates the size of the patient's little finger. The following guidelines for tube size may also be useful: newborns, 1.5–3.5 mm; 1 month, 3.5 mm; 1 year, 4 mm; 2–3 years, 4.5 mm; 4–5 years, 5–6 mm; 6–8 years, 6–6.5 mm; 10–12 years, 7 mm; and 14 years, 7.5–8.5 mm. Uncuffed tubes are used for children under 7–8 years of age.

d. Cricothyroidotomy is indicated in children over 3 years in very rare circumstances where acute airway obstruction cannot be otherwise relieved.

C. Breathing: Check for spontaneous breathing by observing movement of the chest and abdomen or by feeling air movement at the mouth.

1. If the patient is not breathing, begin ventilation by mouth-to-mouth resuscitation, covering both the nose and mouth in infants or pinching the nostrils closed in children (Fig 8–1).

2. Initially, give 4 quick breaths to check for airway patency.

3. Continue ventilating at a cardiac compression to ventilation ratio of 5:1 in infants and children.

4. Subsequently—or initially, if equipment is available—use a self-inflating resuscitation bag (Fig 8–3). Effective positive pressure ventilation can be achieved by applying the mask firmly over the nose and mouth and squeezing the bag, which expands spontaneously when released. Oxygen should be administered by attaching the tubing to the air intake valve at the end of the bag.

D. Circulation: Assess circulation by checking brachial, femoral, or carotid pulses. If there is no pulse, begin external chest compression. Pulses and

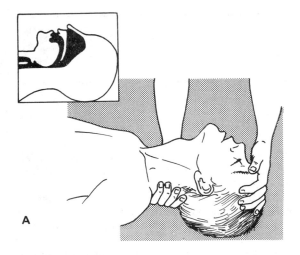

A

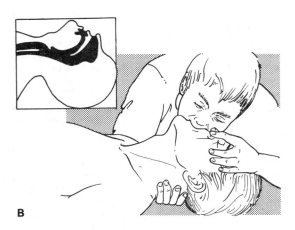

B

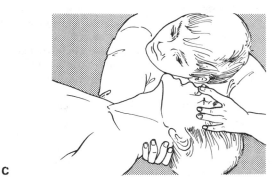

C

Figure 8–1. Proper performance of mouth-to-mouth resuscitation. **A:** Open airway by positioning neck anteriorly in extension. Inserts show airway obstructed when the neck is in resting flexed position and opening when neck is extended. **B:** Rescuer should close victim's nose with fingers, seal mouth around victim's mouth, and deliver breath by vigorous expiration. **C:** Victim is allowed to exhale passively by unsealing mouth and nose. Rescuer should listen and feel for expiratory air flow.

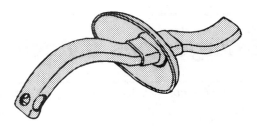

Figure 8–2. Airway for use in mouth-to-mouth insufflation. The larger airway is for adults. The guard is flexible and may be inverted from the position shown for use with infants and children.

blood pressure should be monitored during compression.

1. For children under 1 year of age, draw an imaginary horizontal line between the nipples and compress the sternum one finger-breadth below this line. Deliver 100 compressions per minute with a 5:1 ratio of compressions to ventilations.

2. For children over 1 year of age, use the heel of the hand to compress the lower third of the sternum (Fig 8–4), displacing the sternum 1–1½ inches in children 1–8 years of age and 1½–2 inches in older children. Deliver 60–80 compressions per minute with a 5:1 ratio of compressions to ventilations.

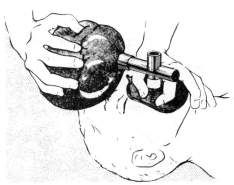

(1) Lift the victim's neck with one hand.
(2) Tilt head backward into maximum neck extension. Remove secretions and debris from mouth and throat, and pull the tongue and mandible forward as required to clear the airway.
(3) Hold the mask snugly over the nose and mouth, holding the chin forward and the neck in extension as shown in diagram.
(4) Squeeze the bag, noting inflation of the lungs by the rise of the chest wall.
(5) Release the bag, which will expand spontaneously. The patient will exhale, and the chest will fall.
(6) Repeat steps 4 and 5 approximately 12–20 times per minute depending on the patient's age.

Figure 8–3. Self-inflating resuscitation bag.

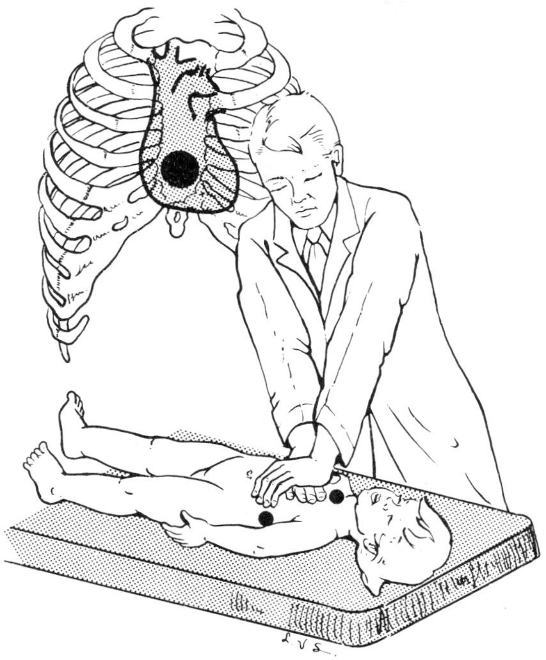

Figure 8–4. Technique of closed chest cardiac massage. (Heavy circle in heart drawing shows area of application of force. Circles on supine figure show points of application of paddles for defribillation.)

E. Intravenous Access and Fluids: Intravenous cannulation must be achieved rapidly. The size and type of catheter depend on the expertise of the clinician and the availability of sites. If venous access is difficult, an intraosseous needle can be inserted for immediate venous access while more permanent routes using central lines or venous cutdown are achieved. Initial fluid management should reflect the cause of cardiopulmonary arrest. If there is any question of hypovolemia, give a rapid infusion of normal saline solution or lactated Ringer's injection, 20 mL/kg over 20–30 minutes. If there is no response and the patient remains in shock following restoration of volume, rhythm, and ventilation, consider administering vasopressor agents (see below).

F. Medications: All patients should receive oxygen, and those who do not respond to relief of airway obstruction should receive one or more of the following:

1. Sodium bicarbonate—Give 1 meq/kg intravenously, while monitoring arterial blood gases and assuring adequate ventilation. Acidosis should be corrected, because it has a negative effect on cardiac function and efficacy of adrenergic drugs. Following cardiac arrest, the reduction of $Paco_2$ levels by adequate ventilation may partially reduce acidosis. Hyperventilation of the patient will further improve the pH.

2. Sympathomimetic drugs—These drugs stim-

ulate the α- and β-adrenergic receptors; their effects vary depending upon the relative balance of stimulation achieved. The primary effect of α-adrenergic drugs is vasoconstriction; of β_1-adrenergic drugs, tachycardia and increased myocardial contraction; and of β_2-adrenergic drugs, vasodilatation and bronchodilatation. The following drugs are commonly used:

a. Epinephrine—Give epinephrine (1:10,000 solution), 0.1 mL/kg intravenously or intratracheally every 5–10 minutes as needed. Epinephrine stimulates both α- and β-adrenergic receptors and increases heart rate, force of myocardial contraction, and vascular resistance. It is utilized in cases of ventricular standstill or fine ventricular fibrillation to convert the latter to coarse fibrillation.

b. Dopamine—Give 5–20 μg/kg/min intravenously by continuous drip. Dopamine stimulates α- and β-adrenergic receptors as well as specific dopaminergic receptors that maintain renal and mesenteric blood vessel dilatation at low doses (< 20 μ/kg/min). At higher doses, α-adrenergic effects become prominent. The drug is particularly useful for treatment of carciogenic shock as well as for maintenance of renal perfusion. It is not indicated for treatment of hypovolemic shock.

c. Isoproterenol—Initially, give 0.1 μg/kg/min intravenously by continuous drip, and increase slowly in increments up to 1.5 μg/kg/min as required. Isoproterenol is a pure β-receptor agonist. It increases heart rate and myocardial contraction and produces vasodilation. The blood pressure is usually maintained by greater cardiac output. It is particularly useful in cases of bradycardia unresponsive to atropine.

3. Atropine—Give 0.01–0.03 mg/kg (minimum, 0.1 mg per dose; maximum, 0.5 mg per dose) intravenously or intratracheally every 5 minutes as needed. Atropine has vagolytic action, causing increased sinoatrial node discharges and increased atrioventricular node conduction, and is useful in cases of symptomatic severe bradycardia as well as in cases of organophosphate overdose.

4. Calcium chloride—Give a 10% solution of calcium chloride, 20–30 mg/kg (0.02–0.03 mL/kg; maximum, 500 mg per dose) intravenously every 10 minutes as needed. Administer the drug slowly and monitor the patient. Calcium chloride is rarely used at present because of its lack of efficacy. Give with caution in patients receiving digitalis. Do not mix with sodium bicarbonate.

5. Antiarrhythmic drugs—These are rarely needed in children, since the incidence of dysrhythmia is relatively low.

a. Lidocaine—Give a loading dose of 1 mg/kg intravenously, followed by 20–50 μg/kg/min by intravenous infusion. Lidocaine is indicated for ventricular dysrhythmia and for cardiac arrest secondary to ventricular fibrillation.

b. Bretylium—Give a loading dose of 5 mg/kg intravenously, followed by 10 mg/kg intravenously every 10 minutes as needed (maximum, 30 mg/kg total dose). Bretylium is used if the patient with dysrhythmia fails to respond to lidocaine.

G. Defibrillation: Defibrillation, employing a shock of 1–2 J/kg as needed, is indicated primarily for ventricular fibrillation. One electrode is placed in the second intercostal space of the right sternal border, and a second electrode is placed in the fourth intercostal space of the left midaxillary line (Fig 8–4). Adequate electrode paste should be applied, and personnel should be warned not to touch the patient or the bed at the time of defibrillation. If a single shock is ineffective, a second shock in rapid succession may be successful. Defibrillation is used for ventricular fibrillation, whereas synchronized cardioversion is appropriate for ventricular tachyarrhythmias.

Chameides L (editor): *Textbook of Pediatric Advanced Life Support.* American Heart Association, 1988.

Kanter RK et al: Pediatric emergency intravenous access. *Am J Dis Child* 1986;**140:**132.

Mayer TA: Emergency pediatric vascular access: Old solutions to an old problem. *Am J Emerg Med* 1986;**4:**98.

SHOCK

Shock occurs when there is acute circulatory dysfunction associated with inadequate tissue perfusion to meet metabolic requirements. Compensatory mechanisms initially sustain cellular function, but with progression of shock, cellular metabolic changes result in further tissue injury and cell death.

Clinical Findings

Compensated shock, the early stage of shock, is marked by maintenance of normal vital signs through intrinsic mechanisms. The effectiveness of these mechanisms depends on the preexisting cardiac and pulmonary status and on the volume and rate of blood loss. Orthostatic changes are the most sensitive indicators of volume status, and acidosis may be the earliest sign of impaired tissue perfusion.

Uncompensated shock follows compensated shock and is characterized by cardiovascular dysfunction and impairment of microvascular perfusion. Hypotension, tachycardia, and decreased cardiac output commonly progress to cardiovascular collapse.

Newborns in shock appear lethargic, with pale, mottled, and slightly gray skin. Late shock is manifested by a decrease in skin temperature, particularly of the extremities.

Classification

Three major types of shock may occur, each requiring a different management approach:

Hypovolemic shock is due to a reduction in circulating blood volume and represents the most common underlying process.

Cardiogenic shock is secondary to depressed cardiac output from myocardial insufficiency or obstruction of venous return or cardiac outflow.

Vasogenic (distributive) shock is due to abnormal distribution of blood secondary to vasomotor paralysis and increased venous capacitance. Typically, vasogenic shock is anaphylactic, septic, or neurogenic in origin.

General Principles of Management

(1) Establish a stable airway; administer oxygen by mask, hood, or cannula; and ensure ventilation.

(2) Give a fluid push of normal saline solution or lactated Ringer's injection, 20 mL/kg, unless the patient is hypervolemic, as determined by clinical examination or central venous pressure measurement. This fluid bolus may be repeated once if hypervolemia is not present.

(3) Establish a central venous pressure monitor if the patient does not respond to the initial fluid push.

(4) Insert a urinary catheter to monitor output.

(5) Measure electrolytes and pH and obtain a complete blood count. Correct fluid and electrolyte imbalance as outlined in Chapter 36.

(6) Insert a nasogastric tube.

Treatment of Specific Types of Shock

A. Hypovolemic Shock:

1. Administer normal saline solution or lactated Ringer's injection intravenously at a rate of 20 mL/kg over 20–30 minutes. If there is no response, repeat the infusion while continuing to monitor urine output, blood pressure, pulse, and perfusion rates.

2. If there is no response after 2 infusions, measure central venous pressure and consider other causes of shock, such as pericardial tamponade or tension pneumothorax.

3. If hemorrhage is the cause of hypovolemia, give type-specific or cross-matched blood following the initial crystalloid infusion. Whole blood is useful for massive acute bleeding; packed red blood cells may be used if there has been extensive infusion of crystalloid solution in the relatively stable patient or if bleeding is chronic.

4. Following massive blood transfusions, give fresh frozen plasma and platelets if indicated. Monitor coagulation.

5. Colloid is not indicated in severe capillary leak syndromes such as burns, sepsis, or terminal shock. It may be useful in hypovolemia accompanied by renal, cardiac, or respiratory failure.

6. After the patient's condition is stable, replace fluid losses and deficits as discussed in Chapter 36. Replacements must reflect the type and degree of dehydration.

7. Crystalloid solution is the initial fluid of choice in burn therapy, as discussed below.

8. Vasopressor agents are not indicated in the treatment of hypovolemic shock. Fluids are the treatment of choice.

B. Cardiogenic Shock:

1. A fluid push may improve cardiac output by increasing filling pressure, particularly if the central venous pressure is 15 cm of water or below. Give normal saline solution or lactated Ringer's injection carefully (because of salt load) at a rate of 5 mL/kg over 30 minutes, and monitor the response.

2. Sodium bicarbonate, 1 meq/kg intravenously, is often indicated either empirically or by acid-base measurements.

3. An ECG and chest x-ray film are mandatory. Echocardiography is also a useful tool in assessing function as well as excluding cardiac tamponade.

4. Dysrhythmia requires emergency treatment. Predisposing factors, including electrolyte abnormalities, acidosis, alkalosis, drugs, fever, pericardial disease, ischemia, and hypoxia, should be excluded.

5. Inotropic agents are usually indicated, optimally following evaluation of preload and ejection time by echocardiography or central venous pressure measurement. If peripheral perfusion is poor and quantitative measurements are not possible, consider giving a crystalloid fluid push to test the response prior to initiating pharmacologic therapy with dopamine, 5–20 μg/kg/min intravenously by continuous drip.

6. Vasodilators are indicated if there is peripheral hypoperfusion and the patient is hypervolemic or if there is outflow obstruction secondary to arteriolar vasoconstriction. Give nitroprusside, 0.5–10 μg/kg/min intravenously by continuous drip, and monitor the blood pressure closely because of the drug's potent vasodilator effect. Nitroprusside is sensitive to light.

7. Pericardiocentesis may be used to exclude pericardial tamponade. Thoracentesis may be used to treat tension pneumothorax.

8. Measurement of central venous pressure or pulmonary artery wedge pressure (by Swan-Ganz catheter) is usually necessary to monitor fluids and efficacy of pharmacologic therapy.

C. Vasogenic (Distributive) Shock:

1. Septic shock—The patient with septic shock presents with fever, toxicity, and concurrent shock. There is often a history of infection preceding shock. Complete blood count, platelet count, and blood cultures should be obtained.

a. Crystalloid solution should be infused to maintain an adequate central venous pressure but is rarely adequate as the only therapy.

b. Inotropic agents are usually required. Dopamine, 5–20 μg/kg/min intravenously by continuous drip, should be given.

c. Corticosteroids may be initiated, although their effects may be detrimental and are not routinely employed. Either hydrocortisone sodium succinate or methylprednisolone sodium succinate may be used. The dosage of hydrocortisone (Solu-Cortef) is 50 mg/kg intravenously; that of methylprednisolone (Solu-Medrol) is 30–50 mg/kg intravenously.

d. Antibiotics should be initiated after appropriate cultures are obtained. The choice may be determined by a specific clinical presentation (eg, meningcoccemia), or broad-spectrum antibiotics may be given initially as follows; ampicillin, 200–300 mg/kg/24 h every 4 hours intravenously plus chloramphenicol, 100 mg/kg/24 h every 6 hours intravenously or a third-generation cephalosporin, eg, cefotaxime (150 mg/kg/24h every 6–8 hours intravenously) or ceftriaxone (75–200 mg/kg/24 h every 12 hours intravenously).

e. Coagulopathies should be treated appropriately.

2. Anaphylactic shock—Anaphylactic shock is an extreme reaction to allergy or hypersensitivity. Anaphylaxis represents a wide spectrum of reactions, ranging from only mild distress to true respiratory insufficiency and cardiovascular collapse. Upper airway laryngospasm and lower airway bronchospasm may be present in association with urticaria.

a. Initial attention must be focused on the airway. Oxygen is always required, and intubation is rarely necessary.

b. In the presence of shock, epinephrine (1:10,000 solution), 0.1 mL/kg, should be administered intravenously.

c. Diphenhydramine (Benadryl), 2 mg/kg parenterally, is given initially, followed by a parenteral dose of 5 mg/kg/24 h every 6 hours.

d. Corticosteroids should be given, although the benefits are delayed. Either hydrocortisone sodium succinate (Solu-Cortef), 4–5 mg/kg, or methylprednisolone sodium succinate (Solu-Medrol), 1–2 mg/kg, may be given intravenously every 6 hours.

e. Hypotension is treated with fluids and dopamine.

f. If possible, a tourniquet should be applied proximal to the site of injection.

3. Neurogenic shock—Neurogenic shock is usually due to interruption of normal neuronal control, resulting in impaired vascular tone. There is usually a history of exposure to anesthetic agents; spinal cord injuries; or ingestion of barbiturates, narcotics, or tranquilizers.

a. Fluids should be administered to maintain a central venous pressure of 5–8 cm of water.

b. Vasopressors are usually required. Many prefer norepinephrine (Levophed), 0.1–1 μg/kg/min intravenously by continuous drip, because of its prominent vasoconstrictive action.

D. Refractory Shock: Shock unresponsive to normal therapy is unusual in children but requires a rapid evaluation of potential complicating conditions, including multiple organ failure, outflow or filling obstruction (eg, tension pneumothorax or pericardial tamponade), coagulopathy, sepsis, respiratory failure, and exsanguinating blood loss.

EVALUATION & STABILIZATION OF THE TRAUMATIZED CHILD

The traumatized patient requires expert medical care combined with reassurance and a special sensitivity to the emotional support needed by the child and family. Establishment of appropriate treatment priorities is crucial to the management of such patients.

An aggressive and deliberate approach must be the basis for caring for the patient and should be individualized to reflect the extent of injury. Victims of major accidents should be considered to be seriously injured until their condition is proved stable. Treatment must often be initiated on the basis of clinical findings and cannot be delayed until diagnostic confirmation is obtained. The assessment and management must be individualized, but the multiply traumatized patient will benefit from the following approach.

Primary Assessment

Primary assessment must focus on the airway, ventilation, adequacy of circulation and perfusion, and management of cervical spine injury or exsanguinating hemorrhage.

A. Airway: Assure patency of the airway by clearing debris (especially chewing gum) and positioning the head to minimize any obstruction. In all patients with head trauma or multiple injuries, specific attention must be directed toward stabilizing the cervical spine to avoid further injury.

B. Ventilation: Ventilation must be assessed to determine its adequacy and ensure that breath sounds are symmetric, with consideration given to the presence of pneumothorax, hemothorax, flail chest, or pulmonary contusion. Evaluate for evidence of respiratory distress, cyanosis, tracheal deviation, and bony crepitus.

C. Cervical Spine Injuries: Cervical spine injuries should be considered in all multiply traumatized patients as well as those with head injuries or impaired sensorium. If there is any question of injury, the head should be immobilized with sandbags and secured in position until a series of x-ray films of the cervical spine can be completed. A cross-table lateral neck film will detect 80–90% of injuries.

D. Circulation: Circulation may be rapidly assessed by determining adequacy of perfusion and by measuring blood pressure. Up to 25% of blood volume may be lost before hypotension is detected in patients in the supine position. Orthostatic changes occur early. In the absence of external trauma, the major body cavities that require evaluation are the chest, abdomen, and retroperitoneum.

Major blood loss may occur secondary to orthopedic injuries.

Head trauma does not cause shock unless there is massive bleeding with spreading of sutures in the infant or avulsion of the scalp. Other causes of post-traumatic shock to consider are cardiac contusion or rupture, lacerations, vascular injury, and underlying disease; these causes should be detectable on physical examination.

Initial Resuscitation

Initial management must focus on eliminating life-threatening conditions and ensuring that a number of technical activities are completed as appropriate.

(1) Oxygen should be administered to all patients. If there is any question of airway patency, the patient should be intubated. Nasotracheal intubation is preferred if cervical spine injury is suspected and no facial injuries are present. If there is no evidence of spinal injury or if the cross-table lateral x-ray film shows negative results, oral intubation may be attempted. Cricothyroidotomy is rarely indicated.

(2) Active intervention may be necessary to control ventilation following stabilization of the airway. If there is evidence of pneumothorax or hemothorax, a chest tube should be inserted, often on the basis of clinical examination in the unstable patient.

(3) External hemorrhage must be controlled, usually by direct pressure. Be careful of pressure over the neck or eyes, because pressure may cause an increase in vagal tone.

(4) An intravenous line must be placed; the number and size of lines should reflect the severity of the injury. If shock is present, a bolus of normal saline solution or lactated Ringer's injection (20 mL/kg) should be given intravenously as rapidly as possible. Subsequent administration of crystalloid solution and blood must reflect the response to this initial infusion. In general, once a total of 40–50 mL of crystalloid solution per kilogram has been given, blood is required if hypovolemic shock is still present. Type- and cross-matched blood should be given if possible.

(5) If significant shock is present, pediatric pneumatic antishock trousers should be inflated after the

lower extremities, back, and abdomen have been examined for injury. Once inflated, pneumatic trousers should not be removed until some stability has been achieved. At that time, the compartments of the trousers should be deflated one at a time, starting with the abdomen, and vital signs and acid-base status should be carefully monitored.

(6) If blood is present at the urethral meatus, immediate urologic consultation is necessary, and radiologic examination is required. Urinary catheters should usually be inserted after ensuring that there is no blood at the urethral meatus. Dipstick tests should be done; if they are positive, a microscopic examination should follow.

(7) A nasogastric tube should be inserted after the cervical spine is proved stable. Aspirate should be obtained and tested for blood.

(8) Cardiac monitoring should be initiated and an ECG done.

(9) Immediately after intravenous catheters are placed, blood should be drawn for hematocrit, complete blood count, typing and cross-matching, and arterial blood gas measurements. Electrolyte, glucose, and blood urea nitrogen determinations and urine and serum toxicology screens should be ordered if appropriate.

(10) A complete series of cervical spine films as well as chest and pelvic films should be obtained. X-ray films of the abdomen and extremities may be obtained, if indicated, after the patient's condition is stable. Portable radiographic equipment is useful in the unstable patient.

(11) All of the patient's clothing should be removed so that no injury is overlooked. A complete examination is necessary; do not stop the examination when one major injury has been detected.

(12) The initial history must be sufficient to determine the nature of the injury, with particular attention to measures of severity (eg, in the case of an accident, the extent of damage to the automobile and its speed) as well as the time elapsed since the accident. Past medical problems, allergies, use of medications, and other relevant medical data should be ascertained rapidly.

(13) Once the priority areas have been evaluated and treatment initiated, the patient should be reassessed. If no further immediate therapy is required, a more complete secondary examination can be initiated and a detailed history obtained.

Secondary Assessment & Treatment

The secondary assessment must include a systematic examination and initiation of appropriate therapeutic procedures.

A. Head and Nerve Injuries: A rapid but complete neurologic examination should be performed (see Chapter 24). The following should be assessed:

1. Level of consciousness.

2. Movement of the body—Determine symmetry, position, and posturing.

3. Pupils—Dilated, fixed pupils are a reliable sign of the site of the lesion unless drug ingestion has occurred. For example, ipsilateral dilatation of the pupil with contralateral hemiparesis indicates cerebral mass lesions.

4. Extraocular movement—A hemispheric lesion causes the eyes to deviate toward the lesion, but a brain stem lesion causes the eyes to deviate away from the lesion.

5. Reflexes.

6. Tympanic membrane and nose—Determine if hematotympanum or otorrhea is present.

7. Rectal examination—Determine muscle tone. Absence of rectal tone in a comatose patient may be the only evidence of spinal cord injury.

8. Head and scalp.

Frequent serial examinations of neurologic function are indicated to determine progression of deficits.

Diagnostic procedures include cervical spine x-ray films, as discussed above. The cross-table lateral spine x-ray film is an excellent screening mechanism that detects 80–90% of injuries. It is indicated in any patient with decreased sensorium, neck trauma, or tenderness of the neck following trauma, as well as in patients with major trauma and an unknown or unreliable medical history.

Skull x-ray films are indicated in patients with an abnormal sensorium following trauma if there has been a significant loss of consciousness, a neurologic defect, or increasing or persistent headache; in patients with head trauma, especially trauma due to a depressing force, such as a blow from a shoe or hammer; and in cases in which CT scans are necessary and a delay in obtaining their results is anticipated.

CT scanning is the definitive test and should be done following trauma if there is a localized neurologic defect, deteriorating neurologic status, evidence of skull depression on x-ray or clinical examination, or any evidence of increased intracranial pressure.

B. Face and Mouth Injuries: The patient should be assessed for lacerations, fractures, malocclusion, and loose teeth.

Most linear lacerations or punctures of the buccal mucosa, tonsillar pillars, or posterior pharynx in children result from falling with a lollipop stick, pencil, ruler, or other object in the mouth. These injuries usually require no therapy beyond antibiotics. They heal as well without sutures as they do with them. The specific indications for examination and possible suturing under anesthesia are (1) deep puncture of the soft palate, (2) the presence of a flap of mucoperiosteum lifted off the hard palate, and (3) crepitus of the neck, indicating deep puncture.

Tongue lacerations usually result from penetration

by the incisors. These, too, will heal without sutures in most cases. Lacerations through the edge of the tongue, producing a triangular flap, are best sutured with an absorbable suture.

Traumatic injuries to the teeth are treated according to how great the displacement or mobility is and whether primary or secondary teeth are involved. In general, displacement or evulsion of a permanent tooth requires emergency care after the patient's condition is stable. The tooth should be reinserted and held in place until a dentist can see the patient. Injuries to primary teeth also should be seen but are less urgent.

C. Neck Injuries: The patient should be assessed for tracheal deviation, vein distention, ecchymosis, and evidence of penetrating injuries. Injuries may be indicative of chest disorders or cervical spine damage. Lesions that penetrate the platysma usually require surgical exploration.

D. Chest Injuries: The chest should be reexamined more thoroughly, and response to initial measures for stabilization should be evaluated. Chest x-ray films and determination of arterial blood gases may be indicated if the patient is stable and findings on examination remain equivocal.

1. Rib fracture—Pleuritic pain (sharp pain exacerbated with breathing), localized severe pain with pressure at the fracture site, crepitus with respiration, pain with compression of the sternum or lateral chest, or pleural friction rub may be present. Patients should be examined for hemothorax or pneumothorax. Rib fractures are unusual in younger children and indicate a severe traumatic injury. Fractures of ribs 1 and 2 may be associated with a vascular injury. Fractures of ribs 10–12 often accompany abdominal injuries.

2. Flail chest—If 3 or more adjacent ribs are fractured at 2 points, the chest may move paradoxically with respiration—ie, the chest moves inward with inspiration and outward with expiration. Flail chest is characterized by pain, dyspnea, and respiratory distress. The respiratory distress is primarily due to the underlying pulmonary injury. Stabilization of the flail chest is necessary, often by mechanical means. Intubation may be required if respiratory distress is present or there are massive injuries with accompanying pathologic disorders. Positive pressure ventilation will stabilize the chest.

3. Pulmonary contusion—Contusion results when there is lung parenchymal damage. Chest trauma causes hemorrhage over the contused area of lung, often with a rapid deceleration injury. Respiratory distress develops with significant hypoxia, usually within 4–6 hours of the injury. Increased pulmonary shunting leads to a progressive rise in $Paco_2$ and fall in Pao_2 levels. Chest films demonstrate alveolar infiltrates progressing on occasion to consolidation. The findings may be delayed.

Patients with pulmonary contusion require oxygen by mask and pulmonary support. Intubation and ventilation may be necessary, with accompanying use of positive end-expiratory pressure.

4. Pneumothorax—Pneumothorax is classically characterized by dyspnea, cyanosis, and absence of breath and voice sounds on the involved side. In cases of tension pneumothorax, pulsus paradoxus is seen.

a. Spontaneous pneumothorax—In older children, there is usually rupture of a bleb, with leakage of air into the pleural cavity; the source of the leak usually heals spontaneously. Spontaneous pneumothorax is characterized by the sudden onset of dyspnea, pleuritic pain, hyperresonance, and absent breath and voice sounds over the involved lobe. Symptoms and signs do not progress. The condition may complicate an asthmatic attack or cystic fibrosis.

b. Tension pneumothorax—Failure of the lung leak to seal may produce a one-way valve effect leading to an increase of air in the pleural space with each breath. This results in mediastinal shift, rapidly progressive dyspnea and cyanosis, and typical physical findings. Tension pneumothorax may result from trauma, such as a penetrating or blunt injury, or may accompany spontaneous pneumothorax. This is a life-threatening condition and requires immediate decompression by needle or chest tube (usually preceding chest radiography).

c. Open pneumothorax—Open pneumothorax is characterized by the presence of an open wound and severe respiratory distress with cyanosis and audible sucking sounds. The opening should be closed at once and covered with an occlusive dressing (eg, petrolatum gauze). A chest tube is required.

5. Hemothorax—Signs of pleural fluid include absent fremitus, loss of resonance, absent breath and voice sounds, and tracheal shift, together with evidence of hemorrhage into the chest. Hemothorax is often associated with pneumothorax. Use of a chest tube is definitive therapy and should follow chest radiography if the patient is stable.

6. Penetrating wounds of the chest.

a. Closed wounds—A minute point of entry may be associated with extensive intrathoracic damage. The patient should be assessed for pneumothorax, hemothorax, subcutaneous or mediastinal emphysema, cardiac contusion, or cardiac tamponade and treated appropriately on the basis of findings.

b. Open wounds—Open wounds inevitably produce critical pneumothorax (see above).

E. Cardiac Injuries: Patients should be examined for evidence of anterior chest wall trauma, which may be the only evidence of cardiac contusion. If present, tachycardia is consistent with cardiac contusion or evidence of ischemia. Fullness of the jugular vein should be ascertained and the point of maximal impulse determined.

1. Cardiac contusion—Cardiac contusion results from blunt trauma to the anterior mid chest. Chest pain may be present initially or may be delayed. Findings on ECG demonstrate tachycardia or nonspecific ST–T wave changes. Dysrhythmia may be present.

2. Pericardial tamponade— Tamponade results from penetrating wounds of the chest and accumulation of blood in the pericardial sac, progressing to limitation of diastolic filling of the heart and subsequent narrowing of pulse pressure, increased pulse rate, paradoxic pulse, engorged neck veins with high central venous pressure, and hypotension. Pericardiocentesis is the treatment of choice (see Chapter 35).

F. Abdominal Injuries: In children, abdominal injuries are primarily blunt in origin. The ability to obtain an accurate history is often compromised by the clinical condition of the patient, the age of the child, the presence of intracranial injuries, or drug or alcohol use. Tenderness is usually present in patients with abdominal disorders and alert mental status. It may be localized or diffuse. Bowel sounds may be absent, and distention may develop. After consultation and with the advice and assistance of a surgical consultant, peritoneal lavage should be performed if indicated. A modified open technique is usually preferred. Helpful x-ray studies that may be done, depending on the stability of the patient, include plain films, contrast studies, a liver-spleen scan, and a CT scan.

1. Nonpenetrating abdominal injuries— Injuries accompanied by significant hypotension and cardiovascular collapse usually require immediate laparotomy. Stable patients with equivocal examination results may be observed or undergo peritoneal lavage, depending on the condition of the child and the facilities and expertise available to care for the patient.

a. Splenic rupture—Manifestations are due to hemorrhage and shock. Splenic rupture is characterized by a history of injury followed immediately or with some delay (subcapsular hemorrhage) by left upper quadrant and shoulder pain, rebound tenderness, muscle rigidity, signs of bleeding, a mass in the left upper quadrant, and shock. Spontaneous rupture may occur with leukemia, infectious mononucleosis, or malaria.

b. Liver rupture—Manifestations are due to hemorrhage, shock, and possibly bile peritonitis. Liver rupture is characterized by a history of injury followed immediately or after a few hours by right upper quadrant pain, tenderness, and signs of hemorrhage. Shock and rapid exsanguination may occur.

c. Pancreatic and duodenal injuries—Because pancreatic and duodenal injuries are retroperitoneal, signs and symptoms are often obscure and delayed. Pancreatic injuries may be associated with diffuse midepigastric, abdominal, or back pain. Amylase levels may be elevated. Pancreatic pseudocysts may

develop. Intramural duodenal hematomas cause proximal intestinal obstruction.

d. Intestinal rupture—Manifestations are due to localized peritonitis, anemia, or gangrene of the bowel following injury or mesenteric tear and impairment of blood supply. Upright x-ray films show free air under the diaphragm and ileus and free fluid in the abdomen. Amylase levels may be elevated.

e. Kidney rupture—Manifestations are due to perirenal bleeding and urinary extravasation or intrarenal bleeding. Kidney rupture is characterized by a history of bleeding or injury followed by flank pain, hematuria, local costovertebral angle tenderness, swelling, muscle spasms, a palpable mass, nonshifting flank dullness, shock, and ecchymoses. An intravenous urogram is important for confirmation and determination of the extent of injury. Hematuria may not be present with renal vascular thrombosis, renal pedicle injury, or complete transection of the ureter.

f. Bladder rupture—Bladder rupture occurs from blunt trauma. Whether it is intraperitoneal or extraperitoneal determines the nature of the signs and symptoms. The trauma usually occurs when the patient has a full bladder. Patients develop persistent pain, suprapubic tenderness, ileus, and inability to void. Signs of free fluid in the peritoneal cavity may be present, and a boggy suprapubic mass may be felt if the diagnosis is delayed. Radiologic examination is the most dependable test for bladder injury and should include a pelvic x-ray film to rule out concurrent fractures.

g. Urethral rupture—Manifestations depend on the segment of the urethra involved. Urine or blood extravasates around the bladder, prostate, or perineum or in the anterior perineal wall. An abdominal or perineal injury followed by pain, blood at the urethral meatus, difficulty in voiding, and signs of extravasation requires immediate evaluation. Urologic consultation should be obtained immediately (before a urinary catheter is inserted).

2. Penetrating abdominal injuries—Penetrating injuries must be explored locally and the patient examined thoroughly. Minute wounds may mask extensive internal damage. If there is any evidence of intraperitoneal penetration on local wound exploration, peritoneal lavage should be performed if the patient is stable and laparotomy if the patient is deteriorating.

G. Perineal Injuries: Perineal injuries most often result from falls on a bicycle (impact of the bicycle seat), falls in the bath tub, or sexual assault.

Injuries to the labia often cause bruising, edema, and urinary retention. Have the child attempt to urinate while sitting in a tub of warm water. Catheterization is rarely necessary.

Vaginal injuries in the young child require examination under sedation or anesthesia.

Penile, scrotal, and testicular injuries reflect the

nature of the insult. A urologist should usually be consulted. Superficial lacerations may be closed with absorbable sutures. Deeper wounds require operative exploration.

H. Orthopedic Injuries: See Chapter 23.

Committee on Trauma, American College of Surgeons: *Advanced Trauma Life Support Course.* American College of Surgeons, 1981.

German JC: Multiple-system injured children. *Top Emerg Med* 1984;**6**:46.

Gratz JR: Accidental injury in childhood: A literature review on pediatric trauma. *J Trauma* 1979;**19**:551.

Jorden RJ: Evaluation and stabilization of multiply traumatized patients. In: *Emergency Pediatrics,* 3rd ed. Barkin RM, Rosen P (editors). Mosby, 1989.

ENVIRONMENTAL INJURIES*

BURNS

Initial assessment and management of the patient with a burn are the most important determinants of morbidity and ultimate survival.

Initial Assessment

Initial evaluation must include information about the nature of the injury and the patient's age, weight, and underlying medical problems. Special attention must be paid to the presence and extent of associated injuries, eg, evidence of significant smoke inhalation associated with hoarseness, cough, singed nasal hairs, oral burns, carbonaceous sputum, wheezing, rhonchi, and cyanosis. Burns should be classified according to their depth and extent.

A. Classification by Depth of Burn:

1. First-degree burns—Superficial partial-thickness (first-degree) burns involve the epidermis only. The skin area is pink or red, blanches with pressure, and is painful to touch. Causes include sunburn, scalds, and distant flash fires.

2. Second-degree burns—Partial-thickness (second-degree) burns involve the epidermis and corium. The skin is red, blistered, or moist with exudate and is painful to pinprick or touch. Causes include scalds and flash fires.

3. Third-degree burns—Full-thickness (third-degree) burns involve the entire dermis and sometimes fat, muscle, or bone. The skin is white, dry or charred, and painless. Causes include scalds from steam, open flame burns, and contact with chemicals or electric current.

B. Classification by Extent of Burn: The body surface area affected in infants and children can be

---

*Drowning is discussed in Chapter 9.

estimated using the percentages depicted in Fig 8–5. In adults, the "rule of nines" is easy to remember: head and neck (9%), anterior trunk (18%), posterior trunk (18%), each leg (18%), each arm (9%), and anorectal area (1%).

1. Major burns—Burns are classified as major if any of the following are present: (a) partial-thickness burns involving more than 25% of the body surface area in adults or more than 20% in children; (b) full-thickness burns involving more than 10% of the

Infant Less Than One Year of Age

Name _____ Age _____ Ward _____

1st-degree erythema not to be included   2nd-degree   3rd-degree

Variations From Adult Distribution in Infants and Children (in Percent).

	New-born	1 Year	5 Years	10 Years
Head	19	17	13	11
Both thighs	11	13	16	17
Both lower legs	10	10	11	12
Neck	2			
Anterior trunk	13			
Posterior trunk	13			
Both upper arms	8	These percentages		
Both lower arms	6	remain constant at		
Both hands	5	all ages.		
Both buttocks	5			
Both feet	7			
Genitalia	1			
	100			

Figure 8–5. Lund and Browder modification of Berkow's scale for estimating extent of burns. (The table under the illustration is after Berkow.)

body surface area; (c) burns involving the hands, face, eyes, ears, feet, or perineum; (d) inhalation injuries, electrical burns, or burns complicated by fractures or other major trauma; and (e) burns in poor-risk patients.

2. Moderate uncomplicated burns—Moderate burns include (a) partial-thickness burns involving 15–25% of the body surface area in adults or 10–25% in children; and (b) full-thickness burns involving less than 10% of the body surface area.

3. Minor burns—Minor burns include (a) partial-thickness burns involving less than 15% of the body surface area in adults or less than 10% in children; and (b) full-thickness burns involving less than 2% of the body surface area.

Initial Management
A. Minor Burns and Rare Moderate Burns:

1. Initially, place a cool cloth on the burned area. Burns should be debrided where appropriate. Intact blisters should be left unbroken unless they are present in flexion creases. Partial-thickness burns should be treated with 1% silver sulfadiazine cream (Silvadene) if they involve more than 5% of the body surface area. Smaller burns may be similarly treated, or a fine-mesh gauze impregnated with water-soluble cream or antibiotic cream may be applied. Very small burns may be left exposed.

2. Have the patient return in 24 hours for a dressing change and then every 2–3 days unless the affected areas become malodorous, painful, hot, or red.

B. Major Burns and Most Moderate Burns:

1. Assess the airway and ventilation, and administer oxygen to all patients. Pulmonary complications may be delayed up to 24 hours.

2. Immediately begin fluid replacement with lactated Ringer's injection containing 5% dextrose, given intravenously by 1 or 2 large-bore catheters. The amount is calculated as follows: 4 mL of fluid × the patient's weight (in kilograms) × the percentage of body surface area involved. This is given over a 24-hour period, with half infused over the first 8 hours. Maintenance requirements are given in addition to the amount calculated. No potassium should be added to the fluid.

3. Monitor urine output and specific gravity; the latter is one of the most sensitive indicators of adequacy of fluid therapy.

4. Insert a nasogastric tube.

5. Monitor electrolyte, hematocrit, and arterial blood gas levels.

6. Treat the wounds as follows:

a. Using sterile technique (gown, gloves, cap, and mask), remove burned clothes and examine the patient. Gently scrub the wound with povidone-iodine (Betadine) soap diluted in saline or water. All dead material should be debrided. Intact blisters

should not be touched unless they are present in flexion creases.

b. Obtain surgical consultation immediately.

c. Apply 1% silver sulfadiazine cream liberally to wounds, and cover them with a bulky dressing consisting of several layers of absorbent material held in place with a gauze wrapping. Burns on the face and perineum are usually left open after application of the cream.

d. Consider skin grafting after early (1–4 days) wound excision.

7. Give penicillin if there is evidence of group A streptococcal infection.

8. Give a tetanus toxoid booster if the child is immunized, or give tetanus immunoglobulin if the child is unimmunized.

9. Give antacid therapy.

10. Pain medication may be used once vital signs have stabilized.

11. Emotional support of the family should be initiated early. Child abuse must be considered.

Barkin RM: Burns. In: *Emergency Pediatrics,* 3rd ed. Barkin RM, Rosen P (editors). Mosby, 1989.
Demling RH: Burns. *N Engl J Med* 1988;**313:**1389.
Dimick HR: Triage of burn patients. *Top Emerg Med* 1981;**3:**17.
Moncrief JA: Burns. 1. Assessment. 2. Initial management. *JAMA* 1979;**242:**72, 179.

ANIMAL BITES

Animal bites are common in children, dog bites being the most frequently encountered. *Pasteurella multocida* is the most common pathogen, and *Staphylococcus aureus* is often a secondary invader. Rabies is an unusual pathogen but must be considered in any case of animal bite (see Chapter 27). Rodents (rats, mice, gerbils, hamsters, squirrels, etc) rarely carry rabies.

Treatment

Irrigation and debridement of the wound are of paramount importance. Local or regional anesthesia may be required. Irrigation should be done extensively with 1% povidone-iodine (Betadine) solution. All devitalized tissue should be excised to give clear, square edges.

Suturing is indicated for cosmetic or functional reasons and should be done only after thorough irrigation and debridement. Hand injuries and puncture wounds should never be sutured. The wound should be left open if there is any question about the extent of the wound and the adequacy of irrigation or if follow-up difficulties are anticipated.

The risk of infection in patients with animal bites is very high, particularly if wounds are on the hands or feet or if wounds have been sutured. Antibiotics (penicillin or a cephalosporin) should be given in these specific cases.

If indicated, tetanus toxoid should be administered (see Chapter 28) and rabies prophylaxis initiated (see Chapter 27).

Marcy SM: Infections due to dog and cat bites. *Pediatr Infect Dis* 1982;**1**:351.

HUMAN BITES

Human bites usually cause more tissue damage and carry a higher risk of infection than do bites inflicted by other animals. The most common injury results from a clenched fist striking an opponent's teeth.

Treatment

Irrigation and debridement are of primary importance, as in other bites. The wound should never be sutured but should be soaked and debrided regularly during the healing phase. Antibiotic (cephalosporin) therapy should be initiated, and tetanus immunization should be given if needed. Close follow-up is essential.

HYPERTHERMIA

Exposure to environmental heat without appropriate preparation and protective equipment may lead to one of several preventable illnesses, including heat cramps, exhaustion, and stroke.

Heat Cramps

Heat cramps are caused by prolonged or excessive exercise in an environment with high temperatures and low humidity. The patient sweats profusely and may try to relieve thirst by drinking fluids that do not contain salt. The condition is characterized by severe cramps in skeletal muscles that were subjected to intense work, most commonly those of the legs. Patients are alert and oriented, with normal or slightly elevated temperatures.

If cramps are mild, an oral salt solution (1 tsp of salt in 500 mL of water) can be given. If they are severe, normal saline solution (20 mL/kg) may be given intravenously over 1–2 hours.

Heat Exhaustion

Heat exhaustion results from exposure to high temperatures and continued sweating in the absence of appropriate replenishment of water and salt. The condition is liable to occur in children with unusual salt losses, eg, those with cystic fibrosis or salt-losing renal disease. It may occur in healthy active children who replace sweat losses with inappropriate fluids.

With water depletion, patients develop hypernatremic dehydration and are thirsty, irritable, fatigued, and disoriented. Salt depletion is more common and presents with fatigue, headache, nausea, vomiting, diarrhea, and muscle cramps. Temperatures are normal with either water or salt depletion.

Treatment must correspond to the underlying cause. The patient should be removed from heat and sun, and the extracellular fluid volume should be restored, usually after normal saline solution, 20 mL/kg, is given intravenously over 45 minutes.

Heat Stroke

Although rare, heat stroke results from the inability of the body to dissipate heat. Factors associated with heat stroke include underlying diseases (eg, cystic fibrosis), large body surface areas (eg, in the newborn), and ingestion of drugs (eg, phenothiazines, anticholinergic agents, beta-blockers, and ethanol). Although strenuous activity may produce heat stroke, the condition may occur without excess exertion.

Patients present with headache, dizziness, fatigue, confusion, or disorientation, which may progress to coma. The skin is red, hot, and dry, and temperatures over 40 °C (104 °F) are common.

Multiple complications may occur, including coma, acute tubular necrosis, acidosis, dysrhythmia, hepatic damage, and disseminated intravascular coagulation.

Treatment must be initiated immediately, because heat stroke is life-threatening. After the patient is removed from the heat source, the airway should be stabilized, clothing removed, and the patient immersed in cool water. Use of cold compresses may be necessary. The patient should be placed in an ice bath until the temperature reaches 38.5 °C (about 101 °F), and extremities should be massaged. Fluids should be given intravenously to maintain the fluid and electrolyte balance after normal saline solution, 20 mL/kg intravenously, is administered initially over 45–60 minutes. Patients with heat stroke require meticulous medical support and intensive monitoring of vital signs, input and output, and urine specific gravity.

HYPOTHERMIA

Hypothermia is characterized by an internal (core) temperature of 35 °C (95 °F) or less. In children, it usually results from prolonged exposure to the cold. Special rectal thermometers are needed for reading of low temperatures.

Clinical Findings

Patients must be carefully examined for underlying medical problems and trauma associated with or preceding the exposure. The severity of clinical findings reflects the degree and duration of hypothermia and the nature of the exposure. There may be progressive deterioration in mental status, with eventual loss of consciousness, dysrhythmia, coma, and cardiopulmonary arrest. Infants with hypothermia have decreased appetite; lethargy; and cold, erythematous, and scleremic (hardened) skin. Bradycardia and abdominal distention may be observed. Metabolic acidosis, hypoglycemia, and hyperkalemia are usually present.

Frostbite may develop in patients with hypothermia. The severity depends on the following factors: (1) the intensity of exposure to cold (a function of temperature and wind velocity) as well as increased rates of heat loss from the tissues owing to contact with water or metal and restrictive or tight clothing proximal to the involved areas; (2) the duration of exposure to cold; and (3) the rate of rewarming. Frostbite injury is characterized by loss of sensation of affected parts and white, cold skin over affected areas.

Classification of Cold Injury

A. First-Degree Injury: Erythema of the skin and edema of the affected part but without blister formation. No significant tissue damage.

B. Second-Degree Injury: Formation of blisters and bullae.

C. Third-Degree Injury: Necrosis of the thick layers and subcutaneous tissues without loss of the affected part.

D. Fourth-Degree Injury: Complete necrosis with gangrene and loss of the affected part.

Complications

Complications include necrosis of the affected area and bacterial infection through broken skin. Late sequelae involving frostbitten areas and lasting months to years have included persistent pain, hyperhidrosis, skin tenderness, cold sensitivity, and retarded epiphyseal growth.

Treatment

A. Superficial and Deep Frostbite:

1. Loosen any garments that restrict blood flow.
2. Remove any wet garments in contact with the skin.
3. Cover the involved area with dry, bulky garments.
4. Elevate the affected area.
5. Protect the part from trauma. Do not rub frostbitten tissue or pack with snow, because this macerates the area and causes further damage.
6. Transport the patient to a warm environment, and rewarm the frostbitten area by immersion in a large volume of water preheated to 38–41 °C (about 100–105 °F) for about 20 minutes. Do not rewarm if there is any chance of refreezing during transport. Rewarming with an oven, fire, or other source of dry heat should *not* be attempted, since unequal exposure will result in tissue burns. Analgesics may be required during the rewarming period.

7. Place the patient at bed rest with the part elevated.
8. Avoid all surgical procedures on cold-injured skin. Do not remove or puncture bullae or blisters.

B. Hypothermia:

1. Initial stabilization must focus on the priorities of airway, breathing, and circulation. The patient should be moved to a warm environment. Treat the underlying disease.
2. Patients with temperatures above 32 °C (89.6 °F) should be rewarmed with external passive measures, such as application of blankets. If there is no increase in temperature, the patient should be evaluated for underlying disease.
3. Temperatures below 32 °C require active rewarming at about 0.5 °C/h.

a. If the cardiovascular system is stable, active external rewarming by means of warmed blankets and water bottles is appropriate.

b. If the cardiovascular system is unstable, spinal injury exists, or diabetic ketoacidosis is present, initiate active external rewarming combined with the use of humidified heated (40.5 °C [104.9 °F]) oxygen, warmed intravenous fluids, and, last, hemodialysis. (Hemodialysis is controversial.) Dysrhythmias should be aggressively treated.

Reuler JB: Hypothermia: Pathophysiology, clinical setting and management. *Ann Intern Med* 1978;**89**:519.
Stine, RJ: Heat illness. *JACEP* 1979;**8**:154.
Zell SC, Kurtz KJ: Severe exposure hypothermia: A resuscitation protocol. *Ann Emerg Med* 1985;**14**:339.

ELECTRIC SHOCK & ELECTRIC BURNS

The danger of injury from electric shock depends on the voltage and the frequency. Alternating current is more dangerous than direct current. At a frequency of 25–300 cycles, voltages below 230 volts can produce ventricular fibrillation. High voltages (which may be encountered in television circuits) produce respiratory failure. Faulty wiring of home appliances may lead to electric shock. In homes with young children, it is advisable to install occlusive safety outlets in the play area.

Electric Shock

Consciousness is rapidly lost. If the current continues, death from asphyxia due to ventricular fibrillation or respiratory arrest occurs within a few minutes.

Interrupt the power source or knock the wire away from the skin with a dry piece of wood or other nonconducting material, and institute external cardiac massage or mouth-to-mouth respiration, depending on whether asphyxia is cardiac or respiratory. Supply oxygen if available, and institute appropriate treatment for shock.

Electric Burns

Momentary contact, particularly with a high-voltage outlet, will lead to localized, sharply demarcated, painless gray areas without associated inflammation of the skin. The examiner should search for a second area of grayness where the current has left the body. Sloughing occurs after a few weeks. With simple burns, the skin should be cleansed and a dry dressing applied. Deeper burns should be treated with 1% silver sulfadiazine cream (Silvadene) under an occlusive dressing. Management is the same as for other types of burns. Infection occurs less often with electric burns, but reconstructive surgery for scarring after healing may be required.

Toddlers and young children often sustain electric burns of the mouth by biting an electric cord. They are rarely electrocuted, because the circuit is completed locally in the mouth. There is a local slough of tissue that may lead to brisk bleeding. The defect should be allowed to heal by scarring and the corner of the mouth revised later. Hospitalization is usually indicated.

Baker MD, Chiarello C: Household electrical injuries in children. *Am J Dis Child* 1989;**143:**59.

Orgel MG, Brown HC, Woolhouse FM: Electrical burns of the mouth in children: A method for assessing results. *J Trauma* 1975;**18:**285.

SELECTED REFERENCES

Barkin RM: *The Emergently Ill Child.* Aspen Publications, 1987.

Barkin RM, Rosen P (editors): *Emergency Pediatrics* 3rd ed. Mosby, 1989.

Mills J et al (editors): *Current Emergency Diagnosis & Treatment,* 3rd ed. Lange, 1990.

Rosen P et al: *Emergency Medicine: Concepts and Clinical Practice,* 2nd ed. Mosby, 1988.

Critical Care

9

Malcolm Packer, MD, and Kurt R. Stenmark, MD

Role of the Pediatric Intensivist

Since the 1960s increasing attention has been focused on the special needs of critically ill or injured children. This has led to development of the highly sophisticated pediatric intensive care unit (PICU), where all severely ill children other than newborns are cared for. PICUs are and should remain relatively scarce, because the needs for tertiary pediatric critical care beds within a given region are relatively small and the costs are extremely high. Once PICUs became established, the need for specialists to conduct research and provide medical care for these children was recognized. This void has been filled by the pediatric intensivist or critical care pediatrician.

All aspects of care of critically ill children are in the domain of the pediatric intensivist. This care may include serving as a consultant for prehospital care, arranging transport of the child, and then remaining primarily responsible for care provided during the child's stay in the PICU. Intensive care should be delivered in a team-oriented approach. Critical care nurses, medical and surgical subspecialists, respiratory therapists, social workers, and the pediatric intensivists need open communication and close coordination to provide the best care for the child and family.

This chapter is the first on pediatric critical care in the Lange Series. It contains basic overviews of several of the diseases intensivists commonly encounter and the management approaches currently in vogue.

Frankel LR: The evaluation, stabilization and transport of the critically ill child. In: *The Critically Ill Child: Diagnosis and Medical Management.* Dickerman JD, Lucey JR (editors). Saunders, 1985.

Glass WL, Pollack MA, Ruttiman UE. Pediatric intensive care: Who, why and how much. *Crit Care Med* 1986; **14**:222.

Pollack MM: Improving the outcome and efficiency of intensive care: The impact of an intensivist. *Crit Care Med* 1988;**16**:11.

Rogers MC: Introduction: Development of pediatric intensive care. In: *Textbook of Pediatric Intensive Care.* Rogers MC (editor). Williams and Wilkins, 1987.

ACUTE RESPIRATORY FAILURE

Respiratory failure is common in infants and children and accounts for approximately 50% of all deaths of children under 1 year of age. Infants are at higher risk for respiratory failure because of physiologic, anatomic, and mechanical differences between their respiratory systems and those of adults. In infants the thoracic cage is soft and therefore provides an unstable base for the ribs. Intercostal muscles are poorly developed, and therefore children cannot achieve the classic bucket handle motion that characterizes adult breathing. Further, the diaphragm is less effective in infants because it is relatively flat and short and has fewer type I muscle fibers. During REM sleep, the ventilatory movements of the rib cage become uncoordinated and out of phase with those of the diaphragm. The infant's trachea is small, only one-third the diameter of the adult trachea. Therefore, according to Poiseuille's law, a 1-mm thickening of the respiratory mucosa in an infant causes a 75% reduction in cross-sectional area in the infant airway, compared to only a 20% reduction in the adult airway. Last, children's alveoli are smaller and have fewer or no pores of Kohn.

Respiratory failure exists when the lungs are unable to exchange sufficient amounts of oxygen and carbon dioxide. Children with respiratory failure generally fall into 2 groups: patients with type I respiratory failure generally have a low Pao_2 with a normal-to-low $Paco_2$; type II patients have a low Pao_2 with a high $Paco_2$. Type I is the failure of the lung to oxygenate the blood and occurs in 3 situations. (1) The most frequent cause is a **ventilation perfusion defect** (V/Q mismatch), which occurs when blood flows to parts of the lung that are poorly ventilated or underventilated, ie, blood flow and alveolar ventilation are mismatched. (2) **Diffusion defects** result from disturbances such as a thickened alveolar membrane or a buildup of interstitial fluid at the alveolar-capillary junction. (3) **Intrapulmonary shunt** occurs when blood flows through areas of the lung that are never ventilated. Type II respiratory failure, characterized by a high $Paco_2$ and a low Pao_2, is generally the result of alveolar hypoventilation and not of a primary disease of the lung. Numerous disease processes can contribute to this hypoventilation (Table 9–1). It is important to remember that hypoxemia is not always related to respiratory failure. Right-to-left cardiac shunts, high altitude with its low ambient oxygen concentration, and the production of methemoglobin all may produce severe hypoxemia with normal respiratory function.

Table 9–1. Types of respiratory failure

Findings	Causes	Examples
Type I Hypoxia Decreased Pao_2 nl $Paco_2$	Ventilation perfusion defect	Positional (supine in bed), ARDS atelectasis, pneumonia, pulmonary embolus, bronchopulmonary dysplasia
	Diffusion impairment	Pulmonary edema, ARDS, interstitial pneumonia
	Shunt	Pulmonary arteriovenous malformation, congenital adenomatoid malformation
Type II Hypoxia Hypercarbia Decreased Pao_2 Increased $Paco_2$	Hypoventilation	Neuromuscular disease (polio, Guillain-Barré), head trauma, sedation, chest wall dysfunction (burns), severe reactive airways

Table 9–2. Clinical criteria for respiratory failure.

Respiratory
  Wheezing
  Expiratory grunting
  Decreased or absent breath sounds
  Flaring of alae nasi
  Retractions of chest wall
  Tachypnea, bradypnea, or apnea
  Cyanosis
Cerebral
  Restlessness
  Irritability
  Headache
  Mental confusion
  Convulsions
  Coma
Cardiac
  Bradycardia or excessive tachycardia
  Hypotension or hypertension
General
  Fatigue
  Sweating

Clinical Findings

A. Symptoms and Signs: The clinical criteria of respiratory failure are determined by the adverse effects of disturbances in arterial blood gas tensions (Pao_2 and $Paco_2$) and pH on the function of susceptible organ systems, chiefly the lung, heart, and brain. As the respiratory pump becomes fatigued, either as a result of intrinsic pulmonary disease or as a consequence of changes in blood gas tensions, several findings, eg, tachypnea, increased work in breathing, and cyanosis, are seen (Table 9–2). The hypoxemia that results from ventilatory inadequacy may interfere with brain metabolism, depress the myocardium, and cause pulmonary hypertension. Hypercapnia depresses the central nervous system, and acidemia depresses myocardial function. Thus, patients in respiratory failure can exhibit significant changes in central nervous system and cardiac function (Table 9–2). It is important to realize that the manifestations of respiratory failure are not always clinically evident and that some signs or symptoms may be due to nonrespiratory causes. Further, a strictly clinical assessment of arterial hypoxemia or hypercapnia is not reliable. Thus, precise assessment of oxygenation and ventilatory adequacy must be based on both clinical and laboratory data.

B. Laboratory Findings: Laboratory findings are often helpful in gauging the severity and acuity of respiratory failure. **Arterial blood gases** give information on the acid-base status (with a measured pH and calculated bicarbonate level) as well as information on the status of oxygenation (Pao_2) and ventilation ($Paco_2$) in the patient. The $Paco_2$ is a sensitive measure of ventilation and is inversely related to

the minute ventilation (Fig 9–1). Knowing the arterial blood gas value and the inspired oxygen concentration enables one to calculate several parameters that may be helpful in deciding the efficiency of gas exchange. The difference between alveolar oxygen concentration and the arterial oxygen value is the **alveolar-arterial oxygen difference** ($Aado_2$). The $Aado_2$ is less than 15 mm Hg under normal conditions, and it increases with increasing inspired oxygen concentrations to about 100 mm Hg in patients breathing 100% oxygen. Diffusion impairment, shunts, and ventilation perfusion mismatches all cause increased $Aado_2$ (Table 9–3). In addition to the

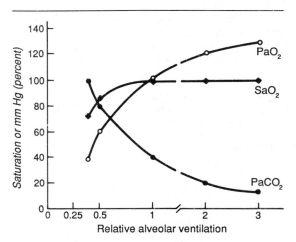

Figure 9–1. Relationship between alveolar ventilation, arterial oxygen saturation (Sao_2), and the partial pressures of oxygen and CO_2 in the arterial blood (Pao_2 and $Paco_2$). (Reproduced, with permission, from Pagtakhan RD, Chernicic V: Respiratory failure in the pediatric patient. *Pediatr Rev* 1982;**3**:244.

Table 9–3. Pulmonary status equations.

Pio_2	=	(barometric pressure $- 47$) $\times$ % inspired oxygen concentration
$Aado_2$	=	$Pio_2 - (Paco_2/R) - Pao_2$ (Normal = $5 - 15$ mm Hg)
Co_2	=	$(1.34 \times$ hemoglobin $\times Sao_2) + (.003 \times Pao_2)$
Do_2	=	$Cao_2 \times CI \times 10$ (Normal 620 ;pm 50 mL/min/m²)
Oxygen consumption (Vo_2) = $(Cao_2 - Cvo_2) \times CI \times 10$ (normal 120 to 200 mL/min/m²)		

$$\frac{Qs}{Qt} = \frac{Cco_2 - Cao_2}{Cco_2 - Cvo_2} \qquad \text{(Normal} < 5\%)$$

$$Vd = \frac{(Paco_2 - Peco_2)}{(Pcco_2)} \qquad \text{(Normal approximately 2 mL/kg)}$$

$$\text{Compliance} = \frac{\text{Volume (Tidal volume)}}{\text{Pressure (PIP} - \text{PEEP)}} \qquad \text{(Normals vary with age)}$$

$Aado_2$	=	Alveolar-arterial oxygen difference (mm Hg).
Cao_2	=	Oxygen content of arterial blood (mL/dL).
Cco_2	=	Oxygen content of pulmonary capillary blood (mL/dL).
CI	=	Cardiac index.
Co_2	=	Oxygen content of the blood (mL/dL).
Cvo_2	=	Oxygen content of mixed venous blood (mL/dL).
Do_2	=	Oxygen delivery.
$Paco_2$	=	Partial pressure of carbon dioxide in arterial blood (mm Hg).
Pao_2	=	Partial pressure of oxygen in arterial blood.
$Pcco_2$	=	Partial pressure of carbon dioxide in capillary blood.
$Peco_2$	=	Partial pressure of carbon dioxide in expired air (mm Hg).
Pio_2	=	Partial pressure of oxygen in inspired air (mm Hg).
Qs/Qt	=	Intrapulmonary shunt (in patients without cardiac shunt) (%).
R	=	Respiratory quotient (usually = 0.8).
Sao_2	=	Arterial oxygen saturation (%).
Vd	=	Physiologic dead space (anatomic dead space + alveolar dead space) (mL).
Ve	=	Expiratory minute volume L/min.
Vo_2	=	Oxygen consumption per minute.

calculation of the $Aado_2$, assessment of the intrapulmonary shunting of blood may be helpful. The intrapulmonary shunt is that percent of pulmonary blood flow not involved in respiration and occurs in an area of lung parenchyma that is not being ventilated. It has the same effect as a right-to-left cardiac shunt in that oxygen saturations are lowered as shunting increases. Normal individuals have less than a 5% physiologic shunt. When the calculated intrapulmonary shunt exceeds 15%, the patient often needs very aggressive respiratory support.

Oxygen content is simple to derive. When the cardiac output is known, one can calculate oxygen transport, oxygen consumption, and oxygen extraction, all variables that are affected in different ways by different disease states.

Dead space ventilation is that part of the breath in the conducting air passages plus the alveolar volume that is not actively involved in gas exchange. Dead space ventilation is increased in bronchopulmonary dysplasia, V/Q mismatches, pulmonary interstitial emphysema, and many other entities. It can be decreased by improving aeration of collapsed alveoli in patients with acute adult respiratory distress syndrome (ARDS) or by such methods as tracheostomy in patients with chronic pulmonary failure.

Treatment

A. Oxygen Supplementation: Patients with hypoxemia induced by respiratory failure may respond to supplemental oxygen administration alone (Table 9-4). Those with hypoventilation and diffusion defects respond better than patients with shunts or V/Q mismatches. Severe V/Q mismatches often do not respond to anything but aggressive airway management and mechanical ventilation. Patients with a decreased functional residual capacity (FRC)—the amount of air left in the lungs at the end of passive expiration—often respond to the delivery of continuous positive airway pressure (CPAP), 5–10 cm H_2O by mask and oxygen. This improves oxygenation by increasing FRC to above closing capacity (closing capacity is the combination of the expiratory reserve volume and closing volume and represents the volume that the FRC must exceed during tidal breathing to prevent closure of airways). Patients with severe hypoventilation or apnea require assistance with bag and mask ventilation until the airway is intubated. Ventilation may be maintained for some time with a mask of the proper size, but gastric distention, emesis, and inadequate tidal volumes are possible complications. In those patients who fail to respond to simple oxygen supplementation, establishment of an artifical airway is often life saving.

B. Intubation: Intubation of the trachea in infants and children requires experienced personnel and the right equipment. Details of the steps in-

Table 9–4. Supplemental oxygen therapy.

Source	Maximum % O$_2$	Range of Flow Rates	Advantages	Disadvantages
Nasal cannula	35–40%	⅛–4 L/min	Easily applied, relatively comfortable	Uncomfortable at higher flow rates, requires open nasal airways, easily dislodged, lower % O$_2$, nosebleeds
Simple mask	50–60%	5–10 L/min	Higher % O$_2$, good for mouth breathers	Uncomfortable, dangerous for patients with poor airway control and at risk for emesis, hard to give airway care, unsure of % O$_2$
Face tent	40–60%	8–10 L/min	Higher % O$_2$, good for mouth breathers, less restrictive	Uncomfortable, dangerous for patients with poor airway control and at risk for emesis, hard to give airway care, unsure of % O$_2$
Rebreathing mask	80–90%	5–10 L/min	Higher % O$_2$, good for mouth breathers, highest O$_2$ concentration by mask	Uncomfortable, dangerous for patients with poor airway control and at risk for emesis, hard to give airway care, unsure of % O$_2$
Oxyhood	90–100%	5–10 L/min (mixed at wall)	Stable and accurate O$_2$ concentration	Temperature regulation, hard to give airway care

volved are included in all the advanced life support courses and are outlined only briefly here. A patient in respiratory failure whose airway must be stabilized requires many interventions before the actual intubation. The patient must be properly positioned to facilitate air exchange while supplemental oxygen is given. The sniffing position is used in infants. Head extension with jaw thrust is used in older children without neck injuries. If obstructed by secretions or vomitus, the airway must be cleared by suction. When not obstructed by a foreign body or epiglottitis, airways should open with proper positioning and placement of an oral or nasopharyngeal airway of the correct size. Nasal airways are better tolerated than oral airways by conscious patients. As each step is taken, it is imperative to monitor changes in chest movement, airway and breath sounds, skin color, and mental status. In patients with a normal airway, an intravenous anesthesia induction for intubation may be performed by those experienced with the drugs and the intubation procedure (Table 9–5). Patients with obstructed upper airways (eg, patients with croup, epiglottitis, obstructions by foreign bodies, or subglottic stenosis) should be awake when intubated unless trained airway specialists decide otherwise.

Insertion of an endotracheal (ET) tube of the correct size is of critical importance in pediatrics. A tube that is too large for a pediatric patient may cause pressure necrosis of the tissues in the subglottic region (the subglottic region is the narrowest portion of the upper airway in children, in contrast to

Table 9–5. Drugs commonly used for controlled intubation.

Drug	Dose (mg/kg)	Advantages	Disadvantages
Atropine	0.02; minimum of 0.1	Blocks bradycardia, dries secretions	Tachycardia, fever, histamine-release seizures, coma
Thiopental	3–5	Fast onset, short duration of action	Vascular irritant, negatively inotropic, no analgesic properties, histamine release (avoid in asthma), induces porphyria
Ketamine	1–2 IV 4–8 IM	Fast onset, positively inotropic	Increased bronchorrhea, increased pulmonary and systemic vascular resistance, increased intracranial pressure, emergence problems
Succinylcholine (depolarizing muscle relaxant)	1–2	Fast onset, short duration of action	Bradycardia (premedicate with atropine); fasciculations; contraindicated in burns, hyperkalemia, massive trauma, and various neurologic disorders
Pancuronium (nondepolarizing muscle relaxant)	0.1	Lasts 40–60 min, can be given by continuous infusion, reversible	Slow onset (2–3 min), tachycardia
Vecuronium (nondepolarizing muscle relaxant)	0.1	Lasts 20–30 min, can be given by continuous infusion, reversible	Slow onset (2–3 min)

the glottis in adults). Insertion of ET tubes of inappropriate size has been associated with scarring and in some cases permanent stenosis of the subglottic region, requiring tracheostomy or cricoid split for repair. There are many ways to calculate the size of endotracheal tube that is appropriate for a child. A useful method is the following: tube size = (16 + age in years)/4. Patients less than 8 years old should have uncuffed endotracheal tubes. After placement of the endotracheal tube, breath sounds should be evaluated for bilateral equality. One should then check for a leak between the ET tube and the larynx. To do this, connect a pressure-monitored anesthesia bag to the circuit and allow it to inflate, giving positive pressure. Check for the leak by auscultating over the throat, noting the pressure at which air escapes around the endotracheal tube. Leaks of 15–20 cm H_2O are acceptable. Larger leaks (> 20 cm H_2O) are acceptable only in patients having severe lung disease and poor compliance and requiring high pressures to achieve ventilation. In this situation, one must be aware of the possible postextubation complications of subglottic stenois in the patient. A chest x-ray film is necessary for final assessment of endotracheal tube placement.

Guiterrez G, Pohl RJ: Oxygen consumption is linearly related to O_2 supply in critically ill patients. *J Crit Care* 1986;**1**:45.

Heffner JE: Tracheal intubation in mechanically ventilated patients. *Clin Chest Med* 1988;**9**:23.

Katz R, Pollack M, Spady D: Cardiopulmonary abnormalities in severe acute respiratory failure. *J Pediatr* 1984; **104**:357.

Kelly HW: Pharmacotherapy of pediatric lung disease: Differences between children and adults. *Clin Chest Med* 1987;**8**:681.

Newth CJL: Respiratory disease and respiratory failure: Implications for the young and the old. *Br J Dis Chest* 1986;**80**:209.

Pagtakhan RD, Chernick J: Respiratory failure in the pediatric patient. *Pediatr Rev* 1982;**3**:247.

Prevoznik SJ: Intubation of the trachea. In: *Introduction to Anesthesia*, 7th ed. Dripps RD, Eckenhoff JE, Vandam LD (editors). Saunders, 1988.

Raphaely RC: Acute respiratory failure in infants and children. *Pediatr Ann* 1986;**15**:315.

Schumaker PT, Cain SM: The concept of a critical oxygen delivery. *Intensive Care Med* 1987;**13**:223.

Steward DJ: Anesthesia in children. In: *Textbook of Pediatric Clinical Pharmacology*. MacLeod, SM, Radde IC (editors). PSG Publishing, 1985.

Steward DJ: *Manual of Pediatric Anesthesia*. Churchill Livingston, 1985.

Ward CF: Pediatric head and neck syndromes. In: *Anesthesia and Uncommon Pediatric Diseases*. Katz J, Steward DJ (editors). Saunders, 1987.

MECHANICAL VENTILATION

Proper mechanical ventilation in infants and children requires knowledge of normal developmental pulmonary physiology and anatomy and of the effects on these by disease. The increased compliance of an infant's chest wall, the growing number of alveoli until approximately the age of 8, and the small size of the airways make pediatric ventilation challenging. Mechanical ventilators are designed to (1) facilitate movement of air into and out of the lungs and (2) deliver oxygen. The two types of commonly used ventilators, pressure ventilators and volume ventilators, provide for both ventilation and oxygen delivery to the lungs.

Pressure Ventilators

Pressure-limited, time-cycled ventilators are usually reserved for neonates and infants. In pressure-limited ventilators, increased air flow is generated at the start of the inspiratory cycle and continues until a preset pressure is reached. Pressure is maintained for a preset inspiratory time usually (0.3–0.6 seconds), and at the end of the inspiratory time, the exhalation valve opens. Pressure ventilators provide intermittent mandatory ventilation (IMV); for example, at a setting of 15 breaths per minute, the machine delivers a breath every 4 seconds. Spontaneous respirations may interfere with the mandatory cycle when the patient's own exhalation coincides with the ventilator's inspiratory phase and causes the peak inspiratory pressure to be reached prematurely. The advantages of pressure-limited ventilators lie with their ability to support spontaneous respirations with continuous gas flow, their avoidance of barotrauma by limiting the pressure of breaths, and their relatively simple operation. The main disadvantages are the possibility of inadequate tidal volumes (especially during periods of rapidly changing lung compliance), the inability to measure compliance, and the possible interference with spontaneous respirations.

Volume Ventilators

Volume ventilators may be used in patients of all ages. With these ventilators, a standard tidal volume is set (10–15 mL/kg), and the inspiratory time is set either to an absolute value (0.3–1.5 second) or to a percentage of the respiratory cycle. Thus, in contrast to pressure-limited ventilators, they always deliver the preset tidal volume. The pressure that is generated in response to a preset tidal volume may change, and this ratio of pressure to volume is an index of compliance in the lung. These ventilators may function in either an intermittent (IMV) or synchronized (SIMV) fashion. SIMV allows a window of time during which a patient's inspiratory effort will initiate the delivery of a tidal volume and is often helpful in spontaneously breathing patients. Volume ventilators are volume-limited and either volume- or time-cycled. Volume ventilators may have either continuous flow through the system or flow that is held in check until an inspiratory effort opens a valve. Volume ventilators also may have an inspiratory hold or pressure support as added variables. The advantages of volume ventilators include ensured delivery of a preset volume, compliance measurements, and availability of SIMV. Disadvantages of some volume ventilators include barotrauma from an excessive delivery pressure and lack of a continuous flow system.

Positive End Expiratory Pressure

All mechanical ventilators open their expiratory limb at the end of inspiration until a preset pressure is achieved; this is the positive end expiratory pressure (PEEP) value. During ventilation of normal lungs, PEEP may be set from 2–4 cm H_2O, mimicking a closed glottis at end expiration in a normal child. In disease states, a higher PEEP may increase the functional residual capacity, open previously closed alveoli, and improve oxygenation. A higher PEEP, although often valuable, may cause carbon dioxide retention, barotrauma with extrapleural air leaks, decreased venous return, decreased cardiac output, and increased intracranial pressure. The term **continuous positive airway pressure** (CPAP) refers to the lowest expiratory pressure that a spontaneously breathing patient achieves. PEEP and CPAP have an optimal setting for each individual patient, maximally improving FRC and ventilation perfusion mismatches while not causing the previously mentioned problems associated with excessive intrathoracic pressure. Multiple parameters have been proposed, with varying success, to define "optimal PEEP." Among these are QS/QT and Pao_2/Fio_2 ratios and respiratory system compliance; even an attempt at computer titration of PEEP has been made.

Ventilator Management

Mechanical ventilators affect both ventilation and oxygenation. Ventilation is related to alveolar minute volume. On a pressure ventilator, the minute volume is directly related to rate and peak inspiratory pressure, on a volume ventilator, it is related to rate and tidal volume. In both ventilators changing the ratio of inspiration to expiration affects ventilation. Changes in oxygenation, other than those due to the concentration of delivered oxygen, depend in part on the variables that determine mean airway pressure (MAP), or the average of all the pressures experienced by the lung in one respiratory cycle. These include PEEP and inspiratory time on both types of ventilators as well as peak inspiratory pressure on a pressure ventilator and tidal volume on a volume ventilator. By increasing any of these settings, one achieves an elevation in MAP and, up to a point, an increase in oxygenation. One must remember that increasing these settings can worsen ventilation perfusion mismatches, decrease cardiac output, and decrease oxygen delivery to the tissue. Therefore, the changes resulting in elevated MAP do not always improve arterial oxygenation or O_2 delivery.

The intubated patient deserves attention directed toward improving comfort and decreasing anxiety.

Chloral hydrate, benzodiazepines, and narcotics have been used. Continuous infusions of certain drugs create a steady state of sedation. Occasionally patients are so agitated that ventilation and oxygenation suffer. In these cases, muscle paralysis may facilitate oxygenation and ventilation. Pancuronium bromide and vecuronium bromide are most commonly used for this purpose. They may be given as necessary or as continuous infusions. When giving muscle relaxants, one must be prepared to provide ventilation and oxygenation by completely mechanical means to the patient who previously breathed spontaneously; in many cases, ventilation support must be increased.

Monitoring the Ventilated Patient

Monitoring of the ventilated patient starts with a physical examination. Respiratory rate and activity, chest wall movement, and quality of breath sounds must be noted. Next, the gas exchange should be measured. Although arterial blood gases are the standard, oxygenation can also be measured by transmission oximetry with lightweight digital or earlobe probes. O_2 (Pto_2) or CO_2 ($Ptco_2$) can be measured transcutaneously with sufficient accuracy in younger patients with good skin perfusion. $Paco_2$ may also be assessed by monitoring end-tidal CO_2. This is done by placing a gas sampling port on the endotracheal tube. Expired gas is analyzed for $Petco_2$, and alveolar $Paco_2$, which is usually several points lower than $Petco_2$, can be estimated. This technique appears more valuable in patients with large tidal volumes and its accuracy improves with more proximal sampling, ie, closer to the airways. $Petco_2$ values may be 5–20 mm Hg lower than $Paco_2$ values and are most useful for trending.

The ventilator itself has many variables. The most common are tidal volume, minute volume, peak inspiratory pressure, inspiratory and expiratory time, compliance, and resistance. Work of breathing may be measured as well as oxygen consumption; these measurements may be helpful in making ventilator changes in chronically ventilated patients. Ways to obtain measurements by computer at the bedside and evaluate all these measurements are becoming available. These technologic advances offer more information but do not eliminate the need for good clinical judgment and instinct.

Alternative Methods of Ventilation

New techniques of ventilating the patient in respiratory failure are now available. High-frequency jet ventilation with passive expiration (60–300/min) and high-frequency oscillation with active expiration (300–1800/min) have been used to manage select groups of patients, including those suffering from major pulmonary barotrauma (air leaks, pulmonary interstitial emphysema), infant or adult respiratory distress syndrome, and congenital diaphragmatic hernia. These techniques have also been used to manage postoperative airway surgery patients. Reports that patients with these conditions are being supported with adequate oxygenation and CO_2 removal at lower MAPs have spurred several large controlled studies. Results from such trials are mixed, and specific recommendations for use of such ventilation techniques cannot be made at this time. Negative pressure ventilators are occasionally used for patients whose respiratory efforts are hindered by muscle or nerve damage.

Beemer GH: Continuous infusions of muscle relaxants: Why and how. *Anaesthes Intensive Care* 1987;**15**:83.

Biondi JW, Schullman DS, Matthay RA: Effects of mechanical ventilation on right and left ventricular function. *Clin Chest Med* 1988;**9**:55.

Clark RH: Pulmonary interstitial emphysema treated by high frequency oscillatory ventilation. *Crit Care Med* 1986;**14**:926.

Doriwsky PM, Hamlin RL, Gadek JE: Alterations in regional blood flow during positive end expiratory pressure ventilation. *Crit Care Med* 1987;**15**:106.

East TD: Computer-controlled positive end-expiratory pressure filtration for effective oxygenation without frequent blood gases. *Crit Care Med* 1988;**16**:252.

Fanconi S: Pulse oximetry in pediatric intensive care: Comparison with measured saturations in transcutaneous oxygen tension. *J Pediatr* 1985;**107**:362.

Gioia FR, Stephenson RL, Alterwitz SA: Principles of respiratory support and mechanical ventilation. In: *Textbook of Pediatric Intensive Care*. Rogers MC (editor). Williams and Wilkins, 1987.

Kanak R, Fahey PJ, Vanderwarf C: Oxygen cost of breathing: Changes dependent upon mode of mechanical ventilation. *Chest* 1985;**87**:126.

Marini JJ: Monitoring during mechanical ventilation. *Clin Chest Med* 1988;**9**:73.

McWilliams BC: Mechanical ventilation in pediatric patients. *Clin Chest Med* 1987;**8**:597.

Nelson LD, Civetia JM, Hudson-Civetia J: Titrating positive end expiratory pressure therapy in patients with early moderate arterial hypoxemia. *Crit Care Med* 1987;**15**:14.

Shapiro BA, Cane RD, Harrison RA: PEEP therapy in adults with special reference to acute lung injury: A review of the literature and suggested clinical correlation. *Crit Care Med* 1984;**12**:127.

Vyas H, Helms P, Cheriyan G: Transcutaneous oxygen monitoring beyond the neonatal period. *Crit Care Med* 1988;**16**:844.

Weinger MB, Brimon JE: End-tidal carbon dioxide as a measure of arterial carbon dioxide during intermittent mandatory ventilation. *J Clin Monitoring* 1987;**3**:73.

Wetzel RC, Gioia FR: High frequency ventilation. *Pediatr Clin North Am* 1987;**34**:15.

Willats SM: Alternative modes of ventilation. (2 parts.) *Intensive Care Med* 1985;**11**:51 and 115.

ADULT RESPIRATORY DISTRESS SYNDROME (ARDS)

ARDS is a syndrome of acute respiratory failure characterized by increased pulmonary capillary permeability and pulmonary edema that results in refractory hypoxemia, decreased lung compliance, and bilateral diffuse alveolar infiltrates on chest radiography.

ARDS starts with the breakdown of the capillary-alveolar membranes from either pulmonary or nonpulmonary causes. Because of the increased permeability, pulmonary edema develops. ARDS may be precipitated by a variety of insults or events (Table 9–6); however, the clinical presentation is remarkably similar in most cases.

According to Nichols, 4 findings are common to all patients with ARDS:

1. Severe event in a patient with previously normal lungs.
2. Findings of respiratory distress with hypoxemia, increased right-to-left intrapulmonary shunt, and decreased pulmonary compliance.
3. Radiologic appearance of diffuse infiltrates.
4. Cardiac disease and congestive heart failure not the initiating events.

Pathophysiology

ARDS accounts for around 1% of pediatric ICU admissions. The mortality rate in this population is 45–60%. The cause of death is more likely to be related to sepsis and multiple organ failure than irreversible respiratory failure. Although much time and research effort have been expended, the pathophysiologic mechanisms operating in ARDS remain unclear. Several reports suggest that the leukocyte plays a significant role in the pathogenesis of ARDS. Studies show increased neutrophil accumulation in the lungs of patients with ARDS. Activated leukocytes produce several toxic products, including oxygen radicals, proteolytic enzymes, and eicosanoids (the prostaglandins PGG_2, PGI_2, and PGE_2 and thromboxane). These neutrophil products may be responsible for the cell breakdown, vasoconstriction, and bronchoconstriction observed in the lungs of ARDS patients. Current research on ARDS centers on endothelial-neutrophil interaction and ways to improve endothelial barrier function and decrease leukocyte-mediated injury. For the clinician, the management of this disease remains most challenging and its outcome most exasperating.

Treatment

A. Ventilatory Support: Because the hypoxemia of ARDS is related to pulmonary edema, V/Q

Table 9–6. ARDS risk factors.

Direct Lung Injury	Indirect Lung Injury
Aspiration of gastric contents	Sepsis syndrome
Inhalation of toxic fumes	Multiple trauma
Near-drowning	Multiple transfusions
Oxygen toxicity	Fat embolism
Pulmonary contusion	
Pneumonia—bacterial, viral, other	

mismatch, decreased functional residual capacity, and increased dead space, it does not respond simply to an increase in inspired oxygen concentration. Also, high concentrations of oxygen (Fio_2 levels greater than 50% over 24 hours) can cause additional lung injury to these patients, who have already altered barrier function. To decrease the potentially injurious effects of high oxygen concentrations, physicians may use positive pressure ventilation and PEEP to improve oxygenation under the least injurious conditions. Ventilation is best maintained on a volume ventilator because of the rapidly changing compliance of the lungs. Because of poor compliance, high peak inspiratory pressure may result from the required preset tidal volume. PEEP is used to open collapsed alveoli, reduce shunting, and increase FRC above the closing volume. All these measures decrease dead space ventilation and may improve oxygenation. PEEPs of 15–25 cm H_2O have been used successfully in some patients. The PEEP that provides the best combination of oxygenation, lung compliance, cardiac output, and lowered intrapulmonary shunt is found by increasing the PEEP by increments (2–3 cm H_2O every 30 minutes) until pulmonary and hemodynamic measurements fit the patient's requirements. Before increasing PEEP, one should optimize conditions by making sure that the intravascular volume is appropriate, the endotracheal tube fits well and has no significant leak, and the patient is well sedated or paralyzed. A QS/QT of less than 15%, oxygen saturations greater than 90% on a Fio_2 of less than 60%, and a good cardiac output may signal the end point of PEEP adjustments.

B. Hemodynamic Support: Hemodynamic support is directed toward increasing perfusion and oxygen delivery. Volume expansion is achieved by giving packed red blood cells to patients with a hematocrit less than 40% and either colloid or crystalloid to nonanemic volume-depleted patients. There is no one recommendation on the type of fluid to give the nonanemic patient. Certainly, colloids should be used in patients with low intravascular oncotic pressure as estimated by reduced total protein or albumin concentrations. In all other ARDS patients, however, the optimal fluid resuscitation has not been well established. Use of inotropic drugs is often necessary. The most effective inotropic dosages should be determined by monitoring blood pressure, urinary output, cardiac output, pulmonary and systemic vascular resistances, and the patient's gas exchange.

C. Pharmacotherapy: Drug therapies have not proved particularly successful in ARDS. Clinical research has been directed at blocking the host's inflammatory response to injury. Steroids could work by stabilizing lysosomal membranes, preventing aggregation of platelets, and inhibiting phospholipase A_2, resulting in decreased eicosanoid production. However, clinical studies have not demonstrated steroid therapy to be of any benefit in ARDS patients. Ibuprofen and indomethacin block synthesis of eicosanoids and have been tried without clear results. Vasodilators such as nitroglycerin, sodium nitroprusside, PGE_1, and PGI_2 have all been used to battle pulmonary vasoconstriction. As yet, there is no clear evidence suggesting that these drugs have beneficial effects.

D. Monitoring: Multiorgan system monitoring is needed in patients with ARDS. Ventilation can be assessed by monitoring arterial blood gases, oxygen saturation, and end-tidal CO_2. Lung compliance should be known as increases in PEEP or tidal volume are made. Obtaining chest films daily is important for patients receiving vigorous support because severe ARDS is associated with a 40–60% incidence of air leaks. Hemodynamic monitoring should include, at the least, central venous monitoring to determine trending volume status; if PEEPs greater than 12 cm H_2O are used, a pulmonary artery catheter is recommended. Surveillance for infection or sepsis is important because secondary infections are common and increase mortality greatly. Renal, liver, and gastrointestinal function need close attention because the likelihood of multiple organ dysfunction is very possible in the ARDS patient.

E. Alternative Management: New techniques have evolved in the respiratory treatment of ARDS. High-frequency ventilation has proved helpful only in patients with large air leaks. Pediatric patients with severe ARDS who received extracorporeal membrane oxygenation (ECMO) have better survival rates than historical controls. Criteria for selecting which patients should receive these new therapies have not been decided.

F. Follow-up: The follow-up of pediatric ARDS patients is limited. One report of 10 children followed from 1 to 4 years after severe ARDS showed 3 still symptomatic and 7 with hypoxemia at rest. Until further information is available, all patients with a history of ARDS need close follow-up of their pulmonary function.

Andreadis N, Petty TL: Adult respiratory distress syndrome: Problems and progress. *Am Rev Respir Dis* 1985;**132**:1344.

Annant G: Oxygen delivery and uptake in the adult respiratory distress syndrome. *Am Rev Respir Dis* 1986; **133**:999.

Bersten A, Sibald WJ: Acute lung injury in septic shock. *Crit Care Clin* 1989;**5**:49.

Fanconi S: Long-term sequences in children survivors of adult respiratory distress syndrome. *J Pediatr* 1985; **106**:218.

Fein A, et al: Pathophysiology of the adult respiratory distress syndrome. What have we learned from human studies? *Crit Care Clin* 1986;**2**:429.

Holcroft JW, Vassar MJ, Weber CJ: Prostaglandin E and survival in patients with the adult respiratory syndrome. *Ann Surg* 1986;**203**:371.

Katz R: Adult respiratory distress syndrome in children. *Clin Chest Med* 1987;**8:**635.

Katz R, Pollack M, Spady D: Cardiopulmonary abnormalities in severe acute respiratory failure. *J Pediatr* 1984;**104:**357.

Luce JM, et al: Ineffectiveness of high-dose methylprednisolone in preventing paryenchymal lung injury and improving mortality in patients with septic shock. *Am Rev Respir Dis* 1988;**136:**62.

Nichols DG, Rogers MC: Adult respiratory distress syndrome. In: *The Textbook of Pediatric Intensive Care.* Roger MC (editor). Williams and Wilkins, 1987.

Potkiw RT: Effect of PEEP on right and left ventricular function in patients with the adult respiratory distress syndrome. *Am Rev Respir Dis* 1987;**135:**307.

Royal JA, Levin DL: Adult respiratory distress syndrome in pediatric patients. 1. Clinical aspects, pathophysiology, and mechanisms of lung injury. *J Pediatr* 1988;**112:**169.

Royal JA, Levin DL: Adult respiratory distress syndrome in pediatric patients. 2. Management. *J Pediatr* 1988;**112:**335.

Zucker AR: Therapeutic strategies for acute hypoxemic respiratory failure. *Crit Care Clin* 1989;**4:**813.

DROWNING

Drowning is defined as death in less than 24 hours after submersion; **near-drowning** is survival for more than 24 hours after this submersion. Drowning was the third leading cause of death in 1988 for the age group of 1–14 years. Fresh-water drownings account for 98% of the drownings; salt water, for the remaining 2%. In the age group of 1–4 years, in which the incidence of drowning is greatest, 85% of children who drown do so after falling into swimming pools or natural bodies of water. **Prevention** is the key to reducing mortality and morbidity due to drownings.

Pathophysiology

Damage to alveolar capillary membranes and surfactant occurs in both fresh- and salt-water drownings. Pulmonary edema develops as a result of this damage. The difference between fresh- and salt-water drownings is the direction of alveolar fluid shifts. The increased tonicity of salt water (similar to 3% saline) causes some movement of free water into the alveolus and a drop in intravascular volume. In fresh-water drownings, fluid movement is toward the higher tonicity of pulmonary capillaries, with a resultant increase in interstitial fluid. The volume shifts are usually small and resolve quickly.

The initial response to submersion is usually laryngospasm. After 1–2 minutes the laryngospasm in 90% of the submersions resolves, and water is aspirated. In 10% of the cases, laryngospasm persists, and no aspiration occurs. Pulmonary damage is caused by the reperfusion of hypoxic tissues, ie, ischemia reperfusion injury, and by aspiration.

Treatment

A. Pulmonary Support: Early and effective resuscitation of a near-drowning patient improves the clinical outcome. Patients who are apneic or have signs of respiratory failure should be intubated and ventilated. If pulmonary edema and poor pulmonary compliance exist, mechanical ventilation should be used. Hypoxemia usually responds to incremental increases (2–3 cm H_2O) in PEEP, which help reduce the intrapulmonary shunt (QS/QT to < 15%) and increase oxygenation.

B. Hemodynamic Support: After CPR, near-drowning patients may have low cardiac output and high systemic vascular resistance. These findings, combined with severe pulmonary abnormalities, signal the need for aggressive ventilatory support and arterial and central venous monitoring. Signs of a depressed cardiac output or large intrapulmonary shunt suggest the need for a pulmonary arterial catheter. Inotropic drugs must often be used to improve tissue and cerebral perfusion.

C. Neurologic Evaluation and Support: Prognostic signs based on history and initial emergency room examination in near-drowning patients are helpful in planning therapy and predicting prognosis. Patients who required CPR and arrive in the ICU with a score of 3 on the Glasgow coma scale generally have a very poor outcome. Patients also can be scored by Orloski's system, which includes 5 unfavorable prognostic factors (Table 9–7). Patients with scores ≤ 2 have a 90% chance of good recovery, whereas those with scores ≥ 3 have a 5% chance of good recovery. Cold-water submersions (< 10°C) often have better results than expected. Any near-drowning patient with a history of neurologic or pulmonary symptoms should be admitted, evaluated completely, and observed.

Neurologic support may be required because of anoxic brain damage. Initial evaluation should include neck and skull films, especially in unwitnessed drownings, so that unstable injuries do not go undetected. Modell distinguishes among 3 groups of patients according to neurologic evaluation in the ICU: (A) awake, (B) blunted, and (C) comatose. Groups A and B generally did very well. Comatose and flaccid patients had the worst prognosis. A comatose near-drowning patient in the ICU who is not improving or is worsening may need continuous measurement of intracranial pressure (ICP) and corresponding cerebral perfusion pressure (CPP) (CPP = mean

Table 9–7. Orlowski score.[1]

Unfavorable Prognostic Factors

Age less than 3 years
Estimated submersion time over 5 minutes
No resuscitation attempts for at least 10 minutes after rescue
Comatose upon admission to emergency department
Arterial blood gas pH ≤ 7.10

[1]One point is assigned for each item present. If information is not available, no point is assigned.

arterial pressure (MAP) − intracranial pressure (ICP)]. Sustained ICP > 20 or CPP < 50 cm H_2O is a poor prognostic sign. The neurologic treatment regimen should include head elevation, hyperventilation, and mild restriction of fluids. Dexamethasone administration, hypothermia, and barbiturate coma, all directed at CNS resuscitation, have not been associated with improved survival rates. Barbiturates are useful when the intent of their administration is to reduce ICP. However, because the hypoxic/ischemic injury has already occurred in the near-drowning patient, this specific injury may not be amenable to currently recommended manipulations.

D. Infectious Complications: Secondary infection in near-drowning victims can be a significant problem. Obtaining serial tracheal aspirates and blood cultures through indwelling lines and via peripheral venipuncture is recommended in place of starting antibiotic therapy on admission. Antibiotic coverage should be instituted when clinically appropriate. Neutropenia indicates a very poor prognosis.

E. Follow-up: Follow-up in near-drowning victims is important. Although many appear grossly intact, neuropsycologic testing reveals mild residual gross motor and coordination deficits. Pulmonary follow-up reveals that, months after a near-drowning, 90% of ''asymptomatic'' children had bronchial hypersensitivity elicited on pulmonary function testing.

Allman FD: Outcome following cardiopulmonary resuscitation in severe pediatric near-drowning. *Am J Dis Child* 1986;**140**:571.

Bell TS, Ellenberg L, McComg JG: Neuropsychological outcome after severe pediatric near-drowning. *Neurosurgery* 1985;**17**:604.

Bohn OJ: Influence of hypothermia, barbiturate therapy and intracranial pressure monitoring on morbidity and mortality after near drowning. *Crit Care Med* 1986;**14**:529.

Brooks JG: Near drowning. *Pediatr Rev* 1988;**10**:5.

Frewen TC: Cerebral resuscitation therapy in pediatric near-drowning. *J Pediatr* 1985;**106**:615.

Hildegrand CA: Cardiac performance in pediatric near-drowning. *Crit Care Med* 1988;**16**:331.

Laughlin JJ, Eilen H: Pulmonary function abnormalities in survivors of near drowning. *J Pediatr* 1982;**100**:26.

Modell JH: Treatment of near-drowning: Is there a role for H.Y.P.E.R. therapy? (Editorial.) *Crit Care Med* 1986; **14**:593.

Nussbaum E: Prognostic variables in nearly drowned, comatose children. *Am J Dis Child* 1985;**139**:1058.

Nussbaum E, Galant SP: Intracranial pressure monitoring as a guide to prognosis in the nearly drowned, severely comatose child. *J Pediatr* 1983;**102**:215.

Nussbaum E, Maggi JC: Pentobarbital therapy does not improve neurologic outcome in nearly drowned flaccid-comatose children. *Pediatrics* 1988;**81**:630.

Orloski JP: Drowning, near drowning and ice water submersion. *Pediatr Clin North Am* 1987;**34**:75.

Orloski JP, Dedhat MA, Phillips JM: Effects of tonicities of saline solutions on pulmonary injury in drowning. *Crit Care Med* 1987;**15**:126.

Robinson MD, Seward PN: Submersion injury in children. *Pediatr Emerg Care* 1987;**3**:44.

ASTHMA (LIFE-THREATING)

Status asthmaticus may be defined as asthma that is refractory to sympathomimetic agents and that may progress to respiratory failure unless prompt and aggressive intervention is taken. Life-threatening asthma is caused by severe bronchospasm, excessive mucous secretions, and inflammation and edema of the airways. Reversal of these mechanisms is the key to successful treatment. Status asthmaticus remains a common diagnosis among children admitted to the ICU, and asthma continues to be associated with a surprisingly high mortality rate. Among adolescents, the mortality rate associated with asthma has actually increased over the last decade. Possible explanations for this increase include undertreatment, overtreatment, overuse of over-the-counter medicines, increased steroid use, and an increase in environmental pollutants.

The physical examination helps determine the severity of illness. Respiration marked by sternocleidomastoid contractions correlates well with a forced expiratory volume of 1 second and maximum expiratory flow rates of less than 50% of normal predicted values. Pulsus paradoxicus of over 22 has been correlated with elevated $Paco_2$ levels. The absence of wheezing may be misleading because, in order to produce a wheezing sound, the patient must take in a certain amount of air. Patients with severe respiratory distress, signs of exhaustion, alterations in consciousness, elevated $Paco_2$, acidosis, or a history of severe exacerbations should be admitted to the ICU.

Treatment

A. Pharmacotherapy: Severe asthmatics are almost always hypoxemic and should be placed immediately on supplemental humidified oxygen. The cornerstone of treatment is **beta-agonist** therapy. First-line drugs are albuterol and terbutaline, which may be delivered by nebulization with oxygen. If the tidal volume appears severely decreased, thus precluding good inspiratory flow rates and preventing adequate delivery of nebulized medication, subcutaneous injection of epinephrine or terbutaline may be required. Terbutaline or albuterol can be given continuously by nebulization, usually without serious side effects. The heart rate and other vital signs of these patients must be closely monitored to keep the heart rate at less than 180 and to detect ventricular ectopy.

The use of **theophylline** in the initial emergency management of asthma has been recently critically reviewed. It is thought to increase toxicity without improving pulmonary function during the first 4–6 hours of treatment. Later in the course, theophylline can and often needs to be added to the treatment regimen because it not only acts as a bronchodilator but also lessens diaphragmatic fatigue. **Corticosteroids** are necessary in treating almost all hospitalized asthmatics. Complications of corticosteroids include GI bleeding or perforations. Nebulized anticholinergic agents are also recommended, at least as a trial, in severe asthmatics. In some patients cholinergic-related bronchoconstriction is more marked than in others, and so not all patients respond. Intravenous infusion of beta-agonists is recommended as a trial in the severe asthmatic who is slowly entering respiratory failure. Terbutaline has fewer cardiac side effects than isoproterenol and is becoming more widely used. Isoproterenol has also been used successfully but with the well-known cardiac complications of ischemia and arrhythmias.

B. Treatment of Severe Asthmatics

1. Give humidified oxygen. Try to keep O_2 saturations $\geq 94\%$.
2. Begin beta-sympathomimetic (albuterol or terbutaline) therapy by nebulization (albuterol 0.1mg/kg per nebulization up to 2.5 mg or terbutaline 0.1–0.2 mg/kg per nebulization up to 4 mg). This may be given continuously.
3. Give corticosteroids (methylprednisolone 2 mg/kg IV load then 1 mg/kg IV every 6 hours).
4. Give theophylline. Be conservative in dosing and watch for toxicities. Follow levels closely.
5. Institute anticholinergic therapy (atropine 0.025–0.075 mg/kg per dose up to 2 mg every 6–8 hours) by nebulization (most useful in only a select group of patients).
6. Begin beta-sympathomimetic (terubutaline and isoproterenol) therapy by continuous intravenous infusion. This should be used only in patients who have not responded to the above steps and have worsening respiratory failure. (Terbutaline: Load with 10 μg/kg for 10 min, then start infusion at 0.1 μg/kg/min, increasing 0.1 μg/kg/min every 30 min to a maximum of 0.4 μg/kg/min. (Isoproterenol: Give 0.1 μg/kg/min, increasing 0.1 μg/kg/min to a maximum of 1.0 μg/kg/min).

If the above aggressive management regimen fails to result in significant improvement, mechanical ventilation may be necessary. Mechanical ventilation in asthmatics is difficult and by no means simplifies treatment. Intubation should be done by experienced personnel once the patient is sedated and paralyzed. Airway obstruction from persistent bronchoconstriction remains a major problem because the constricted bronchus is lined with smooth muscle, and paralyzing drugs affect only skeletal muscle. The patient, once intubated, should remain paralyzed and sedated. A volume ventilator is necessary to deliver a reasonable tidal volume in patients with poor compliance. Expiratory time should be prolonged to avoid air trapping. The IMV rate may need to be lowered to allow proper expiration time. PEEP should be kept low. There are isolated reports of patients who require greater PEEP, but these are the exception. Aerosolized beta-agonists may be given through the ventilator circuit and should be administered as close to the endotracheal tube as possible.

Weaning the very ill asthmatic from ICU therapy should begin with ventilator support and then with the aggressive aspects of the drug regimen. The actual therapy changes should be made very slowly because patients can rebound and worsen quickly.

C. Metabolic Changes in the Severe Asthmatic: Metabolic disorders may occur in the severe asthmatic. Hypercarbia, hypoxia, and poor perfusion may lead to acidosis. Slow intravenous sodium bicarbonate therapy (1 meq/kg for a pH less than 7.20) in the ventilated patient is a reasonable treatment and allows a better metabolic milieu. The physician must keep in mind that the arterial CO_2 may climb because of sodium bicarbonate therapy. Hypokalemia is also a complication of beta-agonist therapy, and serum potassium needs to be monitored, especially in patients receiving nebulized beta-agonist drugs continuously.

D. Monitoring: Monitoring the severe asthmatic should include obtaining values for oxygen saturation, arterial blood gases, and, if the patient is ventilated, end-tidal CO_2. Ventilator monitoring must be carefully done because increases in peak inspiratory pressure or decreases in pulmonary compliance may signal worsening bronchoconstriction or an extrapleural air leak. Chest films of ventilated asthmatics must be obtained daily.

Benatar SR: Fatal asthma. *N Engl J Med* 1986;**314**:423.

Bierman MI: Prolonged isoflurane anesthesia in status asthmaticus. *Crit Care Med* 1986;**14**:832.

Faata CH, Rossing TH, McFadden: Treatment of acute asthma: Is combination therapy with sympathomimetics and methylxanthinics indicated? *Am J Med* 1986;**80**:5.

Jeene JW, Murphy S: Drug therapy for asthma: Research and clinical practice. In: *Lung Biology in Health and Disease*. Vol 5: *Asthma*. Marcel Dekker, 1987.

Kolski GB: Hypokalemia and respiratory arrest in an infant with status asthmaticus. *J Pediatr* 1988;**112**:304.

Moler FW, Hurwitz ME, Custer JR: Improvement in clinical asthma score and Paco2 in children with severe asthma treated with continuously nebulized terbutaline. *J Allergy Clin Immunol* 1988;**81**:1101.

Sly RM: Increases in deaths from asthma. *Ann Allergy* 1984;**53**:20.

Weinberger M: Corticosteroids for exacerbations of asthma: Current status of the controversy. *Pediatrics* 1988;**81**:726.

POSTOPERATIVE CARDIAC VENTILATORY SUPPORT

The outcome of pediatric cardiac surgery patients has been improved not only by advances in surgical technique and myocardial preservation but also by better postoperative care and ventilator management in the ICU. Ventilator support of the postoperative patient is now specifically tailored for individual patients after a consideration of such variables such as pulmonary hypertension, pulmonary edema, and cardiopulmonary bypass time.

Treatment

Optimizing ventilation starts in the operating room with good anesthetic care. On arrival in the PICU, most patients are intubated, although after simple repairs, eg, repair of an atrial septal defect (ASD), stable patients may be extubated in the operating room by experienced cardiac anesthesiologists. Once in the PICU, patients are placed on a volume ventilator with a tidal volume of 12–15 mL/kg and a rate dependent on individual need. The use of PEEP is dictated not only by the pulmonary fluid status but also by the need in some cases to keep pulmonary vascular resistance as low as possible. The primary cardiac lesion often dictates the duration and method of ventilation following surgical repair. Special care should be given to patients who are sensitive to decreases in pulmonary blood flow or who are at risk for pulmonary hypertensive crises (the sudden elevation of pulmonary blood pressures to or near systemic levels). Extreme caution should be taken to avoid manipulations that cause decreases in functional residual capacity, pH, and Pao_2 or increases in $Paco_2$, since any of these may contribute to significant elevations in pulmonary vascular resistance and lead to a worsening of their condition. Manipulations of PEEP, tidal volume, ventilation rate, and Fio_2 almost always allow one to achieve normal oxygenation ($Pao_2 > 80$ mm Hg), ventilation ($Paco_2 \leq 40$ mm Hg), and FRC yet not increase mean airway pressure to levels that can decrease pulmonary blood flow.

Knowledge of the patient's primary lesion and recognition of postoperative pulmonary complications also dictate how aggressively the patient can be weaned from the ventilation. For example, patients with ventricular septal defects and high pulmonary-to-aortic pressure and resistance ratios require mechanical ventilation significantly longer than those with lower ratios. Patients with pulmonary edema, hematomas, or significant effusions after surgery require longer ventilation. Premature extubation decreases FRC, pH, and Pao_2 and significantly increases pulmonary vascular resistance.

Close monitoring of the postoperative cardiac patient is important. Physical assessment of heart and breath sounds is helpful in detecting cardiac tamponade, pneumothorax, hemothorax, and signs of congestive heart failure. Endotracheal tube placement and pulmonary status are checked with a chest film. Knowledge of the amount, level, and direction of residual intracardiac shunt helps in deciding appro-

priate oxygenation values. Otherwise, low O_2 saturation values must be considered as pulmonary in etiology and suggest the need for more aggressive therapy. Close monitoring of physical examination data, laboratory data, and ventilation promotes a faster and safer recovery.

Heard GG: Early extubation after surgical repair of congenital heart disease. *Crit Care Med* 1985;**13**:830.

Jenkins J: Effects of mechanical ventilation on cardiopulmonary function in children after open heart surgery. *Crit Care Med* 1985;**13**:77.

Kanter RK: Prolonged mechanical ventilation of infants after open heart surgery. *Crit Care Med* 1986;**14**:211.

Lister G: Management of the pediatric patient after cardiac surgery. *Yale J Biol Med* 1984;**57**:7.

Murray JP, Lynn AM, Mansfield PB: Effect of pH and Pao_2 on pulmonary and systemic hemodynamics after surgery in children with congenital heart disease and pulmonary hypertension. *J Pediatr* 1988;**113**:474.

Yamaki S, Huriuchi T, Takahashi T: Pulmonary changes in congenital heart disease with Down's syndrome: Their significance as a cause of postoperative respiratory failure. *Thorax* 1985;**40**:380.

SHOCK

Shock may be defined as a failure of the cardiovascular system to deliver critical substrates and to remove toxic metabolites. This failure leads to anaerobic metabolism in cells and ultimately to irreversible cellular damage. Shock has been categorized into a series of recognizable stages: compensated, uncompensated, and irreversible. Patients in compensated shock have relatively normal cardiac output and normal blood pressures but have alterations in the microcirculation. Because of these alterations, certain tissue beds receive decreased flow while others receive increased flow. The pediatric patient in this state of shock exhibits several compensatory mechanisms. In infants, compensatory increases in cardiac output are achieved primarily by tachycardia rather than increases in stroke volume (cardiac output = stroke volume × heart rate). In young infants in compensated shock, heart rates of 190–210 beats/min are not uncommon, but heart rates over 220 raise the possibility of supraventricular tachycardia. In older patients, cardiac contractility (stroke volume) and heart rate increase to improve cardiac output. Blood pressure remains normal initially because of peripheral vasoconstriction and increased systemic vascular resistance. Thus, hypotension occurs late and is more characteristic of the uncompensated stage of shock. In the uncompensated stage, there is further deterioration of the oxygen and nutrient supply to the cells with subsequent cellular breakdown and release of toxic substances, causing further redistribution of flow. At this point, the patient is hypotensive with poor cardiac output.

Irreversible shock involving organ damage of the brain and heart is considered terminal.

The causes of shock fall into 3 general categories: hypovolemic, cardiogenic, and distributive. In many clinical situations, one can see a combination of 2 or perhaps all 3 categories. **Hypovolemic shock** is caused by a decreased circulating blood volume. This may result from the loss of whole blood or plasma or from excess renal and intestinal fluid losses. These patients usually have intact compensatory mechanisms with increased cardiac output, normal blood pressure, and a shunting of blood away from certain organs. All these responses serve to protect blood flow to the heart and brain. Obviously, if untreated, hypovolemic shock can progress to an irreversible stage.

Cardiogenic shock is an ominous state of decreased substrate delivery secondary to "pump failure." The causes include congenital heart disease, cardiac surgery (following cardioplegia and ventriculotomy), cardiomyopathy secondary to infection or toxins, and ischemic-reperfusion injuries. The patient's compensatory efforts (eg, release of catecholamines with increases in blood pressure, heart rate, and systemic vascular resistance) often have deleterious effects on an already stressed and injured myocardium.

"Distributive shock" is a catch-all phrase for those cases that involve arterial and capillary shunting past tissue beds with an increase in venous capacitance. Examples include anaphylaxis and septic shock. Gram-negative septic shock appears to be mediated by endotoxins (lipopolysaccharides) and subsequent formation of lymphokines (eg, tumor necrosis factor), eicosanoid products, bradykinin, and endorphins. Early on, these humoral mediators cause arteriolar dilation with a drop in systemic vascular resistance. Because the skin remains well perfused and warm during this phase, the phrase "warm shock" has come into use to describe this phase. As septic shock progresses, vascular tone and resistance increase due to increases in sympathetic tone and endogenous catecholamines. The perfusion worsens as the shock progresses, and the extremities become cool. The speed with which the distributive shock progresses varies according to the cause; it can be quite fast in anaphylaxis, and insidious in cases associated with gram-positive cocci.

Clinical Findings

Both noninvasive and invasive monitoring of the patient in shock provide information on the severity, progression, and response to treatment. The physical examination is the cornerstone of noninvasive monitoring. Extremely valuable information can be derived from examination of the cardiovascular, central nervous, renal, musculoskeletal, and mucocutaneous systems.

A. Symptoms and Signs: Heart rate and blood pressure are the easiest **cardiovascular** parameters to measure at the bedside. Tachycardia is an early sign, but it is nonspecific and not always present even in profound hypotension. Hypotension is specific but a late sign in pediatric shock. An important part of the cardiovascular examination is a simultaneous palpation of distal and proximal pulses. An increase in the amplitude difference of pulses between proximal (carotid, brachial, femoral) and distal (radial, posterior tibial, dorsalis pedis) arteries can be palpated in early shock and reflects increased systemic vascular resistance. Distal pulses may be thready or absent even in the presence of normal blood pressure due to poor stroke volume compensated by tachycardia and increased systemic vascular resistance. In uncompensated shock, hypotension is present and proximal pulses are also diminished. Early shock causes peripheral cutaneous vasoconstriction, which preserves flow to vital organs. Thus, the **skin** is gray or ashen in newborns and pale in older groups. Capillary refilling after blanching is slow (greater than 3 seconds). Mottling of the skin may also be observed. Decreased oxygen delivery to the **musculoskeletal system** produces hypotonia. Decreased spontaneous motor activity, flaccidity, and prostration are observed. Measurement of urinary output gives important information about the perfusion of an essential organ system because output is directly proportional to renal blood flow and glomerular filtration rate. Catheterization of the bladder is necessary to give accurate and continuous information. (Normal urine output $\geq$ 1mL/kg/h; outputs < 0.5 mL/kg/h are considered significantly decreased.) Assessment of the **central nervous system** also provides valuable information. The patient's level of consciousness reflects the adequacy of cortical perfusion. When cortical perfusion is severely impaired, the infant or child fails to respond first to verbal stimuli, then to light touch, and finally to pain. Lack of motor response and failure to cry in response to venipuncture or lumbar puncture should alert the clinician to the severity of the situation. In uncompensated shock in the presence of hypotension, brain stem perfusion may be decreased. Poor thalamic perfusion can result in loss of sympathetic tone. Finally, poor medullary flow produces irregular respirations followed by gasping, apnea, and a respiratory arrest. Thus, the physical exam can be performed quickly and provide invaluable information on the physiologic state of the child.

B. Invasive Monitoring: Patients identified as being significantly hypovolemic with poor cardiac output often need invasive monitoring for diagnostic and therapeutic reasons. Intravascular arterial catheters give constant blood pressure readings, and, to an experienced interpreter, the shape of the wave form is helpful in evaluating cardiac output. Central venous pressure (CVP) monitoring, accomplished by placing any intravenous catheter within the thorax, gives useful information about changes in volume status as therapy is given. CVP monitoring does not give useful information about absolute volume status because volume status, which is considered preload, is most accurately inferred from left ventricular end diastolic pressure. Therefore, volume status is more accurately assessed by monitoring pulmonary capillary wedge pressure or left atrial pressure. Pulmonary capillary wedge pressure can be obtained with a pulmonary artery catheter. The pulmonary artery (PA) catheter provides additional valuable information on volume and cardiac status but is associated with a higher complication rate than CVP lines are. This clinical tool provides other information (Table 9–8), including cardiac output (CO), systemic and pulmonary vascular resistances, and right and left ventricular work indexes. Measurements of arterial and mixed venous oxygen saturations, along with CO data, are useful in calculating oxygen delivery, consumption, and extraction. Patients receiving significant inotropic or ventilatory support may benefit from the placement of a PA catheter.

New developments in the monitoring of shock in adults include constant esophageal echocardiographic evaluation of cardiac contractility and volume status as well as doppler cardiac outputs. A suprasternal doppler method of measuring cardiac output is available for infants. In infants and children, cardiac output can be measured via throracic bioimpedance. Along with these less invasive measurements, direct oximetry of mixed venous blood appears useful for detecting changes in oxygen consumption and delivery. These and other new tools need careful evaluation in a pediatric setting before they become part of standard care.

Treatment

A. Fluid Resuscitation: The treatment of shock should begin with a logical, stepwise, and quickly instituted plan that takes into account both physical and laboratory assessment as well as the natural history of the disease. A timely infusion of fluids may reverse the shock in patients with hypovolemic and distributive shock. Patients with cardiogenic shock, however, may worsen when given intravenous fluids unnecessarily because of the diminished ability of the left ventricle to handle volume.

Knowing the pathophysiology of the disease helps the clinician decide the proper fluid regimen for each case of shock. Initially, most patients tolerate crystalloid (salt solution), which is readily available and inexpensive. However, after a crystalloid infusion, only 20% of the solution remains in the intravascular space 4 hours after administration. Patients with serious capillary leaks and ongoing plasma losses (eg, burn cases) should initially receive crystalloid, because in these cases colloid (protein and salt solution) leaks into the interstitium. The protein draws intravascular fluid into the interstitium, thus increasing ongoing losses. Those patients with hypoalbuminemia or with intact capillaries who need to retain volume in the intravascular space (eg, patients at risk for cerebral edema) probably benefit from colloid infusions. Experience with dextran (a starch compound dissolved in salt solution) is limited. The amount of fluids given should be governed by physical exam, cardiovascular status, and lab results. Patients with normal heart function tolerate increased volume better than those with poor function.

B. Pharmacotherapy: Patients with inadequate cardiac function may need early inotropic support. Patients with failing hearts may require beta-adrenergic agents to increase contractility and heart rate while slightly decreasing the systemic vascular resistance. Patients with significant decreases in systemic vascular resistance may require a combination of beta- and alpha-sympathomimetics, eg, epinephrine and norepinephrine. Patients with increased sys-

Table 9–8. Hemodynamic parameters[1]

Parameter	Formula[2]	Normal Values	Units
Cardiac output	$CO = HR \times SV$	Wide age-dependent range	L/min
Cardiac index	$CI = CO/BSA$	3.5–5.5	L/min/m^2
Stroke index	$SI = SV/BSA$	30–60	mL/m^2
Systemic vascular resistance	$SVR = 79.9 \dfrac{(MAP - CVP)}{CI}$	800–1600	dyne sec/cm^5/m^2
Pulmonary vascular resistance	$PVR = 79.9 \dfrac{(MPAP - PCWP)}{CI}$	80–240	dyne sec/cm^5/m^2

[1]Formulas and normals from Katz RW, Pollack M, Weibley R: Pulmonary artery catheterization in pediatric intensive care. Adv Pediatr 1984;**30**:169.
[2]HR = Heart rate, SV = Stroke volume, BSA = Body surface area.
MAP = Mean arterial pressure, CVP = Central venous pressure.
MPAP = Mean pulmonary artery pressure, PCWP = Pulmonary capillary wedge pressure.

temic vascular resistance receiving cardiotonic drugs may benefit from a direct vasodilator to reduce the systemic vascular resistance or afterload and increase cardiac contractility (Table 9–9).

New techniques for treating shock are under trial. These include naloxone administration, to reverse the endorphin-mediated component of shock; endotoxin antibodies, to treat septic shock; and extracorporeal membrane oxygenation, to help treat shock in patients with recoverable cardiac and pulmonary function who require both pulmonary and cardiac assistance. The therapeutic role of these techniques remains uncertain.

Complications

Organ dysfunction during and after an episode of shock is common. Systems most often affected include the kidney, the blood coagulation system, the lungs, the central nervous system, the liver, and the gastrointestinal tract. The kidney responds to hypotension by increasing plasma renin and angiotensin concentrations, causing a decrease in glomerular filtration rate and urine output. This can progress to damage of the energy-consuming renal parenchyma, causing acute tubular necrosis. Coagulopathies may exist in any type of shock but are especially common in septic shock. This is the result of the release of

Table 9–9. Pharmacologic support of the shock patient.

Drug	Dose	Alpha[1]	Beta[1]	Vasodilator	Actions and Advantages	Disadvantages
Dopamine	1–20 µg/kg/min	− to + + +; dose related	+ to + + +; dose related	At low doses, renal vasodilation occurs (dopaminergic receptors)	Moderate inotrope, wide and safe dosage range, short half-life	May cause worsening of pulmonary vasoconstriction
Dobutamine	1–10 µg/kg/min	−	+ + +		Moderate inotrope, less chronotropic, fewer dysrhythmias than with isoproterenol or epinephrine	Marked variation among patients
Amrinone	Bolus, 0.75 mg/kg over 3 min; Infusion 5–10 mcg/kg/min	−	−	Direct smooth-muscle relaxant	Non-beta-adrenergic inotrope, afterload reduction	Arrhythmias, thrombocytopenia, gastrointestinal complaints
Epinephrine	.05–1.0 µg/kg/min	+ + to + + +; dose related	+ + +		Significant increases in inotropy, chronotropy, and SVR[2]	Tachycardia, dysrhythmias, renal ischemia, SVR and PVR increases
Isoproterenol	.05–1.0 µg/kg/min	−	+ + +	Peripheral vasodilation	Significant increase in inotropy and chronotropy. SVR can drop, and PVR[2] should not increase and may decrease	Significant myocardial oxygen consumption increases, tachycardia, dysrhythmia
Norepinephrine	.05–1.0 µg/kg/min	+ + +	+ + +		Powerful vasoconstrictor (systemic and pulmonary); rarely used except possibly in patients with very low SVR or in conjunction with vasodilator	Reduced CO if afterload is too high, renal ischemia
Nitroprusside	0.5–8.0 µg/kg/min	−	−	Arterial and venous dilation (smooth muscle relaxation)	Decreases SVR and PVR, very short acting. Blood pressure returns to previous levels within 1 to 10 minutes after stopping infusion	Toxicities (thiocyanate and cyanide), increased intracranial pressure and V/Q mismatch, methemoglobinemia, increased ICP

[1]− no effect, + small effect, + + moderate effect, + + + potent effect.
[2]SVR = systemic vascular resistance, PVR = pulmonary vascular resistance.

mediators that activate the clotting cascade, leading ultimately to a consumptive coagulopathy. The central nervous system dysfunction is related to decreased cerebral perfusion pressure and thus to decreased substrate delivery to the brain. Liver dysfunction commonly occurs after shock and may be manifested by increases in liver enzymes or a bleeding diathesis. Gastrointestinal problems include ileus, bleeding (eg, gastritis and ulcers), and necrosis with sloughing of intestinal mucosa. These organ system complications should be aggressively searched for after an episode of shock. When multiple organ system failure exists secondary to shock, the mortality rates increase dramatically. Therefore, the goal of resuscitation efforts should be not only improving cardiac and volume status but also maintaining and preserving organ function.

Balk RA, Bone RC: The septic syndrome: Definition and clinical implications. *Crit Care Clin* 1989;**5**:129.

Ball HA, Cook JA, Halushka PV: Role of thromboxane, prostaglandins and leukotrienes in endotoxic and septic shock. *Intensive Care Med* 1986;**12**:116.

Billhardt RA, Rosenbush SW: Cardiogenic and hypovolemic shock. *Med Clin North Am* 1986;**70**:853.

Cunnion RE, Parillo JE: Myocardial dysfunction in sepsis. *Crit Care Clin* 1989;**5**:1.

Fields AI: Invasive hemodynamic monitoring in children. *Clin Chest Med* 1987;**8**:611.

Fripp RR, Berman W: A noninvasive assessment of cardiopulmonary function in critically ill infants and children. *Clin Chest Med* 1987;**8**:619.

Hirshl RB, Bartlett RH: Extracorporeal membrane oxygenation support in cardiorespiratory failure. *Ad Surg* 1987;**21**:189.

Introna RPS: Use of transthoracic bioimpedance to determine cardiac output in pediatric patients. *Crit Care Med* 1988;**16**:1101.

Karakusis PH: Considerations in the therapy of septic shock. *Med Clin North Am* 1986;**70**:933.

Katz RW, Pollack MM, Weibly RE: Pulmonary artery catheterization in pediatric intensive care. *Ad Pediatr* 1984;**30**:169.

Kaufman BS, Kalkow EC, Falk JL: The relationship between oxygen delivery and consumption during fluid resuscitation of hypovolemic and septic shock. *Chest* 1984;**85**:336.

Lucking SE, Pollack MM, Fields AI: Shock following generalized hypoxic-ischemic injury in previously healthy infants and children. *J Pediatr* 1986;**108**:359.

Nicholson DP: Review of corticosteroid treatment in sepsis and septic shock: Pro or con. *Crit Care Clin* 1989; **5**:123.

Perkin RM, Levin DL: Shock in pediatric patients. (2 parts.) *J Pediatr* 1982;**101**:163 and 319.

Pollack MM, Fields AI, Ruttiman UE: Sequential cardiopulmonary variables of infants and children in septic shock. *Crit Care Med* 1984;**12**:554.

Shoemaker WC: Relationship of oxygen transport patients to the pathophysiology and therapy of shock states. *Intensive Care Med* 1987;**13**:230.

Simpson SQ, Casey LC: The role of tumor necrosis factor in sepsis and acute lung injury. *Crit Care Clin* 1989; **5**:137.

Ward CK: An update on pediatric monitoring. *J Clin Monit* 1985;**1**:172.

Worthley L, Tyler P, Moran JL: A comparison of dopamine, dobutamine and isoproterenol in the treatment of shock. *Intensive Care Med* 1985;**11**:13.

Sanford TJ: An anesthesiologist's view: The right internal jugular vein. *J Clin Monit* 1985;**1**:58.

Stenzel JP: Percutaneous femoral venous catheterizations: A prospective study of complications. *J Pediatr* 1989; **114**:411.

Venkataraman ST, Orr RA, Thompson AE: Percutaneous infraclavicular subclavian vein catheterization in critically ill infants and children. *J Pediatr* 1988;**113**:480.

VASCULAR CATHETER PLACEMENT

Placement of catheters into the central circulation is important both for evaluation of volume and cardiac status and for improving ease and comfort of care. The following is a description of methods and general rules for the placement of intravascular lines.

General Rules

These are general rules for the placement of central venous lines using the Seldinger technique: (1) open the kit and test all the equipment. This includes feeding the wire through the needle and filling all lines with normal saline to prevent air from entering the system. (2) *Sterilize* and drape the area around the point of entry. (3) Use local anesthetic as needed. (4) Using the needle, find the vein. (5) Once there is a free flow of venous blood into the syringe, take the syringe off and feed the wire into the vein. The wire should pass easily into the vein. (6) Withdraw the needle over the wire and clean the wire of blood. (7) Make a nick with an 11 blade at a point where the skin and wire meet and place the introducer and intravascular catheter over the wire. (8) With the catheters in place, remove the wire along with the introducer. (9) Check that blood can be drawn easily through the new line. (10) Verify the position of the line by obtaining an x-ray film.

Points of Entry for Line Placement

After placing a line through any of the following points, be sure to obtain an x-ray film to verify placement and search for complications.

A. External Jugular: Place a shoulder roll beneath the patient and turn the head to the contralateral side (Fig 9–2). If central venous line is attempted, use a soft J-wire to prevent perforation of the tortuous vein. For patients needing only a simple IV placement, an intravenous catheter is appropriate.

B. Internal Jugular: Once the patient has been prepared, draped, and positioned as shown (Fig 9–3), feel for the trachea halfway between the angle of the jaw and the suprasternal notch and then feel lateral to the trachea for the carotid artery. At that point, at a 30-degree angle from horizontal, insert a

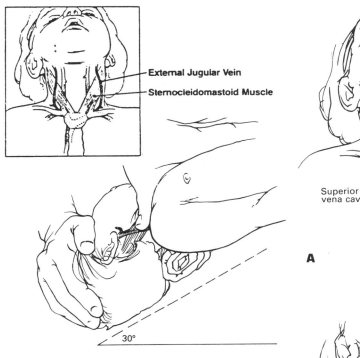

Figure 9–2. External jugular vein technique. (Reproduced, with permission, from Chameides, L: *Textbook of Pediatric Advanced Life Support.* American Heart Association, 1988).

finder needle (25-gauge) over the carotid artery, aiming for the ipsilateral nipple. Once venous return is established, remove the finder needle and repeat the procedure using the Seldinger technique.

C. Subclavian Entry: After the patient has been prepared, draped, and positioned (Fig 9–4), move the needle flat along the chest, entering along the inferior edge of the clavicle and over the first rib just lateral to the midclavicular line and aiming for the suprasternal notch. Once venous return is established, use the Seldinger technique.

D. Femoral Approach: With the patient's leg slightly abducted (Fig 9–5), find the femoral artery 3–4 cm below the inguinal ligament. The femoral vein should be found along the path of the artery, but medial to it. Insert the needle at a 30- to 45-degree angle. Once venous return is established, use the Seldinger technique.

CENTRAL NERVOUS SYSTEM

COMA

This subject is covered in detail in Chapter 24. The workup of the comatose patient is complex and

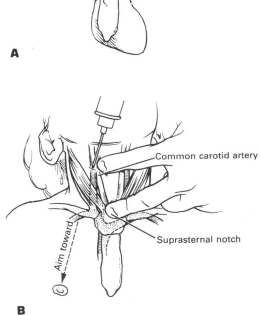

B

Figure 9–3. *A:* The internal jugular vein and its relationship to the surrounding anatomy. *B:* Technique, anterior internal jugular cannulation. (Reproduced, with permission, from Chameides, L: *Textbook of Pediatric Advanced Life Support.* American Heart Association, 1988.)

needs to be carried out quickly. Patients with known causes of coma should be treated appropriately for the underlying cause. Occasionally coma is induced in certain patients, eg, those with extreme and recalcitrant status epilepticus requiring pentobarbital coma therapy.

The comatose patient most often requires basic support, including the maintenance of the airway by intubation and ventilation. Nutritional support is important and should be started early. Monitoring the comatose child is important, and a convenient scale, such as the Glasgow coma scale, should be applied to monitor neurologic status. Many pediatric centers have adapted a version of this scale for their patients.

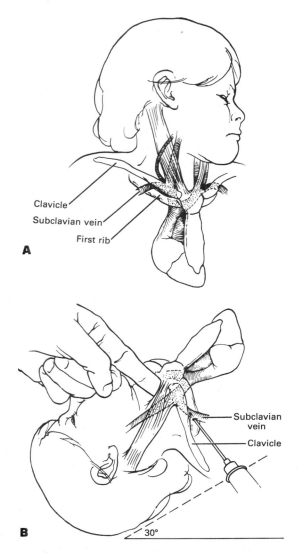

Figure 9–4. Subclavian vein. **A:** Anatomy. **B:** Technique. (Reproduced, with permission, from Chameides, L: *Textbook of Pediatric Advanced Life Support.* American Heart Association, 1988.)

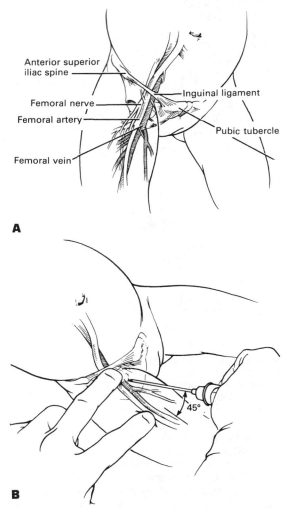

Figure 9–5. Femoral vein. **A:** Anatomy. **B:** Technique. (Reproduced, with permission, from Chameides, L: *Textbook of Pediatric Advanced Life Support.* American Heart Association, 1988.)

CEREBRAL EDEMA

Cerebral edema is a major cause of morbidity and mortality in the PICU. Three mechanisms or categories of cerebral edema have been defined. **Cytotoxic edema** is caused by direct cellular injury, usually as a consequence of hypoxia or anoxia. Cellular energy stores are depleted, and ionic pumps of the cell cease activity, causing fluid to accumulate in the cell. **Vasogenic edema** is the result of direct injury to the blood-brain barrier. The normally tight junctions of capillary endothelium are injured, allowing extravasation of water and protein into the interstitium of the brain. Traumatic head injury characteristically

results in this type of edema. **Interstitial edema** is caused by overproduction of cerebrospinal fluid (CSF) or impaired ability to drain CSF.

Cerebral edema from traumatic head injury may lead to increased ICP, which causes cerebral dysfunction and damage; therefore, treatment of the elevated ICP may be helpful. Cerebral edema associated with already-resolved hypoxic-ischemic injury may not be responsive to ICP treatment. It remains to be determined which patients respond to treatment of elevated cerebral pressures and which treatment is most effective.

Clinical Findings

A. Symptoms and Signs: Patients with elevations in ICP may develop headaches, vomiting, impaired vision with diplopia, seizures, and coma. Physical examination may demonstrate an enlarged head circumference (in infants prior to suture fusion), papilledema, hyporeflexia, or hyperreflexia, depending on the location of the lesion and the length of time it has been present. The young patient may not demonstrate the Cushing reflex (increase in blood pressure and bradycardia). These signs and symptoms may be quite subtle, especially in patients with longstanding, mild-to-moderate cerebral edema. A complete history and physical are often the most useful tools.

B. ICP Monitoring (Table 9–10): The decision to monitor the ICP of a patient is not always clear. Patients with acute closed head injury, acute noncommunicating hydrocephalus, and Reye's syndrome appear to benefit most from ICP monitoring. Patients with cerebral hemorrhage, meningitis, encephalitis, and cerebral mass lesions may also benefit from ICP monitoring. Patients with hypoxic-ischemic injuries (eg, due to near-drowning or respiratory arrest) have not been shown to benefit from ICP monitoring.

Treatment

It is not always necessary to know the ICP before starting treatment. The natural history of the patient's disease often gives sufficient indication to institute treatment early. The following steps outline the approach to treating patients with elevations in ICP.

1. The head of the bed should be elevated to a 30-degree angle and the patient's head kept in the midline to facilitate venous drainage.
2. Ventilation should be used in maintaining the airway (Po_2 greater than 80 torr and Pco_2 25–30 torr) to reduce cerebral blood flow.
3. Proper circulation and blood pressure must be maintained to provide a good cerebral perfusion pressure (CPP = mean arterial pressure − intracranial pressure). This pressure, which should be 50–60 mm Hg, is maintained by volume resuscitation or by improving the cardiac status with inotropic drugs if necessary. If the patient is significantly hypertensive, a trial of short-acting hypotensive agents may be necessary to determine if the elevated blood pressure is causing a secondary elevation of ICP.
4. Patients often must be paralyzed to control ventilation and reduce the agitation induced by ICU procedures. Most relaxants need to be stopped at least once every 24 hours for reevaluation of neurologic status.
5. Sedation is controversial and if used should be tailored to each patient realizing that many of the agents can lower blood pressure and therefore the cerebral perfusion pressure. Sedatives also may mask neurologic changes that are important indicators of changing CNS status.
6. Fluid therapy needs early control. In those patients not requiring intravascular volume repletion, some restriction is helpful. In patients who can withstand a reduction of intravascular volume, administering mannitol and furosemide reduces the intravascular volume. Raising the osmolality of the blood to between 300–310 mosm/dL helps to keep the ICP as low as possible. Osmolality and the electrolyte status must be monitored constantly, because the syndrome of inappropriate antidiuretic hormone (SIADH) or diabetes insipidus (DI) may develop at any time. Nutrition needs should be addressed early to ensure adequate glucose supply. Physicians must keep in mind that certain patients have very high caloric requirements.
7. Lidocaine or thiopental loading before painful procedures is often helpful in blunting ICP elevation. More aggressive therapies, such as pentobarbital coma, hypothermia, and decompressive craniotomy, may be helpful in a very limited patient group and all have very serious complications.

Baethmann A: Mediators of brain edema and secondary brain damage. *Crit Care Med* 1988;**16**:972.

Table 9–10. Comparison of intracranial pressure monitoring techniques.[1]

Type of Monitor	Placement	Advantages	Disadvantages
External (pressure-sensitive)	Over the skin of open anterior fontanelle	Noninvasive Useful as trending device	Very indirect measurement Useful in limited age group
Epidural (fiberoptic, hydraulic, & pneumatic)	Between skull and dura	Easy placement Low risk of infection Difficult to occlude	Unable to draw off CSF fluid May create epidural bleeding
Subarachnoid (hydraulic or fiberoptic)	Between dura and brain substance	Easy placement Low risk of infection	May be occluded by debris Unable to draw off CSF fluid May give falsely low readings
Intraventricular (hydraulic and/or fiberoptic)	Inside the lateral ventricle	Most direct measurement Therapeutic if able to draw off CSF	Requires adequately sized lateral ventricles Increased risk of bleeding and infection

Culditz PB: Fontanelle pressure and cerebral perfusion pressure: Continuous measurements in neonates. *Crit Care Med* 1988;**16**:876.

Dean JM, Rogers MC, Traystman RJ: Pathophysiology and clinical management of intracranial vault. In: *Textbook of Pediatric Intensive Care*. Rogers MC (editor). Williams and Wilkins, 1987.

Duck SC, Wyatt DT: Factors associated with brain herniation in the treatment of diabetic ketoacidosis. *J Pediatr* 1988;**113**:10.

Guertin SR: Cerebral fluid shunts: Evaluation, complications, and crisis management. *Pediatr Clin North Am* 1987;**34**:203.

Heffnen JE, Sahn SA: Controlled hyperventilation in patients with intracranial hypertension: Application and management. *Arch Intern Med* 1983;**143**:837.

Kaner RK: Infectious complications and duration of intracranial pressure monitors. *Crit Care Med* 1985;**13**:837.

McGillicuday JE: Cerebral protection: Pathophysiology and treatment of increased intracranial pressure. *Chest* 1985;**87**:85.

Rogers MC, Traystman RJ: An overview of the intracranial vault. *Crit Care Clin* 1985;**1**:195.

BRAIN RESUSCITATION

The critical care literature is filled with new information regarding mechanisms of cerebral injury during hypoxic-ischemic damage. Attempts to reverse this damage have generally met with little success. The role of hypoxia and ischemia in causing damage is related both to the metabolic breakdown caused by intracellular hypoxia and by the cascade of events that follows the cell reperfusion. Researchers are aggressively investigating reperfusion injury, looking at the involvement of such agents as oxygen radicals, lactic acid, calcium, and products of arachidonate metabolism. Cerebral resuscitation in the future could involve calcium channel blockers, blockage of the production of free oxygen radicals, and inhibition of prostaglandin synthesis. One must keep in mind that respiratory arrest in the research setting causes more brain damage than does the global ischemia caused by circulatory arrest. This finding is worrisome because the typical arrest in pediatrics is respiratory.

Dean JM: Theories of brain resuscitation. In: *Textbook of Pediatric Intensive Care*. Rogers MC (editor). Williams and Wilkins, 1987.

Hoff JT: Cerebral protection. *J Neurosurg* 1986;**65**:579.

Kochanek PM: Novel pharmacologic approaches to brain resuscitation after cardiorespiratory arrest in the pediatric patient. *Crit Care Clin* 1988;**4**:661.

Koehler RC, Michael JR: Cardiopulmonary resuscitation, brain blood flow, and neurologic recovery. *Crit Care Clin* 1985;**1**:205.

Krause GS: Brain cell death following ischemia and reperfusion: A proposed biochemical sequence. *Crit Care Med* 1988;**16**:714.

Safar P: Resuscitation from clinical death: Pathophysiologic limits and therapeutic potentials. *Crit Care Med* 1988;**16**:923.

STATUS EPILEPTICUS

Status epilepticus exists when a child has a single seizure lasting over 30 minutes or a series of seizures lasting over 30 minutes without regaining consciousness (see Chapter 24). Several reviews of status epilepticus document mortality rates of 6–11%. The longer the duration of status epilepticus, the greater the morbidity and mortality. Status epilepticus requires, in addition to routine ICU monitoring, electroencephelographic monitoring, if possible. EEGs obtained at the bedside (compressed spectral analysis), although not as accurate as 21-channel EEGs, may be very helpful in titrating drug therapy.

Treatment

After ensuring the adequacy of the airway and circulation, the physician must assess metabolic conditions and institute appropriate treatment. To control seizures, physicians should first administer a benzodiazepine such as diazepam or lorazepam. These drugs usually work within 10 minutes, and patients receiving them require close observation for respiratory depression. The next drug of choice is phenobarbital, which usually works within 1 hour. This drug also causes sedation and respiratory depression. Phenytoin is not as sedating but does have cardiac side effects. Paraldehyde and valproic acid are available for patients with seizures refractory to the above drugs. For patients with extremely refractory status epilepticus, several therapies are available. These include pentobarbital coma, general anesthesia, and lidocaine infusions.

Dean JM, Singer HS: Status epilepticus. In: *Textbook of Pediatric Intensive Care*. Rogers MC (editor). Williams and Wilkins, 1987.

Delgado-Esaeta AV: Management of status epilepticus. *N Engl J Med* 1982;**306**:1337.

Ferry PC, Banner W, Wolf RA: *Seizure Disorders in Children*. Lippincott, 1986.

Lacey DJ: Lorazepam therapy of status epilepticus in children and adolescents. *J Pediatr* 1986;**108**:771.

Orlowski JP: Hypothermia and barbiturate coma for refractory status epilepticus. *Crit Care Med* 1984;**12**:367.

Phillips SA, Shanahan RJ: Etiology and mortality of status epilepticus in children. *Arch Neurol* 1989;**46**:74.

BRAIN DEATH

The declaration of brain death in the hospital almost always occurs in the ICU. The evolution of the guidelines and laws regarding the declaration of brain death in the United States can be traced to the Harvard Ad Hoc Committee, which examined the definition of brain death in 1968. Since then, several studies have refined the standards. Two works are of special relevance to the pediatric population: Ashwal and Schnieder's "Brain Death in Children" and the Special Task Force Guidelines for determination of brain death. Here is a summary of Ashwal and Schnieder's recommendations for the declaration of brain death in children:

1. Normothermic and normotensive child without volume depletion.
2. A state of coma (no response to external stimuli) that is not related to toxins, metabolic influences, or drugs whose effects are potentially reversible.
3. Absent brain stem reflexes and any one of the following:
   a. Clinical exam that shows no improvement in 24 hours.
   b. Adequate cerebral perfusion study showing no flow.
   c. Two EEGs 12 hours apart that are isoelectric.

Each hospital should develop a set of standards specifically reflecting local standards of medical practice and applicable state law.

Ashwal S, Schnieder S: Brain death in children. (2 parts.) *Pediatr Neurol* 1987;**3**:5 and 69.
Freeman JM, Ferry PC: New brain death guidelines in children: Further confusion. *Pediatrics* 1988;**81**:301.
Setzer HA, Rogers MC: Brain death in children. In: *Textbook of Pediatric Intensive Care*. Rogers MC (editor). Williams and Wilkins, 1987.
Task Force Committee Membership: Guidelines for the determination of brain death in children. *Pediatrics* 1987; **80**:298.

NUTRITIONAL SUPPORT AFTER INJURY

Metabolic and Physiologic Responses

Trauma, sepsis, and significant injury are associated with a variety of profound metabolic and physiologic responses (Table 9–11). These responses, in general, result in the catabolism of whole body protein with subsequent negative nitrogen balance, the hallmarks of the metabolic responses to injury.

Plasma hormone levels are generally elevated as a result of injury. Increases in insulin, glucagon, catecholamines, and glucocorticoids have been reported. Insulin causes increased synthesis of triglycerides and inhibits lipoprotein lipase, thus accounting for the low levels of free fatty acids frequently observed in febrile or injured patients. Reduced serum ketone bodies, often observed in the injured patient, may also be accounted for by increased insulin levels. This reduction in ketones is not insignificant because of the usual protein-sparing effect that ketones provide.

Glucose metabolism is significantly altered in critically ill patients. Despite elevated insulin levels, hyperglycemia and glucose intolerance are frequently observed in the critically ill. This problem is partially due to the increased secretion of counterregu-

Table 9–11. Metabolic and physiologic responses to severe illness.

Physiologic
  Muscle function
    Easier fatigability
    Slower relaxation
    Altered force-frequency pattern
  Respiration
    Increased minute ventilation secondary to increased respiratory frequency
    Inefficient gas exchange (increased VD/VT)
    Increased carbon dioxide responsiveness
Metabolic
  Hormone and hormonelike levels
    Increased insulin
    Increased glucocorticoids
    Increased catecholamines
    Increased interleukin-1
    Increased tumor necrosis factor
  Carbohydrate metabolism
    Increased blood sugar
    Increased gluconeogenesis
    Increased glucose turnover
    Glucose intolerance
  Fat metabolism
    Increased lipid turnover and utilization
    Insuppressible lipolysis
    Decreased ketogenesis
  Protein metabolism
    Increased muscle protein catabolism
    Increased muscle branched-chain amino acid oxidation
    Increased serum amino acids
    Increased mitogen losses

latory products, such as glucagon, cortisol, and norepinephrine, which promote glycogenolysis and enhance the synthesis of glucose from noncarbohydrate compounds (ie, gluconeogenesis). Gluconeogenesis in injury is primarily due to mobilization of alanine, glutamine, and other amino acids from muscle and their biosynthesis to glucose and urea by the liver. The gluconeogenesis observed in injury, as opposed to that seen in starvation, is not easily inhibited or decreased by glucose infusions. Insulin resistance may also develop in skeletal muscle and peripheral adipose tissues in postinjury states. Decreased glucose and fatty acid uptake results, and the energy needs of skeletal muscle must be met by the increased oxidation of the branched-chain amino acids (BCAA). Because BCAAs are essential amino acids, their oxidation depletes a valuable pool of precursors required for protein synthesis.

Lipids are the major energy source during periods of stress starvation. Lipolysis occurs despite high levels of insulin. During stress starvation, peripheral tissues, such as skeletal muscle, myocardium, and respiratory muscles, are able to utilize lipids as their major energy source. This is true despite high circulating levels of glucose because of the suppression of glucose use in these tissues. In the stressed patient, lipolysis is much more rapid and efficient and may cause unrelenting depletion of fat stores.

Significant changes in protein metabolism occur in stress. The contribution of protein to total calorie expenditure (protein utilization) increases from 10% in normal children to 15–20% in severely stressed children. There are also marked changes in nitrogen dynamics following injury because of increases in nitrogen excretion. Amino acid levels may be elevated in stressed patients because of the insuppressible gluconeogenesis. Increased levels of alanine and BCAAs have been correlated with survival in septic patients. Studies in burn patients and septic animal models demonstrate both increased protein synthesis and breakdown. Most critically ill patients are in negative nitrogen balance (protein degradation exceeds synthesis). This condition can be reduced or even reversed with increased nonprotein caloric and protein nutrition, and the increased nutrient intake appears to make a difference in the ability of the patient to tolerate periods of stress.

These abnormalities in classic hormone profiles do not entirely explain the breakdown of skeletal muscle protein. Recent work has demonstrated release of interleukin-1 (IL-1) by phagocytes under the stress of sepsis or trauma. Numerous effects of IL-1 have been reported, including release of amino acids from muscle, increased synthesis of acute-phase proteins, fever, neutrophilia, and activation of T and B cells. Another monokine, tumor necrosis factor (TNF), is increased under stress conditions. Among its many effects is the inhibition of lipoprotein lipase. This could contribute to a reduced capacity of peripheral tissues to utilize triglycerides, leading to further muscle wasting. These findings appear to link the metabolic and immunologic reactions to infection and trauma.

Besides loss of tissue mass, muscle function abnormalities are also observed during stress. Among the abnormalities reported are an altered force-frequency pattern, slower relaxation, and easier muscle fatigability. Easier fatigability could contribute to the subjective feeling of weakness that accompanies recovery from surgery or injury. Significant changes in the pattern of ventilation have been reported. These include increased minute ventilation (secondary to increases in respiratory frequency) and increases in the ratio of dead space to tidal volume ventilation.

Nutritional Assessment

The physician assessing the nutritional needs of the injured patient must address 2 major issues: (1) the preexisting nutritional status of the patient and (2) the degree of stress imposed by the disease process.

The pediatric patient appears at a marked disadvantage compared to adults during periods of stress starvation. Not only is there the problem of increased proteolysis that is less responsive to carbohydrate administration alone, but there is an additional caloric requirement for growth. If this extra energy is not available, growth ceases.

Several methods are available for assessing nutritional status (see Chapter 5). The degree of metabolic stress accompanying the injury should also be examined. Resting energy expenditure is elevated by a minimum of approximately 15% in critically ill patients and may be much higher. The energy needs of a patient may be approximated by multiplying the estimated basal metabolic rate (BMR), as derived from the Harris-Benedict equation, by a factor of 1.75:

Male: BMR = $66 + (13.7 \times W) + (5.0 \times H) - (6.8 \times A)$
Female: BMR = $655 + (9.6 \times W) + (1.7 \times H) - (4.7 \times A)$

where BMR = basal metabolic rate in kilo calories; W = weight in kilograms; H = height in centimeters; A = age in years.

Another practical method of evaluating the nutritional stresses on a patient is by computing a catabolic index:

Catabolic index = $UUN - (0.5 \times N_{in} + 3)$

where UUN = 24-hour urine urea nitrogen in grams; N_{in} = 24 hour nitrogen intake in grams.

This equation expresses the level of dietary intake and the extent of protein degradation as a single number. Scores of -5 to 0 indicate no significant stress; 0 to 5, moderate stress; and 5 to 10, severe stress. High scores may predict which patients may benefit from amino acid solution augmented with BCAAs.

Enteral and Parenteral Alimentation

A. Enteral Alimentation: Present evidence suggests that the enteral route of feeding provides a more normal and homeostatic milieu than parenteral feeding does. Several advantages over parenteral nutrition have been demonstrated. Some reports suggest that host response or defense during stress starvation may be improved when the patient is fed via the gastrointestinal tract. Others have demonstrated that malnutrition increased mortality in laboratory animals after septic peritonitis. Further, malnourished animals fed enterally had much higher survival rates after sepsis induced by *Escherichia coli* than septic animals fed parenterally. Both cellular and humoral immunity can be affected by route of feeding. Lymphocyte function and secretory immunoglobulin A levels are better in animals fed enterally than in those fed parenterally. Lower levels of catabolic hormones (cortisol, glucagon, norepinephrine) have been found in injured animals following early institution of enteral feeding than in injured animals receiving parenteral nutrition. Thus, the hypermetabolic state may be reduced by early enteral feeding. Jejunal weight and thickness are also improved by enteral feeding. This increase has beneficial effects on GI function, including potentially decreased translocation of bacteria across the gut, which could reduce the incidence of secondary infections in stressed patients. Enteral nutrition may also protect against stress ulceration, a serious yet not uncommon complication in severely ill patients.

Complications of enteral feeding are relatively common in critically ill children. Nausea and vomiting occur in up to 20% of patients, usually when gastric emptying time is prolonged as a result of paralytic ileus or gastrointestinal edema. Edema may occur postoperatively or in response to trauma, burns, sepsis, or malnutrition. The incidence of diarrhea is high in critically ill patients receiving enteral alimentation. Diarrhea appears to be related to lower serum albumin levels. Hypoalbuminemia is associated with the development of diffuse gastrointestinal edema, resulting in impaired gastrointestinal absorptive capacity. Some patients with acute kwashiorkor-like hypoalbuminemia develop a protein-losing enteropathy. This can be diagnosed by elevated levels of fecal alpha$_1$-antitrypsin. Tolerance to enteral alimentation in hypoalbuminemic patients may be improved by providing peptide-based rather than standard intact protein diets. These diets are composed of protein hydrolysates of varying chain lengths and of varying concentrations of peptides, free amino acids, fat, and carbohydrate. This type of enteral alimentation attenuates protein turnover in the intestine and results in a rise in serum albumin level. It has been reported that this method of feeding avoids the need for parenteral albumin and TPN when intervention occurs early enough to prevent the development of malnutrition. Thus, peptide-based diets could improve nitrogen retention and the nutritional status of critically ill patients.

B. Parenteral Nutrition: When the gastrointestinal tract is not functional and severe stress is present, central intravenous hyperalimentation should be instituted to provide adequate calories and nutrition during the hypermetabolic state. Carbohydrates should be provided at 2–3 mg/kg/min; proteins, at 1.5 g/kg/d; and fat, at approximately 15–33% of the total caloric demand. Rationales for these recommendations and for the provision of a balanced parenteral diet are provided in the Chapter 5. Because several complications and problems occur in patients with central lines, the placement of these lines must not be taken lightly. Placement of central lines is associated with such complications as pneumothorax, arterial injury, and infection. Central venous thrombosis at the catheter site has been documented by venography in up to 24% of patients. This complication may be reduced by the addition of heparin (1–3 units/mL) to the hyperalimentation solution. Hyperglycemia, which may already be present in the stressed patient, can be aggravated by the large amounts of glucose necessary to meet caloric demands. Insulin infusions occasionally may be necessary to control high levels of blood sugars. Last, if fever is present in a patient receiving central

intravenous alimentation, a routine protocol should be followed. In the absence of frank shock or purulent drainage around the catheter site (which would necessitate immediate removal of the catheter) the catheter can be changed over a wire (Seldinger technique). At this time, cultures are obtained on blood drawn through the catheter, on the catheter tip, and on the peripheral blood. Diagnosis and therapy are guided by culture results.

Balistrevi WF, Farrell MK: Enteral feeding: Scientific basis and clinical applications. Report of the Ninety-Fourth Ross Conference on Pediatric Research. Columbus Ohio, Ross Laboratories, 1988.

Hageman JR, Hunt CE: Fat emulsions and lung function. *Clin Chest Med* 1986;7:69.

Kinney JM, Weissman C: Forms of malnutrition in stressed and unstressed patients. *Clin Chest Med* 1986;7:19.

Lemoyne M, Khursheed NJ: Total parenteral nutrition in the critically ill patient. *Chest* 1986;89:568.

Skeie B: Intravenous emulsion and lung function: A revue. *Crit Care Med* 1988;16:183.

Swiwamer DL: Twenty-four hour emergency expenditure in critically ill patients. *Crit Care Med* 1987;15:637.

PAIN AND ANXIETY CONTROL

Anxiety control and pain relief are 2 of the most important responsibilities of the critical care physician. Earlier perceptions that children do not require pain relief have drastically changed in response to documented proof of improved outcomes in children receiving appropriate pain relief. The anxiety of patients in the ICU is well known. For pediatric patients in the ICU, intensivists are using everything from therapeutic recreation to powerful sedatives to reduce the anxiety of such a stressful environment.

The selection of drugs and mode of administration should fit the need. Commonly used pain-relief drugs other than acetaminophen, in order of increasing strength, are codeine, meperidine, morphine sulfate, methadone, and fentanyl. These narcotics are all respiratory depressants and are associated with other special complications (Table 9–12). With careful monitoring, morphine and fentanyl may be given as continuous infusions to improve steady-state pharmacodynamics. Methadone is used for very long term management because its half-life is *very* long (36–72 hours). When given concurrently, acetaminophen often potentiates the effect of the narcotics, which may be given in lower doses. The half-lives of these drugs are organ dependent, and organ dysfunction or failure may greatly prolong the effects of these drugs. Anxiolytic drugs may help pacify the terrified and uncomfortable infant or child. Benzodiazepines, including diazepam, lorazepam, and midazolam, are excellent for this purpose. Complications include respiratory depression and cardiac depression. Patients may receive midazolam as a continuous infusion or intramuscularly.

Table 9–12. Pain and anxiety control

Drug	Dose and Method of Administration[1]	Advantages	Disadvantages	Usual Duration of Effect
Morphine	IV; 0.1 mg/kg Continuous infusion; .01–.05 mg/kg/h	Excellent pain relief, reversible	Respiratory depression, hypotension, nausea, suppression of intestinal motility, histamine release	2–4 hours
Meperidine	IV; 1 mg/kg	Good pain relief, reversible	Respiratory depression, histamine release, nausea, suppression of intestinal motility	2–4 hours
Fentanyl	IV, 1–2 μg/kg; Continuous infusion; 0.5–2 μg/kg/h	Excellent pain relief, reversible, short half-life	Respiratory depression, chest-wall rigidity, severe nausea and vomiting	30 min
Diazepam	IV, 0.1 mg/kg	Sedation and seizure control	Respiratory depression, jaundice, phlebitis	1–3 hours
Lorazepam	IV, 0.1 mg/kg	Longer half-life, sedation and seizure control	Nausea and vomiting, respiratory depression, phlebitis	2–4 hours
Midazolam	IV, 0.1 mg/kg	Short half-life, only benzodiazapine given as continuous infusion	Respiratory depression	30–60 min

[1]IV administration is most common in the ICU. Effects of morphine, meperidine, and fentanyl are reversible by administration of naloxone (opiate antagonist).

Schecter NL, Allen DA, Hanson K: Status of pediatric pain control: A comparison of hospital analgesic usage in children and adults. *Pediatrics* 1986;**77**:11.

Yaster M, Deshpande JK: Management of pediatric pain with opioid analgesics. *J Pediatr* 1988;**113**:421.

COMPLICATIONS IN THE ICU

Because the ICU is home to patients who require the most aggressive of medical and surgical therapy, it is the setting of many serious complications. Knowledge of these complications is helpful in deciding how aggressive and invasive the interventions should be.

Hemodynamic access is a common source of complications. Intravenous infiltrations with such infusions as potassium, calcium, bicarbonate, and thiopental invite phlebitis and even skin necrosis. Arterial lines are occasionally associated with distal ischemia and loss of digits. The insertion of central venous lines is associated with major complications (incidence of 4–10%), including pneumothorax, hemothorax, arterial occlusion, and hemorrhage. Pulmonary artery catheters may knot intravascularly, rupture the pulmonary artery, or cause arrhythmias. All vascular catheters are infection prone and require careful, sterile placement and meticulous care.

Respiratory complications are related to the aggressiveness of the therapy. Intubation involves the risk of malplacement (bronchial and esophageal intubations), subglottic injury, or perforation of the trachea. Once ventilated, patients requiring high inflation pressures or high PEEP have a significant incidence of complications related to air leaks.

Nosocomial infections are rampant in the PICU, especially in patients with vascular catheters, urethral catheters, and endotrachial tubes. Patients should be followed closely for signs of infection, and invasive access should be discontinued as soon as medically prudent. Often the bacteria responsible for many of the nosocomial infections are specific to the ICU. With this knowledge, the help of the infectious disease consultant, and close monitoring, we can greatly decrease the morbidity and mortality from nosocomial infections.

Riggs CD, Lister G: Adverse occurrences in the pediatric intensive care unit. *Pediatr Clin North Am* 1987;**34**:93.

Smith-Wright DL: Complications of vascular catheterization in critically ill children. *Crit Care Med* 1984; **12**:1015.

Streiter RM, Lynch JP: Complications in the ventilated patient. *Clin Chest Med* 1988;**9**:127.

Adolescence

10

David W. Kaplan, MD, MPH, & Kathleen A. Mammel, MD

Adolescence is a unique period of rapid physical, emotional, cognitive, and social growth and development bridging childhood and adulthood. Generally, adolescence begins at age 11–12 years and ends between ages 18 and 21. Most teenagers complete puberty by ages 16–18 years; in Western society, however, for educational and cultural reasons, the adolescent period is prolonged to allow for further psychosocial development before the young person assumes adult responsibilities.

The developmental passage from childhood to adulthood encompasses: (1) completing puberty and somatic growth; (2) developing socially, emotionally, and cognitively—moving from concrete to abstract thinking; (3) establishing an independent identity and separating from the family; and (4) preparing for a career or vocation.

DEMOGRAPHY

In the United States in 1986, there were 18.6 million adolescents between the ages of 15 and 19 years and 20.4 million between 20 and 24 years of age. Adolescents and young adults, 15–24 years, constitute 16% of the US population.

MORTALITY

As with all age groups in the United States, there has been a remarkable decrease in the mortality rate among 15–24-year-olds during this century. Deaths due to infectious diseases such as tuberculosis, influenza, and pneumonia, which were common at the beginning of the century, are rare events today. During the last 20 years, there have been changes not only in the major causes of mortality in the adolescent and young adult population but also in disease-specific mortality rates. Mortality due to motor vehicle crashes, suicide, and homicide have increased between 300 and 400%. For the adolescent population, cultural and environmental rather than organic factors pose the greatest threats of death. For every 15–19-year-old who dies of cancer, 10 die as a result

of an unintentional injury.[1] For every teenager who dies of heart disease, 3.6 die as a result of homicide; for every teenager who dies of kidney disease, 65 commit suicide.

The 3 leading causes of mortality (Fig 10–1) in the adolescent population (ages 15–19 years) in 1986 were unintentional injuries (55.4%–78% of all unintentional injuries were caused by motor vehicle crashes), suicides (11.7%), and homicides (11.5%). These 3 violent causes of death accounted for 78.6% of all adolescent mortality among 15–19-year-olds. An analysis of the causes of mortality by ethnicity emphasizes how strongly socioeconomic factors contribute to adolescent mortality. The unintentional injury rate among white teenagers ages 15–19 years (52.6 in 100,000) is almost twice as high as that among blacks (27.9 in 100,000). This difference re-

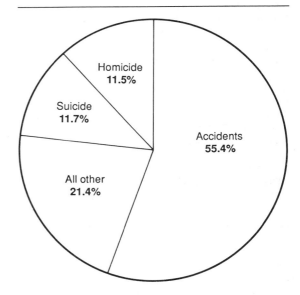

Figure 10–1. Mortality, ages 15–19 years, 1986.

---

[1]The term "injury" is preferable to "accidents," which implies "an act of God" or "bad luck." Injuries during this age period most commonly are related to motor vehicle accidents, drownings, falls, and fires. Injuries comprise 3 elements: the host (who is affected), the agent (the direct cause), and the environment (where, when, and under what conditions).

flects the high rate of mortality due to motor vehicle accidents among white males. By contrast, the homicide rate among black teenagers (31.9 in 100,000) is 5 times greater than that among white teenagers (6 in 100,000). Homicide is the leading cause of death for both male and female black teenagers. Suicide is 2½ times more prevalent among white teenagers (11.3 in 100,000) than black teenagers (4.6 in 100,000). Alcohol plays a significant role not only in mortality due to motor vehicle accidents but also in homicide and suicide. In 1985, 31% of 16-to-19-year-old drivers in fatal motor vehicle crashes had been drinking; 20% were legally intoxicated, with blood alcohol levels of 100 mg/dL or higher. Almost two-thirds of motor vehicle deaths involving young drinking drivers occur on Friday, Saturday, or Sunday, and 70% occur between 8:00 P.M. and 4:00 A.M.

Mortality due to unintentional injury, homicide, and suicide among adolescents and young adults is distressing not only because of its violent nature but also because these are largely preventable problems.

MORBIDITY

During the mid-1970s and 1980s, changes in North American society and the family have had a profound effect on many children and adolescents. Between 1955 and 1980, the divorce rate rose from about 400,000 to nearly 1,200,000 a year. Between 1960 and 1984, the number of children involved in divorce each year increased from 460,000 to 1,100,000. In 1984, nearly 26% of children were living in single-parent homes, compared with 13% in 1970. Over one-half of black children (59%) lived with a single parent, compared to 20% of white children. In 1983, the median income of 2-parent families was $27,286; of single-parent families headed by a man, $21,845; and for single-parent families headed by a woman, $11,789. Fewer than 20% of families headed by women have yearly incomes above $20,000.

The major causes of morbidity during adolescence are primarily psychosocial: unintended pregnancy, sexually transmitted disease, substance abuse, smoking, dropping out of school, depression, running away from home, physical violence, and juvenile delinquency. Early identification of the teenager at risk for these problems is important not only to prevent the immediate complications but also to prevent any future associated problems. High-risk behavior in one area is often associated with or may lead to problems in another area (Fig 10–2). For example, teenagers who live in a dysfunctional family (eg, having problems related to parental alcoholism or perhaps physical or sexual abuse) are much more likely than other teenagers to have emotional problems, such as depression. A depressed teenager is at greater risk for abusing drugs or alcohol, having ac-

ademic difficulties, running away from home, getting involved sexually as a means of seeking the attention and affection they are not receiving at home, acquiring a sexually transmitted disease, and having an unintended pregnancy.

The early indicators of an adolescent at high risk include the following:

(1) Decline in school performance.
(2) Excessive school absences or cutting class.
(3) Frequent or persistent psychosomatic complaints.
(4) Changes in sleeping or eating habits.
(5) Difficulty concentrating or persistent boredom.
(6) Signs or symptoms of depression, extreme stress, or anxiety.
(7) Withdrawal from friends or family, or change to a new group of friends.
(8) Unusually severe violent or rebellious behavior, or radical personality change.
(9) Parent-adolescent conflict.
(10) Sexual acting out.
(11) Conflict with the law.
(12) Suicidal thoughts or preoccupation with themes of death.
(13) Drug and alcohol abuse.
(14) Running away from home.

Centers for Disease Control: Violent deaths among persons 15–24 years of age—United States, 1970–1978. *MMWR* 1983;**32**:453.

Dubowitz H et al: The changing American family. *Pediatr Clin North Am* 1988;**35**:1291.

Irwin CE, Ryan SA: Problem behavior of adolescents. *Pediatr Rev* 1989;**10**:235.

McAnarney ER: Adolescent medicine: Growth of a discipline. *Pediatrics* 1988;**82**:270.

National Highway Traffic Safety Administration: Fatal Accident Reporting System 1985. Department of Transportation Publication No. HS 807–071, Feb 1987.

Wise PH, Meyers A: Poverty and child health. *Pediatr Clin North Am* 1988;**35**:1169.

DELIVERY OF HEALTH SERVICES

How, where, why, and when adolescents seek health care depend on a number of factors: ability to pay for care, distance to health care facilities, availability of transportation, accessibility of services, time out of school, and privacy. Many common teenage health problems—eg, unintended pregnancy, sexually transmitted disease, the need for contraception, substance abuse, and depression and other emotional problems—have moral or ethical implications. Teenagers are often reluctant to confide in their parents for fear of punishment and disapproval.

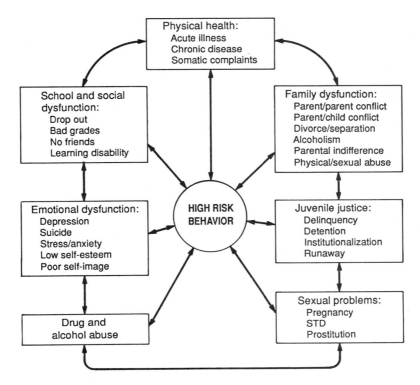

Figure 10–2. Interrelation of high-risk adolescent behavior.

For example, a 15-year-old boy who thinks he has gonorrhea might be reluctant to ask his mother to take him to the doctor. Recognizing this reality, health care providers have set up many specialized programs, eg, teenage family planning clinics, drop-in centers, VD clinics, hot lines, and adolescent clinics. For the physician, establishing a trusting and confidential relationship is basic to meeting an adolescent patient's health care needs. A patient who senses the physician will inform the parents about a confidential problem may lie or fail to disclose information essential for proper diagnosis and treatment.

RELATING TO THE ADOLESCENT PATIENT

Adolescence is one of the physically healthiest periods in an individual's life. The challenge of caring for adolescents does not lie in managing complex organic disease but in accommodating to the changing and developing cognitive, emotional, and psychosocial growth that influences health behavior.

How the physician initially approaches the adolescent may determine the success or failure of the visit. The physician should behave simply and honestly, without an authoritarian or excessively "professional" manner. Because the self-esteem of many

young adolescents is fragile, the physician must be careful not to overpower and intimidate the patient. To establish a comfortable and trusting relationship, the physician should strive to present the image of an ordinary person who has special training and skills.

Because onset and termination of puberty may vary considerably from individual to individual, chronologic age may be a poor indicator of expected physical, physiologic, and emotional development. In communicating with an adolescent, the physician needs to be especially sensitive to the patient's developmental level, recognizing that physical appearance and chronologic age may be misleading as a measure of cognitive development. Talking to a teenager as a child or, at the other extreme, as an adult, may weaken communication and confidence in the provider.

Working with teenagers can be quite draining emotionally. Adolescents have a unique ability to identify hidden emotional vulnerabilities. The physician who has a personal need to control patients or foster dependency may be disappointed caring for teenagers. Because teenagers are consumed with their own emotional needs, they rarely provide the physician with the ego rewards that younger or older patients do.

The physician should be sensitive to the issue of countertransference, the emotional reaction elicited in the physician by the adolescent. How the physician relates to the adolescent patient often depends on many personal characteristics of the physician. This is especially true of physicians treating families with parent-adolescent conflicts. It is common for young physicians to overidentify with the teenage patient and for older physicians to see the conflict from the parents' perspective. Older physicians with adolescent children may carry over many of their own parenting conflicts, dealing with the adolescent patient as they would with their own children. Over-identification with the parents is readily sensed by the teenager, who is likely to view the physician as just another authority figure who cannot understand the problems of being a teenager. Assuming a parental-authoritarian role as a physician and lecturing the adolescent not only is counterproductive but also may seriously jeopardize establishing a working relationship with the patient. In the case of the young physician, overidentification with the teenager may cause the parents to become extremely defensive about their parenting role and discount the experience and ability of the physician.

Meeks JE: *The Fragile Alliance*. Krieger, 1980.

THE SETTING

Adolescents respond positively to a setting and services that communicate a sensitivity to their age. For instance, a pediatrician's waiting room scattered with toddler's toys and exam tables too short for a young adult make adolescent patients feel that they have outgrown the practice. Similarly, a waiting room filled with geriatric or pregnant patients can make a teenager feel out of place. An exam room designed with adolescents in mind and special appointment times may be useful in engaging this age group.

It is not uncommon to see a new teenage patient who has absolutely no interest in being there, especially when the teenager is brought in for an evaluation of drug and alcohol use, parent-adolescent conflict, school failure, depression, or a suspected eating disorder. Even in cases of an acute physical illness, the adolescent may feel anxiety about having a physical examination, especially if the teenager is overly modest, is worried about having blood drawn, or simply fears the unknown. If future visits are to be successful, the physician must spend time on the first visit to give the teenager a sense of trust and an opportunity to feel comfortable.

CONFIDENTIALITY

It is helpful at the beginning of the visit to talk with the adolescent and the parents about what to expect. The physician should address the issue of confidentiality, telling the parents that two meetings—one with the teenager alone and one only with the parents—will take place. Adequate time must be spent with both the patient and the parents, or important information may be missed. At the beginning of the interview with the patient, it is useful to say, "I am likely to ask you some personal questions. This is not because I am trying to snoop into your private life, but because these questions may be important to your health. I want to assure you that what we talk about is confidential, just between the two of us. If there is something I feel we should discuss with your parents, I will ask your permission first, unless I feel it is life-threatening."

THE STRUCTURE OF THE VISIT

Caring for adolescents is a time-intensive process. In many adolescent practices, a 40–50% no-show rate is not unusual, making scheduling complex. In addition, it is not uncommon for an adolescent to come in without an appointment because of a seemingly minor complaint. Because of issues related to confidentiality, teenagers may initially conceal their real concern. For example, a healthy appearing 15-year-old girl may walk in with the chief complaint of a sore throat but actually be worried about being pregnant. What initially appeared to be a 10-minute visit for a throat culture may turn into a 1-hour visit spent counseling an anxious pregnant teenager.

By the age of 11 to 12, patients should be seen alone, without a parent. This gives them an opportunity to ask any questions they may be embarrassed to ask in front of a parent. Because of the physical changes that take place in early puberty, some adolescents are too self-conscious to undress in front of a parent (and sometimes the physician). If an adolescent comes in willingly, either for an acute illness or a routine physical examination, it may be helpful to meet with the adolescent and parent together to obtain the history. In the case of angry adolescents who are brought in against their will, it is useful to meet with the parents and adolescent just long enough to have the parents describe the conflict and state their concerns. This meeting should last no longer than 3 to 5 minutes, and then the adolescent should be seen alone. This approach conveys that the physician is primarily interested in the adolescent patient, yet gives the physician an opportunity to acknowledge the parents' anger and the fact that the patient probably didn't want to come in the first place.

The Interview

The first few minutes of the interview may dictate the success of the visit—whether or not a trusting relationship can be established. Taking a few minutes getting to know the patient is time well spent. For example, immediately asking a teenager who is brought in for suspected marihuana use "Do you smoke marihuana?'' confirms the adolescent's negative preconceptions about the physician and the purpose of the visit.

It is preferable to spend a few minutes asking nonthreatening questions. Examples are: ''Tell me a little bit about yourself so I can get to know you.'' ''What do you like to do best?'' ''What do you like to do least?'' ''What are your friends like?'' Neutral questions help defuse some of the patient's anger and anxiety. Examples are: ''How has your health been?'' ''What kinds of serious accidents or injuries have you had?'' Toward the end of the interview, the physician can ask more directed questions about psychosocial concerns.

Medical history questionnaires for the patient and the parents are very useful in collecting the necessary historical data and making the visit as efficient as possible (Fig 10–3). Although the history questionnaire is helpful, the physician must spend sufficient time to get to know the patient and establish a meaningful relationship.

The history should include an assessment of progress with psychodevelopmental tasks and of behaviors that are potentially detrimental to health. The review of systems should include questions about the following:

(1) Nutrition: number and balance of meals; calcium, iron, cholesterol intake.
(2) Sleep: number of hours, problems with insomnia or frequent waking.
(3) Seatbelt: regularity of use.
(4) Self-care: knowledge of testicular or breast self-exam, dental hygiene, and exercise.
(5) Family relationships: parents, siblings, relatives.
(6) Peers: best friend, involvement in group activities, boy/girlfriend.
(7) School: attendance, grades, activities.
(8) Educational and vocational interests: college, career, short- and long-term vocational plans.
(9) Tobacco: use of cigarettes, snuff, chewing tobacco.
(10) Substance abuse: frequency, extent, and history of alcohol and drug use.
(11) Sexuality: sexual activity, contraceptive use, pregnancies, history of sexually transmitted disease, number of sexual partners, risk for HIV infection.
(12) Emotional health: signs of depression and excessive stress.

The physician's personal attention and interest is likely to be a new experience for the teenager, who has probably experienced medical care only through a parent. The teenager should leave the visit with a sense of having a personal physician.

Physical Examination

During early adolescence many teenagers may be quite shy and modest, especially if examined by a physician of the opposite sex. The examiner should address this concern directly, because it can be allayed by acknowledging the uneasiness verbally and explaining the purpose of the examination, for example, ''Many boys that I see who are your age are embarrassed to have their penis and testes (balls) examined. This is an important part of the exam for a couple of reasons. First, I want to make sure that there aren't any physical problems and second, it helps me determine if your development is proceeding normally.'' This also introduces the subject of sexual development for discussion.

A pictorial chart of sexual development (Figs 10–4 and 10–5) is extremely useful in showing the patient how development is proceeding and what changes to expect in the future. The chart shows the relationship between height, breast development, menstruation, and pubic hair growth in the female and between height, penis and testes development, and pubic hair growth in the male. Although many teenagers do not openly admit that they are interested in this subject, they are usually quite attentive during the discussion. This discussion is particularly useful in counseling teenagers who lag behind their peers in physical development.

Because teenagers are especially sensitive about their changing bodies, it is useful to comment on the findings during the physical exam, for example, ''Your heart sounds fine. I am examining your breasts and feel a small lump under your right breast. This is very common during puberty in boys. It is called gynecomastia and should disappear in 6 months to a year. Don't worry, you are not turning into a girl.''

The question of the appropriate age for the first pelvic examination often arises. The following are indications for a pelvic examination in a teenage girl:

(1) Sexual intercourse. (The pelvic examination should be done for purposes of contraceptive counseling and to rule out sexually transmitted disease.)
(2) Abnormal vaginal discharge.
(3) Menstrual irregularities, eg, amenorrhea, hypermenorrhea, dysmenorrhea.
(4) Suspicion of anatomic abnormalities, eg, diethylstilbestrol exposure, imperforate hymen.
(5) Pelvic pain.
(6) Patient request of an examination.

If a teenage girl has not been sexually active and has no gynecologic complaints or abnormalities, a pelvic examination is usually not necessary until about age 18.

Holder AR: Minors' rights to consent to medical care. *JAMA* 1987;**257**:3400.

Marks A, Fisher M: Health assessment and screening during adolescence. *Pediatrics* 1987;**80(Suppl)**:135.

TEEN HEALTH HISTORY

This information is *strictly confidential.* Its purpose is to help your caregiver give you better care. We request that you fill out the form completely, but you may skip any question that you do not wish to answer.

NAME _____ DATE _____
     FIRST   MIDDLE INITIAL   LAST

BIRTHDATE_____ AGE_____ GRADE_____ Name that you like to be called_____

1. Why did you come to the clinic today? _____
   _____
   _____

STRICTLY CONFIDENTIAL

Medical History
2. Are you allergic to any medicines?   . . . .   YES NO
   Name of medicine _____
3. Are you taking any medicines now?   . . . .   YES NO
   Name of medicine _____
4. Do you have any longterm health conditions? . . . .   YES NO
   Condition _____
5. Date or age at your last tetanus (or dT) shot) _____

School Information
6. What grade do you usually make in English? _____
   (Example: A, B, C, D, E, F)
7. What grade do you usually make in Math? _____
8. How many days were you absent from school last semester?_____
9. How many days were you absent last semester due to illness?_____
10. How do you get along at school? _____

| 1 | 2 | 3 | 4 | 5 | 6 | 7 |
| TERRIBLE | | | | | | GREAT |

11. Have you ever been suspended?   . . . .   YES NO
12. Have you ever dropped out of school?   . . . .   YES NO
13. Do you plan to graduate from high school?   . . . .   YES NO

Job/Career Information
14. Are you working?   . . . .   YES NO
    If YES, What is your job?_____
    How many hours do you work per week? _____
15. What are your future plans or career goals? _____

Family Information
16. Who do you live with? (Check all that apply.)
    _____Both natural parents   _____Stepmother   _____ Brother(s)-ages:___
    _____Mother   _____Stepfather   _____ Sister(s)-ages: ___
    _____Father   _____Guardian   _____Other: explain ____
    _____Adoptive parents   _____Alone
17. Have there been any changes in your family such as: (Check all the changes that apply.)
    _____a. Marriage   _____d. Serious illness   _____g. Births
    _____b. Separation   _____e. Loss of job   _____h. Deaths
    _____c. Divorce   _____f. Move to a new house _____i. Other
18. Father's/stepfather's occupation or job: _____
    Mother's/stepmother's occupation or job: _____

Figure 10–3. Adolescent medical history questionnaire.

19. How do you get along at home?

1	2	3	4	5	6	7
TERRIBLE						GREAT

20. Have you ever run away from home? .... YES NO
21. Have you ever lived in foster care or an institution? .... YES NO

Self Information

22. On the whole, how do you like yourself?

1	2	3	4	5	6	7
NOT VERY MUCH						A LOT

23. What do you do best? _____
24. If you could, what would you like to change about your life or yourself? _____

_____

25. List any habits you would like to break. _____

_____

26. Do you feel people expect too much of you? .... YES NO
27. How do you get along with your friends/peers?

1	2	3	4	5	6	7
TERRIBLE						GREAT

28. Do you feel you have any friends you can count on? .... YES NO
29. Have you ever felt really sad or depressed for more than 3 days in a row? . YES NO
30. Have you ever thought of suicide as a solution to your problems? ...... YES NO
31. Have you gotten into any trouble because of your anger/temper? ...... YES NO

Health Concern

32. On a scale of 1–7, how would you rate your general health?

1	2	3	4	5	6	7
TERRIBLE						GREAT

33. Do you have questions or concerns about any of the following? (Check those that apply.)

___Height/Weight
___Blood pressure
___Head/headaches
___Dizziness/passing out
___Eyes/vision
___Ears/hearing/earaches
___Nose/frequent colds
___Mouth/teeth
___Neck/Back
___Chest/breathing/coughing
___Breasts
___Heart
___Stomach/pain/vomiting
___Diarrhea/constipation

___Skin rash
___Arms, legs/muscle or joint pain
___Frequent or painful urination
___Wetting the bed
___Sexual organs/genitals
___Trouble sleeping
___Tiredness
___Diet food/appetite
___Eating disorder
___Smoking, drugs, alcohol
___Future plans/jobs
___Worried about parents

___Family violence/physical abuse
___Feeling down or depressed
___Dating
___Sex
___Worried about VD/STD
___Masturbation
___Sexual abuse/rape
___Having children/parenting/ adoption
___Cancer or dying
___Other (explain) _____
_____

Health Behavior Information

34. Do you ever drive after drinking or when high?...................... YES NO
35. Do you ever smoke cigarettes? .... YES NO
36. Do you ever smoke marijuana? .... YES NO
37. Do you ever drink alcoholic beverages? .... YES NO
38. Do you ever use street drugs (speed, cocaine, acid, crack, etc.)? .... YES NO
39. Does anyone in your household smoke? .... YES NO
40. Does anyone in your family have a problem with drugs or alcohol? .... YES NO
41. Have you ecer been in trouble with the law? .... YES NO
42. Have you begun dating? .... YES NO

Figure 10–3 (cont'd.). Adolescent medical history questionnaire.

STRICTLY CONFIDENTIAL

43. Do you currently have a boyfriend or girlfriend? .... YES NO
    If YES, how old is he/she?.. YES NO
44. Do you think you might be gay/lesbian/homosexual)? .... YES NO
45. Have you ever had sex (sexual intercourse)? .... YES NO
46. Are you interested in receiving information on preventing pregnancy? .... YES NO
47. If you have had sex, are you (or your partner) using any kind of birth control? . YES NO
48. If you have had sex, have you ever been treated for gonorrhea or chlamydia
    or other sexually transmitted disease? .... YES NO

For males only
49. Have you been taught how to use a condom correctly? .... YES NO
50. If you have had sex, do you use a condom every time or almost every time?.. YES NO
51. Have you ever fathered a child? .... YES NO

For females only
52. How old were you when your periods began? .... _____
53. What date did your last period start? .... _____
54. Are your periods regular (once a month)? .... YES NO
55. Do you have painful or excessively heavy periods? .... YES NO
56. Have you ever had a vaginal infection or been treated for a female disorder? . YES NO
57. Do you think you might be pregnant? .... YES NO
58. Have you ever been pregnant? .... YES NO

Everyone
59. Do you have any other problems you would like to discuss with the caregiver? YES NO

Past Medical History
60. Were you born prematurely or did you have any serious problems as an infant? YES NO
61. Are you allergic to any medicines? vs Do you have any allergies? .... YES NO
    If YES, what? _____
    _____

62. List any medications that you are taking and the problems for which the
    medication was given:
    MEDICATION   REASON   HOW LONG
    _____   _____   _____
    _____   _____   _____
    _____   _____   _____

63. Have you ever been hospitalized? .... YES NO
    If YES, describe the problem and your age at the time.
    AGE   PROBLEM
    _____ _____
    _____ _____
    _____ _____

64. Have you had any injuries? .... YES NO
    If YES, describe the injury and your age when it occurred.
    AGE   KIND OF INJURY
    _____ _____
    _____ _____

65. Have you had any serious illnesses? .... YES NO
    If YES, State the kind of illness and your age when it started.
    AGE   ILLNESS
    _____ _____
    _____ _____

Figure 10–3 (cont'd.). Adolescent medical history questionnaire.

STRICTLY CONFIDENTIAL

Family History
Have any members of your family, alive or dead, (parents, grandparents, uncles, aunts, brothers or sisters) had any of the following problems? If the answer is YES, please state the age of the person when the condition occurred and this person's relationship to you.

PROBLEM	YES	NO	DON'T KNOW	AGE	RELATIONSHIP
A. Seizure disorder Epilepsy					
B. Mental retardation Birth defects					
C. Migraine headaches					
D. High blood pressure High cholesterol					
E. Heart attack or stroke at less than age 60					
F. Lung disease Tuberculosis					
G. Liver or intestinal disease					
H. Kidney disease					
I. Allergies, Asthma, Eczema					
J. Arthritis					
K. Diabetes					
L. Endocrine-Gland					
M. Obesity					
N. Cancer					
O. Blood disorders Sickle cell anemia					
P. Emotional problems Suicide					
Q. Alcoholism Drug problems					

Figure 10–3 (cont'd.). Adolescent medical history questionnaire.

BOYS

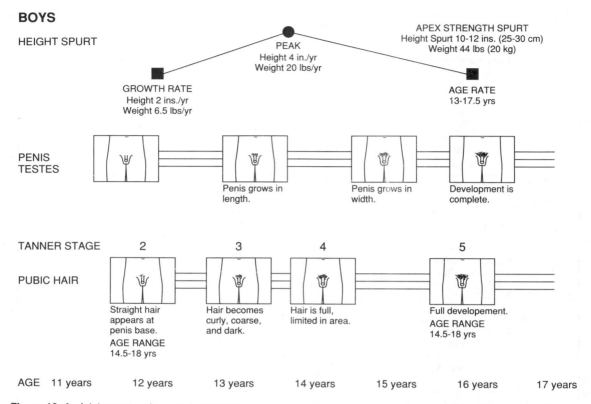

Figure 10—4. Adolescent male sexual maturation and growth. (Adapted and reproduced, with permission, from Tanner JM: *Growth at Adolescence.* Blackwell, 1962.)

GROWTH & DEVELOPMENT

PUBERTY

Pubertal growth and physical development are a result of activation of the hypothalamic-pituitary gonadal axis in late childhood. Before the onset of puberty, pituitary and gonadal hormones remain at very low levels. With the onset of puberty, the inhibition of gonadotropin-releasing hormone (GnRH) in the hypothalamus is removed, allowing pulsatile production and release of the gonadotropins, luteinizing hormone (LH) and follicle-stimulating hormone (FSH). In early to middle adolescence, there is an increase in pulse frequency and amplitude of LH and FSH secretion, which stimulates the gonads to produce sex steroids (estrogen or testosterone). In the female, FSH stimulates ovarian maturation, granulosa cell function, and estradiol secretion. LH is important in ovulation and is also involved in corpus luteum formation and progesterone secretion. Initially, estradiol has an inhibitory effect on the release

of LH and FSH. Eventually, estradiol becomes stimulatory, and the secretions of LH and FSH become cyclic. There is a progressive increase in estradiol, resulting in maturation of the female genital tract and breast development.

In the male, LH stimulates the interstitial cells of the testes, which produce testosterone. FSH stimulates the production of spermatocytes in the presence of testosterone. The testes also produce inhibin, a Sertoli-cell protein that also inhibits the secretion of FSH. During puberty, circulating testosterone increases more than 20-fold. Levels of testosterone correlate with the physical stages of puberty and the degree of skeletal maturation.

PHYSICAL GROWTH

During adolescence, a teenager's weight doubles, and height increases by 15–20%. During puberty, major organs double in size, with the exception of lymphoid tissue, which decreases in mass. Before puberty, there is little difference in muscular strength between boys and girls. The body's musculature increases both in size and strength during puberty,

GIRLS

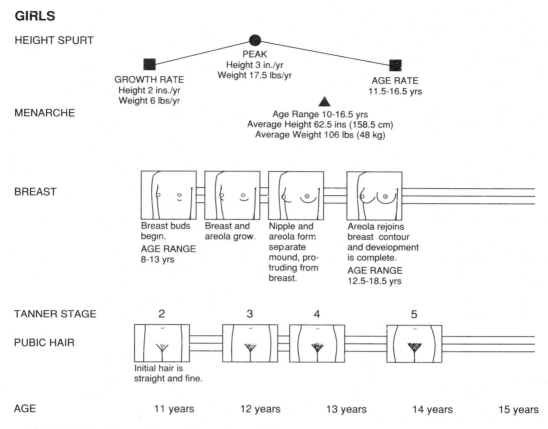

Figure 10–5. Adult female sexual maturation and growth. (Adapted and reproduced, with permission, from Tanner JM: *Growth at Adolescence.* Blackwell, 1962.)

with maximal strength lagging behind the increase in size by many months. Boys attain greater strength and mass, and strength continues to increase into late puberty. Although motor coordination lags behind growth in stature and musculature, it continues to improve as strength develops.

The pubertal growth spurt begins nearly 2 years earlier in girls than in boys. Girls reach their peak height velocity (PHV) between 11.5–12 years of age; boys, between 13.5–14 years of age. Linear growth at peak velocity is 9.5 cm/year +/− 1.5 cm for boys and 8.3 cm/year +/− 1.2 cm for girls. Pubertal growth usually takes 2–4 years and is longer in boys than girls. By age 11 years in girls and age 12 in boys, 83–89% of ultimate height has been attained. An additional 18–23 cm (7–9 inches) in females and 25–30 cm (10–12 inches) in males will be achieved during further pubertal growth. Following menarche, growth is rarely more than 5–7.5 cm. (2–3 inches).

Boys increase the quantity of body fat before beginning the height spurt. They then lose fat until the growth spurt has finished and then gradually again increase in fat. Muscle mass doubles between ages 10–17 years. Girls, by contrast, gradually store fat from about age 6 and do not decrease the quantity of fat, although its location changes, with an increase of subcutaneous fat in the region of the pelvis, breasts, and upper back.

SEXUAL MATURATION

Tanner's scale of sexual maturation is useful clinically to categorize genital development. Tanner staging includes age ranges of normal development and specific descriptions for each stage of pubic hair growth, penis and testes development in boys, and breast maturation in girls. Figs 10–4 and 10–5 graphically represent this chronologic development with reference to each Tanner stage. Tanner stage I is prepuberty; stage V, adult maturity. In stage II there is sparse, fine, nonpigmented, downy pubic hair; in stage III, the hair becomes pigmented and curly and increases in amount; and in stage IV, the hair is adult in texture, but limited in area. The appearance of pubic hair precedes that of axillary hair by more than a year. Male genital development begins with stage II, in which the testes become larger and the scrotal skin reddens and coarsens. In III, the penis lengthens; and in stage IV, the penis enlarges in general size, and the scrotal skin becomes pigmented. Female breast development follows a predictable sequence. Small, raised breast buds appear in stage II. In stage III, there is general enlargement and raising of breast and areolar tissue. The areola and papilla (nipple) form a separate mound from the breast in stage IV, and in stage V the areola is in the same contour as the breast. Great variability exists in the timing and onset of puberty and growth, and psychosocial development does not necessarily parallel physical change. Because of this variability, chronologic age is a poor indication of physiologic and psychosocial development during adolescence. Skeletal maturation correlates well with biologic maturity and pubertal development.

Teenagers have been entering puberty at increasingly earlier ages during the last century because of better nutrition and improved socioeconomic conditions. The age of menarche has decreased by about 4 months per decade during the last century. In the United States, the average age of menarche is 12¾ years. Frisch has shown that among girls reaching menarche, the average weight is 48 kg (106 lbs), and the average height is 158.5 cm (62.5 inches). However, menarche may be delayed until age 16 or begin as early as age 10. Although the first measurable sign of puberty in girls is the beginning of the height spurt, usually the first conspicuous sign is development of breast buds between the ages of 8 to 11 years. Although breast development usually antedates the growth of pubic hair, in some normal girls the reverse may occur. A common concern for girls at this time is whether the breasts will be of the right size and shape, especially since it is not unusual for one breast to grow faster than the other. Among girls, the growth spurt starts at about age 9 years and reaches a peak at age 11½, usually at stage 3–4 breast development and stage 3 pubic hair development. However, the height spurt may start as early as age 8 years in early maturers or as late as age 11½ in late maturers. The spurt usually ends by age 14. Girls who mature early will reach their PHV sooner and attain their final height earlier. Girls who mature late will attain a greater final height due to the longer period of growth before the growth spurt. Final height is related to skeletal age at onset of puberty as well as genetic factors. The height spurt correlates more closely with breast developmental stages than with pubic hair stages.

The first sign of puberty in the male, usually between the ages of 10 to 12, is scrotal and testicular growth. The appearance of pubic hair is usually an early event in puberty but can occur any time between ages 10 and 15 years. The penis begins to grow significantly a year or so after the onset of testicular and pubic hair development, usually between the ages of 10 and 13½. The first ejaculation is a notable event and usually occurs about a year after testicular growth, but its timing is highly variable. About 90% of boys have this experience between the ages of 11 and 15 years. Gynecomastia, a hard nodule under the nipple, occurs in a majority of boys, with a peak incidence between ages 14–15 years. Gynecomastia usually disappears within 2 years. The height spurt begins at age 11 but increases rapidly between the ages of 12 and 13, with the PHV reached at age 13½ years. However, the height spurt may start at age 10 in early maturers or as late as age 13–14 in late maturers. The period of pubertal development lasts much longer in boys and may not be completed until age 18 years. The height velocity is higher in males (8–11 cm/y) than females (6½–9½ cm/y). The development of axillary hair, deepening of the voice, and the development of chest hair in boys usually occurs in middle puberty, about 2 years after the growth of pubic hair. Facial and body hair begin to increase at ages 16–17 years.

Katchadourian H: *The Biology of Adolescence*. Freeman, 1977.
Rosenfeld, RG: Evaluation of growth and maturation in adolescence. *Pediatr Rev* 1982;**4**:175.
Tanner, JM: *Growth at Adolescence*. Blackwell, 1962.
Tanner, JM, Davies PW: Clinical longitudinal standards for height and height velocity for North American children. *J Pediatr* 1985;**107**:317.

PSYCHOSOCIAL DEVELOPMENT

Adolescents are struggling to find out who they are, what they want to do in the future, and, in relation to that goal, what their personal strengths and weaknesses are. These questions arise primarily because teenagers are in the process of establishing their own identity. Adolescence is a period of progressive individuation and separation from the family. Because of the rapid physical, emotional, cognitive, and social growth occurring during adolescence, it is useful to divide the period into 3 sequential phases of development. Early adolescence occurs roughly between ages 10–13; middle adolescence, between ages 14–16; and late adolescence, at age 17 and later.

Early Adolescence

Early adolescence (ages 10–13) is characterized by rapid growth and development of secondary sex characteristics. Young adolescents are often preoccupied with the physical changes taking place in their bodies. Because of these rapid physical changes, body image, self-concept, and self-esteem fluctuate dramatically. Concerns about how their growth and development deviate from that of their friends may be a great worry, especially short stature in boys and delayed breast development or delayed menarche in girls. Although there is a certain curiosity about sexuality, young adolescents tend to feel much more comfortable with members of the same sex. As the young teenager begins to become more independent and family ties loosen, allegiance shifts from parents to peers, who become much more important. Young teenagers still think concretely and cannot easily conceptualize about the future. They may have vague and unrealistic professional goals, such as becoming a lead singer in a rock group or a famous movie star. Only through the experiences encountered in later adolescence do they become more realistic.

Middle Adolescence

During middle adolescence (14–16 years), as the rapid pubertal growth of early adolescence decreases, teenagers begin to adjust and become more comfortable with their "new" bodies. Intense emotions and wide swings in mood are typical. Although some teenagers go through this experience relatively peacefully, other struggle desperately. Cognitively, teenagers move from concrete thinking to formal operations and develop the ability to think abstractly. With this new mental power comes a sense of omnipotence and a belief that the world can be changed by merely thinking about it. Sexually active teenagers may believe they don't need to worry about using contraception because they "can't get pregnant—it won't happen to me." Sixteen-year-old drivers believe that they are the best drivers in the world and think the insurance industry is conspiring against them by charging such high rates for automobile insurance. With the onset of the ability to think abstractly, teenagers begin to see themselves as others see them and may become extremely self-centered. Because they are establishing their own identities, relationships with other people, including peers, are primarily narcissistic, and experimenting with different images is quite common. Peers determine the standards for identification, behavior, activities, and fashion and provide emotional support, intimacy, empathy, and the sharing of guilt and anxiety during the struggle for autonomy. The struggle for independence and autonomy is often a difficult and stressful period for both the teenager and the parents.

As sexuality increases in importance, mid adolescents may begin dating and experimenting with sex. Relationships usually tend to be one-sided and narcissistic. By age 18, nearly one-half of American females and two-thirds of males have had intercourse.

Late Adolescence

Late adolescents (17 years and older) are much less self-centered and begin caring much more about others. Social relationships shift from the peer group

to the individual. Dating becomes much more intimate. The older adolescent becomes more independent from the family. The ability to think abstractly allows older adolescents to think more realistically in terms of future plans, actions, and careers. Older adolescents have very rigid concepts of what is right and what is wrong. This is a period of idealism.

Homosexuality in Adolescence

Homosexual characteristics appear to be established before adolescence. Sexual orientation develops during early childhood. One's gender identity is established by age 2, and a sense of masculinity or femininity usually solidifies by age 5 or 6. Homosexual adults describe homosexual feelings during late childhood and early adolescence, years before engaging in overt homosexual acts.

Although between 5 and 10% of American youth acknowledge homosexual experiences and 5% feel that they are or could be gay, homosexual experimentation is common, especially during early and middle adolescence. Experimentation may include mutual masturbation and fondling the genitals and does not by itself cause or lead to adult homosexuality. Theories about the etiology of homosexuality include genetic, hormonal, environmental, and psychologic models; however, there is no definitive explanation for the development of homosexual behavior.

The development of homosexual identity in youth commonly progresses through 3 stages. The adolescent feels "different," develops a crush on a person of the same sex without clear self-awareness of a gay identity, and then goes through a "coming-out" phase in which the homosexual identity is defined for the individual and revealed to others. The coming-out phase may be a very difficult period for the young person and the family. The young adolescent is afraid of society's bias and seeks to reject homosexual feelings. This struggle with identity may include episodes of both homosexual and heterosexual promiscuity, sexually transmitted disease, depression, substance abuse, attempted suicide, school avoidance and failure, running away from home, and other crises.

In a clinical setting, the issue of homosexual identity most often surfaces as a result of a teenager being seen for a sexually transmitted disease, family conflict, school problem, attempted suicide, or substance abuse rather than as a result of a consultation about sexual orientation. Pediatricians should be aware of the psychosocial and medical implications of homosexual identity and be sensitive to the possibility of these problems in gay adolescents. The successful management of these problems depends on the physician's ability to gain the trust of the gay adolescent and on a knowledge of the wide range of medical and psychologic problems for which gay adolescents may be at risk. Pediatricians must be nonjudgmental in posing sexual questions if they are to be effective in encouraging the teenager to share concerns. Physicians who for religious or other personal reasons cannot be objective must refer the patient to another professional for treatment and counseling.

Greydanus DE, Dewdney D: Homosexuality in adolescence. *Semin Adolesc Med* 1985;**1**:117.

Kreipe RE, McAnarney ER: Psychosocial aspects of adolescent medicine. *Semin Adolesc Med* 1985;**1**:33.

Orr DP, Ingersoll GM: Adolescent development: A biopsychosocial review. *Curr Probl Pediatr* 1988;**18**:441.

Remafedi G: Adolescent homosexuality: Psychosocial and medical implications. *Pediatrics* 1987;**79**:331.

Sussman EJ et al: Hormonal influences on aspects of psychological development during adolescence. *J Adolesc Health Care* 1987;**8**:492.

BEHAVIOR & PSYCHOLOGIC HEALTH

It is not unusual for adolescents to seek medical attention for seemingly minor complaints. During early adolescence, teenagers may worry about normal developmental changes such as gynecomastia. Teenagers may present with vague symptoms—the hidden agenda may be concerns about pregnancy or a sexually transmitted disease. Adolescents with emotional disorders often present with somatic symptoms, eg, abdominal pain, headaches, dizziness or syncope, fatigue, sleep problems, chest pain, that appear to have no biologic cause. The emotional basis of such a complaint may be varied: somatoform disorder, depression, or stress and anxiety.

PSYCHOPHYSIOLOGIC SYMPTOMS & CONVERSION REACTIONS

General Considerations

The most common somatoform disorders during adolescence are conversion disorders or conversion reactions. (A conversion reaction is a psychophysiologic process in which unpleasant feelings, especially anxiety, depression, and guilt, are communicated through a physical symptom.) Psychophysiologic symptoms result when anxiety activates the autonomic nervous system, resulting in tachycardia, hyperventilation, and vasoconstriction. The emotional feeling may be threatening or unacceptable to the individual, who expresses it as a physical symptom rather than verbally. This process is unconscious, and the anxiety or unpleasant feeling is dissipated by the somatic symptom. The degree to which the conversion symptom lessens anxiety, depression, or the unpleasant feeling is referred to as "primary gain." Conversion symptoms not only di-

minish unpleasant feelings but also remove the adolescent from conflict or an uncomfortable situation. This removal is referred to as "secondary gain." Secondary gain may intensify the symptoms, especially with increased attention from concerned parents and friends. Adolescents with conversion symptoms tend to have overprotective parents and become increasingly dependent on their parents as the symptom becomes the major focus of both the parents' and adolescent's life.

Clinical Findings

The symptom may appear at times of stress, eg, parental conflict, serious illness in a parent or grandparent, or change in school. Nervous, gastrointestinal, and cardiovascular systems are frequently involved, eg, parethesias, anesthesia, paralysis, dizziness, syncope, hyperventilation, abdominal pain, nausea, and vomiting. Specific symptoms may reflect existing or previous illness (eg, pseudoseizures in adolescents with epilepsy) or modeling of a close relative's symptom (eg, chest pain in a boy whose grandfather died of a heart attack).

Conversion symptoms tend to be more common in girls than boys. They occur in children and adolescents from all socioeconomic levels; however, the complexity of the symptom may vary with the sophistication and cognitive level of the patient.

Differential Diagnosis

In cases of suspected conversion reaction, history and physical findings are usually inconsistent with anatomic and physiologic concepts. Conversion symptoms are exhibited most frequently at times of stress and in the presence of individuals meaningful to the patient. The patient often exhibits a characteristic personality pattern, including egocentricity, labile emotional states, and dramatic and attention-seeking behaviors.

Conversion reactions are differentiated from hypochondriasis, which is a preoccupation with the fear of having, or the belief that one has, a serious illness. In hypochondriacal patients, despite medical reassurance that there is no evidence of disease, the patient's (or parents') fear persists. Although adolescents generally regard their symptoms (even minor complaints) with great concern, adolescents with hypochondriasis cannot be reassured that they are healthy. Over time, the fear of one disease may be replaced with concern about another. In contrast to patients with conversion symptoms, who seem relieved if an organic cause is considered, patients with hypochondriasis become more anxious when such a cause is considered.

Malingering is uncommon during adolescence. The malingering patient consciously and intentionally produces false or exaggerated physical or psychologic symptoms. Such patients are motivated by external incentives, such as avoiding work, evading criminal prosecution, obtaining drugs, or obtaining financial compensation. These patients may be hostile and aloof. Parents of patients with conversion disorders and malingering have a similar reaction to illness. They have an unconscious psychologic need to have sick children and reinforce their child's behavior.

Somatic delusions are physical symptoms that accompany other signs of mental illness. Examples are visual or auditory hallucinations, delusions, incoherence or loosening of associations, rapid shifts of affect, and confusion. The symptoms are often peculiar or unusual.

Treatment

Because the symptom is perceived as being physical, pediatricians are often the most appropriate professional to care for a patient with a conversion symptom. The physician must plan what further tests need to be done to complete the physical evaluation. It is critical from the onset for the physician to emphasize to the patient and the family that both physical and emotional causes of the symptom need to be considered. The relationship between physical causes of emotional pain and emotional causes of physical pain needs to be described to the family, using examples such as stress causing an ulcer or making a severe headache worse. The patient should be encouraged to understand that the symptom may persist and that at least a short-term goal is to continue normal daily activities in school and with friends. Medication is rarely helpful in relieving or resolving the symptom. If the family is accepting of psychologic referral as part of the evaluation, this is often the initial step for psychotherapy. If the family resists psychiatric or psychologic referral, the pediatrician may need to begin to deal with some of the emotional factors responsible for the persistent symptom while building rapport with the patient and family so that they accept psychologic referral in the future. Regular weekly appointments should be set up with the patient and parents. During the sessions, the teenager should be seen first and encouraged to talk about school, friends, the relationship with the parents, and the stresses and pressures of life. Discussion of the symptom itself should be minimized; however, the physician should be supportive and never suggest that the pain is not real. As the parents gain further insight into the cause of the symptom, they will become less indulgent of the complaints, facilitating the resumption of normal activities. If management is successful, the adolescent will acquire increased coping skills and become more independent, with decreasing secondary gain.

If the symptom continues to interfere with daily activities, school attendance, participation in extracurricular activities, and involvement with peers and if the patient and parents feel that no progress is being made, psychologic referral is definitely indicated. A psychotherapist experienced in treating ad-

olescents with conversion reactions has the greatest probability of establishing a strong therapeutic relationship with the patient and family. After referral is made, the pediatrician should continue to follow the patient to ensure compliance with psychotherapy.

American Psychiatric Association: *Diagnostic and Statistical Manual of Mental Disorders,* 3rd rev ed. American Psychiatric Association, 1987.

Friedman SB: Conversion symptoms in adolescents. *Pediatr Clin North Am* 1973;**20**:873.

Orr D: Adolescence, stress and psychosomatic issues. *J Adolesc Health Care* 1986;**7(Suppl)**:97.

Prazer G: Conversion reactions in adolescents. *Pediatr Rev* 1987;**8**:279.

DEPRESSION
(See also Chapter 25.)

General Considerations

Symptoms of clinical depression—eg, lethargy, loss of interest, sleep disturbances, decreased energy, feelings of worthlessness, and difficulty concentrating—can be quite common during the normal emotional mood swings of adolescence. The intensity of feelings, often to seemingly trivial events such as a poor grade on an examination or not being invited to a party, makes it difficult to differentiate a serious depression from normal sadness or dejection. In a less serious depression, sadness and unhappiness associated with everyday life is generally short-lived. The symptoms usually result in only minor impairment in school, social activities, and relationships with others. With reassurance the teenager should return to a normal affect within a few days.

Clinical Findings

Serious depression in adolescents may present in several ways. The presentation may be similar to that in adults, with vegetative signs such as depressed mood nearly every day, crying spells or inability to cry, discouragement, irritability, sense of emptiness and meaninglessness, negative expectations of self and the environment, low self-esteem, isolation, helplessness, markedly diminished interest or pleasure in most activities, significant weight loss or weight gain, insomnia or hypersomnia, fatigue or loss of energy, feelings of worthlessness, and diminished ability to think or concentrate. However, it is not unusual for a serious depression to be masked because the teenager cannot tolerate the severe feelings of sadness. Such a teenager may present with recurrent or persistent psychosomatic complaints, such as abdominal pain, chest pain, headache, lethargy, weight loss, dizziness and syncope, or other nonspecific symptoms. Other behavioral manifestations of a masked depression include truancy, running away from home, defiance of authorities, self-destructive behavior, drug and alcohol abuse, sexual acting out, and delinquency.

Differential Diagnosis

The pediatrician must first recognize that the teenager may be suffering from an affective disorder. A complete history and physical examination, including a careful review of the patient's past medical and psychosocial history, should be performed. The family history should be explored for psychiatric problems.

The teenager should be questioned directly about any specific symptoms of depression, such as extreme lethargy, decreased energy, feelings of worthlessness, problems sleeping, changes in eating habits, difficulty concentrating, periods of uncontrollable crying, prolonged sadness and unhappiness, suicidal thoughts, or preoccupation with death. The history should include an assessment of the student's school performance. The physician looks for signs of academic deterioration, excessive absences or cutting class, changes in work or other outside activities, and changes in the family (eg, separation, divorce, serious illness, loss of employment by a parent, a recent move to a new house, increasing quarrels or fights with parents, or death of a close relative). The teenager may have withdrawn from friends or family, or changed to a new group of friends. The physician questions to discover a history of drug and alcohol abuse, conflict with the law, sexual acting out, running away from home, unusually violent or rebellious behavior, or radical personality change. Patients with vague somatic complaints (eg, headaches, abdominal pain, dizzy spells, chest pain, joint pains, concerns about having a fatal illness, or a "positive review of systems") often have an underlying affective disorder.

Because a number of physical disorders can mimic, cause, or exacerbate major depression, adolescents presenting with significant symptoms of depression deserve a thorough medical evaluation to rule out any contributing or underlying medical illness. Among the medical conditions associated with affective disorders are eating disorders (anorexia nervosa and bulimia), organic disorders of the central nervous system (tumors, vascular lesions, closed head trauma, and subdural hematomas), metabolic and endocrinologic disorders (systemic lupus erythematosus, hypothyroidism, hyperthyroidism, Wilson's disease, hyperparathyroidism, Cushing's syndrome, Addison's disease, premenstrual syndrome), infections (mononucleosis, syphilis), and mitral valve prolapse. In addition, over 200 drugs have been reported to cause depressive symptoms. Marihuana use, phencyclidine abuse, amphetamine withdrawal, and excessive caffeine intake can cause symptoms of depression. Common prescription medications used by this age group (eg, birth control pills) and anticonvulsants may be responsible for depressive symptoms.

The majority of physical disorders presenting with symptoms of depression are usually evident by history, past medical history, and physical examination. However, some routine laboratory studies are indicated, including: complete blood count and determination of sedimentation rate; urinalysis; serum electrolytes; BUN; calcium; thyroxine and thyroid-stimulating hormone; VDRL or RPR; and liver enzymes. Although metabolic markers such as abnormal secretion of cortisol, growth hormone, and thyrotropin-releasing hormone have been useful in confirming major depression in adults, these neurobiologic markers are less reliable in adolescents.

The risk of depression appears to be greatest in families with a history of depression of early onset and a chronicity of depressive symptoms. Depression of early onset and bipolar illness are more likely to occur in families with a strong multigenerational history of depression. The lifetime risk of depressive illness in first-degree relatives of adult depressed patients has been estimated to be between 18 and 30%.

Treatment

The primary care physician may be able to counsel adolescents and parents if an underlying depression is mild or seems to be the result of an acute identifiable personal loss or frustration and if the patient is not contemplating suicide or at risk for other life-threatening behaviors. If there is evidence of a long-standing depressive disorder, suicidal thoughts, psychotic thinking or if the physician does not feel competent or has no interest in counseling the patient, a psychologic referral should be made. In uncomplicated depressions that are a reaction to life stresses or interpersonal conflicts, helping the adolescent put things in proper perspective may be enormously beneficial. Encouraging the adolescent to verbalize thoughts, understand emotional responses, and examine unrealistic attitudes and beliefs can help the patient find an appropriate solution to the problem that led to the depression.

Counseling involves establishing and maintaining a positive supportive relationship; following the patient at least weekly; remaining accessible to the patient at all times; encouraging the patient to express emotions openly, defining the problem and clarifying negative feelings, thoughts, and expectations; setting realistic goals; helping to negotiate interpersonal crises; teaching assertiveness and social skills; reassessing the depression as it is expressed; and staying alert to the possibility of suicide.

Patients with a clinical course consistent with bipolar disease should be referred for psychiatric evaluation for a trial with lithium. Patients whose depression is unresponsive to supportive counseling or who appear to have a more moderate depression should be referred to a psychiatrist for evaluation of antidepressant medication.

Gourash L, Puig-Antich J: Medical and biologic aspects of adolescent depression. *Semin Adolesc Med* 1986;**2**:299.

Greydanus DE: Depression in adolescence: A perspective. *J Adolesc Health Care* 1986;**7(Suppl)**:109.

ADOLESCENT SUICIDE
(See also Chapter 25.)

General Considerations

In 1986, there were over 5000 suicides among people 15–24 years of age: 2000 suicides among those 15–19 and over 3000 among those 20–24 (a suicide rate of 10.2 per 100,000 in the group 15–19 and 15.8 per 100,000 in the group 20–24). In the younger group, males had a rate 400% higher than females, and white males had the highest rate, 18.2 per 100,000. The incidence of unsuccessful suicide attempts is 3 times higher in females to males. The estimated ratio of attempted suicides to actual suicides is estimated to be 50:1 to 100:1. Among actual suicides, firearms are the leading cause of death for both males and females, used in over 60% of the suicides.

With the normal mood swings of adolescence, short periods of depression are common. At some time, a teenager may have thoughts of suicide. Normal depressive mood swings during this period rarely interfere with sleeping, eating, or participating in normal activities. Acute depressive reactions (transient grief responses) to the loss (death or separation) of a close family member or friend may result in depression lasting for weeks or even months. An adolescent who is unable to work through this grief can become increasingly depressed. A teenager who is unable to keep up with schoolwork, does not participate in normal social activities, withdraws socially, has sleep and appetite disturbances, and has feelings of hopelessness and helplessness should be considered to be at increased risk for suicide. These are signs of a major depression.

Another group of suicidal adolescents is composed of angry teenagers attempting to affect their environment. They may be only mildly depressed and may not have a longstanding wish to die. Teenagers in this group, usually females, may "attempt" or "gesture" suicide as a way to get back at someone or gain attention by scaring another person.

The last group of adolescents at risk for suicide is made up of teenagers with a serious psychiatric problem such as acute schizophrenia or a true psychotic depressive disorder.

Risk Assessment

The physician must determine the extent of the teenager's depression and risk of inflicting self-harm. The evaluation should include interviews with both the teenager and the family. The history should include the medical, social, emotional, and academic background. (See Table 25–15, Clinical Interview to Assess Suicide Risk.) The physician should inquire about (1) common signs of depression; (2) recent events that could be at the root of an underlying depression; (3) evidence of long-standing problems in the home, at school, or with peers; (4) drugs or substance use and abuse; (5) signs of psychotic thinking, such as delusions or hallucinations; (6) evidence of masked depression, such as rebellious behavior, running away from home, reckless driving, or other acting out behavior. When seeing depressed patients, the physician should always inquire about thoughts of suicide: "Are things ever so bad that life doesn't seem worth living?" If the response is positive, a more specific question should be asked: "Have you thought of taking your life?" If the patient has thoughts of suicide, the immediacy of risk can be assessed by determining if there is a concrete, feasible plan. Although the patients who are at greatest risk have a concrete plan that can be carried out in the near future, especially if they have rehearsed the plan, the physician should not dismiss the potential risk of suicide in the adolescent who does not describe a specific plan. The physician should pay attention to "gut feelings." There may be subtle nonverbal signs that the patient is at greater risk than is apparent on the surface.

Treatment

The primary care physician is often in a unique position to identify an adolescent at risk for suicide, because many teenagers who attempt suicide seek medical attention in the weeks preceding the attempt. These visits are often for vague somatic complaints or subtle signs of depression. If there is evidence of depression, the physician must assess the severity of the depression and suicidal risk. The pediatrician should always seek emergency psychologic consultation for any teenager who is severely depressed, psychotic, or acutely suicidal. It is the psychologist's or psychiatrist's responsibility to assess the seriousness of suicidal ideation and decide whether hospitalization or outpatient treatment is most appropriate. Adolescents with mild depression and at low risk for suicide should be followed closely, and the extent of the depression should be assessed on an ongoing basis. If at any point it appears that the patient is worsening or the teenager is not responding to supportive counseling, referral should be made.

American Academy of Pediatrics, Committee on Adolescence: Suicide and suicide attempts in adolescents and young adults. *Pediatrics* 1988;**81**:322.

Brent DA: Suicide and suicidal behavior in children and adolescents. *Pediatr Rev* 1989;**10**:269.

Centers for Disease Control: Youth suicide—United States, 1970–1980. *MMWR* 1987;**36**:87.

Shaffer D et al: Preventing teenage suicide: A critical review. *J Am Acad Child Adolesc Psychiatry* 1988; **27**:675.

SUBSTANCE ABUSE

Substance abuse is a growing problem in a society that seeks quick fixes for complex problems. Seventy-one percent of American adolescents 12–17 years of age have smoked cigarettes, 93% have used alcohol, 57% have used marijuana, and 35% have used stimulants (Table 10–1). Use of all of the major substances abused, except for cocaine and prescribed psychoactive drugs, has been initiated in 90% of abusers by age 21. Although there has been a slight decline in adolescent substance abuse during the 1980s, increasingly younger children are experimenting with drugs. The percentage of students using drugs by the sixth grade has tripled since 1975. In addition, cocaine is now seen as readily available by almost half of high school seniors, and epidemic use of "crack" has been reported among adolescents. The primary pediatrician, then, plays an important role in prevention of substance abuse through anticipatory guidance, identification, and early intervention.

Risk Factors

The causes of substance abuse are multifactorial, including personality characteristics, genetic influences, peer pressure, and parental and cultural influences. Characteristics of normal adolescents, such as a love of danger and risk-taking behavior, the need to belong, and the need for immediate gratification make them vulnerable to initiation of drug use. In addition, low self-esteem, loneliness, inadequate communication and coping skills, and inadequate bonding to family and society have been shown to increase an adolescent's risk for substance abuse.

Adoption and twin studies show that a family history of substance abuse is a strong predictor of substance abuse in the offspring. Both genetic and environmental factors play a role. Sons of alcoholics, whether raised by their biologic parent or by a nonalcoholic foster parent, are 4 times more likely to be alcoholics than sons of nonalcoholics. Parental modeling of smoking, drinking, or other drug use and parental attitudes toward drugs are factors as well. In addition, denial and rationalizations by family members ("enabling" behavior that overprotects the user) foster substance abuse. Inconsistent parental discipline, excessive permissiveness, and severe parental discipline have all been associated with higher rates of substance abuse. Peer pressure is particularly important in preadolescents; whether the adolescent's friends use drugs may be the greatest predictor of substance abuse.

Protective factors include parents who give clear messages against drugs and provide consistent discipline involving warmth and discussion, peers who

Table 10–1. Alcohol and drug use among high school seniors, by substance and frequency of use: 1975–1986.[1]

Substance and frequency of use	Class of 1975	Class of 1980	Class of 1981	Class of 1982	Class of 1983	Class of 1984	Class of 1985	Class of 1986
	Percentage reporting having ever used drugs							
Alcohol	90.4	93.2	92.6	92.8	92.6	92.6	92.2	91.3
Any illicit drug	55.2	65.4	65.6	64.4	62.9	61.6	60.6	57.6
Marihuana only	19.0	26.7	22.8	23.3	22.5	21.3	20.9	19.9
Any illicit drug other than marihuana[2]	36.2	38.7	42.8	41.1	40.4	40.3	39.7	37.7
Use of selected drugs:								
Cocaine	9.0	15.7	16.5	16.0	16.2	16.1	17.3	16.9
Heroin	2.2	1.1	1.1	1.2	1.2	1.3	1.2	1.1
LSD	11.3	9.3	9.8	9.6	8.9	8.0	7.5	7.2
Marihuana/hashish	47.3	60.3	59.5	58.7	57.0	54.9	54.2	50.9
PCP[3]	—	9.6	7.8	6.0	5.6	5.0	4.9	4.8
	Percentage reporting use of drugs in the past 30 days							
Alcohol	68.2	72.0	70.7	69.7	69.4	67.2	65.9	65.3
Any illicit drug	30.7	37.2	36.9	32.5	30.5	29.2	29.7	27.1
Marihuana only	15.3	18.8	15.2	15.5	15.1	14.1	14.8	13.9
Any illicit drug other than marihuana[2]	15.4	18.4	21.7	17.0	15.4	15.1	14.9	13.2
Use of selected drugs:								
Cocaine	1.9	5.2	5.8	5.0	4.9	5.8	6.7	6.2
Heroin	0.4	0.2	0.2	0.2	0.2	0.3	0.3	0.2
LSD	2.3	2.3	2.5	2.4	1.9	1.5	1.6	1.7
Marihuana/hashish	27.1	33.7	31.6	28.5	27.0	25.2	25.7	23.4
PCP[3]	—	1.4	1.4	1.0	1.3	1.0	1.6	1.3

[1]Modified and reproduced from US Department of Health and Human Services, Alcohol, Drug Abuse, and Mental Health Administration, *National Trends in Drug Use and Related Factors Among American High School Students, 1975–1986* and US Department of Education, Office of Educational Research and Improvement, *Youth Indicators 1988*, p. 98.
[2]Other illicit drugs include hallucinogens, cocaine, and heroin, or any other opiates, stimulants, sedatives, or tranquilizers not prescribed by a doctor.
[3]Data for the class of 1975 not available.

do not use drugs, knowledge of the consequences of substance abuse, and a personal value system in which health and achievement are regarded highly.

Stages of Substance Abuse

Chemical dependency is the result of a gradual process. Donald Ian Macdonald, MD, has suggested 5 stages of substance abuse, 0–4, which are outlined in Table 10–2. Progression through these stages occurs at a variable rate, and not every user progresses to stage 4; however, the younger the user, the greater the risk for chemical dependency.

Substances Abused

Although tobacco and alcohol are considered "gateway" drugs, marijuana is also commonly used during adolescence. Of particular concern is the dra-

matic increase in cocaine and "crack" use during the last decade. This is largely a consequence of their lower cost and ready availability. Table 10–3 lists drugs and their effects.

Anticipatory Guidance

The clinician should clearly communicate that alcohol and other drugs can be discussed at any time. Anticipatory guidance on substance abuse can begin during grade school. The physician can ask questions such as "What have you learned about drugs in school?" and "Has anyone ever tried to get you to use drugs?" Follow-up discussion can focus on the harmful effects of drugs and ways to resist drug use. Adolescents should be questioned nonjudgmentally and in a private setting about smoking, drinking, or other drug use by classmates, friends, and the pa-

Table 10–2. The 5 stages of substance abuse.[1]

Stage	Drugs	Sources	Frequency	Feelings	Behavior	Treatment
Stage 0: Curiosity	None	Available—but not used	—	Curiousity	Risk taking, desire for acceptance	Optimal time; anticipatory guidance to develop good coping skills and strong self-esteem; clear family guidelines on drug and alcohol use; drug education
Stage 1: Experimentation	Tobacco, alcohol, marihuana	House supply, friends, siblings	Weekend use for recreational purposes	Excitement, pleasure, few consequences, Learning how easy it is to feel good	Lying, little change	Drug education; attention to societal messages; reduction of supply; strict, loving rules at home; establishment of drug-free alternative activities
Stage 2: Regular use	As above, plus hashish or hash oil, tranquilizers, sedatives, amphetamines	Buying	Progresses to midweek use. Purpose is to get high	Excitement followed by guilt	Mood swings, faltering school performance, truancy, changing peer groups, changing style of dress	Drug-free self-help groups (Alcoholics or Narcotics Anonymous); family involvement; psychiatric counseling unhelpful unless family therapy and aftercare provided
Stage 3: Psychologic or chemical dependency	As above, plus stimulants, hallucinogens	Selling to support their habit; possibly stealing or prostitution in exchange for drugs	Daily	Euphoric highs followed by depression, shame, guilt, and perhaps suicidal thoughts	Pathologic lying; school failure; family fights; involvement with the law over curfew, truancy, vandalism, shoplifting, driving under the influence, breaking and entering, violence	Inpatient or foster care programs that require family involvement and provide aftercare
Stage 4: Using drugs to feel "normal"	As above. Any available drug, including opiates	Any way possible	All day	Euphoria rare and harder to achieve; chronic depression	Drifting, with repeated failures and psychologic symptoms of paranoia and aggression; frequent overdosing, blackouts, amnesia; Chronic cough, fatigue, malnutrition	Inpatient or foster care programs that require family involvement and provide aftercare

[1]Source: MacDonald DI: Substance abuse. *Pediatr Rev* 1988;**10**:89.

Table 10–3. Subjective, objective, and adverse effects of commonly abused drugs.

Drug	Street Names	Subjective Effects	Objective Effects	Adverse/Overdose Reactions
Cannabis Marihuana Hashish Hash oil THC	Pot Grass Weed Maryjane Hash Tea Reefer Joint	Sedation Tranquilization Mild hallucination or pleasurable change in perception	Tachycardia Conjunctival irritation Impaired abstract thinking, reading comprehension, verbal ability, short-term memory, counting, color discrimination Impaired driving ability	Acute anxiety Serious reaction uncommon unless adulterated with hallucinogens
Alcohol	Booze	Stimulation as blood level rises Subsequent sedation, release of inhibitions	Slurred speech Ataxia Impaired driving performance	Poor judgment Impaired cognitive and motor abilities Emotional changes Respiratory depression Decrease in temperature Coma, shock, death
CNS Stimulants Cocaine Amphetamines	Cocaine Coke Snow Dust Crack Rock Amphetamines Uppers Speed Meth Crystal Bennies Dexies	Euphoric effects: exhilaration, calmness, sense of power; omnipotence and unlimited energy in high doses Perception of decrease in appetite, thirst, fatigue Dysphoria or "wired" irritability after euphoric phase.	Local anesthetic Sympathomimetic: mydriasis, hypertension, tachycardia, tachypnea, temperature elevation, tremor, agitation	Anxiety Elevated temperature Seizures Respiratory arrest Arrhythmia Death Hallucinations and paranoia
CNS Depressants Group I Sedatives Tranquilizers	Downers Quaaludes, Ludes Blues, Bluebirds Reds, Red devils Yellows, Yellow jackets	Relaxation Facilitation of social behavior With higher doses, loss of inhibitions, sedation, drowsiness	Nystagmus on lateral gaze Slurred speech, ataxia Impulsiveness	Coma Death
GROUP II Nitrous oxide Toluene Trichlorethylene Methanol Acetone Gasoline Fluorinated hydrocarbons		Sedation Heightened visual imagery Hallucination Euphoria	Drowsiness Rhinitis, bronchitis Odor of inhalant on breath Metabolic abnormalities	Coma (rare) Idiosyncratic reaction to fluorinated hydrocarbons resulting in sudden death by cardiac arrhythmia
Nitrites Amyl nitrite Isobutyl nitrite	Rush Lockerroom Poppers Bolt	Sudden, transient, pleasurable tingling Headache Pounding heart	Tachycardia Hypotension	Exacerbation of preexisting cardiac disease, syncope Elevated intraocular pressure Coma, (rarely) sudden death Methemoglobinemia
Hallucinogens Group I Lysergic acid diethylamide Mescaline Psilocybin	Acid LSD Peyote Button Mesc Mushrooms	Vivid sensory stimulation and distortion Introspection Awareness of drug-induced state	Dizziness, nausea Paresthesias Sympathomimetic effects Varying mental status as changes from hallucinating to coherent recountings	Idiosyncratic "bad trips" or panic reactions with terrifying hallucinations that may last from hours to more than a day
GROUP II Phencyclidine	PCP Angel dust Hog Horse Rocket Fuel	Low doses (1–5 mg) produce floating euphoria or numbness Doses of 5–15 mg cause confusion, agitation, impairment of communication, and distorted body perception Higher doses may cause psychotic reactions lasting from days to months	Sympathomimetic effects Drooling Rotatory nystagmus Decreased response to pain Combative and aggressive or silent and withdrawn	Muscle rigidity, opisthotonus, seizures, coma Toxic psychosis (rotatory nystagmus and fever may be the only signs to differentiate from nontoxic psychosis) Hypertensive crises with CNS hemorrhage and death

Table 10–3 (cont'd). Subjective, objective, and adverse effects of commonly abused drugs.

Drug	Street Names	Subjective Effects	Objective Effects	Adverse/Overdose Reactions
Opiates Heroin Morphine Meperidine Propoxyphene Methadone Codeine	Dope H Horse Smack Meth	With IV use: a sudden "rush" and sensation similar to orgasm occurs With other routes: euphoria, drowsiness, decreased appetite and libido Nausea, vomiting, and dizziness may occur in novices	Oriented but indifferent Slurred speech, unsteady gait Slowed heart and respiratory rates Pinpoint pupils Needle tracks in IV users	CNS and respiratory depression responsive to naloxone (Narcan) Pulmonary edema 24–36 h out, not responsive to naloxone Death

tient. In addition, adolescents can be asked how they would handle various situations, such as being offered drugs or riding in an automobile with someone who has been drinking or using drugs. Information on the immediate and long-term health effects of tobacco and other drugs, effects on the fetus during pregnancy, and the dangers of driving while high should be made available to all adolescents.

Diagnosis

History is the key to the diagnosis of substance abuse, and a history obtained in a nonjudgmental manner may be highly enlightening. In later stages of involvement, however, denial may cause the adolescent to minimize use. Clues to diagnosis include episodes of acute drug abuse (such as overdose or suicide gestures), deteriorating school performance, personality changes (mood swings, lack of motivation), worsening family relationships, change of peer groups, trouble with the law, or persistent regular drug use despite parental or physician discussion with the teenager. When substance abuse is suspected or established in an adolescent, an assessment of the adolescent's involvement with the drug (age at onset, drugs used, duration of use, frequency of use, attitude toward use), involvement with a drug-using peer group, relationship with the family, and psychologic profile (any preexisting psychiatric or developmental or educational difficulties) can guide decisions on appropriate management. Information should also be obtained from the parents, who may suspect substance abuse or may be manifesting "enabling" behavior, therefore denying the significance of the problem.

The physical examination provides few clues other than nonspecific signs, eg, red eyes, signs of an upper respiratory infection, avoidance of eye contact, or evidence of trauma. Laboratory tests are generally helpful only with acute intoxication, when a blood alcohol and urine toxin screen should be obtained. When it is known that one substance has been used at the time of acute intoxication, a drug screen should be obtained. The purpose of this screen is to detect other substances, since more than one drug may have been used, or the drug may have been

adulterated or misrepresented to the user. Drug testing, unless performed during an episode of acute intoxication or in the context a drug-free maintenance program, is generally of little help and may endanger the patient-physician relationship.

Treatment

Prevention and early intervention during experimental use are most effective. By offering assistance to quit tobacco use, the clinician can promote a drug-free posture and often intervene before other substances are abused. When other substances are abused, management depends on the stage of involvement. With experimental use, education on short-term and long-term effects and a contract between patient and physician with interval monitoring may be useful. With higher levels of use, parental involvement is necessary, because the family plays a crucial role in resolution of adolescent chemical dependency. The pediatrician, although rarely in a position to treat the higher levels of involvement, plays a key role in providing referral and ongoing support. To enlist parental support and ensure that referral is completed, the physician must convince the parent of the severity of the situation. It may be necessary to alleviate parental guilt first, since enabling behavior often arises out of guilt. The goal is to stop the adolescent from using drugs and restore a healthful pattern of living. A short-term hospitalization may be useful to interrupt ongoing substance use. This hiatus permits a careful appraisal of factors contributing to drug use and the level of dysfunction. Treatment modalities include drug-free self-help groups (Alcoholics or Narcotics Anonymous), individual or family psychotherapy, inpatient adolescent psychiatric hospitalization, or residential treatment programs (see Table 10–2). In addition to requiring drug-free status, the chosen modality must include exploration of associated psychologic issues, eg, depression, ineffective coping styles, or poor family communication, that may contribute to the substance abuse. Emphasis is then placed on the development of the social skills, positive self-esteem, and academic and work skills needed to remain abstinent. The family is helped to understand the nature of substance abuse and to find patterns of behavior that facilitate abstinence. Sufficient duration of treatment and follow-up care are necessary to prevent recidivism.

American Academy of Pediatrics Policy Statement: Screening for drugs of abuse in children and adolescents, *AAP News*, March 1989, p. 9.

Hawkins JD et al: Childhood predictors of adolescent substance abuse: Toward an empirically grounded theory. *J Child Contemp Society* 1986;**18**:1.

Johnston LD, O'Malley PM, Brachman JG: National trends in drug use and related factors among American high school students and young adults, 1975–1986. National Institute on Drug Abuse Publication No. (ADM)87–1535, 1987.

Kandel DB, Logan JA: Patterns of drug use from adolescence to young adulthood: I. Periods of risk for initiation, continued use, and discontinuation. *Am J Public Health* July 1984, **74**:660.

Macdonald DI: *Drugs, Drinking, and Adolescents*. Yearbook, 1984.

Macdonald DI: Substance abuse, *Pediatr Rev* 1988;**10**:89.

Miller JD, Cisen IH, Abelson HI: National survey on drug abuse: Main findings, 1982. National Institute on Drug Abuse Publication No. (ADM)83–1263, 1983.

Schonberg SK (editor): *Substance Abuse: A Guide for Health Professionals*. American Academy of Pediatrics, 1988.

Smith DE, Schwartz RH, Martin DM: Heavy cocaine use by adolescents. *Pediatrics* 1989;**83**:539.

EATING DISORDERS
(See also Chapter 25.)

General Considerations

It is estimated that 5–10% of adolescent girls and young women have an eating disorder. Although eating disorders may occur in males, 90–95% of patients are female. Most are middle or upper-middle class, but this trend appears to be changing.

The incidence of anorexia nervosa has doubled over the past 2 decades, and the mortality rate is as high as 9%, excluding suicide. The prevalence of the symptom bulimia ranges from 4.5 to 18% among female high school and college students. The causes of eating disorders remain unclear. There are contributing psychosocial and cultural factors, eg, the current emphasis on thinness and the "superwoman" image in today's society. The genetic component and the neuroendocrine/hypothalamic role is being investigated.

A teenager with anorexia is unlikely to present to the physician of her own accord, because denial of illness is one of the components of the syndrome. Often a school nurse or coach becomes suspicious after observing weight loss, excessive concern with weight, or unusual eating and exercise behaviors. Parents, too, have become knowledgeable about eating disorders from the lay press. But often, the patient presents with abdominal pain, nausea, fainting spells, hair loss, or amenorrhea, and it is the clinician who discovers the true diagnosis. Bulimics, however, may present on their own and may feel relieved to share their burden with someone.

Clinical Findings

A. Symptoms and Signs: The diagnosis of anorexia nervosa or bulimia nervosa is largely based on history; specific diagnostic criteria are given in Table 10–4. The history needs to include the presenting symptoms; weight history, including desired weight; dietary intake, unusual eating behaviors, or avoided foods; history of any purging behaviors, eg, vomiting, excessive exercise, or use of diet pills, diuretics, emetics, or laxatives; and menstrual history for irregular cycles, secondary amenorrhea, or delay in menarche when otherwise expected. Social history may provide clues to a perfectionistic drive in anorexics, impulsiveness in bulimics (eg, substance abuse or sexual promiscuity), or family dysfunction. Review of systems should focus on symptoms of possible complications of the above behaviors and on symptoms of other diseases in the differential diagnosis. Table 10–5 lists associated features of eating disorders. The use of the Eating Attitudes Test (EAT) and the Eating Disorder Inventory (EDI) may aid in diagnosis.

The physical examination is most often normal, but this does not rule out the diagnosis of an eating disorder. The anorexic may hide under layers of bulky clothing, but the loss of subcutaneous tissue becomes apparent when the patient disrobes. The anorexic's weight is the indicator of actual loss; however, bulimics are usually of normal weight or within 10 pounds of normal (under or over). Hypothermia, bradycardia, or hypotension may be evident

Table 10–4. Diagnostic criteria for eating disorders.

Anorexia Nervosa

Weight loss or failure to gain weight during growth such that weight is 15% below that expected for age and height.

Fear of weight gain or fatness despite being underweight.

Distorted body image—feels all or part of the body is fat even when severely underweight.

For females, interruption of menstrual cycles for at least 3 months (secondary amenorrhea) or failure to menstruate when expected (primary amenorrhea).

Bulimia Nervosa

Repeated binge eating (large number of calories in short period of time) with a frequency of at least twice a week for 3 or more months.

Perception by patient that eating behavior is out of control.

Recurrent purging behavior to prevent weight gain (self-induced emesis; use of laxatives, diuretics, or emetics), excessive exercise, or severely restricted intake.

Excessive preoccupation with body image.

Modified and reproduced from American Psychiatric Association: *Diagnostic and Statistical Manual of Mental Disorders*, 3rd rev ed. American Psychiatric Association, 1987.

Table 10–5. Associated features of eating disorders.

Anorexia Nervosa	Bulimia Nervosa
Onset at age 12 to mid 30s; bimodal 13–14, 17–18	Onset at age 17–25, but may not present for many years
Extreme weight loss, refusal to maintain minimal normal weight for age	Weight fluctuations
Intense fear of becoming obese	Possible fear of fatness but a greater fear of loss of control of eating
Distorted body image	Overconcern with body shape/weight
Amenorrhea (in females)	Possible menstrual irregularities
Intense preoccupation with food	Intense preoccupation with food
Severe caloric restriction (restrictive anorexia nervosa) or severe restriction alternating with binging/purging (bulimic anorexia nervosa)	Secretive binge-eating episodes, high-carbohydrate foods
	Self-induced vomiting, purging (laxatives, diuretics, emetics), vigorous exercise
Excessive physical activity	Other impulsive behaviors (alcohol/drug use)
Isolation, asexuality	Outgoing personality, heterosexual relationships
Denial of illness	Distress, willingness to accept help

when the anorexic's vital signs are assessed. Other findings in anorexia include dry skin, presence of fine, downy hair on the body or an increase in pigmentation of body hair, limpness and loss of sheen in the scalp hair, excoriation over the sacral spine from excessive sit-ups, prominent ribs, atrophied breasts, scaphoid abdomen, palpable hard stool in the rectal vault, cold extremities, squaring off of the convergence of the thighs, or edema of the extremities. In patients with self-induced emesis, there may be loss of tooth enamel, particularly on the posterior aspect of the front teeth, or calluses on the dorsum of the fingers.

B. Laboratory Findings: The goal of laboratory tests is to exclude other diagnoses and assess the patient's status. Most laboratory studies do not change until late in the disease. It is useful to obtain a complete blood count to assess nutritional status, a determination of sedimentation rate to help exclude inflammatory bowel disease or collagen vascular disease, and electrolyte studies to detect the presence of hypochloremic alkalosis and hypokalemia due to vomiting or of metabolic acidosis due to laxative abuse. A urinalysis may show concentrated urine, or late in anorexia nervosa, the loss of the concentrating ability. Serum total protein and albumin are usually normal until late, and low serum phosphorus and magnesium values are ominous signs. Other laboratory studies, such as thyroid function tests, chest x-ray, upper gastrointestinal series, or CT scan of the head need only be done as indicated by the presentation.

Differential Diagnosis

The causes of weight loss are legion. Causes such as cancer, collagen vascular disease, diabetes mellitus, hyperthyroidism, malabsorptive syndromes, inflammatory bowel disease, or chronic renal, pulmonary, or cardiac disease warrant consideration in the suspected anorexic; however, in patients with these disorders there may be weight loss but no associated disturbance of body image or fear of obesity. Several psychiatric disturbances, including depression, may be associated with loss of appetite and weight loss. Some unusual central nervous system disorders may present like bulimia, but again there is no distorted body image or overconcern with body shape or weight.

Complications

Eating disorders can result in severe consequences to nearly every system of the body (Table 10–6). The most common complications, however, are fluid and electrolyte abnormalities or constipation. In addition, there may be long-term difficulties with eating and weight management.

Treatment

First, the diagnosis must be discussed with the patient and her parents. The patient needs to know that the clinician appreciates her struggle, aims to restore her to health, won't let her become fat, and will help her to regain control. The parents need to

Table 10–6. Complications of eating disorders.

CNS	Gastrointestinal
↓ REM and short-wave sleep	Dental erosion
Cortical atrophy	Parotid swelling
Thermoregulatory abnormalities, eg, hypothermia	Esophagitis, esophageal tears
	Delayed gastric emptying
Endocrine	Gastric dilatation (rarely rupture)
↓ LH, FSH	Pancreatitis
↓ T3, ↑ rT3, normal T4, TSH	Constipation
Irregular menses	Diarrhea (laxative abuse)
Amenorrhea (primary or secondary)	Superior mesenteric artery syndrome
	Hypercholesterolemia
Metabolic	Mild ↑ liver function tests
Dehydration	
Acidosis	**Renal**
Hypokalemia	Hematuria
Hypochloremia	Proteinuria
Hypochloremic alkalosis	↓ Renal concentrating ability
Hypocalcemia	
Hypophosphatemia	**Hematologic**
Hypomagnesemia	Leukopenia
Osteoporosis	Anemia
Hypercarotenemia	Thrombocytopenia
Cardiovascular	
Bradycardia	
Postural hypotension	
Dysrhythmia, sudden death	
Congestive heart failure (during refeeding)	

understand that eating disorders are symptoms of underlying issues, often a family problem, and that the family is very important to the solution. They need to see that although the presenting symptoms are physical, eating disorders are psychiatric disorders and require the intervention of mental health practitioners. With this age group, it is important to have a mental health practitioner who is skilled in family therapy and has experience with adolescents (see Chapter 25).

A complete medical and physical evaluation should be obtained early to ensure stabilization of the patient's physical status and to get a better understanding of the direction therapy should take. The participation of a dietitian in this evaluation may also be important. Restoration of the nutritional and physiologic state is an early goal, because the patient may need to gain weight before she can deal effectively with her fear of fatness or other issues. The patient may not be in any metabolic danger at the time of presentation, and provided the weight can be

stabilized, she may not require hospitalization but rather regular outpatient visits with the medical and mental health practitioners. An individualized contract can be drawn up and signed by the patient. This contract addresses such issues as long-term weight goals, rate of weight gain, amount of exercise, frequency of visits and of lab tests, minimal weight signaling the need for hospitalization, and consequences of failed weight goals. At each medical visit, the patient should be weighed in a gown only after she voids. The long-term goal is to achieve a weight at which menstruation can take place (Figure 10–6); however, it may be less than ideal body weight. Vital signs and chest and abdominal exams should also be conducted at each visit, and height and triceps skinfold monitored over time.

Most often, the patient can eat sufficient amounts to replace nutrient deficits and to gain weight. High-calorie fluid supplements may be added if weekly weight goals are missed. It is best not to tell the patient that she must take in a certain number of cal-

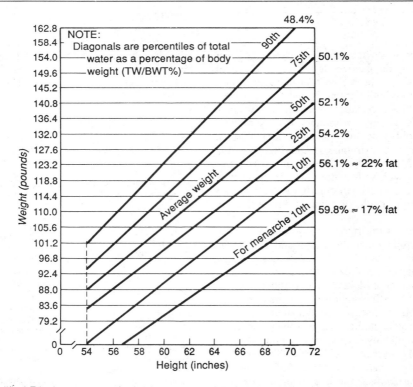

Figure 10–6. Modified Frisch nomogram for minimum weight necessary for normal menstrual cycles. The bottom line shows the minimum weight necessary for menarche. The 10th percentile line shows the minimum weight for correcting secondary amenorrhea in a mature woman. For example, according to the nomogram, an amenorrheic woman 65 inches tall would have to reach at least 103 pounds before menstruation would resume. The top 5 diagonal lines indicate percentiles of total water as a percentage of body weight—which is an index of fatness—for fully grown, mature women in a normal sample. The bottom line represents the 10th percentile for the same sample at menarche. (The 50th percentile line indicates the normal weight for height of mature women who are from 18 to 25 years old. (Reproduced, with permission, from Frisch RE: Fatness and fertility. *Sci Am* (March) 1988;**258**:88.

ories, because she is already fixated on calories. Rather, plans can be developed with the assistance of the dietitian; the planned diets contain sufficient calories for weight .gain. In extremely malnourished and noncompliant hospitalized patients, nasogastric tube feedings or hyperalimentation may initially be necessary. With severe anorexics, one must be on the watch for congestive heart failure caused by refeeding too rapidly. In addition, serum phosphate levels should be followed, because there may be a shift from serum to cells during conversion to anabolic metabolism.

Drug therapy, including appetite stimulants/suppressants, antidepressants, antianxiolytics, and anticonvulsants, has been investigated in a number of studies, but the results to date are equivocal.

Hospitalization may become necessary for medical or psychiatric reasons (Table 10–7). In addition, the patient may require hospitalization not because she is medically unstable or in emotional crisis but because she is out of control or making no progress as an outpatient and thus requires more intensive treatment.

Prognosis

Outcome is difficult to predict because there have been few long-term studies and there is little standardization of criteria and variables. It appears that 40–60% of significantly ill anorexics will make a good physical and psychosocial recovery, and that 75% gain weight. The mortality rate ranges from 0–19% and is at least 5% in those receiving therapy. For bulimia, the literature is even younger, and the outcome appears less favorable. As few as 40–50% of treated bulimics are felt to be cured, and there is a greater likelihood of serious medical complications, death, and risk of suicide than for anorectics who do not manifest bulimic behavior. Recently, however, more attention has focused on eating disorders, and the lay public is becoming more aware of them. For this reason, the disease is being recognized earlier than before.

Table 10–7. Criteria for hospitalization of eating disorder patients.

Medical
Weight loss greater than 30% of body weight over 3 months
Severe metabolic disturbance
  Heart rate < 40
  Temperature < 36 °C (96.8 °F)
  Systolic blood pressure < 70 mm Hg
  Serum K+ < 2.5 despite oral K+ replacement
  Severe dehydration
Severe binging and purging

Psychiatric
Severe depression or risk of suicide
Psychosis
Family crisis
Failure to comply with a therapeutic contract, or inadequate response to outpatient treatment

American Psychiatric Association: *Diagnostic and Statistical Manual of Mental Disorders,* 3rd rev ed. American Psychiatric Association, 1987.
Commerci GD: Eating disorders in adolescents. *Pediatr Rev* 1988;**10**:37.
Garner DM, Garfinkel PE: The eating attitudes test: An index of the symptoms of anorexia nervosa. *Psychol Med* 1979;**9**:273.
Herzog DB, Copeland PM: Eating disorders. *N Engl J Med* 1985;**313**:295.
Palla B, Litt IF: Medical complications of eating disorders in adolescents. *Pediatrics* 1988;**81**:613.
Powers PS: Inpatient treatment of anorexia nervosa. *Pediatrician* 1983–85;**12**:126.
Vandereycken W: Outpatient management of anorexia nervosa. *Pediatrician* 1983–85;**12**:118.
Williams RL: Use of the Eating Attitudes Test and Eating Disorder Inventory in adolescents. *J Adolesc Health Care* 1987;**8**:266.

EXOGENOUS OBESITY

Obesity is the presence of excessive body fat, or weight 20% above desirable weight if the excess weight is due to fat. Body weight is most commonly used to quantitate obesity; however this is a function of age, sex, height, frame, and Tanner stage. In children under 6–7 years of age, body weight tends to underestimate fatness, and in adolescents it overestimates fatness. Weight index, the ratio of actual to ideal weight, may also be used, and an index greater than 1.2 is considered to signal obesity. Although underwater weights may be the most accurate measure of lean body mass, this weighing procedure is not frequently available. Triceps skinfold thickness is the most practical way to measure obesity in children and teenagers, but reproducibility is in question. A triceps skinfold measurement more than one standard deviation above the mean (85th percentile) defines obesity, and one at the 95th percentile indicates superobesity (Fig 10–7).

Background

Obesity is the most common nutritional disorder of children in America, and the prevalence of obesity increases significantly between the elementary and high school years. If a child enters adolescence obese, the odds are 4 to 1 against later achievement of normal weight; but if a child leaves adolescence obese, the odds are 28 to 1 against later normal weight. The National Children and Youth Fitness Study, parts I and II, completed in 1987, demonstrated a decline in fitness of fifth through twelfth graders and first through fourth graders, respectively. When these results were compared to those of a 1960s National Center for Health Statistics study, an increase in skinfold measurements was found. The reduction in fitness has paralleled a rise in hours of TV watched by children. Factors known to increase the risk of a child being obese include having obese parents and being an only child. The associ-

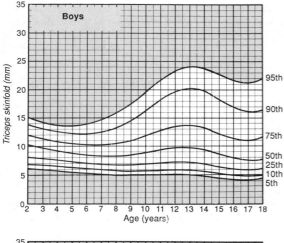

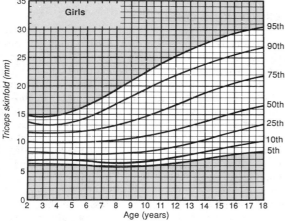

Figure 10–7. Triceps skinfold thickness in boys and girls 2–18 years. (Reproduced, with permission, from Ross Laboratories. Adapted from Johnson CL et al: Basic data on anthropometric measurements and angular measurements of the hip and knee joints for selected age groups, 1–74 years of age, United States, 1971–1975. *Vital and Health Statistics* Series 11, No. 219. [PHS] 81-1669, 1981. © 1983 Ross Laboratories, Columbus, OH 43216. May be copied for individual patient use.)

ated medical risks of obesity include pediatric and adult hypertension, elevated triglyceride levels, cerebrovascular accidents, diabetes mellitus, gallbladder disease, slipped capital-femoral epiphyses, degenerative arthritis, and pregnancy complications. The psychosocial hazards of obesity tend to be the greatest consequence for adolescents, who may experience alienation, distorted peer relations, poor self-esteem, guilt, depression, or distorted body image.

Diagnosis

As stated above, a triceps skinfold measurement

more than one standard deviation above the mean or weight 20% over ideal body weight indicates obesity. Patients can be identified as at risk for obesity based on current weight relative to height, growth and weight trend, and weight of family members. History should include onset of obesity, eating and exercise habits, amount of time spent in sedentary activities such as watching television, previous successful and unsuccessful attempts at weight loss, and family history of obesity. In addition, one needs to assess patients' readiness to lose weight, ie, whether patients are aware of or deny a weight problem; recognize the relationship between food, activity, and weight, and recognize factors that they could change in their own lives. When obesity is diagnosed, the following database can be collected: height; weight; blood pressure; triceps skinfold measurement; fat distribution; examination of the skin, thyroid, heart, and abdomen; hematocrit; and urinalysis. This database helps the physician assess the patient's status and exclude endocrine causes of obesity. Endocrine causes, eg, hypothyroidism or Cushing's disease, can generally be excluded on the basis of history and physical exam.

Treatment

For poorly motivated patients, it is probably best to provide some basic information about weight control and make oneself available for future visits, so as not to set the patient up for failure. For the more motivated patient, treatment should be appropriate to age and developmental level and produce a significant reduction in body weight. The adolescent should be taught appropriate eating and exercise habits to maintain a weight reduction yet meet nutrition needs for growth and development.

Anorectic drugs, fasting, and bypass surgery do not have a role in the management of obese adolescents. An age-appropriate behavior modification program incorporating good dietary counseling and exercise is optimal (Table 10–8). Diet or exercise alone is not nearly as effective. Guidelines that group foods in categories according to their caloric density may be appreciated by adolescents who hate to count calories. Life-style activity, such as walking and taking the stairs, may be more effective in the long run than regimented exercise programs. Behavior-modification components—eg, recording one's eating and activity in a notebook, receiving systematic reinforcement for behavior changes, and restructuring how one sees oneself or plans for success—are especially helpful. One must recognize, however, that no program has the high success rate desired, and that the problem of adolescent obesity must be examined further.

Brownell KD, Stunkard AJ: Behavioral treatment of obesity in children. *Am J Dis Child* 1978;**132:**403.
Brownell KD, Wadden TA, Foster GD: A comprehensive

Table 10–8. Program components for weight control interventions.[1]

Component	Specific Aspects
Physical Activity: Cardiovascular fitness High-calorie equivalent	Frequency: 3–4 times per week Intensity: 50–60% maximal ability (55–65% max heart rate) Duration: 15 min at start, building to 30–40 min Mode: use of large muscle activity, eg, walking, jogging, swimming, cycling Interest: encourage a wide variety of recreational activities Enjoyment: focus on the fun of movement and the enjoyment of being physically active
Nutrition Education	Teach critical aspects of quality nutrition, i.e., food groups, serving requirements, and variety Develop understanding for calorie balance: calories in versus calories out Alert children to pressures of media advertising Instruct on role of snacks and ideas for 'good' snacking Assist children on balancing fast-food eating and calorie intake Teach children to reduce intake of high-calorie, low-nutrition treats
Behavior Modification: Change eating habits Increase habitual physical activity	Identify those cues which affect eating, eg, location of meals, size of plates, food in easy-to-see places Identify behavior that negatively affects weight control: speed of eating, chronic second portions, high-calorie food choices, "pickiness" Contract for increased levels of activity using record cards or activity contracts Develop strategies for more functional activity, eg, walking to school, taking stairs, sitting rather than lying Develop interest in a variety of recreational areas: tennis, dance, skating. Identify cues that lead to inactivity: frequent TV watching, lying down after school or meals, friends who do not like active play

[1]Modified and reproduced, with permission, Ward DS, Bar-Or: Role of the physician and physical education teacher in the treatment of obesity at school. *Pediatrician* 1986;**13**:44. (S Karger AG, Basel.)

treatment plan for obese children and adolescents: Principles and practice. *Pediatrician* 1983–85;**12**:89.

Epstein LH, Wing RR, Valoski A: Childhood obesity. *Pediatr Clin North Am* 1985;**32**:363.

Raithel KS: Are American children really unfit? *Physician Sportsmed* 1988;**16**:146.

SCHOOL AVOIDANCE

General Considerations

Teenagers who have missed more than one week of school for a physical illness or symptom—and whose clinical picture is inconsistent with a serious illness—should be suspected of having primary or secondary emotional factors contributing to the prolonged absence. Investigation of absences may show a pattern, eg, missing morning classes or missing the same days at the beginning or end of the week. Emotional factors for school absenteeism are usually attributed to physical symptoms in this age group.

School avoidance should be suspected in children who are consistently absent in spite of parents' and professionals' attempts to encourage school attendance. Adolescents with school avoidance often have a history of excessive absences or separation difficulties as a younger child. There also may be a record of recurrent somatic complaints. Parents of a school avoider often feel at a loss about how to compel their adolescent to attend school, may lack the sophistication to distinguish malingering from illness, or may have their own underlying need to keep their teenager at home.

A complete history and physical should be performed carefully, reviewing the past medical, educational, and psychiatric history. Signs of emotional problems should be explored. After obtaining permission from the patient and parents, the physician may find it helpful to speak directly with school officials and some key teachers. There may be problems with particular teachers or subjects; environmental factors at the school (eg, fears of physical violence, or problems with intimidation). Some students get so far behind academically that they see no way of catching up and feel overwhelmed. The adolescent may have a long history of separation anxiety, dating back to a traumatic separation from the mother. Separation anxiety may persist and be manifested in subconscious worries that something may happen to the mother while the teenager is at school.

The school nurse may give useful information, including the number of visits to the nurse during the last school year. An important part of the history is how the parents respond to the absences and somatic complaint. There may be a subconscious attempt to keep the adolescent at home, which may be coupled with secondary gains (increased parental attention) for remaining at home.

Treatment

The importance of going back to school in the next 2 to 3 days needs to be emphasized. The pediatrician should facilitate this process by offering to speak with school officials to excuse missed examinations, homework, and papers. The pediatrician should speak directly with teachers who are punitive. The object is to make the transition back to school as easy as possible. The longer adolescents stay out of school, the more anxious they may become about returning, and the more difficult the return becomes. If an illness or symptoms become so severe that an adolescent cannot go to school, both the patient and the parents are informed that a visit to the doctor's office is necessary. The physician focuses visits on the parents as much as the adolescent to alleviate any parental guilt about sending the child to school. If the adolescent cannot stay in school, hospitalization should be recommended for an in-depth medical and psychiatric evaluation. Parents should be cautioned about the possibility of relapse after school holidays, summer vacation, or an acute illness.

Klerman LV: School absence: A health perspective. *Pediatr Clin North Am* 1988;**35**:1253.

SCHOOL FAILURE

General Considerations

When children graduate from grade school to middle school or junior high school, the amount and complexity of coursework increase significantly.

This occurs at about the same time as the rapid physical, social, and emotional changes of puberty. To perform well academically, young adolescents must have the needed cognitive ability, study habits, concentration, motivation, interest, and emotional focus. Academic failure presenting at adolescence has a broad differential: (1) limited intellectual abilities, (2) specific learning disability, (3) depression or emotional problems, (4) physical causes such as visual or hearing problems, (5) excessive school absenteeism secondary to chronic disease such as asthma or neurologic dysfunction, (6) lack of ability to concentrate, (7) attention-deficit disorder, (8) lack of motivation, and (9) drug and alcohol problems. Each of these possible causes must be explored in depth (Table 10–9).

A thorough history, physical examination, appropriate laboratory studies, and educational and psychologic testing should be performed. A detailed medical history is taken to look for the presence of chronic disease or sensory deficits. School avoidance

Table 10–9. A classification of common developmental dysfunctions in adolescence.[1]

Dysfunction	Subtypes	Frequent Manifestations[2]
1. Attention deficits	a. Primary b. Secondary (to anxiety or poor information processing) c. Situational (only evident in certain settings)	Weak attention to detail; distractibility; impulsivity, restlessness; task impersistence; performance inconsistency; organizational problems; reduced working capacity
2. Memory impairments	a. Generalized retrieval problems b. Modality-specific retrieval problems c. Attention-retention deficiencies	Deficient, undependable, or slow recall of data from long- or short-term memory Problems with revisualization or auditory, motor, or sequential recall Poor recall associated with superficial initial registration
3. Language disorders	a. Receptive b. Expressive	Poor verbal and reading comprehension; poor listening; trouble following directions and explanations Problems with word finding, sentence formulation Difficulty with written expression
4. Higher order cognitive disabilities	a. Inferential weakness b. Poor verbal reasoning c. Poor nonverbal reasoning d. Difficulty with abstraction, symbolization e. Weak generalization and rule application	Problems understanding and assimilating new concepts; tendency to think "concretely" delays in mathematics, reading comprehension, science, social studies
5. Fine motor incoordination	a. Eye:hand coordination problems b. Impaired propriokinesthetic feedback c. Dyspraxia d. Motor memory impairment	Slow, labored, sometimes illegible writing; awkward pencil grip; dyssynchrony between cognitive tempo and writing speed; output failure—reduced productivity
6. Organizational deficiencies	a. Temporal-sequential disorientation b. Material disarray c. Integrative dysfunction d. Resynthesis problems e. Attentional disorganization	Problems with time allocation, schedules, planning, arranging ideas in writing Tendency to lose, misplace, forget books, papers; trouble organizing notebook Varying inability to integrate data from multiple sources or sensory modalities Trouble extracting most salient details, retelling and adapting data to current demands Impulsivity, erratic tempo, poor self-monitoring, careless errors
7. Socialization disabilities	a. Wide range of subtypes, including conduct disorder, social impulsivity, impaired social cognition or feedback, egocentricity	Antisocial behaviors; delinquency; withdrawal; excessive dependency on peer support

[1]Modified and reproduced, with permission, from Levine MD, Zallen BG: Learning disorders of adolescence. *Pediatr Clin North Am* 1984;**31**:2.
[2]Manifestations are likely to vary somewhat depending upon compensatory strengths, quality of educational experience, and motivation.

(see the previous section) should be ruled out. A history of an attention-deficit disorder or use of stimulant medication in the past may be an indication of ongoing problems with concentration. Educational records, including previous educational and intelligence testing, are important background information. The emotional history may reveal past episodes of counseling for depression or other significant psychiatric problems. The presence of conflict in the family, eg, divorce or alcoholism, may play an important role, distracting the adolescent from academic responsibilities. There may be a family history of school problems in other siblings or family members.

Treatment

Treatment depends on cause. Management must be individualized to address specific needs, foster strengths, and implement a feasible program. For children with specific learning disabilities, an individual prescription for regular and special educational courses, teachers, and extracurricular activities is important. Counseling helps these adolescents gain coping skills, raise self-esteem, and develop socialization skills. If there is a history of hyperactivity or attention-deficit disorder along with poor ability to concentrate, a trial of stimulant medication (eg, methylphenidate hydrochloride or dextroamphetamine sulfate) may be useful. If the teenager appears to be depressed or if other serious emotional problems are uncovered, further psychologic evaluation should be recommended.

Levine MD, Zallen BG: The learning disorders of adolescence: Organic and nonorganic failure to strive. *Pediatr Clin North Am* 1984;**31**:345.

BREAST DISORDERS

The breast exam should become part of the routine physical exam in females as soon as breast budding occurs. The preadolescent comes to see breast examination as a routine part of health care, and it provides an opportunity to reassure her about any concerns she may have. The breast examination begins with inspection of the breasts for symmetry and Tanner stage. Asymmetric breast development is common in adolescents, who need reassurance that the asymmetry usually becomes less apparent as development progresses. Unusual causes of breast asymmetry that may require further intervention include unilateral breast hypoplasia or amastia, or absence of the pectoralis major muscle. In addition, unilateral virginal hypertrophy (massive enlargement of the breast during puberty) may result in significant asymmetry.

Palpation of the breasts can be performed with the patient in the supine position and the patient's ipsilateral arm placed under her head. The examiner palpates the breast tissue with the flat of the fingers in widening circles from the areola out to the sternum, clavicle, and axilla. The areola should be gently compressed to check for discharge.

Instructions for breast self-exam and its purpose can be given to older adolescents during this portion of the physical exam, and the patient should be encouraged to begin monthly self-exam after each menstrual flow.

BREAST MASSES

Most breast masses in adolescents are benign (Table 10–10); however, approximately 150 cases of adenocarcinoma are reported each year in the USA in women under 25 years of age. Fibroadenomas account for 90% of breast lumps in teenagers seen in referral clinics; the remainder are cysts. In practice, cysts may account for as many as 50% of breast masses in adolescents, but they are readily diagnosed, and many resolve spontaneously.

Fibroadenoma

Fibroadenoma presents as a rubbery, well-demarcated, slowly growing, nontender mass that may occur in any quadrant but is most commonly found in the upper outer quadrant of the breast. Most are less than 5 cm in diameter. In 25% of cases, there are multiple or recurrent lesions. Quiescence can be expected after the teenage years.

Cysts

Breast cysts are generally tender and spongy, with exacerbation of symptoms premenstrually and abatement just after. Often they are multiple. Spon-

Table 10–10. Diagnoses of female patients seen for a breast-related complaint in an adolescent medicine clinic.[1]

Clinical Diagnosis	Patients (*n* = 130)	Total(%)
Fibrocystic disease	66	50.8
Fibroadenoma	19	14.6
Normal breasts	17	13.1
Mastalgia	6	4.6
Unknown	6	4.6
Abscess/mastitis	5	3.9
Breast asymmetry	3	2.3
Breast hypertrophy	2	1.5
Early pregnancy	2	1.5
Hematoma	2	1.5
Granular cell myoblastoma	1	0.8
Lymphadenopathy	1	0.8
Carcinoma	0	0

[1]Modified and reproduced, with permission, from Diehl T, Kaplan DW: Breast masses in adolescent females. *Sexually Active Teenagers* 1988;**2**:151.

taneous regression occurs over 2 to 3 menstrual cycles in about half of cases.

It is reasonable to follow breast masses that are consistent with fibroadenoma or cyst in adolescents for 2 to 3 menstrual cycles. About one-quarter of fibroadenomas become smaller, and about one-half of cysts resolve. If there is no change in a presumed fibroadenoma after this time, an ultrasound study will differentiate a solid tumor from a cyst. Patients with solid tumors should be referred for excisional biopsy. Persistent cystic lesions may be drained by needle aspiration. Patients with suspicious lesions should be referred immediately to a breast surgeon (Table 10–11).

Fibrocystic Breasts

Fibrocystic breasts (or fibrocystic breast disease) is sometimes seen in older adolescents but is more common in women in their third and fourth decades. It is characterized by cyclical tenderness and nodularity bilaterally and is believed to be influenced by the estrogen-progesterone balance.

Reassuring the young woman about the benign nature of the disease and emphasizing the importance of breast self-exam may be all that is needed. Oral contraceptives reduce the risk of fibrocystic breasts and may be appropriate for the sexually active female with a personal history of breast cyst or family history of fibrocystic breasts. Recent studies have shown no association between methylxanthines and fibrocystic breasts; however, some women report reduced symptoms when they discontinue caffeine intake. The efficacy of vitamin E also remains unknown.

Table 10–11. Breast lesions.

Adenocarcinoma: Hard, nonmobile, well-circumscribed, painless mass; generally indolent clinical course; occurs also in males but less frequently

Cystosarcoma phylloides: Firm, rubbery mass that may suddenly enlarge; associated skin necrosis; most often benign

Giant juvenile fibroadenoma: Remarkably large fibroadenoma with overlying dilated superficial veins; accounts for 5–10% of fibroadenomas in adolescents; benign but requires excision to prevent breast atrophy and for cosmetic reasons

Intraductal papilloma: A cylindrical tumor arising from the duct epithelium; often subareolar but may be in the periphery of the breast in adolescents, with associated nipple discharge; most are benign but require excision for cytologic diagnosis

Fat necrosis: Localized, inflammatory process in one breast; follows trauma in about half of cases; subsequent scarring may be confused with cancer

Virginal or juvenile hypertrophy: Massive enlargement of both breasts or, less often, one breast; attributed to end-organ hypersensitivity to normal hormonal levels just before or within a few years after menarche

Miscellaneous: Fibroma, galactocele, hemangioma, intraductal granuloma, interstitial fibrosis, keratoma, lipoma, granular cell myoblastoma, papilloma, sclerosing adenosis

Breast Abscess

The female with a breast abscess usually complains of unilateral breast pain, and examination reveals overlying inflammatory changes. Often the exam is misleading in that the infection may extend much deeper than suspected. A palpable mass is found only late in the course. Although breast-feeding is the most common cause of mastitis, trauma and eczema involving the areola are frequent factors in teenagers. *Staphylococcus aureus* is the most common cause, but other aerobic and anaerobic organisms have also been implicated.

Cyclic mastodynia, fibrocystic disease, or chest wall pain may also be causes of breast pain, but there should be no associated inflammatory signs.

Fluctuant abscesses should be surgically incised and drained. Oral antibiotics with appropriate coverage (dicloxacillin or a cephalosporin) should be given for 2 to 4 weeks. In addition, ice packs for the first 24 hours and heat thereafter may relieve symptoms.

GALACTORRHEA

General Considerations

In teenagers, galactorrhea, or inappropriate nipple discharge, is most often benign; however, a careful history and workup are necessary.

Galactorrhea may be present after spontaneous or induced abortions as well as postpartum. Numerous prescribed and illicit drugs are associated with galactorrhea (Table 10–12). In addition, stimulation of the intercostal nerves (following surgery or due to herpes zoster), stimulation of the nipples, endocrine disorders (hypothyroidism, pituitary prolactinoma), CNS disorders (hypothalamic injury), or significant emotional distress may produce galactorrhea (Table 10–13).

Clinical Findings

If there is no history of pregnancy or drug use, thyroid-stimulating hormone (TSH) and prolactin levels should be determined. An elevated TSH confirms the diagnosis of hypothyroidism. An elevated prolactin and normal TSH, often accompanied by amenorrhea, suggest a hypothalamic or pituitary tumor, and CT scan is indicated. When the prolactin level is normal, uncommon causes such as adrenal, renal, or ovarian tumors should be considered. For those with a negative workup and persistent galactorrhea, careful follow-up is required. In many cases, symptoms resolve spontaneously, and no diagnosis is made.

Treatment

Treatment of galactorrhea depends on the underlying cause. Prolactinomas may be surgically removed or suppressed with bromocriptine. Bromocriptine

Table 10–12. Drugs associated with breast symptoms (galactorrhea, gynecomastia, pain, mass).[1]

Street Drugs (Illicit or Abused)
Marijuana
Opiates
   Codeine
   Heroin
   Morphine
Amphetamines
Meprobamate

Hormones or Related Drugs
Oral contraceptives
Estrogens
Tamoxifen
Bromocriptine withdrawal
Methyltestosterone
Human chorionic gonadotropin

Cancer Drugs
Vincristine
Busulfan

Prescription Medications
Isoniazid
Cimetidine
Diazepam
Chlordiazepoxide
Phenothiazines
Chlorpromazine
Haloperidol
Tricyclic antidepressants
Amitriptyline
Imipramine
Fluphenazine
Mesoridazine
Perphenazine
Thiethylperazine
Trifluoperazine
Trimeprazine
Thioxanthenes
Reserpine
Methyldopa
Spironolactone
Digoxin

[1]Modified and reproduced, with permission, from Beach RK: Routine breast exams: A chance to reassure, guide, and protect. *Contemp Pediatr* 1987;**4**:70.

Table 10–13. Causes of galactorrhea.[1]

Hypothalamic disorders
  Functional
    Postpartum
    Without pregnancy
  Pathologic
    Infiltrative
      Sarcoid
      Histiocytosis X
      Hypothalamic tumors
    Section of pituitary stalk
Drug therapy
  Tranquilizers
  Tricyclic antidepressants
  Methyldopa
  Rauwolfia alkaloids
  Oral contraceptives
  Estrogens
Neoplasms
  Pituitary tumors
    Prolactin secretion only
    Prolactin and ACTH secretion (Cushing's disease)
    Growth hormone secretion with or without prolactin
      secretion (acromegaly)
  Ectopic prolactin-secreting tumors
Hypothyroidism
Neurogenic stimulation
  Breast stimulation
  Chest wall lesions (herpes zoster, thoracotomy)

[1]Modified and reproduced, with permission, from Fraser WM, Blackard WG: Medical conditions that affect the breast and lactation. *Clin Obstet Gynecol* 1975;**18**:51.

may also be beneficial to some amenorrheic females with normal prolactin levels.

GYNECOMASTIA

General Considerations

Gynecomastia is a common concern of male adolescents, the majority of whom (60–70%) develop transient subareolar breast tissue during Tanner stages II–III. Proposed causes include testosterone-estrogen imbalance, increased prolactin level or abnormal serum binding protein levels.

Clinical Findings

In type I idiopathic gynecomastia, the adolescent presents with a unilateral (20% bilateral), tender, firm mass beneath the areola. More generalized breast enlargement is classified as type II. Pseudo-gynecomastia refers to excessive fat tissue or prominent pectoralis muscles.

Differential Diagnosis

Gynecomastia may be drug-induced (see Table 10–12). Klinefelter's syndrome; testicular, adrenal, or pituitary tumors; or thyroid or hepatic dysfunction may also be associated with gynecomastia (Table 10–14).

Treatment

If gynecomastia is idiopathic, reassurance of the common and benign nature of the process is given. Resolution may take several months to 2 years. Medical reduction has been achieved with pharmacotherapeutic agents, eg, dihydrotestosterone heptanoate, danazol, clomiphene citrate, and tamoxifen citrate, but these should be reserved for those with no decrease in breast size after 2 years. Surgery is reserved for those with significant psychologic trauma or severe breast enlargement.

Beach RK: Routine breast exams: A chance to reassure, guide, and protect. *Contemp Pediatr* (Oct) 1987;**4**:70.

Diehl T, Kaplan DW: Breast masses in adolescent females. *Sexually Active Teenagers* 1988;**2**:151.

Dudgeon DL: Pediatric breast lesions: Take the conservative approach. *Contemp Pediatr* (Jan) 1985;**2**:61.

Table 10–14. Disorders associated with gynecomastia.

Klinefelter's syndrome
Traumatic paraplegia
Male pseudohermaphroditism
Testicular feminization syndrome
Reifenstein's syndrome
17-Ketosteroid reductase deficiency
Endocrine tumors (seminoma, Leydig cell tumor, teratoma,
    feminizing adrenal tumor, hepatoma, leukemia, hemo-
    philia, bronchogenic carcinoma, leprosy, etc)
Hypothyroidism
Hyperthyroidism
Cirrhosis
Herpes zoster
Friedreich's ataxia

Eberle AJ, Sparrow JT, Keenan BS: Treatment of persistent pubertal gynecomastia with dihydrotestosterone heptanoate. *J Pediatrics* 1986;**109**:144.

Fraser WM, Blackard WG: Medical conditions that affect the breast and lactation. Clin *Obstet Gynecol* 1975;**18**:51.

Rohn RD: Galactorrhea in the adolescent. *J Adolesc Health Care* 1984;**5**:37.

GYNECOLOGIC DISORDERS IN ADOLESCENCE

MENSTRUAL PHYSIOLOGY

The menstrual cycle is divided into 3 phases: follicular, ovulatory, and luteal. During the follicular phase, pulsatile gonadotropin-releasing hormone (GnRH) stimulates anterior pituitary secretion of follicle-stimulating hormone (FSH) and luteinizing hormone (LH). Under the influence of FSH and LH, a dominant follicle emerges by day 5–7 of the menstrual cycle, and the others become atretic. Rising estradiol levels cause proliferation of the endometrium. By midfollicular phase, FSH is beginning to decline secondary to estradiol-mediated negative feedback, while LH continues to rise due to estradiol-mediated positive feedback.

There has been a proliferation of LH receptors on the follicle, and it secretes more estradiol in the periovulatory phase, resulting in further proliferation of the endometrium. The rising LH initiates progesterone secretion and the luteinization of the granulosa cells of the follicle. Progesterone in turn stimulates LH and FSH further. This leads to the LH surge, which causes the follicle to rupture and expel the oocyte.

During the luteal phase, the pulsatile release of GnRH occurs less frequently, and LH and FSH gradually decline. The corpus luteum secretes progester-

one and 17-OH progesterone. The endometrium enters the secretory phase in response to rising levels of estrogen and progesterone, with maturation 8–9 days after ovulation. If there is no pregnancy or placental human chorionic gonadotropin (hCG), luteolysis begins; estrogen and progesterone levels decline; and the endometrial lining is shed as menstrual flow (Figure 10–8).

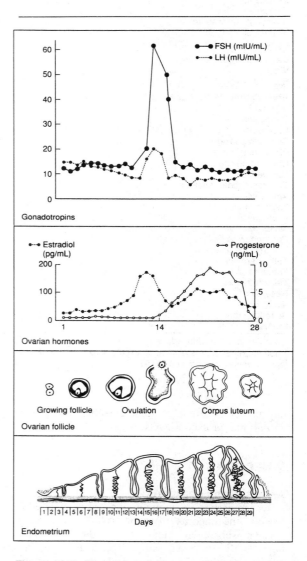

Figure 10–8. Physiology of the normal ovulatory menstrual cycle; gonadotropin secretion, ovarian hormone production, follicular maturation, and endometrial changes during one cycle. FSH = follicle-stimulating hormone; LH = luteinizing hormone. (Reproduced, with permission, from Emans SJH, Goldstein DP: *Pediatric & Adolescent Gynecology*, 2nd ed. Little, Brown, 1982.)

PELVIC EXAM

A pelvic exam may be indicated to evaluate abdominal pain or menstrual disorders, or to detect a suspected sexually transmitted disease in the adolescent. In addition, by approximately 16–18 years of age, a pelvic examination should be performed to obtain the first Papanicolaou smear and ensure normal reproductive anatomy if annual pelvic examination has not yet been initiated. The adolescent may be apprehensive about the first exam. It should not be rushed, and an explanation of the procedure and its purpose should precede it. The patient can be encouraged to relax by slow, deep breathing and by loosening her lower abdominal and inner thigh muscles. A young adolescent may wish to have her mother present during the exam, but the history should be taken privately. A female chaperon should be present for male examiners.

The pelvic exam begins by placing the patient in dorsal lithotomy position after equipment and supplies are ready (Table 10–15). The examiner inspects the external genitalia, noting the pubic hair maturity rating, the size of the clitoris (2–5 mm is normal), the Skene's glands just inside the urethral meatus, and the Bartholin's glands at 4 o'clock and 8 o'clock outside the hymenal ring. In cases of alleged sexual abuse or assault, the horizontal measurement of the relaxed prepubertal hymenal opening should be taken, and the presence of any lacerations, bruises, scarring, or synechiae about the hymen, vulva, or anus should be noted.

Next a vaginal speculum of the appropriate size is inserted at a 45-degree twist and angled 45 degrees down. (A medium Pederson speculum is most often used in sexually experienced patients; a narrow Pederson is used for virginal patients. A pediatric speculum may be necessary in examining children.) The vaginal walls are inspected for estrinization, inflammation, or lesions. The cervix should be dull pink, and a cervical ectropion is commonly seen in adolescents; the columnar epithelium extends outside the cervical os onto the face of the cervix until later adolescence, when it recedes.

At this time specimens are obtained, including wet prep for WBCs, trichomonads, and "clue cells"; potassium hydroxide prep for yeast; cervical swab for gonorrhea culture; endocervical and cervical (transition zone from columnar to squamous epithelium) samples for Papanicolaou smear, and last, cervical swab for *Chlamydia* antigen-detection test.

The speculum is then removed, and the bimanual exam is performed to assess uterine size and position, adnexal enlargement or tenderness, or cervical motion tenderness. Rectovaginal exam may be helpful in assessing uterine size or detecting beading from endometriosis.

MENSTRUAL DISORDERS

1. AMENORRHEA

Amenorrhea is the lack of menses when otherwise expected to occur. **Primary amenorrhea** refers to delay in menarche such that there are no menstrual periods or secondary sex characteristics by 14 years of age or no menses in the presence of secondary sex characteristics by 16 years of age. **Secondary amenorrhea** is defined as the absence of menses for at least 3 cycles after regular cycles have been present. In some instances, evaluation should begin immediately, without waiting for the specified age or duration of lapsed periods, eg, in patients with suspected pregnancy, short stature with the stigmata of Turner's syndrome, or an anatomic defect.

Evaluation for Primary Amenorrhea

Primary amenorrhea may be the result of anatomic abnormalities (imperforate hymen, transverse vaginal septum, vaginal agenesis, agenesis of the cervix, absent uterus), chromosomal deviations (Turner's syndrome XO, mosaicism, testicular feminization), or physiologic delay (hypogonadotropic hypogonadism, familial delay, chronic disease, stress, obesity, or weight loss) (Table 10–16).

During the history, the physician should determine whether puberty has commenced and the age of menarche for other female relatives. A careful physical exam should be done. The examiner keeps in mind that adrenal androgens are largely responsible for axillary and pubic hair and that estrogen is responsible for breast development; maturation of the external genitalia, vagina, and uterus; and menstruation. Tanner stage and percent of ideal body weight should be noted. The stigmas of Turner's syndrome should also be looked for: height less than 60 inches, shieldlike chest, widely spaced nipples, increased carrying angle of the arms, webbed neck, etc. If pelvic exam

Table 10–15. Items for pelvic exam tray.

Medium and virginal speculums (warm)
Gloves
Applicator sticks, sterile
Sigmoidoscopy swabs to remove excess discharge
Cervical spatulas
Microscope slides and cover slips (frosted and labeled)
Centrifuge tube or test tube (if swab is to be placed in drop of saline and slide prepared later)
NaCl dropper bottle
KOH dropper bottle
Slide container to send to lab
Gonorrhea culture plate (room temperature)
Chlamydia culture tube or antigen detection kit
Lubricant
Kleenex
Hemoccult cards
pH paper

Table 10–16. Causes of amenorrhea.

Hypothalamic Pituitary Axis
Hypothalamic repression
  Emotional stress
  Depression
  Chronic disease
  Weight loss
  Obesity
  Severe dieting
  Strenuous athletics
  Drugs (post–birth control pills, phenothiazines)
CNS lesion
  Pituitary lesion: adenoma, prolactinoma
  Craniopharyngioma and other brainstem, parasellar
    tumors
  Head injury with hypothalamic contusion
  Infiltrative process (sarcoidosis)
  Vascular disease (hypothalamic vasculitis)
Congenital conditions[1]
  Kallmann's syndrome
Ovaries
Gonadal dysgenesis[1]
  Turner's syndrome (XO)
  Mosaic (XX/XO)
Injury to ovary
  Autoimmune disease (may include thyroid, adrenal, islet
    cells)
  Infection (mumps, oophoritis)
  Toxins (alkylating chemotherapeutic agents)
  Irradiation
  Trauma, torsion (rare)
Polycystic ovary syndrome (Stein-Leventhal) (virilization may
  be present)
Ovarian failure
  Premature menopause (may result from causes of ovarian
    injury)
  Resistant ovary
  Variant of gonadal dysgenesis (mosaic)
Uterovaginal Outflow Tract
Müllerian dysgenesis[1]
  Congenital deformity or absence of uterus, fallopian
    tubes, or vagina
  Imperforate hymen, transverse vaginal septum, vaginal
    agenesis, agenesis of the cervix[1]
Testicular feminization (absent uterus)[1]
Uterine lining defect
  Asherman's syndrome (intrauterine synechiae
    postcurettage or endometritis)
  TB, brucellosis
Defect in Hormone Synthesis/Action (virilization may be
  present)
Adrenal hyperplasia[1]
Cushing's disease
Adrenal tumor
Ovarian tumor (rare)
Drugs (steroids, ACTH)

[1]Indicates condition that usually presents as primary amenorrhea.

reveals normal female external genitalia and pelvic organs, the physician may order a vaginal smear for estrogen influence or a challenge of progesterone (Provera, 10 mg orally twice daily for 5 days) (Figure 10–9). If the vaginal smear shows estrogen influence or withdrawal bleeding occurs after Provera, normal anatomy and adequate estrogen effect are implied. A determination of serum LH level helps to rule out polycystic ovary syndrome; if this test is normal, reassurance may be given and the developmental process followed every few months. If estrogen is insufficient (atrophic vaginal smear or no withdrawal bleeding), serum gonadotropin (FSH and LH) levels should be determined. Low levels of gonadotropins indicate a more severe hypothalamic suppression, possibly due to anorexia nervosa, chronic disease, or a CNS tumor. Involvement of a gynecologist and endocrinologist is helpful at this point. If gonadotropin levels are high, ovarian failure or gonadal dysgenesis is implied, and a karyotype should clarify the cause. Absence of any sign of puberty by 14 years of age indicates inadequate estrogen, and the physician should check FSH, LH, and karyotype first before testing for estrogen effect.

If signs of virilization are present (Figure 10–10), the first step is to determine the LH level to rule out polycystic ovaries. If the LH level is low in the presence of virilization, an adrenal disorder is the most likely diagnosis. Endocrinologic and gynecologic consultations may assist in determining the diagnosis.

If physical exam reveals an absent uterus (see Figure 10–9), karyotyping should be performed to differentiate testicular feminization from müllerian duct defect, because these 2 entities are managed differently.

Evaluation and Treatment of Secondary Amenorrhea

Secondary amenorrhea results when there is unopposed estrogen, maintaining the endometrium in the proliferative phase. The most common causes are pregnancy, stresses (fever, emotional turmoil, significant weight change, significant exercise, anorexia nervosa, or chronic disease), or Stein-Leventhal syndrome (polycystic ovaries). History should focus on issues of stress, weight change, strenuous exercise, sexual activity, and contraceptive use. Review of systems should include questions about headaches, visual changes, and galactorrhea. Physical exam should include a careful funduscopic exam, examination of visual fields, palpation of the thyroid, determination of blood pressure and heart rate, compression of the areola to check for galactorrhea, and a search for signs of androgen excess (eg, hirsutism, clitoromegaly, severe acne, or ovarian enlargement).

The first laboratory study obtained is a pregnancy test, even if the patient denies sexual activity. If there is no pregnancy, vaginal smear for estrogen or progesterone challenge (Provera 10 mg orally twice daily for 5 days) should be done to determine if the patient has an estrogen-primed uterus that will respond with withdrawal bleeding (Figure 10–11 and Table 10–17).

Generally, progesterone will not induce a period in a patient with hypopituitarism due to a tumor,

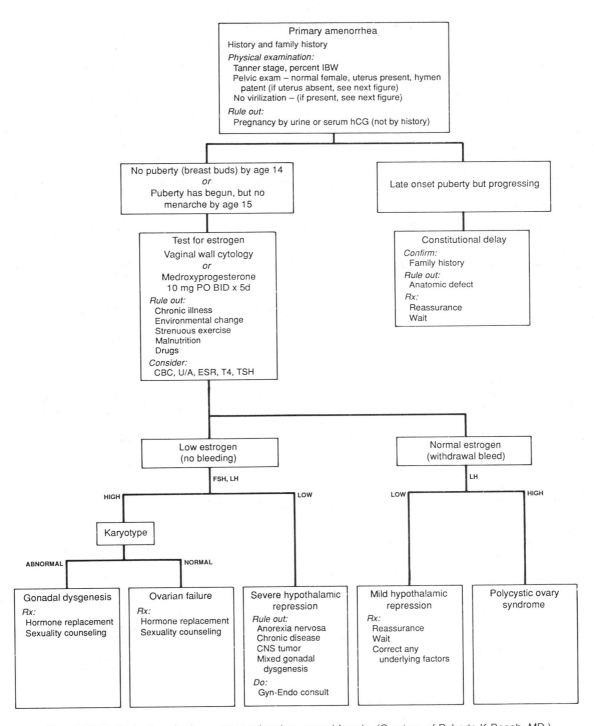

Figure 10–9. Evaluation of primary amenorrhea in a normal female. (Courtesy of Roberta K Beach, MD.)

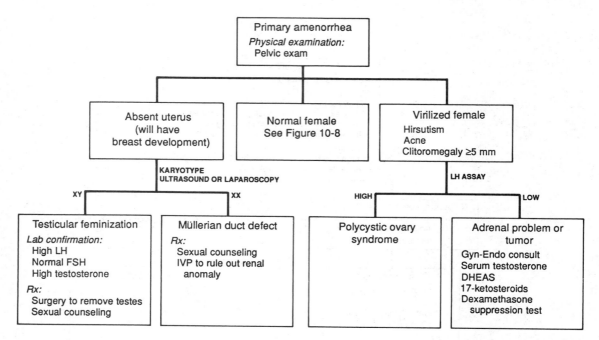

Figure 10–10. Evaluation of primary amenorrhea in a female without a uterus or with virilization. (Courtesy of Roberta K Beach, MD.)

profound hypothalamic suppression due to anorexia nervosa, or a massive weight gain. Most patients who have withdrawal flow to progesterone have hypothalamic amenorrhea due to weight change, athletics, stress, or illness; however, disorders such as polycystic ovaries, adrenal disorders, ovarian tumors, thyroid disease, and diabetes mellitus should be excluded by history and physical exam and appropriate laboratory studies.

If there is no withdrawal flow after the progesterone challenge (see Figure 10–11), serum levels of estradiol, FSH, LH, and prolactin should be checked. An elevated FSH level accompanied by a low estrogen level implies ovarian failure, and antiovarian antibodies and laparoscopy should be considered. If gonadotropin levels are low or normal and estradiol level is normal, hypothalamic amenorrhea is possible, but one must consider the possibilities of a CNS tumor (prolactinoma), pituitary infarction from postpartum hemorrhage or sickle cell anemia, uterine synechia, or chronic disease. Further evaluation may be necessary.

The entity polycystic ovaries is a spectrum of disorders and is not necessarily accompanied by the classic symptoms of obesity, hirsutism, oligomenorrhea, and infertility. The LH level is usually elevated above 30 mIU/mL, and the FSH slightly suppressed. Because of insufficient FSH, androstenedione cannot be converted to estradiol in the ovarian follicle, and anovulation and production of excess androgens re-

sult. These patients can be given progesterone each month to allow a withdrawal flow if there is no evidence of progressive hirsutism and the ovaries are normal in size. Oral contraceptive pills are an alternative treatment. If the patient wishes to become pregnant, she should be referred to a gynecologist for clomiphene or an ovarian wedge resection.

2. DYSMENORRHEA

Dysmenorrhea is the most common gynecologic complaint of adolescent girls, with an incidence of about 60%. Yet many teenage girls will not seek help from their physician, instead relying on female relatives, friends, and the media for advice. Therefore, the physician should ask about menstrual cramps when taking a review of systems. In this era of prostaglandin inhibitors, much can be done to alleviate suffering.

Dysmenorrhea can be divided into primary and secondary dysmenorrhea on the basis of whether or not there is underlying pelvic pathology.

Primary Dysmenorrhea

Primary dysmenorrhea, in which no pelvic pathology is detectable, can be further subdivided into primary spasmodic dysmenorrhea and psychogenic dysmenorrhea. Primary spasmodic dysmenorrhea accounts for 80% of adolescent dysmenorrhea and

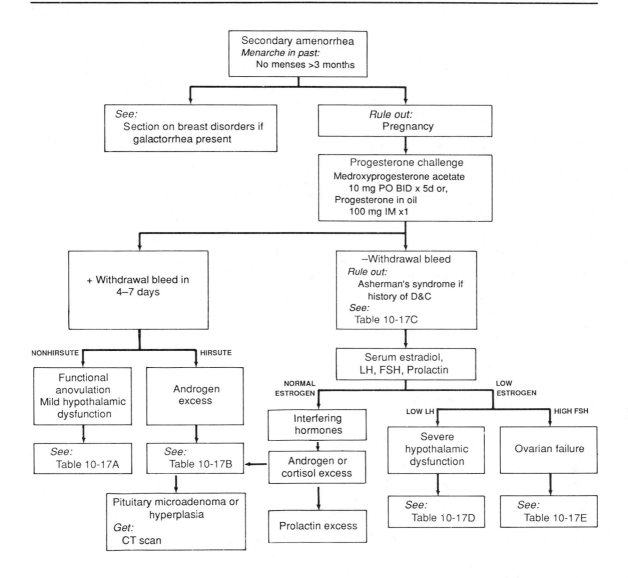

Figure 10–11. Evaluation of secondary amenorrhea. (Courtesy of Roberta K Beach, MD.)

most often affects women under 25 years of age. It results from the release of excessive amounts of prostaglandin $F_{2\alpha}$, which attaches to myometrial receptor sites, causing uterine contractions, hypoxia, and ischemia. In addition, prostaglandins also directly sensitize pain receptors and lower the pain threshold. As most of the prostaglandin release is in the first 48 hours of menses, the pain generally starts with the onset of flow or just prior and lasts 1–2 days. Primary spasmodic dysmenorrhea does not typically begin until 6–18 months after menarche

when the cycles become ovulatory; endometrial production of prostaglandins is higher in the luteal phase, which doesn't exist unless ovulation occurs. Symptoms consist of lower abdominal cramps, which may radiate to the lower back and thighs. Associated symptoms of nausea, vomiting, diarrhea, and urinary frequency may be present and are also due to prostaglandin release.

Psychogenic dysmenorrhea typically starts at menarche. Pain begins with the anticipation of menses and lasts throughout the flow. These patients may

Table 10–17. Management of secondary amenorrhea by cause.

	Cause	Lab	Management
Mild hypothalamic dysfunction	Recent pregnancy Physical illness Weight loss Obesity Emotional stress Environmental change Strenuous athletics Drugs (post birth control pills, phenothiazines)	CBC, urinalysis ESR T_4, TSH, etc. (as indicated)	Reassurance; assessment of birth control needs Repeat of progesterone test every 3 months (after ruling out pregnancy) LH, FSH, prolactin if no menses for 1 year
Androgen excess	Polycystic ovary syndrome (PCO) Cushing's syndrome Adrenal hyperplasia Adrenal tumor Ovarian tumor Drugs (steroids, ACTH)	LH, FSH (high LH suggests PCO); consultation with endocrinologist to help evaluate adrenals	If PCO, birth control pills (Demulen) to control hirsutism and menses Treatment of underlying problem
Asherman's syndrome	Uterine synechiae post TAb or D&C	No bleeding after 1 cycle of combination oral contraceptive (Ovulen)	Referral to gynecologist
Severe hypothalamic dysfunction	Anorexia nervosa Severe emotional stress Chronic systemic disease CNS tumor Pituitary infarction	Low estrogen Low LH Check T_4, TSH, ESR, neurologic exam	Treatment of cause; slow hormone recovery expected
Ovarian failure	Variant of gonadal dysgenesis (mosaicism XX/XO) Postirradiation Postchemotherapy Autoimmune oophoritis Resistant ovarian syndrome Premature menopause	Chromosomes Antiovarian antibodies Laparoscopy Ovarian biopsy	Referral to gynecologist; hormone replacement therapy

have a history of sexual abuse or may be having difficulty adjusting to womanhood. There may be secondary gain from school or work avoidance.

The pelvic exam, when done, is normal in females with primary spasmodic or psychogenic dysmenorrhea. The pelvic exam has diagnostic benefits and provides an opportunity to educate and reassure the patient about her normal reproductive function. However, if the patient has never been sexually active and the history is consistent with primary spasmodic dysmenorrhea, a trial of a prostaglandin inhibitor is reasonable. If the patient is sexually active, or there is no response to a prostaglandin inhibitor, a pelvic exam is indicated.

The patient should be educated about normal menstrual function and reassured that the pain does not indicate disease. Exercise and positive feelings about her body can be encouraged. Relaxation techniques and biofeedback may be helpful for patients with psychogenic dysmenorrhea, but counseling may be necessary to understand underlying issues. Application of a heating pad, warm baths, and nonprescription analgesics may be sufficient for mild primary spasmodic dysmenorrhea. For moderate to severe spasmodic dysmenorrhea, prescription prostaglandin inhibitors, or oral contraceptive pills in sexually active patients, are appropriate. Either of these medications will relieve symptoms in about 90% of patients. The patient should be instructed to begin prostaglandin inhibitors (Table 10–18) with the first sign of pain or menstrual flow. Side effects are rare since prostaglandin inhibitors are used for only 1–4 days but may include epigastric pain, nausea, vomiting, headache, dizziness, tinnitus, or pruritus. They may decrease renal function. Relative contraindications include chronic gastrointestinal inflammation, reactive airways disease, hypersensitivity, or bleeding diathesis.

Secondary Dysmenorrhea

Secondary dysmenorrhea refers to menstrual pain due to an underlying pelvic lesion. Although uncommon in adolescents, when present it is most often due to infection or endometriosis. In the patient with

Table 10–18. Prostaglandin inhibitors used for dysmenorrhea.

Generic Name	Trade Name	Dose (mg)[1]
Aspirin		
Ibuprofen	Motrin, Rufen, Advil, Nuprin, Medipren	200, 300, 400, 600, 800
Mefenamic acid	Ponstel	250
Naproxen	Naprosyn	250, 375, 500
Naproxen sodium	Anaprox	275

[1]It is recommended that 2 tablets be taken at onset of menstrual cramps or flow, then 1 every 6 to 8 hours thereafter.

infection, there may be pelvic cramps of recent onset, excessive bleeding or intermenstrual spotting, or vaginal discharge. The patient is generally sexually active. The pain of endometriosis generally starts more than 2 years after menarche. Two-thirds of those with endometriosis will feel tenderness on exam, particularly during the late luteal phase. This disease is not limited to adults as once thought; in one study of adolescent females with chronic pelvic pain, more than 40% who had not received a definitive diagnosis by the third visit were found to have endometriosis. If the patient has a delay in menses, a complication of pregnancy (eg, spontaneous abortion or ectopic pregnancy) should be suspected. If menstrual cramps start at menarche, congenital anomalies (eg, a transverse vaginal septum, septate uterus, or cervical stenosis) should be suspected. Intrauterine devices may cause dysmenorrhea or may increase the risk of pelvic infections and thereby cause pain. Lastly, pelvic adhesions may be responsible for pelvic pain; a history of abdominal surgery should, therefore, be elicited.

The clinician evaluating a patient with secondary dysmenorrhea should take a sexual history and conduct a pelvic exam, even if the patient is not sexually active. Gonorrhea culture, test for *Chlamydia,* complete blood count, and erythrocyte sedimentation rate should be obtained to look for infection. A gynecologic consultation is indicated to look for endometriosis or congenital problems by ultrasound, hysteroscopy, or laparoscopy.

Treatment depends on cause. Infections can be treated with the appropriate antibiotics (see the sections on sexually transmitted diseases and pelvic inflammatory disease). Hormonal suppression can be achieved with the use of estrogen or danazol in endometriosis, but surgery may be necessary for extensive disease. Prostaglandin inhibitors may be used for the menstrual cramps caused by intrauterine devices once infection is ruled out; mefenamic acid may be the drug of choice for these patients, since it also reduces menorrhagia. Complications of pregnancy require an immediate gynecologic consultation.

3. DYSFUNCTIONAL UTERINE BLEEDING

General Considerations

Dysfunctional uterine bleeding may be referred to as hypermenorrhea or polymenorrhea. It results when an endometrium that has proliferated under unopposed estrogen stimulation finally begins to slough, but incompletely, causing irregular, painless bleeding. The unopposed estrogen stimulation occurs during anovulatory cycles, common in younger adolescents who have not been menstruating for long, but also seen in older adolescents during times of stress or illness.

Clinical Findings

Typically, the adolescent has had several years of regular cycles and then begins to have menses every 2 weeks, or complains of bleeding for 2–3 weeks after 2–3 months of amenorrhea. A past history of painless, irregular periods at intervals of less than 3 weeks may also be elicited. Bleeding for more than 10 days should be considered abnormal.

Differential Diagnosis

Dysfunctional uterine bleeding must be considered a diagnosis of exclusion. The possibility of pelvic inflammatory disease or a complication of pregnancy, eg, ectopic pregnancy or threatened, incomplete, or missed abortion, must be considered in sexually active teenagers. In patients taking birth control pills, breakthrough bleeding is a consideration. Blood dyscrasias such as iron deficiency anemia, thrombocytopenia, coagulopathy, von Willebrand's disease, or leukemia should also be considered. In addition, endocrine disorders such as hypothyroidism, hyperthyroidism, diabetes mellitus, adrenal disease, or hyperprolactinemia are also in the differential diagnosis. Trauma or foreign body are also possible and can be ruled out by history and physical exam. Uterine, vaginal, or ovarian abnormalities (eg, carcinoma, fibroids, adenosis secondary to diethylstilbestrol use, or premature menopause) are less likely causes in teenagers.

Treatment

A pregnancy test and pelvic exam with appropriate cultures should be performed in sexually active patients. A complete blood count, including platelets, should also be obtained. The history and physical findings may suggest the need for additional coagulation or hormonal studies. Management depends on the severity of the problem. If the patient has a history of shortened intervals between cycles or somewhat heavier flow and normal hemoglobin levels, she can be asked to keep a menstrual calendar, and reassurance can be given. Mefenamic acid (500 mg three times a day) may be beneficial for the patient's heavy flow, and an iron supplement may be considered, since anemia can both contribute to dysfunctional uterine bleeding and result from it.

For the patient with moderate dysfunctional uterine bleeding, mild anemia, moderately heavy and prolonged cycles, or persistently short intervals between menses, medroxyprogesterone acetate (10 mg once or twice a day for 10 days starting day 14 of the cycle) may be used for 3 to 6 months. To stop bleeding in progress, one cycle of Ovral may be given, followed by cycling with medroxyprogesterone acetate for 3 to 6 months. Bleeding generally stops in a few days, but the dose of Ovral can be increased to twice a day until bleeding stops. A withdrawal flow should be expected several days after the last dose. Iron supplements should also be given.

Patients with severe dysfunctional bleeding, a low

hemoglobin count, and orthostatic symptoms in conjunction with heavy vaginal bleeding and disruption of menstrual cycles require hospitalization. Clotting studies should be obtained. Premarin (25 mg intravenously) may be given for its hemostatic effect. Ortho-Novum or Norinyl (2 mg) should be given every 4 hours until bleeding stops, then once a day for 21 days. This should be followed by cycling on Ovral or Demulen for 3 to 4 months and iron therapy. Gynecologic consultation should be obtained, because dilatation and curettage may be necessary if there is no improvement in 24 hours.

4. MITTELSCHMERZ

Mittelschmerz refers to the pain caused by irritation of the peritoneum due to spillage of fluid from the ruptured follicular cyst at the time of ovulation. The patient presents with a history of midcycle, unilateral dull or aching abdominal pain lasting a few minutes or as long as 8 hours. This pain rarely mimics the acute abdominal findings of appendicitis, torsion or rupture of an ovarian cyst, or ectopic pregnancy. The patient should be reassured and treated symptomatically. If the findings are severe enough to warrant consideration of the above diagnoses, a laparoscopy may be done to rule them out.

5. PREMENSTRUAL SYNDROME

Premenstrual syndrome (PMS) has received much attention in the lay press. It refers to a cluster of physical and psychologic symptoms that are temporally related to the week preceding menstruation and are alleviated by the onset of menses. There are no established diagnostic criteria, and the symptoms may vary from patient to patient, or from month to month in the same patient. These symptoms include weight gain, edema, breast engorgement, fatigue, headache, backache, and mood swings. This is typically a disorder of adult women and is uncommon in adolescence. Although a number of causes have been proposed (progesterone deficiency, hyperprolactinemia, estrogen excess or an imbalance of the estrogen: progesterone ratio, vitamin B_{12} deficiency, fluid retention, endorphins, hypoglycemia, and psychosomatic factors), none have been proved. There may be some hormonal role; women who have undergone hysterectomy but not oophorectomy may have cyclic symptoms resembling PMS, whereas postmenopausal women have no such symptoms. Several treatments have been advocated, none with consistent benefits. Education is the most indicated measure at this time. The patient can keep a calendar of symptoms for several months, and proper eating, exercise, and sleep can be stressed. Salt restriction or mild diuretics can be used for those with fluid

retention. Tricyclic antidepressants do not have a role in the treatment of this disorder.

6. OVARIAN CYSTS

Functional cysts account for 20–50% of ovarian tumors in adolescents and are a variation of the normal physiologic process. They may be asymptomatic or may cause menstrual irregularity, constipation, or urinary frequency. Functional cysts, unless large, rarely cause abdominal pain; however, torsion or hemorrhage of an ovarian cyst may present as an acute or subacute abdomen. **Follicular cysts** account for the majority of ovarian cysts. They are produced every cycle but occasionally are not resorbed. Follicular cysts are unilateral, usually less than or equal to 4 cm in diameter, and resolve spontaneously. If the patient is asymptomatic, she can be given oral contraceptives containing 50 μg of estrogen for suppression and examined monthly. The patient should be referred to a gynecologist for laparoscopy if (1) she is premenarcheal; (2) the cyst has a solid component or is larger than 5 cm by ultrasound; (3) there are symptoms or signs suggestive of hemorrhage or torsion; or (4) the cyst fails to regress after 2 to 3 menstrual cycles. **Lutein cysts** occur less commonly and may be 5 to 10 cm in diameter. The patient may have associated amenorrhea or, as the cyst becomes atretic, heavy vaginal bleeding. The patient may be monitored on suppression with oral contraceptives for 3 months, but should have a laparoscopy if the cyst is larger than 5 cm or if there is pain or hemorrhage of the cyst.

7. ENDOMETRIOSIS

(See Secondary Amenorrhea, above.)

Beach RK: Relieving the pain of menstrual cramps. *Contemp Pediatr* 1986;**3**:115.

Emans SJH, Goldstein DP: *Pediatric and Adolescent Gynecology*, 2nd ed. Little, Brown, 1982.

Grumbach MM: The neuroendocrinology of puberty. *Hosp Pract* (March) 1980;**15**:51.

Litt IF: Menstrual problems during adolescence. *Pediatr Rev* 1983;**4**:203.

Shangold MM: Causes, evaluation, and management of athletic oligo-/amenorrhea. *Med Clin North Am* 1985;**69**:83.

Strasburger VC (editor): Adolescent gynecology. *Pediatr Clin North Am* 1989;**38**:3.

CONTRACEPTION

Sexually active adolescent females wait an average of one year before seeking contraception; however, one-half of teen pregnancies in the United States occur in the first 6 months after sexual intercourse is begun. Sexuality, contraception, and pregnancy prevention are areas with which the pediatrician has become familiar out of necessity.

Abstinence & Decision Making

Adolescents may have poorly formulated skills for making decisions of any kind and often benefit from a decision-making framework that can be applied to a variety of situations, particularly those involving peer pressure. For younger adolescents, this framework can be made more concrete by providing written materials on which the adolescent fills in alternatives and their consequences.

Many adolescents have given little thought to how they feel about their developing sexuality or how they would handle sexual situations. As a result, sexual intercourse may be initiated because they were ill-prepared to handle a situation. By talking with teenagers about their alternatives to sexual intercourse and its implications (unintended pregnancy; sexually transmitted diseases; possible emotional trauma; effects on education, career, and income; and responsibilities if a pregnancy occurs) physicians can help them make informed decisions before they find themselves in a dilemma.

Teenagers need to be aware that half of all teenagers have not engaged in sexual intercourse. Abstinence is the most commonly used method of birth control. If an adolescent chooses to remain abstinent, the clinician should reinforce the decision. It is also prudent to encourage adolescents to use contraception at the time they do initiate sexual intercourse.

Barrier Methods

Condoms as a method of contraception also offer protection against sexually transmitted diseases by preventing the passage of *Gonococcus, Chlamydia,* spirochetes, hepatitis virion particles, and possibly the human immunodeficiency virus. Spermicides containing nonoxynol-9 have viricidal and bactericidal effects. Aside from the diaphragm and cervical cap, barrier methods do not require a medical visit or prescription, and are widely available (Table 10–19).

Oral Contraceptives

Oral contraceptives have a 3-pronged mechanism of action: (1) suppression of ovulation; (2) thickening of the cervical mucus, thereby making sperm penetration more difficult; and (3) atrophy of the endometrium, which diminishes the chance of implantation. The latter 2 actions are progestin effects.

A. Combination Oral Contraceptives: Combination oral contraceptives are birth control pills containing both estrogen and progestin. Ethinyl estradiol and mestranol (which is converted to ethinyl estradiol by the liver before it is pharmacologically active) are the 2 estrogens currently used in oral contraceptives in the USA. An oral contraceptive containing 30 to 35 μg of ethinyl estradiol is most often prescribed to adolescents beginning birth control pills. A number of different progestins are used in oral contraceptives and differ in their estrogenic, antiestrogenic, and androgenic effects. Triphasic oral contraceptives were introduced in the USA in 1984. Their main advantage is a 35–39% lower progestin dose over the course of the month, resulting in fewer progestin-related metabolic effects such as those on lipids, blood pressure, and carbohydrate metabolism. Disadvantages include confusion due to the multiple pill colors and a breakthrough bleeding rate that is comparable or somewhat greater than that of low-dose biphasic counterparts.

B. Minipill: Minipills contain progestins found in

Table 10–19. Lowest expected, typical, and lowest reported failure rates during the first year of use of a method of contraception, United States. Percentage of women experiencing an accidental pregnancy in the first year of use.[1]

Method	Lowest Expected[2]	Typical[3]	Lowest Reported[4]
Chance	89	89	
Spermicides[5]	3	21	0
Sponge	5 nulliparous > 8 parous	18 nulliparous > 28 parous	14 nulliparous 28 parous
Cervical cap[6]	5	18	8
Diaphragm[6]	3	18	2
Condom[7]	2	12	4

[1]Modified and reproduced, with permission, from Breedlove B, Judy B, Martin N (editors): *Contraceptive Technology 1988–1989,* 14th rev ed. Irvington Publishers, 1988.
[2]Among couples who initiate use of a method (not necessarily for the first time), and who use it perfectly (both consistently and correctly), the authors' best guess of the percentage expected to experience an accidental pregnancy during the first year if they do not stop use for any other reason.
[3]Among typical couples who initiate use of a method (not necessarily for the first time), the percentage who experience an accidental pregnancy during the first year if they do not stop use for any other reason.
[4]In the literature on contraceptive failure, the lowest reported percentage who experienced an accidental pregnancy during the first year following initiation of use (not necessarily for the first time) if they did not stop use for any other reason.
[5]Foams, creams, jellies, and vaginal suppositories.
[6]With spermicidal cream or jelly.
[7]Without spermicides.

combination oral contraceptives, but in smaller doses, and no estrogen. Their chief use is in women who experience unacceptable estrogen-related side effects with combination oral contraceptives. Their lack of estrogen, however, is also responsible for the main side effect, that of less predictable menstrual patterns. For this reason, and because minipills are not quite as effective as combination oral contraceptives, they are a poor choice for adolescents. Their mechanism of action relies on the progestin-mediated actions, and ovulation is suppressed in only 15–40% of cycles.

C. Indications and Contraindications: Combined oral contraceptives may be the method of choice for sexually active adolescents who frequently have unplanned intercourse; however, the patient must be able to comply with a daily dosing regimen. Most states allow oral contraceptives to be prescribed to minors confidentially. Ideally, it is best to wait until 6 to 12 regular menstrual cycles have occurred before beginning oral contraceptives; however, if the teenager is already sexually active, the medical and social risks of pregnancy probably outweigh the risks of oral contraceptives.

Oral contraceptives may also be used to treat dysmenorrhea (see above).

Contraindications to combined oral contraceptives can be categorized as absolute and relative (Table 10–20). When use of estrogenic agents is contraindicated, progestin only pills are an alternative.

D. Beginning Birth Control Pills and Follow-Up: Before a patient begins taking oral contraceptives, a careful menstrual history, medical history, and family medical history should be taken. In addition, baseline weight and blood pressure should be established, breast and pelvic examination should be

---

Table 10–20. Contraindications to combined birth control pills.[1]

Absolute Contraindications
History of thrombophlebitis, thromboembolic disorder, cerebrovascular disorder, ischemic heart disease
Known or suspected carcinoma of the breast or estrogen-dependent neoplasia
Known or suspected pregnancy
History of benign or malignant liver tumor
Undiagnosed abnormal vaginal bleeding

Strong Relative Contraindications
Severe vascular or migraine headaches
Hypertension
Diabetes
Active gallbladder disease
Mononucleosis, acute phase
Sickle cell disease or sickle C disease
Upcoming major surgery
Long leg cast or major injury to lower leg
Known impaired liver function at present time
Completion of term pregnancy within past 10–14 days

[1]Modified and reproduced, with permission, from Breedlove B, Judy B, Martin N (editors): *Contraceptive Technology 1988–1989*, 14th rev ed. Irvington Publishers, 1988.

---

performed, and specimens for urinalysis, Papanicolaou smear, gonorrhea culture, and *Chlamydia* culture or antigen-detection test obtained.

If there are no contraindications (see Table 10–20), the patient may begin her first pack of pills with her next menstrual period (either the first Sunday after flow begins or the first day of flow, depending on the brand). A triphasic or a low-dose combined oral contraceptive is used for those without contraindications to use of estrogen. With adolescents, it is wise to use 28-day packs rather than 21-day packs to reduce the chance of missing pills. The patient should be instructed on the use of her type of pills, and on possible risks and side effects and their warning signs. To ensure protection, she should use a back-up method, such as condoms and foam, for the first 2 weeks. A follow-up visit in 1 month and then every 2–3 months for the first year may improve compliance, since teenagers often discontinue birth control pills because of nonmedical reasons or minor side effects.

E. Management of Side Effects: A different type of combined oral contraceptive should be tried if a patient has a persistent minor side effect for more than the first 2–3 months. Adjustments should be made on the basis of hormonal effects (Table 10–21). Changes are most often made for persistent breakthrough bleeding not related to missed pills.

Intrauterine Devices

Because of the liability costs associated with intrauterine devices (IUDs) in recent years, most have been withdrawn from the market. Because of the risk of sexually transmitted diseases and pelvic inflammatory disease and its serious sequelae (infertility, ectopic pregnancy), IUDs are not a good method for teenagers who frequently have multiple partners and have their childbearing years ahead of them.

A number of mechanisms of action have been suggested for IUDs, including prevention of implantation through a local inflammatory response and local production of prostaglandins.

IUDs must be inserted and removed by a physician trained to do so.

Injectable Hormonal Contraceptives

Medroxyprogesterone acetate (Depo-Provera) is approved and available in the USA for other indications but is not yet approved as a contraceptive. It must be injected in doses of 100–150 mg every 3 months. A recent World Health Organization case-control study concluded there was no increased risk of liver or breast cancer among users of medroxyprogesterone acetate, and the risk of endometrial and ovarian cancers was lower among users than among other women in the study. Consideration might be given to this method for severely retarded female adolescents at risk for unintended pregnancy.

Table 10–21. Pill side effects: hormone etiology.[1]

Estrogen Excess	Progestin Excess	Androgen Excess	Estrogen Deficiency	Progestin Deficiency
1. Nausea, dizziness	1. Increased appetite and weight gain (noncyclic)	1. Increased appetite and weight gain (noncyclic)	1. Irritability, nervousness	1. Late breakthrough bleeding and spotting
2. Edema and abdominal or leg pain with cyclic weight gain, bloating	2. Tiredness, fatigue, and weakness	2. Hirsutism	2. Hot flushes, vaso- motor symptoms	2. Heavy menstrual flow and clots
3. Leukorrhea	3. Depression	3. Acne	3. Uterine prolapse, pelvic relaxation symptoms	3. Delayed onset of menses
4. Increased leiomyoma size	4. Decreased libido	4. Oily skin, rash	4. Early and midcycle spotting	4. Dysmenorrhea
5. Chloasma	5. Oily scalp, acne	5. Increased libido	5. Decreased amount of menstrual flow	5. Weight loss
6. Uterine cramps	6. Loss of hair	6. Cholestatic jaundice	6. No withdrawal bleeding	
7. Irritability, depression	7. Cholestatic jaundice	7. Pruritus	7. Decreased libido	
8. Increased fat deposition	8. Decreased length of menstrual flow		8. Diminished breast size	
9. Cervical extrophia	9. Hypertension?		9. Dry vaginal mucosa, atrophic vaginitis, and dyspareunia	
10. Poor contact lens fit	10. Headaches between Pill packages		10. Headaches	
11. Telangiectasia	11. Monilial vaginitis/ cervicitis		11. Depression	
12. Vascular-type headache	12. Increased breast size (alveolar tissue)			
13. Hypertension?	13. Breast tenderness			
14. Lactation suppression	14. Decreased carbohy- drate tolerance			
15. Headaches while taking the Pill	15. Dilated leg veins			
16. Cystic breast changes	16. Pelvic congestion syndrome			
17. Breast tenderness				
18. Increased breast size (ductal and fatty tissue and fluid retention)				
19. Thrombophlebitis				
20. Cerebrovascular acci- dents				
21. Myocardial infarction				
22. Hepatic adenoma				
23. Cyclic weight gain				

[1]Adapted and reproduced, with permission, from: Dickey RP: Medical approaches to reproductive regulation: The pill. ACOG Semin Fam Plan 1974; Table II:21; Dickey RP: *Managing Contraceptive Pill Patients,* 4th ed. Creative Infomatics, 1984; and Hatcher RA et al: *Contraceptive Technology, 1986–1987,* 13th rev ed. Irvington, 1987.

Progestin-containing nonbiodegradable implants, which are placed under the skin of the upper or lower arm, are approved and marketed in a number of countries and may soon be available in the USA. Their effects last 3 to 5 years.

Miscellaneous Methods

Adolescents should understand the menstrual cycle and be taught either that there is no "safe" period or that ovulation occurs 2 weeks before the next menstrual period and may be difficult to predict. Because teenagers frequently have irregular cycles and because sexual intercourse is often spontaneous and unplanned, the rhythm or calendar method is not very effective for them. Adolescents also need to be educated that withdrawal is not a method of contraception. Sterilization should be viewed as a permanent method of contraception and therefore is not suitable for teenagers.

Hatcher RA et al: Combined oral contraceptives. In: *Con-*

traceptive Technology 1988–1989. Breedlove B, Judy B, Martin N (editors). Irvington Publishers, 1988.
Liskin L, Blackburn R: Hormonal contraception: New long-acting methods. *Popul Rep [K]* 1987;(3).
Reinhart W: Minipill: A limited alternative for certain women. *Popul Rep [A]* 1975;(3).

PREGNANCY

More than 1 million teenage girls become pregnant in the USA each year. Of these pregnancies, about 40% result in abortion, 13% in miscarriage, and 47% in live births (Table 10–22). About 45% of 15–19-year-old females are sexually active, and more than one-third of these become pregnant within 2 years of onset of sexual intercourse. More than 80% of these pregnancies are unintended, and about 60% of pregnancies to women less than 20 years old are out of wedlock (Figure 10–12).

Young maternal age and associated maternal risk factors have been linked to adverse neonatal out-

Table 10–22. Estimated pregnancies to adolescents, by pregnancy outcome and age of mother, 1983.

Number and Percent	Age of Mother			
	Under 15	15–17	18–19	Total Under 20
Estimated pregnancies	29,000	383,320	639,050	1,051,370
Percent to each age	2.8%	36.5%	60.8%	100.0%
Number ending in:				
Abortion	15,730	160,100	235,560	411,390
Miscarriage	3,518	50,547	86,877	140,942
Birth	9,752	172,673	316,613	499,038
Percent of estimated pregnancies to age group ending in:				
Abortion	54.2%	41.8%	36.9%	39.1%
Miscarriage	12.1%	13.2%	13.6%	13.4%
Birth	33.6%	45.0%	49.5%	47.5%
	100.0%	100.0%	100.0%	100.0%
Estimated rates per 1000 female adolescents				
	Under 15	15–17	18–19	15–19[2]
Pregnancy rate	16.2	71.0	157.6	108.1
Abortion rate	8.8[2]	29.6	58.1	41.8
Birth rate	1.1	32.0	78.1	51.7

[1]Reproduced, with permission, from Pittman K, Adams G (editors): Teenage pregnancy: An advocate's guide to the numbers. Children's Defense Fund, Jan/March 1988.
[2]Rates for all women under 20 are not available. Abortion rates for women under age 14 are based on the population of women aged 14.

come, including higher rates of low birth weight babies (< 2500 g) and neonatal mortality. The psychosocial consequences for the teenage mother and her infant are shown in Table 10–23. Teenagers who are pregnant require additional support from their caregivers, and young mothers' clinics may be the ideal providers.

Presentation

Adolescents may present with delayed or missed menses or may even request a pregnancy test, but often they present with an unrelated concern or have a hidden agenda. Because of the high level of denial, they may come in for abdominal pain, urinary frequency, dizziness, or other nonspecific symptoms and have no concern about pregnancy. A history for symptoms such as weight gain, engorged breasts, an unusually light or mistimed period, and urinary frequency can be sought, but the adolescent may not have noted these. Denial also contributes to the delay in seeking prenatal care. Only about one-third of adolescents receive prenatal care in the first trimester. Clinicians need to have a low threshold for suspecting pregnancy. If there is *any* suspicion, a urine pregnancy test should be obtained.

Diagnosis

History, as above, and physical examination may assist in making the diagnosis of pregnancy. Bluish coloring and softening of the cervix may be noted on speculum exam. The uterine fundus may be palpable

on abdominal exam if sufficient time has lapsed. If uterine size on bimanual exam does not correspond to dates, one must consider ectopic pregnancy, incomplete or missed abortion, twin gestation, or inaccurate dates.

Laboratory tests for human chorionic gonadotropin (hCG) are simple to perform and are usually diagnostic. Enzyme-linked immunoassay test kits specific for the beta-hCG subunit and sensitive to < 50 mIU/mL of hCG can be performed on urine (preferably the first morning void because it is more concentrated) in less than 5 minutes, and are accurate within 12 days after conception. Serum radioimmunoassay is also specific for the beta subunit, is accurate within 7 days after conception, and is helpful in ruling out ectopic pregnancy or threatened abortion. Serum radioreceptorassay may cross-react with LH, is accurate within 14 days after conception, and may be used to confirm a normal pregnancy. Slide agglutination tests are more difficult to read, less sensitive than the above tests, and cross-react with LH. Home pregnancy tests are relatively accurate, particularly when positive; however, they are expensive and have fairly complex instructions, which many teenagers have difficulty following. Also, they may preclude obtaining counseling, early entry into prenatal care, or detection of ectopic pregnancy or threatened abortion. The timing of pregnancy tests is important, since hCG levels initially rise after conception, peak at about 60–70 days, then drop to levels not detected by routine office slide tests after 16–20 weeks.

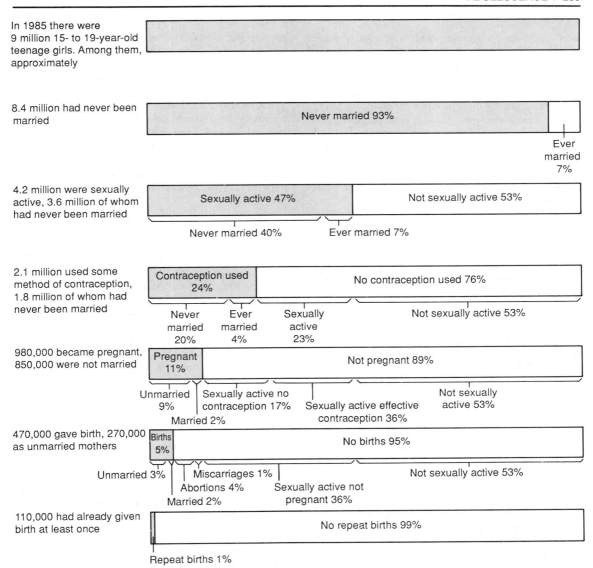

In 1985 there were 9 million 15- to 19-year-old teenage girls. Among them, approximately

8.4 million had never been married

Never married 93%

Ever married 7%

4.2 million were sexually active, 3.6 million of whom had never been married

Sexually active 47%   Not sexually active 53%

Never married 40%   Ever married 7%

2.1 million used some method of contraception, 1.8 million of whom had never been married

Contraception used 24%   No contraception used 76%

Never married 20%   Ever married 4%   Sexually active 23%   Not sexually active 53%

980,000 became pregnant, 850,000 were not married

Pregnant 11%   Not pregnant 89%

Unmarried 9%   Sexually active no contraception 17%   Sexually active effective contraception 36%   Not sexually active 53%

Married 2%

470,000 gave birth, 270,000 as unmarried mothers

Births 5%   No births 95%

Unmarried 3%   Miscarriages 1%   Abortions 4%   Sexually active not pregnant 36%   Not sexually active 53%

Married 2%

110,000 had already given birth at least once

No repeat births 99%

Repeat births 1%

Figure 10–12. A snapshot profile of 15- to 19-year-old teenage women in 1985: sexual activity, pregnancy, childbearing, and related behaviors. (Reproduced, with permission, from Pittman K, Adams G (editors): *Teenage pregnancy: An advocate's guide to the numbers.* Children's Defense Fund, Adolescent Pregnancy Prevention Clearing House, Jan/Mar, 1988.)

Special Issues in Management

When an adolescent presents for pregnancy testing, it is wise to find out what she hopes the results will be and what she thinks she will do before performing the test. If she wants to be pregnant and the test is negative, further counseling about the implications of teen pregnancy should be undertaken. For those who do not wish to be pregnant, this is a good time to begin contraception.

If the adolescent is pregnant, discuss her support systems and her options with her. Many teenagers need help in telling and involving their parents. It is important to remain available for further assistance with decision making. If she knows what she wants to do, refer her to the appropriate resources. Since teenagers are often ambivalent about their plans and

may have a high level of denial, it is prudent to follow up with her in a week to be certain that a decision has been made and to help her obtain prenatal care if she has chosen to continue the pregnancy.

Maternal age alone is not responsible for low birth weight and poor fetal outcome; rather, low maternal prepregnancy weight, poor weight gain, delay in prenatal care, low socioeconomic status, and black race are contributing factors. The poor nutritional status of some teenagers and their erratic diets, smoking, drinking, or substance abuse, and high prevalence of sexually transmitted diseases play a role. Teenagers are also at greater risk of toxemia of pregnancy, iron deficiency anemia, cephalopelvic disproportion, prolonged labor, premature labor, and maternal death. Early prenatal care and good nutrition can make a difference with a number of these.

Because of the high risk of a second unintended pregnancy within the next 2 years, postpartum contraceptive counseling and follow-up are imperative. Pregnancy prevention is the most cost-effective means of reducing the consequences of teenage pregnancy. Sexual decision making, contraceptive counseling, and close follow-up of sexually active male and female adolescents can make a difference. Adolescents who receive sexuality and contraceptive education are not more likely to have intercourse but are less likely to get pregnant than their counterparts who do not receive such instruction.

VULVOVAGINITIS

Vaginitis has two main causes: pathogens, or indigenous flora after a change in milieu of the vagina. *Monilia* vulvovaginitis and bacterial vaginosis (formerly referred to as *Gardnerella, Haemophilus,* or

Table 10–23. Psychosocial consequences of pregnancy for the adolescent mother and her infant.

Mother	Infant
Increased morbidity related to pregnancy	Greater health risks
Greater risk of toxemia, anemia, prolonged labor, premature labor	Increased chance of low birth weight or prematurity
Increased chance of miscarriages, stillbirths	Increased risk of infant death
Increased chance of maternal mortality	Increased risk of injury and hospitalization by age 5
Decreased educational attainment	Decreased academic achievement
Less likely to get high school diploma, go to college, or graduate	Lower cognitive scores
	Decreased development
Lower occupational attainment and prestige	Greater chance of being behind grade or needing remedial help
Less chance of stable employment (some resolution over time)	Lower chance of advanced academics
Lower job satisfaction	Lower academic aptitude as a teenager and perhaps a higher probability of dropping out of school
Lower income/wages	
Greater dependence on public assistance	
Less stable marital relationships	Psychosocial consequences
Higher rates of single parenthood	Greater risk of behavior problems
	Poverty
Earlier marriage (though less common than in the past)	Higher probability of living in a nonintact home while in high school
Accelerated pace of marriage, separation, divorce, and remarriage	Greater risk of adolescent pregnancy
Faster pace of subsequent childbearing	
High rate of repeat unintended pregnancy	
More births out of marriage	
Closer spacing of births	
Larger families	

nonspecific vaginitis) may be found in patients who are not sexually active. These are examples of indigenous flora that may cause infection. Bacterial vaginosis, however, is more prevalent in those who are sexually active. In sexually active patients, *Trichomonas* infection or cervicitis due to sexually transmitted pathogens must be considered (see section on sexually transmitted diseases, below). For this reason, sexually active patients or suspected victims of sexual abuse should have appropriate specimens taken to detect sexually transmitted disease even if yeast or bacterial vaginosis is identified.

1. PHYSIOLOGIC LEUKORRHEA

This refers to the normal vaginal discharge that begins just prior to or around the time of menarche. The discharge is typically clear or whitish, and consistency may vary according to cyclic hormonal influence. There should be no odor. Girls in early adolescence may have concerns about such a discharge and need reassurance that it is normal. This may be a good time to tell girls that there is no need for douching. If a vaginal wet prep is examined a few squamous epithelial cells may be revealed, but there should be fewer than 5 polymorphonuclear cells per high-power field.

2. *MONILIA* VULVOVAGINITIS

General Considerations

Monilial or candidal vulvovaginitis is caused by yeast. It typically occurs after a course of antibiotics, after which the normal perineal flora are altered and yeast is allowed to proliferate. Diabetics, those with compromised immunity, and those who are pregnant or on oral contraceptives are more prone to monilial infections.

Clinical Findings

The patient usually complains of vulvar pruritus or dyspareunia and a cheesy vaginal discharge, frequently beginning the week prior to menses. Examination of the vulva reveals an erythematous mucosa, sometimes with excoriation, and a thick, white, cheesy discharge. The discharge may be adherent to the walls of the vagina, which will also be inflamed if the infection is internal. Leukocytes may be seen on wet prep, and potassium hydroxide prep may reveal budding yeast or mycelia. No "clue cells" should be seen. Often the vaginal preps are unhelpful, and the patient should be treated on the basis of the clinical exam. Vaginal culture for yeast is usually unnecessary.

Treatment

Nystatin, clotrimazole, or terconazole vaginal creams or suppositories designed for 3 nightly or 7 nightly doses are effective in the majority of patients. Some patients require a longer course of treatment and a vinegar douche at the conclusion of treatment to restore the vaginal pH. Patients with recurrent episodes should be given prophylactic treatment whenever they take antibiotics. It may be helpful to simultaneously treat the partners of sexually active patients with recurrent monilial infections.

3. BACTERIAL VAGINOSIS

Bacterial vaginosis may be caused by any of the indigenous vaginal flora, eg, *Gardnerella, Bacteroides, Peptococcus,* or lactobacilli.

Clinical Findings

The patient generally complains of malodorous mild discharge. On examination, a thin, homogeneous, grayish-white discharge is found adherent to the vaginal wall with diffuse vaginal erythema. A whiff test, in which a drop of potassium hydroxide is added to a smear of the discharge on a slide, results in the release of amines, causing a fishy odor. Wet prep reveals an abundance of ''clue cells'' (vaginal epithelial cells stippled with adherent bacteria) and small pleomorphic rods.

Treatment

Treatment is with metronidazole (500 mg orally twice a day for 7 days). Ampicillin (500 mg orally 4 times a day for 7 days) is the alternative for pregnant patients.

4. OTHER

Sexually Transmitted Diseases

See the next section for cervicitis. It behooves one to do appropriate cultures even if the cervix appears normal, since sexually transmitted diseases may otherwise be missed.

Foreign Body Vaginitis

Foreign bodies, most commonly retained tampons, cause extremely malodorous vaginal discharges. Treatment consists of removal, for which ring forceps may be useful. Further treatment is generally not necessary.

Allergic or Contact Vaginitis

Bubble baths, feminine hygiene sprays, or vaginal contraceptive foams or suppositories may cause chemical irritation of the vaginal mucosa. Discontinuing use of the offending agent is indicated.

Carey B, McCann-Sanford T, Davidson EC: Adolescent age and obstetric risk. In: *Premature Adolescent Pregnancy and Parenting.* McAnarney E (editor). Grune & Stratton, 1983.

Hayes CD (editor): *Risking the Future: Adolescent Sexuality, Pregnancy, and Childbearing.* Vol 1. National Academy Press, 1987.

McAnarney ER: Young maternal age and adverse neonatal outcome. *Am J Dis Child* 1987;**141**:1053.

Teenage pregnancy: An advocate's guide to the numbers. Children's Defense Fund, Jan/March 1988.

Zuckerman B et al: Neonatal outcome: Is adolescent pregnancy a risk factor? *Pediatrics* 1983;**71**:489.

SEXUALLY TRANSMITTED DISEASES & PELVIC INFLAMMATORY DISEASE

The groups aged 15–19 and 20–24 years have the highest incidence of sexually transmitted diseases (STD) as a result of multiple sexual partners, failure to use barrier methods of contraception, and delay in seeking treatment. Their inexperience in communicating with their partner about sexual matters further contributes to high rates when one partner develops symptoms of an STD.

Chlamydia, an obligate intracellular body half the size of the gonococcus, is the most common STD, with 2–3 million new cases per year in the USA and peak incidence in 15-to-20-year-olds. One quarter to one-half of those infected are asymptomatic, and one-quarter to one-half are coinfected with gonorrhea. Forty-two percent of the cases of nongonococcal urethritis (NGU) in one study were caused by *Chlamydia,* and *Chlamydia* accounts for 20–30% of the 170,000 cases of pelvic inflammatory disease (PID) per year and is responsible for more than 60% of PID cases in women less than 20 years old.

Gonorrhea is the second most common STD, with peak incidence in the 15-to-25-year-old age group. Five to twenty-five percent of cases are associated with another STD, and more than 50% of those infected are asymptomatic. Although syphilis is less prevalent than gonorrhea and chlamydial infection, its peak incidence is in 15-to-35-year-olds.

Sexually transmitted viruses are also prevalent in the adolescent population. The 1970s saw a dramatic rise in the number of cases of herpes simplex virus. More recently, an association has been established between the human papillomavirus (HPV) responsible for genital warts (condylomata acuminata) and cancer of the cervix and possibly the penis.

In view of the prevalence of STD in the adolescent population and the reluctance of teenagers to speak about them, the clinician must routinely ask adolescents about sexual activity, number of partners, and symptoms of STD when they present for routine physical exams or sexually related symptoms (dysuria, penile or vaginal discharge, genital lesion, or abdominal pain). Because females are frequently asymptomatic, obtaining specimens for wet prep, gonorrhea culture, and *Chlamydia* test at the time of the annual Papanicolaou smear in sexually active females is advised. Although males are usually symptomatic, a significant number of those with *Chlamy-*

dia are asymptomatic. Also, symptoms of gonorrhea may resolve, and the male adolescent may fail to seek treatment.

When an STD is diagnosed, the adolescent and his or her partner(s) should be treated simultaneously with the appropriate antibiotic regimen. They should be followed closely, because poor compliance with treatment is common in this age group. A culture to test cure of gonorrhea should be obtained no sooner than 4–5 days after completion of treatment to allow clearing of serum antibiotic levels. Serology will need to be repeated in patients with syphilis. It is essential to emphasize abstinence until both partners complete treatment to avoid reinfection or spread, and to advise use of barrier methods of contraception to prevent future infections. Possible complications and the implications of recurrent infections with regard to fertility and ectopic pregnancy should also be discussed. Adolescents should also be made aware of transmission of STD to the fetus.

URETHRITIS

General Considerations

Urethritis may be caused by gonorrhea, *Chlamydia, Ureaplasma, Mycoplasma,* and *Trichomonas.*

Clinical Findings

A. Symptoms and Signs: Males may experience dysuria and a clear, white, or purulent penile discharge, or they may be asymptomatic. Females may also develop urethritis, most often in association with a cervicitis, and may complain of dysuria.

The male genital exam may be normal, or there may be a penile discharge. A clear or white discharge is more frequently found in nongonoccal urethritis (NGU), and a purulent discharge in gonorrhea; however, appearance is not diagnostic. Examination of the female may reveal cervicitis (see the next section.)

B. Laboratory Findings: Urinalysis may show a moderate amount of white blood cells without bacteriuria. A moderate pyuria with a negative urine culture, with or without symptoms of urethritis or cervicitis, should cause the clinician to suspect these diagnoses and perform the appropriate pelvic exam and cultures. Gram's stain of the penile discharge shows polymorphonuclear white blood cells and may show gram-negative intracellular diplococci if gonorrhea is the cause. The penile discharge should be cultured for gonorrhea on chocolate agar or Thayer-Martin medium, and a diagnostic test for *Chlamydia* (culture, enzyme-linked immunoassay, or monoclonal antibody immunofluorescence test) performed.

Complications

Urethritis caused by gonorrhea or *Chlamydia* may cause nontender penile edema or ascend to result in prostatitis, epididymitis, or orchitis.

Treatment

See Table 10–24.

CERVICITIS

General Considerations

Cervicitis may be caused by *Chlamydia* or gonorrhea. There may also be involvement of the cervix with *Trichomonas* vaginitis, and herpes may cause characteristic cervical ulcerations.

Clinical Findings

A. Symptoms and Signs: Most females with uncomplicated gonococcal or chlamydial cervicitis are asymptomatic, but about one-third note a vaginal discharge. Dysuria may be present if there is an associated urethritis.

In typical cases of gonococcal cervicitis, the cervical os is erythematous and produces a mucopurulent discharge. Cervical abnormalities may be subtle in patients with chlamydial cervicitis. Although 19–32% of females with chlamydial cervicitis have hypertrophic cervicitis (intensely erythematous, irregular, raised surface that is friable or bleeds easily when touched) and 40% have a mucopurulent or purulent cervical discharge, 20% have a completely normal cervical exam. The findings on physical exam in about 90% of women with cervicitis and positive culture for herpes virus are typically diffuse friability, occasionally frank ulcers, or necrosis. *Tri-*

Table 10–24. Treatment of urethritis or cervicitis in adolescents.[1]

	Drug of Choice	**Alternatives**
Gonorrhea	Ceftriaxone 125–250 mg IM once, **followed by** treatment for *Chlamydia*, below	Spectinomycin 2 g IM once **or** Ciprofloxacin[2] 500 mg orally once **or** Amoxicillin[3] 3 g orally once **plus** probenecid 1 g orally once **Plus** treatment for *Chlamydia*
Chlamydia trachomatis	Doxycycline[4] 100 mg orally twice daily for 7 days **or** tetracycline[4] 500 mg orally 4 times daily for 7 days	Erythromycin 500 mg orally 4 times daily for 7 days

[1]Modified and reproduced, with permission, from Treatment of sexually transmitted diseases. *Med Lett Drugs Ther* 1990;**32**:5.
[2]Quinolones, such as ciprofloxacin, are contraindicated during pregnancy and in children 16 years of age or younger.
[3]May be used for infections proved *not* to be penicillin-resistant gonorrhea.
[4]Contraindicated during pregnancy.

chomonas may cause petechiae of the cervix and upper vaginal vault, the so-called flea-bitten appearance.

B. Laboratory Findings: A wet prep of the vaginal discharge reveals more than 10 white blood cells per high power field. There tend to be greater numbers of white blood cells with gonorrhea than with *Chlamydia;* however, this finding is not diagnostic. Gram-negative intracellular diplococci may be seen on Gram's stain if gonorrhea is the cause. A culture of the cervical discharge for gonorrhea should be obtained on Thayer-Martin medium or chocolate agar. A *Chlamydia* culture or direct antigen-detection test should also be performed.

Complications

Cervicitis caused by *Chlamydia* or gonorrhea may progress to PID with its attendant complications. Infection of Bartholin's glands is also a potential consequence.

Treatment

See Table 10–24.

GENITAL LESIONS

Infectious causes of genital lesions in adolescents include condylomata acuminata, herpes simplex virus, and syphilis.

Condylomata Acuminata

Condylomata acuminata, or genital warts, are caused by human papillomavirus (HPV). The peak incidence is in the 18-to-24-year-old age group. Transmission may occur to 30–60% of one's partners, with an incubation period of 1–8 months. Warts typically occur at the site of minute skin trauma, with 50% occurring on the glans penis or corona in males and 75% at the posterior introitus in females. Diagnosis is based on the clinical appearance of a verrucous skin lesion, which would have a negative darkfield exam.

HPV on the cervix or the penis, however, may be indiscernible to the unaided eye. Colposcopy is valuable in such circumstances and should be performed whenever HPV effects are noted on Papanicolaou smear and perhaps in any patient with condylomata. It is now accepted that HPV is the most important etiologic agent in the development of cervical intraepithelial neoplasia and invasive cervical cancers. It also appears to be associated with penile cancer. Types 6, 11, and 42 are the most common strains found in condylomata. Types 16, 18, 31, 33, 35, and 39 are associated with neoplasia.

Treatment is by application to the wart of 20–25% podophyllin in tincture of benzoin after petroleum jelly is applied to the surrounding normal skin; the solution is washed off in 4 hours. Reapplication at weekly intervals may be necessary. Podophyllin

should not be applied to vaginal or anal mucosa because it may cause a chemical burn and because the vascularity of these areas increases the risk of hematologic or neurologic toxicity. It should not be used in pregnant patients. Additional treatments include application of liquid nitrogen, removed by laser, administration of 5-fluorouracil, surgical excision, or administration of interferon. Abnormalities detected on colposcopy are biopsied. Laser removal is often the treatment of choice for warts on the cervix, because it removes them with minimal tissue damage. It is unlikely that HPV can be eliminated entirely from the genital tract. Repeated treatments will be necessary over time, and the patient should be counseled to use condoms.

Herpes Simplex Virus

Eighty to 95% of cases of genital herpes are due to herpes simplex virus type 2 (HSV-2); the remainder are due to HSV-1. Fifty percent of new cases may be asymptomatic. The primary episode is generally more symptomatic and prolonged than recurrences and is characterized by systemic symptoms such as fever, headache, malaise, and myalgias as well as a cluster of painful papules that progress to vesicles, pustules, ulcers, and finally crusts. HSV remains dormant in the dorsal root ganglion between episodes and migrates down the axon to the same dermatome at the time of recurrences. Recurrences may be preceded by prodromal tingling of the skin, and lesions last about 11 days. If acyclovir (200 mg orally 5 times a day for 7–10 days) is initiated within 6 days of onset of the primary episode, the mean duration of eruptions may be shortened by 3–5 days, and systemic symptoms may be reduced. Acyclovir does not affect the risk, rate, or severity of recurrences. Minimal benefit can be expected for recurrences from episodic use of acyclovir (200 mg orally 5 times a day for five days), preferably instituted at the time of prodromal symptoms or within 2 days of onset. A primary episode of genital herpes in a pregnant woman may increase the risk of spontaneous abortion, prematurity, and congenital infection. With recurrent episodes, however, there is probably no greater risk of miscarriage, prematurity, or even congenital herpes.

Syphilis

Primary syphilis typically presents with a painless chancre that appears as a clean ulcer with an erythematous, indurated border. Diagnosis is by immediate darkfield exam of a microscope slide that has been pressed to the base of the lesion. A drop of saline is added to the slide. A VDRL can be done for further investigation but may be negative early in the course of the disease. The chancre may be self-limited. After a latency period of 4–6 weeks, the disease may resurface in its secondary stage, characterized by a diffuse, nonpruritic, maculopapular rash that is seen on the palms and soles as well, mucous patches on the mucosal surfaces, generalized lymphadenopathy, constitutional symptoms, and the presence of condyloma lata (broad-based, flat, mucoid lesions) on the genitals. At this stage, diagnosis is by VDRL. The tertiary stage is divided into early latent and late benign and may include the cardiovascular and central nervous system complications of dissection of the ascending aorta, seizures, stroke, optic atrophy, and tabes dorsalis. All stages may be treated with penicillin (Table 10–25.) The VDRL should be repeated 3, 6, and 12 months after treatment. It will return to negative during the 2 years after treatment, hence a subsequent rise in the VDRL titer should be interpreted as a treatment failure or a reinfection. The fluorescent treponemal antibody-absorption test remains positive for life unless syphilis is treated very early.

PARASITES

Trichomonas Vaginalis

Trichomonas vaginalis causes vaginitis in females and urethritis in males. Females may be asymptomatic or complain of a pruritic vaginal discharge. Diagnosis is by examination of a vaginal wet prep in females, or a spun urinalysis in males, for the motile trichomonad. The organism is about the size of a white blood cell but is pointed at its flagellated end. The organisms may be missed in a full field of white blood cells unless one looks carefully for the beating motion of the flagellum jolting the neighboring cells. Metronidazole (2 g orally once, or 250 mg orally 3 times a day for 7 days) is the treatment of choice. A warning should be given not to drink alcohol during treatment. In pregnant patients, clotrimazole (100 mg intravaginally at bedtime for 7 days) is used instead.

Arthropods

Phthirus pubis, or crab lice, live a sedentary, 45-day life cycle on the pubic hair and are transmitted during intimate contact. The patient experiences a pruritic rash, and on physical exam, the opalescent nits (eggs) are found securely anchored to the pubic hairs. *Sarcoptes scabiei,* or scabies, are round, flat, motile organisms. The females embed themselves in the skin and deposit 2–3 eggs per day. Scabies also results in an intensely pruritic rash, which is located on the groin, thighs, or abdomen in the case of sexual transmission. Findings on physical exam are the scabietic burrows and an erythematous, maculopapular rash with some scaliness and the tendency to impetiginize. Treatment is with topical application from neck to toe of lindane, remaining on the skin for 8 hours, or application, on 2 separate ocassions, of crotamiton at bedtime, remaining on the skin for 24 hours. (Lindane should not be applied to infants or pregnant or breast-feeding women.) The patient is no longer contagious 24 hours after treatment; however, symptoms may not abate for 2 weeks. Close contacts and fomites also need to be treated.

PELVIC INFLAMMATORY DISEASE

General Considerations

Acute pelvic inflammatory disease (PID), or salp-

Table 10–25. Treatment of syphilis.[1]

Stage	Drug of Choice	Dosage	Alternative Treatments
Early (primary, secondary, or latent less than one year)	Penicillin G benzathine	2.4 million units IM once	Tetracycline 500 mg orally 4 times daily for 15 days Erythromycin 500 mg orally 4 times daily for 15 days
Late (more than one year's duration, cardiovascular)	Penicillin G benzathine	2.4 million units IM weekly for 3 weeks	Tetracycline 500 mg orally 4 times daily for 30 days Erythromycin 500 mg orally 4 times daily for 30 days
Neurosyphilis	Penicillin G or Penicillin G procaine plus probenecid either one followed by penicillin G benzathine	2–4 million units IV every 4 h for 10 days 2.4 million units IM daily 500 mg 4 times daily orally both for 10 days 2.4 million units IM weekly for 3 weeks	Tetracycline 500 mg orally 4 times daily for 30 days Erythromycin 500 mg orally 4 times daily for 30 days
Congenital	Penicillin G or Penicillin G procaine	25,000 units/kg IM or IV twice daily for at least 10 days 50,000 units/kg IM daily for at least 10 days	

[1]Modified and reproduced, with permission, from Treatment of sexually transmitted diseases. The *Med Lett Drugs Ther* (Jan 15) 1988;**30:**5.

ingitis, is the most common serious infection occurring in young women. The adolescent age group has the highest rate of PID, with an annual rate of 1.5% of females aged 15–19 years. PID results from mucosal spread of sexually transmitted organisms from the cervix, through the uterus (where a transient endometritis may occur), to the fallopian tube.

Gonorrhea and *Chlamydia* account for more than 75% of cases of PID; however, normal vaginal aerobic and anaerobic flora have also been recovered from tubal infections and are felt to be secondary invaders. Whereas gonococcal infection may be limited to the tubal mucosa, *Chlamydia* and other organisms may invade the basement membrane and involve the subepithelial connective tissue and muscularis and serosal surfaces in the inflammatory process, thereby producing greater tubal damage. Organisms recovered from the cervix are not necessarily predictive of those causing infection in the tube, since gonorrhea becomes more difficult to isolate later in the disease, and since *Chlamydia* has been isolated from the fallopian tubes of women with or without this organism in the cervix.

Risk factors for PID include sexual activity, multiple partners (5 times greater risk than for one partner), age less than 25, presence of an intrauterine device (2–4 times greater risk than for nonusers), nulliparity, prior history of PID (2 times greater risk), prior history of uncomplicated STD, and prior induced abortion.

Clinical Findings

A. Symptoms and Signs: Abdominal pain is the most common complaint of women with PID, although 3% have no pain despite laparoscopic verification, and half of those with tubal occlusion from PID may report minimal pain. In patients with gonococcal PID, pain often begins with menses. Seventy-five percent report vaginal discharge of recent onset; 40% have excessive menstrual bleeding or intermenstrual spotting; 40% have fever; and 15% experience dysuria. In patients with chlamydial PID, the duration of pain is typically longer but pain is less intense and there is less fever and a higher sedimentation rate.

On physical exam, only one-third of patients with laparoscopically confirmed salpingitis will have fever above 38 °C (100.4 °F). Many have lower abdominal tenderness, or uterine, adnexal, or cervical motion tenderness on pelvic exam. Only half have a grossly abnormal cervical discharge, but many have excessive white blood cells on wet prep.

B. Laboratory Findings: Of patients with laparoscopically confirmed salpingitis, only 45% had a white blood count over 7900 and only 75% had a sedimentation rate above 15 mm/h. Although Gram's stain is positive for gonorrhea in only 67% of cases in which the cervical culture is positive, it may be helpful if positive. Cervical cultures for both gonorrhea and *Chlamydia* should be obtained. Cultures for other flora are not helpful. Culdocentesis may be helpful if it yields white blood cells or non-clotting blood (indicating peritonitis from salpingitis or other causes—eg, appendicitis—versus ectopic pregnancy or ruptured ovarian cyst), but is of no help if negative.

Differential Diagnosis

Sweet has suggested the criteria in Table 10–26 as a diagnostic guideline. Gynecologic consultation for evaluation or laparoscopy is indicated in uncertain cases. Laparoscopy remains the gold standard for the diagnosis of salpingitis, and points out the difficulty in making an accurate clinical diagnosis. Adherence to rigid diagnostic criteria results in diagnosis of only the most overt cases of PID. The diagnosis of acute PID was confirmed by laparoscopy in only 65% of patients felt to have it prior to the procedure; however, another diagnosis was established in 15%, including benign ovarian cysts, ectopic pregnancy, appendicitis, and endometriosis (Table 10–27). Nonetheless, if only women with moderate or severe symptoms are considered, most women with tubal occlusion will be missed. Pelvic ultrasonography may be helpful in diagnosing tubovarian abscess before it is clinically apparent, and increased adnexal volume on ultrasound may suggest the diagnosis of PID.

Complications

The sequelae of acute PID are significant, hence the prudent use of antibiotics. Tubovarian abscess is not uncommon. Twenty to 25% of patients develop subsequent unrelated episodes of PID. Thirteen per-

---

Table 10–26. Criteria for the diagnosis of acute salpingitis.[1]

All 3 must be present:
1. History of lower abdominal pain and the presence of lower abdominal tenderness; with or without evidence of rebound
2. Cervical motion tenderness
3. Adnexal tenderness

Plus

One of these must be present:
1. Temperature of > 38 °C
2. Leukocytosis with > 10,500 white blood cells/μL
3. A culdocentesis that yields peritoneal fluid containing white blood cells and bacteria
4. Presence of an inflammatory mass noted on pelvic examination or sonography
5. Elevated erythrocyte sedimentation rate
6. A gram stain from the endocervix revealing gram-negative intracellular diplococci suggestive of *Neisseria gonorrhoeae* or a monoclonal directed smear from endocervical secretions revealing *Chlamydia trachomatis*
7. Presence of > 5 white blood cells per oil-immersion field on Gram's stain of endocervical discharge

[1]Reproduced, with permission, from Sweet RL: Pelvic inflammatory disease. *Sex Transm Dis* 1986;**13(Suppl 3)**:192.

Table 10–27. Differential diagnosis of pelvic inflammatory disease.

Acute appendicitis
Mesenteric lymphadenitis
Cholecystitis
Ectopic pregnancy
Intrauterine pregnancy
Ovarian cyst
Ovarian tumor
Endometriosis
Urinary tract infection
Renal calculus

cent of women with acute PID have chronic abdominal pain felt to be related to adhesions around the fallopian tubes.

The Fitz-Hugh-Curtis syndrome, or perihepatitis, is found in 5–10% of women with salpingitis and is felt to be due to direct, hematogenous, or lymphatic spread of bacteria from the fallopian tubes to the liver surface. The woman may experience right upper quadrant pain and hepatic tenderness without liver enlargement and usually has normal liver function tests. A friction rub may be present, and on laparoscopy a fibrinous or purulent exudate may be seen over the liver capsule and later result in "violin string" adhesions between the liver capsule and the abdominal wall.

Occlusion of the fallopian tubes after salpingitis accounts for 30–40% of infertility and half of the cases of ectopic pregnancy. Twelve percent of women with one episode, 35% with 2 episodes, and over 73% with 3 or more episodes of PID are infertile because of tubal occlusion. Age is inversely related to risk of infertility due to tubal occlusion after PID. The risk of ectopic pregnancy is 7 to 10 times greater for women who have had salpingitis than for those who have not, and 5% who have had one or more cases of PID will have an ectopic pregnancy.

Treatment

Appropriate cultures from the cervix should be obtained, and consideration should be given as to whether gynecologic consultation or laparoscopy is needed. The patient should be hospitalized if she exhibits significant fever or toxicity, is unable to tolerate oral medication and fluids, has not responded to outpatient therapy or is unlikely to comply with it, is a younger adolescent, or is concerningly ill with unclear diagnosis. If there is the slightest concern for P.I.D., the patient should be treated with appropriate antibiotics to cover *Chlamydia,* gonorrhea, and anaerobes, while cultures are pending (Table 10–28.) The patient should be reevaluated in 48–72 hours and hospitalized if there is no improvement. Appropriate management includes treatment of the male partner(s), regardless of whether urethritis is present.

HIV INFECTION

The human immunodeficiency virus (HIV) is transmitted in blood and semen, and potentially other body fluids, through sexual contact and sharing of needles.

About 75% of cases in the USA have been in homosexual or bisexual men, and 15% in intravenous substance abusers. Although to date few cases have occurred in adolescents, they are at significant potential risk due to their propensity for multiple sexual partners and their limited use of barrier contraceptives, as well as the use of drugs by some. A large number of young adults 20 to 29 years old with HIV infection acquired the infection as adolescents.

Preventive measures need to be taken to ensure that adolescents have the necessary knowledge to protect themselves from HIV infection in current and future relationships and to eliminate hysteria. They need to be instructed in risk factors for HIV infection, modes of transmission, means of protection,

Table 10–28. Treatment of pelvic inflammatory disease.[1]

	Drug of Choice	**Dosage**	**Alternatives**
Hospitalized patients	Cefoxitin or cefotetan either one plus doxycycline followed by doxycycline[2]	2 g IV every 6 hours 2 g IV every 12 hours 100 mg IV every 12 hours until improved 100 mg orally twice daily to complete 10–14 days	Clindamycin 600 mg IV every 6 hours plus gentamicin 2 mg/kg IV once followed by gentamicin 1.5 mg/kg IV every 8 hours until improved followed by doxycycline[2] 100 mg orally twice daily to complete 10–14 days
Outpatients	Cefoxitin plus probenecid or ceftriaxone either one followed by doxycycline[2]	2 g IM once 1 g orally once 250 mg IM once 100 mg orally twice daily for 10–14 days	

[1]Modified and reproduced, with permission, from Treatment of sexually transmitted diseases. *Med Lett Drugs Ther* 1990;**32**:5.
[2]Contraindicated during pregnancy.

Table 10–29. Safer sex practices.

Abstinence: greatest protection against HIV infection
Sexual activity without intercourse: hugging, massaging, masturbation
Sexual activity only in the context of a monogamous relationship
Limiting the number of sexual partners
Using condoms and spermicide for each sexual encounter, including oral and anal intercourse. (Hold rim of condom closed during withdrawal to prevent spilling semen.)
Refraining from anal intercourse
Refraining from oral sex when mouth sores or open wounds are present
Refraining from vaginal or oral sex during menstruation or when vaginal or vulvar sores or infections exist

and availability of confidential testing. The safer sex practices (Table 10–29) promoted as a result of HIV infection can reduce the rate of all kinds of STD. Adolescence is an ideal time to promote these practices because intimate relationships are beginning and sexual decisions become important.

American Academy of Pediatrics Committee on School Health: Acquired immunodeficiency syndrome education in the schools. *Pediatrics* 1988;**82**:278.

Corey L, Holmes KK: Genital herpes simplex virus infections: Current concepts in diagnosis, therapy, and prevention. *Ann Intern Med* 1983;**98**:973.

Fraser JJ Jr, Rettig PJ, Kaplan DW: Prevalence of cervical *Chlamydia trachomatis* and *Neisseria gonorrhoeae* in female adolescents. *Pediatrics* 1983;**71**:3.

Golden N, Neuhoff S, Cohen H: Pelvic inflammatory disease in adolescents. *J Pediatr* 1989;**114**:138.

Hillard PJA et al: Cervical dysplasia and human papillomavirus: Evaluation in an adolescent dysplasia clinic. *Adolesc Pediatr Gynecol* 1989;**2**:32.

Martinez J et al: High prevalence of genital tract papillomavirus infection in female adolescents. *Pediatrics* 1988; **82**:604.

Med Lett Drugs Ther (Jan 15) 1988;**30**:5.

Nicholas SW et al: Human immunodeficiency virus infection in childhood, adolescence, and pregnancy: A status report and national research agenda. *Pediatrics* 1989; **83**:293.

Rosenfeld WD, Litman N: Urogenital tract infections in male adolescents. *Pediatr Rev* 1983;**4**:8.

Strunin L, Hingson R: Acquired immunodeficiency syndrome and adolescents: Knowledge, beliefs, attitudes, and behaviors. *Pediatrics* 1987;**79**:825.

Sweet RL: Pelvic inflammatory disease. *Sexually Transmitted Diseases* 1986;**13(Suppl)**:192.

Washington AE, Sweet RL, Shafer MB: Pelvic inflammatory disease and its sequelae in adolescents. *J Adolesc Health Care* 1985;**6**:298.

Wolner-Hanssen P et al: Clinical manifestations of vaginal trichomoniasis. *JAMA* 1989;**261**:571.

SELECTED REFERENCES

Blos P: *The Adolescent Passage: Developmental Issues.* International Universities Press, 1979.

Blum RW (editor): *Chronic Illness and Disabilities in Childhood and Adolescence.* Grune & Stratton, 1984.

Coates TJ, Petersen AC, Perry C: *Promoting Adolescent Health: A Dialog on Research and Practice.* Academic Press, 1982.

Dickey RP: *Managing Contraceptive Pill Patients.* Creative Infomatics, 1987.

Elkind D: *Children and Adolescents: Interpretive Essays on Jean Piaget.* Oxford Univ Press, 1974.

Emans SJH, Goldstein DP: *Pediatric and Adolescent Gynecology.* Little, Brown, 1982.

Erickson EH: Identity: *Youth and Crisis.* WW Norton, 1968.

Furstenberg FF Jr, Lincoln R, Menken J: *Teenage Sexuality, Pregnancy and Childbearing.* University of Pennsylvania Press, 1981.

Hatcher RA et al: *Contraceptive Technology: 1988–1989.* Irvington Publishers, 1988.

Hoffman A: *Adolescent Medicine.* Appleton & Lange, 1989.

Holder AR: *Legal Issues in Pediatrics and Adolescent Medicine.* Yale University Press, 1985.

Holmes KK et al (editors): *Sexually Transmitted Diseases.* McGraw-Hill, 1984.

Kagan J, Coles R: *Twelve to Sixteen: Early Adolescence.* WW Norton, 1972.

Katchadourian H: *The Biology of Adolescence.* Freeman, 1977.

Levine M et al (editors): *Developmental Behavioral Pediatrics.* Saunders, 1983.

Levine MD, McAnarney ER: *Early Adolescent Transitions.* Lexington Books, 1988.

Malmquist CP: *Handbook of Adolescence.* J Aronson, 1985.

McAnarney ER: *Premature Adolescent Pregnancy and Parenthood.* Grune & Stratton, 1983.

Meeks JE: *The Fragile Alliance.* Krieger, 1980.

Miller D: *The Age Between: Adolescence and Therapy.* J Aronson, 1983.

Muuss RE: *Theories of Adolescence,* 3rd ed. Random House, 1975.

Neinstein LS: *Adolescent Health Care: A Practical Guide.* Urban & Schwarzenberg, 1984.

Speroff L, Glass RH, Kase NG: *Clinical Gynecologic Endocrinology and Infertility.* Williams & Wilkins, 1989.

Strasburger, VC (editor): Adolescent gynecology. *Pediatr Clin North Am* 1989;**38**:3.

Tanner JM: *Growth at Adolescence.* Blackwell, 1962.

11

Skin

William L. Weston, MD

GENERAL PRINCIPLES OF DIAGNOSIS

Examination of the skin requires that the entire surface of the body be inspected in good light and palpated. The skin offers many clues to internal disorders and must be carefully scrutinized. The onset and duration of each symptom should be recorded.

Examination of the Skin

Examination of the skin should consist of identification of a primary lesion followed by description of secondary changes, color, configuration, and distribution of the lesions. The sometimes difficult language of dermatology prevents many students of medicine from accurately describing cutaneous eruptions. The word "rash" is too vague to be useful and should be qualified appropriately. The following terminology should be mastered by all practitioners.

A. Primary Lesions (the First to Appear):

1. Macule—Any circumscribed color change in the skin that is flat. *Examples:* White (vitiligo), brown (café au lait spot), purple (petechia).

2. Papule—A solid, elevated area < 1 cm in diameter whose top may be pointed, rounded, or flat. *Examples:* Acne, warts, small lesions of psoriasis.

3. Plaque—A solid, circumscribed area > 1 cm in diameter, usually flat-topped. *Example:* Psoriasis.

4. Vesicle—A circumscribed, elevated lesion < 1 cm in diameter and containing clear serous fluid. *Example:* Blisters of herpes simplex.

5. Bulla—A circumscribed, elevated lesion > 1 cm in diameter and containing clear serous fluid. *Example:* Bullous erythema multiforme.

6. Pustule—A vesicle containing a purulent exudate. *Examples:* Acne, folliculitis.

7. Nodule—A deep-seated mass with indistinct borders that elevates the overlying epidermis. *Examples:* Tumors, grauloma annulare. If it moves with the skin on palpation, it is intradermal; if the skin moves over the nodule, it is subcutaneous.

8. Wheal—A circumscribed, flat-topped, firm elevation of skin resulting from tense edema of the papillary dermis. *Example:* Urticaria.

B. Secondary Changes:

1. Scales—Dry, thin plates of keratinized epidermal cells (stratum corneum). *Examples:* Psoriasis, ichthyosis.

2. Lichenification—Induration of skin with exaggerated skin lines and a shiny surface resulting from chronic rubbing of the skin. *Example:* Atopic dermatitis.

3. Erosion and oozing—A moist, circumscribed, slightly depressed area representing a blister base with the roof of the blister removed. *Examples:* Burns, bullous erythema multiforme. Most oral blisters present as erosions.

4. Crust—Dried exudate of plasma on the surface of the skin following acute dermatitis. *Examples:* Impetigo, contact dermatitis.

5. Fissure—A linear split in the skin extending through the epidermis into the dermis. *Example:* Angular cheilitis.

6. Scar—A flat, raised, or depressed area of fibrotic replacement of dermis or subcutaneous tissue. *Examples:* Acne scar, burn scar.

7. Atrophy—Depression of the skin surface due to thinning of one or more layers of skin.

C. Color: The lesion should be described as red, yellow, brown, tan, or blue. Particular attention should be given to the blanching of red or brown lesions, eg, petechiae.

D. Configuration of Lesions: Clues to diagnosis may be obtained from the characteristic morphologic arrangement of primary or secondary lesions.

1. Annular (circular)—Annular nodules represent granuloma annulare; annular papules are more apt to be due to dermatophyte infections.

2. Linear (straight line)—Linear papules represent lichen striatus; linear vesicles, incontinentia pigmenti; linear papules with burrows, scabies.

3. Grouped—Grouped vesicles occur in herpes simplex or zoster.

4. Discrete—Discrete lesions are independent of each other.

E. Distribution: It is useful to note whether the eruption is generalized, acral (hands, feet, buttocks, or face), or localized to a specific skin region.

F. Description of Skin Lesions: Skin lesions are described in reverse order from that of their identification. One begins with distribution, configuration, color, secondary changes, and then primary lesion; eg, guttate psoriasis could be described as generalized discrete, red, scaly papules.

GENERAL PRINCIPLES OF TREATMENT OF SKIN DISORDERS

TOPICAL THERAPY

Treatment should be simple and aimed at preserving or restoring the physiologic state of the skin. It is essential to keep in mind that one is treating the child and not the anxious parent or grandparent. Topical therapy is often preferred because medication can be delivered in optimal concentrations at the exact site where it is needed.

Water is an important therapeutic agent that is often forgotten (it is the active ingredient in Burow's solution, calamine lotion, potassium permanganate, and tannic acid soaks). When the skin is optimally hydrated, it is soft and smooth (Table 11–1). This occurs at approximately 60% environmental humidity. Because water evaporates readily from the cutaneous surface, the skin (stratum corneum of the epidermis) is dependent on the water concentration in the air, and sweating contributes little. However, if sweat is prevented from evaporating (eg, in the axilla, groin), the environmental humidity is increased and so is the hydration of the skin. As environmental humidity falls below 15–20%, the stratum corneum shrinks and cracks; the epidermal barrier is lost and allows irritants to enter the skin and induce an inflammatory response. Replacement of water will correct this condition if the water is not allowed to evaporate. Therefore, in treating dry and scaly skin, one would soak the skin in water for 5 minutes and then add a barrier to prevent evaporation. Oils and ointments prevent evaporation for 8–12 hours. Thus, oils and ointments must be applied once or twice a day. In areas already occluded (axilla, diaper area), ointments or oils will merely increase retention of water and should not be used.

Overhydration (maceration) can also occur. As environmental humidity increases to 90–100%, the number of water molecules absorbed by the stratum corneum increases and the tight lipid junctions between the cells of the stratum corneum are gradually replaced by weak hydrogen bonds (water); the cells eventually become widely separated, and the epidermal barrier falls apart. This occurs in immersion foot, diaper areas, axillas, etc. It is desirable to enhance evaporation of water in these areas. Exposure to less humidity and air drying are useful strategies.

Table 11–1. Bases used for topical preparations.

Base	Combined With	Uses
Liquids		Wet dressings: relieve pruritus, vasoconstrict.
	Powder	Shake lotions, drying pastes: relieve pruritus, vasoconstrict.
	Grease and emulsifier; oil in water	Vanishing cream: penetrates quickly (10–15 minutes) and thus allows evaporation.
	Excess grease and emulsifier; water in oil	Emollient cream: penetrates more slowly and thus retains moisture on skin.
Grease		Ointments: occlusive (hold material on skin for prolonged time) and prevent evaporation of water.
Powder		Enhances evaporation.

(1) Most greases are triglycerides (eg, Aquaphor, petrolatum, Eucerin).
(2) Oils are fluid fats (eg, Alpha Keri, olive oil, mineral oil).
(3) True fats (eg, lard, animal fats) contain free fatty acids that increase in amount upon standing and cause irritation.
(4) Ointments (eg, Aquaphor, petrolatum) should not be used in intertriginous areas such as the axillas, between the toes, and in the perineum, because they increase maceration. Lotions or creams are preferred in these areas.
(5) Oils and ointments hold medication on the skin for long periods of time and are therefore ideal for barriers or prophylaxis and for dried areas of skin. Medication gets into the skin more slowly from ointments.
(6) Creams carry medication into skin and are preferable for intertriginous dermatitis.
(7) Solutions, gels, or lotions should be used for scalp treatment.

WET DRESSINGS

By placing the skin in an environment where the humidity is 100% and allowing the moisture to evaporate to 60%, pruritus is relieved. Evaporation of water stimulates cold-dependent nerve fibers in the skin—thereby, theoretically, tying up the circuits so that the itching sensation coming through the pain fibers will not reach the central nervous system. It also is vasoconstrictive, thereby helping to reduce the erythema and also decreasing the inflammatory cellular response.

Gauze of 20/12 mesh is commonly used for wet dressings. Parke-Davis 4-inch gauze comes in 100-yard rolls, and 5 yards is usually sufficient for application to the extremities. Curity 18-inch gauze can be used for application to the trunk. An alternative is to use the "2 long johns" technique, in which a pair of wet cotton long-sleeved and long-legged underwear is covered by a dry pair.

Warm but not hot water is used, and the gauze or long johns are soaked in the water and then wrung out until no more drops come out. The dressings are then wrapped around the extremities and fastened with a safety pin. The wet dressings are then covered with dry flannel or dry long johns, thereby slowing down the evaporation process but not completely retarding it, so that the wet dressings need only be changed every 3 or 4 hours.

TOPICAL GLUCOCORTICOIDS

The mainstay of treatment of all forms of dermatitis is application of topical glucocorticoid preparations twice daily (Table 11–2). Topical steroids can also be used under wet dressings. Wet dressings are removed every 4–6 hours and topical steroid applied; then the skin is covered again with wet dressings. If treatment is applied throughout the 24-hour period, maximum benefit is obtained after 72 hours; if treatment is applied only at night, maximum benefit is obtained after 7 days. When the condition has improved, the wet dressings are discontinued and a steroid ointment applied twice daily. Daily application of steroids is not to be continued for more than one month. Only low-potency steroids (Table 11–2) are applied to the face or intertriginous areas.

Weston WL: Use and abuse of topical steroids. *Contemp Pediatr* 1988;**5**:57.

DISORDERS OF THE SKIN IN NEWBORNS

TRANSIENT DISEASES IN THE NEWBORN

No treatment is required for any of these disorders, though treatment may be given as noted below.

Milia

Multiple white papules 1 mm in diameter scattered over the forehead, nose, and cheeks are present in up to 40% of newborn infants. Histologically, they represent superficial epidermal cysts filled with keratinous material associated with the developing pilosebaceous follicle. Their intraoral counterparts are called Epstein's pearls and are even more common than facial milia. All of these cystic structures spontaneously rupture and exfoliate their contents.

Sebaceous Gland Hyperplasia

Prominent yellow macules at the opening of each pilosebaceous follicle, predominantly over the nose, represent overgrowth of sebaceous glands in response to the same androgenic stimulation that occurs in adolescence.

Table 11–2. Topical glucocorticoids.

	Concentrations (Percent)
Low potency = 1–9 Hydrocortisone	0.5 and 1.0
Desonide	0.05
Moderate potency = 10–99 Mometisone	0.1
Hydrocortisone valerate	0.2
Fluocinolone acetonide	0.025
Triamcinolone acetonide	0.01
Amcinonide	0.1
High potency = 100–499 Desoximetasone	0.25
Fluocinonide	0.05
Halcinonide	0.1
Super potency = 500–7500 Betamethasone dipropionate	0.05
Clobetasol propionate	0.05

Acne Neonatorum

Open and closed comedones, erythematous papules, and pustules identical in appearance to adolescent acne may occur in infants over the forehead, cheeks, and chin. The lesions may be present at birth but usually do not appear until 3–4 weeks of age. Spontaneous resolution occurs over a period of 6 months to a year. Rarely, neonatal acne may be a manifestation of a virilizing syndrome.

Harlequin Color Change

A cutaneous vascular phenomenon unique to neonates occurs when the infant (particularly one of low birth weight) is placed on one side. The dependent half develops an erythematous flush with a sharp demarcation at the midline, and the upper half of the body becomes pale. The color changes usually subside within a few seconds after the infant is placed supine but may persist for as long as 20 minutes.

Mottling

A lacelike pattern of dilated cutaneous vessels appears over the extremities and often the trunk of neonates exposed to lowered room temperature. This feature is transient and usually disappears completely upon rewarming.

Erythema Toxicum

Up to 50% of term infants develop erythema toxicum. Usually at 24–48 hours of age, blotchy erythematous macules 2–3 cm in diameter appear, most prominently on the chest but also on the back, face, and extremities. These are occasionally present at birth. Onset after 4–5 days of life is rare. The lesions vary in number from 2–3 up to as many as 100. Incidence is much higher in term infants than in premature ones. The macular erythema may fade within

24–48 hours or may progress to develop urticarial wheals in the center of the macules or, in 10% of cases, pustules. Examination of a Wright-stained smear of the lesion will reveal numerous eosinophils. This may be accompanied by peripheral blood eosinophilia of up to 20%. All of the lesions fade and disappear by 5–7 days. A similar eruption in black newborns has a neutrophilic predominance and leaves hyperpigmentation.

Sucking Blisters

Bullae, either intact or in the form of an erosion representing a blister base without inflammatory borders, may occur over the forearms, wrists, thumbs, or upper lip. These presumably result from vigorous sucking in utero. They resolve without complications.

Miliaria

Obstruction of the eccrine sweat ducts occurs often in neonates and produces one of 2 clinical pictures depending upon the level of obstruction. **Miliaria crystallina** is characterized by tiny (1–2 mm) superficial grouped vesicles without erythema over intertriginous areas and adjacent skin (eg, neck and upper chest). Obstruction occurs in the stratum corneum portion of the eccrine duct. More commonly, obstruction of the eccrine duct deeper in the epidermis results in erythematous grouped papules in the same areas and is called **miliaria rubra.** Rarely, these may progress to pustules. Heat and high humidity predispose to eccrine duct pore closure. Removal to a cooler environment is the treatment of choice.

Subcutaneous Fat Necrosis

Reddish or purple, sharply circumscribed, firm nodules occurring over the cheeks, buttocks, arms, and thighs and occurring between day 1 and day 7 in infants represent subcutaneous fat necrosis. Cold injury is thought to play an important role. These lesions resolve spontaneously over a period of weeks, although, like all instances of fat necrosis, they may calcify.

Sclerema

Premature newborns, especially those who suffer metabolic alterations (eg, metabolic acidosis, hypoglycemia, hypothermia), are susceptible to a diffuse hardening of the skin that makes the skin look shiny and feel tight. Severe cold injury in undernourished infants is assumed to be the cause.

Treatment consists of protecting the infant from undue exposure to cold and repairing metabolic and nutritional deficiencies.

Lane AT: Development and care of the premature infant's skin. *Pediatr Dermatol* 1987;**4**:1.

Storrer J et al: Neonatal skin and skin disorders. Pages 267–303 in: *Pediatric Dermatology.* Schachner L, Hansen R (editors). Churchill Livingstone, 1988.

BIRTHMARKS

Birthmarks may involve an overgrowth of one or more of any of the normal components of skin: pigment cells, blood vessels, lymph vessels, etc. A nevus is a hamartoma of highly differentiated cells that retain their normal function.

Note: All tissue excised should be submitted for pathologic examination.

1. PIGMENT CELL BIRTHMARKS

Mongolian Spot

A blue-black macule found over the lumbosacral area in 90% of American Indian, black, and Asian infants is called a mongolian spot. These spots are occasionally noted over the shoulders and back and may extend over the buttocks. Histologically, they consist of spindle-shaped pigment cells located deep in the dermis. The lesions fade somewhat with time, but some traces may persist into adult life.

Café au Lait Spot

A café au lait spot is a light brown, oval macule (dark brown on black skin) that may be found anywhere on the body. Ten percent of white and 22% of black children have café au lait spots greater than 1.5 cm in their longest diameter. These lesions persist throughout life and may increase in number with age. The presence of 6 or more café au lait macules greater than 1.5 cm in their longest diameter may represent a clue to neurofibromatosis. Patients with Albright's syndrome also have increased numbers of café au lait macules. Although it has been suggested that the melanocytes of café au lait macules in neurofibromatosis contain giant pigment granules, this is not often the case in children, and their absence does not rule out neurofibromatosis.

Junctional Nevus & Compound Nevus

Dark brown or black macules, usually few in number at birth but becoming more numerous with age, represent junctional nevi. Histologically, these lesions are large clones of melanocytes at the junction of the epidermis and dermis. With aging, they may become raised (papules) and contain intradermal melanocytes, creating a compound nevus. Often the surface becomes irregular and roughened.

There is controversy about whether junctional and compound nevi are precancerous. Seventy to 80% of melanomas arise on skin that previously contained no pigmented lesion, so the question is not whether junctional nevi are more likely to produce melanoma than normal skin but whether the pigmented lesion really is a junctional nevus or has been a melanoma all along.

Lesions with variegated colors (red, white, blue),

notched borders, and nonuniform, irregular surfaces should arouse a suspicion of melanoma. Ulceration and bleeding are advanced signs of melanoma.

If melanoma is a possibility, excisional biopsy for pathologic examination should be done as the treatment of choice.

Brown to blue solitary papules with smooth surfaces represent intradermal nevi. When pigmentation is present deeper in the dermis, the lesions appear blue or blue-black and are called blue nevi.

Spindle & Epithelioid Cell Nevus (Juvenile Melanoma)

A reddish-brown solitary nodule appearing on the face or upper arm of a child represents a spindle and epithelioid cell nevus. The name melanoma is misleading because this tumor is biologically benign. Histologically, it consists of pigment-producing cells of bizarre shape with numerous mitoses.

Treatment consists of excision.

Giant Pigmented Nevus (Bathing Trunk Nevus)

An irregular dark brown to black plaque over 10 cm in diameter represents a giant pigmented nevus. Often the lesions are of such size as to cover the entire trunk (bathing trunk nevi). Histologically, they are compound nevi. Transformation to malignant melanoma has been reported in as many as 10% of cases in some series, although the true incidence is probably somewhat less. Malignant change may occur at birth or at any time thereafter.

Tissue expanders may be useful in excision of large lesions. The risk of melanoma and the potential for cosmetic improvement should be carefully evaluated for each patient.

Bauer BS et al: An approach to excision of congenital giant pigmented nevi in infancy and early childhood. *J Pediatr Surg* 1988;**23**:509.

Gari LM et al: Melanomas arising in large congenital nevocytic nevi: A prospective study. *Pediatr Dermatol* 1988;**5**:151.

Hurwitz S: Pigmented nevi. *Semin Dermatol* 1988;**7**:17.

2. VASCULAR BIRTHMARKS

Flat Hemangioma

Flat vascular birthmarks can be divided into 2 types: those that are orange or light red (salmon patch) and those that are dark red or bluish red (port wine stain).

A. Salmon Patch: The salmon patch (nevus flammeus) is a light red macule found over the nape of the neck, upper eyelids, and glabella. Fifty percent of infants have such lesions over their necks. Eyelid lesions fade completely within 3–6 months and glabellar lesions by age 5 or 6; those on the nape of the neck fade somewhat but may persist into adult life. Salmon patches are usually bilateral, whereas port wine stains are unilateral.

B. Port Wine Stain: Port wine stains are dark red or purple macules appearing unilaterally on the side of the face or an extremity. A port wine stain over the face may be a clue to **Sturge-Weber syndrome,** which is characterized by seizures, mental retardation, glaucoma, and hemiplegia. Most infants with unilateral port wine stains do not have Sturge-Weber syndrome. If the angioma is in the distribution of the ophthalmic branch of the trigeminal nerve or hemihypertrophy of that side of the face exists, Sturge-Weber syndrome is more likely.

Similarly, a port wine hemangioma over an extremity may be associated with hypertrophy of the soft tissue and bone of that extremity (**Klippel-Trenaunay syndrome**).

The pulsed dye laser is the treatment of choice for infants and children with port wine stains.

Paller A: The Sturge-Weber syndrome. *Pediatr Dermatol* 1987;**4**:300.

Tan OT et al: Laser therapy for selected cutaneous vascular lesions in the pediatric population: A review. *Pediatrics* 1988;**82**:652.

Strawberry Hemangioma

A red, rubbery nodule with a roughened surface is a strawberry nevus. The lesion is often not present at birth but is represented by a permanent blanched area on the skin that is supplanted at 2–4 weeks of age by red nodules. Histologically, these are often mixtures of capillary and venous elements, and although a deep nodule (cavernous hemangioma) may be part of the strawberry lesion, the biologic behavior is the same. Fifty percent resolve spontaneously by age 5; 70% by age 7; 90% by age 9; and the rest by adolescence.

Strawberry hemangiomas resolve, leaving only redundant skin, and uncomplicated ones are best treated by watchful waiting. Complications include superficial ulceration and secondary pyoderma, which are treated by topical antiseptics and observation.

Complications that require treatment are (1) thrombocytopenia due to platelet trapping within the lesion (**Kasabach-Merritt syndrome**); (2) airway obstruction (hemangiomas of the head and neck are often associated with subglottic hemangiomas); (3) visual obstruction (with resulting amblyopia); and (4) cardiac decompensation (high-output failure). In these instances, the treatment of choice is prednisone, 1–2 mg/kg orally daily or every other day for 4–6 weeks.

Metzler A: Congenital vascular lesions. *Semin Dermatol* 1988;**7**:9.

Lymphangioma

Lymphangiomas are rubbery, skin-colored nodules occurring in the parotid area (**cystic hygromas**) or on the tongue. They often result in grotesque enlargement of soft tissues.

Surgical excision is the only treatment available, although the results are not satisfactory.

3. EPIDERMAL BIRTHMARKS

Epidermal Nevus

Linear or groups of linear, warty, papular, unilateral lesions represent overgrowth of epidermis since birth. These areas may range from dirty yellow to brown or may be darkly pigmented. The histologic features of the lesions include thickening of the epidermis and elongation of the rete ridges and hyperkeratosis. Clinically, the lesions may be associated with focal motor seizures, mental subnormality, and skeletal anomalies.

Treatment once or twice daily with topical tretinoin 0.05% (retinoic acid [Retin-A]) will keep the lesions flat.

Rogers M et al: Epidermal nevi and the epidermal nevus syndrome. *J Am Acad Derm* 1989;**20**:476.

Nevus Comedonicus

The lesion known as nevus comedonicus consists of linear groups of widely dilated follicular openings plugged with keratin, giving the appearance of localized noninflammatory acne. The treatment of choice is surgical removal. If this is not feasible, topical retinoic acid is helpful.

Nevus Sebaceus

The nevus sebaceus of Jadassohn is a hamartoma of sebaceous glands and underlying apocrine glands that is diagnosed by the appearance at birth of a yellowish, hairless, smooth plaque in the scalp or on the face. The lesion may be contiguous with an epidermal nevus on the face and constitute part of the linear epidermal nevus syndrome.

Histologically, nevus sebaceus represents an overabundance of sebaceous glands without hair follicles. At puberty, with androgenic stimulation, the sebaceous cells in the nevus divide, expand their cellular volume, and synthesize sebum, resulting in a warty mass.

Because 15% of these lesions become basal cell carcinomas after puberty, excision is recommended before puberty.

4. CONNECTIVE TISSUE BIRTHMARKS (JUVENILE ELASTOMA, COLLAGENOMA)

Connective tissue nevi are smooth, skin-colored papules 1–10 mm in diameter that are grouped on the trunk. A solitary, larger (5–10 cm) nodule is called a **shagreen patch** and is histologically indistinguishable from other connective tissue nevi that show thickened, abundant collagen bundles with or without associated increases of elastic tissue. Although the shagreen patch is a cutaneous clue to tuberous sclerosis, the other connective tissue nevi occur as isolated events.

These nevi remain throughout life, and no treatment is necessary.

Uitto J, Santa Cruz DJ, Eisen AZ: Connective tissue nevi of the skin. *J Am Acad Dermatol* 1980;**3**:441.

HEREDITARY SKIN DISORDERS

The Ichthyoses

Ichthyosis is a term applied to several heritable diseases characterized by the presence of excessive scales on the skin. Major categories are listed in Table 11–3. X-linked ichthyosis is related to cholesterol sulfatase deficiency.

Control scaling with Lac-Hydrin 12% applied

Table 11–3. Four major types of ichthyosis.

Name	Age at Onset	Clinical Features	Histology	Inheritance
Ichthyosis with normal epidermal turnover				
Ichthyosis vulgaris	Childhood	Fine scales, deep palmar and plantar markings	Decreased to absent granular layer, hyperkeratosis	Autosomal dominant
X-linked ichthyosis	Birth	Palms and soles spared; thick scales that darken with age; corneal opacities in patients and carrier mothers; cholesterol sulfase deficiency	Hyperkeratosis	X-linked
Ichthyosis with increased epidermal turnover				
Epidermolytic hyperkeratosis	Birth	Verrucous, yellow scales in flexural areas and palms and soles	Hyperkeratosis, vacuolated reticular spaces in epidermis	Autosomal dominant
Lamellar ichthyosis	Birth; collodion baby	Erythroderma, ectropion, large coarse scales; thickened palms and soles	Hyperkeratosis, many mitotic figures	Autosomal recessive

Table 11–4. Types of epidermolysis bullosa.

Name	Age at Onset	Clinical Features	Histology	Inheritance
Nonscarring types Epidermolysis bullosa simplex	Birth	Hemorrhagic blisters over the lower legs; cooling prevents blisters	Disintegration of basal cells	Autosomal dominant
Recurrent bullous eruption of the hands and feet (Weber-Cockayne syndrome)	First few years of life	Blisters brought out by walking	Cytolysis of suprabasal cells; keratotic cells	Autosomal dominant
Junctional bullous epimatosis (Herlitz's disease)	Birth	Erosions on legs, oral mucosa; severe perioral involvement	Separation between plasma membrane of basal cells and PAS-positive basal lamina	Autosomal recessive
Scarring types Epidermolysis bullosa dystrophica, dominant	Infancy	Numerous blisters on hands and feet; milia formation	Separation of PAS-positive basal lamina; anchoring fibrils lost	Autosomal dominant
Epidermolysis bullosa dystrophica, recessive	Birth	Repeated episodes of blistering, secondary infection and scarring—"mitten hands and feet"	Separation below PAS-positive basal lamina; anchoring fibrils lost	Autosomal recessive

once daily. Restoring water to the skin is also very helpful.

Finlay AY: Major autosomal recessive ichthyoses. *Semin Dermatol* 1988;**7**:26.

Williams ML et al: Diagnostic tests for recessive X-linked ichthyosis. *Pediatr Dermatol* 1988;**5**:211.

Epidermolysis Bullosa

The diagnostic feature of this group of diseases is the formation of hemorrhagic blisters in response to slight trauma. They can be divided into scarring and nonscarring types (Table 11–4).

Treatment usually consists of systemic antibiotics for infection, protective dressings of petrolatum or zinc oxide, and cooling the skin. If hands and feet are involved, reducing skin friction with 5% glutaraldehyde every 3 days is helpful. In recessive dystrophic epidermolysis bullosa, phenytoin (Dilantin), 3 mg/kg/d, has reduced new blister formation in most cases.

Incontinentia Pigmenti

Linear blisters in the newborn represent incontinentia pigmenti. These are replaced by hypertrophic, linear, warty bands within several months, followed by swirling brown hyperpigmentation. Most cases are thought to be X-linked dominant, lethal to the male. Mental retardation and seizures were reported in as many as 30% of cases in one series, but the true incidence is probably much less.

Lecher-Gruskay D. et al: Nutritional and metabolic profile of children with epidermolysis bullosa. *Pediatr Dermatol* 1988;**5**:22.

Pearson RW: Clinicopathologic types of epidermolysis bullosa and their nondermatologic complications. *Arch Dermatol* 1988;**124**:718.

COMMON SKIN DISEASES IN INFANTS, CHILDREN, & ADOLESCENTS

ACNE

Essentials of Diagnosis

- Seen in newborns and adolescents.
- Inflammatory papules, open and closed comedones on surface.
- Face, upper chest, and back involvement common.

Clinical Findings

The common forms of acne in pediatric patients occur at 2 ages: in the newborn period and in adolescence. Neonatal acne is a response to maternal androgen, first appearing at 4–6 weeks of age and lasting until 4–6 months of age. It is characterized by inflammatory papules with all lesions in the same stage at the same time. The lesions are primarily on the face, upper chest, and back, in a distribution similar to that seen in adolescent acne. It has been hypothesized but not proved that infants who have severe neonatal acne will develop severe adolescent acne.

The onset of adolescent acne is between ages 8 and 10 in 40% of children. The early lesions are usually limited to the face and are primarily closed comedones (whiteheads; see below). Eventually, 85% of adolescents will develop some form of acne.

Acne occurs in sebaceous follicles, which, unlike hair follicles, have large, abundant sebaceous glands and usually lack hair. They are located primarily on the face, upper chest, back, and penis. Obstruction of the sebaceous follicle opening produces the clinical lesion of acne. If the obstruction occurs at the follicular mouth, the clinical lesion is characterized by a wide, patulous opening filled with a plug of stratum corneum cells. This is the open comedo, or blackhead. Open comedones are the predominant clinical lesion in early adolescent acne. The black color is due not to dirt but to oxidized melanin within the stratum corneum cellular plug. Open comedones do not often progress to inflammatory lesions. Closed comedones, or whiteheads, are caused by obstruction just beneath the follicular opening in the neck of the sebaceous follicle, which produces a cystic swelling of the follicular duct directly beneath the epidermis. The stratum corneum produced accumulates continuously within the cystic cavity. The resultant lesion is an enlarging sphere just beneath the skin surface. Most authorities believe that closed comedones are precursors of inflammatory acne. If open or closed comedones are the predominant lesions on the skin in adolescent acne, it is called **comedonal acne.**

In typical adolescent acne, several different types of lesions are present simultaneously, eg, open and closed comedones and inflammatory lesions such as papules, pustules, and cysts. Inflammatory lesions may also rarely occur as interconnecting, draining sinus tracts. Adolescents with cystic acne require prompt medical attention, since ruptured cysts and sinus tracts result in severe scar formation. New acne scars are highly vascular and have a reddish or purplish hue. Such scars return to normal skin color after several years. Acne scars may be depressed beneath the skin level, raised, or flat to the skin. In adolescents with a tendency toward keloid formation, keloidal scars can occur following acne lesions, particularly over the sternal area.

Differential Diagnosis

Consider rosacea, nevus comedonicus, flat warts, the angiofibromas of tuberous sclerosis, miliaria, and molluscum contagiosum.

Pathogenesis

The primary event in acne formation is obstruction of the sebaceous follicle. Ordinarily the lining of such follicles contains one or 2 layers of stratum corneum cells, but in acne the stratum corneum is overproduced. This phenomenon is androgen-dependent in adolescent acne. The sebaceous follicles contain an enzyme, testosterone 5α-reductase, which converts plasma testosterone to dihydrotestosterone. This androgen is a potent stimulus for nuclear division of the follicular germinative cells and subsequently of excessive cell production. Thus, obstruction requires the presence of both circulating androgens and the converting enzyme. After the production or the administration of androgens, there is

a delay until cellular proliferation occurs and follicular obstruction subsequently appears.

The pathogenesis of inflammatory acne is not well understood. Undoubtedly, physical manipulation of a closed comedo could lead to rupture of the cavity contents into the dermis with a subsequent inflammatory response. Spontaneous inflammation also occurs in obstructed follicles, but the reason for this is unclear. An attractive hypothesis is that overgrowth of gram-positive bacteria in the obstructed follicle (either *Propionibacterium acnes* or *Staphylococcus epidermidis*) might produce enzymes or other factors that initiate inflammation. Overproduction of sebum and free fatty acid formation seem unlikely as causes of inflammation in acne as presently understood.

Adolescent acne may result from several external causes. Frictional acne due to headbands, football helmets, or tight-fitting brassieres or other garments occurs predominantly underneath the area where the garment is worn. Oil-based cosmetics may be responsible for predominantly comedonal acne, and hair sprays may produce acne along the hair margin.

Drug-induced acne should be suspected in teenagers if all lesions are in the same stage at the same time and if involvement extends to the lower abdomen, lower back, arms, and legs. Drugs responsible for acne include corticotropin (ACTH), glucocorticoids, androgens, hydantoin, and isoniazid.

Treatment

A. Topical Keratolytic Agents: The mainstay of acne therapy is the use of potent topical keratolytic agents applied to the skin to relieve follicular obstruction. Two classes of potent keratolytic agents are available: retinoic acid and benzoyl peroxide gel. These have been found to be the most efficacious agents in the treatment of acne. Either agent may be used once daily, or the combination of retinoic acid cream applied to acne-bearing areas of the skin once daily in the evening and a benzoyl peroxide gel applied once daily in the morning may be used. This regimen will control 80–85% of adolescent acne.

B. Topical Antibiotics: Topical antibiotics are used to avoid the side effects caused by systemic antibiotics. Topical antibiotics are less effective than systemic antibiotics and at best are equivalent in potency to 250 mg of tetracycline orally once a day. One percent clindamycin phosphate solution is the most efficacious of all topical antibiotics. Some percutaneous absorption may occur rarely with this drug, resulting in diarrhea and colitis; 1.5% and 2% topical erythromycin solutions are effective; 1% topical tetracycline solution is minimally effective.

C. Systemic Antibiotics: Antibiotics that are concentrated in sebum, such as tetracycline and erythromycin, are very effective in inflammatory acne. The usual dose is 0.5–1 g taken once or twice daily on an empty stomach (nothing to eat 1 hour before or after the medication). Tetracycline or erythromycin should be continued for 2–3 months until the acne lesions are suppressed.

D. Oral Retinoids: An oral retinoid, 13-*cis*-retinoic acid (isotretinoin; Accutane), offers the most efficacious treatment of severe cystic acne. The precise mechanism of its action is unknown, but decreased sebum production, decreased follicular obstruction, decreased skin bacteria, and general anti-inflammatory activities have been described. The initial dosage is 40 mg once or twice daily. This drug is not effective in comedonal acne or other mild forms of acne. Side effects include dryness and sca-liness of the skin, dry lips, and, occasionally, dry eyes and dry nose. Up to 10% of patients experience mild, reversible hair loss. Elevated liver enzymes and blood lipids have rarely been described. Isotretinoin is teratogenic. Use in young women of childbearing age is not recommended unless strict adherence to manufacturer's guidelines is ensured.

E. Other Acne Treatments: There is no convincing evidence that dietary management, mild drying agents, abrasive scrubs, oral vitamin A, ultraviolet light, cryotherapy, or incision and drainage have any beneficial effects in the management of acne.

F. Avoidance of Cosmetics and Hair Spray: Acne can be aggravated by a variety of external factors that result in further obstruction of partially occluded sebaceous follicles. Discontinuing the use of oil-based cosmetics, face creams, and hair sprays may alleviate the comedonal component of acne within 4–6 weeks.

Patient Education & Follow-Up Visits

It is important to explain the mechanism of acne and the treatment plan to adolescent patients. Time should be set aside at the first visit to answer the patient's questions. Explain that there will not be much improvement for 4–8 weeks. Establish guidelines for ideal control, and explain that the best the patient might achieve is one or 2 new pimples a month. No drug is available that will prevent an adolescent from ever having another acne lesion. A written education sheet is most useful.

Follow-up visits should be made every 4–6 weeks. The criterion for ideal control is a few lesions every 2 weeks. Explain again what medications are being used and what the treatment is intended to achieve, and question the patient to determine whether the medications are being used properly.

Buxton PK: Acne and rosacea. *Br Med J* 1988;**296**:41.
Lucky AW: Endocrine aspects of acne. *Pediatr Clin North Am* 1983;**30**:395.

BACTERIAL INFECTIONS OF THE SKIN

Impetigo

Erosions covered by honey-colored crusts are di-agnostic of impetigo. Staphylococci and group A streptococci are important pathogens in this disease, which histologically consists of superficial invasion of bacteria into the upper epidermis, forming a sub-corneal pustule.

Although topical antibiotics may effect a clinical cure, parenteral penicillin or oral penicillin for 10 days is necessary to eradicate streptococci. The risk of nephritogenic strains varies considerably from area to area, but active treatment of patients and contacts with systemic penicillin will significantly reduce the incidence of acute glomerulonephritis in endemic areas. Dicloxacillin or other antistaphylo-coccal antibiotics are used when staphylococcal infection is suspected.

Barton LL et al: Impetigo; A reassessment of etiology and therapy. *Pediatr Dermatol* 1987;**4**:185.
Barton LL et al: Impetigo contagiosa: A comparison of erythromycin and dicloxacillin therapy. *Pediatr Dermatol* 1988;**5**:88.

Ecthyma

Ecthyma is a firm, dry crust, surrounded by erythema, that exudes purulent material. It represents deep invasion by the streptococcus through the epidermis to the superficial dermis.

Treatment is with systemic penicillin.

Cellulitis

Cellulitis is characterized by erythematous, hot, tender, ill-defined plaques accompanied by regional lymphadenopathy. Histologically, this disorder represents invasion of microorganisms into the lower dermis and sometimes beyond, with obstruction of local lymphatics. *Haemophilus influenzae*, *Streptococcus pneumoniae* and *S pyogenes* are the most common offending organisms.

Septicemia is common, and treatment with the appropriate systemic antibiotic is indicated.

Howe PM et al: Etiologic diagnosis of cellulitis: Comparison of the aspirates obtained from the leading edge and the point of maximal inflammation. *Pediatr Infect Dis J* 1987;**6**:685.
Powell CR et al: Periorbital cellulitis. *Am J Dis Child* 1988;**142**:853.

Folliculitis

A pustule at a follicular opening represents folliculitis. If the pustule occurs at eccrine sweat orifices, it is correctly called **poritis.** Staphylococci and streptococci are the most frequent pathogens.

Treatment consists of measures to remove follicular obstruction—either cool wet compresses for 24 hours or keratolytics such as are used for acne.

Abscess

An abscess occurs deep in the skin, at the bottom of a follicle or an apocrine gland, and is diagnosed as an erythematous, firm, acutely tender nodule with ill-defined borders. Staphylococci are the most common organisms.

Treatment consists of incision and drainage and systemic antibiotics.

Scalded Skin Syndrome

This entity consists of the sudden onset of bright red, acutely painful skin, most obvious periorally, periorbitally, and in the flexural areas of the neck, the axillas, the popliteal and antecubital areas, and the groin. The slightest pressure on the skin results in severe pain and separation of the epidermis, leaving a glistening layer (the stratum granulosum of the epidermis) beneath. The disease is due to a circulating toxin (exfoliatin) elaborated by group II staphylococci (types 71, 55, 3A, 3B, and 3C). The site of action of exfoliatin is the intracellular area of the granular layer, resulting in a separation of cells.

Scalded skin syndrome includes **Ritter's disease** of the newborn, toxic epidermal necrolysis, toxic shock syndrome, and the mildest form, staphylococcal scarlet fever. (See also Bullous Impetigo, below.) In all of the forms of this entity, the causative staphylococci may not be isolated from the skin but rather from the nasopharynx, an abscess, blood culture, etc.

Treatment consists of systemic administration of antistaphylococcal drugs, eg, dicloxacillin, 25–50 mg/kg/d orally, or methicillin, 200–300 mg/kg/d intravenously. No topical therapy is necessary or warranted except in the newborn, where silver sulfadiazine or other burn therapy is used.

Bullous Impetigo

A fifth form of scalded skin syndrome is bullous impetigo. All impetigo is bullous, with the blister forming just beneath the stratum corneum, but in "bullous impetigo" there is, in addition to the usual erosion covered by a honey-colored crust, a border filled with clear fluid. Staphylococci may be isolated from these lesions, and systemic signs of circulating exfoliatin are absent. "Bullous varicella" is a disorder that represents bullous impetigo in varicella lesions.

Treatment with dicloxacillin, 25–50 mg/kg/d orally for 5–6 days, is effective. Application of cool compresses to debride crusts is a helpful symptomatic measure.

Hansen RC: Staphylococcal scalded skin syndrome, toxic shock syndrome and Kawasaki disease. *Pediatr Clin North Am* 1983;**30:**533.

FUNGAL INFECTIONS OF THE SKIN

1. DERMATOPHYTE INFECTIONS

Essentials of Diagnosis

- Red, scaly, round lesions.
- Hair loss with or without scaling in tinea capitis.

General Considerations

Dermatophytes become attached to the superficial layer of the epidermis, nails, and hair, where they proliferate. They grow mainly within the stratum corneum and do not invade the lower epidermis or dermis. Release of toxins from dermatophytes, especially those whose natural host is animals or soil, eg, *Microsporum canis* and *Trichophyton verrucosum,* results in dermatitis. Fungal infection should be suspected with any red and scaly lesion.

Classification & Diagnosis

A. Tinea Capitis: Thickened, broken-off hairs with erythema and scaling of underlying scalp are the distinguishing features (Table 11–5). In epidemic ringworm, hairs are broken off at the surface of the scalp, leaving a black dot appearance. Pustule formation and a boggy fluctuant mass on the scalp occur in *M canis* and *Trichophyton tonsurans* infections. This mass, called a **kerion,** represents an exaggerated host response to the organism. Fungal culture should be performed in all cases of suspected tinea capitis.

B. Tinea Corporis: Tinea corporis presents either as annular marginated papules with a thin scale and clear center or as an annular confluent dermatitis. The most common organisms are *Trichophyton mentagrophytes* and *M canis.* The diagnosis is made by scraping thin scales from the border of the lesion, dissolving them in 20% KOH, and examining for hyphae.

C. Tinea Cruris: Symmetric, sharply marginated lesions in inguinal areas are seen with tinea cruris. The most common organisms are *Trichophyton rubrum, T mentagrophytes,* and *Epidermophyton floccosum.*

D. Tinea Pedis: The diagnosis of tinea pedis in a prepubertal child must always be regarded with skepticism; atopic feet or contact dermatitis is a more likely diagnosis in this age group. Tinea pedis is seen most commonly in postpubertal males with

Table 11–5. Clinical features of tinea capitis.

Most Common Organisms	Clinical Appearance	Microscopic Appearance in KOH
Trichophyton tonsurans (60%)	Hairs broken off 2–3 mm from follicle; "black dot"; no fluorescence	Hyphae and spores within hair
Microsporum canis (39%)	Thickened broken-off hairs that fluoresce yellow-green with Wood's lamp[1]	Small spores outside of hair; hyphae within hair
Microsporum audouini (1%)	Thickened broken-off hairs that fluoresce yellow-green with Wood's lamp[1]	Small spores outside of hair; hyphae within hair

[1]Select fluorescent hairs for examination in KOH and culture.

blisters on the instep of the foot. Fissuring between the toes is occasionally seen.

E. Tinea Ungulum (Onychomycosis): Loosening of the nail plate from the nail bed (onycholysis), giving a yellow discoloration, is the first sign of fungal invasion of the nails. Thickening of the distal nail plate then occurs, followed by scaling and a crumbly appearance of the entire nail plate surface. *T rubrum* and *T mentagrophytes* are the most common causes. The diagnosis is confirmed by KOH examination and fungal culture. Usually one or 2 nails are involved. If every nail is involved, psoriasis or lichen planus is a more likely diagnosis than fungal infection.

Treatment

The treatment of dermatophytosis is quite simple: *If hair or nails are involved, griseofulvin is the treatment of choice.* Topical antifungal agents do not enter hair or nails in sufficient concentration to clear the infection. The absorption of griseofulvin from the gastrointestinal tract is enhanced by a fatty meal; thus, whole milk or ice cream taken with the medication increases absorption. The dosage of griseofulvin is 10–20 mg/kg/d. With hair infections, it should be continued for a minimum of 6 weeks; in nail infections, for a minimum of 3 months. It is supplied in capsules containing 250 mg or as a suspension containing 125 mg/5 mL. The side effects are few, and the drug has even been used successfully in the newborn period.

Tinea corporis, tinea pedis, and tinea cruris can be treated effectively with topical medication after careful inspection to make certain that the hair and nails are not involved. Treatment with clotrimazole (Lotrimin), miconazole (MicaTin), econazole (Spectazole) or haloprogin (Halotex) applied twice daily for 3 or 4 weeks is recommended.

Gan VN et al: Epidemiology and treatment of tinea capitis: Ketoconazole vs. griseofulvin. *Pediatr Infect Dis J* 1987; **6**:46.
Hebert AA: Tinea capitis. *Arch Dermatol* 1988;**124**:1554.
Jacobs A et al: Tinea in tiny tots. *Am J Dis Child* 1986; **140**:1034.

2. TINEA VERSICOLOR

Tinea versicolor is a superficial infection caused by *Pityrosporon orbiculare* (also called *Malassezia furfur*), a yeastlike fungus. It characteristically causes polycyclic connected hypopigmented macules and very fine scales in areas of sun-induced pigmentation. In winter, the polycyclic macules appear reddish-brown.

Treatment consists of application of selenium sulfide (Selsun), 2.5% suspension, or 25% sodium thiosulfate (Tinver). Selenium sulfide should be applied to the whole body and left on overnight. Treatment can be repeated again in a week and then monthly thereafter. It tends to be somewhat irritating, and the patient should be warned about this difficulty.

Nanda A et al: Pityriasis (tinea) versicolor in infancy. *Pediatr Dermatol* 1988;**5**:260.

3. *CANDIDA ALBICANS* INFECTIONS

In addition to being a frequent invader in diaper dermatitis, *Candida albicans* also infects the oral mucosa, where it appears as thick white patches with an erythematous base (**thrush**); the angles of the mouth, where it causes fissures and white exudate (**perlèche**); and the cuticular region of the fingers, where thickening of the cuticle, dull red erythema, and distortion of growth of the nail plate suggest the diagnosis of candidal paronychia. *C albicans* is able to penetrate the stratum corneum layer and locally activate the complement system.

Nystatin (Mycostatin) is the drug of first choice for *C albicans* infections. It is supplied as an ointment or a cream, as an oral suspension, and as vaginal tablets. In diaper dermatitis, the cream form can be applied every 3–4 hours. In oral thrush, the suspension should be applied directly to the mucosa with the parent's finger or a cotton-tipped applicator, since it is not absorbed and acts topically. In candidal paronychia, nystatin is applied over the area, covered with occlusive plastic wrapping, and left on overnight after the application is made airtight.

Haloprogin, miconazole, econazole nitrate, or clotrimazole is an effective alternative.

Butler KM et al: Candida: An increasingly important pathogen in the nursery. *Pediatr Clin North Am* 1988; **35**:543.

VIRAL INFECTIONS OF THE SKIN

Herpes Simplex

Grouped vesicles or grouped erosions suggest herpes simplex. The microscopic finding of epidermal giant cells after scraping the vesicle base with a No. 15 blade, smearing on a slide, and staining with Wright's stain (Tzanck smear) suggests herpes simplex or varicella-zoster. In infants, lesions due to herpes simplex type 1 are seen on the gingiva and lips, periorbitally, or on the thumb in thumb suckers. Recurrent erosions in the mouth are usually aphthous stomatitis in children rather than recurrent herpes simplex. Herpes simplex type 2 is seen on the genitalia and in the mouth in adolescents. Herpes simplex infection of the genitalia is now the second most common venereal disease. Cutaneous dissemination of herpes simplex occurs in patients with atopic dermatitis (**eczema herpeticum, Kaposi's varicelliform eruption**).

In severe disseminated infection, oral acyclovir may be helpful.

Arvin AM: Oral therapy with acyclovir in infants and children. *Pediatr Infect Dis J* 1987;**6**:56.

Kibrick S: Herpes simplex infection at term: What to do with mother, newborn, and nursery personnel. *JAMA* 1980;**243**:157.

Spruance SL et al: The natural history of recurrent herpes labialis. *N Engl J Med* 1977;**297**:69.

Varicella-Zoster

Grouped vesicles in a dermatome on the trunk or face suggest herpes zoster. Zoster in children is not painful and usually has a mild course. In patients with compromised host resistance, the appearance of an erythematous border around the vesicles is a good prognostic sign. Conversely, large bullae without a tendency to crusting imply a poor host response to the virus. Varicella-zoster and herpes simplex lesions undergo the same series of changes: papule, vesicle, pustule, crust, slightly depressed scar. Varicella appears in crops, and many different stages of lesions are present at the same time.

Itching is usually the only symptom, and cool baths as frequently as necessary or drying lotions such as calamine lotion are sufficient to relieve symptoms. In immunosuppressed children, intravenous or oral acyclovir should be considered.

Huff JC: Herpes zoster. *Curr Prob Dermatol* 1988;**1**:5.

HIV Infection

The onset of skin lesions in perinatally acquired HIV infection is 4 months, 11 months in transfusion-acquired HIV infection. Persistent oral candidiasis and recalcitrant candidal diaper rash are the most frequent cutaneous manifestations of infantile HIV infection. Severe herpetic gingivostomatitis, herpes zoster, and molluscum contagiosum are seen. Recurrent staphylococcal pyodermas, tinea of the face, and onychomycosis are also observed. A generalized dermatitis with features of seborrhea is extremely common. In general, persistent, recurrent, or extensive skin infections should make one suspicious of HIV infection.

Prose NS et al: Pediatric human immunodeficiency virus infection and its cutaneous manifestations. *Pediatr Dermatol* 1987;**4**:67.

Virus-Induced Tumors

A. Molluscum Contagiosum: Molluscum contagiosum consists of umbilicated, white or whitish-yellow papules in groups on the genitalia or trunk. They are common in sexually active adolescents as well as in infants and preschool children. Crushing a lesion between glass slides followed by microscopic examination after staining with Wright's stain will demonstrate epidermal cells with inclusions. Molluscum contagiosum is a poxvirus that induces the epidermis to proliferate, forming a pale papule.

Removal of the lesion with a sharp curet or knife is curative. This therapy may leave a small scar, and one must weigh the advantage of removal of lesions that will disappear in 2 or 3 years.

B. Warts: Warts are skin-colored papules with irregular (verrucous) surfaces. They are intraepidermal tumors caused by infection with human papilloma virus. This DNA virus induces the epidermal cells to proliferate, thus resulting in the warty growth. If the wart virus stimulus is small, the result is a flat wart. If the stimulation is great, the cells proliferate and thicken, causing the skin to fold upon itself and giving rise to an irregular (verrucous) surface—as seen on the isolated wart on the body (verruca vulgaris), the plantar wart (verruca plantaris), and, often, the venereal wart (condyloma acuminatum).

No therapy for warts is ideal, and some types of therapy should be avoided because the recurrence rate of warts is high. Flat warts generally require no treatment. They may be considered a mild wart virus infection, and since they usually disappear within 6–9 months they are best left alone. This holds true especially for all flat warts on the face. A good response to 0.05% tretinoin (Retin-A) cream, applied once daily for 3–4 weeks, has been reported.

The best treatment for the solitary **common ("vulgaris") wart** is to freeze it with liquid nitrogen. The liquid nitrogen should be allowed to drip from the cotton-tipped applicator onto the wart without pressure. Pressure exaggerates cold injury by causing vasoconstriction and may produce a deep ulcer and scar. Liquid nitrogen is applied by drip until the wart turns completely white and stays white for 20–25 seconds. Small plantar warts usually need not be treated. Large and painful ones are treated most effectively by applying 40% salicylic acid plaster cut with a scissors to fit the lesion. The sticky brown side of the plaster is placed against the lesion, taped on securely with adhesive tape, and left on for 5 days. The plaster is then removed, and the white necrotic warty tissue can be gently rubbed off with the finger and a new salicylic acid plaster applied. This procedure is repeated every 5 days, and the patient is seen every 2 weeks. Most plantar warts resolve in 2–4 weeks when treated in this way.

Sharp scalpel excision, electrosurgery, and radiotherapy should be avoided, since the resulting scar often becomes a more difficult problem than the wart itself and there may be recurrence of the wart in the area of the scar.

Condyloma acuminatum is best treated with 25% podophyllum resin (podophyllin) in alcohol. This should be painted on the lesions and then washed off after 4 hours. Re-treatment in 7–10 days may be necessary. A condyloma not on the vulvar mucous membrane but on the adjacent skin should be treated as a common wart and frozen.

For isolated warts and periungual warts, cantharidin (Cantharone) is effective and painless in children. It causes a blister and sometimes is difficult to control. An undesirable complication is the appearance of warts along the margins of the cantharidin blister. Cantharidin is applied to the skin, allowed to dry, and covered with occlusive tape such as Blenderm for 24 hours.

No wart therapy is immediate and definitive, and recurrences are reported in 20–30% of cases even with the best care.

Bennett RS et al: Human papillomaviruses: Association between laryngeal papillomas and genital warts. *Pediatr Infect Dis J* 1987;**6**:229.

Douglas MC et al: Management of warts in children. *Pediatr Dermatol* 1987;**4**:36.

Highet AS: Viral warts. *Semin Dermatol* 1988;**7**:53.

INSECT INFESTATIONS (ZOONOSES)

Essentials of Diagnosis

- Discrete red papules, nodules, and S-shaped burrows on skin.
- Hand and foot involvement common.

Scabies

Scabies is suggested by the appearance of linear burrows about the wrists, ankles, finger webs, areolas, anterior axillary folds, genitalia, or face (in infants). Often, there are excoriations, honey-colored crusts, and pustules from secondary infection. Identification of the female mite or her eggs and feces is necessary to confirm the diagnosis. Slice off an unscratched papule or burrow with a No. 15 blade and examine microscopically in either immersion oil or 10% KOH to confirm the diagnosis. In a child who is often scratching, scrape under the fingernails. Examine the parents for unscratched burrows.

Lindane (gamma benzene hexachloride; Kwell) is an excellent scabicide. However, since lindane is concentrated in the central nervous system and central nervous system toxicity from systemic absorption in infants has been reported, the following restricted use of this agent is recommended: (1) For adults and older children, one treatment of lindane lotion or cream applied to the entire body and left on for 4 hours, followed by shower, is sufficient. (2) Infants tend to have more organisms and many more lesions and may have to be re-treated in 7–10 days. All family members should be treated simultaneously. Crotamiton (Eurax) may be substituted for lindane in infants.

Hunig PJ: Bites and parasites. *Pediatr Clin North Am* 1983;**30**:563.

Pediculoses (Louse Infestations)

Excoriated papules and pustules with a history of severe itching at night suggest infestation with the human body louse. This louse may be discovered in the seams of underwear but not on the body. In the scalp hair, the gelatinous nits of the body louse adhere tightly to the hair shaft. The pubic louse may be found crawling among pubic hairs, or blue-black macules may be found dispersed through the pubic region (maculae ceruleae). The pubic louse is often seen in the eyelashes of newborns.

Lindane (gamma benzene hexachloride; Kwell) has been the treatment of choice. Since this agent is concentrated in the central nervous system and central nervous system toxicity from systemic absorption in infants has been reported, the following modification in its use is recommended: For head lice, a shampoo preparation is left on the scalp for 5 minutes and rinsed out thoroughly. The hair is then combed with a fine-tooth comb to remove nits. This may be repeated in 7 days. Lindane cream or lotion applied to the body for 4 hours may be necessary for body lice, but washing the clothing in boiling water followed by ironing the seams with a hot iron usually eliminates the organisms. Permethrin 1% creme rinse is also efficacious for the elimination of lice.

Lindane cream or lotion applied to the pubic area for 24 hours is sufficient to treat pediculosis pubis. It may be repeated in 4–5 days.

Bowerman JG et al: Comparative study of permethrin 1% creme rinse and lindane shampoos for the treatment of head lice. *Pediatr Infect Dis J* 1987;**6**:252.

Sarov B et al: Evaluation of an intervention program for head lice infestation in school children. *Pediatr Infect Dis J* 1988;**7**:176.

Papular Urticaria

Papular urticaria is characterized by grouped erythematous papules surrounded by an urticarial flare and distributed over the shoulders, upper arms, and buttocks in infants. These lesions represent delayed hypersensitivity reactions to stinging or biting insects and can be reproduced by patch testing with the offending insect. Fleas from dogs and cats are the usual offenders. Less commonly, mosquitoes, lice, scabies, and bird and grass mites are involved. The sensitivity is transient, lasting 4–6 months.

The logical therapy is to remove the offending insect. Topical corticosteroids and oral antihistamines will control symptoms.

DERMATITIS* (ECZEMA)

Essentials of Diagnosis

- Red skin with disruption of skin surface.
- Vesicles, crusting, or lichenification may be present.

---

*From the perspective of a dermatologist. See also the discussion of atopic dermatitis in Chapter 32.

General Considerations

The terms dermatitis and eczema are currently used interchangeably in dermatology, although the etymologic implication of eczema is "a boiling over" and the term originally denoted an acute weeping dermatosis. All forms of dermatitis, regardless of cause, may present with acute edema, erythema, and oozing with crusting, mild erythema alone, or lichenification. Lichenification is diagnosed by thickening of the skin with a shiny surface and exaggerated, deepened skin markings. It is the response of the skin to chronic rubbing or scratching.

Although the lesions of the various dermatoses are histologically indistinguishable, clinicians have nonetheless divided the disease group called dermatitis into several categories based on known causes in some cases and differing natural histories in others.

Atopic Dermatitis

Atopic dermatitis is not a clearly defined clinical entity but a general term for chronic superficial inflammation of the skin that can be applied to a heterogeneous group of patients. Many (not all) patients go through 3 clinical phases. In the first, infantile eczema, the dermatitis begins on the cheeks and scalp and frequently expresses itself as oval patches on the trunk, later involving the extensor surfaces of the extremities. The usual age at onset is 2–3 months, and this phase ends at age 18 months to 2 years. Only one-third of all infants with atopic eczema progress to phase 2—childhood or flexural eczema—in which the predominant involvement is in the antecubital and popliteal fossae, the neck, the wrists, and sometimes the hands or feet. This phase lasts from age 2 years to adolescence. Some children will have involvement of the soles of their feet *only,* with cracking, redness, and pain—the so-called **atopic feet.** Only a third of children with typical flexural eczema will progress to adolescent eczema, which is usually manifested by hand dermatitis only. Atopic dermatitis is quite unusual after age 30.

Atopic dermatitis has no known cause, and despite the high incidence of asthma and hay fever in these patients (30%) and their families (70%), evidence for allergy beyond this hereditary association is limited to testimonials. The case for food and inhalant allergens as specific causes of atopic dermatitis is not strong.

A few patients with atopic dermatitis have immunodeficiency with recurrent pyodermas, unusual susceptibility to herpes simplex and vaccinia virus, hyperimmunoglobulinemia E, defective neutrophil and monocyte chemotaxis, and impaired T lymphocyte function.

A faulty epidermal barrier may predispose the patient with atopic dermatitis to itchy skin. Inability to hold water within the stratum corneum results in rapid evaporation of water, shrinking of the stratum corneum, and "cracks" in the epidermal barrier.

Such skin forms an ineffective barrier to the entry of various irritants—and, indeed, it may be clinically useful to regard atopic dermatitis as a primary irritant contact dermatitis and simply tell the patient, "You have sensitive skin." Chronic atopic dermatitis is frequently secondarily infected with *Staphylococcus aureus* or *Streptococcus pyogenes.*

A. Treatment of Acute Stages: Application of wet dressings and topical corticosteroids is the treatment of choice for acute, weeping atopic eczema. A topical steroid preparation is applied 4 times daily and covered with wet dressings as outlined at the beginning of this chapter. Systemic antibiotics chosen on the basis of appropriate skin cultures may be necessary, since lesions in the acute stages are often secondarily infected with *S aureus* or streptococci.

B. Treatment of Chronic Stages: Treatment is aimed at avoiding irritants and restoring water to the skin. No soaps or harsh shampoos should be used, and the patient should avoid woolen clothing or any rough clothing. Restoring water to the skin is important in atopic dermatitis. This can be accomplished by 2 "drip-dry" baths daily, less than 5 minutes each, after which lubricating oils or ointments are applied. Moisturel is a useful lubricant. Plain petrolatum and lards are often too greasy and may cause considerable sweat retention. Liberal use of Cetaphil lotion as a soap substitute 4 or 5 times a day is also satisfactory as a means of lubrication. A bedroom humidifier is often helpful. Topical corticosteroids should be limited to the less potent ones (see Table 11–2). Hydrocortisone ointment, 1% twice daily, is often sufficient. There is *never* any reason to use super- or high-potency corticosteroids in atopic dermatitis. In superinfected atopic dermatitis, systemic antibiotics for 10–14 days (erythromycin, 40 mg/kg/d; dicloxacillin, 50 mg/kg/d) are necessary.

Treatment failures in chronic atopic dermatitis are most often due to patient noncompliance. This is a frustrating disease for parent and child.

Graham-Brown RAI: Atopic dermatitis. *Semin Dermatol* 1988;**7:**37.

Lever R et al: Staphylococcal colonization in atopic dermatitis and the effect of topical mupirocin therapy. *Br J Dermatol* 1988;**119:**189.

Morelli JG et al: Soaps and shampoos in pediatric practice. *Pediatrics* 1987;**80:**634.

Turpeinen M: Influence of age and severity of dermatitis on the percutaneous absorption of hydrocortisone in children. *Br J Dermatol* 1988;**118:**517.

Nummular Eczema

Nummular eczema is characterized by numerous symmetrically distributed coin-shaped ("nummular") patches of dermatitis, principally on the extremities. These may be acute, oozing, and crusted or dry and scaling. The disease lasts 9 months to 2 years. The differential diagnosis should include tinea corporis and atopic dermatitis.

The same topical measures should be used as for atopic dermatitis, though treatment is often more difficult.

Primary Irritant Contact Dermatitis (Diaper Dermatitis)

Contact dermatitis is of 2 types: primary irritant and allergic eczematous. Primary irritant dermatitis develops within a few hours, reaches peak severity at 24 hours, and then disappears. Allergic eczematous contact dermatitis (see below) has a delayed onset of 18 hours, peaks at 48–72 hours, and often lasts as long as 2 or 3 weeks, even if exposure to the offending antigen is discontinued.

Diaper dermatitis, the most common form of primary irritant contact dermatitis seen in pediatric practice, is due to prolonged contact of the skin with urine and feces, which contain irritating chemicals such as urea and intestinal enzymes. The diagnosis of diaper dermatitis is based on the picture of erythema and thickening of the skin in the perineal area and the history of skin contact with urine or feces. In 80% of cases of diaper dermatitis lasting more than 4 days, the affected area is colonized with *Candida albicans* even before the classic signs of a beefy red, sharply marginated dermatitis with satellite lesions appear.

Treatment consists of changing diapers frequently. Because rubber or plastic pants serve as occlusive dressings and prevent the evaporation of the contactant and enhance its penetration into the skin, they should be avoided as much as possible. Air drying is useful. Streptococcal perianal cellulitis should be included in the differential diagnosis.

Treatment of long-standing diaper dermatitis should include application of nystatin (Mycostatin) cream with each diaper change. In extremely inflammatory diaper dermatitis, 1% hydrocortisone cream may be alternated with nystatin cream at every other diaper change.

Campbell RL et al: Effects of diaper types on diaper dermatitis associated with diarrhea and antibiotic use in children in day care centers. *Pediatr Dermatol* 1988; 5:83.

Jordan WE et al: Diaper dermatitis: Frequency and severity among a general population. *Pediatr Dermatol* 1986; 3:198.

Rehder PA et al: Perianal cellulitis: Cutaneous group A streptococcal disease. *Arch Dermatol* 1988;**124**:702.

Lichen Simplex Chronicus (Localized Neurodermatitis)

Lichen simplex chronicus is a sharply circumscribed single patch of lichenification, usually found on the back of the neck in adolescent girls. The patients produce the morphologic skin changes by chronic rubbing and scratching.

Treatment of the thickened lesions is with topical corticosteroids. Because the epidermal barrier has thickened, penetration of topical corticosteroids is poor. Penetration can be enhanced in several ways. Airtight occlusion with plastic dressings (eg, Saran Wrap) overnight over topical corticosteroids is useful, or flurandrenolide (Cordran) tape impregnated with corticosteroids will penetrate the lesion. Covering the lesion will also prevent scratching of the area.

Allergic Eczematous Contact Dermatitis (Poison Ivy Dermatitis)

Children often present with acute dermatitis with blister formation, oozing, and crusting. Blisters are often linear and of acute onset. Plants such as poison ivy, poison sumac, and poison oak cause most cases of allergic contact dermatitis in children.

Allergic contact dermatitis has all the features of delayed type (T lymphocyte-mediated) hypersensitivity. Although many substances may cause such a reaction, nickel sulfate (metals), potassium dichromate, and neomycin are the most common causes. The true incidence of allergic contact dermatitis in children is not known.

Treatment of contact dermatitis in localized areas is with topical corticosteroids. In severe generalized involvement, prednisone, 1–2 mg/kg/d orally for 14–21 days, can be used.

Weston WL: Prevalence of positive epicutaneous tests among infants, children and adolescents. *Pediatrics* 1986;**78**:1070.

Seborrheic Dermatitis

Seborrheic dermatitis consists of an erythematous scaly dermatitis accompanied by overproduction of sebum occurring in areas rich in sebaceous glands, ie, the face, scalp, and perineum. This common condition occurs predominantly in the newborn and at puberty, the ages at which hormonal stimulation of sebum production is maximal. Although it is tempting to speculate that the overproduction of sebum causes the dermatitis, the exact relationship is unclear.

Seborrheic dermatitis on the scalp in infancy is often confused with atopic dermatitis, and only after other areas are involved or flexural involvement occurs is it clear that the diagnosis is atopic dermatitis. Psoriasis also occurs in seborrheic areas in older children and should always be considered in the differential diagnosis.

Seborrheic dermatitis responds well to topical corticosteroids; 1% hydrocortisone cream 3 times daily is often sufficient to control this disorder.

Dandruff

Physiologic scaling or mild seborrhea, in the form of greasy scalp scales, can easily be treated by daily or alternate-day shampoos with cream rinse shampoos or selenium sulfide.

Dry Skin (Asteatotic Eczema, Xerosis)

Newborns and older children who live in arid climates are susceptible to dry skin, characterized by large cracked scales with erythematous borders. The stratum corneum is dependent upon environmental humidity for its water, and below 30% environmental humidity the stratum corneum loses water, shrinks, and cracks. These cracks in the epidermal barrier allow irritating substances to enter the skin, predisposing to dermatitis.

Treatment consists of increasing the water content of the skin's immediate external environment. House humidifiers are very useful. Two 5-minute baths a day with immediate application of oils (Alpha Keri) or ointments (petrolatum) after the bath will allow the skin to retain water. Frequent soaping of the skin impairs its water-holding capacity and serves as an irritating alkali, and all soaps should therefore be avoided. Frequent use of emollients (eg, Moisturel, Cetaphil, Eucerin, Lubriderm) should be a major part of therapy.

Keratosis Pilaris

Follicular papules containing a white inspissated scale characterize keratosis pilaris. Individual lesions are discrete and may be red. They are prominent on the extensor surfaces of the upper arms and thighs and on the buttocks and cheeks. In severe cases, the lesions may be generalized. Such lesions are seen frequently in children with dry skin and have also been associated with atopic dermatitis and ichthyosis vulgaris.

Treatment is with keratolytics such as topical retinoic acid cream followed by skin hydration.

Pityriasis Alba

White, scaly macular areas with indistinct borders are seen over extensor surfaces of extremities and on the cheeks in children. Suntanning exaggerates these lesions. Histologic examination reveals a mild dermatitis. These lesions may be confused with tinea versicolor.

There is no satisfactory treatment.

Polymorphous Light Eruption

The appearance of vesicular, eczematous, or urticarial lesions in sun-exposed areas (cheeks, nose, chin, dorsum of the hands and arms) in the springtime should suggest a diagnosis of polymorphous light eruption. Confirmation can be made by skin biopsy demonstrating dense lymphocytic infiltrates in the dermis or by reproducing the lesion by daily exposure to artificial ultraviolet light. In American Indians, it is inherited as an autosomal dominant. Onset is usually at age 5 or 6, and spontaneous improvement occurs at puberty. The first rays of sunlight of sufficient energy reaching the earth's surface in early spring induce the disease. As summer progresses, the skin thickens in response to sunlight, less ultraviolet energy enters the skin, and the disease subsides. The differential diagnosis includes erythropoietic protoporphyria, in which patients experience severe pain and itching after 5 or 10 minutes of exposure to the sun but do not develop significant skin lesions except for small papules over the dorsum of the hand; and photodermatitis from plants (psoralens) or drugs, eg, thiazide diuretics, antihistamines, phenothiazine tranquilizers, tetracyclines, and sulfonamides.

Treatment of the dermatitis with topical corticosteroids, eg, 1% hydrocortisone cream to the face 3 times daily, and daily use of a sunscreen applied at bedtime and each morning are sufficient.

Poh-Fitzpatrick M et al: Photodermatoses in infants and children. *Pediatr Dermatol* 1988;**5**:189.

COMMON SKIN TUMORS

If the skin moves with the nodule on lateral palpation, the tumor is located within the dermis; if the skin moves over the nodule, it is subcutaneous. Table 11–6 lists the tumors according to these categories.

Knight BJ et al: Superficial lumps in children: What, when and why? *Pediatrics* 1983;**72**:147.

Epidermal Inclusion Cysts

Epidermal inclusion cysts are smooth, dome-shaped nodules in the skin that may grow to 2 cm in diameter. In infants they may be found about the eyes and in older children and adolescents on the chest, back, or scalp. They are the most common superficial lumps in children.

Treatment, if desired, is surgical excision.

Granuloma Annulare

Circles or semicircles of nontender intradermal nodules found over the lower legs and ankles, the dorsum of the hands and wrists, and the trunk, in that order, suggest granuloma annulare. Histologically, the disease appears as a central area of tissue

Table 11–6. Common skin tumors.

Intradermal
  Epidermal inclusion cyst
  Pilomatricoma
  Dermatofibroma
  Melanocytic nevus
  Pyogenic granuloma
  Neurofibroma
  Hemangioma
  Granuloma annulare
Subcutaneous
  Lipoma
  Rheumatoid nodule

death (necrobiosis) surrounded by macrophages and lymphocytes.

No treatment is necessary. Lesions resolve spontaneously within 1 or 2 years.

Muhlbauer JE: Granuloma annulare. *J Am Acad Dermatol* 1980;**3**:217.

Pyogenic Granuloma

Rapid growth of a dark red papule with an ulcerated and crusted surface over 1–2 weeks following skin trauma suggests pyogenic granuloma. Histologically, this represents excessive new vessel formation with or without inflammation (granulation tissue). It is neither pyogenic nor granulomatous but should be regarded as an abnormal healing response.

Excision is the treatment of choice.

Leyden JJ, Master GH: Oral cavity pyogenic granuloma. *Arch Dermatol* 1973;**108**:226.

Keloids

Keloids are scars raised above the skin surface with many radial projections of scar tissue. They continue to enlarge over several years. They are often found on the face, earlobes, neck, chest, and back. Keloids show no racial predilection. Treatment includes intralesional injection with triamcinolone acetonide, 20 mg/mL, or excision and injection with glucocorticosteroids.

Murray JC et al: Keloids: A review. *J Am Acad Dermatol* 1981;**4**:461.

PAPULOSQUAMOUS ERUPTIONS
(See Table 11–7.)

Pityriasis Rosea

Erythematous papules that coalesce to form oval plaques preceded by a large oval plaque with central clearing and a scaly border (the herald patch) establish the diagnosis of pityriasis rosea. The herald patch has the appearance of ringworm and is often treated as such. It appears 1–30 days before the onset of the generalized papular eruption. The oval plaques are parallel in their long axis and follow Langer's lines of skin cleavage. In whites, the lesions are primarily on the trunk, accentuated in the

Table 11–7. Papulosquamous eruptions in children.

Psoriasis
Pityriasis rosea
Secondary syphilis
Lichen planus
Chronic parapsoriasis
Pityriasis rubra pilaris
Tinea corporis
Dermatomyositis
Lupus erythematosus

axillary and inguinal areas. In blacks, lesions are primarily on the extremities. This disease is common in school-age children and adolescents and is presumed to be viral in origin. It lasts 6 weeks and may be pruritic the first 7–10 days. The major differential diagnosis is secondary syphilis, and a VDRL test should be done if syphilis is suspected. A chronic variant of this disease may last 2 or 3 years and is called **chronic parapsoriasis or pityriasis lichenoides chronicus.**

Exposing the skin to sunlight until a mild sunburn occurs (slight redness) will hasten the disappearance of lesions. Ordinarily, no treatment is necessary.

Arndt KA et al: Treatment of pityriasis rosea with ultraviolet radiation. *Arch Dermatol* 1983;**119**:381.

Psoriasis

Psoriasis is characterized by erythematous papules covered by thick white scales. Guttate (droplike) psoriasis is a common form in children that often follows an episode of streptococcal pharyngitis by 2–3 weeks. The sudden onset of small (3–8 mm) papules, which are seen predominantly over the trunk and quickly become covered with thick white scales, is characteristic of guttate psoriasis. Chronic psoriasis is marked by thick, large (5–10 cm) scaly plaques over the elbows, knees, scalp, and other sites of trauma. Pinpoint pits in the nail plate are seen as well as yellow discoloration of the nail plate resulting from onycholysis. Thickening of all 20 fingernails and toenails is an uncommon feature. The sacral and seborrheic areas are commonly involved. Psoriasis has no known cause and demonstrates active proliferation of epidermal cells with a turnover time of 3–4 days versus 28 days for normal skin. These rapidly proliferating epidermal cells are producing excessive stratum corneum, giving rise to thick opaque scales. Papulosquamous eruptions that present problems of differential diagnosis are listed in Table 11–7.

All therapy is aimed at diminishing epidermal turnover time. Sunlight or artificial ultraviolet light (UVL) alone will produce some improvement. Coal tar enhances the effect of UVL and hastens the disappearance of psoriatic lesions. Bathing with a bath product containing tar (eg, Balnetar) at night, followed by UVL the next day, may be sufficient in mild cases. In more severe psoriasis, 2% crude coal tar in petrolatum should be applied after the bath. The newer tar gels (Estar gel, psoriGel) do not cause staining and are most efficacious. They are applied twice daily for 6–8 weeks.

Crude coal tar therapy is messy and stains bedclothes, and patients may prefer to use topical corticosteroids. Penetration of topical corticosteroids through the enlarged epidermal barrier in psoriasis requires that more potent preparations be used, eg, fluocinonide (Lidex, Topsyn), 0.05%, or triamcinolone (Aristocort, Kenalog), 0.5%, 4 times daily. A successful alternative is to add a keratolytic agent to the topical corticosteroid to help remove scales and enhance penetration of the steroid. A cream consisting of salicylic acid, 2%, in fluocinonide, 0.05%, 4 times daily, is effective.

Anthralin therapy is also useful. Anthralin is applied to the skin for a short contact time (eg, 20 minutes once daily) and is then washed off with a neutral soap (eg, Dove). A 6-week course of treatment is recommended.

Scalp care using a tar shampoo (Polytar, Zetar, many others) requires leaving the shampoo on for 5 minutes, washing it off, and then shampooing with commercial shampoo to remove scales. It may be necessary to shampoo daily until scaling is reduced.

More severe cases of psoriasis are best treated by a dermatologist using the Goeckerman regimen.

Lowe, NJ: Psoriasis. *Semin Dermatol* 1988;**7**:43.

Lichen Planus

Lichen planus consists of pruritic, light purple, flat-topped, many-sided papules, predominantly on the lower legs, penis, wrists, and arms. A white lacy pattern in the buccal mucosa is often seen. Pruritus may be severe.

If pruritus is mild, no treatment is necessary, and the disease will disappear in 6–12 months. With severe pruritus, a trial of antihistamines, eg, diphenhydramine, 5 mg/kg/d, or hydroxyzine, 2 mg/kg/d orally, is warranted. Rapid relief of pruritus and disappearance of the lesions can be achieved by administering prednisone, 1 mg/kg/d orally for 3–4 weeks.

Kwee DJ et al: Childhood bullous lichen planus. *Pediatr Dermatol* 1987;**4**:325.

HAIR LOSS (ALOPECIA)

Hair loss in children (Table 11–8) imposes great emotional stress on the parent and doctor—often more so than on the child. A 60% hair loss in a single area is necessary before hair loss can be detected clinically. Examination should begin with the scalp to determine if there are color changes or infiltrative changes. Hairs should be examined microscopically for breaking and structural defects and to see if growing or resting hairs are being shed. Placing removed hairs in mounting fluid (Permount) makes them easy to examine. Three diseases account for most cases of hair loss in children: alopecia areata, tinea capitis, and trichotillomania.

Alopecia Areata

Loss of every hair in a localized area is called alopecia areata. This is the most common cause of hair loss in children. An immunologic pathogenic

Table 11–8. Other causes of hair loss in children.

Hair loss with scalp changes
  Nodules and tumors:
    Nevus sebaceus
    Epidermal nevus
  Thickening:
    Linear scleroderma (morphea) (en coup de sabre)
    Burn
  Atrophy:
    Lupus erythematosus
    Lichen planus
Hair loss with hair shaft defects (hair fails to grow out enough to require haircuts):
  Monilethrix—alternating bands of thin and thick areas
  Trichorrhexis nodosa—nodules with fragmented hair
  Trichorrhexis invaginata (bamboo hair)—intussusception of one hair into another
  Pili torti—hair twisted 180 degrees, brittle
  Pili annulati—alternating bands of light and dark pigmentation

mechanism is suspected because dense infiltration of lymphocytes precedes hair loss. Ninety-five percent of children with alopecia areata completely regrow their hair within 12 months, though as many as 40% may have a relapse in 5 or 6 years. A rare and unusual form of alopecia areata begins at the occiput and proceeds along the hair margins to the frontal scalp. This variety, called **ophiasis,** often results in total scalp hair loss (**alopecia totalis**). The prognosis for regrowth in ophiasis is poor.

No treatment is indicated for alopecia areata. Systemic corticosteroids given to suppress the inflammatory response will result in hair growth, but the hair will fall out again when the drug is discontinued. In children with alopecia totalis, a wig is most helpful.

Barth JH: Normal hair growth in children. *Pediatr Dermatol* 1987;**4**:173.
Thiers BH et al: Alopecia areata symposium. *Pediatr Dermatol* 1987;**4**:136.

Trichotillomania

Traumatic hair pulling causes the hair shafts to be broken off at different lengths, an ill-defined area of hair loss, petechiae around follicular openings, and a wrinkled hair shaft on microscopic examination. This may be merely habit or the result of severe anxiety in the child. Eyelashes and eyebrows rather than scalp hair may be pulled out. Such episodes are best considered a nervous habit. Oiling the hair to make it slippery is an aid to behavior modification.

Nail Disorders

Nail biting and *Candida* paronychia are the two most common nail disorders. Onychomycosis is uncommon. Nail pitting is seen in psoriasis and alopecia areata.

Barth JH et al: Diseases of the nails in children. *Pediatr Dermatol* 1987;**4**:275.

REACTIVE ERYTHEMAS

Erythema Multiforme

Erythema multiforme begins with papules that later develop a dark center and then evolve into lesions with central blisters and the characteristic target lesions (iris lesions) with 3 concentric circles of color change. Primary injury is to endothelial cells, with later destruction of epidermal basal cells and blister formation. Erythema multiforme has sometimes been diagnosed in severe mucous membrane involvement, but **Stevens-Johnson syndrome** is the usual term for severe involvement of conjunctiva, oral cavity, and genital mucosa.

Many causes are suspected, particularly herpes simplex virus, sulfonamide drugs, and *Mycoplasma* infections. Recurrent erythema multiforme is usually associated with reactivation of herpes simplex virus. In the mild form, spontaneous healing occurs in 10–14 days, but Stevens-Johnson syndrome may last 6–8 weeks if untreated.

Treatment is symptomatic in uncomplicated erythema multiforme. Removal of offending drugs is an obvious necessary measure. Oral antihistamines such as hydroxyzine, 2 mg/kg/d orally, are useful. Cool compresses and wet dressings will relieve pruritus.

Huff JC: Therapy and prevention of erythema multiforme with acyclovir. *Semin Dermatol* 1988;**7**:212.

Erythema Nodosum

Erythema nodosum consists of painful, erythematous nodules on the anterior lower legs. In streptococcal infections, coccidioidomycosis, histoplasmosis, and tuberculosis, the onset of erythema nodosum parallels the appearance of cell-mediated immunity. Streptococcal infections and birth control pills are the most common causes of this panniculitis in the USA.

Table 11–9. Common drug reactions.

Erythema multiforme/toxic epidermal necrolysis
Sulfonamides
Non-steroidal anti-inflammatory drugs
Anticonvulsants
Urticaria
Penicillins
Cephalosporins
Aspirin
Insulin
Opiates/narcotics
Morbilliform
Penicillins
Thiazides
Sulfonamides
Anticonvulsants
Photodermatitis
Psoralens
Tetracyclines
Thiazides
Antihistamines

Treatment consists of removal of the offending drug or eradication of infection. Topical corticosteroids afford some relief, but prednisone, 1–2 mg/kg/d orally, may be necessary for 2–3 weeks.

Weston WL: Nodular diseases. Pages 849–851 in: *Pediatric Dermatology*. Schachner L, Hansen R (editors). Churchill Livingstone, 1988.

Drug Eruptions

Drugs may produce urticarial, morbilliform, scarlatiniform, or bullous skin eruptions. Urticaria may appear within minutes after drug administration, but most reactions begin 7–14 days after the drug is first administered. Drugs commonly implicated in skin reactions are listed in Table 11–9.

MISCELLANEOUS SKIN DISORDERS ENCOUNTERED IN PEDIATRIC PRACTICE

Aphthous Stomatitis

Recurrent erosions on the gums, lips, tongue, palate, and buccal mucosa are often confused with herpes simplex. A smear of the base of such a lesion stained with Wright's stain will aid in ruling out herpes simplex by the absence of epithelial giant cells. A culture for herpes simplex is also useful in this difficult differential diagnostic problem. It has been shown that recurrence of aphthous stomatitis correlates positively with lymphocyte-mediated cytotoxicity.

There is no specific therapy for this condition. Rinsing the mouth with liquid antacids will provide relief in most patients. Topical corticosteroids in a gel base (eg, Lidex gel) may provide some relief. In severe cases that interfere with eating, prednisone, 1 mg/kg/d orally for 3–5 days, will suffice to abort an episode.

Schachner L, Press S: Vesicular, bullous, and pustular disorders in infancy and childhood. *Pediatr Clin North Am* 1983; **30**:609.

Corns & Calluses

Thickened areas of epidermis in response to repeated or prolonged friction or pressure are called either corns or calluses. Corns are clearly demarcated and painful, whereas calluses have ill-defined margins and are not tender. A painful corn may overlie an exostosis, and one should get an x-ray film of that digit.

Treatment begins with removing the cause of friction or pressure, if possible, such as ill-fitting shoes. Local therapy consists of paring down the lesion with a razor blade or No. 15 knife blade and covering it with a cut-to-size piece of 40% salicylic acid plaster. Cover firmly with adhesive tape to prevent loosening due to sweating. The plaster should not be allowed to get wet. It can be removed every 5 days and the dead skin gently removed. The plaster may then be put in place.

Morphea (Linear Scleroderma)

Morphea is characterized by the appearance, anywhere on the body, of well-circumscribed, shiny, white, firmly adherent skin. It is particularly cosmetically deforming on the face. A light purple border is indicative of an early lesion or continuing activity. Skin biopsy reveals replacement of subcutaneous fat with thickened collagen fibers. The lesions tend to burn themselves out in 3–5 years. It may be difficult to differentiate morphea from lichen sclerosis et atrophicus, which has similar white patches that occur primarily on the upper back and genitalia. Histopathologic differentiation is often necessary and may be difficult. *Borrelia* infections have recently been implicated in morphea. It has been noted that linear scleroderma in children may progress to severe systemic lupus erythematosus after several years.

Lesions that are not cosmetically disturbing should not be treated. Lesions on the face may be cleared by injections of repository corticosteroids, eg, triamcinolone acetonide diluted 1:4 with saline to make 2.5 mg/mL and injected through a 30-gauge needle. Less than 1 mL should be injected. Complications of local corticosteroid injection include atrophy, depigmentation, ulceration, and infection; therefore, this therapy should be reserved for unusual circumstances.

Necrobiosis Lipoidica Diabeticorum

A depressed yellow area with telangiectasia surrounded by an erythematous nodular border found on the anterior lower leg is diagnostic of necrobiosis lipoidica diabeticorum. Histopathologic findings include atrophy of the epidermis and a palisading granuloma of lymphocytes and macrophages surrounding an area of homogenized devitalized dermis. Lesions are most often found in diabetics but can be seen in nondiabetic children. There is no satisfactory treatment.

SELECTED REFERENCES

Hurwitz S: *The Skin and Systematic Disease in Children.* Year Book, 1985. [A detailed source for skin manifestations of systemic disease.]

Schachner L, Hansen R: *Pediatric Dermatology.* Churchill Livingstone, 1988. [The encyclopedia of pediatric dermatology.]

Weston WL, Lane, AT: *Pediatric Dermatology: A Color Textbook.* Mosby–Yearbook, 1990. [Good for common skin problems.]

12

Eye

Philip P. Ellis, MD

GROWTH & DEVELOPMENT OF THE EYE

Although the eye is not completely developed at birth, it is a relatively large functioning sensory organ in the newborn. The postnatal growth of the eye and the brain are comparable. By the end of the fourth year, the eye has attained about 70% of its adult volume. Subsequent growth is much slower, until about age 10–12 years, when adult proportions are reached.

The average anteroposterior diameter of the newborn infant's eye is approximately 16.5 mm (the average adult diameter of the eye is slightly over 24 mm). The cornea is comparatively large, with an average transverse diameter of 10 mm; by the second year of life, the average adult corneal diameter of 12 mm is reached. The cornea in the newborn is relatively flat, and the iris contains little pigment and appears to have a bluish color. As pigment forms, the color of the iris becomes more distinct. By the age of 6 months, it is usually possible to determine whether the irides will become brown or remain blue.

The lens in the newborn infant's eye is quite spherical compared to that in the adult eye. This feature helps to overcome some of the hyperopia (farsightedness) resulting from the comparative shortness of the eyeball and the relative flatness of the cornea. At birth, approximately 75–80% of children are hyperopic. Hyperopia may increase for the first 7 or 8 years of life and then frequently diminishes. This contrasts to myopia (nearsightedness), which does not usually develop until age 8–10 and then increases until 20–30 years of age.

The macula in the retina is poorly developed at birth, and this characteristic is a major factor in the poor vision of newborns. Full development of the macula does not occur until about 6 months of age. The periphery of the retina is not as well developed as the remainder. Peripheral vascularization is not complete until about the time of term delivery.

Myelinization of the optic nerve is incomplete at birth; further myelinization continues until about the fourth month of life. The sclera is relatively thin, and the underlying uvea is what causes the blue color of the newborn sclera. Scleral fibers soon thicken to give a whiter appearance to the eye.

The orbit is almost round at birth. By the first year of life, orbital volume is doubled, and by the sixth year it is redoubled. The lacrimal gland is poorly developed at birth, a fact which accounts for the paucity of tears when the newborn cries. Tear production does not occur until 4 weeks of life. The nasolacrimal duct is usually patent at birth, but in many infants the distal end remains plugged for several months (see discussion under lacrimal apparatus).

Coordinated movement of the eyes is not well developed for the first few months of life, although many full-term infants establish ocular alignment within 4 weeks of birth. Binocular visual responses begin to develop between the ages of 2 and 6 months and become firmly established during the second 6 months of life. Ocular deviations that persist beyond age 6 months should always be investigated by an ophthalmologist.

Visual acuity in infants is much better than previously estimated. At the age of 5 months, it is about 20/100; at 2 years, about 20/60; and at 4–5 years, almost 20/20.

Harley RD (editor): *Pediatric Ophthalmology,* 2nd ed. 2 vols. Saunders, 1983.
Hoyt CS, Nickel B, Billson FA: Ophthalmological examination of the infant: Developmental aspects. *Surv Ophthalmol* 1982;**26:**177.
Isenberg SJ (editor): *The Eye in Infancy.* Year Book, 1988.
Norcia AM et al: Visual acuity development in normal and abnormal preterm human infants. *J Pediatr Ophthalmol Strabismus* 1987;**4:**70.

GENERAL PRINCIPLES OF DIAGNOSIS

A careful history is essential in establishing an accurate diagnosis of an ocular disorder. The history should include time and rate of onset of the presenting symptoms, associated symptoms, past history of eye disorders and treatment, and pertinent family and social history. However, many eye problems, such as poor vision in one eye, are asymptomatic and are discovered only on testing of visual acuity or other objective diagnostic methods.

COMMON NONSPECIFIC SYMPTOMS & SIGNS

Redness

Redness is a common finding in many ocular disorders. It is produced by dilatation of conjunctival and superficial scleral vessels in response to inflammation, infection, or irritation. The differential diagnosis of redness of the eye is presented in Table 12–1.

Tearing

In infants, tearing is usually due to nasolacrimal duct obstruction. Tearing may also be associated with local inflammatory, allergic, and viral diseases and with congenital glaucoma.

Discharge

Purulent discharge is usually associated with bacterial infections. Mucoid discharge is usually associated with chemical irritations, some viral infections, or allergic conditions; it may be secondary to obstructions of the nasolacrimal duct.

Pain

Pain in or about the eye may be due to foreign bodies in the cornea or conjunctiva, corneal abrasions, acute infections of the lid, orbital cellulitis, acute dacryocystitis, acute iritis, or glaucoma. Refractive errors seldom produce headaches in young children. Large refractive errors or poor convergence may produce headaches in older children, particularly those who read a good deal.

Poor Vision (Amblyopia)

In infants, poor vision is usually due to a serious ophthalmologic or neurologic disorder such as congenital nystagmus, corneal or lenticular opacities, disorders of the retina, optic nerve and central nervous system abnormalities, or very high myopia. In older children, the development of poor vision is often associated with refractive errors.

Amblyopia is a unilateral or bilateral reduction in vision, uncorrectable with glasses, that occurs in an eye that is normal on ophthalmoscopy. It is found in 2–4% of the general population. In children, most amblyopia is unilateral and secondary to strabismus. It is the result of a long, continued deviation in one eye with suppression of the retinal image in the deviating eye to avoid diplopia. Amblyopia also may occur when there is a large difference in refractive errors between the 2 eyes (anisometropia). Usually

Table 12–1. Differential diagnosis of redness of the eye in pediatric patients.

	Acute Conjunctivitis	Acute Iritis	Acute Glaucoma[1]	Corneal Abrasion
Incidence	Very common.	Uncommon.	Rare.	Fairly common.
Etiology	Usually bacterial; may be viral, fungal, or allergic.	Usually unknown; may be associated with juvenile rheumatoid arthritis.	Developmental defects or obstruction of aqueous drainage channels.	Foreign body; abrasion.
Redness	Diffuse injection of conjunctiva; greater toward fornices.	Purple-red; circumcorneal injection.	Often diffuse injection of bulbar conjunctiva.	Diffuse injection of conjunctiva.
Discharge	Moderate to heavy; mucoid or mucopurulent.	None.	None; tearing.	Watery.
Visual acuity	Normal.	Decreased.	Decreased.	Decreased.
Corneal transparency	Clear.	Clear or some haze.	Hazy; cornea enlarged in congenital form.	Variable haze.
Anterior chamber depth	Normal.	Normal; cloudy.	Shallow; deep in congenital form.	Normal.
Pupil size	Normal.	Constricted.	Dilated.	Normal.
Intraocular pressure	Normal.	Usually normal; may be low or elevated.	Elevated.	Normal.
Conjunctival smear results	Causative organisms identified; numerous polymorphonuclear neutrophils found in bacterial infection; numerous mononuclear cells found in viral infection.	Normal.	Normal.	Normal.

[1]Primary narrow-angle glaucoma is very rare in children. Congenital glaucoma may not produce redness of the eye.

the eye with the greatest refractive error does not develop a clear retinal image, and as a consequence vision fails to develop fully.

Leukocoria

A white spot in the pupil is a serious finding that may be due to congenital cataract, retrolental fibroplasia, retinal dysplasia, intraocular infection, retinoblastoma, or persistence and hyperplasia of primary vitreous (see Fig 12–1).

EXAMINATION

Visual Acuity

Routine testing of visual acuity should be part of every general physical examination. It is the single most important test of visual function. In children 4 years of age or older, satisfactory visual acuity tests can usually be obtained with the use of Snellen test charts. In children 2½–3 years old, vision can often be tested with the use of Allen or E cards. Objects familiar to the child (eg, animals, trees, houses) are depicted on the Allen cards in graduated sizes. When E cards are used, the child is asked to point in the direction of the "feet" of the figure E. Because of distractions in the office, children are sometimes unable to perform this test adequately; special illiterate E cards may be sent home so that the parents can test the vision at home under better circumstances. The parent can repeat the test at leisure, and the final result is usually more accurate than that obtained from testing done in the office by the pediatrician or the nurse.

Visual acuity is difficult to evaluate in infants.

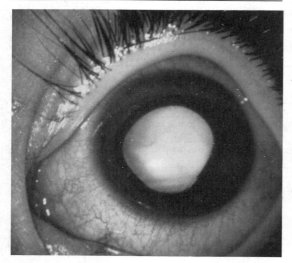

Figure 12–1. Retinoblastoma presenting with leukocoria (white reflex in pupil).

One can observe whether an infant will follow a light or a bright attractive toy in different directions of gaze. The examiner's face is an excellent target to elicit ocular fixation and following movements. Each eye is tested separately. If the infant fails to respond to such testing, one can observe the pupillary responses for reaction to direct light stimulus. These responses depend upon a functioning retina and optic nerve. However, cortical blindness can exist with preservation of pupillary light reflexes. The demonstration of optokinetic nystagmus (slow pursuit movements in the direction of a moving stimulus and quick saccadic movements in the reverse direction or "railway nystagmus") indicates that there are functioning neural receptors in the retina and intact neural pathways.

Infants can also be tested by alternately covering each eye. If visual acuity is poor in one eye, the infant will resist actively when the good eye is covered and vision is disturbed but will be much less affected when the eye with decreased vision is covered.

Poor visual acuity due to refractive errors in older children can be differentiated from poor vision due to other diseases by a pinhole test. If the reduced visual acuity is due to a refractive error, placement of a pinhole before this eye in line with the pupil will result in improved vision.

External Examination

External examination should include general inspection of the lids and eyeballs, noting their prominence, size, and position as well as any growths, inflammations, discharge, or vascular injection. Forward protrusion (exophthalmos) or retraction (enophthalmos) of the globe should be noted. Unusual size of the globes as indicated by megalocornea or microphthalmos should be noted. The positions of the lids in relation to the globe and the coverage of the lids over the closed eyes should be observed. Normally, with the eyes open, the lower lid margin is at the lower border of the cornea in the forward position of gaze, and the upper lid should cover approximately 2 mm of the cornea. Any drooping of the upper lid (ptosis) or retraction of the eyelids should be noted. The lid margins should be inspected to see if they are in proper alignment against the globes or if there is ectropion (turning outward of the lid margins) or entropion (turning inward). The distribution of the lashes and their position should be studied. The lid margins should be inspected for inflammation, crusting, and patency of the lacrimal puncta.

If a conjunctival foreign body is suspected, the lids should be everted and the palpebral and bulbar conjunctivae inspected. The upper lid may be everted by pulling the lid forward (grasping the lashes), placing a small applicator behind the tarsal area, and gently pressing down on the lid (Fig

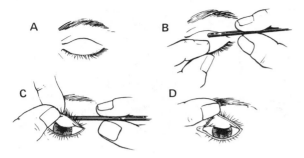

Figure 12–2. Eversion of the upper lid. **A:** The patient looks downward. **B:** The fingers pull the lid down, and a rod is placed on the upper tarsal border. **C:** The lid is pulled up over the rod. **D:** The lid is everted. (Redrawn and reproduced, with permission, from Liebman SD, Gellis SS [editors]: *The Pediatrician's Ophthalmology.* Mosby, 1966.)

12–2). The maneuver is facilitated if the patient looks downward. If a corneal abrasion or foreign body is suspected or if there is sudden unexplained pain in the eye, sterile fluorescein solution should be instilled into the conjunctival cul-de-sac and the cornea observed to see if there is any staining. Observation of staining is enhanced with the use of a blue light. Pupillary light reflexes should be tested for each eye, and both direct and consensual reflexes should be noted.

Corneal sensitivity may be tested by touching the cornea gently with a fine wisp of cotton. If corneal sensation is intact, a brisk blink reflex will result.

Extraocular Muscles

The position of the eyes should be observed by inspection. As a rule, there is little difficulty in telling whether gross strabismus is present. A quick estimation of the alignment of the eyes can be made by the corneal light reflection technique (Hirschberg test). The light reflection should come from corresponding parts of each cornea when a light is shone

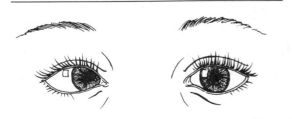

Figure 12–3. Lateral displacement of light reflection showing esotropia (internal deviation) of the right eye. Nasal displacement of the reflection would show exotropia (outward deviation).

into the eyes. If there is lateral displacement of the light reflection, esotropia (internal deviation) of the eye is present (Fig 12–3). If the light reflection is displaced nasally, exotropia (outward deviation) is present. A more refined method of judging alignment of the eyes is by means of the cover test. In this test, the patient is instructed to look at any target, and one eye is then covered. If the uncovered eye has been looking straight forward at the object, there will be no shift in movement of this eye. If, however, the eye has been turned either inward or outward, then a corresponding corrective movement will be made with this eye to align the object in the visual gaze (Fig 12–4). The other eye is then similarly tested. The eye under cover should also be observed to see whether there is inward or outward movement, indicating the presence of a phoria, or a tendency for ocular deviation. If the eye remains in the deviated position after removing the occluder, a tropia (deviation of the eyes not corrected by the fusion mechanism) rather than a phoria (deviation that is corrected by the fusion mechanism) is present.

The cardinal positions of gaze should be checked. An object or light is shown to the infant, and the ability to follow the movement of the object in different directions is tested. If marked strabismus or muscle paralysis is present, there may be limitation of movement in one direction of gaze. To determine if true paresis of an extraocular muscle is present, the nondeviating eye should be covered and the ocular movement of the uncovered eye tested in all directions of gaze. In small infants, extraocular muscle function may be checked by rapidly turning the infant in different directions and observing whether the eyes turn to the side opposite to which the head was turned (doll's head phenomenon).

Nystagmus

If nystagmus is present, its characteristics should be observed and the movements classified, first by rate or variation in rate of movement and then by direction. **Pendular (undulatory) nystagmus** consists of excursions that are equal in each direction of gaze; this type of nystagmus is usually observed in children with poor vision and is usually ocular in origin. **Jerking (rhythmic) nystagmus** is characterized by a slow component followed by a quick corrective component; it may be congenital, physiologic (at the extreme positions of gaze), due to inner ear disease, or secondary to central nervous system disease. **Congenital nystagmus** is a type of jerking nystagmus that is usually not associated with other neurologic disorders. The nystagmus is present in all directions of gaze, but it is usually minimized when the patient's eyes are turned slightly to one side or the other. This type of nystagmus usually decreases when the eyes converge. **Latent nystagmus** is manifest only when one eye is covered.

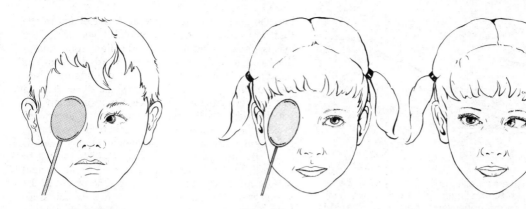

The eyes of a child with severe amblyopia may not be able to fixate an object even when the good eye is covered. Vision of such an eye is 20/200 or less.

If the child with an amblyopic eye will fixate an object only when the good eye is covered but does not hold fixation when the cover is removed, vision of the poor eye is usually from 20/100 to 20/50.

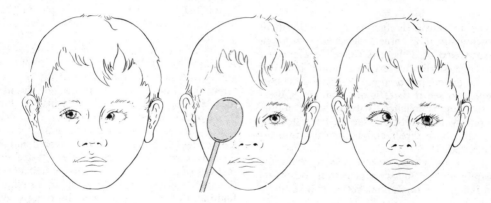

If covering the fixing eye causes fixation with the other eye, and if this second eye maintains fixation for some time even when the cover is removed, the second eye will usually have vision between 20/50 and 20/30.

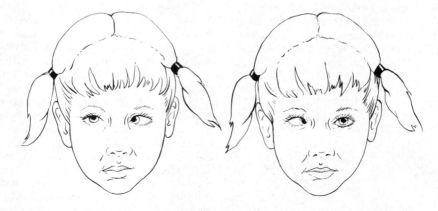

Spontaneous alternation of fixation between the 2 eyes occurs if vision is equal (no suppression amblyopia).

Figure 12–4. Estimation of visual acuity in amblyopia. (Modified slightly. Redrawn and reproduced, with permission, from Havener WH: *Synopsis of Ophthalmology*, 5th ed. Mosby, 1979.)

Nystagmus is further classified according to the direction of movement (horizontal, rotatory, vertical, or mixed). Rotatory and vertical nystagmus result from brain stem disorders. Spasmus nutans is a rare disorder in which vertical head nodding is associated with nystagmus; the nystagmus is usually horizontal but may be vertical. An anomalous head tilt is often present. The condition occurs in small infants and usually disappears within the first 2 years of life. Rarely, spasmus nutans is associated with a central nervous system disorder.

Measurement of Intraocular Pressure

The only satisfactory method of measuring ocular pressure is with a tonometer. Tactile tension, particularly in infants, is totally unreliable.

If glaucoma is suspected because of unexplained tearing or enlarged and hazy corneas, the patient should be referred to an ophthalmologist. Intraocular pressures should be measured with any enlarged or hazy corneas or traumatic hyphema (blood in the anterior chamber).

Ophthalmoscopic Examination

Satisfactory ophthalmoscopic examination of the infant eye can be accomplished only after pupillary dilation. The combination of 1% tropicamide (Mydriacyl) or 2–5% homatropine with 2.5% phenylephrine or that of 0.2% cyclopentolate with 1% phenylephrine (Cyclomydril) instilled 2–3 times at intervals of 10–15 minutes usually gives satisfactory pupillary dilatation. In children 2 years of age and older, 1% cyclopentolate (Cyclogyl) gives good pupillary dilatation; a second dose may be necessary in children with dark irides.

When an ophthalmoscope is held 30–45 cm (12–18 inches) in front of the eye and the eye is observed through a plus 10 or 15 lens, an orange-red reflection of light (the "red reflex") is observed through the pupil. If the red reflex is not present or dark spots are noted in the reflected light, an opacity of the cornea, lens, or vitreous is probably present. If red reflexes from both eyes are different (eg, irregular or distorted), refractive errors in one or both eyes should be suspected.

Ophthalmoscopic study should include all structures of the eye, such as the cornea, lens, vitreous, optic disk, and retina. In the infant, the optic disk appears paler than in the adult. The foveal light reflection is absent. The periphery of the fundus is gray. The peripheral retinal vessels are not well developed.

Refraction Test for Glasses

Cycloplegia is necessary to perform satisfactory refractions in infants and small children. The topical instillation of 1% cyclopentolate (Cyclogyl) or 5% homatropine is usually adequate. More complete cy-

cloplegia can be obtained with 0.5–1% atropine instilled 2–3 times a day for 3 days, but this is seldom necessary. Retinoscopy is used to determine the refractive error in children up to 7–8 years of age. Subsequently, subjective methods of refraction are also used.

Visual Fields

It is virtually impossible to judge visual fields in infants. One can sometimes estimate gross restriction of peripheral visual fields by covering one eye and directing the infant's gaze to an object. A second object is brought in from the side, and the infant is observed to see when the direction of the gaze is first shifted to the new object. Different types of toys and colored lights can be used for the visual test objects.

Perimetry examination of visual fields in children is easier to perform than tangent screen examination. At age 6 or 7 years, satisfactory perimetry examinations can usually be performed. Attractive toys and large objects are brought in along the perimetry arm.

Fielder AR, Moseley MJ: Do we need to measure the vision of children? *J R Soc Med* 1988;**81**:380.

Fulton AB, Hansen RM, Manning KA: Measuring visual acuity in infants. *Surv Ophthalmol* 1981;**25**:325.

Harley RD (editor): *Pediatric Ophthalmology,* 2nd ed. 2 vols. Saunders, 1983.

Helveston EM, Ellis FD: *Pediatric Ophthalmology Practice,* 2nd ed. Mosby, 1983.

Hoyt CS, Nickel B, Billson FA: Ophthalmological examination of the infant: Developmental aspects. *Surv Ophthalmol* 1982;**26**:177.

Lavery MA et al: Acquired nystagmus in early childhood: A presenting sign of intracranial tumor. *Ophthalmology* 1984;**91**:425.

Mayer DL, Fulton AB, Rodier D: Grating and recognition acuities of pediatric patients. *Ophthalmology* 1984;**91**: 947.

von Noorden GK et al: Latent nystagmus and strabismic amblyopia. *Am J Ophthalmol* 1987;**103**:87.

GENERAL PRINCIPLES OF TREATMENT OF OCULAR DISORDERS

For diseases of the anterior segment of the eye, topical medication is effective. For diseases of the posterior segment of the eye and of the orbit, systemic medication is necessary. In many instances (eg, severe intraocular infections or uveitis), a combination of topical and systemic medications is required.

The intraocular penetration of topically applied drugs depends upon their solubility in fat and water. The epithelium of the cornea presents a barrier to medications that are not fat-soluble. The alkaloids, the corticosteroids, and some of the anesthetics penetrate the eye quite easily after topical application to the cornea. Most antibiotics do not penetrate the eye in therapeutic concentrations when topically applied.

The degree of intraocular penetration of systemically administered drugs depends upon their ability to pass the blood-aqueous and blood-vitreous barriers. In the normal eye, most systemically administered antibiotics do not penetrate the barriers. In the inflamed eye, the barriers are broken down, and drugs penetrate in much better concentrations. Systemically administered corticosteroids penetrate the eye quite easily. Certain drugs such as mannitol and glycerol do not cross the blood-aqueous barrier and therefore are valuable in the temporary treatment of acute glaucoma because an osmotic gradient is produced in which the blood is hypertonic to the aqueous and vitreous.

Solutions Versus Ointments

Topical ophthalmic preparations may be administered either as solutions or as ointments. In children, ointments have several advantages over solutions: They are not washed away with the tears; they are quite comfortable upon initial instillation; there is less absorption into the lacrimal passage; and since the contact time in the eye is much longer, they can be used less frequently. The chief disadvantage of ointments is that they produce a film over the eye and thus interfere with vision. The advantages of solutions are that they do not interfere with vision and they cause fewer contact dermatitis reactions than ointments; the chief disadvantage is that they must be instilled frequently.

Topical Corticosteroids

The corticosteroids are effective in many eye diseases, including allergic blepharitis and conjunctivitis, vernal conjunctivitis, phlyctenular keratoconjunctivitis, mucocutaneous conjunctival lesions, contact dermatitis of the eyelid and conjunctiva, interstitial keratitis, and many forms of iritis and iridocyclitis. Weaker corticosteroid preparations such as 1% medrysone, 0.5–1.5% hydrocortisone, and 0.125% prednisolone are usually adequate for the management of allergic reactions of the conjunctiva and eyelid.

Many complications follow long- and short-term administration of topical corticosteroids. Among these are increased incidence or aggravation of herpes simplex keratitis and fungal ulcers of the cornea, decreased healing of corneal abrasions and wounds, glaucoma, and cataract formation. The incidence of complications increases with the use of the more potent corticosteroid preparations such as 0.1% dexamethasone, 1% prednisolone, 0.1% triamcinolone, and 0.1% betamethasone. The use of these agents generally should be reserved for the treatment of severe intraocular inflammation. Any eye disorder severe enough to require prolonged topical corticosteroid therapy should be treated by an ophthalmologist.

Topical Antibiotics & Chemotherapeutic Agents

Ideally, the infecting organism should be identified and its antibiotic sensitivity established before specific antibiotic therapy is started. This is often impractical, however, and topical antibiotics are in most cases instituted empirically. Topical use of antibiotics that are seldom employed systemically will decrease the risk of hypersensitivity reactions. For this reason, neomycin, bacitracin, and polymyxin (or mixtures) are frequently used in the treatment of conjunctivitis. Broad-spectrum antibiotics and sulfacetamide or sulfisoxazole seldom produce sensitivity. Topical penicillin therapy should be avoided if possible.

In Tables 12–2 and 12–3 are listed the commonly used topical chemotherapeutic and antibiotic ophthalmic agents.

Mydriatics & Cycloplegics

Mydriatics are agents that dilate the pupil without paralyzing the ciliary muscle of accommodation. They are useful for ophthalmoscopic examination and in preventing and breaking posterior synechiae (adhesions of the iris to the lens). The commonly used mydriatics are phenylephrine, 2.5–10%, and hydroxyamphetamine, 1%. The duration of effect of the mydriatics is only a few hours.

Cycloplegic drugs are agents that produce paralysis of accommodation as well as pupillary dilatation. They are used in refraction and in the treatment of acute inflammatory conditions of the iris and ciliary body. The more commonly used cycloplegics are atropine, 0.25–2%; homatropine, 2–5%; scopolamine, 0.2%; cyclopentolate, 1–2%; and tropicamide, 1%.

Atropine is the most powerful cycloplegic; its effect may last for as long as 14 days. Scopolamine has an effect that lasts 2–5 days, whereas the effects of homatropine are usually gone within 48 hours. Cyclopentolate and tropicamide produce more rapid cycloplegia than the other agents, but their effect is usually gone within 24 hours.

Topical Anesthetics

The most commonly used local anesthetics are proparacaine, 0.5%; benoxinate, 0.4%; and tetracaine, 0.5%. Topical anesthetics may be used before the removal of a conjunctival or corneal foreign body. They may be necessary to relieve the blepharospasm induced by a chemical injury before satisfactory irrigation and examination of the eye can be accomplished. They should never be prescribed for home use, since they might mask a serious ocular disorder or result in corneal ulceration.

Table 12–2. Topical chemotherapeutic and antibiotic agents.

Drug	Trade Name	Solution	Ointment
Amphotericin B	Fungizone	0.5–1.5 mg/mL[1]	
Bacitracin	Baciguent	2000–10,000 units/mL[2]	500 units/g
Chloramphenicol	Chloromycetin, many others	1.6–5 mg/mL	10 mg/g
Colistin	Coly-Mycin S	1.2–5 mg/mL[1]	
Erythromycin	Ak Mycin, Ilotycin	5 mg/mL[1]	5 mg/g
Gentamicin	Garamycin, many others	3 mg/mL	3 mg/g
Neomycin	Myciguent	1.75–3.5 mg/mL[2]	5 mg/g
Natamycin	Natacyn	50 mg/mL	
Polymyxin B		5000–16,250 mg/mL[2]	5000–10,000 units/g[2]
Streptomycin		50 mg/mL[1]	
Sulfacetamide sodium	Many	100–300 mg/mL	100 mg/g
Sulfisoxazole	Gantrisin	40 mg/mL	40 mg/g
Tetracycline group	Many	5–10 mg/mL	10–30 mg/g
Tobramycin	Tobrex	3 mg/mL	3 mg/g

[1]Not commercially available.
[2]Available commercially only in combined drug preparations.

Sterility of Topical Medication

Any ophthalmic medication may become contaminated. This is particularly true of solutions of fluorescein, which frequently become infected with *Pseudomonas aeruginosa*. It is well to discard all old ophthalmic solutions and any container whose tip has been touched by the examiner's hand or by the patient's eyelids. In the case of fluorescein, single-use disposable solution or impregnated filter paper strips should be employed.

Systemic Absorption of Topical Medication

Since absorption of topical eye medication into the circulation may occur in sufficient quantity to produce systemic side effects, the total dosage should be carefully considered. For example, each drop of 1% atropine contains 0.5 mg of atropine. If 1% atropine drops were instilled into each eye and total absorption occurred, a toxic reaction would result in children. Other drugs most likely to produce toxicity include scopolamine, cyclopentolate, echothiophate iodide, and 10% phenylephrine (the latter should never be used in infants and small children).

When medication is instilled into the eye of an infant, pressure should be exerted over the lacrimal sac for a minute or two to prevent the drug from reaching the nasal mucosa, where it could be absorbed. Alternatively, the head may be tipped temporally to the side of the treated eye so that the excess medication will run out of the outer corner of the eye.

Ellis PP: *Ocular Therapeutics and Pharmacology*, 7th ed. Mosby, 1985.
Fraunfelder FT, Roy FH (editors): *Current Ocular Therapy*, 3. Saunders, 1989.
Palmer EA: How safe are ocular drugs in pediatrics? *Ophthalmology* 1986;**93**:1038.

OCULAR INJURIES

FOREIGN BODIES

Conjunctival Foreign Body

A conjunctival foreign body can usually be removed with a moist cotton applicator. A common site for foreign bodies is the furrow immediately behind the margin of the upper lid. Eversion of the upper lid, as described above, is necessary to visualize these foreign bodies.

Corneal Foreign Body

Superficial corneal foreign bodies usually can be

Table 12–3. Combinations of anti-infective drugs.

Drugs	Trade Name
Bacitracin and polymyxin B	Ak-Poly-Bac, Ocumycin, Polysporin
Bacitracin (gramicidin), neomycin, and polymyxin B[1]	Neosporin, many others
Chloramphenicol and polymyxin B	Chloromyxin
Oxytetracycline and polymyxin B	Terramycin-Polymyxin B
Neomycin and polymyxin B	Statrol

[1]Some commercial preparations utilize gramicidin in place of bacitracin.

removed without difficulty. A sterile topical anesthetic should be instilled into the eye and an attempt made to wipe away the foreign body with a moist cotton applicator. If this is not successful, a blunt spud or small, sterile, dull hypodermic needle (No. 20) can be used. Care must be taken not to injure the deeper layers of the cornea; if the foreign body is deeply embedded in the stroma, the patient should be referred to an ophthalmologist. Rust rings from foreign bodies should be removed primarily. An antibiotic ointment should be instilled, and the eye should be patched until epithelialization of the cornea has occurred. The patient should be reexamined within 24 hours to make certain that infection has not occurred.

Intraocular Foreign Body

Intraocular foreign bodies are serious injuries that may not be suspected on initial examination. The usual history is that the patient was pounding on a metallic object with a hammer when something flew up into the eye. Eye injuries caused by foreign bodies projected from power lawnmowers are becoming more frequent. Examination may show a perforating wound of the cornea, a hole in the iris, an irregular or ''peaked'' pupil, and an opaque lens. However, the foreign body may be so small that little evidence of penetration is seen. X-rays of the eye may be necessary to rule out the possibility of foreign body. If there is any question of a foreign body, the patient should be referred to an ophthalmologist because removal of these foreign bodies is extremely difficult. The visual prognosis is guarded.

Benson WE: Intraocular foreign bodies. Chapter 15 in: *Clinical Ophthalmology*, Vol 5. Duane TD (editor). Harper & Row, 1987.

Cinotti AA: *Handbook of Ophthalmologic Emergencies*, 3rd ed. Medical Examination Publishing Co., 1985.

De Juan E Jr, Sternberg P Jr, Michels RG: Penetrating ocular injuries: Types of injuries and visual results. *Ophthalmology* 1983;**90**:1318.

Deutsch TA, Feller DB: *Paton & Goldberg's Management of Ocular Injuries*, 2nd ed. Saunders, 1985.

Roper-Hall MJ: *Eye Emergencies*. Churchill Livingstone, 1987.

INJURIES OF THE EYELIDS

Ecchymosis

Severe ecchymosis of the eyelids should be treated first with cold compresses to reduce hemorrhage and swelling. After 24–48 hours, hot packs will speed absorption of extravasated blood. It is important to rule out any concurrent injury to the globe.

Lacerations

Lacerations of the eyelids should be sutured primarily. When the laceration involves the lid margin,

particularly the lower lid, it is imperative that the margins be sutured as evenly as possible to prevent development of a notch. In such cases, the patient should be referred to an ophthalmologist. Lacerations involving the medial portion of the eyelids should be examined to rule out injury to the lacrimal canaliculi. If the canaliculi are cut, they should be repaired at the time of primary closure of the lid laceration, since delayed attempts to repair cut canaliculi are less successful.

Cinotti AA: *Handbook of Ophthalmologic Emergencies*, 3rd ed. Medical Examination Publishing Co., 1985.

Deutsch TA, Feller DB: *Paton & Goldberg's Management of Ocular Injuries*, 2nd ed. Saunders, 1985.

Roper-Hall MJ: *Eye Emergencies*, Churchill Livingstone, 1987.

CORNEAL INJURIES

Corneal Abrasions

Corneal abrasions usually produce severe discomfort. The diagnosis is made by instilling fluorescein into the eye and observing the cornea for staining.

Treatment consists of the instillation of a mild cycloplegic such as 5% homatropine or 1% cyclopentolate (Cyclogyl), the application of antibiotic ointments, and firm patching of the eye for 24–48 hours or until the epithelium has healed.

Corneal Lacerations

Patients with corneal lacerations should be referred to an ophthalmologist for primary suturing. The patient should be observed for the development of intraocular infection. Systemic antibiotics and tetanus toxoid are indicated if the perforation occurred with a contaminated object.

Cinotti AA: *Handbook of Ophthalmologic Emergencies*, 3rd ed. Medical Examination Publishing Co., 1985.

Deutsch TA, Feller DB: *Paton & Goldberg's Management of Ocular Injuries*, 2nd ed. Saunders, 1985.

Roper-Hall MJ: *Eye Emergencies*, Churchill Livingstone, 1987.

HYPHEMA

Hyphema (blood in the anterior chamber) is a common contusion injury in children (Fig 12–5). It is a serious injury, often requiring hospitalization. Secondary bleeding is frequent and occurs usually within 6 days after the primary bleeding. Patients with hyphema should be examined for the development of glaucoma. Ophthalmoscopy should also be attempted to ascertain whether there has been more extensive injury to the posterior part of the eye. Black children with hyphema should be tested for sickle cell disease, because if the disease is present, they are more likely to develop complications.

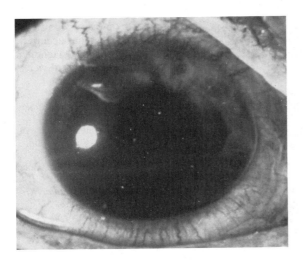

Figure 12–5. Hyphema (blood in anterior chamber).

Treatment consists of bed rest, eye bandages, and sedatives. Binocular bandages are advisable, but they may be omitted if they produce excitement. Recent studies have suggested that bed rest and monocular patches are as effective as binocular patches in mild or moderate hyphemas. However, in severe hyphemas, binocular patches are preferred. No pupillary dilating (mydriatic) or pupillary constricting (miotic) drops should be used. If glaucoma develops, the use of carbonic anhydrase inhibitors, intravenous urea or mannitol, or oral glycerol is indicated initially. If this does not control the glaucoma, surgical removal of the blood clot by irrigation or with a cryoprobe or vitrectomy instrument is indicated. To reduce the incidence of rebleeding, some authors have recommended the use of systemic aminocaproic acid (Amicar) for 5 days after the initial hemorrhage.

Another complication of hyphema is blood staining of the cornea. This occurs only if the hemorrhage remains for a long period; it may occur whether or not glaucoma develops.

Agapitos PJ, Leon-Paul N, Clarke WN: Traumatic hyphema in children. *Ophthalmology* 1987;**94**:1238.

Cinotti AA: *Handbook of Ophthalmologic Emergencies,* 3rd ed. Medical Examination Publishing Co., 1985.

Deutsch TA, Feller DB: *Paton & Goldberg's Management of Ocular Injuries,* 2nd ed. Saunders, 1985.

McGetrick JJ et al: Aminocaproic acid decreases secondary hemorrhage after traumatic hyphema. *Arch Ophthalmol* 1983;**101**:1031.

Uusitalo RJ, Ranta-Kemppainen L, Tarkkanen A: Management of traumatic hyphema in children: An analysis of 340 cases. *Arch Ophthalmol* 1988;**106**:1207.

Wilson FM II: Traumatic hyphema: Pathogenesis and management. *Ophthalmology* 1980;**87**:910.

BURNS

Burns of the eyelids should be treated in essentially the same way as burns of the skin elsewhere. It is important to protect the eyeballs from infection and exposure. Since burns frequently become contaminated with *Pseudomonas* organisms that can produce severe corneal ulceration, an antibiotic preparation containing either colistin, gentamicin, tobramycin, or polymyxin B should be instilled into the eyes 3–4 times a day. As the burns begin to heal, cicatricial ectropion with corneal exposure may develop. To prevent corneal exposure, ointments should be applied inside the eyelids. Plastic surgery often is necessary to correct cicatricial ectropion.

Chemical burns of the cornea and conjunctiva should be treated initially with thorough irrigation with any clean nonirritating fluid. This may be tap water, saline or boric acid solution, or whatever is available. In no case should a delay occur because of attempts to obtain a particular irrigating solution. It may be necessary to instill topical anesthetics into the eye to relieve blepharospasm before irrigation can be accomplished. Adequacy of the irrigation can be judged by testing the conjunctival fluid for neutrality with pH test paper. After irrigation, the eye should be inspected for retained chemical particles, which can be removed with a moist cotton applicator. The extent of the damage is then determined. If the burn involves the cornea, the pupil should be dilated with 1% atropine or 5% homatropine after irrigation to provide comfort. An antibiotic ointment should be instilled and the eye patched. Any patient who has suffered a severe chemical burn of the eye should be hospitalized and should be seen by an ophthalmologist.

Ultraviolet burns of the cornea usually cause severe pain and tearing. There is a history of exposure to ultraviolet light (eg, a welder's arc, snow on the ski slopes, sunlamp or treatment lamp). Symptoms develop 10–12 hours after exposure. Examination shows superficial corneal edema and pinpoint areas that stain with fluorescein. Treatment consists of the application of a topical anesthetic every 5–10 minutes until the pain is relieved. After pain has subsided, an antibiotic or an antibiotic-corticosteroid ointment is instilled into the eye and the eye is patched. Systemic analgesics and sedatives are then prescribed. Recovery is usually prompt and complete within 48 hours. (*Note:* Topical anesthetics should never be sent home with the patient.)

Retinal burns with permanent loss of vision may occur as a result of exposure to strong infrared light such as that received from observing an eclipse. this condition is suspected, the patient should be ferred to an ophthalmologist.

Deutsch TA, Feller DB: *Paton & Goldberg's Manag of Ocular Injuries,* 2nd ed. Saunders, 1985.

Guy RJ et al: Three-years' experience in a regional burn center with burns of the eyes and eyelids. *Ophthalmic Surg* 1982;**13**:383.

Pfister RR: Chemical injuries of the eye. *Ophthalmology* 1983;**90**:1246.

Spoor TC, Nesi FA (editors): *Management of Ocular, Orbital and Adnexal Trauma,* Raven Press, 1988.

FRACTURES OF THE ORBIT

Fractures of the orbit with any degree of displacement of the bones should be surgically reduced. The techniques of surgery depend upon the location and extent of the fracture. If the fractures are not satisfactorily reduced, complications occur that include displacement of the globe, enophthalmos, and diplopia. Any injury severe enough to cause an orbital fracture may cause further skull fractures and intracranial and intraocular damage. The patient should be studied for these possibilities.

Blowout fractures generally result from blunt injury such as a blow from a ball or fist. The bones of the orbital rim usually remain intact, but there is a blowout of the floor of the orbit (rarely, the medial wall of the orbit) with herniation of the orbital contents into the blowout site. Blowout fractures should be suspected if there is evidence of diplopia in any direction of gaze or if there is limitation of ocular movement, particularly upward. Hypesthesia of the skin in the distribution of the infraorbital nerve is present in about 30% of patients. Subcutaneous emphysema may be present. Weakness of ocular movement, particularly downward gaze, and enophthalmos may be present initially or develop later. Blowout fractures are not always seen on routine x-ray films of the orbit. Tomograms and other special diagnostic radiologic techniques, including CT scans, are sometimes necessary to demonstrate this fracture. Surgical treatment is often required.

Hawes MJ, Dortzbach RK: Surgery on orbital floor fractures: Influence of time of repair and fracture size. *Ophthalmology* 1983;**90**:1066.

Spoor TC, Nesi FA (editors): *Management of Ocular, Orbital and Adnexal Trauma.* Raven Press, 1988.

Wilkins RB, Havins WE: Current treatment of blow-out fractures. *Ophthalmology* 1982;**89**:464.

ɔNTUSIONS OF THE GLOBE

ɔddition to the hyphema mentioned above, con-
of the globe may result in dislocation of the
ɔorrhage into the vitreous, retinal edema
ɔhage, retinal detachment, choroidal hem-
ɔoidal rupture, and rupture of the eye-
ɔosis of these conditions is based upon
visual acuity and (2) direct observa-
phthalmoscope and slit lamp. If the
ɔisualized well and if visual acuity is

good, there is little likelihood that any significant damage to the posterior part of the eye has occurred. However, complications such as retinal detachment or dislocation of the lens may not appear until weeks after the initial injury.

Cinotti AA: *Handbook of Ophthalmologic Emergencies,* 3rd ed. Medical Examination Publishing Co., 1985.

Eagling EM: Ocular damage after blunt trauma to the eye: Its relationship to the nature of the injury. *Br J Ophthalmol* 1974;**58**:126.

Holt JE, Holt GR, Blodgett JM: Ocular injuries sustained during blunt facial trauma. *Ophthalmology* 1983;**90**:14.

Spoor TC, Nesi FA (editors): *Management of Ocular, Orbital and Adnexal Trauma.* Raven Press, 1988.

NONACCIDENTAL TRAUMA

A wide range of injuries to the eye and eyelids may occur in children who suffer from nonaccidental trauma (battered child syndrome, shaken baby syndrome, etc). Most common among these are lid ecchymoses, conjunctival hemorrhages, hyphema, and retinal hemorrhages. These last are quite common. Careful ophthalmoscopic examination should be performed in all children suspected of suffering from nonaccidental trauma. Retinal and vitreal hemorrhages may persist long after the child has recovered from other injuries and may lead to the development of amblyopia.

Friendly DS: Ocular manifestations of physical child abuse. *Trans Am Acad Ophthalmol Otolaryngol* 1971; **75**:318.

Gaynon MW et al: Retinal folds in shaken baby syndrome. *Am J Ophthalmol* 1988;**106**:423.

Harcourt B, Hopkins D: Ophthalmic manifestations of the battered-baby syndrome. *Br J Ophthalmol* 1971;**3**:398.

REFRACTIVE ERRORS

Myopia (nearsightedness) is easily diagnosed; distant objects are blurred. Near vision is not usually impaired except in very high myopia. Frequently, the patient squints in order to form a physiologic pinhole to improve visual acuity.

The diagnosis of **hyperopia (farsightedness)** in children is more difficult. Children are able to accommodate much more effectively than adults and thus overcome their hyperopia. Sometimes there are associated symptoms of eyestrain or headaches after prolonged periods of close work. Children with severe farsightedness may have internal deviations of the eyes (accommodative esotropia).

Astigmatism produces distorted vision. Children

will attempt to overcome the blurry vision by squinting their eyes and forming a pinhole. Children with severe astigmatism may complain of eyestrain and headaches.

Anisometropia is a difference in refractive errors of the 2 eyes. Severe anisometropia may cause amblyopia.

Treatment of significant refractive errors consists of the proper fitting of lenses. Small degrees of hyperopia need not be corrected in children. Full correction of myopia is indicated. The use of bifocals in myopic children does not appear to prevent the progressive type of myopia. Other forms of treatment such as the use of ''eye exercises'' or certain diets do not appear to influence the progression of myopia. Long-term use of atropine drops may reduce progression of myopia, but this therapy is impractical and not usually recommended. Amblyopia secondary to anisometropia should be treated with occlusion (patching) of the better seeing eye in addition to correction of the refractive error.

Contact lenses are seldom indicated in children. The exception is the child with unilateral aphakia (absence of the lens), severe anisometropia, corneal scarring producing an irregular astigmatism, or keratoconus. Contact lenses have been purported to reduce the progression of myopia, but there is little evidence to support this view.

Chrousos GA et al: Accommodation deficiency in healthy young individuals. *J Pediatr Ophthalmol Strabismus* 1988;**25**:176.

Kivlin JD, Flynn JT: Therapy of anisometropic amblyopia. *J Pediatr Ophthalmol Strabismus* 1981;**18**:47.

Michaels DD: *Visual Optics and Refraction: A Clinical Approach,* 3rd ed. Mosby, 1985.

Saunders RA, Ellis FD: Empirical fitting of hard contact lenses in infants and young children. *Ophthalmology* 1981;**88**:127.

STRABISMUS (SQUINT)

Approximately 5% of children have strabismus. The eyes may deviate inward (esotropia), outward (exotropia), upward (hypertropia), or downward (hypotropia). Strabismus is comitant if the same degree of deviation exists in all fields of gaze and noncomitant if the angle of deviation changes in the various directions of gaze. The terms tropia and phoria are both used to describe abnormal positions of the eye; tropias are manifest deviations, whereas phorias are latent deviations that become manifest only if fusion or binocular vision is blocked.

Nonparalytic strabismus is usually first observed either shortly after birth or at the age of 2–3 years;

rarely, the onset is at a later age. Infants do not develop coordinated eye muscle movements until about 3–5 months of age. An occasional infant is observed to have temporary deviation of the eyes, and realignment subsequently occurs. Any child who has a deviation that persists for several weeks or who develops a deviation after the age of 6 months should be investigated for the cause of the strabismus.

The diagnosis of strabismus is frequently made by simple inspection. If the eyes are deviated considerably, the diagnosis is evident. If there is only a slight deviation or if there is a questionable deviation because of wide epicanthal folds (pseudostrabismus) with more of the white of the eye being exposed temporally than nasally, the diagnosis is established by the corneal light reflection technique (Fig 12–3) or the cover test (Fig 12–4), as described above. Strabismus may also be suspected on the basis of marked reduced visual acuity in one eye. Children with a persistent head tilt or face turn may have strabismus with very little apparent displacement of the eyes.

During visual development, diplopia occurs if alignment of the eyes is such that the object viewed does not fall on corresponding parts of the retina. To avoid diplopia, the child learns to suppress the vision in the deviating eye. If one eye continually deviates, then suppression is always in this eye, with the result that macular vision never develops. This condition is called **amblyopia ex anopsia** or **suppression amblyopia.** Visual screening examination of preschool children is important in diagnosing early suppression amblyopia.

Paralytic or noncomitant strabismus may result from central nervous system diseases or anatomic maldevelopments of the ocular muscles. The sudden onset of paralytic strabismus in any child should prompt examination for central nervous system disease.

Treatment

Children do not outgrow strabismus. Early treatment is important and should be given by an ophthalmologist. Treatment is directed toward the development of good visual acuity in each eye, realignment of the eyes in good cosmetic position, and functional cures with the establishment of binocular vision. The following steps are considered in the treatment of strabismus: (1) careful ophthalmoscopic examination to rule out an organic intraocular cause for the deviation, eg, congenital cataracts, tumors, optic nerve atrophy; (2) cycloplegic refraction and prescription of lenses; (3) occlusion of the good eye to develop macular vision in the bad eye; and (4) surgery to align the eyes if glasses are unsuccessful in correcting the deviation.

Early surgery (ages 4–24 months) with alignment of the eyes is more likely to result in a functional cure than surgery performed at age 4–5 years or later.

Orthoptic exercises are of value in establishing binocular vision if the visual axes are nearly aligned. They are also of value in certain forms of intermittent strabismus.

Dickey CF, Scott WE: The deterioration of accommodative esotropia: Frequency, characteristics and predictive factors. *J Pediatr Ophthalmol Strabismus* 1988;**25**:172.

Ing MR: Early surgical alignment for congenital esotropia. *J Pediatr Ophthalmol Strabismus* 1983;**20**:11.

Mohindra I et al: Development of acuity and stereopsis in infants with esotropia. *Ophthalmology* 1985;**92**:691.

Nelson LB et al: Congenital esotropia. *Surv Ophthalmol* 1987;**31**:363.

Reinecke RD, Parks MM: *Strabismus: A Programmed Text*, 3rd ed. Appleton & Lange, 1987.

von Noorden GK: *Burian-von Noorden's Binocular Vision and Ocular Motility*, 3rd ed. Mosby, 1983.

PTOSIS

Ptosis is a drooping of the upper eyelid. It may be congenital or acquired and unilateral or bilateral. Ptosis may be associated with anisometropia.

Congenital ptosis usually results from incomplete development of the levator muscle. Occasionally, it is associated with third cranial nerve trauma at the time of birth or congenitally misdirected third cranial nerve fibers, in which case other abnormalities of ocular movement are often present.

Acquired ptosis may be traumatic in origin, may follow inflammation or scarring of the eyelids, or may present as a sign of some neurologic disorder. When ptosis is a sign of myasthenia gravis, an injection of edrophonium chloride (Tensilon) will produce prompt improvement. (See discussion of myasthenia gravis in Chapter 24.)

The treatment of congenital ptosis is surgical. The operation is usually performed at the age of 3–4 years. Rarely, the surgery should be done earlier if the eyelid covers the pupil completely and prevents development of normal vision. Unequal refractive errors between eyes may be associated with ptosis. The treatment of acquired ptosis depends upon the origin, but primary consideration should be directed toward treating any basic underlying disease.

Beard C: *Ptosis*, 3rd ed. Mosby, 1980.

Crawford JS, Iliff CE, Stasior OG: Symposium on congenital ptosis. *J Pediatr Ophthalmol Strabismus* 1982;**19**:245.

Hornblass A (editor): *Oculoplastic Orbital and Reconstructive Surgery*, Vol I: *Eyelids*. Williams & Wilkins, 1988.

GLAUCOMA

Primary Glaucoma

Primary congenital glaucoma (hydrophthalmos) is due to an abnormal development of the aqueous drainage structures; it may be present at birth or may develop within the first 2 years of life. Diagnosis is based upon (1) enlarged corneas that are frequently edematous and show linear white opacities (breaks in Descemet's membrane; see Fig 12–6), (2) symptoms

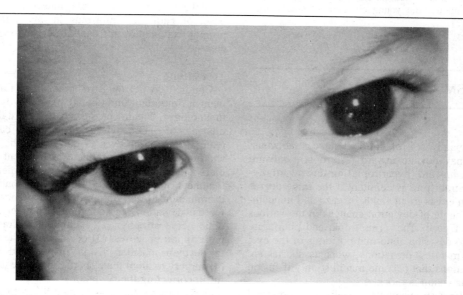

Figure 12–6. Congenital glaucoma. Enlarged, hazy corneas are present. (Reproduced, with permission, from Eichenwald, HF, Stroder J (editors): *Current Therapy in Pediatrics–2*, B.C. Decker, Inc., 1989.)

of photophobia and tearing, (3) increased intraocular pressure, and (4) enlarged cupping of the optic disk. Because the coats of the eye of an infant are not as rigid as those of an adult, increased intraocular pressure results in stretching of the corneal and scleral tissues.

Early surgery is essential. Medical therapy is of little value. Surgery is successful in controlling intraocular pressure in about 75% of cases. Without treatment, permanent blindness occurs at an early age.

Glaucoma may be associated with other developmental anomalies. These include aniridia, posterior embryotoxon (failure of reabsorption of the mesodermal tissue in the periphery of the iris and drainage angle), Sturge-Weber disease, Lowe's syndrome, Marfan's syndrome, Hurler's syndrome, Pierre Robin syndrome, Rubinstein-Taybi syndrome, neurofibromatosis, homocystinuria, congenital rubella syndrome, and trisomy 13 (D) or 18 (E_1).

Secondary Glaucoma

Secondary glaucoma may be due to many causes. The mechanism of this type of glaucoma is usually an obstruction of the aqueous outflow channels. The various causes include lens dislocation, hemorrhage into the eye, iritis, tumors (including retinoblastoma), retrolental fibroplasia, and xanthogranulomas in the iris. Treatment of these conditions is complicated, and the patient should be referred to an ophthalmologist.

Epstein DL (ed): *Chandler & Grant's Glaucoma*, 3rd ed. Lea & Febiger, 1986.

Goethals M, Missotten L: Intraocular pressure in children up to five years of age. *J Pediatr Ophthalmol Strabismus* 1983;**20**:49.

Hodapp E, Heuer DK: A simple technique for goniotomy. *Am J Ophthalmol* 1986;**102**:537.

Luntz MH, Schenker HI (editors): *Glaucoma Surgery*. Williams & Wilkins, 1984.

Quigley HA: Childhood glaucoma: Results with trabeculotomy and study of reversible cupping. *Ophthalmology* 1982;**89**:219.

temic diseases such as diabetes mellitus, galactosemia, atopic dermatitis, Marfan's syndrome, or Down's syndrome. They may also be due to long-term systemic corticosteroid therapy.

The symptoms vary considerably according to location and extent. Vision may be affected very slightly, or considerable reduction in vision can occur. White spots may be observed in the pupil. In a few cases, strabismus or pendular nystagmus is present.

The diagnosis is made by inspection with a flashlight or by examination with an ophthalmoscope or slit lamp. In some cases, cataracts can be observed only when the pupils are dilated.

Surgical lens extraction (within the first few weeks of life) is indicated if the cataracts are bilateral and sufficiently dense that vision cannot develop. If cataracts are not dense enough to interfere with visual development, surgery should be deferred, because some congenital cataracts do not progress. Surgery is indicated when visual loss is a serious handicap to the child.

In the past, the results of surgical treatment of unilateral congenital cataracts were poor. There has been an attempt to improve results with early surgery (as soon as the diagnosis is made) and fitting of contact lenses within a few days after surgery. Most ophthalmologists do not favor intraocular lens implantation in children.

Birch EE, Stager DR: Prevalence of good visual acuity following surgery for congenital unilateral cataract. *Arch Ophthalmol* 1988;**106**:40.

Gelbart SS et al: Long-term visual results in bilateral congenital cataracts. *Am J Ophthalmol* 1982;**93**:615.

Hiles DA: Infantile cataracts. *Pediatr Ann* 1983;**12**:(Aug)556.

Jaffe NS: *Cataract Surgery and Its Complications*, 4th ed. Mosby, 1984.

Parks MM: Visual results in aphakic children. *Am J Ophthalmol* 1982;**94**:441.

Robb RM, Mayer DL, Moore BD: Results of early treatment of unilateral congenital cataracts. *J Pediatr Ophthalmol Strabismus* 1987;**4**:178.

CATARACTS

A cataract is an opacity of the lens; it consists of precipitated lens protein. Cataracts may be unilateral or bilateral and partial or complete; considerable variation exists in the extent, position, shape, and density of cataract formation. They may be congenital and associated with other congenital anomalies. They can occur as a result of maternal rubella during the first trimester of pregnancy. Cataracts may be secondary to ocular trauma or associated with sys-

DISLOCATED LENS

Dislocation (luxation) or partial dislocation (subluxation) of the lens may result from blunt trauma to the eye and orbit. It may also be observed in patients with genetic dwarfism, scleroderma, Rieger's syndrome, and other hereditary disorders, including Marfan's syndrome and Marchesani's syndrome (with the lens usually dislocated superiorly) and homocystinuria (lens usually dislocated inferiorly).

Glaucoma is a common complication of dislocated lenses. All children with dislocated lenses should be evaluated by an ophthalmologist.

Crawford JS, Morin JD (editors): *The Eye in Childhood.* Grune & Stratton, 1983.

Nelson LB, Maumenee IH: Ectopia lentis. *Surv Ophthalmol* 1982;**27**:143.

Seetner AA, Crawford JS: Surgical correction of lens dislocation in children. *Am J Ophthalmol* 1981;**91**:106.

DISEASES OF THE EYELIDS

HORDEOLUM

External hordeolum (sty) is a staphylococcal abscess of the sebaceous glands of the lid margin. Symptoms consist of localized tenderness, redness, and swelling. Internal hordeolum is an acute infection of the meibomian glands that usually points conjunctivally.

Treatment of both types consists of warm moist compresses 3–4 times a day. Instillation of an antibiotic or sulfonamide ophthalmic ointment 4–5 times a day is useful during the acute stage. To reduce the likelihood of a recurrence, treatment should be continued for several days after the lesion has subsided.

Spontaneous rupture frequently occurs, but if it does not, the lesion should be incised when it becomes large and pointed. The removal of an eyelash may promote drainage of an external hordeolum.

Fedukowicz HB, Stenson S: *External Infections of the Eye,* 3rd ed. Appleton-Century-Crofts, 1985.

Vaughan D, Asbury T, Tabbara K: *General Ophthamology,* 12th ed. Appleton & Lange, 1989.

CHALAZION

Chalazion is a granulomatous inflammation of the meibomian glands. The cause is not known. Symptoms consist of slight discomfort in the eyelid and a slight redness and a lump on the conjunctival surface of the lid overlying the involved meibomian gland. Local excision is often necessary, but chalazia may disappear after treatment with warm moist compresses. Corticosteroid injection into the chalazion is often effective.

Epstein GA, Putterman, AM: Combined excision and drainage with intralesional corticosteroid injection in the treatment of chronic chalazia *Arch Ophthalmol* 1988; **106**:514.

Perry HD, Serniuk RA: Conservative treatment of chalazia. *Ophthalmology* 1980;**87**:218.

Vaughan D, Asbury T, Tabbara KF: *General Ophthalmology,* 12th ed. Lange, 1989.

BLEPHARITIS (GRANULATED EYELIDS)

Chronic inflammation of the lid margins may be seborrheic (nonulcerative), staphylococcal (ulcerative), or a combination of the 2 types. Symptoms are redness, burning, itching, and crusting of the lid margins. In the staphylococcal type, the scales are dry; small ulcerative lesions of the skin are observed; and the eyelashes may fall out. In the seborrheic type, the scales are oily; seborrhea of the scalp is usually present as well. Blepharitis is especially common in children with Down's syndrome and eczema.

Treatment of staphylococcal blepharitis consists of the instillation of antibiotic or sulfonamide ophthalmic ointment into the eye twice a day. Treatment should be continued for a week or so after all symptoms have disappeared. The crusts on the lids should be gently removed with a moist cotton applicator before the ointment is instilled. Occasionally, systemic antibiotics are required in severe cases of staphylococcal blepharitis.

The treatment of seborrheic blepharitis consists of controlling scalp seborrhea if it exists, removing the scales along the lid margins with a moist cotton applicator, and instilling sulfacetamide or an antistaphylococcal antibiotic ophthalmic ointment.

Seborrheic blepharitis can often be controlled by scrubbing the edge of the eyelids twice a day with a cotton applicator moistened in a bland, half-strength baby shampoo that does not irritate the eye.

Fedukowicz HB, Stenson S: *External Infections of the Eye,* 3rd ed. Appleton-Century-Crofts, 1985.

Tabbara KF, Hyndiuk RA (editors): *Infections of the Eye,* Little, Brown, 1986.

DISEASES OF THE CONJUNCTIVA

CONJUNCTIVITIS

Conjunctivitis is the most common of all pediatric ocular disorders. It is usually due to bacterial, viral, or fungal infections. Less commonly, it may result from an allergic reaction or physical or chemical irritation. Symptoms consist of redness of the conjunctiva, foreign body sensation, a mucoid or purulent discharge, and sticking together of the eyelids in the morning. (See Table 12–4.) Vision is not affected. The cornea, anterior chamber, and intraocular pressure are normal.

Bacterial Conjunctivitis

The most common causes of bacterial conjunctivitis are the pneumococcus, *Staphylococcus aureus*, Koch-Weeks bacillus, and hemolytic streptococci. There may be associated bacterial infections elsewhere in the body. Conjunctival membranes (diphtheritic conjunctivitis) or pseudomembranes (streptococcal conjunctivitis) may be present. Discharge, usually a prominent feature of bacterial conjunctivitis, is purulent or mucopurulent in character.

The causative organism should be identified, if possible, by obtaining smears and cultures. Empiric treatment with broad-spectrum antibiotics or sulfonamide ophthalmic ointments instilled into the eye 4–5 times a day usually results in improvement within 48–72 hours. If improvement does not occur, it is important to make an etiologic diagnosis if this has not been done earlier. Bacterial conjunctivitis is usually a self-limited disease, but secondary corneal infection and ulceration occur rarely.

Inclusion Conjunctivitis

This disease is caused by the same chlamydial organism that produces inclusion conjunctivitis in the newborn. It is characterized by conjunctival redness, clear or mucoid discharge, and follicles in the lower palpebral conjunctiva. Treatment consists of the systemic administration of a tetracycline (but not to infants or young children) or erythromycin. Topical application of these drugs is not as effective as systemic treatment.

Chlamydial infection should be considered in any sexually active teenager with chronic conjunctivitis. Examination and treatment of the sexual partner should be undertaken.

Trachoma

Trachoma is infection of the conjunctiva with a bacterium formerly thought to be a large atypical virus but now reclassified as a bacterium of the genus *Chlamydia*. The disease is usually associated with poor hygiene and poor economic conditions. It is a major cause of blindness in the world but is rare in the USA except among American Indians.

In the early stages, trachoma is characterized by a catarrhal type of reaction with diffuse redness, mild irritation, and a thin watery discharge. Subsequently, the conjunctiva becomes thickened, with papillary hypertrophy and formation of follicles, particularly in the tarsal region of the upper lids. Scarring of the conjunctiva develops later, and there is corneal vascularization and opacification.

Local therapy can probably control trachoma adequately, but systemic therapy is usually recommended also. Systemic sulfonamides, tetracyclines, and erythromycin are the agents most commonly used. For children over 9 years of age in whom dentition is complete, a 3- to 4-week course of oral tetracycline is given. Doxycycline is preferred, since administration is required only once a day. For children under age 9, the drug of choice is sulfisoxazole (Gantrisin), 100 mg/kg/d orally in 4 divided doses for 1 week, followed by 60 mg/kg/d for an additional 2 weeks. It is sometimes necessary to repeat this treatment after 1 week without medication. Alternatively, a 3- to 4-week course of oral erythromycin may be given. The local treatment of choice is 1% tetracycline ointment applied twice a day, 6 days a week for 10 weeks. Since recurrences are common, follow-up evaluation is important.

Viral Conjunctivitis

Viral conjunctivitis is frequently due to infection with adenovirus type 3, 4, or 7 and may be associated with pharyngitis and preauricular adenopathy. The conjunctiva is quite hyperemic and shows folli-

Table 12–4. Clinical and laboratory features of conjunctivitis.

	Viral	Bacterial	Chlamydial	Allergic
Itching	Minimal	Minimal	Minimal	Severe
Hyperemia	Generalized	Generalized	Generalized	Generalized
Tearing	Profuse	Moderate	Moderate	Moderate
Exudation	Minimal, mucoid	Profuse, purulent	Profuse, mucoid or mucopurulent	Minimal, sl. mucus
Preauricular adenopathy	Common	Uncommon	Common only in inclusion conjunctivitis	None
Stained conjunctival smears and scrapings	Lymphocytes, plasma cells, multinucleated giant cells, eosinophilic intranuclear inclusions	Neutrophils, bacteria	Neutrophils, plasma cells, basophilic intracytoplasmic inclusions	Eosinophils
Associated sore throat and fever	Occasionally	Occasionally	Never in inclusion conjunctivitis. Often present in neonatal conjunctivitis	Never

Modified from Vaughan D, Asbury T: *General Ophthalmology*, 11th ed. Appleton-Century Crofts, 1986.

cular reaction. There is a thin watery discharge. The condition usually lasts 12–14 days. No treatment is of value. Sulfonamide preparations or broad-spectrum antibiotics are instilled locally to prevent secondary infection.

Epidemic keratoconjunctivitis is highly contagious, is usually due to infection with adenovirus type 8 or 19, and is often spread by the fingers of physicians during their examination of the eye or through contaminated instruments or eye drops. Conjunctivitis is followed in 5–14 days by photophobia and epithelial keratitis. Corneal subepithelial opacities may persist for months but will eventually fade without sequelae. While corticosteroids may relieve acute symptoms, their use should be avoided because of their many potential complications.

Measles conjunctivitis is characterized by a catarrhal reaction with mucopurulent discharge and, frequently, a swelling of the semilunar fold. Measles conjunctivitis may precede the skin eruption. If a secondary infection is present, it should be treated with antibiotics; otherwise, no specific treatment is indicated, because the disease is self-limited. Varicella-zoster conjunctivitis is characterized by vesicular lesions of the lids and lid margins and a hyperemia and infiltrative reaction of the conjunctiva. Preauricular lymph nodes are frequently present; secondary corneal involvement may occur.

Allergic Conjunctivitis

Allergic conjunctivitis produces symptoms of itching, lacrimation, mild redness, and a stringy mucoid discharge. Eosinophils may be seen on scrapings from the conjunctiva. For acute cases of conjunctivitis, use of topical weak ophthalmic corticosteroid drops (eg, 0.125% prednisolone) instilled 5–6 times a day or use of 1.5% hydrocortisone ophthalmic ointment or its equivalent instilled 3–4 times a day is quite effective. For chronic forms of allergic conjunctivitis, an attempt should be made to isolate the offending allergen and to eliminate contact with it. Desensitization to the allergen can be carried out if elimination of contact is not possible. Temporary symptomatic relief may be obtained with the use of topical ophthalmic solutions containing vasoconstricting agents and antihistamines.

Phlyctenular Keratoconjunctivitis

Phlyctenular keratoconjunctivitis appears as elevated clear nodules, situated near the limbus, with surrounding hyperemia. The disease has been associated with a hypersensitivity reaction to tuberculin; phlyctenules may also develop as a hypersensitivity reaction to other bacterial products or other antigens.

Treatment consists of the local application of corticosteroids. Systemic tuberculosis should be ruled out.

Vernal Conjunctivitis

This form of conjunctivitis is seen in patients ages 5–20. It tends to be seasonal and becomes less severe with age. Symptoms consist of lacrimation, itching, stringy discharge, and giant "cobblestone" papillary hypertrophy in the tarsal conjunctiva or grayish elevated areas at the limbus. (See Fig 12–7.) Many eosinophils are seen in the scraping of the lesions.

Treatment consists of the local application of corticosteroid ointment several times a day. Topical solutions of 4% cromolyn sodium (Opticrom) applied several times a day often provide relief from symptoms. Severe cases may require more extensive therapy, but this should be conducted by an ophthalmologist.

Ophthalmia Neonatorum

Ophthalmia neonatorum is inflammation of the conjunctiva of the newborn. It may be due to bacterial (gonococcal, staphylococcal, pneumococcal), chlamydial, or herpes simplex infections or to chemical irritation (silver nitrate). Bacterial conjunctivitis appears 2–5 days after birth; chlamydial conjunctivitis appears 5–10 days after birth. Herpes simplex conjunctivitis may be present within 2 weeks of birth. Conjunctivitis associated with silver nitrate usually is evident within the first 24–48 hours after birth. A definite diagnosis is established by smears and cultures of the material taken from the conjunctiva. Conjunctivitis due to silver nitrate is sterile, although secondary bacterial infections may occur.

Chlamydia is the most common cause of infectious neonatal conjunctivitis. Almost 50% of infants born to mothers with chlamydial cervicitis develop neonatal conjunctivitis. Because pneumonitis, otitis media, and vulvovaginitis often accompany the conjunctivitis, systemic antibiotic treatment is necessary.

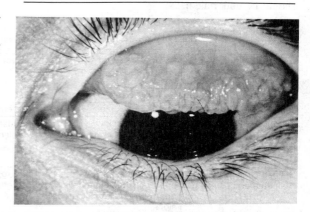

Figure 12–7. Vernal conjunctivitis. "Cobblestone" papillae in superior tarsal conjunctiva. (Courtesy of P Thygeson.) In: *General Ophthalmology,* 12th ed. Vaughan D, Asbury T. Appleton & Lange, 1989.

In most states in the USA, chemical (1% silver nitrate) or antibiotic prophylaxis of the newborn eye is required. These laws are highly variable in the different states. Various antibiotics such as penicillin, tetracyclines, or bacitracin are currently used for prophylaxis of gonococcal ophthalmia.

It is most important to treat gonococcal conjunctivitis vigorously because corneal ulceration and perforation can occur in untreated or inadequately treated cases. Topical antibiotic therapy is unnecessary when systemic antibiotic therapy is given. However, normal saline may be used to irrigate the purulent discharge from the conjunctiva. The treatment of gonococcal conjunctivitis consists of administering penicillin 100,000 units/kg/d intravenously in 4 divided doses for 7 days. Penicillinase-producing strains should be treated with intramuscular ceftriaxone, 25–50 mg/kg/d for 7 days or intramuscular gentamicin 5 mg/kg/d in 2 divided doses for 7 days.

Other types of bacterial conjunctivitis of the newborn should be treated by the instillation of appropriate antibiotic ointments 4 times a day. Chlamydial conjunctivitis should be treated with erythromycin syrup, 50 mg/kg/d orally in 4 divided doses for 14 days. Herpes simplex infections should be treated with 1% trifluridine drops every 2 hours for 7 days.

In all cases of conjunctivitis, treatment should be continued for a few days after the symptoms have subsided; this will prevent early recurrences.

Chandler JW: Ophthalmia neonatorum: An update. *Trans Pac Coast Otoophthalmol Soc Annu Meet* 1982;**63:**161.

Darrell RW: *Viral Diseases of the Eye.* Lea & Febiger, 1985.

Foster CS: The Cromolyn Sodium Collaborative Study Group: Evaluation of topical cromolyn sodium in the treatment of vernal conjunctivitis. *Ophthalmology* 1988; **95:**194.

Isenberg SJ et al: Source of the conjunctival flora at birth and implications for ophthalmia neonatorum prophylaxis. *Am J Ophthalmol* 1988;**106:**458.

Sandström I: Treatment of neonatal conjunctivitis. *Arch Opthalmol* 1987;**105:**925.

Stenson S, Newman R, Fedukowicz H: Conjunctivitis in the newborn: Observations on incidence, cause and prophylaxis. *Ann Ophthalmol* 1981;**13:**329.

MUCOCUTANEOUS DISEASES

Conjunctival lesions may be associated with mucocutaneous diseases, including erythema multiforme, Stevens-Johnson syndrome, Reiter's syndrome, Behçet's syndrome, and mucocutaneous lymph node syndrome (Kawasaki disease). The conjunctival involvement consists of erythema, vesicular lesions that frequently rupture, membrane formation, and the development of symblepharon (adhesion) between the raw edges of the bulbar and palpebral conjunctivae. Goblet cells in the conjunctiva are destroyed in the cicatricial process. This de-

creases the mucus secretion that is essential for the spread of tears over the cornea. Keratitis sicca (corneal drying) may result.

Treatment of the conjunctival lesions associated with these conditions is symptomatic, ie, soothing eye drops and compresses. Topical corticosteroids are helpful in the acute stages in diminishing the intensity and complications of the acute inflammatory phase. Antibiotics are of no benefit except for prevention of secondary infection. Erythema multiforme and Stevens-Johnson disease may be precipitated by sulfonamide and antibiotic therapy. Topical antibiotic therapy may be used when secondary bacterial infection occurs; care must be taken to choose an antibiotic to which the patient is not sensitive. The use of topical lubricants and the application of soft contact lenses may prevent corneal drying and ulceration.

Grayson M: *Diseases of the Cornea,* 2nd ed. Mosby, 1983.

Smolin G, O'Connor GR: *Ocular Immunology,* 2nd ed. Little, Brown, 1986.

DISEASES OF THE CORNEA

CORNEAL ULCERS

Corneal ulcers are serious ocular disorders. They may follow corneal injury or conjunctivitis or may be associated with systemic infections. Corneal ulcers are usually diagnosed by simple inspection. There is loss of anterior substance of the cornea, with surrounding opaque gray or white necrosis. Corneal ulcers may be peripheral or central. Several ulcers may be present in the same eye. The area of ulceration stains with fluorescein. A serious effort should be made to determine the etiology of any corneal ulcer. Cultures and scrapings should be taken, and sensitivity tests should be performed if bacterial organisms are found.

Bacterial Corneal Ulcers

Central bacterial corneal ulcers are due to infections with pneumococci, hemolytic streptococci, *P aeruginosa,* and, less commonly, gram-positive and gram-negative rods. Marginal corneal ulcers may develop as a result of bacterial sensitivity, most commonly to staphylococcal infections.

Treatment should be started immediately, before sensitivity tests are completed. Subsequently, the antibiotic can be changed if necessary. For mild superficial bacterial ulcers, the topical use of antibiotic drops or ointment at frequent intervals is usually satisfactory. Until the susceptibility of the organism is known, treatment can be started with an ophthalmic antibiotic preparation that includes neomycin, bacitracin, and polymyxin B or with a broad-spectrum antibiotic. Cycloplegic drops should be used to relieve the iridocyclitis that accompanies bacterial ulcers. In more severe corneal ulcers that involve the deeper portions of the stroma, more intensive antibiotic therapy should be given. Antibiotics should also be given subconjunctivally and systemically. Corticosteroids should not be given topically in these cases, since they interfere with the healing process and might exaggerate an infection that was not susceptible to the treatment being used.

Marginal corneal ulcers respond to topical corticosteroids. If a staphylococcal infection of the conjunctiva or eyelid is present, it should be treated with appropriate antibiotics.

Viral Corneal Ulcers

A. Herpes Simplex Ulcer (Dendritic): Herpes simplex keratitis is becoming a more common corneal disease in children. Lesions in the cornea may or may not be associated with herpes labialis. Corneal involvement is frequently precipitated by the topical application of corticosteroids and less commonly with the systemic use of corticosteroids. In the initial infection, the lesion has the appearance of a dendrite (Fig 12–8) that may be easily identified after the instillation of fluorescein. There are one or more branching vesicular lesions involving the anterior part of the cornea. These vesicles rupture. Subsequently, deeper involvement of the cornea may occur. Iritis may also develop as a complication.

Treatment of acute herpes infections of the cornea consists of topical application of antiviral medica-

tion: idoxuridine (IDU), vidarabine, or trifluridine. Idoxuridine is applied in 0.5% ointment (Stoxil) 4 times a day or in 0.1% solution (Herplex, Stoxil) hourly during the day and every 2 hours at night. Vidarabine in 3% ointment (Vira-A) is applied 5 times a day. Trifluridine is applied in 1% solution (Viroptic) every 2 hours up to 9 times a day. Acyclovir in 3% ointment is effective, but no commercial preparation for ophthalmic use is available in the USA.

Mechanical denuding of the infected corneal epithelium is also an effective method of treating fresh cases of superficial herpes simplex keratitis. This procedure should be performed by an ophthalmologist. Deeper involvement of the cornea may represent a hypersensitivity reaction, and the use of topical corticosteroids in conjunction with an antiviral medication sometimes improves the condition. Because the use of corticosteroids in an active herpes infection can lead to rapid deterioration of the cornea, this treatment should be conducted only by an ophthalmologist.

B. Herpes Zoster Infection: Herpes zoster keratitis is associated with zoster infection of the first branch of the trigeminal nerve. Corneal involvement may be superficial or deep and accompanied by uveitis. Topical and systemic acyclovir are often effective. Topical corticosteroids are used for the management of deep corneal involvement with uveitis. Relief is obtained with the use of topical corticosteroids. Cycloplegic drops should be used for relieving the iridocyclitis that accompanies herpes zoster infection. The physician must be certain of the diagnosis of herpes zoster before employing topical corticosteroids, since other viral diseases of the cornea are aggravated by these agents.

Fungal Corneal Ulcers

Mycotic corneal infections are difficult to diagnose. There is usually a history of recent trauma or foreign body. Frequently, the ulcerated cornea shows surrounding satellite lesions; hypopyon (pus in the anterior chamber) may be present. Fungal corneal ulcers are rare, but their incidence seems to be increasing, possibly from the widespread use of topical corticosteroid and broad-spectrum antibiotic medications. Whenever a diagnosis of mycotic corneal ulceration is suspected, cultures and sensitivity tests should be obtained.

The management of fungal corneal ulcers is difficult and should always be conducted by an ophthalmologist. Topical antifungal drugs such as 5% natamycin, 1% miconazole, 0.05–0.15% amphotericin B, and 2% ketoconazole may be employed, but systemic antifungals and surgical procedures are sometimes necessary in complicated cases.

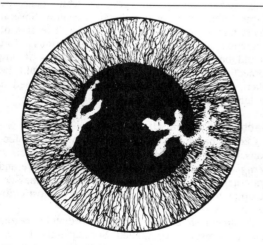

Figure 12–8. Dendritic type of lesion seen in herpes simplex keratitis. (Reproduced, with permission, from Vaughan D, Asbury T: *General Ophthalmology*, 8th ed. Lange, 1977.)

Baum J, Barza M: Topical vs subconjunctival treatment of bacterial corneal ulcers. *Ophthalmology* 1983;**90:**162.

Jones DB: Initial therapy of suspected microbial corneal ulcers. 2. Specific antibiotic therapy based on corneal smears. *Surv Ophthalmol* 1979;**24**:97.

Kaufman HE: Update on antiviral agents. *Ophthalmology* 1985;**92**:533.

Leibowitz HM: *Corneal Disorders: Clinical Diagnosis and Management.* Saunders, 1984.

Liesegang TJ: Corneal complications from herpes zoster ophthalmicus. *Ophthalmology* 1985;**92**:316.

Smolin G, Thoft RA (editors): *The Cornea: Scientific Foundations and Clinical Practice,* 2nd ed. Little, Brown, 1987.

Tabbara KF, Hyndiuk RA (editors): *Infections of the Eye.* Little, Brown, 1986.

ALLERGIC REACTIONS

Allergic reactions in the cornea may involve either the superficial epithelial or deeper stromal layers. Most forms of deep keratitis probably represent hypersensitivity reactions. The allergen may be airborne, or it may enter the cornea by way of the circulation in the limbus. Treatment consists of determining the offending agent, if possible, and then eliminating its contact with the patient. Topical corticosteroids usually are required. They should be used only under the supervision of an ophthalmologist.

Interstitial Keratitis

Interstitial keratitis is an acute immune reaction in the cornea, usually associated with congenital syphilis. Symptoms consist of intense photophobia, tearing, pain, and decreased vision. On examination, the cornea has a diffuse opaque appearance. Fine vessels may be noted in the stroma. There may be aggregates of these vessels, which appear as orange-red areas (salmon patches). Other evidence of congenital syphilis may also be present. Serologic tests are often negative.

Interstitial keratitis may be associated with other diseases such as tuberculosis and the autoimmune disorders, and any such contributing condition should be ruled out.

Treatment consists of the use of topical corticosteroids and cycloplegics for relief of symptoms. If active syphilis is present, it should be appropriately treated.

Grayson M: *Diseases of the Cornea,* 2nd ed. Mosby, 1983.

Smolin G, O'Connor GR: *Ocular Immunology,* 2nd ed. Little, Brown, 1986.

Theodore FH, Bloomfield SE, Mondino BJ: *Clinical Allergy and Immunology of the Eye.* Williams & Wilkins, 1983.

CORNEAL DRYING & EXPOSURE

Keratoconjunctivitis Sicca

This condition is rare in children and results from a lacrimal gland insufficiency. The treatment of choice is tear replacement with artificial tear solutions as necessary to keep the cornea moist. Bland ophthalmic ointments (Duolube, Duratears, Lacri-Lube) may also be used, particularly at bedtime.

Xerophthalmia

Severe vitamin A deficiency reduces conjunctival secretion of mucus, and this leads to conjunctival and corneal drying and keratinization. The cornea may become soft and necrotic (keratomalacia), and corneal perforation may occur. The conjunctival changes are characterized by a foamy, triangular lesion that is usually on the temporal side and has its base at the limbus (Bitot's spot). The conjunctival and corneal changes together are known as xerophthalmia.

Patients are treated with systemic vitamin A. Topical antibiotic drops may be indicated to prevent secondary infection.

Exposure & Neuroparalytic Keratitis

Exposure keratitis may develop after facial nerve palsies or after a period of unconsciousness during which the eyes are exposed. Treatment is similar to that described above.

Familial Dysautonomia (Riley-Day Syndrome)

In this condition, there is a deficiency of tears, and corneal drying can occur. Tear replacement (see Keratoconjunctivitis Sicca, above) is indicated.

Levine MR: Medical and surgical treatment of the dry eye. *Int Ophthalmol Clin* (Fall) 1978;**18**:101.

Smolin G, Thoft RA (editors): *The Cornea: Scientific Foundations and Clinical Practice.* Little, Brown, 1987.

Sommer A, Sugana T: Corneal xerophthalmia and keratomalacia. *Arch Ophthalmol* 1982;**100**:404.

Wilson LA (editor): *External Diseases of the Eye.* Harper & Row, 1979.

CORNEAL INVOLVEMENT IN OTHER SYSTEMIC DISEASES

The cornea is involved in many systemic diseases. Small calcium deposits may be observed in the corneas of patients with hyperparathyroidism. Cystine crystals are observed in patients with renal rickets (cystinosis). Excessive intake of vitamin D may lead to calcification of the anterior part of the cornea in a band opacity of the exposed portion of the cornea. Deficiency of vitamin A may lead to drying (xerosis) and softening (keratomalacia) of the cornea. Corneal ulceration may occur in patients with severe debilitating diseases such as dysentery. Corneal opacities may occur in children with Hurler's disease (gargoylism) and other mucopolysaccharide disorders.

In all of these conditions, it is important to recognize the underlying disease and treat appropriately.

Grayson M: *Diseases of the Cornea,* 2nd ed. Mosby, 1983.

Smolin G, Thoft RA (editors): *The Cornea: Scientific Foundations and Clinical Practice.* Little, Brown, 1987.

Sugar J: Corneal manifestations of systemic mucopolysaccharidoses. *Ann Ophthalmol* 1979;**11**:531.

UVEITIS

Inflammation of the uveal tract may present anteriorly as iritis or cyclitis (inflammation of the ciliary body) or as posterior inflammations (choroiditis). Uveitis may be associated with other ocular diseases, such as corneal ulceration, keratitis, hypermature cataracts, necrotic intraocular tumors, or optic neuritis.

Uveitis may be classified as exogenous or endogenous. Exogenous uveitis follows the accidental introduction of pathogenic organisms or a foreign substance into the eye. Endogenous uveitis is a result of various systemic processes.

Uveitis may also be classified as suppurative or nonsuppurative according to the type of tissue reaction. Nonsuppurative uveitis, which is the more common form, may further be divided into granulomatous and nongranulomatous types. Nongranulomatous uveitis usually involves the iris and ciliary body and produces symptoms of photophobia, pain, redness, and blurred vision. The pupil is small and often irregular. There is circumcorneal injection. On examination with a slit lamp, cells in the anterior chamber and fine precipitates on the posterior surface of the cornea may be observed. Granulomatous uveitis may involve the iris, ciliary body, or choroid. Pain, redness, and photophobia are not so prominent as in the nongranulomatous form. Vision may be markedly disturbed, particularly if the involvement is in the macular area. On ophthalmoscopy, the vitreous may be quite hazy. Active lesions of choroiditis may be seen as swollen, white, indistinct irregular patches. As the choroiditis subsides, pigmentary changes may take place.

Uveitis presents a complex problem. The endogenous nonsuppurative form may be associated with systemic disease. In children, the most common associated disease is juvenile rheumatoid arthritis, usually the pauci articular form. Iritis may antedate joint symptoms. Other common associated diseases are toxoplasmosis; histoplasmosis; tuberculosis; sarcoidosis, polyarteritis, rheumatoid arthritis, and other collagen diseases; bacterial infections of the sinuses or teeth; food and pollen allergies; and viral diseases such as mumps, measles, chickenpox, influenza, herpes simplex, and herpes zoster. The relationship between systemic disease and uveitis may be incidental. There is pathologic evidence that the choroid and retina may be invaded with *Toxoplasma* and *Mycobacterium tuberculosis.* However, aside from these specific instances, causative organisms have not been found to enter the uveal tissue. There is accumulating evidence that most cases of uveitis are due to an immune reaction.

Treatment

If systemic disease is present, it should be appropriately treated. However, successful treatment of systemic disease does not always result in a cure of the uveitis. Nonspecific treatment of uveitis consists of the use of cycloplegics to dilate the pupil and to relieve the ciliary and iris spasm. Atropine, 1–2% solution, or scopolamine, 0.25% solution, should be used 2–3 times daily. In addition, the topical use of 10% phenylephrine hydrochloride to dilate the pupil widely is indicated. Corticosteroids should be used unless they are contraindicated by the presence of a specific bacterial or viral infection. For inflammations of the anterior uveal tract, topical and subconjunctival corticosteroids are useful in reducing the inflammation. For posterior uveitis, systemic corticosteroids should be used.

The management of uveitis is difficult. Many complications can occur, including glaucoma, cataract, and retinal detachment. Therefore, these cases should be managed by an ophthalmologist.

Nussenblatt RB, Palestine AG: *Uveitis: Fundamentals and Clinical Practice.* Year Book, 1989.

Schlaegel TF: Etiologic diagnosis of uveitis. Chapter 41 in: *Clinical Ophthalmology.* Vol 4. Duane TD (editor). Harper & Row, 1987.

Smith RE, Nozik A: *Uveitis: A Clinical Approach to Diagnosis and Management,* 2nd ed. Williams & Wilkins, 1988.

Smolin G, O'Connor GR: *Ocular Immunology,* 2nd ed. Little, Brown, 1986.

Wolf MD, Lichter PR, Ragsdale CG: Prognostic factors in the uveitis of juvenile rheumatoid arthritis. *Ophthalmology* 1987;**94**:1242.

SYMPATHETIC OPHTHALMIA

Sympathetic ophthalmia is a special form of bilateral granulomatous uveitis. It follows a penetrating ocular injury of the uveal tract. It may occur at any time from 10 days after injury to many years later, but it usually presents within the first 2–4 months after initial injury. The etiology of sympathetic ophthalmia is not understood, but it probably represents a hypersensitivity response to uveal pigment. The diagnosis is based on a history of an injury to one (exciting) eye with the subsequent development of uveitis in the other (sympathizing) eye.

Treatment consists of the use of systemic and topical corticosteroids and topical cycloplegics. Immunosuppressive agents also are employed in resistant cases. Long-term therapy is usually necessary, and maintenance doses of corticosteroids are usually indicated to prevent a flare-up of this condition. The disease can be averted by early enucleation of the eye that has received a severe injury to the ciliary body and has become visually useless.

Nussenblatt RB, Palestine AG: *Uveitis: Fundamentals and Clinical Practice.* Year Book, 1989.
Smolin G, O'Connor GR: *Ocular Immunology,* 2nd ed. Little, Brown, 1986.

DISEASES OF THE RETINA

HEREDITARY RETINAL DISORDERS

Hereditary retinal disorders may be evident shortly after birth or not until the second decade of life. Many of these disorders involve primarily one layer of the retina (eg, the pigment epithelium, the rod and cone layer, or the ganglion cell layer), but other layers of the retina are usually secondarily involved.

Retinitis pigmentosa is a bilateral hereditary disease involving chiefly the retinal rods or the retinal pigment epithelium. Symptoms of night blindness usually begin early in the second decade. Restriction of visual fields subsequently occurs; this generally progresses, so that by middle age the visual fields are markedly contracted and the visual acuity severely depressed. However, certain forms of the disease are less severe, especially in the early stages. Ophthalmoscopic examination may reveal only some incipient pigmentary abnormalities in the midperiphery of the ocular fundus. The diagnosis may be confirmed by electroretinography, which shows markedly reduced or unrecordable activity. As the disease progresses, additional changes occur: narrowing of the retinal arteries and veins, waxy appearance of the optic disk, and "bone corpuscle" pigment deposits. Retinitis pigmentosa may be associated with many systemic diseases: renal abnormalities, deafness, convulsions and obesity, hypogenitalism, polydactyly, mental retardation (Laurence-Moon-Biedl syndrome), and abetalipoproteinemia. There is no satisfactory treatment for retinitis pigmentosa. The mode of inheritance varies. Genetic counseling is advisable for prospective parents with this disorder.

Fundus flavimaculatus consists of multiple round and fishtail-like yellow-white lesions of the posterior and midperipheral fundus. The onset is in the first or second decade of life. Some patients with this disorder develop atrophic changes in the macula with severe visual loss (Stargardt's disease); others may retain good macular function and visual acuity.

Coats's disease is an exudative retinopathy characterized by hemorrhagic and exudative lesions and by telangiectatic vessels. The onset is usually within the first few years of life; males are affected more often than females. Usually only one eye is involved; vision is often severely impaired. The disorder may cause a white pupillary reflex (leukocoria) and must be differentiated from other causes of leukocoria, such as cataracts, persistent hyperplastic primary vitreous, and retinoblastoma.

Vitelliruptive degeneration (Best's disease) is a disorder of the retinal pigment epithelium that occurs in the macular region at or shortly after birth. Ophthalmoscopically, the macula has a yellow deposit resembling a "sunny side up" fried egg. During the first or second decade of life, the lesion changes; the sunny side up egg yolk becomes scrambled, and scarring and pigmentary changes may lead to loss of central vision.

Leber's congenital amaurosis is characterized by congenital blindness or reduced vision. Initially, the ocular fundus appears normal or there may be some mild pigmentary changes. With time, the disk becomes atrophic, and pigmentary changes become more obvious. Electroretinographic testing shows changes similar to those seen in retinitis pigmentosa.

Color vision abnormalities are common, with approximately 7% of males and 0.5% of females affected. Many of the tests used clinically are not sensitive enough to detect small changes. Color vision is a retinal cone function; each cone has 3 distinct photosensitive pigments, with spectral sensitive patterns maximal at red, green, or blue. Hereditary color vision defects result from a deficiency or absence of one or more of the 3 cone photosensitive pigments.

Breton ME, Nelson LB: What do color blind children really see? Guidelines for clinical prescreening based on recent findings. *Surv Ophthalmol* 1983;**27**:306.
Heckenlively JR et al: Clinical findings and common symptoms in retinitis pigmentosa. *Am J Ophthalmol* 1988;**105**:504.
Schroeder R et al: Leber's congenital amaurosis. Retrospective review of 43 cases and a new fundus finding in two cases. *Arch Ophthalmol* 1987;**105**:356.
Silodor SW et al: Natural history and management of advanced Coats' disease. *Ophthalmic Surg* 1988;**19**:89.
Tasman W, Shields JA: *Disorders of the Peripheral Fundus.* Harper & Row, 1980.

RETINOPATHY OF PREMATURITY (RETROLENTAL FIBROPLASIA)

Retinopathy of prematurity is a primary bilateral retinal vascular disorder of premature infants. The disease occurs most frequently in those with a birth weight under 1500 g who have received excessive amounts of oxygen therapy during the first 10–14 days of life. Infants at highest risk are those born under 32 weeks' gestation and with a birth weight under 1250 g. For several years, after the role of oxygen in the development of retinopathy of prematurity was established, the disease became almost extinct with restricted oxygen therapy. However, therapy employing high concentrations of oxygen to treat respiratory distress syndrome in premature infants has again been used and, possibly as a result, retinopathy of prematurity is being seen with increasing frequency.

In general, peripheral vascularization of the retina is not complete until about 2 weeks after full-term birth. However, this is variable; some eyes have complete vascularization at 8 months' gestational age. Until retinal vascularization is complete, the peripheral immature vessels, which are immediately posterior to the demarcation site of vascular to avascular retina, are extremely sensitive to hyperoxia and respond by vasoconstriction and obliteration. A vasoproliferative substance is released from the ischemic retina. When oxygen concentrations are subsequently reduced, the retinal vessels in the posterior pole often dilate as a result of peripheral vascular shunts formed near the site of vaso-obliteration. These shunts may take the form of neofibrovascular membranes on the surface of the retina or may extend into the vitreous cavity. Tractional retinal detachments may occur. In advanced stages, the retrolental space is filled with fibrovascular and retinal tissues, the anterior chambers are shallow, and the eyes are small and blind. In incomplete forms, myopia and strabismus are often observed; retinal detachment may occur as a late complication in the teenage years. Up to 85% of acute cases of retinopathy of prematurity regress as vascularization to the peripheral aspect of the retina is completed in a nearly normal manner.

It is essential that pediatricians be aware of the relationship of oxygen therapy to the development of retinopathy of prematurity—not only the concentration of oxygen but also the duration of oxygen treatment and the degree of prematurity. The generally accepted safe concentration of oxygen is less than 40%, but this is subject to the other variables noted above. Many experts believe an arterial blood oxygen level over 70 mm Hg is inadvisable.

All premature infants receiving high concentrations of oxygen therapy should be followed as closely as possible to make certain that arterial blood oxygen levels do not remain excessively high for any period of time. Changes in the immature retinal vessels appear to be related not only to high arterial blood oxygen levels but also to the duration of hyperoxia. The value of the early administration of vitamin E (an antioxidant) in diminishing the severity

of retinopathy of prematurity or in preventing its occurrence is under investigation.

All premature infants should have careful ophthalmoscopy performed by a skilled examiner by the sixth week of life, at which time severe forms of retinopathy are more common. If signs of the disease are present, a follow-up ophthalmoscopic examination is needed after discharge, and the parents should be counseled. Refraction should be an essential part of this follow-up examination, since amblyopia (associated with strabismus and refractive errors) is common and treatable. Surgical treatment of retinal detachment is sometimes indicated. Cryotherapy of the retina in rapidly advancing cases appears to be of benefit in halting progression of the disease.

Flynn JT et al: Retinopathy of prematurity. Diagnosis, severity and natural history. *Ophthalmology* 1987;**94**:620.

Multicenter Trial of Cryotherapy for Retinopathy of Prematurity: Preliminary results. *Arch Ophthalmol* 1988; **106**:471.

Patz A: Current therapy of retrolental fibroplasia: Retinopathy of prematurity. *Ophthalmology* 1983;**90**:425.

Sira IB, Nissenkorn I, Kremer I: Retinopathy of prematurity. *Surv Opthalmol* 1988;**33**:1.

RETINAL DETACHMENT

Detachment of the retina in children is usually associated with severe ocular trauma or with high myopia. In the latter condition, there are degenerative changes in the periphery of the retina that lead to subsequent separation of the retina. The diagnosis is established by a history of progressively more severe blurred vision. The visual disturbance may start with the sensation of flashing lights, or the patient may observe a dark cloud coming in from one section of the visual field. On ophthalmoscopy, the area of detachment appears elevated and gray. The retinal vessels appear darker, and the retina is seen with increased convex dioptric power in the ophthalmoscope.

The only treatment is surgical repair.

Benson WE: *Retinal Detachment,* 2nd ed. Lippincott, 1988.

Rosner M, Treister G, Belkin M: Epidemiology of retinal detachment in childhood and adolescence. *J Pediatr Ophthalmol Strabismus* 1987;**24**:42.

RETINOBLASTOMA

Retinoblastoma is a comparatively rare, malignant tumor of children; it affects approximately one infant in 20,000 live births. A family history of retinoblastoma is found in less than 10% of the cases. However, about 30% of the cases may have a predisposition to tumor formation that can be inherited as an autosomal dominant trait. The remaining 70% of cases occur as a sporadic mutation and are not inherited. Mutations in a specific locus of chromosome 13 correlate with the development of retinoblastoma. Approximately 25% of cases are bilateral. Patients who survive bilateral retinoblastoma or who have a family history of retinoblastoma have about a 50% chance of transmitting the disease to their offspring. Genetic counseling is complex but advisable for survivors of retinoblastoma as well as for parents of children with retinoblastoma.

The presenting symptom is usually a white spot in the pupil (see Fig 12–1). Strabismus may be present. If the tumor becomes very large, glaucoma may occur, with a steamy cornea and red eye. Occasionally, retinoblastoma ruptures through the globe and results in a painful red eye. The diagnosis is usually made by ophthalmoscopic examination. To accomplish ophthalmoscopy, wide pupillary dilatation is essential; general anesthesia is often necessary. The tumor appears as a solid yellow or white elevated mass. A small section of the eye may be involved, or the entire eye may be filled with tumor.

Treatment consists of enucleation of the involved eye in unilateral cases, although in selected cases small tumors are sometimes treated with x-ray or cryotherapy. If there is involvement of both eyes, the more severely involved eye should be enucleated and the other eye treated with x-ray therapy together with chemotherapy. Cryotherapy is sometimes employed for treatment of small peripheral lesions.

For parents who have an affected child but no previous family history of retinoblastoma, the risk of retinoblastoma in a second child is 1–6%. However, if 2 or more siblings are affected, the chances are approximately 50% that the next child will be affected. Approximately 16% of patients with bilateral retinoblastoma, almost all of which are hereditary, will develop a second primary neoplasm later in life, usually osteogenic sarcoma.

Abramson DH et al: The management of unilateral retinoblastoma without primary enucleation. *Arch Ophthalmol* 1982;**100:**1249.
Ellsworth RM: Retinoblastoma. Chapter 35 in: *Clinical Ophthalmology.* Vol 3. Duane TD (editor). Harper & Row, 1987.
Kopelman JE, McLean IW, Rosenberg SH: Multivariate analysis of risk for metastasis in retinoblastoma treatment by enucleation. *Ophthalmology* 1987;**94:**371.
Seidman DJ et al: Early diagnosis of retinoblastoma based on dysmorphic features and karotype analysis. *Ophthalmology* 1987;**94:**663.
Shields JA: *Diagnosis and Management of Intraocular Tumors.* Mosby, 1983.
Wiggs JL, Dryja TP: Predicting the risk of hereditary retinoblastoma. *Am J Ophthalmol* 1988;**106:**346.

OPTIC NEURITIS

Optic neuritis may involve only the head of the nerve (papillitis) or the orbital portion of the nerve (retrobulbar neuritis). Optic neuritis may occur in association with generalized infectious diseases, demyelinating diseases, blood dyscrasias, or metabolic diseases or may be due to exposure to toxins or drugs or extension of inflammatory disease such as sinusitis or meningitis. Clinically, there is an acute loss of vision. Involvement may be of one or both eyes; in children, the disease is frequently bilateral. Central visual defects are present. There may be some discomfort in the eyes on movement of the globes. On ophthalmoscopic examination, papilledema may be present or the disks may appear normal.

Optic neuritis in children often follows viremia and is usually a self-limited disease. The visual prognosis is generally favorable. If the cause can be determined, it should be treated. Systemic corticosteroid therapy has been advocated, but its effectiveness has not been established.

The presence of papilledema may be a sign of increased intracranial pressure. The differentiation between optic neuritis and papilledema secondary to increased intracranial pressure is not always easy. In general, papilledema due to increased intracranial pressure does not produce a severe loss of vision, and there often are associated neurologic signs.

Hess RF, Plant GT (editors): *Optic Neuritis.* Cambridge University Press, 1986.
Miller NR: *Walsh and Hoyt's Clinical Neuro-Ophthalmology,* 4th ed. 3 vols. Williams & Wilkins, 1987.
Repka MX, Miller NR: Optic atrophy in children. *Am J Ophthalmol* 1988;**106:**191.
Walsh TJ: *Neuro-Ophthalmology: Clinical Signs and Symptoms,* 2nd ed. Lea & Febiger, 1985.

DISEASES OF THE ORBIT

ORBITAL CELLULITIS

Orbital cellulitis is a serious illness characterized by proptosis; swelling, redness, and congestion of the eyelids, orbital tissues, and bulbar conjunctiva; discomfort; and, frequently, fever. A distinct magenta discoloration of the skin of the eyelids is present in cases of *Haemophilus influenzae* infection. In children, orbital cellulitis is usually due to bacterial infection. There may be associated infections elsewhere in the body, particularly in the sinuses. Treatment consists of hot packs and the vigorous use of systemic (primarily intravenous) antibiotics; a favorable response is usually obtained within 48–72 hours.

Macy JI, Mandelbaum SH, Minckler DS: Orbital cellulitis. *Ophthalmology* 1980;**87**:1309.

Rootman J: *Diseases of the Orbit: A Multidisciplinary Approach.* Lippincott, 1988.

Weiss A et al: Bacterial periorbital and orbital cellulitis in childhood. *Ophthalmology* 1983;**90**:195.

ENDOCRINE EXOPHTHALMOS

Endocrine exophthalmos is relatively uncommon in children. It may be unilateral or bilateral. In addition to exophthalmos, there may be retraction of the upper lids or swelling of the lids. Injection and swelling of the conjunctiva may be present, and there may also be some extraocular muscle weakness.

Treatment consists of management of the underlying thyroid disturbance. Severe ocular involvement in the form of exposure keratitis, glaucoma, or decreased visual acuity should be treated by an ophthalmologist.

Chumbley LC: *Ophthalmology in Internal Medicine.* Saunders, 1981.

Renie WA (editor): *Goldberg's Genetic and Metabolic Eye Disease,* 2nd ed. Little, Brown, 1986.

Rootman J: *Diseases of the Orbit: A Multidisciplinary Approach.* Lippincott, 1988.

ORBITAL TUMORS & PSEUDOTUMORS

Orbital tumors are rare in children. The most common primary tumors are hemangiomas, neurofibromas, gliomas of the optic nerve, dermoids, rhabdomyosarcomas, and tumors of the lacrimal gland. Neuroblastoma and lymphoma may spread into the orbit. The presenting symptoms are exophthalmos, congestion and ecchymosis of the globe and lids, extraocular muscle weakness, and displacement of the globe. Optic nerve gliomas may show enlargement of the optic foramen on x-ray examination.

Each case should be carefully evaluated. Treatment includes surgical removal, x-ray therapy, or the use of chemotherapy in certain cases. For certain benign tumors, it is often better not to attempt total removal of the lesion.

Pseudotumor of the orbit is uncommon in children. It is an inflammation of the orbital tissues, sometimes granulomatous in character but usually unrelated to any specific granulomatous disease. As a rule, only one orbit is affected, but in about 25% of the cases the other orbit also is involved. The symptoms may develop suddenly or slowly over a period of months. Swelling of the eyelid and conjunctiva often precedes the proptosis and diplopia. The diagnosis is usually made by exclusion of other causes of swelling and proptosis. Spontaneous remission often occurs. However, dramatic improvement usually follows systemic corticosteroid therapy.

Mottow LS, Jakobiec FA: Idiopathic inflammatory orbital pseudotumor in childhood. *Arch Ophthalmol* 1978;**96**:1410.

Rosenthal AR: Ocular manifestations of leukemia: A review. *Ophthalmology* 1983;**90**:899.

Rush JA et al: Optic glioma: Long-term follow-up of 85 histopathologically verified cases. *Ophthalmology* 1982;**89**:1213.

Shields JA: *Diagnosis and Management of Orbital Tumors.* Saunders, 1989.

DISEASES OF THE LACRIMAL APPARATUS

DACRYOSTENOSIS

In a significant number of infants, the nasolacrimal duct fails to completely canalize at the time of birth; the obstruction is usually at the nasal end of the duct. Symptoms consist of persistent tearing and, often, mucoid discharge in the inner corner of the eye.

Most cases subside without treatment. The obstruction usually opens spontaneously, and relief of symptoms occurs. Massage over the lacrimal sac with expression toward the nose may be helpful in establishing the patency. If a purulent discharge is evident, manual expression of the sac should be performed, followed by instillation of topical antibiotics. If a cure does not result within the first few months of life, probing of the nasolacrimal duct should be performed by an ophthalmologist.

El-Mansoury J et al: Results of late probing for congenital nasolacrimal duct obstruction. *Ophthalmology* 1986;**93**:1052.

Kushner BJ: Congenital nasolacrimal system obstruction. *Arch Ophthalmol* 1982;**100**:597.

Paul TO: Medical management of congenital nasolacrimal duct obstruction. *J Pediatr Ophthalmol Strabismus* 1985; **22**:68.

Sevel D: Development and congenital abnormalities of the nasolacrimal apparatus. *J Pediatr Ophthalmol Strabismus* 1981;**18**:13.

DACRYOCYSTITIS

Inflammation of the tear sac (dacryocystitis) is usually secondary to obstruction of the nasolacrimal duct. There is resultant stasis of the tears in the sac, with secondary bacterial infection. Symptoms consist of tearing and mucopurulent discharge. There may be acute inflammation in the region of the lacrimal sac. Fever and leukocytosis may be present. Occasionally, the sac may rupture to the skin surface.

If possible, cultures should be obtained and the organism identified. For mild cases, expression of the contents of the lacrimal sac followed by instillation of topical antibiotics in the region of the lacrimal puncta may be effective. More severe cases should also be treated with systemic antibiotics. Irrigation of the canaliculi and lacrimal sac with antibiotic solution is a more successful method of delivering adequate concentrations of antibiotics to the area of infection. Once the infection has subsided, an attempt should be made to establish the passage of tears. The nasolacrimal duct should be probed under general anesthesia if the system does not permit passage of fluid irrigated through the canaliculi.

Harris GJ, Di Clementi D: Congenital dacryocystocele. *Arch Ophthalmol* 1982;**100:**1763.

Isenberg SJ (editor): *The Eye in Infancy.* Year Book, 1988.

DACRYOADENITIS

Inflammation of the lacrimal gland may be associated with systemic disorders such as mumps or sarcoidosis. More rarely, infections of the lacrimal gland may be secondary to tuberculosis or syphilis.

Treatment should be directed toward the specific disease, if present; otherwise, symptomatic treatment should be used. Local applications of heat or cold over the lacrimal gland may give relief. Bed rest and salicylate analgesics are also useful. Systemic corticosteroids may reduce inflammation, but the use of corticosteroids in any viral infection is risky.

Darrell RW: *Viral Diseases of the Eye.* Lea & Febiger, 1985.

Harris GJ, Snyder RW: Lacrimal gland abscess. *Am J Ophthalmol* 1987;**104:**193.

Rootman J: *Diseases of the Orbit: A Multidisciplinary Approach.* Lippincott, 1988.

VISUAL FUNCTION IN LEARNING DISABILITIES

Learning disabilities are almost never associated with ocular disorders. However, a complete ophthalmologic examination is justified in children with learning disabilities. The examination should include measurement of near and distant vision, near point of accommodation, convergence amplitudes and near points of convergence, and a cycloplegic refraction. Gross ocular problems may cause poor or double vision, which may be significant factors in learning disabilities. Weakness of accommodation or convergence or significant hyperopia (farsightedness) may be related to the comfort of reading, which rarely can be a factor in learning disabilities.

SELECTED REFERENCES

Apt L, Gaffney WL: The eyes. In: *Pediatrics,* 18th ed. Rudolph AM, Hoffman JIE (editors). Appleton & Lange, 1987.

Crawford JS, Morin JD (editors): *The Eye in Childhood.* Grune & Stratton, 1983.

Duane TD (editor): *Clinical Ophthalmology.* 5 vols. Harper & Row, 1987.

Ellis PP: *Ocular Therapeutics and Pharmacology,* 7th ed. Mosby, 1985.

Ernest JT, Deutsch TA (editors): *Year Book of Ophthalmology.* Year Book, 1988.

Fraunfelder FT, Roy FH (editors): *Current Ocular Therapy 3.* Saunders, 1989.

Gittinger JW Jr: *Ophthalmology: A Clinical Introduction.* Little, Brown, 1984.

Harley RD (editor): *Pediatric Ophthalmology,* 2nd ed. 2 vols. Saunders, 1983.

Helveston RM, Ellis FD: *Pediatric Ophthalmology Practice,* 2nd ed. Mosby, 1983.

Isenberg SJ (editor): *The Eye in Infancy.* Year Book, 1988.

Miller NR: *Walsh and Hoyt's Clinical Neuro-Ophthalmology,* 4th ed. 3 vols. Williams & Wilkins, 1988.

Moses RA, Hart WM (editors): *Adler's Physiology of the Eye: Clinical Applications,* 8th ed. Mosby, 1987.

Nelson LB: *Pediatric Ophthalmology.* Saunders, 1984.

Newell FW: *Ophthalmology: Principles and Concepts,* 6th ed. Mosby, 1986.

Vaughan D, Ashbury T, Tabbara K: *General Ophthalmology,* 12th ed. Appleton & Lange, 1989.

Teeth & Periodontium

Gary K. Belanger, DDS, & Paul S. Casamassimo, DDS, MS

THE ORAL CAVITY

Included in the oral cavity are the teeth (20 primary; 32 permanent), the maxillary and mandibular jaws, hard and soft palates, tongue, and salivary glands (major and minor). Each tooth is composed of an enamel crown; a dentin body and roots, with cementum covering the root surfaces; and a pulp cavity containing connective tissue, nerves, lymphatics, and blood vessels that branch off larger structures in the jaw and enter the root tip in a bundle. (See Fig 13–1.)

The teeth are supported in bone via ligaments that connect the cementum-covered root surfaces to the bone. Like the teeth, the periodontal ligament is innervated. The gingivae are attached to alveolar bone and to the teeth on the alveolar process. The area where gingiva meets tooth is called the gingival epithelial attachment, which is usually at the neck of the tooth. Attached gingiva is normally pink and stippled in children.

Primary teeth are usually smaller, whiter, and more bulbous than permanent ones. Below each primary tooth normally rests a permanent successor in a crypt of bone. The developing permanent tooth is susceptible to systemic disorders and to local problems affecting the overlying primary tooth, such as dental caries and trauma.

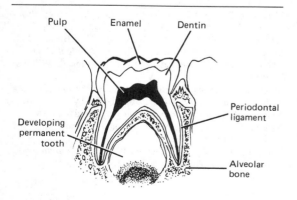

Figure 13–1. Cross-sectional view of a primary tooth and underlying tooth bud.

ERUPTION OF TEETH

Cellular development of primary teeth begins during the sixth week of embryogenesis, with calcification beginning during the second trimester. A few permanent teeth also begin to develop by birth, but very little calcification occurs. Table 13–1 summarizes the timing of calcification, eruption, and exfoliation of primary and permanent teeth.

Although the pattern of tooth eruption is easily observed, it is not a good predictor of general growth and development or other physical parameters. Many local factors influence eruption of teeth, and the pattern can be affected by normal variation, systemic conditions, and genetic tendencies.

Normal Patterns of Eruption

Primary teeth should erupt within 6 months of their average expected time. According to the "rule of 4s," 4 teeth will erupt beginning at about 7 months of age, and 4 more will erupt approximately every 4 months thereafter. Another general guide is that there will be no teeth at 6 months, 6 teeth at 12 months, and 12 teeth at 18 months of age. Primary teeth erupt in the following sequence: central incisors, lateral incisors, first molars, cuspids, and second molars. The exfoliation sequence is more variable (Table 13–1).

As the primary teeth near gingival penetration, infants begin **teething.** They may become more restless and irritable, and they drool and place their fingers in their mouths more frequently. Most studies have discounted teething as a cause of systemic disturbances, diarrhea, fever, seizures, or an altered hematocrit. Although the incidence of fever, rhinitis, gastrointestinal upset, upper respiratory tract infections, and dermatitis may increase coincidentally with tooth eruption, a causal relationship is equivocal. Many normal changes in the infant's environment are thought to contribute to these illnesses, including diet changes, increased exposure to infections, and loss of maternal antibodies; these changes may also hasten the eruption process.

Use of a soft cloth, a teething ring, or dry, abrasive toast may hasten eruption and provide relief of pain. Gingival incision is rarely indicated to allow eruption of primary teeth, although some extremely delayed permanent teeth may benefit from this pro-

Table 13–1. Dental growth and development.

Primary (Deciduous) Teeth						
	Crown Calcification Begins At	Root Completed At	Maxillary Teeth Erupt At	Mandibular Teeth Erupt At	Maxillary Teeth Exfoliate At	Mandibular Teeth Exfoliate At
Central incisor	14 weeks in utero	18 months	6–10 months	5–8 months	6–7½ years	6–7 years
Lateral incisor	16 weeks in utero	18–24 months	8–12 months	8–13 months	7–8½ years	7–8 years
Cuspid	17 weeks in utero	39 months	16–20 months	16–20 months	10–12 years	9–11 years
First molar	15½ weeks in utero	27–30 months	12–18 months	12–18 months	9–11 years	9–11 years
Second molar	18 weeks in utero	36 months	20–30 months	20–30 months	11–13 years	11–13 years

Secondary (Permanent) Teeth				
	Crown Calcification Begins At	Root Completed At	Maxillary Teeth Erupt At	Mandibular Teeth Erupt At
Central incisor	3–4 months	9–10 years	7–8 years	6–7 years
Lateral incisor	Maxilla: 10–12 months Mandible: 3–4 months	10–11 years	8–9 years	7–8 years
Cuspid	4–5 months	12–15 years	11–12 years	9–11 years
First premolar	18–24 months	12–14 years	10–11 years	10–12 years
Second premolar	24–30 months	12–14 years	10–12 years	11–13 years
First molar	Birth	9–10 years	6–7 years	6–7 years
Second molar	2½–3 years	14–16 years	12–14 years	12–14 years
Third molar	7–10 years	18–25 years	17–25 years	17–25 years

cedure. Tooth eruption is a process associated with gingival inflammation that may be made worse as oral bacteria inoculate soft tissues surrounding the erupting tooth. Molars occasionally erupt with a tissue flap of gingiva over them, and this operculum can trap food debris and cause localized discomfort.

Since plaque forms on all teeth—including newly erupted ones—parents should be encouraged to initiate an oral hygiene program as soon as the first tooth erupts. Oral hygiene is reviewed in the section on dental caries (see below).

Abnormal Eruption

A. Precocious Eruption: Teeth present at birth are called **natal teeth,** and teeth erupting within the first month of life are called **neonatal teeth.** Their precocious eruption has been attributed to hormonal imbalances and to their development immediately below the gingival surface rather than deep in bone. They occur in about one out of 2000–3000 infants and most frequently are found in the lower incisor region. Most are the normal mandibular primary incisors, but rarely they may be extra (supernumerary) teeth. A dental radiograph is necessary to make this distinction and usually also shows very little or no root development of the erupted teeth. Natal and neonatal teeth are typically hypermobile and have

the potential of being detached. Supernumerary teeth should definitely be removed because they may be aspirated, may contribute to nursing difficulties, or may cause traumatic ulceration of the ventral surface of the tongue (Riga-Fede disease). These same concerns are present for normal primary incisors that have erupted early, but their removal may lead to later dental arch collapse. Hemostatic screening tests (see Chapter 17) should be performed before natal or neonatal teeth are removed.

B. Delayed Eruption: Premature loss of a primary tooth can cause either accelerated or delayed eruption of the underlying secondary tooth. Early eruption occurs if the permanent tooth is beginning its active eruption and the overlying primary tooth is removed. This generally occurs when the primary tooth is within 1 year of its normal time of exfoliation. If, however, loss of the primary tooth occurs more than a year from expected exfoliation, the permanent tooth will likely be delayed in its eruption, owing to healing that results in filling in of bone and gingiva over the permanent tooth. The loss of a primary tooth may cause adjacent teeth to tip into the space and impact the underlying permanent tooth. A space maintainer should be placed by a dentist to prevent this possibility.

Other local factors delaying or preventing eruption

include supernumerary teeth, cysts, tumors, over-retained primary teeth, ankylosed primary teeth, and impaction. A generalized delay in eruption may be due to endocrinopathies (hypothyroidism, hypopituitarism) or other systemic conditions (cleidocranial dysplasia, rickets, trisomy 21).

C. Ectopic Eruption: Ectopic eruption occurs if the position of an erupting tooth is abnormal. In severe instances, the order in which teeth erupt is affected. If the dental arch provides insufficient room for permanent teeth, they may erupt abnormally. In the mandible, lower incisors may be lingually placed to such an extent that the primary incisors do not exfoliate. The parents' concern about a "double row of teeth" may be the reason for the child's first dental visit. If the primary teeth are not loose, they should be removed by the dentist. If they are loose, they should be allowed to exfoliate naturally. In the maxilla, inadequate room for eruption of the permanent first molar may cause abnormal resorption of the distal root structures of the second primary molar. If the problem is severe, the permanent molar may even become caught under the unresorbed enamel crown of the deciduous molar and thus require extraction of the primary tooth and orthodontic repositioning of the permanent first molar after it has erupted. If it is not repositioned, the second premolar is likely to become impacted. If problems are detected early, the dentist may be able to redirect favorably the permanent molar's eruption pathway so that the permanent first molar correctly erupts and the second primary molar is not lost.

D. Impaction: Impaction occurs when a tooth is prevented from erupting for any reason. The teeth most often affected are the third molars and the maxillary canines. Because patients with impacted third molars are at risk for developing ameloblastomas or dentigerous cysts if these teeth are not surgically removed, the impacted third molar (along with its opposing third molar) should be removed after it has been determined that eruption will not be possible. Maxillary canines, however, should not be extracted, because of their aesthetic importance and key role in dental occlusion. They can often be brought into correct alignment through surgical exposure and orthodontic treatment.

E. Other Variations: Failure of teeth to develop—a condition sometimes called **congenitally missing teeth**—is quite rare in the primary dentition. However, it occurs in about 5% of permanent dentitions (exclusive of third molars), and one or more of the third molars is missing in about 25% of all individuals. The incidence of congenitally missing teeth varies among different genetic groups, but the most frequently missing are maxillary lateral incisors and mandibular second premolars.

Occasionally, there are **extra teeth,** most typically an extra (fourth) molar or extra (third) bicuspid. **Mesiodentes,** which are peg-shaped supernumerary teeth situated at the maxillary midline, are seen in about 5% of individuals and may interfere with eruption of permanent incisors. Mesiodentes should be considered for removal even if they do not erupt.

HYPERTROPHY OF THE MAXILLARY FRENUM

Hypertrophy of the maxillary midline frenum may appear to be the cause of spacing between central incisors. However, this spacing (diastema) is normal in primary dentition (before 6 years of age) and in mixed dentition (6–11 years of age). The flaring of all 4 maxillary permanent incisors is not abnormal and may contribute to spacing between these teeth. The frenum often appears to diminish with age as a consequence of its insertion remaining fixed while the maxilla grows vertically. Surgical intervention is indicated only if the hypertrophied frenum and diastema persist after eruption of the maxillary canines (around 12 years of age). Even after a maxillary frenectomy, orthodontic closure of the diastema may be necessary. The condition is more prevalent among blacks.

DISCOLORATION OF TEETH

Staining of teeth can occur on the outside surface of enamel (extrinsic) or within the tooth structure (intrinsic).

Certain foods and other agents taken orally can cause **extrinsic staining,** and poor oral hygiene (inadequate plaque removal) exacerbates the problem. In young children, plaque adhering to the gingival third of the teeth may take on a greenish-gray, black, or orange discoloration. Regular doses of iron can produce a tenacious black external staining. In almost all cases, professional polishing can remove the stain. If the stain reflects chronic neglect of oral hygiene, there may be areas of decalcification under the stained plaque.

Agents that can be incorporated directly into the tooth structure and cause **internal discoloration** include tetracycline, fluoride in excess amounts, bilirubin, and hemolytic breakdown products. Genetic disorders and environmental conditions affecting developing teeth can cause extra dentin to be deposited in the pulp or can cause hypoplasia or hypomineralization of enamel. Very little can be done to prevent internal discoloration due to the above causes—with the notable exception of tetracycline administration. Extreme care should be taken to avoid prescribing any form of the drug from birth until age 12 years. Pregnant women should not be treated with tetracycline, since the drug can traverse the placenta and be deposited in the calcifying teeth of the fetus. In some patients with tetracycline-stained teeth, dental bleaching procedures result in cosmetic improvement. In others, veneering or complete crowning of affected teeth may be the only satisfactory treatment.

MALOCCLUSION

Classification

Edward Angle's system for classifying molar occlusion (Fig 13–2) was developed at the beginning of this century and still serves as the foundation for describing malocclusions. In class I ("normal") occlusion, the first (mesiobuccal) cusp of the upper first permanent molar is aligned in the major (buccal) groove of the lower first permanent molar. In class II occlusion (distal occlusion), the lower molar aligns in a posterior position, usually signifying lower jaw retrognathia. In class III occlusion (mesio-occlusion), the lower molar aligns in an anterior po-

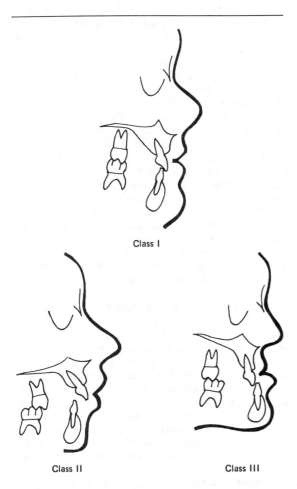

Class I

Class II   Class III

Figure 13–2. Angle's classification of malocclusion based on first permanent molar position. Facial profile is straight in class I, retrognathic in class II (receding chin), and prognathic in class III (jutting chin).

sition, usually signifying lower jaw prognathism.

Very few individuals develop an "ideal" dental occlusion or bite. Other features occurring independently or in combination can contribute to malocclusion and should be noted in the clinical description: skeletal interrelationships of the cranium and upper and lower jaws; position of teeth relative to the supporting jaws; vertical relationship of teeth (open or deep bite); spacing or crowding of teeth; position of individual teeth (rotated in any direction, overlapping, etc); muscular imbalances; and habits that may affect alignment of teeth (eg, sucking the thumb or fingers).

Management

Malocclusion does not carry with it the potential for grave consequences if left untreated. Nonetheless, most individuals want to present the best possible appearance, and measures can be taken to prevent, intercept, or correct common problems related to inadequate room for proper alignment of permanent teeth.

A. Preventive Orthodontics: The fundamental goal of preventive orthodontics is to maintain normal occlusion by detecting and treating abnormalities in the eruption and exfoliation of teeth (eg, over-retained primary teeth, ectopic eruption, extra teeth, impaction) before they contribute to malocclusion. A critical component of preventive orthodontics is the placement of space maintainers to prevent tipping of adjacent teeth into spaces left by large interproximal cavities, such as occurs when primary teeth are lost early.

The elimination of deleterious oral habits (eg, sucking the thumb, fingers, or lips; thrusting the tongue) can prevent or minimize some malocclusion problems. Thumb-sucking is not considered a serious dental problem until the maxillary permanent central incisors begin to erupt. At this point, irreversible bone movement and poor alignment of the teeth can occur. Dental appliances, myofunctional exercises, or both may help some children stop these habits, but each child should be professionally evaluated before such measures are taken.

B. Interceptive Orthodontics: Interceptive orthodontic treatment is indicated if there are factors whose elimination would result in a return to normal occlusion. The interceptive procedures produce maximum benefit for the growing child before complete establishment of the permanent dentition at about age 12 years. Some of the more common treatments include (1) restoring teeth to their proper position if they have drifted and will prevent other teeth from assuming their intended positions; (2) using headgear to move teeth or to inhibit growth of the maxilla (to allow mandibular growth to "catch up"); (3) correcting crossbites in anterior or posterior teeth; (4) eliminating pernicious oral habits; (5) sequentially extracting certain primary teeth or reducing their width to allow space for erupting permanent teeth; and (6) directing forces to counter undesirable jaw relationships that may be developing.

Various mechanical appliances can be used to change the position of the teeth, jaws, or oral musculature. Traditional orthodontic braces, extraoral appliances (eg, headgear), or removable acrylic appliances with orthodontic wires can be used successfully to make minor tooth movements. In the USA, there is a developing popularity for the use of a functional appliance that evolved in Europe after World War II. Bands around teeth have generally been supplanted by plastic brackets bonded to the teeth with resin.

C. Corrective Orthodontics: It is preferable to prevent or intercept developing malocclusion, but this is not always possible. Some children do not have the benefit of preventive services at the most effective time, and others have sufficiently severe problems that can only be treated by corrective orthodontics.

Corrective orthodontics employs many of the treatment methods used in interceptive orthodontics, but treatment is more aggressive and comprehensive. In many instances, all teeth will require treatment. In some patients with small dental arches, there may not be sufficient area to accommodate the permanent teeth. Extraction of permanent teeth is becoming increasingly controversial, and strategies to expand dental arches without extraction are gaining popularity.

DENTAL CARIES

Dental caries is one of the most common infectious diseases. It affects both primary and permanent dentitions and can occur at any age. The disease is characterized by decalcification of the tooth, beginning with the enamel and progressing to the dentin and pulp, and can cause severe tooth pain and abscess formation.

The initiation of dental caries requires 3 factors: (1) acidogenic bacteria, eg, *Streptococcus mutans;* (2) a source of nutrient carbohydrate, usually sugar; and (3) a tooth that is susceptible to decalcification. Research has identified a genetic component to dental caries, but the infectious nature of the disease makes environment far more significant than heredity.

The human body's natural protection against dental caries rests mainly in the saliva. Immunoglobulins, minerals, and the cleansing effect of saliva contribute some degree of natural resistance. The process involved is described as remineralization, a dynamic equilibrium in which new carious lesions are constantly developing and being arrested by the action of saliva. Low levels of fluoride seem to push the equilibrium to the side of recalcification.

Prevention

Public health measures such as water fluoridation, improved access to care, better public education, and better diets have caused a general decrease in the rate of caries in children and adolescents. A vaccine against caries is currently being developed, but large-scale human application is far in the future.

A. Oral Hygiene: Oral hygiene is directed at removing plaque from teeth before it becomes cariogenic. The bacteria in plaque require 18–24 hours to produce acid to decalcify teeth.

Parents should be encouraged to start cleaning the child's teeth as soon as they erupt. A toothbrush and toothpaste are not necessary, because a washcloth, piece of cotton gauze, or cotton-tipped applicator is adequate for wiping away plaque on newly erupted teeth. Subsequent tooth cleaning is best done with a soft toothbrush, and parents should take responsibility for tooth cleaning until the child demonstrates proficiency. A basic scrub technique suffices for primary dentition and mixed dentition, and its aim is mechanical removal of plaque and gentle stimulation of gingivae. Whether or not a child's teeth should be flossed will depend on the presence of interdental caries, tight contact between teeth, and the efficacy of toothbrushing alone for that child. Flossing removes plaque between teeth where toothbrush bristles cannot reach. Parents should assist in flossing because a child may not have the desire to floss or the dexterity to prevent injury to gingivae.

Irrigating devices ("water picks") tend to remove loose food debris but not plaque. Therefore, they are of limited value for tooth cleaning in children. Gingival damage has been noted when irrigation devices are used improperly with the spray directed into the gingival sulci. They may be a useful adjunct to regular brushing procedures in individuals wearing orthodontic appliances.

Devices to clean teeth can be adapted with extensions or special grips to meet the individual needs of the physically handicapped child. Adult participation is crucial to success.

Toothbrushing is mainly responsible for the removal of plaque. Dentifrice itself plays a minor role in tooth cleaning in the young child, but the fluoride in it is beneficial. Some children find the taste of toothpaste offensive. The preparation used should be one approved by the American Dental Association, should contain fluoride to provide maximal topical benefit, and should be pleasant-tasting to encourage the child to brush. Since toothpaste is often ingested by young children, only a small amount is recommended for brushing. Regular professional cleaning is recommended when calculus (tartar) or stain develops on the teeth.

B. Diet and Nutrition: Removal or lessening of carbohydrate substrate prevents bacteria from producing the mucopolysaccharides that form plaque and the acid that decalcifies teeth. Studies in animals have shown that dental caries cannot occur without fermentable carbohydrate. Although no consistent relationship exists between the total amount of carbohydrate consumed and the rate of caries, research has demonstrated that the frequency of carbohydrate ingestion, the consistency of the carbohydrate ingested (eg, stickiness, liquid form), and the timing of carbohydrate ingestion in relation to ingestion of other foods are important factors in the process of caries formation.

A nutritious diet of essential nutrients contributes to the development of healthy teeth and helps prevent caries. Control of refined carbohydrate in the diet is the major aspect of dietary control of dental caries. Restriction of the amount of sugar consumed is a general dietary goal. Several aspects of controlled sugar intake benefit dental health: (1) Decreasing the frequency of carbohydrate ingestion reduces the number of exposures of oral plaque to fermentable substrate and consequently reduces the time teeth are exposed to acid. (2) Ingestion of liquid rather than solid or sticky carbohydrate allows more rapid clearance of sugar from the oral cavity. (3) If carbohydrate ingestion is followed by brushing the teeth, by drinking noncariogenic liquids, or by eating fibrous foods, the time teeth are exposed to acid is decreased. (4) Control of carbohydrate intake by changes in the way these foods are consumed rather than by food substitution is preferred in children, because alternative snacks or foods may be high in sodium, fat, and artificial additives. Current nutritional counseling should approach sugar restriction with attention to overall diet, energy requirements, family resources, and cooperation of the parents and child.

C. Fluoride: Fluoride is the single most effective anticariogenic measure known. It has 3 important mechanisms of action: (1) its incorporation into the developing tooth's enamel, which makes apatite more resistant to acid demineralization by bacteria; (2) its interference in bacterial metabolism; and (3) its enhancement of remineralization, which arrests developing carious lesions. Systemic fluoride can benefit children while teeth are developing, and topical fluoride is helpful after teeth have erupted.

1. Systemic fluoride—Fluoride contained in water, food, and prescribed supplements is absorbed in the blood and distributed to the bones and developing teeth. Fluoride is deposited in the enamel as fluorapatite, which has a greater resistance to acid demineralization.

Both primary and permanent dentitions benefit from systemic fluoride. Fluoride present in water at a level of 0.7–1.2 parts per million (ppm) is considered optimal. There is no proved efficacy of prenatal fluoride therapy, in which a pregnant woman ingests fluoride to benefit her child's primary dentition; therefore, this is not an accepted procedure. Fluoride supplementation in children can begin at birth or as late as 6 months of age to provide protection to the primary and permanent teeth. The average child requires a fluoride intake of 0.05 mg/kg/d for fluoride to provide maximum benefit. If the child's water supply provides less than 0.7 ppm of fluoride, supplementation should be considered.

Table 13–2 shows supplemental fluoride dosage recommendations for children under 15 years of age. At 15 years, systemic fluoride is no longer considered beneficial. As indicated in the table, dosages are based on the level of fluoride in the local water. Well water or water from municipal supplies of unknown fluoride content should be tested by a public health department or private laboratory. Breast-fed infants and infants receiving premixed formula (formula not made to be mixed with tap water) should be assumed to be receiving no fluoride. The appropriate form of supplemental fluoride (vitamin-fluoride compound, tablet, or drop) is based on the child's age and life-style. Supplementation should be reassessed annually.

2. Topical fluoride—Topical fluoride benefits teeth as long as they are subject to decay. Dentifrice and water containing fluoride, foods processed or prepared with fluoridated water, and topical fluoride treatment all help reduce susceptibility to dental caries. Factors to be considered in determining the need for professionally applied fluoride treatments include the child's overall fluoride exposure, extent of dental caries, and presence of risk factors such as a handicapping condition or orthodontic appliances. The combination of topical and systemic fluoride treatment offers increased protection against dental caries.

Over-the-counter topical fluoride rinses can also supplement a systemic treatment program. Inadvertent ingestion of these products and fluoridated dentifrices can result in fluorosis, a white or brown in-

Table 13–2. Supplemental fluoride dosage recommendations.[1]

Fluoride Content of Drinking Water	Dosage of Oral Fluoride		
	Age 0–2 Years	Age 2–3 Years	Age 3–14 Years
< 0.3 ppm	0.25 mg/d	0.5 mg/d	1 mg/d
0.3–0.7 ppm	0 mg/d	0.25 mg/d	0.5 mg/d

[1]Approved by the American Academy of Pediatrics and the American Dental Association. Fluoride supplementation is unnecessary if the fluoride content of drinking water is over 0.7 ppm or if the patient is 15 years of age or older.

trinsic staining of teeth. A dentist should be consulted to determine the fluoride program for a child, based on all sources of fluoride.

D. Sealants: Sealants are plastic coatings designed to be applied by dental professionals on newly erupted or caries-susceptible teeth, usually recently erupted permanent or primary molars and permanent premolars. They are applied to the pits and fissures of the biting surfaces of teeth, which are areas in which fluoride has little effect. Sealants form a barrier to bacterial penetration. Ten-year follow-up studies have shown a high rate of protection. The decision to apply sealant to a tooth should be based on the child's susceptibility to caries, the length of time the tooth has been in the mouth, and the presence of decay on other surfaces of the tooth.

Diagnosis & Treatment

A. Specific Types of Dental Caries: Dental caries can occur any time after eruption of the first primary tooth. "Baby Bottle Tooth Decay" is caused by prolonged access to the bottle, usually at night or nap time. The carbohydrate-containing liquid (milk, formula, carbonated beverage, or fruit juice) pools on the teeth and is metabolized by bacteria to form acid. The decreased saliva flow and the oral muscular activity during sleep contribute to the process. Oral hygiene practices are often lacking. Characteristically, maxillary primary incisors are decayed (with or without abscesses) and mandibular anterior teeth minimally affected. Tooth cleaning, topical fluoride application, restoration or extraction of teeth, and sedation or general anesthesia may be needed to treat the infant. Prevention of "Baby Bottle Tooth Decay" involves either eliminating use of the bottle at night and nap time or substituting water for other liquids in the bottle.

Incipient (beginning) caries involves the early decalcification of enamel. Opaque white areas are the result of changes in the light-transmitting qualities of enamel. Incipient caries often occurs at the gum line under long-standing plaque. Good hygiene and fluoride application can often stop the process before cavitation occurs.

Rampant caries is characterized by rapidly progressing tooth decay in a child or adolescent who may have been free of or minimally affected in the past. The teeth are often cavitated or decayed to the alveolar ridge. Painful abscesses may be present. The dentin is often soft, indicating active decay. Therapy involves extensive restoration, pulpal treatment, dietary measures, and fluoride supplementation.

Radiation caries can occur in children who have head and neck neoplasia and have undergone irradiation of salivary glands. The decay pattern is much like rampant decay. These children should receive care by a dentist prior to irradiation, then careful follow-up.

Caries associated with bulimia is a generalized process that often results in enamel erosion due to regurgitation of acidic stomach contents. Teeth may have a frosted rather than glossy look and may appear to be ground down. There may be gingival recession and areas of dark tooth decay, frequently at the gum line. Treatment is often difficult; therefore, prevention is critical.

B. General Guidelines for Dental Referral: Dark staining of grooves, large accumulations of plaque with or without white decalcification, dark pits, and a history of discomfort to hot, cold, or sweets suggest caries. Frank cavitation, destruction of crowns of teeth, gingival swelling, significant and prolonged pain with or without facial swelling, and broken fillings indicate the need for professional dental attention.

The prognosis for untreated dental caries is poor. Some carious lesions may turn black as exposed dentin picks up food stains. Most often, the caries process progresses to the pulp of the tooth, causing pain, pulpitis, abscess, and loss of the tooth through coronal destruction or extraction.

Secondary prevention involves early intervention by a dental professional. Professional pediatric organizations recommend an initial preventive and educational visit within 6 months of eruption of the first primary tooth, especially if the child has known or suspected developmental delays, lives in a community without fluoridated water, or has a family history of poor dental health. Data indicate that up to 50% of 2-year-olds have some tooth decay, so an initial exam by 18–24 months of age should be beneficial.

The dentist's treatment of dental caries has remained essentially the same, with use of silver amalgam, steel crowns, and plastic fillings as the main elements. Current data support the safety of mercury–silver amalgam as a filling material. Tooth-colored composite resins can also be used for some anterior and posterior teeth; prior to bonding them, the tooth surface is treated with mild acid, which creates microscopic porosities that aid in the binding process.

TOOTHACHE

The most common cause of toothache is pulpal stimulation due to dentin exposure or direct pulpal exposure secondary to dental caries. In some cases, pain is related to infection in the space between the tooth and supporting bone. Toothache secondary to caries or periodontal infection is usually accompanied by one or more of the following: swelling of adjacent gingival tissues, purulence from the gingival sulcus, mobility, elevation from the socket, and a large cavity. If these are lacking, the physician or dentist should suspect a traumatic injury, either chronic (eg, bruxism, or grinding of teeth) or acute (eg, a blow to the teeth); systemic illness; sinusitis; neoplasia; or referred pain. In children, most tooth pain is related to dental caries and subsequent infection.

TRAUMATIC INJURIES

Traumatic injuries to the primary and permanent teeth of children often cause the immediate problems of pain and hemorrhage and can cause long-term sequelae, including loss of damaged teeth, malposition of injured primary teeth or their permanent successors, discoloration of the crowns of injured teeth (due to hemolytic pigments), destruction of the enamel of permanent successors to injured primary teeth, delayed exfoliation of the primary teeth, and possible displacement of an underlying permanent tooth bud.

Factors of concern in cases of traumatic injury are whether the affected teeth are primary or permanent, the type of injury, the time elapsed since the injury occurred, and whether or not any treatment was rendered in that interim. Injuries may involve the teeth or the alveolar bone and tooth-supporting structures. In traumatic injuries, the physician should render immediate care to ensure retention of the teeth (Table 13–3) and make an appropriate dental referral.

Tooth injuries most often involve some type of fracture of the crown, with or without exposure of pulp. When pulpal tissues are exposed, time becomes an important element in management. The longer the pulpal tissues are exposed to the environment, the more likely it is that necrosis and death of the pulp will occur and result in ultimate loss of the tooth. Referral is urgent in these cases.

Injuries that involve dislocation or avulsion of the tooth from the socket are even more urgent. As time elapses, repositioning of dislocated teeth becomes more difficult owing to swelling and clot formation. Although an intruded tooth should be repositioned only by the dentist, other dislocated teeth should be repositioned immediately and stabilized.

An avulsed permanent tooth should be treated as an emergency because immediate reinsertion is critical to saving the tooth. The tooth should be located, placed in the socket, and stabilized until the patient can reach a dentist. Stabilization can be achieved by having the patient bite on a piece of gauze or by having the patient or someone else hold the tooth in the proper position. If the tooth cannot be reinserted owing to poor visibility or the presence of foreign material, it should be placed in milk, saliva, or normal saline solution and then transported with the patient to the dentist. Under no circumstances should the tooth be washed or scrubbed prior to reimplantation. Cleaning should be confined to gentle rinsing in an isotonic solution. Critical to successful reimplantation is maintenance of the viability of the cells on the root surface, and cleaning the root with other than osmotically neutral fluid causes death of these cells.

Reimplantation of primary teeth is usually not recommended. It is difficult to keep the reinserted tooth stable in a young child; thus, reimplantation is unsuccessful.

Antibiotics are not usually required for reimplantation and do not appear to affect the outcome of reimplantation when they are used for other related injuries.

GINGIVAL & PERIODONTAL CONDITIONS

Gingivitis & Periodontitis

Gingivitis is caused by accumulations of plaque and is a common condition in children, especially when oral hygiene is poor. The disease is by definition confined to soft tissues and does not involve loss of alveolar bone supporting the teeth. Clinical findings include redness around the gingival margins

Table 13–3. Management of traumatic injuries of the teeth and supporting bone.

	Tooth Fracture	Tooth Dislocation or Avulsion
Primary teeth	**No pulp exposed:** Refer to dentist within 24 hours. **Pulp exposed:** Refer to dentist immediately.	**Intrusion:** Do not reposition the tooth. Refer to dentist immediately. **Dislocation:** Reposition the tooth and refer to dentist immediately. **Avulsion:** Do not reinsert the tooth. Refer to dentist immediately.
Permanent teeth	**No pulp exposed:** Refer to dentist within 24 hours. **Pulp exposed:** Refer to dentist immediately.	**Intrusion:** Do not reposition the tooth. Refer to dentist immediately. **Dislocation:** Reposition the tooth and refer to dentist immediately. **Avulsion:** Either (1) reinsert the tooth and refer to dentist immediately; or (2) place the tooth in milk, saliva, or normal saline solution and transport it with the patient to the dentist (urgent).

and swelling of the interdental papillae. The disease can occur at any age and does not necessarily progress to periodontitis.

Periodontitis is an infection of the supporting periodontal ligament and bone. Unlike gingivitis, which is reversible with improved hygiene, periodontitis causes irreversible destruction of tissues. Young children are rarely affected by periodontitis. Prepubescent children with **juvenile periodontitis** have rapid and severe loss of supporting bone, usually around permanent molars and incisors. *Actinobacillus actinomycetemcomitans* is thought to be the cause. Diagnosis without radiographs is difficult, because the bone destruction occurs below the gingival margin and inflammation is often lacking. Teeth may or may not be loose.

Both gingivitis and periodontitis are considered infections, and both are caused by bacterial plaque, which produces toxins that destroy tissue. Thus, prevention and treatment are based on removal of the bacterial plaque and calculus (tartar) and institution of good oral hygiene practices (tooth cleaning, gingival stimulation, and flossing). In cases of juvenile periodontitis, tetracycline is prescribed. Some patients with periodontitis also require surgery to remove the diseased tissue and restore tissue to its normal contour so that plaque is less likely to accumulate. The teeth may need to be splinted together for support.

Acute Necrotizing Ulcerative Gingivitis

Acute necrotizing ulcerative gingivitis, also called trench mouth, is thought to be caused by spirochete-fusiform symbiosis. The classic signs and symptoms are fetid breath, pain, and necrotic desquamation of interdental gingival papillae with pseudomembrane formation over the areas of destruction. The infection is often related to stress and tends to occur in the adolescent age group. Treatment consists of gentle debridement of affected tissues and administration of an antibiotic such as penicillin. Oxygenating agents applied topically can also help. Acute necrotizing ulcerative gingivitis can be differentiated from herpetic stomatitis by its odor and classic lesions and by its predilection for older children.

Premature Bone Loss

Bone loss in primary dentition is a rare occurrence. If primary teeth become loose well ahead of their scheduled exfoliation, the following causes should be considered: mercury poisoning, radiation toxicity, juvenile periodontitis, Papillon-Lefèvre syndrome, scurvy, acatalasia, hypophosphatasia, diabetes mellitus, Gaucher's disease, leukemia, neutropenia, histiocytosis X, Wiskott-Aldrich syndrome, and neutrophil dysfunction.

OTHER INTRAORAL LESIONS

A **mucocele** is a benign whitish or light blue swelling that most often occurs on the lower lip but is sometimes seen on the palate, cheek, or floor of the mouth. The lesion, which indicates a blocked minor salivary gland, can rupture and re-form. Treatment is excision.

A **parulis,** or **gumboil,** is the intraoral manifestation of a periapical (pulpal) infection of a tooth. The parulis is the site of fistulation of an abscess at the root tip, which is usually either the result of dental caries that has progressed to the pulp and caused its necrosis or the consequence of a traumatic injury. The lesion can appear as a finely pointed white pimple or a larger yellowish-red elevation, usually on the buccal gingiva at a level approximating the location of the tooth's root. The adjacent tooth often has a large cavity. The parulis may or may not be associated with gingival swelling, pain, or tooth mobility, depending on its duration. Treatment is directed at the offending infection.

An **eruption cyst** is a purple swelling (hematoma) that occurs over the crown of an erupting tooth. Tooth eruption is accompanied by the rupture of small vessels that hemorrhage into the eruption capsule. No treatment is needed, because the cyst will resolve spontaneously.

Gingival overgrowth is common in children whose seizure disorders are being treated with phenytoin. The growth represents both hypertrophy and hyperplasia of gingival cells. Although the response to phenytoin therapy is variable, children tend to have more overgrowth than adults do. Meticulous oral hygiene may lessen the extent of overgrowth, but discontinuance of the medication is the only sure way to prevent it. Surgery is required to remove excess tissue.

Cellulitis of the face can result from disseminated tooth abscess and should be treated with antibiotics. Extraction of the offending tooth may also be indicated. Hot packs to the face are contraindicated because they may cause external pointing of the abscess and result in scarring. Untreated cellulitis can progress to a more severe problem such as brain abscess, cavernous sinus thrombosis, or Ludwig's angina.

SELECTED REFERENCES

American Dental Association: *Accepted Dental Therapeutics,* 40th ed. American Dental Association, 1984.

Andreasen JO: *Traumatic Injuries to the Teeth,* 2nd ed. Saunders, 1981.

Baer PN, Benjamin SD: *Periodontal Disease in Children and Adolescents.* Lippincott, 1974.

McDonald RE: *Dentistry for the Child and Adolescent,* 5th ed. Mosby, 1987.

Moyers RE: *Handbook of Orthodontics,* 4th ed. Year Book, 1988.

Pinkham JR (editor): *Pediatric Dentistry: Infancy Through Adolescence.* Saunders, 1988. ,

Proffit WR: *Contemporary Orthodontics.* Mosby, 1986.

Stewart RE, Barber TK (editors): *Pediatric Dentistry.* Mosby, 1981.

Wei SHY: *Pediatric Dentistry: Total Patient Care.* Lea & Febiger, 1988.

14

Ear, Nose, & Throat

Stephen Berman, MD, & Barton D. Schmitt, MD

THE EAR: DISEASES & DISORDERS

OTITIS MEDIA

Otitis media, defined as an inflammation of the middle ear, is usually associated with an effusion or collection of fluid in the middle ear space. Otitis media with effusion is classified by its duration (acute if present < 6 weeks; subacute if present from 6 weeks to 3 months; and chronic if present > 3 months) and by the characteristics of the effusion. The effusion is purulent in acute otitis media, is a transudate in serous otitis media, and is thick and tenacious in mucoid (secretory) otitis media. Chronic effusions may be purulent, serous, or mucoid, and it is often difficult to identify the type of effusion by otoscopy. Chronic effusions may develop by multiple pathways. The purulent effusion of acute otitis media may persist through the subacute phase or may evolve into a serous or mucoid effusion. Serous effusions may persist, evolve into mucoid effusions, or become reinfected and present as another episode of acute purulent otitis media. Mucoid effusions generally persist but can also become reinfected.

In clinical practice, about one-fourth of the pediatrician's time is spent in the diagnosis and management of otitis media. By the time children reach 3 years of age, more than two-thirds of them have experienced one episode of otitis media, and one-third have had 3 or more episodes. More children present with otitis media in the winter months, when respiratory syncytial virus and other viruses are present in the community. These upper respiratory tract infections adversely affect **auditory tube** function and predispose the child to middle ear effusion. Since young children have shorter, more compliant and more horizontally placed auditory tubes than older children and adults, colds in young patients will produce more severe auditory tube dysfunction. This dysfunction prevents middle ear secretions from draining and results in negative pressure in the middle ear space. Negative pressure predisposes the patient to periodic aspiration of contaminated nasopharyngeal secretions, which causes bacterial infection.

The diagnosis of otitis media with effusion is based on specific otoscopic findings, which include the appearance of the tympanic membrane and an assessment of its mobility. In recent years, tympanometry has also become a useful technique in documenting middle ear effusions in children and infants older than 7 months. Unfortunately, it does not identify early acute otitis media prior to the development of an effusion. In pediatric practice, tympanometry is useful for screening patients uncooperative to examination, clarifying questionable otoscopic findings, and providing an objective measurement to follow the course of persistent effusions. Otoscopy and tympanometry are discussed on p. 327.

Bluestone CD: State of the art: Definitions and classifications. In: *Proceedings of the Third International Symposium: Recent Advances in Otitis Media With Effusion.* Lim DJ (editor). Decker & Co., 1984.

Henderson FW et al: A longitudinal study of respiratory viruses and bacteria in the etiology of acute otitis media with effusion. *N Engl J Med* 1982;**306:**1377.

Howie VM, Schwartz RH: Acute otitis media: One year in general pediatric practice. *Am J Dis Child* 1982;**137:** 155.

1. ACUTE OTITIS MEDIA

Essentials of Diagnosis
- Earache.
- Ear discharge.
- Red, bulging, immobile tympanic membrane.

General Considerations
Bacteriologic findings in middle ear aspirates can be summarized as follows: *Streptococcus pneumoniae,* 30% of cases; *Haemophilus influenzae,* 21%; *Morexella catarrhalis,* 12%; group A streptococci, 3%; *Staphylococcus aureus,* 2%; and others (including enteric gram-negative organisms and anaerobic organisms), 4%. In 20% of cases, aspirates are sterile, and 18% grow presumed nonpathogens such as *Staphylococcus epidermidis* and diphtheroids.

Recently, *M catarrhalis* has been more commonly recognized as a causative agent of acute purulent otitis media. *H influenzae* remains an important pathogen in cases throughout childhood and into early adulthood. In many areas, the prevalence of β-lactamase-producing isolates for *H influenzae* is 30%; that for *M catarrhalis* is 80%. These findings indicate that 1 in 4 cases of acute otitis will be resistant to amoxicillin.

Attempts to isolate respiratory viruses or *Mycoplasma pneumoniae* from ear aspirates have generally been unsuccessful. However, using enzyme-linked immunosorbent assay (ELISA) techniques, investigators have reported that viral antigens (usually of respiratory syncytial virus) are identified in one-fourth of 53 cases of acute purulent otitis media.

In about 5% of cases, multiple pathogens are isolated from a single specimen of middle ear effusion. In children with bilateral acute otitis media, different pathogens can be recovered from each ear in 5–10% of cases.

The microbiologic causes of acute otitis media in early infancy differ from those in later life. The risk of gram-negative enteric infection is especially high in infants who are under 6 weeks of age and have been hospitalized in a neonatal intensive care nursery. In normal infants seen during the first 3 months of life, acute otitis media can often be caused by *S aureus* and *Chlamydia trachomatis*, as well as *S pneumoniae*, *H influenzae*, and *B catarrhalis*.

Clinical Findings

A. Symptoms and Signs: Acute otitis media often presents with pain in association with symptoms of upper respiratory tract infection (eg, rhinorrhea, stuffy nose, and cough) or purulent conjunctivitis. While older children may complain of earache, young children demonstrate pain by crying, increased irritability, or difficulty in sleeping. Irritability may be related to hearing loss as well as pain. Tugging at the ears, is often falsely positive. Fever is present in less than half of cases. Facial palsy or ataxia may occur in the rare case.

The tympanic membrane appears either red or yellow, depending on the degree of inflammation and the amount of purulent material in the middle ear space. White exudate may be visible on the membrane. In early cases, bulging may be limited to the pars flaccida. Later, the entire eardrum bulges outward, giving a doughnutlike appearance. Tympanic membrane mobility is absent or markedly diminished. If the eardrum has spontaneously ruptured, cloudy to purulent discharge will be present in the ear canal, making examination of the tympanic membrane difficult. Cerumen that has melted with high fever or tears and is present in the ear canal can cause confusion with middle ear discharge.

Occasionally, bullae form between the outer and middle layers of the tympanic membrane and produce acute bullous myringitis. This entity should be considered a form of acute purulent otitis media and is described in detail in the next section.

B. Laboratory Findings: Nasopharyngeal and throat cultures are not useful, because *S pneumoniae* and nontypeable *H influenzae* are often present in well children and thus of no significance. If perforation has occurred, it may be useful to culture the discharge, using a nasopharyngeal culture swab. If the discharge has been present for over 8 hours, the likelihood of demonstrating the organism is small, because it frequently is overgrown with saprophytes.

Beyond the neonatal period, acute otitis media infrequently presents with signs of systemic toxicity; therefore, blood cultures, urine culture, and lumbar puncture are indicated in the child with acute purulent otitis media who also appears toxic or has signs of meningeal irritation.

Differential Diagnosis

Not all earaches are caused by acute otitis media. Mumps, toothaches, otitis externa, a foreign body in the ear canal, an ear canal furuncle, ear canal trauma, hard cerumen, and temporomandibular joint dysfunction, can all present with a chief complaint of earache. Injected vessels at the drum periphery and along the malleus are frequently overdiagnosed as "early otitis media." An injected tympanic membrane as well as a flushed face can occur with fever or crying. Cleaning wax from the ear canal can cause reactive hyperemia of the same vessels. Such an eardrum may be red, but it will be mobile and not require treatment. Because acute otitis media is the most common complication of a cold, an infant with a cold and fever should never be sent home without examination of the eardrums. Cerumen removal (see below) will often be necessary.

Complications

The most common complication associated with acute otitis media is a hearing loss of 20–35 dB, which may persist for several months. The tympanic membrane may rupture spontaneously because of pressure necrosis and produce a sizable perforation. Acute otitis media may also cause labyrinthitis and ataxia, facial paralysis, cholesteatoma, mastoiditis, ossicular necrosis, pseudotumor cerebri (otitic hydrocephalus), or cerebral thrombophlebitis.

Treatment

An algorithm for the management of acute purulent otitis media is shown in Fig 14–1.

A. Specific Measures:

1. Systemic antibiotics—In areas where β-lactamase-producing pathogens are common, the initial treatment for acute otitis media should be 10 days of trimethoprim, 10 mg/kg/d, with sulfamethoxazole, in 2 divided doses; or erythromycin, 40 mg/kg/d, plus sulfisoxazole, in 4 divided doses. Otherwise, the drug of choice for acute otitis media in children of all ages is amoxicillin, 50 mg/kg/d in 3 divided doses, continued for 10 days.

Patients allergic to penicillin can be treated ade-

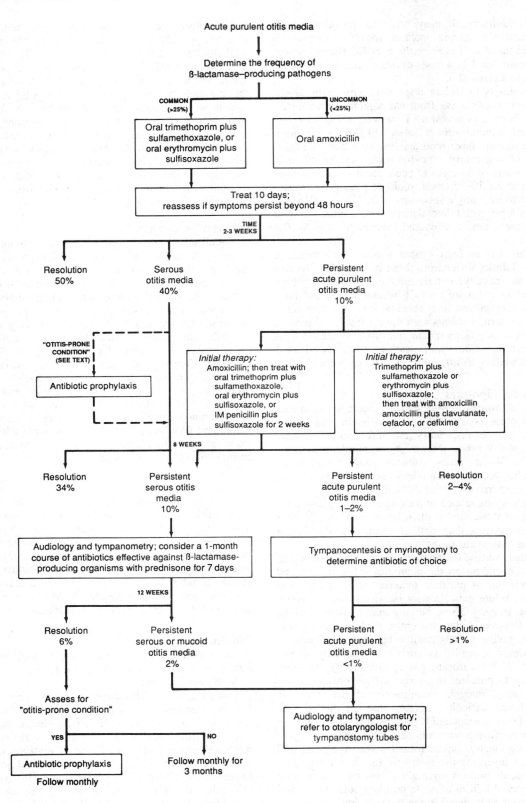

Figure 14–1. Algorithm for the management of otitis media with effusion. For prophylaxis in children with recurrent acute purulent otitis media, see text.

quately with erythromycin plus sulfisoxazole or with trimethoprim plus sulfamethoxazole. Tetracyclines are contraindicated for ear infections because about 50% of pneumococci and streptococci are resistant to these drugs and because they cause staining of the tooth enamel. Trimethoprim prescribed in combination with sulfamethoxazole is not effective against *Streptococcus pyogenes* and should not be used if there is a suspected streptococcal pharyngitis.

If symptoms such as fever, earache, irritability, vomiting, or lethargy persist beyond 48 hours of therapy, the patient should be reevaluated. After 2–3 weeks, about 50% of children are cured, 40% still have residual middle ear effusion, and 10% still have persistent acute infection. Teele (1981), reported that the majority (57%) of children who failed to respond after 36–48 hours of initial therapy with either amoxicillin, trimethoprim plus sulfamethoxazole, or erythromycin plus sulfisoxazole had sterile effusions. Organisms resistant to initial therapy were identified in 19% of repeated cultures of middle ear aspirates. Resistant isolates from children initially treated with amoxicillin were sensitive to trimethoprim plus sulfamethoxazole or erythromycin plus sulfisoxazole and vice versa. Children with an infection that persists after a 10-day course of amoxicillin should receive a full 14-day course of trimethoprim plus sulfamethoxazole or erythromycin plus sulfisoxazole. If the physician is concerned about compliance, the patient can be treated with an intramuscular injection of penicillin G benzathine and procaine combined (Bicillin C-R) and oral sulfisoxazole. Children with an infection that persists after a course of trimethoprim plus sulfamethoxazole should receive amoxicillin, cefaclor 40 mg/kg/d in 3 divided doses, amoxicillin plus clavulanate 40mg/kg/d in 3 divided doses, or cefixime (8 mg/kg/d, in 1 or 2 divided doses).

If the acute symptomatic infection still persists after this second course of antibiotics, myringotomy or tympanocentesis should be performed and middle ear secretions cultured to determine the most appropriate antibiotic therapy. Failure of acute otitis media to resolve after a third course of antibiotic therapy requires referral to an otolaryngologist for possible placement of tympanostomy tubes.

Acute otitis media in infants less than 6 weeks of age with a complicated neonatal course requiring prolonged hospitalization is often caused by gram-negative enteric organisms. These infants require tympanocentesis, blood culture, and a lumbar puncture and should receive intravenous ampicillin plus either gentamicin or cefotaxime in the hospital pending culture results. Acute otitis in infants under 3 months without additional risk factors or signs of serious illness can be treated on an outpatient basis with erythromycin plus sulfamethoxazole, cefaclor, or amoxicillin plus clavulanate (Augmentin). These children should be reexamined at 24 and 48 hours. If their condition worsens during this time period, they should be hospitalized. Infants who present with systemic symptoms or who fail to respond to outpatient management require tympanocentesis, blood culture, and usually a lumbar puncture. Ampicillin plus either gentamicin or cefotaxime should be initiated pending results of culture.

2. Antibiotic ear drops—If the eardrum has been perforated, there is usually a cloudy to watery material in the ear canal, and antibiotic ear drops are not required. However, the child with considerable purulent drainage from the ear may profit from this adjunctive therapy. The purulent material can be removed by gentle suction, using a syringe and a short plastic tubing such as can be made by cutting a scalp vein needle set. Normal saline solution can be instilled without force and then removed. After this type of cleansing has eliminated the pus, antibiotic-corticosteroid ear drops (eg, Cortisporin Otic suspension) can be instilled 3 times a day. The child should be held with head sideways and stationary for a few minutes after drops are instilled. Cotton plugs are contraindicated.

B. General Measures:

1. Analgesics and antipyretics—An irritable child with an earache requires acetaminophen or even codeine in order to sleep through the first night while on treatment. Young children can be given codeine, 0.5 mg/kg/dose, up to 4 times a day. Codeine is available in several cough medicines in a concentration of 10 mg/tsp. Antipyretics for fever control may be required during the first 1 or 2 days.

2. Oral decongestants—Antihistamine-decongestant combinations are ineffective in the treatment of otitis media.

3. Reassurance—Some parents are overly concerned about ear infections and their complications. Reassurance should be given as required. There is little danger of permanent hearing loss as long as the prescribed medicines are taken as directed. The child can be allowed to go outside, and the ears need not be covered. Mountain travel is permitted. Swimming is permitted if perforation is not present.

4. Unwarranted measures—Vasoconstrictor nose drops are of no value, because it is nearly impossible to deliver them to the entrance of the auditory tube. Analgesic ear drops have not proved effective for the relief of pain and have the disadvantage of obscuring the field of vision if the tympanic membrane needs to be reexamined.

C. Myringotomy and Tympanocentesis: A common pitfall in therapy is not performing myringotomy or tympanocentesis when it is indicated (see p 324). In a child with an acutely bulging eardrum, myringotomy is indicated if the patient has severe pain (as evidenced by inconsolable screaming) or if recurrent vomiting or ataxia is associated with the ear infection. In these circumstances, myringotomy is more effective than analgesics or antiemetics. Unfortunately, myringotomy does not appear to prevent the development of persistent residual effusions.

Prognosis

With treatment, suppurative complications such as mastoiditis are rare. Temporary hearing loss is common, permanent conductive hearing loss is less common, and permanent sensorineural hearing loss is rare.

Berman SA, Balkany TJ, Simmons MA: Otitis media in infants less than 12 weeks of age: Differing bacteriology among in-patients and out-patients. *J Pediatr* 1978; **93:**453.

Berman SA, Lauer BA: A controlled trial of cefaclor versus amoxicillin for treatment of acute otitis media in early infancy. *Pediatr Infect Dis* 1983;**2:**30.

Bluestone CD: Management of otitis media in infants and children: Current role of old and new antimicrobial agents. *Pediatr Infect Dis J* 1988;**7:**512.

Blumer JL, Bertino JS, Husak MP: Comparison of cefaclor and trimethoprim-sulfamethoxazole in the treatment of acute otitis media. *Pediatr Infect Dis* 1984;**3:**25.

Boder FF: Conjunctivitis-otitis syndrome. *Pediatrics* 1982;**69:**695.

Cantekin EI et al: Lack of efficacy of a decongestant-antihistamine combination for otitis media with effusion in children. *N Engl J Med* 1983;**308:**297.

Chang MJ et al: *Chlamydia trachomatis* in otitis media in children. *Pediatr Infect Dis* 1982;**1:**95.

Harrison CJ, Marks MI, Welch PF: Microbiology of recently treated acute otitis media compared with previously untreated acute otitis media. *Pediatr Infect Dis J* 1985;**4:**61.

Klein BS, Dollete FR, Yolken RH: The role of respiratory syncytial virus and other viral pathogens in acute otitis media. *J Pediatr* 1982;**101:**16.

Marchant CD et al: A randomized controlled trial of amoxicillin plus clavulanate compared with cefaclor for treatment of acute otitis media. *J Pediatr* 1986;**109:**891.

Marchant CD et al: A randomized controlled trial of cefaclor compared to trimethoprim-sulfamethoxazole for treatment of acute otitis media. *J Pediatr* 1984;**105:**63.

Odio CM et al: Comparative treatment trial of Augmentin versus cefaclor for acute otitis media with effusion. *Pediatrics* 1985;**75:**819.

Rodriguez WJ et al: Erythromycin-sulfisoxazole for persistent acute otitis media due to ampicillin-resistant *Haemophilus influenzae*. *Pediatr Infect Dis* 1983;**2:**27.

Schaefer C et al: Illnesses in infants born to women with *Chlamydia trachomatis* infection. *Am J Dis Child* 1985;**139:**127.

Schwartz RH, Rodriguez WJ, Schwartz DM: Office myringotomy for acute otitis media: Its value in preventing middle ear effusion. *Laryngoscope* 1981;**91:**616.

Shurin PA et al: *Branhamella catarrhalis* in otitis media. *Pediatr Infect Dis* 1983;**2:**34.

Teele DE et al: Bacteriology of acute otitis media unresponsive to initial antimicrobial therapy. *J Pediatr* 1981; **98:**537.

2. ACUTE BULLOUS MYRINGITIS

In acute bullous myringitis, bullae form between the outer and middle layers of the tympanic membrane. In the past, this was considered to be always due to viral infections. Studies demonstrate that 50–75% of affected patients have an underlying acute purulent otitis media. The organisms isolated in cases of acute bullous myringitis are similar to those found in acute otitis media. A causative role for *Mycoplasma pneumoniae* or viruses in cases of bullous myringitis has not been confirmed.

The patient usually complains of ear pain on the involved side. Examination of the ear reveals 1–3 bullae that may cover 20–90% of the drum surface. They are thin-walled and often sagging in appearance, and they often contain a straw-colored fluid. There is minimal erythema.

Antibiotics are prescribed as for acute otitis media. Analgesics are sometimes indicated. The bullae do not have to be opened unless they are causing significant pain. They can be easily opened by nicking with a myringotomy knife or spinal needle.

Follow-up care is the same as that described for acute purulent otitis media.

Klein JO, Teele DW: Isolation of viruses and *Mycoplasma* from middle ear effusions: A review. *Ann Otol Rhinol Laryngol* 1976;**85:**140.

Roberts DB: The etiology of bullous myringitis and the role of *Mycoplasma* in ear disease: A review. *Pediatrics* 1980;**65:**761.

3. SEROUS OTITIS MEDIA

Essentials of Diagnosis

- Painless hearing loss of 15–20 dB.
- Dull, immobile tympanic membrane.

General Considerations

Serous otitis media results when the auditory tube fails to clear secretions present in the middle ear space. The effusion resembles serum transudate, and histopathologic examination of the middle ear shows subepithelial edema. The effusion is usually associated with a low-grade (15–20 dB) conductive hearing loss. Serous effusions may either precede or follow purulent otitis media. Acute serous otitis media can occur in association with transient auditory tube dysfunction in the absence of a middle ear infection. This phenomenon usually occurs during colds or bouts of allergic rhinitis. It can also follow overly vigorous nose blowing. In older children and adolescents, the serous effusion usually resolves in 4–7 days. Residual serous otitis media following appropriate antibiotic therapy for acute otitis media occurs in 40–50% of children. These residual effusions clear spontaneously within 2 months in 85% of cases.

Persistent serous effusions may be associated with a low-grade bacterial infection, especially infection with β-lactamase-producing organisms such as *Haemophilus influenzae*, *Branhamella catarrhalis*, *Staphylococcus aureus*, and penicillin-resistant

Streptococcus pneumoniae. Clinical resolution of acute otitis media may not correlate well with bacteriologic cure. In aspirates of serous effusions obtained during the surgical placement of tympanoplasty tubes, organisms are isolated in about 50% of cases. The most common pathogenic organisms isolated are *H influenzae* (25% of cases), *S pneumoniae* (10%), and *S aureus* (7%). Many of the *H influenzae* strains (45%) are β-lactamase-positive.

Clinical Findings

Children with serous otitis media are usually asymptomatic and have hearing loss. The patient may complain of a feeling of fullness in the ear. An older patient may compare the feeling with "talking inside a barrel." In the preverbal child, hearing loss should be suspected if irritability, inattentiveness, or increased behavior problems are noted. Unlike acute purulent otitis media, there is minimal pain.

The tympanic membrane may appear mildly injected and dull or have a normal appearance. Mobility is diminished or absent. When fluid levels or air bubbles are visualized, the effusion is in a stage of resolution, with auditory tube function improving. When auditory tube dysfunction results in persistent negative pressure in the middle ear space, the tympanic membrane appears retracted, and the position of the short process of the right malleus changes from 7 o'clock to 9 o'clock. Tympanic membrane mobility is altered; ie, the membrane may move only when negative pressure is applied.

The most common complication of serous otitis media is conductive hearing loss, which may adversely affect language development, intellectual functioning, and academic performance. The presence of a serous effusion predisposes the child to another episode of acute otitis media. In some children with recurrent acute otitis media, effusion persists in the middle ear between episodes and causes a cycle of acute otitis media alternating with serous otitis media.

Treatment

Management of serous otitis media is outlined in Fig 14–1. When serous otitis media has persisted longer than 6 weeks, consider a trial of prednisone 1 mg/kg/d in 2 divided doses for 7 days combined with a 28-day course of one of the following regimens to treat β-lactamase-producing organisms: trimethoprim · plus sulfamethoxazole; erythromycin plus sulfisoxazole; cefaclor alone; or ampicillin plus clavulanic acid.

The efficacy of oral decongestants and antihistamines in preventing or treating serous effusions is controversial. Most studies report that these drugs are not effective.

Chan KH et al: A comparative study of amoxicillin-clavulanate and amoxicillin. *Arch Otolaryngol Head Neck Surg* 1988;**114**:142.

Healy GB: Antimicrobial therapy for chronic otitis media with effusion. In: *Proceedings of the Third International Symposium: Recent Advances in Otitis Media With Effusion.* Lim DJ (editor). Decker & Co., 1984.

Lim DJ: Pathogenesis of otitis media with effusion. *Pediatr Infect Dis J* 1982;**1(Suppl 5)**:S14.

Mandel EM et al: Efficacy of amoxicillin with and without decongestant antihistamine for otitis media with effusion in children. *N Engl J Med* 1987;**316**:432.

Marks NJ, Mills RP, Shaheen OH: A controlled trial of cotrimoxazole therapy in serous otitis media. *J Laryngol Otol* 1981;**95**:1003.

4. MUCOID OTITIS MEDIA

Essentials of Diagnosis

- Dull, immobile tympanic membrane.
- Hearing loss of 25–50 dB.
- Type B pattern on tympanogram (Fig 14–3).

General Considerations

Pathogenic bacteria have been isolated from approximately one-third of mucoid effusions at the time of insertion of tympanoplasty tubes. The most common pathogenic organisms isolated from these effusions are *Haemophilus influenzae* (15% of cases), *Morexella catarrhalis* (9%), *Streptococcus pneumoniae* (7%), *Staphylococcus aureus* (3%), *Pseudomonas aeruginosa* (2%), and *Streptococcus pyogenes* (1%). Many of the *H influenzae* strains (34%) and *M catarrhalis* strains (82%) are β-lactamase-positive. *Staphylococcus epidermidis* and diphtheroids are isolated in 33% of effusions. Evidence supporting the pathogenic role of these organisms includes the findings of type-specific antibody in middle ear fluid; studies in animals also suggest that the middle ear space should be sterile. Pathogenic factors that may contribute to the persistence of middle ear effusions include the adverse effects of gram-negative endotoxins on the middle ear space as well as the chronic inflammatory response secondary to persistent bacterial infection.

Mucoid (secretory) otitis media is characterized by a thick and tenacious middle ear effusion that contains high levels of immunoglobulin. The otitis appears to be related to type 1 and type 3 allergic reactions associated with recurrent low-level exposure to bacterial antigens. Evidence supporting a type 1 reaction includes the documentation of a higher level of IgE in mucoid effusions than in blood and the presence of IgE plasma cells in effusions. A type 3 reaction is supported by findings of B cells, specific antibacterial antibody, and depressed total hemolytic complement levels in mucoid effusions.

Most cases of mucoid otitis media are due to primary congenital auditory tube dysfunction. Risk factors that may contribute to a persistent mucoid effusion include the following:

(1) Allergic rhinitis can precipitate mucoid otitis media and is diagnosed by the presence of frequent episodes of clear nasal discharge, sneezing, nasal itching, and over 20% eosinophils on a stained smear of nasal discharge.

(2) Onset of acute otitis in the first 2 months of life and recurrent bilateral episodes of acute otitis predispose the child to develop persistent effusions.

(3) Bottle-feeding in a supine position predisposes the child to persistent serous and mucoid otitis media. Bottle propping should be discontinued and the child fed in a more erect posture.

(4) Certain congenital malformations can lead to recurrent ear problems. Chronic mucoid otitis media is seen in 90% of children with cleft palate and 40% of children with submucous clefts. Cystic fibrosis, trisomy 21, hypothyroidism, and Turner's syndrome also predispose children to recurrent ear problems.

(5) Marked adenoidal hyperplasia can occasionally block the exit of the auditory tubes.

(6) Nasopharyngeal neoplasms can also produce auditory tube obstruction.

(7) The child's risk of developing mucoid effusion may be increased if the parents smoke.

(8) Day care outside the home appears to increase the risk of recurrent and persistent otitis media.

Clinical Findings

Like patients with serous otitis media, those with mucoid otitis media usually are asymptomatic or complain of a feeling of fullness in the ear. The tympanic membrane commonly appears dull and opaque; in severe cases, it may have a bluish tint. Tympanic membrane mobility is usually markedly diminished.

Complications

Children with mucoid otitis media are at increased risk of developing retraction pockets, which predispose them to cholesteatoma and other complications such as necrosis of the ossicles and cholesterol granuloma.

Mucoid otitis media is associated with a hearing loss of 25–50 dB, which may persist for a prolonged period of time. A persistent, moderate hearing loss early in life is likely to result in delays in language development and adversely affect intellectual functioning.

Treatment

A. Medical Measures: If mucoid otitis media has persisted longer than 8 weeks despite 2 courses of antibiotic therapy, consider a trial of prednisone 1 mg/kg/d in 2 divided doses for 7 days combined with a 28-day course of one of the following regimens to treat β-lactamase-producing organisms: trimethoprim plus sulfamethoxazole; erythromycin plus sulfisoxazole; cefaclor alone; or ampicillin plus clavulanic acid.

Oral decongestants and antihistamines have not proved to be effective for treatment.

B. Surgical Treatment: If manifestations of mucoid otitis media (ie, documented effusion, hearing loss > 20 dB, and abnormal findings on tympanogram) have failed to resolve after a 3-month period despite a trial of antibiotics plus prednisone, the patient should be referred to an otolaryngologist for insertion of tympanoplasty tubes. A child with signs of partial resolution noted on otoscopy, audiogram, or tympanogram should be followed for another month prior to referral. A child whose tympanic membrane is severely retracted and whose tympanogram shows a peak at negative pressure should be followed for the development of persistent retraction pockets. Persistent retraction pockets should also be treated with tympanoplasty tubes.

Myringotomy followed by insertion of tympanoplasty tubes (polyethylene flanged ventilation tubes) has given excellent results in this disorder as long as the tubes are in place. The tubes permit pressure equalization and drying of the middle ear cavity without a functional auditory tube. The hearing returns to normal with the tube in place. This procedure can be done in an outpatient surgical setting by an otolaryngologist. The long-term efficacy of tympanoplasty tubes has not been well evaluated. One study from Great Britain with bilateral chronic serous otitis media failed to show a significant postsurgical difference in hearing after 6 months to 5 years between the ear in which a tube was inserted and the control ear. Possible side effects of tympanoplasty tubes are persistent perforations, cholesteatoma, secondary infection, mastoiditis, tympanic membrane scarring or atrophy, retraction pockets, dislocation of the tube into the middle ear cavity, and the risks of anesthesia.

Removal of the adenoids is rarely helpful. Adenoidectomy should be reserved for patients who have not benefited from ventilating tubes or who have signs of upper airway obstruction. Apparently, the extent of the benefit derived from this procedure is not related to adenoid size; therefore, accurate identification of patients who will benefit from this surgery is not possible.

Berman S, Grose K, Zerbe GO: Medical management and chronic middle ear effusion. *Am J Dis Child* 1987; **141**:690.

Gates GA et al: Effectiveness of adenoidectomy and tympanostomy tubes in the treatment of chronic otitis media with effusion. *N Engl J Med* 1987;**317**:1444.

Giebink GS et al.: A controlled trial comparing three treatments for chronic otitis media with effusion. *Pediatr Infect Dis J 1990*;**9**:33.

Mandel et al: Efficacy of myringotomy with and without tympanostomy tube insertion in the treatment of chronic otitis media with effusion in infants and children: Results for the first year of a randomized clinical trial. Pages 308–312 in: *Recent Advances in Otitis Media with Effusions*. Lim DJ et al (editors). BC Decker, 1984.

Paradise JL et al: Efficacy of adenoidectomy for recurrent otitis media in children previously treated with tympanostomy-tube placement. *JAMA* 1990;**263**:2066.

5. RECURRENT OR PERSISTENT OTITIS MEDIA WITH EFFUSION (THE "OTITIS-PRONE CONDITION")

Essentials of Diagnosis

- Two episodes of acute otitis media in a patient under 12 months of age.
- Three episodes of acute otitis media within a 6-month period in a patient over 12 months of age.
- Middle ear effusion persisting 3 months or longer.

General Considerations

Specific conditions that cause auditory tube dysfunction and predispose children to early and recurrent otitis media include viral upper respiratory tract infections, allergic and vasomotor rhinitis, trisomy 21, cystic fibrosis, hypothyroidism, and anatomic abnormalities such as cleft palate, obstructing adenoids, and nasopharyngeal tumors. It is likely that auditory tube dysfunction and abnormalities in immune response are interrelated and that a primary disturbance in one area results in a secondary disorder in the other.

Infants who experience their initial episode of otitis media in the first 2 or 3 months of life are more likely to have bilateral persistent otitis media or recurrent episodes of acute otitis media during the first year. Bottle propping, passive exposure to smoking, and day care outside the home appear to predispose the child to recurrent or persistent otitis media with effusion. Recurrence or persistence of disease places infants and children at risk for permanent ear damage and fluctuating or persistent hearing loss. Studies have shown that the amount of time the effusion is present during the first 6–12 months of life has the strongest correlation with delays in language development at 3 years of age. Therefore, early identification of otitis-prone infants and children is essential for prevention of adverse sequelae.

Management

A. Identification and Monitoring of Otitis-Prone Infants and Children: The criteria for identifying otitis-prone children are listed above (see Essentials of Diagnosis). Because episodes of acute otitis media in infancy are frequently asymptomatic, high-risk infants require close monitoring and monthly follow-up. Tympanometry can be used as an adjunctive method to monitor those over 7 months of age. Audiologic testing should be performed, and patients with conductive hearing loss that persists for longer than 3 months should be referred to an oto-laryngologist. Language development should be evaluated at 18, 24, and 36 months by use of the Early Language Milestone (ELM) scale. An appropriate home language stimulation program and guidelines for the management of behavior problems related to conductive hearing loss should be instituted for all infants and children with impaired hearing. (See Detection and Management of Hearing Deficits, below.)

B. Antibiotic Prophylaxis: Prophylaxis should be started following the resolution of the third episode within a 6-month period. Antibiotics shown to be effective include sulfisoxazole 70 mg/kg/d, amoxicillin 20 mg/kg/d, or erythromycin 20 mg/kg/d, all given in 2 divided doses. One daily dose may also be effective.

Sulfisoxazole should be continued for 3 months. During the next 3–6 months, it is often helpful to advise parents to restart the antibiotic at the first sign of a cold and give it for a minimum of 2 weeks or until cold symptoms resolve. This program of prophylaxis has reduced the frequency of recurrent acute otitis by 50%. Failure to prevent a second breakthrough infection on continuous prophylaxis is an indication that the patient should be referred to an otolaryngologist for the insertion of ventilating tubes. Occasionally, patients with ventilating tubes continue to have recurrent acute otitis media and benefit from antibiotic prophylaxis.

C. Management of Chronic Effusions: Patients in whom middle ear effusion has persisted for 2 months and who have not received a second course of antibiotics should be given appropriate antibiotic treatment to cover β-lactamase-producing organisms. Treatment consists of a 14-day course of one of the following regimens: erythromycin plus sulfisoxazole; trimethoprim plus sulfamethoxazole; ampicillin plus clavulanic acid; or cefaclor alone.

A trial of prednisone 1 mg/kg/d in 2 divided doses in combination with an antibiotic appears to promote resolution of the effusion and obviate the need for surgical insertion of ventilating tubes. After the effusion is cleared with medical therapy, the patient should receive prophylactic therapy for 3 months. If hearing loss with middle ear effusion persists for 3 months, the patient should be referred to an otolaryngologist for insertion of tympanoplasty tubes.

Berman S: Otitis media with effusions: Its relationship to language development, intellectual functioning and academic performance. *Adv Behav Pediatr* 1981;**2**:129.

Berman S, Murphy JR: Persistent and recurrent otitis media: A review of the "otitis-prone" condition. *Prim Care* 1984;**11**:407.

Biedel CW: Modification of recurrent otitis media by short-term sulfonamide therapy. *Am J Dis Child* 1978; **132**:681.

Howie WM et al: Use of pneumococcal polysaccharide vaccine in preventing otitis media in infants: Different results between racial groups. *Pediatrics* 1984;**73**:79.

Lampe RM, Weir MR: Erythromycin prophylaxis for recurrent otitis media. *Clin Pediatr (Phila)* 1986;**25**:510.

Liston TE et al: The bacteriology of recurrent otitis media and the effect of sulfisoxazole chemoprophylaxis. *Pediatr Infect Dis* 1984;**3**:20.

Marchant CD et al: Course and outcome of otitis media in early infancy: A prospective study. *J Pediatr* 1984; **104**:826.

Teele DW et al: Otitis media with effusion during the first three years of life and development of speech and language. *Pediatrics* 1984;**74**:282.

Varsano I et al: Sulfisoxazole prophylaxis of middle ear effusion and recurrent acute otitis media. *Am J Dis Child* 1985;**139**:632.

ACUTE BAROTITIS

Sudden changes in barometric pressure, as can occur with diving or flying, can lead to an acute serous effusion into the middle ear cavity. The history itself is diagnostic. The patient presents with complaints of severe pain and loss of hearing in the affected ear. Otoscopic examination usually reveals a hemorrhagic tympanic membrane.

The process is self-limited, lasting for 2–3 days. The principal therapeutic agent is an analgesic, usually codeine. Decongestants are also prescribed, but antibiotics are not necessary. The prognosis is excellent. The patient should be taught techniques for prevention, such as use of a nasal decongestant spray before descent and autoinflation maneuvers during descent.

ACUTE TRAUMA TO THE MIDDLE EAR

Head injuries, a blow to the ear canal, sudden impact with water, blast injuries, or the insertion of pointed instruments into the ear canal can lead to perforation of the tympanic membrane or hematoma of the middle ear. One study reported that 50% of serious penetrating wounds of the tympanic membrane were due to parental use of a cotton-tipped swab.

Treatment of middle ear hematomas consists mainly of watchful waiting. Prophylactic antibiotics are not necessary unless signs of superimposed infection appear. The prognosis for unimpaired hearing depends upon whether or not the ossicles are dislocated or fractured in the process. The patient needs to be followed by audiometrics until hearing has returned to normal.

Traumatic perforations of the tympanic membrane often do not heal spontaneously and should be referred to an otolaryngologist. Perforations caused by a foreign body must be seen immediately, whereas those due to impact can be seen within 24 hours.

Early debridement and placement of a graft virtually ensure closure.

Silverstein H et al: Penetration wounds of the tympanic membrane and ossicular chain. *Trans Am Acad Ophthalmol Otolaryngol* 1973;**77**:125.

CHRONIC PERFORATION OF THE TYMPANIC MEMBRANE

Essentials of Diagnosis
- Painless otorrhea, intermittent or persistent.
- Perforated tympanic membrane.
- Conductive hearing loss of 20–40 dB.

General Considerations
A perforation of the tympanic membrane can be considered chronic if it lasts for longer than 1 month. Most perforations seen with acute otitis media heal within 2 weeks. Chronic perforations usually can be prevented by aggressive early treatment of acute otitis media. Reinfections of the exposed middle ear cavity are the most common finding in this disorder.

Clinical Findings
A. Symptoms and Signs: A perforation is always present. If no infection is present, the middle ear cavity is seen to contain thickened, inflamed mucosa. If superimposed infection is present, serous or purulent drainage will be seen, and the middle ear cavity may contain granulation tissue or even polyps. A conductive hearing loss will usually be present depending on the size of the perforation.

The site of perforation is important. Central perforations are usually relatively safe from cholesteatoma formation. Peripheral perforations, especially in the pars flaccida, impose a risk for development of cholesteatoma because the ear canal epithelium adjacent to the perforation may invade it. The condition is almost always painless.

B. Laboratory Findings: Any discharge present should be cultured before treatment is initiated. Sensitivity tests are often necessary because the most common organisms are *Pseudomonas* and *S aureus*. The role of anaerobic organisms is unclear. A PPD test should be done to rule out tuberculosis.

C. Imaging: Mastoid films are helpful if a superimposed mastoiditis is suspected.

Complications
This disorder can have serious complications, but they are rare with proper therapy. They occur mainly in unattended cases of superinfected, chronically perforated eardrums. Cholesteatoma is the most common complication and can be suspected if the discharge is foul-smelling and if a white, oily mass is seen within the perforation. The associated perforation may be pinpoint in size. If the discharge does

not respond to 2 weeks of aggressive therapy, mastoiditis or cholesteatoma should be suspected. Serious central nervous system complications such as extradural abscess, subdural abscess, brain abscess, meningitis, labyrinthitis, or lateral sinus thrombophlebitis can occur with extension of this process. Therefore, patients with facial palsy, vertigo, or other central nervous system signs should be referred immediately to an otolaryngologist. Otogenous tetanus is another possible sequela.

Treatment

A. Specific Measures: If a serous or purulent discharge is present, antibiotic-corticosteroid ear drops (eg, Coly-Mycin S Otic, Cortisporin Otic suspension) should be instilled 3 times daily for 1 week. Both products contain polymyxin and neomycin. *Pseudomonas* is sensitive to the former. Caution is advised because of the potential of toxicity of these agents. Gentamicin ear drops are also useful. The ear drops will not be effective unless the ear canals are aspirated before the drops are instilled. If the discharge is purulent or foul-smelling or if systemic signs are present, systemic antibiotics should also be prescribed. A cephalosporin can be given at the outset and another drug substituted depending on the culture results. This therapy can be continued for 2 weeks. If there is any recurrence of discharge, antibiotic ear drops should be instilled immediately.

Chronic suppurative otitis media with *Pseudomonas* is often resistant to outpatient therapy. If daily outpatient aspiration of discharge is unsuccessful, it may be necessary to hospitalize the patient for parenteral therapy with a β-lactam antipseudomonad antibiotic.

B. Surgical Treatment: Repair of the defect in the tympanic membrane is rarely successful during the time period when children have frequent colds and recurrent auditory tube dysfunction. Therefore, tympanoplasty is usually deferred until age 9–12. The perforated eardrum can be repaired earlier if the nonperforated one remains free of infection and effusion for a year. If drainage persists despite treatment, the patient must be referred to an otologist to rule out cholesteatoma, mastoiditis, or other complication.

C. Follow-Up Care: The patient should be seen once a week until the discharge has cleared and about once every 3 months until surgery has been done. This follow-up is imperative to prevent any serious complications.

D. Prevention of Recurrences:

1. Prophylactic ear drops—For the 1-month period following any flare-ups of otorrhea, ear drops consisting of povidone-iodine solution (not tincture) should be instilled in each ear once daily.

2. Bathing—Before bathing and hair washing, cotton plugs should be put in the ear and the surface completely covered with petrolatum ointment.

3. Swimming—Swimming should be discouraged unless it is a matter of great importance to the patient, in which case it can be continued using custom-fitted ear molds plus a bathing cap for girls or a scuba cap for boys. Diving, jumping into the water, and underwater swimming are absolutely forbidden.

4. Unwarranted measures—The constant use of a cotton plug in the ear canal will increase the risk of superinfection. Exposure to air is helpful in the treatment.

Prognosis

With treatment, 80–90% of perforations heal spontaneously by 1 year. The remainder require careful follow-up. With proper care, these patients will be in good condition for tympanoplasty at age 9–12.

Bluestone CD: Current management of chronic suppurative otitis media in infants and children. *Pediatr Infect Dis J* 1988;**7:**5137.
Fairbanks DN: Antibiotic ear drop use in the nonintact tympanic membrane. *Pediatr Ann* 1984;**13:**411.
Felder H: Chronic otitis media in children. *Pediatr Ann* 1976;**5:**474.
Fischer GW et al: Otogenous tetanus: Sequelae of chronic ear infections. *Am J Dis Child* 1977;**131:**445.
MacAdam AM et al: Tuberculous otomastoiditis in children. *Am J Dis Child* 1977;**131:**152.

MASTOIDITIS

Infection of the mastoid antrum and air cells may follow an episode of untreated or improperly treated acute otitis media. The most common etiologic agents are *Streptococcus pyogenes, Streptococcus pneumoniae,* and *Staphylococcus aureus. Haemophilus influenzae* causes mastoiditis much less frequently than expected. Other agents that can cause this disease include *Pseudomonas, Mycobacterium,* enteropathic gram-negative rods, and *Branhamella catarrhalis.* Anaerobic organisms appear to play a role in chronic mastoiditis; however, there are no data on how frequently they cause acute mastoiditis.

Mastoiditis is unusual before age 2, when air cells begin to develop.

Clinical Findings

The principal complaints are usually postauricular pain and fever. On examination, the mastoid area is often swollen and reddened. In the late stage, it may be fluctuant. The earliest finding is severe tenderness upon mastoid percussion. Acute otitis media is almost always present. Late findings are a pinna that is pushed forward by postauricular swelling and an ear canal that is narrowed in the posterior superior wall because of pressure from the mastoid abscess.

In infants less than 1 year of age, the swelling occurs superior to the ear and pushes the pinna downward rather than outward.

Mastoiditis is a clinical diagnosis. It cannot be diagnosed on the basis of x-rays alone. In the acute phase, there is diffuse inflammatory clouding of the mastoid cells as in every case of acute purulent otitis media. Only later is there evidence of bony destruction and resorption of the mastoid air cells.

Complications

Meningitis is a complication in up to 9% of cases of acute mastoiditis. This infection should be suspected when a child has high fever, stiff neck, severe headache, or other meningeal signs. A lumbar puncture should be performed to diagnose this condition. Brain abscess occurs in 2% of cases and may be associated with persistent headache, recurring fever, or changes in sensorium. A CT scan should be performed.

Treatment & Prognosis

The patient must be hospitalized because this disorder represents osteitis. Before therapy is initiated, myringotomy (see below) should be performed in order to obtain material for culture and also to relieve the pressure in the middle ear-mastoid space.

The initial management of uncomplicated acute mastoiditis includes intravenous antibiotic therapy and possibly surgery. Results of gram-stained smears taken during tympanocentesis may help in the choice of antibiotics. Ampicillin and nafcillin appear to be a reasonable initial choice. Indications for immediate surgery include the clear evidence of a major complication such as meningitis, brain abscess, cavernous sinus thrombosis, acute suppurative labyrinthitis, or facial palsy. Some otolaryngologists consider the destruction of septal bone (osteitis) and resorption of the mastoid air cells an indication for surgery.

Oral antibiotics should be continued for 4–6 weeks after the patient is discharged.

The prognosis is good if treatment is started early and continued until the process is inactive.

Brook I: Aerobic and anaerobic bacteriology of chronic mastoiditis in children. *Am J Dis Child* 1981;**135**:478.

Macadam AM, Rubio T: Tuberculous otomastoiditis in children. *Am J Dis Child* 1977;**131**:152.

Meyerhoff WL, Gates GA, Montalbo PJ: *Pseudomonas* mastoiditis. *Laryngoscope* 1977;**87**:483.

Ogle JW, Lauer BA: Acute mastoiditis: Diagnosis and complications. *Am J Dis Child* 1986;**140**:1178.

Ostfeld E, Rubinstein E: Acute gram-negative bacillary infections of middle ear and mastoid. *Ann Otol Rhinol Laryngol* 1980;**89**:33.

Palva T, Virtanen H, Makinen J: Acute and latent mastoiditis in children. *J Laryngol Otol* 1985;**99**:127.

Venezio FR et al: Complications of mastoiditis with special emphasis on venous sinus thrombosis. *J Pediatr* 1982;**101**:509.

CONGENITAL EAR MALFORMATIONS

Agenesis of the external ear canal results in deafness that requires evaluation in the first month of life by hearing specialists and an otolaryngologist.

"Lop ears" (Dumbo ears) lead to much teasing and ridicule. To prevent the secondary emotional problems, these can be corrected at age 5 or 6 by plastic surgery. The ear is of approximately adult size by then, and there is little risk of affecting growth.

An ear is low-set if the upper pole is below eye level. This condition is often associated with renal malformations (eg, Potter's syndrome), and an ultrasound or intravenous urogram is helpful.

Preauricular tags, ectopic cartilages, fistulas, sinuses, or cysts require surgical correction, mainly for cosmetic reasons. Most preauricular pits are asymptomatic. If one should become infected, it should be treated with antibiotics and referred to an otolaryngologist for eventual resection. Children with any of the above findings should have their hearing tested.

Brown FE et al: Correction of congenital auricular deformities by splinting in the neonatal period. *Pediatrics* 1986;**78**:406.

Jaffe BF: Pinna anomalies associated with congenital conductive hearing loss. *Pediatrics* 1976;**57**:332.

OTITIS EXTERNA

Otitis externa is an inflammation of the skin lining the ear canals. The most common cause is accumulation of water in the ear, leading to maceration and desquamation of the lining and conversion of the pH from acid to alkaline (eg, from swimming or frequent showers). Swimming pools are worse than lakes because the chlorine kills the normal ear flora. Other causes are trauma to the ear canal from using cotton-tipped applicators to clean it or poorly fitted ear plugs for swimming; contact dermatitis due to hair sprays, perfumes, or self-administered ear drops; and chronic drainage from a perforated tympanic membrane. The superimposed infections are often due to *Staphylococcus aureus* or *Pseudomonas aeruginosa*.

Clinical Findings

There is pain and itching in the ear, especially with chewing or pressure on the tragus. Movement of the pinna or tragus causes considerable pain. Drainage is minimal. The ear canal is grossly swollen, and the patient resists any attempt to insert an ear speculum. Debris is noticeable in the canal. It is often impossible to visualize the tympanic membrane. Hearing is normal unless complete occlusion has occurred.

Treatment

Topical treatment usually suffices. The crucial initial step is removal of the desquamated epithelium and moist cerumen. This debris can be irrigated out or suctioned out using warm half-strength white vinegar or Burow's solution (1 packet of Domeboro Powder to 250 mL tap water). Once the ear canal is open, a combination of antibiotic-corticosteroid ear drops (eg, Cortisporin Otic) is given 3–4 times daily. The corticosteroid is needed to reduce the severe inflammatory response. The insertion of a wick is painful and usually unnecessary. A follow-up visit in 1 week to document an intact tympanic membrane is imperative.

Oral antibiotics are indicated if any signs of invasiveness are present, such as fever, cellulitis of the auricles, or tender postauricular lymph nodes. Penicillin is an appropriate initial drug while awaiting the results of culture of the ear canal discharge. Systemic antibiotics alone without topical treatment will not clear up otitis externa. Analgesics—sometimes codeine—may be required temporarily. Children predisposed to this problem should instill 2–3 drops of 1:1 white vinegar/70% ethyl alcohol into their ears before and after swimming. During the acute phase, swimming should be avoided if possible. A cotton earplug is not helpful and may be harmful.

Marcy SM: Infections of the external ear. *Pediatr Infect Dis J* 1985;**4**:192.

EAR CANAL FOREIGN BODY

Numerous objects can be inserted into the ear canal by a child. An insect in the ear should be killed with alcohol solution (gin will do for telephone advice). The patient should be immobilized on a papoose board with the head firmly grasped by an assistant.

An attempt should be made first to remove a foreign body by straightening the ear canal by pulling on the pinna and gently shaking the child's head. If a smooth object such as a bead is present, a cotton-tipped applicator with warmed dental wax or collodion should be inserted and placed against the object for 1–2 minutes, after which time it can be removed. An object with an irregular surface can perhaps be removed with a bayonet forceps. A steel object (eg, ball bearing) can sometimes be removed with a magnetic probe. A right-angled hook or custom-designed paper clip can sometimes be inserted past the object and withdrawn, pushing the object ahead of it.

If these methods fail, irrigation can be attempted. The tube should be inserted past the object so the stream rebounds against the tympanic membrane and flushes the object out. Another approach for smooth objects is to use a suction machine. The end of the rubber tubing forms a better seal with the foreign body if it is first coated with petrolatum.

Irrigation with water is contraindicated with vegetable materials because they swell on contact with water. They can be irrigated with a 70% alcohol solution. Wet tissue paper is also difficult to remove.

If the object is large or wedged in place, the patient should be referred to an otolaryngologist early rather than risk damage to the eardrum or ossicles.

Cunningham DG, Zanga JR: Myiasis of the external auditory meatus. *J Pediatr* 1974;**84**:857.

Stool SE, McConnell CS: Foreign bodies in pediatric otolaryngology: Some diagnostic and therapeutic pointers. *Clin Pediatr (Phila)* 1973;**12**:113.

EAR CANAL FURUNCLE

A furuncle in the outer cartilaginous portions of the ear canal is most often caused by *Staphylococcus aureus*. The patient usually complains of pain in the outer part of the ear opening and resists insertion of a speculum. A small red lump will be noticed by simply looking through the otoscope with a large speculum that is not inserted. Treatment consists of topical bacitracin ointment. When the furuncle has pointed, incision and drainage should be carried out, usually with a needle. Spread of this infection is rare; if it occurs, dicloxacillin, 25 mg/kg/d orally, should be added to the regimen. Recurrences point to manipulation of the ear canal (eg, with dirty fingernails, paper clips, hairpins, or cotton swabs).

EAR CANAL TRAUMA

Children may insert sticks or other objects into the ear canal. This normally results in abrasion of the ear canal, with more bleeding than might be suspected. Parents cause similar injuries by overzealous attempts to remove earwax. It is mandatory that the tympanic membrane be examined. If it is free of injury, no treatment is necessary because the abrasions heal readily.

HEMATOMA OF THE PINNA

Trauma to the earlobe can result in the formation of a hematoma between the perichondrium and cartilage. The hematoma appears as a boggy purple swelling of the upper half of the earlobe. If this is unattended, it can cause pressure necrosis of the underlying cartilage and result in a boxer's "cauliflower ear." To prevent this cosmetic handicap, physicians should refer patients to a surgeon for aspiration and the application of a carefully molded pressure dressing.

PIERCED EAR PROBLEMS

The most common complication of ear piercing is superimposed infection, usually with *Staphylococcus aureus*. A small abscess develops at the site, and purulent material drains from both sides of the perforation. The infection usually stems from the use of contaminated needles or posts (eg, keeping the channel open with a piece of straw). This localized infection can occasionally progress to life-threatening staphylococcal septicemia. Other potential complications are viral hepatitis, erysipelas, and keloid formation.

Treatment of a primary infection requires removal of the foreign body (the earring); administration of dicloxacillin, 25 mg/kg/d orally for 5 days while culture is being performed; and use of local bacitracin ointment. Infections acquired later can often be aborted with bacitracin ointment applied to the posts and reinserted 3 times a day.

Earrings, especially if they are made of nickel, can occasionally cause dermatitis of the earlobe. If this condition is suspected, the earrings should be removed and replaced with 14 K gold or stainless steel earrings and topical corticosteroids applied to the posts several times a day.

A serious problem associated with pierced ears occurs when the earring post is grasped by a child in play and completely pulled through the earlobe, leaving a jagged laceration. The scar that develops can lead to deformity of the earlobe and may require plastic surgery. Another hazard is the possibility that an infant or young child may remove the earring and put it in the mouth, causing choking or aspiration. For this reason, the ears should not be pierced until the child is at least 8 years of age. Ideally, ear piercing should be performed on teenagers able to give informed consent to this procedure. The physician can train the office nurse to pierce ears under aseptic conditions with equipment purchased from a surgical supply house. This would prevent the majority of primary infections that occur.

Cortese TA, Dickey RA: Complications of ear piercing. *Am Fam Physician* (Aug) 1971;**4**:66.

Johnson CJ et al: Earpiercing and hepatitis. *JAMA* 1974; **227**:1165.

Lovejoy FH: Life-threatening staphylococcal disease following ear piercing. *Pediatrics* 1970;**46**:301.

THE EAR: DIAGNOSTIC & THERAPEUTIC PROCEDURES

DETECTION & MANAGEMENT OF HEARING DEFICITS*

Hearing deficits are classified as conductive, sensorineural, or mixed. Conductive hearing loss results from a blockage of the transmission of sound waves from the external auditory canal to the inner ear and is characterized by normal bone conduction and reduced air conduction hearing. In children, conductive losses are most often caused by middle ear effusion. Sensorineural hearing loss occurs when the auditory nerve or cochlear hair cells are damaged. Mixed hearing loss is characterized by components of both conductive and sensorineural loss. The criteria for normal hearing levels in children are lower than those in adults, since children are in the process of learning language. In children, a hearing loss of 15–30 dB is considered mild, 31–50 dB moderate, 51–80 dB severe, and 81–100 dB profound.

Conductive Hearing Loss

About 70% of children under 3 years of age will have one or more episodes of otitis media, and by far the greatest number of conductive hearing losses during childhood are caused by otitis media and its sequelae. Other causes include atresia, stenosis, or collapse of the ear canal; furuncle, cerumen, or foreign body in the ear; aural discharge; bony growths; otitis externa; perichondritis; middle ear anomalies (eg, stapes fixation, ossicular malformation); and cleft palate.

The average hearing loss due to middle ear effusion (whether serous, purulent, or mucoid) is 27–31 dB, the equivalent of a mild hearing loss. This loss may be intermittent in nature and may occur in one or both ears, and this accounts for the wide variability of the effects of ear disease on language development in children. A large-scale prospective study documented a correlation between the presence of middle ear effusion in the first 6–12 months of life and lower language scores at 3 years of age. The effect of effusion on language was more severe when the first attack of otitis media occurred before 6 months of age.

The American Academy of Pediatrics recommends that hearing be assessed and language development skills be monitored in children who have frequently recurring acute otitis media or middle ear effusion persisting longer than 3 months. The effects of hearing loss may be insidious and may not be discernible until the explosive phase of expressive language development occurs between 16 and 24 months of age; therefore, the optimal times for screening very young children are 18 and 24 months. An acceptable tool for language screening at these ages is the Early Language Milestone (ELM) scale. Children 3, 4, and 5 years of age should also be screened for language delays.

To mitigate the likelihood of a communication disorder developing, the physician should inform the

---

*Contributed by Dewey Walker, MD, Marion Downs, MA, and Jerry Northern, PhD.

parents of a child with middle ear disease that the child's hearing may not be normal and should instruct the parents to (1) turn off sources of background noise (eg, televisions, radios, dishwashers) when speaking to the child; (2) focus on the child's face and gain his or her direct attention before speaking; (3) speak slightly louder than usual; and (4) have the teacher place the child in the front of the classroom.

Sensorineural Hearing Loss

Sensorineural hearing loss arises from a lesion in the cochlear structures of the inner ear or in the neural fibers of the auditory nerve (cranial nerve VIII). Most sensorineural losses in children are congenital, with an incidence of one in 750 live births. Causes of congenital deafness include perinatal infections, problems related to premature birth, and autosomal recessive and dominant inheritance of various deafness syndromes. In some hereditary diseases (eg, Alport's syndrome), hearing loss is progressive and becomes apparent later in childhood. The incidence of acquired sensorineural loss in children has decreased since the advent of effective immunization programs (eg, against rubella and mumps) and the control of erythroblastosis fetalis with $Rh_O(D)$ immune globulin. Meningitis remains the most common cause of acquired hearing loss, with deafness occurring in 10.3% of children with bacterial meningitis.

In the past, the effect of unilateral deafness on school performance was thought to be insignificant. However, studies now show that more than one-third of affected children fail one or more grades in school. Therefore, merely recommending preferential classroom seating for these children is no longer sufficient; they should be referred for full evaluation of their hearing needs.

Learning language skills is more severely affected by bilateral than unilateral sensorineural hearing loss. The earlier the deafness occurs, the graver the consequences for language development; the earlier a sensorineural loss is detected and treated (by sound amplification and language habilitation), the better the chances of a good outcome. For example, detection of deafness in a 3-month-old infant and treatment by 4 months of age will result in an optimal outcome. Unfortunately, an average of 2.7 years lapses between the time a hearing loss is recognized and treatment is instituted. The alert physician can eliminate this time lag by utilizing the screening techniques described below.

Screening for Hearing Deficits

Screening procedures are essential for early detection and diagnosis of hearing deficits. The procedures used will vary according to the child's age.

A. Screening of Newborns: During either the hospital stay or the infant's first office visit, records of the infant's neonatal course and family history should be reviewed to determine if the infant is at risk for hearing deficits. According to the Joint Committee on Infant Screening, the following factors place infants at high risk: (1) a family history of childhood hearing impairment; (2) perinatal infections (eg, cytomegalovirus, rubella, herpes simplex, toxoplasmosis, syphilis); (3) anatomic malformations involving the head or neck (eg, dysmorphic appearance, including syndromic and nonsyndromic abnormalities of the pinna); (4) birth weight less than 1500 g; (5) hyperbilirubinemia at levels exceeding indications for exchange transfusion; (6) bacterial meningitis; and (7) signs of severe asphyxia at birth (eg, Apgar scores of 0–3, failure to show spontaneous respiration by 10 minutes after birth, hypotonia persisting to 2 hours of age). If any of these risk factors are present, the infant should be screened by an audiologist, preferably prior to 3 months of age but not later than 6 months after birth. The ideal screening test utilizes brain stem-evoked response audiometry. If results of the screening test are positive for hearing deficit, the audiologist should do further diagnostic testing.

B. Screening of Infants: In the past, the parents' report of their infant's behavior was considered an adequate assessment of the infant's hearing. However, a deaf infant's behavior can appear normal and mislead the parents as well as the professional, especially if the infant has autosomal recessive deafness and is the firstborn child of carrier parents. The following office screening techniques should identify gross hearing losses, but they may or may not detect less severe hearing losses due to otitis media.

1. From birth to 4 months—In response to a sudden loud sound (70 dB or more) produced by a horn, clacker, or special electronic device, the infant should show a startle reflex or blink the eyes.

2. From 4 months to 2 years—While the infant is distracted with a toy or bright object, a noisemaker is sounded softly outside of the field of vision at the child's waist level. Normal responses are as follows: at 4 months, there is a widening of the eyes, a cessation of previous activity, and possibly a slight turning of the head in the direction of the sound; at 6 months, the head turns toward the sound; at 9 months or older, the child should usually be able to locate a sound originating from below as well as turn to the appropriate side; after 1 year, the child should be able to locate sound whether it comes from below or above. After responses to these soft sounds are noted, a loud horn or clacker should be used to produce an eye blink or startle reflex. This last maneuver is necessary because deaf children are often very visually alert and scan the environment so actively that their scanning can be mistaken for an appropriate response to the softer noise test. A deaf child will not blink in response to the loud sound. Children who fail to respond appropriately should be referred for audiologic assessment.

C. Screening of Older Children: When children reach 3 years of age, their hearing can be tested by earphones and pure tone audiometry. The test frequencies for screening are 1000 Hz, 2000 Hz, and 4000 Hz, with the same tone presented at each frequency. Normally, the screening level is 20 dB. If a soundproof room is not available, the screening may be done at 25 dB. If the child does not respond at any one of the test frequencies in either ear, the test should be repeated within 1 week. Failures on rescreening should be referred for audiologic evaluation.

High-risk categories in older children include osteogenesis imperfecta and syndromes associated with deafness, such as Waardenburg's syndrome, Hurler's syndrome, Alport's syndrome, Treacher Collins syndrome, Klippel-Feil syndrome, and fetal alcohol syndrome. Children with these disorders should receive an audiologic evaluation as part of the complete workup. In addition, before any child is labeled as having mental retardation, autism, or severe behavior problems, the adequacy of his or her hearing must be determined. If a developmental speech delay is diagnosed, hearing should be tested as the first step in evaluating the language problem.

Referral

In addition to the referrals for audiologic testing described above, a child with confirmed hearing loss should be referred to an otolaryngologist for evaluation and further management. Any child failing the language screen should be referred to a speech pathologist for language evaluation. Home language enrichment programs for children with mild language delays can be directed by the physician or by a speech pathologist. Programs for the deaf child vary from aural to total communication; the latter includes elements of aural programs plus signing. Each program should be thoroughly scrutinized for its relevance to the deaf child's age and hearing level.

Prevention

Appropriate pediatric care may help prevent many causes of hearing deficits. Erythroblastosis fetalis can be prevented by the use of $Rh_O(D)$ immune globulin, and hyperbilirubinemia can be controlled by phototherapy and exchange transfusions. Congenital rubella infections can be prevented by the use of rubella vaccine, and immunizations for other childhood diseases (eg, mumps) effectively prevent hearing losses from those conditions.

Aminoglycosides are potentially ototoxic and should be used judiciously and monitored carefully, especially in premature infants and in patients with renal insufficiency.

Reduction of exposure to loud noise in the child's environment will prevent high-frequency hearing losses. Repeated exposure to loud music, firecrackers, or shots from guns or cap pistols can impair hearing.

American Academy of Pediatrics: Policy statement by the Joint Committee on Infant Hearing. *Pediatrics* 1982; **70**:496.
Bess FH, Tharpe AM: Unilateral hearing impairment in children. *Pediatrics* 1984;**74**:206.
Committee on Audiometric Evaluation, American Speech and Hearing Association: Guidelines for identification audiometry. *ASHA* (Feb) 1985;**17**:94.
Gerkin KP: The high-risk register for deafness. *ASHA* (March) 1984;**26**:17.
Northern JL, Downs MP: *Hearing in Children,* 3rd ed. Williams & Wilkins, 1984.
Roeser RJ, Downs MP: *Auditory Disorders in School Children,* Thieme-Stratton, 1981.
Teele DW et al: Otitis media with effusion during the first three years of life and development of speech and language. *Pediatrics* 1984;**74**:282.

CERUMEN REMOVAL

Cerumen removal is an essential skill for anyone who treats ear problems. Cerumen often prevents adequate visualization of the tympanic membrane. Impacted cerumen can also cause itching, pain, hearing loss, or otitis externa. If cerumen impinges on the eardrum, a chronic cough may be triggered and will persist until the cerumen is removed. The most common cause of impacted cerumen is the use of cotton-tipped swabs by parents in misguided attempts to clean the ear canal. Parents should be advised that earwax protects the ear (cerumen contains lysozymes and immunoglobulins that curtail infection) and will come out by itself; therefore, they should never put anything into the ear canal to hurry the process.

The technique of removal depends on the consistency of the earwax. All the procedures described below require careful immobilization to prevent injury of the ear canal. The physician should remove cerumen under direct visualization through an operating head of an otoscope. Frequently, cerumen that obstructs a view of the tympanic membrane can be pushed aside, the pneumatic seal reestablished, and mobility assessed without removing the speculum.

(1) Very soft/average cerumen: Sticky cerumen will adhere to an ear curet. A piece of this consistency can sometimes be removed by embedding the ear curet in it. If this technique fails, irrigation as described below should be instituted.

(3) Hard cerumen: Very hard cerumen may adhere to the ear canal wall and cause considerable pain or bleeding if one attempts to remove it with a curet. This type of wax should be softened with Cerumenex or a few drops of detergent before irrigation is attempted. After 20 minutes, irrigation can be started with water warmed to 35–38 °C (95–100.4 °F) to prevent vertigo.

An easy-to-assemble ear syringe consists of a 12-mL plastic syringe plus a piece of small plastic tubing. The tubing can be made from any scalp vein needle set by cutting off the needle about 3 inches from the female connector. The front end of the tubing is placed in the canal, behind the cerumen if possible, and the water is ejected with maximal pressure on the syringe plunger. The advantage of this technique is that the very small tubing may be inserted into the ear canal itself and the water stream is thus directed in the proper direction without interfering with reflux.

A commercial Water Pik is also an excellent device for removing cerumen, but it is important to set it at a low power (2 or less) to prevent any damage to the intact tympanic membrane.

A perforated tympanic membrane is a contraindication to any form of irrigation.

Kravitz H et al: The cotton-tipped swab: A major cause of ear injury and hearing loss. *Clin Pediatr (Phila)* 1974;**13**:965.

OTOSCOPY

Removal of cerumen (see above) may be necessary for adequate visualization of the ear and for assessment of the mobility of the tympanic membrane by pneumatic otoscopy.

The tympanic membrane is divided into 4 sections, based on the position of the long process of the malleus and the umbo, as shown in Fig 14–2. The anterosuperior quadrant contains the short process of the malleus; the posterosuperior quadrant, the incus and pars flaccida; the posteroinferior quadrant, the round window; and the anteroinferior quadrant, the pars tensa and light reflex. To assess mobility of the tympanic membrane, a pneumatic otoscope with a rubber suction bulb and tube is used. The speculum inserted into the patient's ear canal must be large enough to provide an airtight seal. When the rubber bulb is squeezed, the tympanic membrane will flap briskly if no fluid is present (normal finding); however, if fluid is present in the middle ear space, the mobility of the tympanic membrane will be diminished.

TYMPANOMETRY

Tympanometry utilizes an electroacoustic impedance bridge to measure tympanic membrane compliance and display it in graphic form. Compliance is determined at specific air pressures (from $+200$ to -400 mm H_2O air pressure) that are created in the hermetically sealed external ear canal. The existing middle ear pressure can be measured by determining the ear canal pressure at which the tympanic membrane is most compliant. Because total visualization of the tympanic membrane is not necessary, tympanometry does not require removal of cerumen unless the canal is completely blocked.

Tympanograms can be classified into 3 major patterns, as shown in Fig 14–3. The type A pattern, characterized by maximum compliance at normal atmospheric pressure (0 mm H_2O air pressure), indicates a normal tympanic membrane, good auditory tube function, and absence of effusion. The type B pattern identifies a nonmobile tympanic membrane, which may be associated with middle ear effusion, perforation, patent ventilation tubes, or excessive and hardpacked cerumen. The type C pattern indicates an intact mobile tympanic membrane with poor auditory tube function and excessive negative pressure (> -150 mm H_2O air pressure) in the middle ear. Middle ear effusion is present in about 20% of patients with a type C pattern.

Northern JL: Advanced techniques for measuring middle ear function. *Pediatrics* 1978;**61**:761.

MYRINGOTOMY & TYMPANOCENTESIS

Tympanocentesis (placement of a needle through the tympanic membrane) is mainly a diagnostic procedure, because the hole closes over quickly and provides little sustained drainage. Tympanocentesis is helpful in (1) acute otitis media in a hospitalized newborn, because the pathogens may be gram-negative; (2) acute otitis media in a patient with compromised host resistance, because the organism may be unusual; (3) painful bullae of the tympanic

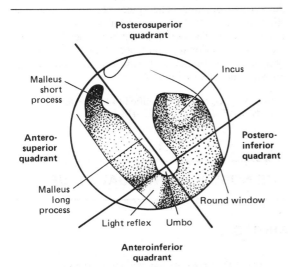

Figure 14–2. Schematic diagram of the left tympanic membrane. (Courtesy of the Department of Otolaryngology, University of Pittsburgh School of Medicine, and Eli Lilly and Co.)

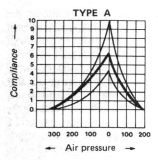
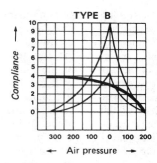
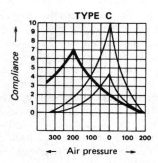

Figure 14–3. Type A tympanograms are characterized by maximum compliance at normal atmospheric pressure (0 mm H$_2$O air pressure). Type B tympanograms show little or no change in compliance of tympanic membrane as air pressure in external ear canal is varied. Type C tympanograms show near-normal compliance with significant negative middle ear pressures (typically more severe than -150 mm H$_2$O). (Reproduced, with permission, from Northern JL. Advanced techniques for measuring middle ear function. *Pediatrics* 1978;**61**:761.)

membrane; (4) a complete workup for presumed sepsis or meningitis; and (5) acute purulent otitis media that is unresponsive to therapy after courses with 2 different antibiotics.

Myringotomy involves incision of the drum with a myringotomy knife, leaving a flap through which drainage fluid may escape. This procedure is helpful for both diagnostic and therapeutic purposes. Myringotomy is indicated (1) when a patient on an initial visit with bulging acute purulent otitis media has severe pain or vomiting, because both symptoms are relieved by myringotomy; (2) when pain and fever fail to resolve after 48 hours of appropriate antibiotic treatment, because a middle ear abscess or resistant organism may exist; and (3) for acute mastoiditis, because it is important to permit drainage as well as to identify the particular organism.

Technique of Myringotomy

A. Premedication: In the conditions mentioned, the pain from a myringotomy is only slightly greater than the pain that already exists from acute inflammation of the tympanic membrane. Therefore, no premedication is generally indicated. The patient who is extremely difficult to hold may be premedicated with meperidine, 1 mg/kg intramuscularly. Some recommend applying Bonain's solution (equal parts cocaine, phenol, and menthol) to the tympanic membrane with a calcium alginate swab.

B. Restraint: The patient must be completely immobile while the incision is being made. A papoose board or a sheet can be used to immobilize the body. An extra attendant is required to hold the patient's head steady.

C. Site: With an open-headed operating otoscope, the operator carefully selects a target. This is generally in the posteroinferior quadrant. This site prevents disruption of the ossicles during the procedure.

D. Incision: The knife is lowered slowly until it touches the surface of the tympanic membrane at the chosen site. A quick 2- to 3-mm incision in the anterior direction is then made, leaving a curved flap in the area indicated (eg, from 8 o'clock to 4 o'clock on the right eardrum).

E. Culture: The myringotomy knife tip should be wiped on a cotton swab moistened with a few drops of normal saline. The material is then placed on a sheep blood agar plate, chocolate agar plate, and a slide for Gram staining.

Technique of Tympanocentesis

Steps A, B, and C are as described above.

In this procedure, the operator needs an assistant to hold the patient's head immobile. An 8.8-cm spinal needle (No. 18 or No. 20) with a short bevel is attached to a 1-mL syringe. The plunger is removed from the syringe, and a suction tube is placed over the syringe opening. The spinal needle is bent at a slight angle so that its end is out of the operator's line of vision. The operator moves the needle toward the posteroinferior quadrant, inserting it through the tympanic membrane, and aspirates the middle ear effusion into the syringe.

Kaplan SL, Feigen RD: Simplified technique for tympanocentesis. *Pediatrics* 1978;**62**:418.

THE NOSE & PARANASAL SINUSES

RHINITIS

1. ACUTE VIRAL RHINITIS (COMMON COLD)

The common cold is the most frequent infectious disease of humans, and the incidence is higher in early childhood than in any other period of life. Children under age 5 have 6–12 colds per year. Closely similar upper respiratory infections may be caused by perhaps 100 different viruses such as rhinovirus, coronavirus, adenovirus, influenza virus, parainfluenza virus, respiratory syncytial virus, coxsackievirus, etc. Minor epidemics occur during the winter months and spread rapidly among susceptible people. The peak month (September) coincides with the opening of schools.

Clinical Findings

The patient usually experiences a sudden onset of clear or mucoid rhinorrhea plus a fever. The main symptoms are usually profound congestion of the nose and sinuses. Mild sore throat and cough also frequently develop. Although the fever is usually low-grade in older children, in the first 5 or 6 years of life it can be as high as 40.6 °C (105 °F). The nose and throat are usually inflamed. Several members of a family are often sick simultaneously.

Complications

Acute otitis media is the most common complication and is often heralded by return of fever or crying. Other complications due to superinfection are purulent sinusitis, purulent conjunctivitis, pneumonia, and pyogenic adenitis.

The onset or presence of a cold or upper respiratory tract infection in a child scheduled for surgery may require postponement of the operation. The primary physician can use the following guidelines when screening children for elective surgery: Surgery is usually postponed if fever or cough is present. Surgery can proceed if the child has only a runny nose, sore throat, or ear infection. If anesthesia will not require intubation (eg, as for placement of tympanoplasty tubes), surgery can be permitted even if the child has a cough (provided that findings on chest film are normal).

Treatment

Treatment is largely symptomatic. Acetaminophen is helpful for fever, sore throat, or muscle aches. A stuffy, congested nose can be treated with normal saline nose drops (mix ¼ teaspoon table salt with 4 oz water), 3 drops in each nostril; the patient should be in the supine position with the neck hyperextended. After several minutes, a suction bulb can be used to remove the secretions of the infant unable to blow its nose. If this procedure fails and the stuffy nose still interferes with feeding or sleep, phenylephrine (Neo-Synephrine), 0.125%, or xylometazoline (Otrivin, Afrin), 0.05%, 2 drops every 4 hours as necessary, can be used in children 6 months to 2 years of age. Children over 2 years of age can use 0.25% phenylephrine drops. Drops should be discontinued after 1 week to prevent a rebound chemical rhinitis. Antihistamines are probably not effec-

tive in relieving cold symptoms. In rhinoviral colds, increased levels of histamine are related to symptoms.

Antibiotics do not prevent superinfection and should not be used. Vaporizers and humidifiers have no proved value and should not be routinely prescribed, especially if the parents cannot easily afford them.

Colds account for many unnecessary visits to the physician. Parents are often unduly worried about how many colds their children have or are overconcerned about noisy breathing, which they fear indicates pneumonia. Parents should be instructed that fast breathing or difficult breathing with chest indrawing is a sign of a lower respiratory infection such as bronchiolitis or pneumonia. Most colds can be assessed and treated by telephone.

The prognosis is excellent. In the usual cold, the fever lasts for less than 3 days and the other symptoms persist for 1–2 weeks.

Doyle W et al: A double-blend, placebo-controlled clinical trial of the effect of chlorpheniramine on response of nasal airway, middle ear and eustachian tube to provocative phenovirus challenge. *Pediatr Infect Dis J* 1988; **7:**229.

Gaffey M, Kaiser DL, Hayden FG: Ineffectiveness of oral terfenadine in natural colds: Evidence against histamine as a mediator of common cold symptoms. *Pediatr Infect Dis J* 1988;**7:**223.

Lampert RP et al: A critical look at oral decongestants. *Pediatrics* 1977;**55:**550.

Naclero RM et al: Is histamine responsible for symptoms of rhinovirus colds? A look at the inflammatory mediators following infection. *Pediatr Infect Dis J* 1988; **7:**215.

2. ACUTE PURULENT RHINITIS

Purulent yellow discharge that persists for several days usually represents purulent sinusitis or other bacterial superinfection of a common cold. Any purulent discharge that is profuse and continuous for over 3 days probably should be treated. The common cold may also be associated with some mucopurulent discharge, but discharge is usually intermittent and worse upon awakening in the morning. The most likely organisms are pneumococci, *Haemophilus influenzae*, β-hemolytic streptococci, and *Staphylococcus aureus*. Rare causes are diphtheria and syphilis. The β-hemolytic streptococci are the most likely organisms if there is crusting around the nares that resembles impetigo, redness of the skin below the nares, or a blistering distal dactylitis.

Oral amoxicillin or trimethoprim plus sulfamethoxazole, administered for 10 days will cure most of these patients. Occasionally, dicloxacillin will be needed because of culture results. The purulent material should be removed as completely as possible with a suction bulb or cotton-tipped applicators and a washcloth and soap. Bacitracin ointment should be applied if nasal impetigo exists.

If the problem recurs after adequate treatment, the patient should be referred to an otolaryngologist to rule out the possibility of a foreign body. If the discharge is foul-smelling and unilateral, this possibility becomes especially likely. The response to treatment is excellent in the majority of cases.

Hays GC, Mullard JE: Can nasal bacterial flora be predicted from clinical findings? *Pediatrics* 1972;**49**:596.

3. PERSISTENT RHINITIS IN NEWBORNS

Rhinorrhea or nasal congestion in a young infant may be due to various causes.

About half of newborns are obligate nasal breathers, and if the nose becomes congested, they have difficulty with air exchange and may become irritable and dyspneic. The problem is worse during feeding because the infant's oral airway is then completely useless. These infants gradually learn to become mouth breathers as well as nasal breathers by age 5 or 6 months.

Differential Diagnosis & Treatment

A. Transient Idiopathic Stuffy Nose of the Newborn: Many infants have unexplained, transient (about 3 weeks) stuffy noses with mucoid or clear discharge that bubbles during feeding. The cause is not known. The diagnosis is made by exclusion. Normal saline nose drops can be instilled and, after several minutes, removed with cotton-tipped applicators or gentle suction on a rubber bulb syringe. If the problem interferes with feeding, this can be preceded by 2 drops of 0.05% xylometazoline no more than 4 times a day for no more than 3 days.

B. Reserpine Side Effects: If the mother is taking reserpine and the drug is in her blood at an effective level during labor, the newborn may have a profoundly stuffy nose. Treatment is as above.

C. Chemical Rhinitis: Chemical rhinitis may be due to overtreatment of idiopathic stuffy nose with topical vasoconstrictors. The irritative nose drops should be discontinued. The patient can be helped with oral decongestants or beclomethasone nasal spray for one week.

D. Pyogenic Rhinitis: Infants with pyogenic rhinitis can have a clear or mucoid discharge rather than the purulent discharge seen in older children. The diagnosis is based on cultures of nasal discharge. Treatment is as outlined above.

E. Congenital Syphilis: The onset is usually before 6 weeks of age. The diagnosis is established by checking the serology done on the mother during the prenatal period. If other signs besides the nasal discharge exist, such as an unresponsive skin rash or hepatosplenomegaly, additional serologic testing

should be performed on the infant. Treatment is discussed in Chapter 28.

F. Hypothyroidism: See Chapter 26.

G. Choanal Atresia: Choanal atresia occurs bilaterally in 25% of affected children and unilaterally in 75%. Bilateral cases can cause severe respiratory distress—even apnea at birth if the child is an absolute nasal breather. Both types eventually present with a chronic nasal discharge because the normal sinus and nasal secretions can escape only anteriorly. A No. 8 soft rubber catheter should be passed through the nose and visualized in the oropharynx. If this procedure cannot be accomplished, a diagnosis of choanal atresia should be confirmed by radiographic study.

An oral airway should be placed immediately if the infant has bilateral choanal atresia. A dentist can fashion a comfortable airway to tide the patient over until mouth breathing is established. Feeding by syringe or medicine dropper is preferred. An otolaryngologist should decide on the optimal timing for definitive surgery, but it is usually 1 year of age.

H. Nasal Fracture Secondary to Birth Trauma: Physical examination should reveal subluxation of the nasal septum occluding the nasal passages. The infant should be referred to an otolaryngologist for reduction.

I. Allergic Rhinitis Associated with Cow's Milk: An allergic reaction to cow's milk can cause noisy breathing and increased production of nasal and oral mucus in infants 1–2 months of age. The symptoms resolve 24–48 hours after eliminating cow's milk from the diet, and they return promptly if the infant is rechallenged with milk.

Myer CM, Cotton RT: Nasal obstruction in the pediatric patient. *Pediatrics* 1983;**72**:766.

4. RECURRENT RHINITIS IN THE OLDER CHILD

This problem is all too frequent in the office practice of pediatrics. A child is brought in with the chief complaint that he or she has "one cold after another," has "constant colds," or "is always sick." Such a patient may be in the office on almost a weekly basis. Although the problem is frustrating, the differential diagnosis is rather simple.* Approximately two-thirds of these children have recurrent colds, and another one-third have allergic rhinitis.

Note: An excessively ordered test is serum immunoelectrophoresis. Children with immune defects do not have an increased number of colds. Therefore, immune globulin tests are worthless unless the patient suffers from recurrent pneumonia, recurrent sinusitis, recurrent adenitis, or other recurrent severe infections.

Differential Diagnosis & Treatment

A. Common Cold: The most common cause of recurrent runny nose is repeated viral upper respiratory infections. The onset is usually after 6 months of age. The bouts of rhinorrhea are usually accompanied by fever. Cultures are negative for bacteria. There is some evidence for contagion within the family or peer group in most of these cases. The nasal mucosa during attacks is often inflamed.

The most common reason for presentation is that the parents are overly concerned because they do not understand that the average child has approximately 6–12 colds a year in the preschool period. Or, the patient may be overly exposed to viruses as a result of close contact with a sibling at school who brings home many pathogens or by frequently being left with large numbers of children at a day-care center or with a baby-sitter.

Treatment consists of specific reassurance and concerned follow-up. The parents can be told that their child's general health is good, as evidenced by adequate weight gain and a robust activity level; that the prognosis is good in that this number of colds will not persist for more than a few years; that the body's exposure and response to colds is building up an antibody supply; and that this problem is not their fault and that they are doing a good job as parents.

B. Allergic Rhinitis: The onset of "hay fever" is usually after 2 years of age—after the child has had adequate exposure to allergens. There is no fever or contagion among close contacts. The attacks include frequent sneezing, rubbing of the nose, and a profuse clear discharge. The nasal turbinates are swollen. The nasal smear demonstrates over 20% of the cells to be eosinophils. (Nasal eosinophilia may be normal during the first 3 months of life.) Nasal secretions should be collected only when the patient is symptomatic. Between attacks or after receiving antihistamines, the eosinophil smear may be falsely negative.

Oral decongestants and antihistamines should be tried until the right drug and dosage are found to give the optimal effect. Avoidance of allergens (especially pets) should be encouraged and environmental controls initiated. If the symptoms persist, the patient should be referred to an allergist for evaluation and possibly for treatment with cromolyn nasal spray, beclomethasone nasal spray, or hyposensitization.

A full discussion of allergic rhinitis is found in Chapter 32.

C. Chemical Rhinitis: Prolonged use of vasoconstrictor nose drops beyond 7 days results in a rebound reaction and secondary nasal congestion (rhinitis medicamentosa). The offending nose drops should be discontinued.

D. Vasomotor Rhinitis: Some children react to sudden changes in environmental temperature with prolonged congestion and rhinorrhea. Air pollution (especially tobacco smoke) may be a factor. Oral decongestants can be used periodically to give symptomatic relief.

Complications

Because this problem is such a nuisance, iatrogenic overtreatment is the most common complication.

Giving immune globulin injections is the most common error made in treating this disorder. The injections may be initiated without determining the serum IgG level or as a consequence of misinterpreting the results by comparing them with adult levels rather than with norms for age. Many studies show that immune globulin injections do not benefit patients with frequent upper respiratory infections. In addition to being painful and expensive, they may cause anaphylaxis or isoimmunization. Other worthless approaches to this problem include bacterial vaccines, prophylactic antibiotics, and tonsillectomy and adenoidectomy. The effectiveness of high doses of vitamin C in reducing the symptoms and duration of colds is still controversial. Patients are not infrequently kept home from school, trips, athletic practices, parties, etc, with little indication. As long as they do not have a fever or severe symptoms, they can attend these functions. They should be given suitable medications for symptomatic relief of mild symptoms so that they can participate normally in these important events of childhood. The risk to other children is almost irrelevant because these infections are contagious even during the incubation period and the best time to have them and develop immunity is during childhood.

Coulehan JL et al: Vitamin C prophylaxis in a boarding school. *N Engl J Med* 1974;**290**:6.

McCammon RW: Natural history of respiratory tract infection patterns in basically healthy individuals. *Am J Dis Child* 1971;**122**:232.

Miller RE et al: The nasal smear for eosinophils: Its value in children with seasonal allergic rhinitis. *Am J Dis Child* 1982;**136**:1009.

Shapiro G: Understanding allergic rhinitis. *Pediatr Rev* 1986;**7**:212.

MOUTH BREATHING SECONDARY TO NASAL OBSTRUCTION

A child is sometimes brought in with the complaint that "He always breathes through his mouth," "He snores," etc. With the mouth covered, each nostril should be tested individually for patency. One or both nostrils may be so severely occluded that adequate air exchange cannot occur. Even when the nasal passages are not completely occluded, the patient may prefer to breathe through the mouth because it is more comfortable. With complete obstruction, a constant nasal discharge ensues because the normal sinus and nasal secretions can escape only anteriorly. The sense of smell is also reduced.

Differential Diagnosis

A. Large Adenoids: Large adenoids can be suspected if the soft palate is depressed or has limited elevation, the patient has hyponasal speech, or possibly if the tonsils are huge. They can be diagnosed more precisely by digital palpation or by lateral soft tissue films of the nasopharynx.

B. Nasal Polyps: Polyps appear as glistening, gray to pink, jellylike masses that are prominent just inside the anterior nares and occur singly or in clusters. They are most common in severe allergic rhinitis. They also occur in cystic fibrosis. One must be careful not to mistake the turbinates for polyps.

C. Recurrent Sinusitis: See below.

D. Allergic Rhinitis: See above.

E. Chemical Rhinitis: See above.

F. Other Causes: Persistent mouth breathing may be due to obstruction by nasopharyngeal tumor or by meningocele or encephalocele herniated into the nasal cavity. If unilateral nasal obstruction and epistaxis are frequent, juvenile angiofibroma should be suspected.

Complications

Most children with prolonged mouth breathing eventually develop dental malocclusion and what has been termed an adenoidal facies. The face is pinched and the maxilla narrowed because the molding pressures of the orbicularis oris and buccinator muscles are unopposed by the tongue. If nasopharyngeal tumors, meningoceles, or encephaloceles are not diagnosed early, they can cause considerable destruction or may even become incurable. Children with severe snoring may also develop sleep apnea or pulmonary hypertension.

Treatment

Allergic rhinitis usually responds to antihistamines or to intranasal cromolyn or corticosteroids. Sinusitis usually resolves with antibiotics. All other patients with documented chronic mouth breathing should be referred to an otolaryngologist for definitive evaluation and treatment. Polyps should never be removed until a meningocele has been ruled out.

Bresolin D et al: Facial characteristics of children who breathe through the mouth. *Pediatrics* 1984;**73**:622.
Myer CM et al: Nasal obstruction in the pediatric patient. *Pediatrics* 1983;**72**:766.
Sessions RB et al: Juvenile nasopharyngeal angiofibroma. *Am J Dis Child* 1981;**135**:535.

SINUSITIS

1. ACUTE SINUSITIS

Essentials of Diagnosis
- Purulent rhinorrhea or postnasal drip.
- Rhinorrhea and daytime cough persisting beyond 10 days.
- Malodorous breath.
- Facial pain or percussion tenderness.
- Periorbital swelling.
- Headache.

General Considerations

Acute inflammation of the paranasal sinuses, or sinusitis, may complicate up to 5% of upper respiratory infections. The maxillary and ethmoidal sinuses are most commonly involved because of poor drainage related to anatomic features. When mucociliary clearance and drainage are further compromised by an upper respiratory infection, the risk of secondary bacterial infection increases. Sinusitis is also commonly seen during pollen season in children with allergic rhinitis. In cases in which superinfection occurs, the organisms are usually *Streptococcus pneumoniae, Haemophilus influenzae* (nontypeable), *Morexella catarrhalis,* and β-hemolytic streptococci. Rarely, anaerobic bacterial infections can cause fulminant frontal sinusitis. Viruses can be isolated in 10% of sinus aspirates, but their pathogenic role is unclear. Anaerobic and staphylococcal organisms are often responsible for chronic sinusitis.

The ethmoidal sinus is the only one that is significantly developed at birth. The maxillary sinus is rudimentary at birth and visible on x-ray film by 6 months. The frontal sinus is not visible until 3–9 years of age. Clinical ethmoiditis does not usually occur until 6 months of age. About half of cases occur between 1 and 5 years of age, during which time the most common presenting sign is periorbital cellulitis. Maxillary sinusitis is seen clinically after 1 year of age. Frontal sinusitis is unusual before 10 years of age.

Clinical Findings

A. Symptoms and Signs: The most common clinical presentation in children is persistence of nasal discharge or postnasal drip and daytime cough longer than 7–10 days. Persistent, low-grade fever is often present. Malodorous breath or intermittent, painless morning periorbital swelling is often noted. Older patients may complain of acute onset of headache, a sense of fullness, or facial pain overlying the involved sinus. Ethmoiditis causes retro-orbital pain; maxillary sinusitis causes upper molar or zygomatic pain; and frontal sinusitis causes pain above the eyebrow. These signs are often associated with a high fever.

Physical examination reveals injected nasal mucosa, usually associated with nasal or postnasal mucopurulent discharge. Occasionally there is percussion tenderness overlying the sinusitis. In ethmoiditis, the tenderness is elicited by pressing medially on the inner canthus of the eye. Tenderness of the eyeball may also be present. Maxillary sinusitis reveals percussion tenderness on the maxillary bone. Frontal sinusitis reveals percussion tenderness when the physician presses upward on the floor of the supraorbital ridge. Periorbital swelling or mild discoloration may be present. The examination should identify exudative tonsillitis, a nasal foreign body, or dental caries and poor dental hygiene. Transillumination of the sinuses is difficult to perform and not very helpful unless it is grossly asymmetric. The chest should be auscultated for wheezing. Sinusitis precipitates intractable wheezing in some children with reactive airway disease. Vigorous treatment of the sinusitis eliminates the wheezing and the need for bronchodilators in many of these children.

B. Laboratory Findings: Sinus aspiration should be performed for diagnostic purposes in patients with complications and in those with an immunosuppressive disease. Gram's stain or culture of nasal discharge is unnecessary as the type of discharge (thin, mucoid, or purulent) is not a useful predictor of sinusitis and does not correlate with cultures of sinus aspirates. If the patient is hospitalized because of complications, a blood culture should be obtained.

C. Imaging: In most cases, the clinical findings are so classic that x-rays are not needed. Positive x-ray films in children over one year will show opacification of the involved sinuses, air-fluid levels if the obstruction is intermittent, or mucosal thickening of greater than 5 mm. It is notable that x-ray findings positive for sinusitis may be found in asymptomatic patients with colds or nasal allergies.

Sinus x-rays are indicated mainly in children with (1) facial swelling of unknown cause; (2) acute sinusitis that is unresponsive to 48 hours of therapy; (3) undocumented chronic or recurrent sinusitis; and (4) chronic asthma. A CT scan should be performed if bony erosions are present. Ultrasonography can also be used to document sinusitis. Sinus views include the anteroposterior (Caldwell) for the frontal and ethmoidal sinuses, occipitomental (Waters) for the maxillary sinuses, and submental-vertex and lateral for the sphenoidal sinus. A Waters view is usually sufficient.

Differential Diagnosis

Similar clinical presentations are associated with viral upper respiratory infection, allergic rhinitis and reactive airway disease, *Streptococcus pyogenes* infection during infancy and early childhood, and nasal foreign body. In older children, the main diagnostic problem is confusion with headaches due to other causes. An uncommon cause of maxillary sinusitis is extension of a periapical abscess of an upper molar.

Complications

The most frequent complication of paranasal sinusitis is preseptal periorbital cellulitis secondary to ethmoiditis. Less frequently, orbital cellulitis or abscess develops. These are associated with decreased extraocular movement, proptosis, edema, and altered visual acuity. The most common complication of frontal sinusitis is osteitis of the frontal bone, called Pott's puffy tumor. Additional serious intracranial complications include cavernous sinus thrombosis, subdural empyema, brain abscess, and meningitis. The most common maxillary complication is cellulitis of the cheek. Rarely, osteomyelitis of the maxilla can develop.

Treatment

A. Specific Measures:

1. Oral antibiotics—Treat acute sinusitis with oral antibiotics for 2–3 weeks to achieve more prompt relief of symptoms and more rapid resolution of inflammation. The usual antibiotic is amoxicillin 15 mg/kg, 3 times a day. In areas where β-lactamase-positive pathogens are common or when the patient is allergic to penicillin, use trimethoprim plus sulfamethoxazole 0.5 cc/kg twice daily, or erythromycin plus sulfamethoxazole 10 mg/kg/dose (E) 4 times a day or amoxicillin clavulanate, 15 mg/kg, 3 times a day. Failure to improve after 48 hours suggests a resistant organism or potential complication. Assess the patient for a central nervous system complication. If none is found, consider drainage or parenteral therapy. Continue antibiotic treatment for another week if the patient has improved but is not totally asymptomatic.

2. Topical and oral decongestants and antihistamines—Topical decongestants and oral combinations are frequently used in acute sinusitis to promote drainage. Their effectiveness has not been evaluated, and concern has been raised about potential adverse effects related to impaired ciliary function, decreased blood flow to the mucosa, and reduced diffusion of antibiotic into the sinuses. Patients with underlying allergic rhinitis may benefit from intranasal cromolyn or corticosteroid nasal spray. Vasoconstrictor nose drops and sprays are all associated with rebound edema if used for more than 5–7 days.

3. Treatment of complications—Patients with evidence of invasive infection or any of the complications listed above should be immediately hospitalized. Intravenous therapy with nafcillin or clindamycusmycin plus cefotaxime or with chloramphenicol alone should be initiated until culture results become available.

B. General Measures: A patient will often need acetaminophen or even codeine temporarily to permit sleep until drainage of the obstructed sinus is achieved. The application of ice over the sinus may help to relieve pain.

Dryness of the mucous membranes—as occurs in many overheated homes in the winter if adequate humidification is not provided—can contribute to the obstruction. A humidifier in the patient's room and periodic warm showers may be of value. A child with sinusitis can be permitted to swim. Diving should be temporarily restricted unless nose plugs are used.

C. Surgical Treatment:

1. Lavage of the sinuses—If there is incapacitating initial pain or persistence of significant pain beyond several days, refer the patient to an otolaryngologist for lavage of the involved sinus.

2. External drainage—In complicated cases admitted to the hospital, an otolaryngologist should always be consulted. Sinus aspiration is helpful in many cases. For sinus intraorbital or intracranial complications, some feel that external drainage of the abscess is as important as antibiotic therapy.

D. Follow-Up Care: The patient should be seen in 48 hours if there is no improvement with antibiotic therapy and at the end of the 2-week course. Obtain a confirmatory x-ray film if symptoms persist at 2 weeks. Chronic or recurrent sinus infections suggest an underlying anatomic malformation, an allergy, cystic fibrosis, immotile-cilia syndrome, or an immunodeficiency disorder.

Arruda L.K. et al: Abnormal maxillary sinus radiographs in children: do they represent bacterial infection. *Pediatr* 1990;**85**:553.

Brook I et al: Complications of sinusitis in children. *Pediatrics* 1980;**66**:568.

Feder HM Jr, Cates KL, Cementina AM: Pott puffy tumor: A serious occult infection. *Pediatrics* 1987;**79**:625.

Kovatch AL et al: Maxillary sinus radiographs in children with nonrespiratory complaints. *Pediatrics* 1984;**73**:306.

Rachelefsky GS, Katz RM, Siegel SC: Chronic sinus disease with associated reactive airway disease in children. *Pediatrics* 1984;**73**:526.

Sable NS, Hengerer A, Powell KR: Acute frontal sinusitis with intracranial complications. *Pediatr Infect Dis J* 1984; **3**:58.

Siegel JD: Diagnosis and management of acute sinusitis in children. *Pediatr Infect Dis J* 1987;**6**:95.

Wald ER: Management of sinusitis in infants and children. *Pediatr, Infect Dis J* 1988;**7**:449.

Wald ER, Chiponis D, Ledesma-Medina J: Comparative effectiveness of amoxicillin and amoxicillin-clavulanate potassium in acute paranasal sinus infections in children: A double-blind, placebo-controlled trial. *Pediatrics* 1986;**77**:795.

2. RECURRENT SINUSITIS

Frequent episodes of sinusitis occur in a small group of patients. The most common cause is allergic rhinitis. The second most common cause—especially of frontal sinusitis—is diving or jumping into water feet first. The remaining cases are caused by pressure against the ostia by a septal deviation, nasal malformation, a polyp, or a foreign body. In cases of recurrent pyogenic pansinusitis, poor host resistance (eg, an immune defect, Kartagener's syndrome, or cystic fibrosis) must be ruled out by immunoglobulin studies, cilia studies, and a sweat

chloride test. If allergies and diving do not offer a sufficient explanation for the problem, the patient should be referred to an otolaryngologist for complete evaluation.

Jaffe BF: Chronic sinusitis in children. *Clin Pediatr (Phila)* 1974;**13**:944.

Rachelefsky GS et al: Chronic sinus disease associated with reactive airway disease in children. *Pediatrics* 1984;**73**:526.

RECURRENT EPISTAXIS

Most children have a few isolated nosebleeds, but recurrent nosebleed usually warrants a visit to the pediatrician. The nose is a very vascular structure. In most cases, epistaxis is due to mild trauma to the anterior portion of the nasal septum (Kiesselbach's area), sometimes as a result of falls or fistfights but usually due to vigorous nose rubbing, nose blowing, or nose picking.

Clinical Findings

A. Symptoms and Signs: The frequency of nosebleeds may be once a month to several times a day. If they are profuse, subsequent hematemesis or tarry stools may be reported. Examination of Kiesselbach's area reveals a red, raw surface with fresh clots or old crusts. There will often be blood under the fingernails.

B. Laboratory Findings: A baseline hematocrit is indicated in most patients. The true degree of anemia following a severe nosebleed may not be evident until 6–12 hours after bleeding has ceased.

Most patients do not need a bleeding workup, but bleeding tests are indicated if any of the following are present: a family history of a bleeding disorder, a past medical history of easy bleeding, spontaneous bleeding at other sites, bleeding that lasts for over 20 minutes or will not clot with direct pressure by the physician, onset before age 2, or a drop in the hematocrit due to epistaxis.

Differential Diagnosis

Although most cases of epistaxis occur following trauma to the normal nose, several contributing factors must be ruled out. If they are present, specific treatment will be needed.

A. Allergic Rhinitis: Boggy, inflamed mucosa is predisposed to epistaxis. This diagnosis is confirmed by a nasal smear for eosinophils. In such a case, antihistamines or cromolyn may help to decrease the amount of nasal pruritus and subsequent rubbing.

B. Chronic Bleeding Disorder: Numerous bleeding disorders (eg, von Willebrand's disease, thrombocytopenia) may present as recurrent epistaxis. A history of easy bleeding with circumcision, tonsillectomy, lacerations, venipuncture, or tooth eruption points to this type of disorder. A family history of hemophilia or other bleeding tendencies is suggestive. A history of spontaneous bleeding at other sites—gastrointestinal tract, hemarthrosis, menorrhagia, petechiae with crying, etc—or current physical findings of bleeding at other sites is suggestive. The presence of hepatomegaly or splenomegaly is also suggestive. These patients require bleeding screens.

C. Aspirin: Recent studies reveal that ingestion of normal doses of aspirin can interfere with platelet aggregation or adhesiveness and cause prolonged bleeding. The abnormal bleeding time is confirmatory.

D. Vascular Malformation: Kiesselbach's area must be carefully examined for telangiectasia, hemangiomas, or varicosities.

E. Hypertension: High blood pressure may predispose to prolonged nosebleeds.

F. Nasopharyngeal Angiofibroma: This tumor of adolescent males often presents with epistaxis. Bleeding confined to the back of the throat makes the elimination of this diagnosis mandatory. Lateral soft tissue films of the nasopharynx are diagnostic.

Complications

Unless an underlying bleeding disorder exists, the only complication of nosebleed is mild anemia. The latter is unusual and responds to iron therapy.

Treatment

A. Immediate Treatment: The following approach can be carried out in the office or given as phone advice: The patient should sit up and lean forward so as not to swallow the blood. The nose is pinched, with pressure over the bleeding site being maintained for 10 minutes by the clock. If bleeding continues, pressure is not being applied to the right spot, and it should be changed.

If this is not effective, clots should be removed by suction or blowing the nose. A pledget wet with 0.25% phenylephrine (Neo-Synephrine) nose drops, 1% lidocaine (Xylocaine) with 1:1000 epinephrine—or the most potent topical vasoconstrictor of all, 1% cocaine—is inserted into the nose. Pressure is again applied for 10 minutes. Rarely does this technique fail.

Two different approaches involve the insertion of a small piece of gelatin sponge (Gelfoam) or topical thrombin over the bleeding site or the insertion of a wedge of salt pork into the bleeding nostril.

B. Preventive Treatment: The friability of the nasal vessels can be decreased with daily application of petrolatum by cotton-tipped applicator. The lubricant is applied daily until 5 days have passed without a nosebleed, then weekly for 1 month, and resumed only if the nosebleeds recur. In a very dry environment, humidification of the patient's room may be helpful. Aspirin should be avoided.

C. Reassurance: Parents need reassurance regarding the amount of blood lost. It always looks like more than it actually is. A normal hematocrit is usually comforting to the parents. The child should not be blamed regarding this problem. The parents should be told that simply rubbing a blocked nose or picking out dried mucus can cause nosebleeds.

D. Unwarranted Treatment: Electrocautery is contraindicated because it is painful and frightening to the child. Both electrocautery and chemical cautery can cause destruction of the septal tissue, resulting in scarring and an increased tendency for later bleeding.

Prognosis

Once home treatment and prophylaxis are mastered, nosebleeds become an insignificant problem for most families. In unusual cases where posterior bleeding occurs, the child must be referred to an otolaryngologist for a posterior pack, evaluation for nasopharyngeal lesions, and possibly a transfusion.

Kirchner JA: Epistaxis. *N Engl J Med* 1982;**307**:11.

NASAL FURUNCLE

A nasal furuncle is an infection of a hair follicle in the anterior nares. Hair plucking or nose picking can provide a route of entry. The most common organism is *Staphylococcus aureus*. The diagnosis is made by finding an exquisitely tender, firm, red lump in the anterior naris. Treatment includes dicloxacillin, 50 mg/kg/d orally for 5 days, to prevent spread. The lesion should be gently incised and drained as soon as it points, usually with a needle. Topical bacitracin ointment may be of additional value. Since this lesion is in the drainage area of the cavernous sinus, the patient should be followed closely until healing is complete. Parents should be advised never to pick or squeeze a furuncle in this location, nor should the physician. Associated cellulitis or spread requires hospitalization for intravenous antibiotics.

Some patients with recurrent skin abscesses as well as nasal furuncles are nasal carriers of *S aureus*. The skin problem will often not resolve until the nasal carrier state is eradicated by systemic antibiotics, topical antibiotics, and recolonization of the nasal mucosa with nonpathogenic staphylococci.

NASAL SEPTUM SUBLUXATION

About 5% of newborn infants have a subluxation of the quadrangular cartilage of the septum. The tip of the nose deviates to one side, and the inferior septal border deviates to the other. There is also leaning of the columella and instability of the nasal tip. In the delivery room, reduction should be accomplished by lifting up the inferior border of the septum and replacing it in the septal groove of the floor of the nose. If any question regarding the procedure exists, an otolaryngologist should be consulted. This disorder must be distinguished from the more common transient flattening of the nose caused by the birth process.

Kent SE: Nasal septal deviation. *J R Soc Med* 1988; **81**:132.
Silverman SH et al: Dislocation of the triangular cartilage of the nasal septum. *J Pediatr* 1975;**87**:456.

NASAL FRACTURE

Most blows to the nose result in swelling and hematoma without a fracture. A persistent nosebleed after trauma suggests nasal fracture. Crepitus or instability of the bones in the nasal bridge is diagnostic of fracture, as is marked deviation of the nose to one side. However, septal injury can only be ruled out by a careful intranasal examination. If the parents feel that the appearance of the nose remains abnormal after the edema has resolved (usually 3–4 days), this should be taken as strong evidence for fracture. X-rays are not usually helpful because they are negative in half of fractures. In general, they are warranted only in patients who have clinical suggestion of a fracture.

Patients with suspected nasal fractures should be referred to an ear, nose, and throat surgeon for definitive therapy. Resetting of the nasal fracture can be postponed up to 1 week without causing difficulty.

Olsen KD, Carpenter RJ, Kern EB: Nasal septal trauma in children. *Pediatrics* 1979;**64**:32.

NASAL SEPTUM HEMATOMA

After nasal trauma, it is essential to examine the inside of the nose with a nasal speculum. Hematoma of the nasal septum imposes a considerable risk of pressure necrosis and resorption of the cartilage, leading to septal perforation or a saddle-back nose in adulthood. This diagnosis is confirmed by the abrupt onset of nasal obstruction following trauma and the presence of a widened nasal septum.

Treatment consists of prompt referral to an otolaryngologist for evacuation of the hematoma and packing of the nose.

Myers EN: Finding the cause of nasal obstruction. *J Respir Dis* 1981;**2**:107.

NASAL SEPTUM ABSCESS

A nasal septal abscess usually follows nasal trauma or a nasal furuncle. The symptoms include fever, nasal tenderness, and nasal occlusion. Physical findings reveal a fluctuant gray septal swelling, usually bilateral. The possible complications are the same as for nasal septal hematoma plus septicemia, meningitis, or cavernous sinus thrombosis.

Treatment consists of immediate hospitalization, incision and drainage by an otolaryngologist, and intravenous antibiotics.

Segal S et al: Bacterial meningitis secondary to abscess of the nasal septum. *Pediatrics* 1977;**60**:102.

FOREIGN BODIES IN THE NOSE

Most objects inserted into the nose are detected by the parent soon after insertion, and the child is brought in immediately. Occasionally, a nasal foreign body is detected only after unilateral purulent rhinitis occurs. Commonly inserted objects are pussy willow buds, beads, buttons, bullets, nuts, and marbles. In preparation for the object's removal, the nose should be suctioned and opened fully with a topical vasoconstrictor. The child's head should be held firmly to prevent movement and secondary injury during the removal. The position of the head should be forward to prevent aspiration of the foreign body into a bronchus. A nasal speculum is sometimes helpful. Suction can be used to remove the layer of mucus that hides the object.

There are many ways to remove nasal foreign bodies. The obvious first maneuver is vigorous nose blowing if the child is old enough. If the object is round, such as a bead, collodion on a cotton-tipped applicator can be placed against it and left there for 1 or 2 minutes, after which it will usually be dry enough to remove the object. Irregular objects can sometimes be grasped with a bayonet forceps. If there is room to go past the object, a right-angled hook can be inserted and withdrawn, pushing the object ahead of it. If these techniques are not successful and there is some space between the object and the side of the nose, a lubricated No. 8 Bardex Foley catheter can be inserted. When the balloon is past the object, it can be inflated and then used to extract the object.

While the child's head remains tilted over a large basin, the noninvolved nostril can be flushed rapidly with normal saline from a nasal bulb syringe. The wave of fluid will wash around to the involved side and in most cases will force the object out. Closing the uninvolved nostril and placing one's mouth over the patient's mouth to administer a sudden blast of air will force the foreign body out if enough pressure is exerted. If the object seems inaccessible, is wedged in, or is quite large, the patient should be referred to an otolaryngologist without worsening its position through futile attempts.

Baker MD: Foreign bodies of the ears and nose in childhood. *Pediatr Emerg Care* 1987;**3**:67.

Goff WE: "Tip of the Month." *Consultant* (Jan) 1973; **13**:144.

Rees AC: "Tip of the Month." *Consultant* (Feb) 1970; **10**:12.

Stool SE, McConnell CS: Foreign bodies in pediatric otolaryngology. *Clin Pediatr (Phila)* 1973;**12**:113.

THE THROAT

ACUTE STOMATITIS

Recurrent Aphthous Stomatitis ("Canker Sore")

The main finding is multiple (1–4) small (3–10 mm) ulcers on the inside of the lips and throughout the remainder of the mouth. There is usually no associated fever or cervical adenopathy. The ulcers are very painful and last 1–2 weeks. They may recur numerous times throughout a patient's life span. The cause is not known, although an allergic or autoimmune basis is suspected. It is important to rule out any offending agents that could be avoided (chocolate, nuts, tomatoes, etc). These lesions are commonly misdiagnosed as herpes simplex.

Treatment consists of topical corticosteroids, either in a dental paste—eg, triamcinolone acetonide, 0.1% (Kenalog in Orabase)—or in a mouthwash administered 4 times a day. Pain can be symptomatically improved by a bland diet, avoiding salty or acid foods, switching from a bottle to a cup in infants, 2% viscous lidocaine (Xylocaine) prior to meals, and aspirin or even codeine at bedtime. In children not old enough to expectorate the lidocaine, it must be used sparingly to prevent side effects. Some patients gain pain relief from chemical cautery of the ulcers (eg, with silver nitrate). Measures that are unwarranted and sometimes harmful are smallpox vaccine, systemic antibiotics, and *Lactobacillus*-containing agents.

Herpes Simplex Gingivostomatitis

Approximately 1% of children who have their first encounter with the herpes simplex organism develop multiple (10 or more) small (1–3 mm) ulcers of the buccal mucosa, anterior pillars, inner lips, tongue, and especially the gingiva, with associated fever, tender cervical nodes, and generalized inflammation of the mouth. The children are commonly under 3 years of age. This disorder lasts 7–10 days. Severe dysphagia interferes with eating and drinking. The primary disorder does not recur; herpes simplex recurs only in the form of cold sores that are found mainly at the labial mucocutaneous juncture.

Treatment is symptomatic as described for recurrent aphthous stomatitis (see above), with the exception that corticosteroids are contraindicated because they may result in spread of the infection. The efficacy of oral acyclovir prescribed within 36 hours of onset is being studied. The patient must be followed closely. Dehydration occasionally ensues despite liberal offerings of cold fluids, in which case the patient must be hospitalized so that intravenous fluids can be administered. Herpetic laryngotracheitis is a rare complication.

Stevens-Johnson Syndrome

The bullous form of erythema multiforme should be considered whenever there are vesicles and ulcers of the lips and oral mucosa with similar lesions on the conjunctivae and genitalia. In addition, most affected patients have a generalized erythema multiforme rash plus high fever and severe prostration. (For full discussion, see Chapter 11).

Thrush of Mouth

Oral candidiasis mainly affects bottle-fed infants and occasionally older children in a debilitated state. *Candida albicans* is a saprophyte that normally is not invasive unless the mouth is abraded. The use of broad-spectrum antibiotics may be a contributing factor. The symptoms include soreness of the mouth and refusal of feedings. Lesions consist of white curd-like plaques predominantly on the buccal mucosa. These plaques cannot be washed away after a water feeding.

Specific treatment consists of use of nystatin (Mycostatin) oral suspension, 1 mL 4 times a day for 1 week. This should be preceded by attempts to remove any large plaques with a moistened cotton-tipped applicator. The child should be fed temporarily with a spoon and cup to eliminate pain or continued abrasion.

Oral Syphilis

The primary chancre can occur on the lips or in the oral cavity. Secondary syphilis can present as mucous patches on any part of the oral cavity. These have a gray, slimy, concentric appearance and can occur in various sizes. Both of these lesions can be diagnosed by darkfield examination. By the time mucous patches are present, the serologic test for syphilis will be positive. Syphilis is discussed more fully in Chapter 28.

Traumatic Oral Ulcers

Ulcers are a nonspecific response of the oral mucosa to trauma. Mechanical trauma most commonly occurs on the buccal mucosa secondary to accidentally biting it with the molars. Thermal trauma, eg, from very hot foods, can also cause ulcerative lesions. Chemical ulcers can be produced by mucosal contact with aspirin, caustics, etc. Oral ulcers can also occur with leukemia or on a recurrent basis with cyclic neutropenia.

These lesions usually need no treatment. The pain subsides in 2 or 3 days.

Dilley DH, Blozis GG: Common oral lesions and oral manifestations of systemic illnesses and therapies. *Pediatr Clin North Am* 1982;**29**:585.

Fermaglich DR, Fermaglich LF: Tracheostomy in primary herpetic gingivostomatitis. *J Pediatr* 1973;**82**:884.

Goldberg MP: The oral mucosa in childhood. *Pediatr Clin North Am* 1978;**25**:239.

Wright JM: A review of the oral manifestations of infections in pediatric patients. *Pediatr Infect Dis J* 1984; **3**:80.

ACUTE VIRAL PHARYNGITIS & TONSILLITIS

Over 90% of cases of sore throat and fever in children are due to viral infections. Most children develop associated rhinorrhea and mild cough and in fact are having a cold and nothing more. The findings seldom give any clue to the particular viral agent, but 6 types of viral pharyngitis are sufficiently different to permit the clinician to make an educated guess about the specific cause.

Clinical Findings

A. Infectious Mononucleosis: The findings are an exudative tonsillitis, generalized cervical adenitis, and fever, usually in a teenage patient. A palpable spleen or axillary adenopathy adds weight to the diagnosis. The presence of more than 20% atypical lymphocytes on a peripheral blood smear or a positive mononucleosis spot test (Monospot) confirms the diagnosis, although the Monospot is frequently negative in children under 5 years old. This diagnosis is often not considered until a patient with a presumptive diagnosis of streptococcal pharyngitis has failed to respond to 48 hours of treatment with penicillin.

B. Herpangina: Herpangina ulcers, 2–3 mm in size, are found on the anterior pillars and sometimes on the soft palate and uvula. There are no ulcers in the anterior mouth as seen in herpes simplex. Fever is present. The disease lasts up to a week. Herpangina is caused by several members of the coxsackie A group of viruses, and a patient can have up to 5 bouts of herpangina in a lifetime.

C. Lymphonodular Pharyngitis: The classic finding is small, yellow-white nodules in the same distribution as the small ulcers in herpangina. In this condition, which is caused by coxsackievirus A10, the nodules do not ulcerate.

D. Hand, Foot, and Mouth Disease: This entity is caused by coxsackieviruses A5, A10, and A16. Ulcers occur on the tongue and oral mucosa. Vesicles, which usually do not ulcerate, are found on the palms, soles, and interdigital areas.

E. Pharyngoconjunctival Fever: This disorder is caused by an adenovirus. Exudative tonsillitis, conjunctivitis, and fever are the main findings.

F. Rubeola: The prodrome of measles looks like any nonspecific viral respiratory infection until one closely examines the buccal mucosa and the inner aspects of the lower lip. Small white specks the size of salt granules on an erythematous base (Koplik's spots) found at these sites are pathognomonic of measles.

Treatment

The treatment of acute viral pharyngitis is strictly symptomatic. Older children can gargle with warm hypertonic salt solution. Younger children can suck on hard candy (especially butterscotch). Analgesics and antipyretics are sometimes helpful. Antibiotics are contraindicated.

ACUTE STREPTOCOCCAL PHARYNGITIS & TONSILLITIS

Approximately 10% of children with sore throat and fever have a streptococcal infection. Untreated streptococcal pharyngitis can result in acute rheumatic fever, glomerulonephritis, and suppurative complications (eg, cervical adenitis, peritonsillar abscess, otitis media, cellulitis, and septicemia). Vesicles and ulcers are suggestive of viral infection, whereas cervical adenitis, petechiae, a beefy-red uvula, and a tonsillar exudate are suggestive of streptococcal infection; the only way to make a definitive diagnosis is by obtaining a throat culture or a rapid identification test. A throat culture can be read 18 hours after being placed in an incubator. The bacteriology involved is simple, and an inexpensive office incubator is available. Office throat cultures or rapid identification tests are essential to the rational treatment of pharyngitis.

Treat cases of suspected or proved *S pyogenes* infection with a 10-day course of oral penicillin V or an intramuscular injection of penicillin G benzathine. Use erythromycin for patients with penicillin allergy. In unresponsive cases, switch to an antibiotic effective against β-lactamase-producing organisms, such as amoxicillin plus clavulanate or a cephalosporin. The presence of these organisms in the throat may protect *S pyogenes*. Treatment failure after 10 days of penicillin V administered 3 times daily varies from 6–23%. Approximately 5% of *S pyogenes* are resistant to erythromycin. Remember that trimethoprim prescribed in combination with sulfamethoxazole is not an acceptable antibiotic for *S pyogenes*.

When the child has a history of recurrent streptococcal infection, document the presence of *S pyogenes* in an asymptomatic patient following a course of therapy. If either compliance or the dose of antibiotic therapy was questionable, treat with intramuscular penicillin; otherwise, treat with an antibiotic effective against β-lactamase-producing organisms ([amoxicillin plus clavulanate], a cephalosporin, or erythromycin). If this therapy fails to eradicate the organism, consider a course of clindamycin or intramuscular penicillin G benzathine plus oral rifampin. Attempt to eradicate the carrier state when the patient or another family member has frequent streptococcal infections or when a family member or patient has a history of rheumatic fever or glomerulonephritis. If the patient had 3 or more documented infections within 6 months, consider instituting daily penicillin prophylaxis during the winter season. Refer patients for tonsillectomy when they continue to have frequent episodes or when persistently enlarged tonsils result in chronic upper airway obstruction. See Fig 14–4.

Other rare causes of acute pharyngitis are *Corynebacterium diphtheriae*, *Neisseria gonorrhoeae*, group C streptococci, meningococci, *Chlamydia*, and *Mycoplasma pneumoniae*.

Berwick DM et al: Impact of rapid antigen tests for group A streptococcal pharyngitis on physician use of antibiotics and throat cultures. *Pediatr Infect Dis J* 1987; **6:**1095.

Denny FW: Current problems in managing streptococcal pharyngitis. *J Pediatr* 1987;**111:**797.

Putto A: Febrile exudative tonsillitis: Viral or streptococcal. *Pediatrics* 1987;**80:**6.

Radetsky M, Solomon JA, Todd JK: Identification of streptococcal pharyngitis in the office laboratory: Reassessment of new technology. *Pediatr Infect Dis J* 1987; **6:**556.

RECURRENT PHARYNGITIS

School-age children are occasionally brought to a physician with a complaint of recurrent or persistent sore throat. Fever and other systemic manifestations are usually absent. There are 3 common causes of this problem: mouth breathing, postnasal drip, and school phobia.

Mouth breathing leads to dryness and irritation of the throat, especially in areas of low humidity. Occasionally, children will even complain upon awakening that their lips are stuck to their teeth. The causes of mouth breathing should be investigated. Symptomatic treatment consists of good hydration and environmental humidification.

Postnasal drip due to chronic sinusitis can lead to continuous irritation of the throat. Examination reveals mucopurulent secretions descending from the nasopharynx after the patient sniffs. The irritation is largely due to repeated clearing of the throat.

Children with **school phobia** are brought in repeatedly for sore throats, but physical examination reveals a normal oropharynx and tonsillar area. The diagnosis is made by asking the parent if the problem has been interfering with the child's school attendance. The answer will be affirmative and completely out of keeping with the degree of symptoms. Management is described in Chapter 25.

PERITONSILLAR ABSCESS (QUINSY)

Tonsillar infection occasionally penetrates the tonsillar capsule, spreads to the surrounding tissues, and causes peritonsillar cellulitis. If untreated, necrosis occurs and a tonsillar abscess forms. This can occur at any age. The most common cause is β-hemolytic streptococci. Other pathogens are group D streptococci, α-hemolytic streptococci, *S pneumoniae* and anaerobes.

The patient complains of a severe sore throat even before the physical findings become marked. A high fever is usually present. The process is almost always unilateral. The tonsil bulges medially, and the anterior pillar is prominent. The soft palate and uvula on the involved side are edematous and displaced medially toward the uninvolved side. In severe cases, there is trismus, dysphagia, and, finally, drooling. The quality of the voice is severely impaired by the fixation of the soft palate. On palpation, the tonsil is firm and exquisitely tender. A serious complication of inadequately treated peritonsillar abscess is a lateral pharyngeal abscess. This leads to fullness and tenderness of the lateral neck, as well as torticollis. Without intervention, the abscess eventually threatens life by airway obstruction or carotid artery erosion.

Aggressive treatment in early cases of peritonsillar cellulitis will usually abort the process and prevent suppuration. The treatment of choice is procaine penicillin by daily injection plus oral penicillin 4 times a day in high doses. Consider adding clindamycin for better coverage of β-lactamase-producing anaerobes. Daily follow-up is critical to detect possible abscess. If the initial swelling is marked, fluctuation develops, a neck mass develops, the patient appears toxic, or symptoms fail to respond to 48 hours of antibiotics, the patient should be hospitalized for intravenous penicillin or clindamycin. An otolaryngologist should be consulted to perform incision and drainage. Recurrent peritonsillar abscesses are so uncommon (7%) that routine tonsillectomy for a single bout is not indicated. Hospitalized patients can be discharged on oral antibiotics when the fever is resolved for 24 hours and they can swallow easily.

Shoemaker M, Lampe R, Weir MR: Peritonsillitis: Abscess or cellulitis? *Pediatr Infect Dis J* 1986;**5:**43.

Stringer SP et al: Outpatient management of peritonsillar

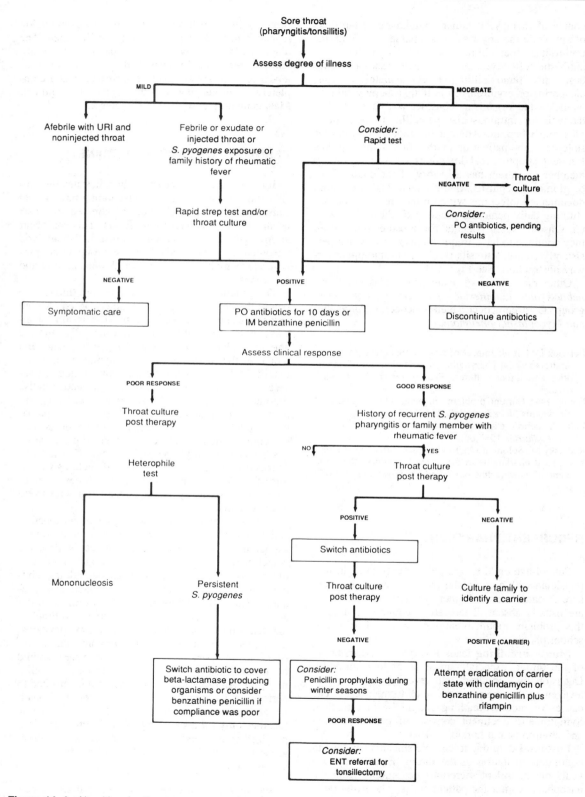

Figure 14–4. Algorithm for the management of streptococcal infection. (Modified and reproduced, with permission, from Berman S: *Pediatric Decision Making.* Decker, 1990).

abscess. *Arch Otolaryngol Head Neck Surg* 1988; **114**:296.

RETROPHARYNGEAL ABSCESS

Retropharyngeal nodes drain the adenoids and nasopharynx and can become infected. The most common cause is β-hemolytic streptococci and *S aureus*. If this pyogenic adenitis goes untreated, a retropharyngeal abscess forms. The process occurs most commonly during the first 2 years of life. Beyond this age, retropharyngeal abscess usually results from superinfection of a penetrating injury of the posterior wall of the oropharynx.

The diagnosis should be strongly suspected in an infant with fever, respiratory symptoms, and neck hyperextension. Dysphagia, drooling, dyspnea, and gurgling respirations are also found and are due to the impingement by the abscess. Prominent swelling on one side of the posterior pharyngeal wall confirms the diagnosis. Swelling usually stops at the midline because a medial raphe divides the prevertebral space. Lateral neck soft tissue films provide additional confirmation if needed.

Retropharyngeal abscess is a surgical emergency. Immediate hospitalization is required. A surgeon should incise and drain the abscess to prevent its extension. The head should be kept down during incision to prevent aspiration of purulent material. Intravenous hydration and antibiotics should be instituted before surgery. A semisynthetic penicillin is the drug of choice pending the results of stained smear examination.

Janecka IP, Rankow RM: Fatal mediastinitis following retropharyngeal abscess. *Arch Otolaryngol* 1971;**93**:630.
McCook TA, Felman AH: Retropharyngeal masses in infants and young children. *Am J Dis Child* 1979;**133**:41.

LUDWIG'S ANGINA

Ludwig's angina is a rapidly progressive cellulitis of the submandibular space. The submandibular space extends from the mucous membrane of the tongue to the muscular and fascial attachments of the hyoid bone. The initiating factor in over half of cases is dental disease, including abscesses and extraction. Some patients have a history of lacerations and injuries to the floor of the mouth. Group A streptococci are the most common organisms identified, but other pathogens have been recovered.

The presenting symptoms are fever and tender swelling of the floor of the mouth. The tongue can become enlarged as well as tender and erythematous. Upward displacement of the tongue may cause dysphagia and drooling. Laboratory evaluation includes

blood cultures and hypopharyngeal aspiration to attempt to identify the specific pathogen.

Treatment consists of giving high dosages of intravenous ampicillin and methicillin until the results of cultures and sensitivity tests are available. Since the most common cause of death in Ludwig's angina is sudden airway obstruction, the patient must be followed closely in the intensive care unit and intubation provided for any progressive respiratory distress.

Barkin RM et al: Ludwig angina in children. *J Pediatr* 1975;**87**:563.
Gross SJ et al: Ludwig angina in childhood. *Am J Dis Child* 1977;**131**:291.

ACUTE UVULITIS

Infections involving the uvula are uncommon. In children under 5 years of age, the cause is usually *Haemophilus influenzae* type b. In children over 5 years of age, group A streptococcus is the usual pathogen. Associated bacteremia is common.

The main symptoms are fever, dysphagia, and drooling. The prominent physical finding is an erythematous, swollen uvula. Laboratory studies should include a complete blood count and blood culture. A lateral neck radiograph should be obtained to rule out associated epiglottiditis. Patients with acute uvulitis should be admitted to the hospital and treated with intravenous antibiotics.

Li KI et al: Isolated uvulitis due to *Haemophilus influenzae* type b. *Pediatrics* 1984;**74**:1054.

ACUTE CERVICAL ADENITIS

Essentials of Diagnosis

- Large, tender, unilateral cervical mass.
- Fever.
- Moderate to marked leukocytosis.

General Considerations

Local infections of the ear, nose, and throat can spread to the regional node and cause a secondary inflammation there. The most commonly involved node is the jugulodigastric node, which drains the tonsillar area. The problem is most prevalent among preschool children.

A classic case involves a large, unilateral, solitary, tender node. About 70% of these cases are due to β-hemolytic streptococci, 20% are due to staphylococci, and the remainder may be due to viruses. *Haemophilus influenzae* or anaerobes have rarely been reported as the cause. Surgeons report a higher incidence of staphylococcal infection, but they see a greater proportion of atypical cases that have failed to respond to penicillin therapy and thus require incision and drainage.

The most common site of invasion is from pharyngitis or tonsillitis. Other entry sites for pyogenic adenitis are periapical dental abscess (usually producing a submandibular adenitis), facial impetigo (infected cuts or bug bites), infected acne, and otitis externa (usually producing a preauricular adenitis).

Clinical Findings

A. Symptoms and Signs: The patient is brought in with the chief complaint of a swollen neck or face. There is usually sustained high fever, especially in staphylococcal infections. The mass is often the size of a walnut or even an egg. It is taut, firm, and exquisitely tender. If left untreated, it may develop an overlying erythema. The exact size of the node should be measured for future follow-up. Each tooth should be examined for a periapical abscess and percussed for tenderness. A protective torticollis is sometimes present.

B. Laboratory Findings: The white blood cell count is usually about 20,000/μL with a shift to the left. The combination of leukocytosis and a positive throat culture or an elevated ASO titer identifies streptococci in about two-thirds of streptococcal cases. A tuberculin skin test should be given. Aspirated material from fluctuant nodes should be gram-stained and cultured.

Differential Diagnosis

The causes of cervical adenopathy are numerous. Five general categories can be distinguished on the basis of the clinical findings.

A. Acute Unilateral Cervical Adenitis: See above.

B. Acute Bilateral Cervical Adenitis: Painful and tender nodes are present on both sides, and the patient usually has fever.

1. Infectious mononucleosis—This diagnosis can be aided by the findings of splenomegaly, over 20% atypical cells on the white blood cell smear, and a positive mononucleosis spot test (Monospot). Toxoplasmosis and cytomegalovirus infections can imitate this disorder.

2. Tularemia—There will be a history of wild rabbit or deerfly exposure.

3. Diphtheria—This occurs only in nonimmunized children.

C. Subacute or Chronic Adenitis: In this condition, an isolated node usually exists, but it is smaller and less tender than the acute pyogenic adenitis described previously.

1. Nonspecific viral pharyngitis—This accounts for about 80% of cases in this category.

2. β-Hemolytic streptococcal infection—Streptococci can occasionally cause a low-grade cervical adenitis; staphylococci never do.

3. Cat-scratch fever—Cat-scratch fever accounts for over 70% of cases of chronic cervical adenopathy. The diagnosis is aided by the finding of a primary papule in approximately 60% of cases. Cat contact or scratches are present in over 90% of cases. The node is usually mildly tender. The cat-scratch skin test is helpful and relatively safe.

4. Atypical mycobacterial infection—The node is generally nontender and submandibular (occasionally preauricular). The nodes become fluctuant after several months. Affected patients are usually 1–5 years of age. A history of drinking unpasteurized milk is helpful. A mildly positive PPD is suggestive. A PPD-standard gives 5–10 mm of induration, whereas the PPD–Battey gives greater than 10 mm of induration. If skin tests for atypical mycobacteria are not available, the OT (old tuberculin) test can be substituted for screening.

D. Cervical Node Tumors: Malignant tumors usually are not suspected until the adenopathy persists despite treatment. Classically, the nodes are painless, nontender, and firm to hard in consistency. They may occur as a single node, unilateral multiple nodes in a chain, bilateral cervical nodes, or generalized adenopathy. Cancers that may present in the neck are Hodgkin's disease, lymphosarcoma, fibrosarcoma, thyroid cancer, leukemia, and cancers with an occult primary in the nasopharynx (eg, rhabdomyosarcoma). A benign tumor that presents as enlarged cervical nodes is sinus histiocytosis.

E. Imitators of Adenitis: Several structures in the neck can become infected and resemble a node. The first 3 masses are of congenital origin and are listed in order of frequency.

1. Thyroglossal duct cyst—When superinfected, this congenital malformation can become acutely swollen. Helpful findings are the fact that it is in the midline, located between the hyoid bone and suprasternal notch, and moves upward on sticking out the tongue or swallowing. Occasionally, the cyst develops a sinus tract and opening just lateral to the midline.

2. Branchial cleft cyst—When superinfected, this can become a tender mass, 3–5 cm in diameter. Aids to diagnosis are the fact that the mass is located along the anterior border of the sternocleidomastoid muscle and is smooth and fluctuant as a cyst should be. Occasionally, it is attached to the overlying skin by a small dimple or a draining sinus tract.

3. Cystic hygroma—Most of these lymphatic cysts are located in the posterior triangle just above the clavicle. The mass is soft and compressible and can be transilluminated. Over 60% are noted at birth, and the remainder usually present by 2 years of age. If cysts become large enough, they can compromise swallowing and breathing.

4. Mumps—The most common pitfall in diagnosis is mistaking mumps for adenitis. However, mumps crosses the angle of the jaw, is associated with preauricular percussion tenderness, and is bilateral in 70% of cases, and there is frequently a history of exposure to mumps. Submandibular mumps can present a diagnostic dilemma.

5. Ranula—This sublingual retention cyst can be mistaken for a submental mass.

6. Sternocleidomastoid muscle hematoma—This cervical mass is noted at 2–4 weeks of age. On close examination it is found to be part of the muscle body and not movable. An associated torticollis is usually confirmatory.

Complications

The most common complication in the untreated case is suppuration of the node, with eventual pointing and exterior drainage. In the preantibiotic era, extension sometimes occurred internally, resulting in jugular vein thrombosis, carotid artery rupture, septicemia, and compression of the esophagus or larynx. Poststreptococcal acute glomerulonephritis and bacteremia have also been reported.

Treatment

A. Specific Measures: Unless the patient has recently been exposed to β-hemolytic streptococci, dicloxacillin or cephalexin is usually started initially. The antibiotic can be changed to penicillin if it is not well tolerated and the throat culture is positive for streptococci. An antistaphylococcal must be started initially if the patient is under 6 months of age or the node is already fluctuant or erythematous. The patient should be referred to a dentist if a periapical abscess is suspected. These dental patients should also be given prophylactic penicillin therapy to prevent associated facial cellulitis or submandibular adenitis.

B. General Measures: Analgesics (even codeine) are necessary during the first few days. Patients may receive significant relief from application of cold compresses or an ice cube to the inflamed node.

C. Surgical Treatment: Early treatment with antibiotics prevents many cases of pyogenic adenitis from progressing to suppuration. However, once fluctuation occurs, antibiotic therapy alone is not sufficient treatment. When fluctuation or pointing is present and the PPD skin test is negative, the primary physician should incise and drain the abscess. This can easily be done as an office procedure or in an ambulatory surgery unit. Hospitalization is required only if the patient is toxic, dehydrated, dysphagic, dyspneic, or less than 6 months of age.

D. Follow-Up Care: The patient must be seen daily. A good response includes resolution of the fever and improvement in the tenderness after 48 hours of treatment. Reduction in size of the nodes may take several more days. The antibiotic should be continued for 10 days. If there is no improvement in 48 hours and the PPD test is negative, the node should be aspirated with an 18-gauge needle and 0.5 mL of normal saline in the syringe to obtain material for gram-stained smear, culture, and sensitivity tests. Aspirated material should be cultured aerobically and anaerobically.

E. Treatment of Nonpyogenic Adenitis:

1. Cat-scratch fever and atypical mycobacterial infection—Treatment is described in Chapter 28.

2. Persistent unexplained node—As previously mentioned, cancer of the cervical node is usually asymptomatic. The patient with a cervical node that has been enlarging for more than 2 weeks despite treatment or is still large and unchanged in size for more than 2 months should be referred to a surgeon for biopsy.

3. Branchial cleft cyst and thyroglossal duct cyst—If superinfected, these lesions should be treated with penicillin for 10 days. After the infection clears, the patient should be referred to a surgeon for definitive excision of the cyst.

Prognosis

With appropriate treatment, the prognosis is excellent. After the infection clears, the node may remain palpable for several months but will gradually decrease in size unless it is scarred. Recurrent pyogenic adenitis is rare. When it occurs, it is usually due to diseases such as chronic granulomatous disease of childhood or an immunologic disorder.

Buckingham JM, Lynn HB: Branchial cleft cysts and sinuses in children. *Mayo Clin Proc* 1974;**49:**172.

Caruthers HA: Cat scratch disease: An overview based on a study of 1200 patients. *Am J Dis Child* 1985;**139:**1124.

Jaffe BF, Jaffe N: Head and neck tumors in children. *Pediatrics* 1973;**51:**731.

Knight PJ, Mulne AF, Vassy LE: When is lymph node biopsy indicated in children with enlarged perpheral nodes? *Pediatrics* 1982;**69:**391.

Marcy SM: Infections of lymph nodes of head and neck. *Pediatr Infect Dis J* 1983;**2:**397.

Pounds LA: Neck masses of congenital origin. *Pediatr Clin North Am* 1981;**28:**841.

Zitelli BJ: Neck masses in children: Adenopathy and malignant disease. *Pediatr Clin North Am* 1981;**28:**813.

TONSILLECTOMY & ADENOIDECTOMY (T&A)

Removal of the tonsils and adenoids has been described as a North American ritual. Although about 30% of children in the USA have their tonsils and adenoids removed, only 1–2% of children have adequate medical indications for this procedure.

Besides being usually unnecessary, the procedure is costly and carries considerable risk. The mortality rate under good conditions is still one death per 15,000 operations. Postoperative bleeding on the fifth to eighth day occurs in approximately 5% of cases and requires transfusion or suturing of the tonsillar bed. Some children with previously normal speech develop hypernasal speech. The emotional hazards of hospitalization and surgery in a child under 5 years of age have been well documented. There are still questions regarding the role of tonsils in immunologic response and disease prevention.

Invalid Reasons for T&A

The following conditions account for the removal of over 95% of tonsils and adenoids.

A. "Large Tonsils": Many parents feel that large tonsils mean bad tonsils. It is unfortunate that the peak incidence of infections correlates so well with tonsillar size. Normal lymphoid atrophy occurs spontaneously after age 8. The parent should be reassured that the patient's tonsils are within normal range. It is very important at well child checkups not to call a child's tonsils "big" or "bad."

B. Recurrent Colds and Sore Throats: T&A does not decrease the incidence of viral respiratory infections. Parents must be reassured that these infections are a natural event at this age and that contacts eventually give the patient increased immunity.

C. Recurrent Streptococcal Pharyngitis: At one time, repeated episodes of "strep throat" were considered an indication for tonsillectomy. However, it has been shown in several studies that the incidence of streptococcal infections does not decrease after the tonsils have been removed unless 7 or more attacks occur per year. Moreover, the future diagnosis of streptococcal infections is made difficult by the lack of tonsillar exudates.

D. Recurrent Otitis Media: Most cases of recurrent purulent otitis media can be treated with prophylactic antibiotics. Most cases of chronic serous otitis media eventually resolve or require tympanoplasty tubes. An adenoidectomy may be helpful if the child also has symptoms of nasal obstruction.

E. Parental Pressure: Some parents place great demands on their doctor for a T&A and must be skillfully reeducated.

F. School Absence: For the child who misses school for vague symptoms, removing the tonsils will not relieve the school phobia.

G. "Chronic Tonsillitis": It is unclear whether this condition even exists. If it does, it is certainly very rare. The tonsil is allegedly so diseased that even antibiotics cannot eliminate the infections.

H. Miscellaneous Conditions: Poor appetite, allergic rhinitis, asthma, unexplained fevers, and halitosis are not indications for tonsillectomy.

Indications for Adenoidectomy

A. Persistent Nasal Obstruction and Mouth Breathing: Mouth breathing can have many causes, however, if this problem is due to large adenoids, they should be removed to prevent an adenoidal facies. Removal should be preceded by a 2-week trial of penicillin to rule out enlargement from subacute adenoiditis.

B. Snoring: The adenoids should be removed if they appear to be the cause of continual nighttime snoring and daytime snorting.

C. Hyponasal Speech: Large adenoids can cause hyponasal speech that leads to poor communication as well as teasing. On examination, large adenoids are found to be preventing the uvula from moving upward normally.

Indications for Tonsillectomy

A. Persistent Oral Obstruction and Dysphagia: Intermittent oral obstruction and dysphagia can occur as a result of inflammation and swelling of the tonsils. If the problem is persistent and the tonsils are seen to almost touch in the midline, tonsillectomy should be performed. This is especially likely to happen in people who have small oral cavities.

B. Recurrent Peritonsillar Abscess: This problem implies that the tonsil is no longer inhibiting the spread of infection and needs to be removed. About 7% of peritonsillar abscesses recur.

C. Recurrent Pyogenic Cervical Adenitis: Again, the tonsil is no longer acting as an effective barrier to the spread of infection.

D. Suspected Tonsillar Tumor: The prominent unilateral tonsil, especially if it is rapidly enlarging, may be removed with the presumptive diagnosis of tonsillar neoplasm. On palpation, these tumors are usually firm and fixed. This is a grave diagnosis to miss.

Indications for Combined T&A

A. Cor Pulmonale: A patient with adenoidal hypertrophy can develop chronic hypoxia that leads to pulmonary hypertension and finally to cor pulmonale and right-sided heart failure. This is a rare but serious complication that is definitely helped by T&A, sometimes on an emergency basis.

B. Sleep Apnea Syndrome: Affected children all have loud snoring interrupted by 30- to 60-second apneic and cyanotic episodes. Many are referred because of excessive daytime sleepiness and worsening school performance. Acquired pectus excavatum has also been reported in some of these children. Their symptoms are reversed by T&A.

C. Recurrent Aspiration Pneumonia: The patient with huge tonsils, muffled speech, and gurgling respirations may occasionally present with repeated aspiration pneumonia.

Contraindications to T&A

A. Short Palate: Adenoids should not be removed in a child with a cleft palate, submucous cleft palate, or bifid uvula, because of the risk of aggravating the velopharyngeal incompetence and causing hypernasal speech and nasal regurgitation.

B. Bleeding Disorder: If a chronic bleeding

disorder is present, it must be diagnosed and compensated for before a T&A.

C. Acute Tonsillitis: T&A should be postponed until an acute tonsillitis is resolved. This guideline may prevent a superinfection of the wound.

D. Polio Season: T&A during polio season in a susceptible population leads to an increased risk of bulbar poliomyelitis. Wide-scale use of poliovaccine can eliminate this hazard.

Management of Parental Pressure

If parents are dissatisfied with the kind of treatment they are receiving, they can "doctor-shop" until they find someone who will remove their child's tonsils. This can be prevented by the following approach:

The parents' complaint must be taken seriously. All of the reasonable indications for T&A must be competently investigated. The ear, nose, and throat examination must be performed carefully, and the parents must be assured that there are some valid reasons to take out the tonsils but only when the benefit outweighs the risk, discomfort, inconvenience, and expense.

The parents can then be reassured that their child is basically healthy. The prognosis for spontaneous involution of the tonsils and adenoids and a lower incidence of respiratory infections in years to come can be offered. In addition, it can be mentioned that the risk of taking the tonsils out is considerably greater than the risk of leaving them in.

If the parents are still unconvinced, a consultation is in order. Since it is in the child's best interest, an otolaryngologist should be chosen who shares the pediatrician's viewpoint on this subject.

Guilleminault C et al: Sleep apnea in eight children. *Pediatrics* 1976;**58**:23.

Paradise JL: Tonsillectomy and adenoidectomy. *Pediatr Clin North Am* 1981;**28**:881.

Paradise JL et al: Efficacy of tonsillectomy for recurrent throat infection in severely affected children. *N Engl J Med* 1984;**310**:674.

Ridgway D et al: Unsuspected non-Hodgkin's lymphoma of the tonsils and adenoids in children. *Pediatrics* 1987;**79**:399.

Shaikh W et al: A systematic review of the literature on evaluative studies of tonsillectomy and adenoidectomy. *Pediatrics* 1976;**57**:401.

DISORDERS OF THE LIPS*

Labial Sucking Tubercle

A small baby may present with a small callus in the mid upper lip. It usually is asymptomatic and disappears after cup feeding is initiated.

---

*Herpetic lesions are discussed in Chapter 27.

Swollen Lip

Allergy can cause the sudden onset of angioedema of the lip. Possible causes include foods, contact dermatitis to lipstick, and insect bites. Treatment includes avoidance of the cause, cold compresses, and oral antihistamines.

Cheilitis

Dry, cracked, scaling lips are usually due to sun or wind exposure. Contact dermatitis from mouthpieces of various woodwind or brass instruments has also been reported. Licking the lips accentuates the process, and the patient should be warned of this. Liberal use of lip balms gives excellent results.

Perlèche

The angle of the mouth may become fissured and raw. This most commonly happens in children who drool or lick the sides of the mouth, establishing a macerated area. The most common pathogen is *Candida albicans*. Sores at the corners of the mouth can also be due to use of wide teething rings with rough edges. Riboflavin deficiency is a rare cause. The lesions respond well to nystatin (Mycostatin) cream. Occasionally, a corticosteroid must be added.

Inclusion Cyst

Inclusion cysts, or retention cysts, are due to the obstruction of mucous glands or other mucous membrane structures. In the newborn, they occur on the hard palate or gums and are called Epstein's pearls. These small cysts resolve spontaneously in 1–2 months. In older children, inclusion cysts usually occur on the palate, uvula, or tonsillar pillars. They appear as taut, yellow sacs varying in size from 2 to 10 mm. They spontaneously resolve in several months to a year without requiring incision and drainage. They can be rechecked in 1 month to confirm that they are not enlarging rapidly and thereafter reevaluated only during regular visits. Occasionally, a mucous cyst on the lower lip (mucocele) will require drainage for cosmetic reasons. Minor salivary glands are present at this site, and biting the lip may sever their ducts and initiate the problem.

DISORDERS OF THE TONGUE

Geographic Tongue (Benign Migratory Glossitis)

This condition of unknown cause is marked by circular or elliptical smooth areas on the tongue devoid of papillae and surrounded by a narrow ring of hyperkeratosis. The pattern can change from day to day. The lesions are painless and may last months to years. This puzzling disorder is benign, uncommon after age 6, and requires no treatment.

Fissured Tongue
(Scrotal Tongue)

This condition is marked by numerous irregular fissures on the dorsum of the tongue. It occurs in approximately 1% of people and is usually a dominant trait. It is also frequently seen in children with trisomy 21 and other retarded patients who have the habit of chewing on a protruded tongue.

Coated Tongue
(Furry Tongue)

The tongue normally becomes coated if mastication is impaired and the patient is on a liquid or soft diet. Mouth breathing, fever, or dehydration can accentuate the process.

Macroglossia

Tongue hypertrophy and protrusion may be a clue to Beckwith's syndrome, glycogen storage disease, cretinism, Hurler's syndrome, lymphangioma, or hemangioma. In trisomy 21, the normal-sized tongue protrudes because the oral cavity is small.

Acute Bacterial Glossitis

Reported causes of acute suppurative glossitis include *Haemophilus influenzae* type b, *Streptococcus pyogenes,* and *Pseudomonas.* This rare disease is characterized by fever and rapid swelling and tenderness of the tongue. Intravenous antibiotics are required.

Edwards MS, Reynolds GES: Acute glossitis due to *Hemophilus influenzae* type b. *J Pediatr* 1978;**93**:532.

ORAL TRAUMA

Puncture wounds of the floor of the mouth and soft palate are not uncommon in children. Most could be prevented if children were forbidden to play with sticks or pencils in their mouths. Treatment includes a tetanus booster if one has not been given in the previous 5 years. Prophylactic antibiotics are not helpful, but the patient should be seen after 48 hours to rule out the possibility of superinfection. Puncture wounds of the anterior pillar or posterior pharynx should be followed closely for carotid thrombosis or retropharyngeal abscess, respectively.

Lacerations of the lip require precise closure and alignment of the mucocutaneous juncture. Lacerations of the buccal mucosa usually heal without suturing. Most tongue lacerations heal without suturing; if they involve the edges of the tongue and are large enough to cause gaping of the wound, black silk sutures must be placed, sometimes under general anesthesia.

HALITOSIS

"Bad breath" is a puzzling and distressing complaint. In most cases, it is due to acute stomatitis,

pharyngitis, or sinusitis. In children, there are 2 common causes of chronic halitosis: continual mouth breathing and thumb-sucking or blanket-sucking. Unusual causes of foul breath are a nasal foreign body, esophageal diverticulum, gastric bezoar, bronchiectasis, and lung abscess. In older children, the presence of orthodontic devices or dentures can cause halitosis if good dental hygiene is not maintained. Also, offensive skin odors (eg, dirty feet) of long duration can become absorbed and excreted through the lungs. Mouthwashes and chewable breath fresheners give limited improvement. The cause must be uncovered to help the patient with chronic halitosis.

SALIVARY GLAND DISORDERS*

Suppurative Parotitis Pyogenic parotitis is an unusual clinical disorder found predominantly in newborns and debilitated older patients. The parotid gland is swollen, tender, and often reddened. The diagnosis is made by expression of purulent material from Stensen's duct. The material should be smeared and cultured. Fever and leukocytosis may be present.

Treatment includes hospitalization and intravenous methicillin because the most common causative organism is *Staphylococcus aureus.* If fluctuation occurs and drainage through Stensen's duct is impaired, aspiration of the pus with an 18-gauge needle can avoid the necessity for incision and drainage. This procedure may have to be repeated 3 or 4 times.

Recurrent Idiopathic Parotitis

Some children experience repeated episodes of parotid swelling that lasts 1–2 weeks and then resolves spontaneously. There is usually mild pain and often no fever. The process is most often unilateral, a fact that weighs heavily against an autoimmune process as the underlying cause and points instead to some sort of obstructive process. Serum amylase is normal, a fact that speaks against a diagnosis of viral parotitis as can occur with mumps, parainfluenza, and other viral infections. As many as 10 episodes may occur from age 2 on. The problem usually resolves spontaneously at puberty.

Treatment includes analgesics if pain is present. A 4-day course of corticosteroids can be recommended if it can be initiated early in an attack. A second attack of parotid swelling without fever should result in referral to an otolaryngologist for a sialogram to rule out calculus of Stensen's duct. The usual finding is sialectasis. The sialogram seems to improve as the recurrence rate diminishes.

Pneumoparotitis

Children with pneumoparotitis complain of a sud-

---
*Mumps is discussed in Chapter 27.

den onset of pain and swelling in the parotid area. A history of playing a musical wind instrument or blowing up balloons confirms the diagnosis. The cause of this transient condition is inflation of the parotid gland secondary to sudden increased intraoral pressure.

Tumors of the Parotid

Mixed tumors, hemangiomas, and leukemia can present in the parotid gland as a hard or persistent mass. The patient should be referred to a surgeon.

Ranula

A ranula is a retention cyst of a sublingual salivary gland. It is found on the floor of the mouth to one side of the lingual frenulum. Ranula has been described as resembling a frog's belly, because it is thin-walled and contains a clear bluish fluid. Referral to an otolaryngologist for exclusion of the cyst and associated sublingual gland is the treatment of choice.

Crysdale WS: Ranulas and their treatment. *Laryngoscope* 1988;**98**:296.
David RB et al: Suppurative parotitis in children. *Am J Dis Child* 1970;**119**:332.
Leake D et al: Neonatal suppurative parotitis. *Pediatrics* 1970;**46**:202.
Saunders HF: Wind parotitis. *N Engl J Med* 1973;**289**:689.

ORAL CONGENITAL MALFORMATIONS

Tongue-Tie

The tightness of the lingual frenulum varies greatly among normal people. A short frenulum prevents both protrusion and elevation of the tongue. A puckering of the midline of the tongue occurs with tongue movement. The condition in no way interferes with the ability to nurse. It is unlikely that it interferes with the ability to speak, because even children with ankyloglossia have normal speech.

Treatment consists of reassurance. Although there is no evidence to support it, clipping of the frenulum is sometimes recommended if the tongue does not protrude beyond the teeth or gums. If this degree of tongue-tie is associated with impairment of rapid articulation, the patient should be referred to an otolaryngologist for correction. Casual frenulum clipping can result in significant bleeding from a cut lingual artery or injury to the orifices of Wharton's duct.

Catlin FI, DeHaan V: Tongue-tie. *Arch Otolaryngol* 1971;**94**:548.

Cleft Lip & Cleft Palate

Cleft lip, cleft palate, or both conditions are found in one in 800 live births. They are readily diagnosed in the newborn nursery. Treatment requires a multidisciplined team approach—plastic surgeons, otolaryngologists, audiologists, speech therapists, orthodontists, and prosthodontists. Cleft lip repair is usually withheld until the child weighs over 5 kg. Cleft palate repair is usually performed at 18 months of age; this is essential to permit normal speech development, which should begin at this time. Occasionally, the palate is short and results in nasal speech. A permanently constructed flap of tissue from the posterior pharyngeal wall may be of benefit.

Cleft palate causes eating problems and poor weight gain due to nasal regurgitation or lung aspiration of milk. Best results are obtained by feeding the baby with a cup or special compressible feeder (see Paradise reference, below). The sitting position is optimal for feeding. Cleft palate nipples are usually no more effective than standard nipples. Approximately 90% of children with cleft palate have chronic otitis media and must be carefully followed for this problem. Some otolaryngologists recommend prophylactic tympanoplasty tubes.

Bergstrom L, Hemenway WG: Otologic problems in submucous cleft palate. *South Med J* 1971;**64**:1172.
Paradise JL, McWilliams BJ: Simplified feeder for infants with cleft palate. *Pediatrics* 1974;**53**:566.
Schilli W et al: A general description of 315 cleft lip and palate patients. *Cleft Palate J* 1970;**7**:573.

Bifid Uvula & Submucous Cleft Palate

A bifid uvula can be a normal finding. However, there is a close association between this and submucous cleft palate. A submucous cleft can be diagnosed by a translucent zone in the middle of the soft palate. Palpation of the hard palate reveals the absence of the posterior bony portion. Affected children have a 40% risk of developing chronic serous otitis media. They also are at risk of incomplete closure of the palate, resulting in hypernasal speech. During feeding, many of these infants experience nasal regurgitation of food. Children with a submucous cleft palate that causes symptoms need referral to a plastic surgeon for repair.

High-Arched Palate

A high-arched palate is usually a genetic trait of no consequence. It is also seen in children who are chronic mouth breathers and in premature infants who undergo prolonged oral intubation. Some rare causes of high-arched palate are congenital disorders such as Marfan's syndrome, Treacher Collins syndrome, and Ehlers-Danlos syndrome.

Pierre Robin Syndrome

This congenital malformation is characterized by the triad of micrognathia, cleft palate, and glossoptosis. Affected children present as emergencies in the newborn period because of infringement on the airway by the tongue. The main objective of treatment is to prevent asphyxia until the mandible becomes large enough to accommodate the tongue. In some cases, this objective can be achieved by leaving the child in a prone position while unattended. In severe cases, a custom-fitted oropharyngeal airway or large suture through the base of the tongue that is anchored to the soft tissue in front of the mandible is required. The child requires close observation until the problem is outgrown.

Gunter G et al: Early management of the Pierre Robin syndrome. *Cleft Palate J* 1970;**7:**495.

Hawkins DB, Simpson JV: Micrognathia and glossoptosis in the newborn. *Clin Pediatr (Phila)* 1974;**13:**1066.

Shprintzen JJ: Morphologic significance of bifid uvula. *Pediatrics* 1985;**75:**553.

SELECTED REFERENCES

Bluestone CD: *Pediatric Otolaryngology.* 2 vols. Saunders, 1983.

Bluestone CD, Klein JO: *Otitis Media in Infants and Children.* Saunders, 1988.

Stool SE, Belafsky ML: *Pediatric Otolaryngology: Current Problems in Pediatrics.* Year Book, 1971.

Strome M: *Differential Diagnosis in Pediatric Otolaryngology.* Little, Brown, 1976.

Respiratory Tract & Mediastinum 15

Gary L. Larsen, MD, Steven H. Abman, MD, Leland L. Fan, MD, Carl W. White, MD, & Frank J. Accurso, MD

Respiratory disorders are among the most common acute and chronic problems encountered by physicians who care for children. Pediatric pulmonary diseases account for slightly less than one-half of deaths under one year of age and are responsible for approximately 20% of all hospitalizations of children under 15 years of age. Furthermore, it is estimated that approximately 7% of children suffer some sort of chronic disorder of the lower respiratory system.

Understanding the physiologic and pathologic consequences of these diseases in this age group requires an appreciation of the normal growth and development of the lung. In addition, the physician must be familiar with the common diagnostic aids and therapeutic options used in approaching these problems. These general subjects form the foundation of this chapter and are followed by discussions of congenital and acquired diseases of the respiratory tract and mediastinum.

Mellins RB, Stripp B, Taussig LM: Pediatric pulmonology in North America: Coming of age. *Am Rev Respir Dis* 1987;**134**:849.

US Department of Health and Human Services, National Institutes of Health: *Pediatric Respiratory Disorders.* Department of Health and Human Services Publication No. (NIH) 86–2107, 1986.

GROWTH & DEVELOPMENT OF THE LUNG

Understanding the growth and development of the respiratory system requires understanding changes in its anatomy, mechanical properties, and metabolic and defense functions. In addition to traditional approaches, the techniques of molecular and cellular biology are now being used to investigate the normal growth and development of the respiratory system, as well as the response to injury, at different stages of development.

The lung derives from the foregut during the fourth week of gestation. Subsequent branching leads to the development of the conducting airways (bronchial tree) by about 16 weeks of gestation. The terminal respiratory units, the gas-exchanging portion of the lung, undergo development from the latter third of gestation through the first few months after birth, when alveoli morphologically similar to those in adults are formed. It is clear that alveoli increase in number throughout childhood, but the age at which this increase normally stops is a controversial topic, with estimates ranging from 2 years to adolescence. The development of the pulmonary arterial system in general occurs with the development of the airways, while capillary proliferation in the terminal respiratory units occurs with the development of the alveoli.

With birth, the lung assumes the gas-exchanging function served by the placenta in utero, placing immediate stress on all components of the respiratory system. Abnormalities in the lung, respiratory muscles, chest wall, airway, respiratory controller, or pulmonary circulation may therefore present at birth. Postnatal survival depends, for example, on the development of the surfactant system to maintain airway stability and allow gas exchange. Immaturity of the surfactant system, seen often in infants of less than 35 weeks of gestation, can result in severe respiratory morbidity in the immediate neonatal period as well as subsequent chronic lung disease in infancy. Persistent pulmonary hypertension of the newborn, the failure of the normal transition to a low-resistance pulmonary circulation at birth, can complicate a number of neonatal respiratory diseases.

Several mechanical properties of the respiratory system in infants increase the risk of respiratory compromise in this age group. The upper airway in infants is smaller and less firm than the upper airway in adults; therefore, obstruction in response to infection, inflammation, or foreign body is more likely. The chest wall of the infant is more compliant than that of the adult. For this reason, respiratory efforts encountered in some disease states can result in collapse and more labored breathing. In addition, the infant has fewer fatigue-resistant diaphragmatic muscle fibers, a fact suggesting that respiratory muscle fatigue may occur earlier in response to an increased load.

The development of airways reactivity, ie, acute changes in airways resistance in response to a given stimulus, has been controversial. Earlier studies suggested that infants lack the airway smooth muscle morphologically similar to that in adults; this finding would imply that bronchoconstriction cannot occur in infants. The weight of evidence now suggests that infants can exhibit airways reactivity. The mechanisms of airways reactivity in infancy are not completely understood but likely include some contractile elements in the airway that respond to neural stimuli. Recent studies also suggest that genetic factors play a role in the development of airways reactivity.

Defense mechanisms of the lung, including cough, mucociliary clearance, and local and circulating components of the immune system, are present at birth. However, specific defects in immunity may present over variable time periods after birth. This time lapse possibly reflects passive immunity from the mother and the timing of infectious challenges to the respiratory tract.

Bernfield M: Matrix regulation of cell proliferation: Implications for growth of the embryo. *Semin Perinatol* 1984; **8**:117. [Review of biochemical processes during embryonic growth.]

Cagle PT, Thurlbeck WM: Postpneumonectomy compensatory lung growth. *Am Rev Respir Dis* 1988;**138**:1314.

Langston C et al: Human lung growth in late gestation and in the neonate. *Am Rev Respir Dis* 1984;**129**:607.

Laros CD, Westermann CJJ: Dilatation, compensatory growth, or both following pneumonectomy during childhood and adolescence. *J Thorac Cardiovasc Surg* 1987; **93**:570. [Demonstrates good functional outcome in humans following pneumonectomy.]

Murray JF: *The Normal Lung: The Basis for Diagnosis and Treatment of Pulmonary Disease.* Saunders, 1986.

Reid LM: The pulmonary circulation: Remodeling in growth and disease. The 1978 J Burns Amberson Lecture. *Am Rev Respir Dis* 1978;**119**:531.

DIAGNOSTIC AIDS

PHYSICAL EXAMINATION OF THE RESPIRATORY TRACT

The physical examination is done to corroborate findings obtained from the history, to assess severity of illness and adequacy of gas exchange, and to localize disease processes. The traditional approach of inspection, palpation, percussion, and auscultation remain important, although these techniques have limitations in small infants. Assessing the rate, depth, ease, symmetry, and rhythm of respiration is critical to the detection of pulmonary disease. Attention should be given to tracheal position and thoracic configuration. Auscultation should be done to assess the quality of breath sounds and to detect the presence of abnormal sounds. Although there is confusion in the literature, the American Thoracic Society recommends classifying abnormal breath sounds as interrupted (fine or coarse crackles) or continuous (wheezing or rhonchi) sounds.

Extrapulmonary manifestations of pulmonary disease include growth failure, altered mental status (with hypoxemia or hypercarbia), cyanosis, clubbing, and osteoarthropathy. Evidence of cor pulmonale (loud pulmonic component of the second heart sound, hepatomegaly, elevated neck veins, and, rarely, peripheral edema) signifies advanced lung disease.

It is critical to establish whether respiratory derangements are (1) the primary abnormality, (2) secondary to some other disease process, or (3) part of a more generalized condition. Therefore, the physician should perform a complete physical examination to look for evidence of other conditions such as congenital heart disease (murmur, gallop), neuromuscular disease (muscle wasting, scoliosis), immunodeficiency (rash, diarrhea), and collagen-vascular disease or occult malignancy (arthritis, hepatosplenomegaly).

Scarpelli EM: Examination of the lung (physiologic and anatomic basis). In: *Pulmonary Disease of the Fetus, Newborn, and Child.* Scarpelli EM, Auld PAM, Goldman HS (editors). Lea & Febiger, 1978.

Waring WW: The history and physical examination. In: *Disorders of the Respiratory Tract in Children,* 4th ed. Kendig EL Jr, Chernick V (editors). Saunders, 1983.

PULMONARY FUNCTION TESTS

An assessment of lung function in pediatric patients with either an acute or chronic respiratory disorder can aid in diagnosis, quantitate disease severity, define precipitants of symptoms, evaluate therapy, and chart the course of a disease. In addition, a preoperative evaluation of pulmonary function in patients with lung disease can help define the risks of anesthesia and surgery and assist in the planning of respiratory care in the postoperative period. Balanced against these potential benefits of assessing lung function are several limitations, which must also be kept in mind. For example, the range of normal values for a test may be quite wide, and the predicted normal values change dramatically with growth. For this reason, serial determinations of lung function are often more informative than a single determination, especially when dealing with a disease in which values may vary as a reflection of disease severity (asthma) or progression (cystic fibrosis). In addition, patient cooperation is essential for almost all physiologic assessments. Most children are not able to perform the necessary maneuvers before 5 to 7 years of age. Therefore, tests for use in infants and small children are not widely available and, at this time, are more of a research tool than a clinical adjunct to care. Despite these problems, tests of lung function may still contribute in a positive way to the care of children.

The pulmonary function equipment most often available in an office or clinic is a spirometer, on which a forced vital capacity maneuver is recorded as either a volume-time tracing (spirogram) or a flow-volume curve. The maneuver consists of the patient's performing a slow, full inhalation of air to maximum inflation, holding the breath for a short period of time, and then performing a sudden, sustained maximal exhalation that lasts a minimum of 3 seconds. From the tracing of the exhalation can be obtained the forced vital capacity (FVC), the total amount of air that is exhaled from maximum inspiration, and the forced expiratory volume in the first second of the exhalation (FEV_1). The maximum midexpiratory flow rate (MMEF or $FEF_{25-75\%}$), the mean flow rate during the middle portion of the FVC maneuver, is also commonly calculated. In addition to obtaining the absolute values for these 3 tests and comparing them to normal values, medical personnel may also determine the FEV_1/FVC ratio. A value greater than 0.8 in children and young adults is consistent with normal airflow, without limitation.

An important use of these basic tests of lung function is differentiating an obstructive from a restrictive process. Examples of obstructive processes include asthma, chronic bronchitis, and cystic fibrosis, whereas restrictive problems include chest wall deformities that limit lung expansion and interstitial processes due to collagen-vascular diseases, hypersensitivity pneumonitis, and interstitial fibrosis. Classically, diseases that obstruct airflow decrease the FEV_1 more than the FVC, so that the FEV_1/FVC ratio is low. In restrictive problems, however, the decreases in the FEV_1 and FVC are proportional; thus, the ratio of FEV_1 to FVC is either normal or high. Clinical suspicion of a restrictive disease is usually an indication for referral of the patient to a tertiary care center for a more complete evaluation of lung function and disease process.

An additional test of lung function, which can be readily measured in both the office and at home, is the peak expiratory flow rate (PEFR), the maximal flow recorded during an FVC maneuver. The test can be assessed by a number of hand-held devices specifically made for this one test of pulmonary function. Patients can measure the PEFR at home at regular intervals and record the results in a diary, a practice that may be helpful in following the course of various pulmonary disorders, especially those that are difficult to control and require multiple medications (eg, steroid-dependent asthma). These devices can also be used to give patients with poor perception of their disease an awareness of a decrease in

lung function, thus facilitating earlier therapeutic intervention.

Lemen RJ: Pulmonary function testing in the office and clinic. In: *Disorders of the Respiratory Tract in Children,* 4th ed. Kendig EL Jr, Chernick V (editors). Saunders, 1983.
Wilson MC, Larsen GL: The assessment of lung function: Pulmonary function tests. In: *Allergic Disease of Infancy, Childhood and Adolescence,* 2nd ed. Bierman CW, Pearlman DS (editors). Saunders, 1988.

ARTERIAL BLOOD GASES & NONINVASIVE ASSESSMENT OF OXYGEN TENSION & SATURATION

Arterial blood gas determinations are the best indicators of how well the respiratory system is performing its gas-exchanging function and how well acid-base homeostasis is being maintained. Assessment of blood gases is essential in critically ill children but also may be used in determining the severity of lung involvement in chronic conditions. Abnormalities in blood gas tensions may be seen with dysfunction of any part of the respiratory system, including the respiratory controller, the conducting airways, the gas-exchanging portions of the lung, the pulmonary circulation, the respiratory muscles, and the chest wall. In pediatrics, hypoxia (low Pao_2) most commonly results from mismatching of ventilation and perfusion. Hypercarbia (elevated $Paco_2$) often results from increased work of breathing secondary to increased pulmonary resistance, decreased compliance, or an abnormal chest wall. Hypercarbia may also occur with normal lungs and chest wall if there is a depressed respiratory controller or weakened respiratory muscles. Blood gases may be sampled by intermittent arterial puncture or through indwelling arterial lines. The techniques of sampling are reviewed in Chapter 35. Table 15–1 gives normal values for arterial pH, Pao_2, and $Paco_2$ at sea level and at an altitude of 5000 feet.

The noninvasive, transcutaneous techniques of measuring oxygen saturation and Po_2 allow on-line monitoring in many different settings. Monitoring oxygen saturation in the intensive care unit is vital to anticipating respiratory failure in critically ill patients. As another example, desaturation during sleep is an important finding in patients with upper airway obstruction. The importance of evaluating the gas-exchanging portions of the lung make arterial blood gas measurements or noninvasive measurements of

Table 15–1. Normal arterial blood gas values on room air.

	pH	Pao_2 (torr)	$Paco_2$ (torr)
Sea level	7.38–7.42	85–95	36–42
5000 feet	7.36–7.40	65–75	35–40

oxygen saturation an important part of the evaluation of any pediatric patient with suspected lung disease.

Gregory GA: Respiratory care of the child. *Crit Care Med* 1980;**8**:582.

Huch R, Lubbers DW, Huch A: Reliability of transcutaneous monitoring of arterial Po$_2$ in newborn infants. *Arch Dis Child* 1974;**49**:213. [Pioneering work in the area of noninvasive estimation of arterial blood gas tensions.]

Levison H et al: Arterial blood gases, alveolar-arterial oxygen difference, and physiologic deadspace in children and young adults. *Am Rev Respir Dis* 1970;**101**:972. [Early report of the use of arterial blood gases in children.]

Yahav J, Mindorff C, Levison H: The validity of transcutaneous oxygen tension method in children with cardiorespiratory problems. *Am Rev Respir Dis* 1981;**124**:586. [Demonstrates the reliability of transcutaneous monitoring in patients with cardiorespiratory disorders without shock.]

CULTURE OF MATERIAL FROM THE RESPIRATORY TRACT

Expectorated sputum is rarely available from patients under 5–6 years of age, but in older children, a sputum Gram stain showing significant numbers of organisms within neutrophils may indicate the pathogen present. Stains and cultures for bacteria from nasopharyngeal secretions are frequently misleading.

Cultures from the lower respiratory tract can be obtained by (1) tracheal aspiration through an endotracheal tube or through a rigid or fiberoptic bronchoscope, (2) transtracheal percutaneous aspiration, (3) lung puncture, or (4) the double-brush technique through the fiberoptic bronchoscope. The latter technique can be used to obtain endobronchial secretions in older critically ill or debilitated children large enough to accommodate the large (4.9 mm) bronchoscope required for the procedure.

Complications are most likely to occur with transtracheal percutaneous aspiration or lung puncture. These complications are related to a lack of experience by most physicians in utilizing these techniques in children. The other methods, however, are more likely to produce samples contaminated with oropharyngeal flora and may not be the best guide to therapy. Lung puncture, directed to a consolidated area using physical examination, radiographic studies, or ultrasound, is the favored approach in the child who deteriorates after initial antibiotic treatment or in the critically ill or immunocompromised child. Pneumothoraces (1–10%) that follow lung puncture are usually small. Open lung biopsy, although a major intervention, should be considered in the worsening or critically ill child when other approaches have not been productive. Thoracentesis should be performed when pleural fluid is present, and complete cultures should be obtained. Blood glucose and lactate dehydrogenase should be drawn simultaneously for comparison with pleural fluid chemistries. Blood cultures provide specific diagnoses and must be obtained in children with acute pneumonia.

If indeed a specimen is obtained through invasive means, it is critical that appropriate studies be obtained for the following: (1) viruses, (2) *Mycoplasma pneumoniae*, (3) chlamydia, (4) *Legionella pneumophila*, (5) *Bordetella pertussis*, (6) fungi, (7) acid-fast bacteria, and (8) anaerobes or other bacteria. In addition, these specimens should be studied for potential pathogens using rapid diagnostic techniques, such as immunofluorescent antibody and enzyme-linked immunosorbent assay (ELISA), when available. Counterimmunoelectrophoresis performed on pleural fluid, serum, or concentrated urine may help identify disease due to *Streptococcus pneumoniae* or *Haemophilus influenzae*. Because these tests can be performed quickly, they may obviate further, more invasive studies.

Bromberg K, Hammerschlag MR: Rapid diagnosis of pneumonia in children. *Semin Respir Infect* 1987;**2**:159.

Peter G: The child with pneumonia: Diagnostic and therapeutic considerations. *Pediatr Infect Dis J* 1988;**7**:453.

IMAGING OF THE RESPIRATORY TRACT

The plain chest radiograph remains one of the most important techniques of investigating suspected lung disease. Both frontal and lateral views should be obtained in most instances. Hyperaeration, best demonstrated in the lateral projection as flattening of the diaphragm, is a common finding because of the propensity of young children to develop small airways obstruction and also because of the prevalence of asthma in all pediatric age groups. Parenchymal changes may be manifested by increased interstitial markings, consolidation, air bronchograms, or loss of diaphragm or heart contours. When pleural fluid is suspected, lateral decubitus films may be helpful in determining the extent and mobility of the fluid. When foreign body is suspected, forced expiratory films may demonstrate focal air trapping and shift of the mediastinum to the contralateral side. Lateral neck films can be useful in assessing the size of adenoids and tonsils and also in differentiating croup from epiglottitis, the latter being associated with the "thumbprint" sign.

Barium swallow is indicated for patients with suspected aspiration so that the physician can look for swallowing dysfunction, tracheoesophageal fistula, gastroesophageal reflux, and achalasia. This technique is also very important in detecting vascular rings and slings, because most (though not all) are also associated with esophageal compression. Airway fluoroscopy is another important tool to assess both fixed airways obstruction (ie, subglottic stenosis) and dynamic airways obstruction (ie, tracheomalacia). Fluoroscopy of the diaphragm can detect paralysis by demonstrating paradoxical movement of the involved hemidiaphragm.

Computed tomography has improved the radiologist's ability to evaluate metastatic disease, mediastinal masses, and complex parenchymal or chest wall disease. Magnetic resonance imaging is also proving to be useful in detecting subtle abnormalities or defining complicated abnormalities. Ventilation and perfusion scans can provide information about regional ventilation and perfusion and can be helpful in detecting vascular malformations and pulmonary emboli (rare in children). Pulmonary angiography is occasionally necessary to define the pulmonary vascular bed more precisely. Bronchograms are rarely done in this country but can be useful in the specific circumstance when lobectomy is contemplated for suspected localized bronchiectasis.

Effmann EL, Kirks DR: Chest computed tomography in children. *Pediatr Clin North Am* 1985;**32:**1383.

Eggleston DE, Slovis TL, Watts FB: Update on pediatric chest imaging. *Pediatr Pulmonol* 1988;**5:**158.

Kirchner SG, Horev G: Diagnostic imaging in children with acute chest and abdominal disorders. *Pediatr Clin North Am* 1985;**32:**1363.

BRONCHOSCOPY

Pediatric patients with potential airway problems become candidates for laryngoscopy or bronchoscopy (or both) when less invasive modalities fail to define the lesion adequately. The diagnostic indications for laryngoscopy include hoarseness, stridor, and symptoms of obstructive sleep apnea; those for bronchoscopy include wheezing, suspected foreign body, pneumonia, atelectasis, chronic cough, hemoptysis, and placement of an endotracheal tube and assessment of patency. In general, the more specific the indication, the higher the diagnostic yield.

Currently, pediatric bronchoscopy can be done with either flexible, fiberoptic instruments or rigid, open-tube instruments. Recent advances in fiberoptic technology and the development of flexible, ultrathin bronchoscopes have greatly expanded the physician's ability to explore the pediatric airway. The advantages of using a flexible bronchoscope include the following: (1) the procedure can be done at the bedside with sedation and topical anesthetics and requires no general anesthesia; (2) the evaluation of the upper airway can be done with very little risk in patients who are awake; (3) the distal airways of intubated patients can be examined without removing the endotracheal tube; (4) the instrument can be used as an obturator to intubate a patient with a difficult upper airway; (5) endotracheal tube placement and patency can be checked; (6) assessment of airway dynamics is generally better; and (7) it is possible to examine more distal airways. The advantages of using a rigid instrument are the following: (1) easier removal of foreign bodies (for this reason, rigid bronchoscopy remains the procedure of choice for suspected foreign body aspiration); (2) better airway control, which allows the patient to be ventilated through the bronchoscope; and (3) superior optics. The choice of procedures depends largely on the expertise available, but in general, pediatric airway evaluation is optimal with a multidisciplinary approach involving pediatric anesthesia, surgery, otolaryngology, and pulmonology.

Fan LL, Flynn JW: Laryngoscopy in neonates and infants: Experience with the flexible fiberoptic bronchoscope. *Laryngoscope* 1981;**91:**451.

Fan LL, Sparks LM, Dulinski JP: Applications of an ultrathin flexible bronchoscope for neonatal and pediatric airway problems. *Chest* 1986;**89:**673.

Fan LL, Sparks LM, Fix EJ: Flexible fiberoptic endoscopy for airway problems in a pediatric intensive care unit. *Chest* 1988;**93:**556.

Godfrey S et al: Is there a place for rigid bronchoscopy in the management of pediatric lung disease? *Pediatr Pulmonol* 1987;**3:**179.

Wood RE: Endoscopy of the airway. *J Pediatr* 1988;**112:**1.

Wood RE: Spelunking in the pediatric airways: Explorations with the flexible fiberoptic bronchoscope. *Pediatr Clin North Am* 1984;**31:**785.

GENERAL THERAPY OF PEDIATRIC LUNG DISEASES

OXYGEN THERAPY

Oxygen therapy refers to the administration of supplemental oxygen at concentrations greater than that of room air (21%) in order to increase arterial oxygen tension. Supplemental oxygen can be administered through an endotracheal tube during mechanical ventilation or through an inflatable anesthesia bag with a mask. In spontaneously breathing patients, delivery can be achieved by nasal cannula, head hood, or mask (including simple, rebreathing, nonrebreathing, or Venturi). The general goal of oxygen therapy is to correct for hypoxemia by attempting to achieve an arterial oxygen tension of 65–90 torr or an oxygen saturation above 92%. The actual oxygen concentration achieved by nasal cannula or mask depends on flow rate, the type of mask used, and the patient's age. For example, small changes in flow rate during oxygen administration by nasal cannula can lead to substantial changes in inspired oxygen concentration in young infants. In addition, the amount of oxygen required to correct hypoxemia may vary according to the child's activity. It is not unusual, for example, that an infant with chronic lung disease may require ¾ L/min while awake but need 1 L/min while asleep or feeding.

Although the head hood is an efficient mode to maintain oxygen delivery in young infants during hospitalization, the nasal cannula is used more often because it allows the infant greater activity. The cannula generally has nasal prongs that are inserted in the nares, but it can be modified by removing the prongs. This nasal catheter can then be taped under the nose or inserted in the nasopharynx, as has been recently described. The flow through nasal cannula should generally not exceed 3 L/min to avoid excessive drying of the nasal mucosa. In general, administration of supplemental oxygen by nasal cannula, even at high flow rates, can rarely achieve inspired oxygen concentrations greater than 40–45%. In contrast, partial rebreathing and nonrebreathing masks or head hoods can be used to achieve inspired oxygen concentrations as high as 90–100%.

Because the physical findings of cyanosis can be subtle, especially with milder degrees of hypoxemia, the adequacy of oxygenation must be assessed by measuring arterial oxygen tension via arterial blood gas or transcutaneous Po_2 monitor. In addition, oxygen saturation can be determined by oximetry. The advantages of the noninvasive methods (transcutaneous Po_2 and oximeter) include the ability to obtain continuous measurements during various normal activities and to avoid artefact caused by crying or breath holding during attempts at arterial puncture. For children with chronic cardiopulmonary disorders that may require supplemental oxygen therapy (such as bronchopulmonary dysplasia or cystic fibrosis), frequent noninvasive assessments are essential to ensure the safety and adequacy of treatment. In addition, long-term follow-up of children with chronic oxygen requirements should include serial electrocardiogram or echocardiogram assessments at regular intervals to monitor for early signs of pulmonary hypertension and cor pulmonale, which may suggest that therapy has been inadequate.

Abman SH et al: Pulmonary vascular response to oxygen in infants with BPD. *Pediatrics* 1985;**75**:80.

Fan LL et al: Determination of inspired oxygen delivery by nasal cannula in infants with chronic lung disease. *J Pediatr* 1983;**103**:923.

National Conference on Oxygen Therapy. *Chest* 1984;**86**:236.

INHALATION OF BRONCHODILATORS & OTHER MEDICATIONS

Various diseases in pediatric patients give rise to airways obstruction that may be reversed by an inhaled bronchodilator. Airways obstruction may be encountered in cystic fibrosis, bronchiolitis, and bronchopulmonary dysplasia, as well as in acute and chronic asthma. Of the classes of inhaled drugs used in the treatment of these disorders, the β-adrenergic agonists and parasympatholytic agents may lead to the most prompt reversal of the obstruction. Other classes of inhaled drugs that may be beneficial, especially in the treatment of asthma, include corticosteroids and sodium cromoglycate. Inhalation therapy with these classes of drugs are discussed below. The cystic fibrosis section contains a discussion of the use of inhaled antibiotics.

The β-adrenergic agonists may be delivered by either a prepackaged, pressurized canister (metered-dose inhaler, or MDI) or a reusable nebulizer, in which a solution of the medication is aerosolized by the flow of gas from a portable gas compressor or a source of compressed gas (such as 100% oxygen). The MDIs are convenient to use and easy to carry and can be combined with spacing devices for younger children who lack the ability to coordinate actuation of the MDI with proper inhalation technique. On the other hand, the nebulizer is a more effective method of delivering medication to infants and young children—perhaps to patients of all ages. Several inhaled $β_2$-adrenergic agents that are more selective for the respiratory tract and have longer durations of action are now available (see Chapter 32 and discussion on asthma). In the treatment of acute episodes of airways obstruction, the inhaled adrenergic agents have been shown to be as effective as the injectable adrenergic agonists. In addition, delivery of the drug by the aerosol route has been associated with fewer side effects. Although concern has been raised about the safety of delivering this class of medication directly to the airways, most authorities believe that these drugs are safe when both physician and family realize that a poor response to the agents may signify the need for corticosteroids to help restore β-adrenergic responsiveness.

Anticholinergic agents may also acutely decrease airways obstruction. Furthermore, they may yield a longer duration of bronchodilation than do many adrenergic agents. Selected patients may benefit from receiving both β-adrenergic and anticholinergic agents. In general, this class of drugs is most effective in the treatment of chronic bronchitis.

Other classes of inhaled medications used primarily to treat asthma include corticosteroids and sodium cromoglycate. Currently in the United States, corticosteroids are available only in MDIs, whereas cromolyn may be prescribed as either an MDI or a solution for nebulization. Although these medications are not effective in acutely relieving airways obstruction, long-term use may lead to decreases in airways reactivity. In addition, corticosteroids may help maintain or restore responsiveness of the airways to adrenergic drugs.

Gross NJ: The use of anticholinergic agents in the treatment of airways disease. *Clin Chest Med* 1988;**9**:591.

Kerrebijn KF, van Essen-Zandvliet EEM, Neijens HJ: Effect of long-term treatment with inhaled corticosteroids and beta-agonists on the bronchial responsiveness in children with asthma. *J Allergy Clin Immunol* 1987; **79**:653.

König P: Inhaled corticosteroids: Their present and future role in the management of asthma. *J Allergy Clin Immunol* 1988;**82**:297.

Levison H, Reilly PA, Worsley GH: Spacing devices and metered-dose inhalers in childhood asthma. *J Pediatr* 1985;**107**:662.

Nelson HS: Beta-adrenergic therapy. In: *Allergy: Principles and Practice,* 3rd ed. Middleton E et al (editors). Mosby, 1988.

Ruddy RM et al: Aerosolized metaproterenol compared to subcutaneous epinephrine in the emergency treatment of acute childhood asthma. *Pediatr Pulmonol* 1986;**2**:230.

Shapiro GG et al: Double-blind evaluation of nebulized cromolyn, terbutaline, and the combination for childhood asthma. *J Allergy Clin Immunol* 1988;**81**:449.

Desmond KJ et al: Immediate and long-term effects of chest physiotherapy in patients with cystic fibrosis. *J Pediatr* 1983;**103**:538.

Reisman JJ et al: Role of conventional physiotherapy in cystic fibrosis. *J Pediatr* 1988;**113**:632.

PULMONARY PHYSIOTHERAPY

Chest physical therapy (PT), including postural drainage with percussion and forced expiratory maneuvers, has been widely employed in an attempt to improve the clearance of secretions in patients with impaired clearance. However, there are few studies of the efficacy of techniques of chest PT. Studies have suggested that chest PT is not helpful in adults with uncomplicated pneumonias. However, data indicating that postural drainage can be beneficial in children with cystic fibrosis are accumulating. A recent 3-year study indicates that there is less decline in pulmonary function of children treated with traditional postural drainage and percussion than with directed coughing alone. The experience of many pediatric pulmonary centers now suggests that chest PT is an important adjunct to other therapies.

Postural drainage requires positioning of the patient to favor emptying each of the segmental bronchi. Percussion or vibration is used to loosen secretions and facilitate drainage. Physicians should carefully review the positions and the technique of percussion to perform this mode of therapy properly. In general, the patient spends 1–2 minutes in each of 9 body positions (ie, 10–20 minutes for the duration of a treatment). Treatments may be given 1–4 times a day at home and sometimes more frequently in the hospital setting. Patients are encouraged to cough regularly during the procedure. Children who cannot be encouraged to cough may require pharyngeal suctioning by trained personnel.

"Blow bottles" that provide the patient feedback about respiratory efforts may also encourage deep breathing. This technique is particularly useful in patients recovering from surgery.

DISORDERS OF THE CONDUCTING AIRWAYS

GENERAL PRINCIPLES

The conducting airways consist of the nose, mouth, pharynx, larynx, trachea, bronchi, and bronchioles. These airways direct inspired air to the gas exchange units of the lung; they do not participate in gas exchange themselves. Airflow obstruction in the conducting airways occurs by any of 3 mechanisms: (1) external compression (eg, vascular ring, tumor), (2) abnormalities of the airway structure itself (eg, congenital defects, thickening of an airway wall due to inflammation), or (3) material in the airway lumen (eg, foreign body, mucus).

Airway obstruction can be fixed (airflow limited in both the inspiratory and expiratory phases of respiration) or variable (airflow limited more in one phase of respiration than the other). Variable obstruction is common in children because their airways are more compliant and susceptible to dynamic compression. With variable extrathoracic airway obstruction (eg, croup), airflow limitation is greater during inspiration, leading to inspiratory stridor. With variable intrathoracic obstruction, limitation is greater during expiration, producing expiratory wheezing. Thus, determining the phase of respiration in which obstruction is greatest may be helpful in localizing the site of obstruction.

CLINICAL FINDINGS IN EXTRATHORACIC AIRWAYS OBSTRUCTION

Patients with abnormalities of the extrathoracic airway may present with snoring and other symptoms of obstructive apnea, hoarseness, brassy cough, or stridor. When taking the history, the physician should obtain the following information: (1) the onset of symptoms; (2) the nature of the course of the illness, ie, acute (eg, infectious croup), recurrent (eg, spasmodic croup), chronic (eg, subglottic stenosis), or progressive (eg, laryngeal papillomatosis); and (3) risk factors (eg, difficult delivery, ductal ligation, intubation). A careful physical examination should determine if obstructive symptoms are present at rest or with agitation, if they are positional, or if they are related to sleep. The presence of agitation, air hunger, severe retractions, cyanosis, lethargy, or coma should alert the physician to a potentially life-threatening condition that may require immediate airway intervention. Helpful diagnostic studies in the evaluation of upper airway obstruction include chest and lateral neck films, airway fluoroscopy, and barium swallow. An electrocardiogram can provide evidence of pulmonary hypertension in patients with chronic obstruction. Patients with symptoms of obstructive sleep apnea may benefit from polysomnography (measurements during sleep of the motion of the chest wall, airflow at the nose and mouth, heart rate, oxygen saturation, and selected electroencephalographic leads to stage sleep), which can help define the severity of the illness. In older children, pulmonary function tests can differentiate fixed from variable airflow obstruction and determine the site of variable obstruction. Direct laryngoscopy and bronchoscopy remain the procedures of choice to establish the precise diagnosis. Treatment should be directed at relieving airway obstruction and correcting the underlying condition (if possible).

CLINICAL FINDINGS IN INTRATHORACIC AIRWAYS OBSTRUCTION

Patients with abnormalities of the intrathoracic airways usually present with wheezing that is most prominent during expiration. The history should include the following: (1) age of onset; (2) precipitating factors (exercise, upper respiratory illnesses, allergens, choking while eating, etc); (3) course, ie, acute (bronchiolitis, foreign body), chronic (tracheomalacia, vascular ring), recurrent (reactive airways disease), or progressive (cystic fibrosis, bronchiolitis obliterans); (4) presence and nature of cough; (5) production of sputum; (6) previous response to bronchodilators; (7) symptoms with positional changes (vascular rings); and (8) involvement of other organ systems (malabsorption in cystic fibrosis).

Physical examination should include growth measurements and vital signs. The examiner should look for cyanosis or pallor, barrel-shaped chest, retractions and use of accessory muscles, and presence of clubbing. Auscultation should be done to define the pattern and timing of respiration, to detect the presence of crackles and wheezing, and to determine if findings are localized or generalized.

Routine laboratory tests include plain chest films, sweat test, and pulmonary function tests in older children. Other diagnostic studies are dictated by the history and physical findings. Treatment should be directed toward the primary cause of the obstruction but generally includes a trial of bronchodilators.

CONGENITAL DISORDERS OF THE EXTRATHORACIC AIRWAY

LARYNGOMALACIA

Laryngomalacia is a benign, congenital disorder in which the cartilaginous support for the supraglottic structures is underdeveloped. It is the most common cause of persistent stridor in infants and usually presents in the first 6 weeks of life. Stridor has been reported to be worse in the supine position, with increased activity, with upper respiratory infections, and during feeding; however, the clinical presentation can be variable. The condition usually improves with age and resolves by 2 years of age, but symptoms may persist for many years in some. The diagnosis is established by direct laryngoscopy, in which inspiratory collapse of an "omega-shaped" epiglottis (with or without long, redundant arytenoids) is visualized. In mildly affected patients with a typical presentation (those without stridor at rest or retractions), this procedure may not be necessary. No treatment is needed except in the extremely rare circumstance of severe obstruction that requires airway intervention. A recent observation suggests that these patients may have slight desaturation during sleep, the clinical importance of which is unknown.

Belmont JR, Grundfast K: Congenital laryngeal stridor (laryngomalacia): Etiologic factors and associated disorders. *Ann Otol Rhinol Laryngol* 1984;**93**:430.

Macfarlane PI, Olinsky A, Phelan PD: Proximal airway function 8 to 16 years after laryngomalacia: Follow-up flow-volume loop studies. *J Pediatr* 1985;**107**:216.

McCray PB et al: Hypoxia and hypercapnia in infants with mild laryngomalacia. *Am J Dis Child* 1988;**142**:896.

Phelan PD et al: The clinical and physiological manifestations of the "infantile" larynx: Natural history and relationship to mental retardation. *Aust Paediatr J* 1971;**7**:135.

OTHER CONGENITAL PROBLEMS

Other congenital lesions of the larynx are quite rare. These include laryngeal atresia, laryngeal web, laryngocele and cyst of the larynx, subglottic hemangioma, and laryngeal cleft. All these disorders are best diagnosed by direct laryngoscopy. Laryngeal atresia obviously presents immediately after birth with severe respiratory distress and is most often fatal, although a few survivors have been reported.

Laryngeal web, representing fusion of the anterior portion of the true vocal cords, is associated with hoarseness, aphonia, and stridor. Surgical correction may be necessary, depending upon the degree of airway obstruction.

Congenital cysts and laryngoceles are believed to have similar origin. Cysts are more superficial, whereas laryngoceles communicate with the interior of the larynx. Cysts are generally fluid-filled, whereas laryngoceles may be air- or fluid-filled. Airway obstruction is usually prominent and requires surgical intervention. Laser therapy is commonly employed for this purpose.

Subglottic hemangiomas usually present in infancy with signs of upper airway obstruction and are often associated with similar lesions of the skin. Although these lesions tend to regress spontaneously over time, airway obstruction may require surgical treatment with laser or even tracheostomy.

Laryngeal cleft is a very rare condition resulting from failure of posterior cricoid fusion. Patients with this condition may have stridor but always aspirate severely, resulting in recurrent or chronic pneumonia and failure to thrive. Barium swallow is always positive for severe aspiration, but diagnosis can be very difficult even with direct laryngoscopy. Patients often require tracheostomy and gastrostomy, because surgical correction is not always successful.

Gatti WM, MacDonald E, Orfei E: Congenital laryngeal atresia. *Laryngoscope* 1987;**97**:966.

Richardson MA, Cotton RT: Anatomic abnormalities of the pediatric airway. *Pediatr Clin North Am* 1984;**31**: 821.

Smith RJH, Catlin FI: Congenital anomalies of the larynx. *Am J Dis Child* 1984;**138**:35.

ACQUIRED DISORDERS OF THE EXTRATHORACIC AIRWAY

CROUP SYNDROME

1. VIRAL CROUP

Croup describes a series of acute inflammatory diseases of the larynx including viral croup (laryngotracheobronchitis), epiglottitis (supraglottitis), and bacterial tracheitis. In patients presenting with acute stridor, these entities form the main differential diagnosis, although spasmodic croup, angioneurotic edema, laryngeal or esophageal foreign body, and retropharyngeal abscess should be considered.

General Considerations

Viral croup generally affects younger children in the fall and early winter and is most often caused by parainfluenza virus type 1. Other responsible organisms include parainfluenza virus types 2 and 3, respiratory syncytial virus, influenza virus, rubeola virus, adenovirus, and *Mycoplasma pneumoniae*. Although inflammation of the entire airway is usually present, edema formation in the subglottic space accounts for the predominant signs of upper airway obstruction.

Clinical Findings

A. Symptoms and Signs: There is usually a prodrome of upper respiratory tract symptoms followed by the development of a barking cough and stridor. Fever is usually absent or low-grade but may on occasion be as high as in patients with epiglottitis. More mildly affected patients may exhibit only stridor when agitated, but as obstruction worsens, symptoms may progress to stridor at rest, accompanied by retractions, air hunger, and cyanosis in severe cases. On examination, the presence of cough and the absence of drooling tend to favor the diagnosis of viral croup over epiglottitis.

B. Imaging: Lateral neck films can be diagnostically helpful by showing subglottic narrowing and a normal epiglottis. It is important to confirm that the epiglottis is normal by direct laryngoscopy, because the presentation of epiglottitis may be similar to that of croup. Although controversy exists regarding the safety of such a procedure, a recent study suggests that it is reasonably safe in patients with suspected viral croup. Direct inspection is necessary because some patients with suspected croup actually prove to have epiglottitis.

Treatment

Treatment of viral croup is supportive. Patients without stridor at rest may be managed as outpatients with mist therapy, oral hydration, and minimal handling. Although mist is believed to be helpful in relieving symptoms, the only clinical study done to date failed to demonstrate its effectiveness. Patients with stridor at rest require hospitalization. Appropriate hospital management includes the same therapy given to outpatients. Additionally, oxygen should be administered with careful observation to patients demonstrating desaturation by pulse oximetry. Nebulized racemic epinephrine (0.5 mL of a 2.25% solution diluted with 1.5–3.5 mL of sterile water) has been shown to relieve airway obstruction for up to 2 hours, presumably by reducing edema. Other, more pure α-agonists are also effective but are shorter acting. The use of steroids remains controversial; all controlled studies to date have had methodologic shortcomings. Nonetheless, the efficacy demonstrated in some studies, coupled with the lack of identified side effects, seems to justify a short course in severe cases (those patients not responding to racemic epinephrine). Dexamethasone (0.5–1 mg/kg up to 10 mg, given orally or parenterally as a single dose or repeated in 12 hours) is appropriate.

Patients with impending respiratory failure require an artificial airway. Although there are controversies regarding the choice between intubation and tracheostomy, recent studies suggest that intubation with an endotracheal tube of slightly smaller diameter than would ordinarily be used is reasonably safe. Extubation should be accomplished within 2–3 days to minimize the risk of laryngeal injury. If the patient fails extubation, tracheostomy should be performed.

Prognosis

Most children with viral croup have an uneventful course and improve within a few days. Recent studies suggest that patients with a history of croup may have airway hyperreactivity. However, it has not been determined if this was present prior to the croup episode or if the croup episode itself altered airway function. Recurrence of croup occurs in some instances, implying airway hyperreactivity.

Bourchier D, Dawson KP, Ferguson DM: Humidification in viral croup: A controlled trial. *Aust Paediatr J* 1984; **20**:289.

Couriel JM: Management of croup. *Arch Dis Child* 1988; **63**:1305.

Denny FW et al: Croup: An 11-year study in a pediatric practice. *Pediatrics* 1983;**71**:871.

Fogel JM et al: Racemic epinephrine in the treatment of croup: Nebulization alone versus nebulization with intermittent positive pressure breathing. *J Pediatr* 1982; **101**:1028.

Mauro RD, Poole SR, Lockhart CH: Differentiation of epiglottitis from laryngotracheitis in the child with stridor. *Am J Dis Child* 1988;**142**:679.

Tunnessen WW, Feinstein AR: The steroid-croup controversy: An analytical review of methodologic problems. *J Pediatr* 1980;**96**:751.

Zulliger JJ, Schuller DE, Beach TP: Assessment of intubation in croup and epiglottitis. *Ann Otol Rhinol Laryngol* 1982;**91**:403.

2. EPIGLOTTITIS

General Considerations

Epiglottitis represents a true medical emergency. It is almost always caused by *Haemophilus influenzae* type B, although other organisms such as *Streptococcus pneumoniae* and groups A and C *Streptococcus pyogenes* have been implicated. Resulting inflammation and swelling of the supraglottic structures (epiglottis and arytenoids) can develop rapidly and lead to life-threatening upper airway obstruction.

Clinical Findings

A. Symptoms and Signs: Typically, patients present with a rather sudden onset of fever, dysphagia, drooling, muffled voice, inspiratory retractions, cyanosis, and soft stridor. They often sit in a "sniffing dog" position, which gives them the best airway possible under the circumstances. Progression to total airway obstruction may occur and result in respiratory arrest.

B. Imaging: Diagnostically, lateral neck films may be helpful in demonstrating a classic "thumbprint" sign. However, obtaining films may delay important airway intervention. The definitive diagnosis is made by direct inspection of the epiglottis, a procedure that should be done by an experienced airway specialist under controlled conditions (usually the operating room). The typical findings are a cherry-red and swollen epiglottis and arytenoids.

Treatment

Once the diagnosis is made, endotracheal intubation should be performed immediately. Most anesthesiologists favor the use of general anesthesia (but not muscle relaxants) to facilitate intubation. Once an airway is established, cultures of the blood and epiglottis should be obtained and the patient started on appropriate intravenous antibiotics to cover *Haemophilus influenzae* (ceftriaxone sodium, 150 mg/kg/d in 2 divided doses or equivalent cephalosporin; chloramphenicol, 100 mg/kg/d in 4 divided doses; or ampicillin, 200 mg/kg/d in 4 divided doses). Ampicillin should probably not be used alone unless cultures are positive and demonstrate a sensitive organism.

Careful attention should be given to respiratory care of the intubated patient to prevent accidental extubation and tube obstruction. This includes adequate restraint, humidification, and frequent suctioning. Extubation can usually be accomplished in 24–48 hours, when direct inspection shows significant reduction in the size of the epiglottis. Some centers use the resolution of fever as a criterion for extubation. Intravenous antibiotics should be continued for 2–3 days, followed by oral antibiotics to complete a 10-day course.

If a physician who has little experience in treating airway disorders and is located far from a tertiary pediatric facility encounters a patient with epiglottis, the following is recommended. Start the patient on oxygen, and obtain all the airway equipment available. Manipulate the patient as little as possible, and allow the child to remain sitting up. Mobilize the most experienced airway person available, or call a transport team. Carefully start an intravenous line, and give antibiotics. If the patient obstructs completely and suffers a respiratory arrest, attempt to establish an airway by any means possible. This includes intubation, bag and mask ventilation, transtracheal ventilation with a large-bore angiocatheter attached to a 3-mm endotracheal tube adaptor and resuscitation bag, or tracheostomy.

Complications

Complications related to *Haemophilus influenzae*

disease in other sites include pneumonia, cervical adenitis, and septic arthritis. Meningitis is extremely rare.

Prognosis

Prompt recognition and appropriate treatment usually results in rapid resolution of swelling and inflammation. Recurrence is unusual.

Barker GA: Current management of croup and epiglottitis. *Pediatr Clin North Am* 1979;**26**:565.

Battaglia JD, Lockhart CH: Management of acute epiglottitis by nasotracheal intubation. *Am J Dis Child* 1975; **129**:334.

Butt W et al: Acute epiglottitis: A different approach to management. *Crit Care Med* 1988;**16**:43.

3. BACTERIAL TRACHEITIS

General Considerations

Bacterial tracheitis (pseudomembranous croup) represents a severe form of laryngotracheobronchitis that has received increased attention in the recent literature. It is not a new condition but one that has been "rediscovered." The organism most often isolated is *Staphylococcus aureus,* but organisms such as *H influenzae,* group A *Streptococcus pyogenes, Neisseria* species, and others have been reported. The disease probably represents localized, mucosal invasion of bacteria in patients with primary viral croup, resulting in inflammatory edema, purulent secretions, and pseudomembranes. Although cultures of the tracheal secretions are frequently positive, blood cultures are virtually always negative.

Clinical Findings

A. Symptoms and Signs: The early clinical picture is similar to that of viral croup. However, instead of gradual improvement, patients develop high fever, toxicity, and progressive upper airway obstruction that is unresponsive to standard croup therapy. The incidence of sudden respiratory arrest or progressive respiratory failure is very high; in such instances, airway intervention is required.

B. Laboratory Findings: The white count is usually elevated, with left shift. Cultures of tracheal secretions usually demonstrate one of the causative organisms.

C. Imaging: Lateral neck films show a normal epiglottis but often severe subglottic and tracheal narrowing. Frequently, irregularity of the contour of the proximal tracheal mucosa and pseudomembrane formation in the airway are present.

Treatment

Patients with suspected bacterial tracheitis should be managed in a similar fashion to those with epi-

glottitis. Because of the high incidence of respiratory arrest or progressive respiratory failure, intubation is almost always necessary. Once intubated, patients often have thick, purulent, obstructive tracheal secretions. Therefore, extreme care (adequate humidification, frequent suctioning, intensive care monitoring) is required to prevent endotracheal tube obstruction. Appropriate intravenous antibiotics to cover *S aureus, H influenzae,* and the other organisms are indicated. Because thick secretions persist for several days, the period of intubation required is longer for bacterial tracheitis than for epiglottis.

Prognosis

Despite the severity of this illness, the reported mortality rate is very low. Therefore, appropriate management is generally associated with a excellent outcome.

Han BK, Dunbar JS, Striker TW: Membranous laryngotracheobronchitis (membranous croup). *AJR* 1979;**133**:53.

Hen J: Current management of upper airway obstruction. *Pediatr Ann* (April) 1986;**15**:274.

Jones R, Santos JI, Overall JC: Bacterial tracheitis. *JAMA* 1979;**242**:721.

Liston SL et al: Bacterial tracheitis. *Am J Dis Child* 1983; **137**:764.

Nelson WE: Bacterial croup: A historical perspective. *J Pediatr* 1984;**105**:52.

VOCAL CORD PARALYSIS

Unilateral or bilateral vocal cord paralysis may be a congenital condition or, more commonly, a condition acquired from injury to the recurrent laryngeal nerves. Risk factors that predispose patients to acquired paralysis include difficult delivery (especially face presentation), neck and thoracic surgery (eg, ductal ligation, repair of tracheoesophageal fistula), trauma, mediastinal masses, pulmonary hypertension, and central nervous system disease (eg, Arnold-Chiari malformation). Patients usually present with varying degrees of hoarseness, aspiration, or high-pitched stridor. Unilateral cord paralysis is more likely to occur on the left because of the longer course of the left recurrent laryngeal nerve and its proximity to major thoracic structures. Patients with unilateral paralysis are usually hoarse but rarely have stridor. With bilateral cord paralysis, the closer to midline the cords are positioned, the greater the airway obstruction; the more lateral the cords are positioned, the greater the tendency to aspirate and experience hoarseness or aphonia. With partial function (paresis), the adductor muscles tend to operate better than the abductors, with a resultant high-pitched inspiratory stridor and normal voice. Airway intervention (intubation, tracheostomy) is rarely indicated in unilateral paralysis but is often necessary for bilateral paralysis. Recovery is related to the severity of nerve injury and the potential for healing.

Cohen SR et al: Laryngeal paralysis in children: A long-term retrospective study. *Ann Otol Rhinol Laryngol* 1982;**91**:417.
Emery PJ, Fearon B: Vocal cord palsy in pediatric practice: A review of 71 cases. *Int J Pediatr Otorhinolaryngol* 1984;**8**:147.
Fan LL et al: Paralyzed left vocal cord associated with patent ductus arteriosus ligation. *J Thorac Cardiovasc Surg* 1989;**98**:611.

SUBGLOTTIC STENOSIS

Subglottic stenosis can be a congenital condition or, more commonly, a lesion acquired from endotracheal intubation. Neonates and infants are particularly vulnerable to subglottic injury from intubation: the subglottis is the narrowest part of an infant's airway, and the cricoid cartilage, which supports the subglottis, is the only cartilage that completely encircles the airway. The clinical presentation may vary from patients who are totally asymptomatic to those who have typical evidence of severe upper airway obstruction. Patients with signs of stridor who fail extubation repeatedly are likely to have subglottic stenosis. As with other conditions, diagnosis is ultimately established by direct laryngoscopy and bronchoscopy. Tracheostomy is often required when airway compromise is severe. Although a number of surgical approaches to correct this problem have been tried, the failure rate is high. The most promising procedures are the "cricoid split," in which the cricoid cartilage is surgically opened (better for acquired than congenital lesions), and the laryngotracheoplasty, in which a cartilage graft from another source (eg, rib) is used to expand the framework.

Fan LL: Complications of intubation in children. *Prob Anesth* 1988;**2**:250.
Pashley NRT, Fan LL: Laryngeal injury from endotracheal intubation in the neonate. In: *Bronchopulmonary Dysplasia*. Bancalari E, Stocker JT (editors). Hemisphere Publishing, 1988.

LARYNGEAL TRAUMA

Injury to the larynx may result from external trauma, such as automobile accidents, snowmobile accidents (clothesline injury), and hanging, or internal trauma, such as noxious inhalation (burns and caustic substances) and intubation (already discussed). External trauma can cause laryngeal fracture, which requires an emergency tracheostomy to prevent death. After appropriate airway intervention, attention should be directed to debridement and closure of lacerations. Reduction of laryngeal fractures

should be performed as soon as the patient is stabilized.

Myers EN: Assessing and repairing laryngeal injuries. *J Respir Dis* 1982;**3**:43.

LARYNGEAL PAPILLOMATOSIS

Papillomas of the larynx are benign, warty growths that are difficult to treat. The presumed cause is human papilloma virus. A substantial percentage of mothers of patients with laryngeal papillomas have a history of genital condylomas at the time of delivery, a fact suggesting that the virus is acquired at birth during passage through an infected birth canal.

The age of onset is usually 2 to 4 years, but the disease may present at any age. Patients usually develop hoarseness, croupy cough, or stridor that can lead to life-threatening airway obstruction. Diagnosis is established by direct laryngoscopy.

Treatment is directed at relieving airway obstruction, usually by surgical removal of the lesions. Occasionally, tracheostomy is necessary when life-threatening obstruction or respiratory arrest occurs. Although a number of surgical procedures (laser, cup forceps, cryosurgery) have been used to remove papillomas, none is satisfactory: recurrences are the rule, and repeated operations at frequent intervals to prevent airway compromise are required. Occasionally, the lesions will spread down the trachea and bronchi, making surgical removal more difficult. Fortunately, spontaneous remissions do occur, usually by puberty, so that the goal of therapy is to maintain an adequate airway until remission occurs.

McDonald GA, Strong MS: Respiratory papillomatosis: Keeping it under control. *J Respir Dis* 1984;**5**:36.

CONGENITAL DISORDERS OF THE INTRATHORACIC AIRWAYS

TRACHEOMALACIA

Tracheomalacia exists when the cartilaginous framework of the trachea is inadequate to maintain airway patency. Because cartilage of the infant airway is normally "soft," all infants may have some degree of dynamic collapse of the trachea during expiration, when pressure outside the trachea exceeds intraluminal pressure. In tracheomalacia, whether congenital or acquired, dynamic collapse leads to airway obstruction. The congenital variety may be isolated or associated with another developmental defect, such as tracheoesophageal fistula or vascular ring. It may be localized to part of the trachea or, more commonly, involve the entire trachea as well as the remainder of the conducting airways. In severe cases, cartilage in the involved area may be missing or underdeveloped. The acquired variety has been associated with long-term ventilation of premature newborns that results in chronic tracheal injury.

Patients present with coarse wheezing, a prolonged expiratory phase, and a croupy cough, all of which increase with agitation and upper respiratory tract infections. Diagnosis can be made by cinefluoroscopy or bronchoscopy. Barium swallow may be indicated to rule out coexisting conditions. Usually, no treatment is indicated for the isolated condition, which generally improves over time. Coexisting lesions such as tracheoesophageal fistulas and vascular rings need primary repair. In severe cases of tracheomalacia, airway intervention by intubation or tracheostomy may be necessary; but this procedure alone is seldom satisfactory, because airway collapse continues to exist below the tip of the artificial airway. The application of continuous positive airway pressure through an artificial airway has occasionally been successful in stabilizing the collapsing airway.

Cogbill TH et al: Primary tracheomalacia. *Ann Thorac Surg* 1983;**35**:538.
Kanter et al: Treatment of severe tracheobronchomalacia with continuous positive airway pressure (CPAP). *Anesthesiology* 1982;**57**:54.
Sotomayor JL et al: Large-airway collapse due to acquired tracheobronchomalacia in infancy. *Am J Dis Child* 1986;**140**:367.

VASCULAR RINGS & SLINGS

Vascular anomalies of the aorta and its branches and the pulmonary arteries may compress the trachea or esophagus. The most common varieties include double aortic arch, right aortic arch with left ligamentum arteriosum or patent ductus arteriosus, pulmonary sling, anomalous innominate or left carotid artery, and aberrant right subclavian artery.

All but the aberrant right subclavian artery are associated with tracheal compression and, therefore, present in infancy with symptoms of chronic airway obstruction including stridor, course wheezing, and croupy cough. Symptoms are often worse in the supine position. Respiratory compromise is most severe with double aortic arch and may lead to apnea, respiratory arrest, or even death. Esophageal compression, present in all but anomalous innominate or carotid artery, may result in feeding difficulties, including dysphagia and vomiting. Therefore, barium swallow demonstrating this esophageal compression forms the mainstay of establishing the diagnosis. In the case of anomalous innominate or carotic artery,

diagnosis is best established by cinefluoroscopy or bronchoscopy.

Patients with significant symptoms require surgical correction, especially those with double aortic arch. Some controversy exists regarding whether angiography is necessary to define the anatomy prior to surgery. Patients usually improve following correction but may have persistent but milder symptoms of airway obstruction due to associated tracheomalacia.

Ashraf H, Subramanian S: Identifying the hallmarks of vascular rings in children. *J Respir Dis* 1985;**6**:31.
Keith HH: Vascular rings and tracheobronchial compression in infants. *Pediatr Ann* (Aug) 1977;**6**:91.

BRONCHOGENIC CYSTS

Bronchogenic cysts generally occur in the middle mediastinum (see Mediastinal Masses) near the carina and adjacent to the major bronchi but can be found elsewhere in the lung as well. Sizes are variable, ranging between 2 and 10 centimeters. Cyst walls are thick and may contain pus, mucus, or blood. These develop from abnormal lung budding of the primitive foregut. They do not contain distal lung parenchyma and generally do not communicate with the airway.

Clinically, respiratory distress can appear acutely in early childhood or present as chronic wheezing, chronic cough, tachypnea, recurrent pneumonia, or stridor, depending on location, size, and the degree of airway compression. On physical examination, tracheal deviation away from the midline may be noted, and the percussion note over involved lobes may be hyperresonant. Breath sounds over such areas will also be decreased. Air trapping and hyperinflation of the affected lobe(s) is found on chest x-ray film. Smaller lesions or those detected early may not be appreciated on chest x-ray film or may appear spherical. Initial assessment of a suspected bronchogenic cyst usually includes a barium swallow to demonstrate the presence of a mass. This study also helps determine whether the lesion communicates with the gastrointestinal tract. CT scans or ultrasound can differentiate solid versus cystic mediastinal masses and define the cyst's relationship to the rest of the lung.

Treatment involves surgical resection of the bronchogenic cyst. Vigorous pulmonary physiotherapy is indicated in the postoperative period to prevent complications of the surgery (atelectasis, infection of lung distal to the site of resection of the cyst).

Stocker JT et al: Cystic and congenital lung disease in the newborn. In: *Perspectives in Pediatric Pathology.* Vol 4. Rosenberg H, Bolande T (editors). Yearbook, 1978.
Turcios NL et al: When a neonate has cystic lung disease. *J Respir Dis* 1987;**8**:85.

ACQUIRED DISORDERS
OF THE INTRATHORACIC AIRWAYS

FOREIGN BODY ASPIRATION

1. FOREIGN BODIES IN THE UPPER RESPIRATORY TRACT

Essentials of Diagnosis

Upper airway obstruction:
- Acute onset of cyanosis and choking, with the inability to vocalize or cough (complete obstruction) or drooling and stridor (partial obstruction).

General Considerations

Foreign body aspiration contributes significantly to morbidity and mortality of early childhood, with many deaths resulting from upper airway obstruction each year. Most commonly, children between 6 months and 4 years of age are at particularly high risk for foreign body aspiration.

Clinical Findings

Foreign bodies lodged within the esophagus may compress the airway and cause respiratory distress. More typically, the foreign body lodges in the supraglottic airway, triggering protective reflexes that attempt to dislodge the object and causing laryngospasm. Onset is generally abrupt, with a history of the child running with food or other object in the mouth or playing with seeds, small coins, toys or other objects. Poor ''child proofing'' in the home and cases in which an older sibling feeds age-inappropriate foods (peanuts, hard candy, carrot slices, etc) to the younger child are typical. If the obstruction is only partial, coughing, stridor, and the ability to vocalize may persist. If complete, an inability to cough or vocalize and cyanosis with marked distress are observed. If untreated, progressive cyanosis, loss of consciousness, seizures, bradycardia, and cardiopulmonary arrest follow.

Treatment

The emergency treatment of upper airway obstruction due to foreign body aspiration is somewhat controversial. In general, it is recommended that if partial obstruction is present, children should be allowed to use their own cough reflex to extrude the foreign body. If after a brief observation period, the obstruction persists or the patient becomes completely obstructed, acute intervention is required. The American Academy of Pediatrics and the American Heart Association distinguish between children less than or greater than one year of age. In the choking infant less than one year, the child should

be placed in a face down position over the rescuer's arm, with the head positioned below the trunk. Four measured back blows are delivered rapidly between the infant's scapulas with the heel of the rescuer's hand. If still obstructed, the infant should be rolled over and 4 rapid chest compressions performed (in a fashion similar to CPR). This sequence is repeated until the obstruction is relieved. In children over 1 year, abdominal thrusts (the ''Heimlich maneuver'') may be performed, with special care taken in younger children because of concern regarding potential risks for intra-abdominal organ injury.

In both groups, blind probing of the airway to dislodge a foreign body is discouraged because of possible impaction. The airway may be opened by jaw thrust, and if the foreign body can be directly visualized, careful removal with the fingers or available instruments (Magill forceps) can be attempted. Patients with persistent apnea and the inability to achieve adequate ventilation may require emergency intubation, tracheostomy, or needle cricothyroidectomy, depending on the setting and the rescuer's skills.

Abman SH et al: Emergency treatment of foreign body obstruction of the upper airway in children. *J Emerg Med* 1984;**2**:7.

American Heart Association: Standard guidelines for CPR and emergency cardiac care. *JAMA* 1986;**255**:2959.

Committee on Accident and Poison Prevention, American Academy of Pediatrics: First aid for the choking child. *Pediatrics* 1981;**67**:744.

Greensher J, Mofenson HC: Emergency treatment of the choking child. *Pediatrics* 1982;**70**:110.

Heimlich JH: First aid for choking children: Back blows and chest thrusts cause complications and death. *Pediatrics* 1982;**70**:124.

2. FOREIGN BODIES IN THE LOWER RESPIRATORY TRACT

Essentials of Diagnosis

Lower airway obstruction:
- Sudden onset of coughing, wheezing, or respiratory distress.
- Asymmetric physical findings of decreased breath sounds or localized wheezing.
- Asymmetric radiographic findings, especially with forced expiratory view.

General Considerations

The problem with diagnosing foreign body aspiration of the lower respiratory tract is the lack of parental observations documenting an acute aspiration. The abrupt onset of cough, choking or wheezing, especially in children between 6 months and 4 years who have access to high-risk objects such as peanuts, hard candy, small toys, and other objects, should heighten suspicion.

Clinical Findings

A. Symptoms and Signs: Clinically, the range of respiratory symptoms and signs varies, depending on the site of obstruction and the duration following the acute episode. For example, a large or central airway obstruction may cause marked distress and prompt early intervention. In contrast, if the foreign object remains in the lower respiratory tract, the acute cough or wheezing may diminish over time, only to recur later and present as chronic cough or persistent wheezing. Thus, foreign body aspiration should be suspected in children with chronic cough, persistent wheezing, or recurrent pneumonia. Long-standing foreign bodies may lead to bronchiectasis or lung abscess. On physical examination, asymmetric breath sounds or localized wheezing also suggest the presence of a foreign body.

B. Imaging: A physician who suspects foreign body aspiration should obtain inspiratory and forced expiratory chest x-rays. The latter study can be obtained in young children by manually compressing the abdomen during expiration. The initial inspiratory view may show localized hyperinflation due to the ball-valve effect of the foreign body, causing distal air trapping. A positive forced expiratory study shows a mediastinal shift away from the affected side. If airway obstruction is complete, atelectasis and related volume loss will be the major radiologic findings. Chest fluoroscopy is an alternative approach for detecting air trapping and mediastinal shift.

Treatment

If positive findings are absent but clinical suspicion persists, further evaluation with bronchoscopy is indicated. Rigid, not flexible, bronchoscopy is the recommended diagnostic and therapeutic approach to managing suspected or proved foreign body aspiration. Flexible bronchoscopy may be helpful for follow-up evaluations (after the foreign object has been removed).

Children with suspected acute foreign body aspiration should be admitted to the hospital for evaluation and treatment. Chest postural drainage was often performed in the past, prior to technologic improvements in bronchoscopy; however, postural drainage is no longer recommended because the foreign body may become dislodged and obstruct a major central airway. Rigid bronchoscopy under general anesthesia is the current treatment for foreign body aspiration. Bronchoscopy should not be delayed in children with respiratory distress but should be performed as soon as possible once the diagnosis is made, even in children with more chronic symptoms. Following the removal of the foreign body, β-adrenergic nebulization treatments followed by chest physiotherapy are recommended to help clear related mucus or bronchospasm. Current bronchoscopy skills facilitate foreign body removal with little

risk. The relative dangers of missing a foreign body in the lower respiratory tract are much greater; these include the development of bronchiectasis and lung abscess over time. This risk justifies an aggressive approach to suspected foreign bodies in undocumented but suspicious cases.

Kosloske AM: Tracheobronchial foreign bodies in children: Back to the bronchoscope and a balloon. *Pediatrics* 1980;**66**:321.

Law D, Kosloske AM: Management of tracheobronchial foreign bodies in children: A reevaluation of postural drainage and bronchoscopy. *Pediatrics* 1976;**58**:362.

Wood RE, Gauderer MWL: Flexible fiberoptic bronchoscopy in the management of tracheobronchial foreign bodies in children: The value of a combined approach with open tube bronchoscopy. *J Pediatr Surg* 1984;**19**:693.

BRONCHITIS

Essentials of Diagnosis

- Cough that usually progresses from dry to productive.
- Rhonchi appearing predominantly during expiration.

General Considerations

Bronchitis refers to inflammation of the major conducting airways within the lung. As an isolated entity, this problem is probably unusual in children. However, inflammation within this section of the airways commonly occurs as part of disease processes involving other areas of the respiratory tract. From a temporal standpoint, bronchitis may be acute, chronic, or recurrent. In adults, the diagnosis of chronic bronchitis is based on a history of at least 3 months of productive cough occurring for 2 or more years, but no generally acceptable criteria for this diagnosis exist in children. However, if cough with sputum production persists in a child for a period of at least 3–4 weeks, the physician should consider the diagnoses discussed below (see Differential Diagnosis).

Clinical Findings

A. Symptoms and Signs: An acute bronchitis usually begins as a dry, nonproductive cough that may be associated with other features of an upper respiratory illness of viral origin. The longer the cough persists, the more likely the cough will become productive. In general, children with uncomplicated acute bronchitis appear nontoxic, and fever, if present, is low-grade. On examination of the chest, diffuse rhonchi appearing predominantly during expiration are noted. In uncomplicated acute bronchitis, mucus production decreases, and the cough disappears over a period of 7–10 days.

B. Laboratory Findings: The white blood count is usually normal and, if elevated, may suggest a viral infection. Pulmonary function tests may reveal variable degrees of airway obstruction.

C. Imaging: An x-ray examination of the chest may be normal or show a mild increase in bronchovascular markings.

Differential Diagnosis

Most attacks of acute bronchitis are caused by viral infections. Although episodes are usually self-limited, certain viral pathogens, such as the adenovirus, can produce a more severe clinical picture that resembles a pertussislike illness. Bacteria that may produce disease in which bronchitis is a prominent symptom include *Bordetella pertussis, Mycobacterium tuberculosis, Corynebacterium diphtheriae,* and *Mycoplasma pneumoniae.*

Noninfectious diseases need to be considered in the evaluation of an acute bronchitis that differs from the clinical picture described above and in cases of chronic bronchitis or recurrent bronchitic episodes. Asthma may present as a persistent cough with little or no wheezing. Sinus infections may provide a source of persistent irritation to the respiratory tract and lead to a chronic cough. Cystic fibrosis, an immunodeficiency, or an immotile cilia syndrome must also be considered if the bronchitic syndrome persists or recurs and if bronchiectasis is present or suspected. In the younger child, respiratory tract anomalies, foreign bodies, and recurrent aspiration must also be considered. Tobacco or marijuana smoking may contribute to this process in older children. In patients of all ages, the potential role of irritants within their environment must also be evaluated.

Complications

In otherwise healthy children, complications of an acute bronchitis secondary to a viral infection are few but include otitis media, sinusitis, and pneumonia. When the bronchitic syndrome is secondary to other underlying problems outlined in the differential diagnosis, the prognosis depends on the primary problem.

Treatment

When bronchitis is secondary to an uncomplicated acute viral infection, supportive therapy (stressing adequate hydration, rest, and patience) is all that is necessary. Expectorants and cough suppressants, although commonly used, are seldom indicated. Avoidance of irritants during the viral infection may also decrease symptoms and morbidity. When the bronchitic syndrome is due to other underlying problems, the treatment must address the primary process.

Florman AL, Cushing AH, Umland ET: Rapid noninvasive techniques for determining etiology of bronchitis and pneumonia in infants and children. *Clin Chest Med* 1987;**8**:669.

Loughlin GM: Bronchitis. In: *Disorders of the Respiratory Tract in Children,* 4th ed. Kendig EL, Jr, Chernick V (editors). Saunders, 1983.

Morgan WJ, Taussig LM: The chronic bronchitis complex in children. *Pediatr Clin North Am* 1984;**31**:851.

Taussig LM, Smith SM, Blumenfeld R: Chronic bronchitis in childhood: What is it? *Pediatrics* 1981;**67**:1.

BRONCHIOLITIS

Essentials of Diagnosis

- Young infant with acute onset of tachypnea, cough, rhinorrhea, and expiratory wheeze.
- Chest x-ray with streaky infiltrates and hyperaeration.

General Considerations

Bronchiolitis is a common cause of acute hospital admissions in young infants (under 2 years), especially during the winter months. Although respiratory syncytial virus (RSV) is by far the most common pathogen, other viral agents include parainfluenza, influenza, and adenovirus. *Mycoplasma, Chlamydia, Ureaplasma,* and *Pneumocystis* are other potential causes of wheezing-associated respiratory illness during early infancy. Major concerns include not only the acute effects of bronchiolitis but also the possibility of long-term airway injury and the development of chronic airways hyperreactivity (asthma). In addition, RSV bronchiolitis contributes substantially to morbidity and mortality in children with underlying cardiopulmonary disorders, including bronchopulmonary dysplasia, cystic fibrosis, and congenital heart disease, especially when pulmonary hypertension is present.

Clinical Findings

A. Symptoms and Signs: The usual course of RSV bronchiolitis includes 1–2 days of fever, rhinorrhea, and cough, followed by wheezing, tachypnea, and respiratory distress. Typically, the breathing pattern is shallow with rapid respirations. Nasal flaring, cyanosis, retractions, and rales may be present, along with prolongation of the expiratory phase and wheezing, depending on the severity of illness. Some young infants present with apnea and little auscultatory findings but may subsequently develop rales, rhonchi, and expiratory wheezing. Otitis media, superimposed bacterial pneumonia, and bacteremia may be observed.

B. Laboratory Findings: The peripheral white blood cell count may be normal or show a mild lymphocytosis.

C. Imaging: Chest x-ray findings typically include hyperinflation with mild interstitial infiltrates, but segmental atelectasis is not uncommon.

Treatment

Although most children infected with RSV are

readily managed as outpatients with supportive therapy, hospitalization is required in children less than 2 months of age and in patients with hypoxemia in room air, a history of apnea, moderate tachypnea with feeding difficulties, marked respiratory distress with retractions, and underlying chronic cardiopulmonary disorders. Initial management includes an assessment of oxygenation and ventilation with an arterial blood gas and, if hypoxemia is present, the administration of supplemental oxygen. Noninvasive measurements of oxygenation by oximeter or transcutaneous Po_2 monitor should be used to assess the response to therapy and provide early warning of impending respiratory failure in infants. In one series, 7% of normal children admitted for viral bronchiolitis subsequently required mechanical ventilation; infants with bronchopulmonary dysplasia and cystic fibrosis hospitalized with RSV develop respiratory failure at higher rates. Progressive respiratory distress (including progressive hypoxemia and hypercarbia) and apnea are common indications for admission to the intensive care unit and mechanical ventilation.

Medical staff should also administer intravenous hydration to correct losses and poor intake, while carefully monitoring intake, output, and urinary specific gravity to avoid overhydration and the risk of fluid overload and pulmonary edema. Although β-adrenergic therapy, theophylline, and steroids may attenuate airways obstruction, their use remains controversial and empiric, and patients should be assessed individually to determine the degree of responsiveness to pharmacologic interventions.

The availability of rapid diagnostic testing for RSV may allow for early intervention with antiviral therapy (ribavirin), especially in children with marked respiratory distress or chronic cardiopulmonary disease. Although ribavirin's efficacy remains unclear, its use is currently recommended for hospitalized infants with severe disease or with coexistent congenital heart disease, bronchopulmonary dysplasia, cystic fibrosis, immunodeficiencies, and other chronic lung disorders, as well as recent transplant recipients and patients undergoing chemotherapy. In addition, children less than 6 weeks of age and those with underlying metabolic, neurologic, or congenital abnormalities should be considered for ribavirin therapy.

Prognosis

Although the outcome following bronchiolitis is good for the overall population, the mortality rate in patients with congenital heart disease has been reported to be near 50%. In addition, recurrent episodes of wheezing may follow acute infection in almost half of the hospitalized infants, a fact suggesting the possibility that early infection may contribute to the subsequent development of chronic reactive airways disease.

Abman SH et al: Role of RSV in early hospitalizations for respiratory distress of young infants with cystic fibrosis. *J Pediatr* 1988;**113**:826.

Groothius J et al: RSV in children with bronchopulmonary dysplasia. *Pediatrics* 1988;**82**:199.

MacDonald NE et al: RSV in infants with congenital heart disease. *N Engl J Med* 1982;**307**:397.

Outwater KM, Crone RK: Management of respiratory failure in infants with acute viral bronchiolitis. *Am J Dis Child* 1984;**138**:1071.

Volovitz B, Faden H, Ogra PL: Release of leukotriene C_4 in respiratory tract during acute viral infection. *J Pediatr* 1988;**112**:218.

Wohl MEB, Chernick V: Bronchiolitis. *Am Rev Respir Dis* 1978;**118**:758.

BRONCHIECTASIS

Essentials of Diagnosis

- Chronic cough with sputum production.
- Persistent abnormalities on physical examination of the chest.
- Persistent abnormalities on chest x-ray.

General Considerations

The term bronchiectasis means dilatation of bronchi. The dilatation may be regular, with the airway continuing to have a smooth outline (cylindric bronchiectasis); irregular, with areas of dilatation and constriction (varicose bronchiectasis); or marked, with destruction of structural components of the airway wall (saccular bronchiectasis). Although the incidence of the disease in the general population is low (less than 0.5%), the morbidity associated with the more severe forms of bronchiectasis is significant. For this reason, an appreciation for the pathogenesis of the problem is important; medical intervention can halt the progression of a potentially reversible form of the problem (cylindric bronchiectasis) to an irreversible form of destructive airway disease (saccular bronchiectasis).

In terms of pathogenesis, 2 factors appear to be important in the acquisition of bronchiectasis. First, obstruction of the airway resulting in poor drainage is a feature of many disease processes that lead to this disorder (cystic fibrosis, foreign bodies). In addition, infection must also be present to damage the airway. Thus, in the healthy airway, either self-limited infection without significant obstruction or obstruction without infection is unlikely to lead to the more severe forms of bronchiectasis. However, the combination of the 2 for a period of time favor the development of bronchiectatic areas of lung.

Clinical Findings

A. Symptoms and Signs: The clinical manifestations of bronchiectasis vary widely from the healthy-appearing child whose only symptom may be chronic cough with early morning sputum production to chronically ill children with recurrent pneumonia with or without hemoptysis. There may be a history of recurrent respiratory infections, dyspnea on exertion, and a productive cough precipitated by exercise. In addition, some children present with a history of recurrent fevers. Chronic cough, persistent atelectasis, and failure of a chest x-ray to clear after a respiratory infection should raise the possibility of bronchiectasis in the physician's mind. On physical examination, digital clubbing may be present, and there may be evidence of sinusitis suggested by sinus tenderness or postnasal drainage of purulent secretions. Persistent adventitious sound (moist rales, rhonchi) and decreased air entry are often noted over the bronchiectatic area when saccular changes are present.

B. Laboratory Findings and Imaging: Cultures from the respiratory tract usually reveal mixed flora; *Haemophilus influenzae* is one of the more common isolates. Because of coexistent sinus disease in many patients, cultures of secretions from the upper airway may also assist in determining antimicrobial therapy.

Chest x-ray films may show mildly abnormal findings with slightly increased bronchovascular markings or areas of atelectasis, or they may demonstrate cystic changes in one or more areas of the lung. The anatomy of the airways is best defined by a high-resolution CT scan of the lung, which often reveals far more extensive disease (in terms of involvement of other areas of lung) than expected from the plain chest x-ray. Although bronchograms have been used in the past to determine whether a disease is localized or diffuse and to determine if varicose or saccular bronchiectasis is present, the bronchogram may lead to significant morbidity and has been replaced by the radiologic studies. However, bronchograms may still be of assistance when surgery is seriously considered as a therapeutic option.

An assessment of lung function often reveals an obstructive pattern, even in the absence of asthma, cystic fibrosis, or other disease processes leading to airways obstruction. This obstruction may reflect difficulty in handling airway secretions or a more generalized pulmonary problem involving both large and small airways. Evaluation of lung function before and after inhalation of a bronchodilator is helpful in assessing the potential contribution of this class of medications to therapy. In addition, serial assessments of lung function help define the progression or resolution of the disease.

Differential Diagnosis

Infectious diseases have always been important factors predisposing to bronchiectasis. Both rubeola and pertussis were prominently associated with bronchiectasis in older reports of this disorder. In addition, tuberculosis continues to lead to significant airways damage. More recently, adenoviral infections have been noted to lead to bronchiectasis. From a

practical point, however, any viral or bacterial infection of the lung that leads to significant obstruction and persistent inflammation has the potential to damage the airway wall.

Bronchiectasis also develops in patients with cystic fibrosis, immunodeficiencies involving humoral immunity, and abnormal mucociliary clearance (immotile-cilia syndromes). Recurrent aspiration has also been associated with this disorder. Aspiration of a foreign body must also be considered, especially when bronchiectatic changes are confined to one area of the lung.

Although congenital causes of bronchiectasis are relatively uncommon compared to the predisposing factors listed above, they must still be considered in the differential diagnosis. Bronchiectasis may result from a developmental arrest of bronchial cartilage in which the involved areas give rise to cysts that are prone to infection. In addition, defective development of bronchial cartilage (Williams-Campbell syndrome) and developmental failure of elastic and muscular tissues of the trachea and bronchi (tracheobronchomegaly or Mounier-Kuhn syndrome) have been associated with bronchiectasis. Bronchial stenosis, either congenital or acquired, also predisposes to bronchiectasis.

Complications

Several complications may develop as a consequence of the more severe forms of bronchiectasis. The major concerns include severe pneumonia, hemoptysis, and cor pulmonale. More unusual complications include abscesses of the lung or central nervous system, as well as empyema and bronchopleural fistula.

Treatment

The initial approach to almost all children with bronchiectasis is medical and consists of identifying bacterial pathogens present in the bronchiectatic area(s) of lung. Based on the severity of the airway damage, antibiotics can be delivered either systemically (for saccular changes) or orally. Coupled with use of antibiotics is optimal pulmonary physiotherapy, which consists of inhalation of bronchodilators followed by postural drainage and chest percussion to affected areas of lung. If present, sinusitis must also be vigorously treated.

Surgical removal of an area of lung that has severe saccular bronchiectasis is considered when the response to several months of optimal medical therapy has been poor. Other indications include extensive or repeated hemoptysis and recurrent pneumonia in one area of lung. In general, surgery is best performed when the bronchiectatic area(s) is well localized and the rest of the lung appears to be normal. This clinical description is most likely to be found in a child who has saccular bronchiectasis due to foreign body aspiration or a congenital defect. In general, children with more serious underlying disorders (cystic fibrosis, hypogammaglobulinemia) are likely to have bronchiectatic changes in several areas of the lung and are not good candidates for surgery.

Prognosis

The outlook for patients with bronchiectasis depends on the underlying cause of the problem, the severity of the bronchiectatic changes, and the extent of lung involvement. As noted, good pulmonary hygiene and avoidance of infectious complications in the involved areas of lung may reverse cylindric bronchiectasis.

Barker AF, Bardana EJ Jr: Bronchiectasis: Update of an orphan disease. *Am Rev Respir Dis* 1988;**137**:969.

Lewiston NJ: Bronchiectasis in childhood. *Pediatr Clin North Am* 1984;**31**:865.

Nemir RL: Bronchiectasis. In: *Disorders of the Respiratory Tract in Children*, 4th ed. Kendig EL Jr, Chernick V (editors). Saunders, 1983.

BRONCHIOLITIS OBLITERANS (Bronchiolitis Fibrosa Obliterans)

Essentials of Diagnosis

- Airways obstruction unresponsive to therapy.

General Considerations

Bronchiolitis obliterans is a disease characterized by obstruction of bronchi and bronchioles by fibrous tissue after an insult to the lower respiratory tract. The disorder can be precipitated by inhalation of toxic gases, infections of the lower respiratory tract (adenovirus, influenza, rubeola, pertussis, mycoplasma), connective tissue diseases, transplantation, and aspiration. Many episodes of bronchiolitis obliterans are idiopathic (no definable cause can be identified). Studies of adenovirus-induced bronchiolitis obliterans indicate that the disease occurs more frequently in the American Indian population in Canada and in Polynesian children in New Zealand, suggesting that racial or socioeconomic factors predispose to this process.

Clinical Findings

A. Symptoms and Signs: Bronchiolitis obliterans should be considered when there is persistent cough or wheezing after an acute pneumonia. Prolonged rales or wheezing or persistent exercise intolerance following a pulmonary insult should also suggest this disease. Sputum production may accompany these complaints.

B. Laboratory Findings and Imaging: Chest x-ray abnormalities include evidence of localized or generalized air trapping, as well as possibly nodular densities and alveolar opacification. Scattered areas of matched decreases in ventilation and perfusion are seen when the lung is scanned. Pulmonary angiograms reveal decreased vasculature in the area of lung involvement, whereas bronchograms demonstrate marked pruning of the bronchial tree. An assessment of lung function demonstrates an obstructive process that may be combined with evidence of restriction. Administration of an inhaled bronchodilator both before and after courses of corticosteroids leads to little improvement in lung function.

Differential Diagnosis

Poorly treated asthma, cystic fibrosis, and bronchopulmonary dysplasia must be considered in the pediatric patient with evidence of persistent airways obstruction and ruled out on the basis of the history and appropriate diagnostic tests. A trial of medications (including corticosteroids) employed in the treatment of asthma may help to define the reversibility of the process when the primary differential is between asthma and bronchiolitis obliterans. Although the laboratory findings outlined above are very suggestive of the correct diagnosis, the most definitive way to establish the diagnosis is by an open lung biopsy with proper histologic assessment of the specimen.

Complications

Sequelae of bronchiolitis obliterans include persistent airways obstruction, recurrent wheezing, bronchiectasis, chronic atelectasis, recurrent pneumonia, and unilateral hyperlucent lung syndrome.

Treatment

Supplemental oxygen should be given to patients with oxygen desaturation during normal activities or sleep. In addition, early treatment should be directed at preventing ongoing airway damage due to problems such as aspiration, which may be either the primary insult or an acquired problem secondary to marked hyperinflation. Other forms of treatment may be more difficult to evaluate in terms of effectiveness. Oral and inhaled bronchodilators may be helpful in reversing any airways obstruction produced by a reactive component to the disease. Many children also receive at least one course of corticosteroid treatment in an attempt to reverse the obstruction or prevent ongoing damage. Antibiotics should be used as clinically indicated for pneumonia.

Prognosis

Prognosis may depend in part on the underlying cause of the bronchiolitis obliterans, as well as the age of the patient when the insult to the airways took place. The course varies from mild asthmalike symptoms to rapidly fatal deterioration despite the therapy outlined above.

Hardy KA, Schidlow DV, Zaeri N: Obliterative bronchiolitis in children. *Chest* 1988;**93**:461.

Wohl MEB: Bronchiolitis. In: *Disorders of the Respiratory Tract in Children,* 4th ed. Kendig EL Jr, Chernick V (editors). Saunders, 1983.

BRONCHOPULMONARY DYSPLASIA

Essentials of Diagnosis

- Acute respiratory distress in first week of life.
- Required oxygen therapy or mechanical ventilation.
- Persistent respiratory abnormalities, including physical signs, radiographic findings and O_2 requirement, after 1 month of age.

General Considerations

As mortality rates for premature newborns have fallen dramatically over the past 2 decades, bronchopulmonary dysplasia (BPD) remains one of the most significant sequelae following the management of acute respiratory distress in the neonatal intensive care unit, with an estimated incidence ranging between 10–40% (depending on the exact criteria used for definition and the gestational age of the population base). This disease was first characterized in 1967 when Northway and coworkers reported the clinical, radiologic, and pathologic findings in a group of premature newborns who required prolonged mechanical ventilation and oxygen therapy to treat hyaline membrane disease. The progression from acute hyaline membrane disease to chronic lung disease was divided into 4 stages: acute respiratory distress shortly after birth, usually hyaline membrane disease (Stage I); clinical and radiographic worsening of the acute lung disease, often due to increased pulmonary blood flow secondary to a patent ductus arteriosus (Stage II); and progressive signs of chronic lung disease (Stages III and IV). Although some of the clinical features of bronchopulmonary dysplasia (BPD) have changed over the past 20 years along with changes in therapeutic interventions, this seminal paper provided an important framework for understanding the evolution of this problem and also provided an initial recognition of the potential risk factors: immaturity, oxygen toxicity, barotrauma, and inflammation.

The precise definition of BPD remains somewhat controversial. For most purposes, however, BPD can be defined clinically as a chronic respiratory disorder of infancy which follows therapeutic intervention during the first week of life for acute respiratory distress and which subsequently is associated with persistent physical signs of respiratory distress, a requirement for supplemental oxygen, and radiographic abnormalities beyond 30 days of age. This definition is broad and does not reflect some key issues, including the following: (1) although most of these children were premature and had hyaline membrane disease, full-term newborns with such disorders as meconium aspiration or persistent pulmonary hypertension can also develop BPD; (2) some severely preterm newborns require minimal ventilator support yet subsequently develop a prolonged oxygen requirement despite the absence of severe acute manifestations of respiratory failure; (3) newborns dying within the first weeks of life can already have the aggressive, fibroproliferative pathologic lesions that resemble BPD; and (4) physiologic abnormalities (increased airway resistance) and biochemical markers of lung injury (altered protease and antiprotease ratios, increased inflammatory cells and mediators), which are predictive of BPD, are already present in the first week of life.

Although the exact mechanisms leading to chronic lung disease are not completely understood, BPD represents the consequences of lung injury caused by oxygen toxicity, barotrauma, and inflammation superimposed on a susceptible, generally immature, lung. The premature lung often lacks the ability to make adequate amounts of functional surfactant; furthermore, the antioxidant defense mechanisms are not sufficiently mature to protect the lung from the toxic oxygen metabolites generated from hyperoxia, which cause further lung injury. Thus, abnormal lung mechanics due to structural immaturity, surfactant deficiency, atelectasis, and pulmonary edema, plus lung injury secondary to hyperoxia and mechanical ventilation, lead to further abnormalities of lung function, causing increases in ventilator and oxygen requirements, leading to a vicious cycle that compounds the progression of lung injury. Other factors, such as excessive fluid administration, patent ductus arteriosus, pulmonary interstitial emphysema, pneumothorax, infection, and inflammatory stimuli secondary to lung injury or infection, also play important roles in the pathogenesis and pathophysiology of BPD.

Differential Diagnosis

The radiologic differential diagnosis includes meconium aspiration syndrome, congenital infection (such as cytomegalovirus or *Ureaplasma*), cystic adenomatoid malformation, recurrent aspiration, pulmonary lymphangiectasia, total anomalous pulmonary venous return, overhydration, or idiopathic pulmonary fibrosis.

Clinical Course & Treatment

The clinical course of infants with BPD is extremely variable, ranging from patients with a mild oxygen requirement that gradually resolves over a few months to more severely affected children who require chronic tracheostomy and mechanical ventilation throughout the first 2 years of life. In general, BPD patients show slow, steady improvements in oxygen or ventilator requirements but can have frequent respiratory exacerbations leading to frequent or prolonged hospitalizations. Clinical management generally includes careful attention to growth, nutrition, metabolic status, development, neurologic status, and related problems, along with the various cardiopulmonary abnormalities described below.

Because increased airways resistance and bronchial hyperreactivity are common in BPD infants, various combinations of β-adrenergic agonists, theophylline, steroids and cromolyn are commonly part of the treatment plan. Part of the rationale for the use of steroids in BPD infants is to decrease lung inflammation and enhance responsiveness to the β-adrenergic therapy, as in the treatment of infants with severe asthma. Because thick secretions are common and may contribute to airway obstruction or recurrent atelectasis, chest physiotherapy following the administration of β-adrenergic agonists is commonly part of the regimen.

Although bronchial hyperreactivity in BPD infants is well recognized, structural lesions (such as subglottic stenosis, vocal cord paralysis, tracheal stenosis, tracheomalacia, bronchial stenosis, granulomatous bronchial polyps, and others) often contribute to airflow limitation. This possibility suggests the need for careful bronchoscopic evaluations in children with significant BPD.

Infants with BPD often have recurrent pulmonary edema, which may be due to increased permeability of the injured pulmonary circulation or to increases in hydrostatic pressure if left ventricular dysfunction is present. In addition, salt and water retention secondary to chronic hypoxemia, hypercarbia, or other stimuli may be present. Chronic or intermittent diuretic therapy with furosemide, hydrochlorothiazide, and spironolactone, is commonly used to treat BPD infants with rales or signs of persistent pulmonary edema, with acute improvement in lung function demonstrated by clinical studies. Unfortunately, diuretics often cause important side effects, including severe volume contraction, hypokalemia, alkalosis, and hyponatremia. Potassium and arginine chloride supplements are commonly required.

Infants with BPD often have pulmonary hypertension, and in many children, even mild hypoxia can cause significant elevations of pulmonary artery pressure. To minimize the harmful effects of hypoxia, medical staff must constantly maintain Pao_2 above 55–60 torr. Because even intermittent hypoxia contributes to the development or progression of pulmonary hypertension and cor pulmonale, noninvasive assessments of oxygenation must be made during all activities, including the infant's waking, sleeping, and feeding periods. Serial electrocardiogram and echocardiogram studies monitor the development of right ventricular hypertrophy (RVH). If RVH persists or develops where it previously was not present, intermittent hypoxia should be considered and further assessments of oxygenation pursued, especially while the infant sleeps. In addition, barium swallow, esophageal pH probe studies, bron-

choscopy, and cardiac catheterization may reveal previously unsuspected cardiac or pulmonary lesions, such as aspiration, tracheomalacia, obstructive sleep apnea, anatomic cardiac lesions, and others, that contribute to the underlying pathophysiology. In addition, long-term care should include monitoring systemic hypertension and the development of left ventricular hypertrophy.

Nutritional problems leading to poor growth in BPD infants are not uncommon and may be due to increased O_2 consumption, feeding difficulties, gastroesophageal reflux, and chronic hypoxia. Hypercaloric formulas and gastrostomies are often required to ensure adequate intake while avoiding overhydration. In addition, influenza vaccine is recommended. With the onset of acute wheezing secondary to suspected viral infection, rapid diagnostic testing for RSV may facilitate early treatment, which may diminish the late morbidity of RSV bronchiolitis in BPD.

For BPD children who remain ventilator-dependent, the authors believe that arterial CO_2 should be maintained below 60 torr, even when pH is normal, because of the potential adverse effects of hypercarbia on salt and water retention, cardiac function, and perhaps pulmonary vascular tone. Changes in ventilator settings in children with severe lung disease should be slow, because the effects of many of the changes may not be manifested for days. These signs may include poor feeding, irritability, weight loss, vomiting, increased retractions, wheezing, and CO_2 retention. Medical staff should frequently meet with the parents to review progress and changes in treatment plans and thereby decrease some of the family stresses involved in caring for children with chronic severe disease. Patience, continued family support, attention to developmental issues, and speech and physical therapy help to improve the long-term outlook.

Prognosis

Although mortality is high in infants with severe (Stage IV) BPD, the long-term outlook is generally favorable for most BPD patients. However, more time and further study is needed to assess fully the impact in adolescence and early adulthood of such sequelae as persistent airways hyperreactivity, exercise intolerance, and perhaps abnormal lung growth. The potential role of new therapeutic approaches such as surfactant replacement and high-frequency ventilation have not yet been shown to attenuate the severity or incidence of BPD, but these therapies are still under study. The possible impact of antioxidant therapy or specific antiinflammatory agents must be pursued.

Abman SH et al: Pulmonary vascular response to oxygen in infants with severe bronchopulmonary dysplasia. *Pediatrics* 1985;**75**:80.

Bancalari E, Stocker JT (editors): *Bronchopulmonary Dysplasia.* Hemisphere Publishing, 1988.

Gerhardt T et al: Serial determination of pulmonary function in infants with chronic lung disease. *J Pediatr* 1987;**110**:448.

Kao LC et al: Effects of oral diuretics on pulmonary mechanics in infants with BPD: Results of a double-blind cross-over sequential trial. *Pediatrics* 1984;**74**:37.

Koops BL et al: Outpatient management and follow-up of BPD. *Clin Perinatol* 1984;**11**:101.

Northway WH, Rosan RC, Porter DY: Pulmonary disease following respiratory therapy of hyaline membrane disease: Bronchopulmonary dysplasia. *N Engl J Med* 1967;**276**:357.

O'Brodovich HM, Mellins RM: Bronchopulmonary dysplasia. Unresolved neonatal acute lung injury. *Am Rev Respir Dis* 1985;**132**:694.

Smyth JA et al: Pulmonary function and bronchial hyperreactivity in long-term survivors of bronchopulmonary dysplasia. *Pediatrics* 1981;**68**:336.

Tepper RS et al: Expiratory flow-limitation in infants with bronchopulmonary dysplasia. *J Pediatr* 1986;**109**:1040.

CYSTIC FIBROSIS

Essentials of Diagnosis

- Sweat chloride greater than 70 mmol/L.
- Pulmonary, gastrointestinal, or hepatic dysfunction or injury.

General Considerations

Cystic fibrosis (CF) is the most common lethal genetic disease in the United States, with an incidence of 1:2000 whites. It is a major cause of pulmonary and gastrointestinal morbidity in children and a leading cause of death in early adulthood. Although CF causes abnormalities in the hepatic, gastrointestinal, and male reproductive systems, the lung disease is the major cause of morbidity and mortality. Almost all patients develop obstructive lung disease associated with chronic infection that leads to progressive loss of pulmonary function. The prognosis in CF has, however, improved dramatically and steadily over the past 20 years; the median survival is now 28 years. Use of antibiotics, better treatment of the concomitant malabsorption, and the development of a network of special CF care centers are possible explanations for the increased longevity. The CF centers usually employ a multidisciplinary approach to patient care with physicians, nurses, social workers, nutritionists, and physical or respiratory therapists experienced in the care of patients with CF. This network of centers is funded and reviewed by the Cystic Fibrosis Foundation, also a major driving force in basic and clinical research in CF.

Cystic fibrosis follows an autosomal recessive inheritance pattern. Restriction fragment length polymorphisms applied to large kindreds of patients with CF have demonstrated that the abnormal gene is located on the long arm of the seventh chromosome, but the exact location and the nature of the gene is not known. Patch clamp studies indicate that the basic defect is abnormal control of chloride channels, primarily in epithelial cells of mucosal surfaces. However, the precise cellular abnormality is also unknown. Clinically, the disease is expressed primarily in the exocrine glands. (See Addendum p 411.)

Clinical Findings & Treatment

A. Clinical Presentations and Diagnosis: Fifteen percent of infants with CF present at birth with an intestinal obstruction known as meconium ileus. Abdominal distention and the presence of a thick, sticky meconium throughout the large colon on meglumine diatrizoate (Gastrografin) enema examination suggest the diagnosis. In the past, surgical removal of the meconium often leading to resection of bowel was common. However, improved techniques of enema administration under radiologic observation have reduced the need for surgery.

Roughly half of patients with CF present classically in infancy with failure to thrive, respiratory compromise, or both. However, the age at presentation can be quite variable; some patients are not diagnosed until adulthood. Neonatal screening based on elevations of immunoreactive trypsinogen in the blood of infants with CF has recently received attention as an alternative method of case identification. Newborn screening has facilitated studies of early abnormalities in CF, but the long term benefits of early diagnosis are still uncertain.

Whether the clinical suspicion of CF is based on meconium ileus, failure to thrive, recurrent respiratory infections, or elevated immunoreactive trypsinogen in infancy, the diagnosis is made only after a positive sweat test. The sweat of individuals with CF contains elevated levels of chloride and sodium. Although elevated sweat electrolytes are associated with other conditions, a positive sweat test coupled with the clinical picture usually confirms the diagnosis. Laboratories routinely performing sweat tests give more reliable results than those that perform them only occasionally. The Gibson-Cooke quantitative technique is the only acceptable method. Measurements of electrical conductivity alone can be unreliable.

B. Gastrointestinal and Nutritional Findings and Treatment: Untreated patients with CF have abdominal distention and discomfort, large, bulky, greasy stools and increased flatulence secondary to exocrine pancreatic insufficiency and malabsorption. Some infants present with hypoalbuminemia, anemia, edema, and hepatomegaly. These infants with severe protein calorie malnutrition have particularly difficult courses, with a high rate of morbidity and mortality. Older patients with CF are subject to intestinal blockages from inspissated stool. This "meconium ileus equivalent" is now most often treated with cathartics and enemas and only rarely requires surgery. Patients with CF are more prone to intussuception (especially of the appendix) than are normal individuals.

The cornerstone of gastrointestinal treatment in CF is pancreatic enzyme supplementation. Patients are required to take the enzyme capsules with each meal and with snacks. Newer enzyme preparations contain more lipase per capsule than older preparations; therefore, patients take fewer capsules, making administration easier. Occasionally, enzyme supplementation alone does not control the malabsorption, and antacids are added to the regimen.

Individuals with CF may demonstrate abnormalities in nutritional status, including fat-soluble vitamin deficiency, hypoalbuminemia, and poor growth with decreased stores of body fat. In the past, fat-restricted diets were recommended. It is now recognized that patients with CF need all the calories they can take, and, therefore, unrestricted diets are now the norm in most centers. Moreover, caloric supplements, such as starches (eg, dextromaltose), medium-chain triglycerides, or high-calorie formulas, are often added to the patient's diet. In patients who do not respond to oral supplementation, nighttime nasogastric feeding or feeding by means of gastrostomy or jejunostomy has been tried. Although there is general agreement that quality of life is enhanced by improved nutrition, whether aggressive nutritional treatment increases longevity is unknown.

C. Pulmonary Findings and Treatment: Infants with CF frequently have respiratory compromise. Cough, tachypnea, rales, and wheezing are common findings. Respiratory syncytial virus infection is associated with marked morbidity in early infancy. Some patients develop cough only later in childhood or adolescence, but by adulthood almost all patients with CF have productive coughs. In more advanced disease, hemoptysis due to bronchiectasis, exercise limitation, and cor pulmonale may be present. Rales may be heard on physical exam. Clubbing also develops as the lung disease progresses.

Pulmonary function abnormalities initially show obstructive patterns with diminished flow rates and increased lung volumes. As the disease progresses, vital capacity is also affected. The incidence of airways reactivity in CF has been estimated at between 25 and 50%, several times the incidence in the general population. Initially, the airway is colonized with *Staphylococcus aureus,* but in most patients, *Pseudomonas aeruginosa* becomes predominant at some point. The acquisition of the characteristic mucoid *Pseudomonas* is associated with a more rapid decline in pulmonary function. In addition, infection with *Pseudomonas cepacia* has been associated with rapid deterioration and death. Pathologically, the earliest lesions involve hyperplasia of the mucous glands of the bronchial epithelium and mucosal and submucosal cellular infiltrates. Bronchiolectasis and bronchiectasis follow most often throughout all lung fields.

Treatment for the pulmonary disease in CF includes chest physical therapy, antibiotics, bronchodilators, and (more recently) anti-inflammatory agents. Each of these treatments is controversial. A recent study of postural drainage (PD) and percussion has demonstrated benefit over a 3-year period in those patients receiving the therapy compared to those patients not receiving it. This study has put the use of PD on firmer ground. Although controlled trials have yielded ambiguous results, there is general agreement that antibiotics play a major role in pulmonary treatment. Antibiotics are used liberally in outpatient treatment (eg, with a change in cough or respiratory symptoms) and are used extensively during inpatient admissions. Recent studies have suggested a benefit from inhaled antibiotics. The high incidence of airways reactivity suggests an important treatment role for bronchodilators, yet some studies have shown paradoxical responses to these medications. The paradoxical responses may be related in part to the fact that the increasing compliance of large airways leads to earlier airway closure.

Current speculation on the development of lung disease in CF includes not only the effects of the bacterial pathogens but also the host response to such pathogens. If activated neutrophils or immune complexes are important in the genesis of the airway injury, then anti-inflammatory agents may be helpful. There is one study suggesting clinical benefit from long-term alternate-day steroid treatment. A large multicenter trial funded by the Cystic Fibrosis Foundation to evaluate steroid therapy further is currently underway.

A subgroup of patients with CF have frequent pulmonary exacerbations characterized by difficult breathing, increased sputum production, decreased exercise tolerance, and diminished pulmonary function. These patients often benefit from hospital treatments including intensive physical therapy, intravenous antibiotics, bronchodilators, and concentrated efforts at nutritional rehabilitation. The length of hospitalization is determined by following the improvement in pulmonary function; discharge is planned once the pulmonary functions have plateaued. Increasingly, outpatient intravenous therapy is being used to shorten the duration of hospitalization.

D. Hepatic Disease: Although the majority of patients with CF at autopsy demonstrate cirrhosis, only a small percentage develops portal hypertension. In these individuals, however, the clinical manifestations of the liver disease may be severe, with esophageal varices leading to life-threatening gastrointestinal bleeding and hypersplenism requiring splenic embolization.

E. Reproductive Tract Involvement: More than

95% of males with CF are infertile, a condition secondary to the failure of wolffian tract structures such as the vas deferens to develop. CF is occasionally diagnosed through infertility evaluations in adult males with relatively mild involvement of the respiratory and gastrointestinal tracts. In general, females with CF are fertile, but pregnancy may place considerable stress on patients with limited pulmonary function.

Prognosis

The rate of progression of lung involvement determines length of survival in the majority of patients with CF. Most patients now survive into adulthood. Recent reports of successful lung transplantation in patients with CF have been encouraging.

Davis PA, di Sant'Agnese PA: Diagnosis and treatment of cystic fibrosis: An update. *Chest* 1984;**85**:802.

Doring G, Albus AM, Hoiby N: Immunologic aspects of cystic fibrosis. *Chest* 1988;**94(Suppl 2)**:109S.

Lloyd-Still JD: *Textbook of Cystic Fibrosis.* Hohn Wright-PSG Inc, 1983.

Reardon MC et al: Nutritional deficits exist before 2 months of age in some infants with cystic fibrosis identified by screening test. *J Pediatr* 1984;**105**:271.

Redding G et al: Serial changes in pulmonary function in children hospitalized with cystic fibrosis. *Am Rev Respir Dis* 1982;**126**:31.

Scott J et al: Heart-lung transplantation for cystic fibrosis. *Lancet* 1988;**2**:192.

Taussig LM: *Cystic Fibrosis.* Thieme-Stratton, 1984.

Wang EEL et al: Association of respiratory viral infections with pulmonary deterioration in patients with cystic fibrosis. *N Engl J Med* 1984;**311**:1653.

CONGENITAL DISEASES INVOLVING ALVEOLI

The clinical spectrum of congenital lung disorders can vary widely, ranging from severe, life-threatening respiratory distress in the neonate (which typically occurs with cystic adenomatoid malformation and most cases of congenital lobar emphysema) to chronic cough, wheezing, or stridor in the older child (with bronchogenic cyst, for example) to incidental radiologic findings in patients with very mild symptoms. The following is a limited discussion of selected congenital structural lesions that involve or compromise alveoli.

PULMONARY AGENESIS & HYPOPLASIA

General Considerations

Pulmonary agenesis or hypoplasia represents absent or incomplete lung development, which generally reflects an intrauterine interruption or alteration of the normal sequence of embryologic events, and may be associated with other congenital abnormalities. With unilateral pulmonary agenesis (the complete absence of one lung), the trachea continues into a main bronchus and often has complete tracheal rings. The left lung is affected more often than the right. With compensatory postnatal growth over time, the remaining lung often herniates into the contralateral chest. Chest x-ray study shows a mediastinal shift toward the affected side, and vertebral abnormalities may be present. The outcome is primarily related to the severity of associated congenital lesions. About 50% of patients survive; the mortality is higher in those with agenesis of the right lung than in those with agenesis of the left lung. This difference is probably not related to the greater incidence of associated anomalies but rather may be due to a greater shift in the mediastinum that leads to tracheal compression and distortion.

Hypoplasia is the incomplete development of the lung, resulting in the reduction of the number of bronchial branchings or a decrease in expected lung weight, volume, or DNA content. It is part of a spectrum with a gradual transition. Pulmonary hypoplasia may be present in up to 10–15% of perinatal autopsies. The pathogenesis of hypoplasia is multifactorial and includes the presence of an intrathoracic mass, resulting in lack of space for the lungs to grow, decreased size of the thorax, decreased fetal breathing movements, decreased blood flow to the lungs, or possibly a primary mesodermal defect affecting multiple organ systems. Congenital diaphragmatic hernia is the most common cause of pulmonary hypoplasia, with an incidence of 1:2200 births. Other causes include extralobar sequestration, diaphragmatic eventration or hypoplasia, thoracic neuroblastoma, fetal hydrops, and fetal hydrochylothorax. Chest cage abnormalities, diaphragmatic elevation, oligohydramnios, chromosomal abnormalities, severe musculoskeletal disorders, and cardiac lesions also may lead to hypoplastic lungs. In addition, postnatal factors may play important roles; for example, infants with advanced BPD can have pulmonary hypoplasia.

Clinical Findings

A. Symptoms and Signs: The clinical presentation is highly variable and is related to the severity of hypoplasia as well as associated abnormalities. Frequently, lung hypoplasia is associated with pneumothorax. Some newborns present with perinatal stress, severe acute respiratory distress, and persistent pulmonary hypertension of the newborn secondary to primary pulmonary hypoplasia (without associated anomalies). Children with milder degrees of hypoplasia may present with chronic cough, tachypnea, wheezing, and recurrent pneumonia.

B. Laboratory Findings and Imaging: Chest x-ray findings include variable degrees of volume loss in a small hemithorax with mediastinal shift. Ventilation-perfusion scans, angiography, and bronchoscopy are often helpful in the clinical evaluation. The degree of respiratory impairment is defined by an analysis of arterial blood gases.

Treatment & Prognosis

Treatment is primarily supportive and directed at the symptoms produced by the hypoplastic lung. The overall outcome is determined by the severity of underlying medical problems and the extent of the hypoplasia.

Askenazi SS, Perlman M: Pulmonary hypoplasia: Lung weight and radial alveolar count as criteria of diagnosis. *Arch Dis Child* 1979;**54**:614.

Langston C, Thurlbeck WM: Conditions altering normal lung growth and development. In: *Neonatal Pulmonary Care*. Thibeault DW, Gregory GA (editors). Appleton-Century-Crofts, 1986.

Stocker JT et al: Cystic and congenital lung disease in the newborn. In: *Perspectives in Pediatric Pathology*. Vol 4. Rosenberg H, Bolande T (editors). Yearbook, 1978.

PULMONARY SEQUESTRATION

Pulmonary sequestration is a localized mass of disorganized growth that is classified as either extralobar or intralobar. Extralobar sequestration (ELS) is a mass of pulmonary parenchyma anatomically separate from the normal lung, with a distinct pleural investment. Its blood supply derives from either the systemic circulation (more typical), pulmonary vessels, or both. Although it can rarely communicate with the esophagus or stomach, it does not communicate directly with the tracheobronchial tree. Pathologically, ELS appears as a solitary thoracic lesion near the diaphragm. Abdominal sites are rare. Size varies between 0.5 and 12 cm. Histologic findings include uniformly dilatated bronchioles, alveolar ducts, and alveoli. Occasionally, the bronchial structure appears normal; often, however, the cartilage in the wall is deficient, or no cartilage-containing structures can be found. On occasion, lymphangiectasia is found within the lesion. ELS can be associated with other anomalies, including bronchogenic cysts, heart defects, and diaphragmatic hernia.

Intralobar sequestration (ILS) is an isolated segment of lung within the normal pleural investment but without connection to the tracheobronchial tree. The arterial supply is often provided by one or more arteries arising from the aorta or its branches. ILS is usually found within the lower lobes (98%) and is rarely associated with other congenital anomalies (less than 2% versus 50% with ELS). ILS is rarely seen in the newborn period (unlike ELS). Some have hypothesized that ILS is an acquired lesion secondary to chronic infection. Clinical presentation includes chronic cough, wheezing or "recurrent pneumonias." Rarely, ILS can present with hemoptysis. Treatment is by surgical resection.

Alivizatos P et al: Pulmonary sequestration complicated by anomalies of pulmonary venous return. *J Pediatr Surg* 1985;**20**:76.

Savic B et al: Lung sequestrations: Report of 7 cases and review of 540 published cases. *Thorax* 1979;**34**:96.

CONGENITAL LOBAR EMPHYSEMA

General Considerations

Congenital lobar emphysema (also known as infantile lobar emphysema, congenital localized emphysema, unilobar obstructive emphysema, or congenital hypertrophic lobar emphysema) presents in most patients as severe neonatal repiratory distress or as progressive respiratory impairment during the first year of life. Rarely, the mild or intermittent nature of the symptoms in older children or young adults results in a delayed diagnosis. Most patients are white males. Although the cause of congenital lobar emphysema is not well understood, some lesions exhibit bronchial cartilaginous dysplasia due to abnormal orientation or distribution of the bronchial cartilage. This leads to expiratory collapse, producing obstruction and the symptoms outlined below.

Clinical Findings

A. Symptoms and Signs: Clinical features include tachypnea, cyanosis, wheezing, retractions, and cough. Physical exam reveals decreased breath sounds on the affected side, perhaps with hyperresonance to percussion, mediastinal displacement, and bulging of the chest wall on the affected side.

B. Imaging: Radiologic findings include overdistention of the affected lobe, with wide separation of bronchovascular markings, collapse of adjacent lung, shift of the mediastinum away from the affected side, and a depressed diaphragm on the affected side. Other diagnostic studies include chest x-ray with fluoroscopy, ventilation-perfusion study, and perhaps CT scan followed by bronchoscopy with or without bronchography, angiography, and exploratory thoracotomy.

Differential Diagnosis

The differential diagnosis of congenital lobar emphysema includes pneumothorax, pneumatocele, atelectasis with compensatory hyperinflation, diaphragmatic hernia, and congenital cystic adenomatoid malformation. The most common site of involvement is the left upper lobe (42%) or right middle lobe (35%). Evaluation must differentiate regional obstructive emphysema from lobar hyperinflation secondary to an uncomplicated ball-valve mechanism due to extrinsic compression from a mass (bronchogenic cyst, tumor, lymphadenopathy, foreign body, "pseudotumor" or plasma cell granuloma, vascular compression, etc) or intrinsic obstruction from a mucus plug due to infection and inflammation from various causes.

Treatment

Management generally involves surgery, especially when respiratory distress is marked, with either segmental or complete lobectomy. Conservative management in less symptomatic, older children may lead to an outcome not different from those treated surgically with lobectomy.

Eigen H et al: Congenital lobar emphysema: Long-term evaluation of surgically and conservatively treated children. *Am Rev Respir Dis* 1976;**113**:823.

Luck SR et al: Congenital bronchopulmonary malformations. *Curr Probl Surg* (April) 1986;**23**:245.

Man DWK et al: Congenital lobar emphysema: Problems in diagnosis and management. *Arch Dis Child* 1983; **58**:709.

McBride JT et al: Lung growth and airway function after lobectomy in infancy for congenital lobar emphysema. *J Clin Invest* 1980;**66**:962.

Michelson E: Clinical spectrum of infantile lobar emphysema. *Ann Thorac Surg* 1977;**24**:182.

CONGENITAL CYSTIC ADENOMATOID MALFORMATION

General Considerations

Congenital cystic adenomatoid malformations (CCAM) are unilateral, hamartomatous lesions that generally present as marked respiratory distress within the first days of life. CCAM accounts for most cases of congenital cystic lung disease (95%). Right and left lungs are involved with equal frequency. These lesions appear as glandlike, space-occupying masses or with an "adenomatoid" increase in terminal respiratory structures, forming intercommunicating cysts of various sizes, lined by cuboidal or ciliated pseudostratified columnar epithelium. They may have polypoid formations of mucosa, with focally increased elastic tissue in the cyst wall beneath the bronchial type of epithelium. Air passages appear malformed and tend to lack cartilage.

There are 3 types of CCAM. Type 1 consists of single or multiple large (1–5 cm in diameter) cysts with features of mature lung tissue. Type 1 is most common (75%) and is amenable to surgical resection. A mediastinal shift is evident on exam or chest x-ray film in 80% of patients and can mimic infantile lobar emphysema. Approximately 75% of type 1 lesions are right-sided. A survival rate of 90% is generally reported. Type 2 lesions represent 20% of patients with CCAM. These consist of multiple small (0.5–1.5 cm) cysts resembling dilatated simple

bronchioles and are often associated with other anomalies (60%), especially renal agenesis or dysgenesis, cardiac malformations, and intestinal atresia. Approximately 60% of type 2 lesions are on the left side. Mediastinal shift is evident less often than in type 1 (10%), and the survival rate is worse (40%). Type 3 lesions are the rarest (only 5% of CCAM) and consist of small cysts (less than 0.5 cm). They appear as a bulky, firm mass. The survival rate is reported at 50%.

Clinical Findings

A. Symptoms and Signs: Clinically, respiratory distress is noted soon after birth. Expansion of the cysts occurs with the onset of breathing and produces compression of normal lung areas with mediastinal herniation. Breath sounds are decreased. With type 3 lesions, dullness to percussion may be present.

B. Imaging: The chest x-ray film of type 1 CCAM shows an intrapulmonary mass of soft-tissue density with scattered radiolucent areas of varying sizes and shapes, usually with a mediastinal shift and pulmonary herniation. Placement of a radiopaque feeding tube into the stomach helps differentiate CCAM from diaphragmatic hernia. Type 2 lesions appear similar, with the exception that the cysts are smaller. Type 3 CCAM may appear as a solid homogeneous mass filling the hemithorax and causing a marked mediastinal shift.

Treatment

Treatment of types 1 and 3 is surgical removal of the affected lobe. Because type 2 CCAM is often associated with other severe anomalies, management may be more complex. Unlike congenital lobar emphysema, segmental resection is not a possibility because smaller cysts may expand after removal of the more obviously affected area.

Adzick NS, Harrison MR, Glick PC: Fetal cystic adenomatoid malformation: Prenatal diagnosis and natural history. *J Pediatr Surg* 1985;**20**:483.

Stocker JT, Madewell JE, Drake RM: Congenital cystic adenomatoid malformation of the lungs: Classification and morphologic spectrum. *Hum Pathol* 1977;**8**:155.

ACQUIRED DISORDERS INVOLVING ALVEOLI

BACTERIAL PNEUMONIA

Essentials of Diagnosis

- Fever of acute onset.
- Respiratory signs: cough, dyspnea, tachypnea, grunting, or retractions.

■ Abnormal chest examination (rales or decreased breath sounds) or abnormal chest radiograph.

General Considerations

Bacterial pneumonia is an inflammation of the lung categorized by the bacterial pathogen causing the disease. It usually develops when one or more of the defense mechanisms normally protecting the lung is inadequate. Patients with the following problems are particularly predisposed to this disease: aspiration, immunodeficiency or immunosuppression, congenital anomalies (intrapulmonary sequestration, tracheoesophageal fistula, cleft palate), abnormalities in mucus clearance (cystic fibrosis, ciliary dysfunction, tracheomalacia, bronchiectasis), congestive heart failure, and perinatal contamination.

Clinical Findings

A. Symptoms and Signs: The bacterial pathogen, severity of disease, and age of the patient may cause substantial variations in the presenting manifestations of acute bacterial pneumonia. Infants may manifest few or nonspecific findings on history and physical examination. Immunocompetent older patients may not be extremely ill. Some patients may present only with fever or signs of generalized toxicity. Others may have additional symptoms or signs of (1) lower respiratory tract disease (evidence of respiratory distress, cough, sputum production), (2) pneumonia (rales, decreased breath sounds, dullness to percussion, abnormal tactile or vocal fremitus), or (3) pleural involvement (splinting, pain, friction rub, dullness to percussion). Some patients may manifest additional extrapulmonary findings, such as meningismus or abdominal pain, due to pneumonia itself. Others may have evidence of infection at other sites due to the same organism causing their pneumonia: meningitis, otitis media, sinusitis, pericarditis, epiglottitis, or abscesses.

B. Laboratory Findings: Elevated white blood cell counts ($> 15,000/\mu L$) frequently accompany bacterial pneumonia. However, a low white blood count ($> 5000/\mu L$) can be an ominous finding in this disease.

C. Imaging: Chest radiographic findings (lateral and frontal views) define bacterial pneumonia. Patchy infiltrates, atelectasis, hilar adenopathy, or pleural effusion may be observed. Films in the lateral decubitus position should be taken to identify pleural fluid. Complete lobar consolidation is not a common finding in infants and children. Disease in infants may not correlate with radiographic findings. Clinical resolution precedes resolution by chest x-ray.

D. Special Examinations: Invasive diagnostic procedures (transtracheal aspiration, bronchial brushing or washing, lung puncture, or open biopsy) should be undertaken in critically ill patients when other means do not adequately define etiology (see Culture of Material from the Respiratory Tract).

Differential Diagnosis

The differential diagnosis of bacterial pneumonia also varies with the age and immunocompetence of the host. The full spectrum of potential pathogens that includes aerobic and anaerobic bacteria, acid-fast bacteria including tuberculosis, Chlamydia *(trachomatis* and *psittaci), Rickettsia* (Q fever), *Pneumocystis carinii, Bordetella pertussis, Mycoplasma pneumoniae,* and respiratory viruses needs to be considered in each host.

Noninfectious pulmonary disease (including gastric aspiration, foreign body aspiration, atelectasis, congenital malformations, congestive heart failure, malignant growths, tumors such as plasma cell granuloma, chronic interstitial lung diseases, and pulmonary hemosiderosis) should be considered in the differential diagnosis of localized or diffuse infiltrates. When effusions are present, additional noninfectious disorders such as collagen diseases, neoplasm, and pulmonary infarction should also be considered.

Complications

Empyema may occur frequently with staphylococcal and group A β-hemolytic streptococcal disease. Pneumococcal effusions have a more benign course. Distal sites of infection—meningitis, otitis media, sinusitis (especially of the ethmoids) and septicemia—may be present, particularly with disease due to *Streptococcus pneumoniae* or *Haemophilus influenzae.* Certain immunocompromised patients, such as those who have undergone splenectomy or who have hemoglobin SS or SC disease or thalassemia, are especially prone to overwhelming sepsis with these organisms. Distal infection of the bones, joints, or other organs (eg, liver abcess) may occur in certain hosts with specific organisms.

Treatment

Appropriate antimicrobial therapy varies according to which organisms are the likely cause of the bacterial pneumonia. Treatment should be guided by (1) Gram stain of sputum, tracheobronchial secretions, or pleural fluid if available; (2) radiographic findings; and (3) age and known or suspected immunocompetence of the host. For initial coverage in a patient with an unknown pathogen, the physician should consider (1) appropriate penicillins or cephalosporins (or both) to cover gram-positive organisms including *Staphylococcus aureus;* (2) an aminoglycoside to cover gram-negative enteric organisms (especially in the newborn or immunocompromised host); (3) suitable coverage for *H influenzae* in patients at risk; and (4) erythromycin to cover *M pneumoniae, L pneumophila, Chlamydia,* and *Ureaplasma.* Therapy is also guided by results of studies for bacterial and viral pathogens (see Culture of Material from the Respiratory Tract) and is based on other diagnostic studies (see below).

Additional therapeutic considerations include (1) oxygen, (2) humidification of inspired gases, (3) hydration and electrolyte supplementation, (4) oral hygiene, and (5) nutrition. Removal of pleural fluid for diagnostic purposes is indicated initially to guide antimicrobial therapy. Many feel that early chest tube drainage of empyema fluid due to *S aureus* is indicated. Empyema due to group A β-hemolytic streptococcus or *H influenzae* may also necessitate chest tube drainage, whereas pleural effusions due to *S pneumoniae* rarely do. Repeated pleural taps should be considered in the patient who has persistent high fever for more than 10 days in association with significant pleural effusion(s). The persistence of organisms in this fluid or the persistence of toxicity, malaise, anorexia, and wasting in the patient suggests the potential need for pleural decortication.

Endotracheal intubation or mechanical ventilation may be indicated in patients with respiratory failure or those too debilitated or overwhelmed to handle their secretions.

Prognosis

For the immunocompetent host in whom bacterial pneumonia is adequately recognized and treated, survival is high. For example, mortality from uncomplicated pneumococcal pneumonia is less than 1%. If the patient survives the initial illness, persistently abnormal pulmonary function following empyema is surprisingly uncommon, even when therapies are delayed or inappropriate.

Bromberg K, Hammerschlag MR: Rapid diagnosis of pneumonia in children. *Semin Respir Infect* 1987;**2**:159.
Long SS: Treatment of acute pneumonia in infants and children. *Pediatr Clin North Am* 1983;**30**:297.
Peter G: The child with pneumonia: Diagnostic and therapeutic considerations. *Pediatr Infect Dis J* 1988;**7**:453.
Timmons OD et al: Association of respiratory syncytial virus and *Streptococcus pneumoniae* infection in young infants. *Pediatr Infect Dis J* 1987;**6**:1134.
Wald ER: Management of pneumonia in outpatients. *Pediatr Infect Dis J* 1984;**3**(**Suppl 3**):S21.

VIRAL PNEUMONIA

Essentials of Diagnosis

- Upper respiratory infection prodrome (fever, coryza, cough, hoarseness).
- Wheezing or rales.
- Myalgia, malaise, headache (older children).

General Considerations

Viral pneumonia constitutes the vast majority of pediatric pulmonary infections. Respiratory syncytial virus (RSV), parainfluenza (1, 2, and 3) viruses, and influenza (A and B) viruses are responsible for more than 75% of the infections. Neither severity of disease or fever, radiographic findings, nor characteristics of cough or lung sounds reliably differentiate viral from bacterial pneumonias. Substantial pleural effusions, pneumatoceles, abscesses, lobar consolidation with lobar volume expansion, and "round" pneumonias are generally inconsistent with viral disease.

Clinical Findings

A. Symptoms and Signs: An upper respiratory infection frequently precedes the onset of lower respiratory disease due to viruses. Although wheezing or stridor may be prominent in viral disease, cough, signs of respiratory difficulty (retractions, grunting, nasal flaring) and physical findings (rales, decreased breath sounds) may not be distinguishable from those in bacterial pneumonia.

B. Laboratory Findings: The peripheral white blood cell count may be normal or slightly elevated and is not useful in distinguishing viral from bacterial disease. A markedly elevated white count, however, indicates that viral disease is less likely.

Rapid viral diagnostic tests, such as fluorescent antibody (FA) tests or ELISA for RSV, are increasingly available and should be performed to confirm this diagnosis in high-risk patients and for purposes of epidemiology or infection control. Rapid diagnosis of RSV does not preclude the possibility of concomitant infection with additional pathogens.

C. Imaging: Chest radiographs frequently show perihilar streaking, increased interstitial markings, peribronchial cuffing, or patchy bronchopneumonia. However, lobar consolidation, as in bacterial pneumonia, may occur. Patients with adenovirus disease may have severe necrotizing pneumonias, resulting in the development of pneumatoceles. Hyperinflation of the lungs may occur when small airways involvement is prominent.

Differential Diagnosis

Considerations for the differential diagnosis of viral pneumonia are the same as those for bacterial pneumonia. In patients in whom wheezing is a prominent feature, the physician should consider asthma, airways obstruction due to foreign body aspiration, acute bacterial or viral tracheitis, and parasitic disease.

Complications

Bronchiolitis obliterans or severe chronic respiratory failure may follow adenovirus pneumonia. Bronchiolitis or viral pneumonia may contribute to persistent reactive airways disease in some patients. Bronchiectasis, persistent interstitial lung diseases (fibrosis and desquamative interstitial pneumonitis), and unilateral hyperlucent lung (Swyer-James syndrome) may follow measles, adenovirus, and influenza pneumonias. Viral pneumonia or laryngotracheobronchitis may predispose the patient to subsequent bacterial tracheitis or pneumonia as immediate sequelae. Plasma cell granuloma may develop as a rare sequela of viral or bacterial pneumonia.

Treatment

General supportive care for viral pneumonia does not differ from that for bacterial pneumonia. Patients can be quite ill and should be hospitalized according to the level of their illness. Because bacterial disease frequently cannot be definitively excluded, appropriate concomitant antibiotic coverage is often indicated.

Patients at risk for life-threatening RSV infections, such as those with bronchopulmonary dysplasia (BPD) or other severe pulmonary conditions, congenital heart disease, or significant immunocompromise, should be hospitalized and treated with ribavirin. Rapid viral diagnostic tests may be a useful guide for such therapy. These high-risk patients should be immunized annually against influenza A and B viruses. Despite immunization, however, influenza infection can still occur. When available epidemiologic data indicate an active influenza A infection in the community, amantadine hydrochloride should be considered early in treating high-risk infants and children who appear to be infected.

Children with suspected viral pneumonia should be placed in respiratory isolation, and careful attention should be given to good handwashing practices.

Prognosis

Although most children with viral pneumonia recover uneventfully, worsening reactive airways disease, abnormal pulmonary function or chest radiographs, persistent respiratory insufficiency, and even death may occur in high-risk patients such as newborns or those with underlying lung, cardiac, or immunodeficiency disease. Patients with adenovirus infection or those concomitantly infected with RSV and second pathogens such as influenza, adenovirus, cytomegalovirus or *Pneumocystis carinii* also have a poorer prognosis.

Brasfield DM et al: Infant pneumonitis associated with cytomegalovirus, *Chlamydia, Pneumocystis,* and *Ureaplasma:* Follow-up. *Pediatrics* 1987;**79**:76.

Glezen WP: Viral pneumonia as a cause and result of hospitalization. *J Infect Dis* 1983;**147**:765.

Hall CB: Hospital-acquired pneumonia in children: The role of respiratory viruses. *Semin Respir Infect* 1987; **2**:48.

Khamapirad T, Glezen WP: Clinical and radiographic assessment of acute lower respiratory tract disease in infants and children. *Semin Respir Infect* 1987;**2**:130.

Tristram DA et al: Simultaneous infection with respiratory syncytial virus and other respiratory pathogens. *Am J Dis Child* 1988;**142**:834.

CHLAMYDIAL PNEUMONIA

Essentials of Diagnosis

- Cough, tachypnea, rales, few wheezes, and no fever (most patients).
- Appropriate age: 2–12 weeks.
- With or without inclusion conjunctivitis.
- With or without peripheral eosinophilia.
- Elevated immunoglobulins: IgM > IgG >> IgA.

General Considerations

Disease due to *Chlamydia trachomatis* usually evolves gradually as the infection descends the respiratory tract. Infants may appear quite well despite the presence of significant pulmonary illness. Infant infections are now at epidemic proportions in urban environments worldwide. Other sexually transmitted organisms, such as *Ureaplasma urealyticum* may also be widespread and contribute to lung disease in infants. Unlike bacteria, the chlamydiae are unable to synthesize their own ATP and are sometimes called "energy parasites."

Clinical Findings

A. Symptoms and Signs: About half of patients with chlamydial pneumonia have active inclusion conjunctivitis or a history of it. A rhinopharyngitis with nasal discharge or otitis media may have occurred or be present. Female patients may have vulvovaginitis.

Cough is usually present. It can have a staccato character and resemble that accompanying pertussis. The infant is usually tachypneic. Scattered inspiratory rales are commonly heard; wheezes are rarely present. Significant fever suggests another or additional diagnosis.

B. Laboratory Findings: Although patients may frequently be hypoxemic, CO_2 retention is not common. Absolute peripheral blood eosinophilia (> 400 cells/μL) has been observed in about 75% of patients. Serum immunoglobulins are usually abnormal. IgM is virtually always elevated, IgG is high in many, and IgA is less frequently abnormal.

C. Imaging: Chest radiographs may reveal diffuse interstitial and patchy alveolar infiltrates, peribronchial thickening, or focal consolidation. A small pleural reaction can be present. Despite the usual absence of wheezes, hyperexpansion is commonly present. *C trachomatis* can usually be identified in nasopharyngeal washings employing a fluorescent antibody (FA) or culture techniques.

Differential Diagnosis

Bacterial, viral, and parasitic (*P carinii*) pneumonias should be considered. Premature infants and those with BPD may also have chlamydial or associated pneumonias.

Treatment

Erythromycin or sulfisoxazole therapy should be administered for 14 days. Hospitalization may be required for infants with significant respiratory distress, coughing paroxysms, or posttussive apnea. Oxygen therapy may be required for prolonged periods in some patients.

Prognosis

An increased incidence of obstructive airways disease and abnormal pulmonary function tests may occur for at least 7–8 years following the initial infection.

Brayden RM et al: Apnea in infants with *Chlamydia trachomatis* pneumonia. *Pediatr Infect Dis J* 1987; **6:**423.

Hammerschlag MR et al: Comparison of enzyme immunoassay and culture for diagnosis of chlamydial conjunctivitis and respiratory infections in infants. *J Clin Microbiol* 1987;**25:**2306.

Paisley JW et al: Rapid diagnosis of *Chlamydia trachomatis* pneumonia in infants by direct immunofluorescence microscopy of nasopharyngeal secretions. *J Pediatr* 1986;**109:**653.

Rettig PJ: Chlamydial infections in pediatrics: Diagnostic and therapeutic considerations. *Pediatr Infect Dis J* 1986;**5:**158.

Weiss et al: Pulmonary assessment of children after chlamydial pneumonia of infancy. *J Pediatr* 1986;**108:** 659.

MYCOPLASMAL PNEUMONIA

Essentials of Diagnosis

- Fever (usually > 39 °C).
- Cough.
- Appropriate age: over 5 years old.

General Considerations

Mycoplasma pneumoniae is a common cause of symptomatic pneumonia in older children. Endemic and epidemic infection can occur. The incubation period is long (2–3 weeks), and onset of symptoms is slow. Although the lung is the primary infection site, a variety of extrapulmonary complications can arise.

Clinical Findings

A. Symptoms and Signs: Fever, cough, headache, and malaise are common symptoms as the illness evolves. Although cough is usually dry at the onset, sputum production may develop as the illness progresses. Sore throat, otitis media, otitis externa, and bullous myringitis may occur. Rales are frequently present on chest examination; decreased breath sounds or dullness to percussion over the involved area may be present.

B. Laboratory Findings: The peripheral blood leukocyte count and differential white blood cell count are usually normal. The cold hemagglutinin titer should be determined, because it may be elevated during the acute presentation. A titer greater than or equal to 1:64 supports the diagnosis. Acute and convalescent titers for *M pneumoniae* demonstrating a 4-fold or greater rise in specific antibodies confirm the diagnosis.

C. Imaging: Chest radiographs usually demonstrate interstitial or bronchopneumonic infiltrates, frequently in the middle or lower lobes. Pleural effusions are extremely uncommon.

Complications

Extrapulmonary involvement of the blood, central nervous system, skin, heart, or joints can occur. Direct Coombs'-positive autoimmune hemolytic anemia, occasionally a life-threatening disorder, is the most common hematologic abnormality that can accompany *M pneumoniae* infection. Coagulation defects and thrombocytopenia can also occur. Cerebral infarction, meningoencephalitis, Guillian-Barré syndrome, cranial nerve involvement, and psychosis all have been described. A wide variety of skin rashes, including erythema multiforme and Stevens-Johnson syndrome, can occur. Myocarditis, pericarditis, and a rheumatic fever-like illness can occur.

Treatment

Antibiotic therapy with erythromycin for 7–10 days usually shortens the course of illness. Supportive measures, including hydration, antipyretics, and bed rest, are helpful.

Prognosis

In the absence of the less common extrapulmonary complications, the outlook for recovery is excellent. However, the extent to which *M pneumoniae* can initiate or exacerbate chronic lung disease is not well understood.

Broughton RA: Infections due to *Mycoplasma pneumoniae* in childhood. *Pediatr Infect Dis J* 1986;**5:**71.

Isles AF et al: Obliterative bronchiolitis due to *Mycoplasma pneumoniae* infection in a child. *Pediatr Radiol* 1987;**17:**109.

Leigh MW, Clyde WA Jr: Chlamydial and mycoplasmal pneumonias. *Semin Respir Infect* 1987;**2:**152.

McCracken GH Jr: Current status of antibiotic treatment for *Mycoplasma pneumoniae* infections. *Pediatr Infect Dis J* 1986;**5:**167.

TUBERCULOSIS

Essentials of Diagnosis

- Positive tuberculin skin test *or* anergic host.
- Positive culture for *Mycobacterium tuberculosis*.
- With or without history of contact.

General Considerations

The clinical spectrum of pulmonary infection with tuberculosis includes a positive tuberculin skin test without evident disease, asymptomatic primary infection, the Ghon complex, bronchial obstruction with secondary collapse or obstructed airways, segmental lesions, calcified nodules, pleural effusions, progressive primary cavitating lesions, contiguous spread into adjacent thoracic structures, acute miliary tuberculosis, adult respiratory distress syndrome (ARDS), overwhelming reactivation infection in the immunocompromised host, occult lymphohematogenous spread, and metastatic extrapulmonary involvement at almost any site.

Clinical Findings

A. Symptoms and Signs: The most important aspect of the history is that of contact with an individual with tuberculosis. Frequently, this contact may be made through an elderly grandparent, a caretaker, or a person previously residing in a region with endemic tuberculosis or by travel of the patients themselves to such an area. In suspected cases, the patient, immediate family, and suspected carrier(s) of the disease should be tuberculin tested. The route of contagion is through inhalation. Thus, isolated pulmonary parenchymal tuberculosis constitutes more than 95% of presenting cases. The primary focus, which is usually single, and the nodal involvement may or may not be radiographically visible. Because healing, rather than progression, is the usual course in the uncompromised host, a positive tuberculin test may be the only manifestation of disease.

The tuberculous complications listed above most often occur during the first year of infection. Thereafter, infection remains quiescent until adolescence, when reactivation of pulmonary tuberculosis is common. At any stage, chronic cough, anorexia, weight loss or failure to gain weight, or fever are useful clinical signs if present. Except in cases with complications or advanced disease, physical findings are few.

B. Laboratory Findings: A positive tuberculin skin test is defined as 10 mm or more of induration 48–72 hours after *intradermal* injection of 5 tuberculin units (TU) of PPD. Appropriate control skin tests, such as those for hypersensitivity to diphtheria/tetanus, mumps, *Candida albicans,* or dermatophyton/trichophyton, should be applied at the same time the PPD is applied. If the patient fails to respond to PPD and all of the controls, the possibility of tuberculosis is not excluded.

Chest radiographs, both anteroposterior and lateral views, should be obtained in all suspected cases. Culture for *M tuberculosis* is critical for proving the diagnosis and for defining drug susceptibility. Early-morning gastric lavage following an overnight fast should be performed on 3 occasions in infants and children with suspected active pulmonary tuberculosis prior to the onset of drug therapy when the severity of illness allows. Although stains for acid-fast bacilli on this material are of little value, this is the ideal culture site.

Sputum cultures from older children and adolescents are similarly useful. Stains and cultures of bronchial secretions are useful if bronchoscopy is performed in the patient's evaluation. When pleural effusions are present, pleural biopsy for cultures and histopathologic examination for granulomas or organisms most consistently provide diagnostic information. Meningeal involvement is a real possibility in young children, and lumbar puncture should be considered in their initial evaluation.

Differential Diagnosis

Fungal diseases that primarily affect the lungs such as histoplasmosis, coccidiomycosis, cryptococcosis, and North American blastomycosis may resemble tuberculosis and should be excluded by appropriate serologic studies if the diagnosis is uncertain. Atypical tuberculous organisms may involve the lungs, especially in the immunocompromised patient. Depending on the presentation, diagnoses such as lymphoreticular and other malignancies, collagen-vascular disorders, or other pulmonary infections may be considered.

Complications

In addition to those listed above (see General Considerations), lymphadenitis, meningitis, osteomyelitis, arthritis, enteritis, peritonitis, and renal, ocular, middle ear, and cutaneous disease may occur. The infant born to tuberculous parent(s) is at great risk for developing illness. The possibility of life-threatening airway compromise must always be considered in patients with large mediastinal/hilar lesions.

Treatment

Because the risk of hepatitis due to isoniazid is extremely low in children, this drug is indicated in patients with inactive primary tuberculosis or children with a positive tuberculin skin test who have not received BCG vaccination. This greatly reduces the risk of subsequent active disease and complications with minimal morbidity. Isoniazid plus rifampin is commonly used in active pulmonary disease. Additional drugs that may be used include ethambutol hydrochloride, streptomycin, and ethionamide. In general, the more severe tuberculous complications are treated with a larger number of drugs. Recommendations for antituberculous chemotherapy, based on disease stage, are continuously being updated. The most current edition of *The Red Book* of the American Academy of Pediatrics is a reliable source for these protocols.

Corticosteroids are used to control inflammation

in selected patients with (1) potentially life-threatening airway compression by lymph nodes, (2) acute pericardial effusion, (3) massive pleural effusion with mediastinal shift, and, possibly, (4) miliary tuberculosis with respiratory failure.

Prognosis

In patients with an intact immune system, modern antituberculous therapy provides an excellent potential for recovery. The outlook for patients with immunodeficiencies, organisms resistant to multiple drugs (rare), poor drug compliance, or advanced complications is guarded.

Hsu KHK: Isoniazid in the prevention and treatment of tuberculosis. *JAMA* 1974;**229**:528.

Kendig EL Jr.: The routine tuberculin test: A neglected pediatric procedure. *J Pediatr* 1952;**40**:813.

Snider D: Pregnancy and tuberculosis. *Chest* 1984;**86** **(Suppl 3)**:10S.

Steinhoff MC, Lionel J: Treatment of tuberculosis in newborn infants and their mothers. *Indian J Pediatr* 1988; **55**:240.

Woodring JH et al: Intrathoracic lymphadenopathy in postprimary tuberculosis. *South Med J* 1988;**81**:992.

ASPIRATION PNEUMONIA

Essentials of Diagnosis

- Patient at risk.
- Fever.
- Cough.

General Considerations

The risk of aspiration pneumonia occurs in patients when anatomic defense mechanisms are impaired. These include patients with (1) seizures, (2) depressed sensorium, (3) recurrent gastroesophageal reflux, (4) neuromuscular disorders with suck-swallow dysfunction, (5) anatomic abnormalities (laryngeal cleft, tracheoesophageal fistula), and (6) debilitating illnesses. Acute disease is commonly caused by bacteria present in the mouth (especially gram-negative anaerobes), and multiple organisms may concomitantly cause infection in many patients. Chronic aspiration often causes recurrent bouts of acute febrile pneumonia. It may also lead to chronic focal infiltrates, atelectasis, or illness resembling asthma or interstitial lung disease.

Clinical Findings

A. Symptoms and Signs: Acute onset of fever, cough, respiratory distress, or hypoxemia in a patient at risk suggests aspiration pneumonia. Chest physical findings, such as rales, rhonchi, or decreased breath sounds, may initially be limited to the lung region into which aspiration occurred. Although any region may be affected, the right side, especially the right upper lobe in the supine patient, is commonly affected. In patients with chronic aspiration, diffuse wheezing may occur. Generalized rales may also be present. Such patients may not develop acute febrile pneumonias.

B. Laboratory Findings and Imaging: Chest radiographs may reveal lobar consolidation or atelectasis and focal or generalized alveolar or interstitial infiltrates. In some patients with chronic aspiration, perihilar infiltrates with or without bilateral air trapping may be seen.

In severely ill patients with acute febrile illnesses, a bacteriologic diagnosis should be made. In addition to blood cultures, cultures of tracheobronchial secretions and transtracheal or lung puncture specimens may be desirable (see Culture of Material from the Respiratory Tract).

In patients with chronic aspiration pneumonitis, solid documentation of aspiration as the cause of illness may be elusive. Barium contrast studies may provide evidence of suck-swallow dysfunction, laryngeal cleft, occult tracheoesophageal fistula, or gastroesophageal reflux. Overnight or 24-hour esophageal pH probe studies may also help establish the latter. Although radionuclide scans are commonly employed, the yield from such studies is disappointingly low. Rigid bronchoscopy in infants or flexible bronchoscopy in older children, can be useful in (1) more definitively excluding tracheoesophageal fistula and (2) obtaining bronchoalveolar lavage specimens to search for lipid-laden macrophages as evidence of chronic aspiration.

Differential Diagnosis

In the acutely ill patient, routine bacterial, viral, or mycoplasmal pneumonias should be considered. In the chronically ill patient, the differential diagnoses may include disorders causing (1) recurrent pneumonia (immunodeficiencies, ciliary dysfunction, foreign body, etc), (2) chronic wheezing, or (3) interstitial lung disorders (see below), depending on the presentation.

Complications

Empyema or lung abscess may result from acute aspiration pneumonia. Chronic disease may result in bronchiectasis.

Treatment

Antimicrobial therapy for acute aspiration pneumonia includes appropriate coverage for gram-negative anaerobic organisms. In the hospital setting, coverage for nosocomial infection by gram-negative enteric and other multiply resistant bacteria should be provided.

Treatment of recurrent and chronic aspiration pneumonia may include the following: (1) surgical correction of anatomic abnormalities, (2) improved oral hygiene, (3) improved hydration, and (4) inhaled bronchodilators, chest physical therapy, and suctioning. In patients with compromise of the central nervous system, exclusive feeding by gastrostomy and (in some) tracheostomy may be required to control airway secretions. Gastroesophageal reflux, often requiring surgical correction, is commonly present in such patients.

Prognosis

The outlook for patients with aspiration pneumonia is directly related to the disorder causing their aspiration.

Colombo JL, Hallberg TK: Recurrent aspiration in children: Lipid-laden alveolar macrophage quantitation. *Pediatr Pulmonol* 1987;**3**:86.

Fawcett HD et al: How useful is gastroesophageal reflux scintigraphy in suspected childhood aspiration? *Pediatr Radiol* 1988;**18**:309.

Marks JD, Brooks JG: Sleep-associated airway problems in children. *Pediatr Clin North Am* 1984;**31**:907.

Moran JR et al: Lipid-laden alveolar macrophage and lactose assay as markers of aspiration in neonates with lung disease. *J Pediatr* 1988;**112**:643.

PNEUMONIA IN THE IMMUNOCOMPROMISED HOST

Essentials of Diagnosis

- Immunodeficiency disease, HIV infection, leukemia, lymphoma, cancer chemotherapy, chronic corticosteroid or ACTH therapy, postsplenectomy, sickle hemoglobinopathies, or splenic dysfunction states.
- Fever.
- Cough.

General Considerations

The immunocompromised host with pneumonia may be infected with any common organism (pneumococcus, streptococcus, staphylococcus, *M pneumoniae*) or less common organism of several classes. These include (1) parasites (*Pneumocystis carinii, Toxoplasma gondii*), (2) fungi (*Aspergillus* species, mucormycosis, *Candida* species, *Cryptococcus neoformans, Cryptosporidium*), (3) viruses (cytomegalovirus, varicella-zoster, herpes simplex, influenza, respiratory syncytial virus, adenovirus), and (4) bacteria (gram-negative enteric and anaerobic bacteria, *Nocardia* and *Actinomyces* species, and *Legionella pneumophila*). Multiple organisms and types of organisms are commonly present.

Clinical Findings

A. Symptoms and Signs: Patients often present with subtle signs such as mild cough, tachypnea, or low-grade fever. Unfortunately, these are commonly overlooked until a predictable, rapid progression manifested by worsening cough, fever, respiratory

distress, and hypoxemia occurs. An obvious portal of infection, such as an intravascular catheter, may predispose a patient to bacterial or fungal infection and should be suspected as the cause.

B. Laboratory Findings and Imaging: Fungal, parasitic, or bacterial infection, especially with antibiotic-resistant bacteria, should be suspected in the neutropenic child. Cultures of peripheral blood, sputum, tracheobronchial secretions, urine, nasopharynx or sinuses, bone marrow, pleural fluid, biopsied lymph nodes, or skin lesions or cultures through intravascular catheters should be obtained as soon as infection is suspected.

Invasive methods are commonly required to make an adequately early diagnosis. The results of these procedures do appear, in the majority of cases, to lead to important changes in empiric preoperative therapy. Sputum is frequently unavailable. Transtracheal aspiration has a high complication rate in children. Percutaneous lung puncture has a very high false-negative rate in *P carinii* pneumonia, and this is a very common organism. Bronchoalveolar lavage frequently provides the diagnosis of one or more organisms and should be done *early* in evaluation. The combined use of a wash, brushing, and lavage has given a particularly high yield in such patients. In patients with very rapidly advancing or advanced disease, open lung biopsy becomes more urgent. However, the morbidity and mortality of this procedure in this setting is high. Because of the multiplicity of organisms that may cause disease, a comprehensive set of studies should be done on lavage or biopsy material. These consist of (1) rapid diagnostic studies, including fluorescent antibody studies for *Legionella*, ELISA for RSV, etc; (2) Gram, acid-fast, fungal, and methenamine silver stains; (3) cytologic examination for viral inclusions; and (4) cultures for viruses, anaerobic and aerobic bacteria, fungi, mycobacteria, and *Legionella*. If available, newly developed rapid immunofluorescent studies for *P carinii* should be obtained.

Chest radiographs may be useful. However, dyspnea and hypoxemia may be marked despite minimal radiographic abnormalities in *P carinii* pneumonia (PCP).

Differential Diagnosis

The organism(s) causing disease vary with the type of immunocompromise present. For example, the splenectomized patient may be overwhelmed by infection with *Pneumococcus* or *H influenzae*. The infant on ACTH therapy likely has PCP infection. The febrile, neutropenic child who has been receiving adequate doses of intravenous broad-spectrum antibiotics may have fungal disease or PCP. However, the key to diagnosis is to remain open to all infectious possibilities and to neglect no diagnostic study.

Depending on the form of immunocompromise,

perhaps only half to two-thirds of new pulmonary infiltrates in such patients represent infection. Such infiltrates may also represent the following: (1) pulmonary toxicity of radiation, oxygen, chemotherapy, or other drugs; (2) pulmonary disorders, including hemorrhage, embolism, atelectasis, aspiration, or adult respiratory distress syndrome; (3) recurrence or extension of primary malignant growths or immunologic disorders; (4) transfusion reactions, leukostasis, or tumor cell lysis; or (5) interstitial lung disease, such as lymphocytic interstitial pneumonitis with HIV infection or Epstein-Barr virus infection.

Complications

Respiratory failure, shock, multiple organ damage, disseminated infection, and death commonly occur in the infected, immunocompromised host.

Treatment

Broad-spectrum intravenous antibiotics are indicated early in febrile, neutropenic, or immunocompromised children. Trimethoprim-sulfamethoxazole and erythromycin are also indicated early in the treatment of immunocompromised children. Further therapy should be based on studies of specimens obtained from bronchoalveolar lavage or lung biopsy.

Prognosis

Prognosis is guarded and based upon the severity of the underlying immunocompromise, appropriate early diagnosis and treatment, and the infecting organism(s) present.

Barbour SD: AIDS of childhood. *Pediatr Clin North Am* 1987;**34**:247.
de Blic J et al: Value of bronchoalveolar lavage in the management of severe acute pneumonia and interstitial pneumonitis in the immunocompromised child. *Thorax* 1987;**42**:759.
Frankel LR et al: Bronchoalveolar lavage for diagnosis of pneumonia in the immunocompromised child. *Pediatrics* 1988;**81**:785.
Hughes WT: Pneumonia in the immunocompromised child. *Semin Respir Infect* 1987;**2**:177.
Hughes WT et al: Successful intermittent chemoprophylaxis for *Pneumocystis carinii* pneumonitis. *N Engl J Med* 1987;**316**:1627.
Martin WJ et al: Role of bronchoalveolar lavage in the assessment of opportunistic pulmonary infections: Utility and complications. *Mayo Clin Proc* 1987;**62**:549.
Prober CG et al: Open lung biopsy in immunocompromised children with pulmonary infiltrates. *Am J Dis Child* 1984;**138**:60.
Springmeyer SC et al: Use of bronchoalveolar lavage to diagnose acute diffuse pneumonia in the immunocompromised host. *J Infect Dis* 1986;**154**:604.
Valteau D et al: Nonbacterial nonfungal interstitial pneumonitis following autologous bone marrow transplantation in children treated with high-dose chemotherapy without total-body irradiation. *Transplantation* 1988;**45**:737.

HYPERSENSITIVITY PNEUMONIA

Essentials of Diagnosis

- History of exposure (birds, organic dusts or molds, etc).
- Interstitial infiltrates on chest radiograph or diffuse rales.
- With or without recurrent cough, fever, wheezing, and/or weight loss.

General Considerations

Hypersensitivity pneumonitis is a disease involving peripheral airways, interstitium, and alveoli. Both acute and chronic forms may occur. In children, the most common forms are brought on by exposure to birds or bird droppings (pigeons, parakeets, parrots, doves, etc). However, inhalation of almost any organic dust (moldy hay, compost, logs or tree bark, sawdust, or aerosols from humidifiers) can cause disease. Although uncommon in children, many of the latter present as occupational lung diseases in adults.

Clinical Findings

A. Symptoms and Signs: Episodic cough and fever can occur with acute exposures. Chronic exposure results in weight loss, fatigue, dyspnea, cyanosis, and, ultimately, respiratory failure.

B. Laboratory Findings: Acute exposures may be followed by polymorphonuclear leukocytosis with eosinophilia and evidence of airways obstruction on pulmonary function testing. Chronic disease results in a restrictive picture on lung function tests. Arterial blood gases may reveal hypoxemia with a decreased $paco_2$ and normal pH (respiratory alkalosis, compensated).

The serologic key to diagnosis is the finding of precipitins (precipitating IgG antibodies) to the organic dusts that contain avian proteins or fungal or bacterial antigens. However, exposure without related disease may cause the presence of precipitions.

Differential Diagnosis

Patients with primarily acute symptoms must be differentiated from patients with atopic asthma. Those with chronic symptoms must be distinguished from those with collagen-vascular, immunologic, or primary interstitial pulmonary disorders.

Complications

Prolonged exposure to offending antigen(s) may result in pulmonary hypertension due to chronic hypoxemia, cor pulmonale, irreversible restrictive lung disease due to pulmonary fibrosis, or respiratory failure.

Treatment

Complete elimination of exposure to the offending

antigen(s) is required. Corticosteroids may hasten recovery.

Prognosis

With appropriate diagnosis and avoidance of offending antigens, the prognosis is excellent. However, a good prognosis is dependent on early diagnosis before irreversible pulmonary damage has occurred.

Barker PM, Warner JO: "Atypical pneumonia" due to parakeet sensitivity: Bird fancier's lung in a 10-year-old girl. *Br J Dis Chest* 1984;**78**:404.

Chiron C et al: Lung function in children with hypersensitivity pneumonitis. *Eur J Respir Dis* 1984;**65**:79.

Fink JN et al: Interstitial lung disease due to contamination of forced air systems. *Ann Intern Med* 1976;**84**:406.

Shimazu K et al: Hypersensitivity pneumonitis induced by *Trichosporon cutaneum. Am Rev Respir Dis* 1984;**130**:407.

Stiehm ER et al: Pigeon breeder's lung in children. *Pediatrics* 1967;**39**:904.

INTERSTITIAL LUNG DISEASE

Essentials of Diagnosis

- Tachypnea, dyspnea, retractions, or hypoxemia.
- Cough or rales.
- Bilateral pulmonary infiltrates.

General Considerations

Interstitial lung disorders (ILD) in children may have a wide variety of presentations, and these are often subtle and gradual in onset. ILD in the child, unlike the adult, is commonly caused by infection, immunodeficiency, aspiration, cardiac disease, or pulmonary vascular disease. Also unlike adults, children with ILD less commonly have primary pulmonary interstitial lung disorders (desquamative, usual, or lymphocytic interstitial pneumonitis, etc), hypersensitivity pneumonitis, or collagen-vascular diseases.

Clinical Findings

A. Symptoms and Signs: Children with ILD may present with a chronic, dry cough or a history of dyspnea on exertion. The child with more advanced disease may have increased tachypnea, dyspnea, retractions, cyanosis, clubbing, failure to thrive, or weight loss. Physical examination may reveal these findings, and dry ("velcro") rales may be present on chest auscultation, especially at the lung bases.

B. Laboratory Findings and Imaging: Chest radiographs may be normal in up to 10–15% of patients. More commonly, diffuse or perihilar bilateral reticular interstitial infiltrates are present. Nodular and reticulonodular diseases are uncommon in children except in cases of HIV infection. Although infiltrates may show a unilateral predominance, bilat-

eral disease is the rule except in cases of infection and aspiration-related disorders.

On pulmonary function testing, interstitial disorders often show a restrictive pattern of decreased lung volumes, compliance, and diffusing capacity for carbon monoxide, whereas FEV_1/FVC may be normal or increased. However, exercise-induced hypoxemia is often the earliest detectable abnormality of lung function. Blood gas abnormalities, if present, are the same as those in chronic hypersensitivity pneumonitis.

Whereas acute fulminant illness requires immediate, definitive diagnosis, a methodical, staged approach can be used in many chronically ill patients. This consists of (1) "serologic," (2) bronchoscopic, and (3) biopsy stages. Although bronchoalveolar lavage may be useful in identifying patients with pulmonary hemosiderosis (hemosiderin-laden macrophages), aspiration (lipid-laden macrophages), and infectious disorders, lung biopsy is the most reliable method for definitive ILD diagnosis.

During the initial phase, x-rays, barium swallow, tests of pulmonary function, skin tests (see Tuberculosis), complete blood count, erythrocyte sedimentation rate, sweat test for cystic fibrosis, electrocardiogram or echocardiogram, serum immunoglobulins, IgE, and other immunologic evaluations, sputum studies (see Pneumonia in the Immunocompromised Host), and serologic studies for Epstein-Barr virus, cytomegalovirus, *M pneumoniae, Chlamydia, Pneumocystis,* and *Ureaplasma urealyticum* may appropriately be considered and performed.

During the second phase, rigid bronchoscopy should be performed to exclude anatomic abnormalities and obtain multiple specimens of the tracheobronchial wall for evaluation of cilia. At the same procedure, bronchoalveolar lavage, preferably through a flexible bronchoscope and an endotracheal tube if the patient is sufficiently large, should be done. Material for stains and cultures for microorganisms and for cytologic studies should be processed. In patients with static or slowly progressing disease, one can await results of bronchoscopic studies before proceeding further. In patients with more rapidly progressive disease, this stage should be combined with open lung biopsy. Studies of lung tissue, including histopathology, cultures, stains, immunofluorescence for immune complexes, and electron microscopy, should be processed. Although transbronchial biopsy may be useful in diagnosing a few disorders (eg, sarcoid), its overall usefulness in pediatrics is limited.

Differential Diagnosis

Malignant disorders (histiocytosis X, disseminated carcinoma), congenital disorders (Gaucher's disease, neurofibromatosis, tuberous sclerosis, familial ILD), pulmonary hemosiderosis, pulmonary telangiectasia or lymphangiectasia, bronchiolitis obliterans, sarcoidosis, and ciliary dyskinesia should be considered in addition to the groups of disorders mentioned above.

Complications

Respiratory failure or pulmonary hypertension with cor pulmonale may occur.

Treatment

Therapy of ILD due to infection, aspiration, or cardiac disorders should be directed at the primary disorder. The majority of primary pulmonary interstitial disorders are treated initially with daily prednisone (2 mg/kg/d) therapy for a period of 6 weeks to 6 months, depending on the intensity of disease and response. Many patients require even more prolonged therapy with alternate-day prednisone. Chloroquine (5–10 mg/kg/d) may be useful in selected disorders such as desquamative interstitial pneumonitis. Use of additional cytotoxic drugs (azathioprine, cyclophosphamide) has not been shown in a controlled fashion to be more beneficial than prednisone alone.

Prognosis

The prognosis is guarded in children with interstitial lung disease due to collagen-vascular and primary pulmonary interstitial diseases, immunodeficiency diseases, and cancer.

Crystal RG et al: Interstitial lung disease: Current concepts of pathogenesis, staging, and therapy. *Am J Med* 1981; **70**:542.

Falloon J et al: Human immunodeficiency virus infection in children. *J Pediatr* 1989;**114**:1.

Laraya-Cuasay LF, Hughes WT: *Interstitial Lung Diseases in Children.* Vols 1–3. CRC Press, 1988.

Springer C et al: Chloroquine treatment in desquamative interstitial pneumonia. *Arch Dis Child* 1987;**62**:76.

Stagno S et al: Infant pneumonitis associated with cytomegalovirus, *Chlamydia, Pneumocystis,* and *Ureaplasma:* A prospective study. *Pediatrics* 1981;**68**:322.

EOSINOPHILIC PNEUMONIA

Essentials of Diagnosis

- Pulmonary infiltrates, often migratory, on chest radiograph.
- Persistent cough; wheezes or rales on chest auscultation.
- Excessive eosinophils in peripheral blood or in lung biopsy specimens.

General Considerations

A spectrum of diseases including (1) transient pulmonary infiltrates with eosinophilia (Löffler's syndrome), (2) tropical eosinophilia, (3) pulmonary eosinophilia with asthma (allergic bronchopulmonary aspergillosis [ABPA] and related disorders), (4) hypereosinophilic mucoid impaction, (5) bronchocentric granulomatosis, and (6) collagen-vascular disorders should be considered under the heading of eosinophilic pneumonia. Many may occur in children with personal or family histories of allergies or asthma. These disorders may be related to hypersensitivity to migratory parasitic nematodes (*Ascaris, Strongyloides, Ancylostoma, Toxocara, Trichuris*), larval forms of filariae (*Wuchereria bancrofti*), or fungi (*Aspergillus, Candida*).

Clinical Findings

A. Symptoms and Signs: Patients may present with a recent onset or exacerbation of asthma (Löffler syndrome) or exacerbation of more severe, longstanding asthma or cystic fibrosis (ABPA). In most, cough, wheezing, or dyspnea are presenting complaints. In Löffler syndrome, fever, malaise, sputum production, and, rarely, hemoptysis may be present. In ABPA, patients may present all of these findings and commonly produce brown mucus plugs. Anorexia, weight loss, night sweats, and clubbing can also occur.

B. Laboratory Findings and Imaging: Elevated absolute peripheral blood eosinophil counts (greater than 3000 cells/μL and often exceeding 50% of leukocytes) are present in Löffler syndrome, tropical eosinophilia, and ABPA. Elevated serum IgE levels (often as high as 1000–10,000 IU/mL or more) are commonly present. In ABPA, the serum IgE concentration appears to correlate with activity of the disease. Stools should be examined for ova and parasites, often several times, to clarify the diagnosis. Isohemagglutinin titers are often quite elevated in Löffler syndrome.

In ABPA and related disorders, patients may have central bronchiectasis demonstrable by chest radiograph ("tramlines") or CT scan. Saccular proximal bronchiectasis of the upper lobes is pathognomonic. Although the chest radiograph may be normal, peribronchial haziness, focal or platelike atelectasis, or patchy to massive consolidation can occur. Positive immediate skin tests, serum IgG precipitating antibodies, or IgE specific for the offending fungus are present.

Differential Diagnosis

These disorders must be differentiated from exacerbations of asthma, cystic fibrosis, or other underlying lung disorders that can be manifested by infiltrates on chest x-ray films.

Complications

Although Löffler syndrome is usually self-limited, delayed recognition and treatment of ABPA may cause progressive lung damage and bronchiectasis. Lesions of the conducting airways in bronchocentric granulomatosis can extend into adjacent lung parenchyma and pulmonary arteries, resulting in a secondary vasculitis.

Treatment

Therapy for parasites causing Löffler syndrome

should be given, and corticosteroids may be required when illness is severe. Treatment of disease due to microfilariae is both diagnostic and therapeutic. ABPA and related disorders are treated with prolonged courses of oral corticosteroids, bronchodilators, and chest physical therapy. Antifungal agents are not useful in these latter disorders.

Ahmad M et al: Thoracic aspergillosis. 2. Primary pulmonary aspergillosis, allergic bronchopulmonary aspergillosis, and related conditions. *Cleve Clin Q* 1984; **51**:631.

Christensen WN, Hutchins GM: Hypereosinophilic mucoid impaction of bronchi in 2 children under 2 years of age. *Pediatr Pulmonol* 1985;**1**:278.

Howard WA: Löeffler syndrome (pulmonary infiltrates with eosinophilia). In: *Disorders of the Respiratory Tract in Children.* Kendig EL Jr, Chernick V (editors). Saunders, 1983.

Ivanick MJ, Donohue JF: Chronic eosinophilic pneumonia: A cause of adult respiratory distress syndrome. *South Med J* 1986;**79**:686.

Lee TM et al: Allergic bronchopulmonary candidiasis: Case report and suggested diagnostic criteria. *J Allergy Clin Immunol* 1987;**80**:816.

LUNG ABSCESS

Essentials of Diagnosis

- Fever.
- Cavitary mass on chest radiograph.
- With or without cough, chest pain, dyspnea, sputum production, or hemoptysis.

General Considerations

Lung abscesses are most likely to occur in immunocompromised patients, in those with severe infections elsewhere (embolic spread), or in those with recurrent aspiration. Although organisms such as *Staphylococcus aureus, Haemophilus influenzae,* and *Streptococcus viridans* and *pneumoniae* more commonly affect the previously normal host, anaerobic and gram-negative organisms as well as *Nocardia* and fungi *(Candida, Aspergillus)* should also be considered in the immunocompromised.

Clinical Findings

A. Symptoms and Signs: High fever, malaise, and weight loss are often present. Symptoms and signs referable to the chest may or may not be present. In infants, evidence of respiratory distress can be present.

B. Laboratory Findings and Imaging: Elevated peripheral white blood cell count with a neutrophil predominance or an elevated erythrocyte sedimentation rate may be present. Blood cultures are rarely positive except in the overwhelmed host.

Chest radiographs usually reveal single or multiple thick-walled lung cavities. Air-fluid levels can be present. Local compressive atelectasis, pleural thickening, or adenopathy may also occur.

In patients producing sputum, stains and cultures may provide the diagnosis. Direct percutaneous aspiration of material for stains and cultures directed by fluoroscopy or ultrasound should be considered in the severely compromised or ill.

Differential Diagnosis

Loculated pyopneumothorax, Echinococcus cyst, neoplasms, plasma cell granuloma, and infected congenital cysts and sequestrations should be considered in the differential diagnosis.

Complications

Although complications due to abscesses are now rare, mediastinal shift, tension pneumothorax, and spontaneous rupture can occur. Diagnostic maneuvers such as lung puncture may also cause complications (pneumothorax).

Treatment

Because of the risks of lung puncture, uncomplicated abscesses are frequently treated in the uncompromised host with appropriate broad-spectrum antibiotics directed at *S aureus, H influenzae,* and streptococci. Additional coverage for anaerobic and gram-negative organisms should be provided for others. Prolonged therapy (3 weeks or more) may be required. Attempts to drain abscesses via bronchoscopy have caused life-threatening airway compromise. Surgical drainage or lobectomy is occasionally required, primarily in immunocompromised patients. However, such procedures may themselves cause life-threatening complications, and surgical intervention must be judicious and well planned.

Prognosis

Although radiologic resolution may be very slow, resolution occurs in most patients without propensity to lower respiratory tract infections or loss of pulmonary function. Nonetheless, in the immunocompromised host, the outlook is guarded and dependent on the underlying disorder.

Asher MI et al: Primary lung abscess in childhood: The long-term outcome of conservative management. *Am J Dis Child* 1982;**136**:491.

Bujak JS et al: Nocardiosis in a child with chronic granulomatous disease. *J Pediatr* 1973;**83**:98.

Hammer DL et al: Massive intrabronchial aspiration of contents of pulmonary abscess after fiberoptic bronchoscopy. *Chest* 1978;**74**:306.

Johnson JF et al: Concealed pulmonary abscess: Diagnosis by computed tomography. *Pediatrics* 1986;**78**:283.

Kosloske AM et al: Drainage of pediatric lung abscess by cough, catheter, or complete resection. *J Pediatr Surg* 1986;**21**:596.

Lewin S et al: Legionnaire's disease. A cause of severe abscess-forming pneumonia. *Am J Med* 1979;**67**:339.

Siegel JD, McCracken GH: Neonatal lung abscess. *Am J Dis Child* 1979;**133**:947.

PULMONARY TUMORS

Essentials of Diagnosis
■ Mass identified on chest x-ray or by direct visualization on bronchoscopy.

General Considerations
Primary tumors of the airway and parenchyma of the lung are unusual in pediatrics. Most intrathoracic tumors occur in or close to the mediastinum (see Mediastinal Masses). Other pulmonary tumors may be classified as benign, malignant, or metastatic. Benign pulmonary tumors include plasma cell granulomas, hamartomas, adenomas, papillomas, angiomas, leiomyomas, lipomas, and neurogenic tumors. The most common malignant tumor in children is a bronchogenic carcinoma, but this is again very rare. Other malignant tumors include fibrosarcomas and leiomyosarcomas. Metastatic tumors in childhood include Wilms's tumor, hepatoblastoma, osteogenic sarcoma, chondrosarcoma, Ewing's tumor, reticulum cell sarcoma, and soft tissue sarcomas. Because metastatic pulmonary tumors are more common than primary malignant growths in the lungs of children, patients with symptoms and roentgenographic or other data suggesting a pulmonary cancer should be thoroughly evaluated for nonpulmonary malignant tumors.

Clinical Findings
A. Symptoms and Signs: When tumors produce symptoms, they may include pain, fever, cough, wheezing, weight loss, malaise, anemia, anorexia, and hemoptysis. On physical examination, signs of volume loss or consolidation may be present if the tumor has led to significant airways obstruction. Physical findings consistent with pleural effusions may also be present.

B. Laboratory Findings and Imaging: In addition to frontal and lateral chest x-rays, fluoroscopy, CT scans, and angiography may be helpful in defining and delineating the tumor. In approaching the differential diagnosis (below), sputum cultures and cytology, as well as tuberculin and fungal skin tests plus fungal serology, may be of benefit in ruling out conditions that may appear to be mass lesions.

Differential Diagnosis
The differential diagnosis includes acute, recurrent, or persistent viral and bacterial pneumonia, tuberculosis, and pulmonary infiltrates due to fungal infections. In infants, congenital malformations (pulmonary sequestration, cystic adenomatoid malformation) may also present as mass lesions.

Treatment & Prognosis
Both the appropriate therapy and the response to therapy depend on the type and location of the tumor. Benign lesions may be cured with surgical re-

section, but the prognosis is more guarded with both primary and metastatic malignant lesions.

Brooks JW: Tumors of the chest. In: *Disorders of the Respiratory Tract in Children,* 4th ed. Kendig EL Jr, Chernick V (editors). Saunders, 1983.
Hartman GE, Shochat SJ: Primary pulmonary neoplasms in childhood: A review. *Ann Thorac Surg* 1983;**36**:108.
Monzon CM et al: Plasma cell granuloma of the lung in children. *Pediatrics* 1982;**70**:268.

DISEASES OF THE PULMONARY CIRCULATION

PULMONARY HEMORRHAGE

General Considerations
Acute pulmonary hemorrhage can be defined as bleeding within the lungs, with or without hemoptysis, and is usually accompanied by alveolar-filling infiltrates on chest x-ray. Hemosiderin-laden macrophages are found in the sputum and tracheal or gastric aspirate. Many cases are secondary to infection (bacterial, mycobacterial, parasitic, viral, or fungal), lung abscess, bronchiectasis (cystic fibrosis or other causes), foreign body, coagulopathy (often with overwhelming sepsis), or elevated pulmonary venous pressure (secondary to congestive heart failure or anatomic heart lesions). Structural lesions including arteriovenous fistula, multiple telangiectasia, pulmonary sequestration, agenesis of a single pulmonary artery, and esophageal duplication or bronchogenic cyst are other related causes. Lung contusion from trauma and such tumors as bronchial adenoma or left atrial myxoma are other causes. Pulmonary infarction secondary to pulmonary embolus is another uncommon cause in pediatrics.

In addition, alveolar hemorrhage syndromes, ie, alveolar bleeding that occurs as a primary manifestation, includes several uncommon disorders or uncommon manifestations of systemic disease. Disorders associated with pulmonary hemorrhage include Goodpasture's syndrome, idiopathic, rapidly progressive glomerulonephritis, drug-related and systemic vasculitides (often associated with such collagen-vascular diseases as systemic lupus erythematosus, rheumatoid arthritis, Wegener's granulomatosis, polyarteritis nodosa, Schönlein-Henoch purpura, and Behçet's disease). Idiopathic pulmonary hemosiderosis refers to the accumulation of hemosiderin in the lung, especially the alveolar macrophage, as a result of chronic or recurrent hemorrhage (usually from pulmonary capillaries) that is not associated with the causes listed above. Children and young adults are primarily affected, with the age at onset ranging between 6 months and 20 years. This group of disorders includes young infants with milk allergy (Heiner's syndrome).

Clinical Findings

A. Symptoms and Signs: Idiopathic pulmonary hemosiderosis usually presents with nonspecific respiratory symptoms (cough, tachypnea, retractions), with or without hemoptysis, poor growth, and fatigue. Some children or young adults may present with massive hemoptysis, marked respiratory distress, stridor, or a pneumonialike syndrome. Fever, abdominal pain, digital clubbing, and chest pain may be reported. Jaundice and hepatosplenomegaly may be present with chronic bleeding. Physical exam often reveals decreased breath sounds, rales, rhonchi, or wheezing. Laboratory studies demonstrate an iron-deficiency anemia, and heme-positive sputum. Nonspecific findings may include lymphocytosis and an elevated erythrocyte sedimentation rate. Peripheral eosinophilia is present in up to 25% of patients.

B. Laboratory Findings and Imaging: Chest x-ray findings include a range of findings, from transient perihilar infiltrates to large, fluffy alveolar infiltrates, with or without atelectasis and mediastinal adenopathy. Pulmonary function testing generally reveals a restrictive impairment, with low lung volumes and poor compliance. Hemosiderin-laden macrophages are found in bronchial or gastric aspirates. The usefulness of lung biopsy in reaching the diagnosis is controversial. Suspected cases of cow's milk-induced pulmonary hemosiderosis can be confirmed by laboratory findings that include high titers of serum precipitins to multiple constituents of cow's milk and positive intradermal skin tests to various cow's milk proteins. Improvement after an empiric trial of a diet free of cow's milk also supports the diagnosis.

Differential Diagnosis

In contrast to idiopathic pulmonary hemosiderosis, Goodpasture's syndrome presents in a slightly older age group (15–35 years), tends to have a more aggressive pulmonary course, and has renal involvement (crescentic proliferative glomerulonephritis and circulating anti-glomerular basement membrane antibody). Wegener's granulomatosis also has renal involvement (granulomatous glomerulitis with necrotizing vasculitis, but renal biopsy may be nonspecific) and other systemic manifestations, especially with upper and lower respiratory tract inflammation. Upper tract involvement includes sinusitis, rhinitis, recurrent epistaxis, otitis media, saddle nose deformity, and subglottic stenosis.

Treatment

Therapy should be aimed at direct treatment of the underlying disease. Supportive measures, including iron therapy, supplemental oxygen, and blood transfusions, are provided as clinically indicated. In selected cases, a trial of cow's milk-free diet should be tried. The usefulness of steroids or cytotoxic agents is unproved in idiopathic pulmonary hemosiderosis but appears to be beneficial in Wegener's granulomatosis and perhaps Goodpasture's syndrome.

Prognosis

The outcome of idiopathic pulmonary hemosiderosis is markedly variable, typically characterized by a waxing and waning course of intermittent intrapulmonary bleeds and the gradual development of chronic lung disease over time. The severity of the underlying renal disease contributes to the mortality of Goodpasture's syndrome and Wegener's granulomatosis.

Bradley JD: Pulmonary hemorrhage syndromes. *Clin Chest Med* 1982;**3:**593.

Hall SL et al: Wegener granulomatosis in pediatric patients. *J Pediatr* 1985;**106:**739.

Kjellman B et al: Idiopathic pulmonary hemosiderosis in Swedish children. *Acta Paediatr Scand* 1984;**73:**584.

Leatherman JW et al: Alveolar hemorrhage syndromes. *Medicine (Baltimore)* 1984;**63:**343.

Miller RW et al: Pulmonary hemorrhage in pediatric patients with systemic lupus erythematosus. *J Pediatr* 1986;**108:**576.

PULMONARY EMBOLISM

General Considerations

Although apparently rare in children, the incidence of pulmonary embolism is probably underestimated in pediatrics because it is often not considered in the differential diagnosis of respiratory distress. It occurs most commonly in pediatrics in sickle cell anemia as part of the "acute chest syndrome" and in rheumatic fever, infective endocarditis, schistosomiasis, bone fracture, dehydration, polycythemia, nephrotic syndrome, atrial fibrillation, "complicated" pneumonia, and other settings. The emboli may be single or multiple, large or small, with the clinical signs and symptoms dependent on the severity of pulmonary vascular obstruction.

Clinical Findings

A. Symptoms and Signs: Most often, pulmonary embolism presents clinically as the acute onset of dyspnea and tachypnea. Heart palpitations or "a sense of impending doom" may be reported. Pleuritic chest pain and hemoptysis may be present (but are not common), along with splinting, cyanosis, and tachycardia. Massive emboli may present with syncope and cardiac dysrhythmias. Physical examination is usually normal (except for tachycardia and tachypnea) unless the embolism is associated with an underlying disorder. Mild hypoxemia, rales, focal wheezing, or a pleural friction rub may be noted.

B. Laboratory Findings and Imaging: Radiologic findings may be normal, but a peripheral infiltrate, small pleural effusion, or elevated hemidiaphragm can be present. If the emboli are massive, differential blood flow and pulmonary artery enlargement may be appreciated. The electrocardiogram is usually normal unless the pulmonary embolus is massive. Ventilation-perfusion scans show localized areas of ventilation without perfusion. If this study is normal, pulmonary embolus is virtually excluded. Further evaluation may include radiofibrinogen leg scanning and impedance plethysmography to search for findings of significant deep venous thrombosis. Coagulation studies, including assessments of antithrombin III and protein C or S deficiencies, or defective fibrinolysis may be indicated. However, 90% of adult patients with venous thromboembolism have no identified coagulopathy.

Treatment

Acute treatment includes supplemental oxygen, sedation, and anticoagulation. Although controversial, current recommendations include heparin administration to maintain an activated partial thromboplastin time at a value of 1.5 or more times the control value. Thrombolytic therapy with streptokinase and urokinase may be necessary if the pulmonary embolus is massive. In patients with identifiable deep venous thrombosis of the lower extremities and significant pulmonary emboli (with hemodynamic compromise despite anticoagulation), inferior vena caval interruption may be necessary. However, long-term prospective data is lacking.

Malik AR, Johnson A: Role of humoral mediators in the pulmonary vascular response to pulmonary embolism. In: *Pulmonary Vascular Physiology and Pathophysiology.* Weir EK, Reeves JT (editors). Dekker, 1989.

Moser KM: Pulmonary embolism. In: *Textbook of Respiratory Medicine.* Murray JF, Nadel JA (editors). Saunders, 1988.

PULMONARY EDEMA

General Considerations

The morbidity of many cardiopulmonary disorders appears to be directly related to the severity of pulmonary edema, defined as the excessive accumulation of extravascular fluid in the lung. This occurs when fluid is filtered into the lungs faster than it can be removed, leading to detrimental changes in lung mechanics, eg, decreased lung compliance, worsening hypoxemia from ventilation-perfusion mismatch, bronchial compression, and, if advanced, decreased surfactant function. In the normal lung, the rate of fluid filtration is determined by the balance of hydrostatic and oncotic pressures in the microcirculation and interstitium, as well as vascular permeability,

surface area, and lymphatic function. In general, there are 2 basic types of pulmonary edema: increased pressure (cardiogenic or hydrostatic) and increased permeability (noncardiogenic or "primary"). Hydrostatic pulmonary edema is usually due to excessive increases in pressure, which is most commonly due to congestive heart failure from multiple causes. In contrast, many lung diseases, especially the adult respiratory distress syndrome (ARDS; see below) are characterized by the development of pulmonary edema secondary to changes in permeability due to injury to the alveolocapillary barrier. In these settings, pulmonary edema formation occurs primarily, independent of the elevations of pulmonary venous pressure.

Clinical Findings

A. Symptoms and Signs: Clinical findings depend on the underlying cause and clinical setting. In general, cyanosis, tachypnea, tachycardia, and respiratory distress are present. Physical findings include rales, diminished breath sounds, and (in young infants) expiratory wheezing. More severe disease is characterized by progressive respiratory distress with marked retractions, dyspnea, and severe hypoxemia.

B. Imaging: Chest x-ray findings are dependent on the cause of the edema. Typically, pulmonary vessels appear prominent, often with diffuse interstitial or alveolar infiltrates. Heart size is usually normal in permeability edema but enlarged when hydrostatic causes underlie the problem.

Treatment

Although specific therapy depends on the underlying cause of the pulmonary edema, supplemental oxygen therapy and, if needed, ventilator support for respiratory failure are instituted. Diuretics, digoxin, and vasodilators may be indicated for congestive heart failure, along with restriction of salt and water. Recommended interventions for permeability edema are reducing vascular volume and maintaining the lowest central venous or pulmonary arterial wedge pressure, without sacrificing cardiac output or causing hypotension (see below).

Malik AR: Mechanisms of neurogenic pulmonary edema. *Circ Res* 1985;**57**:1.

Staub NC: Pathogenesis of pulmonary edema. *Prog Cardiovasc Dis* 1980;**23**:53.

ADULT RESPIRATORY DISTRESS SYNDROME
(Shock Lung Syndrome)

Essentials of Diagnosis

- Progressive respiratory distress following an acute catastrophic event such as shock.
- Low lung compliance, marked hypoxemia.

- Chest x-ray demonstrating bilateral fluffy infiltrates, usually with normal heart size.
- Normal pulmonary artery wedge pressure (as measured by pulmonary artery catheter).

General Considerations

Adult respiratory distress syndrome (ARDS) is a clinical syndrome characterized by the progressive development of respiratory failure associated with acute lung injury. The inciting insult may be indirect (septic or hemorrhagic shock, head trauma and other causes of neurogenic pulmonary edema, burns, drug overdose, pancreatitis, massive blood transfusion, and many others) or direct (smoke or chemical inhalation, aspiration, lung infection, emboli, contusion, radiation pneumonitis). First reported by Ashbaugh in 1967, the term ''adult'' respiratory distress syndrome was derived from histologic and physiologic similarities with the respiratory distress syndrome observed in premature newborns. Despite its name, ARDS can be observed at any age. Its pathophysiologic hallmark is the presence of nonhydrostatic pulmonary edema due to increased pulmonary capillary permeability secondary to acute lung injury, in contrast to pulmonary edema secondary to elevated pulmonary venous pressures more typical of congestive heart failure. The exact mechanisms contributing to lung injury are not completely understood and may vary according to the type of insult involved. Several studies, however, have implicated a central role for the accumulation of activated neutrophils within the pulmonary circulation, leading to the release of injurious mediators, including toxic oxygen metabolites, eicosanoids, and proteinases. These agents may directly damage the endothelium, causing the loss of its barrier function, leading to increased permeability and resultant pulmonary edema. The acute inflammatory response associated with ARDS and its experimental models may also include contributions from alveolar macrophages, platelets, lymphocytes, and fibroblasts. Along with cellular infiltration, early histologic findings include microthrombi within the pulmonary circulation, intra-alveolar proteinaceous material, alveolar septal edema, and type I epithelial cell damage. Later findings (a few days after the initial injury) include increased interstitial and alveolar inflammation, type II cell proliferation, interstitial thickening with early collagen accumulation, and increased fibroblasts.

Clinical Findings

The classic clinical course of ARDS consists of progressive cyanosis and respiratory distress associated with stiff lungs (low compliance) and diffuse pulmonary infiltrates after an acute catastrophic event. The rate of development of acute respiratory failure is variable, but often there may be little sign of respiratory distress in its earliest stages, with progressive hypoxemia appearing within the period of 6–48 hours following the acute event. Early chest x-ray films may appear normal, but serial studies subsequently reveal patchy alveolar infiltrates, air bronchograms, and loss of lung volume, with the progression of increasing tachypnea, dyspnea, and hypoxemia. Rales are common on auscultation. Although initially responsive to supplemental oxygen, hypoxemia often becomes refractory to treatment because of marked ventilation-perfusion mismatching (intrapulmonary shunting) and low lung compliance with loss of lung volume. At this stage, mechanical ventilation is required, often with high-peak positive end-expiratory pressure (PEEP) and mean airway pressure (MAP).

Treatment

Therapy is primarily supportive. The first step lies in recognizing patients at risk, thereby anticipating and monitoring for the earliest signs of acute respiratory failure. Along with treating the underlying disorder (antibiotics for sepsis, blood products for hemorrhagic shock, etc), appropriate monitoring should be established early. This includes placement of a systemic arterial line for frequent assessments of arterial pH and blood gas tensions and for continuous measurements of arterial blood pressure. Pulse oximetery or transcutaneous Po_2 measurements provide serial, continuous determinations of oxygenation. Assessments of fluid status require placement of a Foley catheter. Dependable peripheral and central venous lines provide access for the administration of medications, blood products, and fluids and for assessing volume status by central venous pressures. In some cases, placement of a pulmonary arterial catheter allows essential determinations of pulmonary capillary wedge pressure, cardiac output, and mixed venous oxygen tensions and saturations (see Chapter 9).

The overall goal of acute therapy is to maximize tissue oxygen delivery, which is determined by the oxygen content of arterial blood (reflecting hemoglobin concentration, percent saturation, and arterial oxygen tension) and the cardiac index. Therefore, treatment typically includes maintaining hematocrit above 40%, cardiac index over 4.5 L/min/m^2, and oxygen saturation over 90–92%. Because of the severity and rapidity of the progression of lung disease, volume-limited ventilators are generally recommended to ensure the constant delivery of adequate tidal volume in the face of changing respiratory system compliance. With advanced disease, high levels of PEEP and MAP are needed to treat severe hypoxemia. In addition, this may allow the Fio_2 to be lowered below 1, thereby decreasing the potential risk of superimposed hyperoxic lung injury which, if prolonged, may paradoxically contribute to a worse outcome of ARDS (see below). High PEEP appears to improve the clinical course in ARDS by attenuating the alterations of lung mechanics caused by pulmonary edema (especially the loss of lung volumes, thereby decreasing the magnitude of intrapulmonary shunt), but does not appear to decrease the amount of edema fluid present within the lung itself. The amount of PEEP required to improve oxygenation will vary considerably, from 4–6 cm H_2O for mild ARDS to levels over 20 cm H_2O for more advanced disease. The potential harmful effects of high PEEP include barotrauma, increased pulmonary hypertension, and decreased cardiac output, potentially leading to worse O_2 delivery. Paralysis and sedation often facilitate more effective ventilation. Clinical studies have failed to demonstrate beneficial effects of corticosteroids in treating ARDS. Inotropic support, careful fluid management, prophylaxis against gastrointestinal bleeding, early antibiotic therapy with suspected secondary sepsis, close attention to nutritional needs, and exact guidelines for the onset and duration of mechanical ventilation are important aspects of intensive care unit management of ARDS (see Chapter 9).

Prognosis

Mortality rates of 50–60% are commonly reported. Death is often due to multiple organ system failure associated with secondary infection and progressive respiratory failure. As in the premature newborn who develops BPD, therapeutic efforts to support and treat underlying acute respiratory failure (with hyperoxia and high airway pressure) may paradoxically contribute to subsequent irreversibility or to the progression of the lung injury to chronic stages. Although tracheostomy and prolonged mechanical ventilation are required in some patients with chronic lung disease after the acute course of ARDS, most adults who survive ARDS have little respiratory sequelae at follow-up.

Ashbaugh et al: Acute respiratory distress in adults. *Lancet* 1967;**2**:319.
Demling RH: Role of mediators in human adult respiratory distress syndrome. *J Crit Care* 1988;**3**:56.
Royall JA, Levin DL: Adult respiratory distress syndrome in pediatric patients. 1. Clinical aspects, pathophysiology, pathology, and mechanisms of lung injury. 2. Management. *J Pediatr* 1988;**112**:169,335.

CONGENITAL PULMONARY LYMPHANGIECTASIA

General Considerations

Structurally, congenital pulmonary lymphangiectasia appears as dilated subpleural and interlobular lymphatic channels and may present as part of a generalized lymphangiectasis (in association with obstructive cardiovascular lesions, especially total anomalous pulmonary venous return) or as an isolated, idiopathic lesion. Pathologically, the lung appears firm, bulky, and noncompressible, with prominent cystic lymphatics visible beneath the pleura. On cut section, dilatated lymphatics are present near the hilum, along interlobular septae, around bronchovascular bundles, and beneath the pleura. Histologically, dilatated lymphatics have a thin endothelial cell lining overlying a delicate network of elastin and collagen.

Clinical Findings

Congenital pulmonary lymphangiectasia is a rare, usually fatal disease that generally presents as acute or persistent respiratory distress at birth. Although most patients do not survive the newborn period, some survive longer, and there are isolated case reports of its diagnosis later in childhood. It may be associated with features of Noonan's syndrome, asplenia, total anomalous pulmonary venous return, septal defects, atrioventricularis communis, hypoplastic left heart, aortic arch malformations, and renal malformations. Chylothorax has been reported. Chest x-ray findings include a ''ground glass'' appearance, prominent interstitial markings suggesting lymphatic distention, diffuse hyperlucency of the pulmonary parenchyma, and hyperinflation with depression of the diaphragm.

Prognosis

The outcome is poor. Although the onset of symptoms may be delayed for as long as the first few months of life, prolonged survival is extremely rare; most deaths occur within weeks of birth.

Gardner TW et al: Congenital pulmonary lymphangiectasis. *Clin Pediatr* 1983;**22**:75.
Noonan JA et al: Congenital pulmonary lymphangiectasis. *Am J Dis Child* 1970;**120**:314.

DISORDERS OF THE CHEST WALL

EVENTRATION OF THE DIAPHRAGM

Eventration of the diaphragm is characterized on x-ray film by elevation of part or all of the diaphragm. Degrees of clinical symptomatology vary. Pathologically, the layers of the diaphragm are incompletely formed, with fibrous or loose connective tissue found where striated muscle is normally located. This congenital disorder is thought to represent incomplete formation of the diaphragm in utero. When defects are small, there is no paradoxical movement of the diaphragm and little symptomatology. Small eventrations may be detected on a chest x-ray film taken for another reason. When defects are large, there may or may not be paradoxical movement of the diaphragm, depending upon the nature of the tissue replacing the normal diaphragm.

The degree of respiratory distress depends in large part upon the amount of paradoxical motion of the diaphragm. When the diaphragm moves upward during inspiration, instability of the inferior border of the chest wall increases the work of breathing and can lead to respiratory muscle fatigue. Treatment for respiratory distress is surgical plication, which stabilizes the diaphragm.

The differential diagnosis of an eventration includes phrenic nerve injury and partial diaphragmatic hernia. The former can result from birth or other trauma and may also be seen following cardiac surgery. Usually, only one phrenic nerve is involved. An elevated hemidiaphragm is noted on chest x-ray film, and paradoxical motion of the diaphragm may be seen by fluoroscopy or ultrasound. Often, patients cannot be extubated or have persistent respiratory compromise, particularly with feeding. If symptoms persist for 2–4 weeks, the diaphragm is surgically plicated as described above. Function returns to the diaphragm in about 50% of cases of phrenic nerve injury whether or not plication was performed. Recovery periods of up to 100 days have been reported in these cases.

Obara H et al: Eventration of the diaphragm in infants and children. *Acta Paediatr Scand* 1987;**76**:654. [Compares histologic changes in diaphragm and lung in patients with congenital eventration of the diaphragm and phrenic nerve injury.]

SCOLIOSIS

Scoliosis, or lateral curvature of the spine, can, if uncorrected, lead to severe restrictive lung disease and death from cor pulmonale. Most cases of idiopathic scoliosis occur in adolescent females and are corrected before there is significant pulmonary impairment. Congenital scoliosis of a severe degree or with other major abnormalities carries a more guarded prognosis. Scoliosis may also occur in patients with progressive neuromuscular disease, such as Duchenne's muscular dystrophy, and can be a major contributor to respiratory failure.

DiRocco PJ, Vaccaro P: Cardiopulmonary functioning in adolescent patients with mild idiopathic scoliosis. *Arch Phys Med Rehabil* 1988;**69**:198.
Szeinberg A et al: Forced vital capacity and maximal respiratory pressures in patients with mild and moderate scoliosis. *Pediatr Pulmonol* 1988;**4**:8. [Describes the loss of vital capacity seen in patients with moderate scoliosis.]

PECTUS EXCAVATUM

Pectus excavatum is an anterior depression of the chest wall that may be symmetric or asymmetric with respect to the midline. Reports of exercise testing and pulmonary function testing in patients with pectus excavatum have not clearly demonstrated any marked abnormalities. Therefore, the decision to repair the deformity is usually based on cosmetic considerations. Postoperative care of patients following pectus excavatum requires mechanical ventilation and careful respiratory monitoring because of the weak chest wall following surgery.

Peterson RJ et al: Noninvasive assessment of exercise cardiac function before and after pectus excavatum repair. *J Thorac Cardiovasc Surg* 1985;**90**:251.

PECTUS CARINATUM

Pectus carinatum is a bowing out of the sternum. This problem is usually apparent at birth. In addition, this abnormality may be associated with some systemic diseases such as the mucopolysaccharidoses. As with pectus excavatum, abnormalities of pulmonary function testing in the absence of other disorders is unusual. The decision to repair this deformity is based primarily on cosmetic grounds. Postoperative care similarly requires careful monitoring because of chest wall instability produced by the repair.

Cahill JL, Lees GM, Robertson HT: A summary of preoperative and postoperative cardiorespiratory performance in patients undergoing pectus excavatum and carinatum repair. *J Pediatr Surg* 1984;**19**:430.

NEUROMUSCULAR DISORDERS

Many neuromuscular diseases are associated with chronic or recurrent pulmonary problems secondary to weakness of the respiratory and pharyngeal muscles. These difficulties are manifested as chronic or recurrent pneumonia secondary to aspiration and infection, atelectasis, hypoventilation, and respiratory failure in severe cases. Scoliosis, which frequently accompanies long-standing neuromuscular disorders, may further compromise respiratory function. Typical physical findings include weak cough, decreased air exchange, rales, wheezing, and dullness to percussion. Signs of cor pulmonale (loud pulmonary component to the second heart sound, hepatomegaly, elevated neck veins) may be evident in advanced cases. Chest films generally show small lung volumes. If chronic aspiration is present, increased interstitial infiltrates and areas of atelectasis or consolidation may be present. Arterial blood gases demonstrate hypoxemia in the early stages and compensated respiratory acidosis in the late stages. Typical pulmonary function abnormalities include low lung volumes and decreased inspiratory force generated against an occluded airway. Treatment is supportive and includes vigorous pulmonary toilet, antibiotics with infection, and oxygen to correct hypoxemia. Unfortunately, despite aggressive medical therapy, many neuromuscular conditions progress to respiratory failure and death. The decision to intubate and ventilate is a difficult one; it should be made only when there is real hope that deterioration, though acute, is potentially reversible or when chronic ventilation has been deemed a therapeutic option.

Brooks JG, Swisher CN: Respiratory dysfunction in pediatric neurologic disorders. In: *Respiratory Dysfunction in Primary Neurologic Disease.* Weiner WJ (editor). Futura, 1980.

Gioia FR: Neuromuscular disease and respiratory failure. In: *Textbook of Pediatric Intensive Care.* Rogers MC (editor). Williams & Wilkins, 1987.

DISORDERS OF THE PLEURA AND PLEURAL CAVITY

The pleural membranes cover the outer surface of the lungs (visceral pleura) and the inner surface of the chest wall (parietal pleural). Because they are normally in intimate contact, the "space" between them is more of a potential space. However, disease processes can lead to accumulation of air or fluid in the pleural space. Classically, pleural effusions have been classified as transudates or exudates. Transudates occur when there is imbalance between hydrostatic and oncotic pressure, so that fluid filtration exceeds reabsorption (eg, congestive heart failure). Exudates form as a result of inflammation of the pleural surface leading to increased capillary permeability (eg, parapneumonic effusions). Other forms of pleural effusions include chylothorax and hemothorax.

Thoracentesis is helpful in characterizing the fluid and providing definitive diagnosis. Recovered fluid is considered an exudate (as opposed to a transudate) if any of the following are found: a pleural fluid to serum protein ratio of greater than 0.5, a pleural fluid to serum lactic dehydrogenase (LDH) ratio of greater than 0.6, or a pleural fluid LDH greater than 200 IU. Important additional studies on pleural fluid include cell count; pH and glucose; Gram, acid-fast, and fungal stains; cultures; counterimmune electrophoresis (CIE) for specific organisms; cytology; and, occasionally, amylase.

Sahn SA: Pleural manifestations of pulmonary disease. *Hosp Pract* (March) 1981;**16**:73.

PARAPNEUMONIC EFFUSION & EMPYEMA

General Considerations

Bacterial pneumonia is often accompanied by pleural effusion. Some of these effusions contain infection, and others represent inflammatory reaction to pneumonia. The nomenclature in this area is somewhat confusing. Some use the term empyema for grossly purulent fluid and parapneumonic effusion for nonpurulent fluid. However, it is clear that some nonpurulent effusions will also contain organisms and represent either partially treated or early empyema. Therefore, it is probably best to refer to all effusions associated with pneumonia as parapneumonic effusions, some of which are infectious and some of which are not.

The organism most commonly associated with empyema is *Streptococcus pneumoniae*. Other common organisms include *Haemophilus influenzae* and *Staphylococcus aureus* (formerly the most common). Less common causes are group A streptococcus, gram-negative organisms, and anaerobic organisms. Effusions associated with tuberculosis are almost always sterile and represent an inflammatory reaction.

Clinical Findings

A. Symptoms and Signs: Patients usually present with typical signs of pneumonia, including fever, tachpynea, and cough. In addition, they may have chest pain, decreased breath sounds, and dullness to percussion on the affected side. They may prefer to lie on the affected side. With large effusions, there may be tracheal deviation to the contralateral side.

B. Laboratory Findings: The white blood count will often be elevated with left shift. Blood cultures will sometimes be positive. Tuberculin skin test will be positive in most cases of tuberculosis except when anergy is present or when the disease process is in a very early stage. Thoracentesis reveals findings consistent with an exudate. Pleural fluid cell count usually reveals predominantly polymorphonuclear cells in bacterial disease and lymphocytes in tuberculous effusions. In bacterial disease, the pleural fluid pH and glucose is often low. Although in adults the presence of low pH and glucose necessitates aggressive and thorough drainage procedures, the prognostic significance of these findings in children is not known. Gram stain, cultures, or CIE is often positive for the offending organism.

C. Imaging: The presence of pleural fluid is suggested by a homogeneous density that obscures the underlying lung. Large effusions may cause a shift of the mediastinum to the contralateral side. Small effusions may only blunt the costophrenic angle. Lateral decubitus films may help to detect freely movable fluid by demonstrating a "layering-out" effect. If the fluid is loculated, no such effect is appreciated. Ultrasonography can be extremely valuable in localizing the fluid and detecting loculations, especially when thoracentesis is contemplated.

Treatment & Prognosis

Appropriate intravenous antibiotics for at least 14

days and adequate drainage of the fluid remain the mainstay of therapy. Although there is a trend toward conservative management (no chest tube) of smaller pneumococcal empyemas, most larger effusions require chest tube drainage. More aggressive procedures such as thoracotomy with open drainage or decortication are rarely indicated except for less common causes of this disorder such as group A streptococcus and gram-negative and anaerobic organisms.

Prognosis is related to severity of disease but is generally excellent, with complete or nearly complete recovery expected in most instances.

Foglia RP, Randolph J: Current indications for decortication in the treatment of empyema in children. *J Pediatr Surg* 1987;**22**:28.

McLaughlin FJ et al: Empyema in children: Clinical course and long-term follow-up. *Pediatrics* 1984;**73**:587.

Murphy D, Lockhart CH, Todd JK: Pneumococcal empyema: Outcome of medical management. *Am J Dis Child* 1980;**134**:659.

Solak H, Yuksek T, Solak N: Methods of treatment of childhood empyema in a Turkish university hospital. *Chest* 1987;**92**:517.

HEMOTHORAX

Accumulation of blood in the pleural space can be caused by surgical or accidental trauma, coagulation defects, and pleural or pulmonary tumors. With blunt trauma, hemopneumothorax may be present. Symptoms are related to blood loss and compression of underlying lung parychema. There is some risk of secondary infection resulting in empyema. Drainage of a hemothorax is required when significant compromise of pulmonary function is present, as with hemopneumothorax. In uncomplicated cases, observation is indicated, because blood is readily absorbed spontaneously from the pleural space.

Rowe MI, Marchildon MB: Pediatric trauma. In: *Critical Care: State of the Art.* Vol 2. Shoemaker WC, Thompson WL (editors). Society of Critical Care Medicine, 1981.

CHYLOTHORAX

The accumulation of chyle in the pleural space usually results from accidental or surgical trauma to the thoracic duct. In the newborn, chylothorax can be congenital or secondary to birth trauma. This condition also occurs as a result of superior vena cava obstruction secondary to central venous lines. Symptoms of chylothorax are related to the amount of fluid accumulation and degree of compromise of underlying pulmonary parynchema. Thoracentesis reveals typical milky fluid (unless the patient has been fasting) containing predominantly T lymphocytes.

Treatment should be conservative because many chylothoraces resolve spontaneously. This includes the use of oral feedings with medium-chain triglycerides to reduce lymphatic flow through the thoracic duct. Drainage of chylous effusions should be performed only in the event of respiratory compromise because the fluid often rapidly reaccumulates. Repeated or continuous drainage may lead to protein malnutrition and T cell depression, rendering the patient relatively immunocompromised. If reaccumulation of fluid persists for a prolonged period, surgical ligation of the thoracic duct or sclerosis of the pleural space can be attempted, although the results may be less than satisfactory.

Dhande V, Kattwinkel JA, Alford B: Recurrent bilateral pleural effusions secondary to superior vena cava obstruction as a complication of central venous catheterization. *Pediatrics* 1983;**72**:109.

McWilliams BC, Fan LL, Murphy SA: Transient T-cell depression in post-operative chylothorax. *J Pediatr* 1981; **99**:595.

Puntis JWL, Roberts KD, Handy D: How should chylothorax be managed? *Arch Dis Child* 1987;**62**:593.

PNEUMOTHORAX & RELATED AIR LEAK SYNDROMES

General Considerations

Pneumothorax can occur spontaneously in newborns and in older children or, more commonly, as a result of birth trauma, positive pressure ventilation, underlying obstructive or restrictive lung disease, and rupture of a congenital or acquired lung cyst. Pneumothorax can also occur as an acute complication of tracheostomy. Usually, air dissects from the alveolar spaces into the intersitial spaces of the lung. Migration to the visceral pleura ultimately leads to rupture into the pleural space. Associated conditions include pneumomediastinum, pneumopericardium, pneumoperitoneum, and subcutaneous emphysema. These conditions are more commonly associated with dissection of air into the interstitial spaces of the lung with retrograde dissection along the bronchovascular bundles toward the hilum.

Clinical Findings

A. Symptoms and Signs: The clinical spectrum can vary from patients who are asymptomatic to those with severe respiratory distress. Associated symptoms include cyanosis, chest pain, and dyspnea. Physical examination may reveal decreased breath sounds and hyperresonance to percussion on the affected side with tracheal deviation to the opposite side. When the pneumothorax is under tension, cardiac function may be compromised, resulting in hypotension or narrowing of the pulse pressure. Pneumopericardium is a life-threatening condition that presents with muffled heart tones and shock.

Pneumomediastinum rarely causes symptoms by itself.

B. Imaging: Chest films usually demonstrate the presence of free air in the pleural space. If the pneumothorax is large and under tension, compressive atelectasis of the underlying lung and shift of the mediastinum to the opposite side may be demonstrated. Cross-table lateral and lateral decubitus films can aid in the diagnosis of free air. Pneumopericardium is identified by the presence of air completely surrounding the heart, whereas in patients with pneumomediastinum, the heart and mediatinal structures may be outlined with air but the air does not involve the diaphragmatic cardiac border.

Differential Diagnosis

When a patient on a ventilator acutely deteriorates, one must consider not only tension pneumothorax but also obstruction or dislodgement of the endotracheal tube and failure of the mechanical ventilator. Radiographically, pneumothorax must be distinguished from diaphragmatic hernia, lung cysts, congenital lobar emphysema, and cystic adenomatoid malformation, but this task is usually not difficult.

Treatment

Small or asymptomatic pneumothoraces usually do not require treatment and can be managed with close observation. Larger or symptomatic ones require drainage. Needle aspiration should be used to relieve tension acutely, followed by chest tube placement. Pneumopericardium requires immediate identification and needle aspiration to prevent death, followed by pericardial tube placement.

In older patients with spontaneous pneumothorax, recurrences are common; sclerosing and surgical procedures are required.

Fan LL et al: Giant pulmonary cyst simulating a pneumothorax. *Am J Dis Child* 1988;**142:**189.

Ogata ES et al: Pneumothorax in the respiratory distress syndrome: Incidence and effect on vital signs, blood gases, and pH. *Pediatrics* 1976;**58:**177.

Yaster M, Haller JA: Multiple trauma in the pediatric patient. In: *Textbook of Pediatric Intensive Care.* Rogers MC (editor). Williams & Wilkins, 1987.

DISORDERS OF THE MEDIASTINUM

MEDIASTINITIS

Essentials of Diagnosis

- Toxic child in whom esophageal perforation has occurred.

General Considerations

An acute infection involving the mediastinum in pediatric patients is usually due to perforation of the esophagus secondary to trauma. The trauma may be self-induced (foreign body, puncture injury to the pharynx with a sharp object) or iatrogenic (endoscopy, attempted endotracheal intubation). Spontaneous esophageal perforation leading to mediastinitis can accompany vomiting, but this is rare. In addition, acute suppurative mediastinitis without trauma does occur but is unusual.

Clinical Findings

A. Symptoms and Signs: The early symptoms and signs of an acute mediastinitis may be vague in nature and include the gradual onset of fever, chills, and dysphagia with substernal pain. Dyspnea and cough may also be present. Inspiration may be accompanied by discomfort due to stretching of inflamed mediastinal structures, leading to a pattern of spasmodic or "halting" inspiration. On physical examination, evidence of obstruction of venous return may be present, with substernal pain elicited on palpation of the structures of the thorax. In addition, subcutaneous emphysema may be appreciated in the thoracic and cervical areas.

B. Laboratory Findings and Imaging: The white blood count of the patient with mediastinitis is usually high, with neutrophils and band forms prominent on the differential. The frontal view of the chest x-ray may reveal widening of the upper mediastinum; the lateral view shows anterior displacement of the trachea and the esophagus. Mediastinal emphysema, pleural effusions, and pyopneumothorax may also be present.

Differential Diagnosis

The differential diagnosis includes diseases that lead to the toxic appearance of an infant or child. A primary bacterial pneumonia as well as septicemia must be considered. Retropharyngeal abscesses may also lead to the pattern of respiratory distress seen with a suppurative mediastinitis.

Complications

If not recognized and rapidly treated, this disease can progress rapidly and lead to death. Death may result from the infection or tracheal obstruction. The formation of a mediastinal abscess may also complicate the clinical course of the disease.

Treatment

As soon as the diagnosis is made, parenterally administered broad-spectrum antibiotics need to be given. If significant tracheal obstruction is present, an airway must be provided. Drainage of abscesses in the mediastinum may also be indicated.

Feldman R, Gromisch DS: Acute suppurative mediastinitis. *Am J Dis Child* 1971;**121:**79.

North J, Emanuel B: Mediastinitis in a child caused by performation of pharynx. *Am J Dis Child* 1975;**129:** 962.

Templeton JM: Thoracic emergencies. In: *Textbook of Pediatric Emergency Medicine,* 2nd ed. Fleisher GR, Ludwig S (editors). Williams & Wilkins, 1988.

MEDIASTINAL MASSES

Essentials of Diagnosis

■ Identification of a mass within the mediastinum on radiographic studies.

General Considerations

Mediastinal masses may come to attention because of symptoms produced by pressure on the esophagus, airways, nerves, or vessels within the mediastinum or may be discovered unexpectedly on a routine chest x-ray. Once the mass is identified, localization to one of 4 mediastinal compartments aids in the differential diagnosis (Fig 15–1). The superior mediastinum is the area above the pericardium that is bordered inferiorly by an imaginary line from the manubrium to the fourth thoracic vertebra. The anterior mediastinum is bordered by the sternum anteriorly and the pericardium posteriorly, whereas the posterior mediastinum is defined by the pericardium and diaphragm anteriorly and the lower 8 thoracic vertebrae posteriorly. The middle mediastinum is surrounded by these 3 compartments.

Clinical Findings

A. Symptoms and Signs: When present, respiratory symptoms are due to pressure on an airway and may include cough, wheezing, and complaints consistent with an infectious process caused by partial or complete obstruction of an airway (unresolving pneumonia in one area of lung, bronchitis). Hemoptysis can also occur but is an unusual presenting symptom. Dysphagia may occur secondary to compression of the esophagus. Encroachment of the

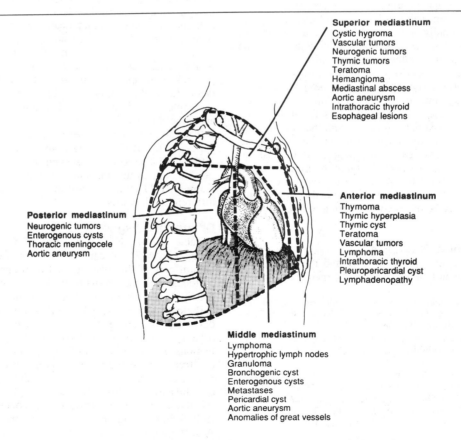

Superior mediastinum
Cystic hygroma
Vascular tumors
Neurogenic tumors
Thymic tumors
Teratoma
Hemangioma
Mediastinal abscess
Aortic aneurysm
Intrathoracic thyroid
Esophageal lesions

Anterior mediastinum
Thymoma
Thymic hyperplasia
Thymic cyst
Teratoma
Vascular tumors
Lymphoma
Intrathoracic thyroid
Pleuropericardial cyst
Lymphadenopathy

Posterior mediastinum
Neurogenic tumors
Enterogenous cysts
Thoracic meningocele
Aortic aneurysm

Middle mediastinum
Lymphoma
Hypertrophic lymph nodes
Granuloma
Bronchogenic cyst
Enterogenous cysts
Metastases
Pericardial cyst
Aortic aneurysm
Anomalies of great vessels

Figure 15–1. Anatomic compartments within the mediastinum. The differential diagnosis for mediastinal masses is based on location within these 4 compartments.

mass on the recurrent largyngeal nerve can cause hoarseness due to paralysis of the left vocal cord. Superior vena caval obstruction can lead to dilatation of neck vessels as well as other signs and symptoms of obstruction of venous return from the upper part of the body (superior mediastinal syndrome).

B. Laboratory Findings and Imaging: The mass is initially defined by frontal and lateral chest x-rays together with thoracic CT scans and, possibly, magnetic resonance imaging. A barium swallow may also help define the extent of a mass. Other studies that may be required include angiograms (to define the blood supply to large tumors), electrocardiogram, echocardiogram, ultrasound of the thorax, fungal and mycobacterial skin tests, and urinary catecholamine assays. A myelogram may be necessary in children suspected of having a neurogenic tumor in the posterior mediastinum.

Differential Diagnosis

The differential diagnosis classified by the mediastinal compartment housing the mass is shown in Fig 15–1. Several general points should be kept in mind. In some series, more than 50% of mediastinal tumors occur in the posterior mediastinum and are mainly neurogenic tumors or enterogenous cysts. Most neurogenic tumors in children less than 4 years of age are malignant (neuroblastoma, neuroganglioblastoma), whereas a benign ganglioneuroma is the most common histologic type in older children. In the middle and anterior mediastinum, tumors of lympathatic origin (lymphomas) are the primary concern. Bulky anterior mediastinal tumors that compress the trachea and the great vessels can lead to a superior mediastinal syndrome, and the children can present difficult diagnostic problems because of anesthesia hazards. Definitive diagnosis in most instances relies on surgery to obtain the mass or a part of the mass for a histologic assessment. In cases of lymphoma, the scalene nodes may also contain tumor and may be biopsied in an attempt to establish a diagnosis.

Treatment & Prognosis

Both the appropriate therapy and the response to therapy depend on the cause of the mediastinal mass.

Brooks JW: Tumors of the chest. In: *Disorders of the Respiratory Tract in Children,* 4th ed. Kendig EL Jr, Chernick V (editors). Saunders, 1983.

Filler RM, Simpson HS, Ein SH: Mediastinal masses in infants and children. *Pediatr Clin North Am* 1979; **26:**677.

Halpern S et al: Anterior mediastinal masses: Anesthesia hazards and other problems. *J Pediatr* 1983;**102:**407.

Templeton JM: Thoracic emergencies. In: *Textbook of Pediatric Emergency Medicine,* 2nd ed. Fleisher GR, Ludwig S (editors). Williams & Wilkins, 1988.

DISORDERS OF THE CONTROL OF BREATHING

ACUTE LIFE-THREATENING EPISODES IN INFANCY (ALTE)

Essentials of Diagnosis

■ A sudden unexpected episode of cyanosis, pallor, or apnea.

General Considerations

A substantial number of infants are brought to medical attention following apparently acute life-threatening episodes (ALTE) of cardiorespiratory instability involving cyanosis, pallor, or apnea. In one-half of cases, a well-recognized medical entity that accounts for the episode can be found after a thorough and careful evaluation. The infants in whom no explanation for the episode can be found are said to have apnea of infancy. Initial interest in these infants was sparked in part by the observation that some died suddenly, leading some to speculate that ALTE may provide a clue to the identification of infants at risk for the sudden infant death syndrome (SIDS). After almost 2 decades of study, the picture emerging is that of a weak relationship between apnea of infancy and SIDS, with only a small percentage of patients with apnea of infancy at risk for sudden death. In addition, only a small percentage of infants succumbing to SIDS have identifiable episodes of apnea beforehand.

The following section describes an approach to the patient with ALTE, taking note of the very broad differential diagnosis in this syndrome and uncertainties in both evaluation and treatment. The clinical features of ALTE are discussed in relationship to the differential diagnosis.

Differential Diagnosis

Table 15–2 lists a classification of disorders associated with ALTE. A careful history is often the most helpful part of the evaluation. Much attention must be focused on the details of the episode or episodes. It is useful to determine whether the infant has been chronically ill or essentially well. A report of several days of poor feeding, temperature instability, or respiratory or gastrointestinal symptoms suggests an infectious process. Reports of ''struggling to breathe'' or ''trying to breathe'' imply airway obstruction. Association of the episodes with feeding implies discoordinated swallowing, gastroesophageal reflux (GER), or airway obstruction. Episodes that typically follow crying may be related to breath holding. Association of episodes with sleeping may also suggest GER or apnea of infancy. Attempts should be made to determine the duration of the episode, but

Table 15–2. Differential diagnosis of acute life-threatening episodes (ALTE).

Infectious	Viral: respiratory syncytial virus and other respiratory viruses Bacterial: sepsis, pertussis
Gastrointestinal	Gastroesphageal reflux with or without obstructive apnea
Respiratory	Airway abnormality: vascular rings, pulmonary slings, tracheomalacia Pneumonia
Neurologic	Seizure disorder CNS infection: meningitis, encephalitis Vasovagal response Leigh's encephalopathy Brain tumor
Cardiovascular	Congenital malformation Arrhythmia Cardiomyopathy
Nonaccidental trauma	Battering Drug overdose Munchausen-by-proxy syndrome
No definable cause	Apnea of infancy

this is often difficult. It is helpful to role-play the episode with the family. Details regarding the measures taken to resuscitate the infant and the infant's recovery from the episode are often useful in determining the severity of the episode.

The physical examination provides further direction in pursuing the differential diagnosis. The presence of fever or hypothermia suggests infection. An altered state of consciousness implies a post-ictal state or drug overdose. Respiratory distress implies cardiac or pulmonary lesions.

Most patients with ALTE are hospitalized for observation in order to reduce stress on the family and allow prompt completion of the evaluation. Laboratory evaluation includes a complete blood count for indications of infection. Serum electrolytes are usually obtained. Elevations in serum bicarbonate suggest chronic hypoventilation, whereas decreases suggest acute acidosis, possibly due to hypoxia during the episode. A chronic acidosis is suggestive of an inherited metabolic disorder. The chest x-ray film is examined for infiltrates suggesting acute infection or chronic aspiration and for cardiac size with respect to intrinsic cardiac disease. An arterial blood gas is helpful in several respects. It provides an initial assessment of the infant's oxygenation and acid-base status. Low Pao_2 or elevated $Paco_2$ (or both) implies cardiorespiratory disease. A significant base deficit suggests that the episode was accompanied by hypoxia or circulatory impairment. On-line oxygen saturation measurements in the hospital assess the infant's oxygenation status during different activities

and are more comprehensive than a single arterial blood gas sample.

Because apnea has been associated with respiratory infections, diagnostic studies for respiratory syncytial virus in particular but also other viruses and pertussis may contribute to the diagnostic process. The apnea seen with infection often precedes other physical findings. If there is any possibility that the episode involved airway obstruction, a barium swallow and air laryngotracheogram should be done. Vascular rings, pulmonary slings, and other intrathoracic lesions impinging upon the trachea are often best demonstrated on barium swallow. The air laryngotracheogram also aids in identifying structural lesions or tracheomalacia. Fiberoptic bronchoscopy may also be used to evaluate the airway. The barium swallow is not done to identify gastroesophageal reflux, because it is presumed that the majority of normal infants demonstrate reflux. If reflux is suspected to be the cause of the apnea, it should be documented by esophageal pH monitoring coupled with respiratory pattern recording. In general, most infants with reflux and apnea can be treated with medical antireflux measures. Those infants with reflux and repeated episodes of apnea may benefit from a surgical antireflux procedure.

There are several neurologic causes of ALTE. Apnea as the sole manifestation of a seizure disorder is unusual but may occur. In cases of repeated episodes, 24-hour EEG monitoring may be helpful in detecting a seizure disorder. Leigh syndrome, a brain stem disorder characterized pathologically by neuronal dropout, may present with apneic episodes.

Apneic episodes have been linked to child abuse in several ways. Head injury following nonaccidental trauma may be first brought to medical attention because of apnea. Other signs of abuse are usually immediately apparent in these cases. Drug overdose, either accidental (eg, mistakes in application of anticolic medications containing barbiturates) or intentional, may also present with apnea. Several series document that apneic episodes may be falsely reported by parents seeking attention—one of the instances of Munchausen-by-proxy syndrome. In addition, parents may physically interfere with respiratory efforts. Pinch marks on the nares are sometimes found in these cases.

Treatment

If an underlying cause is found, therapy in ALTE is directed at the cause. After blood cultures are taken, antibiotics should be administered to those infants appearing toxic. Seizure disorders are treated with anticonvulsants. Vascular rings and pulmonary slings must be corrected surgically because of severe morbidity and mortality in uncorrected cases.

The approach to care in apnea of infancy is controversial. These are infants presenting with ALTE who have no definable cause for the episode. Treatment in this group of patients has centered around the use of electronic monitors for the detection of apnea or bradycardia in the home. Parents are then taught cardiopulmonary resuscitation so that they may intervene in the event of a serious episode. The rationale for the use of monitors implies that infants who are at risk for subsequent severe episodes can be identified. Medical personnel have made a number of attempts to predict which of these infants are at risk for subsequent severe episodes. These attempts have included hypoxic and hypercarbic challenges and determinations of the frequency of periodic breathing or apnea, usually through the use of pneumograms. None of these techniques is sufficiently specific or selective to be useful in prediction. In addition, the efficacy of home monitoring has never been demonstrated in controlled trials.

The decision to monitor these infants involves the participation of the family as well as the physician. Infants with severe initial episodes or repeated severe episodes are now thought to be at significant increased risk for sudden death and should probably be monitored in the home despite the uncertainty of their effectiveness of this step. Episodes in these children are so severe that the parents want to know their infant's condition at all times. Monitoring is not indicated in patients who have isolated episodes of less severity unless the parents express a clear wish for it. Pneumograms can be used to determine whether apnea is occurring if there is uncertainty. However, pneumograms are not predictive and play no role in the decision to monitor or when to stop monitoring. Discontinuing the monitor is usually based on the infant's ability to go several months without triggering the alarm. Theophylline has been suggested as a treatment for apnea of infancy, but controlled trials are lacking; at this point, it is not recommended.

Kahn A, Montauk L, Blum D: Diagnostic categories in infants referred for an acute event suggesting near-miss SIDS. *Eur J Pediatr* 1987;**146**:458. [Study of a large number of patients illustrating the breadth of the differential diagnosis in ALTE.]

National Institutes of Health Consensus Development Conference Statement: Infantile apnea and home monitoring. Sept 29 to Oct 1, 1986. *Pediatrics* 1987;**79**:292. [This report defines ALTEs and apnea of infancy, describes the limitations of pneumograms, and provides recommendations for home monitoring.]

Southall DP: Role of apnea in the sudden infant death syndrome: A personal view. *Pediatrics* 1988;**81**:73. [Examines the potential role of apnea in the sudden infant death syndrome and points out limitations in the links between the 2 diseases.]

SUDDEN INFANT DEATH SYNDROME

Essentials of Diagnosis

- Sudden and unexpected death in infancy.
- Adequate post mortem examination excluding known causes of death.

General Considerations

The sudden infant death syndrome (SIDS) is a poorly understood disorder encompassing cases of sudden and unexpected death of previously well or nearly well infants that remain unexplained after an adequate postmortem examination. The postmortem examination is an important feature of the definition because approximately 20% of cases of sudden death can be explained by autopsy findings. The incidence of SIDS in the United States (1–2:1000) makes it the leading cause of death in infancy outside the neonatal period. The overall incidence of SIDS has steadily declined over the past few decades.

Epidemiologic and pathologic data constitute most of what is known about SIDS. The number of deaths peaks at age 2 months, and most deaths occur in infants a few weeks of age to 6 months of age. There is an increase in deaths during the peak respiratory virus season, and most deaths occur between midnight and 8:00 A.M. The syndrome is more common among minorities and socioeconomically disadvantaged populations. There is a 3:2 male predominance in most series. Other risk factors include low birth weight, teenage or drug-addicted mothers, maternal smoking, and a family history of SIDS. Most of these risk factors are associated with a 2- or 3-fold elevation of incidence but are not specific enough to be useful in predicting which infants will die unexpectedly. Recent immunization is not a risk factor.

The most consistent pathologic findings are intrathoracic petechiae and mild inflammation and congestion of the respiratory tract. Subtler pathologic findings include brain stem gliosis, extramedullary hematopoiesis, and increases in periadrenal brown fat. These latter findings suggest that infants who succumb to SIDS have had intermittent or chronic hypoxia before death.

The mechanism or mechanisms of death in SIDS are unknown. For example, it is not known whether the initiating event at the time of death is cessation of breathing or cardiac dysrhythmia or asystole. Hypotheses put forth have included upper airway obstruction, catecholamine excess, brain stem immaturity or injury, and increased fetal hemoglobin. It has been recognized that some infants who presented with apneic episodes subsequently died from SIDS; however, study of these infants and prospective studies of large numbers of newborns have indicated that most infants with apnea do not die from SIDS and that most infants with SIDS have no identifiable episodes of apnea (see discussion of ALTE).

A history of mild symptoms of upper respiratory infection before death is not uncommon, and SIDS victims are sometimes seen by physicians the day or so before death. When infants are discovered blue, cold, and motionless by parents or caretakers they are most commonly taken to the emergency room, where resuscitative efforts are almost uniformly to no avail. Families must then be supported following the death. The National Sudden Infant Death Syndrome Foundation provides information about psychosocial support groups and counseling for families of SIDS victims. The postmortem examination can be of value to the family; when the diagnosis of SIDS is established, lingering questions about other possible causes of death are resolved. For this reason, as well as for ascertaining causes of death in infancy, the postmortem examination should always be recommended. Some recent reports have suggested that a death scene investigation may also be important in determining the cause of sudden, unexpected deaths in infancy.

Bentele KH, Albani M: Are there tests predictive for prolonged apnoea in SIDS? A review of epidemiological and function studies. *Acta Paediatr Scand* [**Suppl**] 1988;**342**:1. [Comprehensive review of attempts to predict infants at risk for SIDS, with the conclusion that no physiologic testing at this time is predictive of SIDS.]

Giulian GG, Gilbert EF, Moss RL: Elevated fetal hemoglobin levels in sudden infant death syndrome. *N Engl J Med* 1987;**316**:1122.

Hoffman HJ et al: Risk factors for SIDS: Results of the National Institute of Child Health and Human Development SIDS Cooperative Epdemiological Study. *Ann N Y Acad Sci* 1988;**533**:13.

Southall DP, Talbert DG: Mechanisms for abnormal apnea of possible relevance to the sudden infant death syndrome. *Ann N Y Acad Sci* 1988;**533**:329.

Valdes-Dapena M: A pathologist's perspective on possible mechanisms in SIDS. *Ann N Y Acad Sci* 1988;**533**:31.

ADDENDUM: CYSTIC FIBROSIS

The cystic fibrosis gene has recently been located. The area of interest on the long arm of human chromosome 7 spans approximately 250,000 base pairs of genomic DNA. Its messenger RNA codes for a 1,480 amino acid protein, the cystic fibrosis transmembrane regulator (CFTR). The function of CFTR is presently undefined but the subject of intense investigation. Approximately 75 percent of the mutations in cystic fibrosis patients correspond to a specific deletion of three base pairs which results in the loss of a phenylalanine residue at amino acid position 508 of the putative product of the cystic fibrosis gene. The remainder of the CF mutant gene pool consists of multiple, different mutations.

Iannuzzi MC, Collins FS: Reverse genetics and cystic fibrosis. *Am J Respir Cell Mol Biol* 1990;**2**:309.

Kerem B-S et al: Identification of the cystic fibrosis gene: Genetic analysis. *Science* 1989;**245**:1073.

Riordan JR et al: Identification of the cystic fibrosis gene: Cloning and characterization of complementary DNA. *Science* 1989;**245**:1066.

Rommens JM et al: Identification of the cystic fibrosis gene: Chromosome walking and jumping. *Science* 1989;**245**:1059.

16 Cardiovascular Diseases

Robert R. Wolfe, MD, & James W. Wiggins, Jr, MD

Cardiovascular disease is a significant cause of death and chronic illness in the pediatric population. In North America, more than 1% of newborn infants have congenital heart disease, usually due to multifactorial causes. It is becoming obvious that the prevention of adult heart disease must begin in childhood (eg, prevention of atherosclerosis by diet modification). Preventive medicine is the most important aspect of pediatric practice; indeed, the goal of prevention pervades all aspects of cardiovascular disease. But prevention requires an understanding of the causes of disease, and in this there are wide discrepancies, ranging from significant accomplishments in the case of rheumatic fever to the very tentative steps being taken to understand the causes of congenital heart disease, atherosclerosis, and essential hypertension.

CLUES TO THE PRESENCE OF HEART DISEASE

Although there are traditional signs and symptoms suggesting the presence of heart disease in an infant or child, it is necessary to know how to weigh clinical findings to determine which are significant and require immediate attention and which are insignificant. The presence of a heart murmur, for example, may suggest the possibility of heart disease in an infant, or the murmur may be a functional or innocent murmur (see p 414). Not all serious cardiovascular disorders are accompanied by an easily detectable murmur.

The most important clues to the presence of heart disease requiring prompt attention are congestive heart failure and cyanosis. These clinical conditions will be discussed in more detail in subsequent sections.

DIAGNOSTIC EVALUATION

Sequence of evaluation:
(1) History
(2) Physical examination

(3) Electrocardiogram
(4) Chest x-ray
(5) Echocardiogram
(6) Cardiac catheterization (with angiography)

HISTORY

In obtaining the history from the family or the patient, one must keep in perspective the age and relative activity of that patient. A history of increasing feeding difficulties and diaphoresis is the most common feature of early congestive heart failure.

Family History
Because most cardiac diseases are familial, one of the first clues to the cause of cardiovascular disease in the child is a history of heart disease in a first-degree relative. A careful history should include details of early adult cardiovascular problems. These details might suggest the need to evaluate the child for hyperlipidemia.

Pregnancy
The history of pregnancy should elicit information regarding first-trimester exposure to illness or medications, which places infants at high risk for congenital heart disease. A history of significant problems related to labor and delivery, such as perinatal stress or asphyxia at birth, suggests causes of myocardial dysfunction in the neonate.

Growth & Development
Major cardiac problems frequently affect a child's ability to grow. There may be a history of poor feeding (early fatigue, vomiting, lethargy) or of failure to thrive despite adequate caloric intake. Gross motor development may also be delayed in children with significant congestive heart failure or cyanosis, although other aspects of development are less frequently affected.

Tachypnea
Parents frequently notice rapid or abnormal breathing in the child. Although infants at rest rarely breathe faster than 40 respirations per minute, infants in congestive heart failure usually have respiratory rates in excess of 60 (and often as rapid as

80–100). Tachypnea may be considered the cardinal sign of left-sided heart failure in the pediatric patient.

Cyanosis

The physiologic basis of cyanosis and the medical and surgical approaches to the cyanotic patient will be discussed later. What should be noted here is that, curiously, many parents do not readily recognize cyanosis—nor do many physicians. The infant with a cyanotic heart lesion may be more gray than blue (and may have no heart murmur). Cyanotic heart disease may go unrecognized because of lack of appreciation of the subtleties of diagnosing cyanosis.

Hypoxemic Spells

It is important to determine if the patient with a cyanotic heart lesion such as tetralogy of Fallot is having hypoxemic spells, because prompt surgical intervention may be required. These spells usually occur on morning awakening or after a feeding or bowel movement; the infant begins breathing fast, becomes progressively more gray or blue, and cries as if having severe pain. Such a spell rarely may progress to unconsciousness, paresis, or even death.

Other Clinical Clues

Orthopnea, dyspnea, easy fatigability, growth failure, sweating, squatting, and pneumonia are frequent clues to the presence of various forms of heart disease.

PHYSICAL EXAMINATION

Careful and thorough examination of the patient frequently offers the best clues to significant cardiac problems. A systematic approach to the entire child will frequently lead to the probable diagnosis. The presence of other congenital abnormalities, particularly chromosomal disorders, increases the probability of congenital heart disease.

The examination should begin with a careful general inspection to note activity (agitation, lethargy) and skin perfusion and color. Vital signs, including temperature, pulse rate, respiratory rate, and particularly blood pressure (in all 4 extremities in symptomatic infants), can reflect the overall status of the patient. Auscultation of the heart and lungs should be performed early in the overall examination, because the infant's crying limits the physician's ability to hear even pronounced cardiac sounds. Abdominal examination for position and size of organs is also important.

1. CARDIOVASCULAR EXAMINATION

Inspection & Palpation

Conformation of the chest can give clues to past or present cardiomegaly. Prominence of the precordial chest wall is frequently seen in infants and children with cardiomegaly. Increased cardiac activity is often noted on inspection.

Palpation may reveal the presence of precordial activity, right ventricular lift, or left-sided heave; a diffuse point of maximal impulse; or the presence of a thrill due to a loud murmur. Thrills are typically located where the murmur is most intense and can sometimes be felt at the point of radiation, as in a suprasternal notch or carotid thrill with aortic stenosis. In patients with severe pulmonary hypertension, palpable pulmonary closure is frequently noted, usually at the mid to upper left sternal border.

Auscultation

To detect and differentiate abnormal heart sounds, one must be familiar with the pattern and timing of normal heart sounds.

A. Normal Heart Sounds: S_1 (the first heart sound) is the sound of atrioventricular valve closure. It is best heard at the lower left sternal border and is usually medium-pitched. Although 4 components of S_1 can be detected by phonocardiography, only one or 2 of these are usually heard when a stethoscope is used.

S_2 (the second heart sound) is the sound of semilunar valve closure. It has a higher pitch than S_1 and is best heard along the lower and upper left sternal border. S_2 has 2 component sounds, A_2 and P_2 (aortic and pulmonary valve closure). A_2 is best appreciated at the mid and lower left sternal border, whereas P_2 is best heard at the upper left sternal border and is normally softer than A_2. Splitting of S_2 varies with respirations, widening with inspiration and narrowing with expiration, and is best heard at the second left intercostal space at the sternal border.

S_3 (the third heart sound) is the sound of rapid filling of the left ventricle. It occurs in early diastole, after S_2, and is a medium- to low-pitched thud. When heard in normal children, the sound will diminish or disappear when there is a change from the supine to the sitting or standing position; it is usually also intermittent.

S_4 (the fourth heart sound) is associated with atrial contraction and increased atrial pressure and has a low pitch similar to that of S_3. It occurs just prior to S_1 and is not normally audible.

B. Abnormal Heart Sounds: Findings of abnormalities in splitting or intensity of the component sounds of S_2 can be helpful in the diagnosis of major heart problems. With inspiration, there is a decrease in the intrathoracic pressure; this decrease causes increased filling of the right side of the heart, thereby prolonging the ejection time and delaying closure of the pulmonary valve. Normal intrathoracic pressure changes have little effect on the filling of the left side of the heart. Widening of splitting can be a clue to right-sided volume overload, whereas narrowing may indicate increased pulmonary artery pressure. A single S_2 is often heard in cases of malposition of the great vessels or severe pulmonary hypertension.

Ejection clicks are high-pitched and are usually related to dilated great vessels or valve abnormalities (or both). They can be heard throughout the ventricular systole and are classified as early, mid, or late. Early ejection clicks at the upper left sternal border are usually of pulmonary origin. Aortic clicks are heard in a wider distribution but best at the apex. Widespread clicks originating or loudest at the apex can be mitral or aortic in origin. The mid to late ejection click at the apex is most typically mitral valve prolapse. Early clicks may also be heard in spontaneous closure of ventricular septal defects.

S_3 can be a functional sound in childhood, although it often is associated with cardiac abnormalities.

S_4 is not normally audible; its finding on auscultation is almost always associated with cardiac abnormalities.

C. Murmurs: Murmurs are the most common cardiovascular finding. The presence of a murmur in a child almost always causes alarm in the parents, who associate murmurs with major heart disease. However, most children have murmurs, and, fortunately, these are usually normal functional or innocent murmurs.

1. Characteristics—Murmurs can be evaluated on the basis of the following characteristics:

a. Location and radiation—Where the murmur is best heard and where the sound extends.

b. Relationship to cardiac cycle and duration—Systolic (with the pulse), diastolic, continuous, or to-and-fro.

c. Intensity—Classified as grade I, soft and heard with difficulty; grade II, soft but easily heard; grade III, loud but without a thrill; grade IV, loud and associated with a precordial thrill; grade V, loud, with thrill, and audible with the edge of the stethoscope; or grade VI, very loud and audible with the stethoscope off the chest or with the naked ear.

d. Quality—Harsh, musical, or rough; high, medium, or low in pitch.

e. Variation with position—Audible when patient is supine, sitting, standing, or squatting.

2. Functional murmurs—Most functional murmurs change or disappear with a change in position. The 7 most common functional murmurs heard in childhood can be classified as follows:

a. Newborn murmur—As the name implies, this murmur is frequently heard within the first few days of life. Typically, it is located at the lower left sternal border, without significant radiation. Newborn murmur is a soft, short, vibratory grade I–II/VI early systolic murmur that often subsides when mild pressure is applied to the abdomen. Newborn murmur usually disappears by 2–3 weeks of age.

b. Functional murmur of peripheral arterial pulmonary stenosis—This murmur is frequently heard in the premature infant, often after closure of a patent ductus arteriosus. It is secondary to branching of the pulmonary artery. Typically, the murmur is heard with equal intensity at the upper left sternal border, back, and in both axillas. It is a soft, short, high-pitched, grade I–II/VI systolic ejection murmur and usually disappears by 6 months of life. This murmur must be differentiated from true peripheral arterial pulmonary stenosis (rubella syndrome), coarctation of the thoracic aorta, valvular pulmonary stenosis, and atrial septal defect. These entities should, however, have other findings to suggest their organic nature.

c. Still's murmur—Probably the most common murmur of early childhood, this murmur can be heard in infancy, although it is most typically heard from the age of 2 years until adolescence. Classically, Still's murmur is loudest midway between the apex and the lower left sternal border, and often it may be transmitted (depending on loudness) to the remainder of the precordial area. Still's murmur is a musical or vibratory, short, high-pitched, grade I–III early systolic ejection murmur. It is loudest when the patient is in the supine position; it diminishes or disappears when the patient sits or stands or during Valsalva's maneuver. Still's murmur may be louder in patients with fever or tachycardia.

d. Pulmonary outflow ejection murmur—This murmur may be heard throughout childhood. It is usually a soft, short, systolic ejection murmur, grade I–II in intensity and well localized to the upper left sternal border. The murmur becomes louder when the patient is in the supine position or when cardiac output is increased and softens with standing or during Valsalva's maneuver. Pulmonary outflow ejection murmur must be differentiated from other murmurs, such as that of pulmonary stenosis, which radiates to the back and has an associated click; atrial septal defect, which is characterized by a persistently split S_2 and tricuspid flow rumble; and peripheral arterial pulmonary stenosis, which is transmitted throughout the entire chest.

e. Venous hum—This very common murmur of childhood is usually heard after 3 years of age. The murmur is located at the upper right and left sternal borders and in the lower neck. It is described as a continuous musical hum of grade I–II intensity, and it may be accentuated in diastole and with inspiration. This murmur always disappears when the patient is placed in a supine position or when the jugular vein is compressed. Venous hum is thought to be produced by turbulence in the subclavian and jugular veins.

f. Innominate or carotid bruit—This murmur is more common in the older child and adolescent. It is heard in the right supraclavicular and neck areas. This is a long systolic ejection murmur, somewhat harsh and of grade II–III intensity. The bruit can be accentuated by light pressure on the carotid artery and must be differentiated from all types of aortic stenosis.

g. Hemic murmur—Hemic murmurs are heard whenever anemia, fever, stress, or any increase in cardiac output is present. Typically, they are heard best in the aortic and pulmonary areas. These systolic ejection murmurs are of grade I–II intensity and are high-pitched. They disappear with normalization of cardiac output.

Frequently, an experienced listener is able to ascertain that a murmur is functional without performing extensive and expensive laboratory evaluations. When functional murmurs are found in a child, the physician should assure the parents that these are normal heart sounds of the developing child and that they represent no abnormality of the heart.

3. Organic murmurs—Organic murmurs are evaluated on the basis of the characteristics outlined above (location, intensity, etc). These murmurs will be discussed in relationship to specific lesions later in this chapter.

2. NONCARDIAC EXAMINATION

Arterial Pulse

A. Rate and Rhythm: Cardiac rate and rhythm are usually determined by palpation of the radial or brachial pulse. Throughout infancy and childhood, the rate is subject to great variation. Multiple determinations must be made under properly evaluated conditions before conclusions can be drawn about their significance. This cautious approach is particularly important in infants.

Marked variations in heart rate occur with activity; therefore, the resting heart rate may be most accurately determined during sleep. In older children, exercise and emotional factors have a marked effect upon the heart rate. All of these factors should be taken into account when examining the child, because many children are apprehensive and may react emotionally to the initial phases of the examination. It is possible for normal infants to have heart rates of 180 or 190 during the activity associated with a physical or electrocardiographic examination. Average resting heart rates range from 120 in infants to 80 in older children.

In the pediatric age group, the rhythm may be regular, or there may be a phasic variation in the heart rate (sinus dysrhythmia). Variations occasionally occur without relation to the respiratory cycle. Sinus dysrhythmia is a normal finding.

B. Quality and Amplitude of Pulse: Examination of the cardiovascular system should always include a careful examination and comparison of the pulses of the upper and lower extremities. A bounding pulse is characteristic of patent ductus arteriosus or aortic regurgitation. Narrow or thready pulses are

found in patients with congestive heart failure or severe aortic stenosis.

Examination of the suprasternal notch should always be included. A visible pulsation in the suprasternal notch is usually abnormal, although it may be seen in patients who are emotionally excited. A prominent pulsation is found in aortic insufficiency, patent ductus arteriosus, and coarctation of the aorta. A palpable thrill in the suprasternal notch is characteristic of aortic stenosis and is occasionally found with valvular pulmonary stenosis, coarctation of the aorta, and patent ductus arteriosus.

Assessment of the femoral pulse is an essential part of the physical examination of every infant and child. The femoral pulse should be readily palpable and equal in amplitude and time of appearance with the brachial pulse. A femoral pulse that is absent or weak or one that is delayed in comparison with the brachial pulse suggests coarctation of the aorta. An absent or diminished femoral pulse may be the only clue to the cause of a life-threatening problem.

Arterial Blood Pressure

Blood pressures should be obtained in the upper and lower extremities. Systolic pressure in the lower extremities determined by the auscultatory technique is usually higher than that found in the upper extremities in patients *over age 1 year*. In normal infants, the pressure in the arms may be higher. The cuff must cover the same relative area of the arm and leg; for this reason, a larger cuff usually must be used for the leg than for the arm.

A. Procedures: Because of variation of blood pressure with respiration and slower rhythmic variations (Mayer or Traube-Hering waves), pressure obtained by any method should be repeated several times.

1. Auscultatory method—The auditory recognition of Korotkoff's sounds by means of a stethoscope and sphygmomanometer is the most commonly used method of obtaining blood pressure in children and correlates well with direct intra-arterial measurements. However, despite its widespread application as the standard method of indirect blood pressure measurement, many factors grossly affect its accuracy. Among these are the dimensions of the inflatable bag within the cuff. The length of the bag should be 100% and the width 50% of the circumference of the limb. A cuff that is too narrow or too short will produce a blood pressure reading that is higher than the true pressure.

2. Palpatory method—This method can be used when the application of a stethoscope head to a small limb is awkward or impossible. Palpation of the pulse characteristics distal to the occluding cuff provides an approximation of the systolic blood pressure in the infant.

3. Flush method—The flush method is also useful in small infants. The distal foot or hand is blanched by manual squeezing or application of an elastic bandage, and the cuff is inflated above the systolic pressure. The extremity is then observed as the cuff pressure is slowly reduced. The observed flush corresponds to a value approximating that of the systolic pressure. A useful technique for assessing coarctation of the aorta is to apply the cuffs to the upper and lower extremities simultaneously and observe flushing.

4. Doppler ultrasonic method—The combination of a small ultrasound transducer and a sphygmomanometer has proved to be especially applicable to the small infant. Considerations of cuff dimensions are still critical, however.

B. Pulse Pressure: Pulse pressure is determined by subtracting the diastolic pressure from the systolic pressure. Normally, the pulse pressure is less than 50 mm Hg or less than half the systolic pressure. A widened pulse pressure (which is associated with a bounding pulse) is present in aorticopulmonary shunt (eg, patent ductus arteriosus), aortic insufficiency, fever, anemia, and complete heart block. A narrow pulse pressure is seen in congestive heart failure, severe aortic stenosis, and pericardial tamponade.

Venous Pressure & Pulse

The level of the distended jugular vein above the suprasternal notch when the patient is at a 45-degree angle is a determinant of venous pressure in older children and adults. Normally, one may observe the level of the transition between collapse and distention of the jugular vein approximately 1–2 cm above the notch. This technique frequently is not too helpful in examining infants and young children, however, because their necks are short and fat. In addition to the level of the pulse, the wave pattern should be observed. Two waves can frequently be seen: (1) The *a* wave, due to right atrial contraction, is a rather sharply rising wave and therefore occurs immediately before or with the first heart sound or point of maximum impulse. (2) The *v* wave, caused by filling of the right atrium during ventricular systole, is a more slowly rising wave and occurs toward the end of ventricular systole.

Extremities

Cyanosis of the extremities usually indicates congenital heart disease, but severe pulmonary disease must be excluded. Cyanosis is characterized by a bluish discoloration of the nails, but the entire distal portion of the extremity may be involved.

A. Clubbing of Fingers and Toes: Clubbing implies fairly severe cyanotic congenital heart disease. It usually does not appear until approximately age 1, although occasionally, in patients with severe cyanosis, it may occur earlier. The first sign of clubbing is softening of the nail beds, followed by rounding of the fingernails and then by thickening

and shininess of the terminal phalanx, with loss of creases.

Cyanosis is by far the most common cause, but clubbing occurs also in patients with infective endocarditis, severe liver disease, and lung abscess.

B. Edema: Edema of the lower extremities is characteristic of right ventricular heart failure in older children and adults. However, in infants and younger children, peripheral edema is more likely to affect first the face, then the presacral region, and eventually the extremities.

Abdomen

Hepatomegaly is the cardinal sign of right heart failure in the infant and child. Presystolic pulsation of the liver may occur with right atrial hypertension and systolic pulsation with tricuspid insufficiency. Congestive splenomegaly may be present in patients who have had long-standing congestive heart failure. Enlargement of the spleen is one of the characteristic features of subacute infective endocarditis. Ascites is occasionally present in right heart failure.

Nelson WP, Egbert AM: How to measure blood pressure accurately. *Primary Cardiol* (Sept) 1984;**10**:14.

Nora JJ: Etiologic aspects of heart diseases. Chap 1, pp 2–10, in: *Heart Disease in Infants, Children, and Adolescents.* 3rd ed. Adams FH, Emmanouilides GC (editors). Williams & Wilkins, 1983.

Rosenthal A: How to distinguish between innocent and pathologic murmurs in childhood. *Pediatr Clin North Am* 1984;**31**:1229.

ELECTROCARDIOGRAM & VECTORCARDIOGRAM (ECG & VCG)

Certainly the ECG is to be considered an essential part of the evaluation of the cardiovascular system, and frequently the information gained from this study is very useful. The ECG is the sine qua non for the diagnosis of dysrhythmias and may offer the best clue to the specific diagnosis of congenital lesions (eg, left axis deviation in a blue baby, suggesting tricuspid atresia). Conversely, the ECG may provide little or no help (as in assessing right ventricular hypertrophy in the newborn or left ventricular hypertrophy in the child with congenital aortic stenosis).

It is not possible, within the limitations of this presentation, to teach the interpretation of the ECG, but a few basic facts and definitions should help to orient the student.

A. Propagation of Electrical Force: As shown in Fig 16–1, a wave of electrical force traveling toward an electrode inscribes a positive (upward) deflection; away from an electrode, a negative deflection; and perpendicular to an electrode, a low-voltage, isodiphasic complex. These forces are inscribed as loops on the VCG, and abnormalities are manifested as alterations in direction and duration of force or as increased or decreased electrical force

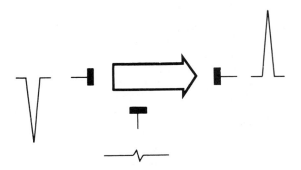

Figure 16–1. Depolarization of the myocardium. The arrow represents the wave of electrical force. As it travels toward the electrode, it inscribes a positive (upward) deflection; away from the electrode, a negative (downward) delfection; perpendicular to the electrode, a low-voltage, isodiphasic deflection.

(amplitude of QRS complex on ECG or loop on VCG).

B. Age-Related Variations: The ECG and VCG evolve with the age of the patient. The rate gradually decreases and intervals generally increase with age. There is also progressive change in dominance of ventricles from right ventricular dominance in the young infant to left ventricular dominance in the older infant, child, and adult. The normal ECG of the 1-week-old would be highly abnormal for a 1-year-old, and the ECG of a 5-year-old would not be normal for an adult.

C. ECG Interpretation: Fig 16–2 defines the events recorded on the ECG. The sequence of recording the findings of the ECG is usually as follows: rate, rhythm, P wave, PR interval, QRS complex (including axis, amplitude, and duration), QT interval, ST segment, T wave, and impression.

1. Rate—The paper speed at which ECGs are usually taken is 25 mm/s. Each small square is 1 mm and each large square 5 mm. Therefore, 5 large squares represent 1 second, one large square 0.2 second, and one small square 0.04 second. A common method of estimating the ventricular rate is to count the number of large squares between 2 QRS complexes: If QRS complexes appear at a rate of one per large square (5/s), the ventricular rate is 300; if QRS complexes appear every 2 squares, the ventricular rate is 150, etc. The formula is to divide the number of large squares between QRS complexes into 300 and roughly interpolate for fractions of large squares.

2. Rhythm—Cardiac rhythm is a difficult subject that does not yield easily to oversimplification. However, a working definition of normal sinus rhythm must be offered even if it is not entirely satisfactory: a normal P wave followed by a normal PR interval and a normal QRS complex.

3. P wave—The P wave represents atrial depolar-

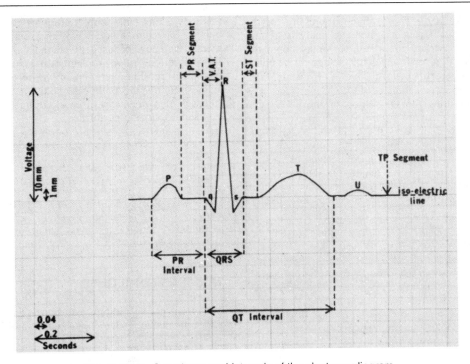

Figure 16–2. Complexes and intervals of the electrocardiogram.

ization. In the pediatric patient, it is normally not taller than 2.5 mm or more than 0.08 second in duration.

4. PR Interval—This interval is measured from the beginning of the P wave to the beginning of the QRS complex. It increases with age and with slower rates. The PR interval ranges from a minimum of 0.11 second in infants to a maximum of 0.18 second in older children with slow rates. The PR interval is commonly prolonged in rheumatic heart disease and by digitalis.

5. QRS complex—This represents ventricular depolarization, and its amplitude and direction of force (axis) reveal the relative size of (viable) ventricular mass in hypertrophy, hypoplasia, and infarction. Abnormal ventricular conduction (eg, right bundle branch block, anterior fascicular block) is also revealed. Interpretation of the QRS complex is one of the most important aspects of cardiologic diagnosis.

6. QT Interval—This interval is measured from the beginning of the QRS complex to the end of the T wave. The QT duration is affected by drugs such as digitalis and electrolyte imbalances such as hypocalcemia and hypokalemia (really QU interval prolongation). The normal duration is rate-related.

7. ST segment—This short segment lying between the end of the QRS complex and the beginning of the T wave is affected by drugs and electrolyte imbalances and reflects myocardial injury.

8. T wave—The T wave represents myocardial repolarization and is altered by electrolytes, myocardial hypertrophy, and ischemia.

9. Impression—The ultimate impression of the ECG is derived from a systematic analysis of features such as those described above as compared with expected normal values for the age of the child.

D. VCG Interpretation: The VCG reveals much of the same information as the ECG. In fact, it is possible to draw the QRS loop of the VCG with considerable accuracy from QRS complexes of the ECG. Fig 16–3 displays the ECG and VCG of the same patient. The vector interpretation of the ECG (eg, direction and shape of loop) derived by looking at the ECG is perhaps the major contribution of vectorcardiography. It is usually not necessary to obtain an actual VCG to know what the loops look like.

Garson A Jr, Gillette PC, McNamara DC: *A Guide to Cardiac Dysrhythmias in Children.* Grune & Stratton, 1980.
Goldman MJ: *Principles of Clinical Electrocardiography,* 12th ed. Lange, 1986.
Liebman J, Plonsey R, Gillette PC: *Pediatric Electrocardiography.* Williams & Wilkins, 1982.

CHEST X-RAY

The chest x-ray, along with all other tests performed in pediatric patients, requires systematic

evaluation. Accurate conclusions about the presence or absence of congenital heart defects and bone abnormalities can only be drawn if the proper procedures were followed—eg, the penetration of x-ray was adequate, and the films were obtained on adequate inspiration (distortions due to inadequate inspiration may look like cardiomegaly and increased vascular markings). The size of the heart, as seen on the chest x-ray film, must be evaluated in relationship to the age and size of the patient. Chest films of the normal newborn will show a greater heart size and more pronounced vascular markings than those of the normal older child. These factors must all be taken into consideration in evaluating heart size and configuration and lung fields. The standard posteroanterior and left lateral chest films are usually adequate for this evaluation (Fig 16–4). If there is suspicion of vascular ring or mediastinal mass, multiple-view films with barium swallow are indicated.

Daves ML: *Cardiac Roentgenology.* Year Book, 1981.

ECHOCARDIOGRAPHY & DOPPLER ULTRASONOGRAPHY

Echocardiography is now the major noninvasive method for diagnosis of congenital heart defects and is used to define anatomy, function, chamber and vessel size, and valve abnormalities. The use of M mode and 2-dimensional echocardiography will in most instances allow accurate diagnosis. These methods, along with doppler ultrasonography (color, pulsed, or continuous wave ultrasound measurements) can now be used to predict cardiac output, flow direction, valve gradients, and pulmonary artery pressure. Interpretation of the results of these studies requires the skill of the pediatric cardiologist. In cases of major heart disease, cardiac catheterization should also be performed.

Feigenbaum H: *Echocardiography,* 4th ed. Lea & Febiger, 1986.
Goldberg SJ, Allen HD, Sahn DJ: *Pediatric and Adolescent Echocardiography: A Handbook,* 2nd ed. Year Book, 1980.
Meyer RA: Echocardiography. Chap 4, pp 58–82, in: *Heart Disease in Infants, Children, and Adolescents,* 3rd ed. Adams FH, Emmanouilides GC (editors). Williams & Wilkins, 1983.

NUCLEAR CARDIOLOGY

Current use of radionuclide tracers in infants and children includes detection and quantification of left-to-right and right-to-left intracardiac shunting, quantification of cardiac output at rest and during exercise using gated blood pool scintigraphy, and

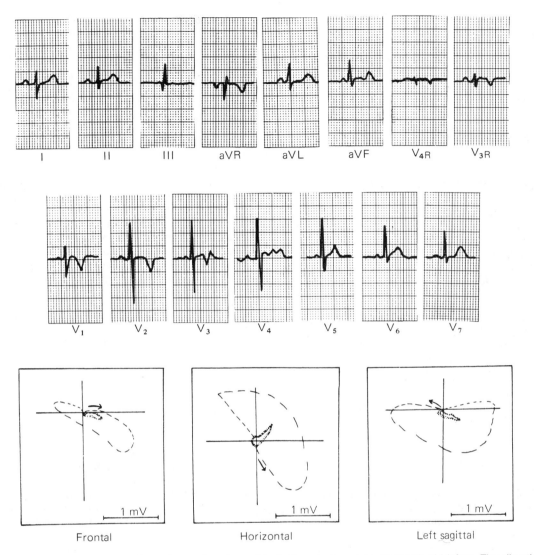

Figure 16–3. Electrocardiographic and vectorcardiographic findings in the same 10-month-old infant. The direction, duration, and magnitude of electrical force are comparable in each tracing.

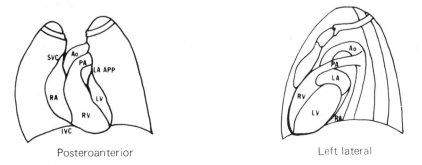

Figure 16–4. Position of cardiovascular structures in principal x-ray views. RV = right ventricle; LA = left atrium; LA APP = left atrial appendage; LV = left ventricle; Ao = aorta; PA = pulmonary artery; SVC = superior vena cava; IVC = inferior vena cava.

myocardial imaging with thallium-201 for ischemia or infarction. In the older child, the latter method can be enhanced by exercise stress testing. These tests yield more objective data for evaluation of children with heart disease.

Hurwitz PA, Treves ST: Nuclear cardiology. Chap 6, pp 101–107, in: *Heart Disease in Infants, Children, and Adolescents,* 3rd ed. Adams FH, Emmanouilides GC (editors). Williams & Wilkins, 1983.

MAGNETIC RESONANCE IMAGING

Magnetic resonance imaging (MRI) techniques, which are just being introduced in pediatric medicine, provide yet another method for noninvasive imaging of normal and abnormal cardiovascular structures. ^{31}P magnetic resonance spectroscopy appears to hold great promise as a clinical research tool for investigation of myocardial metabolism.

Boxer RA et al: Cardiac magnetic resonance imaging in children with congenital heart disease. *J Pediatr* 1986; **109**:460.

Friedman BJ et al: Comparison of magnetic resonance imaging and echocardiography in determination of cardiac dimensions in normal subjects. *J Am Coll Cardiol* 1985; **5**:1369.

Leonard JC et al: Nuclear magnetic resonance. *J Pediatr* 1985;**106**:756.

ERGOMETRY

Pediatric ergometry is a newly evolving technique. It has long been hampered by lack of appreciation of its applications and availability of normal data. Most children with heart disease are capable of normal activity, and exercise data are essential to prevent overprotection. The response to exercise is valuable in determining the need for cardiovascular surgery and its timing. Bicycle ergometers or treadmills can often be employed to test children as young as 6 years. Important exercise parameters include stress ECGs, conditioning, and performance data. Significant stress ischemia or dysrhythmias warrant physical restrictions or appropriate therapy. Children demonstrating poor performance with suboptimal conditioning benefit from an exercise prescription. The pre- and postoperative child can then be objectively guided into appropriate recreational and competitive activities and given prevocational guidance.

James FW: Ergometry. Chap 7, pp 107–115, in: *Heart Disease in Infants, Children, and Adolescents,* 3rd ed. Adams FH, Emmanouilides GC (editors). Williams & Wilkins, 1983.

ARTERIAL BLOOD GASES (ARTERIAL Po₂, SYSTEMIC O₂ SATURATION)

Because cyanosis is difficult to measure (and sometimes to recognize) by inspection of the patient, objective laboratory determinations are required. The quantitative response of arterial Po_2 or O_2 saturation (eg, by pulse oximetry) to administration of 100% oxygen is one of the most useful methods of distinguishing cyanosis produced by heart disease from cyanosis related to lung disease in sick infants. In cyanotic heart disease, Pao_2 increases very little from values obtained while breathing ambient room air as compared with values during 100% oxygen administration. However, there is usually a very significant increase in Pao_2 when oxygen is administered to a patient with lung disease. Continuous noninvasive methods for monitoring arterial Po_2 include the transcutaneous O_2 monitor. Inherent limitations have prevented the general substitution of these noninvasive methods for direct arterial sampling in this evaluation, but they are valuable in overall cardiopulmonary care of the sick infant. Table 16–1 illustrates the sort of response one might expect following at least 10 minutes of 100% oxygen administration to cyanotic infants with heart disease versus lung disease.

OTHER NONINVASIVE LABORATORY STUDIES

In children of all ages, but particularly in the infant and newborn, many metabolic abnormalities can have a major influence on the performance of the cardiovascular system. In evaluating the symptomatic infant, it is important to rule out infection, hypoglycemia, hypocalcemia, hypovolemia, hyperkalemia, inborn errors of metabolism, anemia, etc. Likewise, severe cardiovascular problems may be accompanied by some of these abnormalities.

CARDIAC CATHETERIZATION & ANGIOCARDIOGRAPHY

The definitive anatomic and physiologic study of infants and children with heart disease is cardiac

Table 16–1. Examples of responses to 10 minutes of 100% oxygen in lung disease and heart disease.

	Lung Disease		Heart Disease	
	Room Air	100% O₂	Room Air	100% O₂
Color	Blue	→ Pink	Blue	→ Blue
Oximetry	60%	→ 99%	60%	→ 62%
Pao₂ (mm Hg)	35	→ 120	35	→ 38

catheterization. It is essential for the primary physician to distinguish those infants and children who require the specialized diagnostic and therapeutic facilities of the pediatric cardiac center from those who may be safely managed without such facilities and consultation. On the basis of the preceding steps of diagnostic evaluation—history, physical examination, ECG, chest x-ray, and other noninvasive laboratory studies—the consulting pediatric cardiologist has a rather precise assessment of the anatomic and physiologic abnormalities in simple malformations and considerable useful information about complex malformations.

Indications & Objectives

A. Infants:

1. Indications—

a. All infants with cyanosis presumed to be cardiovascular in origin should be catheterized as soon as a reasonably stable clinical condition can be achieved—not only for diagnosis of the anatomic and physiologic abnormality but also for possibly lifesaving procedures such as the Rashkind balloon septostomy and balloon valvuloplasty (which take place in the cardiac catheterization laboratory).

b. Infants with severe congestive heart failure that does not respond promptly and satisfactorily to anticongestive measures.

c. Infants in whom early operation for congenital heart disease is contemplated.

d. Infants in whom the anatomic and physiologic abnormality is sufficiently vague that appropriate medical management is not possible.

e. Infants who have evidence of complicating or potentially progressive problems, such as pulmonary hypertension.

2. Objectives—(In descending order of importance.)

a. To perform the study with the lowest possible rate of death or serious complications. Pediatric cardiologists and pediatric cardiac catheterization laboratories with experience in studying infants are required so that these objectives can be met: to gain meaningful information promptly; to care for the critically ill infant with temperature and pH control, fluid management, and all essential pediatric treatment; and to anticipate and handle life-threatening crises.

b. To gain information which is not available by other methods and which will provide the basis for therapeutic decisions (medical or surgical).

c. To provide therapeutic intervention (eg, Rashkind septostomy, balloon valvuloplasty).

d. To obtain sufficient physiologic and anatomic data so that repeat catheterization to complete the study will not be necessary.

B. Children:

1. Indications—

a. All children for whom heart surgery is contemplated (with the occasional exception of children with unequivocal patent ductus arteriosus or atrial septal defect [or both] and no evidence of an associated cardiovascular problem).

b. All children in whom there is question about the anatomic or physiologic abnormality which would significantly influence management and which cannot be completely answered by noninvasive methods.

c. Children with progressive lesions that require careful physiologic monitoring (such as pulmonary hypertension).

d. Children who have had cardiovascular surgery and require assessment of the adequacy of the repair.

e. Children with mild to moderate cardiovascular lesions when important information about the natural history is required. This procedure should be done only in the setting of a well-designed protocol and fully informed consent.

2. Objectives—It goes without saying that conducting the study with the lowest possible risk is the most important objective of cardiac catheterization of the child as well as the infant; and the risk to the child ($< 0.2\%$) is certainly much less than to the sick infant (2%). Complete anatomic and physiologic data are more important objectives of catheterization in children than in infants. No physician or laboratory should undertake the catheterization of a child unless prepared to obtain a completely informative study and unless physicians and surgeons are available who are capable of proceeding with whatever medical or surgical therapy may be indicated.

Contraindications

Cardiac catheterization is contraindicated in infants and children who present with no clinical urgency and none of the indications listed above. It should not be done if personnel and facilities fail to meet high standards of patient safety and clinical diagnostic and therapeutic expertise.

Cardiac Catheterization Data

Fig 16–5 shows oxygen saturation (in percent) and pressure (in mm Hg) values obtained at cardiac catheterization from the chambers and great arteries of the heart. These values would be within the normal range for a child.

A. Oxygen Content and Saturation; Pulmonary and Systemic Blood Flow (Cardiac Output): In most laboratories, evidence of left-to-right shunt is determined by changes of blood oxygen content or saturation during passage of the catheter through the right side of the heart. A significant increase in oxygen content or oxygen saturation from one chamber to another indicates the presence of a left-to-right shunt at the site of the increase. The oxygen saturation of the peripheral arterial blood should always be determined during cardiac catheterization. Normal arterial oxygen saturation is 91–

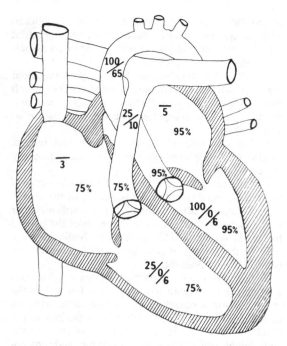

Figure 16–5. Pressures (in mm Hg) and oxygen saturation (in percent) obtained by cardiac catheterization in a normal child. 3 = mean pressure of 3 mm Hg in right atrium; 5 = mean pressure of 5 mm Hg in left atrium.

97%. A decrease (at sea level) below 91% suggests the presence of a right-to-left shunt, underventilation, or pulmonary disease.

The size of a left-to-right shunt is usually expressed as a ratio of the pulmonary to systemic blood flow or as liters per minute as determined by the Fick principle:

$$\text{Cardiac output (L/min)} = \frac{\text{Oxygen consumption (mL/min)}}{\text{Arteriovenous difference (mL/L)}}$$

B. Pressures: Pressures should be determined in all chambers and vessels entered. Pressures should always be recorded when a catheter is pulled back from a distal chamber or vessel into a more proximal chamber. It is not normal for systolic pressure in the ventricles to exceed systolic pressure in the great arteries or mean diastolic pressure in the atria to exceed end-diastolic pressure in the ventricles. If a "gradient" in pressure does exist, it means that there is obstruction, and the severity of the gradient is one criterion for the necessity of operative repair. A right ventricular systolic pressure of 100 mm Hg and a pulmonary artery systolic pressure of 20 mm Hg yield a gradient of 80 mm Hg. In this case, the patient would be classified as having severe pulmonary stenosis requiring repair.

C. Pulmonary and Systemic Vascular Resistance: The vascular resistance is calculated from the following formula and reported in units or in dynes-sec-cm^{-5}/m^2:

$$\text{Resistance} = \frac{\text{Pressure}}{\text{Flow}}$$

Pulmonary vascular resistance equals mean pulmonary artery pressure divided by pulmonary blood flow per square meter of body surface area. (Pulmonary blood flow is determined from the Fick principle, as noted previously.) **Systemic vascular resistance** equals mean systemic arterial pressure divided by systemic blood flow.

Normally, the pulmonary vascular resistance ranges from 1 to 3 units or 80 to 240 dynes · sec · cm^{-5}/m^2. If pulmonary resistance is above 10 units or the pulmonary/systemic resistance ratio is above 0.7, all other diagnostic findings should be reviewed carefully to confirm the presence of pulmonary hypertension that is so severe as to render the patient inoperable.

D. Special Techniques: Special techniques are frequently employed during the course of cardiac catheterization. These include the following:

1. Hydrogen electrode catheter—Used to determine the presence of very small left-to-right shunts, this technique enables the operator to detect such shunts even in the absence of any increase in oxygen saturation.

2. Indicator dilution curves—This involves injection of an indicator, such as indocyanine green (Cardio-Green), at specific places in the heart and detection of the dye downstream, usually in a peripheral artery. This technique permits the detection of both right-to-left and left-to-right shunts at the specific points within the cardiovascular system. Cardiac output is frequently determined by this method.

3. Selective angiocardiography and cineangiocardiography—In this technique, contrast material is injected in a specific chamber or vessel and the course of the contrast material followed by serial large film x-rays (angiocardiography) or by motion pictures (cineangiocardiography).

4. Contrast echocardiography—Saline or indocyanine green is rapidly injected via the cardiac catheter, and downstream "clouding" is imaged with either M mode or 2-dimensional echocardiography. Dynamic spatial or structural relationships of chambers, valves, and vessels are visualized; this procedure may be done repetitively without the risk of radiation.

5. Interventional catheterization—Specially designed catheters are now used for dilatation of stenotic valves and vascular structures. Balloon valvuloplasty/angioplasty is now the treatment of choice for valve pulmonary stenosis, recurrent coarctation of the thoracic aorta, and pulmonary arterial stenoses. Other valve and vascular stenoses are being evaluated along with special occluding devices for closing patent ductus arteriosus and atrial septal defects. Many simple defects are now treated effectively through these and other procedures.

Jarmakani JM: Catheterization in angiocardiography. Chap 5, pp 83–100, in: *Heart Disease in Infants, Children, and Adolescents,* 3rd ed. Adams FH, Emmanouilides GC (editors). Williams & Wilkins, 1983.

Lock JE, Keane JF, Fellows KE (editors): The use of catheter intervention procedures for congenital heart disease. *J Am Coll Cardiol* 1986;7:1420.

PRENATAL & NEONATAL CIRCULATION

Fetal Circulation

In the fetus, the placenta serves as the organ of respiration and for exchange of waste products for nutritive material. Oxygenated blood (approximately 80% saturated) passes from the placenta through the umbilical vein to the heart. As it flows toward the heart, it mixes with blood from the inferior vena cava and from the portal vein, so that blood entering the right atrium is approximately 65% saturated. A considerable amount of this blood is shunted immediately across the foramen ovale into the left atrium. The venous blood derived from the upper part of the body is much less saturated (approximately 30%), and most of it enters the right ventricle through the tricuspid valve. Thus, the blood in the right ventricle is a mixture of both relatively highly saturated blood from the umbilical vein and desaturated blood from the venae cavae. This mixture results in a blood oxygen saturation of approximately 50% in the right ventricle.

The blood in the left atrium is derived from the blood shunting across the foramen ovale and the blood returning from the pulmonary veins. A great deal of the left ventricular output goes to the head, whereas the lower portion of the body is supplied by blood both from the right ventricle, through the patent ductus arteriosus, and from the left ventricle.

Physiologic Changes at Birth & in the Neonatal Period

At birth, 2 dramatic events that affect the cardiovascular and pulmonary system occur: (1) the umbilical cord is clamped, removing the placenta from the circulation; and (2) breathing commences. As a result, marked changes in the circulation occur. During fetal life, the placenta offers little resistance to the flow of blood, so that the systemic circuit is a low-resistance one. On the other hand, the pulmonary arterioles are markedly constricted and offer strong resistance to the flow of blood into the lung. Clamping the cord causes a sudden increase in resistance to flow in the systemic circuit. As the lung becomes the organ of respiration, the oxygen tension (Po_2) increases in the vicinity of the small pulmonary arterioles, resulting in a release of the constriction and thus a significant decrease in the pulmonary arteriolar resistance. Indeed, the pulmonary vascular resistance shortly after birth is less than that of the systemic circuit.

Because of the changes in resistance, the great majority of the right ventricular outflow now passes into the lung rather than through the ductus arteriosus into the descending aorta. In fact, functional closure of the ductus arteriosus begins to develop shortly after birth. Recent studies have demonstrated that the ductus arteriosus remains patent for a variable period, usually 24–48 hours. During the first hour after birth, there is a small right-to-left shunt (as in the fetus). However, after 1 hour, bidirectional shunting occurs, with the left-to-right direction predominanting. In most cases, right-to-left shunting completely disappears by 8 hours. However, in patients with severe hypoxia (eg, in respiratory distress syndrome), the pulmonary vascular resistance remains quite elevated, resulting in a continued right-to-left shunt. The cause of the functional closure of the ductus arteriosus is not completely known. However, evidence indicates that the increased Po_2 of the arterial blood causes spasm of the ductus. Anatomically, however, the ductus arteriosus does not close until approximately age 3 months.

In fetal life, the foramen ovale serves as a one-way valve, permitting shunting of blood from the inferior vena cava through the right atrium into the left atrium. At birth, because of the changes in the pulmonary and systemic vascular resistance and the increase in the quantity of blood returning from the pulmonary veins to the left atrium, the left atrial pressure rises above that of the right atrium. This functionally closes the flap of the one-way valve, essentially preventing flow of blood across the septum. It has been shown, however, that a small right-to-left shunt does continue for the first week of life. Although the foramen ovale remains functionally closed throughout life, it remains patent in about 25% of patients.

A clinical syndrome has been recognized that is characterized in term infants by onset of tachypnea, cyanosis, and clinical evidence of pulmonary hypertension during the first 8 hours after delivery. These infants have massive right-to-left ductal or foramen shunting or both for 3–7 days because of the high pulmonary vascular resistance. The clinical course is generally one of progressive cor pulmonale, hypoxia, and acidosis, terminating in early death unless the pulmonary resistance can be lowered. The resistance can usually be reversed by instituting appropriate means to increase alveolar Po_2: hyperventilation (to produce respiratory alkalosis) and intravenous administration of vasoactive drugs. At postmortem, the only findings are increased thickness of the pulmonary arteriolar media, which is believed to represent persistence of the fetal circulation.

Changes in the First Year of Life

The most significant changes occur at birth and within the neonatal period. However, pulmonary vascular resistance and the pulmonary arterial pressure continue to fall during the first year of life. This phenomenon results from the involution of the pulmonary arteriole from a relatively thick-walled, small-lumen vessel to a thin-walled, large-lumen vessel. Adult levels of resistance and pressure are usually achieved by age 6 months to 1 year.

Adams FH: Fetal and neonatal circulation. Chap 2, pp 11–17 in: *Heart Disease in Infants, Children, and Adolescents*, 3rd ed. Adams FH, Emmanouilides GC (editors). Williams & Wilkins, 1983.

Fox WW, Shahnag D: Persistent pulmonary hypertension in the neonate: Diagnosis and management. *J Pediatr* 1983;**103**:505.

MAJOR CLUES TO HEART DISEASE IN INFANTS & CHILDREN

CONGESTIVE HEART FAILURE

There are many levels of definition of congestive heart failure. At the clinical level, a simple definition is failure of the heart to meet the circulatory and metabolic needs of the body. Congestive heart failure is one of the 2 major clues to the presence of important heart disease. (The other is cyanosis; see below.) It has been estimated that congestive heart failure begins before age 1 year in over 90% of infants and children who ever develop the disorder in the pediatric age period—and most of these patients are less than 6 months of age.

Congestive heart failure beginning in infancy may persist throughout childhood until operation relieves the underlying malformation (unless surgery is not possible). Other infants with moderately severe heart failure in the first few months of life may gradually compensate (for a variety of reasons) and not require medical intervention after age 12 or 18 months even though their congenital heart lesions are still unrepaired.

Clinical Findings

The symptoms and signs of congestive heart failure have been discussed in the preceding sections on history and physical examination. Certain findings will be reviewed again here for purposes of emphasis and organization.

The 3 cardinal signs of congestive heart failure in the pediatric patient are cardiomegaly (the sine qua non), tachypnea (left side), and hepatomegaly (right side).

Cardiomegaly represents a homeostatic (compensatory) mechanism that maintains adequate cardiac output by enlarging the capacity of the pump. This mechanism is frequently referred to as Starling's law of the heart. Up to a point, the enlarging heart can deliver a greater stroke volume output, but limits are soon reached (the descending limb of Starling's curve). Fig 16–6 shows a family of ventricular performance curves. The curve at the right depicts a damaged myocardium; the curve in the center, a normal myocardium; and the curve at the left, a myocardium under inotropic stimulation. One should be very cautious about the diagnosis of congestive heart failure in the absence of an enlarged heart (an exception being a condition such as total anomalous venous return below the diaphragm, which will for a short period of time be characterized by other signs of congestive heart failure without an enlarged heart). Cardiomegaly without other signs of congestive failure may well be taken as early or homeostatically compensated congestive heart failure.

Tachypnea may be considered the cardinal sign of left-sided heart failure. It may be present for a short time before hepatomegaly occurs, although pure left-sided or pure right-sided heart failure does not commonly exist independently for long.

Hepatomegaly is the cardinal sign of right-sided heart failure. The liver is capable of trapping relatively large amounts of edema fluid in the infant that would be more evident as peripheral edema in the older child and adult. It is therefore common rather than unusual for the infant in moderately severe heart failure to have an enlarged liver with no pretibial or even presacral or facial edema. Peripheral edema is found in infants only in the most severe cases of congestive heart failure.

Additional signs and symptoms of congestive

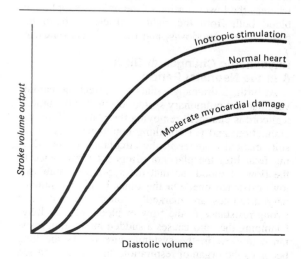

Figure 16–6. Ventricular performance curves.

heart failure are feeding difficulties, dyspnea, restlessness, easy fatigability, weak pulses, pallor, rales, peripheral edema, weight gain from fluid accumulation, tachycardia, sweating, pneumonia, orthopnea, and growth failure.

Underlying Causes of Heart Failure in the Pediatric Age Group

By far the most common cause of congestive heart failure in the pediatric patient is congenital heart disease. Causes in infancy and childhood appear in the outline below:

A. Heart Failure in Infancy:

1. Cardiovascular causes—Congenital heart disease (producing volume overload, outflow obstruction, myocardial impairment), congenital vascular disease (eg, coarctation of the aorta, an outflow-obstruction disorder, peripheral arteriovenous shunts, a volume overload disorder), acquired myocardial disease (eg, myocarditis), dysrhythmias, rheumatic fever (very rare in infants in the USA).

2. Noncardiovascular causes—Acidosis, respiratory disease, central nervous system disease, anemia, sepsis, hypoglycemia.

B. Heart Failure in Childhood: Cardiovascular causes are potentially the same as in infancy except that rheumatic fever plays a more important role in childhood. Noncardiovascular causes become less important with increasing age—especially such mechanisms as acidosis and hypoglycemia.

Treatment

The physician undertaking the responsibility of caring for children must have facility with routine measures and familiarity with some emergency measures for treating congestive heart failure.

A. Routine Measures:

1. Digitalis—Digitalis is the keystone of the treatment of congestive heart failure. The major effect that is sought is improvement in myocardial performance (inotropic effect). This may be visualized as shifting the patient to a more efficient ventricular performance curve in the family of curves shown in Fig 16–6. The preparation most widely used in pediatrics is digoxin, which may be administered (in order of rapidity of onset of effect) intravenously, intramuscularly, or orally. The clinical urgency of the individual case dictates how quickly digitalization should be accomplished. Although there are general guidelines, the ultimate dosage (on a milligram per kilogram basis) must be individualized for each patient.

a. Protocols for digitalization—

(1) In hospital—

Age	Parenteral	Oral
Premature	0.035 mg/kg	0.04 mg/kg
2 weeks to 2 years	0.05 mg/kg	0.07 mg/kg
Under 2 weeks or over 2 years	0.04 mg/kg	0.06 mg/kg

Use of the elixir (0.05 mg/mL) is advisable even in older children because the bioavailability of the tablet preparations is unreliable.

The routine schedule consists of giving one-fourth the digitalizing dose intramuscularly or orally every 6 hours for 4 doses. For rapid digitalization, give half the digitalizing dose intravenously or intramuscularly and repeat in 4–6 hours. For very rapid digitalization, give the full digitalizing dose intravenously with very close monitoring. For maintenance, give one-fourth to one-third the oral digitalizing dose daily (divided into morning and evening doses).

(2) Digitalization of outpatients—Give the maintenance dose of digoxin (see above) divided in morning and evening doses. In less than a week, adequate digitalization is obtained without running the risk of a parent inadvertently failing to revert to a maintenance dosage schedule and continuing a high digitalizing dose to the point of toxicity (even death).

b. Digitalis toxicity—Slowing of the heart rate below 100 in infants, below 80 in young children, and below 60 in older children is often taken as a guide to reducing the dosage of digoxin. Any dysrhythmia that occurs during digitalis therapy should be attributed to the drug until proved otherwise, although ventricular bigeminy and various degrees of atrioventricular block are characteristic of digitalis toxicity. Age-specific serum levels suggestive of toxicity during maintenance therapy are as follows: newborn, over 4 ng/mL; 1 month to 1 year, over 3 ng/mL; after 1 year, over 2 ng/mL.

c. Digitalis poisoning—This is an acute emergency that must be treated *without delay*. The sooner the stomach is emptied, the better the prognosis, but even if many hours have passed, the stomach should still be emptied. Attention must then be paid to maintaining an adequate cardiac rate and output and to controlling the dysrhythmia. A useful basic intravenous solution is 10% glucose in water to which KCl (3 meq/kg/d) and regular insulin (20 units/1000 mL) have been added. KCl must be used with caution in patients with electrocardiographic high-grade block. It should be given in amounts not to exceed the maintenance requirement per 24 hours for the weight or surface area of the patient. To this solution may be added isoproterenol (in the calibrated administration set) titrated in quantities appropriate to maintain adequate heart rate and output in the face of complete heart block. Phenytoin may be administered through the intravenous tubing to treat dysrhythmias by beginning with a 1-mg/kg slow intravenous push followed every 5–10 minutes with doubling doses to a maximum total combined dose of 15 mg/kg. In severe cases, digoxin-specific Fab fragments should be used (given intravenously). If these are not available, a temporary transvenous pacemaker may be required to control dysrhythmias.

2. Diuretics—If digitalis alone is inadequate to

achieve satisfactory compensation, diuretics may be required. For rapid inpatient diuresis, give furosemide intravenously or intramuscularly; for maintenance therapy, give thiazides or furosemide orally daily along with spironolactone.

The dosages are as follows:

a. Furosemide—

(1) Intravenously or intramuscularly, 1 mg/kg as a single dose. Do not repeat more than once in a day, and be cautious about using on consecutive days.

(2) Orally, 2–5 mg/kg/d.

b. Thiazides—These drugs should be given daily with spironolactone (which helps to prevent excessive potassium loss). Do not give daily for prolonged periods unless spironolactone is being given also and serum electrolytes are being monitored periodically.

(1) Chlorothiazide suspension (250 mg/tsp), 20 mg/kg/d.

(2) Hydrochlorothiazide tablets, 2 mg/kg/d.

c. Spironolactone—Give 2–4 mg/kg/d in 2 divided doses.

3. Rest and sedation—The decompensated and mildly distressed patient requires rest; the severely distressed and anxious infant or child requires sedation. Parenteral morphine, 0.1 mg/kg, is useful for sedation as well as for control of acute pulmonary edema, but it should only be given with good airway control.

4. Oxygen—Oxygen will not make a patient with cyanotic heart disease pink, but it will raise the systemic Pao_2 in patients with severe congestive heart failure, overcoming the capillary-alveolar block of pulmonary edema and alleviating the hypoxemic contribution to congestive failure.

5. Salt restriction—Salt restriction must be approached with caution in infants and children. Treatment of the disease entity known as low-salt congestive heart failure is one of the more hazardous undertakings in medical management. Our feeling is that there is no place for salt-free formulas in the treatment of congestive failure in infants. Standard SMA or Similac 60/40 has about the same sodium content as human milk and about half the sodium content of cow's milk and other prepared formulas. Most cases of "low-salt failure" are largely due to overly vigorous salt restriction (sometimes combined with the other major factor, overly vigorous diuretic therapy). Clearly salty foods such as potato chips and bacon should be avoided, and no salt should be used beyond what is normally used in cooking. It is important that food be palatable enough to eat for a child, who may already be undernourished as a consequence of chronic, poorly compensated heart failure.

B. Emergency and Heroic Measures: The acute emergencies of congestive heart failure are usually related to fluid retention with pulmonary edema and low cardiac output. Some emergency therapeutic measures that may be lifesaving include the following:

1. Morphine—For acute pulmonary edema, give 0.1 mg/kg intravenously or subcutaneously.

2. Diuretics—Furosemide or ethacrynic acid may be given intravenously in an initial dosage of 1 mg/kg to produce a rapid diuresis.

3. Positive pressure breathing—Pulmonary edema may sometimes be managed by intubation or mask with bag-breathing or a respirator to raise the alveolar pressure above pulmonary capillary pressure.

4. Peritoneal dialysis—Although furosemide has largely met the need for the extremely rapid relief of fluid retention, there are 3 specific instances where peritoneal dialysis with a hypertonic solution may be indicated: (1) when fluid retention (especially pulmonary edema) is life-threatening and diuretics are unsuccessful; (2) in low-salt congestive heart failure when both the fluid retention and the electrolyte imbalance require correction; and (3) in the early postoperative care of an infant who may have transient renal failure with both fluid retention and hyperkalemia.

The advantages of hypertonic peritoneal dialysis are that the procedure promptly (within minutes) draws fluid into the peritoneal cavity, where it is subject to immediate removal, while simultaneously correcting the electrolyte imbalance, whether it is low-sodium, high-potassium, or both. For methods of dialysis, see Chapter 22, Kidney & Urinary Tract. If the major problem is electrolyte imbalance, such as potassium retention, a hypertonic solution is not required and the usual "isotonic" dialyzing fluid is indicated.

5. Afterload reduction—A relatively new form of therapy for "pump" failure is to effect afterload reduction by decreasing systemic vascular resistance with an intravenous infusion of vasodilators. Experience in children is limited. The procedure has been used largely in postoperative patients with reduced cardiac output and peripheral vasoconstriction. Agents such as nitroprusside have been lifesaving but must be used in a setting where central venous pressure, arterial pressure, cardiac output, etc, can be carefully monitored.

Arnold SB et al: Long-term digitalis therapy improves left ventricular function in heart failure. *N Engl J Med* 1980; **303:**1443.

Beckman RH, Rocchini AP, Rosenthal A: Hemodynamic effects of nitroprusside in infants with a large ventricular septal defect. *Circulation* 1981;**64:**553.

Beckman RH et al: Vasodilator therapy in children. *Pediatrics* 1984;**73:**43.

Driscoll D et al: Dopamine in children. *J Pediatr* 1978; **92:**309.

Epstein SE (editor): Calcium channel blockers: Present and future directions. *Am J Cardiol* 1985;**55:**1. [Entire issue.]

Smith TW: Digitalis in the management of heart failure. *Hosp Pract* (March) 1984;**19:**67.

Zaritsky A, Chernow B: Use of catecholamines in pediatrics. *J Pediatr* 1984;**105:**341.

CYANOSIS

One of the 2 major clues to the presence of heart disease in the infant and child is cyanosis. (The other is congestive heart failure; see above.)

Cyanosis represents an increased concentration (4–5 g/dL) of reduced hemoglobin in the blood. Bluish discoloration is usually, but not always, a sign. Patients with anemia and cyanosis may not appear blue; patients with polycythemia may appear cyanotic, even though true cyanosis and inadequate blood oxygen content are not present. Visible cyanosis accompanies low cardiac output, hypothermia, and systemic venous congestion, even in the presence of adequate oxygenation.

In patients with true central cyanosis, the cause of cyanosis (cardiac, pulmonary, hematologic, or central nervous system disorder) must be determined. Most often, the physician is faced with differentiating between cardiac and pulmonary problems. Evaluation of arterial blood gases (see above) is one of the easiest ways to differentiate between lung and heart disease. Cyanosis in heart disease is also related to pulmonary blood flow. In some "cyanotic" congenital heart defects, the decrease in pulmonary blood flow is minimal and results in minimal cyanosis. Presence of pulmonary hypertension also influences pulmonary blood flow, and thus oxygen therapy may cause a partial increase in oxygen saturation; the increase is usually much less in patients with heart disease than in those with pulmonary disease.

Evaluation for methemoglobinemia may be necessary to rule out hematologic causes of cyanosis. If the cause of cyanosis is a disease of the central nervous system, the patient will usually respond to oxygen therapy.

Cyanotic heart disease is usually a medical emergency, most often requiring palliative or corrective surgery.

CONGENITAL HEART DISEASE

Congenital heart disease is present in about 1% of studied North American and British populations, making this the most common category of congenital structural malformation. Curative or palliative surgical correction is now available for over 90% of patients with congenital heart disease.

The customary division of congenital heart diseases into noncyanotic and cyanotic types is useful if one understands the basis for it. By convention, patients with right-to-left shunts fall into the cyanotic category whether they have readily recognizable cyanosis or not; patients who do not have right-to-left shunts—even if they are cyanotic for other reasons, such as low cardiac output—are placed in the noncyanotic category. The physiologic basis of cyanosis has been discussed above. It should be remembered that whatever brings 4–5 g of reduced hemoglobin to the capillary bed produces cyanosis; if 4–5 g of reduced hemoglobin are not present (as in a patient with a cyanotic heart lesion, but with anemia), cyanosis is not present.

Etiologic Considerations

The incidence of congenital heart disease is high (1% of live births). Only 8% of all congenital heart defects are known to be associated with single mutant gene or chromosome abnormalities, and the remainder are due to various other causes. Multiple environmental factors, including diabetes, alcohol consumption, progesterone use, certain viruses, and other teratogens, are now associated with an increased incidence of malformations. These factors probably represent environmental triggers in persons susceptible or predisposed to congenital heart defects. The effect of rubella virus is probably independent of hereditary factors and consequently predisposes to patent ductus arteriosus and pulmonary artery branch stenosis. Acquired heart diseases, such as rheumatic fever, appear to have much stronger environmental influence. Atherosclerosis clearly can have distinct familial patterns but in some circumstances can be influenced by diet, drugs, or lifestyle.

In dealing with families of children with congenital heart disease, the physician must often answer the question of risk to future pregnancies. Table 16–2 outlines the risk for certain lesions in patients with

Table 16–2. Observed and expected recurrence risks in siblings of 1478 probands with congenital heart lesion.[1]

Anomaly	Probands	Affected Siblings		
		No.	Percent	Exp. ($\sqrt{p}$)
Ventricular septal defect	212	24/543	4.4	5.0
Patent ductus arteriosus	204	17/505	3.4	3.5
Tetralogy of Fallot	157	9/338	2.7	3.2
Atrial septal defect	152	11/342	3.2	3.2
Pulmonary stenosis	146	10/345	2.9	2.9
Aortic stenosis	135	7/317	2.2	2.1
Coarctation of aorta	128	5/272	1.8	2.4
Transpositions of great vessels	103	4/209	1.9	2.2
Atrioventricular canal	73	4/151	2.6	2.0
Tricuspid atresia	51	1/96	1.0	1.4
Ebstein's anomaly	42	1/96	1.1	0.7
Truncus arteriosus	41	1/86	1.2	0.7
Pulmonary atresia	34	1/77	1.3	1.0
Total	1478	95/3376		

[1]Reproduced, with permission, from Nora JJ: Etiologic factors in congenital heart disease. *Pediatr Clin North Am* 1971; **18**:1059.

one affected first-degree relative. Studies indicate that the incidence in children of affected mothers may be as high as 10–15%. With more than one affected first-degree relative, recurrence is also much higher, and some families may have a hereditary predisposition to congenital heart disease.

Nora JJ, Nora AH: *Genetics and Counseling in Cardiovascular Diseases.* Thomas, 1978.

Whittemore R, Hobbins JC, Engle MA: Pregnancy and its outcome in women with and without surgical treatment of congenital heart disease. *Am J Cardiol* 1982;**50**:641.

NONCYANOTIC HEART DISEASE

ATRIAL SEPTAL DEFECT OF THE OSTIUM SECUNDUM VARIETY

Essentials of Diagnosis

- S_2 widely split and usually fixed.
- Grade I–III/VI ejection systolic murmur at pulmonary area.
- Widely radiating systolic murmur mimicking peripheral pulmonary artery stenosis (common in infancy).
- Diastolic flow murmur at lower left sternal border (if shunt is significant in size).
- ECG with rsR′ in lead V_1.

General Considerations

An atrial septal defect is an opening in the atrial septum permitting the shunting of blood between the 2 atria. There are 3 major types: (1) The ostium secundum type (discussed here) is the most common and is in an intermediate position. (2) The sinus venosus type is positioned high in the atrial septum, is the least common, and is frequently associated with partial anomalous venous return. (3) The ostium primum type is low in position and is a form of atrioventricular septal defect; it is discussed in that section.

Atrial septal defect of the ostium secundum variety occurs in approximately 10% of patients with congenital heart disease and is twice as common in females as in males. Diagnosis in infancy is becoming more common.

Pulmonary hypertension and growth failure are increasingly recognized in infancy and childhood. After the third decade, an increased pulmonary vascular resistance develops, the left-to-right shunting decreases, and right-to-left shunting begins.

Clinical Findings

A. Symptoms and Signs: Infants may present with congestive heart failure often unresponsive to medical management, necessitating early total corrective surgery. However, children with atrial septal defects often have no cardiovascular symptoms. Some patients remain asymptomatic throughout life; others develop easy fatigability as older children or adults. Cyanosis does not occur until pulmonary hypertension develops. This may never occur; if it does, it is not seen until after the third decade of life. Congestive heart failure is uncommon in infants and young children.

The arterial pulses are normal and equal throughout. In the usual case, the heart is hyperactive, with a heaving impulse felt best at the lower left sternal border and over the xiphoid process. There are usually no thrills. S_2 at the pulmonary area is widely split and sometimes fixed. The pulmonary component is normal in intensity. A grade I–III/VI, blowing, ejection type systolic murmur is heard best at the left sternal border in the second intercostal space. An additional murmur of relative peripheral pulmonary artery stenosis may be heard, more commonly in infants. A middiastolic murmur can often be heard in the fourth intercostal space at the left sternal border. This murmur is due to increased blood flow across the tricuspid valve during diastole (tricuspid flow murmur). The presence of this murmur suggests a high flow (pulmonary to systemic blood flow ratio greater than 2:1).

B. Imaging: Chest x-ray films usually demonstrate cardiac enlargement. The main pulmonary artery may be dilated. The pulmonary vascular markings are increased as a result of increased pulmonary blood flow.

C. Electrocardiography and Vectorcardiography: The usual ECG shows right axis deviation with a clockwise loop in the frontal plane. In the right precordial leads, there is usually an rsR′ pattern.

D. Echocardiography: M mode echocardiography shows (1) paradoxic motion of the ventricular septal wall (moving in the same direction rather than the direction opposite to that of the free left ventricular wall) and (2) dilated right ventricular cavity with increased tricuspid valve excursion. Direct visualization of the atrial septal defect by 2-dimensional echocardiography, plus demonstration of a left-to-right shunt through the defect by color flow doppler, confirms the diagnosis and may eliminate the need for cardiac catheterization.

E. Cardiac Catheterization: Oximetry reveals evidence of a significant increase in oxygen saturation at the atrial level. The pulmonary artery pressure is usually normal. The right ventricular pressure is occasionally greater than the pulmonary artery pressure, owing to "flow." Pulmonary vascular resistance is usually normal. The ratio of pulmonary to systemic blood flow may vary from 1.5:1 to 4:1. A catheter can easily be passed across the atrial septum into the left atrium.

Treatment

Surgical closure is generally recommended for ostium secundum type atrial septal defects in which the ratio of pulmonary to systemic blood flow is greater than 2:1. Operation is usually performed electively in patients between ages 2 and 4 years. The death rate for surgical closure is less than 1%. When surgical intervention is early, late complications of right ventricular dysfunction and significant dysrhythmias may be avoided or diminished. Early surgery is also indicated in infants presenting with congestive heart failure or significant pulmonary hypertension.

Course & Prognosis

Patients with atrial septal defects usually tolerate them very well in the first 2 decades of life, and an occasional patient may live a completely normal life without symptoms. Frequently, however, pulmonary hypertension and reversal of the shunt develop by the third or fourth decade. Heart failure may also occur at this time. Subacute infective endocarditis is a very rare complication. Spontaneous closure occurs and is sometimes associated with an aneurysm of the atrial septum. Exercise tolerance and oxygen consumption in surgically corrected children are generally normal, and physical limitations are unnecessary.

Cockerham JT et al: Spontaneous closure of secundum atrial septal defect in infants and young children. *Am J Cardiol* 1983;**52**:1267.

Fukazawa M, Fukushige J, Ueda K: Atrial septal defects in neonates with reference to spontaneous closure. *Am Heart J* 1988;**116**:123.

Mahoney LT et al: Atrial septal defects that present in infancy. *Am J Dis Child* 1986;**140**:1115.

Marx GA et al: Transatrial septal velocity: Measurement by Doppler echocardiography in atrial septal defect. *Am J Cardiol* 1985;**55**:1162.

Meyer RA et al: Long-term follow-up study after closure of secundum atrial septal defects in children. *Am J Cardiol* 1982;**50**:143.

Pollick C et al: Doppler color flow imaging assessment of shunt size in atrial septal defect. *Circulation* 1987;**78**:522.

VENTRICULAR SEPTAL DEFECTS

Essentials of Diagnosis

Small- to moderate-sized left-to-right shunt without pulmonary hypertension:
- Acyanotic, relatively asymptomatic.
- Grade II–IV/VI pansystolic murmur, maximal along the lower left sternal border.
- P_2 not accentuated.

Large left-to-right shunt:
- Acyanotic.
- Easy fatigability.
- Congestive heart failure in infancy (often).
- Hyperactive heart; biventricular enlargement.

- Grade II–V/VI pansystolic murmur, maximal at lower left sternal border.
- P_2 usually accentuated.
- Diastolic flow murmur at apex.

Insignificant left-to-right shunt or bidirectional shunt with pulmonary hypertension:
- Quiet precordium with right ventricular lift.
- Palpable P_2.
- Short ejection systolic murmur along left sternal border; single accentuated S_2.
- Systemic arterial oxygen desaturation may be present; pulmonary arterial pressure and systemic arterial pressures are equal; little or no oxygen saturation increase at right ventricular level by catheterization.

General Considerations

Simple ventricular septal defect (without other lesions) is the single most common congenital heart malformation, accounting for about 25% of all cases of congenital heart disease. Defects in the ventricular septum can occur both in the membranous portion of the septum (most common) and in the muscular portion.

There are 5 different courses that patients with ventricular septal defect may follow:

A. Spontaneous Closure: Thirty to 50% of all ventricular septal defects close spontaneously. The small defects close in 60–70% of cases. Larger defects may occasionally also close spontaneously, and there are many documented examples of spontaneous closure of ventricular septal defects in the second and third decades of life. Half of the defects that do not close become functionally or anatomically smaller.

B. Shunts Too Small to Justify Repair: Asymptomatic patients with hearts normal in size (as seen on x-ray film) and without pulmonary hypertension are generally not subjected to surgical repair. In those who have had cardiac catheterization, the ratio of pulmonary to systemic blood flow is usually found to be less than 2:1, and serial cardiac catheterizations demonstrate that the shunts get progressively smaller.

C. Disease Severe Enough to Require Surgery: The time of surgery depends upon the nature of the disease. Patients may require surgery in infancy because of intractable congestive heart failure; surgery before 2 years of age because of progression of pulmonary hypertension; or surgery between 2 and 5 years of age as an elective procedure.

D. Defect Inoperable Because of Pulmonary Hypertension: The vast majority of patients with inoperable pulmonary hypertension will develop this condition progressively. The combined data of the multicenter National History Study indicate that most cases of irreversible pulmonary hypertension can be prevented by surgical repair of the defect before 2 years of age.

E. Development of Infundibular Pulmonary

Stenosis: Approximately 5% of infants with large left-to-right shunts will develop progressive infundibular obstruction effecting an outflow gradient and diminution of the shunt. A small proportion of these infants have precyanotic tetralogy of Fallot, as evidenced by coexistent right aortic arch or abnormal spatial orientation of the infundibulum.

Clinical Findings

A. Symptoms and Signs: Patients with small or moderate left-to-right shunts usually have no cardiovascular symptoms. There may be a history of frequent respiratory infections in infancy and early childhood. Patients with large left-to-right shunts frequently are sick early in infancy. Such patients have frequent respiratory infections, including bouts of pneumonitis. They grow slowly, with very poor weight gain. Dyspnea, exercise intolerance, and fatigue are quite common. Congestive heart failure may develop between 1 and 6 months of age. Patients who survive the first year usually improve, although easy fatigability may persist. With severe pulmonary hypertension (Eisenmenger's syndrome), cyanosis is present.

1. Small left-to-right shunt—There are usually no lifts, heaves, thrills, or shocks. The first sound at the apex is normal, and the second sound at the pulmonary area is split physiologically. The pulmonary component is normal. A grade II–IV/VI, medium- to high-pitched, blowing pansystolic murmur is heard best at the left sternal border in the third and fourth intercostal spaces. There is slight radiation over the entire precordium. No diastolic murmurs are heard.

2. Moderate left-to-right shunt—Slight prominence of the precordium is common. There is a moderate left ventricular thrust. A systolic thrill is palpable at the lower left sternal border between the third and fourth intercostal spaces. The second sound at the pulmonary area is most often split but may be single. A grade IV/VI, harsh pansystolic murmur is heard best at the lower left sternal border in the fourth intercostal space. A diastolic flow murmur is heard and indicates that the pulmonary venous return across the mitral valve is large and that the pulmonary to systemic blood flow ratio is at least 2:1.

3. Very large ventricular septal defects with pulmonary hypertension—The precordium is prominent, and the sternum bulges. A left ventricular thrust and a right ventricular heave are palpable. A shock of the second sound can be felt at the pulmonary area. A thrill may or may not be present at the lower left sternal border. A second heart sound is usually single or narrowly split, with accentuation of the pulmonary component. The murmur ranges from grade II to grade V/VI and is usually harsh and pansystolic. Occasionally, when the defect is large, very little murmur can be heard. A diastolic flow murmur may or may not be heard, depending on the size of the shunt.

B. Imaging: X-ray findings of the chest vary, depending upon the size of the shunt. In patients with small shunts, x-ray findings may be normal. The heart is normal in size, and the pulmonary vascular markings may be just beyond the upper limits of normal. Patients with large shunts usually show significant cardiac enlargement involving both the left and right ventricles and the left atrium. The aorta is usually small to normal in size, and the main pulmonary artery segment is dilated. The pulmonary vascular markings are significantly increased in patients with large shunts.

C. Electrocardiography: There is some correlation between the electrocardiographic and the hemodynamic findings. The ECG is normal in patients with small left-to-right shunts and normal pulmonary arterial pressures. Left ventricular hypertrophy is usually found in patients with large left-to-right shunts and normal pulmonary vascular resistance. Combined ventricular hypertrophy (both right and left) is found in patients with pulmonary hypertension due to increased flow, increased resistance, or both. Pure right ventricular hypertrophy is found in patients with pulmonary hypertension due to pulmonary vascular obstruction.

D. Echocardiography: Two-dimensional echocardiography provides visualization of defects that are 4 mm or larger in about 65–75% of cases and often can pinpoint the anatomic location. Addition of color flow doppler, however, allows detection of smaller defects.

E. Cardiac Catheterization and Angiocardiography: Oxygen saturation is increased at the right ventricular level. The pulmonary artery pressure may vary from normal to that in the systemic arteries. Left atrial pressure (pulmonary capillary pressure) may be normal to increased. Pulmonary vascular resistance varies from normal to markedly increased. The ratio of pulmonary to systemic blood flow may vary from 1.1:1 to 4:1. Hydrogen electrode curves and dye dilution curves may indicate a shunt at the ventricular level. Angiocardiographic examination defines the number, size, and location of the defects.

Treatment

A. Medical Management: Patients who develop congestive heart failure should be treated vigorously with anticongestive measures (see Congestive Heart Failure, above). If the patient does not respond to vigorous anticongestive measures or shows signs of progressive pulmonary hypertension, surgery is indicated without delay. Transcatheter closure of ventricular septal defects is being evaluated as an experimental procedure.

B. Surgical Treatment: The age for elective surgery is becoming progressively younger in most centers (range, < 2 years to 5 years). Patients with cardiomegaly, poor growth, poor exercise tolerance, or other clinical abnormalities who have cardiac catheterization findings of significant shunt ($\geq$ 2:1) without significant pulmonary hypertension (> 10 units of resistance) are candidates for surgery. In general, patients with mean pulmonary artery pressures equal to systemic pressure who are unresponsive to oxygen administration, with little or no left-to-right shunt or bidirectional shunting, and pulmonary resistance calculated to be greater than 10 resistance units (or pulmonary/systemic resistance ratios > 0.7) are considered inoperable. There are patients who have pulmonary hypertension of lesser degree who remain operable, but there is a progressively greater risk with increasing pulmonary hypertension (from 1% risk for patients without pulmonary hypertension to 25% for those at the upper limits of operability).

In order to prevent pulmonary hypertension from reaching inoperable levels, early surgical intervention is recommended for patients who have increased pulmonary vascular resistance. In centers with the capability of doing total correction on infants with or without deep hypothermia, complete repair before 2 years of age is recommended. The presence of multiple muscular defects in a tiny symptomatic infant is still considered to be an indication for pulmonary artery banding as an initial palliative procedure.

Course & Prognosis

Significant late dysrhythmias are uncommon. Functional exercise capacity and oxygen consumption are usually normal, and physical restrictions are unnecessary.

Cheatham JP, Latson LA, Gutgesell HP: Ventricular septal defect in infancy: Detection with two-dimensional echocardiography. *Am J Cardiol* 1981;**47**:85.

Lock JE et al: Transcatheter closure of ventricular septal defects. *Circulation* 1988;**78**:361.

Moller JH et al: Predictive value of lung biopsy in ventricular septal defect: Long-term follow up. *J Am Coll Cardiol* 1986;**8**:1113.

Ramaciollit C, Keven A, Silverman NH: Importance of perimembranous ventricular septal aneurysm in the natural history of isolated permembranous ventricular septal defect. *Am J Cardiol* 1986;**57**:268.

Yeager SB et al: Primary surgical closure of ventricular septal defect in the first year of life: Results in 128 infants. *J Am Coll Cardiol* 1984;**3**:1269.

ATRIOVENTRICULAR SEPTAL DEFECT

Essentials of Diagnosis
- Murmur often inaudible in neonates.
- Loud pulmonary component of S_2.
- Common in infants with Down's syndrome.
- ECG with left axis deviation.

General Considerations

An atrioventricular septal defect is a congenital cardiac abnormality that results from incomplete fusion of the embryonic endocardial cushions. The endocardial cushions help to form the lower portion of the atrial septum, the membranous portion of the ventricular septum, and the septal leaflets of the tricuspid and mitral valves. These defects are not very common. They account for about 4% of all cases of congenital heart disease. The incidence of this abnormality is 20% in patients with Down's syndrome.

Atrioventricular septal defects may be divided into incomplete and complete forms. The complete form, also known as persistent common atrioventricular canal, consists of a high ventricular septal defect, a low atrial septal defect of the ostium primum variety that is continuous with the ventricular septal defect, and a cleft in both the septal leaflet of the tricuspid valve and the anterior leaflet of the mitral valve. In the incomplete form, any one of these components may be present. The most common partial form of atrioventricular septal defect is the ostium primum type of atrial septal defect with a cleft in the mitral valve.

The complete form (persistent common atrioventricular canal) results in large left-to-right shunts at both the ventricular and atrial levels, tricuspid and mitral regurgitation, and marked pulmonary hypertension, usually with some increase in pulmonary vascular resistance. When the latter is present, the shunts may be bidirectional. The hemodynamics in the incomplete form are dependent upon the lesions present.

Clinical Findings

A. Symptoms and Signs: The clinical picture varies depending upon the severity of the defect. In the incomplete form, these patients may be indistinguishable from patients with the ostium secundum type of atrial septal defect. They are often asymptomatic. On the other hand, patients with atrioventricular canal usually are severely affected. Congestive heart failure often develops in infancy, and recurrent bouts of pneumonitis are common.

In the complete form, the murmur may be inaudible in the neonate. After 4–6 weeks, a nonspecific systolic murmur develops; the murmur is usually not as harsh as that of an isolated ventricular septal defect. The heart is significantly enlarged (both right and left sides), and a systolic thrill may be palpated at the lower left sternal border. The second heart sound is split, with an accentuated pulmonary component. A pronounced diastolic flow murmur may be heard at the apex and lower left sternal border.

When severe pulmonary vascular obstruction is present, there is evidence of dominant right ventricular enlargement. A shock of the second sound can be palpated at the pulmonary area. No thrill is felt. The second sound is markedly accentuated and single. A nonspecific short systolic murmur is heard at the lower left sternal border. No diastolic flow murmurs are heard. Cyanosis is detectable in severe cases with predominant right-to-left shunts.

The physical findings in the incomplete form depend upon the lesions. In the most common variety (ostium primum atrial septal defect with mitral regurgitation), the findings are similar to those of the ostium secundum type of atrial septal defect with or without findings of mitral regurgitation.

B. Imaging: As indicated on x-ray film, cardiac enlargement is present depending on the degree of specific anatomic defect and the severity. In the complete (canal) form, there is enlargement of all 4 chambers. The pulmonary vascular markings are increased. In patients with pulmonary vascular obstruction, only the main pulmonary artery segment and its branches are prominent. The peripheral markings are usually decreased.

C. Electrocardiography: In all forms of atrioventricular septal defect, left axis deviation with a counterclockwise loop in the frontal plane is present. The mean axis varies from approximately -30 to -90 degrees. Since left axis deviation is present in all patients with this defect, the ECG is a very important diagnostic tool. First-degree heart block is present in over 50% of cases. Right, left, or combined ventricular hypertrophy is present depending upon the particular type of defect and the presence or absence of pulmonary vascular obstruction.

D. Echocardiography: On M mode echocardiography, excursion of the atrioventricular valve through the plane of the interventricular septal defect is characteristic. The anatomy can be directly visualized by 2-dimensional echocardiography; the sensitivity of this method is equal to that of selective cineangiography.

E. Cardiac Catheterization and Angiocardiography: The results of cardiac catheterization vary depending upon the type of defect present. When catheterization is performed from the leg, the catheter is easily passed across the atrial septum in its lowest portion and frequently enters the left ventricle directly. This catheter course is a result of the very low atrial septal defect and the cleft in the mitral valve. Increased oxygen saturation in the right ventricle or right atrium identifies the level of the shunt. Angiocardiography reveals a characteristic "gooseneck" deformity in the complete canal form. Two-dimensional doppler color flow echocardiography is extremely useful in identifying the subgroups of endocardial cushion defects.

Treatment

Treatment consists of anticongestive measures and eventual surgical correction. In the incomplete form, surgery is associated with a relatively low death rate (2–5%). The complete form is associated with a significantly higher death rate (about 15–25%), but complete correction in the first year of life, prior to the onset of irreversible pulmonary hypertension, is advisable.

Pulmonary artery banding procedures are contraindicated in infants with shunts predominantly at the atrial level. They are less effective in patients with predominantly ventricular level shunts than in patients with simple ventricular septal defect.

Hawort SG: Pulmonary vascular bed in children with complete atrioventricular septal defect: Relation between structure and hemodynamic abnormalities. *Am J Cardiol* 1986;**57**:833.

Kawashima Y et al: Surgical treatment of complete atrioventricular canal defect with an endocardial cushion prosthesis. *Circulation* 1983;**68**:1421.

Sato B et al: Angiography of atrioventricular canal defects. *Am J Cardiol* 1981;**48**:492.

PATENT DUCTUS ARTERIOSUS

Essentials of Diagnosis

- Variable murmur, with active percordium and full pulses, in newborn premature infants.
- Continuous murmur and full pulses in older infants.

General Considerations

Patent ductus arteriosus is the persistence in extrauterine life of the normal fetal vessel that joins the pulmonary artery to the aorta. It closes spontaneously in normal term infants by 4 days of age. It is a common abnormality, accounting for about 12% of all cases of congenital heart disease. It is very common in children born to mothers who had rubella during the first trimester of pregnancy. There is a higher incidence of patent ductus arteriosus in infants born at high altitudes (over 10,000 feet). It is twice as common in females as in males. In intensive care premature nurseries in infants weighing less than 1500 g, the frequency of patent ductus arteriosus may be as high as 20–60%.

The defect occurs as an isolated abnormality, but associated lesions are not infrequent. Coarctation of the aorta, patent ductus arteriosus, and ventricular septal defect are commonly associated. Even more important to recognize are those patients with murmurs of patent ductus but without readily apparent findings of other associated lesions who are being kept alive by the patent ductus (eg, a patient with patent ductus with asymptomatic pulmonary atresia).

Clinical Findings

A. Symptoms and Signs: The clinical findings and the clinical course depend on the size of the shunt and the degree of pulmonary hypertension.

1. Typical patent ductus arteriosus—The pulses are bounding, and pulse pressure is widened (pulse pressure is greater than half of the systolic pressure). The first heart sound is normal. The second heart sound is usually narrowly split and very rarely (when the shunt is maximal) paradoxically split (ie, the second sound closes on inspiration and splits on expiration). The paradoxic splitting is due to the maximal overload of the left ventricle and the prolonged ejection of blood from this chamber.

The murmur is quite characteristic. It is a very rough "machinery" murmur that is maximal at the second intercostal space at the left sternal border and inferior to the left clavicle. It begins shortly after the first heart sound, rises to a peak at the second heart sound, and passes through the second heart sound into diastole, where it becomes a descrescendo murmur and fades or disappears before the first heart sound. The murmur tends to radiate fairly well over the lung fields anteriorly but relatively poorly over the lung fields posteriorly. A diastolic flow murmur is often heard at the apex. Depending on the pulmonary artery pressure, the murmur may be only systolic in time. This characteristic should be fully appreciated when trying to reach a diagnosis of patent ductus arteriosus in infants. If the shunt is small, congestive failure is absent; if the shunt is large, congestive failure becomes important.

2. Patent ductus arteriosus with pulmonary hypertension—The physical findings depend upon the cause of the pulmonary hypertension. If pulmonary hypertension is due primarily to a marked increase in blood flow and only a slight increase in pulmonary vascular resistance, the physical findings are similar to those listed above. The significant difference is the presence of an accentuated pulmonary component of S_2. Bounding pulses and a loud continuous heart murmur are present. In patients with pulmonary vascular resistance and predominant right-to-left shunt, the findings are quite different. There may be evidence of cyanosis. The second heart sound is single and quite accentuated, and there is no significant heart murmur. The pulses are normal rather than bounding.

3. Patent ductus arteriosus in the premature neonate with associated RDS—A premature neonate during or after the clinical course of respiratory distress syndrome (RDS) may have a significant associated patent ductus arteriosus that is paradoxically difficult to detect clinically but is often threatening in magnitude. A soft, nonspecific systolic murmur or no murmur is more common than the classic continuous murmur. The peripheral pulse and precordium are often bounding but typically are not characteristic for several days after the onset of a large left-to-right shunt. An early sign indicating the presence of a significant left-to-right shunt with concomitant congestive heart failure is increasing dependence on oxygen and respiratory support. In addition, increasing radiographic cardiomegaly and pulmonary edema plus increasing echocardiographic evidence of a left-to-right shunt differentiate this clinical and laboratory picture from bronchopulmonary dysplasia.

B. Imaging: In simple patent ductus arteriosus, the x-ray appearance depends upon the size of the shunt. If the shunt is relatively small or moderate in size, the heart is not enlarged. If the shunt is large, there is evidence of both left atrial and left ventricular enlargement. In both cases, the aorta is prominent, as is the main pulmonary artery segment.

C. Electrocardiography: The ECG may be normal or may show left ventricular hypertrophy, depending on the size of the shunt. In patients with pulmonary hypertension due to increased blood flow, there is usually biventricular hypertrophy. In those with pulmonary vascular obstruction, there is pure right ventricular hypertrophy. An anterior ST depression (V_1) of 2 mm suggests subendocardial ischemia due to a diastolic "steal" from the coronary arteries via the ductus; this finding indicates the need for closure.

D. Echocardiography: Enlargement of the left atrium as measured by M mode echocardiography is an important clue to the presence of congestive heart failure and is especially useful in diagnosing patent ductus arteriosus in the premature infant. A left atrial to ascending aorta ratio of less than 1.2 or 1.3 is considered evidence of a sizable left-to-right ductal shunt. Premature infants with patent ductus arteriosus who are undergoing medical or surgical therapy for closure should have a complete 2-dimensional echocardiographic evaluation to rule out associated heart disease, especially ductus-dependent lesions. The use of color flow pulsed doppler ultrasonography and 2-dimensional echocardiography can provide visualization of the ductus and confirmation of the direction and degree of shunting and may eliminate the need for a diagnostic cardiac catheterization.

E. Cardiac Catheterization and Angiocardiography: Cardiac catheterization will reveal increased oxygen content or saturation at the level of the pulmonary artery. Hydrogen electrode curves are positive in the pulmonary artery and negative in the right ventricle. The catheter can often be passed through the ductus from the pulmonary artery into the descending thoracic aorta. Arteriograms taken following injection of contrast material into the aortic arch show a shunt at the level of the ductus. If catheterization is not performed, the cardiologist must be completely satisfied that there is neither an associated lesion nor pulmonary hypertension. Transcatheter closure of patent ductus arteriosus is once again being evaluated in selected centers staffed by personnel with expertise in interventional cardiology in older children.

Patients with patent ductus arteriosus and pulmonary hypertension due to large left-to-right shunts show a marked increase in oxygen saturation at the pulmonary artery level and normal systemic arterial saturation. Those with marked pulmonary vascular obstruction show little or no increase in oxygen content at the pulmonary artery and a decrease in systemic arterial saturation. In both cases, a catheter may be passed through the ductus into the descending thoracic aorta.

Cardiac catheterization is rarely indicated in the premature infant with symptomatic ductus.

Treatment

Treatment consists of surgical correction except in patients with pulmonary vascular obstruction. Patients with large left-to-right shunts and pulmonary hypertension should be operated on very early (even under the age of 1 year) to prevent the development of progressive pulmonary vascular obstruction. Simple patent ductus arteriosus should be corrected after the child reaches age 1, though the operation may be delayed until later without increasing the risk of death.

Patients with nonreactive pulmonary vascular obstruction who have resistance greater than 10 units and a pulmonary/systemic resistance ratio greater than 0.7 should not be operated upon. These patients are made worse by closure of the ductus, because the ductus serves as an escape route and limits the degree of pulmonary hypertension.

The premature infant with symptomatic ductus presents a special and controversial problem. At some institutions, it is customary to operate on virtually all premature infants weighing under 1200 g. At other institutions, surgery is rarely done, and most infants receive a maximum of 3 doses of either oral indomethacin (0.1–0.3 mg/kg every 8–24 hours) or parenteral indomethacin (0.1–0.3 mg/kg every 12 hours) if adequate renal, hematologic, and hepatic function are demonstrated. Contraindications to indomethacin treatment include hyperbilirubinemia of 12 mg/100 mL or greater, renal failure, shock, necrotizing enterocolitis, intracranial hemorrhage, hemorrhagic disease, and evidence of a spontaneously closing ductus. Efficacy and safety of indomethacin use are enhanced by the careful monitoring of serum levels of indomethacin. A serum level of less than 250 ng/mL is associated with treatment failure. Conventional conservative management includes fluid restriction with or without diuretics and ligation only if these fail. Factors to be considered in making a rational decision on modality of therapy include a high rate of spontaneous ductus closure without therapy and an extremely low surgical risk in experienced centers; the inability of a laboratory to monitor serum levels of indomethacin may influence the decision.

Course & Prognosis

Patients with simple patent ductus arteriosus and small to moderate shunts usually do quite well even without surgery. However, in the third or fourth decade of life, symptoms of easy fatigability, dyspnea on exertion, and exercise intolerance appear, usually

as a consequence of the development of pulmonary hypertension or congestive heart failure.

Spontaneous closure of a patent ductus arteriosus may occur within the first 2 years of life. This is especially true in infants who were born prematurely. After age 2, spontaneous closure is rare. Because subacute infective endocarditis is a potential complication, surgical ligation is recommended if the defect persists beyond age 2 years.

Patients with large shunts or pulmonary hypertension do much less well. Poor growth and development, frequent episodes of pneumonitis, and the development of congestive heart failure are not uncommon in patients with large left-to-right shunts. If these patients do not succumb to congestive heart failure in early infancy, they frequently go on to develop pulmonary vascular obstruction in later childhood or adolescence. Life expectancy is markedly reduced, and these patients often die in their second or third decade. Those rare patients with pulmonary vascular obstruction from very early infancy are actually less symptomatic than those with pulmonary hypertension without obstruction.

Dudell GG, Gersony WM: Patent ductus arteriosus in neonates with severe respiratory disease. *J Pediatr* 1984;**104**:915.

Gersony WM et al: Effects of indomethacin in premature infants with patent ductus arteriosus: Results of a national collaborative study. *J Pediatr* 1983;**102**:895.

Goldberg SJ: Response of the patent ductus arteriosus to indomethacin treatment. *Am J Dis Child* 1987;**141**:250.

Rashkind WJ et al: Nonsurgical closure of patent ductus arteriosus. *Circulation* 1987;**75**:583.

Reller MD et al: Duration of ductal shunting in healthy preterm infants: An echocardiographic color flow Doppler study. *J Pediatr* 1988;**112**:441.

Valdez-Cruz M et al: Real-time Doppler color flow mapping for detection of patent ductus arteriosus. *J Am Coll Cardiol* 1986;**8**:1105.

Way GL et al: ST depression suggesting subendocardial ischemia in neonates with respiratory distress syndrome and patent ductus arteriosus. *J Pediatr* 1979;**95**:609.

MALFORMATIONS ASSOCIATED WITH OBSTRUCTION TO BLOOD FLOW ON THE RIGHT SIDE OF THE HEART

1. VALVULAR PULMONARY STENOSIS WITH INTACT VENTRICULAR SEPTUM

Essentials of Diagnosis

- No symptoms with mild and moderately severe cases.
- Cyanosis and a high incidence of right-sided congestive heart failure in very severe cases.

- Right ventricular lift; systolic ejection click at the pulmonary area in mild to moderately severe cases.
- S_2 widely split with soft to inaudible P_2; grade I–VI/VI obstructive systolic murmur, maximal at the pulmonary area.
- Dilated pulmonary artery on posteroanterior chest x-ray film.

General Considerations

Obstruction of right ventricular outflow at the pulmonary valve level accounts for about 10% of all cases of congenital heart disease. In the usual case, the cusps of the pulmonary valve are fused to form a membrane or diaphragm with a hole in the middle that varies from 2 mm to 1 cm in diameter. Occasionally, there may be a fusion of only 2 cusps, producing a bicuspid pulmonary valve. Very frequently, especially in the more severe cases, there is secondary infundibular stenosis. The pulmonary valve ring is usually small. There is usually moderate to marked poststenotic dilatation of both the main and left pulmonary arteries. Patent foramen ovale is fairly common.

Obstruction to blood flow across the pulmonary valve results in an increase in pressure developed by the right ventricle to maintain an adequate output across that valve. Pressures greater than systemic are potentially life-threatening and are associated with ''critical'' obstruction. As a consequence of the increased work required of the right ventricle, severe right ventricular hypertrophy and eventual right ventricular failure can occur. In contrast to patients with right ventricular outflow obstruction, patients with this obstruction who also have a large ventricular septal defect (ie, tetralogy of Fallot) are not at great risk for heart failure; because of the septal defect, there is communication between the ventricles, which limits the amount of pressure developed in the right ventricle (pressure is equal to systemic pressure) and thereby makes heart failure extremely uncommon.

When the obstruction is severe and the ventricular septum is intact, a right-to-left shunt will often occur at the atrial level through a patent foramen ovale. Accordingly, patients with this condition may have a varying degree of cynosis. The presence of cyanosis indicates a relatively severe degree of valvular obstruction.

Clinical Findings

A. Symptoms and Signs: The history depends upon the severity of the obstruction. Patients with a mild or even a moderate degree of valvular pulmonary stenosis are completely asymptomatic throughout infancy, childhood, and adolescence. Patients with a more severe type of valvular obstruction may develop cyanosis and congestive heart failure very early—even in the neonatal period. Hypoxemic spells characterized by a sudden onset of marked cyanosis and dyspnea are much less common than in tetralogy of Fallot.

Patients with mild to moderate obstruction are acyanotic. Patients with severe or critical stenosis usually show evidence of central cyanosis. These patients are usually well developed and well nourished. They often have a round face and widely spaced eyes. The pulses are normal and equal throughout. Clubbing may occur in severe cases in which cyanosis has persisted for a long time. On examination of the heart, there may be prominence of the precordium. A heaving impulse of the right ventricle can frequently be palpated. A systolic thrill is often palpated in the pulmonary area and occasionally in the suprasternal notch. The first heart sound is normal. In patients with mild to moderate stenosis, a prominent ejection click of pulmonary origin is heard best at the second left intercostal space. This click varies with respiration. It is much more prominent during expiration than inspiration. In patients with severe stenosis, the click tends to merge with the first heart sound. The second heart sound also varies with the degree of stenosis. In mild valvular stenosis, the second heart sound is normally split and the pulmonary component is normal in intensity. In moderate degrees of obstruction, the second heart sound is more widely split and the pulmonary component is softer. In severe pulmonary stenosis, the second heart sound is single, since the pulmonary component cannot be heard. An ejection type, rough, obstructive systolic murmur is best heard at the second interspace at the left sternal border. It radiates very well to the back. No diastolic murmurs are audible. In older children, a prominent ''A'' wave is seen in the jugular venous pulse. If there is congestive heart failure, the liver is enlarged.

B. Imaging: In the mild form of pulmonary stenosis, the heart may be normal in size. Poststenotic dilatation of the main pulmonary artery segment and the left pulmonary artery is often present. In moderate to severe cases, there may be a slight right ventricular enlargement, and there may or may not be poststenotic dilatation of the main pulmonary artery. In patients who are cyanotic, the pulmonary vascular markings are decreased; otherwise, they are normal.

C. Electrocardiography: Electrocardiographic findings are usually normal in patients with mild obstruction. Right ventricular hypertrophy is present in patients with moderate to severe valvular obstruction. In severe obstruction, right ventricular hypertrophy and the right ventricular strain pattern (deep inversion of the T wave) are seen in the right precordial leads. In the most severe form, right atrial hypertrophy is also present. Right axis deviation is also seen in the moderate to severe forms. Occasionally, the axis is greater than +180 degrees.

D. Echocardiography: M mode echocardiography reveals atrial contraction and elevated right ventricular diastolic pressure causing early opening of the pulmonary valve (ie, opening prior to the onset of ventricular systole). The pulmonary valve appears to be unusually echo-dense. The pulmonary valve image on 2-dimensional echocardiography shows a thickened structure with less than normal excursion. The transvalvular pressure gradient can be noninvasively and accurately estimated by echo doppler technique.

E. Cardiac Catheterization and Angiocardiography: There is no increase in oxygen saturation or oxygen content in the right side of the heart. In the more severe cases, there is a right-to-left shunt at the atrial level. Pulmonary artery pressure is normal in milder cases and quite low in moderately severe to severe cases. Right ventricular pressure is always higher than pulmonary artery pressure. The gradient across the pulmonary valve varies from 10 to 200 mm Hg. In severe cases, the right atrial pressure is often elevated, with a predominant "A" wave. Cineangiocardiography with injection of contrast material into the right ventricle shows thickening of the pulmonary valve and the very narrow opening of the pulmonary valve. This produces a "jet" of contrast from the right ventricle into the pulmonary artery. Infundibular hypertrophy may be present. This is seen as a marked narrowing of the right ventricular outflow track during ventricular systole followed by a widening during diastole.

Treatment

Elective valvotomy is recommended for children with right ventricular pressures of greater than 50 mm Hg or higher than two-thirds of systemic pressure. Immediate correction is indicated for patients with systemic or greater right ventricular pressure. Percutaneous balloon valvuloplasty can also be performed to relieve the valvular obstruction.

The need for additional surgical resection of associated infundibular hypertrophy is controversial. Because additional surgery increases the risk and because the outflow obstruction usually regresses, many centers perform only the valvotomy.

Course & Prognosis

Patients with mild pulmonary stenosis live a normal life and have a normal life span. Those with stenosis of moderate severity usually show symptoms of easy fatigability and dyspnea on exertion, which may be progressive. Those with severe valvular obstruction may develop severe cyanosis and congestive heart failure in early life.

Postoperative follow-up suggests that most patients with right ventricular pressure equal to or less than systemic pressure who were treated surgically early in life have good voluntary maximum exercise capacity. If relief of valvular obstruction occurs prior to 20 years of age, longevity is essentially the same as that of the general population. Physical restriction is unwarranted in these patients.

Edwards BS et al: Morphologic changes in the pulmonary arteries after percutaneous balloon angioplasty for pulmonary artery stenosis. *Circulation* 1985;**71**:195.

Griffith BP et al: Pulmonary valvulotomy alone for pulmonary stenosis: Results in children with and without muscular infundibular hypertrophy. *J Thorac Cardiovasc Surg* 1982;**83**:577.

Kan JS et al: Percutaneous balloon valvuloplasty: A new method for treating congenital pulmonary valve stenosis. *N Engl J Med* 1982;**307**:540.

Kopecky SL et al: Long term outcome of patients undergoing surgical repair of isolated pulmonary valve stenosis. *Circulation* 1988;**78**:1150.

Marantz PM et al: Results of balloon valvuloplasty in typical and dysplastic pulmonary valve stenosis: Doppler echocardiographic follow up. *J Am Coll Cardiol* 1988; **12**:476.

Rey C et al: Percutaneous transluminal balloon valvuloplasty of congenital pulmonary valve stenosis, with a special report on infants and neonates. *J Am Coll Cardiol* 1988;**11**:815.

2. INFUNDIBULAR PULMONARY STENOSIS WITHOUT VENTRICULAR SEPTAL DEFECT

Pure infundibular pulmonary stenosis is rare. One should suspect infundibular pulmonary stenosis where there is evidence of mild to moderate pulmonary stenosis and intact ventricular septum and (1) no pulmonary ejection click is audible and (2) the murmur is maximal in the third and fourth intercostal spaces rather than in the second intercostal space. Otherwise, the clinical picture may be identical.

3. DISTAL PULMONARY STENOSIS

Supravalvular Pulmonary Stenosis

Supravalvular pulmonary stenosis, a relatively rare condition, is due to coarctation of the body of the main pulmonary artery. The clinical picture may be identical with that of valvular pulmonary stenosis, although the murmur is maximal in the first intercostal space at the left sternal border and in the suprasternal notch. No ejection click is audible. A second heart sound is usually narrowly split, and the pulmonary component is quite loud as a result of closure of the pulmonary valve under high pressure. The murmur radiates extremely well into the neck and over the lung fields.

Peripheral Pulmonary Branch Stenosis

In peripheral pulmonary branch stenosis, there are multiple small coarctations of the branches of the pulmonary artery in the periphery of the lung. Systolic murmurs may be heard over both lung fields, both anteriorly and posteriorly. The transient pulmonary branch stenosis murmurs of infancy (previously described under heart murmurs) are innocent. Pulmonary artery branch stenosis murmurs may be the most audible murmurs in atrial septal defects in infancy and early childhood. The most common cause of significant pulmonary artery branch stenosis is maternal rubella. Several types of supravalvular aortic stenosis syndromes may be found in association with this condition.

Surgery is often unsuccessful. Transvenous angioplasty is currently being assessed but does not appear to be as efficacious in patients with peripheral pulmonary branch stenosis as in patients with pulmonary valvular stenosis.

Absence of a Pulmonary Artery

Absence of a pulmonary artery may be an isolated malformation or may occur in association with other congenital heart diseases. It is occasionally seen in patients with tetralogy of Fallot.

Dunkle LM, Rowe RD: Transient murmur simulating pulmonary artery stenosis in premature infants. *Am J Dis Child* 1972;**124:**666.

Lock JE et al: Balloon dilatation angioplasty of hypoplastic and stenotic pulmonary arteries. *Circulation* 1983; **67:**962.

MALFORMATIONS ASSOCIATED WITH OBSTRUCTION TO BLOOD FLOW ON THE LEFT SIDE OF THE HEART

1. COARCTATION OF THE AORTA

Essentials of Diagnosis

- Pulse lag in lower extremities.
- Blood pressure of 20 mm Hg or pressure greater in upper than in lower extremities.
- Blowing systolic murmur in left axilla.

General Considerations

Coarctation is a common cardiac abnormality accounting for about 6% of all cases of congenital heart disease. Three times as many males as females are affected. In the vast majority of cases, coarctation occurs in the thoracic portion of the descending aorta. The abdominal aorta is very rarely involved. Coarctations are usually in the juxtaductal position rather than the pre- or postductal position. The term **coarctation of aorta syndrome** is a useful concept, because most symptomatic infants will have associated patent ductus arteriosus, tubular hypoplasia of the aortic isthmus (frequently erroneously termed a coarctation), ventricular septal defect, and bicuspid aortic valve. The tubular hypoplasia of the aortic

isthmus is probably related to paucity of blood flow in the fetus and often spontaneously enlarges with postnatal growth.

Clinical Findings

A. Symptoms and Signs: Patients with coarctation may or may not have cardiovascular symptoms in infancy, childhood, and adolescence. Congestive heart failure may develop in early infancy, and symptoms of decreased exercise tolerance and fatigability may appear in childhood.

The important physical finding is diminution or absence of femoral pulses. However, a significant number of infants will initially have equal upper and lower extremity pulses until the coexistent patent ductus arteriosus closes. Normally, the blood pressure in the upper extremities is slightly higher than in the lower extremities during the first few months of life. After 1 year of age, blood pressure higher in the arms than in the legs is suggestive of coarctation of the aorta. The actual level of blood pressure in the arms may be only moderately elevated, even in severe coarctation, or it may be significantly elevated. In the presence of severe congestive heart failure, the differences in pulses in the upper and lower extremities may not be readily apparent, but with compensation, the pulses in the arms are palpably stronger than those of normal infants; the pulses in the legs remain diminished or absent in affected infants. The left subclavian artery is occasionally involved in the coarctation, in which case the left brachial pulse is weak. If the coarctation is uncomplicated, the heart sounds are normal. The aortic component of the second heart sound is occasionally increased in intensity. An ejection systolic murmur of grade II/VI intensity is often heard at the aortic area and the lower left sternal border. The pathognomonic murmur of coarctation is heard in the interscapular area of the back, over the area of the coarctation. This murmur is usually systolic in timing. If the coarctation is complicated by other malformations, murmurs associated with these other abnormalities will be audible.

B. Imaging: In the older child, x-ray findings may indicate a heart normal in size, although there is usually some evidence of left ventricular enlargement. The ascending aorta is usually normal in size. On barium swallow, the esophagus has a characteristic E shape. The first arc of the E is due to dilatation of the aorta just proximal to the coarctation. The second arc is due to poststenotic dilatation of the aorta. The middle bar of the E is due to the coarctation itself. In older children, notching or scalloping of the ribs caused by marked enlargement of the intercostal collaterals can be seen.

In infants in congestive heart failure, there is evidence of marked cardiac enlargement and pulmonary venous congestion.

C. Electrocardiography: ECGs in children may

be normal or may show evidence of slight left ventricular hypertrophy. In infants with or without congestive heart failure, the ECG usually demonstrates right ventricular hypertrophy.

D. Echocardiography: M mode echocardiography reveals only secondary evidence of the coarctation. In infants with congestive heart failure, dilated right and left ventricles are noted. A striking posterior displacement of the mitral valve in the left ventricular cavity with poor excursion is common. Real-time 2-dimensional echocardiography may visualize the coarctation directly, and color flow doppler may serve as an accurate predictor of severity.

E. Cardiac Catheterization and Angiocardiography: These studies demonstrate the position, anatomy, and severity of the coarctation and will assess the adequacy of the collateral circulation.

Treatment

Infants with coarctation of the aorta and congestive heart failure require vigorous anticongestive measures. Dilation of the associated patent ductus arteriosus with a constant infusion of prostaglandin E_1 may stabilize the critically ill infant until operation can be performed. Many with isolated coarctation and no associated lesions respond well and do not require surgery in infancy. In infants with striking congestive heart failure and without associated cardiovascular abnormalities, severe systemic hypertension is often a contributing factor. Reduction of afterload with intravenous nitroprusside or propranolol followed by chronic oral propranolol is often lifesaving and allows deferral of definitive correction until a more optimal age.

Infants with associated intracardiac defects sometimes need immediate surgery but frequently require revision of the recoarctation later in life. Modification of the surgical technique utilizing a subclavian flap anastomosis reduces the likelihood of this late complication. This technique has been used successfully in infants weighing as little as 1000 g.

Percutaneous balloon angioplasty has been used successfully as a palliative procedure to stabilize critically ill infants with coarctation of aorta syndrome. It is likely that surgical correction will be necessary after stabilization. Percutaneous balloon angioplasty is also being utilized to dilate recoarctations in postoperative patients.

Patients who do not require surgery early in life may be corrected electively at ages 3–5 years unless significant systemic hypertension develops.

Course & Prognosis

Children who survive the neonatal period without developing congestive heart failure do quite well throughout childhood and adolescence. Fatal complications (eg, hypertensive encephalopathy, intracranial bleeding) occur uncommonly. Subacute infective endocarditis is also rare before adolescence.

School-age children in whom coarctation was corrected during infancy are at significant risk for systemic hypertension and myocardial dysfunction. Careful exercise testing is mandatory prior to their participation in athletic activities.

Starting in the third decade of life, the patient may develop the onset of easy fatigability, dyspnea on exertion, cardiac enlargement, and left ventricular failure. Only one-fourth of these patients may be expected to live through the fourth decade. Death results from subacute infective endocarditis or hypertensive cardiovascular disease.

Hammon JW Jr et al: Operative repair of coarctation of the aorta in infancy: Results with and without ventricular septal defect. *Am J Cardiol* 1985;**55**:1555.

Markel H et al: Exercise-induced hypertension after repair of coarctation of the aorta: Arm versus leg exercise. *J Am Coll Cardiol* 1986;**8**:165.

Morrow WR et al: Balloon dilatation of unoperated coarctation of the aorta: Short- and intermediate-term results. *J Am Coll Cardiol* 1988;**11**:133.

Moss AJ: Coarctation of the aorta: Current status. *J Pediatr* 1983;**102**:253.

Parker BP et al: Preoperative and postoperative renin levels in coarctation of the aorta. *Circulation* 1982;**66**:513.

Rao PS: Balloon angioplasty for coarctation of the aorta in infancy. *J Pediatr* 1987;**110**:713.

Simpson IA et al: Color flow Doppler flow mapping in patients with coarctation of the aorta: New observations and improved evaluation with color flow diameter and proximal acceleration as predictors of severity. *Circulation* 1988;**77**:736.

Stafford MA, Griffiths SP, Gersony WM: Coarctation of the aorta: A study in delayed detection. *Pediatrics* 1982;**69**:159.

2. AORTIC STENOSIS

Essentials of Diagnosis

- Systolic ejection murmur at upper right sternal border.
- Thrill in carotid arteries.
- Systolic click at the apex.
- Dilatation of the ascending aorta on chest x-ray.

General Considerations

Aortic stenosis may be defined from the anatomic or physiologic point of view. Anatomically, it consists of an obstruction to the outflow from the left ventricle at or near the aortic valve. Physiologically, aortic stenosis may be defined as a condition in which a systolic pressure gradient of more than 10 mm Hg exists between the left ventricle and the aorta. Aortic stenosis accounts for approximately 5% of all cases of congenital heart disease. Anatomically, congenital aortic stenosis may be divided into 4 types:

A. Valvular Aortic Stenosis (75%): Critical aortic stenosis presenting in infancy usually consists of a unicuspid diaphragmlike structure without well-defined commissures. Preschool and school-age children more commonly present with a bicuspid valve. Teenagers and young adults characteristically present with tricuspid but partially fused leaflets. This lesion is more common in males than females.

B. Discrete Membranous Subvalvular Aortic Stenosis (20%): This consists of a membranous or fibrous ring just below the aortic valve. The ring forms a diaphragm with a hole in the middle and results in obstruction to left ventricular outflow. The aortic valve itself and the anterior leaflet of the mitral valve are often deformed.

C. Supravalvular Aortic Stenosis: In this variety, there is a constriction of the ascending aorta just above the coronary arteries. This condition is often associated with a family history, abnormal facies, and mental retardation (idiopathic hypercalcemia syndrome).

D. Idiopathic Hypertrophic Subaortic Stenosis (IHSS): In this case, there is a marked hypertrophy of the entire left ventricle and, predominantly, the ventricular septum. With contraction of the ventricle, the hypertrophic portion of the septum, together with the mitral valve, causes obstruction of left ventricular outflow. A family history is often present.

Obstruction to outflow from the left ventricle causes the left ventricle to work harder to maintain an adequate pressure and flow in the systemic arterial circuit, resulting in hypertrophy of the left ventricle and increased oxygen requirement. If the stenosis is severe, the oxygen requirements may exceed the capacity of the coronary arteries to supply oxygen, and relative coronary insufficiency may develop. In critical aortic stenosis, left ventricular failure may occur. The left ventricle is usually able to adapt to the increased pressure load for a considerable period of time before heart failure or coronary insufficiency develops.

Clinical Findings

A. Symptoms and Signs: Most patients with aortic stenosis have no cardiovascular symptoms. Except in the most severe cases, the patient may do well up until the third to fifth decade of life, although some patients have mild exercise intolerance and easy fatigability. A small percentage of patients have significant symptoms within the first decade, ie, dizziness and syncope. Sudden death, although uncommon, may occur in all forms of aortic stenosis, with the greatest risk being idiopathic hypertrophic subaortic stenosis.

Although isolated valvular aortic stenosis seldom causes symptoms in infancy, severe heart failure occasionally occurs when critical obstruction is present. The response to medical management is poor; therefore, an aggressive surgical approach is recommended.

The physical findings vary somewhat depending upon the anatomic type of lesion:

1. Valvular aortic stenosis—Affected patients are well developed and well nourished. The pulses are usually normal and equal throughout. If the stenosis is severe and there is a gradient of greater than 80 mm Hg, the pulses are small with a slow upstroke. Examination of the heart reveals a left ventricular thrust at the apex. A systolic thrill at the right base, the suprasternal notch, and both carotid arteries accompanies moderate disease. If only one carotid artery manifests a thrill, it is the right carotid (usually seen in milder disease).

The first heart sound is normal. A prominent aortic type ejection click or ejection sound is best heard at the apex. Very frequently, this click can be heard at the lower left sternal border and at the aortic area. It is separated from the first heart sound by a short but appreciable interval. It does not vary with respiration. The second heart sound at the pulmonary area is physiologically split. The aortic component of the second heart sound is of good intensity. There is a grade III–V/VI, rough, medium- to high-pitched ejection type systolic murmur, loudest at the first and second intercostal spaces, which radiates well into the suprasternal notch and along the carotids. The murmur also radiates fairly well down the lower left sternal border and can be heard at the apex. The murmur transmits to the neck, and its grade correlates roughly with the severity of the stenosis.

2. Discrete membranous subvalvular aortic stenosis—The findings are essentially the same as those of valvular aortic stenosis. Absence of an aortic ejection click is an important differentiating point, and the thrill and murmur are usually somewhat more intense at the left sternal border in the third and fourth intercostal spaces than at the aortic area. Frequently, however, the murmur is equally intense at both areas. A diastolic murmur of aortic insufficiency is commonly heard after 5 years of age.

3. Supravalvular aortic stenosis—Affected patients often have abnormal facies and are mentally retarded. The thrill and murmur are characteristically best heard in the suprasternal notch and along the carotids, although they are well transmitted over the aortic area and near the mid left sternal border. A difference in pulses and blood pressure between the right and left arms may be found, with the more prominent pulse and pressure in the right arm.

4. Asymmetric septal hypertrophy—The murmur in this case is ejection in quality, grade II–III/VI, and heard from the left sternal border toward the apex and sometimes associated with a murmur of mitral insufficiency. There is often an atrial fourth heart sound with a diastolic murmur. No ejection click is audible. The arterial pulse wave has a rapid upstroke and frequently a bisferious quality.

B. Imaging: In most cases, x-ray findings indicate that the heart is not enlarged. The left ventricle, however, is slightly prominent. In valvular and discrete subvalvular aortic stenosis, dilatation of the ascending aorta is frequently seen (more commonly in the former). The ascending aorta is usually normal in idiopathic hypertrophic subaortic stenosis and in supravalvular aortic stenosis.

C. Electrocardiography: There is some correlation between the severity of the obstruction and the ECG. Patients with mild aortic stenosis have normal ECGs. Patients with severe obstruction frequently demonstrate evidence of left ventricular hypertrophy and left ventricular strain, but many do not. In about 25% of severe cases, the ECG is normal. Progressive increase in left ventricular hypertrophy on serial ECGs indicates a significant degree of obstruction. Left ventricular strain is taken as a potential indication for operation.

D. Echocardiography: This has become a reliable noninvasive technique for the initial diagnosis and follow-up evaluation of idiopathic hypertrophic subaortic stenosis. It also provides clues to the progression of other forms of aortic stenosis. Doppler echocardiographic techniques can now predict transvalvular gradients quite accurately.

E. Cardiac Catheterization and Angiocardiography: Left heart catheterization demonstrates the pressure differential between the left ventricle and the aorta and the level at which the gradient exists. Patients with severe aortic stenosis may be asymptomatic and have normal ECGs and chest x-rays. Serial cardiac catheterization is frequently the only reliable guide to the progression and the severity of the lesion. In the case of valvular aortic stenosis, an asymptomatic patient with a resting gradient of 60–80 mm Hg is considered to require surgery. In the face of symptoms, patients with lesser gradients are surgical candidates. Cineangiocardiography is helpful in demonstrating the level of the obstruction.

Treatment

Because the results of surgery are too frequently unsatisfactory, surgical repair should only be considered in patients with symptoms or a large resting gradient (60–80 mm Hg). In many cases, the gradient can only be moderately to minimally relieved without producing aortic insufficiency (which is potentially more harmful than the lesion for which surgery was undertaken). Percutaneous balloon valvuloplasty is now accepted as standard treatment. Discrete subvalvular aortic stenosis requires a lesser gradient for surgical intervention, because continued trauma to the aortic valve by the subvalvular jet may destroy the valve. Unfortunately, simple resection is followed by recurrence in more than 25% of patients with subvalvular aortic stenosis. Asymmetric septal hypertrophy has even less satisfactory results than muscle resection; therefore, medical management with propranolol should be tried initially.

Patients for whom surgery is not strongly indicated should have close follow-up, and those over age 6 years should undergo yearly exercise testing. If exercise testing is normal, restriction of physical activity may not be necessary in patients with mild to moderate aortic stenosis; in many cases, these patients may participate in competitive sports.

Course & Prognosis

All forms of left ventricular outflow tract obstruction tend to be progressive diseases. However, regression of the obstruction has been documented in a few patients with supravalvular obstruction. Pediatric patients with left ventricular outflow tract obstruction—with the exception of those with critical aortic stenosis of infancy—are usually asymptomatic. Symptoms accompanying severe unoperated obstruction (angina, syncope, and congestive heart failure) are all rare currently because of detection and surgical intervention. The vast majority of children without asymmetric septal hypertrophy are not only asymptomatic but also tend to have the personality and capabilities to compete in sports. There is increasing evidence that pre- or postoperative children whose obstruction is mild to moderate have above-average oxygen consumption and maximum voluntary working capacity. Children in this category with normal findings on resting and exercising ECG and normal heart size may safely participate in vigorous physical activity, including nonisometric competitive sports.

Choy M et al: Percutaneous balloon valvuloplasty for valvar aortic stenosis in infants and children. *Am J Cardiol* 1987;**59:**1010.

Flaker G et al: Supravalvular stenosis. *Am J Cardiol* 1983; **51:**256.

Helgason H et al: Balloon dilatation of the aortic valve: Studies in normal lambs and in children with aortic stenosis. *J Am Coll Cardiol* 1987;**9:**816.

Hsieh KS et al: Long-term follow up of valvulotomy before 1968 for congenital aortic stenosis. *Am J Cardiol* 1986; **58:**338.

Huhta JC et al: Prenatal diagnosis and postnatal management of critical aortic stenosis. Circulation 1987; **75:**573.

Oh JK et al: Prediction of the severity of aortic stenosis by Doppler aortic valve area determination. *J Am Coll Cardiol* 1988;**11:**1227.

Waldman JD et al: The obstructive subaortic conus. *Circulation* 1984;**70:**339.

3. MITRAL VALVE PROLAPSE

Essentials of Diagnosis

- Midsystolic click best heard with patient in standing or squatting position.
- Occasional late systolic murmur.

General Considerations

Mitral valve prolapse is the most common entity to present with abnormal auscultatory findings in pediatric patients. It is secondary to redundant valve tissue or abnormal tissue comprising the mitral valve apparatus. The mitral valve prolapses, moving posteriorly or superiorly into the left atrium during ventricular systole. A systolic click occurs at the time of this movement and is the clinical hallmark of this entity. Mitral insufficiency may occur late in systole, causing an atypical, short, late systolic murmur with variable radiation. It is most commonly found in individuals with the following characteristics: over 6 years of age, female, slender habitus, and bony thoracic abnormalities. Its incidence is estimated to vary from 2 to 20%, with the higher part of the range representing incidence in slender teenage females.

Clinical Findings

A. Symptoms and Signs: The vast majority of patients with mitral valve prolapse are asymptomatic. Chest pain, palpitations, and dizziness are reported, but it is not clear whether or not these symptoms are more common in affected patients than in the normal population. Significant dysrhythmias are uncommon, and true exercise intolerance is rare. The standard approach to auscultation must be modified to diagnose mitral valve prolapse; ie, auscultation should be performed with the patient placed in various positions. Clicks with or without systolic murmur are more commonly elicited in the standing and squatting positions than in the supine and sitting positions. The systolic click occurs earlier in children than in adults; ie, it tends to be midsystolic rather than late systolic. Although it is usually heard at the apex, it may be audible at the left sternal border or even occasionally may be panthoracic. A midsystolic or systolic murmur following the click implies mitral insufficiency and is much less common than isolated prolapse. The murmur tends to be atypical for mitral insufficiency in that it is not pansystolic and radiates to the sternum rather than to the left axilla. A coexistent diastolic murmur of relative or real mitral stenosis is rare. Occasionally, a systolic "honk" is heard.

B. Imaging: In the rare case of significant mitral insufficiency, the left atrium may be enlarged; this is visualized best on lateral film x-ray. Most chest x-rays show normal findings, and their use is therefore largely unwarranted.

C. Electrocardiography: Despite the fact that flat or inverted T waves in precordial lead V_6 have been reported, almost all electrocardiographic findings are normal. Disabling chest pain is rare and should be assessed with ergometric electrocardiography.

D. Echocardiography: Significant posterior systolic movement of the posterior mitral valve leaflet is considered diagnostic. Many false-positive results are due to multiple leaflet images (chevroning) or to the presence of insignificant (small duration and amplitude) posterior systolic valve movement. False-

negative results are also common, partly owing to performance of the procedure when the patient is in the supine position. If the physical findings are typical for isolated prolapse, echocardiography is not warranted.

E. Cardiac Catheterization and Angiography: Invasive procedures are very rarely indicated.

Treatment & Prognosis

Use of oral propranolol may be effective in rare cases of disabling chest pain. Prophylaxis for subacute infectious endocarditis is indicated only in individuals with associated mitral insufficiency.

The natural course of disease is largely unknown. Twenty years of observation indicate, however, that mitral valve prolapse in childhood is a largely benign entity. It merges with a common variation from normal in slender children and is associated with an asthenic body build that presumably results from altered geometry of the left ventricle and mitral valve.

Barlow JB, Pocock WA: Billowing, floppy, prolapsed or flail valves? *Am J Cardiol* 1985;**55**:501.

Barlow JB, Pocock WA, Obel IWP: Mitral valve prolapse: Primary, secondary, both or neither? *Am Heart J* 1981; **102**:140.

Kessler KM: Prolapse paranoia. *J Am Coll Cardiol* 1988; **11**:48.

Levine RA: Reconsideration of echocardiographic standards for mitral valve prolapse: Lack of association between leaf displacement isolated to the epical 4-chamber view and independent echocardiographic evidence of abnormality. *J Am Coll Cardiol* 1988;**11**:1010.

Shamberger RC, Welch KJ, Sanders SP: Mitral valve prolapse associated with pectus excavatum. *J Pediatr* 1987;**111**:404.

Worth DC et al: Prevalence of mitral valve prolapse in normal children. *J Am Coll Cardiol* 1985;**5**:1173.

4. OTHER CONGENITAL VALVULAR LESIONS

Congenital Mitral Stenosis

In this rare disorder, the valve leaflets are thickened and fused to produce a diaphragmlike or funnellike structure with an opening in the center. Frequent associated malformations include subaortic and aortic stenosis and coarctation of the aorta. This lesion complex is known as Shone's syndrome. Most patients develop symptoms early in life. Early symptoms include tachypnea, dyspnea, and severe failure to thrive. Physical examination reveals a regular sinus rhythm. The first heart sound is accentuated, and the pulmonary closure sound is loud. No opening snap can be heard. In most cases, a presystolic crescendo murmur is heard at the apex. Occasionally, only a middiastolic murmur can be heard. Rarely, no murmur at all is heard. Electrocardiography shows right axis deviation, biatrial enlargement, and right ventricular hypertrophy. X-ray reveals evidence of left atrial enlargement and, frequently, pulmonary venous congestion. Echocardiography shows abnormal valve structures with reduced excursion and left atrial enlargement. Cardiac catheterization reveals an elevated pulmonary capillary pressure and wedge pressure and pulmonary hypertension.

Surgical treatment, including valve replacement with a prosthetic mitral valve, has become possible even in infants weighing 3–5 kg.

Cor Triatriatum

This is an extremely rare abnormality in which the pulmonary veins enter a separate chamber rather than pass directly into the left atrium. The chamber communicates with the left atrium through an opening of variable size. The physiologic consequences of this condition are very similar to those of mitral stenosis. The clinical findings depend upon the size of the opening. If the opening is extremely small, symptoms develop very early in life. If the opening is large, patients may be asymptomatic for a considerable period of time. Echocardiography may reveal a hard shadow in the left atrium. Two-dimensional color flow doppler echocardiographic techniques have greatly enhanced the noninvasive accuracy of the diagnosis. Cardiac catheterization may be diagnostic. Finding a high pulmonary capillary pressure (high pulmonary venous pressure) and a low left atrial pressure (if the catheter can be passed through the foramen ovale into the true left atrial chamber) makes the diagnosis certain. Angiocardiographic studies may identify 2 "left atrial" chambers.

Surgical repair is usually successful.

Congenital Mitral Regurgitation

This is a relatively rare abnormality that is usually associated with other congenital heart lesions, including corrected transposition of the great vessels, endocardial cushion defect, and endocardial fibroelastosis. Uncomplicated congenital mitral regurgitation is very rare. It is sometimes present in patients with Marfan's syndrome. Occasionally, there is a congenital dilatation of the valve ring with an otherwise normal valve. In other cases, the chordae tendineae are malformed, resulting in mitral regurgitation.

Congenital Aortic Regurgitation

The most common causes of this disorder are bicuspid aortic valve, either uncomplicated or with coarctation of the aorta; ventricular septal defect and aortic insufficiency; and fenestration of the aortic valve cusp (one or more holes in the cusp).

Absence of the Pulmonary Valve

This rare abnormality is usually associated with ventricular septal defect. In about 50% of cases, severe infundibular pulmonary stenosis is present (tetralogy of Fallot).

Ebstein's Malformation of the Tricuspid Valve

This uncommon abnormality consists of downward displacement of the tricuspid valve such that the greater portion of the valve is attached to the ventricular wall rather than to the fibrous ring. As a result, the upper portion of the right ventricle is within the right atrium. The portion of the ventricle below the apex of the tricuspid valve is very small and represents the true functioning right ventricle. Clinically, there is a wide spectrum of abnormalities ranging from relative absence of symptoms to death in early infancy. The severity depends upon the degree of malattachment of the valve and the associated abnormalities. Echocardiography is useful in diagnosis.

Surgical repair consists of an annuloplasty procedure to modify the level of tricuspid orifice and diminish mitral insufficiency. The procedure's rate of success is highly variable. Late dysrhythmias are common. Postoperative tolerance of exercise is significantly increased compared to preoperative status but decreased compared to normal individuals.

Driscoll DJ, Mottram CD, Danielson GK: Spectrum of exercise intolerance in 45 patients with Ebstein's anomaly and observations on exercise tolerance in 11 patients after surgical repair. *J Am Coll Cardiol* 1988;**11**:831.

Mair DD et al: Surgical repair of Ebstein's anomaly. *Circulation* 1985;**72**:70.

Oh JK et al: Cardiac arrhythmias in patients with surgical repair of Ebstein's anomaly. *J Am Coll Cardiol* 1985;**6**:1351.

Silver MA et al: Late clinical and hemodynamic results after either tricuspid valve replacement or annuloplasty for Ebstein's anomaly of the tricuspid valve. *Am J Cardiol* 1984;**54**:672.

MYOCARDIAL DISEASES

Myocardial diseases are characterized by significant cardiac enlargement. Murmurs may or may not be present. Electrocardiographic changes include left ventricular hypertrophy, ST depression, and T wave inversion.

1. GLYCOGEN STORAGE DISEASE OF THE HEART

At least 10 types of glycogen storage disease are recognized. The type that primarily involves the heart is known as Pompe's disease. The deficient enzyme (acid maltase) is necessary for hydrolysis of the outer branches of glycogen, and its absence results in marked deposition of glycogen within the myocardium. Cardiac glycogenosis is a rare heritable (autosomal recessive) disorder.

Affected infants are usually normal at birth, but

onset commonly begins by the sixth month of life. These children have a history of retardation of growth and development, feeding problems, poor weight gain, and then the findings of heart failure. Physical examination reveals generalized muscular weakness, a large tongue, cardiomegaly, no significant heart murmurs, and, occasionally, evidence of congestive heart failure. Chest x-rays reveal marked cardiomegaly with or without pulmonary venous congestion. The ECG shows a short PR interval with left ventricular hypertrophy and shows ST depression and T wave inversion over the left precordial leads. Echocardiography shows extremely thick ventricular wall structures.

Children with this disease usually die within the first year of life. Death may be sudden or due to progressive congestive heart failure.

2. ANOMALOUS ORIGIN OF THE LEFT CORONARY ARTERY

In this condition, the left coronary artery arises from the pulmonary artery rather than from the aorta. In the neonatal period, while the pulmonary arterial pressure is relatively high, blood is supplied to the left ventricle from the pulmonary artery. Accordingly, during this period the child is asymptomatic and does well. However, within the first 2 months of life, the pulmonary arterial pressure decreases to normal. This phenomenon results in a marked decrease of flow to the left coronary artery. Infarction of the heart usually occurs. If the patient survives, collateral channels appear that join the peripheral branches of the right with the branches of the left coronary artery. As a result, the direction of blood flow in the left coronary artery changes. Whereas previously there was some flow from the pulmonary artery into the myocardium through the left coronary, flow now occurs from the right coronary artery through the collateral into the left coronary artery and then into the pulmonary artery. In essence, then, an arteriovenous fistula is formed that further removes blood from the myocardium, resulting in further myocardial infarction and fibrosis. Death occurs eventually as a result of marked dilatation of the heart and congestive heart failure. At autopsy, the left ventricle is found to be markedly fibrosed and thin.

Clinical Findings

A. Symptoms and Signs: Patients appear to be normal at birth. Growth and development are relatively normal for a few months, although detailed questioning of the parents often discloses a history of intermittent episodes of severe abdominal pain, pallor, and sweating, especially during or after feeding. These episodes are thought to be secondary to "colic," and attacks are similar to anginal attacks in adults.

On physical examination, the patients are usually well developed and well nourished. The pulses are usually weak but equal throughout. The heart is enlarged but not very active. A murmur of mitral regurgitation is frequently present, although no murmur may be heard.

B. Imaging: Chest x-ray films show significant cardiac enlargement with or without pulmonary venous congestion.

C. Electrocardiography: The ECG is usually diagnostic. There are T wave inversions in leads I and aVL. The precordial leads show T wave inversions from V_{4-7}. Deep Q waves are often seen in leads I, aVL, and V_{4-6}. These findings of myocardial infarction are similar to those in adults.

D. Echocardiography: The diagnosis can be made with 2-dimensional techniques by visualizing a single large right coronary artery arising from the aorta.

E. Cardiac Catheterization and Angiocardiography: A small left-to-right shunt (a result of the flow of blood from the right through the left coronary artery into the pulmonary artery) can often be detected at the pulmonary artery level. Frequently, however, the shunt is very small and can be detected only by the most sensitive techniques, eg, by the use of a hydrogen electrode catheter. Cineangiocardiography following injection of contrast material into the root of the aorta shows absence of origin of the left coronary artery from the aorta. A huge right coronary artery fills directly from the aorta, and the contrast material will flow through the right coronary system into the left coronary arteries and finally into the pulmonary artery.

Treatment & Prognosis

Treatment remains controversial. Medical management with anticongestives and afterload reduction is advocated by some. Lengthy operations requiring cardiopulmonary bypass to effect 2 functional coronary arteries from the aorta have a high death rate in critically ill infants. Simple ligation of the left coronary artery or subclavian to coronary artery anastomosis (without cardiopulmonary bypass) should be considered for the most critically ill infants. More complex operations should only be considered for the more stable infants or older children.

The prognosis is guarded. No therapeutic modality has been shown to be superior in follow-up studies of survivors.

Midgley A et al: Repair of anomalous origin of the left coronary artery in the infant and small child. *J Am Coll Cardiol* 1984;**4**:1231.

3. ENDOCARDIAL FIBROELASTOSIS

The incidence of endocardial fibroelastosis has decreased dramatically over the past 2 decades, and this entity is now uncommon. The cause is not known, although intrauterine infection with mumps or coxsackievirus B has been suggested.

Pathologic examination discloses a marked milky white thickening of the endocardium, the subendocardial layers of the left ventricle, and, usually, the left atrium. The mitral valve is frequently involved also. The myocardial fibers themselves are fibrotic and disorganized, and associated hypervascularization is common. Serial sections often show coexistent evidence of myocarditis. Thus, endocardial fibroelastosis appears to be part of a continuum of primary endomyocardial diseases and may be a sequela to myocarditis.

Clinical Findings

A. Symptoms and Signs: Patients appear normal at birth, and growth and development during early infancy are normal. About half develop symptoms within the first 5 months of life, and most are symptomatic by age 1. An occasional patient may have no symptoms until age 5.

The symptoms and signs that do develop are associated with left ventricular heart failure. These include dyspnea, easy fatigability, feeding difficulties, and, eventually, findings of left and right heart failure.

On physical examination, these children are often small and undernourished. The heart is usually enlarged, and the heart tones are poor (when there is evidence of decompensation). A murmur of mitral regurgitation may be present.

B. Imaging: Chest x-ray films show generalized cardiac enlargement with or without pulmonary venous congestion.

C. Electrocardiography: The ECG almost always shows evidence of left ventricular hypertrophy and, quite frequently, ST depression and T wave inversion. If there has been pulmonary hypertension secondary to left heart failure, right ventricular hypertrophy may be present. Right atrial hypertrophy is sometimes present. Complete heart block is occasionally seen.

D. Echocardiography: M mode and 2-dimensional techniques reveal dilatation of cardiac chambers and echo-dense endocardial images indicating decreased myocardial function.

E. Cardiac Catheterization and Angiocardiography: Catheterization reveals the absence of left-to-right shunts. Pulmonary hypertension may be present. Cineangiocardiography demonstrates diminished myocardial contractility. Transcatheter endomyocardial biopsy has become a more common technique in infants and children for primary myocardial disease but seldom reveals a cause.

Treatment & Prognosis

Treatment of endocardial fibroelastosis is medical and consists of adequate and prolonged use of digi-

talis and oral diuretics. If response to the usual dose is not satisfactory, the dosage of both digitalis and diuretics should be increased until a satisfactory response is noted or toxicity occurs. Afterload reduction would appear to be rational therapy for infants with this disease. Continue these agents for several years.

Some children appear to improve initially with treatment but then develop recurrent bouts of heart failure. Complete recovery in such patients is very infrequent, and most eventually die with intractable congestive heart failure. The prognosis is most favorable in patients who present between 6 months and 3 years of age and respond promptly to treatment.

Hutchins GM, Vie SA: The progression of interstitial myocarditis to idiopathic endocardial fibroelastosis. *Am J Pathol* 1972;**66**:483.

Lewis AB et al: Findings on endomyocardial biopsy in infants and children with dilated cardiomyopathy. *Am J Cardiol* 1985;**55**:143.

CYANOTIC HEART DISEASE

TETRALOGY OF FALLOT

Essentials of Diagnosis

- Cyanosis after the neonatal period.
- Hypoxemic spells during infancy.
- Right-sided aortic arch in 25%.
- Systolic ejection murmur at upper left sternal border.

General Considerations

In Fallot's tetralogy, there is a ventricular septal defect and severe obstruction to right ventricular outflow such that the intracardiac shunt is predominantly from right to left. This is the most common type of cyanotic heart lesion, accounting for 10–15% of all cases of congenital heart disease. The ventricular defect is usually located in the membranous portion of the septum but may be totally surrounded by muscular tissue and is usually quite large. Obstruction to right ventricular outflow may be solely at the infundibular level (50–75%), at the valvular level alone (rarely), or at both levels (25% or more). The term tetralogy has been used to describe this combination of lesions, since there is always associated right ventricular hypertrophy and a varying degree of "overriding of the aorta." The overriding is present because of the position of the ventricular septal defect in relation to a dilated and often dextroposed aorta. These 2 factors (right ventricular hypertrophy and overriding aorta) plus the major lesions make up the tetralogy. A right-sided aortic arch is present in 25% of cases and an atrial septal defect in 15%.

Severe obstruction to right ventricular outflow

plus a large ventricular septal defect results in a right-to-left shunt at the ventricular level and desaturation of the arterial blood. The degree of desaturation and the extent of cyanosis depend upon the size of the shunt. This in turn is dependent upon the resistance to outflow from the right ventricle, the size of the ventricular septal defect, and the systemic vascular resistance. The greater the obstruction, the larger the ventricular septal defect, and the lower the systemic vascular resistance, the greater the right-to-left shunt. Although the patient may be deeply cyanotic, the amount of pressure the right ventricle can develop is limited to that of the systemic (aortic) pressure. In other words, right ventricular pressure cannot exceed left ventricular pressure. The right ventricle is usually quite able to maintain this level of pressure without developing heart failure.

Clinical Findings

A. Symptoms and Signs: The clinical findings vary depending upon the degree of right ventricular outflow obstruction. Patients with a mild degree of obstruction are only minimally cyanotic or acyanotic and may even present initially with congestive heart failure. Those with maximal obstruction are deeply cyanotic from birth. However, few children are asymptomatic; most have cyanosis by 4 months of age; and the cyanosis usually is progressive. Growth and development are retarded, and easy fatigability and dyspnea on exertion are common. Squatting is seen when the children become old enough to walk.

Hypoxemic spells (cyanotic spells) are characterized by the following signs and symptoms: (1) sudden onset of cyanosis or deepening of cyanosis; (2) sudden onset of dyspnea; (3) alterations in consciousness, encompassing a spectrum from irritability to syncope; and (4) decrease in intensity or disappearance of the systolic murmur. These episodes may begin in the neonatal period and continue until nearly school age. It is unusual, however, for the initial episode to occur after 2 years of age. Acute treatment of cyanotic spells consists of giving oxygen and placing the patient in the knee-chest position. Acidosis, if present, should be corrected with intravenous sodium bicarbonate. Morphine sulfate should be administered cautiously by a parenteral route in a dosage of 0.1 mg/kg. Propranolol, 0.1–0.2 mg/kg intravenously, has been found to be useful. Chronic (daily) treatment of cyanotic spells with propranolol, 1 mg/kg orally every 4 hours while awake, remains controversial; however, in a significant number of patients, this regimen has prevented subsequent "spells" and made it possible to delay operation until total correction can be performed.

Patients with tetralogy are usually small and thin. The degree of cyanosis is variable. The fingers and toes show varying degrees of clubbing depending upon the age of the child and the severity of the cyanosis.

On examination of the heart, a right ventricular lift is palpable. No thrills are present. The first sound is normal; occasionally, there is an ejection click at the apex that is aortic in origin. The second sound is single and best heard at the lower left sternal border between the third and fourth intercostal spaces. The second heart sound at the pulmonary area is soft; however, aortic closure is loud and heard best in the third and fourth intercostal spaces at the left sternal border. There is a grade I–III/VI, rough, ejection type systolic murmur that is maximal at the left sternal border in the third intercostal space. This murmur radiates over the anterior and posterior lung fields. Diastolic murmurs are not present.

B. Laboratory Findings: The hemoglobin, hematocrit, and red blood count are usually mildly to markedly elevated, depending upon the degree of arterial oxygen desaturation.

C. Imaging: Chest x-rays reveal the overall heart size to be normal, and indeed the x-ray film may sometimes be interpreted as being entirely normal. However, the right ventricle is hypertrophied, and this is often shown in the posteroanterior projection by an upturning of the apex (boot-shaped heart). The main pulmonary artery segment is usually concave, and the aorta in 25% of cases arches to the right. The pulmonary vascular markings are usually decreased.

D. Electrocardiography: The cardiac axis is to the right, ranging from $+90$ to $+180$ degrees. The P waves are usually normal, although there may be evidence of slight right atrial hypertrophy. Right ventricular hypertrophy is always present, but right ventricular strain patterns are rare.

E. Echocardiography: M mode and 2-dimensional techniques reveal thickening of the free right ventricular wall, with overriding of the aorta and a membranous ventricular septal defect. In addition, obstruction at the level of the infundibulum and pulmonary valve may be seen, and the anatomy of the coronary artery may be visualized.

F. Cardiac Catheterization and Angiocardiography: Cardiac catheterization reveals the absence of a significant left-to-right shunt, although the hydrogen electrode curve may be positive in the right ventricle. There is arterial blood desaturation of varying degree. The right-to-left shunt exists at the ventricular level. The right ventricular pressure is at systemic levels, and the pressure contour in the right ventricle is almost identical with that of the left ventricle. The pulmonary artery pressure is extremely low (mean ranges of 5–10 mm Hg). The gradients and pressure may be noted at the valvular level, the infundibular level, or both. The catheter frequently is passed from the right ventricle into the overriding ascending aorta.

Cineangiocardiography is diagnostic. Injection of contrast material into the right ventricle reveals the right ventricular outflow obstruction and the right-to-left shunt at the ventricular level. An aortic root injection or selective coronary angiography may be necessary to demonstrate anomalies of coronary artery distribution that can effect surgical mortality.

Treatment

A. Palliative Treatment: Palliative treatment is recommended for very small infants who are markedly symptomatic (severely cyanotic, frequent severe anoxic spells) and in whom complete correction would be difficult or impossible. It may be medical (chronic oral β-blocking agents) or, more often, surgical (creation of a systemic arterial to pulmonary arterial anastomosis).

The earliest procedure employed for this disease (Blalock-Taussig) consists of an anastomosis between the subclavian artery and the pulmonary artery. It is usually done on the side opposite the aortic arch. A synthetic anastomosis between the ascending aorta and the main pulmonary artery may be performed.

B. Total Correction: Total correction of tetralogy of Fallot is performed under the cardiopulmonary bypass. It involves opening the right ventricle, closing the ventricular septal defect, and removing the obstruction to right ventricular outflow. The surgical death rate varies from 2 to 15%. The major limiting anatomic feature of total correction is the size of the pulmonary artery and its branches. Children who survive the operation are markedly improved. There is complete disappearance of cyanosis, and clubbing disappears shortly thereafter. Growth and development improve markedly, and these patients often become asymptomatic within a short period of time. However, these patients remain at risk for sudden death due to dysrhythmias. Currently, major cardiovascular centers are performing total correction for virtually all infants with this condition, including newborns.

Course & Prognosis

Infants with the most severe form of the disease are usually deeply cyanotic at birth. Hypoxemic spells may occur during the neonatal period. Death is extremely rare during a severe hypoxemic spell. Many patients who survive the first year of life seem to improve. This may be due to the development of systemic-to-pulmonary collateral vessels. Although hypoxemic spells may decrease in severity, these children remain deeply cyanotic and markedly limited in their activity. They seldom survive the second decade of life without surgical treatment.

Infants with moderate obstruction to right ventricular outflow do fairly well. Although cyanosis is present in very early life, it is usually not severe. The cyanosis may progress in severity, and anoxic spells may occur. These patients do fairly well in later childhood, but their condition progressively deteriorates during the second and third decades of life.

Death occurs by the third decade as a result of cerebrovascular accidents, brain abscess, subacute infective endocarditis, anoxia, or pulmonary hemorrhage.

Patients with the mildest form of the disease are said to have the "acyanotic" variety. The degree of obstruction is very mild, and the right-to-left shunt is small. Very frequently, there is a predominant left-to-right shunt. However, the degree of obstruction often increases as the patient gets older. This, combined with the increased activity, results in progressively worsening cyanosis. Many of these patients live relatively normal lives without severe symptoms. Life expectancy, however, is definitely decreased, and death usually occurs by the third to fourth decade.

In school-age children, complete repair usually results in fair to good function, although patients are occasionally subject to sudden death from dysrhythmias.

Berry JM et al: Evaluation of coronary artery anatomy in patients with tetralogy of Fallot by 2-dimensional echocardiography. *Circulation* 1988;**78**:149.
Friedli B, Bolens M, Taktak M: Conduction disturbances after correction of tetralogy of Fallot. *J Am Coll Cardiol* 1988;**11**:162.
Garson A Jr, Gillette PC, McNamara DG: Propranolol: The preferred palliation for tetralogy of Fallot. *Am J Cardiol* 1981;**47**:1098.
Garson A Jr et al: Prevention of sudden death after repair of tetralogy of Fallot. *J Am Coll Cardiol* 1985;**6**:221.
Walsh EP: Late results in patients with tetralogy of Fallot repaired during infancy. *Circulation* 1988;**77**:1062.
Zahka KG et al: Long-term valvular function after total repair of tetralogy of Fallot: Relation to ventricular arrhythmias. *Circulation* 1988;**78(Suppl 3)**:14.

PULMONARY ATRESIA WITH VENTRICULAR SEPTAL DEFECT

This condition consists of complete atresia of the pulmonary valve in association with ventricular septal defect. Essentially, it is an extreme form of tetralogy of Fallot. Since there is no flow outward from the right ventricle into the pulmonary artery, the pulmonary blood flow must be derived either from a patent ductus arteriosus or from collateral channels.

The clinical picture depends entirely upon the size of the ductus or the collateral channels (or both). If they are large, patients may do quite well and actually do better than those with severe tetralogy of Fallot. If effective pulmonary blood flow is small, death occurs secondary to severe anoxia early in life. This may occur suddenly with postnatal closure of a patent ductus arteriosus.

Echocardiography or cardiac catheterization and angiocardiography are diagnostic. If patent ductus arteriosus dependency is established, a prostaglandin E_1 infusion to dilate the patent ductus arteriosus may help stabilize the patient until surgery.

Infants who are severely hypoxemic require urgent systemic to pulmonary anastomosis in order to provide sufficient oxygenated blood to the body.

A corrective surgical procedure that has been successful in patients with adequate-sized pulmonary arteries consists of bypassing the obstructed right ventricular outflow and closing the ventricular septal defect. Success may depend on precise definition of pulmonary arterial and collateral blood supply to the lung and prior unifocalization of segments with dual arterial blood supply. More recently, an approach has been adopted to create initially a central connection between the right ventricle or aorta to the central pulmonary artery.

Edwards WD et al: Pulmonary blood supply in patients with pulmonary atresia and ventricular septal defect. *J Am Coll Cardiol* 1985;**6**:1343.

Sullivan ID et al: Surgical unifocalization in pulmonary atresia and ventricular septal defect: A realistic goal? *Circulation* 1988;**78(Suppl 3)**:55.

PULMONARY ATRESIA WITH INTACT VENTRICULAR SEPTUM

Essentials of Diagnosis

- Cyanosis at birth.
- Continuous murmur.
- Chest x-ray film with concave pulmonary artery segment and apex tilted upward.

General Considerations

In this uncommon condition, the pulmonary valve is absent and is replaced by a small diaphragm consisting of the fused cusps. The ventricular septum is intact. The main pulmonary artery segment is somewhat hypoplastic but almost always patent. In the type 1 deformity (80%), the cavity volume of the right ventricle is extremely small and the wall is thickened and fibrotic. In type 2, the right ventricular cavity is frequently of normal size.

During intrauterine life, if the tricuspid valve is intact and normal, very little blood enters the right ventricle, since there is no outlet for this chamber. Almost all of the blood passes through the foramen ovale directly into the left side of the heart. In the type 2 deformity, there is usually an outlet for the right ventricle (tricuspid valve insufficiency), and the right ventricle receives a sufficient quantity of blood to permit it to develop in a relatively normal fashion.

Following birth, the pulmonary circulation is maintained primarily by a patent ductus arteriosus. Although a bronchial pulmonary collateral network is present, it is usually insufficient to maintain the pulmonary circulation. Accordingly, whether or not the patients live depends upon the patency of the ductus arteriosus. The ductus usually remains open

for only a short period of time. As it closes, hypoxia becomes progressively more severe, and death eventually occurs.

Clinical Findings

A. Symptoms and Signs: Patients may be normal at birth, although they are usually cyanotic. Cyanosis becomes progressively more severe and is associated with severe dyspnea. A blowing systolic murmur due to the associated patent ductus arteriosus may be heard at the pulmonary area and under the left clavicle. In type 2 deformity, a loud pansystolic murmur due to the tricuspid insufficiency is heard at the lower left sternal border. Not infrequently, the liver is pulsating.

B. Imaging: Chest x-rays show a markedly enlarged heart with marked decrease in pulmonary vascular markings. With striking tricuspid insufficiency, right atrial enlargement may be massive and the cardiac silhouette may virtually fill the chest.

C. Electrocardiography: Electrocardiography reveals an axis that is usually normal in the frontal plane. Evidence for right atrial enlargement is usually striking. Voltage criteria for other chamber enlargement are variable.

D. Echocardiography: M mode or 2-dimensional echocardiography shows absence of the pulmonary valve, with varying degrees of hypoplasia of the right ventricular cavity.

E. Cardiac Catheterization and Angiocardiography: The diagnosis can be made on cardiac catheterization and cineangiocardiography. Right ventricular pressure is very high (greater than systemic). A cineangiocardiogram following injection of contrast material into the right ventricle reveals absence of filling of the pulmonary artery from the right ventricle. It also demonstrates the size of the right ventricular chamber and the presence or absence of tricuspid regurgitation, and right ventricular sinusoids that drain into the coronary arteries may fill.

Treatment & Prognosis

As in pulmonary atresia with ventricular septal defect, a prostaglandin E_1 infusion is useful in stabilizing the patient and maintaining patency of the ductus until surgery can be performed. Surgery should be undertaken as soon as the diagnosis is made by cardiac catheterization. A Rashkind atrial septostomy is performed to open up the communication across the atrial septum and permit adequate flow in both directions. Subsequent surgical approaches vary widely. In cases of type 1 deformity, it is necessary to immediately establish a surgical aorticopulmonary anastomosis (usually a Blalock-Taussig shunt). Later in infancy, a communication between the right ventricle and pulmonary artery should be created in an attempt to stimulate right ventricular cavity growth. In cases of type 2 deformity, a closed valvotomy may be all that is necessary initially, with a more definitive reconstruction of the right ventricular outflow tract accomplished at a later date.

The prognosis is unpredictable for patients with type 1 or type 2 deformity who survive the surgery. In type 1 patients, the dimensions of the right ventricle can increase significantly after the initial procedure. Overall, however, this disorder remains one of the least satisfactory forms of cyanotic congenital heart disease, because little progress has been made in surgical management.

Calder AL, Co EE, Sage MD: Coronary artery abnormalities in pulmonary atresia with intact ventricular septum. *Am J Cardiol* 1987;**59**:436.

de Leval M et al: Pulmonary atresia and intact ventricular septum: Surgical management based on a revised classification. *Circulation* 1982;**66**:272.

Fyfe DA, Edward WD, Driscoll DJ: Myocardial ischemia in patients with pulmonary atresia and intact ventricular septum. *J Am Coll Cardiol* 1986;**8**:402.

Leung M et al: Echocardiographic assessment of neonates with pulmonary atresia and intact ventricular septum. *J Am Coll Cardiol* 1988;**12**:719.

TRICUSPID ATRESIA

Essential of Diagnosis

- Marked cyanosis present from birth.
- ECG with left axis deviation, right atrial enlargement, and left ventricular hypertrophy.

General Considerations

This relatively rare condition (< 1% of cases of congenital heart disease) is characterized by complete atresia of the tricuspid valve. As a result, no direct communication exists between the right atrium and right ventricle.

Tricuspid atresia may be divided into 2 types, depending upon the relationship of the great vessels:

Type 1. Without transposition of the great arteries: (a) No ventricular septal defect. Hypoplasia or atresia of the pulmonary artery. Patent ductus arteriosus. (b) Small ventricular septal defect. Pulmonary stenosis. Hypoplastic pulmonary artery. (c) Large ventricular septal defect and no pulmonary stenosis. Normal-sized pulmonary artery.

Type 2. With transposition of the great arteries: (a) With ventricular septal defect and pulmonary stenosis. (b) With ventricular septal defect but without pulmonary stenosis.

Because there is no direct communication between the right atrium and right ventricle, the entire systemic venous return must flow through the atrial septum (either an atrial septal defect or patent foramen ovale) into the left atrium. Accordingly, the left atrium receives both the systemic venous return and the pulmonary venous return. Complete mixing occurs in the left atrium, resulting in a greater or lesser degree of arterial desaturation.

As a result of this lack of direct communication, the development of the ventricle depends upon the presence of a left-to-right shunt at the ventricular level. Therefore, severe hypoplasia of the right ventricle occurs in those forms in which there is no ventricular septal defect or in which the ventricular septal defect is very small.

Clinical Findings

A. Symptoms and Signs: In the great majority of patients with tricuspid atresia, symptoms develop very early in infancy. Except in cases in which the pulmonary blood flow is great, cyanosis is present at birth. Growth and development are very poor, and there is usually easy fatigability on feeding, tachypnea, dyspnea, anoxic spells, and evidence of right heart failure. Patients with marked increase in pulmonary blood flow (types 1c and 2b) will develop evidence of left heart failure as well.

Clubbing is present if the child is old enough. On examination of the heart, a slight bulge on the right side of the sternum may occasionally be seen. The first heart sound is normal. The second heart sound is most often single (owing to aortic closure). A murmur is usually present, although it is variable. It ranges from grade I to grade III/VI in intensity and usually is a harsh blowing murmur heard best at the lower left sternal border.

B. Imaging: Chest x-ray findings are variable. The heart may be slightly to markedly enlarged. The main pulmonary artery segment is usually small or absent. The size of the right atrium varies from huge to only moderately enlarged, depending upon the size of the communication at the atrial level. The pulmonary vascular markings are usually decreased, although in types 1c and 2b they are increased.

C. Electrocardiography: The ECG is usually helpful. It often shows a left axis deviation with a counterclockwise loop in the frontal plane. The P waves are tall and peaked, indicative of right atrial hypertrophy. The size of the P wave depends upon the right atrial pressure, which in turn depends upon the size of the interatrial communication (the taller the P wave, the smaller the communication). Left ventricular hypertrophy or left ventricular preponderance is found in almost all cases. Voltage over the right precordium is usually low.

D. Echocardiography: M mode or 2-dimensional methods are diagnostic and show absence of the tricuspid valve.

E. Cardiac Catheterization and Angiocardiography: This reveals the marked right-to-left shunt at the atrial level and desaturation of the left atrial blood. Because of the complete mixing in the left atrial chambers, oxygen saturation in the left ventricle, right ventricle, pulmonary artery, and aorta is identical to that in the left atrium. The right atrial pressure is increased. Left ventricular and systemic pressures are normal. The catheter cannot be passed through the tricuspid valve from the right atrium to the right ventricle. The course of the catheter is always from right atrium into left atrium and from there into left ventricle.

Cineangiocardiography following injection of contrast material into the right atrium is diagnostic. It reveals the lack of communication of the right atrium with the right ventricle and the right-to-left shunt at the atrial level.

Treatment & Prognosis

In infants with high pulmonary artery flow, conventional anticongestive therapy should be given until the infant begins to outgrow the ventricular septal defect. At that point, a Fontan procedure (connection of right atrium to right ventricle or pulmonary artery) should be considered.

In infants with extremely low pulmonary artery flow, prostaglandin E_1 should be infused until an aorticopulmonary shunt can be performed. The Fontan procedure is rapidly gaining acceptance as the "corrective" procedure of choice. The optimal timing is controversial, but the procedure has been performed successfully in infants under 1 year of age at our institution.

The prognosis for all patients with tricuspid atresia depends on achieving a balance of pulmonary blood flow that permits adequate oxygenation of the tissues without producing intractable congestive heart failure. For children treated by the Fontan procedure, the prognosis is as yet undefined; initial results are moderately encouraging.

Girod DA et al: Long-term results after the Fontan operation for tricuspid atresia. *Circulation* 1987;**75**:605.

Nakazawa M et al: Flow dynamics in the pulmonary artery after the Fontan procedure in patients with tricuspid atresia or single ventricle. *Circulation* 1987;**75**:1117.

Sanders SP et al: Clinical and hemodynamic results of Fontan operation for tricuspid atresia. *Am J Cardiol* 1982;**49**:1733.

HYPOPLASTIC LEFT HEART SYNDROME

Hypoplastic left heart syndrome includes a number of conditions in which there are either valvular or vascular lesions on the left side of the heart, resulting in hypoplasia of the left ventricle.

The lesions that make up this syndrome are mitral atresia, aortic atresia, or both. In all of these conditions, there is severe obstruction to either filling or emptying of the left ventricle. As a result, during intrauterine life, the quantity of blood filling the left ventricle is extremely small, resulting in hypoplasia of this chamber. Following birth, there is marked impairment of the circulation because of the very small size of the left ventricle and the presence of obstructing lesions. Congestive heart failure develops rapidly, in most cases within several days to 3 months of life.

Patients with aortic atresia develop congestive heart failure very early, usually within the first week. Death occurs earliest in this group. Patients with mitral atresia who have large atrial and ventricular communications may live longer. Some patients have lived beyond the first decade. Patients with involvement of the aortic arch usually die within 1 month or less.

The clinical picture depends upon the type of obstructing lesion. Cyanosis is usually present early in life and is usually generalized. Patients with hypoplasia or atresia of the aortic arch may show differential cyanosis. Murmurs may or may not be present and are usually nondiagnostic. Congestive heart failure develops early.

Chest x-ray findings usually are relatively normal at birth. Rapid and progressive cardiac enlargement then occurs, frequently associated with pulmonary venous congestion. These changes occur earliest in patients with aortic atresia.

The ECG usually demonstrates right axis deviation, right atrial hypertrophy, and right ventricular hypertrophy with relative paucity of left ventricular forces and absence of a Q wave in V_6.

Echocardiography is usually diagnostic and often eliminates the need for cardiac catheterization. A diminutive aorta and left ventricle with a poorly defined mitral valve in the presence of a normal and easily definable tricuspid valve are diagnostic.

During the past several years, a 2-stage complex surgical approach to palliation of aortic atresia has been advocated. Although not widely tried, this extremely high-risk approach offers some small hope for patients with aortic atresia.

Lang P, Norwood WI: Hemodynamic assessment after palliative surgery for hypoplastic left heart syndrome. *Circulation* 1983;**68**:104.

COMPLETE TRANSPOSITION OF THE GREAT ARTERIES

Essentials of Diagnosis

- Cyanotic newborn without respiratory distress.
- More common in males.

General Considerations

Complete transposition of the great vessels is the second most common variety of cyanotic congenital heart disease, accounting for about 16% of all cases. The male/female ratio is 3:1. The disorder is due to an embryologic abnormality in the spiral division of the truncus arteriosus.

The aorta is located anterior to the pulmonary artery—either directly anterior or to the left or right. The pulmonary artery usually ascends parallel to the aorta rather than crosses it. In most cases, associated intracardiac abnormalities are present. These include ventricular septal defect, atrial septal defect, pulmonary stenosis, and patent ductus arteriosus. Obstructive changes within the pulmonary arteriolar bed are common in patients past infancy.

Transposition of the great vessels can be classified as follows:

Group 1. Transposition with intact ventricular septum: (a) Without pulmonary stenosis or (b) with pulmonary stenosis, subvalvular or valvular (or both).

Group 2. Transposition with ventricular septal defect: (a) With pulmonary stenosis, (b) with pulmonary vascular obstruction, or (c) without pulmonary vascular obstruction (normal pulmonary vascular resistance).

Since the aorta arises directly from the right ventricle, life would not be possible unless there were mixing between the systemic and pulmonary circulations; oxygenated blood from the pulmonary veins must in some way reach the systemic arterial circuit. In patients with intact ventricular septum (group 1), mixing occurs at the atrial and also at the ductal levels. However, in most patients, these communications are small, and the ductus arteriosus often closes shortly after birth. These patients are therefore severely cyanotic, and congestive heart failure occurs rapidly as a result of the marked increase in cardiac output. Patients with a ventricular septal defect show greater or lesser degrees of cyanosis, depending upon the ratio of the pulmonary to systemic blood flow. Patients with ventricular septal defect and pulmonary stenosis (group 2a) are usually severely cyanotic because of the limited blood flow to the lungs. Patients with ventricular septal defect and pulmonary vascular obstruction (group 2b) show a moderate degree of cyanosis. Patients with ventricular septal defect and normal pulmonary vascular resistance (group 2c) show the least cyanosis but often develop heart failure very early because of the enormous pulmonary blood flow.

Congestive heart failure develops not only because of the high cardiac output but also because of the poor oxygenation of the myocardium and the presence of systemic pressure in both ventricles.

Clinical Findings

A. Symptoms and Signs: Many of the neonates are quite large, some weighing 4 kg (9 lb) at birth, and most are cyanotic at birth, although cyanosis occasionally does not develop until later. Patients in groups 1 and 2a are most cyanotic; those in group 2c are least cyanotic. Retardation of growth and development after the neonatal period is common. Congestive heart failure occurs in patients in groups 1 and 2c. Patients in group 2a show no evidence of congestive heart failure but often have severe anoxic spells in early life; if they survive the

first year of life, retardation of growth and development is common and cyanosis becomes progressively more severe. However, intellectual development may be unaffected.

Although these infants are usually large at birth, growth and development are retarded; thus, when they reach age 6 months to 1 year, they are usually below the third percentile in both height and weight. Cyanosis is marked. Clubbing is present in children over age 1. The findings on cardiovascular examination depend somewhat upon the intracardiac defects. Group 1a patients have only soft murmurs or none at all. The first heart sound is usually normal. The second heart sound is single and accentuated and is best heard at the lower left sternal border. Patients in group 1b have loud obstructive systolic murmurs that are maximal at the second and third intercostal spaces and the left sternal border, radiating well to the first and second intercostal spaces. Group 2a patients have a murmur of pulmonary stenosis (obstructive systolic murmur at the base of the heart, best heard to the right of the sternum). Those in group 2c have a systolic murmur along the lower sternal border and a mitral diastolic flow murmur at the apex.

B. Imaging: In the sick, blue newborn, at a time when any diagnostic clues are greatly appreciated, the chest x-ray in transposition is often very nonspecific. In fact, at any age, the so-called characteristic findings may be lacking.

C. Electrocardiography and Echocardiography: Early in infancy, the ECG is usually of little positive help. It reveals the usual amount of right ventricular hypertrophy expected for age. The absence of positive findings of other lesions, such as left axis deviation of tricuspid atresia, provides some deductive information. Abnormal relationships of the great vessels by echo are suggestive of a lesion in the transposition group.

D. Cardiac Catheterization and Angiocardiography: Cardiac catheterization has a dual purpose in this malformation: diagnosis and therapy. The sequence is usually to enter the right ventricle and immediately record a contrast medium injection on videotape and ciné. As soon as the cardiologist has confidently demonstrated that complete transposition of the great arteries exists and that there are 2 well-developed ventricles, a Rashkind septostomy is performed.

Treatment

It has become increasingly apparent at many pediatric cardiology centers throughout the world that survival of patients with transposition of the great arteries depends on early, aggressive management.

A. Cardiac Catheterization: A routine for all types of transposition is as follows:

1. Newborn period—Diagnostic and therapeutic cardiac catheterization should be performed as soon as the patient achieves as much stability as the clinical course indicates is possible. The therapeutic part of the catheterization is, of course, the Rashkind balloon septostomy, which enlarges the atrial septal communication by repeatedly pulling a dye-filled balloon across the foramen ovale, tearing the septum. In patients with persistent significant hypoxia ($Po_2 < 20$–25 mm Hg), administration of prostaglandin E_1 has been found to cause an immediate improvement in oxygenation, presumably owing to a decrease in pulmonary vascular resistance. We have found, however, that if the arterial pH remains constant, oxygenation virtually always improves spontaneously in several days.

2. At 4–6 months—Repeat the catheterization (with catheterization of the pulmonary artery to assess progression of pulmonary vascular obstruction), determine the presence or absence of left ventricle outflow obstruction, and repeat the Rashkind septostomy if indicated.

3. At 8–10 months—Repeat the catheterization if definitive surgery has not taken place before this time.

B. Complete Surgical Correction:

1. Elective surgery—All patients with favorable anatomic and hemodynamic criteria should be offered corrective surgery by 6 months of age. Surgery currently involves insertion of an intra-atrial baffle (by either a Mustard or a Senning operation) to redirect systemic and pulmonary venous blood to the appropriate pulmonary and aortic ventricles.

2. Early surgery—Certain patients, especially those with rapidly rising pulmonary artery pressures (with or without ventricular septal defect) and those with rapidly progressing left ventricular outflow obstruction, may require surgical intervention as early as 1–2 weeks to 6 months of age (after the second cardiac catheterization). In patients with transposition, it is not uncommon for a ventricular septal defect to close spontaneously, depriving the patient of the necessary mixing of systemic and pulmonary circulations. A patent ductus arteriosus has not proved to be an asset in some cases and has inhibited atrial level mixing (despite an adequate atrial septostomy), necessitating ligation and early intra-atrial baffling.

3. Late surgery—Some patients, especially those in group 2a (ie, patients with ventricular septal defect and pulmonary stenosis), may have had early or relatively late development of severe left ventricular-pulmonary outflow obstruction. This is not ideally amenable to a Mustard correction but may be more suitable for a Rastelli operation (an aortic homograft from left ventricle to pulmonary arteries).

4. Palliative surgical correction—Open atrial septectomy and aorticopulmonary shunts may be used under special circumstances, but the trend is to perform early total correction whenever possible.

5. Anatomic correction—Since 1975, surgical techniques to "switch" the great vessels to their anatomically appropriate locations have undergone a painful and slow evolution. A key feature in the development of techniques has been careful patient selection. The left ventricular musculature in this entity rapidly loses its muscle mass and potential to meet systemic afterload unless a large ventricular septal defect or left ventricular outflow obstruction occurs; consequently, newborns with either of these conditions are appropriate candidates. The incidence of death from this type of surgery has fallen from 25% to approximately 10%. Although the death rate following an intra-atrial baffling procedure is less, there is growing concern about the long-term ability of an anatomic right ventricle to function as a systemic circulation pump. During the past several years, many institutions have begun using anatomic correction techniques in almost all patients. As the use of anatomic correction (vessel switch) techniques has spread to more centers, postoperative complications such as supravalvular pulmonary stenosis and stenoses or kinking of coronary arteries have been noted. The long-term exercise capacity of patients after interatrial rerouting operations has, in some studies, turned out to be better than that projected by early studies. Long-term results for anatomic correction are awaited.

Bove EL et al: Arterial repair for transposition of the great arteries and large ventricular septal defect in early infancy. *Circulation* 1988;**78:(Suppl 3)**:26.

Muewe NN et al: Cardiopulmonary adaption at rest and during exercise 10 years after Mustard atrial repair for transposition of the great arteries. *Circulation* 1988;**77**:1055.

Paillole C et al: Fate of pulmonary artery after anatomic correction of simple transposition of great arteries in newborn infants. *Circulation* 1988;**78**:870.

Rubay J, deLeval M, Bull C: To switch or not to switch? The Senning alternative. *Circulation* 1988;**78(Suppl 3)**:1.

Sidi D et al: Anatomic correction of simple transposition of the great arteries in 50 neonates. *Circulation* 1987;**75**:429.

Wernovsky G et al: Midtown results after the arterial switch operation for transposition of the great arteries with intact ventricular septum. *Circulation* 1988;**77**:1333.

ORIGIN OF BOTH GREAT VESSELS FROM THE RIGHT VENTRICLE

In this rare malformation, the aorta is completely transposed, but the pulmonary artery occupies a relatively normal position. Accordingly, both great vessels arise from the right ventricle. Ventricular septal defect is present in all cases and provides the only outlet for the left ventricle.

This malformation may be divided into 5 types on the basis of the relationship of the ventricular septal defect to the great arteries and the presence or absence of pulmonary stenosis: (1) ventricular septal defect related to the aorta, (2) ventricular septal defect related to the pulmonary artery (Taussig-Bing type), (3) ventricular septal defect committed to both great vessels, (4) ventricular septal defect uncommitted to the great vessels, and (5) ventricular septal defect related to the aorta, with pulmonary stenosis (tetralogy of Fallot type).

The clinical and laboratory features depend on which of the 5 anatomic types occurs. Two-dimensional echocardiography has proved to be extremely important in the diagnosis and classification of this entity.

Surgical correction is most satisfactory in patients with ventricular septal defect related to the aorta and is effected by closing the defect and creating a tunnel from the left ventricle to the aorta via the patch. Correction of uncommitted defects or defects related to the pulmonary artery requires patch closure and directing the blood to the pulmonary artery, thereby creating a transposition of the great vessels and an associated interatrial rerouting procedure. The use of a valued external conduit may be necessary in the complex varieties.

Toussant M et al: Double outlet right ventricle associated with common atrioventricular canal. *J Am Coll Cardiol* 1986;**8**:396.

TOTAL ANOMALOUS PULMONARY VENOUS RETURN WITH OR WITHOUT OBSTRUCTION

Essentials of Diagnosis
- Mild cyanosis.
- Systolic ejection murmur with left sternal border flow rumble and accentuated P_2.
- Right atrial and right ventricular hypertrophy.

General Considerations
This malformation accounts for approximately 2% of all congenital heart lesions. The pulmonary venous blood does not drain into the left atrium but either directly or indirectly (via a systemic venous connection) into the right atrium. Thus, the entire venous drainage of the body drains into the right atrium.

This malformation may be classified according to the site of entry of the pulmonary veins into the right side of the heart.

Type 1 (55%): Entry into the left superior vena cava (persistent anterior cardinal vein) or right superior vena cava.

Type 2: Entry into the right atrium or into the coronary sinus.

Type 3: Entry below the diaphragm (usually into the portal vein).

Type 4: Multiple types of entry.

Since the entire venous drainage from the body drains into the right atrium, a right-to-left shunt is always present at the atrial level. This may take the form either of a large atrial septal defect or a patent foramen ovale. Relatively complete mixing of the systemic and pulmonary venous return occurs in the right atrium, so that the left atrial and hence the systemic arterial saturation levels approximately equal that of the right atrial saturation.

The degree of desaturation of the blood (and thus the degree of cyanosis present) is determined by the ratio of the quantity of pulmonary blood flow to that of the systemic blood flow. If pulmonary vascular resistance is normal, the flow of blood into the pulmonary artery is much greater than that into the left side of the heart. In this case, there is much greater return from the pulmonary than from the systemic venous system, and the saturation within the right atrium is high. Affected patients function very well, with relatively normal pulmonary artery pressures, and at least physiologically are very similar to patients with very large atrial septal defects and normal pulmonary venous return.

If pulmonary vascular resistance is elevated, the ratio of pulmonary to systemic blood flow is much lower. When the pulmonary vascular resistance equals that of the systemic vascular resistance, equal amounts of blood flow in both directions. When this occurs, marked desaturation of the mixed blood develops and the patient is markedly cyanotic. Such patients do much less well and eventually develop severe right heart failure.

Clinical Findings
A. With Normal Pulmonary Vascular Resistance: The great majority of patients in this group have some elevation of the pulmonary artery pressure owing to the marked increase in pulmonary blood flow. In most cases, the pressure does not reach systemic levels.

1. Symptoms and signs—These patients may have a history of mild cyanosis in the neonatal period and during early infancy. Thereafter, they do relatively well except for frequent respiratory infections. They are usually rather small and thin and resemble patients with very large atrial septal defects.

Careful examination discloses duskiness of the nail beds and mucous membranes, but definite cyanosis and clubbing are usually not present. The arterial pulses are normal. The jugular venous pulses usually show a significant V wave. Examination of the heart shows left chest prominence. A right ventricular heaving impulse is palpable.

The pulmonary component of the second sound is usually increased in intensity. A grade II–IV/VI ejection type systolic murmur is heard at the pulmonary area. It radiates very well over the lung fields anteriorly and posteriorly. An early to middiastolic flow murmur is often heard at the lower left sternal border in the third and fourth intercostal spaces (tricuspid flow murmur).

2. Imaging—Chest x-ray reveals evidence of cardiac enlargement primarily involving the right atrium, right ventricle, and pulmonary artery. There is a marked increase in pulmonary vascular markings. There is often a characteristic contour called a "snowman" or "figure of 8," which is seen where the anomalous veins drain into a persistent left superior vena cava.

3. Electrocardiography—Electrocardiography reveals right axis deviation and varying degrees of right atrial and right ventricular hypertrophy. There is often a QR pattern over the right precordial leads.

4. Echocardiography—Demonstration by echocardiography of a chamber posterior to the left atrium is strongly suggestive of the diagnosis. However, echocardiographic discrimination between anomalies of pulmonary venous return and persistence of pulmonary fetal circulation is still difficult. The availability of 2-dimensional echocardiography plus color flow doppler has increased the diagnostic accuracy.

B. With Increased Pulmonary Vascular Resistance: This group includes patients in whom the pulmonary veins drain into a systemic venous structure below the diaphragm. It also includes a small number of patients in whom the venous drainage is into a systemic vein above the diaphragm.

1. Symptoms and signs—These infants are usually quite sick. Half die within the first 6 months; most are dead by age 1 year unless treated surgically. Cyanosis is common at birth and is quite evident by 1 week. Another common early symptom is severe tachypnea. Congestive heart failure develops later.

Cardiac examination discloses a striking right ventricular impulse. A shock of the second sound is palpable. The first heart sound is accentuated. The second heart sound is markedly accentuated and single. A grade I–II/VI ejection type systolic murmur is frequently heard over the pulmonary area with radiation over the lung fields. Diastolic murmurs are uncommon. In many cases, no murmur is heard at all.

2. Imaging—In the most severe and classic cases, the heart is small and pulmonary venous congestion is marked. In less severe cases, the heart may be slightly enlarged or normal in size, with only slight pulmonary venous congestion.

3. Electrocardiography—The ECG shows right axis deviation, right atrial hypertrophy, and right ventricular hypertrophy.

4. Echocardiography—Echocardiography may demonstrate the combination of a small left atrium and a vessel lying parallel and anterior to the descending aorta and to the left of the inferior vena cava. Color flow doppler echocardiographic patterns are useful in establishing the diagnosis.

5. Cardiac catheterization and angiocardiography—These procedures are diagnostic. Cardiac catheterization demonstrates the presence of total anomalous pulmonary venous return and (usually) the site of entry of the anomalous veins. It also demonstrates the ratio of the pulmonary to systemic blood flow and the degree of pulmonary hypertension and pulmonary vascular resistance.

Cineangiocardiography following injection of contrast material into the right ventricle or pulmonary artery demonstrates the presence of anomalous pulmonary venous return and the site of entry of the anomalous veins. In cases of severe obstruction and a right-to-left patent ductus arteriosus, catheter balloon occlusion of the ductus may be necessary to achieve dense opacification of the pulmonary venous return.

Treatment

If immediate surgical intervention is not contemplated, atrial balloon septostomy should be performed during the initial diagnostic cardiac catheterization. This procedure coupled with vigorous medical management may sustain some infants for several months. Until recently, the surgical death rate in infants was greater than 90%. Within the past few years, however, certain centers have reported excellent results employing either cardiopulmonary bypass or deep hypothermia (cooling to 20 °C [68 °F]). A modification of the anastomosis allowing a larger communication has also greatly improved the surgical results. In such centers, the option of immediate surgical correction may be taken.

Course & Prognosis

Patients with normal pulmonary vascular resistance and only modest elevation of pulmonary artery pressures may do quite well through the second or third decade. Eventually, however, progressive increase in pulmonary vascular resistance and pulmonary hypertension does occur. Patients with increased pulmonary vascular resistance and pulmonary hypertension do poorly, and most die unless treated before age 1 year.

Clarke DR, Paton BC, Stewart JR: Surgical treatment of total anomalous pulmonary venous drainage. *Adv Cardiol* 1979;**26**:129.

Newfeld EA et al: Pulmonary vascular disease in total anomalous pulmonary venous drainage. *Circulation* 1980;**61**:103.

Smallhorn JF et al: Two-dimensional and pulsed Doppler echocardiography in the postoperative evaluation of total anomalous pulmonary venous connection. *Circulation* 1987;**76**:298.

Snider AR et al: Evaluation of infradiaphragmatic total anomalous pulmonary venous connection with two-dimensional echocardiography. *Circulation* 1982;**66**:1129.

Ward KE et al: Restrictive interatrial communication in

total anomalous pulmonary venous connection. *Am J Cardiol* 1986;**57**:1131.

PERSISTENT TRUNCUS ARTERIOSUS

Essentials of Diagnosis
- Neonatal cyanosis.
- Systolic ejection click.

General Considerations
Persistent truncus arteriosus probably accounts for less than 1% of all congenital heart malformations. Only one (huge) great vessel arises from the heart and supplies both the systemic and pulmonary arterial beds. It develops embryologically as a result of complete lack of formation of the spiral ridges that divide the fetal truncus arteriosus into the aorta and pulmonary artery. A high ventricular septal defect is always present. The number of valve leaflets varies from 2 to 6, and the valve may be sufficient, insufficient, or stenotic.

The classification most commonly employed is divided into 4 types:

Type 1: One pulmonary artery that arises from the base of the trunk just above the semilunar valve and runs parallel with the ascending aorta (48%).

Type 2: Two pulmonary arteries that arise side by side from the posterior aspect of the truncus (29%).

Type 3: Two pulmonary arteries that arise independently from either side of the trunk (11%).

Type 4: No demonstrable pulmonary artery (12%). Pulmonary circulation is derived from bronchials arising from the descending thoracic aorta. (The existence of this variety of truncus is controversial. Many authorities consider it an extreme form of tetralogy of Fallot with an atretic main pulmonary artery.)

In this condition, blood leaves the heart through a single common exit. Therefore, the saturation of the blood in the pulmonary artery is the same as that in the systemic arteries. The degree of systemic arterial oxygen saturation depends upon the ratio of the pulmonary to systemic blood flow. If pulmonary vascular resistance is normal, the pulmonary blood flow is much greater than the systemic blood flow and the saturation is relatively high. If pulmonary vascular resistance is great, owing either to pulmonary vascular obstruction or to very small pulmonary arteries, pulmonary blood flow is reduced and oxygen saturation is low. The systolic pressures in both ventricles are identical to that in the aorta.

Clinical Findings
A. Symptoms and Signs: The clinical picture varies depending upon the degree of pulmonary blood flow.

1. Large pulmonary blood flow—Patients with large pulmonary blood flow do well and are usually acyanotic, though the nail beds are commonly dusky. They function similarly to patients with large ventricular septal defects and pulmonary hypertension. Examination of the heart reveals a hyperactive impulse, felt both at the apex and over the xiphoid process. A systolic thrill is common at the lower left sternal border. The first heart sound is normal. A loud early systolic ejection click is commonly heard. The second sound is single and accentuated. A grade IV/VI, completely pansystolic murmur is audible at the lower left sternal border. A diastolic flow murmur can often be heard at the apex (mitral flow murmur).

2. Decreased pulmonary blood flow—Patients with decreased pulmonary blood flow have marked cyanosis early and do very poorly. The most common manifestations include retardation of growth and development, easy fatigability, dyspnea on exertion, and congestive heart failure. The heart is not unduly active. The first and second heart sounds are loud. A systolic grade II–IV/VI murmur is heard at the lower left sternal border. No diastolic flow murmur is heard. A continuous heart murmur is very uncommon except in type 4, in which the continuous murmur is due to the large bronchial collateral vessels. A very loud systolic ejection click is commonly heard.

B. Imaging: Most common x-ray findings are a boot-shaped heart, absence of the main pulmonary artery segment, and a large aorta that frequently arches to the right. The pulmonary vascular markings vary, depending upon the degree of pulmonary blood flow.

C. Electrocardiography: The axis is usually normal, though left axis deviation occurs rarely. Evidence of right ventricular hypertrophy or combined ventricular hypertrophy is commonly present. Left ventricular hypertrophy as an isolated finding is rare.

D. Echocardiography: A characteristic tracing would exhibit override of a single great artery (similar to tetralogy of Fallot) without a demonstrable right ventricular infundibulum.

E. Angiocardiography: This procedure is usually diagnostic. Injection of contrast material into the right ventricle demonstrates the presence of a ventricular septal defect and the single vessel arising from the heart. The exact type of truncus, however, may be somewhat difficult to determine even from angiocardiograms. It may occasionally also be difficult to differentiate this condition from pulmonary atresia and ventricular septal defect (pseudotruncus).

Treatment
Anticongestive measures and, in some cases, banding of the pulmonary artery are indicated for patients with high pulmonary blood flow and congestive failure. Aortic homografting for "total correction" of the truncus has been performed in selected patients. During the past several years, the number of severely symptomatic infants undergoing

"total correction" in the first 6 months of life has increased.

Course & Prognosis

The outcome depends to a great extent upon the status of the pulmonary circulation. Patients with a low pulmonary blood flow usually do very poorly and die within 1 year. Those with increased pulmonary blood flow can survive for a variable period. A few cases of survival into the third decade have been reported. Death is usually due to congestive heart failure, hypoxia, subacute infective endocarditis, or brain abscess.

Juanida E, Haworth SG: Pulmonary vascular disease in children with truncus arteriosus. *Am J Cardiol* 1984;**54:** 1315.

Pierpont MEM et al: Cardiac malformations in relatives of children with truncus arteriosus or interruption of the aortic arch. *Am J Cardiol* 1988;**61:**423.

Spicer B et al: Repair of truncus arteriosus in neonates with the use of a valveless conduit. *Circulation* 1984;**70:**26.

DEXTROCARDIA

This lesion consists of right-sided heart with or without reversal of position of other organs (situs inversus). If there is no reversal of other organs, the heart usually has other severe defects. With complete situs inversus, the heart is usually normal.

Apical pulse and sounds are heard on the right side of the chest. X-ray film shows the cardiac silhouette on the right side. On electrocardiography, the P waves are usually inverted in lead I; QRS is predominantly down in lead I; and lead II resembles normal lead III and vice versa. Two-dimensional echocardiography is extremely useful in defining the complex anatomy.

With situs inversus and no heart defects, the prognosis is excellent. If severe heart defects are present, definitive diagnosis is imperative, because corrective surgery is frequently beneficial.

Emmanouilides GC, Baylen BG. Dextrocardia and the cardiosplenic syndromes. Page 245 in: *Neonatal Cardiopulmonary Distress.* Emmanouilides GC, Baylen BG (editors). Year Book, 1988.

Van Praagh R et al: Malposition of the heart. Page 422 in: *Heart Disease in Infants, Children, and Adolescents,* 3rd ed. Adams FH, Emmanouilides GC (editors). Williams and Wilkins, 1983.

ACQUIRED HEART DISEASE

RHEUMATIC FEVER

Rheumatic fever is a disease in transition. Although it is still an important disease in the USA, its frequency has diminished significantly over the past half century. Penicillin is largely responsible, but the decrease in frequency of rheumatic fever was already apparent before the antibiotic era. In the USA and other developed countries in the temperate zone, improvement in standards of living, general hygiene, and opportunities for medical care have greatly reduced the incidence of this disease. However, there has been a startling resurgence of acute rheumatic fever in several regions of the United States (the Midwest in 1984 and the intermountain West in 1987). In addition, the character of the illness is more malignant than that seen in the 1970s, with a high incidence of myocarditis and polyvalvular involvement. The reason for these regional epidemics is not as yet known, but it is clear that the disease is back.

Until the recent epidemic, the symptomatic presentation of the disease had also changed significantly in the USA within the past 2 decades. The frequency with which one encounters severe disabling carditis has greatly diminished, and the attack rate of acute rheumatic fever is considerably less than the original estimate of 0.3% in untreated children. Current manifestations of carditis are often mild and transient and require serial examinations by a skilled auscultator to confirm or rule out the diagnosis. One can only speculate on the reasons for these changes in the epidemiologic characteristics of the disease in different communities and on what role, if any, the liberal use of antibiotics may have played.

Group A β-hemolytic streptococcal infection of the respiratory tract is the essential environmental trigger that acts on predisposed individuals. The latest attempts to define host susceptibility implicate immune response (Ir) genes, which are present in approximately 15% of the population. The immune response triggered by colonization of the pharynx with group A streptococci consists of (1) sensitization of B lymphocytes by streptococcal antigens, (2) formation of antistreptococcal antibody, (3) formation of immune complexes that cross-react with cardiac sarcolemma antigens, and (4) myocardial and valvular inflammatory response.

The peak period of risk in the USA is age 5–15 years. The disease is slightly more common in girls and is now more common in blacks, perhaps reflecting socioeconomic factors. The average annual attack rate in the total North American population is less than one per 10,000, and the presence of rheumatic heart disease in the school-age population is less than one per 1000. The annual death rate from rheumatic heart disease in school-age children (whites and nonwhites) recorded a decade ago was less than one per 100,000.

Jones Criteria (Revised) for Diagnosis of Rheumatic Fever

Major manifestations
    Carditis
    Polyarthritis
    Sydenham's chorea
    Erythema marginatum
    Subcutaneous nodules
Minor manifestations
    Clinical
        Previous rheumatic fever or rheumatic heart disease
        Polyarthralgia
        Fever
    Laboratory
        Acute phase reaction: elevated erythrocyte sedimentation rate, C-reactive protein, leukocytosis
        Prolonged PR interval

Plus

Supporting evidence of preceding streptococcal infection, ie, increased titers of antistreptolysin O or other streptococcal antibodies, positive throat culture for group A *Streptococcus.*

Traditionally, 2 major or one major and 2 minor criteria (plus supporting evidence of streptococcal infection) justified the presumptive diagnosis of rheumatic fever. However, the major modern dilemma regarding diagnosis is that the physical findings may be so subtle and transient that the criteria are marginal. Since improper diagnosis has lifelong and serious consequences, it is justified to hospitalize patients with marginal findings so that serial clinical studies of the patient, including multiple examinations by a pediatric cardiologist, can be performed. If rheumatic fever appears likely on the basis of appropriate and careful evaluation but does not fully meet the Revised Jones Criteria, the diagnosis of suspect acute rheumatic fever is appropriate. This diagnosis mandates anti-infective prophylaxis but attempts to avoid the social and economic sequelae of the full diagnosis.

Major Manifestations of Rheumatic Fever

A. Active Carditis: Any one of the following—

1. A significant *new* murmur that is clearly mitral insufficiency (with or without a transient apical diastolic Carey-Coombs murmur) or aortic insufficiency. It should be remembered that mitral insufficiency, while commonly caused by rheumatic fever, has many other causes in childhood.

2. Pericarditis, manifested by a pericardial friction rub or evidence of pericardial effusion.

3. Evidence of congestive heart failure.

B. Polyarthritis: Two or more joints must be involved; involvement of one joint does not constitute a major manifestation. The joints may be involved simultaneously or (more diagnostically) in a migratory fashion. The most commonly involved joints are the ankles, knees, hips, wrists, elbows, and shoulders. Heat, redness, swelling, severe pain, and tenderness are usually all present. Arthralgia alone without the other signs of inflammation is not sufficient to meet the criterion of polyarthritis.

C. Subcutaneous Nodules: These are usually seen only in severe cases, and then most commonly over the joints, scalp, and spinal column. They vary from a few millimeters to 2 cm in diameter and are nontender and freely movable under the skin.

D. Erythema Marginatum: While this is a specific and major manifestation of acute rheumatic fever, many physicians fail to distinguish it from other skin lesions. It usually occurs only in severe cases and is rarely an essential diagnostic clue. It consists of a macular erythematous rash with a circinate border and appears primarily on the trunk and extremities. The face is usually not involved.

E. Sydenham's Chorea: Sydenham's chorea is characterized by emotional instability and involuntary movements. These findings become progressively more severe and are often followed by the development of ataxia and slurring of speech. Muscular weakness becomes apparent following the onset of the involuntary movements. The individual attack of chorea is self-limiting, although it may last up to 3 months. It is not uncommon to find involvement on only one side. Manifestations may not be apparent for months to years after the acute episode of rheumatic fever.

Minor Manifestations of Rheumatic Fever

A. Fever: The fever is usually low-grade, although occasionally it reaches 39.4–40 °C (103–104 °F).

B. Polyarthralgia: Pain in 2 or more joints without heat, swelling, and tenderness is a minor rather than a major manifestation.

C. Electrocardiographic Changes: Prolongation of the PR interval represents only a minor manifestation and does not qualify as active carditis.

D. Acute Phase Reaction: The sedimentation rate is accelerated and, more specifically, the C-reactive protein is elevated. Congestive heart failure does not influence the C-reactive protein and usually does not affect the sedimentation rate. Leukocytosis is the rule.

E. History: There is a prior history of acute rheumatic fever or the presence of inactive rheumatic heart disease.

Essential Manifestation

Except in cases of rheumatic fever presenting solely as Sydenham's chorea or long-standing carditis, there should be clear supporting evidence of a streptococcal infection such as scarlet fever, a positive throat culture for group A β-hemolytic *Streptococcus,* and increased antistreptolysin O or other streptococcal antibody titers. The antistreptolysin O titer is significantly higher in rheumatic fever than in uncomplicated streptococcal infections.

Other Manifestations

Associated findings may include erythema multiforme; abdominal, back, and precordial pain; and nontraumatic epistaxis, vomiting, malaise, weight loss, and anemia.

Treatment & Prophylaxis

A. Treatment of the Acute Episode:

1. Anti-infective therapy—Eradication of the streptococcal infection is essential. Benzathine penicillin G is the drug of choice. Depending on the age and weight of the patient, give a single intramuscular injection of 0.6–1.2 million units, or give 125–250 mg orally 4 times a day for 10 days. Erythromycin, 250 mg orally 4 times a day, may be substituted if the patient is allergic to penicillin.

2. Anti-inflammatory agents—

a. Aspirin—Patients with the contemporary form of the disease need significantly less aspirin than in the past. Currently, 30–60 mg/g/d is given in 4 divided doses; this dosage is often more than sufficient to effect dramatic relief of the arthritis and fever. In general, higher dosages carry a greater risk of side effects, and there are no proved short- or long-term benefits of giving high doses to effect salicylate blood levels of 20–30 mg/dL. The duration of therapy must be tailored to meet the needs of the patient, but use of aspirin for 2–6 weeks, with reduction in dosage toward the end of the course, is usually sufficient.

b. Corticosteroids—Corticosteroids are rarely indicated in current therapy. However, in the unusual patient with severe carditis and manifestations of congestive heart failure (as evidenced by radiographic findings of cardiomegaly or by cardiopulmonary symptoms or a gallop rhythm), therapy may not only be effective but lifesaving. Corticosteroid therapy may be given as follows: prednisone, 2 mg/kg/d orally for 2 weeks (or comparable doses of other corticosteroids); reduce prednisone to 1 mg/kg/d the third week, and begin aspirin, 50 mg/kg/d; stop prednisone at the end of 3 weeks, and continue aspirin for 8 weeks or until the C-reactive protein is negative and the sedimentation rate is falling.

3. Therapy of congestive heart failure—See Congestive Heart Failure, above.

4. Bed rest and ambulation—Strict bed rest is not required for patients with arthritis and mild carditis without congestive heart failure. It is preferable to maintain a regimen of bed-to-chair with bathroom privileges and meals at the table for patients who are relatively asymptomatic while on aspirin therapy. Asymptomatic patients can be kept in bed only under duress anyway. Patients with severe carditis (congestive heart failure) have no desire to get out of bed and should be at bed rest at least as long as corticosteroid therapy is required. *Gradual* indoor ambulation followed by modified outdoor activity may be ordered when symptoms have disappeared but there is still clinical and laboratory evidence of rheumatic activity. Modified bed rest for 2–6 weeks is generally adequate. Children should not return to school while there is clear evidence of rheumatic activity.

B. Treatment After the Acute Episode:

1. Prevention—The patient who has had rheumatic fever has a greatly increased risk of developing rheumatic fever following the next inadequately treated group A β-hemolytic streptococcal infection. *Prevention is thus the most important therapeutic course for the physician to emphasize.* The purpose of follow-up visits after the acute episode is not so much to evaluate the evolution of mitral insufficiency murmurs as to reinforce the physician's advice about the necessity for antibacterial prophylaxis with benzathine penicillin G. At such times, the physician should stress that greater protection is afforded by administration via the intramuscular route than via the oral route and that, in addition, failure to comply with regular oral medication programs increases the risk for recurrence of rheumatic fever. Thus, patients should be informed that the parenteral route will be favored until they are adults, at which time their internists may elect oral medication.

If myocardial or valvular disease persists, antibacterial prophylaxis is a lifelong commitment. More commonly with transient cardiac involvement, 3–5 years of therapy or discontinuance at adolescence is a practical and effective approach.

The following regimens are in current use:

a. Benzathine penicillin G, 1.2 million units intramuscularly every 28 days, is the drug of choice.

b. Sulfadiazine, 500 mg daily as a single oral dose for patients weighing over 27 kg (60 lb), is the drug of second choice. Blood dyscrasias and a lesser effectiveness in reducing streptococcal infections make this drug less satisfactory than benzathine penicillin G.

c. Penicillin G (buffered), 250,000 units orally twice daily, offers approximately the same protection afforded by sulfadiazine but is much less effective than intramuscular benzathine penicillin G (5.5 versus 0.4 streptococcal infections per 100 patient years).

d. Erythromycin, 250 mg orally twice a day, may be given to those patients who may be allergic to both penicillin and sulfonamides.

2. Residual valvular damage—Chronic congestive heart failure may follow a single severe episode of acute rheumatic carditis or, more commonly, may follow repeated episodes. In children in the USA, the usual manifestations of residual valvular damage are heart murmurs of mitral and aortic insufficiency;

murmurs are not accompanied by congestive heart failure during most of the pediatric age period *as long as repeated attacks are prevented.*

Methods of managing congestive heart failure have been previously discussed. Children with severe valvular damage who cannot be adequately managed on a medical regimen must be considered for valve replacement—and considered before the myocardium is irreversibly damaged.

Congeni B et al: An outbreak of acute rheumatic fever in northeast Ohio. *J Pediatr* 1987;**111:**176.

Hosier DM et al: Resurgence of acute rheumatic fever. *Am J Dis Child* 1984;**141:**730.

Kaplan EL, Hill HR: The return of rheumatic fever: Consequences, implications and needs. *J Pediatr* 1987; **111:**244.

Markowitz M: The decline of rheumatic fever. *J Pediatr* 1985;**106:**545.

Veasy LG et al: Resurgence of acute rheumatic fever in the intermountain west of the United States. *N Engl J Med* 1987;**316:**421.

Zabriskie JB: Rheumatic fever: The interplay between host, genetics, and microbe. *Circulation* 1985;**71:**1077.

RHEUMATIC HEART DISEASE

Mitral Insufficiency

Mitral insufficiency, the most common valvular residual of acute rheumatic carditis, is characterized by a pansystolic murmur that localizes at the apex. In patients with mitral involvement, the murmur appears early in the course of rheumatic carditis, and—depending on the severity of the damage—may disappear over a period of days or months or may persist for life. Although rheumatic fever is a common cause of mitral insufficiency in pediatric patients, the mitral insufficiency murmur cannot be taken as diagnostic of a rheumatic episode.

Among the many other causes of mitral insufficiency, the most common is the mitral dysfunction syndrome, characterized by a mid to late apical systolic murmur introduced by a click.* Other causes are myocarditis, endocardial fibroelastosis, anomalous left coronary artery, and congenital anomalies of the mitral valve, which occur as isolated lesions or as part of a complex of anomalies (eg, endocardial cushion defects). It is thus essential to define the cause of mitral insufficiency in order to provide knowledgeable management—and not to prescribe a lifetime program of rheumatic fever prophylaxis for a patient who has only mitral dysfunction or to fail to provide appropriate surgical treatment if the mitral insufficiency is secondary to an anomalous left coronary artery.

---

*A word of caution about diagnosing the mitral dysfunction syndrome: The echocardiographic finding of prolapse (redundancy) of the mitral valve, which characterizes mitral dysfunction, may also be found in patients with acute rheumatic fever and recently acquired rheumatic heart disease.

Mitral Stenosis

There are murmurs of mitral stenosis which are secondary to structural stenosis of the valve; those which are due to relative excess of flow (in large volumes of regurgitation); and those which are present during acute valvulitis (Carey-Coombs murmur). Mitral stenosis due to structural stenosis is rarely encountered in the USA before 5–10 years following the first episode of acute rheumatic carditis and is much more commonly discovered in adults than in children. Early mitral stenosis murmurs, flow murmurs, and Carey-Coombs murmurs are short and heard in mid diastole. Established mitral stenosis murmurs become progressively longer in duration until they attain the classic crescendo, presystolic configuration.

Aortic Insufficiency

This early decrescendo diastolic murmur—heard maximally at the secondary aortic area—is not commonly encountered as the sole valvular involvement of rheumatic carditis, as is mitral insufficiency. It is the second most frequent valve affected in polyvalvular as well as in single valvular disease. It appears that the aortic valve is involved more often in males and in blacks. A short aortic systolic murmur due to excess flow may accompany the aortic insufficiency murmur.

Aortic Stenosis

Dominant aortic stenosis of rheumatic origin does not occur in pediatric patients. Aortic stenosis in children is congenital. In one large series, the shortest length of time observed for a patient to develop dominant aortic stenosis secondary to rheumatic heart disease was 20 years.

Lembo NJ et al: Mitral valve prolapse in patients with prior rheumatic fever. *Circulation* 1988;**77:**830.

Vardi P et al: Clinical echocardiographic correlations in acute rheumatic fever. *Pediatrics* 1983;**71:**830.

MYOCARDITIS

In the great majority of cases, the cause of myocarditis is not determined. Coxsackievirus B is the commonest infectious agent isolated. Coxsackievirus A, rubella virus, cytomegalovirus, mumps virus, herpes virus, adenovirus, and many other viral agents have been implicated. Virtually every other infectious agent, including bacteria, fungi, rickettsiae, chlamydiae, spirochetes, and parasites, has been suggested as a cause of myocarditis, but laboratory confirmation is seldom possible. It is important to emphasize that myocarditis is part of a spectrum of primary endomyocardial diseases and may be one of the causes of endocardial fibroelastosis.

Clinical Findings

A. Symptoms and Signs: The clinical picture

usually falls into 2 separate patterns: (1) Onset of congestive heart failure is sudden in a newborn who has been in relatively good health 12–24 hours previously. This is a malignant form of the disease and is thought to be solely secondary to overwhelming viremia and tissue invasion of multiple organ systems, including the heart. (2) In the older child, the onset of cardiac findings tends to be much more gradual. There is often a history of an upper respiratory tract infection or gastroenteritis within the month prior to the development of cardiac findings. This is a more insidious form of the disease and may have a late postinfectious or autoimmune component. Recovery from the initial infection is followed by gradual and progressive development of easy fatigability, dyspnea on exertion, and malaise.

In the newborn infant, the signs of congestive heart failure are usually quite apparent. The skin is pale and gray, and peripheral cyanosis may be present. The pulses are rapid, weak, and thready. Edema of the face and extremities may be present. Significant cardiomegaly is present, and the left and right ventricular impulses are weak. On auscultation, the heart sounds may be poor, muffled, and distant. Third and fourth heart sounds are common, resulting in a gallop rhythm. Murmurs are usually absent, though a murmur of tricuspid or mitral insufficiency can occasionally be heard. Moist rales are usually present at both lung bases. The liver is enlarged and frequently tender. The level of the jugular venous pulse is elevated. In the latter group, the signs of congestive heart failure are often quite subtle.

B. Imaging: Generalized cardiomegaly involving all 4 chambers of the heart can be seen on x-ray. There is evidence of moderate to marked pulmonary venous congestion. Pneumonitis is commonly present.

C. Electrocardiography: The ECG is variable. Classically, there is evidence of low voltage of the QRS throughout all frontal and precordial leads and depression of the ST segment and inversion of the T waves in leads I, III, and aVF and in the left precordial leads during the acute malignant stage. Dysrhythmias are common, and atrioventricular and intraventricular conduction disturbances may be present. With the more benign form—or during the recovery phase of the malignant form—high-voltage QRS complexes are commonly seen and are indicative of left ventricular hypertrophy.

Treatment

A. Digitalis: All patients with clinical findings of myocarditis and in congestive heart failure should be started immediately on digitalis. Because the inflamed myocardium is markedly sensitive to digitalis, only about two-thirds of the usual total digitalizing dose should be employed. During the initial phase of therapy, frequent ECGs should be taken. If serious dysrhythmias or other evidence of digitalis

intoxication develops, the drug should be stopped and not reinstituted until all evidence of digitalis toxicity has disappeared. If toxicity is not evident and there is no clinical response, digitalis doses should be increased until one or the other is noted.

B. Diuretics: Diuretics should be administered with caution, since they may potentiate digitalis toxicity.

C. Corticosteroids: The administration of corticosteroids is controversial but seems more rational when used in the treatment of the more benign postinfectious autoimmune cases. If the patient's condition continues to deteriorate despite anticongestive measures, corticosteroids are commonly employed.

Prognosis

The prognosis is related to the age at onset, the response to therapy, and the presence or absence of recurrences. If the patient is less than 6 months of age or older than 3 years, responds poorly to therapy, and manifests multiple recurrences of congestive heart failure, the prognosis is poor. Many patients recover clinically but have persistent cardiomegaly. It is possible that subclinical myocarditis in childhood is the pathophysiologic basis for some of the idiopathic myocardiopathies seen later in life.

Pulido S: Acute and subacute myocarditis. *Cardiovasc Rev Rep* 1984;**5**:912.

Ringel RE et al: Serologic evidence for *Chlamydia trachomatis* myocarditis. *Pediatrics* 1982;**70**:54.

Rozkovec A et al: Natural history of left ventricular function in neonatal coxsackie myocarditis. *Pediatr Care* 1985;**6**:151.

INFECTIVE ENDOCARDITIS

Essentials of Diagnosis

- Preexisting organic heart murmur.
- Persistent fever.
- Increasing symptoms of heart disease (ranging from easy fatigability to heart failure).
- Splenomegaly (70%).
- Embolic phenomena (50%).
- Leukocytosis, elevated erythrocyte sedimentation rate, positive blood culture.

General Considerations

Bacterial infection of the endocardial surface of the heart or the intimal surface of certain arterial vessels (coarcted segment of aorta and ductus arteriosus) is a rare condition that usually occurs when an abnormality of the heart or great vessels exists. It may develop in a normal heart during the course of septicemia.

The incidence of infective endocarditis appears to be increasing owing to many factors, including (1) increased survival rates for children with congenital heart disease, (2) greater use of chronic central venous catheters, and (3) increased use of prosthetic material and valves. Pediatric patients without preexisting heart disease also are at increased risk for infective endocarditis owing to (1) increased survival rates for children with immune deficiencies, (2) greater use of chronic indwelling lines in critically ill newborns, and (3) increased incidence of intravenous drug abuse.

Patients at greatest risk include those with aorticopulmonary shunts, left-sided outflow obstruction, and ventricular septal defects. Predisposing factors can be identified approximately 30% of the time and include dental procedures, nonsterile surgical procedures, and cardiovascular surgery.

Organisms causing endocarditis include *Streptococcus viridans* (about 50% of cases), *Staphylococcus aureus* (about 30%), and fungal agents (about 10%).

Clinical Findings

A. History: Almost all patients have a history of heart disease. There may or may not be a history of infection or a surgical procedure (tooth extraction, tonsillectomy).

B. Symptoms, Signs, and Laboratory Findings: In one large study, the following symptoms, signs, and laboratory findings were reported (in order of decreasing frequency): changing murmurs, fever, positive blood culture, weight loss, cardiomegaly, elevated sedimentation rate, splenomegaly, petechiae, embolism, and leukocytosis. Other findings include hematuria, signs of congestive heart failure, clubbing, joint pains, and hepatomegaly. Echocardiography has become a valuable tool in diagnosing large vegetations.

Prevention

It is recommended that patients at risk for infective endocarditis be given appropriate antibiotics before any type of dental work (tooth extraction, cleaning) and before operations within the oropharynx, gastrointestinal tract, and genitourinary tract. Continuous antibiotic prophylaxis (as in the treatment of rheumatic fever) is *not* recommended in patients with congenital heart disease.

It is economically and logistically easier to give parents a supply of oral penicillin tablets to be used by their school-age children for dental procedures. The following schedule is recommended: for children less than 27 kg, 1 g of penicillin V one hour prior to procedure and then 500 mg 6 hours after initial dose; for children greater than 27 kg, 2 g of penicillin V one hour prior to procedure and then 1 g of penicillin 6 hours after initial dose.

Treatment

In a patient with known heart disease, the presence of an otherwise unexplained fever should alert the physician to the possibility of infective endocarditis. A positive blood culture or other major findings of infective endocarditis confirm the diagnosis. If a positive blood culture is obtained and the organism is identified, specific treatment should be begun immediately. Even if blood cultures are negative after 48 hours, it is advisable to begin penicillin therapy (if there is other evidence of infective endocarditis), because most positive cultures are obtained within the first 48 hours. Penicillin is the drug choice in most cases. Other antibiotics may be added (see Chapter 38). If congestive heart failure occurs and progresses unremittingly in the face of adequate antibiotic therapy, surgical excision of the infected area and prosthetic valve replacement should be considered.

Course & Prognosis

The prognosis depends upon how early in the course of the infectious process treatment is instituted. The prognosis is better in patients in whom blood culture is positive. If congestive heart failure develops, the prognosis is usually poor.

Even though bacteriologic cure of the infectious process is achieved, death may occur as a result of congestive heart failure secondary to severe valvular destruction. Intractable congestive heart failure may occur weeks or months following bacteriologic cure. Embolization may occur following bacteriologic cure when vegetations tear off from the involved area.

The death rate for infective endocarditis is still about 20%.

Allen HD et al: New recommendations for antibiotic prophylaxis of bacterial endocarditis. *Am J Dis Child* 1985; **139:**225.

Brandenburg C et al: Infective endocarditis: A 25-year overview of diagnosis and therapy. *J Am Coll Cardiol* 1983; **1:**280.

Noel GJ et al: Staphylococcus epidermidis right-sided endocarditis. *Pediatrics* 1988;**82:**234.

Shulman ST: Prevention of bacterial endocarditis. *Pediatrics* 1985;**75:**603.

PERICARDITIS

Essentials of Diagnosis

- Retrosternal pain made worse by deep inspiration and decreased by leaning forward.
- Fever.
- Shortness of breath and grunting respirations are common.
- Pericardial friction rub.
- Tachycardia.
- Hepatomegaly and distention of the jugular veins.
- ECG with elevated ST segment.

General Considerations

Involvement of the pericardium rarely occurs as

an isolated event. In the great majority of cases, pericardial disease occurs in association with a more generalized process. Important causes include rheumatic fever, viral pericarditis, purulent pericarditis, rheumatoid arthritis, uremia, and tuberculosis.

In the pediatric age group, pericardial disease usually takes the form of acute pericarditis. In most cases, there is effusion of fluid into the pericardial cavity. The consequences of such effusion depend upon the amount, type, and speed of fluid accumulation. Under certain circumstances, serious compression of the heart occurs. The direct compression and the body's attempt to correct it result in cardiac tamponade. Unless the pericardial fluid is evacuated, death occurs very rapidly.

Clinical Findings

A. Symptoms and Signs: The symptoms depend to a great extent upon the cause of the pericarditis. Pain is common. It is usually sharp and stabbing, located in the mid chest and in the shoulder and neck, made worse by deep inspiration, and considerably decreased by sitting up and leaning forward. Shortness of breath and grunting respirations are common findings in all patients.

The physical findings depend upon whether or not a significant amount of effusion is present: (1) In the absence of significant accumulation of fluid, the pulses are normal and the level of the jugular venous pulse is normal. On examination of the heart, a characteristic scratchy, high-pitched friction rub may be heard. It is often systolic and diastolic and can be located at any point between the apex and the left sternal border. The location and timing vary considerably from time to time. The heart sounds are usually normal, and the heart is not enlarged to percussion. (2) If there is a considerable accumulation of pericardial fluid, the cardiovascular findings are different. The heart is enlarged to percussion, but on inspection of the precordium, it seems to be very quiet. Auscultation reveals distant and muffled heart tones. Friction rub is usually not present. In the absence of cardiac tamponade, the peripheral, venous, and arterial pulses are normal.

Cardiac tamponade is characterized by distention of the jugular veins, tachycardia, enlargement of the liver, peripheral edema, and "paradoxic pulse," in which the systolic pressure drops by more than 10 mm Hg during inspiration. The term paradoxic pulse is a misnomer, since the drop is only an accentuation of a normal event. (Normally, the systolic pressure drops by no more than 5 mm Hg.) This finding is best determined with the use of a blood pressure cuff. At this point, the patient is critically ill and has all the symptoms and signs suggestive of right-sided congestive heart failure.

Not all patients with marked cardiac compression demonstrate all the findings listed above. If the patient appears critically ill and has evidence of pericarditis and effusion, treatment should be instituted even though all the clinical signs of cardiac tamponade are not present.

B. Imaging: In pericarditis without effusion, chest x-ray findings are normal. With pericardial effusion, the cardiac silhouette is enlarged, often in the shape of a water bottle, with blunting of the cardiodiaphragmatic borders. When there is evidence of cardiac tamponade, the lung fields are clear. This is in contrast to patients with myocardial dilatation, who show evidence of pulmonary congestion.

Cardiac fluoroscopy usually demonstrates absence of pulsations of the cardiac borders. This is helpful in differentiating this condition from myocarditis, in which the pulsations, although feeble, are present.

C. Electrocardiography: A number of electrocardiographic abnormalities occur in patients with pericarditis. Low voltage is commonly seen in patients with significant pericardial effusion, although the voltage may be normal. The ST segment is commonly elevated during the first week of involvement. The T wave is usually upright during this time. Following this, the ST segment is normal and the T wave becomes flattened. After about 2 weeks, the T wave inverts and remains inverted for several weeks or months. In contrast to findings in patients with myocardial infarction, there is no reciprocal relationship between the findings in lead I and lead III in the frontal plane and the right and left precordial leads.

D. Echocardiography: Echocardiography has become a most reliable form of noninvasive diagnosis of pericardial effusion. The results must be considered in the light of the clinical picture in deciding whether or not to remove the fluid.

Treatment

Treatment depends upon the cause of the pericarditis. Cardiac tamponade due to any cause must be treated by evacuation of the fluid. It is usually desirable to perform a wide resection of the pericardium through a surgical incision. However, needle insertion into the pericardial sac may be lifesaving in an emergency situation (see Chapter 35).

Prognosis

The prognosis depends to a great extent upon the cause of the pericardial disease. Cardiac tamponade due to any cause will result in death unless the fluid is evacuated.

See references below.

SPECIFIC DISEASES INVOLVING THE PERICARDIUM

Acute Rheumatic Fever

When pericarditis occurs during the course of acute rheumatic fever, it is almost always associated with involvement of the myocardium and endocardium (pancarditis). Thus, heart murmurs are almost always present. The pericarditis is usually of the serofibrinous variety and usually not associated with significant pericardial effusion.

Patients with acute rheumatic fever and pericarditis are usually very ill, with severe cardiac involvement. They respond extremely well to corticosteroid therapy. Pericarditis usually disappears rapidly (1 week) after corticosteroid therapy is started. Constrictive pericarditis almost never occurs secondary to this disease.

Viral Pericarditis

Viral pericarditis is uncommon in children and young adults. The most common cause is the coxsackievirus B4. Influenza virus has also been implicated. There is usually a history of a protracted upper respiratory tract infection.

The pericardial effusion usually lasts for several weeks. Cardiac tamponade is rare. Recurrences of pericardial effusion are quite common even months or years after the initial episode. Constrictive pericarditis has been reported in this disease.

Purulent Pericarditis

The most common causes of purulent pericarditis are pneumococci, streptococci, staphylococci, *Escherichia coli,* and *Haemophilus influenzae.* This disorder is always secondary to infection elsewhere, although occasionally the primary site is not obvious. In addition to demonstrating signs of cardiac compression, patients are quite septic and run extremely high fevers. The purulent fluid accumulating within the pericardial sac is usually quite thick and filled with polymorphonuclear leukocytes. Although antibiotics will sterilize the pericardial fluid, pericardial tamponade commonly develops, and evacuation of the pericardial sac is usually necessary. Wide resection of the pericardium through a surgical incision performed in the operating room is most desirable, but pericardiocentesis is often dramatically effective and lifesaving. Drainage of the purulent fluid is followed by marked improvement of symptoms.

Postpericardiotomy Syndrome

Postpericardiotomy syndrome is characterized by fever, chest pain, friction rub, and elevation of ST segment noted on ECG 1–2 weeks after open heart surgery. It appears to be an autoimmune disease with high titers of antiheart antibody and with detectable evidence of fresh or reactivated viral illness. The syndrome is often self-limited and responds well to short courses of aspirin or corticosteroid therapy. Occasionally, it lasts for months to years and may require pericardiocentesis or pericardiectomy.

Clapp SK et al: Postoperative pericardial effusion and its relation to postpericardiotomy syndrome. *Pediatrics* 1980;**66**:585.

Engle MA et al: Viral illness and the postpericardiotomy syndrome. *Circulation* 1980;**62**:1151.
Fowler NO, Gabel M: The hemodynamic effects of cardiac tamponade. *Circulation* 1985;**71**:154.
Sagrista-Sauleda J, Permanyer-Miralda G, Soler-Soler J: Tuberculous pericarditis: Ten-year experience with a prospective protocol for diagnosis and treatment. *J Am Coll Cardiol* 1988;**11**:724.

HYPERTENSION*

Blood pressure determinations are being more routinely obtained in the examination of infants and children; as a result, systemic hypertension has become more widely recognized as a pediatric problem. Pediatric standards for blood pressure have been published, but the studies from which these standards were derived suffered from 3 methodologic problems. The first and most important is that the widest cuff that would fit between the axilla and antecubital fossa was not routinely used. The use of a wide cuff either has no effect on blood pressure or decreases blood pressure by a maximum of 5 mm Hg. Use of a narrow cuff, however, routinely increases blood pressure by 10–50 mm Hg. The second methodologic problem was lack of an ethnic cross section. Third, the fact that systemic blood pressure decreases with increasing altitude of residence was not taken into consideration.

These 3 problems were addressed in a study of a triracial population at sea level and at an altitude of 10,000 feet. The widest cuff that would fit between the axilla and antecubital fossa was used in each case. Most children from 10–11 years of age needed a standard adult-size cuff (bladder width of 12 cm), and many high school students needed a large adult-size cuff (width of 16 cm) or leg cuff (width of 18 cm). Results of the study are shown in Table 16–3. The 95th percentile value for blood pressure was similar for both sexes and all 3 ethnic groups. Blood pressure varied more with altitude and body weight than with sex or ethnic origin. If the blood pressure taken in a quiet atmosphere and sitting position exceeds the 95th percentile for systolic, diastolic muffle, or diastolic disappearance pressures, it should be repeated twice in 1- to 2-week intervals. If it is abnormal all 3 times, a pediatric hypertension diagnostic center should be consulted.

Essential hypertension is the most common form of pediatric hypertension. Coarctation of the thoracic or abdominal aorta, renal artery stenosis, renal disease, and pheochromocytoma should be ruled out.

Patients with essential hypertension often show improvement with reduction of obesity, reduction of excessive salt intake, institution of an exercise pro-

---

*The diagnostic evaluation of renal hypertension and the treatment of hypertensive emergencies, as well as the ambulatory treatment of chronic hypertension, are discussed in Chapter 22.

Table 16–3. The 95th percentile value for blood pressure (mm Hg) taken in the sitting position.[1]

Age (y)	Sea Level			10,000 Feet		
	S	Dm	Dd	S	Dm	Dd
5				92	72	62
6	106	64	60	96	74	66
7	108	72	66	98	76	70
8	110	76	70	104	80	70
9	114	80	76	106	80	70
10	118	82	76	108	80	70
11	124	82	78	108	80	72
12	128	84	78	108	80	72
13	132	84	80	116	84	76
14	136	86	80	120	84	76
15	140	88	80	120	84	80
16	140	90	80	120	84	80
17	140	92	80	122	84	80
18	140	92	80	130	84	80

[1]Blood pressures: S = systolic (Korotkoff's sound 1; onset of tapping); Dm = diastolic muffling (Korotkoff's sound 4); Dd = diastolic disappearance (Korotkoff's sound 5).

gram, avoidance of cigarette smoking, and avoidance of use of oral contraceptives. The use of antihypertensive drugs in pediatric hypertension is controversial, but thiazide diuretics and propranolol are useful in selected cases.

Burke GL et al: Blood pressure and echocardiographic measures in children: The Bogalusa heart study. *Circulation* 1987;**75**:106.

Fraser GE, Phillips RL, Harris R: Physical fitness and blood pressure in school children. *Circulation* 1983;**67**:405.

Loggie JM et al: Juvenile hypertension. *J Pediatr* 1984;**104**:657.

McCrory WW: Blood pressure in healthy children. *Pediatrics* 1982;**70**:143.

Rocchini AP: Blood pressure in obese adolescents. *Pediatrics* 1988;**82**:16.

Steinfeld L et al: Sphygmomanometry in pediatric patients. *J Pediatr* 1978;**92**:934.

Task force on blood pressure control in children. *Pediatrics* 1987;**79**:1.

Weisman DN: Systolic or diastolic blood pressure. *Pediatrics* 1988;**82**:112.

ATHEROSCLEROSIS AS A PEDIATRIC PROBLEM

Awareness of the importance of coronary artery risk factors in general—and atherosclerosis in particular—has risen dramatically in the general population during the past 25 years. In adults, the incidence of death from ischemic heart disease has been decreasing over the last decade, presumably as a result of modifying the diet or life-style to avoid known risks for heart disease. During this same decade, a large number of serum samples from the pediatric population have been collected and analyzed for lipids, and epidemiologic studies have been performed to determine the relationship of lipid levels to coronary heart disease.

The level of serum lipids in childhood usually remains the same through adolescence. Biochemical abnormalities in the lipid profile appear early in childhood and correlate with higher risk for coronary artery disease in adulthood. High-density lipoprotein has been identified as an antiatherogenic agent through these studies.

The concept of pediatric screening for hyperlipidemia has been evaluated carefully. Currently, only children at high risk—ie, children with a family history of early myocardial infarction (prior to 50–55 years) in parents or grandparents or with known familial hyperlipidemia—are screened routinely. In addition, some researchers consider adolescents with total cholesterol levels of greater than 180 mg/dL or low-density lipoprotein levels of greater than 110 mg/dL to be at risk for coronary artery disease in adulthood.

In the majority of cases, treatment consists of dietary restrictions, exercise, abstinence from smoking, and avoidance of other ischemic heart disease risk factors. In patients with life-threatening familial hyperlipidemia, pharmacologic and surgical intervention (ileal bypass or portacaval shunt) may be considered.

Aristimuño GG et al: Influence of persistent obesity in children on cardiovascular risk factors: The Bogalusa heart study. *Circulation* 1984;**69**:895.

Jacobson MS, Lillienfeld DE: The pediatrician's role in atherosclerosis prevention. *J Pediatr* 1988;**112**:836.

Lauer RM et al: Relationship between childhood and adult cholesterol levels. *Pediatrics* 1988;**82**:309.

Lee J, Lauer RM, Clark WR: Lipoproteins in the progeny of young men with coronary artery disease: Children with increased risk. *Pediatrics* 1986;**78**:330.

Moll PP et al: Total cholesterol and lipoproteins in school children. *Circulation* 1983;**67**:127.

Uauy R: Lovastatin therapy in receptor-negative homozygous familial hypercholesterolemia. *J Pediatr* 1988;**113**:387.

MUCOCUTANEOUS LYMPH NODE SYNDROME

Mucocutaneous lymph node syndrome, also known as Kawasaki disease, was first described in Japan in 1967. The acute illness is characterized by (1) prolonged fever (over 5 days) that is unresponsive to antibiotics; (2) conjunctivitis; (3) cracking and fissuring of the lips, with inflammation of mucous membranes; (4) cervical lymphadenopathy; (5) rash involving the trunk and extremities, with reddened palms and soles of the hands and feet and subsequent desquamation of tips of the toes and fingers; and (6) edema. Patients may also have associated arthritis. Thrombocytosis and increased sedimentation rate are seen on laboratory examination.

Cardiovascular complications during the acute illness include myocarditis, pericarditis, and arteritis that predisposes to aneurysm formation in the coronary arteries in approximately 20% of patients. Aneurysm formation may occur 7–45 days after the onset of illness. Acute myocardial infarction may occur during the acute illness secondary to thrombosis of these aneurysms. Death occurs in 1–2% of patients during this phase of the illness. Long-term followup of patients with aneurysms shows some resolution of aneurysms in half of those affected; the remainder may continue to have aneurysms, may develop stenosis, and, possibly later, may develop myocardial ischemia.

During the acute illness and for 2–3 months after, patients should be monitored closely by serial electrocardiography, chest x-ray, and M mode and 2-dimensional echocardiography. Selective coronary angiography is recommended in those patients with coronary abnormalities detected by echocardiography.

The acute illness is now treated with high doses of intravenous gamma globulin (either 400 mg/kg daily for 4 d or 2 gm/kg once; both regimens appear equally efficacious), and high doses of aspirin, 20 mg/kg/dose given 4 times a day until day 14 of illness, then 3–5 mg/kg/d for 2–3 months from the onset of illness if echocardiogram is normal or indefinitely if coronary abnormalities are present. Evidence of myocardial ischemia or infarction warrants early cardiac catheterization and bypass surgery if obstruction exists.

Burns JC et al: Coagulopathy and platelet activation in Kawasaki syndrome: Identification of patients at high risk for development of coronary artery aneurysms. *J Pediatr* 1984;**105**:206.

Tatara K, Kasakawa S. Long term prognosis of giant coronary aneurysm in Kawasaki disease: an angiographic study. *J Pediatr* 1987;**111**:705.

Management of Kawasaki syndrome: a consensus statement prepared by North American participants of the third international Kawasaki disease symposium, Tokyo, Japan, December 1988. *Pediatr Infect Dis J* 1989;**8**:663.

Newberger JW et al: The treatment of Kawasaki syndrome with intravenous gamma globulin. *N Engl J Med* 1986; **315**:341.

DISORDERS OF RATE, RHYTHM, & ELECTROLYTE IMBALANCE

In normal cardiac conduction, depolarization occurs in the following sequence: sinoatrial node (depolarization cannot be seen on ECG), atria (P wave), atrioventricular node (PR segment), and bundles and ventricles (QRS). Repolarization (T wave) then occurs.

In evaluating cardiac dysrhythmia and abnormal findings on ECG, it is important to keep in mind the normal sequence of cardiac conduction as well as the normal intervals of conduction (PR, QRS, QT, etc) and the normal rates in children. A systematic approach to electrocardiography is essential.

SINUS DYSRHYTHMIA

It is normal to have phasic variation in heart rate (sinus dysrhythmia). Typically, dysrhythmia is associated with the respiratory cycle. Heart rate is accelerated on inspiration and decelerated on expiration. P–QRS–T intervals are normal.

SINUS BRADYCARDIA

Depending on the age of the patient, sinus bradycardia may be a normal finding, particularly when the patient is at rest or asleep. Sleeping infants and children commonly have sinus rates of 80/min or lower. In critically ill patients, common causes of bradycardia include hypoxia, use of medications, and central nervous system damage. Bradycardia is usually not a primary cardiac abnormality.

SINUS TACHYCARDIA

The heart rate normally accelerates in response to stress, eg, fever, hypovolemia, anemia, or congestive heart failure. Tachycardia with decreased cardiac output is more ominous and warrants evaluation for shock or tachyarrhythmia. Treatment may be indicated for correction of the underlying cause of tachycardia (transfusion for anemia, correction of hypovolemia or fever, etc).

PREMATURE ATRIAL CONTRACTIONS

Premature atrial contractions are triggered by an ectopic focus in the atrium. They are one of the most common premature beats seen in the pediatric population, particularly during the newborn period. They may be nonconducted (with associated QRS) (Fig 16–7A) or conducted (with premature P wave) (Fig 16–7B). There is usually some delay until the next normal sinus beat (compensatory pause). Depending on the ectopic focus of the premature contraction, the frontal plane vector of the P wave may be normal (+60 degrees) or abnormal. The PR interval may be short if the focus is close to the atrioventricular node.

As an isolated finding, premature atrial contractions are benign and require no treatment. They may occur more frequently in association with excessive caffeine ingestion. In patients with heart disease, premature atrial contractions are not treated unless

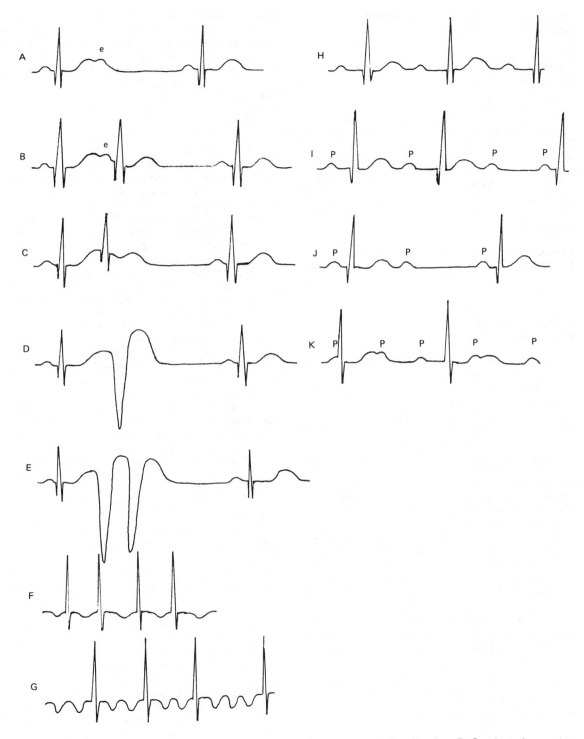

Figure 16–7. Dysrhythmias shown on ECG. **A:** Nonconducted premature atrial contraction. **B:** Conducted premature atrial conduction. **C:** Premature junctional contraction. **D:** Premature ventricular contraction. **E:** Premature ventricular contraction in couplet. **F:** Paroxysmal supraventricular tachycardia. **G:** Atrial flutter with variable conduction. **H:** First-degree atrioventricular heart block. **I:** Mobitz type I (Wenckebach type) second-degree atrioventricular heart block. **J:** Mobitz type II (2:1 type) second-degree atrioventricular heart block. **K:** Complete heart block. e = ectopic atrial premature beat; P = P wave.

they are associated with specific tachyarrhythmias or are frequent and cause decreased cardiac output.

PREMATURE JUNCTIONAL CONTRACTIONS

Premature junctional contractions occur high in the bundle of His and may or may not induce aberrant conduction (wide QRS configuration). Most often, they induce a narrow QRS complex (Fig 16–7C) with no preceding P wave and may have retrograde atrial depolarization (P wave seen on early portion of the T wave). When aberrantly conducted, premature junctional contractions cannot be distinguished from premature ventricular contractions except by invasive (electrophysiologic) study.

As an isolated finding, premature junctional contractions are usually benign and require no specific therapy. When associated with junctional tachycardia, they are one of the most difficult abnormalities to treat.

PREMATURE VENTRICULAR CONTRACTIONS

Premature ventricular contractions may originate in either ventricle and are characterized by a bizarre QRS of greater than 10 ms in duration, an abnormal T wave not preceded by a P wave (Fig 16–7D), and a compensatory pause (interval between 2 beats, including the premature contraction) equal to 2 normal cardiac cycles. Premature ventricular contractions originating from a single ectopic focus all have the same configuration; those of multifocal origin show varying configurations. The consecutive occurrence of more than one beat can result in coupling (Fig 16–7E) or ventricular tachycardia (3 or more consecutive ventricular beats).

Most unifocal premature ventricular contractions in otherwise normal patients are benign. The nature of contractions can be confirmed by having the patient exercise. As the heart rate increases, benign premature contractions disappear. If exercise results in an increase or coupling of contractions, there may be underlying disease. Multifocal premature ventricular contractions are always abnormal and are more dangerous. They may be associated with drug overdosages (cyclic antidepressant, digoxin toxicity, etc). When associated with organic heart disease, they must be thoroughly evaluated and treated if necessary. Phenytoin, propranolol, or quinidine is currently used for treatment.

PAROXYSMAL SUPRAVENTRICULAR TACHYCARDIA

Paroxysmal supraventricular tachycardia, the most common tachyarrhythmia of childhood, often pre-

sents in infancy. It is most often secondary to bypass tracts (accessory pathways between the atria and ventricles) whose conduction times differ from those of the atrioventricular node. With premature stimulation (preexcitation), these tracts can be activated and cause repetitive rapid stimulation of atria and ventricles (''circus phenomenon''). Only rarely is paroxysmal supraventricular tachycardia caused by ectopic foci.

Clinical Findings

A. Symptoms and Signs: Clinical presentation varies with the age of the patient. Infants tend to turn pale and mottled with onset of tachycardia and may become irritable. With long duration of tachycardia, symptoms of congestive heart failure develop. Heart rates can be from 240 to 300 beats per minute. Early diagnosis and prompt therapy are imperative in this group of patients. Older children may complain of dizziness, palpations, fatigue, and chest pain. Heart rates usually range from 240 in the younger child to 150–180 in the teenager. Congestive heart failure is less common in children than in infants. Tachycardia may be associated with either congenital heart defects such as Ebstein's anomaly or acquired conditions such as cardiomyopathies and myocarditis. Complete noninvasive cardiovascular evaluation is indicated in all patients with a first episode of paroxysmal supraventricular tachycardia.

B. Imaging: Findings on chest x-ray are normal during the early course of dysrhythmia. If congestive heart failure is present, the heart is enlarged and there is evidence of pulmonary venous congestion.

C. Electrocardiography: Electrocardiography (Fig 16–7F) is the most important tool in the diagnosis of this condition.

1. The heart rate is very rapid, ranging from 160 to 320/min.

2. The rhythm is extremely regular. There is no variation in the PR interval throughout the entire tracing.

3. P waves may or may not be present. If they are present, there is no variation in the appearance of the P wave or in the PR interval. P waves may be difficult to find because they are superimposed upon the preceding T wave. Furthermore, if the abnormal focus is located within the atrioventricular node, the P waves will not be seen.

4. The QRS complex is usually the same as during normal sinus rhythm. However, the QRS complex is occasionally widened, in which case the condition may be difficult to differentiate from ventricular tachycardia (supraventricular tachycardia with aberrant ventricular conduction). Presence of a delta wave or slurring of the initial portion of the QRS, with a short PR interval during or after paroxysmal supraventricular tachycardia, is indicative of preexcitation.

5. Termination of the tachycardia is characterized

by conversion to normal sinus rhythm. In contrast with atrial flutter, degrees of atrioventricular block do not develop.

Treatment

During initial episodes, all patients (particularly infants) require close monitoring of intravenous blood pressure. In severe failure, intra-atrial blood pressure should be monitored. Correction of acidosis or electrolyte abnormalities is also indicated.

A. Verapamil: Despite medicolegal concerns, the current drug of choice for acute conversion to normal sinus rhythm is verapamil, 0.1 mg/kg given intravenously as a slow push (1–2 minutes). Conversion usually occurs within 1–2 minutes. This dose may be repeated in 20 minutes. Transient hypotension may occur but usually does not require treatment.

B. Digitalis: Digitalis is still the drug of choice for long-term therapy (1–2 years). It can be used with or without verapamil, and conversion should be accomplished within 8–12 hours. Doses used are the same as those for congestive heart failure.

C. DC Cardioversion: DC cardioversion (1–2 J/kg) is also effective in more refractory cases of tachycardia and in critically ill infants. The procedure should be supervised by a cardiologist.

D. Other Drugs and Procedures: Other drugs such as propranolol, quinidine, or procainamide may be used when other measures fail.

The older child who has short episodes of tachycardia can learn Valsalva's maneuver to convert the dysrhythmia during reflex. Also very effective is placing a plastic bag full of ice cold water or crushed ice on the face. Ocular pressure or carotid massage is rarely of great benefit and is particularly dangerous in the infant.

Prognosis

Paroxysmal supraventricular tachycardia that presents during infancy has a low recurrence rate if the patient is treated with digitalis for 1–2 years. If it presents or recurs after infancy, long-term pharmacologic therapy is indicated. If pharmacologic intervention fails to control the tachycardia, surgical ablation should be considered.

ATRIAL FLUTTER & FIBRILLATION

Atrial flutter and fibrillation are quite rare in children and are most often associated with organic heart disease, particularly cardiomyopathies and myocarditis. Atrial flutter (Fig 16–7G) can present in infancy, and if 1:1 conduction of flutter occurs, it can mimic paroxysmal supraventricular tachycardia. Atrial rate is usually greater than 240 and is often 300. Ventricular rate depends on the degree of atrioventricular response and is usually slower. Atrial fibrillation is an irregular rhythm with variable rate.

DC cardioversion, followed by digitalization, is indicated for treatment of either of these entities. Either or both may require the addition of quinidine to the regimen for adequate control. Both forms of dysrhythmia are frequently difficult to control and should be managed under the supervision of a pediatric cardiologist.

VENTRICULAR TACHYCARDIA

Ventricular tachycardia, an uncommon dysrhythmia in children, is often associated with organic heart disease or myocardial tumor. It can be quite regular, although typically there is variation in the RR interval. All QRS complexes are widened and bizarre. The heart rate is usually 120–180 (less than that of paroxysmal supraventricular tachycardia). Intermittent runs of ventricular tachycardia frequently precede sustained tachycardia, which can develop into ventricular fibrillation.

The electrocardiographic pattern of ventricular tachycardia must be differentiated from that of hyperkalemia. Differentiation is accomplished by administering intravenous sodium bicarbonate or an intravenous flush of calcium chloride and continuously monitoring the ECG. If the QRS complexes narrow and T waves return to baseline, the diagnosis of hyperkalemia is suggested and can be confirmed by serum electrolyte evaluation.

Treatment for ventricular tachycardia is lidocaine, 1 mg/kg given as an intravenous bolus. If there is no response to lidocaine, DC cardioversion is indicated. Use of either of these modalities in patients with hyperkalemia can be fatal.

FIRST-DEGREE HEART BLOCK

First-degree heart block is an electrocardiographic diagnosis for prolongation of the PR interval (Fig 16–7H). The block does not in itself cause problems of heart function. However, it is commonly found in association with such congenital heart defects as ostium secundum type atrial septal defect and with such diseases as rheumatic carditis or viral myocarditis. The PR interval may also be prolonged as a result of digoxin therapy. This is a sign of digoxin effect, not toxicity.

SECOND-DEGREE HEART BLOCK

Mobitz type I (Wenckebach type) heart block is recognized by progressive prolongation of the PR interval until there is no QRS associated with a P wave (Fig 16–7I); then the cycle may repeat itself. In Mobitz type II (2:1 type) heart block, every other P wave has a dropped beat or nonconduction to the ventricles (Fig 16–7J).

Second-degree heart block of either type can occur

in the normal heart but is usually associated with organic heart disease or drug intoxication. Treatment is correction of the underlying problem.

COMPLETE HEART BLOCK

In complete heart block, the atria and ventricles beat independently. The atrial rate is usually more rapid than the ventricular rate (Fig 16–7K). Ventricular rates can range from 40 to 80 beats per minute, while atrial rates may be 1½–3 times that rate.

Congenital complete heart block, the most common form of complete heart block, has a very high association with maternal systemic lupus erythematosus (80% at our institution). Serologic screening should be performed in the mother of an infant with complete heart block, even if she has no symptoms of systemic lupus erythematosus. Congenital complete heart block is also associated with corrected transposition of the great vessels, endocardial cushion defect, and endocardial fibroelastosis.

Acquired complete heart block can be secondary to acute myocarditis, digoxin toxicity, and open heart surgery.

Clinical Findings

Prenatal bradycardia is frequently noted in infants with congenital complete heart block. In the past, this finding occasionally indicated the need for emergency delivery of the infant; however, since the advent of fetal monitoring and fetal echocardiography, this is infrequently necessary. An overall assessment of postnatal adaptation to the heart block is important. Adaptation is largely dependent on the heart rate; infants with heart rates less than 60 are at significantly greater risk for low cardiac output and congestive heart failure. Wide QRS complexes and a

rapid atrial rate are also poor prognostic signs. All patients have some heart murmur from increased stroke volume. In more symptomatic patients, the heart can be quite enlarged and pulmonary edema present. In older patients, Stokes-Adams syncope may be the presenting symptom, or heart block may be found on routine physical examination.

Full cardiac evaluation, including echocardiography, is indicated. Holter monitoring is used to assess the patient for evidence of ventricular ectopy and to document the slowest heart rate attained.

Treatment

In patients thought to be at risk for Stokes-Adams attacks or congestive heart failure, the treatment of choice is surgical insertion of a programmable permanent pacemaker. Until surgery is performed, patients can be temporarily assisted by intravenous drip of isoproterenol or by transvenous pacemaker. Permanent transvenous pacemakers are increasingly used in pediatric patients.

ELECTROLYTE IMBALANCE

Potassium, calcium, and, to a lesser extent, magnesium imbalances are reflected on ECG. The electrolyte disturbances of potassium are of greatest concern to the pediatrician, and some familiarity with abnormal tracings found in hyperkalemia and hypokalemia is essential. In hyperkalemia (Fig 16–8), there is gradual progression from tall peaked T waves (5–7 meq/L) through widening of the QRS complex (8–9 meq/L) to a broad, almost sine wave configuration (> 10 meq/L). Hypokalemia (Fig 16–9) is characterized by progressive prominence of the U wave and prolongation of the QT (really QU) interval with ST segment depression.

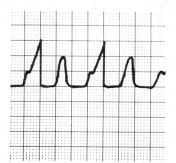 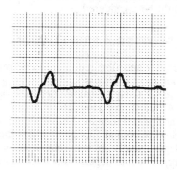

Figure 16–8. Hyperkalemia. **Left:** Serum K$^+$ of 8.5 meq/L. **Right:** Serum K$^+$ of 11 meq/L.

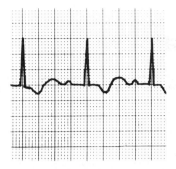 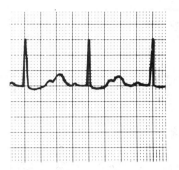

Figure 16–9. Hypokalemia. *Left:* Serum K$^+$ of 2.5 meq/L. *Right:* Serum K$^+$ of 3.5 meq/L.

SELECTED REFERENCES

Benson DW, Dunnigan A, Benditt DG: Follow-up evaluation of infant paroxysmal atrial tachycardia. *Circulation* 1987;**75:**542.

Campbell RM et al: Surgical treatment of pediatric cardiac arrhythmias. *J Pediatr* 1987;**110:**501.

Garson A: Medicolegal problems in the management of cardiac arrhythmias in children. *Pediatrics* 1987;**79:**84.

Garson A et al: Atrial flutter in the young: A collaborative study of 380 cases. *J Am Coll Cardiol* 1985;**6:**871.

Garson A et al: Incessant ventricular tachycardia in infants: Myocardial hamartomas and surgical cure. *J Am Coll Cardiol* 1987;**10:**619.

Liebman J, Plonsey R, Gillette PC: *Pediatric Electrocardiography.* William & Wilkins, 1982.

Wiggins JW et al: Echocardiographic diagnosis and intravenous digoxin management of fetal tachyarrhythmias and congestive heart failure. *Am J Dis Child* 1986; **140:**202.

17

Hematologic Disorders

John H. Githens, MD, & William E. Hathaway, MD

Knowledge of the normal ranges by age is essential in the diagnosis of hematologic disorders of infancy and childhood. The normal values for bone marrow and peripheral blood are shown in Tables 17–1 and 17–2. These values vary significantly with age.

The important changes shown in Table 17–2 include polycythemia in the neonatal period followed by physiologic anemia of infancy, which is maximal at 2½–3 months. Subsequently, there is a gradual rise of the hemoglobin, hematocrit, and red cell count through childhood. Adult levels are not reached until after puberty.

Screening for anemia by microhematocrit should be done at birth, 9 months, 18 months, 5 years, and 14 years of age. (See Chapter 7).

The red blood cells of the newborn are macrocytic (8–9 μm in diameter). There is a gradual change to microcytosis at 3 months, with return to normal diameter (7.4 μm) by 8 months.

The white blood count may normally remain higher than in the adult throughout infancy and childhood. The differential white count shows a predominance of lymphocytes, which may normally comprise as much as 80% of the white blood cells through the first 6 years of life.

Young PC et al: Evaluation of the capillary microhematocrit as a screening test for anemia in pediatric office practice. *Pediatrics* 1986;**78**:206.

I. ANEMIAS

Anemia is always a manifestation of disease or nutritional deficiency. The cause should be determined by appropriate clinical and laboratory investigations or, if necessary, by therapeutic trial with specific replacement therapy. "Shotgun" treatment with multiple drugs is never indicated.

The cell indices that are most useful are the MCHC (mean corpuscular hemoglobin concentration), the MCH (mean corpuscular hemoglobin), and the MCV (mean corpuscular volume). The normal values are shown in Table 17–2.

The primary cause of anemia in infancy is nutri-

Table 17–1. Normal values of cellular elements in bone marrow in older infants and children[1]

	Range (%)	Mean (%)
Myeloblasts	1–5	2
Myelocytes (including promyelocytes)	10–25	20
Nonsegmented polymorphonuclear cells (including metamyelocytes)	15–30	20
Segmented polymorphonuclear cells	5–30	25
Lymphocytes	5–25	13
Nucleated red cells (principally normoblasts)	15–30	20
Megakaryocytes	10–35/μL	
Total nucleated cell count	100,000–200,000/μL	

[1]From Smith CH: *Blood Diseases of Infancy and Childhood,* 2nd ed. Mosby, 1966.

tional iron deficiency. Anemias due to causes other than iron deficiency fall into 2 major groups: (1) those due to impaired red cell production, maturation, or release from the marrow; and (2) those due to acute blood loss or destruction (hemolysis). The studies needed to determine the exact cause are different for these 2 groups.

The essential test in differentiating anemias due to defective production from the hemolytic group is the reticulocyte count. This must be done prior to treatment with drugs or transfusion.

Diagnosis of Anemia

The following scheme for diagnosis of anemia is useful:

(1) Careful history: Duration of symptoms, diet, rate of growth, evidence of acute or chronic hemorrhage, jaundice, and a family history of anemia, jaundice, or gallbladder disease.

(2) Determination of hemoglobin, hematocrit, red blood cell count, MCH, MCV, MCHC, and examination of the smear. The blood smear often provides the clue for the final workup.

(a) If the MCV and MCH are low (microcytosis and hypochromia), evaluate first for iron deficiency—serum ferritin or serum iron and iron-binding capacity. Free erythrocyte protoporphyrin is slightly increased. In children over 3 years of age, stool examination for blood is indicated.

Table 17–2. Normal peripheral blood values at various ages.[1]

	1st Day	2nd Day	6th Day	2 weeks	1 Month	2 Months	3 Months	6 Months	1 Year	2 Years	5 Years	8–12 Years	Adults Males	Adults Females
Red Blood Cells (millions/µL)	5.9 (4.1–7.5)	6 (4.0–7.3)	5.4 (3.9–6.8)	5 (4.5–5.5)	4.7 (4.2–5.2)	4.1 (3.6–4.6)	4 (3.5–4.5)	4.5 (4–5)	4.6 (4.1–5.1)	4.7 (4.2–5.2)	4.7 (4.2–5.2)	5 (4.5–5.4)	5.4 (4.6–6.2)	4.8 (4.2–5.4)
Hemoglobin (g/dL)	19 (14–24)	19 (15–23)	18 (13–23)	16.5 (15–20)	14 (11–17)	12 (11–14)	11 (10–13)	11.5 (10.5–14.5)	12 (11–15)	13 (12–15)	13.5 (12.5–15)	14 (13–15.5)	16 (13–18)	14 (11–16)
White blood cells (per µL)	17,000 (8–38)		13,500 (6–17)	12,000 (5–16)	11,500 (5–15)	11,000 (5–15)	10,500 (5–15)	10,500 (5–15)	10,000 (5–15)	9,500 (5–14)	8,000 (5–13)	8,000 (5–12)	7,000 (5–10)	7,000 (5–10)
PMNs[2] (%)	57	55	50	34	34	33	33	36	39	42	55	60	57–68	57–68
Eosinophils (total) (per µL)	20–1000				150–1150		70–550	70–550					100–400	
Lymphocytes[2] (%)	20	20	37	55	56	56	57	55	53	49	36	31	25–33	25–33
Monocytes[2] (%)	10	15	9	8	7	7	7	6	6	7	7	7	3–7	3–7
Immature white cells (%)	10	5	0–1	0	0	0	0	0	0	0	0	0	0	0
Platelets[2] (per µL)	350,000		325,000	300,000			260,000			260,000		260,000	260,000	
Nucleated red cells/100 white cells[3]	0–10		0–0.3	0	0	0	0	0	0	0	0	0	0	
Reticulocytes (%)	3 (2–8)	3 (2–10)	1 (0.5–5)	0.4 (0–2)	0.2 (0–0.5)	0.5 (0.2–2)	2 (0.5–4)	0.8 (0.2–1.5)	1 (0.4–1.8)	1 (0.4–1.8)	1 (0.4–1.8)	1 (0.4–1.8)	1 (0.5–2)	1 (0.5–2)
Mean diameter of red cells (µm)	8.6				8.1		5–7		7.4		7.4		7.5	
MCV[4] (fL)	85–125		89–101	94–102	90		80	78	78	80	80	82	82–92	
MCHC[4] (%)	36		35	34				33		32	34	34	34	
MCH[4] (pg)	35–40		36	31	30		27	26	25	26	27	28	27–31	
Hematocrit (%)	54 ± 10		51	50	40		35	35	36	37	38	40	40–54	37–47

[1]Modified and reproduced, with permission, from Silver HK et al: *Handbook of Pediatrics*, 15th ed. Lange, 1986.
[2]Usual or average values; considerable individual variation may occur.
[3]Total nucleated red cells: first day, < 1000/µL.
[4]MCV = mean corpuscular volume. MCHC = mean corpuscular hemoglobin concentration. MCH = mean corpuscular hemoglobin.

(b) If normochromia (or hyperchromia) is shown, the reticulocyte count is essential. If the reticulocyte count is low (due to defect in marrow production or release), examine bone marrow; if high (due to hemolytic disease or acute hemorrhage), perform blood smear and Coombs test. If the Coombs is negative, perform red cell saline fragility test, autohemolysis test, hemoglobin electrophoresis, fetal hemoglobin determination, and Heinz body preparation. If spherocytosis or a hemoglobinopathy has not been identified, red cell enzyme studies are indicated.

ANEMIAS DUE TO DEFICIENT PRODUCTION

PHYSIOLOGIC "ANEMIA" OF THE NEWBORN & ANEMIA OF PREMATURITY

Essentials of Diagnosis

- Age 2–3 months.
- Normochromia; microcytosis.

General Considerations

Physiologic "anemia" occurs in all full-term infants and reaches its low point (hemoglobin about 10–11 g/dL) at about age 2½ months. The exact mechanism is not known, although it is recognized that both erythropoietin release and bone marrow production cannot keep pace with somatic growth. The anemia may be more severe in premature infants, in whom the hemoglobin may drop to levels of 6–7 g/dL.

Clinical Findings

A. Symptoms and Signs: Slight pallor may be noted in full-term infants, but usually no other symptoms occur. If the anemia is severe in the premature infant, decreased activity and fatigue with feeding may occur.

B. Laboratory Findings:

1. Blood—Anemia is normocytic (MCV 80 fL); reticuloycte count is low (0.5%) but may rise to 3–4% at 2–3 months of age.

2. Bone marrow—The marrow appears relatively normal but shows slight erythroid hypoplasia; morphologic changes are not indicative of decreased production.

Differential Diagnosis

Iron deficiency anemia usually does not manifest itself until after the age of 2–3 months. Congenital hemolytic anemias that are associated with red cell membrane or red cell metabolic abnormalities (such as hereditary spherocytosis, pyruvate kinase deficiency, etc) are present from birth and should be considered. Congenital pure red cell hypoplastic anemia presents within the first few months of life; an extremely low reticulocyte count should suggest this diagnosis. Hemolysis associated with sepsis or following erythroblastosis fetalis should be considered. Chronic infection may increase the degree of anemia.

Treatment

The only effective treatment is blood transfusion, which should be given in the form of packed red cells in doses of 5–10 mL/kg if the hemoglobin drops below 9 g/dL. The anemia will not respond at this age to iron or folic acid or other hematinics.

Prognosis

Spontaneous recovery is apparent by about 12–14 weeks of age in all infants. Anemia that persists beyond 3 months usually has another cause.

Dallman PR: Anemia of prematurity. *Annu Rev Med* 1981; **32:**143.

Holland BM et al: Lessons from the anemia of prematurity. *Hematol Oncol Clin North Am* 1987;**1:**355.

Joshi A et al: Blood transfusion effect on the respiratory pattern of preterm infants. *Pediatrics* 1987;**80:**79.

Stockman JA III, Garcia JF, Oski FA: The anemia of prematurity: Factors governing the erythropoietin response. *N Engl J Med* 1977;**296:**647.

NUTRITIONAL ANEMIAS

Anemia is the most common manifestation of nutritional deficiency in children in the USA; it is even more frequent in other parts of the world. In the USA, iron deficiency is responsible for the majority of these nutritional anemias. Folic acid and vitamin B_{12} deficiencies are seen principally in economically underprivileged children. The need for exogenous iron is greatly increased during the first 2 years of life and again in adolescence because of the rapid growth of the child.

1. IRON DEFICIENCY ANEMIA

Essentials of Diagnosis

- Pallor, fatigue.
- Good weight gain, poor muscle tone.
- Delayed motor development.
- Poor dietary intake of iron.
- Age 6 months to 2 years.
- Hypochromic microcytic anemia.

General Considerations

The average diet contains 12–15 mg of iron (of which approximately 10% is absorbed), and the normal daily excretion of iron is less than 1 mg/d.

Iron deficiency on a nutritional basis generally occurs between 6 months and 2 years of age and is an extremely rare cause of anemia after age 3 except in adolescence. Because infants rarely outgrow their iron stores prior to the age of 4 months, iron deficiency is almost never a cause of anemia in the first 3 months of life except with severe iron deficiency in the mother or following blood loss by hemorrhage in the infant. It has been demonstrated that iron deficiency is associated with abnormalities of the intestinal mucosa that allow for loss of serum proteins as well as chronic intestinal hemorrhage. In some cases, occult gastrointestinal blood loss may be a major factor. Thus, the exudative enteropathy that may occur secondary to dietary iron deficiency further aggravates the iron depletion in the body. Other primary conditions (eg, cow's milk intolerance) may cause exudative enteropathy and initiate the iron loss.

Iron deficiency is also seen in association with chronic hemorrhage or rapid growth. Infestation with hookworm or *Trichuris trichiura* should be considered as primary cause of chronic gastrointestinal blood loss in endemic areas.

The diagnosis depends largely on a history of a diet low in iron-containing solid foods with a high intake of milk (> 1 quart/d) and evidence of early rapid weight gain during the first 1–2 years of life. Hypochromia with microcytosis, decreased serum ferritin, and decreased serum iron with increased iron-binding capacity are characteristic.

Clinical Findings

A. Symptoms and Signs: Pallor, fatigue, irritability, and delayed motor development are common. The child is often fat and flabby, with poor muscle tone. Beeturia (red urine from the pigment of beets) occurs more frequently in iron-deficient children and may be a clue to the anemia. Nonhematologic manifestations of iron deficiency are caused in part by deficiencies in the cytochrome system. Irritability and decreased intellectual performance and perception have been demonstrated. Other symptoms include anorexia, koilonychia, atrophy of the tongue papillae, gastric achlorhydria, and the alterations in small bowel mucosa noted above. Pica is common in all age groups.

B. Laboratory Findings: The hemoglobin is depressed and may be as low as 3–4 g/dL. The red cell count and hematocrit are proportionately higher, producing a significantly lowered MCHC (< 30%). The red cells on smear are microcytic and hypochromic, with a low MCV and low MCH for age. The reticulocyte count is usually normal, but it may be elevated in severe cases.

Serum iron or ferritin need not be determined in early childhood if the dietary and growth history readily explain the cause of the microcytic hypochromic anemia. If there is doubt regarding the diagnosis

or the cause or if exudative enteropathy is suspected, these studies should be performed. Serum iron is low—usually below 30 μg/dL (normal, 90–150 μg/dL). Total iron-binding capacity is usually elevated to 350–500 μg/dL (normal, 250–350 μg/dL). Iron saturation is under 20% (normal, 30%), and serum ferritin is decreased to less than 10 ng/mL. Free erythrocyte protoporphyrin (FEP) is elevated. An FEP/hemoglobin ratio greater than 2.8 μg/g of hemoglobin usually indicates iron deficiency or lead poisoning. Values greater than 17.5 μg/g of hemoglobin, however, are usually caused by lead intoxication. A hematocrit less than 33% or hemoglobin less than 11 g/dL may be effective screening for iron deficiency during the first 2 years of life. If a trial of iron therapy results in a hemoglobin rise of at least 1 g/dL, mild iron deficiency is confirmed.

Bone marrow examination is usually not useful in infants for the diagnosis of iron deficiency. Even normal children under 2 years of age deposit little or no iron in the form of hemosiderin in the marrow.

The diagnosis is best confirmed by administration of an adequate dose of iron and the demonstration of a reticulocyte rise in 3–5 days and a hemoglobin rise in 7–14 days.

Differential Diagnosis With Iron-Resistant Microcytic Anemias

Iron deficiency anemia must be differentiated from several other hypochromic microcytic anemias caused by defective incorporation of iron into the hemoglobin molecule. These disorders include thalassemia minor, lead poisoning, the anemia of chronic diseases (infectious, inflammatory, or malignant), and the rare hereditary sideroblastic anemias. The laboratory differential diagnosis is summarized in Table 17–3. Homozygous hemoglobin E disease is also characterized by microcytic red cells (see hemoglobinopathy section).

Complications

Children with iron deficiency anemia are more susceptible than others to infection. In severe cases, heart failure may occur. Motor development is often delayed, and cognitive function may be impaired, resulting in diminished achievement. Anorexia and irritability cause additional feeding problems and further malnutrition. Severe iron deficiency interferes with the normal integrity of the gastrointestinal tract; exudative enteropathy associated with protein and additional iron loss may occur.

Prevention

Iron deficiency can be prevented in full-term infants by using iron-fortified infant formulas for 12 months or by the addition of iron-containing solid foods by 4 months of age. Breast-fed infants absorb up to 50% of the iron in the milk, but supplemental iron-fortified solid foods (such as infant cereals) are

Table 17–3. Iron-resistant microcytic, hypochromic anemias: differential with iron deficiency anemia.

	Iron Deficiency	Thalassemic Minor		Lead Poisoning	Chronic Disease	Hereditary Sideroblastic Anemias
		Beta	Alpha			
Hemoglobin range (g/dL)	3–10	9–11	10–12	7–10	8–11	5–10
Serum ferritin	Low	Increased	Increased	Low to increased	Normal to increased	Increased
Serum iron	Low	Increased	Increased	Low to increased	Low	Increased
TIBC[1]	Increased	Normal	Normal	Low to increased	Low	Normal
FEP[2]	Moderately increased	Normal	Normal	Very high	Increased	Increased
Hemoglobin A_2	Low to normal	Increased	Normal	Normal	Normal	Normal
Other features	Smear: microcytic, hypochromic	Smear: targets, stippling	Smear: microcytosis only	Smear: stippling	Smear: normal or microcytic	Marrow: sideroblasts
Treatment	Iron	None	None	Chelate lead	Treatment of disease	Pyridoxine (Vitamin B_6 100 mg)[3]

[1]TIBC = total iron-binding capacity.
[2]FEP = free erythrocyte protoporphyrin.
[3]Hereditary sideroblastic anemias may be pyridoxine-responsive or refractory.

also recommended. Small preterm infants should receive iron-fortified formulas or supplemental iron medication by 2 months of age in a large prophylactic dose (2–4 mg/kg/d) of elemental iron.

Treatment

A. Oral Iron: The recommended oral dose of elemental iron is 1.5–2 mg/kg 3 times daily between meals (4.5–6 mg/kg/d). Although absorption is better if the medication is given between meals, it may cause gastrointestinal irritation; iron can be administered with food or even in milk. Various iron complexes and concentrates are available, but there is little evidence that any one is preferable to the others. Ferrous sulfate remains the drug of choice. Patients should be observed for a reticulocyte rise in 3–5 days and for a hemoglobin increase in 1–2 weeks. Replenish iron stores by continuing therapy for 2 months after the hemoglobin has reached a normal level.

B. Intramuscular Iron: Iron dextran (Imferon) may be given intramuscularly if oral intolerance or malabsorption is present or if parental supervision is inadequate. The total dose can be calculated from the following formula:

$$mg\ Iron = \frac{Desired\ hemoglobin - Initial\ hemoglobin}{100} \times 80 \times Weight\ in\ kg \times 3.4$$

An additional 30% should be given to replace deficient iron stores. Daily doses should be limited to 1 mL (50 mg) in infants and 2 mL (100 mg) in very young children. When administering iron dextran, pull the skin to one side before injecting; this technique will prevent leakage to the skin. The response of the reticulocyte count and the hemoglobin to the intramuscular product is no more rapid than to oral administration of an adequate dose of ferrous sulfate.

C. Ascorbic Acid: Large doses of ascorbic acid increase absorption of iron from food but probably do not affect the efficacy of iron medication.

D. Blood Transfusions: Transfusion therapy is reserved for children with extremely low levels of hemoglobin who are bordering on congestive failure or who have serious acute infections. Packed red cells should be used and administered slowly in a dose not to exceed 10 mL/kg. In the severely ill child with impending or frank congestive failure, a partial exchange transfusion (isovolumetric) with packed red cells should be given.

E. Diet: Ultimate management of iron deficiency anemia requires improvement in the diet, with reduction of milk intake, use of iron-fortified formulas, and an increase in iron-containing foods such as meat, eggs, fortified infant cereals, and green vegetables.

Prognosis

Iron therapy will produce rapid and complete recovery within 2–4 weeks if the anemia is due to nutritional inadequacy. If the anemia persists, other causes must be found and treated.

Committee on Nutrition, American Academy of Pediatrics: Iron supplementation for infants. *Pediatrics* 1976; **58:**765.

Dallman PR et al: Diagnosis of iron deficiency: The limitations of laboratory tests in predicting response to iron treatment in 1-year-old infants. *J Pediatr* 1981;**99:**376.

Lozoff B, Brittenham GM: Behavioral alterations in iron deficiency. *Hematol Oncol Clin North Am* 1987;**1:**499.

Oski FA, Stockman JA III: Anemia due to inadequate iron sources or poor iron utilization. *Pediatr Clin North Am* 1980;**27:**237.

Siimes MA, Jävenpää AL: Prevention of anemia and iron deficiency in very low birth weight infants. *J Pediatr* 1982;**101**:277.

Yip R et al: Declining prevalence of anemia in a middle-class setting: A pediatric success story? *Pediatrics* 1987; **80**:330.

2. MEGALOBLASTIC ANEMIAS

Essentials of Diagnosis

- Pallor, fatigue.
- Macrocytic anemia.
- Megaloblastic marrow.

Megaloblastic anemias are characterized by oval macrocytes and hypersegmented polymorphonuclear neutrophils in the peripheral blood and megaloblasts in the bone marrow. They are due primarily to a deficiency of folic acid or vitamin B_{12} or a combination of both. These 2 substances function as coenzymes in the synthesis of nuclear protein.

Folic acid must be converted to folinic acid with the assistance of ascorbic acid. The gastric intrinsic factor is necessary for the absorption of vitamin B_{12}. Megaloblastic anemias develop in the absence of gastric intrinsic factor or as a result of dietary deficiencies of folic acid or, rarely, vitamin B_{12}, or they may appear in the presence of ascorbic acid deficiency if the folic acid intake is low.

Folic Acid Deficiency

Dietary deficiency of folic acid occurs most frequently in infancy. It appears in an acute form within the first few months of life and is almost always due to the combination of low folic acid intake and ascorbic acid deficiency. Whole cow's milk and human breast milk provide adequate folic acid. However, certain powdered milk products, unless supplemented, contain inadequate folate. Goat's milk is deficient in both folate and vitamin B_{12}, and its use is a major cause of nutritional megaloblastic anemia in infancy. Preterm infants and those with prolonged diarrhea are more likely to become deficient.

Folic acid-deficient megaloblastic anemia also occurs in older children with severe nutritional deficiency or with serious absorption problems such as celiac disease, intestinal bypass, or blind loops of the bowel.

Megaloblastic anemia may also result from infestation with the fish tapeworm (*Diphyllobothrium latum*). The administration of certain anticonvulsant drugs (phenytoin, primidone, phenobarbital) and the use of isoniazid with cycloserine, phenylbutazone, nitrofurantoin, and methotrexate have been reported to cause megaloblastic anemia.

Folate deficiency also occurs secondary to increased utilization of folate in chronic hemolytic anemias such as sickle cell disease.

The characteristic findings are weakness, pallor, and anorexia in infancy. Glossitis and a beefy red tongue are occasionally noted, but the neurologic manifestations of pernicious anemia are not seen. The anemia is frequently severe, with hemoglobin levels below 4 g/dL. The red cell count is low and may be under 1 million/μL in severe cases. The blood smear shows macrocytes and significant anisocytosis and poikilocytosis. The red cells are usually normochromic but may be hypochromic if iron deficiency is also present. Leukopenia with neutropenia is usually present. Polymorphonuclear neutrophils are enlarged and hypersegmented. The platelets are usually moderately reduced. The reticulocyte count is low. Formiminoglutamic acid (FIGLU) is present in the urine in folic acid deficiency after histidine loading. The Schilling test will differentiate folic acid deficiency from defective vitamin B_{12} absorption. Erythrocyte transketolase activity is normal in folate deficiency but elevated in vitamin B_{12} deficiency.

The marrow examination is diagnostic. The smear is characterized by delayed maturation and the presence of the typical megaloblastic forms of the nucleated red cells. Giant metamyelocytes may be seen, and megakaryocyte nuclei may be hypersegmented.

Megaloblastic anemia due to folic acid deficiency responds rapidly to oral or parenteral administration of folic acid in a daily dosage of 5 mg. Two to 3 weeks of treatment are usually sufficient. A significant rise in the reticulocyte count will occur within a few days after therapy is started. Ascorbic acid in a dosage of about 200 mg/d orally should be given at the same time. In generalized malnutrition, vitamin B_{12} should also be given. Dietary changes should be instituted to prevent the recurrence of megaloblastic anemia.

Complete and permanent recovery will follow the administration of folic acid and ascorbic acid. Relapses occur only with dietary deficiencies.

Administration of folic acid in a dose of 25–50 μg/d is recommended for preterm infants under 1700 g during the first 3 months of life, because their absorption of folate is poor.

Chanarin I: Management of megaloblastic anaemia in the very young. *Br J Haematol* 1983;**53**:1.

Dallman PR: Iron, vitamin E, and folate in the preterm infant. *J Pediatr* 1974;**85**:742.

Congenital Megaloblastic Anemias

A few cases of megaloblastic anemia have been reported in infancy in association with a congenital metabolic block in nucleic acid formation. Large quantities of orotic acid appear in the urine because of the inborn error in pyrimidine metabolism. Patients respond well to treatment with uridine but are unresponsive to folic acid or vitamin B_{12}. Therapy must usually be continued throughout life. Other infants with associated homocystinuria have responded to vitamin B_{12}.

Hallam LJ et al: Vitamin B_{12}-responsive neonatal megaloblastic anemia and homocystinuria. *Blood* 1987;**69**:1128.

Smith LH Jr: Pyrimidine metabolism in man. *N Engl J Med* 1973;**288**:764.

Vitamin B_{12} Deficiency & Juvenile Pernicious Anemia Syndromes

Vitamin B_{12} deficiency in childhood is usually due to dietary lack or malabsorption. Because the primary source of vitamin B_{12} is meat, a deficiency can occur in families on a pure vegetarian diet and has been described in breast-fed infants of vegan mothers. Vitamin B_{12} malabsorption may occur in the presence of adequate intrinsic factor, with acquired intestinal lesions, with generalized intestinal malabsorption, and in a familial disease of infants characterized by selective malabsorption of B_{12}.

The pernicious anemia syndromes of childhood are all caused by impaired absorption of vitamin B_{12}. Although pernicious anemia is rare in childhood, a number of different forms have been described. A congenital deficiency of intrinsic factor has been observed, with onset of symptoms in early infancy. Several forms of intrinsic factor defect have been differentiated with onset in the second decade—one type without antibodies, one type with antibodies to parietal cells and intrinsic factor (similar to the disease in adults), and pernicious anemia associated with various endocrinopathies.

The clinical picture is very similar to that in the adult, with anemia resulting in pallor, fatigue, and the development of anorexia and diarrhea. The presence of a beefy red, smooth, sore tongue and the development of neurologic manifestations differentiate this anemia from the other megaloblastic anemias of childhood. The central nervous system involvement includes ataxia, paresthesias of the hands and feet, impaired vibratory perception, a positive Babinski sign, and the absence of tendon reflexes.

Typical laboratory findings include a macrocytic anemia with anisocytosis and poikilocytosis. Neutropenia and thrombocytopenia are common, and the polymorphonuclear neutrophils are hypersegmented. Reticulocytes are within the normal range. The bone marrow is hyperplastic and shows characteristic megaloblastic abnormalities with a delay in maturation. Giant metamyelocytes and hypersegmented megakaryocytes are found.

The serum vitamin B_{12} concentration is usually less than 100 pg/mL (normal, 300–400 pg/mL).

Treatment consists of the administration of vitamin B_{12} (cyanocobalamin) by parenteral injection. In children, a dosage of 15–30 μg intramuscularly given 3–5 times per week for 2–4 weeks (or until blood values return to normal) is usually adequate. In large children or adolescents, the dose may be increased to 100 μg given at the same intervals. A maintenance dose of 100 μg should be administered by injection each month. This therapy usually produces an excellent remission, although it must be continued throughout life. Oral administration of vitamin B_{12}, liver injections, and folic acid therapy are not recommended. Treatment with folic acid alone will allow the neurologic manifestations to progress even though the anemia may be controlled.

Chanarin I: Management of megaloblastic anaemia in the very young. *Br J Haematol* 1983;**53**:1.

Higginbottom MC, Sweetman L, Nyhan WL: A syndrome of methylmalonic aciduria, homocystinuria, megaloblastic anemia, and neurologic abnormalities in a vitamin B_{12}-deficient breast-fed infant of a strict vegetarian. *N Engl J Med* 1978;**299**:317.

Russo CL, Hyman PE, Oseas RS: Megaloblastic anemia characterized by microcytosis: Imerslund-Graesbeck syndrome with coexistent α-thalassemia. *Pediatrics* 1988;**81**:875.

APLASTIC & HYPOPLASTIC ANEMIAS

Congenital Hypoplastic Anemia (Congenital Aregenerative Anemia, Congenital Pure Red Cell Anemia, Primary Erythroid Hypoplasia, Diamond-Blackfan-Syndrome)

Essentials of Diagnosis

- Pallor, weakness, fatigue.
- Onset in first few months of life.
- Normochromic, macrocytic anemia.
- Very low reticulocyte count (often zero).
- Normal white blood cells and platelets.

General Considerations

Congenital pure red cell anemia (Diamond-Blackfan Syndrome) usually manifests itself in the first 4 months of life—often immediately after birth—and should be suspected in an infant with severe normochromic anemia and a very low reticulocyte count in the presence of normal circulating white cells and platelets. The diagnosis is made by bone marrow examination; failure of erythropoiesis without equivalent depression of the white cells or platelets is characteristic. The disorder appears to be caused by a block in the maturation of the erythroid series at the stem cell or earliest erythroblast stage. However, recent studies suggest a possible autoimmune T cell mechanism. Thymoma is not present in the congenital childhood form. Although this is sometimes observed in adults with acquired pure red cell anemia, this form is very rare in childhood.

Clinical Findings

A. Symptoms and Signs: Pallor, fatigue, and

weakness becoming progressively more severe from early infancy are produced by the anemia. Short stature and growth retardation are characteristic (in untreated cases). Occasionally, there are other associated anomalies, particularly of the kidneys.

B. Laboratory Findings:

1. Blood—The anemia is normochromic but macrocytic, with an MCV greater than 90 fL. The hemoglobin is often less than 5 g/dL. The reticulocyte count is characteristically very low and may be zero. The platelet count, white count, and differential count are normal.

2. Bone marrow—The bone marrow is characterized by a striking absence of nucleated red cell precursors without any depression of the granulocytic series or the megakaryocytes. Occasionally, very immature cells of the erythroid series may also be seen.

3. Other tests—Levels of erythropoietin are markedly elevated, and abnormalities of tryptophan metabolites have been described in the urine following a tryptophan loading test.

The erythrocytes have the characteristics of fetal red cells, with increased hemoglobin F, increased i antigen, and elevated levels of glycolytic enzymes. Activity of erythrocyte adenosine deaminase is increased.

Differential Diagnosis

Other conditions occurring in the neonatal period with depressed erythropoiesis in the presence of normal granulocytes and platelets include the anemia of prematurity and the anemia that often follows severe erythroblastosis fetalis. In both of these situations, reticulocytes should be present, and the past history is suggestive.

Congenital pure red cell anemia may occasionally be confused with hemolytic anemia in the first few months of life, when physiologic processes inhibit the normal reticulocyte response to hemolysis.

A variant of pure red cell anemia has been described in infants with triphalangeal thumbs and neutropenia.

Transient erythroblastopenia of infancy may closely mimic congenital hypoplastic anemia. It can be differentiated by a later age of onset, normal MCV (< 80 fL), normal adenosine deaminase activity, and spontaneous recovery.

Complications

The principal complications are associated with therapy. Repeated blood transfusions have resulted in widespread hemosiderosis, at times progressing to hemochromatosis. Therapy with corticosteroids has resulted in marked impairment of physical growth and in osteoporosis.

Treatment

A. Corticosteroids: In many cases, the anemia responds dramatically to therapy with corticosteroids, particularly if therapy is begun before age 3. Oral prednisone is the most frequently used drug, in an initial dose of 2 mg/kg/d. It should be given in divided doses. A significant response of the anemia will usually be seen within 3–4 weeks. Following this initial therapy, the dosage should be reduced to determine the minimal level with which a remission can be obtained. Alternate-day therapy is often possible and may cause less interference with growth.

Other drugs such as testosterone and cobalt have no effect in this condition. Intensive immunosuppressive therapy has been effective in a few resistant cases.

B. Blood Transfusions: Transfusions must be given in the presence of severe anemia and as a chronic supportive measure in the child who does not respond to corticosteroid therapy. Packed cells should be administered every 3–4 weeks to keep the hemoglobin above 11 g/dL.

C. Splenectomy: Splenectomy is occasionally of value but is never curative. Its effect is probably greatest in the child who has developed splenomegaly and has an extracorpuscular hemolytic component that is presumably in the spleen. This condition is confirmed by tagging normal donor red cells with radioactive chromium (^{51}Cr) and noting their shortened survival.

D. Iron Chelation Therapy: Deferoxamine has been used as a chelating agent in patients who require chronic transfusions. Administration by subcutaneous drip over 12 hours has been shown to be most effective. Ascorbic acid aids in mobilizing the iron stores for chelation. (See section on thalassemia.)

E. Bone Marrow Transplantation: This form of therapy has been attempted and may hold promise for the future.

Prognosis

Many children have been maintained in remission throughout childhood with corticosteroid therapy. Markedly impaired growth appears to be the primary complication of this treatment. Repeated packed red cell transfusions in refractory cases prolong life but cause severe iron overload hemosiderosis unless compliance with iron chelation therapy is good. (See section on thalassemia for details.)

Occasionally, children have spontaneous remission during later childhood or at adolescence. The milder cases that show a few red cell precursors in the bone marrow are more apt to have remissions.

Alter BP: Childhood red cell aplasia. *Am J Pediatr Hematol Oncol* 1980;**2**:131.

Ambruso DR et al: Effect of subcutaneous deferoxamine and oral vitamin C on iron excretion in congenital hypoplastic anemia and refractory anemia associated with the 5q-syndrome. *Am J Pediatr Hematol Oncol* 1982; **4**:115.

Chan HS, Saunders EF, Freedman MH: Diamond-

Blackfan syndrome. 1. Erythropoiesis in prednisone responsive and resistant disease. *Pediatr Res* 1982; **16**:474.

Glader BE: Diagnosis and management of red cell aplasia in children. *Hematol Oncol Clin North Am* 1987;**1**:431.

Taniguchi S et al: Demonstration of three distinct immunological disorders on erythropoiesis in a patient with pure red cell aplasia and autoimmune hemolytic anemia associated with thymoma. *Br J Haematol* 1988;**68**:473.

TRANSIENT ERYTHROBLASTOPENIA OF INFANCY

This disorder is characterized by anemia, reticulocytopenia, and absence of erythroid precursors in an otherwise normal marrow. It appears acutely in infants and children, often preceded by an infection. Recovery usually occurs spontaneously within 1–2 weeks. It is differentiated from congenital hypoplastic anemia by the normal size of the red cells (MCV < 80 fL), normal hemoglobin F, and no increase in the i antigen. There is evidence in some cases to suggest an IgG-mediated autoimmune basis, and other cases may be due to viral suppression of erythroblastosis.

Glader BE: Diagnosis and management of red cell aplasia in children. *Hematol Oncol Clin North Am* 1987;**1**:431.

Labotka RJ, Maurer HS, Honig GR: Transient erythroblastopenia of childhood: Review of 17 cases, including a pair of identical twins. *Am J Dis Child* 1981;**135**:937.

Wang WC, Mentzer WC: Differentiation of transient erythroblastopenia of childhood from congenital hypoplastic anemia. *J Pediatr* 1976;**88**:784.

APLASTIC ANEMIA

Essentials of Diagnosis

- Weakness and pallor.
- Purpuras, petechiae, and bleeding.
- Frequent infections.
- Pancytopenia with empty bone marrow.

General Considerations

Aplastic anemia is characterized by a severe pancytopenia with an acellular marrow and normal-sized spleen.

In childhood, aplastic anemia may be of 3 general types.

A. Fanconi's Congenital Pancytopenia: See below.

B. Idiopathic Aplastic Anemia: In at least half of cases in childhood, no etiologic agent or specific congenital cause can be found. Recent studies suggest a T cell autoimmune mechanism in the other 50%.

C. Secondary (Acquired) Aplastic Anemia: Aplastic anemia may occur as a toxic reaction to various chemicals and drugs. Chloramphenicol previously accounted for the majority of cases in childhood. Other antibiotics, sulfonamides, benzene, acetone, toluene, phenylbutazone, mephenytoin, certain insecticides such as DDT, and heavy metals have all been incriminated. Glue sniffing has produced aplastic anemia and has also initiated aplastic crises in patients with sickle cell anemia. Large amounts of radiation and high doses of cytotoxic drugs such as mechlorethamine and the folic acid antagonists will also produce severe aplasia. Aplastic anemia has been observed as a complication of severe infectious hepatitis and may be caused by other viruses also.

Clinical Findings in Idiopathic & Secondary Types

A. Symptoms and Signs: Weakness, fatigue, and pallor are the result of the anemia; purpura and bleeding occur because of the thrombocytopenia; and severe generalized or localized infections are frequently due to neutropenia.

B. Laboratory Findings: Severe normochromic anemia is usually present, with some microcytosis. The reticulocyte count is usually very low, but in early cases with partial marrow destruction, it may be slightly elevated. The white count is usually less than 2000/μL, with a marked neutropenia. The platelet count is usually below 50,000/μL. Thrombocytopenia is often the earliest manifestation.

The bone marrow is practically devoid of normal marrow elements and is replaced with fat. A bone marrow section is indicated for absolute diagnosis.

The fetal hemoglobin level remains elevated in congenital aplastic anemia (Fanconi type) but may or may not rise in acquired forms.

Differential Diagnosis

Other causes of pancytopenia in childhood include infiltration with leukemia, Hodgkin's disease, Niemann-Pick disease, Gaucher's disease, histiocytosis disease, osteopetrosis, myelofibrosis, and various toxic agents. Most of these conditions are associated with splenomegaly.

Complications

The disease is characteristically complicated by overwhelming infection and severe hemorrhage. With long-term transfusion therapy, problems may develop in association with leukoagglutinins, erythrocyte antibodies, and hemosiderosis.

A significant complication of prolonged testosterone therapy in childhood in the development of secondary sex characteristics in boys and evidence of masculinization and hirsutism in girls. Epiphyseal closure and stunting of growth have not been a problem in most cases, but patients should be checked periodically with bone x-rays for epiphyseal maturation.

Treatment

A. General Measures: Severely ill children should be protected from infection in their environment by being placed in "reverse isolation." Specific and appropriate antibiotics should be used for infection.

Transfusions are usually necessary. If bleeding is not present, packed red cells in a dose of 10–20 mL/kg should be used for treatment of the anemia when symptoms develop. For severe hemorrhage, platelet concentrates should be used. White blood cell transfusions are indicated for severe infections that do not respond rapidly to antibiotic therapy. Single donors should be used if possible for both platelet and leukocyte transfusions to reduce the incidence of alloimmunization.

B. Bone Marrow Transplantation: Early marrow transplantation is the treatment of choice when an HLA-matched sibling donor is available. Cure has been achieved in over 50% of patients with the use of homologous bone marrow transplantation using a sibling donor with the same tissue (HLA) type. Isogenic marrow grafting has been consistently successful when an identical twin with unaffected bone marrow is the donor.

C. Drug Therapy:

1. Immunosuppressive therapy—Antithymocyte globulin (ATG) with methylprednisolone is currently considered the therapy of choice for patients with no HLA-matched marrow donor. Corticosteroids have generally not been effective in usual doses. However, up to 20% of patients respond to intravenous high-dose methylprednisolone, and up to 50% respond to therapy with antilymphocyte globulin (ALG) or antithymocyte globulin (ATG). Remissions have occasionally been observed following cyclophosphamide treatment. Data suggesting the presence of overactive suppressor thymocytes in some cases are confirmed by these responses.

2. Androgens—Androgens will produce remissions in a small proportion of both secondary and idiopathic cases of aplastic anemia in childhood. A patient who has a few residual marrow cells will respond more frequently than a patient with a totally empty bone marrow. The remission will frequently not occur until 1–2 months after treatment is started. Once a remission has been achieved, the lowest possible maintenance dose should be determined by gradual reduction of dosage. Temporary cessation of therapy may be indicated because of untoward drug side effects. Oxymetholone (2–4 mg/kg/d orally) has been used widely in the past. Hepatic toxicity and heptomas have been associated with long-term use. Nandrolone decanoate (1–1.5 mg/kg/wk intramuscularly) has proved effective in some cases and has not been associated with hepatic complications. Androgen therapy should probably be reserved for patients for whom a transplant donor is not available and who have not improved with antithymocyte globulin (ATG) therapy. Androgens may be given in conjunction with ATG.

Prognosis

The prognosis for patients with either the second-ary (acquired) or the idiopathic form of aplastic anemia is extremely poor when the bone marrow is totally empty and complete pancytopenia is present. In spite of supportive measures, these patients usually die of infection or hemorrhage within a period of a few months. Very few will respond to testosterone therapy. If some marrow elements remain, however, spontaneous remissions occasionally occur; remissions are sometimes induced with testosterone therapy. In the acquired form, a spontaneous remission may eventually occur 1–2 years after initiating treatment with testosterone or testosterone plus prednisone. Bone marrow transplantation with a histocompatible donor has provided a 50–60% cure rate (especially if done early in the disease), and a similar remission rate may be achieved with immunosuppressive therapy. The recovery with supportive therapy and androgens is only about 20%.

Champlin R, Ho W, Gale RP: Antithymocyte globulin treatment in patients with aplastic anemia: A prospective randomized trial. *N Engl J Med* 1983;**308:**113.

Gordonsmith EC: Treatment of aplastic anemias. *Hosp Pract* (May) 1985;**20:**69.

McGlave PB et al: Therapy of severe aplastic anemia in young adults and children with allogenic bone marrow transplantation. *Blood* 1987;**70:**1325.

Mangan KF: T-cell mediated suppression of hematopoiesis. (Editorial.) *N Engl J Med* 1985;**312:**306.

Najean Y, Girot R, Baumelou E: Prognostic factors and evolution of acquired aplastic anemia in childhood: A prospective analysis of 48 androgen-treated cases. *Am J Pediatr Hematol Oncol* 1982;**4:**273.

Storb R et al: Graft-versus-host disease and survival in patients with aplastic anemia treated by marrow grafts from HLA-identical siblings. *N Engl J Med* 1983;**308:**302.

Workentin PI et al: Immunosuppressive therapy for severe aplastic anemia. *Am J Pediatr Hematol Oncol* 1980;**2:**327.

CONGENITAL APLASTIC ANEMIA WITH MULTIPLE CONGENITAL ANOMALIES
(Fanconi's Anemia)

This is a familial aplastic anemia in which hypoplastic or aplastic bone marrow is associated with a number of other congenital anomalies. Occasionally, pancytopenia occurs in association with a hyperplastic marrow as a result of a delay in maturation. The most common defects are skeletal and include hypoplasia or absence or anomalies of the thumb, the thenar eminence, and the radius. Other skeletal anomalies may include syndactyly, congenital dislocation of the hips, and abnormalities of the long bones. Some affected children have patchy brown pigmentation of the skin, hypogenitalism, microcephaly, short stature, strabismus, ptosis of the eyelids, nystagmus, anomalies of the ears, and mental retardation. The condition may occur in siblings and is probably transmitted as an autosomal recessive trait. The hematologic manifestations rarely are manifested prior to age 1 and may appear at any time between ages 1 and 12. Thrombocytopenia is usually the first abnormality to be noted, followed later by neutropenia and anemia. Although the bone marrow in the typical patient is hypoplastic and progresses to aplasia, in rare cases it may be hyperplastic, with a delay in maturation of marrow elements.

The hematologic disorder is slowly progressive, and severe aplasia will develop in most cases. Death due to infection or bleeding will eventually occur if therapy is not instituted.

The clinical manifestations are principally those of the aplastic anemia (see above).

Fanconi's anemia is characterized by elevated fetal hemoglobin, an increased red cell MCV, and an increased number of chromosomal breaks. These findings are present prior to the onset of the pancytopenia and can aid in early diagnosis. The heterozygotes also have the chromosomal anomalies. Both the patients and the carriers have an increased risk of cancer, both for leukemia and for solid tumors. Prenatal diagnosis can be made by study of amniotic fluid fibroblasts for chromosomal breaks. For these studies, cell cultures must be stressed with alkylating agents such as diepoxybutane.

The majority of patients with Fanconi's anemia will respond to testosterone therapy or testosterone plus prednisone, although relapse will occur when drug therapy is discontinued. (See section on aplastic anemia for details of therapy.) Transfusion should be used in patients who do not respond to either testosterone or a combination of testosterone and prednisone. These children are especially prone to the development of hepatomas with long-term oxymetholone treatment; therefore, nandrolone decanoate treatment should be used instead.

The prognosis is much better since testosterone therapy came into use. However, long-term experience is beginning to suggest that many of these patients may eventually become resistant to testosterone therapy and die of the aplastic anemia in early adult life. Spontaneous recovery has occurred in a few cases during adolescence. Successful bone marrow transplantation using an unaffected histocompatible sibling donor has been reported in this disease.

Auerbach AD, Adler B, Chaganti RS: Prenatal and postnatal diagnosis and carrier detection of Fanconi anemia by a cytogenetic method. *Pediatrics* 1981;**67:**128.

Gastearena J et al: Fanconi's anemia: Clinical study of 6 cases. *Am J Pediatr Hematol Oncol* 1986;**8:**173.

German J et al: A test for Fanconi's anemia. *Blood* 1987;**69:**1637.

ANEMIA OF RENAL FAILURE
(Anemia of Uremia)

A severe normochromic anemia occurs in almost all forms of renal disease that have progressed to renal insufficiency. Although white cell production remains normal and platelet production may be normal, the bone marrow shows significant hypoplasia of the erythroid series.

The marrow hypoplasia is due to decreased circulating erythropoietin, which is normally produced principally in the kidney. Erythropoiesis is also suppressed (in vitro) by the serum of uremic patients.

The anemia of renal disease is frequently complicated by an extracorpuscular hemolytic component that occurs in the presence of significant uremia. Hemolytic-uremic syndrome, a more severe form of hemolytic anemia that occurs occasionally in children in association with renal disease, is discussed in Chapter 22.

Patients on dialysis often require packed red cell transfusions, which should be given in a dose of 10–20 mL/kg to keep the hemoglobin above 8 g/dL. The use of recombinant erythropoietin has been successful in initial trials and may eliminate the need for transfusion in the future. Successful renal transplantation cures the anemia.

Erslev A: Erythropoietin coming of age. *N Engl J Med* 1987;**316:**101.

Wallner SF, Vautrin RM: Evidence that inhibition of erythropoiesis is important in the anemia of chronic renal failure. *J Lab Clin Med* 1981;**97:**170.

ANEMIA OF HYPOTHYROIDISM

Certain patients with hypothyroidism develop fairly severe normochromic anemias. The red cells frequently tend to be macrocytic. However, microcytic hypochromic anemia also has been described. The bone marrow shows hypocellularity of the erythroid series, with a normoblastic pattern.

Replacement therapy with thyroid hormone is effective in treating the anemia of the hypothyroid patient. Some of the hypochromic patients also respond partially to iron.

ANEMIAS ASSOCIATED WITH
MARROW REPLACEMENT
(Myelophthisic Anemias)

Anemias resulting from bone marrow invasion or replacement are known as myelophthisic anemias. The most common cause in childhood is invasion with leukemic cells or lymphosarcoma. The differentiation from aplastic anemia in the hypoplastic form of leukemia can be made only by bone marrow examination. Hodgkin's disease in its advanced form may also be associated with severe marrow involvement. Other malignant tumors (particularly neuroblastoma) may cause diffuse involvement of the marrow. The disseminated acute form of histiocytosis

(Letterer-Siwe disease) may be associated with a diffuse involvement of the marrow. Some lipid storage diseases (eg, Gaucher's disease and Niemann-Pick disease) gradually invade the marrow. Osteopetrosis (Albers-Schönberg disease) in the acute infantile form is associated with severe encroachment on the marrow space by bone and usually presents initially as a myelophthisic anemia. True myelofibrosis with the development of classic agnogenic myeloid metaplasia is rarely seen in childhood.

All of these forms of myelophthisic anemia are characterized by the development of a normochromic anemia and associated thrombocytopenia. The presence of nucleated red cells and immature white cells with an elevated nucleated cell count in the peripheral blood suggests the existence of a myelophthisic process. Immature white and red cells are not always released, and they are probably related to the degree of extramedullary hematopoiesis. Splenomegaly is present in the majority of these conditions. The diagnosis is dependent upon finding the specific infiltrating process, osteopetrosis, or myelofibrosis in the bone marrow.

ANEMIAS DUE TO FAILURE OF RELEASE FROM THE MARROW

PRIMARY REFRACTORY ANEMIA (Refractory Normoblastic Anemia)

This condition is characterized by the paradoxic association of a hypercellular marrow and a moderate to severe chronic anemia, occasionally associated with neutropenia and thrombocytopenia. The reticulocyte count is low to normal. There are usually no other clinical findings, and the spleen is not enlarged. The marrow is markedly hypercellular, with normoblastic hyperplasia. Megaloblastic changes are usually present. Marrow hemosiderin is greatly increased.

The exact cause of this syndrome is not known, although many patients previously given this diagnosis may have had some type of dyserythropoietic anemia associated with intramedullary hemolysis (see next section). Treatment of the primary refractory anemias has been generally without success, and transfusion is usually the only treatment. In rare cases, splenectomy has been of slight value. Occasionally, congenital cases have responded to testosterone therapy. All patients should be given a trial of vitamin B, because the findings in pyridoxine-dependent anemias may be similar.

DYSERYTHROPOIETIC ANEMIAS

The dyserythropoietic anemias are characterized by maturation abnormalities in the bone marrow with associated intramedullary hemolysis. The clinical manifestations include the presence of intermittent scleral jaundice and splenomegaly. Anemia occasionally is not present. Some patients are well compensated, with hemoglobins and hematocrits within the normal range. The majority have a mild to moderate anemia of about 10 g/dL. Occasional patients show intermittent severe anemia associated with increased jaundice. They are frequently not recognized as having a hemolytic process, since the destruction takes place in the marrow and an excessive number of reticulocytes are not released. The reticulocyte count usually ranges from normal to a maximum of about 4%. In most of the reported familial cases, the mode of genetic transmission appears to be autosomal recessive. At least 4 different types have been described.

Additional laboratory findings include the presence of marked anisocytosis and poikilocytosis on the blood smear. There is usually an elevation of the indirect serum bilirubin to approximately 2 mg/dL. The haptoglobin is low or absent. Urobilin and urobilinogen are increased in the urine. The bone marrow pattern is diagnostic, with erythroid hyperplasia and characteristic erythroblasts showing several separate nuclei or with clover leaf-shaped nuclei.

Findings include elevated fetal hemoglobin and increased hemolysis in acidified serum (a positive Ham test) in the presence of a negative sugar water test in type II. A high proportion of cells are agglutinated by anti-i antibody. Osmotic fragility is normal or increased. The autohemolysis test and hemoglobin electrophoresis are normal. Iron stores are increased, and iron kinetics show a rapid plasma clearance.

The exact mechanism of the ineffective erythropoiesis and the intramedullary hemolysis has not been specifically explained.

The differential diagnosis includes Gilbert's disease, because patients with little or no anemia show primarily an elevated unconjugated (indirect reacting) serum bilirubin and intermittent scleral icterus. In patients with anemia, the differential diagnosis includes the other types of mild hemolytic disease.

Treatment is symptomatic.

Alloisio N et al: Alterations of globin chain synthesis and of red cell membrane proteins in congenital dyserythropoietic anemia I and II. *Pediatr Res* 1982;**16**:1016.

Lewis SM, Verwilghen RL: *Dyserythropoiesis.* Academic Press, 1977.

Schwartz CL et al: Preleukemic syndromes and other syndromes predisposing to leukemia. *Pediatr Clin North Am* 1988;**35**:853.

van der Weide et al: Myelodysplastic syndromes: Analysis of clinical and prognostic features in 96 patients. *Eur J Haematol* 1988;**41**:115.

HEMOLYTIC ANEMIAS

The hemolytic anemias of childhood may be classified as hereditary or acquired. The hereditary group is of particular importance, because the manifestations usually present in infancy or childhood. They may be divided first into those associated with a defect of the red cell membrane, such as hereditary spherocytosis, and those due to abnormalities in red cell glycolysis. (This includes the majority of the nonspherocytic hemolytic anemias that are associated with specific red cell enzyme defects and the drug-induced hemolytic anemias.) Second, there is a large group of hemoglobinopathies that includes the anemias with abnormal hemoglobin chains, those with a genetically determined decrease in production of one of the hemoglobin chains, and those with unstable hemoglobin. The majority of the acquired hemolytic anemias are on an "autoimmune" basis; are secondary to drug or chemical poisoning; or are associated with sepsis from hemolytic organisms.

DISORDERS OF RED CELL MEMBRANE

1. HEREDITARY SPHEROCYTOSIS (Congenital Hemolytic Anemia, Congenital Hemolytic Jaundice)

Essentials of Diagnosis
- Anemia.
- Sudden weakness and jaundice.
- Splenomegaly.
- Spherocytosis, increased reticulocytes.
- Increased osmotic fragility, abnormal autohemolysis.
- Negative Coombs test.
- Positive family history of anemia, jaundice, or gallbladder disease.

General Considerations

Hereditary spherocytosis is a common inherited hemolytic anemia that occurs in about one in 5000 persons of Northern European ancestry, as well as in other races. It is caused by an abnormal skeletal structure of the red cell membrane due to deficiencies in spectrin. Instability of the membrane allows fragmentation and loss of surface area. There is also increased influx of water and sodium into the erythrocytes. Increased glycolysis is necessary to prevent the intracellular accumulation of sodium. Spherocytosis and decreased red cell survival occur when the cell is deprived of sufficient glucose. The cells are

sequestered and destroyed in the spleen. Transfused cells from normal donors have a normal survival in the patient with spherocytosis, whereas spherocytic cells transfused into a normal recipient maintain their shortened survival rate. The disease may be mild to severe, depending on the degree of spectrin deficiency. It is characterized by intermittent crises associated with rapid hemolysis and jaundice. Hypoplastic crises occasionally occur in association with decreased erythroid production in the bone marrow. In most instances, the disease is transmitted as an autosomal dominant, and abnormalities can usually be detected in one of the parents of the child even though they are asymptomatic. However, in some families the abnormality cannot be found in other generations, suggesting that it can be transmitted as a recessive. Hereditary spherocytosis may be a cause of neonatal hyperbilirubinemia and may be confused with ABO incompatibility because of the presence of spherocytes in both conditions.

Clinical Findings

A. Symptoms and Signs: Jaundice usually occurs in the newborn period. Splenomegaly without other symptoms characterizes many of the cases in childhood. Chronic fatigue and malaise may be present, and abdominal pain is a frequent complaint. Gallbladder pain may occur in the adolescent.

Hemolytic or aplastic crises may develop and are associated with severe weakness, fatigue, fever, abdominal pain, and jaundice.

B. Laboratory Findings: Mild chronic anemia is characteristic. The hemoglobin usually varies from 9 to 11 g/dL, although a few cases may have almost normal levels of 12–13 g/dL. The red cells are microcytic and hyperchromic (MCV = 70–80 fL, and MCHC = 36–40%). Spherocytes characteristically are seen on the smear but may comprise no more than 10% of the cells prior to splenectomy. A persistently elevated reticulocyte count is characteristic. White cells and platelets are usually normal.

The bone marrow shows typical erythroid hyperplasia of hemolytic anemia (except during the hypoplastic crisis, when there may be marked reduction of erythropoiesis).

Osmotic fragility is increased, particularly after incubation at 37 °C for 24 hours. Autohemolysis of blood incubated for 48 hours is greatly increased. Incubation with glucose or ATP will decrease the hemolysis (usually to normal levels). Serum bilirubin may show elevation of the unconjugated portion. Stool urobilinogen is usually elevated. The Coombs test is negative, and hemoglobin electrophoresis reveals a normal pattern.

Complications

Severe jaundice may occur in the newborn period with the development of kernicterus if exchange transfusion is not performed. Splenectomy in the first 2 years of life is associated with increased susceptibility to overwhelming bacterial infections (particularly pneumococcal sepsis). Gallstones (composed principally of bile pigments) occur in up to 85% of young adults with this disease, and they may even develop during later childhood if splenectomy is not performed by the middle childhood years.

Treatment

There is no satisfactory medical treatment for this condition, but splenectomy is effective.

A. Exchange Transfusions: For hyperbilirubinemia in the neonatal period, exchange transfusion should be performed.

B. Surgical Treatment: Splenectomy is the treatment of choice in hereditary spherocytosis. Except in unusually severe cases, the procedure should be postponed until the child is at least 5 or 6 years of age, because of the increased risk of infection prior to this time. The operation is indicated in older children by the age of 10 years, even though the degree of hemolysis may be mild. Cholecystectomy for cholelithiasis is rarely indicated in childhood, particularly if splenectomy is performed by 10 years of age.

C. Postoperative Anti-infective Prophylaxis: Prophylactic penicillin is recommended following splenectomy in all children. It should be continued throughout childhood and adolescence. Pneumococcal vaccine should be given before splenectomy.

D. Treatment of Hemolytic and Hypoplastic Crises: Crises associated with anemia are frequently precipitated by infection. Therapy should include antibiotics for bacterial infections and packed red cell transfusions for both hemolytic and hypoplastic crises.

Prognosis

Splenectomy will eliminate all signs and symptoms, and the red cell survival usually returns to normal following this procedure. The development of cholelithiasis will also be prevented if splenectomy is performed during childhood. The abnormal red cell morphology, increased osmotic fragility, and the abnormal findings on autohemolysis test persist following splenectomy but are of no clinical significance.

Agre P et al: Inheritance pattern and clinical response to splenectomy as a reflection of erythrocyte spectrin deficiency in hereditary spherocytosis. *N Engl J Med* 1986; **315**:1579.

Marchesi VT: The red cell membrane skeleton: Recent progress. *Blood* 1983;**61**:1.

Young N: Hematologic and hematopoietic consequences of B19 parvovirus infection. *Semin Hematol* 1988;**25**:159.

2. ELLIPTOCYTOSIS (Ovalocytosis)

Hereditary elliptocytosis is characterized primarily by the presence of large numbers of oval and elliptic cells in the peripheral blood. It is usually discovered on routine examination, and the majority of patients are asymptomatic. The morphologic abnormality of the peripheral blood is transmitted as an autosomal dominant and occurs in both sexes. Approximately 12% of the heterozygous cases demonstrate evidence of mild hemolytic disease characterized by slight splenomegaly and reticulocytosis. There may be low-grade anemia, but even in these patients the hemoglobin is frequently within normal limits. Varying clinical manifestations have been explained by different alpha spectrin deficiencies in the red cell membrane associated with various spectrin mutations.

In the more severe forms, a transient poikilocytosis (pyropoikilocytosis) occurs in the newborn period with significant hemolytic anemia and neonatal jaundice.

A few cases of children who are homozygous for the disease have been reported. These children have severe hemolytic anemia, with splenomegaly and hematologic evidence of hemolysis.

Treatment is not usually indicated except in severe cases, for which splenectomy is usually beneficial.

Mentzer WC et al: Modulation of erythrocyte membrane mechanical stability by 2, 3-DPG in neonatal poikilocytosis/elliptocytosis syndrome. *J Clin Invest* 1987; **79**:943.

Palek J, Coetzer T: Clinical expression of spectrin mutants in hereditary elliptocytosis. *Blood Cells* 1987;**13**:237.

3. HEREDITARY PYROPOIKILOCYTOSIS

This is a rare disorder presenting in infancy with severe hemolytic anemia. It is characterized by extreme poikilocytosis with budding red cells, spherocytes, elliptocytes, and bizarrely shaped fragmented cells. The MCV is very low (25–55 fL), and osmotic fragility and autohemolysis are markedly increased. The red cells have unusual sensitivity to heat and will fragment at 45–46 °C (normally at 49 °C). Red cell membrane spectrin is abnormal and unusually heat-sensitive. Pyropoikilocytosis has been reported primarily in black families. Splenectomy results in marked improvement but not complete cure. Pyropoikilocytosis also has been reported to be transient in infancy in some families with mild hereditary elliptocytosis, as noted above.

Coetzer T et al: Molecular determinants of clinical expression of hereditary elliptocytosis and pyropoikilocytosis. *Blood* 1987;**70**:766.

Prchal JT et al: Hereditary pyropoikilocytosis and elliptocytosis: Clinical, laboratory, and ultrastructural features in infants and children. *Pediatr Res* 1982;**16**:484.

4. STOMATOCYTOSIS

A rare form of hemolytic anemia has been described in which the red blood cells have a characteristic cup-shaped appearance. The anemia is mild, and the disease has the characteristics of a hemolytic process with elevated reticulocyte count. The red cells have increased osmotic fragility, increased autohemolysis, and reduced glutathione.

Splenectomy results in improvement.

5. ACANTHOCYTOSIS
(Abetalipoproteinemia)

This rare autosomal recessive disorder is characterized by acanthocytes (thorny cells) in the blood, progressive ataxic neurologic disease, retinitis pigmentosa, malabsorption, and abetalipoproteinemia. Although the red cells are very abnormal, the degree of hemolysis is mild. (See also Chapter 33.)

6. XEROCYTOSIS
(Desiccytosis)

Xerocytosis is a rare autosomal dominant condition characterized by mild to moderate congenital hemolytic anemia. The number of reticulocytes is increased, and the blood smear usually shows shrunken, spicular cells in which hemoglobin is "puddled" on one side. Target cells, stomatocytes, and dense cells may also be present. This disorder is due to a membrane defect that causes loss of water and potassium but little change in intracellular sodium, resulting in intracellular dehydration. Diagnosis is made by measurement of red cell cations and isopyknic centrifugation. Osmotic fragility is usually decreased. Splenectomy has not been of value.

Glader BE et al: Desiccytosis associated with RBC potassium loss: A new congenital hemolytic syndrome. *Pediatr Res* 1973;**7**:350.

7. HYDROCYTOSIS

Hydrocytosis is a rare congenital hemolytic anemia in which the red cells have a primary defect in permeability that leads to cell swelling. Anemia varies from mild to severe, and the inheritance is usually autosomal dominant. The increase in cell water, which produces stomatocytes, can be demonstrated by either isopyknic centrifugation or osmotic gradient ectocytometry. Osmotic fragility is increased, and there is an increase in total red cell cation con-

centration due to increased intracellular sodium. Some patients respond to splenectomy.

Lande WM, Mentzer WC: Haemolytic anaemia associated with increased cation permeability. *Clin Haematol* 1985;**14**:89.

8. ACQUIRED CELL MEMBRANE DEFECTS ASSOCIATED WITH HEMOLYSIS

Infantile Pyknocytosis

A transient hemolytic anemia has been described in newborn infants in association with a high degree of pyknocytosis of their red cells. Pyknocytes bear a close resemblance to acanthocytes. They occur in small numbers in all newborn and premature infants, but in infants with hemolysis, as many as 50% of red cells may be pyknocytes. The exact cause remains unknown. The syndrome is characterized by hemolysis beginning during the first week of life, with jaundice, anemia, reticulocytosis, and splenomegaly. The anemia usually reaches its peak by 3 weeks of age, and recovery is spontaneous.

The diagnosis is based on the presence of large numbers of pyknocytes (> 6%) in association with a Coombs-negative hemolytic anemia.

Exchange transfusion may be necessary for the hyperbilirubinemia of pyknocytosis during the first week. Small transfusions are indicated for increasing anemia after that time.

Vitamin E Deficiency Hemolytic Anemia

Vitamin E deficiency may cause hemolysis and an increase in acanthocytes. It can be differentiated from pyknocytosis by demonstrating an increased hemolysis in hydrogen peroxide and a response to the administration of parenteral vitamin E.

The disorder occurs primarily in preterm infants after the fourth week of life and is due to poor absorption of vitamin E. It is aggravated by the oral administration of iron medication. A dosage of 25 units of vitamin E per day orally is adequate prophylaxis.

Lubin B, Chiu D: Properties of vitamin E-deficient erythrocytes following peroxidant injury. *Pediatr Res* 1982; **16**:928.

Melhorn DK, Gross S: Vitamin E-dependent anemia in the premature infant. 1. Effects of large doses of medicinal iron. *J Pediatr* 1971;**79**:569.

Liver Disease

Red cell membrane changes may occur in liver disease and can be associated with significant hemolytic anemia. The membrane abnormality is associated with changes in serum and membrane lipid involving the cholesterol-phospholipid ratio. The most severe form (usually seen in hepatocellular disease) is characterized by ''spur'' cells. The more common and milder form is characterized by target cells.

Renal Disease

A marked hemolytic anemia may occur secondary to the effect of elevated metabolites and urea in severe uremia. Burr cells are usually present. These changes are corrected by dialysis.

Hemolytic-Uremic Syndrome

Hemolytic anemia may be severe and often is the presenting complaint in this disorder. It is a microangiopathic anemia associated with destruction of red cells in small renal vessels and characterized by fragmented cells. (See Chapter 22.)

Hemolysis With Disseminated Intravascular Coagulation

A microangiopathic hemolytic anemia with fragmented cells is characteristic of this syndrome.

DISORDERS OF RED CELL Glycolysis (The Hereditary Nonspherocytic Hemolytic Anemias)

Essentials of Diagnosis

- Moderate to severe anemia.
- Elevated reticulocyte count.
- Normal osmotic fragility test with abnormal autohemolysis.
- Splenomegaly.
- Present from birth, with neonatal jaundice.
- Negative Coombs test.

General Considerations

The hereditary nonspherocytic hemolytic anemias include a number of different defects in red cell metabolism. A number of specific enzymes necessary for erythrocyte glycolysis have been shown to be deficient in various forms of nonspherocytic hemolytic anemia. These enzyme deficiencies include glucose 6-phosphate dehydrogenase (G6PD), 6-phosphogluconate dehydrogenase, pyruvate kinase, triosephosphate isomerase, hexokinase, hexosephosphate isomerase, phosphoglycerate kinase, adenosinetriphosphatase (ATPase), 2,3-diphosphoglycerate mutase, phosphoglucose isomerase, phosphofructokinase, glyceraldehyde 3-phosphate dehydrogenase, lactate dehydrogenase, glutathione reductase, glutathione peroxidase, glutathione synthetase, and hereditary absence of glutathione. The most frequently encountered are those associated with G6PD or pyruvate kinase deficiency. These will be discussed in more detail in succeeding sections.

The hereditary pattern varies. Deficiency of G6PD is transmitted as an X-linked recessive, whereas pyruvate kinase deficiency and most of the other types occur as autosomal recessives.

1. PYRUVATE KINASE DEFICIENCY HEMOLYTIC ANEMIA

A severe chronic hemolytic anemia is associated with erythrocyte pyruvate kinase deficiency. It is transmitted as an autosomal recessive condition. It presents with splenomegaly and a moderate or severe hemolytic anemia in the immediate neonatal period. Jaundice in the newborn is a common complication, and exchange transfusion is usually required.

The anemia is normochromic, and there is a marked elevation of the reticulocyte count. The blood smear shows some microcytes and a few spherocytes. Differentiation from hereditary spherocytosis is not easy, because spherocytes may be seen in pyruvate kinase deficiency and red cell osmotic fragility may also be slightly increased; the autohemolysis test is markedly increased, as in spherocytosis. The most useful point of differentiation between the 2 diseases is the fact that the red cell fragility is only slightly increased and the autohemolysis test is only partially corrected by glucose in pyruvate kinase deficiency, whereas the latter is markedly corrected in spherocytosis.

Family studies are also helpful in differentiating the 2 conditions because pyruvate kinase deficiency is autosomal recessive, whereas spherocytosis is usually dominant.

Red cell glycolysis and specific enzyme assays for pyruvate kinase are indicated if this condition is suspected. Several different mutant forms of the enzyme have been reported; recently, a mutant enzyme was described in patients with a similar disorder who appear to have adequate pyruvate kinase activity by the usual assay but who are found to have a pathologic isoenzyme that can be detected only by assays using low levels of substrate.

Treatment consists of splenectomy. Significant improvement usually follows this procedure, although complete cure is not achieved. Prior to splenectomy, repeated transfusions are usually necessary every few months. No drugs or other methods of management are effective.

The prognosis following splenectomy is fairly good, although the complications of cholelithiasis should be anticipated.

Max-Audit I et al: Pyruvatokinase synthesis and degradation by normal and pathologic cells during erythroid maturation. *Blood* 1988;**72**:1039.

Miwa S: Pyruvate kinase deficiency and other enzymopathies of the Embden-Meyerhof pathway. *Clin Haematol* 1981;**10**:57.

Valentine WN: Erythrocyte pyruvate kinase (PK): The

variable significance of "nucleotide specificity" in the characterization of mutant variants. *Am J Hematol* 1987;**26**:353.

2. GLUCOSE 6-PHOSPHATE DEHYDROGENASE DEFICIENCY (Drug-Sensitive Hemolytic Anemia, Primaquine-Sensitive Hemolytic Anemia)

Drug-induced hemolytic anemia is most commonly associated with a red cell deficiency of glucose 6-phosphate dehydrogenase (G6PD). The deficiency is due to a labile G6PD enzyme that is present in young cells but rapidly disappears with cell aging. A large number of variant defective enzymes have been found in different racial groups. It is estimated that G6PD deficiency affects more than 125 million persons worldwide. Most persons with a G6PD defect have episodes of hemolysis only after exposure to certain oxidant drugs or fava beans, although the more severe forms may be manifested by a chronic hemolytic anemia.

The disease is transmitted as an X-linked recessive. Full expression occurs also in females who are homozygous for the gene; intermediate expression occurs in the heterozygous female carrier. In the USA, about 10% of black males manifest this enzyme deficiency, whereas only 1–2% of black females tend to be mildly symptomatic when challenged with drugs. This disease occurs also in Chinese, Southeast Asians, Greeks, Italians, Arabs, and Sephardic Jews. The exact mechanism of the enzyme defect is not quantitatively or qualitatively identical in all of these racial groups. The disorder is less severe in blacks than in other racial groups.

Symptoms usually occur only in association with oxidant drug exposure or infections. In the neonatal period, certain racial groups (Greek, Italian, and Chinese) may show increased hyperbilirubinemia, whereas full-term black infants do not. The most common offenders are the antimalarials, sulfonamides, sulfones, nitrofurans, antipyretics, analgesics, synthetic vitamin K, and uncooked fava beans. G6PD deficiency does not affect the course of sickle cell disease in blacks with both disorders.

The clinical picture is characterized by an acute hemolytic episode following exposure to one of these substances. The anemia is normochromic, and Heinz body formation is characteristic. An elevated reticulocyte count will appear within a few days.

Because only the older red cells are susceptible, the process becomes self-limited as a younger red cell population appears in response to the hemolytic process.

A specific laboratory diagnosis may be made by one of several tests, including the glutathione stability test, the dye reduction test using cresyl blue, the methemoglobin reduction test, and a commercially available dye reduction spot test. The G6PD levels and the screening test may be normal immediately after a hemolytic episode because only young cells, which may have normal enzyme activity, remain.

Routine laboratory screening has been recommended for persons in the high-risk racial groups.

Treatment includes discontinuing exposure to the offending agent and transfusion of packed red cells. Vitamin E therapy has been useful in the rare chronic forms.

Corash LM et al: Chronic hemolytic anemia due to G6PD deficiency: The role of vitamin E in its treatment. *Ann N Y Acad Sci* 1982;**393**:348.

HEMOGLOBINOPATHIES: QUALITATIVE DEFECTS

1. SICKLE CELL ANEMIA

Essentials of Diagnosis

- Anemia, elevated reticulocyte count, jaundice.
- Positive sickling test, hemoglobin S and F.
- Splenomegaly in early childhood, with later disappearance.
- Crises with pain in the legs and abdomen.
- Usually black African ethnic origin.

General Considerations

Sickle hemoglobin is found with high frequency in black persons of central African origin. It also occurs in other racial groups in Sicily, Italy, Greece, Turkey, Saudi Arabia, and India and, rarely, in other Caucasians. Sickle cell anemia is seen in about one in 500 blacks in the USA. The incidence is much higher in some parts of Africa.

Sickle cell anemia occurs in individuals who are homozygous for the sickle cell gene. Sickle hemoglobin is characterized by a single amino acid substitution (valine for glutamic acid) at the 6 position in the beta globin chain of adult type (A_1) hemoglobin. The sickling trait is transmitted as a dominant; the carrier shows a combination of hemoglobin A_1 and sickle hemoglobin, whereas the patient with sickle cell anemia has only sickle, A_2, and fetal hemoglobins. The sickling process is often initiated by low oxygen tension and low pH. The sickled cells obstruct small vessels, and infarcts are frequent. Infarction accounts for the abdominal pain, bone pain, and gradual decrease in the size of the spleen ("autosplenectomy"). Functional hyposplenism and splenic sequestration may occur as early as 4 months of age.

Clinical Findings

A. Symptoms and Signs: The onset of symptoms is usually between 4 and 12 months of age, because high levels of fetal hemoglobin prevent sickling in the first few months of life. Functional hyposplenism (often associated with splenomegaly) occurs at this age and is associated with a high risk of sepsis and meningitis due to *Streptococcus pneumoniae* and *Haemophilus influenzae*. Acute splenic sequestration crises are common and result in life-threatening anemia. Pneumonia, urinary tract infections, and osteomyelitis (especially due to *Salmonella*) are also common, with the highest risk of infection occurring between the ages of 1 and 10 years. Moderately severe hemolytic anemia occurs by 1 year of age and causes mild scleral icterus. Hemolytic or hypoplastic crises may occur. Pain crises in the extremities and abdomen occur in varying degrees in most patients who develop the disease in early childhood. Strokes occur in about 10% of children and tend to be recurrent. Physical growth is often retarded; puberty may be delayed; and children are usually asthenic. Older children show enlargement of the facial and skull bones and may develop a "tower skull." During adolescence, leg ulcers may develop and cholelithiasis often occurs. Pulmonary infarctions, priapism, hepatic dysfunction, cardiomegaly, systolic ejection murmur, and even heart failure may occur in older children and adolescents. Chronic sickling in the kidneys results in hyposthenuria (with dilute urine), occasional hematuria, and eventual renal function impairment. Repeated bone infarctions may result in aseptic necrosis (particularly in the hip or shoulder).

B. Laboratory Findings: The hemoglobin usually ranges between 7 and 10 g/dL. It may drop as low as 2–3 g/dL at the time of a sequestration or hypoplastic crisis. The reticulocyte count is markedly elevated. The anemia is normocytic or mildly macrocytic; the smear shows increased numbers of target cells and abnormalities of size and shape. Irreversible sickled cells (ISCs) may be seen on the ordinary blood smear and are common at the time of crisis. The sickling phenomenon can be demonstrated by reducing the oxygen tension in the finger with a small tourniquet prior to obtaining blood or by ringing the coverslip on a slide with petrolatum over a drop of blood. Fresh sodium metabisulfite, 2%, mixed on the slide with the drop of blood will bring out the sickling in a few minutes. The blood "solubility" tests are positive in the presence of sickle hemoglobin. Nucleated red cells are present and may equal the number of white cells. The total nucleated cell count is high. Serum bilirubin usually shows an elevation of unconjugated (indirect) bilirubin. The specific gravity of the urine becomes fixed at about 1.010 in later childhood, and both hemosiderinuria and hematuria may be seen.

The bone marrow shows marked erythroid hyperplasia. X-rays of the skull and spine reveal cortical thinning, enlargement of the marrow spaces, and increased trabecular markings.

Hemoglobin electrophoresis reveals only sickle (S), fetal (F), and A_2 hemoglobin. The fetal component usually varies between 5% and 20%, while A_2 is normal. Techniques for intrauterine diagnosis have been developed using cells from amniocentesis and restriction enzyme fragmentation of DNA.

Differential Diagnosis

The most important differentiation is from the other sickle hemoglobinopathies that are also common in the black population. The differentiation from sickle thalassemia and sickle hemoglobin C disease is made primarily by hemoglobin electrophoresis and determination of fetal and A_2 hemoglobin. The hematuria that occurs with sickle cell anemia must be differentiated from renal bleeding due to other causes. In crisis, the primary differentiation is from acute appendicitis in the presence of abdominal pain and tenderness and from rheumatic fever because of the frequent joint and bone pains and the systolic precordial murmur in sickle cell disease.

Hemoglobins D and G migrate electrophoretically on paper and cellulose acetate at pH 8.4 at the same rate as S and are indistinguishable by this method. They can be differentiated by the negative sickling test with hemoglobin D and G and by electrophoresis on citrate agar at pH 6.2. Study of the entire family is often of importance in determining the exact nature of the hemoglobinopathy.

Sickle cell trait associated with iron deficiency anemia can be differentiated by the presence of a low reticulocyte count, high red cell count, and hypochromia.

Complications

Repeated small vascular infarctions may result in damage to nearly every organ system. The early splenic involvement, with eventual splenic fibrosis, results in increased susceptibility to overwhelming infection. (See also Clinical Findings.)

Treatment

Treatment is instituted primarily for the crises. There is no known effective method for reducing the rate of chronic hemolysis or preventing crises. Both the splenic sequestration and hypoplastic crises should be treated with transfusion. Transfusions are also helpful in terminating prolonged "painful" crises. Packed red cells are usually used. A partial exchange with packed red cells is indicated in pulmonary infarction and other severe crises and prior to surgery. Repeated transfusion every 3–4 weeks is recommended with iron chelation therapy in patients with strokes and other severe complications. The use of oxygen, maintenance of good hydration, and correction of acidosis are the most important measures for management of severe pain crises. Rest, analgesics, and sedatives may be sufficient in mild cases. Corticosteroids have been reported to be helpful in the management of painful swelling of the hands and feet. Clinical trials using testosterone to stimulate marrow production have been associated with an increased incidence of thrombosis. A number of antisickling drugs have been evaluated or are under investigation, but none have yet proved suitable for long-term clinical use. Urea and cyanate are effective but toxic. Hydroxyurea and 5-azacytidine (still under investigation) have been shown to cause moderate increases in fetal hemoglobin but are toxic. Bone marrow transplantation has been successful but would not be indicated in most patients because of the risk of the procedure.

In the young patient, early treatment of suspected sepsis with intravenous antibiotics is essential. Prevention of life-threatening pneumococcal disease may be accomplished by use of prophylactic penicillin throughout childhood. Pneumococcal vaccine is recommended at 1, 2, and 6 years of age in young children and on one occasion in older children and adults. *H influenzae* vaccine should be administered to all children over 2 years of age with sickle cell disease. Folic acid, 1 mg/d, is given to prevent folate deficiency.

Prognosis

Overwhelming infection in early childhood has resulted in a mortality rate of more than 10% in the past. This rate can be reduced by early diagnosis of sickle cell anemia (by 4 months of age) and appropriate preventive and therapeutic measures. Diagnosis can be made by hemoglobin electrophoresis done at both alkaline and acid pH in the newborn or at age 4 months. Sickling or solubility tests will usually be normal during the first few months of life. Early diagnosis and parental counseling regarding complications such as sepsis and acute splenic sequestration can lead to improved medical care with reduced morbidity and mortality rates. In the future, relatively few patients should die in childhood of this disease. Many patients, however, die in early adult life. Progressive renal damage usually occurs, and death from uremia, heart failure, or pulmonary infarction is common. Some patients survive to over 60 years of age.

Ambruso DR et al: Experience with donors matched for minor blood group antigens in patients with sickle cell anemia on chronic transfusion. *Transfusion* 1987;**27**:94.

Castro OL et al: Managing sickle cell emergencies. *Patient Care* (Jan) 1985;**19**:92.

Kapland et al: Revaccination with polyvalent pneumococcal vaccine in children with sickle cell anemia. *Am J Pediatr Hematol Oncol* 1986;**8**:80.

Serjeant GR: *Sickle Cell Disease.* Oxford Univ Press, 1985.

Sprinkle RH et al: Acute chest syndrome in children with sickle cell anemia: A retrospective analysis of 100 hospitalized cases. *Am J Pediatr Hematol Oncol* 1986;**8**:105.

Vichinsky E, Lubin BH: Suggested guidelines for the treatment of children with sickle cell anemia. *Hematol Oncol Clin North Am* 1987;**1**:483.

Vichinsky E et al: Newborn screening for sickle cell disease: Effect on mortality. *Pediatrics* 1988;**81**:749.

2. SICKLE CELL TRAIT

Sickle cell trait occurs in about 8–10% of blacks in the USA and in as much as 40% of the population in certain areas of Africa. The high incidence of the carrier state in African blacks has been attributed to the increased resistance to malaria conferred by the condition; this resistance tends to increase selectively the representation of these individuals in the population. The disorder is generally asymptomatic, and anemia, reticulocytosis, and morphologic red cell changes are not observed. Hematuria is the principal complication and occurs in 3–4% of cases. Progressive impairment in the ability of the kidneys to concentrate urine is sometimes noted. Splenic infarction or sequestration may occur in the presence of low oxygen tension at extremely high altitudes—particularly with flying in unpressurized aircraft. Except for these unusual circumstances, the prognosis is excellent and the life expectancy is normal.

Heller P et al: Clinical implications of sickle-cell trait and glucose-6-phosphate dehydrogenase deficiency in hospitalized black male patients. *N Engl J Med* 1979;**300**:1001.

Lane PA, Githens JH: Splenic crises at mountain altitudes in nonblack persons with sickle trait. *JAMA* 1985;**253**:2251.

Mahony BS, Githens JH: Sickling crises and altitude: Occurrence in the Colorado patient population. *Clin Pediatr* 1979;**18**:431.

Sears DA: The morbidity of sickle cell trait: A review of the literature. *Am J Med* 1978;**64**:1021.

3. HEMOGLOBIN S-C DISEASE

Hemoglobin S-C disease is caused by the double autosomal heterozygous state for both hemoglobin S and C. The incidence in the American black population is about one in 1500. Symptoms are similar to those of homozygous sickle cell disease but are usually less marked. Persons with S-C disease are particularly prone to develop splenic sequestration crises at high altitudes or while flying in unpressurized aircraft. Some patients are prone to vaso-occlusive crises involving the lung, kidney, retina, and femoral head. Target cells are prominent, and a mild anemia with persistent reticulocytosis is usually present. The diagnosis is confirmed by hemoglobin electrophoresis and the sickling test, along with evaluation of other members of the family. The complications and general treatment are similar to those for sickle cell anemia, although most patients require no therapy. However, retinopathy occurs in a high percentage of young adults and may result in blindness from retinal detachment or vitreous hemorrhage. These complications can be prevented by regular ophthalmologic examination and treatment of the characteristic neovascularization with laser beam coagulation or cryotherapy. Although the severity of the disease may vary, the prognosis is much better than in homozygous sickle disease, and the life span is usually not seriously affected.

Githens JH et al: Splenic sequestration syndrome at mountain altitudes in sickle/hemoglobin C disease. *J Pediatr* 1977;**90**:203.

Kim HC: Variants of sickle cell disease. Page 215 in: *Hemoglobinopathies in Children.* Schwartz E (editor). PSG Publishing Co., 1980.

Stevens MCG et al: Haematologic changes in sickle cell-haemoglobin C (SC) disease and in sickle cell-B thalassemia: A cohort study from birth to 6 years. *Br J Haematol* 1985;**60**:279.

4. SICKLE BETA THALASSEMIA

This disease is due to the double heterozygous state for both hemoglobin S and beta thalassemia. In blacks with sickle beta[+] thalassemia, symptoms are similar to those of sickle cell anemia but are less marked. Painful vaso-occlusive crises may occur. Anemia is mild and microcytic—hemoglobin is in the range of 10–12 g/dL. Hemoglobin electrophoresis shows both A_1 and S hemoglobins but with S being over 50% (usually 60–80%). A_2 and fetal hemoglobins are also present and elevated.

Some patients with the Mediterranean beta thalassemia gene (sickle beta[0] thalassemia) have only S, F, and A_2 hemoglobins, making it difficult to differentiate them from patients with sickle cell anemia. The presence of a low MCV and elevated A_2 hemoglobin suggests this diagnosis. Family studies are needed to confirm the diagnosis. Symptomatic treatment may be required for crises. Life expectancy is probably normal in sickle beta[+] thalassemia but reduced in sickle beta[0] thalassemia.

Stevens MCG et al: Haematologic changes in sickle cell-haemoglobin C (SC) disease and in sickle cell-B thalassemia: A cohort study from birth to 6 years. *Br J Haematol* 1985;**60**:279.

5. HEMOGLOBIN C TRAIT & HEMOGLOBIN C DISEASE

Hemoglobin C trait occurs in approximately 2–3% of blacks in the USA. Individuals with the trait are heterozygous for the gene and are essentially asymptomatic; they have a normal life expectancy. The blood smear, however, reveals the presence of large numbers of target cells. Renal hematuria has occasionally been reported.

Hemoglobin C disease is rare and occurs in individuals who are homozygous for the gene. It occurs almost exclusively in blacks. Onset is at about 1 year of age, because the infant is protected by fetal hemoglobin. Patients usually demonstrate a mild hemolytic anemia with a persistently elevated reticulocyte count. Red cell morphology is characterized by many target cells, which are usually normocytic and normochromic. Tetragonal crystals of hemoglobin can be found in the erythrocyte. Osmotic fragility is decreased. The diagnosis is made by hemoglobin electrophoresis, which usually reveals 100% hemoglobin C. Fetal hemoglobin is usually not elevated. Moderate to marked splenomegaly is the only significant clinical finding. There are usually no symptoms, although abdominal pain, arthralgia, and jaundice may occur occasionally.

Treatment is usually not required, and transfusions are rarely needed. Splenectomy is occasionally indicated if anemia is severe.

6. HEMOGLOBIN M DISEASE

The designation M is given to several abnormal hemoglobins associated with methemoglobinemia. Affected individuals are heterozygous for the gene, and it is transmitted as an autosomal dominant. A number of different types have been described in which various abnormal amino acids are substituted in the poplypeptide chain, producing a hemoglobin molecule in which the iron remains in the ferric instead of the ferrous state and cannot combine with oxygen. The defect may be on either the alpha or the beta globin chain. Hemoglobin electrophoresis at the usual pH will not always demonstrate the abnormal hemoglobin, and special techniques are necessary to detect it by electrophoresis as well as spectroscopically.

The patient has marked and persistent cyanosis but is otherwise usually asymptomatic. Exercise tolerance may be normal, and life expectancy is not affected. When the abnormality is on the beta chain, the infant is unaffected for the first few months of life. Some persons with the M hemoglobinopathy of the beta chain may also have mild hemolysis.

This type of methemoglobinemia does not respond to any form of therapy.

Vichinsky EP, Lubin BH: Unstable hemoglobins, hemoglobins with altered oxygen affinity, and m-hemoglobins. *Pediatr Clin North Am* 1980;**27**:421.

7. HEMOGLOBIN E DISORDERS

Hemoglobin E is common in Southeast Asia and has been seen in the USA with increasing frequency. Hemoglobin E trait (heterozygous hemoglobin E) is totally asymptomatic, with no anemia. Occasional microcytes are seen on blood smear. Hemoglobin E disease (homozygous hemoglobin E) is a benign disorder. The blood smear shows many target cells and significant microcytosis, with a low MCV. There may be borderline anemia and mildly elevated reticulocyte levels. Slight splenomegaly occurs rarely.

The double heterozygous state of hemoglobin E and beta thalassemia results in moderate (beta$^+$ thalassemia-hemoglobin E) or severe (beta^0 thalassemia-hemoglobin E) anemia, with microcytosis, hypochromia, hemolysis, and splenomegaly. The more severe cases may be transfusion-dependent.

When hemoglobin E is submitted to electrophoresis at an alkaline pH, it migrates at the same rate as hemoglobin C, but it can be differentiated from hemoglobin C at an acid pH.

Cunningham TM: Hemoglobin E in Indochinese refugees. *West J Med* 1982;**137:**186.

Sanguansermsri T et al: Distribution of hemoglobin E and β-thalassemia in Kampuchea (Cambodia). *Hemoglobin* 1987;**11:**481.

8. ABNORMAL D & G HEMOGLOBINS

Hemoglobins D and G are rare in the USA but occur with a higher incidence in other parts of the world. Hemoglobin D has been reported particularly from the Punjab area of India and in parts of Turkey and Africa, as well as occasionally in North American blacks and Indians. It is generally asymptomatic unless associated with another abnormal hemoglobin such as S. Hemoglobin D-β^0 thalassemia may result in moderate anemia. Hemoglobin G, even in the homozygous form, has not been associated with symptoms but has been described in combination with other abnormal hemoglobins as a cause of mild anemia.

The majority of the other abnormal hemoglobins that have been described occur only in the heterozygous form and are asymptomatic.

Dawod ST et al: Hemoglobin D-β^0 thalassemia: A case report and family study. *Am J Pediatr Hematol Oncol* 1988;**10:**316.

9. THERMOLABILE (Unstable) HEMOGLOBINS

Since the first report in 1960, a number of families have now been described with a mild form of hemolytic anemia due to a hemoglobinopathy in which the hemoglobin is thermolabile. All of these patients with unstable hemoglobins have had mild anemia and scleral jaundice. They frequently report intermittent exacerbations of hemolysis, and in all cases a dark brown urine has been noted. Mild splenomegaly is usually present. The disorders appear to be transmitted as an autosomal dominant, with symptoms occurring in the heterozygous form.

The laboratory findings reveal a typical picture of a hemolytic anemia with a mild to moderate depression of the hemoglobin and hematocrit and a significant elevation of the reticulocyte count. The unconjugated (indirect reacting) serum bilirubin is often slightly elevated, and haptoglobin levels are usually zero, confirming the evidence for hemolysis. The blood smear in some patients has demonstrated marked basophilic stippling. The osmotic fragility test may show both increased fragility and increased resistance. The autohemolysis test is normal. Specific diagnostic studies include the presence of Heinz bodies, particularly after incubation at 37 °C for 48 hours. Hemoglobin electrophoresis in some families has shown an abnormal hemoglobin on paper electrophoresis at pH 8.5. In all cases in which the abnormal hemoglobin was identified on electrophoresis, it has migrated more slowly than hemoglobin A$_1$ and frequently has been more readily identified on starch gel or agar gel. The percentage of abnormal hemoglobin identified has usually been low (in the range of 5–10%). The heat stability test is the best method for identification of the thermolabile hemoglobin. All of the reported hemoglobins precipitate with heating to 50 °C for 1 hour. The dark pigment in the urine has been identified as mesobilifuscin.

At least 50 different unstable hemoglobins have been identified to date. These include Scott, Zurich, Köln, Ubi 1, Summersmith, Dacie, Seattle, St. Mary's, Sydney, King's County, and others.

The differential diagnosis includes all of the hereditary hemolytic anemias such as spherocytosis and the nonspherocytic group as well as the other hemoglobinopathies. The autosomal dominant genetic transmission tends to exclude the majority of these except for spherocytosis. The diagnostic test is a demonstration of a thermolabile hemoglobin in the blood and the presence of mesobilifuscin in the urine.

The prognosis in most patients is probably good, since the anemia appears to be mild. There is no specific treatment.

Vichinsky EP, Lubin BH: Unstable hemoglobins, hemoglobins with altered oxygen affinity, and m-hemoglobins. *Pediatr Clin North Am* 1980;**27:**421.

10. HEMOGLOBINOPATHIES WITH ABNORMAL OXYGEN AFFINITY

Over 20 different hemoglobinopathies have been described in which the primary clinical sign is polycythemia. The individuals have been heterozygous for the abnormal hemoglobins (eg, hemoglobins Chesapeake, Malmö, Yakima, and Rainier), and the condition is usually transmitted as an autosomal dominant. These hemoglobins have an increased oxygen affinity that results in decreased tissue oxygenation and a compensatory erythrocytosis. Most affected individuals have been asymptomatic except for plethora.

At least 3 different hemoglobins with low oxygen affinity have been described. They may demonstrate cyanosis (hemoglobin Kansas) or anemia (hemoglobin Seattle).

THALASSEMIA SYNDROMES

1. BETA THALASSEMIA MINOR (Thalassemia Trait, Cooley's Carrier State)

Essentials of Diagnosis
- Mild hypochromic anemia.
- Unresponsiveness to iron.
- Elevated A_2 hemoglobin.
- Usually in Mediterranean, black, or Asian persons.

General Considerations
Beta thalassemia is due to a genetic defect in the production of beta globin chains of hemoglobin. The patient with thalassemia minor is heterozygous for the gene.

Clinical Findings
A. Symptoms and Signs: There are usually no symptoms, and the only physical sign may be slight enlargement of the spleen.

B. Laboratory Findings: The anemia is usually mild; the hemoglobin is rarely under 9 g/dL and may be within normal limits. The red count and hematocrit are very slightly reduced. The red cells are small and hypochromic, with low MCV and MCH. Target cells are often present, and stippled cells are seen occasionally. Variations in the size and shape of the cells are often noted. The reticulocyte count may be slightly elevated but is frequently within normal limits. Osmotic fragility is markedly decreased.

The diagnosis is confirmed by finding an elevation of the A_2 hemoglobin on electrophoresis in 90% of families; fetal hemoglobin is increased in 10% of families. (In alpha thalassemia—see below—the A_2 hemoglobin is normal.) The serum iron may be normal in infancy but becomes elevated. The bone marrow may show excessive iron deposition in the older child. Free erythrocyte protoporphyrin is normal.

Differential Diagnosis
The primary differentiation is from other mild hypochromic anemias. In childhood, nutritional iron deficiency is readily differentiated by the finding of low serum iron levels and a response to iron therapy. In iron deficiency, free erythrocyte protoporphyrin is elevated, and the hemoglobin A_2 concentration is normal. Lead poisoning and pyridoxine-responsive

anemia may present with a similar hematologic picture.

Several closely related beta thalassemialike carrier states have been described. One of these, the Lepore trait, is characterized by a mild hypochromic anemia and an abnormal hemoglobin, which comprises approximately 10% of the hemoglobin. Delta-beta thalassemia is characterized by low A_2 and high fetal hemoglobins.

Complications
There are no complications of thalassemia trait in childhood. In late adult life, excess accumulation of iron may lead to hemosiderosis.

Treatment
No therapy is indicated. Iron should definitely not be administered.

Ohene-Frempong K, Rappaport E, Schwartz E: Thalassemia syndromes: Recent advances. *Hematol Oncol Clin North Am* 1987;**1**:503.

2. BETA THALASSEMIA MAJOR (Cooley's Anemia, Mediterranean Anemia)

Essentials of Diagnosis
- Moderate to very severe anemia.
- Marked erythroblastemia.
- Splenomegaly and hepatomegaly.
- Elevated fetal hemoglobin.
- Usually Mediterranean, African, Arabian, or Southeast Asian ancestry.

General Considerations
Beta thalassemia major occurs in persons who are homozygous for a beta thalassemia gene or doubly heterozygous for 2 different beta thalassemia genes. The severe anemia is caused both by a quantitative deficiency in production of beta globin chains of adult hemoglobin (hemoglobin A_1) and by hemolysis related to the excess alpha globins in the red cell. Ineffective erythropoiesis and increased intramedullary hemolysis contribute to the anemia. In the beta^0 thalassemias, no beta globin is produced, and the disease is very severe. The disorder is more mild in the beta$^+$ thalassemias where some A_1 hemoglobin is produced.

The beta thalassemia genes are most prevalent in southern Europe, Arabia, the Middle East, Africa, and Southeast Asia. The beta^0 thalassemias occur primarily in the Mediterranean area and Southeast Asia, whereas the beta$^+$ form is most common in Africa but occurs in Asia as well.

Molecular genetic techniques make prenatal diagnosis possible in most families.

Clinical Findings
A. Symptoms and Signs: In the beta^0 thalas-

semias, severe anemia usually does not manifest itself clinically until about age 1, because of the protective effect of normal fetal hemoglobin. However, splenomegaly and mild anemia are often noted by 6 months. Massive splenomegaly and significant hepatomegaly are usually seen by age 2 and continue until the spleen extends into the pelvis. Physical growth and sexual development are markedly impaired, and there is increased susceptibility to infections. As the child approaches the school years, the widening of the flat bones of the face and skull in association with marrow hypertrophy gives all children with thalassemia major a characteristic facies: prominence of the malar eminences, depression of the bridge of the nose, a slightly oblique appearance of the eyes, and an enlargement of the superior maxilla with upward protrusion of the lip. The anemia is severe; after age 1, frequent transfusions are usually required. Jaundice may be present. The clinical manifestations are less severe in the beta$^+$ thalassemias.

B. Laboratory Findings: In the beta^0 thalassemias, the blood smear reveals a severe hypochromic microcytic anemia with marked anisocytosis and poikilocytosis. Target cells are prominent. Nucleated red cells are numerous and often exceed the circulating white blood cells. The hemoglobin is low (5–6 g/dL). The reticulocyte count is significantly elevated. Platelet and white cell counts are frequently high. Serum bilirubin is elevated. The diagnosis is confirmed by hemoglobin electrophoresis, which reveals no abnormal hemoglobin but a marked increase in fetal hemoglobin and in A$_2$ hemoglobin. The exact level of fetal hemoglobin should be determined by the alkali denaturation method. Osmotic fragility is markedly decreased. The bone marrow shows marked erythroid hyperplasia with increased iron deposition. The anemia is less marked in the beta$^+$ thalassemias (hemoglobin 8–10 g/dL).

C. Imaging: Bone x-rays are very characteristic and reveal an increase in the medullary area with thinning of the cortex. The skull has a "hair-on-end" appearance.

Differential Diagnosis

There is usually no problem in the diagnosis of homozygous thalassemia, because essentially no other disease shows the characteristic peripheral blood and hemoglobin electrophoresis findings. The primary clinical differentiation is among the combinations of thalassemia and other abnormal hemoglobins, as in thalassemia-hemoglobin S disease, thalassemia-hemoglobin E disease, etc. These have similar clinical pictures but are usually more mild. They are differentiated by the electrophoretic pattern.

Complications

Patients with beta^0 thalassemia major have multiple complications. They have an increased suscepti-

bility to infections, particularly following splenectomy. Acute benign nonspecific pericarditis is a common problem. Repeated fractures are associated with the thinning of cortical bone. The multiple transfusions that are required are ultimately associated with transfusion reactions and the development of leukocyte antibodies. Growth is impaired, and adolescent development of secondary sex characteristics is delayed. Cholelithiasis and cholecystitis are almost always present in the adolescent or young adult. The major complication, however, is the development of hemochromatosis secondary to excessive absorption and transfusion of iron in these patients. This results in cirrhosis and in heart failure. Cardiac complications are related primarily to the heavy deposition of iron in the myocardium, and death is usually due to heart failure.

Treatment

There is no specific treatment for thalassemia major. Infections should be treated promptly with antibiotics, and heart failure with digitalis and other appropriate therapy.

A. Transfusion: Blood transfusion is the primary therapeutic measure in beta^0 thalassemia major. Packed red cells are indicated (in many cases, every 3–4 weeks) to maintain the hemoglobin level above 12 g/dL. This therapy has been associated with increased vigor and well-being, improved growth, and fewer overall complications. Frequent transfusions reduce gastrointestinal absorption of iron. Hemochromatosis will still develop unless iron chelation is carried out. Life expectancy may be greater if the hemoglobin is maintained at a nearly normal level. Beta$^+$ thalassemia patients are usually not transfusion-dependent.

B. Chelation: The chelating agent deferoxamine (Desferal), when given by slow continuous infusion either intravenously or subcutaneously, has proved effective in removing iron in chronically transfused patients. The subcutaneous route is most practical; the drug is administered by a small portable infusion pump in a dose of 2–4 g over a 12-hour period. Urinary excretion is enhanced by ascorbic acid given orally in a dose of 200–500 mg daily.

C. Folic Acid: A relative folic acid deficiency may develop because of the marked overproduction of bone marrow. Folic acid, 1 mg daily orally, is often of value.

D. Splenectomy: Splenectomy is usually of value in the older child and is definitely indicated if the transfusion requirements become progressively greater. It is also indicated for the abdominal discomfort and distention associated with massive enlargement of the organ. Although splenectomy does not change the basic rate of hemolysis, it will eliminate the hypersplenism, which further shortens survival of the patient's red cells and the transfused red cells. The hazard of severe and overwhelming infection following splenectomy is much greater in patients with thalassemia major than in any other group, and the use of prophylactic penicillin following this procedure is recommended. Pneumococcal and *Haemophilus influenzae* vaccines should also be administered.

E. Testosterone: Testosterone may stimulate bone marrow and enhance the patient's red cell production.

F. Bone Marrow Transplantation: This has been tried with success and may be considered if an HLA-compatible donor is available.

Prognosis

The prognosis has improved significantly in the past decades and should continue to improve with frequent transfusions to maintain a high level of hemoglobin and the use of chelating agents to remove iron and prevent hemosiderosis. Very few patients survived into adult life in the past, although the majority reached adolescence.

Alter BP: Antenatal diagnosis of thalassemia: A review. *Ann N Y Acad Sci* 1985;**445**:393.

Cohen A: Management of iron overload in the pediatric patient. *Hematol Oncol Clin North Am* 1987;**1**:521.

Lucarelli G et al: Marrow transplantation for thalassemia after treatment with busulfan and cyclophosphamide. *Ann N Y Acad Sci* 1985;**445**:428.

Ohene-Frempong K, Rappaport E, Schwartz E: Thalassemia syndromes: Recent advances. *Hematol Oncol Clin North Am* 1987;**1**:503.

Wolfe L et al: Prevention of cardiac disease by subcutaneous deferoxamine in patients with thalassemia major. *N Engl J Med* 1985;**312**:1600.

3. THALASSEMIA VARIANTS

Double heterozygosity of thalassemia with other hemoglobinopathies such as C, S, and E is fairly common in certain parts of the world; these variants manifest themselves clinically as milder forms of thalassemia major. The diagnosis is made by hemoglobin electrophoresis, which shows a predominance of fetal hemoglobin and the other abnormal hemoglobin. Family studies will reveal one parent to be a thalassemia carrier and the other a carrier of C, S, or E.

4. HEREDITARY PERSISTENCE OF FETAL HEMOGLOBIN

Hereditary persistence of fetal hemoglobin occurs most commonly black and Greek families. It is usually found in the heterozygous form and is associated with no symptoms. The blood counts and blood smears are normal. The fetal hemoglobin level is approximately 20% after 2 years of age and higher than normal during infancy. The homozygous form is also asymptomatic. There is usually a deletion of the beta globin gene complex, and the switch from gamma to beta globin chain production does not occur. The double heterozygous state with hemoglobin S is asymptomatic but can mimic homozygous (SS) disease on electrophoresis. Nondeletional forms also occur and have been recognized in individuals with sickle cell anemia and very elevated fetal hemoglobin.

Stamatoyannopoulos G, Nienhuis AW: Hemoglobin switching. In: *The Molecular Basis of Blood Diseases.* Stamatoyannopoulos G et al. Saunders, 1987.

5. ALPHA THALASSEMIA

Defective production of alpha chains also results in anemia. Several different forms of alpha thalassemia have been described. The disorder has been recognized chiefly in Southeast Asia (especially Thailand) and in blacks. Recent evidence indicates that 4 alpha globin genes exist and that different degrees of severity of anemia are related to the number of gene deletions.

The alpha thalassemia carriers who lack one gene ("silent carriers") are completely asymptomatic and have normal blood findings. Those with 2 deleted genes show mild hypochromia and microcytosis on the blood smear. No abnormal hemoglobin is demonstrated in older children with the 2-gene deletion, and there are no compensatory increases in hemoglobin A_2 or fetal hemoglobin. Bart's hemoglobin (4 gamma chains) is present in small amounts at birth. This mild form of alpha thalassemia has been found in 5–7% of blacks in the USA and is common in Southeast Asian and Arabian peoples. Sickle cell disease is less severe in persons with the 2-gene deletion type of alpha thalassemia.

The disorder previously called thalassemia-hemoglobin H disease is now recognized to be a form of alpha thalassemia in which 3 of the 4 genes are deleted. It has been described primarily in Southeast Asia. The patient demonstrates a chronic microcytic anemia that is refractory to iron therapy and tends to resemble an intermediate form of beta thalassemia. Hemoglobin electrophoresis at pH 8.5 reveals a fast hemoglobin (hgb H) that migrates more rapidly than A_1. This hemoglobin is composed of 4 beta chains. Characteristic red cell inclusions are demonstrated by the reticulocyte stain upon incubation. There is no satisfactory treatment. Iron should not be administered to patients with any form of alpha thalassemia unless associated iron deficiency is present.

The most severe type of alpha thalassemia is caused by deletion of all 4 genes and is incompatible with life. These severely anemic and hydropic infants have only Bart's hemoglobin because they are unable to produce any alpha hemoglobin chains. Intrauterine diagnosis of the alpha thalassemias is now possible.

Kulozik AE et al: The molecular basis of thalassemia in India: Its interaction with the sickle gene. *Blood* 1988; **71**:467.

Lie-Injo LE et al: Hb Bart's level in cord blood and deletions of alpha-globin genes. *Blood* 1982;**59**:370.

Ohene-Frempong K, Rappaport E, Schwartz E: Thalassemia syndromes: Recent advances. *Hematol Oncol Clin North Am* 1987;**1**:503.

ACQUIRED HEMOLYTIC ANEMIAS

1. AUTOIMMUNE HEMOLYTIC ANEMIA

Essentials of Diagnosis

- Sudden pallor, fatigue, and jaundice.
- Splenomegaly.
- Positive Coombs test.
- Reticulocytosis and spherocytosis.

General Considerations

Acquired autoimmune hemolytic anemia is rare during the first 4 months of life but is one of the more common causes of acute anemia after the first year. It is caused by antibodies that coat the red cells and are responsible for the positive direct Coombs test. Circulating antibodies are demonstrated by the indirect Coombs test. The "primary" (or idiopathic) cases may be associated with an unrecognized preceding infection. The disease may be "symptomatic" and may occur in association with a known infection such as hepatitis, viral pneumonia, or infectious mononucleosis; or it may occur as a manifestation of a generalized autoimmune disease such as disseminated lupus erythematosus or with a type of cancer such as Hodgkin's disease or leukemia. The antibodies may be of the "cold-reacting" IgM type or "warm" antibodies of the IgG type.

Clinical Findings

A. Symptoms and Signs: The disease usually has an acute onset and is associated with weakness, pallor, and fatigue. Hemoglobinuria may be present. Jaundice and splenomegaly are often present. Occasional cases are chronic and insidious in onset. Clinical evidence of the underlying disease such as infection or lupus erythematosus may be present.

B. Laboratory Findings: The anemia is normochromic and normocytic and may be very severe, with hemoglobin levels as low as 3–4 g/dL. Occasionally, the secondary form of acquired hemolytic anemia may be very mild and may present with evidence of a positive Coombs test but with compensated anemia. Reticulocytes are usually increased but occasionally may be normal or low. Spherocytes are usually present, and within 24 hours nucleated red cells and reticulocytes are present in the peripheral blood. There is usually a significant leukocytosis, and the platelet count may be elevated. Bone marrow shows a marked erythroid hyperplasia. Both the direct and indirect Coombs tests are usually positive. Autoagglutination may be present, and for this reason the patient may be incorrectly typed as AB, Rh-positive. The indirect serum bilirubin may be elevated, and the stool and urine urobilinogen are increased.

Differential Diagnosis

The principal condition to be differentiated in childhood is hereditary spherocytic anemia in crisis, because both diseases present with acute hemolysis and spherocytosis. The Coombs test differentiates the 2 anemias, because it is negative in hereditary spherocytosis. The Coombs test likewise differentiates autoimmune hemolytic anemia from essentially all other anemias except erythroblastosis.

Complications

The anemia may be very severe and result in shock, requiring emergency management. Thrombocytopenia may occur as an associated autoimmune condition. The complications of the underlying disease such as disseminated lupus erythematosus or lymphoma may be present in the symptomatic form.

Treatment

Medical management of the underlying disease is important in symptomatic cases.

A. Transfusion: Transfusion is necessary in the acute disease and may be an emergency procedure. Difficulty in cross-matching will usually be encountered. A search should be made for blood that will provide the best major cross-match. Packed, washed cells are often more compatible. The IgG antibody is often type-specific (particularly to one of the Rh antigens), and cross-matching may be possible, whereas the IgM antibody is usually a panagglutinin (frequently anti-I). Transfusion occasionally must be given in spite of agglutination or a positive Coombs test in the major cross-match. Donor cells may be destroyed at a rapid rate, particularly if compatible blood cannot be found. Donor cells may be tagged with ^{51}Cr to determine their rate of survival in severe cases.

B. Immunosuppressive Therapy: Medical treatment to block the immune process or the reticuloendothelial system is indicated. Corticosteroid therapy in the form of hydrocortisone intravenously in large doses or prednisone, 2 mg/kg/d orally, should be tried initially. If a response is observed, the dose is decreased at weekly intervals until the lowest level that will maintain the patient in remission is reached. Other immunosuppressive drugs such as cyclophosphamide, mercaptopurine, or azathioprine may be tried alone or in conjunction with corticosteroid therapy.

C. Heparin: Heparin may be useful in the IgM type (which binds complement) because of its anti-complementary effect. It may also help prevent intravascular coagulation and the associated secondary renal disease.

D. Exchange Transfusion or Plasmapheresis: Plasma or whole blood exchange transfusion or plasmapheresis will temporarily wash out antibody and may be a lifesaving measure in severe cases.

E. Splenectomy: Splenectomy may be beneficial in cases in which all forms of medical treatment have failed. About 50% of cases may be expected to respond to this procedure, particularly those with an IgG antibody.

F. Intravenous Gamma Globulin: Intravenous gamma globulin has been effective in large doses (400 mg/kg/d or greater for 5 days).

Prognosis

The disease is self-limited in most idiopathic cases in childhood, although hemolysis does not usually cease completely for months to years; the Coombs test often remains weakly positive for years. Most patients will show a response to corticosteroid therapy, and about 50% will improve with splenectomy. In the majority of chronic cases, there is a basic underlying disease or immunologic disorder.

Bussel JB et al: Intravenous treatment of autoimmune hemolytic anemia with gamma globulin. *Pediatr Res* 1984;**12**:237.

Heidemann SM et al: Exchange transfusion for autoimmune hemolytic anemia. *Am J Pediatr Hematol Oncol* 1988;**9**:302.

Salama A, Mueller-Eckhardt C: Autoimmune haemolytic anaemia in childhood associated with non-complement binding IgM autoantibodies. *Br J Haematol* 1987; **65**:67.

Schreiber AD: Autoimmune hemolytic anemia. *Pediatr Clin North Am* 1980;**27**:253.

2. MISCELLANEOUS ACQUIRED (NONIMMUNE) Hemolytic Anemias

A wide variety of extracorpuscular mechanisms can produce hemolysis of a nonimmune type. Hemolysis in association with ingestion of oxidant drugs (eg, antimalarials, sulfonamides) or uncooked fava beans occurs primarily in individuals with a deficiency of G6PD. Certain other chemicals and drugs such as arsenic and benzene may produce hemolysis by their direct effect. Exposure to physical agents such as extreme heat or cold may cause hemolysis. Hemolytic anemia is a common complication of severe burns. Microangiopathic hemolytic anemia, characterized by fragmented cells (schistocytes), is often a major complication of disseminated intravascular coagulation and the hemolytic-uremic syndrome.

Many bacterial infections with hemolytic organisms such as *Bartonella bacilliformis* and *Clostridium perfringens* produce hemolysis. In the neonatal period, hemolytic anemia may be a complication of almost any infection, but it is seen most commonly with hemolytic staphylococcal and *Escherichia coli* infections. Malaria and some other parasitic diseases are characteristically associated with hemolysis. The venom of most poisonous snakes (in particular, the pit vipers of North America) contains a hemolysin, as do the venoms of certain spiders. The management of the majority of the acquired toxic hemolytic anemias is dependent upon the removal of the offending agent or treatment of the toxic disorder. Transfusion may be important in the more severe cases.

Hemolysis in heart disease or after open heart surgery has been reported. This hemolysis has usually occurred in cases of certain congenital valvular defects, in situations where a jet of blood was driven against a Teflon prosthesis, and in cases of prosthetic valve replacement. The hemolysis is on a mechanical basis.

II. POLYCYTHEMIA & METHEMOGLOBINEMIA

PRIMARY ERYTHROCYTOSIS (Benign Familial Polycythemia)

This is the most common type of primary polycythemia of childhood. It differs from polycythemia vera in that it affects only the erythroid series; the white cell count and platelet count are normal. It frequently occurs on a familial basis as an autosomal dominant, although it may also occur as an autosomal recessive. There are usually no physical findings except for plethora and splenomegaly. The hemoglobin may be as high as 27 g/dL, with a hematocrit of 80% and a red cell count of 10 million/μL. There are usually no symptoms other than headache and lethargy. Recent studies in a number of families have revealed (1) an abnormal hemoglobin with increased oxygen affinity, (2) reduced red cell diphosphoglycerate, or (3) autonomous increase in erythropoietin production.

Treatment is not indicated unless symptoms are marked. Phlebotomy is the treatment of choice.

Adamson JW: Familial polycythemia. *Semin Hematol* 1975; **12**:383.

SECONDARY POLYCYTHEMIA
(Compensatory Polycythemia)

Secondary polycythemia occurs in response to hypoxia in any condition that results in a lowered oxygen saturation of the blood. The most common cause of secondary polycythemia is cyanotic congenital heart disease. It also occurs in chronic pulmonary disease such as cystic fibrosis and in pulmonary arteriovenous shunts. Persons living at extremely high altitudes, as well as those with methemoglobinemia and sulfhemoglobinemia, develop polycythemia. It has on rare occasions been described without hypoxia in association with renal tumors, brain tumors, Cushing's disease, or hydronephrosis; in association with cobalt therapy; and in patients with certain unusual hemoglobinopathies.

Polycythemia occurs normally in the neonatal period; it is particularly exaggerated in infants who are preterm or small for gestational age. In these infants, polycythemia is frequently associated with other symptoms. It may occur in infants of diabetic mothers, and it has recently been described as a manifestation of Down's syndrome in the newborn and as a complication of congenital adrenal hyperplasia.

Multiple coagulation and bleeding abnormalities have been described in severely polycythemic cardiac patients. These abnormalities include thrombocytopenia, mild consumption coagulopathy, and elevated fibrinolytic activity. Bleeding at surgery may be severe.

The ideal treatment of secondary polycythemia is correction of the underlying disorder. When this cannot be done, phlebotomy is often necessary to control the symptoms. Adequate hydration of the patient and phlebotomy with plasma replacement are indicated prior to major surgical procedures; these measures prevent the complications of thrombosis and hemorrhage. Isovolumetric exchange transfusion is the treatment of choice in severe cases.

Balcerzak SP, Bromberg PA: Secondary polycythemia. *Semin Hematol* 1975;**12**:353.

METHEMOGLOBINEMIA

Methemoglobin is formed when hemoglobin in a deoxygenated state is oxidized to the ferric form. Methemoglobin is being formed continuously in the red cells and is simultaneously reduced to hemoglobin by enzymes in the erythrocyte. Methemoglobin becomes unavailable for transport of oxygen and causes a shift in the dissociation curve of the residual oxyhemoglobin. Cyanosis is produced with methemoglobin levels of approximately 15% or greater. There are several mechanisms for the production of methemoglobinemia.

Congenital Methemoglobinemia Associated With Hemoglobin M

Congenital and familial methemoglobinemia associated with an abnormal hemoglobin molecule (hemoglobin M) is discussed under the hemoglobinopathies (see above). Affected patients are cyanotic but asymptomatic. They do not respond to any form of treatment.

Congenital Methemoglobinemia Due to Enzyme Deficiencies

Congenital methemoglobinemia is most frequently caused by congenital absence of a reducing factor in the erythrocyte that is responsible for the conversion of methemoglobin to hemoglobin in normal red cells. Most patients with this disease suffer from a deficiency of the reducing enzyme diaphorase I (coenzyme factor I). It is transmitted as an autosomal recessive trait. These patients may have as high as 40% methemoglobin but usually have no symptoms, although a mild compensatory polycythemia may be present.

Patients with methemoglobinemia associated with a deficiency of diaphorase I respond readily to treatment with ascorbic acid and with methylene blue (see below). However, treatment is not usually indicated.

Acquired Methemoglobinemia

A number of compounds activate the oxidation of hemoglobin from the ferrous to the ferric state, forming methemoglobin. These include the nitrites and nitrates (contaminated water), chlorates, and quinones. Common drugs in this group are the aniline dyes, sulfonamides, acetanilid, phenacetin, bismuth subnitrate, and potassium chlorate. Poisoning with a drug or chemical containing one of these substances should be suspected in any infant or child who presents with sudden cyanosis. Methemoglobin levels in cases of poisoning may be extremely high and can produce severe anoxia and dyspnea with unconsciousness, circulatory failure, and death. Young infants and newborns are more susceptible to poisoning because their red cells have difficulty reducing hemoglobin, probably on the basis of a transient deficiency of DPNH-dependent hemoglobin reductase. Infants with diarrhea and dehydration (acidosis) may show elevated levels of methemoglobin.

Patients with the acquired form of methemoglobinemia respond dramatically to methylene blue in a dosage of 2 mg/kg given intravenously. For infants and young children, a smaller dose (1–1.5 mg/kg) is recommended. Ascorbic acid administered orally or intravenously also reduces methemoglobin, but it acts more slowly.

Bricker T, Jefferson LS, Mintz AA: Methemoglobinemia in infants with enteritis. *J Pediatr* 1983;**102**:161.
Jaffé ER: Methaemoglobinaemia. *Clin Haematol* 1981;**10**:99.

III. DISORDERS OF LEUKOCYTES

NEUTROPENIA & AGRANULOCYTOSIS

Essentials of Diagnosis

- Increased frequency of infections.
- Ulceration of oral mucosa and throat.
- Normal red cells and platelets.

General Considerations

Neutropenia in infancy and childhood is usually defined as an absolute neutrophil (granulocyte) count of less than 1500/μL. However, in the first 2 years of life, normal infants may have absolute counts as low as 1000/μL. Most neutropenias in childhood are acquired and frequently caused by viral infections. A few are associated with other primary disorders, and some are congenital and hereditary. Many are physiologic in young children.

Neutropenias may result from absent or defective granulocyte stem cells, ineffective or suppressed myeloid maturation, decreased or absent monocyte production of granulopoietin (colony-stimulating factor), decreased marrow release, increased neutrophil destruction, or an increased neutrophil "marginating pool" (pseudoneutropenia). A classification of neutropenic disorders is shown in Table 17–4.

Benign Neutropenias of Childhood

A. Physiologic Neutropenia: After the first few weeks of life, all infants and young children have neutropenic neutrophil levels in comparison with adult levels. The normal white blood cell count of infants and children may be as low as 5000–6000/μL, and the percentage of neutrophils may normally be as low as 18–20% during the first 3–4 years of life. A diagnosis of neutropenia should be considered in infancy and early childhood only if the absolute neutrophil count is below 1000/μL. (See Table 17–2 for normal values.)

B. Pseudoneutropenia: This term is used for neutropenia that is caused by excessive marginal pooling of neutrophils along vessel walls and in the spleen. Ordinarily, about 50% of neutrophils are in the marginal pool (which equals the circulating pool). Some children have excess margination, but these neutrophils are available when needed, and there is no increased susceptibility to infection. The diagnosis is made by administration of epinephrine, which causes release of marginal neutrophils into the circulation.

C. Chronic Benign Neutropenia of Childhood: Several series of cases have been described in which persistent neutropenia was noted throughout childhood. The bone marrow usually shows nor-

Table 17–4. Neutropenias of childhood.

Acquired neutropenia
 Infection
 Drugs and chemicals (anticonvulsants, antimicrobials
  (chloramphenicol, sulfas), antithyroids, etc)
 Immune
  Drug-induced
  Neonatal alloimmune neutropenia
  Neonatal autoimmune (systemic lupus erythematosus)
  Idiopathic autoimmune neutropenia of childhood
  Secondary: Systemic lupus erythematosus, rheumatoid
   arthritis, infectious mononucleosis
 Hypersplenism
 Bone marrow hypoplasia or infiltration
Congenital and hereditary neutropenia
 Infantile genetic agranulocytosis (Kostmann's syndrome)
 Chronic hypoplastic neutropenia
 Cyclic (periodic) neutropenia
 Reticular dysgenesis
 Familial benign neutropenia
Neutropenia associated with other disorders
 Hypoplastic anemias (Pure red cell hypoplasia, Fanconi's
  anemia, dyskeratosis congenita)
 Pancreatic insufficiency and bone marrow dysfunction
  (Shwachman syndrome)
 Cartilage-hair hypoplasia
 Immunodeficiency syndromes (agammaglobulinemia and
  dysgammaglobulinemia)
 Metabolic disorders
  Hyperglycinemia
  Isovaleric acidemia
  Methylmalonic acidemia
  Type IB glycogen storage disease

mal cellularity but abnormal maturation of granulocytes. In most cases, neutrophils represent about 10% of the circulating leukocytes, and infection is not a serious problem. Spontaneous remission may occur. The neutrophil count usually rises with bacterial infections and in response to administration of endotoxins or cortisone.

Clinical Findings

A. Symptoms and Signs: The symptoms are those of infection, with chills and fever. Sore throat and oral mucosa ulceration are common, and chronic or recurrent staphylococcal skin infection is frequent. In most cases, the spleen and liver are not enlarged. A complete history should be taken, and a physical examination should be performed to look for acquired or congenital causes of the disease. A family history should also be taken.

B. Laboratory Findings: Neutrophils are absent or markedly reduced in the peripheral blood. In the purer forms of neutropenia or agranulocytosis, the monocytes and lymphocytes will be normal and the red cells and platelets not affected. The bone marrow usually shows a normal erythroid series, with adequate megakaryocytes but a marked reduction in the myeloid cells or a significant delay in maturation of this series.

White blood cell counts should be taken for parents and siblings.

If there is no obvious acquired cause such as viral infection or drug ingestion and no other primary disease, tests should be performed as follows: White blood cell counts should be performed twice weekly for 2 months to diagnose cyclic neutropenia. An epinephrine stimulation test will diagnose pseudoneutropenia due to "marginal pooling." The absolute neutrophil count should more than double. Epinephrine, 0.1 mL (1:1000 solution), is given subcutaneously, and neutrophil counts are done at 5, 10, 20, 40, and 60 minutes. Bone marrow aspiration and biopsy are most important. If marrow is normally cellular, marrow release may be measured by stimulation with intravenous hydrocortisone, 50–100 mg, or typhoid vaccine, 0.5 mL subcutaneously. Neutrophil counts are recorded every 30 minutes for 4 hours. Measure immunoglobulins to detect associated dysgammaglobulinemias. Elevated urinary muramidase levels and elevated serum lactoferrin may be found if increased neutrophil destruction is the cause. Other more specific tests to identify the mechanism of neutropenia include chemotactic studies and measurement of neutrophil antibodies if the marrow is highly cellular. Cultures of bone marrow and buffy coat are evaluated for colony-forming units and production of colony-stimulating factor (granulopoietin).

Treatment

Removal of the toxic agent or treatment of the associated disease is essential if one can be identified. Otherwise, treatment consists of administering appropriate antibiotics. Prophylactic antimicrobial therapy is not indicated, and the patient should be managed with specific therapy directed toward the infecting organism.

Marrow stimulation with testosterone or with testosterone plus one of the corticosteroids (see Aplastic Anemia) or a course of antilymphocyte globulin (ALG) may be tried in chronic cases, but there is little evidence that it is effective.

Fresh-frozen plasma has produced remissions in a few cases with immunoglobulin deficiencies, and intravenous immune globulin has helped in the idiopathic autoimmune neutropenia of childhood. Chloramphenicol has been reported to cause maturation of granulocytes in one type of congenital neutropenia.

Prognosis

The prognosis varies greatly with the cause and severity of the neutropenia. In severe cases with persistent agranulocytosis, the prognosis is very poor in spite of antibiotic therapy; in mild or cyclic forms of neutropenia, symptoms may be minimal and the prognosis for normal life expectancy excellent.

Bussel J, Lalezari P, Fikrig S: Intravenous treatment with γ-globulin of autoimmune neutropenia of infancy. *J Pediatr* 1988;**112**:298.

Cairo MS: Neonatal neutrophil host defense. *Am J Dis Child* 1989;**143**:40.

Lange RD, Jones JB: Cyclic neutropenia: Review of clinical manifestations and management. *Am J Pediatr Hematol Oncol* 1981;**3**:363.

Stork LC et al: Pancytopenia in propionic acidemia: Hematologic evaluation and studies of hematopoiesis in vitro. *Pediatr Res* 1986;**20**:783.

Weetman RM, Boxer LA: Childhood neutropenia. *Pediatr Clin North Am* 1980;**27**:361.

MYELOPROLIFERATIVE DISORDER OF DOWN'S SYNDROME

A severe myeloproliferative disorder affecting granulocytes, erythrocytes, platelets, or any combination of these cell lines may be present at birth in infants with Down's syndrome. The granulocytic hyperplasia with immature cells in the blood is the most common and has in the past been confused with acute or subacute myelogenous leukemia. It clears spontaneously and should not be treated with antileukemic therapy. There is a significant mortality rate from bleeding or infection in the first few weeks before the marrow recovers and matures.

Nakagawa T et al: Hyperviscosity syndrome with transient abnormal myelopoiesis in Down syndrome. *J Pediatr* 1988;**112**:58.

Nix WL, Fernbach JD: Myeloproliferative diseases in childhood. *Am J Pediatr Hematol Oncol* 1981;**3**:397.

Wong KY et al: Transient myeloproliferative disorder and acute nonlymphoblastic leukemia in Down syndrome. *J Pediatr* 1988;**112**:18.

GRANULOCYTE FUNCTION DISORDERS

Disorders of neutrophil function include those related to cell movement, adherence, phagocytosis, and bacterial killing. Examples of primary defects in cell movement (chemotaxis) are **Chédiak-Higashi syndrome** (recurrent infections, decreased skin pigment, nystagmus, and giant granules in leukocytes and platelets) and **lazy leukocyte syndrome.** Acquired or transient defects in chemotaxis are associated with diabetes mellitus, burns, malnutrition, and corticosteroid therapy or may occur during the neonatal period. A leukocyte adherence defect called **congenital neutrophil glycoprotein deficiency** is characterized by recurrent bacterial infections, elevated white blood cell count, delayed umbilical cord separation, and severe periodontitis. Disorders of phagocytosis are related to deficient opsonization of bacteria and are seen in patients with antibody deficiencies, lack of complement (C3), or primary cellular abnormality (actin dysfunction). The clinically important defects in microbial killing are related to intracellular oxygen-dependent mechanisms as seen in **chronic granulomatous disease** (X-linked disorder of chronic purulent infections of lymph nodes, skin, liver, lungs), severe G6PD deficiency, and myeloperoxidase deficiency.

Little specific therapy is available for patients with primary defects in granulocyte function. In general, treatment is directed toward management of infections and includes prompt antibiotic therapy with drugs that penetrate cell membranes (eg, chloramphenicol in chronic granulomatous disease), surgical drainage of suppurative lesions, and general supportive care. Ascorbate therapy has been used in Chédiak-Higashi syndrome; sulfisoxazole may help in chronic granulomatous disease. The prognosis is poor in severe disorders such as chronic granulomatous disease and Chédiak-Higashi syndrome. In cases of chemotaxic or opsonization defects, fresh plasma transfusions may be of benefit if a plasma component is deficient (antibody, complement).

Ambruso DR, Johnston RB: *Immunodeficiency Disorders.* Chandra RK (editor). Churchill Livingstone, 1981.
Boxer GJ, Curnutte JT, Boxer LA: Polymorphonuclear leukocyte function. *Hosp Pract* (March) 1985;**20**:69.
Gallin JI et al: Recent advances in chronic granulomatous disease. *Ann Intern Med* 1983;**99**:657.

IV. BLEEDING DISORDERS

Bleeding disorders may be classified as (1) defects in small vessel hemostasis, which include (a) quantitative and qualitative abnormalities of platelets (thrombocytopenia, platelet function defects, and thrombocythemia) and (b) the vascular disorders; and (2) intravascular disorders (defects in blood coagulation).

The initial laboratory workup for screening patients with bleeding disorders should include a careful history and physical examination and all of the following laboratory investigations:

(1) Bleeding time to test small vessel integrity and platelet function.

(2) Platelet count or estimation of platelet number on blood smear.

(3) Partial thromboplastin time (PTT) to measure clotting activity of factors XII, IX, XI, VIII, X, II, V, and fibrinogen.

(4) One-stage prothrombin time (PT) to screen the tissue thromboplastin system of coagulation (factors II, V, VII, X, and fibrinogen).

(5) Thrombin time to measure antithrombin effect of fibrin split products or heparin as well as fibrinogen level and function.

(6) Fibrinogen determination.

With this battery of screening tests, it is usually possible to determine the general area of the defect and proceed with more specific tests in order to make an exact diagnosis.

Katsanis E et al: Prevalence and significance of mild bleeding disorders in children with recurrent epistaxis. *J Pediatr* 1988;**113**:73.
Rapaport SI: Brief review: Preoperative hemostatic evaluation: Which tests, if any? *Blood* 1983;**61**:229.

ABNORMALITIES OF PLATELET NUMBER OR FUNCTION

IDIOPATHIC THROMBOCYTOPENIC PURPURA
(Werlhof's Disease, Purpura Haemorrhagica)

Essentials of Diagnosis

- Petechiae, ecchymoses.
- Decreased platelet count.
- No splenomegaly.
- Normal bone marrow examination.

General Considerations

Acute idiopathic thrombocytopenic purpura is the most common bleeding disorder of childhood. It most frequently follows infections, particularly the common contagious diseases (rubella, varicella, and rubeola). As a rule, it is self-limited; this is particularly true of the postinfectious type, the majority of which cases recover spontaneously within a few months and approximately 90% within a year after onset. Chronic idiopathic thrombocytopenic purpura is rare in childhood.

Most cases of idiopathic thrombocytopenic purpura are felt to be an immunologic disorder, and platelet-associated IgG can usually be demonstrated. The spleen plays a major role by sequestering damaged platelets and by forming antibodies.

Clinical Findings

A. Symptoms and Signs: The onset is usually acute, with the appearance of multiple ecchymoses. Petechiae are often present, and epistaxis is common. There are no other physical findings, and the spleen is not palpable.

B. Laboratory Findings:

1. Blood—The platelet count is markedly reduced (usually < 50,000/μL), and platelets are decreased and frequently of larger size on peripheral blood smear. The white blood count and differential count are normal. Anemia is not present unless hemorrhage has occurred.

2. Bone marrow—The bone marrow usually shows increased numbers of megakaryocytes.

3. Other laboratory tests—The bleeding time is prolonged, and clot retraction is abnormal. PTT and PT are normal. Platelet-associated IgG may be demonstrated in the platelets or serum (platelet antibody testing).

Differential Diagnosis

The presence of a low platelet count immediately differentiates idiopathic thrombocytopenic purpura from all other bleeding disorders except those associated with thrombocytopenia. A normal white blood count and normal precursors in the bone marrow differentiate the idiopathic disease from leukemia and aplastic anemia. The bone marrow is important in making the differential diagnosis. The family history may be helpful in indicating hereditary or familial thrombocytopenia.

Complications

Severe exsanguinating hemorrhage and bleeding into vital organs are the primary complications of idiopathic thrombocytopenic purpura. Intracranial hemorrhage is the most serious. Complications of treatment include those associated with prolonged corticosteroid therapy. Splenectomy, particularly in children under age 2, may be associated with increased incidence of infection.

Treatment

A. General Measures: Avoidance of trauma is important, and in many postinfectious cases no other therapy may be required. In the presence of hemorrhage, blood transfusions may be necessary. Platelet transfusions are usually ineffective and should be reserved for life-threatening hemorrhage. The platelets (platelet concentrate or platelet pack) from 1 unit of blood per 6 kg of body weight are usually required to produce an observable rise in platelet count. Patients must avoid aspirin and aspirin-containing drugs.

B. Corticosteroids: Patients with a significant hemorrhagic tendency or with a platelet count less than $10,000/\mu L$ are treated with prednisone (2 mg/kg orally in divided daily doses) for a period of 2 weeks. The dosage is tapered and stopped during the third week. No further prednisone is given regardless of the level of the platelet count unless significant bleeding recurs, at which time the dosage of prednisone used is the smallest that will give symptomatic relief (usually 2.5–5 mg twice daily). The patient is then followed, using the general measures outlined above, until spontaneous remission occurs or until the patient is a candidate for splenectomy.

C. Intravenous Gamma Globulin (IVGG): As an alternative or adjunct to steroid treatment, intra-venous gamma globulin (IVGG) has been demonstrated to be effective in raising the platelet count in acute and chronic idiopathic thrombocytopenic purpura of childhood. Occasionally, IVGG is effective when the patient is resistant to steroids; responses are prompt and may last for several weeks. Most patients respond to 1 g/kg/d for 1–3 days.

D. Splenectomy: Splenectomy produces permanent remission in most cases of idiopathic thrombocytopenic purpura; however, it is now usually reserved for children who have shown no evidence of spontaneous remission over a period of 6 months to 1 year, because about 90% of children with the disease will recover without surgical intervention within 1 year after onset. If symptoms are not controlled by medical management, splenectomy may be done prior to this time, and in most cases splenectomy is advised if symptoms persist beyond 1 year after onset. Fifty to 75% of chronic cases in childhood respond to the procedure.

Bleeding is rarely a complication of splenectomy, but platelet concentrates should be available during surgery. If the patient has been receiving corticosteroid therapy prior to surgery, the dose should be increased to the full therapeutic level during and after surgery.

Anticoagulant therapy is not indicated postoperatively even though the platelets may rise to levels of approximately 1 million.

The risk of overwhelming infection is low in the older child undergoing splenectomy. It does represent a significant risk in the young child, and the procedure should be postponed if possible until the child is older. Administration of pneumococcal vaccine and prophylactic penicillin following splenectomy is indicated.

Prognosis

Spontaneous remission with permanent recovery occurs in almost 90% of cases of idiopathic thrombocytopenic purpura in childhood. (The incidence of spontaneous remission is much lower in adults.)

Buchanan GR: The nontreatment of childhood idiopathic thrombocytopenic purpura. *Eur J Pediatr* 1987; **146:**107.

Bussel JB et al: Treatment of acute idiopathic thrombocytopenia of childhood with intravenous infusions of gamma globulin. *J Pediatr* 1985;**106:**886.

Imbach P et al: Intravenous immunoglobulin versus oral corticosteroids in acute immune thrombocytopenic purpura in childhood. *Lancet* 1985;**2:**464.

Sartorius JA: Steroid treatment of idiopathic thrombocytopenic purpura in children: Preliminary results of a randomized cooperative study. *Am J Pediatr Hematol Oncol* 1984;**6:**165.

van Hoff J, Ritchey AK: Clinical and laboratory observations: Pulse methylprednisolone therapy for acute childhood idiopathic thrombocytopenic purpura. *J Pediatr* 1988;**113:**563.

THROMBOCYTOPENIA IN THE NEWBORN

Thrombocytopenia is one of the most common causes of purpura in the newborn and should be considered and investigated in any infant with petechiae or a significant bleeding tendency. A platelet count less than 150,000/μL establishes a diagnosis of thrombocytopenia in the neonatal period. A number of specific entities may be responsible (Table 17–5). Management is directed toward alleviation of the specific cause; special situations are discussed below.

Thrombocytopenia Associated with Platelet Alloimmunization

An uncommon cause of thrombocytopenia in the neonatal period is platelet alloimmunization, which is similar to the mechanism responsible for Rh blood group alloimmunization. Alloimmunization occurs when the platelet type of the infant differs from that of the mother and when a significant number of platelets cross from the fetal to the maternal circulation. Platelet antibodies can usually be demonstrated by platelet IgG-binding techniques. Petechiae are usually present shortly after birth, and a male may bleed from circumcision. The bone marrow usually shows normal to increased megakaryocytes. The disease is self-limited; platelets show a spontaneous rise within 2 weeks, with complete recovery by 4–6 weeks. Severe intracranial bleeding can occur in utero or after delivery.

Platelet transfusions may be used in an emergency. In very severe cases, exchange transfusion with fresh whole blood is effective in removing antibody and in replacing platelets temporarily; a platelet concentrate from the mother will be more effective in raising the platelet count. IVGG infusions have been used successfully to raise the platelet count (see p 500).

Thrombocytopenia Associated With Idiopathic Thrombocytopenic Purpura in the Mother

Infants born to mothers with idiopathic thrombocytopenic purpura or systemic lupus erythematosus develop thrombocytopenia as a result of passive transfer of antibody from the mother to the infant. Evaluation of the maternal platelet count is indicated in any infant with thrombocytopenia. The persistence of antibodies in the infant's circulation is temporary, and spontaneous recovery is the rule. In severe cases (platelet count < 20,000/μL), which may be detected prior to delivery by careful sampling of the infant's scalp, cesarean section should be performed. Others have advocated the administration of corticosteroids to the mother for 10–14 days prior to vaginal delivery in order to increase the infant's platelet count. Severely thrombocytopenic infants

(platelet count < 50,000/μL) can also be given a short course of corticosteroids.

Neonatal Thrombocytopenia Associated With Infections

Thrombocytopenia is commonly associated with severe generalized infections of the newborn period, particularly those which develop in utero. Megakaryocytes are decreased and immature, and splenomegaly is usually present. Other intrauterine infections such as syphilis, toxoplasmosis, and cytomegalic inclusion disease are almost invariably associated with thrombocytopenia, and thrombocytopenia is frequently present with bacterial sepsis and generalized infection with herpes simplex virus or other viruses.

In addition to specific treatment for the underlying disease if available, platelet transfusions may be indicated in severe cases. Platelet concentrate in a dos-

Table 17–5. Causes of neonatal thrombocytopenia.

Infection
    Bacterial: Sepsis, congenital syphilis
    Viral: Cytomegalic inclusion disease, disseminated herpes simplex, rubella syndrome, enteroviruses
    Other: Toxoplasmosis
Immune disorders
    Alloimmunization
    Maternal antibody-induced disorders: Systemic lupus erythematosus, idiopathic thrombocytopenic purpura, drug-associated disorders
Bone marrow abnormality
    Congenital megakaryocytic hypoplasia
    Thrombocytopenia-absent radius syndrome
    Fanconi's pancytopenia
    Aplastic anemia
    Myeloproliferative disease (Down's syndrome)
    Osteopetrosis
    Congenital leukemia
Maternal drugs
    Tolbutamide
    Thiazide diuretics
Infant drugs
    Intravenous fat emulsion (eg, Intralipid)
    Tolazoline
Intravascular coagulation syndromes
    Disseminated intravascular coagulation
    Large-vessel thrombosis (renal vein, aorta)
    Necrotizing enterocolitis
    Placental chorioangioma
Excessive peripheral utilization
    Giant hemangioma
    Hyperviscosity syndrome
    Erythroblastosis fetalis
    Congenital heart disease
Other causes
    Postexchange transfusion
    Maternal hyperthyroidism
    Metabolic disorders: Hyperglycinemia, cirrhosis, mucolipidosis
    Thrombotic thrombocytopenic purpura
    Postmature and small-for-gestational-age infants (often with maternal toxemia)
    Neonatal neuroblastoma
    Perinatal pulmonary syndromes
    Neonatal cold injury
    Hereditary thrombocytopenia

age of 10 mL/kg will raise the platelet count by about 75,000/μL.

Thrombocytopenia Associated With Giant Hemangiomas

A rare but important cause of thrombocytopenic purpura in the newborn is giant hemangioma. Platelet sequestration in the tumor results in peripheral depletion of platelets. The bone marrow usually shows marked hyperplasia of megakaryocytes. In the presence of massive hemangiomas, the thrombocytopenia may be associated with disseminated intravascular coagulation and result in fatal hemorrhage.

X-ray treatment of hemangiomas may be indicated. Heparinization is indicated if there is evidence of disseminated intravascular coagulation. Surgery is usually contraindicated because of the risk of hemorrhage. Prednisone therapy has been associated with marked regression of infantile hemangiomas.

Andrew M et al: Clinical impact of neonatal thrombocytopenia. *J Pediatr* 1987;**110**:457.

Bussel JB: Management of infants of mothers with immune thrombocytopenic purpura. *J Pediatr* 1988;**113**:497.

Esterly NB: Kasabach-Merritt syndrome in infants. *J Am Acad Dermatol* 1983;**8**:504.

Management of alloimmune neonatal thrombocytopenia. (Editorial.) *Lancet* 1989;**1**:137.

Reznikoff-Etievant MF: Management of alloimmune neonatal and antenatal thrombocytopenia. *Vox Sang* 1988;**55**: 193.

THROMBOCYTOPENIA ASSOCIATED WITH APLASTIC ANEMIA

Thrombocytopenia is frequently the first manifestation of aplastic anemia and may be present before neutropenia and anemia develop. The child who presents with amegakaryocytic thrombocytopenia in the first few years of life—particularly if there are associated skeletal anomalies—should be considered as a possible case of congenital pancytopenia of the Fanconi type.

Hedberg VA, Lipton JM: Thrombocytopenia with absent radii. *Am J Pediatr Hematol Oncol* 1988;**10**:51.

THROMBOCYTOPENIA IN LEUKEMIA

Thrombocytopenia is almost invariably a major finding in acute leukemia of childhood. This is discussed in Chapter 31.

HEREDITARY THROMBOCYTOPENIAS

At least 3 types of hereditary thrombocytopenia can be recognized based on the mode of inheritance and characteristic clinical and laboratory findings: (1) Wiskott-Aldrich syndrome is characterized by X-linked thrombocytopenia, eczema, recurrent infections, and findings of low levels of IgA and IgM immunoglobulins, impaired delayed hypersensitivity and abnormal lymphocyte function, and decreased numbers of small, poorly functioning platelets with a short life span. Variants of this disorder without the severe immunologic difficulties may be confused with chronic idiopathic thrombocytopenic purpura, and patients with this disorder are at great risk of developing overwhelming infection if splenectomy is performed. (2) Bernard-Soulier giant platelet syndrome is a rare autosomal, incompletely recessive disorder characterized by giant, bizarre platelets of varying numbers but with normal in vitro function except for defective aggregation with ristocetin. (3) A heterogeneous group of thrombocytopenias with failure to release ADP (a release defect similar to that produced by aspirin) may be inherited by either the recessive or the dominant mode and can also be confused with chronic idiopathic thrombocytopenic purpura. Platelet function tests are usually abnormal. Occasionally, these disorders are seen in association with hereditary nephritis.

Bellucci S et al: Inherited platelet disorders. *Prog Hematol* 1983;**13**:223.

Heynen MJ et al: Congenital macrothrombocytopenia, leucocyte inclusions, deafness and proteinuria: Functional and electron microscopic observations on platelets and megakaryocytes. *Br J Haematol* 1988;**70**:441.

Standen GR et al: Inherited thrombocytopenia, elevated serum IgA and renal disease: Identification as a variant of the Wiskott-Aldrich syndrome. *Q J Med* 1986; **59**:401.

DISORDERS OF PLATELET FUNCTION

The hereditary disorders of platelet function are characterized by a bleeding diathesis, usually associated with a prolonged bleeding time in spite of normal numbers of platelets. The findings in these diseases are summarized in Table 17–6. Acquired disorders of platelet function include uremia, cirrhosis, disseminated intravascular coagulation, macroglobulinemias, systemic lupus erythematosus, vitamin B_{12} deficiency, myeloproliferative disorders, acyanotic congenital heart disease, and viral infections. Many pharmacologic agents decrease platelet function. Clinically, the most important of these include aspirin, dipyridamole, phenylbutazone, and synthetic penicillins.

Champion LA et al: The effects of four commonly used drugs on platelet function. *J Pediatr* 1976;**89**:653.

Table 17–6. Hereditary platelet function disorders.[1]

Category	Heredity	Morphology	Platelet-Rich Plasma Aggregation to[2]				Specific Defects
			ADP	Collagen	AA[3]	Ristocetin	
Glanzmann's thrombasthenia	Autosomal recessive	Normal	−	−	−	+	Decreased membrane glycoprotein IIb-IIIa
Bernard-Soulier syndrome	Autosomal dominant	Giant platelets	+	+	+	−	Decreased membrane glycoprotein Ib
Storage pool deficiency syndromes: Dense body deficiency, Hermansky-Pudlak syndrome	Autosomal recessive	Electron microscopy—decreased to absent dense bodies	±	−	±	±	Decreased ADP-ATP, Ca^{2+}, serotonin storage and release
Dense body with α-granule deficiency	Autosomal dominant	Electron microscopy—decreased dense bodies and α-granules	±	−	±	±	Decreased ADP, Ca^{2+}, serotonin, PF_4,[4] fibrinogen, βTG[5] storage and release, decreased PDGF[6]
α-Granule deficiency, gray platelet syndrome	Autosomal recessive	Light gray platelets; Electron microscopy—decreased α-granules	±	±	+	+	Decreased PF_4, βTG, fibrinogen, decreased PDGF storage and release[4]
Wiskott-Aldrich syndrome	X-linked	Tiny platelets; decreased organelles	±	−	+	+	Decreased
Failure to release (aspirin like defect)	Variable	Normal	±	−	−	±	Deficiency of cyclooxygenase or thromboxane synthetase
Isolated platelet factor V deficiency	Autosomal dominant	Normal	?	?	?	?	Decreased platelet factor V function
Pseudo-von Willebrand's disease	Autosomal dominant	Normal	+	+	+	Increased	Intrinsic platelet abnormality of increased reaction with von Willebrand's factor

[1]Modified and reproduced, with permission, from Hathaway WE, Bonnar J: *Hemostatic Disorders of the Pregnant Woman and Newborn Infant.* Elsevier, 1987. Copyright 1987 by Elsevier Science Publishing Co., Inc.
[2]+ signifies yes; − signifies no; ± signifies partial or slight.
[3]AA = arachidonic acid.
[4]PF_4 = platelet factor 4.
[5]βTG = β-thromboglobulin.
[6]PDGF = platelet-derived growth factor.

Depinho RA, Kaplan KL: The Hermansky-Pudlak syndrome: Report of three cases and review of pathophysiology and management considerations. *Medicine* 1985;**64**:192.
Gootenberg JE et al: Severe hemorrhage in a patient with gray platelet syndrome. *J Pediatr* 1986;**109**:1017.

VON WILLEBRAND'S DISEASE

Essentials of Diagnosis

- History of easy bruising and epistaxis from early childhood.
- Prolonged bleeding time with normal platelet count.
- Reduced levels of factor VIII-vWf complex.

General Considerations

Von Willebrand's disease is a familial bleeding disorder that is usually transmitted as a dominant trait and occurs in both sexes. It is associated both with a prolonged bleeding time and with a reduced level of factor VIII and von Willebrand's factor (vWf). The partial thromboplastin test is usually prolonged but may be normal.

Von Willebrand's disease and variants are due to abnormalities of the factor VIII-vWf complex. In severe classic von Willebrand's disease, both the vWf molecule and the factor VIII molecule, which circulate in a complex form, are markedly reduced. Variants or types of von Willebrand's disease are based on the structure (multimeric analysis) and function of the factor VIII-vWf complex.

Clinical Findings

A. Symptoms and Signs: There is usually a history of increased bruising and severe prolonged epistaxis. Increased bleeding will also occur with lacerations or at surgery. Excessive menstrual flow is a problem in the adolescent female. Petechiae are usually not observed, and hemarthrosis is rare.

B. Laboratory Findings: A prolonged bleeding time is present; platelet number and aggregations in platelet-rich plasma are normal except for decreased platelet aggregation with the antibiotic ristocetin. Factor VIII coagulant activity (VIIIc) and vWf antigen are usually decreased but may be normal. Analysis of vWf multimers allows the disorder to be classified into types (I, IIa, IIb, III).

Treatment

The depressed levels of factor VIIIc can be easily corrected with freshly frozen plasma or cryoprecipitates. The VIIIc levels increase both after transfusion of VIIIc and as a result of endogenous production of VIIIc; therefore, VIIIc levels remain elevated longer than in classic hemophilia. Transfusions with cryoprecipitates are more effective than normal plasma in correcting the bleeding time.

In severe von Willebrand's disease (type III), one bag of cryoprecipitate per 6 kg body weight given every 6–12 hours may be necessary to correct the bleeding time adequately. Infusions of desmopressin acetate (DDAVP) have been shown to be effective in raising the factor VIII complex levels in mild to moderate von Willebrand's disease (type I).

However, in type II disease, DDAVP may be ineffective or even harmful. The intravenous dose of DDAVP is 0.3 μg /kg in 30 mL saline given slowly over 20–30 minutes.

When dental extractions are necessary, management consists of systemic correction, local pressure, and use of aminocaproic acid (Amicar).

Prognosis

Patients with mild forms of the disease have a normal life expectancy, and bleeding can be controlled with the measures noted above or may cease spontaneously. In severe cases, it may be difficult to control hemorrhage, although recent methods of therapy with plasma and concentrates have greatly improved the outlook.

Handin RI, Wagner DD: Molecular and cellular biology of von Willebrand factor. *Prog Hemost Thromb* 1989; **9:**261.

Mannucci PM: Desmopressin: A nontransfusional form of treatment for congenital and acquired bleeding disorders. *Blood* 1988;**72:**1449.

Ruggeri ZM, Zimmerman TS: Von Willebrand factor and von Willebrand disease. *Blood* 1987;**70:**895.

VASCULAR DEFECTS

ANAPHYLACTOID PURPURA (Schönlein-Henoch Purpura, Allergic Purpura)

Essentials of Diagnosis
- Purpuric cutaneous rash.
- Urticaria.
- Migratory polyarthritis.
- Gastrointestinal pain and hemorrhage.
- Hematuria.

General Considerations

Anaphylactoid purpura is characterized by a typical purpuric skin rash plus (in any combination) migratory arthritis, gastroenteritis, and nephritis. It is believed to be a vasculitis related to vessel damage by deposits of immune complexes (antigen-antibody). It is characterized by involvement of the small vessels, particularly in the skin, the gastrointestinal tract, and the kidneys. The cause of the allergic reaction is frequently not recognized, although in some parts of the world group A β-hemolytic streptococcal infection may precede the disease in some cases. Other inciting antigens such as drugs, other infections (viruses), food allergens, insect bites, and horse serum have been implicated.

Clinical Findings

A. Symptoms and Signs: Migratory polyarthritis very similar to that of rheumatic fever frequently precedes the onset of the skin rash. Gastrointestinal pain, diarrhea, and gastrointestinal bleeding are common. Nephritis occurs in about 50% of cases, either with symptomless proteinuria or hematuria or with nephrotic syndrome. The skin rash is diagnostic in appearance: It is characteristically distributed on the ankles, buttocks, and elbows; purpuric areas a few millimeters in diameter are present and may progress to form larger hemorrhages ("palpable purpura"). Petechial lesions occur, but the majority of skin or mucous membrane hemorrhages are slightly larger. The rash usually begins on the lower extremities, but the entire body may be involved. Erythematous and urticarial skin eruptions (which may become hemorrhagic) often accompany the hemorrhage. Cardiac involvement is rare.

B. Laboratory Findings: The platelet count, platelet function tests, and bleeding time are usually negative. Blood coagulation is normal except for elevated factor VIII levels and an increase in fibrin split products. Urinalysis frequently reveals hematuria and proteinuria, but casts are unusual. Stool tests may be positive for occult blood, even though gross melena is not observed. The ASO titer is frequently elevated or the throat culture positive for group A β-hemolytic streptococci. Serum IgA globulins may be elevated.

Differential Diagnosis

The hemorrhagic rash of anaphylactoid purpura can be differentiated from thrombocytopenic purpura by the presence of raised skin lesions in the former and by the platelet count. The rash of septicemia (especially meningococcemia) may be very similar, although the distribution tends to be more generalized in sepsis. Blood culture may be necessary for final diagnosis.

Complications

Intussusception of the small bowel occurs in a significant number of patients with intestinal manifestations. The most important complications derive from the renal involvement. About 10% of patients develop renal failure as a result of advancing proliferative glomerulonephritis, and an equal number will have continuing hematuria, proteinuria, and hypertension after 2 years. About 25% have recurring hematuria, and in the remainder the renal disease clears completely. Clinical severity is proportionate to the extent of the lesion histologically; older children are more liable to severe involvement.

Treatment

There is no satisfactory treatment for anaphylactoid purpura. Corticosteroid therapy may be useful in patients with acute gastrointestinal manifestations. If the culture is positive for group A β-hemolytic streptococci or if the ASO titer is elevated, give penicillin in full therapeutic doses for 10 days. Aspirin is useful for the arthritis, and sedatives may benefit the patient with gastrointestinal pain. Immunosuppressive drugs such as cyclophosphamide and azathioprine are now contraindicated in the treatment of the nephritis.

Prognosis

The prognosis for recovery is good, although symptoms frequently recur over a period of several months. In patients who develop renal manifestations, approximately 50% may have persistent abnormal urinary findings. This occasionally progresses to significant impairment of renal function.

Kitchens CS: The anatomic basis of purpura. *Prog Hemost Thromb* 1980;**5**:211.
Saulsbury FT: Henoch-Schönlein purpura. *Pediatr Dermatol* 1984;**1**:195.
Stewart M et al: Long term renal prognosis of Henoch-Schönlein purpura in an unselected childhood population. *Eur J Pediatr* 1988;**147**:113.

Weber TR et al: Massive gastric hemorrhage: An unusual complication of Henoch-Schönlein purpura. *J Pediatr Surg* 1983;**18**:576.

INTRAVASCULAR DEFECTS; COAGULATION FACTOR DEFICIENCIES

Essentials of Diagnosis

- Generalized bleeding tendency.
- Ecchymoses (not petechiae).
- Congenital (family history) or acquired (systemic illness).
- Abnormal partial thromboplastin time or prothrombin time (or both).

General Considerations

A congenital or acquired deficiency of one or more of the coagulation factors in the blood can result in a generalized bleeding diathesis. The bleeding tendency may be mild (bleeding only at time of severe traumas or surgical procedures), moderate, or severe (frequent spontaneous hemarthroses and ecchymoses) depending on the degree of the coagulation factor deficit. Fig 17–1 depicts the interaction of these factors in producing coagulation of the blood. Hemostasis depends upon platelet and vascular factors as well as blood coagulation.

A specific hemorrhagic diathesis has been seen with a deficiency of each of the coagulation factors except Hageman factor (XII), calcium deficiency, prekallikrein, and high-molecular-weight kininogen. These disease entities are discussed below.

The diagnosis and classification of clinical coagulation factor deficiencies depend upon proper performance and interpretation of specific clotting tests that are briefly reviewed below.

Coagulation Tests

A. Whole Blood Coagulation Time (Lee-White): This test is too insensitive to be of value in diagnosis or treatment of patients with mild to moderate coagulation factor deficiencies. The clotting time is influenced by heparin and can therefore be used as a rough guide to heparinization. Although simple to perform, this procedure is not an adequate screening test and should be abandoned as a "routine" test. A more useful test is the activated whole blood clotting time (ACT), which is performed by addition of an activating agent (kaolin, silica) to the clotting tube.

B. One-Stage Prothrombin Time (Quick): This procedure consists of noting the clotting time of citrated plasma after addition of calcium and tissue thromboplastin. Normal adult values are between 10

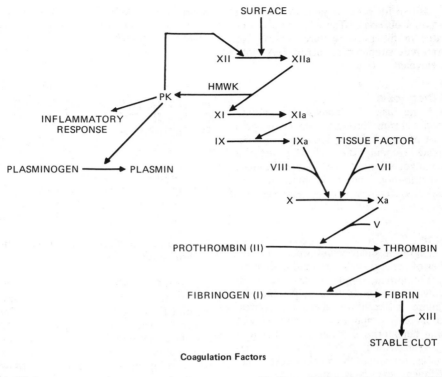

Figure 17–1. Blood coagulation scheme and terminology of coagulation factors.

Coagulation Factors

I Fibrinogen	XI Plasma thromboplastin antecedent (PTA)
II Prothrombin	XIa Activated form
V Ac-globulin, proaccelerin, labile factor	XII Hageman factor
VII Proconvertin, SPCA	XIIa Activated form
VIII Antihemophilic factor (AHF)	XIII Fibrin stabilizing factor, fibrinase
IX Plasma thromboplastin component (PTC)	PK Prekallikrein (Fletcher factor)
IXa Activated form	HMWK High-molecular-weight kininogen
X Stuart-Prower factor	
Xa Activated form	

and 11 seconds (100%). This is an adequate screening test for proconvertin (VII), proaccelerin (V), Stuart-Prower factor (X), and prothrombin (II). It does not measure the factors necessary for the earlier stages of coagulation or fibrinogen levels greater than 75 μg/dL.

C. Partial Thromboplastin Time (PTT): This test is performed much like the prothrombin time except that a phospholipid is added instead of tissue thromboplastin. In addition, a contact activator substance such as kaolin may be added to avert the influence of glass contact. The test is very sensitive, relatively easy to perform, and inexpensive. All coagulation factors except proconvertin are measured.

D. Thrombin Time: Bovine or human thrombin is added to plasma and the clotting time recorded. The normal adult range is 7–15 seconds or more, depending upon the amount of thrombin added. The

test measures the conversion of fibrinogen to fibrin and is dependent upon the concentration and function of fibrinogen or inhibitors such as fibrin split products, antithrombins, and heparin.

E. Specific Factor Assays: Each of the coagulation factors can be assayed by an indirect clotting method using natural or synthetic factor-deficient substrates or chromogenic substrates and compared to the activity of normal plasma (100%).

F. Bleeding Time (Ivy or Template): The bleeding time measures the platelet-vessel interaction (number and function of platelets) and is performed as follows. Place a blood pressure cuff on the upper arm and inflate to 40 mm Hg. With an alcohol sponge, clean an area free of visible veins on the flexor surface of the forearm. In the Ivy method, using a sterile Bard-Parker No. 11 blade, make a punction wound 5 mm deep and 2 mm wide. Note time of puncture; touch wound gently with sterile filter paper to absorb blood every 30 seconds until bleeding stops. Normal bleeding time is 1–7 minutes. A modification of this test using a template to make a cut 1 mm deep and 1 mm long is now frequently used (template bleeding time); the normal range is up to 9 minutes. A commercially available variation of this test (Simplate) is widely used.

Bennett JS: Blood coagulation and coagulation tests. *Med Clin North Am* 1984;**68:**557.

Buchanan GR, Holtkamp CA: A comparative study of variables affecting the bleeding time using two disposable devices. *Am J Clin Pathol* 1989;**91:**45.

AFIBRINOGENEMIA & DYSFIBRINOGENEMIA

There have been reports of several patients with a bleeding tendency and delayed clotting due to an abnormal molecule of fibrinogen (congenital dysfibrinogenemia). Immunologic determinations of fibrinogen are normal, but the thrombin and prothrombin times are often prolonged. Treatment is similar to that outlined for afibrinogenemia.

Congenital absence of fibrinogen produces a definite entity that resembles hemophilia clinically. However, the condition is inherited as an autosomal recessive and affects both sexes. The patients have persistent bleeding from small injuries, hematomas, ecchymoses, and hemarthroses. Although fatal bleeding from the umbilical cord has been reported, most cases are usually much less severe than classic hemophilia.

The principal laboratory finding in afibrinogenemia is complete absence of a fibrin clot by any of the usual clotting tests attempted. Whole blood and plasma are incoagulable even upon the addition of optimal amounts of calcium, thromboplastin, and thrombin. The erythrocyte sedimentation rate is zero. There is an absence of precipitable fibrinogen upon heating of plasma to 56 °C for 10 minutes. Specific assays for other coagulation factors are normal. Hypofibrinogenemia (fibrinogen level < 100 mg/dL) is also rarely seen.

Transfusion with whole blood, fresh plasma, or cryoprecipitate generally controls the acute bleeding episodes. The minimal hemostatic level of circulating fibrinogen is about 60 mg/dL (normal, 250–450 mg/dL). The half-life of transfused fibrinogen is about 4 days. Therefore, 10–20 mL of plasma per kilogram of body weight or one bag of cryoprecipitate per 6 kg should achieve hemostasis. This dose may need to be repeated daily depending upon the type and severity of bleeding and the rate of healing.

Mammen EF: Congenital coagulation disorders. *Semin Thromb Hemost* 1983;**9:**1.

HEMOPHILIA A (Antihemophilic Factor [AHF, Factor VIIIc] Deficiency)

Classic hemophilia (hemophilia A) is a bleeding disorder characterized by decreased activity of circulating antihemophilic factor (AHF or factor VIIIc, the coagulant portion of the factor VIII complex molecule). The disease occurs in males and is inherited in an X-linked recessive manner. All degrees of severity of the disease have been reported.

Clinical Findings

A. Symptoms and Signs: Patients with severe hemophilia, characterized by frequent spontaneous bleeding epidodes involving skin, mucous membranes, joints, muscles, and viscera, have no circulating factor VIIIc activity. However, mild hemophilia is also recognized; these patients bleed only at times of severe trauma or surgery. They have 5–20% factor VIIIc activity. An intermediate group of patients with moderate symptoms (usually no severe joint involvement) have 1–5% factor VIIIc levels.

The most crippling aspect of hemophilia A is the tendency to develop chronic hemarthroses, especially of knees and elbows, which lead to fibrosis and joint contractures.

B. Laboratory Findings: In about 70% of families with this disease, the female carriers will have low levels of factor VIIIc (20–70%) and may occasionally be mildly symptomatic. Otherwise, low levels of factor VIIIc are not seen in a female unless the individual has von Willebrand's disease or a circulating anticoagulant or is the product of the union of a hemophiliac male and a carrier female. Carriers of hemophilia can be detected in most instances by determination of the ratio of factor VIIIc to vWf or by molecular genetic techniques.

Results of tests measuring intrinsic plasma thromboplastin formation (whole blood clotting time, plasma recalcification time, partial thromboplastin time [PTT], and thromboplastin generation test [TGT]) are all abnormal. The bleeding time and one-stage prothrombin time are usually normal. The specific diagnosis is made by specific assays for factor VIIIc. Levels of vWf are normal in classic hemophilia.

Complications

The principle complication of classic hemophilia is the development of an acquired circulating anticoagulant to factor VIIIc. Inhibitors or antibodies to factor VIIIc develop in about 15% of factor VIIIc-deficient hemophiliacs. Patients may have both mild and severe inhibitor states. Mild inhibitor or anticoagulant substances specific to factor VIIIc not uncommonly can be shown in factor VIIIc-deficient patients, but the development of a severe factor VIIIc inhibitor is a rare and dreaded complication.

When this occurs, the patient is often resistant to all attempts at therapy. The inhibitor has been shown to be an antibody but is rarely amenable to immunosuppressive therapy. "Activated" prothrombin complex concentrates (Autoplex, Feiba Immuno) may be of help in stopping hemorrhage in these patients.

Other complications in hemophilia include chronic crippling arthritis due to repeated hemarthroses; development of pseudotumors as a result of multiple bleeding in one site; chronic hepatitis contracted through transfusion; and human immunodeficiency virus (AIDS), which may also be contracted through transfusion.

The majority of hemophilia patients exposed to factor concentrates prior to 1985 have become positive to HIV antibody, and many have progressed to HIV infection. Since 1985, the use of treated products has eliminated this risk; current factor concentrates should be shown by safety testing to be free of HIV and non-A, non-B hepatitis virus.

Treatment

The basis of treatment of classic hemophilia is the administration of a factor VIIIc-containing substance in order to achieve adequate hemostasis. Factor VIIIc is temperature and storage labile in biologic fluids.

The in vitro half-life of infused factor VIIIc is about 12 hours.

The following substances can be used for therapy: (1) fresh-frozen plasma or cryoprecipitates, stored at −30 °C for less than 12 months; and (2) lyophilized concentrates of factor VIIIc, reconstituted and given immediately.

Dosage and duration of therapy depend upon the type of bleeding seen clinically. Bleeding that occurs from lacerations of the skin or mucous membranes, tooth extractions, surgical wounds, or severe traumatic epistaxis usually requires more intense therapy than joint or soft tissue bleeding.

In order to achieve the desired in vivo level of factor VIIIc, use either of the following: (1) cryoprecipitated factor VIIIc, prepared from individual blood donors and supplied frozen in 10- to 20-mL amounts per plastic bag; or (2) commercially prepared factor VIIIc concentrates from large donor pools, supplied in lyophilizied form in vials. Dosages can be calculated as follows:

Units of factor VIIIC = Weight in kilograms ×
Desired in vivo percentage level × 0.5

Cryoprecipitates usually contain 100 units* of factor VIIIc per bag; concentrate potency is designated on the vial. Fresh-frozen plasma, 10 mL/kg, will produce an in vivo level of 15–20% factor VIIIc.

---

*A unit of factor VIIIc is the amount contained in 1 mL of fresh plasma at as 100% factor VIIIc activity level.

Treatment must be continued until adequate healing occurs—ie, 2–5 days for tooth extractions or epistaxis but 7–10 days for lacerations or surgical wounds. The principle of therapy is to rapidly achieve a hemostatic level of factor VIIIc (at least 20%) and to maintain this level until the lesion is adequately healed. For surgical procedures, levels of 30–40% are usually necessary for hemostasis. In mucous membrane bleeding or wounds (tongue, tooth socket), the duration of factor VIIIc therapy can often be reduced to 1–2 days if a fibrinolytic inhibitor, aminocaproic acid (Amicar), is given in a dosage of 100 mg/kg orally every 6 hours until healing is complete. Major surgical procedures and central nervous system bleeding usually require levels of 80–100% for adequate hemostasis.

Bleeding in joints or soft tissue areas can often be controlled by a single infusion of fresh frozen plasma, cryoprecipitates, or factor VIIIc concentrate to reach a single peak of 20%. If bleeding is severe, this dose should be repeated in 12 hours or a higher level achieved initially (ie, 40%). However, if the lesion is a dissecting hematoma that might threaten nerve function or endanger respiration or vision, a level of 20% should be maintained for at least 48 hours.

Corticosteroids may be helpful in instances of recurrent joint bleeding. Patients with renal bleeding have also benefited from corticosteroid therapy. Local hemostatic measures such as pressure or application of Gelfoam soaked in bovine thrombin are often helpful in cases of epistaxis. Patients with mild hemophilia should be treated with fresh-frozen plasma, cryoprecipitates, or desmopressin acetate (DDAVP) (see p 504) in order to avoid complications of concentrate therapy.

Prognosis

With prophylaxis against injury, early treatment of bleeding episodes, careful orthopedic care of joint lesions, and attention to emotional, social, and educational adjustment, the prognosis for a useful normal life is good.

Brettler DB et al: A long-term study of hemophilic arthropathy of the knee on a program of factor VIII replacement given at the time of each hemarthrosis. *Am J Hematol* 1985;**18**:13.

Hargraves MA et al: Hemophiliac patient's knowledge and educational needs concerning acquired immunodeficiency syndrome. *Am J Hematol* 1987;**26**:115.

Horowitz MS et al: Virus safety of solvent/detergent-treated antihaemophilic factor concentrate. *Lancet* 1988;**2**:186.

Kasper CK: Treatment of factor VIII inhibitors. *Prog Hemost Thromb* 1989;**9**:57.

Lillicrap D et al: Carrier detection strategy in haemophilia A: The benefits of combined DNA marker analysis and coagulation testing in sporadic haemophilic families. *Br J Haematol* 1988;**70**:321.

Perkocha LA, Rodgers GM: Hematologic aspects of human immunodeficiency virus infection: Laboratory and clinical considerations. *Am J Hematol* 1988;**29**:94.

Schwartz RS et al: Comparative efficacy of nonheated and heat-treated factor IX complex concentrate in treatment of hemophiliacs with inhibitors. *Am J Hematol* 1989;**30**:22.

HEMOPHILIA B
(PTC [Factor IX] Deficiency)

The mode of inheritance and clinical manifestations of hemophilia B (PTC deficiency, factor IX deficiency, Christmas disease) are the same as those of factor VIIIc deficiency (hemophilia A). Congenital PTC deficiency is 15–20% as prevalent as factor VIIIc deficiency. PTC is made in the liver and is vitamin K-dependent; therefore, acquired deficiencies of factor IX are fairly common.

In hereditary factor IX deficiency, the PTT is prolonged, but prothrombin time and thrombin time are normal. Diagnosis is confirmed by specific coagulation assay. Genetic variants of factor IX deficiency have been described; however, diagnosis and management are the same for all types.

Although factor IX is stable in storage and is not consumed during coagulation, the therapy of bleeding episodes differs little from that outlined above for classic hemophilia. The products that can be used include recently outdated blood bank plasma (approximately 3 weeks old) at 4 °C, plus fresh-frozen plasma or factor IX concentrate. Unlike factor VIII, approximately half of the administered dose of factor IX diffuses into the extravascular space. Therefore, twice the calculated factor VIII dose (see above) should be given as plasma or factor IX concentrate initially. Subsequently, half of the initial dose can be given to achieve the desired in vivo level. (Factor IX has a half-life of 20–22 hours in vivo). Cryoprecipitates and factor VIIIc concentrates do not contain sufficient PTC for use in this disease. The prognosis is good if the bleeding episodes are adequately controlled.

Hoffman C, Hultin MB: Factor IX concentrate therapy and thrombosis: Relation to changes in plasma antithrombin III. *Thromb Res* 1986;**43**:143.

Trent RJ et al: A factor IX gene probe: Its use in carrier detection, antenatal diagnosis and characterisation of the molecular basis for hemophilia B. *Aust N Z J Med* 1985;**15**:721.

HEMOPHILIA C
(PTA [Factor XI] Deficiency)

PTA (factor XI) deficiency is a bleeding diathesis of mild to moderate severity. Inheritance is by the autosomal recessive mode. Heterozygotes rarely show a mild bleeding tendency at surgery or following severe trauma. Homozygous patients may have spontaneous hemorrhage (ecchymoses, epistaxis) in addition to bleeding due to trauma. Only rarely do patients with hemophilia C have spontaneous hemarthroses. Hemophilia C has been found mainly in Jews and comprises less than 5% of all hemophiloid diseases.

The defect may be very mild, and a sensitive coagulation test is required to identify the deficiency. Factor XI is a stable factor found in both serum and plasma and shows increased activity in contact with glass or after storage. Therefore, differentiation from PTC deficiency may be difficult unless tests are done with fresh plasma using known PTA-deficient plasma for assays.

The bleeding defect is mild and requires treatment usually only at times of survery (eg, tooth extractions) or trauma. PTA is a stable factor, and good levels are found in plasma stored for several weeks at 4 °C. Therefore, the principles of treatment outlined for PTC deficiency apply equally well to PTA deficiency.

The prognosis for an average life span is excellent.

Bolton-Maggs PHB et al: Inheritance and bleeding in factor XI deficiency. *Br J Haematol* 1988;**69**:521.

Schnall SF, Duffy TP, Clyne LP: Acquired factor XI inhibitors in congenitally deficient patients. *Am J Hematol* 1987;**26**:323.

DEFICIENCIES OF LIVER-DEPENDENT COAGULATION FACTORS

The following clotting factors are known to be produced in the liver: fibrinogen (I), PTC (IX), prothrombin (II), proconvertin (VII), proaccelerin (V), Stuart-Prower factor (X), PTA (XI), and Hageman factor (XII). Vitamin K is necessary for the synthesis of II, VII, X, and IX. Hereditary bleeding diseases due to isolated deficiencies of prothrombin, proconvertin, proaccelerin, or Stuart-Prower factor are exceedingly rare. Congenital deficiencies of fibrinogen and PTC are discussed above.

Hereditary prothrombin deficiency, proconvertin deficiency, Stuart-Prower factor deficiency, and proaccelerin deficiency have been reported in both males and females and have a recessive mode of transmission. Mild to moderately severe bleeding manifestations can occur. The prothrombin time is uniformly prolonged in these disorders. The diagnosis is suspected when a patient is seen with a history of bleeding manifestations, a prolonged prothrombin time without liver disease, and no response to vitamin K therapy. The diagnosis must be confirmed by specific factor assays.

Treatment consists of transfusion of whole plasma

in dosages sufficient to achieve at least 20–30% correction of the prothrombin time. Fresh plasma must be used for proaccelerin (V) deficiency because this is a relatively unstable factor. Prothrombin complex concentrates (Konyne, Proplex) may be used for therapy of factor II, VII, and X when higher levels are desired.

Ragni MV et al: Factor VII deficiency. *Am J Hematol* 1981;**10**:79.

Rocha E et al: Prothrombin Segovia: A new congenital abnormality of prothrombin. *Scand J Haematol* 1986; **36**:444.

Tracy PB et al: Factor V (Quebec): A bleeding diathesis associated with a qualitative platelet factor V deficiency. *J Clin Invest* 1984;**74**:1221.

HAGEMAN FACTOR (Factor XII) DEFICIENCY; PREKALLIKREIN DEFICIENCY; HIGH-MOLECULAR-WEIGHT KININOGEN DEFICIENCY

Severe deficiencies of the "contact" factors (factor XII, or Hageman factor, prekallikrein, or Fletcher factor; and high-molecular-weight kininogen, or Fitzgerald factor) cause marked prolongation of the PTT but are not associated with a bleeding diathesis. Severe factor XII deficiency has been associated with thrombosis. Mild deficiencies of factor XII and high-molecular-weight kininogen also prolong the PTT and are frequently of clinical importance in the evaluation of a mildly prolonged PTT prior to surgical procedures.

Mannhalter CH (editor): Contact phase coagulation disorders. *Semin Thromb Hemost* 1987;**13**:1. [Entire issue.]

FIBRIN STABILIZING FACTOR (Factor XIII) DEFICIENCY; ALPHA₂ ANTIPLASMIN DEFICIENCY

Two separate but closely related coagulation factor deficiencies are associated with a severe bleeding diathesis characterized by mucous membrane, muscle, and joint hemorrhages. Fibrin stabilizing factor (factor XIII) deficiency and alpha$_2$ antiplasmin deficiency are autosomal recessive. Affected individuals may present with hemorrhage into the umbilical cord at birth. Factor XIII and alpha$_2$ antiplasmin are both necessary for stabilization and persistence of the fibrin clot; therefore, the usual screening tests of hemostasis (bleeding time, PTT, prothrombin time, thrombin time) are normal. Factor XIII deficiency is diagnosed by demonstration of plasma clot lysis in urea, 5 mol/L, and alpha$_2$ antiplasmin deficiency by increased lysis of whole blood and dilute plasma. Specific assays are available for both factors. Treatment consists of plasma transfusions, 10–15 mL/kg, to control acute bleeding episodes.

Daly HM, Haddon ME: Clinical experience with a pasteurised human plasma concentrate in factor XIII deficiency. *Thromb Haemost* 1988;**59**:171.

Miles LA et al: A bleeding disorder due to deficiency of alpha 2-antiplasmin. *Blood* 1982;**59**:1246.

ACQUIRED COAGULATION FACTOR DEFICIENCIES

1. HEMORRHAGIC DISEASE OF THE NEWBORN

A generalized bleeding diathesis can occur in newborn infants who are markedly deficient in vitamin K-dependent coagulation factors (factors II, VII, IX, and X). This clinical syndrome is called hemorrhagic disease of the newborn. It may be present at birth or may occur any time in the first 3 days of life. All newborn infants show a moderate deficiency of these vitamin K-dependent factors at a level of 25–60% of normal adult values. However, when the levels fall below 20% in infants who are vitamin K-deficient, a generalized bleeding tendency can ensue. Ecchymoses, gastrointestinal hemorrhage, hematuria, and cerebral hemorrhages may occur on the second to fourth days of life.

Hemorrhagic disease may also occur at 1–2 months of age in breast-fed infants who have not received prophylactic vitamin K at birth or who have malabsorption syndromes (see below). The prothrombin time is markedly prolonged to a level below 20% of normal. The PTT is also greatly prolonged. Platelet estimation and bleeding times are normal. In this age group, bleeding in association with a greatly prolonged prothrombin time is very suggestive of hemorrhagic disease of the newborn. The diagnosis is confirmed by the response to specific treatment and by demonstration of the precursor protein present *in v*itamin *K* absence (PIVKA) (abnormal prothrombin).

By definition, this disorder is due to severe vitamin K deficiency. Therefore, the disease can be prevented and treated adequately by a single intramuscular injection of 1 mg of vitamin K$_1$ (phytonadione). It is also recommended that this dose be given prophylactically to all newborn infants and to older breast-fed infants with protracted diarrhea. The prothrombin will become essentially normal within 12 hours, and the bleeding will stop within 6 hours after treatment with vitamin K. If life-threatening hemorrhage is present, a transfusion of fresh plasma (10 mL/kg) is indicated.

Infants of mothers receiving hydantoin or warfarin therapy are especially susceptible to vitamin K deficiency.

Hathway WE, Bonnar J: *Hemostatic Disorders of the Pregnant Woman and Newborn Infant.* Elsevier, 1987.

2. VITAMIN K DEFICIENCY IN OLDER CHILDREN

Older infants and children, especially if they were breast-fed, may develop vitamin K deficiency secondary to chronic diarrhea, malabsorption syndrome, obstructive jaundice, and defective synthesis associated with prolonged antibiotic therapy. The clinical and laboratory manifestations are similar to those seen in hemorrhagic disease of the newborn. Treatment is by administration of vitamin K_1 (phytonadione) in doses of 5–10 mg intravenously or intramuscularly.

Lane PA, Hathaway WE: Vitamin K in infancy. *J Pediatr* 1985;**106**:351.

3. SECONDARY HEMORRHAGIC DIATHESIS OF THE NEWBORN

Premature and full-term infants frequently develop generalized bleeding tendencies associated with other illnesses such as respiratory distress syndrome, cyanotic congenital heart disease, cerebral anoxia, and severe sepsis. Factors often present and possibly related to this bleeding syndrome are "physiologic" depression of coagulation factors, hypoxia, acidosis, vascular fragility, defective platelet number and function, and increased fibrinolytic activity. Laboratory tests of bleeding and coagulation are difficult to interpret because results in affected patients overlap with those in normal infants. The values for these tests seen in "normal" full-term and premature infants are shown in Table 17–7. The pathophysiologic mechanisms of these secondary bleeding syndromes (cerebral hemorrhage, pulmonary hemorrhage, generalized bleeding tendency) are related to increased consumption (due to pathologic proteolysis) or decreased synthesis (due to functional impairment of the liver) of clotting factors and platelets.

Treatment consists of correcting the associated conditions and replacing clotting factors and platelets with doses of fresh frozen plasma, 10 mL/kg, or platelet concentrates, 10 mL/kg. Occasionally, exchange transfusion or heparinization is indicated.

Hathaway WE, Bonnar J: *Perinatal Coagulation*. Grune & Stratton, 1978.

4. DISSEMINATED INTRAVASCULAR COAGULATION

Essentials of Diagnosis

■ Presence of disorder known to trigger disseminated intravascular coagulation.
■ Evidence for activation of coagulation (prolonged PTT, prothrombin time, or thrombin time or decreased fibrinogen or platelets).
■ Microangiopathic red cell changes.

General Considerations

Disseminated intravascular coagulation (DIC) is an acquired pathologic process characterized by activation of the coagulation system leading to thrombin generation, intravascular fibrin deposition, and platelet consumption. Microthrombi, composed of fibrin and platelets, may produce ischemic tissue damage as well as fragmentation of erythrocytes. The fibrinolytic system is also frequently activated, producing plasmin-mediated destruction of fibrin, fibrinogen, and other clotting factors (factor V, factor VIII). Degradation or split products of fibrin-fibrinogen are formed and function as anticoagulants and inhibitors of platelet function. Disseminated intravascular coagulation commonly accompanies disorders seen in critically ill infants and children. Conditions known to trigger disseminated intravascular coagulation include endothelial cell damage (endotoxin, virus), tissue destruction (necrosis, physical injuries), hypoxia (acidosis), ischemic and vascular changes (shock, hemangiomas), and release of tissue procoagulants (cancer, placental disorders).

Clinical Findings

Physical signs of the disorder include (1) evidence of a diffuse bleeding tendency (hematuria, melena, purpura, petechiae, persistent oozing from needle punctures or other invasive procedures); (2) circulatory collapse, poor skin perfusion, early ischemic changes; and (3) evidence of thrombotic lesions (major vessel thrombosis, gangrene, purpura fulminans).

The laboratory diagnosis of disseminated intravascular coagulation is outlined in Table 17–8. Tests that are most sensitive, easiest to perform, and best reflect the hemostatic capacity of the patient are the PTT, prothrombin time, platelet count, fibrinogen level, and a test for fibrin-fibrinogen split products (Thrombo-Wellco test for serum fibrin-fibrinogen split products; protamine precipitation test for plasma monomer-fibrin-fibrinogen split product complexes). If these tests are normal or only slightly abnormal, clinically significant disseminated intravascular coagulation is not present. When disseminated intravascular coagulation is present, varying degrees of abnormality may be seen with these screening tests, depending on the triggering event. Patients with infections may have primarily thrombocytopenia, only slight prolongation of PTT and prothrombin time, and mildly elevated fibrin-fibrinogen split products. Platelets may be consumed in bacterial sepsis without any other evidence of activated coagulation. Asphyxia (at any age) may produce significant consumption of fibrinogen and elevated fibrin-fibrinogen split products without depression of platelets. In the neonatal period, the PTT is often prolonged on a physiologic basis and is thus less useful as a screening test for disseminated intravascular coagulation.

Table 17–7. Coagulation factor and test values in normal pregnant women and newborn infants.[1]

| Category | Fibrinogen (mg/dL) | Factors | | | | | | | | | Platelet Count (per µL) | Euglobulin Lysis Time (minutes) | Partial Thromboplastin Time[2] (seconds) | Prothrombin Time (seconds) | Thrombin Time (seconds) |
		II (%)	V (%)	VII (%)	VIII (%)	IX (%)	X (%)	XI (%)	XII (%)	XIII (titer)					
Normal adult or child	190–420	100	100	100	100	100	100	100	100	1/16	200,000–450,000	90–300	37–50	12–14	8–10
Term pregnancy	483	92	108	170	196	130	130	69	...	1/16	290,000	278	44	13	8
Premature infant (1500–2500 g), cord blood	233	25	67	37	100	34	29	30	33	1/8	220,000	214	90	17 (12–21)	14 (11–17)
Term infant, cord blood	216	41	92	56	100	27	55	36	47	1/8	190,000	84	71	13.5 (12–16)	12 (10–16)
Term infant, 48 hours	210	46	105	20	100	→	45	39	25	...	200,000	105	65	16 (12–21)	13 (10–16)

Note: All levels expressed as means or ranges.

[1]Modified and reproduced, with permission, from Hathaway WE: Coagulation problems in the newborn infant. *Pediatr Clin North Am* 1970;**17**:929.

[2]Kaolin PTT.

Table 17–8. Laboratory tests that may be abnormal in disseminated intravascular coagulation.

Test	Mechanism of Abnormality
Prolonged partial thromboplastin time (PTT, APTT)	Decreased procoagulants, increased fibrin-fibrinogen split products.
Prolonged prothrombin time (PT)	Decreased fibrinogen, increased fibrin-fibrinogen split products.
Prolonged thrombin time (TT)	Decreased fibrinogen, increased fibrin-fibrinogen split products.
Prolonged reptilase time	Decreased fibrinogen, increased fibrin-fibrinogen split products.
Decreased platelet count	Platelet consumption.
Decreased fibrinogen level	Fibrinogen consumption.
Increased fibrin-fibrinogen split products	Plasmin degradation of fibrin and fibrinogen.
Prolonged bleeding time	Decreased platelets and decreased platelet function.
Decreased activity of coagulation factors XII, V, VII, VIII, II, and XIII and of prekallikrein, antithrombin III, and plasminogen	See text.

Differential Diagnosis

The differential diagnosis of a diffuse bleeding tendency in a critically ill patient must include other causes as well as disseminated intravascular coagulation. Uremic bleeding (due to a platelet function defect), severe hepatic coagulopathy (due to decreased synthesis of clotting factors), and vitamin K deficiency can all mimic disseminated intravascular coagulation or may be present along with it. Vitamin K deficiency can be easily diagnosed and treated, and uremia is not hard to recognize, but severe liver disease may be more difficult to diagnose. Patients with fulminant hepatitis or advanced cirrhosis often have evidence of both decreased production of liver factors and increased consumption of platelets and fibrinogen.

Treatment

The most important aspects of therapy are identification and treatment of the triggering event. For bacterial sepsis, give antibiotic therapy and provide volume replacement and circulatory support. Relieve hypoxia, and correct acidosis in neonatal asphyxia and respiratory distress syndromes. Restore blood volume in hemorrhagic shock, and give antiviral agents in severe viral infections. If the precipitating event can be quickly treated (eg, hypoxia or shock), often no other therapy is needed. Serial determination with coagulation tests will help in deciding whether further therapy is indicated.

Replacement of depleted coagulation factors and platelets may be necessary in severe disseminated intravascular coagulation, especially with an associated bleeding diathesis or potential severe hemorrhage. Initial stabilization of children suspected of having disseminated intravascular coagulation should include use of fresh frozen plasma whenever volume expanders are indicated in order to replace depleted coagulation factors. Fibrinogen and other clotting factors can be replaced by use of fresh frozen plasma; 10–15 mL/kg will raise the clotting factor level by about 20%. Fibrinogen (and factor VIII) can be given in cryoprecipitates also; one bag of cryoprecipitate per 3 kg in infants or one bag of cryoprecipitate per 5 kg in older children will raise the fibrinogen level by about 75–100 mg/dL. Platelets are replaced by use of platelet concentrates; in the neonate, 10 mL of platelet concentrate per kilogram will raise the platelet count by about 75,000–100,000/μL. In older children, one bag of platelet concentrate per 5–6 kg is the usual dose. The minimal hemostatic levels of procoagulants are estimated by a platelet count of 30,000–50,000/μL, a prothrombin time of 16 seconds, and a fibrinogen level of 100 mg/dL.

In specific instances, interruption of the clotting process by heparin may be necessary when the triggering event cannot be quickly treated and consumptive coagulopathy or tissue necrosis is ongoing (eg, acute promyelocytic or monocytic leukemia, giant hemangioma, hemolytic-uremic syndrome in the patient with frank disseminated intravascular coagulation [infrequent], impending tissue necrosis or gangrene in septic shock, large vessel thrombosis, or purpura fulminans). In these instances, heparin will halt disseminated intravascular coagulation or allow for more effective replacement therapy while the primary disease is being specifically treated. The most effective and safest method of giving heparin is by continuous intravenous administration. A loading dose of 50 units/kg is followed by 10–15 units/kg/h by continuous intravenous infusion. Unless there is significant tissue necrosis, this dose is usually effective, and improvement on coagulation screening tests should occur in 12–24 hours or sooner.

In purpura fulminans, where heparin is absolutely indicated, a higher dose (20–25 units/kg/h) may be needed in order to halt the gangrenous process.

Baker WF: Clinical aspects of disseminated intravascular coagulation. *Semin Throm Hemost* 1989;**15**:1.

Hathaway WE: Haemostatic and thrombotic problems in the fetus and neonate. In: *Haemostasis and Thrombosis in Obstetrics and Gynaecology.* Greer IA (editor). Chapman & Hall Ltd. [In press.]

Hathaway WE, Bonnar J: *Hemostatic Disorders of the Pregnant Woman and Newborn Infant.* Elsevier, 1987.

5. CIRCULATING ANTICOAGULANTS

Acquired anticoagulants or coagulation inhibitors are of 2 types: (1) a blocking inhibitor such as the "lupus" anticoagulant, which prolongs the PTT and is not corrected by 1:1 mixing with normal plasma; and (2) specific coagulation factor inhibitors or antibodies, which progressively destroy a clotting factor (often factor VIII) on incubation with normal plasma at 37 °C. The lupus inhibitor is seen in disseminated lupus erythematosus and other collagen-vascular disorders, in postviral infections, and in patients who have been given certain drugs such as penicillin. Thrombosis rather than hemorrhage may be associated with the occurrence of the lupus anticoagulant. The second type is also found in patients with collagen-vascular disorders or may appear spontaneously postpartum and is associated with a bleeding tendency. Both types tend to disappear with time. Treatment with prednisone or immunosuppressive drugs may occasionally be indicated. Heparin and dicumarol are potent anticoagulants when administered as drugs. Heparin affects the whole blood coagulation time or PTT primarily, whereas dicumarol affects the prothrombin time by inhibiting the utilization of vitamin K.

Brandt JT, Britton A, Kraut E: A spontaneous factor V inhibitor with unexpected laboratory features. *Arch Pathol Lab Med* 1986;**110**:224.

Lottenberg R, Kentro TB, Kitchens CS: Acquired hemophilia. *Arch Intern Med* 1987;**147**:1077.

Triplett DA et al: The relationship between lupus anticoagulants and antibodies to phospholipid. *JAMA* 1988; **259**:550.

6. HEREDITARY THROMBOEMBOLIC DISEASE

Hereditary deficiencies of several physiologic anticoagulants are known to be associated with recurrent thromboembolic disease. Heterozygous deficiencies of antithrombin III-heparin cofactor, protein C, and protein S are expressed in an autosomal dominant fashion. Homozygous protein C deficiency is characterized by severe thrombosis or recurrent and often fatal purpura fulminans in newborn infants. Treatment of acute thrombosis is by systemic anticoagulation with or without replacement of the deficient factor.

Hereditary deficiencies in the amount and function of plasminogen as well as certain dysfibrinogenemias are associated with a lifelong thrombotic tendency.

Collen D: Fibrin-specific thrombolytic therapy. *Thromb Res [Suppl]* 1988;**No. 8**:3.

Comp PC: Hereditary disorders predisposing to thrombosis. *Prog Hemost Thromb* 1986;**8**:71.

Manco-Johnson MJ: The pathophysiology of neonatal disseminated intravascular coagulation and thrombosis. In: *Neonatal and Fetal Medicine: Physiology and Pathophysiology.* Fox WW, Polin RA (editors). Saunders, [In press.]

Schmidt B, Andrew M: Neonatal thrombotic disease: Prevention, diagnosis, and treatment. *J Pediatr* 1988; **113**:410.

V. THE SPLEEN

SPLENOMEGALY

The child with a relatively isolated finding of splenomegaly frequently presents a puzzling diagnostic problem. In the diagnosis of chronic splenomegaly, the following categories of diseases should be considered: congestive splenomegaly, chronic infections, leukemia and lymphomas, hemolytic anemias, reticuloendothelioses, and storage diseases. The clinical findings in these entities and the recommended diagnostic procedures are summarized in Table 17–9.

DEVELOPMENTAL DEFECTS OF THE SPLEEN

Simultaneous injury, at about the 25th day of embryonic life, of the splenic anlage, atrioventricular cushions of the heart, and mesentery may account for the triad of situs inversus, congenital lesions of the heart, and asplenia. Fewer than 10% of cases of congenital absence of the spleen occur without serious heart lesions. Most infants with this triad die within a few weeks. The principal evidence of asplenia in these infants consists of erythrocytic inclusions such as Howell-Jolly bodies, nucleated red cells, and Heinz bodies. A mild reticulocytosis and siderocytosis can be found. The discovery of these red cell inclusions in a patient with congenital heart disease is strong presumptive evidence of this syndrome.

No specific therapy is available.

Freedman RM et al: Development of splenic reticuloendothelial function in neonates. *J Pediatr* 1980;**96**:466.

Table 17–9. Causes of chronic splenomegaly in children.

Cause	Associated Clinical Findings	Diagnostic Investigation
Congestive splenomegaly	History of umbilical vein catheter or neonatal omphalitis. Signs of portal hypertension (varices, hemorrhoids, dilated abdominal wall veins); pancytopenia, history of hepatitis or jaundice.	Complete blood count, platelet count, liver function tests, upper gastrointestinal x-rays, ultrasonography.
Chronic infections	History of exposure to tuberculosis, histoplasmosis, coccidioidomycosis, other fungal disease; chronic sepsis (foreign body in bloodstream; subacute infective endocarditis).	Appropriate cultures and skin tests, ie, blood cultures, PPD, histoplasmin, coccidioidin skin tests; chest film, HIV serology.
Infectious mononucleosis	Fever, fatigue, pharyngitis, rash, adenopathy.	Heterophil antibodies.
Leukemia, lymphoma, Hodgkin's disease	Evidence of systemic involvement with fever, bleeding tendencies, and lymphadenopathy; pancytopenia.	Blood smear, bone marrow examination, spleen biopsy.
Hemolytic anemias	Anemia, jaundice; family history of anemia, jaundice, and gallbladder disease in young adults.	Reticulocyte count, Coombs test, spherocytosis (blood smear, osmotic fragility), autohemolysis test, gallium scan.
Reticuloendothelioses (histiocytosis X)	Chronic otitis media, seborrheic or petechial skin rashes, anemia, infections, lymphadenopathy.	Skeletal x-rays for bone lesions; biopsy of bone, liver, bone marrow, or lymph node.
Storage diseases	Family history of similar disorders, neurologic involvement, evidence of macular degeneration.	Biopsy of rectal mucosa, liver, bone marrow, spleen, or brain in search for storage cells.
Splenic cyst	Evidence of other infections (postinfectious cyst) or congenital anomalies; peculiar shape of spleen.	Radioisotope scans, ultrasonography.

Majeski JA, Upshur JK: Asplenia syndrome: A study of congenital anomalies in 16 cases. *JAMA* 1978;**240:** 1508.

INFECTIONS FOLLOWING SPLENECTOMY

There is good evidence that infants and children who have undergone splenectomy are subsequently more susceptible to septicemia, meningitis, and pneumonia due to pneumococci, group A streptococci, *Haemophilus influenzae,* and enteric organisms. Children under 4 years of age and those with generalized disorders of the reticuloendothelial system are more frequently affected. The increased susceptibility to infection following splenectomy has not been explained, but it is probably related to the role of the spleen in antibody synthesis and phagocytic function. If possible, splenectomy should be delayed until after age 4, and prophylactic antibiotic therapy should be used after splenectomy in susceptible patients in addition to the administration of pneumococcal meningococcal, and *Haemophilus influenzae* vaccines.

Krivit W: Overwhelming postsplenectomy infection. *Am J Hematol* 1977;**2:**193.

Kumpe DA et al: Partial splenic embolization in children with hypersplenism. *Radiology* 1985;**155:**357.

Powell RW et al: The efficacy of postsplenectomy sepsis prophylactic measures: The role of penicillin. *J Trauma* 1988;**28:**1285.

Wadenvik H, Kutti J: The spleen and pooling of blood cells. *Eur J Haematol* 1988;**41:**1.

TRANSFUSION-ASSOCIATED COMPLICATIONS

General Considerations

The incidence of transfusion-associated complications (including acute reactions and disease transmission) is high—estimates range up to 20%. A common form is a febrile reaction which may be related to contamination with bacterial or other pyrogenic products or which may accompany hemolytic reactions or reactions in which transfused leukocytes are destroyed by antileukocyte antibodies present in the recipient. Urticarial reactions have been reported to occur in 1–3% of transfusions and are said to be more common in atopic individuals. Citrate toxicity, manifested largely as tetany and vascular collapse progressing at times to death, is an unusual complication of transfusion therapy.

Transfusion of mismatched blood may have any of the following adverse effects: symptoms and signs of intravascular or extravascular hemolysis; ischemia or bleeding; or a reaction involving antibodies formed to IgA, especially in IgA-deficient recipients. Allergic reactions to mismatched blood may result from passive sensitization of the recipient through blood from a donor sensitive to foods, drugs, inhalants or other allergens or from the infusion of allergen present in donor's plasma to which the recipient is sensitive. Hemolytic reactions are among the most severe transfusion reactions and have a high mortality rate.

Diseases that may be transmissible by blood transfusion include non-A, non-B (NANB) hepatitis, hepatitis B, human immunodeficiency virus infection (HIV-1, HIV-2), cytomegalovirus (CMV), malaria, toxoplasmosis, Chagas' disease, and babesiosis. NANB hepatitis is a chronic illness that frequently results in hepatic cirrhosis and may be transmitted in up to 10% of transfusions. Since 1985, HIV infection has rarely been transmitted by blood transfusions because of antibody testing of all donors; current estimated risk of contracting HIV-1 via blood transfusion is approximately 4 per million. HIV-2, which causes an immunodeficiency syndrome in some parts of Africa, is transmitted by blood containing cells (like CMV) and is also currently being tested for routinely. Newborn infants, particularly prematures, are especially susceptible to CMV-associated disease, which can be prevented by using CMV-seronegative donor blood.

Prevention

A. Reactions: Antihistamines given 1 hour before the blood transfusion may be used prophylactically to decrease the incidence and severity of allergic reactions. Used prophylactically, *antihistamines do not completely eliminate the possibility of a severe transfusion reaction.* Febrile reactions to leukocytes can be avoided by using frozen washed red cells. Problems consequent to the administration of hemolyzed blood can largely be avoided with proper inspection of the blood and equipment prior to transfusion.

B. Infectious Disease Transmission: At present, all blood is tested for elevated alanine aminotransferase (ALT) levels and antibody to Hepatitis B core antigen and Hepatitis C (a major cause of NANB hepatitis). Units positive for any of these have a higher incidence of transmitting NANB hepatitis and are not used. Although hepatitis B is screened for in all blood to be used for transfusion, patients who receive frequent blood transfusions or pooled plasma products should be vaccinated before exposure (see Chapter 6). The majority of blood banks (United States) provide CMV-seronegatigve blood for all neonates. Routine antibody screening for HIV will detect all virus-contaminated blood except for those rare instances of early infection.

Treatment of Acute Transfusion Reactions

Treatment consists chiefly of immediate discontinuance of the transfusion and maintenance of ade-

quate blood volume and pressure with intravenous fluids and pressor amines. Other ancillary measures depend upon the degree and nature of the reaction.

Urticaria with pruritus unaccompanied by other signs or symptoms does not necessarily contraindicate continuing the transfusion, as is the case with mild febrile reactions.

The treatment of urticarial reactions, angioedema, laryngeal edema, asthma, serum sickness, and anaphylactic shock has been described elsewhere.

Epinephrine, 1:1000, 0.2–0.4 mL intramuscularly, remains the most important single drug early in the treatment of severe acute allergic reactions. Antihistamines may also be given intravenously. Corticosteroids have also been recommended for the treatment of allergic and hemolytic transfusion reactions, but their efficacy in acute reactions is questionable.

For citrate toxicity, treatment consists of discontinuance of the transfusion and *slow* administration of calcium chloride (5%) or calcium gluconate (10%), 5–20 mL intravenously.

With hemolytic reactions, recipient and donor blood should be retyped and cross-matched and recipient blood cross-matched against other possible donors. If the hemolytic reaction is severe—and in the absence of cardiac failure, severe dehydration, intracranial bleeding, or renal failure—a 20% solution of mannitol, 0.3 g/kg intravenously over 10–15 minutes, should be given in addition to intravenous fluids to ensure adequate urine flow. Alternatively, furosemide (Lasix) may be used. This may be repeated once in 2 hours if adequate urine flow is not attained.

Plasma expanders may be necessary to treat hypotension due to hypovolemia.

Corticosteroids—eg, hydrocortisone sodium succinate (Solu-Cortef), 4 mg/kg—should be added to intravenous fluids and infused in a 4- to 6-hour period.

Prognosis

The prognosis depends on the nature and degree of the reaction. Hemolytic reactions must be kept in mind, because they are associated with a high fatality rate.

Berkman SA, Groopman JE: Transfusion-associated AIDS. *Transf Med Rev* 1988;**2**:18.

Mollison PL: Blood transfusion. In: *Clinical Medicine,* 7th ed. Blackwell, 1983.

O'Connor JC et al: A near-fatal reaction during granulocyte transfusion of a neonate. *Transfusion* 1988;**28**:173.

Strauss RG, Sacher RA: Directed donations for pediatric patients. *Transf Med Rev* 1988;**2**:58.

Tegtmeier GE: The use of cytomegalovirus-screened blood in neonates. *Transfusion* 1988;**28**:201.

SELECTED REFERENCES

Bloom AL, Thomas DP: *Haemostasis and Thrombosis.* Churchill Livingstone, 1987.

George JN, Nurden AT, Phillips DR: Molecular defects in interactions of platelets with the vessel wall. *N Engl J Med* 1984;**311:**1084.

Hathaway WE, Bonnar J. *Hemostatic Disorders of the Pregnant Woman and Newborn Infant.* Elsevier, 1987.

Miller DR, Baehner RL (editors). *Blood Diseases of Infancy and Childhood.* Mosby, 1989.

Mollison PL: *Blood Transfusion in Clinical Medicine,* 7th ed. Blackwell, 1983.

Montgomery RR, Hathaway WE: Acute bleeding emergencies. *Pediatr Clin North Am* 1980;**27:**327.

Nathan DG, Oski FA: *Hematology of Infancy and Childhood,* 3rd ed. Saunders, 1987.

Oski FA (editor). *Hematol Oncol Clin North Am* 1987;**6.**[Entire issue.]

Oski FA, Naiman JL: *Hematologic Problems of the Newborn,* 3rd ed. Saunders, 1982.

Petz LD, Garratty G: *Acquired Immune Hemolytic Anemias.* Churchill Livingstone, 1980.

Stamatoyannopoulos G et al: *The Molecular Basis of Blood Diseases.* Saunders, 1987.

Stiehm ER, Fulginiti VA: *Immunologic Disorders in Infants and Children,* 3rd ed. Saunders, 1989.

Wintrobe MM et al: *Clinical Hematology,* 8th ed. Lea & Febiger, 1981.

Zimmerman TS, Ruggeri ZM: *Coagulation and Bleeding Disorders: The Role of Factor VIII and von Willebrand Factor.* Marcel Dekker, 1989.

18 Immunodeficiency

Anthony R. Hayward, MD, PhD

Recurrent or severe infection is the most common symptom of immunodeficiency, but most children with recurrent minor infections do not have a definable immunodeficiency. Protection from infection depends primarily on the exclusion of pathogens by intact surfaces, followed by the decontamination of surfaces by mechanical and other nonspecific means. It is only after an organism gains access to the body that specific and nonspecific immune mechanisms are used to achieve its elimination. *Specific* immunity in this context includes antibody and cell-mediated immunity. *Nonspecific* immunity mechanisms include mechanical barriers, complement, phagocytes, and natural killer cells. Nonspecific mechanisms may be endowed with specificity by specific responses, such as the ability of antibody to direct killing by natural killer cells or to promote phagocytosis by opsonizing bacteria.

In deciding whether a patient has an immunodeficiency, the physician must exclude factors that increase local susceptibility to infection, eg, interference with the integrity of skin or mucous membranes, or defective ciliary function, before ordering laboratory tests of specific or nonspecific immunity. Table 18–1 illustrates some of the possibilities that must be considered.

NONSPECIFIC FACTORS IN RESISTANCE TO INFECTION

DEFECTS OF COMPLEMENT

The complement series of proteins are activated by IgG or IgM antibody bound to surfaces. The split products of C3 and C5 activation attract neutrophils, and C3b bound to the surface of bacteria opsonizes for phagocytosis by neutrophils. Deficiencies of individual classical pathway factors (C1–C9) occur as autosomal recessive traits and are rare. The most common clinical association is with immune complex disorders, which include systemic lupus erythematosus, chronic glomerulonephritis, dermatomyosi-

tis, and cutaneous vasculitis. Primary deficiency of C3 interferes with the opsonization of bacteria by the classical and alternate pathways of complement activation and results in recurrent bacterial infections similar to those seen in antibody deficiency. Treatment is with antibiotics. Serum levels of C3 are occasionally low enough in cases of partial lipodystrophy associated with glomerulonephritis to increase susceptibility to infection. Deficiency of properdin and factor D of the alternative pathway factors may also occasionally predispose to severe or recurrent bacterial infection.

C5, C6, C7, and C8 deficiencies are associated with dissemination of *Neisseria* infections, which results in an increased frequency of gonococcal arthritis in those with gonorrhea and in recurrence of meningitis in the survivors of meningococcal meningitis. Complement function should be screened with a hemolytic assay in patients with recurrent meningitis.

Recurrent angioedema without itching or wheals, usually beginning in late childhood, should lead one to suspect **hereditary angioedema.** This disorder is rare and results from C1 esterase inhibitor deficiency. Susceptibility to infection is not increased, and attacks may not start until adolescence. Transmission is autosomal and dominant. Affected individuals typically have recurrent episodes of edema lasting 48–72 hours and affecting the face or a limb. Edema affecting the bowel can be very painful. Patients are at risk for life-threatening laryngeal edema. Diagnosis is by measurement of C1 esterase inhibitor levels in serum; symptomatic individuals have levels below 30%. C4 levels are often low. Danazol, a synthetic androgen, prevents attacks by increasing C1 inhibitor levels. The diagnosis is suggested by decreased activity of whole complement, C4, and C2 and confirmed by direct assay of the C1 inhibitor.

Table 18–1. Host defense mechanisms and examples of nonspecific defects.

Protection by	Example of Defect
Intact skin	Burns, eczema, sinus tracks
Drainage	Auditory tube obstruction, cystic fibrosis, foreign body, urinary tract obstruction
Normal flora	Antibiotic-induced diarrhea, postantibiotic candidiasis

Fries LF, O'Shea JJ, Frank MM: Inherited deficiencies of complement and complement related proteins. *Clin Immunol Immunopathol* 1986;**40**:37.

DEFECTS OF PHAGOCYTE FUNCTION

Chemotaxis Defects

Useful phagocyte function requires the production of adequate numbers of neutrophils by the bone marrow, the migration of these cells to sites of inflammation, and finally the ingestion and killing of bacteria. Defects may exist at one or more of these levels. Neutropenia is described in Chapter 17. Defects of chemotaxis may be due to abnormalities of the cell, either intrinsic or secondary; to a deficiency of complement-derived chemotactic factors; or to increased activity of cell-directed or chemotactic factor-directed inhibitors. Primary cellular abnormalities are rare; they include Chédiak-Higashi syndrome (see Chapter 17) and leukocyte functional antigen-1 (LFA-1) deficiency (see Chapter 17). Burns, infections (eg, HIV, rubella, and influenza), metabolic and nutritional disorders (including diabetes mellitus), hypophosphatemia associated with hyperalimentation, and a wide variety of other conditions can be associated with depressed motility of phagocytic cells. Infections occurring in patients with chemotactic defects include furunculosis, subcutaneous abscesses, oral ulcers, gingivitis, and pneumonia, but the pathogenesis of these associations is obscure. The chemotactic defect itself would be expected to limit the amount of pus produced in response to a bacterial infection.

The association of **impaired neutrophil chemotaxis with hyperimmunoglobulinemia E** (levels are usually > 2000 units IgE/mL), recurrent staphylococcal abscesses of the skin, eczema, and otitis media is clinically recognizable and sometimes described as Job's syndrome. The occurrence is sporadic, and no cause is known. Treatment is symptomatic.

van der Valk P, Herman CJ: Leukocyte functions. *Lab Invest* 1987;**56**:127.

White CJ, Gallin JI: Phagocyte defects. *Clin Immunol Immunopathol* 1986;**40**:50.

Bacterial-Killing Defects

Chronic granulomatous disease (CGD) is described first because it is the best-defined defect of bacterial killing by neutrophils. The disorder is characterized by recurrent infections of the skin with catalase-positive bacteria (mostly staphylococci, sometimes *Serratia* spp or other opportunists) leading to abscesses in the draining lymph nodes. The patients' neutrophils fail to reduce nitroblue tetrazolium in the NBT test, and they fail to kill staphylococci in a bacterial-killing test. Coding defects of the β chain of cytochrome b, which is encoded on the X chromosome, are responsible for most of the cases with X-linked recessive inheritance. The rarer families with autosomal recessive transmission may have defects of the α chain of the same cytochrome, or other undefined defects of the electron transport pathway.

Affected boys usually present in the first months of life with superficial staphylococcal infections followed by recurrent groin, cervical, or axillary abscesses requiring incision and drainage. The infections cause high neutrophil counts and fever and sometimes spread to produce osteomyelitis or liver abscess. Colitis, leading to diarrhea and slow growth, is common. Treatment of abscesses requires drainage and appropriate antibiotic therapy for lengthy courses (3 weeks or more). CGD patients are best maintained on long-term antibiotic treatment with either a trimethoprim-sulfa combination or dicloxacillin. Good dental care is necessary because of the increased risk of gingivitis and periodontitis. Patients are significantly at risk for invasive fungal infections of lung and bone, especially by *Aspergillus* spp. Bone marrow transplantation has been attempted following suppression of specific immunity in several children with CGD. Some recipients have developed chimeric states, but it has been difficult to obtain long-term engraftment of donor neutrophils.

Antenatal diagnosis of X-linked CGD should be possible by analysis of restriction fragment length polymorphisms (RFLPs) using cells obtained by culture of amniotic fluid or sampling of chorionic villus, by direct hybridization for the cytochrome gene, or possibly, using fetal blood, by staining neutrophils with a monoclonal-antibody-to-cell-surface cytochrome.

Many of the other reports of defective bacterial killing by neutrophils (eg, deficiency of leukocyte glucose-6-phosphate dehydrogenase and glutathione dehydrogenase deficiency) will need to be reassessed following the characterization of the defects in chronic granulomatous disease. Their reported severity was variable, and they should be screened for by a bacterial killing test because the NBT test might not be abnormal.

Dinauer MC, Orkin SH: Molecular genetics of chronic granulomatous disease. *Immunodeficiency Rev* 1988;**1**:55.

Mizuno Y, Hara T, Nakamura M, et al: Classification of chronic granulomatous disease on the basis of monoclonal antibody. *J Pediatr* 1988;**113**:458.

Segal AW: The molecular and cellular pathology of chronic granulomatous disease. *Eur J Clin Invest* 1988;**18**:433.

Leukocyte Adhesion Deficiency

Leukocytes, monocytes, and some activated T cells normally express cell surface adhesion molecules—LFA-1 (CD11a), Mac-1 (CD11b), and p150,95 (CD11c). These molecules have a common beta subunit (CD18) encoded on chromosome 21 and cell-specific but related alpha subunits (CD11). Defects or deficiency of the beta subunit alone results in defective expression of all members of this family of proteins.

The most severe cases present in infancy with progressive and necrotic periumbilical infections. A range of organisms is isolated, the neutrophil count is high, but there is relatively little pus formation. In childhood the infections are often around body orifices; they also affect the skin, esophagus, and the respiratory tract. Death in childhood is common. Other patients with a milder phenotype have survived for 20 or more years. Diagnosis is by phenotyping blood mononuclear cells for LFA-1 or Mac-1; this approach can also be used for antenatal diagnosis.

Treatment of infections is by antibiotics, and prophylactic antibiotics may suffice for mildly affected patients. Mixed but stable chimerism, sufficient to reduce the risk of infections, has followed treatment by bone marrow transplantation.

Fischer A, Lisowska-Grospierre B, Anderson DC, Springer TA: Leukocyte adhesion deficiency. *Immunodeficiency Rev* 1988;**1**:39.

PRIMARY DEFICIENCIES OF SPECIFIC IMMUNITY

These disorders are broadly subdivided into defects affecting predominantly antibody formation, those affecting cellular immunity, and those in which both mechanisms are impaired. The classification in Table 18–2 is based on combinations of clinical and laboratory results and includes only the more common conditions. Family studies in which a

Table 18–2. Classification of primary defects of specific immunity.

Immunoglobulin deficiency
All Ig classes: hypogammaglobulinemia
Congenital (see text for varieties)
Acquired
Unclassified (common variable hypogammaglobulinemia)
Selective immunoglobulin deficiency
IgA deficiency
IgG subclass deficiencies
IgM deficiency
Transient hypogammaglobulinemia
Antibody deficiency with immunoglobulins
Defect of cell-mediated immunity
PNP deficiency
DiGeorge syndrome
Cartilage hair hypoplasia
Unclassified (common variable immunodeficiency affecting cell-mediated immunity
Combined antibody and cell-mediated defects
Severe combined immunodeficiency (various types)

mode of inheritance can be shown are the most secure basis of classification, and in a few instances the underlying single gene defect is known, eg, in adenosine deaminase (ADA) and purine nucleoside phosphorylase (PNP) deficiencies. Occasionally, as in ataxia-telangiectasia, the phenotypic features are sufficiently characteristic to facilitate recognition. The fact that most cases of immunodeficiency are still reported as "varied immunodeficiency, largely unclassified" indicates that major advances remain to be made.

IMMUNOGLOBULIN & ANTIBODY DEFICIENCY SYNDROMES

HYPOGAMMAGLOBULINEMIA SYNDROMES

Congenital X-linked agammaglobulinemia occurs in about 1 of 10^5 live births. Other types of hypogammaglobulinemia are slightly more common and may develop at any age. It is helpful to distinguish between the congenital X-linked and other forms of hypogammaglobulinemia for the sake of genetic counseling: the diagnosis, treatment, and complications are similar regardless of the type of antibody deficiency. The different types are summarized in Table 18–2.

Conley ME, Puck JM: Carrier detection in typical and atypical X-linked agammaglobulinemia. *J Pediatr* 1988; **112**:688.

A. Congenital X-linked Agammaglobulinemia: The most common symptoms arise from bacterial infection of the respiratory tract (sinusitis, otitis, pneumonia) or skin (cellulitis, abscesses). Without antibiotic therapy, these infections spread and result in septicemia and meningitis. Infections usually start after 4 months of age, when maternal IgG levels have declined. The organisms responsible for the presenting infections are mostly encapsulated bacteria, but following courses of antibiotics, mycoplasma strains, such as *Ureaplasma urealyticum*, become important. At the time of diagnosis, a few boys have an asymmetric arthritis, most often of the knee or ankle, which usually resolves after adequate IgG replacement is given. There are no very useful physical signs other than a paucity of tonsillar and adenoidal tissue. Because the severity of infections varies very much among individuals, the diagnosis may not be made for many years.

The diagnosis requires that the serum IgG be less than 200 mg/dL; IgA and IgM are generally undetectable. Causes of secondary hypogammaglobulinemia (nephrotic syndrome, HIV infection, and protein-losing enteropathy) should be excluded by measuring serum albumin. Boys with congenital X-linked agammaglobulinemia differ from most other antibody-deficient subjects in that they have few if any B cells in their blood although they have normal blood counts and normal numbers of pre-B cells in their marrow. They lack serum isohemagglutinins and do not make antibody following immunization. The DNA probes that are now becoming available should facilitate the identification of affected boys who do not have affected maternal male relatives.

B. Immunodeficiency With High IgM Levels: This condition affects predominantly boys, who differ from those with congenital agammaglobulinemia by having normal or high serum IgM levels, often with lymphadenopathy. Because the IgM has no useful antibody activity, the treatment is as for hypogammaglobulinemia. The level of IgG is less than 200 mg/dL, and that of IgA is low or absent. Impaired cell-mediated immunity and consequent *Pneumocystis* infections, lymphomas, and neutropenia all occur as complications.

C. Acquired and Unclassified Hypogammaglobulinemia Syndromes: This heading includes patients with congenital or acquired antibody deficiency syndromes not classified elsewhere. It is a heterogeneous group with symptoms developing at any age. Patients with varied hypogammaglobulinemia outnumber patients with all other types of antibody deficiency except selective IgA deficiency. A familial trend in some cases (including relatives with autoimmune disorders) and an excess of affected boys suggest that both multifactorial and single gene causes exist. The circulating B cells of these patients are immature and generally do not differentiate normally in tissue culture, but the pathogenesis of these disorders is not understood. Infections follow the patterns described for other types of antibody deficiency. Some patients have remarkably few infections despite long-standing, very low immunoglobulin levels. The laboratory findings are heterogeneous: low levels of one or more immunoglobulin classes are associated with varying degrees of impairment of cellular immunity (although infants with severe combined immunodeficiency are excluded from this classification). Autoantibody formation, elevated IgE levels, and positive immediate hypersensitivity skin reactions occur. Almost all these patients have B cells in their blood, although their number may be low. Neutropenia is common, and thrombocytopenia occurs sometimes in acquired hypogammaglobulinemia syndromes. Varied immunodeficiency syndromes are too heterogeneous for a confident prognosis.

D. Complications of Hypogammaglobulinemia: Affected boys occasionally develop optic atrophy or ataxia, which evolves slowly or rapidly into fatal encephalitis. Echoviruses have sometimes been isolated from their cerebrospinal fluid or brains at biopsy or necropsy. A smaller proportion develop a dermatomyositis-like syndrome, with prominent peripheral cyanosis and myopathy but little heliotrope coloration. Both of these complications may be less commonly seen now that much higher immune globulin replacements are given. About 10% of patients develop symptoms of diarrhea and malabsorption that resemble Crohn's disease and are generally unresponsive to dietary changes. Infection is the most likely cause of the diarrhea, and efforts should be made to exclude treatable causes such as *Giardia lamblia* or *Cryptosporidium* sp. In adult life, patients with hypogammaglobulinemia often develop gastric achlorhydria and atrophic gastritis, leading to vitamin B_{12} deficiency. The rate of cancer in patients with antibody deficiency is increased, mainly because of an increased incidence of T and B cell lymphomas. Epstein-Barr virus infections may contribute to the B cell lymphomas, and it is important to remember that lymphoreticular proliferations in hypogammaglobulinemia patients are not always malignant.

Buckley R: Humoral immunodeficiency. *Clin Immunol Immunopathol* 1986;**40**:13.

den Hartog G, van der Meer JW, Jansen JB, van Furth R, Lamers CB: Decreased gastrin secretion in patients with late-onset hypogammaglobulinemia. *N Engl J Med* 1988;**318**:1563.

Kim JH, Bedrosian CL, Jain R, Schlossman DM: Peripheral T-cell lymphoma complicating common variable hypogammaglobulinemia. *Am J Med* 1988;**85**:123.

E. Immunoglobulin Replacement: Patients with serum IgG levels of 200 mg/dL or less and who fail to make IgG antibody following immunization should have serum IgG replaced to protect against infection. The testing of antibody responses is important to exclude the small number of infants with transient hypogammaglobulinemia with normal IgM levels who make sufficient antibody to remain free from infection. IgG is usually given by intravenous infusions of specially prepared deaggregated IgG (200–600 mg/kg every 4 weeks of preparations such as Sandoglobulin or Gammimmune-N). A first infusion should be of about 100 mg/kg, given over several hours with acetaminophen pretreatment to reduce fever. Intravenous treatment may be difficult in young children, who may temporarily be managed by giving intramuscular injections of IgG concentrate (0.6 ml/kg every 2–3 weeks). The aim of treatment must be to avoid, or minimize the progression of, chronic lung disease (bronchitis, bronchiectasis). Productive cough and purulent sputum or conjunctivitis must be taken seriously, and antibiotic therapy must be continued until there is radiologic and clinical resolution. Mycoplasma infections of the respiratory or urinary tracts should be sought and treated with erythromycin or doxycycline.

Reactions to immune globulin infusions or injections are relatively common. In patients receiving their first infusion, the reaction may be due to antigen binding by antibody. Reactions to injected IgG concentrates are likely to be due to complement activation by IgG aggregates. Symptoms generally include back and limb pain, anxiety, and tightness of the chest. Signs are tachycardia, shivering, fever, and, in severe cases, shock. The rare patients who have frequent reactions to intravenous immune globulin infusions may have antibodies to IgA, but in most instances reactions are sporadic and not due to hypersensitivity. Skin tests are not helpful. It is important to maintain immune globulin replacement, and attempts should be made to limit the severity of the reactions by premedication with aspirin, an antihistamine, or intravenously administered hydrocortisone immediately before the infusion. Alternative brands of IgG may be tried, some of which contain little if any IgA.

Wedgwood R: Intravenous immunoglobulin. *Clin Immunol Immunopathol* 1986;**40:**147.

TRANSIENT HYPOGAMMAGLOBULINEMIA

Infants' IgG levels fall during the first 4–5 months of life while maternal IgG is diluted and catabolized. The physiologic trough that occurs before the infants' IgG production reaches adult levels is accentuated in premature and dysmature infants. IgG levels of 250–300 mg/dL lie within 2 standard deviations of the mean at 3–4 months of age, and the diagnosis of transient hypogammaglobulinemia is often made in infants with infections and IgG levels in this range. The diagnosis should be made retrospectively, since the transitory nature of the hypogammaglobulinemia can be established only when immunoglobulin levels have returned to normal. The only diagnostic laboratory findings are of low IgG, with or without low IgA and IgM, and subsequent return to normal levels. Salivary IgA is generally detectable, and, despite the low immunoglobulin levels, antibody activity (isohemagglutinin or antidiphtheria or tetanus antibody) is present in serum. IgG antibody is generally made following immunization, and tests for cellular immunity are normal. IgG replacement is not usually required for infants who make antibody following immunization and who do not have severe or invasive infections, because treatment with appropriate antibiotics for bacterial infections should be sufficient. Infants who do not meet these criteria should be given IgG, and their preinfusion levels should be checked every 6 months for a return to normal levels. The prognosis for affected infants

is (by definition) excellent provided they do not succumb to infection before achieving normal immunity.

McGeady SJ: Transient hypogammaglobulinemia of infancy: Need to reconsider name and definition. *J Pediatr* 1987;**110:**47.

SELECTIVE IMMUNOGLOBULIN DEFICIENCIES

A. IgA Deficiency: With a prevalence of 1 in 500 in Caucasian populations, this is by far the most common primary defect of specific immunity. The proportion of IgA-deficient patients who ultimately develop symptoms is uncertain, but it may be at most two-thirds. Most cases appear sporadically, but both dominant and recessive inheritance occurs, and so the syndrome is heterogeneous. Postulated cellular mechanisms include an intrinsic defect of differentiation of B lymphocytes committed to IgA production and failure of IgA production secondary to a defect of T cells. Many patients have no symptoms, perhaps because adequate protection of the mucosa is conferred by IgG and IgM. Failure of antibody responses in the IgG2 subclass is reported in symptomatic patients. Symptoms, if present, are predominantly due to upper respiratory tract infections or diarrhea. There are also strong associations with allergy (mainly respiratory and gut) and autoimmune disorders (eg, thyroiditis, arthritis, vitiligo).

Arbitrary criteria for diagnosis are serum IgA less than 5 mg/dL, absent salivary IgA, normal IgM and IgG, and normal cellular immunity. A search for anti-IgA antibodies may be important, since these can cause transfusion reactions. The selective lack of IgA antibody responses and the presence of normal antibody responses in other immunoglobulin classes serve to distinguish IgA deficiency from unclassified variable immunodeficiency. IgA has a short half life in serum, and replacement is impractical. It is conceivable but unproved that colostrum feeding could modify severe gut symptoms. Treatment of symptomatic patients with IgG injections has been both advocated and condemned on theoretical grounds. Anti-IgA antibodies in the recipient are occasionally responsible for reactions to intravenous IgG preparations (most of which contain small amounts of IgA). Most IgA-deficient patients manage reasonably well with antibiotics only; atopic or autoimmune symptoms should be treated conventionally.

B. Other Selective Subclass Deficiencies: The IgG heavy chain genes are on chromosome 11, where the IgG1 gene is close to the IgG3 gene and the IgG2 gene close to the IgG4 gene. Most serum IgG is IgG1, and most viral and protein antigens elicit antibody of IgG1 and IgG3 subclasses. When IgG1 is deficient, IgG2 and IgG3 are generally also low, resulting in the clinical picture of hypogammaglobulinemia. The

IgG2 subclass has much of the antibody to capsular polysaccharides. IgG2 deficiency is often associated with IgA deficiency and may contribute to the respiratory tract infections seen in IgA deficiency. Deficiency of IgG3 with normal levels of other subclasses is rare but may occasionally be responsible for an antibody deficiency syndrome in subjects with normal IgG or IgG1 levels. The diagnosis of IgG subclass deficiency requires the demonstration of low subclass levels for age. Age-matched controls are required because normal infants produce little IgG2 before the age of 2. A history of significant infections attributable to a subclass deficiency might justify evaluation for IgG replacement; many patients are managed with antibiotics alone.

Selective deficiencies of IgM, IgE, IgG subclasses and kappa or lambda light chains have been described but are rare. IgM deficiency has been associated with marked susceptibility to septicemia. Serum IgM has a short half life, and replacement is not possible. Some protection could probably be provided by IgG infusion, but practitioners rely mainly on antibiotics.

Cunningham-Rundles C: Selective IgA deficiency. *J Pediatr Gastroenterol Nutr* 1988;**7**:482.

Ferreira A, Garcia Rodriguez MC, Lopez-Trascasa M, Pascual Salcedo D, Fontan G: Anti-IgA antibodies in selective IgA deficiency and in primary immunodeficient patients treated with gamma-globulin. *Clin Immunol Immunopathol* 1988;**47**:199.

SELECTIVE DEFECTS OF CELL-MEDIATED IMMUNITY

PURINE NUCLEOSIDE PHOSPHORYLASE DEFICIENCY

Purine nucleoside phosphorylase (PNP) deficiency results in increased intracellular levels of deoxyguanosine triphosphate (dGTP), which inhibits ribonucleotide reductase and interferes with DNA synthesis, especially in T cells. The action of T cells on B cells is not affected, probably because it is not dependent on cell division. The structural locus for PNP is on chromosome 14; transmission is recessive. Presenting features may be neurologic (developmental retardation, behavior disorders, and spasticity) with immunodeficiency (severe varicella, anemia, and failure to thrive) developing later. The age at presentation has ranged from 6 months to 7 years. Investigations show low serum levels of uric acid, low-normal blood lymphocyte counts, absence of delayed hypersensitivity skin responses, and low or absent lymphocyte responses to mitogens. Serum immunoglobulins and antibody responses to injected antigens are normal. In many cases, an autoimmune hemolytic anemia has developed. Diagnosis depends on enzyme measurement, and all patients with severely impaired cellular immunity who make immunoglobulin should probably be tested. Antenatal diagnosis is possible. It has been difficult to achieve stable engraftment following bone marrow transplantation.

Carapella De Luca E, Stegagno M, Dionisi Vici C, Paesano R, Fairbanks LD, Morris GS, Simmonds HA: Prenatal exclusion of purine nucleoside phosphorylase deficiency. *Eur J Pediatr* 1986;**145**:51.

Rijksen G, Kuis W, Wadman SK, Spaapen LJ, Duran M, Voorbrood BS, Staal GE, Stoop JW, Zegers BJ: A new case of purine nucleoside phosphorylase deficiency: Enzymologic, clinical, and immunologic characteristics. *Pediatr Res* 1986;**21**:137.

THYMIC HYPOPLASIA (DiGeorge Syndrome)

The diagnostic criteria are small or absent thymus, lack of parathyroid glands, and major vessel abnormalities, eg, truncus arteriosus, anomalous pulmonary venous drainage, or right-sided aortic arch. Other features include a small jaw, low-set ears, and a short philtrum. A few cases are familial (some with deletions of C22), but a family history is exceptional, and environmental damage to the fetus, probably between 5 and 7 weeks of gestation, seems the most likely cause. The term "partial DiGeorge syndrome" is commonly applied to infants who have impaired rather than absent parathyroid or thymus function. Clinical presentation usually results from cardiac failure or, after 24–48 hours, from hypocalcemia, and the diagnosis is sometimes made during the course of cardiac surgery, when no thymus is found in the mediastinum. Postoperative hypocalcemia can be severe and persistent, requiring both calcium and vitamin D supplementation. Despite receiving fresh blood transfusions during cardiopulmonary bypass, patients do not usually develop graft-versus-host disease. Nevertheless, all blood transfusions to known or suspected immunodeficient patients should be irradiated (1500+ rads; see below). Patients with DiGeorge syndrome have variable susceptibility to infection. A few have died of septicemia, and some have had chronic candidiasis, but many appear to respond normally. This may reflect the tendency for the number of T cells in the patients' blood to rise spontaneously over the course of several years. The differential diagnosis includes hypocalcemia and a small or absent thymus on chest x-ray secondary to infection. Treatment is primarily directed toward correcting the cardiac defects and hypocalcemia. Patients with thymic hypoplasia receiving grafts of fetal thymus or thymic epithelial cells often demonstrate a rapid improvement in the lymphocyte response to mitogens. The improvement is so rapid that thymic humoral factors are thought to be responsible, but factors currently available for treatment have not been useful. Graft treatment is generally reserved for those who do not improve spontaneously and poses a risk for graft-versus-host disease.

Greenberg F, Crowder WE, Paschall V, et al: Familial DiGeorge syndrome and associated partial monosomy of chromosome 22. *Hum Genet* 1984;**65**:317.

Bastian J, Law S, Vogler L, Lawton A, Herrod H, Anderson S, Horowitz S, Hong R: Prediction of persistent immunodeficiency in the DiGeorge anomaly. *J Pediatr* 1989;**115**:391.

OTHER DEFECTS OF CELL-MEDIATED IMMUNITY

Cartilage hair hypoplasia is an autosomal recessively inherited syndrome characterized by disproportionately short stature and fine hair that lacks a central shaft. American kindreds, but not those from Finland, have a moderate degree of lymphopenia, low lymphocyte responses to mitogens, and higher than normal morbidity and mortality rates from herpesvirus and poxvirus infections. There is no established treatment. Short-limbed dwarfs who are immunodeficient should probably be tested for adenosine deaminase deficiency, since this is treatable. Other types of immunodeficiency affecting predominantly cellular immunity exist but are poorly classified. Currently these are included in the "varied immunodeficiency" group. People in this group have infections resembling those described above and frequently also have chronic diarrhea and malabsorption as well as lung infections due to atypical mycobacteria, fungi, and *Pneumocystis carinii*. Treatment is investigational.

COMBINED IMMUNODEFICIENCY DISORDERS

Essentials of Diagnosis

- Hypogammaglobulinemia.
- Defective cell-mediated immunity.

General Considerations

Severe combined immunodeficiency (SCID) comprises a heterogeneous group of conditions that have a primary severe impairment of both antibody- and cell-mediated immunity in common. The term SCID is usually applied only to infants with congenital im-

munodeficiency, but equally severe defects can be caused by acquired immunodeficiency syndrome (AIDS) or lymphocyte loss. The heterogeneity of the congenital forms reflects the range of underlying metabolic defects that may interfere with lymphocyte development at different stages and the varying degrees of engraftment with maternal lymphocytes that can occur during gestation or at birth.

Clinical Findings

A. Symptoms and Signs: Diarrhea, vomiting, and cough are common symptoms due to infection. The diarrhea causes failure to thrive. Although the diarrhea may briefly abate after dietary changes, it recurs after a few days. The cough is usually persistent; it is often due to *Pneumocystis carinii* infection and can cause cyanosis. Skin rashes are common and frequently evanescent, except for rash following blood transfusion, which is due to graft-versus-host disease. A *Candida* diaper rash is usual. Findings initially include absence of tonsils or palpable lymph nodes; later, there is emaciation. The presence of a thymus shadow on chest x-ray suggests another diagnosis.

B. Laboratory Findings: All patients with SCID have some degree of hypogammaglobulinemia and failure of antibody production (though maternal IgG will be present in infants). Lymphopenia is not always present, but, with the exception of patients with HLA-DR deficient SCID, very few or no T (CD3$^+$) cells and normal numbers of natural killer (NK) (CD16$^+$) cells are present in the blood of all patients with SCID. B lymphocytes (with surface IgM) are usually present in the blood. In vitro lymphocyte responses to mitogens are generally absent. Antigen-specific responses (T cell or antibody) are difficult to test for in infancy because of uncertainty about prior experience and generally too time-consuming for clinical purposes.

Variants of Severe Combined Immunodeficiency

A. Adenosine Deaminase Deficiency: ADA converts adenosine and deoxyadenosine to inosine and deoxyinosine, respectively. Its structural locus is on chromosone 20, and individuals homozygous for a null gene account for about 20% of cases of SCID. The biochemical basis for impairment of lymphocyte function is not fully understood but appears to involve raised deoxy-ATP levels, which inhibit ribonucleotide reductase so that T lymphocytes are prevented from dividing. In addition, there is increased DNA fragmentation and interference with methylation reactions. Affected infants may be near-normal at birth (presumably because their mothers maintain low deoxyadenosine levels in utero). Their cellular immunity fails first; they then become antibody-deficient, although they may continue to produce immunoglobulin for months or years. Diagnosis is by assay of adenosine deaminase in red cell lysates. A bone marrow graft from an HLA-matched sibling with normal red cell adenosine deaminase levels is the ideal treatment (see below). ADA-deficient cases have been more prone to reject parental T cell-depleted grafts than others. Some patients may benefit from weekly injections of a stabilized enzyme conjugate, which increases adenosine excretion but does not correct the lymphopenia.

B. SCID With Immunoglobulins: Affected patients have severely impaired cellular immunity, and although they may make small or large amounts of immunoglobulin (usually IgM), they do not make useful antibodies. Their clinical course is therefore similar to those with other types of SCID. The condition is heterogeneous in that both X-linked and autosomal recessive forms exist.

C. SCID With Reticuloendotheliosis: This describes the combination of skin rash, lymphadenopathy, and splenomegaly with SCID, most probably as a consequence of partial engraftment with sufficient maternal T cells to cause graft-versus-host disease in the infant with SCID. Therapy consisting of immunosuppression and marrow ablation followed by area bone marrow transplantation has sometimes been successful under these conditions.

D. SCID With Leukopenia (Reticular Dysgenesis): This describes infants with SCID who also have severe neutropenia, often with reduced numbers of granulocyte precursors in the marrow. Only about 20 cases have been reported. There is a familial trend, but the severity of the neutropenia varies between affected siblings, and so neutropenia may be a secondary feature.

E. SCID With Defective Expression of HLA Antigens: This is a difficult condition to diagnose because affected patients generally make immunoglobulins and have low-to-normal numbers of B and T cells in their blood, together with positive responses to PHA stimulation. Their clinical symptoms are nevertheless those of SCID. The defect is of HLA-D antigen expression. Because the T cells do not make antigen-specific responses, the patients remain antibody-deficient. Diagnosis is by phenotyping blood lymphocytes for HLA-DR antigen expression. Several affected families have been of North African descent.

Diagnosis & Treatment of SCID

Defects of cellular immunity should be suspected in infants (especially females) with antibody deficiency who continue to have diarrhea after IgG replacement. The main differential is between severe varied immunodeficiency and secondary immunodeficiency due to gastrointestinal disease, eg, HIV infection, long-standing gastroenteritis, or intestinal lymphangiectasia. In secondary immunodeficiency, the blood lymphocyte response to phytohemagglutinin is usually not completely absent, and the serum albumin concentration may be low. Antenatal diagnosis is possible by sampling fetal blood at about 15 weeks of gestation and phenotyping the lymphocytes obtained.

Infants in whom the diagnosis is suspected should receive antibiotics for infection and IgG replacement. They should not receive blood transfusions unless the blood has first been irradiated. With confirmation of the diagnosis, they may be started on trimethoprim-sulfamethoxazole for *Pneumocystis* prophylaxis. Bone marrow grafting offers the best hope for cure. If an HLA-matched sibling is available, there is a high chance of success; the treatment can be given without depleting the marrow of T cells or immunosuppressing the recipient. HLA-matched donors cannot be found for most patients with SCID, and SCID patients are now treated with grafts of parental bone marrow from which the T cells are removed by lectins or monoclonal antibodies. Pregraft suppression, with the attendant hazards of thrombocytopenia and neutropenia, may be required. Reconstitution can take 4 months, and the overall rate of T cell engraftment is between 50 and 70%. Reconstitution for antibody responses may not occur even if B cells are produced.

Griscelli C, Fischer A, Durandy A, et al: Defective synthesis of HLA class I and II molecules associated with a combined immunodeficiency. In: *Primary Immunodeficiency Diseases.* Eibl MM, Rosen FS (editors). Elsevier, 1986.

Levy Y, Herschfield MS, Fernandez-Mejia C, et al: Adenosine deaminase deficiency with late onset of recurrent infections: Response to treatment with polyethylene glycol-modified adenosine deaminase. *J Pediatr* 1988; **113**:312.

OTHER DISORDERS ASSOCIATED WITH IMMUNODEFICIENCY

WISKOTT-ALDRICH SYNDROME

Characteristics are thrombocytopenia, eczema, and recurrent infection (initially, draining ears). The incidence is about 1 per 4 million male births. Inheritance is X-linked recessive, and the gene has been localized to the p11 region of the X chromosome. The disorder is associated with deficient expression of a 115 kDa cell surface sialophorin identified as CD43. Common presenting symptoms are bloody diarrhea, cerebral hemorrhage, or septicemia, followed by severe infections with polysaccharide-encapsulated bacteria. Some patients, however, have little if any eczema, and others have few infections. The main causes of death in infancy are bleeding and infections, but lymphomas become increasingly common as survivors grow older. Survival through the teens is rare in untreated patients, although partial syndromes are sometimes diagnosed in adults. The variability of the clinical picture makes diagnosis difficult in the absence of a family history. Laboratory findings helpful in diagnosis include a low platelet count, low or absent isohemagglutinins, and reduced cell surface CD43. Bone marrow transplantation with matched sibling marrow offers the best hope for long-term correction of the defect but suitable donors are available for only a minority of patients. Haploidentical T-depleted grafts often fail to take. The platelet count generally rises following splenectomy, but this operation must be accompanied by life-long antibiotic prophylaxis because of the increased risk of septicemia and sudden death. If the abnormal X chromosome in a family can be identified, then antenatal diagnosis should be possible either by RFLPs or by methylation protection analysis.

Fearon ER, Kohn DB, Winkelstein JA, Vogelstein B, Blaese RM: Carrier detection in the Wiskott-Aldrich syndrome. *Blood* 1988;**72:**P1735.

ATAXIA-TELANGIECTASIA

Characteristics include a cerebellar ataxia (due to degeneration of Purkinje's cells) usually developing between 2 and 5 years of age and followed by the appearance of telangiectases, particularly on the conjunctivae and over exposed areas, eg, the nose, ears, and shoulders. The inheritance pattern is autosomal recessive, but there are 6 or more different complementation groups. The abnormal gene is on chromosome 11—11q22-23 in one study—but its mechanism of action is unknown. Abnormal findings in ataxia-telangiectasia include raised serum alpha fetoprotein levels (useful diagnostically), thymic hypoplasia, low or absent serum IgE in 60%, low IgA in 50%, abnormal carbohydrate tolerance, and defective ability to repair radiation-induced DNA fragmentation. Clinically the most important symptom is the progressive loss of motor coordination, followed by weakness. Respiratory tract infection is the major cause of death, followed by malignancy. About 10% of patients develop lymphomas, the majority of which are T-cell derived. Many of the lymphomas have translocations or inversions at sites where T-cell receptor genes are normally rearranged. Radiotherapy has been followed by skin breakdown, which is presumably the result of the DNA repair defect. The heterozygote frequency is 0.5–5%, depending on geographic and ethnic factors, and heterozygotic individuals have an increased incidence of breast cancer. No specific treatment is known.

Gatti RA, Berkel I, Boder E, et al: Localization of an ataxia-telangiectasis gene to chromosome 11q22-23. *Nature* 1988;**336:**577.

CHRONIC MUCOCUTANEOUS CANDIDASIS

Diagnostic criteria are chronic candidiasis affecting skin or nails and mucous membranes and not attributable to antibiotic treatment or another defined immunodeficiency. Involvement of scalp and flexures is common, usually as erythema and scaling but occasionally as granulomas with skin hypertrophy. The recurrent candidiasis that these patients experience points to an underlying immunodeficiency, although the faulty mechanism has not been identified. Affected patients make anti-*Candida albicans* antibodies, and their in vitro lymphocyte responses may be positive even when skin tests for *Candida* are negative. *Candida* antigens themselves may modulate immune responses to the fungus. Evidence for the complexity of this form of immunodeficiency includes the frequent association with endocrinopathy, sometimes autoimmune (affecting parathyroid, thyroid, pituitary, or gonads) and, less commonly, susceptibility to staphylococcal infections with defective neutrophil mobility. Continuous ketoconazole treatment usually provides some control of the candidiasis.

Domer J, Elkins K, Ennist D, Baker P: Modulation of immune responses by surface polysaccharides of *Candida albicans. Rev Infect Dis* 1988;**10(Suppl 2):**419.

X-LINKED LYMPHOPROLIFERATIVE SYNDROME

This term is applied to boys who develop bone marrow aplasia, hypogammaglobulinemia, or a lymphoproliferative syndrome following Epstein-Barr virus (EBV) infection. The gene responsible has been mapped to Xq2s, and antenatal diagnosis is possible using polymorphisms at DXS42 and DXS37. Affected boys are immunologically normal prior to EBV infection, and during acute mononucleosis they make some antibody to the EBV. In most instances the EBV infection results in a lethal lymphoproliferative syndrome characterized by liver failure, disseminated intravascular coagulation, and multiple monoclonal serum IgM bands. Agents active against EBV are of no clear benefit; alpha interferon and monoclonal anti-B cell antibodies are being investigated as treatments. Only 10–20% of affected boys who are infected with EBV survive to develop hypogammaglobulinemia.

Hayoz D, Lenoir GM, Nicole A, Pugin P, Regamey C: X-linked lymphoproliferative syndrome. Identification of a large family in Switzerland. *Am J Med* 1988;**84:**529.

BIOCHEMICAL DEFECTS SOMETIMES ASSOCIATED WITH IMMUNODEFICIENCY

Several primary errors of metabolism affect immunity adversely. Transcobalamin II deficiency causes a megaloblastic anemia with impaired bacterial killing by neutrophils and reduced serum immunoglobulins of all classes. Biotin-dependent decarboxylase deficiencies may be associated with convulsions, alopecia, candidiasis, low serum IgA, and a reduced number of T cells. Lymphopenia and impaired cell-mediated immunity are reported in hereditary orotic aciduria, with, in one case, response to oral uridine replacement. Chromosomal instability syndromes impair cell-mediated immunity; in Bloom syndrome, this may be severe enough to cause malabsorption. An increased mortality from infection suggests that Down syndrome also impairs immunity.

Alvarado CS, Livingstone LR, Jones ME, et al: Uridine-responsive hypogammaglobulinemia and congenital heart disease in a patient with hereditary orotic aciduria. *J Pediatr* 1988;**113**:867.

SECONDARY IMMUNODEFICIENCY

Secondary immunodeficiency is a common cause of pediatric illness. The mechanisms that may be impaired are summarized in Table 18–3, and the symptoms are generally those that would be anticipated from the combination of the primary disorder and the complicating immunodeficiency. Whenever possible, treatment should be of the primary disorder. Occasionally, immunologic methods may help, eg, zoster immune globulin may prevent varicella in patients with leukemia, and intravenous IgG replacement might provide added protection in patients with diminished antibody production. IgG replacement is unlikely to help when loss (as in nephrotic syndrome) is responsible for hypogammaglobulinemia.

Pinching AJ: Secondary immunodeficiency. *Clin Immunol Allergy* 1985;**5**:469.

GRAFT-VERSUS-HOST DISEASE

Infusion of mature T lymphocytes from an HLA-unmatched donor into a patient with severely impaired or absent cell-mediated immunity (eg, a patient with SCID) is followed after 4 to 5 days by fevers and 1 to 2 days later by a generalized erythematous rash. Diarrhea develops, the rash becomes

Table 18–3. Mechanisms of secondary immunodeficiency.

Mechanism	Example
Loss Immunoglobulin	Renal, in nephrotic syndrome
Immunoglobulin	Skin, from burns
Immunoglobulin and cells	Gut, in intestinal lymphangiectasia
Phagocytes	Following splenectomy
Malnutrition	Kwashiorkor
Zinc deficiency	Impaired cell-mediated immunity, thymic hypoplasia experimentally
Cu/Fe deficiency	Impaired neutrophil function
Drugs	Steroids, immunosuppressive agents, phenytoin (IgA deficiency)
Infections	Human immunodeficiency virus, Epstein-Barr virus, measles, rubella, hepatitis, malaria

macular and may blister, and hepatitis, jaundice and liver failure follow. Graft-versus-host disease is generally fatal in infants with SCID who are inadvertently given transfusions of unmatched, unirradiated blood. In other defects of cell-mediated immunity, and in certain situations after bone marrow transplantation, chronic graft-versus-host disease develops, characterized by symmetric arthritis, chronic skin rash, keratoconjunctivitis sicca, and scleroderma. Graft-versus-host disease is best avoided by irradiating (1500 rads) all blood products given to patients with suspected or known defects in cell-mediated immunity. Acute graft-versus-host disease may be ameliorated with steroids and cyclosporine A; thalidomide has also recently been used experimentally.

Vogelsang GB, Hess AD, Santos GW: Thalidomide for treatment of graft-versus-host disease. *Bone Marrow Transplant* 1988;**3**:393.

HUMAN IMMUNODEFICIENCY VIRUS (HIV) INFECTION & ACQUIRED IMMUNODEFICIENCY SYNDROME (AIDS)

Essentials of Diagnosis

- Serologic evidence for infection with HIV.
- Risk factors for infection.
- Opportunistic infections.

General Considerations

HIV is a retrovirus that infects CD4$^+$ lymphocytes, monocytes, and, in the brain, multinucleated giant cells, macrophages, and microglia. The infection is cytolytic for T cells. It is the resulting loss of cell-mediated immunity that predisposes the patient to infection by opportunists as well as pathogens. Transmission of the virus to infants and children is now mainly by vertical transmission from infected mothers (with a transmission rate of about 50%) who themselves became infected from drug use or from infected partners. Because of the slow progression of this disease patients who were previously infected through blood transfusion or clotting factor concentrates continue to present at the time of writing.

Clinical Findings

A. Symptoms and Signs: The initial infection with HIV can cause a transient febrile illness, but this is often missed. Subsequently the symptoms and signs of HIV infection advance at a variable rate, but in proportion to the progressive immunodeficiency that results from the destruction of CD4 lymphocytes. The major symptoms arise from infections, particularly by opportunists such as *Pneumocystis carinii* in the lung and *Cryptosporidium* spp (causing diarrhea) in the gut. Congenitally infected children may have lymphadenopathy at birth and develop infections in the first month of life. The median age for diagnosis in children infected perinatally is 9 months. Weight loss is common in older children, whereas younger patients often have recurrent bacterial infections with encapsulated organisms, as seen in antibody deficiency syndromes. The signs have little diagnostic specificity. They include lymphadenopathy, hepatosplenomegaly, and wasting together with whatever additional signs may result from infections. The most common opportunistic infections are caused by *Pneumocystis carinii, Mycobacterium avium-intracellulare, Candida albicans,* and cytomegalovirus.

HIV encephalopathy is common. It causes developmental delay and loss of acquired skills, sometimes with weakness, ataxia, and acquired microcephaly. CT scan shows ventricular enlargement. The CSF is normal or shows a mild increase in mononuclear cells and protein. Lymphocytic interstitial pneumonitis results from the infiltration of alveolar septa and peribronchiolar areas by lymphocytes and plasma cells. This is seen on x-ray films as a diffuse bilateral infiltrate, sometimes with micronodules, and may result in impaired oxygenation. Kaposi's sarcoma is rare.

B. Laboratory Findings: Diagnosis is suspected by a positive ELISA test for antibody to HIV. Because the sensitivity of tests is high, there are a significant number of false positive tests. For this reason, positive sera should be tested by Western blot for antibodies to the p17 and p24 (core) and gp160 (envelope) antigens. HIV antibodies take 1 to 2 months to appear following infection and, when present in mothers, are passed across the placenta. Rapid laboratory diagnosis of HIV infection in infants may therefore require the detection of viral DNA in blood following amplification by polymerase chain reaction. Alternatively, patients may be retested at intervals of 1 to 2 months to determine

whether the antibody titer increases. In a minor proportion of HIV-infected infants, the ELISA test is negative but the Western blot test is positive. Additional laboratory abnormalities include reduced numbers of CD4 lymphocytes with normal or raised numbers of CD8 lymphocytes in blood. Serum immunoglobulin levels are usually elevated, even before there are changes in T cell numbers. However, because levels of immunoglobulins may also be normal or low, this finding is not helpful diagnostically. Other common laboratory abnormalities include thrombocytopenia, neutropenia, and elevated transaminase levels.

Differential Diagnosis

Other congenital and acquired immunodeficiencies should be considered. Useful differentiating factors include the presence of risk factors in the child with HIV infection (such as an infected mother or the receipt of blood products) with the presence of normal or high serum immunoglobulin levels.

Criteria for the diagnosis of AIDS, which developed when acquired immunodeficiency was first recognized in children, included a documented opportunistic infection, an AIDS-associated malignancy, or lymphocytic interstitial pneumonitis.

Prognosis

Factors determining the rate of progression to AIDS-related complex (ARC) and then to AIDS (with failure to thrive, encephalopathy, recurrent infections, and lymphopenia) are unknown. Recent analyses suggest that 20% of infants who are infected at birth develop AIDS in the first year of life, and that the rate of diagnosis subsequently falls to about 8% per year. Recently developed, complex classification systems may permit a better prediction of survival. Overall, median survival following diagnosis ranges between 12 months for children developing *Pneumocystis* pneumonia and 31 months for children with other infections, but following the *Pneumocystis* infection survival was only around 3 months. Children diagnosed before the age of 1 generally have a shorter course.

Treatment

Infections require diagnosis and appropriate treatment (see Chapters 27–29). Malnutrition can be a problem requiring caloric supplementation. There is a strong impression of benefit (fewer febrile episodes and documented infections) following IgG replacement at 200–300 mg/kg twice monthly in younger infants and children. This approach may be less helpful in older children, eg, hemophiliacs. Azidothymidine (AZT) is currently available for children (see Chapter 27). Preliminary observations suggest a beneficial effect on HIV encephalopathy. Adverse effects occurring in adults treated with AZT include bone marrow suppression, headaches, and nausea, and up to 30% of patients cannot tolerate the drug. AZT has to be continued indefinitely because it does not eliminate the virus.

Immunizations

Exposure of HIV-positive subjects or their household contacts to oral attenuated polio virus should probably be avoided, and killed vaccine should be given instead. Measles-mumps-rubella vaccine has not had adverse effects and may protect HIV-infected children from severe or fatal measles. Immunization with DPT and *Haemophilus influenzae* type b conjugate vaccine is currently recommended. Administration of immune globulin following exposure to measles or varicella is recommended for children not receiving IgG replacement therapy.

Augur I, Thomas P, De Gruttola V, Morse D, Moore D, Williams R, Truman B, Lawrence CE: Incubation periods for paediatric AIDS patients. *Nature* 1988;**336:**575.

Falloon J, Eddy J, Weiner L, Pizzo PA: Human immunodeficiency virus infection in children. *J Pediatr* 1989; **114:**1.

Immunization of children infected with human immunodeficiency virus: Supplementary ACIP statement. *MMWR* 1988;**37:**181.

INVESTIGATION OF IMMUNODEFICIENCY

Evaluation for a possible underlying immunodeficiency should begin with a thorough history, since this is useful diagnostically. Physical, environmental, and anatomic defects are, as a group, the most common causes of recurrent infections, and recurrence at a single site should prompt a search for a local abnormality. The age at onset of infections can be an important clue. Infections associated with defects of phagocytes, C3, or cellular immunity commonly start in the first months of life, whereas maternal antibody protects infants with hypogamma-globulinemia for 3–6 months. Antibody, complement, and phagocyte defects predispose mainly to bacterial infections; superficial candidiasis and severe herpesvirus and poxvirus infections are typical of cellular immunodeficiency. A simple protocol for testing these mechanisms is presented in Table 18–4, and the level of investigation should reflect the frequency and severity of infections. Thus, it is reasonable to measure serum immunoglobulins in a 14-month-old with recurrent otitis alone, whereas the concurrent presence of failure to thrive should prompt a more comprehensive investigation plan.

Phagocyte Function

Evaluation of phagocyte function should begin with a white blood cell count and differential to rule out neutropenia. A blood film is useful to exclude the Howell-Jolly bodies of asplenia and to ascertain the presence or absence of normal lysosomal granules in neutrophils. Chemotaxis is generally measured in migration chambers in the laboratory and can also be assessed by migration of cells from abraded skin onto a sterile coverslip. Results of chemotaxis tests must be interpreted cautiously, because secondary and transient defects in chemotaxis are common. Quantitation of ingestion and microbicidal activity requires special techniques available chiefly in research laboratories. However, because the chemical reduction of nitroblue tetrazolium by phagocytes requires normal oxidation metabolism, this test screens for chronic granulomatous disease and for leukocyte glucose 6-phosphate dehydrogenase deficiency. Myeloperoxidase deficiency is excluded by histochemical stain available in most pathology laboratories.

Complement

Deficiency of a classical pathway component can be excluded by a normal hemolytic complement titer (CH_{50} assay), for which the patient's serum must be separated within 30 minutes of collection and stored at -70 °C. There is little point in measuring individual complement component levels if the hemolytic titer is normal, unless it is to follow the activity of an immune complex-associated disease in which C4 and C3 may be low. Opsonizing defects can be due to classical or alternative pathway defects or, if yeast is used, to abnormal C5.

Table 18–4. Hierarchy of tests for investigation of primary immunodeficiency.

Test Level	Complement	Phagocytes	Antibody	Cell-mediated Immunity
Screening	CH_{50} assay	Count/morphology	Immunoglobulin measurement	Delayed skin tests
1st level		NBT, LFA-1[1]	IHA, TTab[2]	T cell counts[3]
2nd level	Factor assays	Bactericidal and chemotaxis	Response to immunization	In vitro lymphocyte function tests

[1]Only where chronic granulomatous disease or LFA-1 deficiency is suspected.
[2]IHA = isohemagglutinins, after age 1; TTab = tetanus toxoid antibody.
[3]Identify all T cells with CD3, subsets with CD4 and CD8, CD45R for nonmemory cells.

Antibodies & Immunoglobulins

In patients who are not blood group AB, isohemagglutinins are the easiest naturally occurring antibodies to determine. They are of the IgM class, become detectable by 6 months of age, and reach adult levels about a year later. The titer of anti-O antibodies following immunization with typhoid-paratyphoid vaccine is another measure of IgM antibody production. The importance of antibody tests is illustrated by the inverse correlation between isohemagglutinin titer and susceptibility to meningitis in patients with hypogammaglobulinemia, irrespective of their serum IgM levels. Lack of availability of Schick antigen means that in vitro methods are required to test for IgG antibodies. Tetanus and diphtheria antibody tests are widely available, as are antibodies to pneumococcal polysaccharide, rubella, and mumps.

In practice, it is often easier to measure serum immunoglobulins as a screening procedure than to test for antibodies, but it should be appreciated that some patients with varied immunodeficiency syndromes and some infants with severely impaired cell-mediated immunity make immunoglobulin that does not have useful antibody activity. Because properly performed immunoglobulin estimations are reproducible to +10% for IgG and IgA and +20% for IgM, small changes are of no significance. Measurement of serum IgD is of not generally of diagnostic value in pediatrics. Immunoglobulin concentrations are lower in infants than in adults (Table 18–5), and laboratories may erroneously report the values of normal children as low. Comparisons of results from different laboratories may be difficult, because few commercial kit suppliers calibrate their control sera against the international standard. Simple protein electrophoresis is not sufficiently sensitive to make a confident diagnosis of hypogammaglobulinemia, although it is valuable for identifying the monoclonal excesses seen in macroglobulinemia and the oligoclonal gammopathy of Epstein-Barr virus infections in X-linked lymphoproliferative syndrome. Serum albumin should be measured at least once in patients with hypogammaglobulinemia to exclude secondary deficiencies due to loss. IgG or IgA subclass measurements may be abnormal in patients with varied immunodeficiency syndromes, but they are rarely helpful.

Cell-Mediated Immunity

Positive delayed hypersensitivity tests are good evidence of antigen-specific immunity. Only a positive response is interpretable, particularly in infancy, when prior immunization may not have been adequate to elicit good skin responses.

A bewildering number of antibodies is now available to characterize blood lymphocytes. Some of the more useful, and common deviations from normal,

Table 18–5. Relation of age to serum immunoglobulin (Ig) levels and isohemagglutinin activity (IHA).

	IgG (mg/dL) (Mean ±1 SD and Range)	IgA (mg/dL) (Mean ±1 SD and Range)	IgM (mg/dL) (Mean ±1 SD and Range)	IHA Titer (Mean and Range)
Cord blood	1086 ± 290 (740 − 1374)	2 ± 2 (0 − 15)	14 ± 6 (0 − 22)	0[1]
1–3 months	512 ± 152 (280 − 950)	16 ± 10 (4 − 36)	28 ± 14 (15 − 86)	1:5 0 − 1:10[2]
4–6 months	520 ± 180 (240 − 884)	22 ± 14 (11 − 52)	36 ± 18 (21 − 74)	1:10 0 − 1:160[2]
7–12 months	742 ± 226 (281 − 1280)	54 ± 17 (22 − 112)	76 ± 27 (36 − 150)	1:80 0 − 1:640[3]
13–24 months	945 ± 270 (290 − 1300)	67 ± 19 (9 − 143)	88 ± 36 (18 − 210)	1:80 0 − 1:640[3]
25–36 months	1030 ± 152 (546 − 1562)	89 ± 34 (21 − 196)	94 ± 23 (43 − 115)	1:160 1:10 − 1:640[4]
3–5 years	1150 ± 244 (546 − 1760)	126 ± 31 (56 − 284)	87 ± 24 (26 − 121)	1:80 1:5 − 1:640
6–8 years	1187 ± 289 (596 − 1744)	147 ± 35 (56 − 330)	108 ± 37 (54 − 260)	1:80 1:5 − 1:640
9–11 years	1217 ± 261 (744 − 1719)	146 ± 38 (44 − 208)	104 ± 46 (27 − 215)	1:160 1:20 − 1:640
12–16 years	1248 ± 221 (796 − 1647)	168 ± 54 (64 − 290)	96 ± 31 (60 − 140)	1:160 1:10 − 1:320

[1]IHA is rarely detectable in cord blood.
[2]50% of normal infants have no isohemagglutinins at age 6 months.
[3]10% of normal infants have no isohemagglutinins at age 1.
[4]Beyond age 2, all normal individuals (except those with blood type AB) have isohemagglutinins.

Table 18–6. Antigens used to identify lymphocytes in man.

Antigen	Commercial Antibodies	Cells Stained	Normal Range	Changes seen Clinically
CD2	OKT 11,	T cells, NK cells	70–90%	Falls to 10–20% when T cells lacking
CD3	OKT 3, Leu 4	All T cells	55–85%	Falls when T-cell number reduced, increases to 90% when B cells absent
CD4	OKT 4, Leu 3	HLA-D restricted T cells	35–60%	Selectively reduced in HIV infections; reduced with other T cells by steroids, defect of cell-mediated immunity
CD5		T cells, immature B cells	55–85%	Falls when T-cell number reduced, increases with immature B cells
CD8	OKT 8, Leu 2	HLA-A/B restricted T cells	25–50%	Selectively increased in response to some virus infections, reduced with other T-cell defects
CD11	OKM 1, Mac-1	Monocytes	5–15%	Lacking in LFA-1 deficiency
CD16	Leu 11	NK cells	5–15%	Increased by virus infections
CD19		B cells	4–10%	Increased when T cells lacking
CD20		B cells	4–10%	Lacking in X-linked agammaglobulinemia
CD25		IL2 receptor	<2%	Activated T cells, increased in graft-versus-host disease
CD45RA	2H4	Naive T cells	20–80%	Percentage falls with age

are summarized in Table 18–6. When abnormalities are suspected, it is important to check absolute numbers of lymphocytes and their subsets. Functional tests of T cells are mainly useful to characterize immunodeficiency detected by simpler tests. It is possible to distinguish between defects of cell activa-tion, lymphokine (IL2) production, and proliferation; effector function is measurable in cytotoxicity tests.

Thompson RA (editor): Laboratory investigation of immunological disorders. *Clin Immunol Allerg* 1985;**5**:385.

19

Rheumatic Diseases

J. Roger Hollister, MD

Rheumatic diseases have an autoimmune basis. Unknown factors in the environment act upon the immune system of patients who have inherited a predisposition to these diseases. Expression of disease is rarely seen in a familial pattern, although patients share common immunogenetic traits.

JUVENILE RHEUMATOID ARTHRITIS
(Juvenile Chronic Arthritis)

Essentials of Diagnosis

- Nonmigratory monarticular or polyarticular arthropathy, with a tendency to involve large joints or proximal interphalangeal joints and lasting more than 3 months.
- Systemic manifestations with fever, erythematous rashes, nodules, leukocytosis, and, occasionally, iridocyclitis, pleuritis, pericarditis, and hepatitis.

General Considerations

Juvenile rheumatoid arthritis patients exhibit different immunogenetic traits from adult rheumatoid arthritis patients. In juvenile rheumatoid arthritis, HLA-DR5 is associated with iritis and the production of antinuclear antibodies, whereas HLA-DR4 is found in seropositive, polyarticular disease. These traits may be important in the formation of anti-suppressor cell antibodies, immune complex generation, and consequent chronic inflammatory disease.

Clinical Findings

A. Symptoms and Signs: There are 4 patterns of presentation in juvenile rheumatoid arthritis that provide clues to the prognosis and possible sequelae of the disease. In the acute febrile form, which is most common in children under age 4, an evanescent salmon-pink macular rash, arthritis, hepatosplenomegaly, leukocytosis, and polyserositis characterize the constellation described by George Still. These patients have episodic illness, and remission of the systemic features can be expected within 1 year. They do not develop iridocyclitis.

The polyarticular pattern resembles the adult disease, with chronic pain and swelling of many joints in a symmetric fashion. Both large and small joints are usually involved. Systemic features are less prominent, though low-grade fever, fatigue, rheumatoid nodules, and anemia may be present. These pa-

tients tend to have long-standing arthritis, although the disease may wax and wane. Iridocyclitis is occasionally seen in this group. Older children may have a positive latex fixation test.

The third pattern consists of pauciarticular disease characterized by chronic arthritis of a few joints, often the large weight-bearing joints, in an asymmetric distribution. The synovitis is usually mild and may be painless. Systemic features are uncommon, but there is serious extra-articular involvement with inflammation in the eye. Up to 30% of children with pauciarticular juvenile rheumatoid arthritis develop insidious, asymptomatic iridocyclitis, which may cause blindness if untreated. The activity of the eye disease does not correlate with the activity of the arthritis. Therefore, routine ophthalmologic screening with slit lamp examination must be performed every 6 months until puberty.

The fourth pattern occurs in late childhood mainly in boys, of whom 75% have HLA-B27. The early clinical pattern is of pauciarticular disease involving the lower limbs; later, the sacroiliac joints may be involved, and ultimately the lumbar and thoracic spine.

B. Laboratory Findings: There is no diagnostic test for juvenile rheumatoid arthritis. Rheumatoid factor is positive by the latex fixation test in about 15% of cases, usually when onset of polyarticular disease occurs after age 8 years. Antinuclear antibodies are most often present in pauciarticular disease with iridocyclitis and may serve as an indication of this complication; they are also fairly common in the late-onset rheumatoid factor-positive group. A normal erythrocyte sedimentation rate does not exclude the diagnosis. Synovial fluid examination is rarely performed in childhood but will establish the presence of inflammation or infection, especially in monarticular cases.

C. Imaging: In the early stages of the disease, only soft tissue swelling and regional osteoporosis are seen. Cervical subluxation should be monitored by radiographs in patients with neck pain.

Differential Diagnosis

Monarticular arthritis is the most important differential disorder to establish. Pain in the hip or lower extremity is a frequent symptom with childhood cancer, especially leukemia, neuroblastoma, and rhabdomyosarcoma. Infiltration of bone by tumor and actual joint effusion may be seen. X-rays of the affected site and a careful examination of the blood smear for unusual cells and thrombocytopenia are necessary. In doubtful cases, bone marrow examination is indicated.

Bacterial arthritis is usually acute and monarticular except for arthritis associated with *Haemophilus influenzae* and gonorrhea, both of which may be associated with a migratory pattern. Fever, leukocytosis, and increased sedimentation rate with an acute process in a single joint demand synovial fluid examination and culture to identify the pathogen. An elevated synovial fluid white count and low glucose (relative to plasma glucose) suggest sepsis.

The arthritis of rheumatic fever is migratory, transient, and often more painful than that of juvenile rheumatoid arthritis. Rheumatic fever is very rare under the age of 5 years. The murmur of rheumatic endocarditis should be carefully sought. Evidence of recent streptococcal infection is essential to the diagnosis. The fever pattern in rheumatic fever is low-grade and persistent in comparison to the intermittent fever in the systemic form of juvenile rheumatoid arthritis.

Articular involvement with inflammatory bowel disease, psoriasis, and Reiter's syndrome most often involves the lower extremities and frequently the heel. If there are associated abdominal complaints, weight loss, etc, contrast x-rays are indicated. Other forms of reactive arthritis are associated with enteric bacterial infections, Schönlein-Henoch purpura, toxic synovitis, and rubella immunization. Arthritis is the most frequent symptom in systemic lupus erythematosus; a careful history and examination for multisystem disease will establish the diagnosis. Chondromalacia patellae, which characteristically causes pain when the patient walks up and down stairs, may be confused with juvenile rheumatoid arthritis. There is patellar tenderness with this condition.

Treatment

The objective of therapy is to restore function, relieve pain, and maintain joint motion. Salicylates are the treatment of choice at the outset. Aspirin, 75–100 mg/kg/d in 4 divided doses, will frequently relieve pain and inflammation and allow good physical therapy. A self-limited hepatotoxicity occurs with high-dose salicylate therapy, but most patients can continue to take aspirin. If the patient is exposed to chickenpox or Asian influenza, however, aspirin should be withheld to reduce the risk of Reye's syndrome. Range-of-motion exercises and muscle strengthening should be taught and supervised by a therapist, and a home program should be instituted. Bed rest is to be avoided except in the most acute stages. Joint casting is almost never indicated. In patients who fail to respond to aspirin, there are a number of alternatives. Corticosteroids are of value

as a temporary measure during acute flare-ups and when there is acute systemic disease or iridocyclitis. Gold salts are of proved efficacy. The dose of gold salt (eg, gold sodium thiomalate) is 1 mg/kg/wk intramuscularly. As symptoms are controlled, the frequency of injection can be gradually decreased. White cell counts and urine testing for protein must be done on a regular basis. Auranofin, a recently licensed oral gold preparation, also appears to be safe and efficacious. The dose is 0.15 mg/kg/d. Diarrhea is the most common side effect. Blood counts and urinalysis should be monitored, as with parenteral gold. The newer nonsteroidal anti-inflammatory agents such as tolmetin, ibuprofen, and naproxen cause fewer gastric problems but otherwise appear to offer little advantage over aspirin. Immunosuppressive therapy with cytotoxic drugs is experimental and should be reserved for patients who have failed other therapy.

Iridocyclitis should be treated by an ophthalmologist. Orthopedic consultation on a regular basis is helpful, although surgery is seldom necessary.

Prognosis

In the primarily articular forms, disease activity progressively diminishes with age and ceases in about 95% of cases by puberty. In a few instances, this will persist into adult life. Problems after puberty therefore relate primarily to residual joint damage. Cases presenting in the teen years usually presage adult disease. The children most liable to be permanently handicapped are those with unremitting synovitis, hip involvement, or positive rheumatoid factor tests.

Baum J: Juvenile arthritis. Am J Dis Child 1981;**135**:557.

Glass D et al: Early-onset pauciarticular juvenile rheumatoid arthritis associated with human leukocyte antigen-DRw5, iritis, and antinuclear antibody. J Clin Invest 1980;**66**:426.

Olson NY, Lindsley CB, Godfrey WA: Nonsteroidal anti-inflammatory drug treatment in chronic childhood iridocyclitis. Am J Dis Child 1988;**142**:1289.

Rosenberg AM: Advanced drug therapy for juvenile rheumatoid arthritis. J Pediatr 1989;**114**:171.

Schaller J: Juvenile rheumatoid arthritis. Pediatr Rev 1980;**2**:163.

Vostrejs M, Hollister JR: Muscle atrophy and leg length discrepancies in pauciarticular juvenile rheumatoid arthritis. Am J Dis Child 1988;**142**:343.

SYSTEMIC LUPUS ERYTHEMATOSUS

Essentials of Diagnosis

- Multisystem inflammatory disease of joints, serous linings, skin, kidneys, and central nervous system.
- Antinuclear antibodies must be present in active, untreated disease.

General Considerations

Systemic lupus erythematosus is the prototype of immune complex diseases; its pathogenesis is related to deposition in the tissue of soluble immune complexes existing in the circulation. The spectrum of symptoms in systemic lupus erythematosus appears to be due not to tissue-specific autoantibodies but rather to damage to the tissue by lymphocytes, neutrophils, and complement evoked by the deposition of antigen-antibody complexes. In systemic lupus erythematosus, many such antigen-antibody systems are present, but the best correlation exists between DNA-anti-DNA complexes and the activity of the disease. Laboratory tests of these antibodies and complement components give an objective assessment of disease pathogenesis and response to therapy. The trigger for the formation of immune complexes in systemic lupus erythematosus has not been identified. Autoreactive T lymphocytes that have escaped clonal deletion and unregulated B lymphocyte production of autoantibodies may initiate the disease.

A drug-related syndrome resembling systemic lupus erythematosus may be produced by procainamide, hydantoin compounds, and isoniazid, among others. Affected patients recover on stopping the drug and do not manifest renal disease.

Clinical Findings

A. Symptoms and Signs: The onset is most common in females (8:1) between the ages of 9 and 15 years. The symptoms depend on what organ is involved with immune complex deposition.

1. Joint symptoms are the commonest presenting feature. Nondeforming arthritis may involve any joint, often in a symmetric manner. Myositis may also occur and is more painful than the inflammation in dermatomyositis.

2. Systemic manifestations include weakness, anorexia, fever, fatigue, and loss of weight.

3. Skin lesions include butterfly erythema and induration, small ulcerations in skin and mucous membranes, purpura, alopecia, and Raynaud's phenomenon. The sun sensitivity of the dermal lesions may be striking.

4. Polyserositis may include pleurisy with effusions, peritonitis, and pericarditis. Libman-Sacks endocarditis is rarely seen since corticosteroids became available for treatment.

5. Hepatosplenomegaly and lymphadenopathy may occur.

6. Renal systemic lupus erythematosus produces few symptoms at onset but is often progressive and is the leading cause of death. Renal biopsy is indicated in all patients with evidence of renal involvement, because the course of the renal disease varies with the lesion produced by immune complex deposition in the glomerular basement membrane. Late complications are nephrosis and uremia.

7. Central nervous system involvement produces a variety of symptoms such as seizures, coma, hemiplegia, focal neuropathies, and behavior disturbances, including psychosis. The psychosis may be impossible to distinguish from corticosteroid-induced psychosis.

B. Laboratory Findings: Leukopenia and anemia are frequently found with a low incidence of Coombs positivity. Thrombocytopenia and purpura may be early manifestations even in the absence of other organ involvement. The erythrocyte sedimentation rate is elevated, and hypergammaglobulinemia is often present. Renal involvement is indicated by the presence in the urine of red cells, white cells, red cell casts, and proteinuria.

The antinuclear antibody test is the most sensitive diagnostic test and has supplanted the LE preparation. The antinuclear antibody test is invariably positive in patients with active untreated systemic lupus erythematosus, and a negative antinuclear antibody test effectively excludes the diagnosis. For patients with a positive antinuclear antibody test, a profile identifying individual disease-specific antibodies should be ordered.

In managing the disease, elevated titers of anti-DNA antibody and depressed levels of serum complement (hemolytic, C3, or C4) accurately reflect active disease, especially renal, central nervous system, and skin disease. A CT scan or MRI scan may identify pathologic conditions of the brain in lupus cerebritis, such as infarction, vasculitis, or atrophy.

Differential Diagnosis

Systemic lupus erythematosus may simulate many inflammatory diseases such as rheumatic fever, rheumatoid arthritis, and viral infections. It is essential to review all organ systems carefully to establish a clinical pattern. Renal and central nervous system involvement are unique to systemic lupus erythematosus. A negative antinuclear antibody test excludes the diagnosis of systemic lupus erythematosus. Tests yielding false-positive results are usually of low titer (ie, < 1:320).

An overlap syndrome known as mixed connective tissue disease, with features of several collagen-vascular diseases, has recently been described in adults and children. The symptom complex is diverse and does not readily fit previous classifications. Arthritis, fever, skin tightening, Raynaud's phenomenon, muscle weakness, and rashes are most commonly present. Important factors in recognition of this disease entity are the relative infrequency of renal disease, which implies a better prognosis than systemic lupus erythematosus, and the corticosteroid responsiveness of symptoms, which distinguishes mixed connective tissue disease from scleroderma. The definition of the disease includes the presence of serum antibody to an extractable nuclear antigen. Patients are initially identified by a speckled pattern of immunofluorescence in the antinuclear antibody test. The specialized extractable nuclear antigen test demonstrates very high titers of up to 1:1,000,000 of the antibody. Pulmonary disease in childhood produces major morbidity.

Treatment

The treatment of systemic lupus erythematosus should be tailored to the organ system involved so that toxicities may be minimized. Prednisone, 0.5–1 mg/kg/d orally, has significantly lowered the mortality rate in systemic lupus erythematosus and should be used in all cases with renal, cardiac, or central nervous system involvement. The dose should be varied using clinical and laboratory parameters of disease activity, and the minimum amount of corticosteroid to control the disease should be used. Alternate-day regimens of corticosteroid are frequently possible. Skin manifestations may frequently be treated with antimalarials, eg, hydroxychloroquine, 5–7 mg/kg/d orally. Pleuritic pain or arthritis can often be managed with salicylates alone.

If disease control is inadequate with prednisone or if the dose required produces intolerable side effects, an immunosuppressant should be added. Either azathioprine, 2–3 mg/kg/d orally, or cyclophosphamide, 1–2 mg/kg/d orally, has been most widely used. These drugs are ineffective during acute crises such as seizures.

The toxicities of the regimens must be carefully considered. In life-threatening disease, the choices are easier. Growth failure, osteoporosis, Cushing's syndrome, adrenal suppression, and aseptic necrosis are serious side effects of chronic use of prednisone. When high doses of corticosteroids are used (> 2 mg/kg/d), the risk of sepsis is very real. Cyclophosphamide causes bladder epithelial dysplasia, hemorrhagic cystitis, and sterility. Azathioprine has been associated with liver damage and bone marrow suppression. Immunosuppressant treatment should be withheld if the total white count falls below 3000/μL or the neutrophil count below 1000/μL. Retinal damage from chloroquine derivatives has not been observed in the recommended dosage. Intravenous pulse steroid therapy and monthly pulse cyclophosphamide are treatments that may be useful in selected cases.

Amenorrhea may result from uncontrolled systemic lupus erythematosus but may also be a consequence of prednisone, cyclophosphamide, or azathioprine administration.

Course & Prognosis

The prognosis in systemic lupus erythematosus relates to the presence of renal involvement or infectious complications of treatment. With improved diagnosis, milder cases are now identified. Nonetheless, the survival rate has improved from 51% at 5 years in 1954 to 71% at 10 years in 1979. The disease has a natural waxing and waning cycle, and periods of complete remission are not unusual.

Austen HA et al: Therapy of lupus nephritis: Controlled trial of prednisone and cytotoxic drugs. *N Engl J Med* 1986;**314**:614.

Baron KS et al: Pulse methylprednisolone therapy in diffuse proliferative lupus nephritis. *J Pediatr* 1982; **101**:137.

Celermajer DS et al: Sex differences in childhood lupus nephritis. *Am J Dis Child* 1984;**138**:586.

Chudwin DS et al: Significance of a positive antinuclear antibody test in a pediatric population. *Am J Dis Child* 1983;**137**:1103.

Harisdangkul V et al: Causes of death in systemic lupus erythematosus: A pattern based on age of onset. *South Med J* 1987;**80**:1250.

Oetgen WJ, Boice JA, Lawless OJ: Mixed connective tissue disease in children and adolescents. *Pediatrics* 1981;**67**:333.

DERMATOMYOSITIS (Polymyositis)

Essentials of Diagnosis

- Pathognomonic skin rash.
- Weakness of proximal muscles and occasionally of pharyngeal and laryngeal groups.
- Pathogenesis related to vasculitis.

General Considerations

Dermatomyositis, a rare inflammatory disease of muscle and skin in childhood, is uniquely responsive to corticosteroid treatment. The vasculitis observed in childhood dermatomyositis differs pathologically from the adult disease. Small arteries and veins are involved, with an exudate of neutrophils, lymphocytes, plasma cells, and histiocytes. The lesion progresses to intimal proliferation and thrombus formation. These vascular changes are found in the skin, muscle, kidney, retina, and gastrointestinal tract. Postinflammatory calcinosis is frequent.

The autoimmune pathogenesis of dermatomyositis has been difficult to prove. Recent studies have shown that both cellular and humoral mechanisms may be involved. Lymphocytes from patients are stimulated to undergo blastogenesis in the presence of muscle tissue and will release lymphotoxin, which destroys cultured fetal muscle cells. Biopsies studied with immunofluorescence techniques demonstrate immunoglobulin and complement in a perivascular distribution. The putative antigen has not been identified. Suggestive data relating adult myositis to toxoplasmosis have not been found in children, and results of viral studies have been negative.

Clinical Findings

A. Symptoms and Signs: The predominant symptom is muscular weakness in a proximal distribution affecting pelvic and shoulder girdles. Tenderness, stiffness, and swelling may be found but are not striking. Neurologic findings such as absence of tendon reflexes are not seen until late in the disease. Pharyngeal and respiratory involvement can be life-threatening. Flexion contractures and muscle atrophy produce significant residual deformities. Calcinosis may follow the inflammation in muscle and skin. Vasculitis of the intestine causing hemorrhage or perforation is less frequently seen in recent years, perhaps owing to corticosteroid treatment.

The rash of dermatomyositis is very helpful in the diagnosis of unknown muscle disease. Characteristically, the rash involves the upper eyelids and extensor surfaces of the knuckles, elbows, and knees with a distinctive heliotrope color that progresses to a scaling and atrophic appearance. Periorbital edema is not uncommon. Nailfold capillary abnormalities may identify patients with a poorer prognosis. None of the rashes associated with other childhood rheumatic diseases have these features of distribution. The activity of the rash frequently does not parallel the muscle disease.

B. Laboratory Findings: Determination of muscle enzyme levels is the most helpful tool in diagnosis and treatment. All enzymes, including serum aldolase, should be screened to detect an abnormality that reflects activity of the disease. The blood count, erythrocyte sedimentation rate, and acute phase reactants are frequently normal. No autoantibodies are found. Electromyography is useful to distinguish myopathic from neuropathic causes of muscle weakness. Muscle biopsy is indicated in doubtful cases of myositis without the pathognomonic rash.

Treatment

Prednisone in high doses (1–2 mg/kg/d orally) has been shown to speed recovery. The dose should be maintained or increased until muscle enzymes have returned to normal. Functional recovery will lag somewhat behind laboratory improvement. With improvement, the dose may be cut to that level which maintains disease control and normal muscle enzymes. Treatment must be continued for an average of 2 years. Immunosuppressant agents are occasionally required in childhood dermatomyositis. Intravenous gamma globulin therapy may be tried in refractory cases. Physical therapy is critical to prevent or allay contractures.

Course & Prognosis

Most children will recover and discontinue medications in 1–3 years. Relapses may occur. Functional ability is very good in most patients. Myositis in childhood is not associated with an increased risk of cancer.

Bowyer SL et al: Childhood dermatomyositis and factors predicting functional outcome and development of dystrophic calcification. *J Pediatr* 1983;**103**:882.

Miller G, Heckmatt JZ, Dubowitz V: Drug treatment of juvenile dermatomyositis. *Arch Dis Child* 1983;**58**:445.

Miller LC, Michael AF, Kim Y: Childhood dermatomyositis, clinical course and long-term followup. *Clin Pediatr (Phila)* 1987;**26**:561.

Spencer CH et al: Course of treated juvenile dermatomyositis. *J Pediatr* 1984;**105**:399.

Spencer-Green G, Crowe WE, Levinson JE: Nailfold capillary abnormalities and clinical outcome in childhood dermatomyositis. *Arthritis Rheum* 1982;**25**:954.

POLYARTERITIS NODOSA

Polyarteritis nodosa is a rare disease, but a significant number of cases have been reported in childhood and infancy. No single cause has been found, but evidence of a streptococcal trigger has been found in some series.

Pathologically, the disease is a vasculitis of medium-sized arteries with fibrinoid degeneration in the media extending to the intima and adventitia. Neutrophils and eosinophils comprise the inflammatory reaction. Aneurysms may be palpated or seen radiographically. Thrombosis of diseased arteries may cause infarction in many organs. Fibrosis of vessels and surrounding tissues accompanies the healing stages.

Symptomatology involves many tissues, and diagnosis is difficult. In childhood, unexplained fever, conjunctivitis, central nervous system involvement, and cardiac disease are more prominent than is the case in adult disease. Many cases appear as acute myocarditis, and the peripheral neuropathy so common in the adult is unusual. Diagnosis depends on biopsy-proved vasculitis or characteristic aneurysms on angiography.

The mortality rate is high, especially with cardiac involvement. Treatment consists of prednisone, 1–1.5 mg/kg/d orally, and azathioprine, 1–2 mg/kg/d orally, but controlled studies of the efficacy of therapy of this rare disease are not yet available.

Blau Eb, Morris RF, Yunis EJ: Polyarteritis nodosa in older children. *Pediatrics* 1977;**60**:227.

Fauci AS: Vasculitis. *J Allergy Clin Immunol* 1983;**72**:211.

Fink CW: Vasculitis. *Pediatr Clin North Am* 1986;**33**:1203.

Magilavy DB et al: A syndrome of childhood polyarteritis. *J Pediatr* 1977;**91**:25.

DIFFUSE SCLERODERMA
(Progressive Systemic Sclerosis)

Scleroderma is a rare disease in childhood. Both the generalized systemic type and the more localized benign form (morphea) have been described. The diagnosis is made on a clinical basis with the finding of a skin disease that progresses from an edematous phase to an atrophic, taut, immobile dermis involving some or all of the skin. Systemic involvement may include Raynaud's phenomenon, arthralgias, pulmonary fibrosis, and renal disease. Involvement of the lungs and kidneys leads to rapid demise. Histologically, the diagnosis may not be specific but includes dermal atrophy with increased fibrosis and collagen content. The pathogenesis remains obscure, but studies indicate an increased synthesis of immature collagen by cultured scleroderma fibroblasts.

Penicillamine and newer antihypertensive agents may provide effective treatment in the future. Physical therapy is sometimes helpful in reducing debilitation from contractures and muscle wasting.

Singsen BH: Scleroderma in childhood. *Pediatr Clin North Am* 1986;**33**:1119.
Steen VD et al: Clinical and laboratory associations of anticentromere antibody in patients with progressive systemic sclerosis. *Arthritis Rheum* 1984;**27**:125.

NONRHEUMATIC PAIN SYNDROMES

Reflex Sympathetic Dystrophy

Reflex sympathetic dystrophy is a painful condition that is frequently confused with arthritis. There appears to be both an increased prevalence and recognition of the condition. Severe extremity pain leading to nearly complete loss of function is the hallmark of the condition. Evidence of autonomic dysfunction is demonstrated by color changes, temperature differences, and dyshidrosis in the affected extremity. Foot involvement is more common than hand involvement. A puffy swelling of the entire hand or foot is common. On examination, there is marked cutaneous hyperesthesia to even the most gentle touch. Results of laboratory tests are negative. X-ray findings are normal except for late development of osteoporosis. Bone scans are very helpful and demonstrate either increased or decreased blood supply to the painful extremity.

The cause of this condition remains elusive. Unlike adults, children only occasionally have a history of significant physical trauma at onset. How the autonomic dysfunction causes severe somatic pain is not known, but the pain does provide the basis for treatment. In mild cases, a program of rehabilitative physical therapy in combination with desensitization techniques will restore function and relieve pain. Refractory cases need family counseling and may respond to steroids or ganglionic blocks by local anesthesia. Long-term prognosis is good if recovery is rapid; recurrent episodes imply a less favorable prognosis.

Fibromyalgia

Fibromyalgia is a diffuse pain syndrome in which patients experience pain all over their bodies without objective swelling. Weather changes and fatigue exacerbate symptoms. A sleep disturbance, such as insomnia or prolonged waking periods in the night, is an almost universal symptom; therefore, patients should be carefully questioned in this regard. On examination, patients are normal except for characteristic trigger points at the insertion of muscles, especially along the neck, spine, and pelvis.

Treatment consists of physical therapy and relieving the sleep disorder. Low-dose antidepressant medication (amitryptyline hydrochloride, 25 mg) taken before sleep may produce remarkable benefit in reduction of pain. Physical therapy should emphasize a graded rehabilitative approach to stretching and exercise. Analgesic medications provide poor pain relief and should be avoided because their use leads to escalation of medication, including narcotics. The prognosis is not clear in pediatric patients, and patients may need to adopt long-term strategies to enable them to cope with the condition.

Goldenberg DL: Fibromyalgia syndrome, an emerging but controversial condition. *JAMA* 1987;**257**:2782.
Sherry DD, Weisman R: Psychologic aspects of childhood reflex neurovascular dystrophy. *Pediatrics* 1988; **81**:572.

HYPERMOBILITY SYNDROME

Ligamentous laxity, which previously was thought to occur only in Ehlers-Danlos syndrome or Down syndrome, is now recognized as a frequent cause of joint pain in our increasingly physically competitive society.

Children are now participating in a wide range of physically demanding sports and activities. Patients with hypermobility present with episodic joint pain and occasionally with swelling that lasts a few days after increased physical activity. Depending on the activity, almost any joint may be affected.

Physical examination may reveal joint swelling and tenderness, but the key to diagnosis is the demonstration of ligamentous laxity. Five criteria have been established: (1) passive opposition of the thumb to the flexor surface of the forearm, (2) passive hyperextension of the fingers so that they are parallel to the extensor surface of the forearm, (3) hyperextension of the elbow, (4) hyperextension of the knee (genu recurvatum), and (5) palms on floor with knees extended. Results of laboratory tests are normal. The pain associated with the syndrome is produced by improper joint alignment, due to the laxity, during exercise.

Treatment consists of a graded conditioning program designed to provide muscular support of the joints to compensate for the loose ligaments. Prognosis should be good provided that conditioning before activities is adequate.

Gedalia A et al: Hypermobility of the joints in juvenile episodic arthritis/arthralgia. *J Pediatr* 1985;**107**:873.

20

Gastrointestinal Tract*

Judith M. Sondheimer, MD & Arnold Silverman, MD

GASTROESOPHAGEAL REFLUX & CHALASIA

Forty percent of infants less than one month of age regurgitate some gastric contents after eating. Regurgitation ranges from effortless spitting to forceful vomiting. On fluoroscopy, reflux of barium from stomach into esophagus can be elicited in close to 40% of normal newborns. The cause is not known but may relate to delayed gastric emptying, relaxations of the lower esophageal sphincter, hypotension of the lower esophageal sphincter, increases in intra-abdominal pressure secondary to crying or straining, and the recumbent position. The condition is usually self-limited, resolving at about 6–8 months of age.

Clinical Findings

Effortless postprandial spitting and vomiting is the most common symptom. In some infants, vomiting causes failure to thrive, esophagitis, hematemesis or occult blood loss, iron deficiency anemia, strictures, and inflammatory esophageal polyps. Aspiration pneumonia, chronic cough, wheezing, and asthma-like attacks are reported. Dysphagia, discomfort or colic after feedings, and neck contortions (Sandifer's syndrome) may occur. Ruminative behavior is sometimes a symptom. Apneic spells and sudden infant death syndrome or "near miss" episodes have been ascribed to gastroesophageal reflux. Gastroesophageal reflux is common in neurologically impaired children. Vomiting associated with reflux can mimic pyloric stenosis and gastric outlet obstruction. (See Table 20–1.) An associated sliding hiatal hernia is not rare.

Gastroesophageal reflux is usually diagnosed clinically in thriving infants under 6 months of age. In less typical cases, it can be diagnosed on barium swallow by observing free regurgitation of barium from stomach to esophagus. However, both false-positive and false-negative tests are common. Prolonged monitoring of esophageal pH is a more specific test. Esophageal scintiscanning is sometimes

Table 20–1. Causes of vomiting and regurgitation.

Gastrointestinal tract disorders	
Esophagus	**Intestine**
Achalasia	Atresia and stenosis
Gastroesophageal reflux (chalasia)	Meconium ileus
	Malrotation, volvulus
Hiatal hernia	Duplication
Peptic esophagitis	Intussusception
Atresia with or without fistula	Foreign body, polyposis
	Soy or cow's milk protein intolerance
Congenital vascular or mucosal rings, webs	Gluten enteropathy
Stenosis	Food allergy
Duplication and diverticulum	Hirschsprung's disease
	Chronic intestinal pseudo-obstruction
Foreign body	Appendicitis, perforations
Periesophageal mass	Crohn's disease
Stomach	Gastroenteritis, infestations
Hypertrophic pyloric stenosis	
Pylorospasm	**Other abdominal organs**
Diaphragmatic hernia	Hepatitis
Peptic disease and gastritis	Gallstones
	Pancreatitis
Gastric volvulus, diaphragm	Peritonitis
Duodenum	
Atresia, diaphragm	
Annular pancreas	
Duodenitis and ulcer	
Malrotation	
Mesenteric bands	
Superior mesenteric artery syndrome	

Extra-gastrointestinal tract disorders	
Sepsis	Adrenal insufficiency
Pneumonia	Renal tubular acidosis
Otitis media	Inborn errors
Urinary tract infection	Urea cycle disorders
Meningitis	Phenylketonuria
Subdural effusion	Maple syrup urine disease
Hydrocephalus	
Brain tumor	Lactic acidosis
Reye's syndrome	Organic (propionic) aciduria
Rumination	
Intoxications	Gadacroseme
Alcohol	Fructose intolerance
Aspirin	Tyrosinosis
Acetaminophen	Scleroderma
	Epidermolysis bullosa

---

*Esophageal atresia and tracheoesophageal fistula are discussed in Chapter 4.

helpful in identifying pulmonary aspiration. Esophageal manometry is not diagnostic but may identify the infant with hiatal hernia, reduced lower esophageal sphincter pressure, or motor disorders of the esophagus. Gastroesophageal reflux cannot be diagnosed by esophagoscopy, but esophagitis can be identified.

Treatment & Prognosis

In 85% of patients, gastroesophageal reflux is self-limited, disappearing between 6 and 12 months. Conservative measures such as small, frequent feedings thickened with rice cereal (2–3 teaspoons per ounce of formula) and placing the child in a prone position with the head elevated 30 degrees help reduce frequency of spitting. Cimetidine (20 mg/kg/d in 4 doses) or liquid antacids reduce colicky symptoms and prevent or heal esophagitis. Smooth muscle stimulants, such as metoclopramide (0.1 mg/kg before meals) or bethanechol (0.1 mg/kg before meals), are sometimes helpful.

Indications for surgery include (1) persistent vomiting with failure to thrive after 2–3 months of conservative treatment; (2) esophagitis refractory to medical treatment or persistent esophageal strictures; and (3) reflux causing apneic spells or chronic pulmonary disease. Neurologically handicapped children respond less well to medical therapy for gastroesophageal reflux. Decreased vomiting is almost uniformly noted after a fundoplication. Dysphagia, decreased gastric capacity with early satiety, and retching are sometimes seen after surgery.

Herbst JJ: Gastroesophageal reflux. *J Pediatr* 1981;**98:** 859.

Orenstein SR et al: Gastroesophageal reflux and respiratory disease in children. *J Pediatr* 1988;**112:**847.

Sondheimer JM: Gastroesophageal reflux: Update on pathogenesis and diagnosis. *Pediatr Clin North Am* 1988;**35:**103.

Tunnel WP et al: Gastroesophageal reflux in childhood: The dilemma of surgical success. *Ann Surg* 1983;**197:**560.

ACHALASIA OF THE ESOPHAGUS

Esophageal achalasia is characterized by failure of relaxation of the inferior esophageal sphincter (cardiospasm) and lack of propulsive peristalsis in the body of the esophagus.

Clinical Findings

A. Symptoms and Signs: Achalasia is seen in all age groups but is uncommon under the age of 5 years. The history of difficulty in swallowing solid food is intermittent at first and often goes back for many years. Typical symptoms include retrosternal pain and frequent episodes of food "sticking" in the throat or upper chest. Patients are slow eaters and consume large amounts of fluids while eating. Familial cases have been described. The dysphagia is relieved by repeated swallowing movements (wet or dry) or by vomiting. Bouts of coughing and wheezing, recurrent pneumonitis, anemia, and weight loss may occur.

B. Imaging and Manometric Studies: The barium swallow shows a grossly dilated esophagus (megaesophagus) with a short, narrow segment at the distal end. Cinefluoroscopic examination may show absence of normal peristalsis and failure of relaxation of the gastroesophageal sphincter.

The esophageal motility pattern confirms the abnormal propulsive peristalsis and failure to relax the lower esophageal sphincter during swallowing.

Differential Diagnosis

Reflux esophagitis with or without hiatal hernia is the most common cause of organic esophageal stricture in childhood and must be ruled out by esophagoscopy, x-rays, pH probe, and manometric studies.

Treatment & Prognosis

Balloon (pneumatic) dilation is of value in most cases and can be repeated if symptoms recur. More definitive results can be achieved by surgically splitting the lower esophageal sphincter muscle (Heller myotomy). Because of the shorter duration of the illness in pediatric patients, the prognosis for return of the esophagus to normal caliber after surgical treatment is better than in adults.

Berquist WE et al: Achalasia: Diagnosis, management and clinical course in 16 children. *Pediatrics* 1983;**71:**798.

Nakayama DK et al: Pneumatic dilation and operative treatment of achalasia in children. *J Pediatr Surg* 1987; **22:**619.

CAUSTIC BURNS OF THE ESOPHAGUS

Ingestion of caustic solids or liquids may cause a range of lesions from superficial esophagitis to severe coagulative necrosis, ulceration, or perforation with mediastinitis or peritonitis if the stomach is involved. The severity of oral lesions does not correlate well with the presence or degree of esophageal damage.

Children who have swallowed lye usually present with painful, edematous lesions of the lips, mouth, pharynx, and (sometimes) the larynx. Esophageal or laryngeal obstruction secondary to edema and exudate may occur early. Usually, however, the dysphagia caused by local edema and tissue necrosis resolves over a few hours or days. The child may remain asymptomatic for a few months as an esophageal stricture develops. X-ray findings usually reveal esophageal stricture in the areas of anatomic narrowing, eg, the cervical region, at the point at which the left bronchus crosses the esophagus and at the gastroesophageal junction. Stenosis of the esophagus occurs only if full-thickness necrosis of the deep muscle layers occurs. Single, dense, localized strictures may occur, although in other cases the entire esophagus may become twisted and narrowed. Shortening of the esophagus may lead to a hiatal hernia.

The child with a history of alkali ingestion should have a careful examination of the lips and mouth and evaluation of the airway. Drooling is common. Oral lesions are frequent if solid agents have been ingested. Stricture formation may occur slowly over months. Dysphagia is first manifest for solids and eventually for liquids.

Vomiting should not be induced following alkali ingestion. Hospitalization is recommended even if ingestion is only suspected. Prednisone, 1–2 mg/kg/d (or its equivalent intravenously) is started immediately. Intravenous fluids may be necessary. Esophagoscopy should be done within 24–48 hours after ingestion. Treatment is stopped if there is no visible lesion or if only a first-degree burn is seen. Corticosteroids are continued and a program of bougienage started for more severe cases. In cases where x-rays show evidence of erosion into the mediastinum or peritoneum, antibiotics become mandatory. Intraluminal stenting may be beneficial.

Without early treatment, stricture formation is inevitable. Surgical replacement of the esophagus with a segment of colon may be necessary if dilation fails.

Although other ingestants may cause esophageal irritation (eg, bleach, detergents, or acids), it is rare for any but the strongest acids and detergents to result in the full-thickness necrosis that produces stricture.

Crain FC, Gershel JC, Mezey AP: Symptoms as predictors of esophageal injury. *Am J Dis Child* 1984;**138**:863.

Gaudreault P et al: Predictability of esophageal injury from signs and symptoms. A study of caustic ingestion in 378 children. *Pediatrics* 1983;**71**:767.

Goldman LP, Weigert JM: Corrosive substance ingestion: A review. *Am J Gastroenterol* 1984;**79**:85.

HIATAL HERNIA

Hiatal hernias may be classified as follows: (1) paraesophageal hernia, in which the esophagus is normal up to the esophageal hiatus but the gastric fundus is herniated into the thorax; and (2) sliding hernia, in which the esophagogastric junction is located above the esophageal hiatus. Sliding hernia is the most common type in children. Paraesophageal hernias are rare and present with symptoms of esophageal obstruction or respiratory compromise. Gastroesophageal reflux frequently accompanies sliding hiatal hernias, although many sliding hernias (even those of large size) may be asymptomatic.

PYLORIC STENOSIS

Essentials of Diagnosis

- Vomiting, usually projectile.
- Constipation.
- Poor weight gain or weight loss.
- Dehydration.
- Palpable olive-sized mass in the right upper quadrant.
- Typical hypoechoic mass of 1.5 cm or greater in diameter detected by ultrasonography.
- "String sign" and retained gastric contents on x-ray.

General Considerations

The cause of the increase in the size of the circular muscle of the pylorus is not known. There is a coincidence of the disease in twins or fathers and sons. The disease occurs in one out of 500 births, and males are affected 3–4 times more commonly than females. The reported increased incidence in firstborns and in the spring and fall months is controversial.

Clinical Findings

A. Symptoms and Signs: Vomiting usually begins between 2 and 4 weeks of age and becomes projectile after each feeding; it starts at birth in about 10% of cases. In premature infants, the onset of symptoms is often delayed. The vomitus does not contain bile but may be bloodstreaked. The infant is hungry and nurses avidly, but constipation and failure to thrive occur. Dehydration, fretfulness, and apathy may be present. The upper abdomen is distended, and gastric peristaltic waves from left to right may be seen. An olive-sized tumor can almost always be felt to the right of the umbilicus, especially after the child has vomited.

B. Laboratory Findings: Elevated unconjugated bilirubin occurs in 2–3% of cases. There is hypochloremic alkalosis with potassium depletion. Hemoconcentration is reflected by elevated hemoglobin and hematocrit values.

C. Imaging: An upper gastrointestinal series reveals delay in gastric emptying and an elongated narrowed pyloric channel ("string sign"). On frontal views, the enlarged pylorus causes characteristic semilunar impressions on the gastric antrum. Ultrasonography shows a hypoechoic ring in front of the right kidney and medial to the gallbladder.

Differential Diagnosis

Other causes of vomiting in young infants must be ruled out. (See Table 20–1). In esophageal stenosis or achalasia, the emesis contains no gastric contents, and metabolic alkalosis is not present. With annular pancreas, malrotation, volvulus, and other lesions causing small bowel obstruction, the emesis is bilious. The absence of virilization and hyperkalemia generally rules out congenital adrenal hyperplasia with adrenal insufficiency. Neurologic abnormalities and metabolic acidosis are often associated with other metabolic disorders. Sepsis and urinary tract infections should be checked by culture. In simple cases of "pylorospasm," there may be a delay in gastric emptying, but the elongated narrow pyloric canal is not seen and no tumor is present. Antral webs or diaphragms, duplications, cysts, and channel ulcers of the pyloric canal are rare causes of gastric outlet obstruction.

Treatment & Prognosis

Pyloromyotomy is the treatment of choice and consists of incision down to the mucosa and fully across the pyloric length. Prior to surgery, the necessary time must be taken to repair dehydration and electrolyte abnormalities and to assuage any gastritis by saline gastric irrigations.

The outlook is excellent following surgery. Sometimes there is continued vomiting postoperatively in cases with a long preoperative history. The postoperative barium x-ray remains abnormal despite relief of symptoms.

Khamapirad T, Athey PA: Ultrasound diagnosis of hypertrophic pyloric stenosis. *J Pediatr* 1983;**102**:23.

Moazam F, Kolts BE, Rodgers B: In pursuit of the etiology of congenital hypertrophic pyloric stenosis. *J Pediatr Gastroenterol Nutr* 1982;**1**:97.

NEONATAL PERFORATIONS OF THE GASTROINTESTINAL TRACT

Intrauterine intestinal perforation causes sterile meconium peritonitis. Abdominal x-ray films reveal intraperitoneal calcifications. Causes include perforation of the appendix, intestinal atresia or stenosis, malrotation with volvulus, meconium ileus, internal hernia, idiopathic perforation of the stomach and duodenum, intestinal duplication, intussusception, and Hirschsprung's disease. Postpartum intestinal perforation causes bacterial peritonitis. The most common cause is necrotizing enterocolitis. Other entities include perforated peptic ulcers, Hirschsprung's disease, intestinal atresia, gastroschisis, and malrotation with volvulus. Stress ulcers and necrotizing enterocolitis are manifestations of ischemic necrosis, usually likely to be seen in neonates with asphyxia, sepsis, or hypotension.

Premature infants are more prone to develop idiopathic gastric or intestinal perforation. The syndrome has been observed in identical twins. The affected newborns usually appear normal at birth; the average age at onset of symptoms is the third day of life. Refusal of feedings is followed by vomiting, sometimes bloody. The abdomen becomes distended; dyspnea and cyanosis frequently ensue and are followed by shock. X-ray findings may reveal free air under the diaphragm. The gastric air bubble is usually absent, especially when the perforation is large.

Fluid and electrolyte balance should be corrected while the abdomen is decompressed by nasogastric suction. Plasma volume maintenance and systemic antibiotics are indicated.

Surgery should be carried out as soon as possible. The prognosis is poor.

Emanuel B et al: Perforation of the gastrointestinal tract in infancy and childhood. *Surg Gynecoi Obstet* 1978; **146**:926.

Roy CC et al: Gastrointestinal emergency problems in pediatric practice. *Clin Gastroenterol* 1981;**10**:225.

PEPTIC DISEASE

Essentials of Diagnosis

- Abdominal pain and vomiting.
- Melena or hematemesis (or both).
- Unexplained anemia.
- Vague abdominal complaints in a patient with a strong family history.

General Considerations

Peptic ulcers may occur at any age but are more frequent between the ages of 12 and 18 years. Boys are affected more commonly than girls. Up to age 6, most ulcers are secondary, associated with an underlying illness, toxin, or drug. A positive family history is present in about 30% of cases of primary duodenal ulcer.

Although the pathogenesis of peptic ulcer is multifactorial, the final common pathway appears to be a breakdown in the normal mucosal defense, which permits acid peptic digestion of the mucosa. Causes include (1) reduced mucous protective layer (aspirin, nonsteroidal anti-inflammatory drugs, hypoxia); (2) reduced metabolic activity of the gastric mucosal cell, which allows for the diffusion of hydrogen ions into the cell (hypoxia, hypotension); (3) increased gastric secretion of acid or pepsin (increased parietal cell mass, increased postprandial secretion of gastrin, increased vagal tone); (4) reflux of bile from duodenum to stomach; and (5) decreased neutralizing activity in duodenal secretions. The most common causes of secondary ulcer are toxins (alcohol, aspirin), sepsis, hypotension, burns, and injury of the central nervous system.

Recent clinical research has shown a close association between *Helicobacter pylori* infection of the gastric antrum and the presence of antral gastritis and primary peptic ulcer of both duodenum and stomach. There is no evidence to support a role for

H pylori infection in recurrent abdominal pain of childhood without gastritis.

Clinical Findings

A. Symptoms and Signs:

1. At 0–3 years of age—In infants past the neonatal period up to the age of 3, symptoms of primary ulcers include poor eating, vomiting, crying after meals, and melena or hematemesis. Secondary ulcers are more acute, and hemorrhage perforation may be the first signs.

2. At 3–6 years of age—Vomiting related to eating is usually present. Gastric outlet obstruction may cause protracted vomiting. Periumbilical or generalized abdominal pain is common. The typical "ulcer pain" is rarely present. Melena, hematemesis, and perforation are common in cases of secondary ulcers.

3. At 6–18 years of age—Fewer than 50% of patients have "typical" ulcer symptoms. Melena or hematemesis (or both) is noted in over 50%; occult bleeding and anemia without other symptoms are not uncommon. In addition to the acute illnesses responsible for secondary ulcers, chronic conditions such as chronic lung disease, Crohn's disease, cirrhosis, and rheumatoid arthritis are associated with an increased incidence of peptic disease.

B. Gastric Analysis: The chief value of gastric fluid analysis is to rule out extreme hypersecretion such as that associated with the Zollinger-Ellison syndrome. Gastrin levels after a feeding tend to be higher in children with duodenal ulcers. They should be obtained in cases of recurrent ulcers if no other cause is found.

C. Imaging: Radiologic signs of ulceration or a deformity should be present. The frequency with which the radiologic sign of duodenal irritability is found in normal infants makes this x-ray finding unreliable. In patients with severe degrees of duodenal irritability, a crater may not be demonstrated, because the barium is moved out of the bulb very rapidly.

D. Panendoscopy: Although a barium meal remains a useful diagnostic tool for 85% of active ulcers, endoscopy should be carried out if x-ray findings are negative or equivocal. In the case of a bleeding ulcer, endoscopy takes precedence over x-ray studies if it can be done within 48 hours of cessation of hematemesis or melena. Endoscopy also permits gastric biopsy necessary for the identification of *H pylori* by culture, histology and urease activity. The presence of serum anti-*H pylori* antibody appears to correlate well with infection; titers fall with eradication and rise with relapse.

Differential Diagnosis

The diagnosis of acute secondary ulcers should be suspected in any child with a severe underlying disease who suddenly presents with abdominal disten-

tion, hematemesis, or melena. The differential diagnosis of primary peptic ulcer includes recurrent abdominal pain, irritable colon syndrome, esophagitis, chronic pancreatitis, cholelithiasis, and recurrent midgut volvulus. Suspicion should increase when there is a family history of primary peptic ulcer disease, even if the gastrointestinal complaints are vague.

Treatment

The mainstay of therapy is either antacids or gastric antisecretory medication. Antacids (1–5 mL/kg every 1–2 hours and at bedtime) are given initially. Later, antacids are given 1 and 3 hours after meals and at bedtime for 6 weeks. Cimetidine, a histamine$_2$ receptor antagonist, is administered before meals and at bedtime (5 mg/kg) or, in cases of severe disease, by continuous intravenous infusion. Ranitidine hydrochloride, another H$_2$ receptor antagonist, has higher affinity for the histamine$_2$ receptor and is effective at lower doses, is longer-acting, and has fewer side effects (2.5 mg/kg every 12 hours). Both cause healing in 85% of duodenal ulcers after 6 weeks, and neither is more effective than liquid antacids used in appropriate dosage. Recurrences may be prevented with a single nighttime dose of H$_2$ receptor antagonist. Anticholinergics should be given only in rare cases with significant hypersecretion.

Strict "ulcer diet" is not indicated. Foods that cause pain should be avoided. Caffeine should be avoided because it increases gastric secretion. Three regular meals are recommended; snacks are to be avoided, especially at bedtime. Aspirin and nonsteroidal anti-inflammatory drugs should be avoided.

Surgical treatment is reserved for the complications, eg, perforation, hemorrhage, obstruction, or incapacitating, intractable pain.

Peptic disease associated with *H pylori* recurs less often and may heal more rapidly if the organism is eradicated. The optimal therapeutic regimen is unknown. A course of at least 4 weeks of an oral bismuth preparation plus a 10-day course of an antimicrobial agent (amoxicillin, metronidazole, or tinidazole) are most often prescribed.

Prognosis

Long-term studies show that up to 80% of children with primary duodenal ulcers have recurrent symptoms on long-term follow-up. The prognosis for recurrence is much lower in the younger group (0–6 years). Surgery for duodenal ulcers (pyloroplasty and vagotomy) gives excellent results.

Drum B et al: Association of *Campylobacter pylori* on the gastric mucosa with antral gastritis in children. *N Engl J Med* 1987;**316:**1557.

Marshall BJ et al: Prospective double-blind trial of duodenal ulcer relapse after eradication of *Campylobacter pylori*. *Lancet* 1988;**2:**1437.

Nord KS: Peptic ulcer disease in the pediatric population. *Pediatr Clin North Am* 1988;**35:**117.

CONGENITAL DIAPHRAGMATIC HERNIA

Diaphragmatic hernia may be secondary to a posterolateral defect in the diaphragm (foramen of Bochdalek) or, in about 5% of cases, to a retrosternal defect (foramen of Morgagni). It represents failure of division of the thoracic and abdominal cavities at the eighth to tenth weeks of fetal life.

All degrees of protrusion of the abdominal viscera through the diaphragmatic opening into the thoracic cavity may occur. The extent of herniation determines the severity and the timing of the symptoms. In the posterolateral variety, more than 80% involve the left diaphragm.

Symptoms of mild to severe respiratory distress and cyanosis are usually present from birth, although some patients remain asymptomatic and the finding of a large diaphragmatic hernia with air-filled coils on x-ray is incidental. The abdomen is scaphoid. Breath sounds in the affected hemithorax are absent, with displacement of the point of maximal cardiac impulse.

Fatal cases (about 30%) have circulatory problems secondary to the mediastinal shift, giving rise to stretching and kinking of the great vessels. Pulmonary infections also constitute a major cause of death, along with prematurity, cardiac anomalies, and malrotation. The most frequent cause of death, however, is pulmonary insufficiency. The lung on the affected side is compressed and hypoplastic, with decreased numbers of generations of airways and pulmonary arteries throughout. Extracorporeal membrane oxygenation may decrease the early postoperative mortality rate in patients with poor lung compliance. The long-term follow-up of survivors shows that although hypoperfusion and a preemphysematous state can be identified, hypoplastic lungs remain asymptomatic at least until late in childhood.

In the eventration of the diaphragm, a leaf of the diaphragm containing a diminution of muscular elements is ballooned into the chest and leads to identical but much milder symptoms.

Adzick NS et al: Diaphragmatic hernia in the fetus: Prenatal diagnosis and outcome in 94 cases. *J Pediatr Surg* 1985;**20**:357.

Loe WA et al: Extracorporeal membrane oxygenation for newborn respiratory failure. *J Pediatr Surg* 1985; **20**:684.

Marshall A, Sumner E: Improved prognosis in congenital diaphragmatic hernia: Experience of 62 cases over 2-year period. *J R Soc Med* 1982;**75**:607.

CONGENITAL ATRESIAS & STENOSES OF THE GASTROINTESTINAL TRACT

The usual mode of presentation is neonatal intestinal obstruction or perforation. The presence of atresia or stenosis may produce polyhydramnios prenatally and can be diagnosed before birth by ultrasound. The triad of abdominal distention, bilious vomiting, and obstipation or failure to pass meconium constitutes the most important clue to diagnosis. Prematurity and other congenital anomalies may be present. The localization and relative incidence of atresias and stenoses are given in Table 20–2.

CONGENITAL DUODENAL OBSTRUCTION

Extrinsic duodenal obstruction is usually due to congenital peritoneal bands with or without volvulus associated with intestinal malrotation; to annular pancreas; or, more rarely, to duplication of the duodenum. Intrinsic obstruction is due to stenosis or atresia. The duodenal lumen may be obliterated by a membrane or completely interrupted with a fibrous cord between the 2 segments. Atresia may be proximal or distal to the ampulla of vater.

Clinical Findings

A. Atresia: A history of polyhydramnios is common. Vomiting (usually bile-stained) begins within a few hours after birth, with epigastric distention. Meconium may be normally passed. The association between duodenal atresia and severe congenital anomalies (30%), such as esophageal atresia, atresias elsewhere in the gastrointestinal tract, and cardiac and renal anomalies, is well described. Prematurity (25–50%) and Down's syndrome (20–30%) are other associated conditions.

B. Stenosis: Symptoms of duodenal obstruction are delayed for weeks, months, or years. Although the stenotic area is usually postampullary, the vomitus does not always contain bile. Abdominal x-ray films show gastric and duodenal gaseous distention proximal to the atretic site (''double bubble''). With

Table 20–2. Localization and incidence of gastrointestinal atresias and stenoses.

	Area Involved	Type of Lesion	Relative Frequency
Pylorus		Atresia Web or diaphragm (66%)	1%
Duodenum	Distal to the ampulla of Vater (80%)	Atresia Web or diaphragm (40%)	45%
Jejunoileal	Proximal jejunum and distal ileum (66%)	Atresia (multiple in 6–29%) Stenosis (20%)	50%
Colon	Left colon and rectum (50%)	Atresia (may be associated with atresias of the small bowel)	5–9%

protracted vomiting and dehydration, there may be little air in the stomach; it is then advisable to instill air into the stomach to elicit the typical pattern. Absence of gas in the intestinal tract distal to the obstruction suggests atresia or an extrinsic obstruction severe enough to completely occlude the lumen, whereas air scattered over the lower abdomen may indicate a partial duodenal obstruction of either the intrinsic or extrinsic variety. A barium enema may be helpful in determining the presence of a concomitant malrotation or of atresia lower in the gastrointestinal tract.

Treatment & Prognosis

Thorough exploration is necessary at operation both to find the cause of the obstruction and to make sure no additional pathologic anomalies are present lower in the gastrointestinal tract.

The mortality rate (35–40%) is significantly affected by prematurity, Down's syndrome, and associated congenital anomalies.

CONGENITAL JEJUNAL & ILEAL OBSTRUCTION

Bile-stained or fecal vomiting usually begins in the first 48 hours of life, and distention is frequent. Small amounts of meconium may be passed. Prematurity and severe congenital anomalies often coexist. Atresias, stenoses, and obstructing membranes may affect multiple sites. X-ray features include dilated loops of small bowel and absence of colonic gas. Barium enema will reveal a colon of restricted caliber (microcolon) if the atresia is in the lower small bowel. In over 10% of cases of jejunoileal atresia, there is absence of the mesentery, and the superior mesenteric artery cannot be identified beyond the origin of the right colic and ileocolic arteries. As a result, the ileum coils around one of these 2 arteries, giving rise to the "Christmas tree" deformity. The tenuous blood supply often leads to long areas of gangrenous bowel and compromises surgical anastomoses.

The differential diagnosis should include Hirschsprung's disease, paralytic ileus secondary to sepsis, gastroenteritis or pneumonia, midgut volvulus, and meconium ileus. Ninety percent of infants with meconium ileus will prove to have cystic fibrosis. The remainder of cases are idiopathic or are associated with intestinal atresia (especially ileal atresia) or pancolonic Hirschsprung's disease.

Surgery is mandatory. The prognosis remains guarded.

ANNULAR PANCREAS

Annular pancreas is usually associated with failure of segmental duodenal development. The symptoms are those of partial or complete duodenal obstruction. Down's syndrome and congenital anomalies of the gastrointestinal tract occur frequently. As with other gastrointestinal obstructive lesions of the neonate, polyhydramnios is common. Clinical manifestations can develop late in childhood.

Treatment consists of duodenoduodenostomy or duodenojejunostomy without operative dissection or division of the pancreatic annulus.

Kiernan PD et al: Annular pancreas: Mayo Clinic experience from 1957 to 1976 with review of the literature. *Arch Surg* 1980;**115**:46.

Merrill JR, Raffensperger JG: Pediatric annular pancreas: Twenty years' experience. *J Pediatr Surg* 1976;**11**:921.

MIDGUT MALROTATION WITH OR WITHOUT VOLVULUS

Normally, the midgut (which extends from the duodenojejunal junction to the mid transverse colon and which is supplied by the superior mesenteric artery) returns to the intra-abdominal position during the tenth week of embryonic life, and the root of the mesentery rotates in a counterclockwise direction. This causes the colon to cross ventrally; the cecum moves from the left to the right lower quadrant, and the duodenum crosses dorsally to become partly retroperitoneal. When this rotation is incomplete, the posterior fixation of the mesentery is defective, so that the bowel from the ligament of Treitz to the mid transverse colon may twist, causing a volvulus around the pediclelike mesentery. Duodenal or ileal obstruction may later result through peritoneal bands from the mobile hepatic flexure or cecum. Most cases are asymptomatic.

Clinical Findings

A. Symptoms and Signs: Seventy-five percent of symptomatic cases show high intestinal obstruction within the first 3 weeks of life, with bile-stained vomitus, abdominal distention, and visible peristalsis. The first signs may occur later in life, with symptoms of intermittent intestinal obstruction or, rarely, with malabsorption or intermittent profuse watery diarrhea. Diarrhea may be an early symptom in infants under the age of 6 months. Associated congenital anomalies, especially cardiac, occur in over 25% of symptomatic cases.

B. Imaging: An upper gastrointestinal series may show partial or complete small bowel obstruction. There may be proximal distention with air. The diagnosis of malrotation can be further confirmed by barium enema, which shows a cecum that is mobile and abnormally located.

Treatment & Prognosis

Midgut volvulus is a catastrophic disease of the newborn period. Ischemia usually involves the segment of intestine supplied by the superior mesenteric artery (from the ligament of Treitz to the mid transverse colon). When necrosis is extensive, a second-look operation is recommended 48 hours after reducing the volvulus and dividing Ladd's bands. The prognosis in the newborn period is guarded in view of the incidence of perforation, peritonitis, and extensive intestinal necrosis.

Duke JH Jr, Yar MS: Primary small bowel volvulus. *Arch Surg* 1977;**112**:685.

Janik JS, Ein SH: Normal intestinal rotation with nonfixation: A cause of chronic abdominal pain. *J Pediatr Surg* 1979;**14**:670.

Millar AJW et al: The deadly vomit: Malrotation and midgut volvulus. *Pediatr Surg Int* 1987;**2**:172.

Stewart DR et al: Malrotation of the bowel in infants and children: A 15 year experience. *Surgery* 1976;**79**:716.

MAJOR ABDOMINAL WALL DEVELOPMENTAL DEFECTS

Omphalocele

This is a rare condition (1:10,000 births) associated with variable herniation of intestine and liver into the base of the umbilical cord. There is no defect of the abdominal wall, but cardiac anomalies (20%) and the midline syndromes are common. Primary closure of those less than 5 cm in diameter has a good prognosis. When the defect is large, the abdominal cavity may be small. Reduction of large defects may have to be performed in stages to prevent compression of intra-abdominal and intrathoracic structures.

Gastroschisis

Herniation of bowel and other viscera through a defect in the abdominal wall is twice as frequent as omphalocele. There is no covering membrane, and the eviscerated bowel loops are dark red, edematous, and adherent. They are encased in a thick matrix of fibrinous material. Gangrene may be present. All patients have associated malrotation and some degree of congenital shortening of the small bowel. Associated intestinal atresias are common. Closure is by stages with a prosthetic abdominal wall. Prematurity (40%), the threat of sepsis, and malnutrition remain the long-term challenges of this entity. The postoperative course is usually difficult because of protracted intestinal obstruction and intestinal dysfunction.

Congenital Deficiency of Abdominal Musculature

This disorder, known as the prune-belly syndrome, is apparent from the flaccid and wrinkled appearance of the abdominal wall. Almost all affected infants are males with undescended testes; 50% present with clubfoot. Between 20 and 25%

also have cardiac and gastrointestinal anomalies. Urinary tract anomalies consist of urethral and functional bladder neck obstructions associated with a patent urachus. Corseting counteracts the abdominal wall weakness, but 60% die in infancy as a result of renal insufficiency or respiratory failure.

De Vries PA: The pathogenesis of gastroschisis and omphalocele. *J Pediatr Surg* 1980;**15**:245.

DiLorenzo M et al: Gastroschisis: A 15 year experience. *J Pediatr Surg* 1987;**22**:710.

Moore TC, Nur K: An international survey of gastroschisis and omphalocele (490 cases). *Pediatr Surg Int* 1987;**2**:27.

MECKEL'S DIVERTICULUM & OMPHALOMESENTERIC DUCT REMNANTS

Meckel's diverticulum is present in 1.5% of the population but rarely causes symptoms. Familial cases have been reported. Complications occur 3 times more frequently in males than in females, and in 50–60% of cases within the first 2 years of life. Heterotopic tissue (gastric mucosa mostly, but also pancreatic tissue and jejunal or colonic mucosa) is 10 times as likely to be present within the diverticulum in symptomatic cases. Meckel's diverticulum is usually located within 100 cm of the ileocecal valve on the antimesenteric side and has its own blood supply.

Clinical Findings

A. Symptoms and Signs: In 40–60% of symptomatic cases, massive, painless rectal bleeding or dark red stool is characteristic and may cause shock. Occult bleeding may cause anemia. Gastric mucosa and an ulcer of the ileal mucosa are found in the majority of diverticula that bleed.

Intestinal obstruction occurs in 25% of symptomatic cases. Ileocolic intussusception occurs with intestinal infarction. A mass is palpable.

Volvulus of the bowel around a fibrous remnant of the vitelline duct extending from the tip of the diverticulum to the abdominal wall may occur. In some cases, entrapment of a bowel loop under a band running between the diverticulum and the base of the mesentery has been associated with intestinal obstruction. The diverticulum may be trapped in an inguinal hernia.

Diverticulitis occurs in 10–20% of symptomatic cases and is clinically indistinguishable from acute appendicitis. Perforation and generalized peritonitis may occur. There may be chronic recurrent abdominal pain.

B. Imaging: Diagnosis of this condition is seldom made on barium x-ray. Radionuclide imaging with ^{99m}Tc pertechnetate may demonstrate the diverticulum lined with heterotopic gastric mucosa. Stimulation of ^{99m}Tc pertechnetate uptake by both pentagastrin and cimetidine can reduce the number of false-negative results. Angiography may be useful when bleeding is brisk.

Treatment

A. Diverticulum: Treatment is surgical. At operation, close inspection of the ileum proximal and distal to the diverticulum may reveal ulcerations and heterotopic tissue adjacent to the neck of the diverticulum.

B. Other Remnants of the Omphalomesenteric Duct: Fecal discharge from the umbilicus is evidence of a patent omphalomesenteric duct. The duct may be completely closed, leading to persistence of a fibrous cord joining ileum and umbilicus and potentially the origin of a volvulus. In other instances, a mucoid discharge may be indicative of a mucocele, which can protrude through the umbilicus and be mistaken for an umbilical granuloma, since it is firm and bright red. In all cases, surgical excision of the omphalomesenteric remnant is indicated.

Prognosis

The prognosis for Meckel's diverticulum is good. Marked hemorrhage may occur but is rarely exsanguinating.

Mackey WC, Dineen P: A fifty-year experience with Meckel's diverticulum. *Surg Gynecol Obstet* 1983; **156**:56.
Treves S, Grand RJ, Eraklis AJ: Pentagastrin stimulation of technetium-99m uptake by ectopic gastric mucosa in Meckel's diverticulum. *Radiology* 1978;**128**:711.

DUPLICATIONS OF THE GASTROINTESTINAL TRACT

Duplications of the gastrointestinal tract are congenital malformations most often discovered during infancy. Duplications are spherical or tubular structures of various size that may occur anywhere along the gastrointestinal tract. They usually contain fluid and sometimes blood if necrosis has taken place. Most duplications do not communicate with the intestinal lumen; they are attached to the mesenteric side of the gut and share a common muscular coat. The epithelial lining of the duplication is usually of the same type as that from which it originates; 20–30% contain ectopic gastric mucosa. Some duplications are attached to the spinal cord and are associated with hemivertebrae (neurenteric cysts). Esophageal duplications are rare.

Symptoms usually begin in infancy, with vomiting, abdominal distention, colicky pain, rectal bleeding, partial or total intestinal obstruction, or an abdominal mass. Physical examination reveals a rounded, smooth, freely movable mass, and x-ray films of the abdomen show a noncalcified mass displacing the intestines or compressing the stomach. Scanning with ^{99m}Tc pertechnetate is useful in duplications containing gastric mucosa. Involvement of the terminal small bowel can give rise to an intussusception.

Prompt surgical treatment is indicated.

Favara B, Franciosi RA, Akers DR: Enteric duplications. Thirty-seven cases: A vascular theory of pathogenesis. *Am J Dis Child* 1971;**122**:501.
Pruksapong C et al: Gastric duplication. *J Pediatr Surg* 1979;**14**:83.

NECROTIZING ENTEROCOLITIS (See Chapter 4.)

PERITONITIS

Primary bacterial peritonitis is rare. The most common organisms responsible include *Escherichia coli,* hemolytic streptococci and pneumococci, and (occasionally) viruses. Primary peritonitis occurs in young patients with splenic dysfunction or splenectomy and in patients with ascites (nephrotic syndrome, advanced liver disease, kwashiorkor). Secondary peritonitis usually results from penetrating abdominal trauma or ruptured viscus. (Appendicitis, perforated peptic ulcer, cholecystitis, pancreatitis, inflammatory bowel disease, midgut volvulus, intussusception, and strangulated hernia are some primary events.) Intra-abdominal abscesses may form in pelvic, subhepatic, or subphrenic areas, but localization of infection is less common in young infants than it is in adults.

Symptoms include severe abdominal pain, fever, nausea, and vomiting. Respirations are shallow. The abdomen is tender, rigid, and distended, with involuntary guarding. Bowel sounds may be absent. Tenderness is present on rectal examination. In secondary peritonitis, these signs are accompanied by, and even overshadowed by, the signs and symptoms of the underlying cause of peritonitis. Diarrhea is fairly common in primary peritonitis and less so in secondary peritonitis.

The leukocyte count is initially high (greater than 20,000/mL) and later may fall to neutropenic levels, especially in primary peritonitis. Bacterial peritonitis should be suspected if paracentesis fluid contains more than 500 WBC/mL or more than 32 mg/dl of lactate, has a pH less than 7.34, or if the pH of ascites is more than 0.1 pH unit less than arterial pH. Etiologic diagnosis is made by Gram's stain and culture, preferably of 5–10 mL of fluid for optimal yield.

Antibiotic treatment and supportive therapy for dehydration, shock, and acidosis are indicated. Surgical treatment of the underlying cause of secondary peritonitis is critical. Drainage of localized abscess is often required.

Bell MJ et al: The microbiological flora and anti-microbial therapy of neonatal peritonitis. *J Pediatr Surg* 1980;**15:**569.

Bell MJ: Peritonitis in the newborn: Current concepts. *Pediatr Clin North Am* 1985;**32:**1181.

Emanuel B et al: Perforation of gastrointestinal tract in infancy and childhood. *Surg Gynecol Obstet* 1978;**146:**926.

Garcia-Tsau G, Conn HO, Lerner E: The diagnosis of bacterial peritonitis: Comparison of pH, lactate concentration and leucocyte count. *Hepatology* 1985;**5:**91.

McDougal WS et al: Primary peritonitis in infancy and childhood. *Ann Surg* 1975;**181:**310.

CONGENITAL AGANGLIONIC MEGACOLON (Hirschsprung's Disease)

Essentials of Diagnosis

- Partial or complete intestinal obstruction in the newborn period, with vomiting, diarrhea, abdominal distention, and shock.
- Obstinate constipation, abdominal enlargement, ribbonlike stools, and failure to thrive in infancy or childhood.
- Absence of fecal material on rectal examination.
- Narrowed colonic segment proximal to the anus visible on x-ray film.
- Absence of ganglion cells in the narrowed segment.

General Considerations

Hirschsprung's disease is due to an absence of ganglion cells in the mucosal and muscular layers of the colon. During development of the fetus, there is a failure of neural crest cells to migrate to the mesodermal layers. The rectum alone (30%) or the rectosigmoid (44%) is usually affected. The entire colon is aganglionic in 8% of cases. Segmental aganglionosis is very rare and may be an acquired lesion secondary to ischemia. The denervated segment is narrowed, with dilatation of the proximal uninvolved colon. In long-standing cases, the mucosa of the dilated colonic segment may become thin and inflamed (enterocolitis) with both blood and protein loss.

A familial pattern has been described, particularly in total colonic aganglionosis. The disease is 4 times more common in boys than in girls, and 10–15% of patients have Down's syndrome.

Clinical Findings

A. Symptoms and Signs: Failure of the newborn to pass meconium—followed by vomiting, abdominal distention, and reluctance to feed—suggests the diagnosis. The infant is irritable, and breathing may be rapid and grunting because of abdominal distention. In some cases, symptoms appear later and are those of partial intestinal obstruction, with abdominal distention and bilious vomiting. Bouts of enterocolitis manifested by fever, explosive diarrhea, and prostration are reported in about 50% of newborns with this disease. These episodes may lead to acute inflammatory and ischemic changes in the colon, with perforation (especially cecal) and sepsis. In later infancy, alternating obstipation and diarrhea predominate. The older child is more likely to present with constipation. The stools are offensive and ribbonlike, the abdomen enlarged, and the veins prominent; peristaltic patterns are readily visible, and fecal masses are palpable. Intermittent bouts of intestinal obstruction due to fecal impaction, hypochromic anemia, hypoproteinemia, and failure to thrive are common. Encopresis is rarely seen.

On digital examination, the anal canal and rectum are devoid of fecal material and may feel narrow. If the involved segment is short, there may be a gush of flatus and of pale, liquid, offensive stool as the finger is withdrawn. The presence of fecal colonic impaction associated with an empty rectum is most suggestive of the disease.

B. Laboratory Findings: The diagnosis is based on histologic evidence of aganglionosis and histochemical evidence of increased acetylcholinesterase activity. Rectal biopsies taken at 3, 4, and 5 cm from the anus readily establish the diagnosis, although some prefer a full-thickness rectal biopsy in order to have access to the ganglion cells between the muscular layers (plexus myentericus).

C. Imaging: X-ray examination of the abdomen may reveal dilated colonic loops and absence of gas from the pelvic colon on an erect lateral film. A barium enema, introducing a small amount of radiopaque material through a catheter with the tip inserted barely beyond the anal sphincter, will usually demonstrate the narrowed segment distally with a sharp transition to proximal dilated colon. However, in neonates a "transition zone" may not be seen. Retention of barium for 24–48 hours is not diagnostic of Hirschsprung's disease but can be seen in retentive constipation as well.

D. Special Examinations: Manometric studies can be diagnostic, especially when a short, aganglionic segment is present. Failure of the internal sphincter muscle to relax after balloon distention of the rectum is consistent with Hirschsprung's disease. Interpretation of acetylcholinesterase staining in newborns is sometimes difficult.

Differential Diagnosis

Congenital aganglionic megacolon accounts for 15–20% of cases of neonatal intestinal obstruction. In childhood, this disease must be differentiated from retentive constipation with colon distention. It can also be confused with celiac disease because of the striking abdominal distention and failure to thrive.

Treatment

A colostomy should be performed proximal to the

aganglionic segment. If the entire colon is involved, ileostomy is performed. If enterocolitis is clinically present and radiologically demonstrated by the typical "sawtooth" appearance, saline irrigations should be repeatedly given through a rectal cannula. Plasma expanders and fluid and electrolyte homeostasis are essential before surgery. Resection of the aganglionic segment is delayed until the infant is at least 6 months of age.

During operation, it is essential to ascertain from biopsies of the bowel that ganglion cells are present in the proximal portion of the resected bowel before the final anastomosis is made. The endorectal pull-through (Soave) procedure is the preferred surgical operation. Long-term complications following surgery include fecal incontinence or fecal impaction.

Prognosis

Enterocolitis before or after surgery is associated with a 30% mortality rate, especially in infants with a long aganglionic segment. Hirschsprung's disease has recurred postoperatively in some cases because of the dropping out of ganglion cells secondary to vascular impairment and chronic inflammatory changes.

Dykes EH, Guiney EJ: Total colonic aganglionosis. *J Pediatr Gastroenterol Nutr* 1989;**8:**129.

Klein MD et al: Hirschsprung's disease in the newborn. *J Pediatr Surg* 1984;**19:**370.

Kleinhaus S et al: Hirschsprung's disease: A survey of the members of the Surgical Section of the American Academy of Pediatrics. *J Pediatr Surg* 1979;**14:**588.

Landman GB: A five-year chart review of children biopsied to rule out Hirschsprung's disease. *Clin Pediatr (Phila)* 1987;**26:**288.

Weinberg RJ et al: Acquired distal aganglionosis of the colon. *J Pediatr* 1982;**101:**406.

THE MECONIUM PLUG SYNDROME

Low intestinal obstruction occurs on the second day of life. Little or no meconium is passed, and abdominal distention is followed by bile-stained vomiting and dehydration. On rectal examination, the anal canal may be abnormally small. Occasionally, after the rectal exam, the meconium plug may be passed with large amounts of gas and meconium.

In addition to air distention seen on x-ray film, fluid levels are observed in half of the patients. A barium enema performed under low pressure with a soft-tipped catheter is not only diagnostic, because it reveals a change in the caliber of the colon at the site of obstruction, but can also be therapeutic in dislodging the meconium plug. The finding of a microcolon distal to the plug makes the differentiation from Hirschsprung's disease difficult. Indeed, 10–20% of neonates with meconium plug have Hirschsprung's disease (30–50% of male patients). Rectal

biopsy may be necessary to rule out Hirschsprung's disease if bowel function does not normalize after passage of the meconium plug. The presence of a rubbery meconium plug sometimes indicates the presence of cystic fibrosis, but meconium obstruction of the terminal ileum is a more common problem.

SMALL LEFT COLON SYNDROME

This condition is most often seen in infants of diabetic mothers, infants delivered by cesarean section, premature infants, and twins. It presents with failure to pass meconium in the first 24–48 hours. Plain abdominal x-ray films show air-fluid levels and a dilated colon proximal to the splenic flexure. Meconium is easily evacuated with barium or meglumine diatrizoate (Gastrografin) enema, which is both therapeutic and diagnostic. The descending colon and rectosigmoid are narrow. Hirschsprung's disease must be ruled out, but the outlook for normal colon function is good. Immaturity of the neural plexus with self-limited abnormality of colon motor function may be the cause.

CHYLOUS ASCITES

Chylous ascites due to congenital infection or developmental abnormality of the lymphatic system may be observed at birth. If the thoracic duct is involved, chylothorax may be present. Later in life, chylous ascites may result from congenital lymphatic abnormality, tumors, peritoneal bands, or trauma to major lymphatics.

Clinical Findings

A. Symptoms and Signs: In both congenital and acquired forms, diarrhea and failure to thrive are noted. The abdomen is distended, with a fluid wave and shifting dullness. Unilateral or generalized peripheral lymphedema may be present.

B. Laboratory Findings: Laboratory findings include hypoalbuminemia, hypogammaglobulinemia, and lymphopenia. Ascitic fluid will have the composition of chyle if the patient has been fed; otherwise it is indistinguishable from ascites secondary to cirrhosis.

Differential Diagnosis

Chylous ascites must be differentiated from ascites due to liver failure and, in the older child, from constrictive pericarditis and neoplastic, infectious, or inflammatory diseases causing lymphatic obstruction.

Complications & Sequelae

Severe chylous ascites can be fatal. Chronic loss of albumin and gamma globulin through the gastrointestinal tract may lead to edema and increase the risk of infection. Rapidly accumulating chylous ascites may cause respiratory complications.

Treatment & Prognosis

If there is a congenital abnormality due to hypoplasia, aplasia, or ectasia of the lymphatics, little can be done for the patient. Shunting of peritoneal fluid into the venous system is sometimes effective. Attempts to relieve the ascites by bringing the saphenous vein into the peritoneal cavity have had partial success. A fat-free diet supplemented with medium-chain triglycerides decreases the formation of chylous ascitic fluid. Total parenteral nutrition may be necessary. The congenital form of chylous ascites may spontaneously disappear following paracentesis and a medium-chain triglyceride diet. The prognosis is guarded, although spontaneous cures have been reported.

Cochran WJ et al: Chylous ascites in infants and children: A case report and literature review. *J Pediatr Gastroenterol Nutr* 1985;**4**:668.

Guttman FM, Montupet P, Bloss RS: Experience with peritoneovenous shunting for congenital chylous ascites in infants and children. *J Pediatr Surg* 1982;**17**:368.

CONGENITAL ANORECTAL ANOMALIES

Anorectal anomalies occur once in every 3000–4000 births, and most types are more common in males. Inspection of the perianal area is essential in all newborns.

Classification

A. Anterior Displacement of the Anal Opening: This condition is more common in girls than in boys. It may be associated with a posterior rectal shelf and usually is characterized by constipation that responds poorly to medical management.

B. Anal Stenosis: The anal aperture is very small and filled with a dot of meconium. Defecation is difficult, and there may be ribbonlike stools, fecal impaction, and abdominal distention. This malformation accounts for perhaps 10% of cases of anorectal anomalies.

C. Imperforate Anal Membrane: The infant fails to pass meconium, and a greenish bulging membrane is seen. After excision, bowel and sphincter function are normal.

D. Anal Agenesis: This results from defective development of the anus. The anal dimple is present, and stimulation of the perianal area leads to puckering indicative of the presence of the external sphincter. If there is no associated fistula, intestinal obstruction occurs. Fistulas may be perineal or vulvar in the female and perineal or urethral in the male. A perineal fistula presents as a streak of meconium buried in thickened perineal skin.

E. Rectal and Anal Agenesis: Rectal and anal agenesis accounts for 75% of total anorectal anomalies. Fistulas are almost invariably present. In the female, they may be vestibular or vaginal or may enter a urogenital sinus, which is a common passageway for the urethra and vagina. In the male, fistulas are rectovesical or rectourethral. Associated major congenital malformations are common. Sacral defects, prematurity, and hypoplastic internal and external sphincters significantly influence the prognosis for life and function.

F. Rectal Atresia: The anal canal and lower rectum form a blind pouch that is separated for a variable distance from the blind upper rectal pouch.

Radiologic Findings

Careful radiologic evaluation is indicated immediately so that the anal anomaly and the extent of associated anomalies of the bowel and the urogenital tract can be fully appraised.

Treatment & Prognosis

Dilation of the anus should be undertaken in cases of anal stenosis. Treatment for imperforate anal membrane consists of excision of the membrane and dilation. Colostomy is advocated for all cases of rectal agenesis. In patients with anal agenesis and a visible fistula of sufficient size to pass meconium, treatment can be deferred. The male without a visible fistula may have a urethral fistula; therefore, colostomy is recommended.

Of the patients with "low" defects, 80–90% are continent after surgery; with "high" defects, only 30% achieve continence. Gracilis muscle transplants may improve continence. Levatorplasty may also be used as a secondary operation following surgery for anorectal agenesis.

The mortality rate is about 20%. The prognosis is worse in small premature infants and in infants with associated anomalies.

De Vries PA: The surgery of anorectal anomalies: Its evolution with evaluation of procedures. *Curr Probl Surg* 1984;**21**(5):1.

Ditesheim JA, Templeton JM: Short-term vs. long-term quality of life following repair of high imperforate anus. *J Pediatr Surg* 1987;**22**:581.

Reisner SH et al: Determination of anterior displacement of the anus in newborn infants and children. *Pediatrics* 1984;**73**:216.

Roy CC, Morin CL, Weber AM: Gastrointestinal emergency problems in paediatric practice. *Clin Gastroenterol* 1981;**10**:225.

Smith ED: The bathwater needs changing, but don't throw out the baby: An overview of anorectal anomalies. *J Pediatr Surg* 1987;**22**:335.

ACUTE ABDOMEN

Many disorders must be considered in the differential diagnosis of acute abdomen. Emergency surgery should not be considered until the differential diagnosis has been completed. The patient may be too young to describe symptoms, and the parent's description is a subjective interpretation of what he or she thinks is wrong. A partial etiologic classification of acute abdomen is shown in Table 20–3, with the most common causes noted. Some of the specific entities are discussed in subsequent sections. Reaching a speedy and accurate diagnosis in the patient with an acute abdomen is critical and requires skill in physical diagnosis, intimate acquaintance with the characteristic symptoms of a large number of conditions, and the judicious selection of laboratory and radiologic tests.

Hatch EI: The acute abdomen in children. *Pediatr Clin North Am* 1985;**32**:1151.

ACUTE APPENDICITIS

Essentials of Diagnosis

- Diffuse, crampy abdominal pain, followed by right lower quadrant pain.
- Anorexia, vomiting, and constipation.
- Low-grade fever (38–38.5 °C [100–101.3 °F]).
- Right lower quadrant tenderness with rebound tenderness and, eventually, guarding.
- White blood cell count < 15,000/μL, with raised neutrophil levels.

General Considerations

Acute appendicitis is the most common cause of abdominal surgery in childhood. The frequency increases with age and peaks between 15 and 30 years. Luminal obstruction by fecaliths (25%) or parasites is a predisposing factor.

The incidence of perforation is high (40%) in infants and children. In order to avoid delay in diagnosis, it is important to maintain close communication with parents, perform a thorough physical examina-

tion and sequential examinations of the abdomen over a period of several hours, and interpret correctly the evolving symptoms and signs.

Clinical Findings

A. Symptoms and Signs: The triad of persistent localized right lower quadrant pain, localized abdominal tenderness, and slight fever strongly suggests appendicitis. Anorexia, vomiting, and constipation also occur. The clinical picture is often atypical, ie, generalized pain, tenderness around the umbilicus, and no leukocytosis. Diarrhea can substitute for constipation, and a subsiding upper respiratory tract infection may be found. Rectal examination should always be done and may reveal localized mass or tenderness. Examination of the stool may suggest other diagnoses, such as colitis or intussusception. Because many infections give rise to symptoms mimicking appendicitis and because physical findings are often inconclusive, it is important to repeat examinations of the abdomen. In children under 2 years old, the pain of appendicitis is poorly localized, and perforation before surgery is common.

B. Laboratory Findings: White blood cell counts are seldom higher than 15,000/μL. Fecal leukocytes and blood are rare.

C. Imaging: A radiopaque fecalith is reportedly present in two-thirds of cases of ruptured appendix. A barium enema examination showing a normal appendix and cecum usually rules out appendicitis. However, a positive diagnosis of nonperforated appendicitis cannot be made by barium enema.

Differential Diagnosis

The presence of intrathoracic infection (eg, pneumonia) or urinary tract infection should be kept in mind, along with other medical and surgical conditions leading to acute abdomen (see above).

Treatment & Prognosis

Appendectomy is indicated whenever the diagno-

Table 20–3. Etiologic classification of acute abdomen.[1]

Mechanical Obstruction		Inflammatory Diseases and Infections			
Intraluminal Obstruction	Extraluminal Obstruction	Gastrointestinal Disease	Paralytic Ileus	Blunt Trauma	Miscellaneous
Foreign body	Hernia	Appendicitis	Sepsis	Accident	Lead poisoning
Bezoar	Intussusception	Crohn's disease	Pneumonia	Battered child	Sickle cell crisis
Fecalith	Volvulus	Ulcerative colitis	Pyelonephritis	syndrome	Familial Mediterra-
Gallstone	Duplication	Henoch-Schönlein-	Peritonitis		nean fever
Parasites	Stenosis	purpura and other	Pancreatitis		Porphyria
Meconium ileus	Tumor	causes of vasculi-	Cholecystitis		Diabetic acidosis
equivalent	Mesenteric cyst	tis	Renal and gallblad-		Addisonian crisis
Tumor	Superior mesenteric	Peptic ulcer	der stones		Torsion of testis
Fecaloma	artery syndrome	Meckel's diverticulitis	Pelvic inflammation		Torsion of ovarian
	Pyloric stenosis	Acute gastroenteritis	Lymphadenitis due		pedicle
		Pseudomembranous	to viral or bacterial		
		enterocolitis	infection		

[1]Reproduced, with permission, from Roy CC, Morin CL, Weber AM: Gastrointestinal emergency problems in paediatric practice. *Clin Gastroenterol* 1981;**10**:225.

sis of appendicitis cannot be ruled out after a period of close observation. Postoperative antibiotic therapy directed to the treatment of anaerobes and coliforms is reserved for cases with gangrenous or perforated appendix.

The mortality rate is less than 1% in patients during childhood, despite the high incidence of perforation.

Fedyshin P, Kelvin FM, Rice RP: Nonspecificity of barium enema findings in acute appendicitis. *AJR* 1984; **143**:99.

Gilbert SR: Appendicitis in children. *Surg Gynecol Obstet* 1985;**161**:261.

Harrison MW et al: Acute appendicitis in children: Factors affecting morbidity. *Am J Surg* 1984;**147**:605.

INTUSSUSCEPTION

Essentials of Diagnosis

- Paroxysmal, episodic abdominal pain and vomiting.
- Sausage-shaped mass in upper abdomen.
- Rectal passage of bloody material (mucus and stool).
- Barium enema evidence of intussusception.

General Considerations

Intussusception is the most frequent cause of intestinal obstruction in the first 2 years of life. It is 3 times more common in males than in females. In most cases (85%) the cause is not apparent, although polyps, Meckel's diverticulum, Schönlein-Henoch purpura, lymphomas, lipomas, constipation, parasites, foreign bodies, or adenovirus or rotavirus infections with hypertrophy of Peyer's patches are predisposing factors. Intussusception occurs in patients with cystic fibrosis and celiac disease and usually relates to inspissated fecal material in the terminal ileum and colon. In children older than age 6 years, lymphoma is the most common lesion. Intermittent small bowel intussusception is a rare cause of recurrent abdominal pain.

The intussusception usually starts just proximal to the ileocecal valve, so that invagination is ileocolic. Other forms include ileoileal and colocolic. Swelling, hemorrhage, incarceration with necrosis of the intussuscepted bowel, and eventual perforation and peritonitis occur as a result of impairment of venous return.

Clinical Findings

Characteristically, a thriving infant 3–12 months of age suddenly develops periodic abdominal pain with screaming and drawing up of the knees. Vomiting occurs soon afterward (90% of cases), and bloody bowel movements with mucus appear within the next 12 hours (50%). Severe prostration and fever supervene, and the abdomen is tender and becomes distended. On palpation, a sausage-shaped tumor may be found in the early stages. In rare cases, the onset may be painless or with diarrhea. Some patients show signs of altered consciousness, particularly lethargy between spasms of pain, or may have seizures.

The intussusception can persist for several days when obstruction is not complete, and such cases may present as separate attacks of enterocolitis. In older children, sudden attacks of abdominal pain may be related to chronic recurrent intussusception with spontaneous reduction.

Treatment

A. Conservative Measures: A barium enema is both diagnostic and therapeutic. It is a safe procedure in experienced hands if the following recommendations are observed:

1. No attempt should be made at hydrostatic reduction if there are signs of strangulated bowel, perforation, or severe toxicity.

2. The barium solution should be allowed to drip by gravity through a Foley bag catheter inserted in the rectum from a height not more than 1 meter (3½ feet) above the fluoroscopy table.

3. There should be no manipulation of the abdomen during hydrostatic reduction under fluoroscopic examination, because this may increase intraluminal pressure and thus the risk of perforation.

4. Upon reduction, there should be free reflux of barium into the ileum; this is better elicited in a postevacuation film, which should be repeated in 24 hours.

B. Surgical Measures: For patients not suitable for hydrostatic reduction or in whom it is unsuccessful (25%), surgery is required. This has the advantages of demonstrating any lead point (such as Meckel's diverticulum) and of a lower recurrence rate.

Prognosis

Intussusception is almost uniformly fatal if untreated. The prognosis relates to the duration of the intussusception before reduction. The mortality rate with treatment is 1–2%. The patient should be observed carefully in hospital after hydrostatic reduction because intussusception recurs in 3–4% of patients, usually within 24 hours after reduction.

Bruce J et al: Intussusception: Evolution of current management. *J Pediatr Gastroenterol Nutr* 1987;**6**:663.

Singer J: Altered consciousness as an early manifestation of intussusception. *Pediatrics* 1979;**64**:93.

FOREIGN BODIES IN THE ALIMENTARY TRACT

Most foreign bodies pass through the esophagus and the rest of the gastrointestinal tract without difficulty, although anything longer than 3–5 cm may have difficulty passing the duodenal loop at the region of the ligament of Treitz. Foreign bodies lodged in the esophagus for more than 3 hours require removal. Smooth foreign bodies in the stomach, such as buttons or coins, may be watched without attempting removal for up to several months if the child is free of symptoms. The use of balanced electrolyte lavage solutions containing polyethylene glycol (Golytely) may help the passage of small, smooth foreign bodies lodged in the stomach or intestine. Failure to pass after several weeks suggests the possibility of gastric outlet obstruction. Straight pins, screws, and nails generally pass without incident. Removal of open safety pins or wooden toothpicks is recommended. Camera batteries that contain 45% potassium hydroxide are hazardous and should be removed endoscopically if present in the esophagus or in the stomach after 24 hours.

If a foreign body remains in the small bowel for longer than 5 days, surgical removal should be considered, especially if symptoms occur. Esophagogastroscopy will permit the removal of the majority of foreign bodies lodged in the esophagus and stomach. A Foley catheter introduced into the esophagus may obviate the need for endoscopy, especially for removal of coins.

Bloom RR et al: Foreign bodies of the gastrointestinal tract. *Am Surg* 1986;**52**:618.

Campbell JB, Foley LC: A safe alternative to endoscopic removal of blunt esophageal foreign bodies. *Arch Otolaryngol* 1983;**109**:323.

Litovitz TL: Battery ingestions: Product accessibility and clinical course. *Pediatrics* 1985;**75**:469.

TRAUMATIC INJURIES OF THE GASTROINTESTINAL TRACT (See Chapter 8.)

ANAL FISSURE

Anal fissure consists of a slitlike tear in the anal canal, usually secondary to the passage of large, hard, dry fecal masses. Anal stenosis and trauma can be contributory factors, as can a crypt abscess following gastroenteritis.

The infant or child cries with defecation and will try to hold back stools. Sparse, bright red bleeding is seen on the outside of the stool or on the toilet tissue following defecation. The fissure can often be seen if the patient is held in a knee-chest position and the buttocks spread apart.

When a fissure cannot be identified, it is essential to rule out other causes of rectal bleeding. If there is no history of constipation, the physician should consider juvenile polyp, perianal inflammation (due to group A streptococcal infection), or inflammatory bowel disease.

Anal fissures should be treated promptly, especially in infancy, to break the constipation-fissure-retention-constipation cycle. A stool softener should be given and is usually effective against constipation. The introduction of a gloved, lubricated finger twice daily lessens sphincter spasm. Warm sitz baths after defecation may be helpful. In rare cases, silver nitrate cauterization or surgery is indicated.

INGUINAL HERNIA

A peritoneal sac precedes the testicle as it descends from the genital ridge to the scrotum. The lower portion of this sac envelops the testis to form the tunica vaginalis, and the remainder normally atrophies by the time of birth. Persistence of the processus vaginalis presents as a mass in the inguinal region when an abdominal structure or peritoneal fluid is forced into it. The persistent sac may be very short or may extend into the scrotum. In some cases, peritoneal fluid may become trapped in the tunica vaginalis of the testis (noncommunicating hydrocele). If the processus vaginalis remains open, peritoneal fluid or an abdominal structure may be forced into it (indirect inguinal hernia).

Most inguinal hernias are of the indirect type and occur much more frequently in boys than in girls (9:1). Hernias may be present at birth or may appear at any age thereafter. The incidence in premature infants is close to 5%. In those weighing 1000 g or less, inguinal hernia is reported in 30%. In this weight group, girls are more commonly affected than boys.

Clinical Findings

There are no symptoms associated with an empty hernial sac. In most cases, the hernia is a painless inguinal swelling varying in size. There may be a history of inguinal fullness associated with coughing or long periods of standing; or there may be a firm, globular, and tender swelling, sometimes associated with vomiting and abdominal distention.

Spontaneous reduction frequently occurs while sleeping or with mild external pressure. In some instances, a herniated loop of intestine may become partially obstructed, leading to pain, irritability, and incomplete intestinal obstruction. More rarely, the loop of bowel becomes incarcerated, and signs of complete intestinal obstruction are present. Gangrene of the testis may occur; in the female, the ovary may prolapse into the hernial sac.

Inspection of the 2 inguinal areas may reveal a characteristic bulging or mass. Infants should be observed for evidence of swelling after crying and older children after bearing down.

A suggestive history is often the only criterion for diagnosis, along with the "silk glove" feel of the rubbing together of the 2 walls of the empty hernial sac.

Differential Diagnosis

An inguinal mass may represent lymph nodes. They are usually multiple and more discrete. Hydrocele of the cord transilluminates. An undescended testis may be moved along the canal and is associated with absence of the testicle in the scrotum.

Treatment

Surgery is indicated. There is still controversy about exploring the opposite side. Herniography is helpful in determining the patency of the processus vaginalis, but patency does not necessarily lead to a hernia.

Incarcerated inguinal hernias occur most often in the first 10 months of life and are more common in girls than in boys. Manipulative reduction can be attempted after placing the sedated infant in the Trendelenburg position with an ice bag on the affected side. This is contraindicated if the incarcerated hernia has been present for more than 12 hours or if bloody stools are noted.

McGregor DB et al: The unilateral pediatric inguinal hernia: Should the contralateral side be explored? *J Pediatr Surg* 1980;**15**:313.

Viidik T, Marshall DG: Direct inguinal hernias in infancy and early childhood. *J Pediatr Surg* 1980;**15**:646.

UMBILICAL HERNIA

Umbilical hernias are more common in premature than in full-term infants. This defect is also more common in black infants.

Excessive thinning of the skin distended by the hernia and progressive enlargement of the fascial defects are rarely reported unless there is increased intra-abdominal pressure due to organomegaly or ascites. Incarceration is the only dangerous problem and is limited to smaller hernias.

Most umbilical hernias regress spontaneously if the fascial defect has a diameter of less than 1 cm. Large defects may still disappear without treatment, but seldom before school age. Large defects and smaller hernias persisting up to school age should be treated surgically. Reducing the hernia and strapping the skin do not accelerate the healing process.

Hale DE et al: Umbilical hernia: What happens after age 5 years. *J Pediatr* 1981;**98**:415.

TUMORS OF THE GASTROINTESTINAL TRACT

1. JUVENILE POLYPS

Juvenile polyps are nearly always pedunculated and solitary, with a stalk covered in part by colonic mucosa. The head of the polyp is composed of hyperplastic glandular and vascular elements, often with cystic transformation. These polyps are benign, and 80% occur in the rectosigmoid.

Rarely, there are many polyps present in the colon, causing anemia, diarrhea, and protein loss. There are a few cases of generalized juvenile polyposis involving the stomach and the small and large bowel. These cases are associated with a slightly increased risk of cancer.

Juvenile polyps are rare before age 1, and their incidence is highest between 3 and 5 years of age. They are rare after age 15 because of autoamputation. They are more frequent in boys. Small amounts of bright red blood on the stools, intermittent melena, and occult, painless gastrointestinal bleeding with anemia in otherwise well children are the most frequent manifestations. Abdominal pain is infrequent, but a juvenile polyp can be the lead point for an intussusception. Low-lying polyps may prolapse during defecation.

Flexible fiberoptic colonoscopy is both diagnostic and therapeutic when polyps are suspected. After removal of the polyp by electrocautery, nothing further should be done if histologic findings confirm the diagnosis of juvenile polyp. There is a very slight risk of developing further juvenile polyps.

Erbe RW: Inherited gastrointestinal polyposis syndromes. *N Engl J Med* 1976;**294**:1101.

Haggitt RC, Reid BJ: Hereditary polyposis syndromes. *Am J Surg Pathol* 1986;**10**:871.

2. OTHER POLYPOSIS SYNDROMES (See Table 20–4.)

3. CANCER OF THE SMALL & LARGE INTESTINES

The most common small bowel cancer in children is lymphosarcoma. Intermittent abdominal pain, abdominal mass, intussusception, or a celiaclike picture may be present. Long-term survivals are reported in patients without lymph node involvement at surgery.

Carcinoid tumors of the appendix in children are not aggressive, regardless of the degree of invasion. However, carcinoid tumors of the ileum may metastasize.

Adenocarcinoma of the colon is rare in the pediatric age group. The transverse colon and rectosigmoid are the 2 most commonly affected sites. The low 5-year survival relates to the nonspecificity of presenting complaints and the large percentage of undifferentiated types. Children with a family history of cancer and chronic ulcerative colitis or familial poly-

Table 20–4. Gastrointestinal polyposis syndromes.

	Location	Number	Histology	Extraintestinal Findings	Malignant Potential
Juvenile polyps	Colon	Usually single; rarely multiple	Hyperplastic, hamartomatous	None	None (single) Slight (multiple)
Familial polyposis	Colon; less commonly, stomach and small bowel	Multiple	Adenomatous	None	Very common
Peutz-Jeghers syndrome	Small bowel, stomach, colon	Multiple	Hamartomatous	Pigmented cutaneous and oral macules; ovarian cysts and tumors; bony exostoses	2–3%
Gardner's syndrome	Colon; less commonly, stomach and small bowel	Multiple	Adenomatous	Cysts, tumors, and desmoids of skin and bone; other tumors	Very common
Cronkhite-Canada syndrome	Stomach, colon; less commonly, esophagus and small bowel	Multiple	Hamartomatous	Alopecia; onychodystrophy; hyperpigmentation	Rare
Turcot syndrome	Colon	Multiple	Adenomatous	Thyroid and brain tumors	Possible

posis are at greater risk but seldom develop cancer before age 15.

Aiges HW et al: Adenocarcinoma of the colon in an adolescent with the family cancer syndrome. *J Pediatr* 1979;**94**:632.

Collins RH et al: Colon cancer, dysplasia and surveillance in patients with ulcerative colitis: A critical review. *N Engl J Med* 1987;**316**:1654.

Gray GM et al: Lymphomas involving the gastrointestinal tract. *Gastroenterology* 1982;**82**:143.

4. MESENTERIC CYSTS

These rare tumors may be small or large, single or multiloculated. Invariably thin-walled, they contain either serous, chylous, or hemorrhagic fluid. They are commonly located in the mesentery of the small intestine but may also be seen in the mesocolon.

Most mesenteric cysts are asymptomatic. Traction on the mesentery eventually leads to colicky abdominal pain, which can be mild and recurrent but may present acutely with vomiting. Volvulus is reported, as is hemorrhage into the cyst. A rounded mass can occasionally be palpated or can be seen on x-ray film to displace adjacent intestine. Abdominal ultrasonography is usually diagnostic.

Surgical removal is indicated.

Christensen JA et al: Mesenteric cysts. *Am Surg* 1975; **41**:352.

5. INTESTINAL HEMANGIOMA

Hemangiomas of the bowel may be a source of acute or chronic blood loss and anemia. They may also cause intestinal obstruction by triggering intussusception, by local stricture, or by intramural hematoma formation. Thrombocytopenia and con-

sumptive coagulopathy are occasional systemic complications. Some lesions are telangiectasias (Rendu-Osler-Weber syndrome), and others are capillary hemangiomas. However, the largest group consists of cavernous hemangiomas, which are large, thin-walled vessels arising from the submucosal vascular plexus. They may protrude into the lumen as polypoid lesions or may invade the intestine from mucosa to serosa.

Abrahamson J, Shandling B: Intestinal hemangiomata in childhood and a syndrome for diagnosis: A collective review. *J Pediatr Surg* 1973;**8**:487.

Mestre JR, Andres JM: Hereditary hemorrhagic telangiectasia causing hematemesis in an infant. *J Pediatr* 1982;**101**:577.

ACUTE INFECTIOUS DIARRHEA (Gastroenteritis)

General Considerations

Acute gastroenteritis (AGE) is one of the most common pediatric illnesses and causes great morbidity and mortality in undeveloped countries. Although bacteria (primarily *Shigella, Salmonella,* and *Campylobacter*—see Chapter 28) and parasites (*Entamoeba histolytica*—see Chapter 29) may be etiologic, rotavirus and other viruses (enteric adenovirus, Norwalk-like agents, calicivirus) cause most infections. They are generally hardy agents and are easily spread by fecal-oral transmission. Outbreaks are common; winter rotavirus epidemics and outbreaks in day-care centers and hospitals are well known. See Table 20–5.

Management of most cases of AGE consists of first excluding nonviral causes by clinical assessment and simple laboratory tests, followed by careful rehydration. (See Chapter 36.) In presumed viral AGE, specific etiologic diagnosis is usually unnecessary. Infants, especially those under 6 months old,

Table 20–5. Causes, characteristics, and treatment of acute enteritis.

Cause	Stool Exam	Symptoms	Treatment
Bacterial			
Salmonella	Liquid, foul, positive for white blood cells, positive for gross or occult blood	Fever, abdominal pain	None unless signs of extra-intestinal infection or sepsis; ampicillin, amoxicillin, trimetho-prim-sulfamethoxazole.
Shigella	Small, grossly bloody, frequent	Fever, tenesmus, abdominal pain	None or trimethoprim-sulfamethoxazole.
Campylobacter jejuni	Gross blood and mucus in streaks	Few systemic symptoms	None or erythromycin.
Yersinia enterocolitica	Similar to Salmonella	Similar to Salmonella	None effective for enteric disease.
Aeromonas hydrophila	Watery; mild to moderate	Nausea, vomiting; probably enterotoxin-mediated	Usually self-limited; trimethoprim-sulfamethoxazole.
Plesiomonas shigelloides	Watery	Nausea, vomiting; possible enterotoxin	Usually self-limited; trimethoprim-sulfamethoxazole.
Escherichia coli			
Invasive	Small, grossly bloody, positive for white blood cells	Abdominal pain, tenesmus	Trimethoprim-sulfamethoxazole; ampicillin; gentamycin.
Enterotoxic	Liquid, green, voluminous	Nausea, vomiting; heat labile toxin-mediated	Usually self-limited.
Enteropathogenic	Liquid, green, voluminous	Nausea, vomiting; adherence factors important	Usually self-limited.
Hemorrhagic serotype 0157:H7	Small, grossly bloody, positive for white blood cells	Fever, tenesmus; organism produces shigella-type toxin; may cause hemolytic-uremic syndrome	Trimethoprim-sulfamethoxazole.
Viral			
Rotavirus	Liquid, few white blood cells	Vomiting, nausea	None; fluid management.
Others: Norwalk, enteric adenovirus, enteroviruses	Same as above	As above	None; fluid management.
Parasitic			
Giardia lamblia	Very foul, liquid, negative for blood, negative for white blood cells, Cysts present in 30–60%	Vomiting, nausea, abdominal distension, gas	Furazolidone (5 mg/kg/d for 7 days), metronidazole (15 mg/kg/d for 5 days), quinacrine (6 mg/kg/d for 5 days).
Entamoeba histolytica	Blood and mucus, trophozoites on fresh stool exam	Abdominal pain, tenesmus	Metronidazole (35–50 mg/kg/d for 10 days).
Cryptosporidium	Watery or bloody, depending upon site of infestation	Incidence often in immunodeficient patients but occasionally in healthy children; history of animal exposure	Spiramycin or metronidazole may be tried.
Other toxic diarrheas			
E coli (see above)			
Clostridium difficile	Bloody, positive for white blood cells, cytotoxin present in stool	Abdominal pain, fever; history of prior antibiotic use is typical	Vancomycin (30–40 mg/kg/d for 7 days); metronidazole (25 mg/kg/d for 7 days); oral bacitracin (1,500 u/kg/d for 7 days).
Staphylococcus aureus	Explosive, watery, positive for white blood cells	Nausea, vomiting, history of group outbreaks	Fluid management.
Clostridium perfringens	Explosive, watery, positive for white blood cells	Vomiting; abrupt onset; history of meat ingestion	Fluid management.

are at most risk of severe dehydration and secondary complications.

Clinical Findings

A. History: Although there may have been contacts with others who have gastroenteritis, there usually is no particular exposure to animals, travel, or foods. The incubation period for rotavirus infection is 2–4 days.

B. Symptoms and Signs: Most symptoms derive from the degree of dehydration (see Chapter 36). Fever is variable. Rash and other findings are notably absent in most viral AGE. Occasionally, there is transient abdominal distention due to ileus or dysmotility. The vomiting is initially (and usually remains) nonbloody and nonbilious. Grossly bloody stools are rare.

C. Laboratory Findings: The leukocyte count is variable; marked elevation or left-shift is unusual for viral AGE. Electrolytes reflect the degree of dehydration and bicarbonate loss in the stools. Metabolic acidosis may be due to fecal bicarbonate loss, ketoacidosis from starvation, and lactic acidosis from hypovolemia. Measurement of stool electrolytes is usually unnecessary unless the diarrhea appears to be secretory.

Stool should be tested during the initial evaluation for blood and leukocytes. If positive for either, culture for enteric bacterial pathogens is indicated; examination for ameba may also be done. If neither leukocytes nor blood is present, further testing is not usually needed.

If an etiologic diagnosis is needed for patient isolation, public health requirements, or prolonged or unusual illness, the stool may be tested for rotavirus antigen by a number of commercial methods or by electron microscopy, which is more sensitive and makes diagnosis of other enteric viruses possible.

D. Imaging: X-ray films are rarely needed. A nonspecific gas pattern including air-fluid levels in both large and small bowel is expected.

Differential Diagnosis

Although a common problem, AGE is often a "waste basket" diagnosis for a number of disorders associated with vomiting, abdominal pain, or loose stools. High fever, febrile seizure, or change in mental status is typical of shigellosis. Significant abdominal tenderness or peritoneal signs suggest a more serious problem; a ruptured appendix in an infant is often misdiagnosed as AGE, as are intussusception, volvulus, pancreatitis, lower lobe pneumonia, meningitis, and urinary tract infection. Duration of vomiting longer than 24–48 hours or persistence of vomiting without diarrhea requires consideration of other causes. Elevated intracranial pressure, hepatitis, metabolic disorders (adrenal insufficiency, acidoses), and poisoning are a few possibilities.

Complications & Sequelae

Dehydration and electrolyte abnormalities (eg, severe hypernatremia with cerebral damage) are the most important acute complications; improper attention to nutrition results in most secondary problems. Intractable diarrhea of infancy may follow an AGE-like illness (see below). Inappropriate continuation of a clear-liquid diet, often due to poor medical instruction, may result in persistent, loose "starvation" stools and weight loss. Secondary lactase defi-

ciency is unusual with a brief episode of viral AGE (and most infants may be breast-fed during the illness without ill effect), but it may follow a prolonged bout. Loose, acid stools (pH < 5.5) that are positive for reducing substances are diagnostic of this complication; change to a sucrose- or glucose-based formula is curative. Occasionally, milk protein allergy follows AGE, and the persistent diarrhea responds only to an elemental formula. Small bowel colonization with enteric organisms may follow many intestinal insults, including AGE; this condition may produce a secretory diarrhea.

Systemic spread of enteric viruses that cause AGE essentially never occurs except in the case of the enteroviruses; these, however, are not major causes of dehydrating enteritis (see Chapter 27).

Therapy & Prevention

For management of fluid and electrolyte balance, including oral rehydration regimens, see Chapter 36.

When stooling has markedly diminished, half-strength formula is offered as tolerated for 24–48 hours; full-strength formula must then be given so that secondary caloric deprivation can be avoided. Constipating solids (rice cereal, bananas, carrots, applesauce—not apple juice, which is hyperosmolar) may be given to older infants when feeding resumes. Antidiarrheal agents (in particular, loperamide, which is now available over-the-counter) are usually unnecessary; those that block motility may be dangerous if used in inflammatory enteritis (such as shigellosis). Drugs with significant nonintestinal actions, such as diphenoxylate-atropine (Lomotil), may be fatal in young children. (See Chapter 30.)

Good hygiene reduces fecal-oral spread of these agents. Vaccines for rotavirus are being evaluated. Oral bovine antirotavirus gamma globulin is also being tested. There is no specific antiviral or oral therapy. Immunity is only partial, and repeated attacks may occur.

Guerrant RL, Lohr JA, Williams EK: Acute infectious diarrhea. 1. Epidemiology, etiology, and pathogenesis. *Pediatr Infect Dis J* 1986;**5**:353.

Williams EK, Lohr JA, Guerrant RL: Acute infectious diarrhea. 2. Diagnosis, treatment, and prevention. *Pediatr Infect Dis J* 1986;**5**:455.

CHRONIC DIARRHEA*

Diarrhea may be defined as water and electrolyte malabsorption leading to accelerated excretion of intestinal contents. What constitutes diarrhea is sometimes difficult to define because there are wide vari-

---

*Epidemic diarrhea of the newborn is discussed in Chapter 4; diarrhea due to viral infections, in Chapter 27; diarrhea due to bacterial infections, in Chapter 28; and diarrhea due to parasitic infections, in Chapter 29.

ations in normal bowel habit. Some infants pass one firm stool every second to third day, whereas others may have 5–8 soft small stools daily. A gradual or sudden increase in the number of stools, a reduction in their consistency coupled with an increase in their fluid content (> 15 g/kg/d), and a tendency for the stools to be green are more important factors.

Diarrhea may result from any of the following closely related pathogenetic mechanisms: (1) interruption of normal cell transport processes; (2) decrease in the surface area available for absorption, which may be due to shortening of the bowel or mucosal disease; (3) increase in intestinal motility; (4) presence in the intestine of large amounts of unabsorbable osmotically active molecules; and (5) abnormal increase in gastric or intestinal permeability, leading to increased secretion of water and electrolytes.

The physiologic consequences of diarrhea vary with its severity and duration, the age of the patient and state of nutrition prior to onset, and the presence or absence of associated symptoms. Acute diarrhea may lead to dehydration and acid-base disturbances (see Chapter 36), whereas chronic diarrhea is more likely to be associated with malnutrition as a consequence of malabsorption or insufficient intake of nutrients.

The differential diagnosis of chronic diarrhea is lengthy. Table 20–6 lists some disease categories and specific conditions in which diarrhea is a prominent feature.

Causes of Diarrhea Other Than Infectious

A. Antibiotic Therapy: Antibiotic therapy may be associated with diarrhea. Some antibiotics actually decrease carbohydrate transport and intestinal lactase levels. Eradication of normal gut flora and

Table 20–6. Guide to differential diagnosis of chronic diarrhea.

Disease	Age	Type of Diarrhea	Associated Features
Bacterial infections	Any age	Mucoid, bloody stool with polymorphonuclear leukocytes.	Rarely chronic except in immunocompromised hosts; *Salmonella* and *Yersinia* most likely.
Viral infections	Any age	Watery.	Rarely chronic except in immunocompromised hosts; cytomegalovirus, adenovirus, rotavirus.
Parasitic infestations	Any age	Depends on organism.	*Amoeba, Giardia, Cryptosporidium.*
Dietary factors Overfeeding (especially starches)	< 6 m	Watery.	Colicky behavior without weight loss.
Protein allergy	< 2 m	Watery with or without malabsorption of fat; at times, blood and mucus.	Colic, vomiting (anemia, hypoproteinemia).
Acrodermatitis enteropathica	< 12 m	Voluminous with steatorrhea.	Malnutrition, skin rash; low serum zinc; usually genetic; sometimes secondary to severe dietary zinc deficiency.
Primary bile acid malabsorption	< 1 m	Voluminous with steatorrhea.	Malnutrition; defective ileal transport of bile acids.
Irritable colon/chronic, nonspecific diarrhea	6–36 m	Watery, frequent, with mucus, undigested food; no steatorrhea.	Healthy child; often starts with bout of gastroenteritis.
Toxic diarrhea (Antibiotics, cancer chemotherapy, radiation)	Any age	Loose; sometimes steatorrhea, with occult blood or pus.	Vomiting; anorexia.
Functional tumors (Neuroblastoma, carcinoid, pancreatic cholera, Zollinger-Ellison syndrome)	Any age	Secretory diarrhea, watery; persists when patient fasts.	Hypokalemia; other symptoms depend upon tumor.
Carbohydrate malabsorption Congenital deficiencies			
Sucrase-isomaltase	< 6 m	Watery; low pH; reducing substance-positive after acid hydrolysis; volume varies with sucrose intake.	Abdominal distension; poor growth; deficiency present in 0.8% of North Americans, 10% of Alaskan natives.
Glucose-galactose malabsorption	< 1 m	Intractable diarrhea with feeding; stool pH low; watery; reducing substances present.	Poor growth; defect in glucose transport.
Genetic deficiencies Lactase	> 4 y	Watery diarrhea with lactose; low pH; reducing substances present.	Deficiency develops in 100% of Asians, 80% of American blacks, 15% of American whites.

Table 20–6 (cont'd). Guide to differential diagnosis of chronic diarrhea.

Disease	Age	Type of Diarrhea	Associated Features
Acquired deficiencies			
Lactase and sucrase	Any age	Watery; low pH; reducing substances present.	Follows intestinal injury or infection.
Monosaccharide intolerance	< 6 m	Watery; low pH; reducing substances present.	Rare; follows infection; made worse by malnutrition.
Pancreatic disorders			
Cystic fibrosis	< 6 m	Steatorrhea; bulky, foul, pale.	Respiratory infection; poor weight gain.
Shwachman syndrome	< 2 y	Steatorrhea; bulky, foul, pale.	Neutropenia; short stature; bacterial infections; metaphyseal dysostosis.
Chronic pancreatitis	Any age	Steatorrhea; bulky, foul, pale.	Rare in children; usually associated with alcoholism.
Celiac disease	> 12 m	Steatorrhea; bulky, foul, pale.	Vomiting, distention, irritability, anorexia.
Intestinal lymphangiectasia	3 m	Voluminous: steatorrhea.	Lymphedema, lymphopenia, hypoalbuminemia.
Immune defects			
Hypogammaglobulinemia; IgA deficiency	Any age	Watery; sometimes steatorrhea.	Recurrent cutaneous and respiratory infection.
Combined immunodeficiency	< 1 m	Severe; watery.	Stomatitis, skin rash, recurrent infection, opportunistic infection.
HIV infection	Any age	Steatorrhea.	
Defective cellular immunity	< 2 y		
Genetic-metabolic disorders			
Chloride-losing diarrhea	< 1 m	Watery.	Alkalosis; growth failure.
abeta- and hypobetalipoproteinemia	< 3 m	Profuse; steatorrhea.	Progressive neurologic symptoms; low serum cholesterol; acanthocytosis.
Wolman's disease	< 1 m	Profuse; steatorrhea.	Vomiting; severe growth failure; adrenal calcification; hypercholesterolemia.
Folate malabsorption	< 1 m	Watery.	Anemia, stomatitis, seizures, retardation.
Anatomic abnormalities			
Blind (stagnant) loop/bacterial overgrowth	Any age	Watery; fat and carbohydrate malabsorption.	Caused by surgical adhesions, intestinal duplication, abnormal gastrointestinal motility, partial obstruction.
Short bowel	Any age	Watery; malabsorption of all nutrients.	Rarely congenital; usually secondary to surgical resection.
Intestinal pseudo-obstruction	Any age	Watery; malabsorption of all nutrients.	Distention; May be acquired or congenital; diarrhea secondary to bacterial overgrowth.
Inflammatory bowel disease			
Crohn's disease	Usually > 10 y	Loose with or without steatorrhea.	Pain, fever, abdominal mass, growth failure; joint pain, perianal disease.
Ulcerative colitis	Usually > 10 y	Bloody stools with polymorphonuclear leukocytes.	Tenesmus, anemia, abdominal pain, fever, joint pain; less severe growth failure.
Eosinophilic gastroenteritis	Any age	Watery or bloody, depending upon site of disease.	Intestinal or gastric obstruction, eczema, asthma.
Hirschsprung's disease with enterocolitis	< 1 y	Foul, liquid with white and red blood cells.	Abdominal distention, fever, history of constipation.
Malnutrition	< 1 y	Loose, steatorrhea; sometimes with carbohydrate malabsorption.	Becomes temporarily worse with refeeding.
Endocrine disorders			
Hyperthyroidism	Any age	Frequent, loose stool without malabsorption.	Other signs of hyperthyroidism.

overgrowth of other organisms may cause diarrhea. Of particular importance is *Clostridium difficile,* whose toxin causes pseudomembranous colitis.

B. Parenteral Infections: Infections of the urinary tract and upper respiratory tract (especially otitis media) are at times associated with diarrhea. The actual mechanism remains obscure. In the opinion of several investigators, a concomitant intestinal infection is likely.

C. Malnutrition: Malnutrition may predispose the child to diarrhea because of an increased occurrence of enteral infections, decreased bile acid synthesis, decreased disaccharidase activity, altered motility, or changes in the intestinal flora.

D. Diet: Overfeeding may cause diarrhea, especially in young infants. Some foods seem particularly prone to cause diarrhea in young infants, including fruit juices (because of the infant's relative inability to absorb fructose), eggs, and tomatoes. Intestinal irritants (spices and foods high in roughage) are also frequent offenders.

E. Allergic Diarrhea: Diarrhea caused by gastrointestinal allergy to dietary proteins is a frequently entertained diagnosis but a poorly documented clinical entity except in cases of milk sensitivity (discussed separately).

F. Chronic, Nonspecific Diarrhea: Chronic, nonspecific diarrhea, sometimes called irritable colon syndrome, is the most common type of diarrhea in well and thriving children. The typical patient is a child 6–20 months of age who was a colicky baby and who has 3–6 loose, mucoid stools per day during the waking hours. The child is active, looks healthy, has a good appetite, and is growing normally. The diarrhea worsens with a low-residue, low-fat, or high-carbohydrate diet and during periods of stress and infection. It clears spontaneously at about 3½ years of age (usually coincident with toilet training). No organic disease is discoverable. The pathogenesis of the condition is obscure. Possible causes include abnormalities of bile acid absorption in the terminal ileum, incomplete carbohydrate absorption (excessive fruit juice ingestion seems to worsen the condition), and abnormal motor function. A high familial incidence of functional bowel disease is observed. Stool tests for blood, fat, parasites, and ova are negative.

The following measures are helpful: institution of a high-fat, low-carbohydrate, high-fiber diet; avoidance of between-meal snacks; and avoidance of chilled fluids, especially fruit juices. It may be helpful to give loperamide (Imodium), 0.1–0.2 mg/kg/d in 2–3 divided doses; cholestyramine (Questran), 2–4 g with breakfast; or psyllium agents, 1–2 tsp twice daily.

Greene HL, Ghishan FK: Excessive fluid intake as a cause of chronic diarrhea in young children. *J Pediatr* 1983; **102**:836.

Hyams JS et al: Carbohydrate malabsorption following fruit juice ingestion in young children. *Pediatrics* 1988; **82**:64.

Jonas A, Diver-Haber A: Stool output and composition in the chronic non-specific diarrhoea syndrome. *Arch Dis Child* 1982;**57**:35.

Lloyd-Still JD: Chronic diarrhoea of childhood and the misuse of elimination diets. *J Pediatr* 1979;**95**:10.

THE MALABSORPTION SYNDROMES

Intestinal absorption is affected by the length of the small bowel and the amount of available absorptive surface area. Anatomic abnormalities and impaired motility of the small intestine interfere with normal propulsive movements and mixing of food with pancreatic and biliary secretions. Anaerobic bacteria proliferate under these conditions and impair fat absorption by deconjugation of bile acids. Impaired intestinal lymphatic or venous drainage and mucosal dysfunction secondary to hypoxia also cause malabsorption, as can diseases interfering with pancreatic exocrine function and with the production and flow of biliary secretions. Other causes include disaccharidase deficiency, glucose-galactose malabsorption, abetalipoproteinemia, malnutrition, endocrine conditions, immune deficiencies, celiac disease, and cystic fibrosis.

Clinical Findings

Gastrointestinal symptoms such as diarrhea, vomiting, anorexia, abdominal pain, and bloating are not always present, and the presenting complaints may not refer to the gastrointestinal tract. Certain physical features such as potbelly and wasted buttocks may indicate celiac disease. Personal observation of the stools for abnormal color, consistency, bulkiness, odor, mucus, and blood is important. Microscopic examination of stools for neutral and split fat (fatty acids) is helpful because most malabsorption syndromes involve some fat malabsorption.

The following are the most helpful investigations:

A. Fat Absorption: Qualitative or quantitative (72-hour) fecal fat excretion, serum carotene, and prothrombin time.

B. Protein Absorption or Abnormal Protein Loss: Serum protein electrophoresis and fecal excretion of α_1-antitrypsin.

C. Carbohydrate Absorption: Stool pH and reducing substances, breath hydrogen analysis after carbohydrate ingestion, and disaccharidase levels in intestinal mucosa.

D. Absorption of Folic Acid and Vitamin B$_{12}$: Schilling test and serum folic acid and vitamin B$_{12}$.

E. Bacteriology and Parasitology: Culture and microscopic examination of stool and duodenal juice.

F. Imaging: Upper gastrointestinal series with

small bowel follow-through, barium enema, and bone age.

G. Sweat Test: Chloride determination.

H. Pancreatic Exocrine Function: Examination of duodenal aspirate (volume, viscosity, pH, and bicarbonate, trypsin, lipase, and amylase activity) and bentiromide excretion test.

I. Liver Function Tests: Bilirubin, transaminases, alkaline phosphatase, and prothrombin time.

J. Miscellaneous: Peroral small bowel biopsy, D-xylose absorption, rectosigmoidoscopy and rectal biopsy, immunoglobulin levels, lipoprotein electrophoresis, urine catecholamines, and endocrine function tests.

Differential Diagnosis

The pathophysiologic classification set forth in Table 20–7 may be helpful in view of the considerable variety of disorders giving rise to malabsorption.

Treatment & Prognosis

See specific syndromes (celiac disease, disaccharidase deficiency, etc).

Anderson CM: Malabsorption in children. *Clin Gastroenterol* 1977;**6**:355.

Friedman HI, Nylund B: Intestinal fat digestion, absorption, and transport: A review. *Am J Clin Nutr* 1980; **33**:1108.

Table 20–7. Malabsorption syndromes.

Intraluminal phase abnormalities	**Intestinal phase abnormalities (cont'd)**
Acid hypersecretion; Zollinger-Ellison syndrome	Circulatory disturbances
Gastric resection	Cirrhosis
Exocrine pancreatic insufficiency	Congestive heart failure
Cystic fibrosis	Abnormal structure of gastrointestinal tract
Chronic pancreatitis	Dumping syndrome after gastrectomy
Pancreatic pseudocysts	Malrotation
Shwachman syndrome	Stenosis of jejunum or ileum
Enterokinase deficiency	Small bowel resection; short bowel syndrome
Lipase and colipase deficiency	Polyposis
Malnutrition	Selective inborn absorptive defects
Decreased conjugated bile acids	Congenital malabsorption of folic acid
Liver production and excretion	Selective malabsorption of vitamin B_{12}
Neonatal hepatitis	Cystinuria, methionine malabsorption
Biliary atresia: intrahepatic and extrahepatic	Hartnup disease, blue diaper syndrome
Acute and chronic active hepatitis	Glucose-galactose malabsorption
Disease of the biliary tract	Primary disaccharidase deficiency
Cirrhosis	Acrodermatitis enteropathica
Fat malabsorption in the premature infant	Abetalipoproteinemia
Intestinal malabsorption of bile acids	Congenital chlorioorrhea
Short bowel syndrome	Primary hypomagnesemia
Bacterial overgrowth	Hereditary fructose intolerance
Blind loop	Familial hypophosphatemic rickets
Fistula	Endocrine diseases
Strictures, regional enteritis	Diabetes
Scleroderma, intestinal pseudo-obstruction	Addison's disease
Intestinal phase abnormalities	Hyperthyroidism
Mucosal diseases	Hypoparathyroidism, pseudohypoparathyroidism
Infection, bacterial or viral	Neuroblastoma, ganglioneuroma
Infestations	**Delivery phase defects**
Giardia lamblia	Whipple's disease
Fish tapeworm	Intestinal lymphangiectasis
Hookworm	Congestive heart failure
Malnutrition	Regional enteritis with lymphangiectasis
Marasmus	Lymphoma
Kwashiorkor	Abetalipoproteinemia
Derermatitis herpetiformis	**Miscellaneous**
Folic acid deficiency	Renal insufficiency
Drugs: methotrexate, antibiotics	Carcinoid, mastocytosis
Crohn's disease	Immunity defects
Cow's milk and soy protein intolerance	Familial dysautonomia
Secondary disaccharidase deficiency	Collagen disease
Secondary monosaccharide intolerance	Wolman's disease
Hirschsprung's disease with enterocolitis	Histiocytosis X
Tropical sprue	
Celiac disease	
Radiation enteritis	
Lymphoma	

CONSTIPATION

Constipation is the regular passage of firm or hard stools or the infrequent passage of stool. In the presence of fecal impaction, there may be encopresis (involuntary fecal soiling). Familial, cultural, and social factors influence the genesis, development, and course. Psychologic factors, toilet-training techniques, and diet (particularly excessive milk intake and low-residue diets) may also influence bowel habits. Neurologic (spinal cord lesions) and anatomic (anorectal) disorders, hypothyroidism, and hypercalcemia, are all well-known causes of constipation.

Clinical Findings

Many symptoms, such as fever, convulsions, nervousness, school failure, bad breath, and the like have been improperly attributed to constipation. Normal infants often appear to have difficulty passing a stool. The child's face may turn red and the legs are drawn up on the abdomen even when the stool passed is soft. This pattern may be erroneously viewed as constipation. Similarly, the infant 6–12 months of age may become flushed, draw up the legs, and act as though struggling to pass stool, when in fact the infant is attempting to withhold stool. Failure to appreciate this normal developmental pattern may lead to the unwise use of laxatives or enemas. As children become ambulatory, many new and exciting activities interfere with the response to the "call to stool"; they may pass enough stool to relieve rectal distention while continuing to play, or they may gradually develop the ability to ignore the sensation of rectal fullness. In older children, school, games, social events, and the inadequate privacy and hygiene of school toilets may all interfere

with regular defecation. Fecal retention may lead to impaction of the rectum, with involuntary fecal leakage. Leakage generally stops when impaction is relieved. Occasionally, fecal incontinence is a sign of primary emotional disturbance, especially if no impaction is present.

Differential Diagnosis

Constipation is prevalent among mentally retarded children with associated motor deficits and in those with hypothyroidism. Causes of constipation are listed in Table 20–8.

Distinguishing features from Hirschsprung's disease are summarized in Table 20–9. Rare cases of short-segment aganglionosis may present with symptoms and signs suggestive of chronic constipation.

Treatment

A reduction of milk intake and increase of high-residue foods such as bran, whole wheat, fruits, and vegetables are sometimes sufficient in cases of mild constipation. The use of a barley malt extract such as Maltsupex, 1–2 tsp added to feedings 2 or 3 times daily, is helpful in small infants. Stool softeners such as dioctyl sodium sulfosuccinate (Colace), 5–10 mg/kg/d, prevent excessive drying of the stool and are effective unless there is voluntary stool retention. Cathartics such as standardized extract of senna fruit (Senokot syrup), 1–2 tsp twice daily depending on age, can be used for short periods of time.

If encopresis is present, treatment should start with relieving fecal impaction. Following this step, an effective stool softener should be given in amounts sufficient to induce 3–4 loose stools per day (2–5 mL/kg/d of mineral oil in 2 doses). After sev-

Table 20–8. Causes of constipation.[1]

Functional or retentive causes	Abnormalities of myenteric ganglion cells
Dietary causes	Hirschsprung's disease
Undernutrition, dehydration	Hypo- and hyperganglionosis
Excessive milk intake	Recklinghausen's disease
Lack of bulk	Multiple endocrine neoplasia type IIB
Drug and cathartic abuse	Absence of abdominal musculature
Structural defects of gastrointestinal tract	Spinal cord defects
Anus and rectum	Metabolic and endocrine disorders
Fissure, hemorrhoids, abscess	Hypothyroidism
Anterior location of anus	Hyperparathyroidism
Anal and rectal stenosis	Renal tubular acidosis
Presacral teratoma	Diabetes insipidus (dehydration)
Rectal prolapse	Vitamin D intoxication, hypercalcemia
Small bowel and colon	Idiopathic hypercalcemia
Tumor, stricture	Neurologic and psychiatric conditions
Chronic volvulus	Myotonic dystrophy
Intussusception	Amyotonia congenita
Internal hernia	Brain tumors
Smooth muscle diseases of gastrointestinal tract	Mental retardation
Scleroderma and dermatomyositis	Psychosis
Systemic lupus erythematosus	
Chronic intestinal pseudo-obstruction	

[1]Modified and reproduced, with permission, from Silverman A, Roy CC: *Pediatric Clinical Gastroenterology*, 3rd ed. Mosby, 1983.

Table 20–9. Differentiation of retentive constipation and Hirschsprung's disease.

	Retentive Constipation	Hirschsprung's Disease
Onset	2–3 years	At birth
Abdominal distention	Rare	Present
Nutrition/growth	Normal	Poor
Soiling	Intermittent or constant	Never
Rectal examination	Ampulla full	Ampulla may be empty
Rectal biopsy	Ganglion cells present	Ganglion cells absent
Rectal manometry	Normal rectoanal reflex	Nonrelaxation of internal anal sphincter
Barium enema	Distended rectum	Narrow distal segment with proximal megacolon

eral weeks to months of regular loose stools, the dosage of mineral oil can be tapered and stopped. Mineral oil should not be given to nonambulatory infants, retarded children, or those with gastroesophageal reflux. Aspiration of mineral oil may cause severe lipid pneumonia.

The prevention of stool holding and the establishment of a regular soft bowel movement pattern are accomplished by "toileting" the child at regular times each day and by the daily administration of mineral oil over a period of several months in a reduced dosage. Recurrence of encopresis should be treated promptly with a short course of laxatives or enemas. A multiple vitamin is recommended while mineral oil is administered.

Psychiatric consultation may be indicated for patients with recurrent symptoms or overt, severe emotional disturbances.

Hatch TF: Encopresis and constipation in children. *Pediatr Clin North Am* 1988;**35**:257.

Olness K, McParland FA, Piper J: Biofeedback: A new modality in the management of children with fecal soiling. *J Pediatr* 1980;**96**:505.

Schmitt BD: Encopresis. *Prim Care* 1984;**11**:497.

GASTROINTESTINAL BLEEDING

Vomiting or rectal evacuation of blood is an alarming symptom. The history should provide detailed answers to the following questions:

(1) *Is it really blood and is it coming from the gastrointestinal tract?* A number of substances may simulate hematochezia or melena; therefore, the presence of blood should be confirmed chemically. Information concerning genitourinary problems, coughing, or epistaxis may identify a source of bleeding elsewhere than in the gastrointestinal tract.

(2) *How much blood is there and what is its color and character?* Table 20–10 lists the sites of gastrointestinal bleeding in relationship to the amount and the appearance of the blood in the stools. Tables 20–11 and 20–12 list clinical causes of hematemesis and rectal bleeding.

(3) *Is the child acutely or chronically ill?* The physical examination should be thorough no matter how ill the patient is. Alertness to signs of portal hypertension, intestinal obstruction, or blood dyscrasia is particularly important. The nasal passages should be inspected for signs of recent epistaxis; the vagina for menstrual blood; and the anus for fissures and hemorrhoids.

A systolic blood pressure below 100 mm Hg and a pulse rate above 100/min in an older child suggest at least a 20% reduction of blood volume. A pulse rate increase of 20/min or a drop in systolic blood pressure greater than 10 mm Hg when the patient sits up is also a sensitive index of significant volume depletion.

(4) *Is the child still bleeding?* A determination of vital signs every 15 minutes is essential to assess ongoing bleeding. Serial hematocrits are useful; remember, however, that plasma expansion subsequent to a loss of red cell mass may be delayed for hours or days.

The most important maneuver for the assessment of the origin and severity of gastrointestinal bleeding is the introduction of a naso-gastric tube in the stomach. Detection of blood in the gastric aspirate confirms a bleeding site proximal to the ligament of Treitz. However, its absence does not rule out the duodenum as the source.

Management

A hemorrhagic diathesis should be ruled out, and

Table 20–10. Identification of sites of gastrointestinal bleeding.

Symptom or Sign	Location of Bleeding Lesion
Effortless welling forth of bright red blood from the mouth	Nasopharyngeal or oral lesions; esophageal varices; lacerations of esophageal or gastric mucosa (Mallory-Weiss syndrome).
Vomiting of bright red blood or of "coffee grounds"	Lesion proximal to ligament of Treitz.
Melena	Lesion proximal to ligament of Treitz. Blood loss in excess of 50–100 mL/24 h.
Bright red or dark red blood in stools	Lesion in the ileum or colon. (Massive upper gastrointestinal bleeding may also be associated with bright red blood in stool.)
Streak of blood on outside of a stool	Lesion in the rectal ampulla or anal canal.

Table 20–11. Causes of hematemesis in infants and children.[1]

Entity	Age	Amount of Blood	Clinical Features	Cause
Swallowed maternal blood	Newborn	Variable	No other signs of illness; Apt test shows alkaline denaturation of blood.	Blood swallowed at delivery or during nursing.
Stress ulcer	Any age	Large	Sickliness; pallor; shock.	Central nervous system disease, sepsis, asphyxia, burns.
Hemorrhagic gastritis	Newborn	Large	Sickliness; pallor; shock.	Central nervous system disease, sepsis, asphyxia.
Hemorrhagic disease of newborn	Newborn to 2 months	Variable	Melena, bleeding elsewhere.	Vitamin K deficiency, liver disease, clotting defect.
Gastric volvulus	Newborn, infancy	Small	Intractable vomiting.	Congenital defect, eventration of diaphragm.
Peptic disease	Any age	Variable	Relatively good health, vomiting, pain.	Duodenal or antral ulcer.
Esophageal varices	Any age	Large	May have signs of liver disease.	Portal hypertension secondary to liver disease or portal obstruction.
Esophagitis	Any age	Small	Dysphagia, chronic vomiting.	Peptic; infection (in immunocompromised hosts).
Foreign body	Infancy to later childhood	Small	Dysphagia.	Trauma.
Gastric outlet obstruction	Any age	Small	Vomiting, failure to thrive.	Gastric or esophageal ulcer or mucosal tear.
Erosive gastritis or esophagitis	Any age	Small	Vomiting, pain, dysphagia.	Ingestion of acids, alkali, iron, aspirin.
Gastritis	Any age	Small	Protracted vomiting.	Infection, bile reflux, ingestion.
Mallory-Weiss syndrome	Preschool to adolescence	Moderate to large	Retching, vomiting.	Increased intraesophageal pressure and mucosal tear.
Swallowed blood	Any age	Moderate to large	Nausea, epistaxis.	Bleeding from mouth, gums, ears, nose, or throat.

[1]Modified and reproduced, with permission, from Silverman A, Roy CC: *Pediatric Clinical Gastroenterology*, 3rd ed. Mosby, 1983.

vitamin K should be given intravenously. In severe bleeding, needs for volume replacement are monitored by measurement of central venous pressure. In less severe cases, vital signs, serial hematocrits, and gastric aspirates are sufficient.

If blood is recovered from the gastric aspirate, gastric lavage with saline should be performed for 30–60 minutes, until only a blood-tinged return is obtained. Panendoscopy is then done to identify the bleeding site. Endoscopy is superior to barium contrast study for lesions such as esophageal varices, stress ulcers, and gastritis. Colonoscopy may identify the source of bright red rectal bleeding and should be performed if plain x-ray films show no signs of intestinal obstruction.

Nonobstructing small or large bowel lesions that bleed briskly (> 0.5 mL/min) may be localized by angiography or radionuclide scanning following injection of labeled red cells.

Persistent vascular bleeding (varices, vascular anomalies) may be temporarily relieved using vasopressin (20 units/1.73 m² intravenously over a 20-minute period). Thereafter it may be necessary to sustain the infusion for 24 hours at a rate of 0.2–0.4 units/1.73 m²/min. It is rarely necessary to use a pediatric Sengstaken-Blakemore tube in cases of bleeding esophageal varices. Sclerotherapy of the varices is the treatment of choice.

The challenging patients are those with cirrhosis and abnormal coagulation. Emergency shunt operations are at times inevitable. Surgical treatment is also warranted in peptic disease and stress ulcers when severe ongoing bleeding continues over several days despite conservative management.

Hyams JS, Leichtner AM, Schwartz AN: Recent advances in diagnosis and treatment of gastrointestinal hemorrhage in infants and children. *J Pediatr* 1985;**106**:1.

McKusick KA et al: 99mTc red blood cells for detection of gastrointestinal bleeding. *AJR* 1981;**137**:1113.

Roy CC, Morin CL, Weber AM: Gastrointestinal emergency problems in paediatric practice. *Clin Gastroenterol* 1981;**10**:225.

RECURRENT ABDOMINAL PAIN

About 10% of unselected school children experience at least 3 attacks of recurrent abdominal pain severe enough to affect their activities. An organic

Table 20–12. Differential diagnosis of rectal bleeding in infants and children.

Cause	Usual Age Group	Additional Complaints	Amount of Blood	Color of Blood
Swallowed foreign body	Any age	Rarely, perforation and abscess	Usually small	Melena
Systemic bleeding	Any age	Other evidence of bleeding	Variable	Dark or bright
Hemorrhagic disease of the newborn	Newborn	Other evidence of bleeding	Variable	Dark or bright
Milk intolerance	Infants	Colicky abdominal pain, diarrhea	Moderate to large	Dark or bright; usually with diarrhea
Esophageal varices	> 4 years	Signs of portal hypertension	Variable	Usually dark; bright with massive bleed
Hemangioma or familial telangiectasia	Any age	Telangiectasia elsewhere	Variable	Dark or bright
Peptic ulcer, gastritis	Any age	Abdominal pain	Usually small; can be massive	Dark
Duplication of bowel	Any age	Pain, obstruction, mass	Usually small	Usually dark
Meckel's diverticulum	Any age; rare under 2 months	Anemia, painless bleeding	Small to large; usually large	Maroon
Volvulus	Infant or young child	Abdominal pain, intestinal obstruction	Small to large	Dark or bright
Intussusception	< 18 months	Abdominal pain, mass	Small to large	Dark or bright with "currant jelly" mucus
Ulcerative colitis	> 4 years	Diarrhea, cramps	Small to large	Usually bright, with diarrhea
Bacterial enteritis	Any age	Diarrhea, cramps	Small to large	Usually bright, with diarrhea
Juvenile polyp	2–8 years	None	Small to large	Bright, with normal stool
Inserted foreign body	Child	Pain	Small	Bright with mucus
Anal fissure or proctitis	< 2 years	Pain with defecation	Small	Bright with mucus
Swallowed maternal blood	Newborn	None	Variable	Dark
Esophagitis	Any age	Dysphagia, hematemesis	Usually small	Dark
Schönlein-Henoch purpura	3–10 years	Purpuric rash, arthritis, abdominal pain, hematuria	Variable	Dark or bright
Lymphoid nodular hyperplasia	3–24 months	Loose stools	Small	Bright

cause can be found in fewer than 10% of cases, and there is usually evidence that the pain is a reaction to emotional stress. The age at onset is usually between 5 and 10 years.

Clinical Findings

A. Symptoms and Signs: Attacks of abdominal pain are characteristically of variable duration and intensity. Although the pain is usually located in the periumbilical area, location far from the umbilicus does not rule out recurrent abdominal pain. Nighttime occurrence is not uncommon. Weight loss rarely occurs. Pain may be associated with dramatic reactions; patients may clutch the abdomen, double over, or even throw themselves to the ground. School attendance may suffer. Indeed, reluctance to attend school (school phobia) may be an important

etiologic factor. The pain may be associated with pallor, nausea, vomiting, and slight temperature elevation.

The pain usually bears little relationship to bowel habits and activity, although constipation is present in some. At times, pain may occur during meals or before the child leaves for school. A definite precipitating or particularly stressful situation in the child's life at the time the pains began can sometimes be elicited. A history of functional gastrointestinal complaints is often found in family members.

A thorough physical examination is essential and is usually negative in these children. Abdominal tenderness, if present, is diffuse and mild, although discomfort over the descending colon is common.

B. Laboratory Findings: Complete blood count, sedimentation rate, urinalysis, and stool test for occult blood usually suffice. If the pain is atypical, further testing suggested by symptoms should be done.

Differential Diagnosis

Organic causes relating to the urinary and gastrointestinal tracts, as well as extra-abdominal causes (Table 20–3), should be ruled out by appropriate studies. Oxyuriasis, "mesenteric lymphadenitis," and "chronic appendicitis" are improbable causes of recurrent abdominal pain. Milk intolerance due to lactose intolerance usually manifests itself by both pain and diarrhea. However, abdominal discomfort may at times be the only symptom. Abdominal migraine and abdominal epilepsy are truly rare conditions.

Treatment & Prognosis

Treatment consists of reassurance based on a thorough physical appraisal and a sympathetic explanation of the functional nature of the complaint. Therapy for emotional problems is sometimes required, but drugs should be avoided. The prognosis is good.

Appley J: *The Child With Abdominal Pain,* 2nd ed. Blackwell, 1975.
Liebman WM: Recurrent abdominal pain in children: A retrospective survey of 119 patients. *Clin Pediatr* 1978;**17**:149.
Silverman A, Roy CC: Psychophysiologic recurrent abdominal pain. Pages 418–430 in: *Pediatric Clinical Gastroenterology,* 3rd ed. Mosby, 1983.

PROTEIN-LOSING ENTEROPATHIES

Excessive loss of plasma proteins into the gastrointestinal tract occurs in association with a number of disorders, some of which are listed below.

Disorders Associated With Protein-Losing Enteropathy

A. Vascular Obstruction: Congestive heart failure, constrictive pericarditis, atrial septal defect, primary myocardial disease, increased right atrial pressure.

B. Gastric: Giant hypertrophic gastritis (Ménétrier's disease), polyps.

C. Small Intestine: Celiac disease, intestinal lymphangiectasia, regional enteritis, Whipple's disease, lymphosarcoma, acute gastrointestinal infection, allergic gastroenteropathy, blind loop syndrome, abetalipoproteinemia, chronic mucosal ischemia (eg, from chronic volvulus or radiation enteritis). teritis).

D. Colon: Ulcerative colitis, Hirschsprung's disease, polyposis syndromes, villous adenoma, solitary rectal ulcer.

E. Other: Immunologic deficiency states.

Clinical Findings

The signs and symptoms include edema, chylous ascites, poor weight gain, deficiencies of fat-soluble vitamins, and anemia. Serum albumin is usually less than 2.5 g/dL.

Differential Diagnosis

Hypoalbuminemia may be due to an increased catabolic rate or may be associated with poor protein intake, impaired hepatic protein synthesis, mechanical or functional obstruction of lymph flow, or congenital malformations of lymphatics outside the gastrointestinal tract. It is especially important to rule out malnutrition and to make certain that no significant proteinuria is present. Lymphangiography is useful after age 2 years.

Treatment

Temporary benefits can be derived from albumin infusions in conjunction with diuretics. Treatment must be directed toward the primary underlying cause.

Magazzu G et al: Reliability and usefulness of random fecal alpha-1-antitrypsin concentration: Further simplification of the method. *J Pediatr Gastroenterol Nutr* 1985;**4**:402.
Thomas DW et al: Random fecal alpha-1-antitrypsin concentration in children with gastrointestinal disease. *Gastroenterology* 1981;**80**:776.

CELIAC DISEASE
(Gluten Enteropathy)

Essentials of Diagnosis

- Diarrhea and steatorrhea.
- Failure to thrive; loss of weight involving mostly the limbs and buttocks.
- Abdominal distention.
- Depressed D-xylose absorption.
- Villous atrophy on small bowel biopsy.
- Improvement on gluten-free diet, and histologic relapse following reintroduction of gluten into the diet.
- Normal pancreatic and biliary secretions.

General Considerations

Celiac disease results from intestinal sensitivity to the gliadin fraction of gluten from wheat, rye, barley, and oats. Most cases present during the second year of life, but the age at onset and the severity are both variable. The disease is more common in Europe and in Canada than in the USA and is uncommon in blacks and Asians.

The underlying pathologic process is not yet clearly understood, but it is thought that the intestinal lesion is the result of a cell-mediated immune response in individuals susceptible to gluten—or, more specifically, to gliadin, the alcohol-soluble fraction of gluten. A positive family history is not unusual. Ten percent of first-degree relatives may be affected. The inheritance is probably polygenic, but some have postulated that it results from a single gene in combination with an environmental precipitant such as intestinal adenovirus infection. The adenovirus shares some chemical homology with gliadin.

Clinical Findings

A. Symptoms and Signs:

1. Diarrhea—Affected children present with a history of digestive disturbances starting at 6–12 months of age—the age at which wheat, rye, or oat glutens are first fed. Initially, the diarrhea may be intermittent and related to upper respiratory tract infections. Subsequently, it is continuous, with voluminous, bulky, pale, frothy, greasy, offensive floating stools. During celiac crises, dehydration, shock, and acidosis are commonly seen. Diarrhea is absent in 10% of cases.

2. Constipation, vomiting, and abdominal pain—This triad of symptoms may in a small number of cases dominate the clinical picture and suggest a diagnosis of intestinal obstruction. Constipation generally results from a combination of anorexia, dehydration, muscle weakness, and very thick, fatty stools.

3. Failure to thrive—The onset of diarrhea is usually accompanied by loss of appetite, failure to gain weight, and increased irritability.

4. Wasting and retardation of growth—In established cases, there is a loss of weight, which is most marked in the limbs and buttocks. The face remains plump, and the abdomen becomes distended secondary to poor musculature and accumulation of gas and fluid in the hypotonic intestinal tract with altered peristaltic activity. Growth failure may dominate the clinical picture.

5. Anemia and vitamin deficiencies—Anemia usually responds to iron and is rarely megaloblastic. Deficiencies in fat-soluble vitamins are common. Rickets can be seen when growth has not been completely halted by the disease; however, osteomalacia is more common, and pathologic fractures may occur. Hypoprothrombinemia can be severe, and some patients are known to present with severe intestinal hemorrhages.

B. Laboratory Findings:

1. Fat content of stools—A 3-day collection of stools usually reveals fecal fat levels over 4.5 g/d. However, steatorrhea may be absent in 10–25% of cases. A normal child will excrete 5–10% of ingested fats. The untreated celiac patient, on the other hand, will excrete an excess of 15% of daily fat intake.

2. Impaired carbohydrate absorption—A low oral glucose tolerance curve is seen. Absorption of D-xylose is impaired, with blood levels lower than 20 mg/dL 60 minutes after ingestion.

3. Hypoproteinemia—Hypoalbuminemia can be severe enough to lead to edema. There is evidence of increased protein loss in the gut lumen and poor hepatic synthesis secondary to malnutrition.

C. Imaging: A small bowel series shows a malabsorptive pattern characterized by segmentation, clumping of the barium column, and hypersecretion. These changes are nonspecific, and x-ray films of the small bowel should therefore be taken to rule out structural defects that might cause malabsorption. (See Table 20–7).

D. Biopsy Findings: Peroral intestinal biopsy provides the only reliable evidence for the diagnosis of celiac disease. It is a safe and simple procedure even in infants.

Under the dissecting microscope, the jejunal mucosa lacks the slender, fingerlike projections that characterize normal villi. Under the light microscope, the celiac mucosa is readily recognized by shortened or absent villi, by lengthening of the crypts of Lieberkühn, and by increased round cell infiltration of the lamina propria. Normal to nearly normal appearance of the lamina propria can be expected after withdrawal of gluten from the diet.

E. Serologic Tests: Measurements of gliadin antibody and reticulin antibody may be useful screening tests. IgG antibodies to gliadin are present in 10% of normal children. IgA antibodies are more specific to celiac patients.

Differential Diagnosis

The differential diagnosis includes disorders that cause malabsorption. Strict adherence to 2 diagnostic criteria—ie, the characteristic small bowel microscopic changes and clinical improvement on a gluten-free diet—is essential. Whenever the mucosal lesion is not characteristic or the response to a gluten-free diet is not as good as expected, challenge with a gluten-containing diet is indicated. Biopsy should be performed as soon as the patient becomes symptomatic or after 6 months if the child remains healthy and is growing well on a normal diet.

Treatment

A. Diet: Treatment consists of dietary gluten restriction for life. Dietary supervision is essential. Initially, the diet (Table 20–13) should provide 25% more calories than calculated for expected weight. Lactose is poorly tolerated in the acute stage because the extensive mucosal damage leads to acquired disaccharidase deficiency. Normal amounts of fat are advisable. Supplemental vitamins and minerals are indicated in the acute phase.

In treating a severely affected child, the diet should be tailored to the child's appetite and capacity to absorb. A full gluten-free diet can usually be given after 2–3 weeks. Clinical improvement is usually evident within a week, and histologic repair is complete after 3–12 months.

Table 20–13. Gluten-free diet.[1]

Foods allowed
Milk, cream, and cheese
Eggs
Meat, fish, and poultry (unless breaded or creamed)
Vegetables
Bread made from rice, corn, soy, or gluten-free wheat starch
Cornflakes: cornmeal, puffed rice, or precooked gluten-free cereals
All clear soups
Fruit and fruit juices

Foods to be avoided
Bread, rolls, crackers, cakes, and cookies made from wheat or rye
Cereals, spaghetti, macaroni, and noodles made from wheat or rye
All canned soups except clear broth
Malt flavoring
Prepared mixes and puddings
Commercial candies containing cereal products
Malted milk, beer, ale, and some instant coffees

[1]All possible sources of wheat, rye, barley, and oats must be eliminated from the patient's diet.

B. Corticosteroids: Corticosteroids can hasten clinical improvement but are indicated only in very ill patients with signs and symptoms of celiac crisis.

Prognosis

Improvement and clinical recovery are the rule. However, disappearance of symptoms can be a protracted, intermittent process. Although good gastrointestinal tolerance for gluten may be eventually noted in a number of patients maintained on the gluten-free diet, most patients undergo a histologic relapse on reexposure. Malignant lymphoma of the small bowel is a long-term risk that is not averted by good dietary control.

Aurrichio S et al: Gluten-sensitive enteropathy in childhood. *Pediatr Clin North Am* 1988;**35**:157.
Burgin-Wolff A et al: A reliable screening test for childhood celiac disease: Fluorescent immunosorbent test for gliadin antibodies. *J Pediatr* 1983;**102**:655.
Cacciari E et al: Short stature and celiac disease: A relationship to consider even in patients with no gastrointestinal tract symptoms. *J Pediatr* 1983;**103**:708.
Cooper BT et al: Celiac disease and malignancy. *Medicine* 1980;**59**:249.

DISACCHARIDASE DEFICIENCY

Essentials of Diagnosis

- Watery diarrhea, explosive and frothy.
- Stool pH < 5.5.
- Reducing substances present in stools.
- Flat glucose tolerance test following disaccharide loading.
- A positive breath hydrogen test following an oral test dose of lactose or sucrose.

General Considerations

Carbohydrates account for a substantial proportion of the human diet. The polysaccharide starch and the disaccharides sucrose and lactose are quantitatively the most important and require hydrolysis by intestinal brush border disaccharidases before significant absorption can take place. Disaccharidase levels are higher in the jejunum and in the proximal ileum than in the distal ileum and duodenum. Some substrates can be hydrolyzed by more than one enzyme, and, conversely, some enzymes act on more than one substrate.

In primary disaccharidase deficiency, the enzyme deficit is isolated, the disaccharide intolerance is likely to persist, intestinal histologic findings are normal, and a family history is common.

Because disaccharidases are confined to the outer cell layer of the intestinal epithelium, they are very susceptible to mucosal damage. A number of conditions are now known to give rise to secondary disaccharidase deficiency, which is transient and involves decrease in all mucosal enzymes with lactase usually most severely depressed. Histologic examination reveals changes compatible with the underlying disorder. A familial incidence is uncommon.

Clinical Findings

A. Primary (Congenital):

1. Lactase deficiency—Congenital lactase deficiency is a rare condition leading to diarrhea after lactose is ingested. The stools are frothy and acid; their pH may fall below 4.5 owing to the presence of organic acids that stimulate peristalsis and hypersecretion. The osmotic action of unhydrolyzed lactose leads to catharsis. Vomiting is common. Severe malnutrition may occur. Reducing substances are usually present in the stools, and lactosuria may occur. Infants with lactosuria, aminoaciduria, proteinuria, acidosis, and elevated blood urea nitrogen have been described. An oral lactose tolerance test (2 g/kg) after dietary lactose has been withdrawn is likely to result in symptoms of intolerance within 8 hours; the blood glucose levels show no appreciable rise. A rise in breath hydrogen after oral administration of lactose is also diagnostic.

Patients respond to the exclusion of lactose from their diets.

2. Sucrase and isomaltase deficiency—This is a combined defect that is inherited as an autosomal recessive trait. Diarrhea usually occurs only when sucrose is fed. Abdominal distention, failure to thrive, and chronic diarrhea may be the presenting symptoms. Distaste for and avoidance of sucrose occurs even in young infants. Since sucrase-isomaltase deficiencies have been found in siblings who had few or no symptoms, it is likely that a number of persons with this trait—particularly adults—remain unrecognized.

Because sucrose is not a reducing sugar, the usual 5 drops of stool and 10 drops of water added to a Clinitest tablet will not give a positive reaction unless sucrose is hydrolyzed (1 N HC1 is substituted for the water and the mixture allowed to boil for a few seconds before adding the tablet). A sucrose tolerance test (2 g/kg) is likely to be flat. Breath hydrogen will be elevated after injestion of sucrose. Because many gastric and extraintestinal factors can account for very poor blood glucose rises, it is wise to check the stools for the presence of sucrose and to follow the sucrose tolerance test by the xylose absorption test. Shock may occur owing to osmotic water losses in some patients with lactase or sucrase-isomaltase deficiency with a standard dose of the disaccharide for the tolerance test. In sucrase-isomaltase deficiency, exclusion of sucrose is usually sufficient. Starch intolerance is rarely a problem, because the 1–6 linkages of starch hydrolyzed by isomaltase constitute only a small part of the molecule.

B. Secondary (Acquired):

1. Secondary lactase deficiency—Diarrhea may be produced in normal individuals if a large dose of lactose is ingested. The threshold for lactose tolerance is usually much lower than that for sucrose. There is a high prevalence of lactose intolerance in certain racial groups (70% in North American blacks and nearly 100% in Asian populations) after 3–5 years of age. Disaccharidase deficiency has been described in association with many disorders. Neomycin and kanamycin administration can reduce lactase activity in adults. Celiac disease, giardiasis, malnutrition, viral or bacterial gastroenteritis, abetalipoproteinemia, and immunoglobulin deficiencies, all can decrease intestinal lactase activity.

2. Secondary sucrase deficiency—Intestinal mucosal damage tends to lower the levels of all disaccharidases. Signs of sucrose intolerance are usually masked by the more striking symptoms related to lactose. Infectious diarrhea is the most frequent cause of secondary sucrose intolerance.

Treatment

A. Lactose-Free Diet: Many commercially available infant formulas are lactose-free. Foods containing whey, dry milk solids, and curds should be excluded. It is important to see if labels indicate any lactose content, particularly in canned puréed baby foods. Cheeses (cottage, cheddar, cream), ice cream, sherbet, yogurt, and chocolate milk powders contain variable amounts of lactose, small amounts of which may be well tolerated.

B. Sucrose-Restricted Diet: See Table 20–14.

Prognosis

Primary disaccharidase deficiency is a lifelong defect. However, in both lactase and sucrase deficiencies, tolerance for the disaccharide may increase with age. The prognosis in the secondary or acquired forms of disaccharidase deficiency is that of the underlying illness. Normal tolerance for lactose may not be regained for many months after an acute mucosal injury.

Barilas-Mury C, Solomons NW: Test-retest reproducibility of hydrogen breath test for lactose maldigestion in preschool children. *J Pediatr Gastroenterol Nutr* 1987; **6:**281.

Heitlinger LA, Lebenthal E: Disorders of carbohydrate digestion and absorption. *Pediatr Clin North Am* 1988; **35:**239.

Kilby A et al: Sucrase-isomaltase deficiency: A follow-up report. *Arch Dis Child* 1979;**53:**677.

Lebenthal E et al: Recurrent abdominal pain and lactose absorption in children. *Pediatrics* 1981;**67:**828.

Perman JA et al: Sucrose malabsorption in children: Noninvasive diagnosis by interval breath hydrogen determination. *J Pediatr* 1978;**93:**17.

GLUCOSE-GALACTOSE MALABSORPTION

Glucose malabsorption can also cause osmotic diarrhea. A decreased rate of tubular reabsorption of glucose is often associated with the intestinal cell transport defect.

In the congenital form of the disease, severe diarrhea begins within a few days after birth. Small bowel histologic findings are normal. Glycosuria and aminoaciduria may occur. The glucose tolerance test

Table 20–14. Sucrose restricted diet.[1]

Foods allowed
Milk, cream, butter, cheese, and salad and cooking oils
Eggs, meat, and fish
Potatoes
Asparagus, broccoli, brussels sprouts, cucumbers, spinach, tomatoes, and lettuce
Grapes, cherries, strawberries, cranberries, and blackberries
Homemade bread and pastries containing dextrose; homemade ice cream; and gelatin desserts
Diet carbonated beverages, diet Kool-Aid, unsweetened cocoa, and vegetable juices

Foods to be avoided
Fruits and vegetables not included in the above list, especially peas, beans, and lentils
Breakfast cereals
Commercial ice cream, pies, cookies, and cakes
Jam, honey, jelly, candy, molasses, and maple syrup
Kool-Aid and carbonated beverages
Medicines made up in syrup

[1]The diet described here does contain small amounts of sucrose that are usually well tolerated.

is flat. Fructose is well tolerated. The diarrhea promptly subsides on withdrawal of glucose and galactose from the diet. The stool pH is not as acid as that reported in disaccharidase deficiencies; fecal reducing substances are consistently found. The clinical features associated with acquired disease are the same as those seen with disaccharidase deficiency states. The acquired form is mainly seen in the perinatal period but is also described in older infants, usually following an acute viral or bacterial enteritis. Both disaccharides and monosaccharides, including fructose, are malabsorbed.

In the congenital form, total exclusion of glucose and galactose from the diet is mandatory. A satisfactory formula consists of fructose with a carbohydrate-free formula. The prognosis is good if the disease is diagnosed early, because tolerance for glucose and galactose improves with age. In the secondary form, prolonged parenteral nutrition may be required until intestinal transport mechanisms for monosaccharides return.

Fairclough PD et al: Absorption of glucose and maltose in congenital glucose-galactose malabsorption. *Pediatr Res* 1978;**12**:1112.

Klish WJ et al: Intestinal surface area in infants with acquired monosaccharide intolerance. *J Pediatr* 1978; **92**:566.

Nichols VN et al: Acquired monosaccharide intolerance in infants. *J Pediatr Gastroenterol Nutr* 1989;**8**:51.

INTESTINAL LYMPHANGIECTASIA

This form of protein-losing enteropathy results from a congenital abnormality of the lymphatic system and is often associated with lymphatic aberrations in the extremities. Obstruction to lymphatic drainage of the intestine leads to rupture of the intestinal lacteals with leakage of lymph into the lumen of the bowel. Fat loss may be significant and lead to steatorrhea. Chronic loss of lymphocytes and of immunoglobulins is usual and increases the susceptibility to infections.

Clinical Findings

Peripheral edema, diarrhea, abdominal distention, lymphedematous extremities, chylous effusions, and repeated infections are common. Laboratory findings are low serum albumin, decreased immunoglobulin levels, lymphocytopenia, and anemia. Serum calcium is frequently depressed, and stool fat may be elevated. Lymphocytes may be seen in large numbers on a stool smear. Fecal α_1-antitrypsin is elevated. X-ray studies reveal an edematous small bowel mucosal pattern, and biopsy reveals dilated lacteals in the villi and lamina propria. In certain cases where the disorder involves the submucosa, subserosa, mesentery, and omentum, the mucosal bi-opsy may be normal, and laparotomy is necessary to establish the diagnosis.

Differential Diagnosis

Other causes of protein-losing enteropathy must be considered, although an associated lymphedematous extremity strongly favors this diagnosis.

Treatment & Prognosis

Surgery is needed when the lesion is localized to a small area of the bowel or in cases of constrictive pericarditis or obstructing tumors. This may include placement of a LeVeen or Denver shunt or construction of a saphenous vein-peritoneal anastomosis in intractable cases.

A low-fat diet reduces lymph flow. Medium-chain triglycerides as a fat source are effective only in the mucosal type of lymphangiectasia. Water-soluble vitamin and calcium supplements should be given. Antibiotics are used for specific infections. Total parenteral nutrition is helpful on a temporary basis.

The prognosis at present is not favorable, although there may be remission with age.

Tift WL, Lloyd JK: Intestinal lymphangiectasia: Long-term results with MCT diet. *Arch Dis Child* 1975;**50**:269.

Vardy PA, Lebenthal E, Shwachman H: Intestinal lymphangiectasia: A reappraisal. *Pediatrics* 1975;**55**:842.

COW'S MILK PROTEIN INTOLERANCE

Milk intolerance is more common in males and in children with a family history of allergy. The estimated incidence is 0.5–1%. The gastrointestinal features vary in severity and last from 6 weeks to 12 months of age. In some patients, colic is present. In others, vomiting or diarrhea (or both) predominate. Occult or gross rectal bleeding is common, and colitis is present at sigmoidoscopy. Pneumatosis intestinalis may suggest necrotizing enterocolitis. Eosinophilic gastroenteritis with a protein-losing enteropathy characterized by hypoalbuminemia and hypogammaglobulinemia is less common. A celiaclike syndrome with villous atrophy and malabsorption can occur. Anaphylactic shock is a rare threat.

In most cases, milk protein elimination results in a rapid amelioration of symptoms. Patients with milk protein allergy have an increased incidence of sensitivity to soy protein, with similar symptoms. It is best to use a casein hydrolysate formula as an elimination diet to prove the diagnosis. A normal 1-hour blood xylose level 4–12 weeks after clinical recovery, with a drop below 25 mg/dL 4 days after reintroduction of cow's milk protein, has been shown to be a reliable means of diagnosis.

Patrick MK, Gall DG: Protein intolerance and immunocyte and enterocyte interaction. *Pediatr Clin North Am* 1988;**35**:17.

IMMUNOLOGIC DEFICIENCY STATES WITH DIARRHEA OR MALABSORPTION

Both cellular and humoral mechanisms are important for intestinal function; they prevent adherence and penetration of pathogens and regulate antigen absorption.

Diarrhea is a frequent finding in immunoglobulin deficiency states, but the cause is usually obscure. Standard pathogenic bacteria may not be found in the stools, but giardiasis is common. Fifty to 60% of patients with idiopathic acquired hypogammaglobulinemia have steatorrhea and intestinal villous atrophy. Lymphonodular hyperplasia is a common feature in this group of patients. Congenital or Bruton type agammaglobulinemics uniformly have diarrhea and abnormal intestinal morphology. Patients with isolated IgA deficiency may also present with chronic diarrhea, a celiaclike picture, lymphoid nodular hyperplasia, and giardiasis. Patients with isolated cellular immunity defects, combined cellular and humoral immune incompetence, and HIV infection may have severe chronic diarrhea leading to malnutrition. The cause of diarrhea may be recognized bacterial, viral, or parasitic pathogens, organisms usually considered nonpathogens (*Blastocystis hominis, Candida*), or unusual organisms (cytomegalovirus, *Cryptosporidium*). Often, the cause is not found. There is a high incidence of disaccharidase deficiency. Chronic granulomatous disease may be associated with intestinal symptoms suggestive of chronic inflammatory bowel disease. A rectal biopsy may reveal the presence of typical macrophages.

Treatment must be directed toward correction of the immunologic defect. Gluten-free diets have been disappointing in most cases with villous atrophy. Dramatic improvement may follow the eradication of giardiasis. In patients exhibiting disaccharidase deficiencies, dietary manipulations are helpful.

Frost SS: Gastrointestinal manifestations in AIDS patients. *Contemp Gastroenterol* 1988;**1**:29.

Ogra PL, Bienenstock J (editors): *The Mucosal Immune System in Health and Disease.* 81st Ross Conference on Pediatric Research. Columbus, Ohio, 1981.

INFLAMMATORY BOWEL DISEASE

Crohn's disease and ulcerative colitis are the 2 major idiopathic inflammatory bowel diseases of children. They share many features resulting from bowel inflammation, such as diarrhea, pain, fever, and blood loss, but they differ in important aspects, such as distribution of disease, histologic findings, incidence and type of extraintestinal symptoms, response to medications and surgery, and prognosis. A comparison of these 2 conditions is shown in Table 20–15. The cause is unknown but is probably a genetically determined immunologic response to an environmental antigenic trigger, possibly a virus or bacterium, which may cross-react with antigens in the gastrointestinal tract. There is no indication that diet or emotional factors are a primary cause of these diseases.

Differential Diagnosis

A. Crohn's Disease: When extraintestinal symptoms predominate, Crohn's disease can be mistaken for rheumatoid arthritis, systemic lupus erythematosus, or hypopituitarism. Frequently, the acute onset of ileocolitis is mistaken for acute appendicitis. Symptoms sometimes suggest celiac disease, peptic ulcer, intestinal obstruction, or intestinal lymphoma.

B. Ulcerative Colitis: In the acute stage, bacterial pathogens and toxins causing colitis must be ruled out. These include *Shigella, Salmonella, Yersinia, Campylobacter, Entamoeba histolytica,* invasive *Escherichia coli, Aeromonas hydrophila,* and toxin producers *E coli* serotype 0157:H7 and *Clostridium difficile.* Mild ulcerative colitis mimics irritable bowel symptoms. Connective tissue diseases must be considered. Crohn's disease of the colon is an important differential possibility.

Complications (See Table 20–15.)

A. Crohn's Disease: Intestinal obstruction, fistula, and abscess formation are frequent. Perforation and hemorrhage are rare. Malnutrition is caused by anorexia and compounded by malabsorption, protein-losing enteropathy, disaccharidase deficiency, and diarrhea induced by bile salts. Systemic complications include perianal disease, pyoderma gangrenosum, arthritis, amyloidosis, and growth retardation.

B. Ulcerative Colitis: Arthritis, uveitis, pyoderma gangrenosum, and malnutrition all occur. Growth failure and delayed puberty are less common than in Crohn's disease. Liver disease (chronic active hepatitis, sclerosing cholangitis) is more common. In patients with pancolitis, carcinoma of the colon occurs with an incidence of 1–2% per year after the first 10 years of disease. Cancer risk is a function of disease duration and not age of onset. Mortality with colon cancer is high, because the usual screening tests (occult blood in stool, pain, and abnormal x-ray findings) are less useful in colitis.

Treatment

Medical treatment for these conditions is similar and includes anti-inflammatory, antidiarrheal, and antibiotic medication. No medical therapy has proved uniformly effective.

A. Diet: A high-protein, high-carbohydrate diet with normal amounts of fat is recommended. Decreased amounts of roughage may help decrease symptoms in those with colitis or with partial intestinal obstruction. Lactose is poorly tolerated when

Table 20–15. Features of Crohn's disease and ulcerative colitis.[1]

	Crohn's Disease	Ulcerative Colitis
Age at onset	10–20 years	10–20 years
Incidence	4–6 per 100,000	3–15 per 100,000
Relative incidence in children	2	1
Area of bowel affected	Oropharynx, esophagus, and stomach, rare; small bowel only, 25–30%; colon and anus only, 25%; ileocolitis, 40%; diffuse disease, 5%.	total colon, 90%; proctitis, 10%.
Distribution	Segmental; disease-free skip areas common.	Continuous; distal to proximal.
Pathology	Full-thickness, acute, and chronic inflammation; noncaseating granulomas (50%), extraintestinal fistulas, abscesses, stricture, and fibrosis may be present.	Superficial, acute inflammation of mucosa with microscopic crypt abscess.
X-ray findings	Segmental lesions; thickened, circular folds, cobblestone appearance of bowel wall secondary to longitudinal ulcers and transverse fissures; fixation and separation of loops; narrowed lumen; "string sign"; fistulas.	Superficial colitis; loss of haustra; shortened colon and pseudopolyps (islands of normal tissue surrounded by denuded mucosa) are late findings.
Intestinal symptoms	Abdominal pain, diarrhea (usually loose with blood if colon involved) perianal disease, enteroenteric/enterocutaneous fistula, abscess, anorexia.	Abdominal pain, bloody diarrhea, urgency, and tenesmus.
Extraintestinal symptoms		
Arthritis/arthralgia	15%	9%
Fever	40–50%	40–50%
Stomatitis	9%	2%
Weight loss	90% (mean 5.7 kg.)	68% (mean 4.1 kg.)
Delayed growth and sexual development	30%	5–10%
Uveitis/conjunctivitis	15% (in Crohn's colitis)	4%
Sclerosing cholangitis	—	4%
Renal stones	6% (oxalate)	6% (urate)
Pyoderma gangrenosum	1.3%	5%
Erythema nodosum	8–15%	4%
Laboratory findings	High erythrocyte sedimentation rate; microcytic anemia; low serum iron and total iron-binding capacity; increased fecal protein loss; low serum albumin.	High erythrocyte sedimentation rate; microcytic anemia, high white blood cell count with "left shift."

[1]Source: Kirschner BS: Inflammatory bowel disease in children. *Pediatr Clin North Am* 1988;**35**:189.

disease is active. The main concern should be ensuring adequate caloric intake. Restrictive or "bland" diets are counterproductive because they usually result in poor intake. Vitamin and iron supplements are recommended. Zinc levels are often low in patients with Crohn's disease and should be repleted. Supplemental calories in the form of liquid diets are well tolerated. Total parenteral nutrition for periods of 4–6 weeks may not only improve the patients with severe malnutrition but may also induce a temporary remission of symptoms and stimulate linear growth and sexual development. Enteral administration of low-residue or elemental liquid diets may also be associated with rapid nutritional repletion and temporary remission of symptoms. Home programs of both enteral and parenteral nutritional support have been used in many patients with intractable symptoms or growth failure.

B. Sulfasalazine: This drug is effective in mild cases of ulcerative colitis and possibly in cases of Crohn's disease of the colon. It is recognized to prevent relapse of ulcerative colitis. The drug is not absorbed in the small intestine but is hydrolyzed by colon flora into sulfapyridine and 5-amino salicylate. The sulfa moiety is probably inactive but is responsible for the allergic side effects of the drug. The salicylate moiety probably has a local anti-inflammatory activity in the colon. Side effects are common, including skin rash, nausea, headache, and abdominal pain. More rarely, serum sickness, hemolytic anemia, aplastic anemia, and pancreatitis occur. Response to therapy may be slow.

Two to 3 grams per day in 3 divided doses are recommended for children over 10 or 50 mg/kg/d for those under 10. Half of this dose is used as a maintenance medication for well-controlled ulcerative colitis. Salicylate polymers for both oral and rectal instillation will soon be available. They are no more effective than sulfasalazine, but they have fewer side effects.

C. Corticosteroids: With more severe inflammatory bowel disease, corticosteroids are used.

1. Intravenous steroids—Methylprednisolone, 2 mg/kg/d, or hydrocortisone, 10 mg/kg/d, may be given for up to 10 days when disease is severe. Adrenocorticotropic hormone (ACTH) has more side effects and is no more effective.

2. Prednisone—Prednisone, 1–2 mg/kg/d orally in 2 or 3 divided doses, is given for 6–8 weeks, followed by a gradual tapering. Alternate-day steroids are associated with fewer side effects as the dosage of drug is tapered. There is no evidence that corticosteroids prevent relapses. Prednisone is often given in conjunction with sulfasalazine. The patient or the parents should be warned about the risk of varicella infection while on high-dose prednisone as well as the other numerous side effects of high-dose steroids.

Hydrocortisone in the form of enema or foam can be instilled into the rectum in patients with severe tenesmus or ulcerative proctitis.

D. Azathioprine (Imuran): Azathioprine, 1.5–2 mg/kg/d orally, is used only when a high maintenance dose of corticosteroids is necessary to keep the disease under control and there are serious risks of steroid-induced complications. The results of this therapy may be delayed weeks to months.

E. Metronidazole (Flagyl): This drug is now used routinely in Crohn's disease patients with perianal disease. Disease tends to recur when the drug is discontinued. It may also be effective in Crohn's disease of the colon. The dose of metronidazole is 15–30 mg/kg/d in 3 divided doses. Peripheral neuropathy may be a side effect with prolonged use.

F. Cyclosporine: There are scattered reports that this powerful immunosuppressant may be effective in severe inflammatory bowel disease.

G. Surgery:

1. Crohn's Disease—Crohn's disease is not cured by surgery. However, 70% of patients will eventually require surgery to relieve obstruction, drain abscess, relieve intractable symptoms, or encourage growth and sexual maturation. The relapse rate 6 years after surgery is 60%. The recurrence usually occurs at the site of anastomosis. The recurrence of disease in previously normal bowel is most likely to occur in the first 2 years after surgery. The rate of recurrence may be less in disease limited to the colon. Surgery performed for the alleviation of growth retardation must be performed before puberty.

2. Ulcerative colitis—Surgery is curative in this disease. It is reserved for those with uncontrolled hemorrhage, toxic megacolon, unrelenting pain and diarrhea, high-grade mucosal dysplasia, or malignant growths. There are now several surgical approaches (ileoanal anastomosis, Koch-type continent ileostomy) that allow a near normal life-style after colectomy. Liver disease may not be improved by the removal of the colon.

Prognosis

A. Crohn's Disease: Although the mortality rate is low (2% in the first 7 years), the morbidity is high. The disease is progressive in most cases, and its course is interspersed with both acute and chronic complications, leading to variable degrees of disability. Over 50% of patients experience symptoms that impose limits on the quality of their lives. About 20% have severe disabling disease, and 20% have so few symptoms that they describe themselves as healthy.

B. Ulcerative Colitis: The overall prognosis for ulcerative colitis is good. About 5% of patients present with toxic megacolon and require immediate surgery. Seventy-five percent will have a relapsing remitting course. Twenty-five to 40% of patients will require surgery, especially those with pancolitis, anemia, and hypoalbuminemia at the time of presentation.

Chong SKF et al: Histologic diagnosis of chronic inflammatory bowel disease in childhood. *Gut* 1985;**26**:55.

Greenstein AJ et al: The extraintestinal complications of Crohn's disease and chronic ulcerative colitis: A study of 700 patients. *Medicine* 1976;**55**:401.

Helzer JE et al: A study of the association between Crohn's disease and psychiatric illness. *Gastroenterology* 1984;**86**:324.

Kirschner BS: Inflammatory bowel disease in children. *Pediatr Clin North Am* 1988;**35**:189.

Telander RL, Perrault J: Total colectomy with rectal mucosectomy and ileo-anal anastomosis for chronic ulcerative colitis in children and young adults. *Mayo Clin Proc* 1980;**55**:420.

Wesson DE, Shandling B: Results of bowel resection for Crohn's disease in the young. *J Pediatr Surg* 1981;**16**:449.

SELECTED REFERENCES

Lebenthal E: *Textbook of Gastroenterology and Nutrition in Infancy.* Raven Press, 1981.

Lebenthal E (editor): Pediatric gastroenterology. (2 parts.) *Pediatr Clin North Am* 1988;**35**:1, 215.

Silverman A, Roy CC: *Pediatric Clinical Gastroenterology,* 3rd ed. Mosby, 1983.

Sleisenger MH, Fordtran JS: *Gastrointestinal Disease,* 3rd ed. Saunders, 1983.

Welch KJ et al (editors): *Pediatric Surgery,* 4th ed. Year Book, 1986.

Liver & Pancreas

21

Arnold Silverman, MD, & Ronald J. Sokol, MD

LIVER

PROLONGED NEONATAL CHOLESTATIC JAUNDICE

The main clinical features of the group of disorders causing prolonged neonatal cholestasis are (1) elevated direct-reacting bilirubin fraction (> 2 mg/dL or $> 20\%$ of total bilirubin) (2) elevated serum bile acids (> 10 micromol/L), (3) variably acholic stools, (4) dark urine, and (5) hepatomegaly.

Prolonged neonatal cholestasis may be due to intrahepatic or extrahepatic causes. Though many specific causes of intrahepatic cholestasis have been identified, a specific etiologic origin is found only in about 25% of cases. With rare exceptions, extrahepatic cholestasis is due to anatomic defects that occur without specific known cause.

Attention to specific clinical clues distinguishes these 2 major categories of jaundice in 85% of cases. Histologic examination of tissue obtained by percutaneous liver biopsy increases the accuracy of differentiation to over 95% (Table 21–1).

INTRAHEPATIC CHOLESTASIS

Intrahepatic cholestasis is characterized by patency of the extrahepatic biliary system, despite cholestasis, and abnormalities on liver function tests. A specific cause can be identified in about 25% of cases. Patency of the extrahepatic biliary tract can best be confirmed nonsurgically by hepatobiliary scintigraphy using ^{99m}Tc-diethyliminodiacetic acid (diethyl-IDA, DIDA) or ^{99m}Tc-*p*-isopropylacetanilidoiminodiacetic acid (PIPIDA). Radioactivity in the bowel within 4–14 hours is evidence of patency.

1. PERINATAL OR NEONATAL HEPATITIS DUE TO INFECTION

This diagnosis is justified in infants with jaundice, hepatomegaly, vomiting, lethargy, and other systemic signs if a perinatally acquired viral, bacterial, or protozoal infection can be established. Infection may occur by transplacental spread, via the ascend-

Table 21–1. Differentiating clinical and pathologic features of intra- and extrahepatic neonatal cholestasis.

	Intrahepatic	Extrahepatic
Clinical features	Preterm, small for gestational age, appears ill; hepatosplenomegaly, other organ or system involvement; incomplete cholestasis (stools with some color); associated cause identified (infections, metabolic, familial, etc).	Full-term, seems well, hepatomegaly (firm to hard), complete cholestasis (acholic stools), polysplenia syndrome, equal right and left hepatic lobes.
Pathologic features	Cholestasis, lobular disarray, giant cells, portal inflammation, minimal fibrosis, rare neoductular formation, steatosis, extramedullary hematopoiesis.	Cholestasis, neoductular proliferation, portal fibrosis, bile lakes, normal lobular architecture, rare giant cells.

ing route from vaginal or cervical structures into amniotic fluid; from swallowed contaminated products (maternal blood, urine) during delivery; or from breast milk, contaminated hands, etc. The infectious agents most apt to be associated with neonatal intrahepatic cholestasis include herpesvirus, varicella, coxsackievirus, cytomegalovirus, rubella virus, echoviruses, adenovirus, hepatitis B virus, *Treponema pallidum,* and *Toxoplasma gondii.* The degree of liver cell injury caused by these agents is variable, ranging from massive hepatic necrosis (herpesvirus) to focal necrosis and mild inflammation (cytomegalovirus, hepatitis B virus). Injury to critical hepatocyte organelles is usual, affecting bilirubin uptake, binding, conjugation, and excretion (mixed hyperbilirubinemia). Bile acids, ALT, AST, and alkaline phosphatase are elevated. The infant is jaundiced and generally appears ill.

Clinical Findings

A. Symptoms and Signs: Clinical symptoms usually appear in the first 2 weeks of life but may appear as late as 2–3 months. Jaundice may be noted in the first 24 hours or may develop later. Loss of appetite, poor sucking reflex, lethargy, and vomiting are frequent. Stools may be normal to pale in color but are seldom acholic. Dark urine stains the diaper. Hepatomegaly is present with a uniform, firm consistency. Splenomegaly is variable. Macular, papular, or petechial rashes may occur. In less severe cases, failure to thrive may be the major complaint. Unusual presentations include hypoproteinemia and anasarca (nonhemolytic hydrops) and hemorrhagic disease of the newborn.

B. Laboratory Findings: The blood count often shows neutropenia, thrombocytopenia, and signs of mild hemolysis. Mixed hyperbilirubinemia, elevated transaminases, prolongation of clotting studies, mild acidosis, and elevated cord serum IgM levels suggest congenital infection. Nasopharyngeal washings, urine, stool, and cerebrospinal fluid should be cultured for virus. Specific serologic tests may be useful (TORCH titers), as are long bone x-rays to determine the presence of "celery stalking" in the metaphyseal regions of the humeri, femurs, and tibias. When indicated, CT and MRI scans can be used to identify intracranial calcifications. DIDA scans show decreased hepatic clearance of the circulating isotope with excretion into the gut.

Histologic examination of liver biopsy tissue obtained by the percutaneous route is performed to distinguish intrahepatic from extrahepatic cholestasis rather than to identify a specific infectious agent within the liver tissue. Exceptions to this generalization include the finding of intracytoplasmic inclusions of cytomegalovirus in hepatocytes or bile duct epithelium cells and the finding of intranuclear acidophilic inclusions of herpesvirus. Variable degrees of lobular disarray characterized by focal necrosis, multinucleated giant cell transformation, and ballooned pale hepatocytes with loss of cordlike arrangement of liver cells are usual. Intrahepatocytic and canalicular cholestasis may be prominent. Portal changes are not striking, but modest neoductular proliferation and mild fibrosis may occur.

Differential Diagnosis

Great care must be taken to distinguish infectious causes of intrahepatic cholestasis from genetic or metabolic causes (inborn errors), because the clinical presentations are very similar. Galactosemia, congenital fructose intolerance, and tyrosinemia must be investigated promptly, because specific dietary therapy is available. Alpha-antitrypsin deficiency and cystic fibrosis must also be considered. Specific physical features may be helpful when considering Alagille or Zellweger syndromes.

Unless the bile ducts have spontaneously perforated, infants with extrahepatic cholestasis act well; stools are usually completely acholic, and the liver is enlarged and firm. Histologic findings are shown in Table 21–1.

Treatment

Most forms of viral neonatal hepatitis are treated symptomatically. Infants with herpesvirus may be treated with acyclovir. Fluids and adequate calories are encouraged. The consequences of cholestasis are treated as indicated (Table 21–2). Vitamin K orally or by injection, vitamins D and E orally, and calcium supplementation should be provided. Choleretics (cholestyramine, phenobarbital) are used if cholestasis persists. Corticosteroids are contraindicated. Penicillin for suspected syphilis or specific antibiotics for bacterial hepatitis need to be administered promptly. Infants born to women with hepatitis B should be given hepatitis B immune globulin immediately and subsequently immunized with hepatitis B virus vaccine, as outlined in Chapter 6.

Prognosis

Multiple organ involvement is commonly associated with neonatal infectious hepatitis and has a poor outcome. Death from hepatic or cardiac failure, intractable acidosis, or intracranial hemorrhage is seen, especially in herpesvirus or echovirus infection and occasionally in cytomegalovirus or rubella infection. Hepatitis B virus may cause fulminant neonatal viral hepatitis; however, most infected infants become asymptomatic carriers of hepatitis B. On the other hand, infants with transplacental diseases may recover completely or suffer sequelae, especially neurologic ones. Persistent liver disease results in mild chronic hepatitis, portal fibrosis, or cirrhosis. Chronic cholestasis may lead to dental enamel hypoplasia, biliary rickets, severe pruritus, and xanthoma.

Specific Infectious Agents

A. Neonatal Hepatitis Virus B Disease: Infection with hepatitis B (HB) virus may occur at any time during perinatal life, but the risk is higher when acute maternal disease occurs during the last trimester of pregnancy. However, most cases of neonatal disease are acquired from mothers who are asymptomatic carriers of hepatitis B. Hepatitis B virus has been found in most body fluids besides blood, including breast milk, but it does not seem to be present in feces. In chronic HBsAg carrier mothers, fetal and infant acquisition risk is greatest if the mother (1) is also HBeAg-positive and HBeAb-negative, (2) has detectable levels of serum-specific HB DNA polymerase, or (3) has high serum levels of HBcAb. These findings are markers of high infectivity; however, hepatitis B can be transmitted even if HBsAg is the only marker present.

**Nomenclature for Hepatitis B
Antigens and Antibodies**

HBsAg = Hepatitis B surface antigen
HBsAb = Hepatitis B surface antibody
HBeAg = Hepatitis B e antigen
HBeAb = Hepatitis B e antibody
HBcAb = Hepatitis B core antibody
HBcAb-IgM = Hepatitis B core antibody IgM
HBV-DNA = Hepatitis B virus DNA

Table 21–2. Treatment of complications of chronic liver disease.

Indication	Treatment	Dose	Toxicity
Intrahepatic cholestasis	Phenobarbital	3–10 mg/kg/d	Drowsiness, irritability, interference with vitamin D metabolism
	Cholestyramine/colestipol hydrochloride	250–500 mg/kg/d	Constipation, acidosis, binding of drugs, increased steatorrhea
Pruritis	Phenobarbital or cholestyramine/colestipol (or both)	Same as above	
	Antihistamines: Diphenhydramine hydrochloride Hydroxyzine	5–10 mg/kg/d 2–5 mg/kg/d	Drowsiness
	Ultraviolet light B	Exposure as needed	Skin Burn
	Carbamazepine	20–40 mg/kg/d	Hepatotoxicity, marrow suppression, fluid retention
Steatorrhea	Formula containing medium-chain triglycerides (eg, Pregestimil)	120–150 calories/kg/d for infants	Expensive
	Oil supplement containing medium-chain triglycerides	1–2 mL/kg/d	Diarrhea, Aspiration
Malabsorption of fat-soluble vitamins	Vitamin A	10,000–25,000 units/d	Hepatitis, pseudotumor cerebri, bone lesions
	Vitamin D	800–5000 units/d	Hypercalcemia, hypercalciuria
	25-hydroxycholecalciferol (vitamin D)	3–5 μg/kg/d	
	1,25-dihydroxycholecalciferol (vitamin D_3)	0.05–0.2 μg/kg/d	
	Vitamin E (oral)	25–200 IU/kg/d	Potentiation of vitamin K deficiency
	Vitamin E (intramuscular)	1–2 mg/kg/d	
	Vitamin K (oral)	2.5 mg twice per week to 5.0 mg per day	
	Vitamin K (intramuscular)	2–5 mg each 4 weeks	
Malabsorption of other nutrients	Multiple vitamin	1–2 times the standard dose	
	Calcium	25–100 mg/kg/d	Hypercalcemia, hypercalciuria
	Phosphorus	25–50 mg/kg/d	Gastrointestinal intolerance
	Zinc	1.0 mg/kg/d	Interference with copper absorption
Ascites[1]	Sodium restriction	1–2 meq/kg/d	
	Spironolactone	3–5 mg/kg/d (up to 10 mg)	Gynecomastia, hyperkalemia
	Furosemide	1–2 mg/kg/d	Hyponatremia, hypokalemia
	Intravenous albumin	1 g/kg/dose	
	Paracentesis		Hypotension
	Peritoneovenous (Le Veen) shunt		
Hepatic encephalopathy[1]	Protein restriction	0.5–1.0 g/kg/d	
	Intravenous glucose (10% dextrose)		
	Oral neomycin	2–4 gm/m² BSA in 4 doses	Renal toxicity
	Oral lactulose	1 mL/kg/dose each 4–6 hours	Diarrhea
	High branched-chain amino acid— enteral or parenteral supplements (unproved benefit)	0.5–1.0 g/kg/d	
	Plasmapheresis		
	Hemodialysis		
	Benzodiazepine antagonist (experimental)		

[1] In order of sequential management

Neonatal liver disease due to HB virus is extremely variable. Fulminant hepatic necrosis has rarely been reported, especially in association with intrapartum or postpartum transfusions of infected blood. However, it also can occur from maternally transmitted virus. In such cases, progressive jaundice, stupor, shrinking liver size, and coagulation abnormalities dominate the clinical picture. Respiratory and circulatory failure usually follow. Histologically, the liver shows massive hepatocyte necrosis, collapse of reticulum framework, minimal inflammation, and occasional pseudoacinar structures. Rare survivors are reported with reasonable restitution of liver architecture toward normal.

In less severe cases, focal hepatocyte necrosis is seen with a mild portal inflammatory response. Cholestasis is intracellular and canalicular. Chronic persistent hepatitis may be found for many years, with serologic evidence of persisting antigenemia (HBsAg) and mildly elevated serum transaminases. However, liver disease progressing to cirrhosis is very rare.

Mothers with markers for infectivity (HBsAg, HBeAg, DNA polymerase, HBcAb-IgM) may be chronic carriers, and their infants should receive hepatitis B immune globulin and hepatitis B virus vaccine. All infants of mothers who are HBsAg-positive should be treated prophylactically and immunized (see Chapter 6).

B. Neonatal Bacterial Hepatitis: Most bacterial liver infections in newborns are acquired by transplacental invasion from amnionitis with ascending spread from maternal vaginal or cervical infection. Onset is abrupt, usually within 48–72 hours after delivery, with signs of sepsis and often shock. Jaundice, seen in less than 25% of cases, appears early and is of the mixed type. The liver enlarges rapidly, and the histologic picture is that of a diffuse hepatitis with or without micro- or macro-abscess. The most common organisms are *Escherichia coli, Listeria monocytogenes,* and group B streptococci. Isolated neonatal liver abscess due to *E coli* or *Staphylococcus aureus* is often associated with omphalitis or umbilical vein catheterization. Bacterial hepatitis and neonatal liver abscesses require specific antibiotics in large doses and, rarely, surgical drainage. Deaths are common, but survivors show no long-term consequences of liver disease.

C. Neonatal Jaundice With Urinary Tract Infection: Jaundice in affected infants—usually males—typically appears between the second and fourth weeks of life. The manifestations of this disorder are lethargy, fever, poor appetite, jaundice, and hepatomegaly. Except for mixed hyperbilirubinemia, other liver function tests are not remarkable. Leukocytosis is present, and infection is confirmed by culture techniques. The mechanism for the liver impairment is unknown, though toxic action of

bacterial products (endotoxins) and the inflammatory response have been incriminated.

Treatment of the infection leads to prompt resolution of the cholestasis without hepatic sequelae.

Balistreri WF: Neonatal cholestasis. *J Pediatr* 1985; **106:**171.

Committee on Infectious Diseases, American Academy of Pediatrics: Prevention of hepatitis B virus infections. *Pediatrics* 1985;**75:**362.

Felber S, Sinatra F: Systemic disorders associated with neonatal cholestasis. *Semin Liver Dis* 1987;**7:**108.

Pickering LK: Management of the infant of a mother with viral hepatitis. *Pediatr Rev* 1988;**9:**315.

Spivak WF: Diagnostic utility of hepatobiliary scintigraphy with ^{99m}Tc-DISIDA in neonatal cholestasis. *J Pediatr* 1987;**110:**885.

Stevens CE et al: Perinatal hepatitis B virus transmission in the United States. *JAMA* 1985;**253:**1740.

2. INTRAHEPATIC CHOLESTASIS DUE TO INBORN ERRORS OF METABOLISM, FAMILIAL CAUSES, & "TOXIC" CAUSES

These cholestatic syndromes are caused by specific enzyme deficiencies or other inherited disorders; a positive history of certain precipitants associated with neonatal liver disease; and features of intrahepatic cholestasis—ie, jaundice, hepatomegaly, and normal to completely acholic stools. Some of the specific clinical conditions have characteristic clinical signs.

Enzyme Deficiencies & Other Inherited Disorders

Early specific diagnosis is important because dietary treatment may be available (Table 21–3). Reversal of liver disease and clinical symptoms is prompt and permanent as long as the diet is maintained. As with other genetically inherited inborn errors of metabolism, proper counseling for parents of the affected infant should be done as soon as possible.

Cholestasis due to metabolic diseases such as galactosemia, fructose intolerance, and tyrosinemia may be accompanied by vomiting, lethargy, poor feeding, and irritability. Hepatomegaly is a constant finding. The infants often appear septic; gram-negative bacteria can be cultured from blood in 25–50% of cases, especially in patients with galactosemia.

Other inherited conditions that present with neonatal intrahepatic cholestasis are outlined in Table 21–3.

"Toxic" Causes of Neonatal Cholestasis

A. Neonatal Ischemic/Hypoxic Conditions: Perinatal events that result in hypoperfusion of the gastrointestinal system are sometimes followed in 1–

2 weeks by cholestasis. This is seen in premature infants with respiratory distress, severe hypoxia, hypoglycemia, shock, and acidosis. When these perinatal conditions develop in association with gastrointestinal lesions such as ruptured omphalocele, gastroschisis, or later necrotizing enterocolitis, a subsequent cholestatic picture is common (25–50% of cases).

Liver function studies reveal mixed hyperbilirubinemia, elevated alkaline phosphatase values, and variable elevation of the transaminases. Stools are seldom persistently acholic.

Choleretics (cholestyramine, phenobarbital) and nutritional support are the mainstays of treatment until the cholestasis resolves (see Table 21–2). In some cases, this resolution may take 3–6 months. Complete resolution of the hepatic abnormalities is the rule, but portal fibrosis with perilobular scarring is occasionally seen on follow-up biopsy.

B. Prolonged Parenteral Nutrition: Cholestasis may develop after 1–2 weeks in premature newborns receiving total parenteral nutrition.

The mechanism seems to result from both concentration of amino acids and duration of their use. Diminished stimulation of bile flow from prolonged absence of oral feedings, toxic additives in the solutions, and translocation of intestinal bacteria and of their products have been considered as cholestatic "toxic" factors.

Early introduction of feedings has reduced the frequency of this disorder. The prognosis is generally good. Rare cases of portal fibrosis or stable cirrhosis have been found on follow-up liver biopsy.

C. "Inspissated Bile Syndrome": This is the result of accumulation of bile in canaliculi and in the small and medium-sized bile ducts in hemolytic disease of the newborn (Rh, ABO) and in some infants receiving total parenteral nutrition. The same mechanisms may cause intrinsic obstruction of the common duct. In extreme hemolysis, the cholestasis may be seemingly complete with acholic stools. Levels of bilirubin may reach 40 mg/dL, primarily direct-reacting. If inspissation of bile occurs within the extrahepatic biliary tree, differentiation from biliary atresia may be difficult. A trial of choleretics (cholestyramine, phenobarbital, aluminum hydroxide gel, theophylline) is indicated. Once stools show a return to normal color, patency of the extrahepatic biliary tree is ensured. Small bile-colored plugs in the stools are sometimes reported by parents at the time stool color becomes normal. Though most cases slowly improve over 2–6 months, persistence of complete cholestasis for more than 6–8 weeks requires further studies (ultrasonography, ^{99m}Tc diethyl-IDA scanning, liver biopsy) with possible laparotomy for exploration of the extrahepatic biliary tree. Irrigation of the common duct is sometimes necessary to dislodge the obstructing inspissated biliary material.

Dosi PC et al: Perinatal factors underlying neonatal cholestasis. *J Pediatr* 1985;**106**:471.

Enzenauer RW et al: Total parenteral nutrition cholestasis: A cause of mechanical biliary obstruction. *Pediatrics* 1985;**76**:905.

Merritt RJ: Cholestasis associated with total parenteral nutrition. *J Pediatr Gastroenterol Nutr* 1986;**5**:9.

Mock DM et al: Chronic fructose intoxication after infancy in children with hereditary fructose intolerance: A cause of growth retardation. *N Engl J Med* 1983;**309**:764.

Odievre M et al: Hereditary fructose intolerance in childhood. *Am J Dis Child* 1978;**132**:605.

Singh I et al: Peroxisomal disorders: Biochemical and clinical diagnostic considerations. *Am J Dis Child* 1988;**142**:1297.

Suchy FJ, Mullick FG. Total parenteral nutrition-associated cholestasis. In Balistreri WF, Stocker JT (ed). *Pediatric Hepatology Hemisphere,* New York. 1990. pp 29–40.

3. NEONATAL HEPATITIS (Giant Cell Hepatitis)

This type of cholestatic jaundice of unknown cause presents with the usual features of cholestasis and a typical appearance on histologic examination of biopsied liver tissue; it accounts for up to 75% of cases of neonatal intrahepatic cholestasis. The degree of cholestasis is variable, and the disorder may be indistinguishable from extrahepatic causes (10% of cases).

Intrauterine growth retardation, prematurity, poor feeding, emesis, poor growth, and partially or intermittently acholic stools are typical clinical characteristics of intrahepatic cholestasis.

In cases of suspected idiopathic neonatal hepatitis (absence of infectious, metabolic, and toxic causes), patency of the biliary tree should be verified to exclude extrahepatic "surgical" disorders. ^{99m}Tc-DIDA scanning and ultrasonography may be helpful in this regard. Liver biopsy findings are frequently diagnostic, especially after 6–8 weeks of age (see Table 21–1). Failure to detect patency of the biliary tree, nondiagnostic liver biopsy findings, or persisting complete cholestasis (acholic stools) are indications for minilaparotomy and intraoperative cholangiography by an experienced surgeon. Occasionally, a small but patent (hypoplastic) extrahepatic biliary tree is demonstrated and is probably the result rather than the cause of diminished bile flow; reconstruction of hypoplastic biliary trees should not be attempted.

Once a patent extrahepatic tree is confirmed, therapy should include choleretics (cholestyramine, phenobarbital), a special formula with medium-chain triglycerides (Pregestimil), and supplemental fat-soluble vitamins in water-miscible form. (See Table 21–2.) These are continued as long as significant cholestasis remains.

Eighty percent of patients recover without significant hepatic fibrosis. However, if a relative previously had neonatal hepatitis, there is a 70–80% probability of progression to cirrhosis.

Long-term consequences correlate best with the duration of the cholestasis. In general, failure to resolve the cholestatic picture is associated with progressive liver disease and evolving cirrhosis. This may occur either with normal numbers of interlobular bile ducts or when diminished numbers of ducts (paucity of interlobular ducts) result. Perilobular and intralobular fibrosis both progress, and portal hypertension eventually ensues, with splenomegaly and esophageal varices. Finally, ascites with rising bilirubin levels heralds the onset of hepatic failure. Liver transplantation has been successful when signs of hepatic decompensation are noted (rising bilirubin, intractable ascites).

Dick MC, Mowat AP: Hepatitis syndrome in infancy: An epidemiological survey with 10 year follow-up. *Arch Dis Child* 1985;**60**:512.

Odievre M et al: Long-term prognosis for infants with intrahepatic cholestasis and patent extrahepatic biliary tract. *Arch Dis Child* 1981;**56**:373.

Sokol RJ: Medical management of the infant or child with chronic liver disease. *Semin Liver Dis* 1987;**7**:155.

4. PAUCITY OF INTERLOBULAR BILE DUCTS

Forms of intrahepatic cholestasis caused by decreased numbers of interlobular bile ducts may be classified according to whether or not they are associated with other malformations. The syndromic forms, eg, Alagille syndrome (arteriohepatic dysplasia) are sometimes recognized by identification of the characteristic facies, which becomes more obvious with age. The forehead is prominent, as is the nasal bridge. The eyes are set deep and sometimes widely apart (hypertelorism). Often the chin is small and slightly pointed and projects forward. Cholestasis is usually incomplete, and stool color is normal. Pruritus begins by 3–4 months of age. Firm, smooth hepatomegaly is present, and cardiac murmurs are frequent. Xanthomas are rare early in the disease. Occasionally, early cholestasis is mild and not recognized.

Mild conjugated hyperbilirubinemia is found (up to 2–8 mg/dL). Serum alkaline phosphatase and cholesterol are markedly elevated, especially early in life. Serum bile acids are always elevated. Transaminases are slightly increased, but clotting factors and other liver proteins are usually normal.

The cardiovascular abnormalities include peripheral and valvular pulmonary stenoses (most common), atrial septal defect, coarctation of the aorta, and tetralogy of Fallot.

Vertebral arch defects are common, including incomplete fusion of the vertebral body or anterior arch (butterfly deformity) and diminished interpedicle distance in the thoracolumbar spine. Eye abnor-

malities (posterior embryotoxon) and renal abnormalities (dysplastic kidneys, renal tubular ectasia, single kidney, hematuria) are also associated with this disorder. Growth retardation with normal to increased levels of growth hormone is common. A weak, high-pitched voice may develop. Neurologic disorders due to vitamin E deficiency (areflexia, ataxia, ophthalmoplegia) eventually develop in many children.

In the nonsyndromic form, paucity of interlobular bile ducts is seen in the absence of the extrahepatic malformations. Paucity may also be seen in α_1-antitrypsin deficiency, in Zellweger syndrome, and in association with lymphedema (Aagenaes' syndrome).

High doses (4–8 g/d) of cholestyramine may control pruritus, lower cholesterol, and clear xanthomas. Phenobarbital may lower serum bilirubin. Ursodeoxycholic therapy is now being studied in clinical trials. Nutritional therapy to prevent wasting and deficiencies of fat-soluble vitamins is of particular importance because of the severity of cholestasis (see Table 21–2).

Prognosis is more favorable in the syndromic than in the nonsyndromic varieties. In the former, only 30–40% of patients have severe, progressive disease, whereas over 70% of patients suffering from the latter progress to cirrhosis. In Alagille syndrome, cholestasis usually improves by age 2–4 years, with minimal residual hepatic fibrosis. Survival into adulthood despite raised serum bile acids, transaminases, and alkaline phosphatase is common. Hypogonadism has been noted; however, fertility is not obviously affected. Cardiovascular anomalies may shorten life expectancy. Some patients have persistent, severe cholestasis, rendering their quality of life poor; liver transplant has been performed under these circumstances.

Alagille D et al: Syndromic paucity of interlobular bile ducts (Alagille syndrome or arteriohepatic dysplasia): Review of 80 cases. *J Pediatr* 1987;**110**:195.

Markowitz J et al: Arteriohepatic dysplasia. 1. Pitfalls in diagnosis and management. *Hepatology* 1983;**3**:74.

Riely CA: Familial intrahepatic cholestatic syndromes. *Semin Liver Dis* 1987;**7**:119.

Sokol RJ: Improved neurologic function after long-term correction of vitamin E deficiency in children with chronic cholestasis. *N Engl J Med* 1985;**313**:1580.

EXTRAHEPATIC NEONATAL CHOLESTASIS

Extrahepatic neonatal cholestasis is characterized by complete and persistent cholestasis (acholic stools) in the first 1–4 weeks of life, surgically proved lack of patency of the extrahepatic biliary tree by intraoperative cholangiography, firm to hard hepatomegaly, and typical features on histologic examination of liver biopsy tissue. (See Table 21–1.)

Causes include extrahepatic biliary atresia, choledochal cyst, intrinsic obstruction of the common duct, and spontaneous perforation of the extrahepatic ducts.

Extrahepatic Biliary Atresia

In Caucasians, extrahepatic biliary atresia occurs in 1:8000–1:13,000 births, and the incidence in both sexes is equal. In Asians, the incidence is higher, and the disorder is twice as common in girls. The abnormality found most commonly is complete atresia of all extrahepatic biliary structures, but there are variants. The specific cause is not known, although evidence supports an insult to the biliary structures in the perinatal period that progresses in postnatal life. Extrahepatic atresia has not been found in stillborn fetuses and is rarely seen in premature infants. Meconium and first-passed stools are usually normal in color, suggesting early patency of the ducts. Furthermore, the presence of patent intrahepatic bile ducts near the porta hepatis is not consistent with congenital absence of the primitive bile duct. Evidence obtained from surgically removed remnants of the extrahepatic biliary tree suggests an inflammatory or sclerosing cholangiopathy. Although an infectious cause seems reasonable, no agent has been consistently found in such cases. The role of reovirus type 3 in biliary atresia is controversial. Though other congenital malformations, especially vascular ones, may occasionally be seen in extrahepatic biliary atresia, only polysplenia syndrome (situs inversus, levocardia, absence of the inferior vena cava) is consistently associated with extrahepatic biliary atresia.

Jaundice may be noted in the newborn period but is more often delayed until 2–3 weeks of age. The urine is dark and stains the diaper, and the stools are often pale yellow, buff-colored, gray, or acholic. Seepage of bilirubin products across the intestinal mucosa gives some yellow coloration to the stools. Hepatomegaly is common, and the liver may feel firm to hard; splenomegaly develops later. Pruritus, digital clubbing, xanthomas, and a rachitic rosary may be noted in slightly older patients. Murmurs reflecting increasing cardiovascular output or shunting through bronchial arteries may be heard over the entire precordium and back. By 2–3 months, the growth curves reveal poor weight gain, probably as a result of fat malabsorption, though vomiting and diarrhea are seldom reported. Late in the course, ascites and bleeding complications occur.

No single laboratory test will consistently differentiate this entity from other causes of "complete" obstructive jaundice. A ^{99m}Tc diethyl-IDA excretion study performed early in the course of disease and after pretreatment with phenobarbital (3–5 mg/kg/d for 5–7 days) may distinguish hepatocyte disease from small and large bile duct disease. Although biliary atresia is suggested by persistent elevation of serum γ-glutamyl transpeptidase or alkaline phosphatase levels, high cholesterol levels, and prolonged prothrombin times, these findings have also been reported in severe neonatal hepatitis. Furthermore, these tests will not differentiate the location of the obstruction within the extrahepatic system ("correctable" versus "noncorrectable" lesions). Generally, the transaminases are only modestly elevated in biliary atresia. Serum proteins and blood clotting factors are not affected early in the disease. Routine chest x-ray may reveal abnormalities suggestive of polysplenia syndrome. Ultrasonography of the biliary system should be performed to ascertain the presence of choledochal cyst. Biopsy specimens can differentiate intrahepatic causes of cholestasis from biliary atresia in over 90% of cases.

The major diagnostic dilemma is between this entity and "complete" intrahepatic cholestasis, choledochal cyst, or intrinsic bile duct obstruction (stones, bile plugs). Though spontaneous perforation of extrahepatic bile ducts leads to jaundice and acholic stools, the infants are usually quite ill with chemical peritonitis from biliary ascites, and hepatomegaly is not found.

If the diagnosis of biliary atresia cannot be excluded by the diagnostic evaluation, surgical exploration is necessary. Associated anomalies should be anticipated (malrotation, preduodenal portal vein, situs inversus). Laparotomy must include liver biopsy and an operative cholangiogram if a gallbladder is present. The presence of bile in the gallbladder implies patency of the proximal extrahepatic duct system. Radiographic visualization of dye in the duodenum excludes obstruction to the distal extrahepatic ducts.

In the absence of surgical correction, the following eventually develop: failure to thrive, marked pruritus, portal hypertension, hypersplenism, bleeding diathesis, rickets, ascites, and cyanosis. Bronchitis and pneumonia are common. Eventually, hepatic failure and death occur.

Except for the occasional example of "correctable" biliary atresia where choledocho- or cholecystojejunostomy is feasible, the standard procedure is hepatoportoenterostomy (Kasai procedure). Occasionally, portocholecystostomy may be performed if the gallbladder is present and the passage to the duodenum is patent. These procedures are best done in specialized centers where experienced surgical, pediatric, and nursing personnel are available. It is recommended that surgery be performed as early as possible (age 6–10 weeks); the Kasai procedure should not be undertaken in infants over 4 months of age, because the prognosis in these patients is hopeless.

Orthotopic liver transplantation is now indicated for patients who progress to end-stage biliary cirrhosis despite surgical intervention. The 1- to 2-year survival rate is 60–80%.

Whether or not the Kasai procedure is performed, supportive medical treatment measures consist of vitamin and caloric support (using water-miscible forms of vitamins A, D, K, and E and formulas containing medium-chain triglycerides [Pregestimil]). (See Table 21–2.) Bacterial infections (eg, ascending cholangitis) should be treated promptly and signs of bleeding tendency corrected with intramuscular vitamin K. Ascites can be managed with reduced sodium intake and spironolactone. Choleretics and bile acid-binding products (cholestyramine, aluminum hydroxide gel, phenobarbital) are of little value.

When bile flow is sustained, the 5-year survival rate is 35–50%. Complete surgical failures have the same outcome as nonoperated cases, but patients die sooner (age 8–15 months versus age 18–36 months). Death is usually due to liver failure, sepsis, acidosis, or respiratory failure secondary to intractable ascites. Surprisingly, terminal hemorrhage is unusual.

Barkin R, Lilly JR: Biliary atresia and the Kasai operation: Continuing care. *J Pediatr* 1980;**96:**1015.

Kaufman SS et al: Nutritional support for the infant with extrahepatic biliary atresia. *J Pediatr* 1987;**100:**679.

Kobayashi A, Itabashi F, Ohbe Y: Long-term prognosis in biliary atresia after hepatic portoenterostomy: Analysis of 35 patients who survived beyond 5 years of age. *J Pediatr* 1984;**105:**243.

McClement JW, Howard ER, Mowat AP: Results of surgical treatment for extrahepatic biliary atresia in United Kingdom 1980–1982. *Br Med J* 1985;**290:**345.

Ryckman FC, Noseworthy J: Neonatal cholestatic conditions requiring surgical reconstruction. *Semin Liver Dis* 1987;**7:**134.

Choledochal Cyst

Choledochal cysts causes 2–5% of cases of extrahepatic neonatal cholestasis; the incidence is higher in Asians. In most cases, the clinical manifestations, basic laboratory findings, and histopathologic features on liver biopsy are indistinguishable from those seen in biliary atresia. Neonatal symptomatic cysts are usually associated with atresia of the distal common duct—accounting for the diagnostic dilemma—and may simply be part of the spectrum of biliary atresia. However, a palpable subhepatic mass, positive ultrasound scan, or pressure deformity on the first and second portion of duodenum seen on upper gastrointestinal series promptly resolves the question. Immediate operation is indicated once abnormalities in clotting factors have been corrected. Discovery of such a mass eliminates the need for other studies.

Excision of the cyst and hepatojejunal anastomosis are recommended. In some cases, because of technical problems, only the mucosa of the cyst can be removed with jejunal anastomosis to the proximal bile duct.

The prognosis depends upon the presence or absence of associated evidence of atresia and the appearance of the intrahepatic ducts. If atresia is found, the prognosis is similar to that described above. If an isolated cyst is encountered, the outcome is generally excellent, with resolution of the jaundice and return to normal liver cellular architecture the rule. However, bouts of ascending cholangitis or obstruction of the anastomotic site may occur. The risk of biliary carcinoma developing within the cyst is about 1–3% at adulthood; therefore, cystectomy should be done whenever possible.

Kim SH: Choledochal cyst: Survey of the Surgical Section of the American Academy of Pediatrics. *J Pediatr Surg* 1981;**16:**402.

Saing H et al: Surgical management of choledochal cysts: A review of 60 cases. *J Pediatr Surg* 1985;**20:**443.

Spontaneous Perforation of the Extrahepatic Ducts

The sudden appearance of obstructive jaundice, acholic stools, and abdominal enlargement with ascites in a sick newborn is suggestive of this condition. The liver is usually normal in size, and a yellow-green discoloration can often be discerned under the umbilicus or in the scrotum. Aspiration of ascitic fluid reveals the bilious color and is best performed after intravenous injection of ^{99m}Tc diethyl-IDA. Radioisotope activity is present in the removed fluid, confirming the diagnosis.

Treatment is surgical. Simple drainage is sufficient in primary perforations. A diversion anastomosis is constructed in cases associated with choledochal cyst or stenosis.

The prognosis is generally good.

Haller JO et al: Spontaneous perforation of the common bile duct in children. *Radiology* 1989;**172:**621.

OTHER NEONATAL HYPERBILIRUBINEMIC CONDITIONS (Noncholestatic Nonhemolytic)

This group of disorders associated with hyperbilirubinemia is of 2 types: (1) unconjugated hyperbilirubinemia, consisting of breast milk jaundice, Lucey-Driscoll syndrome, congenital hypothyroidism, upper intestinal obstruction, Gilbert's syndrome, Crigler-Najjar syndrome, and drug-induced hyperbilirubinemia; and (2) conjugated noncholestatic hyperbilirubinemia, consisting of Dubin-Johnson syndrome and Rotor's syndrome.

1. UNCONJUGATED HYPERBILIRUBINEMIA

Breast Milk Jaundice

Persistent elevation of the indirect bilirubin fraction may occur in 1–3% of breast-fed infants. In some cases, it is due to an inhibitor of bilirubin conjugation appearing in mature breast milk. Pregnane-3α,20β-diol and nonesterified fatty acids have been suggested as the inhibitor. Increased intestinal absorption of bilirubin in breast-fed infants, due to β-glucuronidase activity in breast milk or low fecal output, may contribute.

Hyperbilirubinemia does not usually exceed 10–15 mg/dL. The jaundice is noticeable by the fifth to seventh day of breast feeding and may accentuate the underlying physiologic jaundice. Physical examination is normal; urine does not stain the diaper; and the stools are golden-yellow.

The jaundice clears before 3 months in almost all infants, even when breast feedings are continued.

Kernicterus has never been reported in this condition. In special situations, breast feeding may be discontinued and replaced by formula feedings for 2–3 days until serum bilirubin decreases by 2–8 mg/dL. When breast feeding is reinstituted, the serum bilirubin may increase slightly but not to the previous level.

De Carvalho M et al: Fecal bilirubin excretion and serum bilirubin concentrations in breast-fed and bottle-fed infants. *J Pediatr* 1985;**107**:786.

Gourley GR, Aren RA: β-glucuronidase and hyperbilirubinemia in breast-fed and formula-fed babies. *Lancet* 1986;**1**:644.

Poland RL: Breast-milk jaundice. *J Pediatr* 1981;**99**:86.

Congenital Hypothyroidism

Though the differential diagnosis should always include consideration of congenital hypothyroidism as a cause of indirect hyperbilirubinemia, the diagnosis may be obvious from other clinical and physical clues. The jaundice quickly clears with replacement thyroid hormone therapy, though the mechanism is unclear.

Smith DW et al: Congenital hypothyroidism: Signs and symptoms in the newborn period. *J Pediatr* 1975;**87**:958.

Upper Intestinal Obstruction

The association of indirect hyperbilirubinemia with high intestinal obstruction—eg, pyloric stenosis—in the newborn has been observed repeatedly; the mechanism is unknown. Diminished levels of hepatic glucuronyl transferase have been found on liver biopsy.

Treatment is that of the underlying obstructive condition (usually surgical), and jaundice disappears once adequate nutrition is achieved.

Wolley MM et al: Jaundice, hypertrophic pyloric stenosis and hepatic glucuronyl transferase. *J Pediatr Surg* 1974;**9**:359.

Gilbert's Syndrome

This is a common form of familial hyperbilirubinemia associated with a partial reduction of hepatic bilirubin uridine diphosphate glucuronyl transferase activity. Mild fluctuating jaundice, especially with illness, and vague constitutional symptoms are common. A shortened red cell survival has been shown in some patients. Subsidence of hyperbilirubinemia has been achieved in patients by administration of phenobarbital (5–8 mg/kg/d).

The disease is inherited as an autosomal dominant with incomplete penetrance. Males are affected more often than females (4:1). The findings on liver biopsy and most other liver function tests are normal except for prolonged sulfobromophthalein (BSP) retention. An increase in the level of unconjugated bilirubin after a 2-day fast (300 kcal/d) of 1.4 mg/dL or more is consistent with the diagnosis of Gilbert's disease.

Gollan JL et al: Effect of dietary composition on the unconjugated hyperbilirubinemia of Gilbert's syndrome. *Gut* 1976;**17**:335.

Crigler-Najjar Syndrome

Patients with type I disease usually develop rapid severe elevation of unconjugated bilirubin, with neurologic consequences (kernicterus). Some survive without neurologic signs until adolescence and early adulthood, at which time deterioration may suddenly occur. The bile is colorless and contains only traces of conjugated bilirubin. The glucuronyl transferase deficiency is inherited as an autosomal recessive. Phenobarbital is without effect, though phototherapy and cholestyramine may keep bilirubin levels below 25 mg/dL. Liver transplantation may be curative.

Occasionally, a milder autosomal dominant form (type II) without neurologic complications has been found. Hyperbilirubinemia is less severe, and the bile is pigmented and contains bilirubin diglucuronide. Patients with this form usually respond to phenobarbital.

Liver biopsy findings and liver function tests are consistently normal in both types.

Farrell GC et al: Crigler-Najjar type 1 syndrome: Absence of hepatic bilirubin UDP-glucuronyl transferase activity and therapeutic response to light. *Aust N Z J Med* 1982;**12**:280.

Shevell MI et al: Crigler-Najjar syndrome type 1: Treatment by home phototherapy followed by orthotopic liver transplantation. *J Pediatr* 1987;**110**:429.

Drug-Induced Hyperbilirubinemia

Vitamin K_2 may elevate indirect bilirubin levels by causing hemolysis. Other drugs (eg, sulfonamides) may displace bilirubin from albumin, potentially increasing the risk of kernicterus. In the latter case, total measured levels are not altered.

2. CONJUGATED NONCHOLESTATIC HYPERBILIRUBINEMIA (Dubin-Johnson Syndrome & Rotor's Syndrome)

The diagnosis is aided by a positive family history and jaundice that persists or recurs.

The basic defect is impaired hepatocyte excretion of conjugated bilirubin, with a variable degree of impairment in uptake and conjugation complicating the picture. Bile acids are normally handled so that cholestasis does not occur. Bilirubin values range from 2 to 5 mg/dL, and other liver function tests are normal. In Rotor's syndrome, the liver is normal; in Dubin-Johnson syndrome, it is darkly pigmented on gross inspection. Microscopic examination reveals numerous dark-brown pigment granules, especially in the centrilobular regions. However, the amount of pigment varies within families, and some jaundiced members may have no demonstrable pigmentation in the liver. Otherwise, the liver is histologically normal. Oral cholecystography fails to visualize the gallbladder. Differences in the excretion patterns of BSP, in results of ^{99m}Tc-HIDA cholescintigraphy, in urinary coproporphyrin I and III levels, and in the serum pattern of mono- and diglucuronide conjugates of bilirubin can help distinguish these conditions.

The prognosis is excellent, and no treatment is needed.

Bar-Meir S et al: ^{99m}Tc-HIDA cholescintigraphy in Dubin-Johnson and Rotor syndromes. *Radiology* 1982; **142:**743.

Rosenthal P et al: The distribution of serum bilirubin conjugates in pediatric hepatobiliary diseases. *J Pediatr* 1987;**110:**201.

Sotelo-Avila C et al: Cholecystitis in a 17-year-old boy with recurrent jaundice since childhood. *J Pediatr* 1988; **112:**668.

Wolkoff AW et al: Rotor's syndrome: A distinct inheritable pathophysiologic entity. *Am J Med* 1976;**60:**173.

HEPATITIS A

Essentials of Diagnosis

- Gastrointestinal upset (anorexia, vomiting, diarrhea).
- Jaundice.
- Liver tenderness.
- Abnormal liver function tests.
- Local epidemic of the disease.
- Specific antibody rise.

General Considerations

This disease is caused by a virus or strains of related viruses and tends to occur in both epidemic and sporadic fashion. Transmission by the fecal-oral route explains epidemic outbreaks from contaminated food or water supplies. Particles 27 nm in diameter have been found in stools during the acute phase of type A hepatitis and are similar in appearance to the enterovirus group. Sporadic cases usually result from contact with an affected individual. Very rarely, transmission through blood products has occurred. The overt form of the disease is easily recognized by the clinical manifestations, but a large number of affected individuals have an anicteric and unrecognized form of the disease. This has been especially true in outbreaks of hepatitis A reported in day-care centers for children younger than 3 years of age. Both forms probably confer lifelong immunity to hepatitis A virus.

Antibody to this virus appears within 1–4 weeks of clinical symptoms. While the great majority of children with infectious hepatitis are asymptomatic or have mild disease and recover completely, some will develop fulminant hepatitis, or rarely cirrhosis. Children who die during the initial attack of the disease do so from massive hepatic necrosis secondary to overwhelming viremia, an immunologic deficiency state, or perhaps exposure to a completely different strain of virus.

Clinical Findings

A. History: A history of direct exposure to a previously jaundiced individual or of eating seafood or drinking contaminated water in the recent past should be sought. Following an incubation period of 14–50 days, the initial nonspecific symptoms usually precede the development of jaundice by 5–10 days.

B. Symptoms and Signs: Fever, anorexia, vomiting, headache, and abdominal pain are the usual symptoms. Darkening of the urine, suggesting the presence of bile, precedes jaundice. Jaundice reaches a peak in 1–2 weeks and then begins to subside. The stools may become light or clay-colored during this time. Clinical improvement can be noted during the early phase of developing jaundice. Jaundice and liver tenderness are the most consistent physical findings. Splenomegaly may be present.

C. Laboratory Findings: Transaminases and conjugated and unconjugated bilirubin levels are elevated. The leukocyte count is normal to low; the sedimentation rate is elevated. Serum proteins are generally normal, but an elevation of the gamma globulin fraction (> 2.5 g/dL) can occur and indicates a worse prognosis. Hypoalbuminemia, hypoglycemia, and marked prolongation of prothrombin time are serious prognostic findings. Urine bile and urobilinogen are increased. Serologic tests are available for both the specific IgM and IgG antibodies to the type A hepatitis virus. A positive hepatitis A-IgM indicates acute disease, whereas the IgG remains elevated after recovery.

If the diagnosis is in doubt, a percutaneous liver biopsy may be safely performed in most children—provided the partial thromboplastin time, platelet count, and bleeding time are normal and the prothrombin time is greater than 50% of normal. The presence of ascites may increase the risk of percutaneous liver biopsy. "Balloon cells" and acidophilic bodies are characteristic histologic findings. Liver cell necrosis may be diffuse or focal, with accompanying infiltration of inflammatory cells containing polymorphonuclear leukocytes, lymphocytes, macrophages, and plasma cells, particularly in portal areas. Some bile duct proliferation may be seen in the perilobular portal areas alongside areas of bile stasis. Regenerative liver cells and proliferation of reticuloendothelial cells are present. Occasionally, massive hepatocyte destruction is seen with scarcely a normal liver cell visible.

Differential Diagnosis

Before jaundice appears, the symptoms are those of a nonspecific viral enteritis. Other diseases with somewhat similar onset include pancreatitis, infectious mononucleosis, leptospirosis, drug-induced hepatitis, Wilson's disease, and, most often, type B hepatitis or non-A, non-B hepatitis. Acquired cytomegalovirus disease may also mimic hepatitis A.

Prevention

Some attempt at isolation of the patient is indicated, although the majority of patients with type A hepatitis are noninfectious by the time the disease becomes overt. Stool, urine, and blood-contaminated objects should be handled with extreme care for 1 month after the appearance of jaundice.

Passive-active immunization of exposed susceptibles can be achieved by giving standard immune globulin, 0.02–0.04 mL/kg intramuscularly. Illness is prevented in 80–90% of individuals if immune globulin is given within 1–2 weeks of exposure. Individuals traveling to endemic disease areas should receive 0.02–0.06 mL/kg as prophylaxis, depending on length of stay.

Treatment

There are no specific measures. Sedatives and corticosteroids should be avoided.

At the start of the illness, a light diet is preferable. Fruits, vegetables, and plenty of sugars are usually well tolerated. Adequate protein can be supplied by grilled meats or broiled fish with less than normal amounts of fat.

Prognosis

Ninety-five percent of children recover without sequelae. In rare cases of fulminant hepatitis, the patient may die in 5 days or may survive as long as 1–2 months. The prognosis is poor if the signs and symptoms of hepatic coma prevail, with deepening of jaundice and development of ascites; orthotopic liver transplantation may be successful under these circumstances. Incomplete resolution leads to pro-

longed hepatitis, or chronic cholestatic hepatitis. Rare cases of aplastic anemia following acute infectious hepatitis have also been reported. A benign relapse of symptoms may occur in 10–15% of cases after 6–10 weeks of apparent resolution.

Feinstone SM, Purcell RH: New methods for the serodiagnosis of hepatitis A. *Gastroenterology* 1980;**78**:1092.

Hadler SC et al: Risk factors for hepatitis A in day care centers. *J Infect Dis* 1982;**145**:255.

Hoofnagle JH: Type A and type B hepatitis. *Lab Med* 1983;**14**:705.

Noble RC et al: Post transfusion hepatitis A in a neonatal intensive care unit. *JAMA* 1984;**252**:2711.

Tabor E et al: Asymptomatic viral hepatitis types A and B in an adolescent population. *Pediatrics* 1978;**62**:1026.

HEPATITIS B

Essentials of Diagnosis

- Gastrointestinal upset, anorexia, vomiting, diarrhea.
- Jaundice, tender hepatomegaly, abnormal liver function tests.
- Serologic evidence of hepatitis B disease: HBsAg, HBeAg, HBcAb-IgM.
- History of parenteral exposure.

General Considerations

In contrast to hepatitis A, hepatitis B has a delayed onset with an incubation period of 21–135 days. The disease is due to a virus (42-nm Dane particle) that is usually acquired parenterally (eg, perinatal transmission from a carrier mother, blood products, needle sticks, tattoos) or through sexual transmission. Breast milk, urine, and saliva have been shown to contain viral antigen. Transmission via blood products has been almost eliminated by HBsAg donor-screening protocols.

The complete Dane particle is composed of a core (28-nm particle) that is found in the nucleus of infected liver cells and a double-shelled surface particle apparently formed in the cytoplasm where the completed virus particle is synthesized. The surface antigen in blood is termed HBsAg. This particle is found as a 22-nm spherical particle in the serum but occasionally occurs as a filamentous structure as well. The antibody to it is HBsAb. The core antigen is termed HBcAg and its antibody HBcAb. A specific HBcAb-IgM occurs during active viral replication.

Another important antigen-antibody system associated with hepatitis B virus disease is the "e" antigen system. A soluble antigen, HBeAg, appears in the serum of infected patients early and correlates with active virus replication. Persistence of HBeAg is a marker of infectivity, whereas the appearance of

HBeAb generally implies termination of the carrier state. Other serologic markers indicating viral replication include the presence of DNA polymerase and hepatitis B viral DNA (HBV-DNA).

A new hepatitis virus, the delta agent, is a "parasitic" RNA virus that is infective only in patients with preexisting or concurrent hepatitis B infection. Superinfection or coinfection with delta virus in hepatitis B increases the risk of fulminant or chronic hepatitis B.

Clinical Findings

A. Symptoms and Signs: The symptoms are nonspecific, consisting only of slight fever (which may be absent) and mild gastrointestinal upset. Visible jaundice is usually the first significant finding. It is accompanied by darkening of the urine and pale or clay-colored stools. Hepatomegaly is present. Occasionally, a symptom complex of macular rash, urticarial lesions, and arthritis antedates the appearance of icterus.

B. Laboratory Findings: The presence of HBsAg, HBcAb-IgM, or hepatitis B-specific DNA polymerase signifies acute hepatitis virus B disease. HBsAb develops later (months to years) as recovery occurs. Carriers of HBsAg also have detectable levels of HBcAb, and e antigen may also be present in the serum of patients with persistent antigenemia.

Liver function test results are similar to those discussed previously for hepatitis A. Liver biopsy seldom differentiates hepatitis A and B disease, although specific stains may detect HBcAg or HBsAg in liver.

Renal involvement may be suspected by urinary findings suggesting glomerulonephritis.

Differential Diagnosis

The differentiation between hepatitis A and hepatitis B disease is made easier by a history of parenteral exposure and an unusually long period of incubation. The history may suggest a drug-induced hepatitis, especially if a serum sickness prodrome is reported.

Non-A, non-B hepatitis is diagnosed in the absence of serologic markers of hepatitis types A or B.

Prevention

Control of the incidence of hepatitis B in the population is based on screening of blood donors, use of properly sterilized needles and surgical equipment, and avoidance of sexual contact with carriers. The vaccine is highly effective for preexposure prophylaxis (see Chapter 6). Postexposure administration of hepatitis B immune globulin (0.1 mL/kg intramuscularly, given as soon as possible after exposure, up to 7 days) is also effective.

Treatment

Supportive measures such as bed rest and a nutri-

tious diet are used during the active stage of disease. Corticosteroids are contraindicated. For patients with progressive disease (chronic active hepatitis), treatment with antiviral agents and interferon has met with variable success.

Prognosis

The prognosis is good, although fulminant hepatitis, chronic persistent hepatitis, or chronic active hepatitis and cirrhosis may supervene. The course of the disease is variable, but jaundice seldom persists for more than 2 weeks. HBsAg disappears in 95% of cases at the time of clinical recovery. Persistent asymptomatic antigenemia may occur, particularly in children with Down's syndrome or leukemia and those undergoing chronic hemodialysis. Persistence of neonatally acquired HBsAg is common, and the presence of e antigen in the HBsAg carrier patient seems to convey a poorer prognosis. Chronic hepatitis B disease predisposes the patient to developing hepatocellular carcinoma.

Bortolotti F et al: Liver cirrhosis associated with chronic hepatitis B virus infection in childhood. *J Pediatr* 1986; **108**:224.

Centers for Disease Control: Update on hepatitis B prevention: Recommendations of the Immunization Practices Advisory Committee. *Ann Intern Med* 1987;**107**:353.

Dupuy JM et al: Hepatitis B in children. 1. Analysis of 80 cases of acute and chronic hepatitis B. *J Pediatr* 1978; **92**:17.

Hoofnagle JH: Type A and type B hepatitis. *Lab Med* 1983;**14**:705.

Xu Z-Y et al: Prevention of perinatal acquisition of hepatitis B virus carriage using vaccine: Preliminary report of a randomized, double-blind placebo-controlled and comparative trial. *Pediatrics* 1985;**76**:713.

HEPATITIS NON-A, NON-B (NANB)

This disease is caused by at least 3 hepatotropic viruses distinct from those causing hepatitis types A and B. One of the viruses, hepatitis C virus, has recently been isolated, and may be identified by serologic testing. Otherwise, the diagnosis is based on excluding other hepatitis viruses. Ninety percent of cases of posttransfusion hepatitis in North America and Europe are caused by a NANB virus; the risk is about 1 to 2 cases per 100 units transfused. Children with hemophilia who receive concentrated factor VIII prepared from pooled plasma are commonly infected with NANB hepatitis. Finally, an enterically transmitted (ET) NANB hepatitis virus (fecal-oral route of transmission) causes outbreaks in Asia, Africa, USSR, and Mexico; the attack rate is highest in individuals aged 15–40, with very high mortality rate (20%) in pregnant women.

Clinical symptoms are mild in posttransfusion forms; incubation is 5–12 weeks, only 25% of cases becoming icteric. Over 40% of patients develop chronic elevations of ALT (SGPT), with a fluctuating ALT pattern being common. Cirrhosis may develop in up to 10–20% of cases with chronic active hepatitis. ET-NANB hepatitis resembles hepatitis A clinically, although serologic markers are absent; no chronicity has been reported.

Differential diagnosis is similar to that of hepatitis types A and B. Diagnosis rests on excluding other causes of acute hepatitis; history of transfusion or travel is supportive. Immune globulin (0.06 mL/kg intramuscularly) may be given to close contacts or newborn infants born to infected women, although benefit has not been proved. Treatment of acute hepatitis is supportive; interferon may be helpful in chronic hepatitis.

Posttransfusion hepatitis NANB frequently results in chronic active hepatitis and cirrhosis with the expected complications. ET-NANB infection has high mortality in pregnant females; however, chronic disease is negligible. Many cases of fulminant hepatitis are presumably caused by these viruses and may be treated by liver transplantation.

Aplastic anemia occasionally follows NANB hepatitis. The current screening of blood donors for anti-HCV, serum ALT and HBcAb in the USA will reduce the transmission of this virus.

Dienstag JL: Non-A, non-B hepatitis. (2 parts.) *Gastroenterology* 1983;**85**:439, 743.

McGrath KM et al: Liver disease complicating severe haemophilia in childhood. *Arch Dis Child* 1980;**55**:537.

FULMINANT HEPATITIS
(Acute Massive Hepatic Necrosis, Acute Yellow Atrophy)

Fulminant hepatitis has a mortality rate close to 95% in children. An unusual virulence of the infectious agent or peculiar host susceptibility is postulated in these cases. In the first few weeks of life, fulminant hepatic necrosis can be caused by herpesvirus, echovirus, or adenovirus. Metabolic disease may also be responsible. Later, hepatitis B virus and non-A, non-B hepatitis virus are sometimes causative. Hepatitis A virus rarely is responsible for this dreaded disease. Patients with immunologic deficiency diseases and those receiving immunosuppressive drugs are especially vulnerable. In the older child, Wilson's disease and drugs or toxins (eg, mushroom ingestions) must also be considered.

Clinical Findings

In a number of patients, the disease proceeds in a rapidly fulminant course with deepening jaundice, deterioration of laboratory indices, ascites, a rapidly shrinking liver, and progressive coma. Terminally, some laboratory values, such as AST (SGOT) and ALT (SGPT), may improve at the time when the liver is getting smaller (massive necrosis and collapse). Another group of patients start with a course typical of "benign" hepatitis and then suddenly become ill once again during the second week of the disease. Fever, anorexia, vomiting, and abdominal pain may be noted, and worsening of liver function tests parallels changes in sensorium or impending coma. Hyperreflexia and upgoing toes are seen. A characteristic breath odor is present (fetor hepaticus). A generalized bleeding tendency occurs at this time. Impairment of renal function, manifested by either oliguria or anuria, is an ominous sign. The striking laboratory findings include elevated serum bilirubin levels (usually > 20 mg/dL), high AST and ALT (> 5000 IU/L) that may decrease terminally, low serum albumin, hypoglycemia, and prolonged prothrombin time. Blood ammonia levels may be elevated, whereas blood urea nitrogen is often very low initially. Hyperpnea is frequent, and a mixed respiratory alkalosis and metabolic acidosis is apparent from serum electrolyte values. A rise in the polymorphonuclear count often presages acute liver failure.

Differential Diagnosis

Other known causes of fulminant hepatitis, such as drugs and other chemical poisons or naturally occurring plant toxins, may be difficult to exclude. Patients with Reye's syndrome are typically anicteric. A liver biopsy may be helpful. Wilson's disease, acute leukemia, and Budd-Chiari syndrome should be considered.

Complications

Hepatic failure is soon followed by hepatic coma, the depth of which (stage I-IV) corresponds to the prognosis. Cirrhosis of the postnecrotic type is the usual sequela in the rare pediatric survivor, with some cases of chronic active hepatitis evolving from submassive hepatic necrosis. Cerebral edema may be the cause of death in 15–30% of patients. Complete restoration of normal histologic features is more likely in drug-induced hepatic encephalopathy. Sepsis, hemorrhage, renal failure, or cardiorespiratory arrest is a common terminal event.

Treatment

Many regimens have been tried, but controlled evaluation of therapy remains difficult. Exchange transfusion (with fresh heparinized blood) temporarily repairs both the chemical and hematologic abnormalities. Response may be delayed and repeated exchange transfusions necessary. Plasmapheresis with plasma exchange, total body washout, charcoal hemoperfusion, and hemodialysis using a special high-permeability membrane have been used in the treatment of fulminant hepatic failure. Removal of circulating toxins may be of greater benefit to extrahepatic organ function (brain) than to the liver itself.

Reversal of hepatic encephalopathy may follow any of these therapeutic modalities but without improvement in the final prognosis. Survival in adults is not improved over the control group (about 20%). Orthotopic liver transplantation has met with success in approximately 50–60% of cases; however, patients in stage 4 coma may not always recover cerebral function. Criteria for deciding when to perform the transplantation on these patients are not firmly established.

Corticosteroids may actually be harmful. Sterilization of the colon with oral antibiotics such as clindamycin, neomycin, or kanamycin is recommended. An alternative is acidification of the colon with lactulose, 2–3 tablespoons 3 or 4 times daily, which reduces blood ammonia levels and traps ammonia in the colon. There is experimental animal evidence that insulin and glucagon given via the portal vein may be hepatotropic and of some help in fulminant hepatic necrosis. Preliminary studies suggest that intravenous infusions of prostaglandin E may be beneficial.

Close monitoring of fluid and electrolytes is mandatory and requires a central venous line. Maintenance of normal blood glucose levels is important. Diuretics, sedatives, and tranquilizers are to be avoided or used sparingly. Early signs of cerebral edema are treated with dexamethasone and careful infusions of mannitol (0.5–1 g/kg).

Comatose patients are intubated, given mechanical ventilatory support, and monitored for signs of infection. Coagulopathy is treated with fresh-frozen plasma, other clotting factor concentrates, platelet infusions, or exchange transfusion. Plasmapheresis and hemodialysis may help maintain a patient while awaiting liver transplantation. Prophylactic immune globulin, 0.02 mL/kg intramuscularly, should be given to close contacts of the patient with hepatitis A and, perhaps, NANB hepatitis.

Prognosis

The overall prognosis remains very grave. Exchange transfusions or other modes of heroic therapy do not improve survival figures. The presence of nests of liver cells seen on liver biopsy amounting to more than 25% of the total cells and rising levels of clotting factors V and VII coupled with rising levels of serum alpha-fetoprotein may signify a more favorable prognosis for early survival. Only the rare survivor escapes postnecrotic cirrhosis.

Fraser CL, Arieff AI: Hepatic encephalopathy. *N Engl J Med* 1985;**313:**865.

Psacharopoulos HT et al: Fulminant hepatic failure in childhood. *Arch Dis Child* 1980;**55:**252.

Russell GJ et al: Fulminant hepatic failure. *J Pediatr* 1987; **111:**313.

Treem WR, Boyle JT: Severe cardiomyopathy simulating hepatitis in adolescence. *Clin Pediatr (Phila)* 1986; **25:**260.

AUTOIMMUNE CHRONIC ACTIVE HEPATITIS
(Lupoid Hepatitis)

Autoimmune chronic active hepatitis (CAH) is most common in teenage girls, though it does occur at all ages and in either sex. CAH may also follow acute hepatitis B and perhaps hepatitis A or non-A, non-B hepatitis. Rarely, CAH evolves from drug-induced hepatitis or may develop in conjunction with such diseases as ulcerative colitis, Sjögren's syndrome, or autoimmune hemolytic anemia. Wilson's disease and α_1-antitrypsin deficiency may also present as CAH. A positive HBsAg indicates CAH caused by hepatitis type B. Positive antinuclear antibodies, smooth muscle antibodies or liver-kidney-microsomal antibodies, and systemic manifestations (such as arthralgia, acne, and amenorrhea) are characteristic of autoimmune CAH.

A genetic susceptibility to development of this entity is suggested by the increased incidence of the histocompatibility antigens HLA-A1 and HLA-B8. These histocompatibility antigens may code for the defect in suppressor T cell function also noted in patients with chronic active hepatitis. Increased autoimmune disease in families of patients and a high prevalence of seroimmunologic abnormalities in relatives have been noted.

Clinical Findings

Fever, malaise, recurrent or persistent jaundice, skin rash, arthritis, amenorrhea, gynecomastia, acne, pleurisy, pericarditis, or ulcerative colitis may be found in the history of these patients. Cutaneous signs of chronic liver disease may be noted (eg, spider angiomas, liver palms). Hepatosplenomegaly is frequently present. Digital clubbing may be found.

Liver function tests reveal smoldering disease with abnormal values for bilirubin, AST (SGOT), ALT (SGPT), and serum alkaline phosphatase. Serum albumin may be low. Serum gamma globulin levels are strikingly elevated (in the range of 2–6 g/dL), with reports of values as high as 11 g/dL. Low levels of C3 complement have been seen. Antibody to a liver-specific membrane lipoprotein has been found, corresponding to ongoing liver disease activity.

Histologic examination of liver biopsy specimens shows loss of the lobular limiting plate, "piecemeal" necrosis, portal fibrosis, an inflammatory reaction of lymphocytes and plasma cells in the portal areas as well as perivascularly, and some bile duct and Kupffer cell proliferation and pseudolobule formation. Cirrhosis may be present at diagnosis.

Differential Diagnosis

Laboratory and histologic findings differentiate other types of chronic hepatitis (eg, Wilson's disease, chronic persistent hepatitis, α_1-antitrypsin disease, chronic pericholangitis, subacute hepatitis). Wilson's disease and α_1-antitrypsin deficiency must be excluded if hepatitis B studies are negative. Drug-induced (isoniazid, methyldopa) chronic active hepatitis should be ruled out. In acute, severe viral hepatitis, histologic examination may also show an "aggressive" lesion early in the disease (< 3 months).

Complications

Untreated disease that continues for months to years eventually results in postnecrotic cirrhosis. Persistent malaise, fatigue, and anorexia parallel disease activity. Bleeding from esophageal varices and development of ascites usually usher in hepatic failure.

Treatment

Corticosteroids (prednisone, 2 mg/kg/d) decrease the mortality rate during the early active phase of the disease. Azathioprine, 1 mg/kg/d, is of value in decreasing the side effects of long-term corticosteroid therapy but should not be used alone during the "induction" phase of treatment. Treatment of chronic active liver disease after hepatitis B infection may include brief corticosteroid "priming" followed by interferon. Remissions occur in 75–85% of autoimmune cases. Treatment is continued for 1–2 years. Relapses are treated in a similar manner. In doubtful cases, a 3- to 6-month period of observation may be indicated prior to commencement of therapy. Liver transplantation has been used when disease progresses to cirrhosis despite therapy.

Prognosis

The overall prognosis for chronic active hepatitis has been significantly improved by early therapy. Some report cures (normal histologic findings) in 15–20% of cases. Relapses (seen clinically and histologically) occur in 40–50% of cases after cessation of therapy; remissions follow re-treatment. Survival for 10 years is common despite residual cirrhosis. Progressive portal hypertension is seen, and complications (bleeding varices, ascites) require specific therapy.

Davis GL, Czaja AJ, Ludwig J: Development and prognosis of histologic cirrhosis in corticosteroid-treated hepatitis B surface antigen-negative chronic active hepatitis. *Gastroenterology* 1984;**87**:1222.

Fitzgerald JF: Chronic hepatitis. *J Pediatr* 1984;**104**:893.

Larcher V: Chronic active hepatitis and related disorders. *Clin Gastroenterol* 1986;**15**:173.

Maddrey WC: Subdivisions of idiopathic autoimmune chronic active hepatitis. *Hepatology* 1987;**7**:1372.

Maggiore G et al: Treatment of autoimmune chronic active hepatitis in childhood. *J Pediatr* 1984;**104**:839.

CIRRHOSIS

Cirrhosis is a pathologic condition of the liver characterized histologically by the presence of extensive fibrosis associated with regenerating liver nodules. It may be micro- or macronodular in appearance. Although the severity of this process may vary from one area of the liver to the next, the whole liver is typically involved. The architectural distortion is caused by the loss of hepatocytes, replacement by scar tissue (fibrosis), and the regrowth of liver cells, a combination of events that interferes with the flow of blood through this organ. The increased resistance to blood flow produces portal hypertension and its consequences. This also affects the microcirculation to regional hepatocytes, impairing their metabolic function. This latter phenomenon may cause a self-perpetuation of the cirrhotic process by stimulating collagen deposition (fibrogenesis).

Many liver diseases may progress to cirrhosis. However, 30–50% of cases of cirrhosis have no discoverable etiology at the time of diagnosis.

Two major forms of cirrhosis are described, postnecrotic and biliary, with different etiologies, clinical symptomatology, and treatment needs. Both forms can eventually lead to liver failure and death.

In the pediatric population, postnecrotic cirrhosis most often evolves as a consequence of acute liver disease (eg, idiopathic neonatal giant-cell hepatitis, viral hepatitis type B, non-A non-B hepatitis, chronic active hepatitis, drug hepatitis) or certain inborn errors of metabolism (see Table 21–3). Cirrhosis is an exceptional outcome of acute viral hepatitis A disease. The course may be insidious, with no recognized icteric phase, as in some cases of hepatitis B virus disease, Wilson's disease, or α_1-antitrypsin deficiency. The underlying liver disease may be active, with abnormal function test results; or it may be quiescent, with only minimal derangement of liver tests. A stable cirrhosis may exist. Most cases of biliary cirrhosis are due to congenital abnormalities of the bile ducts (biliary atresia, choledochal cyst, common duct stenosis), tumors of the bile duct, Caroli's disease, Byler's disease, sclerosing cholangitis, hypoplasia of the intrahepatic bile ducts, and cystic fibrosis.

Occasionally, the disease may follow a hypersensitivity reaction to certain drugs, such as phenytoin. Parasites (*Clonorchis sinensis*, *Fasciola*, *Ascaris*) may be causative in children living in endemic areas.

Clinical Findings

A. Symptoms and Signs: In postnecrotic causes of cirrhosis, general malaise, loss of appetite, failure to thrive, and nausea are frequent complaints, especially in the anicteric varieties. Easy bruising may be reported. Jaundice may or may not be present. The first indication of underlying liver disease may be ascites, gastrointestinal hemorrhage, or even signs of hepatic encephalopathy. There may be variable hepatosplenomegaly, spider angiomas, warm skin, and red "liver" palms. A small, shrunken liver may be detected by percussion over the right chest wall that

Table 21–3. Metabolic and genetic causes of neonatal cholestasis.

Disease	Inborn Error	Hepatic Pathology	Diagnostic Studies
Galactosemia	Galactose-1-phosphate uridyltransferase	Cholestasis, steatosis, necrosis, pseudoacini, fibrosis	Galactose-1-phosphate uridyltransferase assay of red blood cells
Fructose intolerance	Fructose-1-phosphate aldolase	Steatosis, necrosis, pseudoacini, fibrosis	Liver fructose-1-phosphate aldolase assay
Tyrosinemia	Fumarylacetoacetase	Necrosis, steatosis, pseudoacini, portal fibrosis	Urinary succinylacetone, fumarylacetoacetase assay of red blood cells
Cystic fibrosis	Unknown	Cholestasis, neoductular proliferation, excess bile duct mucus, portal fibrosis	Sweat test
Hypopituitarism	Deficient production of pituitary hormones	Cholestasis, giant cells	Thyroxin, TSH, cortisol levels
Alpha$_1$-antitrypsin deficiency	Abnormal α_1-antitrypsin molecule (Pi ZZ phenotype)	Giant cells, cholestasis, steatosis, neoductular proliferation, fibrosis, PAS-diastase resistant cytoplasmic granules	Serum α_1-antitrypsin phenotype
Gaucher's disease	β-glucosidase	Cholestasis, cytoplasmic inclusions in Kupffer's cells (foam cells)	β-glucosidase assay in leukocytes
Niemann-Pick disease	Lysosomal sphingomyelinase	Cholestasis, cytoplasmic inclusions in Kupffer's cells	Sphingomyelinase assay of leukocytes or liver
Glycogen storage disease type IV	Branching enzyme	Fibrosis, cirrhosis, PAS-diastase resistant cytoplasmic inclusions	Brancher enzyme analysis of leukocytes or liver
Neonatal hemochromatosis	Unknown	Giant cells, portal fibrosis, hemosiderosis, cirrhosis	Histology, iron stains
Peroxisomal disorders (eg, Zellweger syndrome)	Deficient peroxisomal enzymes or assembly	Cholestasis, necrosis, fibrosis, cirrhosis, hemosiderosis	Plasma very long chain fatty acids, qualitative bile acids, plasmalogen, pipecolic acid, liver electron microscopy
Abnormalities in bile acid metabolism	Several enzyme deficiencies defined	Cholestasis, necrosis, giant cells	Urine, serum, duodenal fluid analyzed for bile acids by gas chromatography-mass spectroscopy

reveals resonance rather than expected dullness. Most often, the liver is slightly enlarged, especially in the subxiphoid region, where it has a firm to hard quality and an irregular edge. Ascites may be detected as shifting dullness. Gynecomastia may be noted in males. Digital clubbing is found in 10–15% of cases. Pretibial edema is often seen, reflecting underlying hypoproteinemia. In adolescent girls, irregularities of menstruation and amenorrhea may be early complaints.

In biliary cirrhosis, the patients usually have jaundice, dark urine, pruritus, and sometimes xanthoma in addition to the above clinical findings. Undernutrition and failure to thrive due to steatorrhea may be more apparent in this form of cirrhosis.

B. Laboratory Findings: In postnecrotic cirrhosis, mild abnormalities of transaminases (AST, ALT) are present, while serum protein determinations often reveal a decreased level of albumin and a variable increase in the level of gamma globulins. Prothrombin time is prolonged and usually unresponsive to vitamin K administration. ''Burr'' red cells may be noted on the peripheral blood smear. A mild anemia is present, and thrombocytopenia and leukopenia are present if hypersplenism exists.

In biliary cirrhosis, elevated conjugated bilirubin, bile acids, gamma glutamyl transpeptidase (GGTP), alkaline phosphatase, and cholesterol are commonly found. The prolonged prothrombin time may respond to vitamin K administration (1–5 mg intramuscularly).

C. Imaging: As portal hypertension complicates cirrhosis, esophageal varices may be demonstrated by endoscopy or x-ray. Small amounts of ascitic fluid can be seen by abdominal ultrasound examination. The evaluation process of biliary cirrhosis is often more involved and requires hepatobiliary scintigraphy, ultrasound scans of the biliary system, transhepatic cholangiography, or endoscopic or operative cholangiograms.

D. Pathologic Findings: Because sampling error by percutaneous needle biopsy in cirrhotic patients is high (50%), liver biopsy, preferably by laparoscopy or by surgical means, is advisable for confirmation of cirrhosis. Regenerating nodules and surrounding fibrosis are hallmarks of cirrhosis. These specific histologic features, combined with special stains, may uncover the etiologic origin in cases of posthepatitic cirrhosis. Pathologic features of biliary cirrhosis also include canalicular and hepatocyte cholestasis, as well as plugging of bile ducts. The interlobular bile ducts may be increased or decreased, depending on the cause and the stage of the disease process.

Complications & Treatment

Major complications of cirrhosis in childhood include progressive nutritional disturbances, hormonal disturbances, the evolution of portal hypertension and its vagaries, and hepatic encephalopathy (see Table 21–2). Hepatocarcinoma occurs with increased frequency in the cirrhotic liver, especially in patients with the chronic form of hereditary tyrosinemia. At present, there is no proved treatment for cirrhosis, but wherever a treatable condition is identified (such as Wilson's disease, galactosemia, congenital fructose intolerance) or an offending agent eliminated (drugs, toxins), the disease's progression can be altered; in occasional cases, regression of fibrosis has been noted. Immunosuppressive treatment in autoimmune chronic liver disease also halts the progression of cirrhosis in most cases. Surgical correction of biliary tree abnormalities can stabilize the disease process or lead to a reversal in some situations.

Prognosis

Postnecrotic cirrhosis follows an unpredictable pattern. Death occurs in the majority of patients within 10–15 years of diagnosis, usually from liver failure. A better short-term predictor is a rising bilirubin coupled with diuretic refractory ascites. These observations in a cirrhotic patient portend demise from hepatic decompensation within 6–12 months (or less). The terminal event in some patients may be generalized hemorrhage, sepsis, or cardiorespiratory arrest. For patients with biliary cirrhosis, the prognosis is good only for those with surgically corrected lesions that result in regression or stabilization of the underlying liver condition. For the remainder, this is a progressive, ultimately fatal disease. With the advent of liver transplantation, increased survival figures are to be expected when the timing for liver transplant is optimal.

Conn HO, Atterbury CE: Cirrhosis. In: *Disease of the Liver,* 5th ed. Schiff L, Schiff ER (editors). Lippincott, 1987.

ALPHA₁-ANTITRYPSIN DEFICIENCY LIVER DISEASE

Essentials of Diagnosis

- Serum α_1-antitrypsin level less than 80 mg/dL.
- Identification of specific phenotype (Pi ZZ, SZ).
- Detection of diastase-resistant glycoprotein deposits in periportal hepatocytes.
- Histologic evidence of liver disease.

- Family history of early-onset pulmonary disease or liver disease.

General Considerations

The disease is due to a deficiency in the protease inhibitor system (Pi), predisposing patients to chronic liver disease and an early onset of pulmonary emphysema. It is most often associated with the Pi phenotype ZZ. With the intermediate serum levels of α_1-antitrypsin present in the heterozygote phenotype (MZ), the incidence of liver disease in adults is only slightly greater than that in the general population despite the presence of glycoprotein deposits in hepatocytes. The exact relationship between low levels of serum α_1-antitrypsin and the development of liver disease is unclear. Emphysema develops because of a lack of inhibition of elastase, which destroys pulmonary connective tissue. Inclusion bodies in the liver contain a protein component immunologically cross-reactive with serum α_1-antitrypsin, containing excess mannose but lacking sialic acid. This structural abnormality leads to aggregation in the endoplasmic reticulum and is resistant to sialization by sialyltransferase. Although all patients with the ZZ genotype have antitrypsin inclusions in hepatocytes, it may be the only histologic evidence of liver disease. However, the likelihood of developing severe liver disease in response to hepatic injury is definitely increased in patients homozygous for this condition. From 30 to 50% of adults with α_1-antitrypsin deficiency have been found to have cirrhosis. A few children will have only pulmonary or pulmonary and hepatic involvement.

Clinical Findings

A. Symptoms and Signs: α_1-antitrypsin deficiency should be suspected in all small-for-gestational-age newborns with neonatal cholestasis. Poor appetite, lethargy, slight irritability, and jaundice suggest neonatal hepatitis but are not pathognomonic of any one cause. Hepatosplenomegaly is present. Family history may be positive for emphysema or cirrhosis.

In the older child, hepatomegaly or physical findings suggestive of cirrhosis, especially in the face of a negative history of liver disease, should always lead one to suspect α_1-antitrypsin deficiency. Recurrent pulmonary disease (bronchitis, pneumonia) may be present in a few children.

B. Laboratory Findings: Low levels (< 0.2 mg/dL) of the α_1-globulin fraction may be noted on serum protein fractionation. Specific quantitation of α_1-antitrypsin reveals levels of less than 80 mg/dL in homozygotes (ZZ) deficient in this glycoprotein. Specific Pi genotyping should be done to confirm the diagnosis. Liver function tests often reflect underlying hepatic pathologic changes. Bilirubin (mixed type), transaminases, and liver alkaline phosphatase are elevated in the acute stage, and low albumin and prolonged prothrombin time may occur in the cirrhotic stage. Hematologic assessment may reveal evidence of hypersplenism. The esophagogram or endoscopy frequently shows varices in advanced cases with portal hypertension.

Liver biopsy shows diastase-fast intracellular granules positive to periodic acid-Schiff reaction, with hyaline masses, particularly in periportal zones.

Differential Diagnosis

Other specific causes of neonatal cholestasis need to be considered, as well as causes of insidious cirrhosis in childhood (eg, viral hepatitis A or B, autoimmune chronic active hepatitis, Wilson's disease, cystic fibrosis, glycogen storage disease). If pulmonary symptoms predominate, then cystic fibrosis, immunodeficiency disease, tracheoesophageal anomalies, hiatal hernia, and hypoplastic pulmonary artery and lung disease should be considered.

Complications

Of all infants with Pi ZZ α_1-antitrypsin deficiency, only 20% develop liver disease in childhood. The complications of portal hypertension, cirrhosis, and chronic cholestasis predominate in affected children.

Early-onset pulmonary emphysema occurs in young adults (aged 30–40 years), particularly in smokers. An increased susceptibility to hepatocarcinoma has been noted in cirrhosis with α_1-antitrypsin deficiency.

Treatment

There is no specific treatment for the liver disease of this deficiency disorder. Affected infants who are breast-fed appear to have less severe liver disease. Replacement of the protein by transfusion therapy is successful in preventing pulmonary disease in affected adults. The neonatal cholestatic condition is treated with oral phenobarbital, cholestyramine, medium-chain triglyceride-containing formula, and water-miscible vitamins (see Table 21–2). Portal hypertension, esophageal bleeding, ascites, and other complications are treated as described elsewhere. Genetic counseling is indicated whenever the diagnosis is made. Diagnosis by prenatal screening is possible. Liver transplantation has been shown to cure the deficiency.

Prognosis

From 30 to 50% of patients with liver injury either die from progressive liver disease or develop cirrhosis. A correlation between histologic patterns and clinical course has been documented in the infantile form of the disease. Liver failure can be expected 5–15 years after development of cirrhosis. Decompensated cirrhosis caused by this disease is an excellent indication for liver transplantation; the survival rate is 70–85%.

Nebbia G et al: Early assessment of evolution of liver disease associated with alpha$_1$-antitrypsin deficiency in childhood. *J Pediatr* 1983;**102**:661.

Sharp HL: Alpha$_1$-antitrypsin: An ignored protein in understanding liver disease. *Semin Liver Dis* 1982;**2**:314.

Sveger T: Prospective study of children with alpha$_1$-antitrypsin deficiency: Eight-year old follow-up. *J Pediatr* 1984;**104**:91.

Wewers MD et al: Replacement therapy for alpha$_1$-antitrypsin deficiency associated with emphysema. *N Engl J Med* 1987;**316**:1055.

BILIARY TRACT DISEASE

1. CHOLELITHIASIS

Both calcium bilirubinate and cholesterol gallstones may develop at all ages in the pediatric population. Gallstone formation is a multifactorial process, the evolution of which is favored when the solubility of cholesterol (or calcium bilirubinate) in bile is exceeded. In the presence of poorly defined nucleation factors, cholesterol crystals begin to precipitate, incorporating proteins, mucus, and sometimes calcium bilirubinate as stone formation occurs. For some patients, gallbladder dysfunction is associated with biliary sludge formation, which may evolve into "sludge balls" or tumefaction bile and thence into gallstones. The process may be reversible in many patients.

Clinical Findings

A. History: Most symptomatic gallstones present with acute and recurrent episodes of moderate to severe, sharp epigastric or right upper quadrant pain. The pain may radiate substernally or to the right shoulder. On rare occasions, the presentation may include a history of jaundice, back pain, or generalized abdominal discomfort, where it is associated with pancreatitis, suggesting stone impaction in the common duct or ampulla hepatopancreatica. Nausea and vomiting may occur during attacks. Not infrequently, the pain episodes occur postprandially, and a relationship to the ingestion of fatty foods may be obtained but is not a consistent observation. The groups at risk for gallstones include the following: patients with known or suspected hemolytic disease (congenital spherocytosis, blacks with sickle cell disease); females; teenagers with prior pregnancy; obese individuals; certain racial/ethnic groups, particularly Native Americans (Pima Indians); Hispanics; and infants and children with ileal disease (Crohn's disease) or prior ileal resection. Fasting premature infants on prolonged parenteral hyperalimentation (with or without chronic furosemide therapy) are at particular risk for gallstone formation. Patients with cystic fibrosis or Wilson's disease also have an increased incidence of gallstones. Other, less certain risk factors include a positive family history, use of birth control pills, and diabetes mellitus.

B. Symptoms and Signs: During acute episodes of pain, tenderness in the upper abdomen, especially epigastric and right upper quadrant, can be elicited. Right flank pain may be noted. Referred pain is absent, as are peritoneal signs. The presence of scleral icterus should be sought. Evidence of underlying hemolytic disease in addition to icterus includes pallor (anemia), splenomegaly, tachycardia, and high-output cardiac murmur. Fever is unusual in uncomplicated cases.

C. Laboratory Findings: The white blood cell count is normal or slightly elevated. Liver function test results are not disturbed unless calculi have lodged in the extrahepatic biliary system, in which case elevated serum bilirubin and GGTP (or alkaline phosphatase) are noted. Serum pancreatic amylase may be increased if stone obstruction occurs at the ampulla hepatopancreatica.

D. Imaging: Plain abdominal x-rays are indicated in patients with acute, severe abdominal pain and may show calculi in the region of the gallbladder or bile ducts. Because most gallstones are radiolucent cholesterol stones, ultrasound evaluation is the diagnostic procedure of choice and reveals the presence of abnormal intraluminal contents (stones, sludge), as well as anatomic alterations of the gallbladder or dilatation of the biliary ductal system. The presence of an anechoic acoustic shadow differentiates calculi from intraluminal sludge or sludge balls. Gallbladder function is best assessed by cholescintigraphy methods. Abdominal CT scanning may be helpful if tumor or other neighboring disease is suspected. Endoscopic retrograde cholangiopancreatography (ERCP) is particularly helpful in defining subtle abnormalities of the bile ducts and locating intraductal stones. In selected cases, therapeutic intervention such as sphincterotomy and stone removal can be done by endoscopic means.

Differential Diagnosis

Other abnormal conditions of the biliary system with similar presentation are seen in Table 21–4. Liver disease (hepatitis, abscess, tumor, perihepatitis [Fitz-Hugh-Curtis syndrome]) can cause somewhat similar symptoms or signs. Peptic disease, reflux esophagitis, paraesophageal hiatal hernia, cardiac disease, and pneumomediastinum must be considered when the pain is epigastric or substernal in location. Renal or pancreatic disease is a possible explanation if the pain is located to the right flank or mid back. Subcapsular or supracapsular lesions of the liver (abscess, tumor, hematoma) or right lower lobe infiltrate may also be a cause of nontraumatic right shoulder pain.

Complications

Major problems are related to stone impaction in either the cystic or common duct and lead to stricture formation or perforation. Acute distention and subsequent perforation of the gallbladder may occur when gallstones cause obstruction of the cystic duct.

Exploration and surgical removal of calculi within the extrahepatic ducts requires T-tube drainage, and both procedures predispose the patient to bile duct stricture or ascending cholangitis. Stones impacted at the level of the ampulla hepatopancreatica often cause "gallstone pancreatitis."

Treatment

Symptomatic cholelithiasis is best treated by cholecystectomy. Intraoperative cholangiography via the cystic duct is required so that the physician can be certain the ductal system is free of retained stones. Gallstones developing in premature infants on total parenteral nutrition can be followed by ultrasound exam: most of the infants are asymptomatic, and the stones will resolve in 3–12 months. Gallstone dissolution using modalities such as cholelitholytics or mechanical means (lithotripsy) have not been approved for use in children. Asymptomatic gallstones can be followed expectantly because only 20% will eventually cause problems.

Prognosis

The prognosis is excellent in uncomplicated cases that come to surgery not requiring exploration and T-tube drainage of the common bile duct. Cystic duct "stump pain" is not reported to occur in the pediatric population.

Fromm H: Gallstone dissolution therapy. *Gastroenterology* 1986;**91**:1560.

Holcomb GW Jr et al: Cholecystitis, cholelithiasis and common duct stenosis in children and adolescents. *Ann Surg* 1980;**191**:626.

LaRusso NF: Pathogenesis of gallstones, including predisposing factors. *Pract Gastroenterol* 1981;**5**:21.

Somjen GJ, Gilat T: Changing concepts of cholesterol solubility in bile. *Gastroenterology* 1986;**91**:772.

2. ACUTE HYDROPS, CHOLEDOCHAL CYST, ACALCULOUS CHOLECYSTITIS, SCLEROSING CHOLANGITIS, CAROLI'S DISEASE, CONGENITAL HEPATIC FIBROSIS (See Table 21–4.)

For a schematic representation of the various types of choledochal cysts, see Fig 21–1.

Hydrops
Bowen A: Acute gallbladder dilatation in a neonate: Emphasis on ultrasonography. *J Pediatr Gastroenterol Nutr* 1984;**3**:304.

Suddleson E et al: Hydrops of the gallbladder associated with Kawasakie Syndrome. *J. Pediatr Surg* 1987;**22**:956.

Choledochal Cyst
Kim S: Choledochal cyst: Survey by the Surgical Sec-

tion of the American Academy of Pediatrics. *J Pediatr Surg* 1981;**16:**402.

Sherman P et al: Choledochal cysts: Heterogenicity of clinical presentation. *J Pediatr Gastroenterol Nutr* 1986; **5:**867.

Cholecystitis

Holcomb GW, O'Neill J Jr, Holcomb GW III: Cholecystitis, cholelithiasis and common duct stenosis in children and adolescents. *Ann Surg* 1980;**191:**626.

Sclerosing Cholangitis

LaRusso NF et al: Primary sclerosing cholangitis. *N Engl J Med* 1984;**310:**899.

Sisto A et al: Primary sclerosing cholangitis in children: Study of 5 cases and review of the literature. *Pediatrics* 1987;**80:**918.

Caroli's Disease

Fagundes-Neto U et al: Caroli's disease in childhood: Report of 2 new cases. *J Pediatr Gastroenterol Nutr* 1983;**2:**708.

Congenital Hepatic Fibrosis

Alvarez F et al: Congenital hepatic fibrosis in children. *J Pediatr* 1981;**99:**370.

Table 21–4. Biliary tract abnormalities.

	Acute Hydrops Transient Dilatation of Gallbladder	Choledochal Cyst (See Fig 21–1.)	Acalculous Cholecystitis	Sclerosing Cholangitis	Caroli's Disease (Idiopathic Intrahepatic Bile Duct Dilatation)	Congenital Hepatic Fibrosis (CHF)
Predisposing or associated conditions	Premature infants with prolonged fasting or systemic illness. Hepatitis (giant cell, viral). Abnormalities of cystic duct. Kawasaki disease.	Congenital lesion. Female sex, Asians. Extrahepatic biliary atresia, idiopathic giant cell hepatitis. Rarely with Caroli's disease or congenital hepatic fibrosis.	Systemic illness, sepsis (*Streptococcus, Salmonella, Klebsiella*, etc). Gallbladder stasis, obstruction of cystic duct (stones, nodes, tumor).	Most have chronic ulcerative colitis (70%); 75% are males. Increased incidence of HLA-B8. Sicca syndrome, fibroinflammatory conditions, familial immunodeficiency syndrome.	Congenital lesion. Also found in congenital hepatic fibrosis (CHF) or with choledochal cyst. Female sex. Autosomal recessive polycystic kidney disease.	Familial (autosomal recessive) 25% with autosomal recessive polycystic kidney disease. Choledochal cyst. Caroli's disease.
Symptoms	Absent in prematures. Vomiting, abdominal pain in older children.	Abdominal pain, vomiting, jaundice.	Acute severe abdominal pain, vomiting, fever.	Pruritus, jaundice, abdominal pain, fatigue.	Recurrent abdominal pain, vomiting. Fever, jaundice when cholangitis occurs.	Hematemesis, melena from bleeding esophageal varices.
Signs	Right upper quadrant abdominal mass. Tenderness in some.	Icterus, acholic stools, dark urine in neonatal period. Right upper quadrant abdominal mass or tenderness in older child.	Tenderness in midabdomen and right upper abdomen. Occasional palpable mass in right upper quadrant.	Icterus, hepatomegaly, splenomegaly.	Icterus, hepatomegaly.	Hepatosplenomegaly.
Laboratory abnormalities	Most are normal. Increased WBC count in sepsis (may be decreased in premature infants). Abnormal LFT's in hepatitis.	Conjugated hyperbilirubinemia, elevated GGTP, slightly increased AST. Elevated pancreatic serum amylase if ampulla hepatopancreatica is involved.	Elevated WBC, normal or slight abnormality of LFT's.	Elevated serum bile acids, bilirubin, GGTP. Slight elevation of AST.	Abnormal LFT's. Increased WBC with cholangitis. Urine abnormalities if associated with CHF.	Low platelet and WBC count (hypersplenism), slight elevation of AST, GGTP. Inability to concentrate urine.
Diagnostic studies most useful	Gallbladder ultrasound.	Gallbladder ultrasound, hepatobiliary scintigraphy, and ERCP.	Scintigraphy to confirm nonfunction of gallbladder. Ultrasound or abdominal CT scan to rule out other neighboring disease.	Ultrasound of the biliary tree, ERCP, scintigraphy.	Transhepatic cholangiography, ERCP, scintigraphy, ultrasound, intravenous pyelography.	Liver biopsy (open is best). Ultrasound liver and kidneys. Upper endoscopy, splenoportogram.
Treatment	Treatment of associated condition. Needle or tube cystostomy. Cholecystectomy seldom indicated.	Surgical resection rather than simple drainage.	Broad-spectrum antibiotic coverage, then cholecystectomy or cholecystostomy drainage and definitive surgery 3–4 weeks later.	Cholestyramine, immunosuppressive drugs, methotrexate. Liver transplant.	Antibiotics and surgical drainage for cholangitis. Liver transplant for some. Lobectomy for localized disease.	Endosclerosis of varices, portacaval shunt. Liver transplantation.

Table 21–4. (cont'd). Biliary tract abnormalities.

	Acute Hydrops Transient Dilatation of Gallbladder	Choledochal Cyst (See Fig 21–1.)	Acalculous Cholecystitis	Sclerosing Cholangitis	Caroli's Disease (Idiopathic Intrahepatic Bile Duct Dilatation)	Congenital Hepatic Fibrosis (CHF)
Complications	Perforation with bile peritonitis rare.	Progressive biliary cirrhosis. Increased incidence of cholangiocarcinoma. Cholangitis in some.	Perforation and bile peritonitis, sepsis, abscess or fistula formation. Pancreatitis.	Progressive biliary cirrhosis, portal hypertension, liver failure.	Sepsis with episodes of cholangitis, biliary cirrhosis, portal hypertension. Intraductal stones. Cholangiocarcinoma.	Bleeding from varices. Splenic rupture, severe thrombocytopenia. Progressive renal failure.
Prognosis	Excellent with resolution of underlying condition. Consider cystic duct obstruction if disorder fails to resolve.	Depends upon anatomic type of cyst, associated condition, and success of surgery. Liver transplant may be needed in some.	Good with early diagnosis and treatment.	Guarded; disease progression is expected even with medical treatment. Course not changed by colectomy. No recurrence to date after liver transplant.	Poor, with gradual deterioration of liver function. Multiple surgical drainage procedures expected. Liver transplant should alter long-term prognosis.	Good in absence of serious renal involvement and with control of portal hypertension. Slightly increased risk to cholangiocarcinoma. Liver/kidney transplant for some.

Ultrasound = refers to liver and biliary tract scanning; scintigraphy = refers to hepatobiliary scan using radiolabelled
^{99m}technetium; CHF = congenital hepatic fibrosis; ERCP = endoscopic retrograde cholangiopancreatography; LFT = liver
function test; GGTP = gamma-glutamyl transpeptidase; AST = aspartate aminotransferase (SGOT); WBC = white blood
count.

PYOGENIC & AMEBIC LIVER ABSCESS

Pyogenic liver abscesses are usually secondary to bacterial seeding via the portal vein from infected viscera and occasionally from ascending cholangitis or gangrenous cholecystitis. Solitary or mixed flora of intestinal origin (aerobes and anaerobes) are usually grown from aspirated material. Blood cultures are frequently positive in up to 60% of cases. The

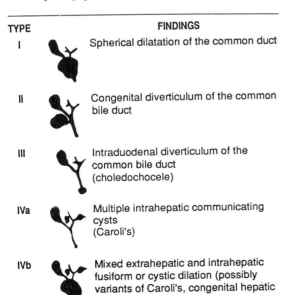

TYPE		FINDINGS
I		Spherical dilatation of the common duct
II		Congenital diverticulum of the common bile duct
III		Intraduodenal diverticulum of the common bile duct (choledochocele)
IVa		Multiple intrahepatic communicating cysts (Caroli's)
IVb		Mixed extrahepatic and intrahepatic fusiform or cystic dilation (possibly variants of Caroli's, congenital hepatic fibrosis)

Figure 21–1. Classification of cystic dilatation of the bile ducts. Types I, II and III are extrahepatic, IVa is solely intrahepatic and IVb is both intra and extrahepatic.

resulting lesion tends to be solitary and located in the right hepatic lobe. Bacterial seeding may also occur from infected burns, pyodermas, and osteomyelitis. Unusual causes include omphalitis, subacute infective endocarditis, pyelonephritis, and perinephric abscess. Multiple pyogenic liver abscesses are associated with severe sepsis. At particular risk are children receiving anti-inflammatory and immunosuppressive agents. Likewise, children with defects in white blood cell function (chronic granulomatous disease) are more prone to pyogenic hepatic abscesses, especially those due to *Staphylococcus aureus*. In adults there is a male preponderance, and the abscesses are usually solitary.

Although amebic liver abscess is still rare in children, an increase in frequency has been noted, presumably as a result of increased travel through endemic areas (Mexico, Southeast Asia). *Entamoeba histolytica* invasion occurs via the large bowel, though a history of diarrhea (colitislike picture) is not always obtained.

Clinical Findings

With pyogenic liver abscess, nonspecific complaints of low-grade to septic fever, chills, malaise, and abdominal pain are frequent. Weight loss is very common, especially in delayed diagnosis. A few patients have shaking chills and jaundice. The dominant complaint is a constant dull pain over an enlarged liver that is tender to palpation. An elevated hemidiaphragm with reduced or absent respiratory excursion may be demonstrated on physical examination and confirmed by fluoroscopy. Laboratory studies show leukocytosis and, at times, anemia. Liver function tests reveal low-grade bilirubin elevation and an elevated alkaline phosphatase. Elevated vitamin B_{12} levels are reported. Amebic liver abscesses are usually heralded by an acute illness with high fever, chills, and leukocytosis. Early in the course, liver tests may suggest mild hepatitis. An occasional prodrome may include cough, dyspnea, and shoulder pain as rupture of the abscess into the right chest occurs. Consolidation of the right lower lobe is common (30%).

Ultrasound liver scan is the most useful diagnostic aid in evaluating pyogenic and amebic abscesses, detecting lesions as small as 1–2 cm. Nuclear scanning with gallium or technetium sulfur colloid or CT imaging may be useful to differentiate tumor or hydatid cyst.

The distinction between pyogenic and amebic abscesses is best made by indirect hemagglutination test (which is positive in more than 95% of patients with amebic liver disease) and the prompt response of the latter to antiamebic therapy (metronidazole). Examination of material obtained by needle aspiration of the abscess using ultrasound guidance is often diagnostic.

Differential Diagnosis

Hepatitis, hepatoma, hydatid cyst, gallbladder disease, or biliary tract infections can mimic liver abscess. Subphrenic abscesses, empyema, and pneumonia may give a similar picture. Inflammatory disease of the intestines or of the biliary system may be complicated by liver abscess.

Complications

Spontaneous rupture of the abscess may occur with extension of infection into the subphrenic space, thorax, peritoneal cavity, and, occasionally, the pericardium. Bronchopleural fistula with large sputum production and hemoptysis can develop in severe cases. Simultaneously, the amebic liver abscess may be secondarily infected with bacteria (10–20% of cases). Metastatic hematogenous spread to the lungs and brain has been reported.

Treatment

When a solitary pyogenic liver abscess is suspected, needle aspiration using ultrasound guidance should be attempted. The decision regarding surgical drainage versus antibiotic treatment alone is best made on clinical grounds. Cultures (aerobic and anaerobic) are taken and specific antibiotic therapy started. Both solitary and multiple pyogenic liver abscesses can be treated by medical means.

Amebic abscesses should be treated promptly. Only those that are sufficiently large and threaten to rupture need to be aspirated. Uncomplicated cases can be treated with oral metronidazole, 30–50 mg/kg/d in 3 divided doses for 10 days. Intravenous metronidazole can be used in patients unable to take oral medication. In severe cases, give dehydroemetine, 1–1.5 mg/kg/d intramuscularly for 5 days, and

chloroquine, 10–20 mg/kg/d in one or 2 divided doses for 21 days. Failure to improve after 72 hours on drug therapy indicates superimposed bacterial infection or an incorrect diagnosis. At this point, needle aspiration or surgical drainage is indicated. Once oral feedings can be tolerated, a 10-day course of diloxanide furoate (20 mg/kg/d in 3 doses) is started as a luminal amebicide. Resolution of the abscess cavity occurs over 3–6 months.

Prognosis

An unrecognized and untreated pyogenic liver abscess is universally fatal. The surgical cure rate is about 75%. Most amebic abscesses are cured with conservative medical management; the mortality rate is less than 3%. If extrahepatic complications occur (empyema, bronchopleural fistula, pericardial complications), 10–15% of patients will succumb.

Berger LA, Osborne DR: Treatment of pyogenic liver abscesses by percutaneous needle aspiration. *Lancet* 1982; **1**:132.

Harrison HR, Crowe CP, Fulginiti VA: Amebic liver abscess in children: Clinical and epidemiologic features. *Pediatrics* 1979;**64**:923.

Herbert DA et al: Pyogenic liver abscesses: Successful nonsurgical therapy. *Lancet* 1982;**1**:134.

Knight R: Hepatic amebiasis. In: *Seminars in Liver Disease: Infectious Agents as Causes of Liver Diseases.* Vol 4. Burke PD, Zuckerman AJ (editors). Thieme-Stratton, 1984.

Thompson JE Jr, Forlenza S, Verma R: Amebic liver abscess: A therapeutic approach. *Rev Infect Dis* 1985; **7**:171.

PREHEPATIC PORTAL HYPERTENSION

Essentials of Diagnosis

- Splenomegaly.
- Esophageal varices with hematemesis or melena.
- Elevated splenic pulp pressure.
- Normal wedge hepatic vein pressure.
- Normal liver histology.
- Impaired patency of splenic and portal veins shown by duplex doppler ultrasound scanning, splenoportography, and venous phase of superior mesenteric or splenic aortography.

General Considerations

Prehepatic portal hypertension from acquired abnormalities of the portal and splenic veins accounts for 5–8% of cases of gastrointestinal bleeding in children. A history of neonatal omphalitis, sepsis, dehydration, and umbilical vein catheterization is present in 30–50% of cases. Less common known causes in older children include local trauma, peritonitis (pylephlebitis), and pancreatitis. Symptoms may occur before 1 year of age, but in most cases the diagnosis is not made until 3–5 years of age.

Those with a positive neonatal history tend to become symptomatic earlier. Splenomegaly is often the first abnormal physical finding. Massive hematemesis or melena occurs within a few years.

A variety of portal or splenic vein malformations, some of which may be congenital, have been described, including valves and atretic segments. "Cavernous" transformation is probably the result of attempted collateralization about the thrombosed portal vein rather than a congenital malformation. The site of the venous obstruction may be anywhere from the hilum of the liver to the hilum of the spleen. Proper studies are necessary to differentiate this condition from those with intrahepatic but presinusoidal portal hypertension (hepatoportal sclerosis, idiopathic portal hypertension, noncirrhotic portal fibrosis, schistosomiasis, congenital hepatic fibrosis).

Clinical Findings

A. Symptoms and Signs: Splenomegaly in an otherwise well child is the most constant physical sign. Recurrent episodes of abdominal distention due to ascites may also be noted. The usual presenting symptoms are hematemesis and melena. An episode of bronchitis, tracheitis, or pneumonia with significant cough can precipitate esophageal bleeding. The presence of prehepatic portal hypertension is suggested by the following: (1) an episode of severe infection in the newborn period or early infancy—especially omphalitis, sepsis, gastroenteritis, severe dehydration, or prolonged or difficult umbilical vein catheterizations; (2) no previous evidence of liver disease; and (3) a history of well-being prior to onset or recognition of symptoms. In addition, transient ascites may occur following a bleeding episode.

B. Laboratory Findings and Imaging: Most other common causes of splenomegaly may be excluded by proper laboratory tests. Cultures, Epstein-Barr virus titers, blood smear examination, bone marrow studies, and liver function tests are necessary. Hypersplenism with mild leukopenia, and thrombocytopenia are present in most cases. Fiberoptic esophagoscopy will reveal varices in symptomatic patients. In addition to normal liver function tests, confirmation of a normal liver is best obtained directly by liver biopsy or indirectly by measurement of wedge hepatic vein pressure (normal, 3–12 mm Hg). The finding of an elevated splenic pulp pressure (normal, 8–12 mm Hg) and demonstration of the block by simultaneous splenic portography confirm the diagnosis of prehepatic portal hypertension. Filling of collateral vessels to stomach and esophagus by the dye is frequently demonstrated. Selective arteriography using the superior mesenteric artery is recommended prior to definitive surgery to determine the patency of the superior mesenteric vein. Hypercoagulability due to antithrombin III, protein C, or protein S deficiency should be considered in the "idiopathic group."

Differential Diagnosis

All causes of splenomegaly must be included in the differential diagnosis, the most common ones being infections, blood dyscrasias, lipidosis, reticuloendotheliosis, cirrhosis of the liver, and cysts or hemangiomas of the spleen. When hematemesis or melena occurs, other causes of gastrointestinal bleeding are possible, ie, gastric or duodenal ulcers, tumors, Meckel's diverticulum, duplications, inflammatory bowel disease, and suprahepatic or hepatic venous obstructions.

Complications

The major manifestation and complication of this condition is bleeding esophageal varices. Fatal exsanguination appears to be uncommon, but hypovolemic shock or resulting anemia may require prompt treatment. Congestive splenomegaly with granulocytopenia and thrombocytopenia occurs but seldom causes major symptoms. Rupture of the enlarged spleen due to trauma is always a threat. Unexplained fluctuating episodes of ascites may develop, and retroperitoneal edema has been reported (Clatworthy's sign).

Treatment

A. Surgical Measures: Except in specialized centers, the surgical treatment of this disease has been disappointing. Portacaval anastomosis would be the most satisfactory procedure, but the portal vein is often involved in the basic disease process, making it unsuitable for anastomosis except in rare cases. Children have previously been treated by means of simultaneous splenectomy and splenorenal shunts. Sustained patency of the shunt is unlikely in children under the age of 8–10 years except when placed by an experienced surgeon. Thrombosis of the shunt is soon followed by recurrent and often more severe hemorrhage from esophageal varices. Splenectomy increases the risk of overwhelming sepsis. More importantly, however, it removes a "safe" group of collateral vessels running from the splenic capsule to the azygos veins, thereby bypassing the esophageal and gastric drainage system. Partial splenectomy or splenic embolization of one-third to one-half of the organ reduces concerns about traumatic rupture and improves the leukopenia and thrombocytopenia.

Other surgical decompression procedures include anastomosis of the superior mesenteric vein to the inferior vena cava (mesocaval shunt), distal splenorenal shunt (Warren procedure), and the interposition mesocaval shunt using knitted Dacron or Teflon for the graft. Esophageal and gastric resection of the varices and transthoracic ligation of the varices have been used as more desperate measures.

B. Medical Treatment: Because a few children with this disease will die as a result of esophageal bleeding, every effort should be made to control the disease medically. The chances for successful surgical shunting procedures improve as the child gets older. In addition, the patient may spontaneously develop a decompressive shunt adequate to prevent major bleeding from the esophageal varices.

Spontaneous cessation of hemorrhage from esophageal varices occurs frequently. Shock must be treated with crystalloid or colloid and then with blood transfusions. Platelet transfusions may be indicated if counts are below 10,000 mm³. Gastric irrigation with iced 0.5% saline solution may help.

Early fiberoptic endoscopy is indicated to confirm the source of hemorrhage and, if possible, permit immediate treatment of ongoing bleeding. Intravariceal or paravariceal injection of a sclerosing agent is otherwise carried out within 2–3 days after cessation of bleeding via the endoscope or via a rigid esophagoscope. Additional sclerosing sessions may be needed to control the acute bleeding. Thereafter, elective sclerotherapy is utilized to attempt obliteration of the varices.

A transient reduction of portal venous pressure may be achieved by the use of intravenous vasopressin. A dose of 0.1–0.3 unit/min given intravenously often stops the bleeding by constricting the splanchnic and hepatic arterioles and lowering portal venous pressure. Hypertension, bradycardia, diminished cardiac output, water retention, hyponatremia, and pulmonary edema may occur with this form of treatment. Careful use of a pediatric Sengstaken-Blakemore tube can effectively stop the bleeding in over 90% of cases. In desperate cases, selective venous embolization can be life-saving but requires a minilaparotomy for access to the vessel in question.

An intravenous H₂ blocking agent is employed during the acute episode to reduce gastric acid output and its erosive effect on the varices by way of gastroesophageal reflux. Antitussive agents (eg, codeine) may be used when cough is excessive. Avoidance of contact sports in the presence of splenomegaly is advisable. Aspirin products should be avoided. Propranolol, a β-adrenergic antagonist, may reduce the risk of subsequent bleeding by lowering venous pressure in the portal drainage system.

Prognosis

The prognosis depends upon the site of the block, the effectiveness of sclerotherapy, the availability of suitable vessels for shunting procedures, and the experience of the surgeon. Each unsuccessful surgical procedure worsens the prognosis for life. In patients managed by medical means, bleeding episodes seem to diminish with adolescence.

The prognosis in patients managed by medical and supportive therapy may be better than in the surgically treated group, especially when surgery is performed at an early age. Portacaval encephalopathy is unusual in the postshunted child except when protein intake is excessive.

Alvarez F et al: Portal obstruction in children. (2 parts.) *J Pediatr* 1983;**103**:696, 703.

Bernard O et al: Portal hypertension in children. *Clin Gastroenterol* 1985;**14**:33.

Mowat AP: Prevention of variceal bleeding. *J Pediatr Gastroenterol Nutr* 1986;**5**:679.

SUPRAHEPATIC & INTRAHEPATIC (NONCIRRHOTIC) PORTAL HYPERTENSION

In the absence of cirrhosis, suprahepatic or intrahepatic causes of portal hypertension are rare. The following entities should be considered:

(1) Suprahepatic vein occlusion or thrombosis (Budd-Chiari syndrome): In most instances, no cause can be demonstrated. Endothelial injury to hepatic veins by bacterial endotoxins has been shown experimentally. The occasional association of hepatic vein thrombosis in inflammatory bowel disease favors the presence of endogenous toxins traversing the liver. Allergic vasculitis leading to endophlebitis of the hepatic veins has been occasionally described. In addition, hepatic vein obstruction may be secondary to tumor, abdominal trauma, hyperthermia, or sepsis, or it may occur following the repair of an omphalocele or gastroschisis. Congenital vena caval bands, webs, membrane, or strictures above the hepatic veins are sometimes causative. Hepatic vein thrombosis may be a complication of oral contraceptive medications. Underlying thrombotic conditions (antithrombin III, protein C, or protein S deficiency) should be considered.

(2) Intrahepatic veno-occlusive disease (acute stage): This entity is often the result of ingestion of pyrrolizidine alkaloids ("bush tea"), which causes widespread occlusion of the small- and medium-sized hepatic veins, with congestion and necrosis of the neighboring parenchymal cells. A familial form of the disease occurs in congenital immunodeficiency states. The disorder may develop after chemotherapy for acute leukemia. Veno-occlusive disease is being seen with increased frequency in patients who have undergone bone marrow transplantation.

The acute form of the disease generally follows a nonspecific respiratory illness. The disease may be rapidly fatal, although about 50% of patients recover. A subacute and chronic form also exists. Increased use of herbal teas in the USA has been responsible for several reported cases.

(3) Congenital hepatic fibrosis: This rare cause of intrahepatic presinusoidal portal hypertension is inherited as an autosomal recessive and usually requires open liver biopsy for diagnosis (see Table 21–4). Splenoportography reveals patency of the portal venous system even though splenic pulp pressure is increased. The intrahepatic branches of the portal vein may be abnormal (duplicated). Renal abnormalities (microcystic disease) are often associated with the hepatic lesion; therefore, renal ultrasound and urography should be routinely performed.

(4) Hepatoportal sclerosis (idiopathic portal hypertension, noncirrhotic portal fibrosis), noncirrhotic nodular transformation of the liver, and schistosomal hepatic fibrosis: These are also rare causes of intrahepatic presinusoidal portal hypertension.

Clinical, Laboratory, & Radiographic Findings

Most patients with suprahepatic portal hypertension present with abdominal enlargement due to ascites. Some have firm hepatomegaly. Abdominal pain and tender hepatosplenomegaly are frequently found. Jaundice is present in about 25% of cases. Vomiting hematemesis, and diarrhea are less common. Cutaneous signs of chronic liver disease are lacking because the obstruction is usually acute. The presence of distended superficial veins on the back and anterior abdomen, along with dependent edema, is usually seen with inferior vena cava obstruction. Absence of hepatojugular reflux (jugular distention when pressure is applied to the liver) is a helpful clinical sign. Liver function tests are not usually helpful; liver function tends to be better preserved in this disorder than in the membranous obstruction of the Budd-Chiari syndrome. Localization is difficult. An inferior venacavogram using catheters from above or below the suspected obstruction may reveal an intrinsic filling defect, an infiltrating tumor, or extrinsic pressure and obstruction of the inferior vena cava by an adjacent lesion. A large caudate lobe of the liver suggests Budd-Chiari syndrome. Care must be taken in interpreting extrinsic pressure defects of the subdiaphragmatic inferior vena cava in the face of significant ascites.

Duplex doppler-assisted ultrasound scanning of the suprahepatic inferior vena cava and the hepatic veins may be diagnostic of intrinsic disease. Simultaneous wedge hepatic vein pressure and hepatic venography are also useful procedures. Obstruction to major hepatic vein ostia and smaller vessels may be demonstrated by this procedure. In the absence of obstruction, reflux across the sinusoids into the portal vein branches can be accomplished. Pressures should also be taken from the right heart and supradiaphragmatic portion of the inferior vena cava. These should eliminate constrictive pericarditis and pulmonary hypertension from the differential diagnosis. Hepatic vein pressure is elevated to a greater degree than portal vein and splenic pulp pressure. In most instances, a liver biopsy should be done. Marked central venous congestion and necrosis without fibrosis are striking. Endothelial thickening of hepatic veins may also be found.

Differential Diagnosis

Because ascites is almost always present, cirrhosis due to any cause must be excluded. Suprahepatic (cardiac and pulmonary) or prehepatic causes of portal hypertension must also be excluded. Although ascites may occur in prehepatic portal hypertension, it is not common.

Complications

Without treatment, complete and persistent hepatic vein obstruction leads to liver failure, coma, and death. A nonportal type of cirrhosis may develop in the chronic form of hepatic veno-occlusive disease in which small- and medium-sized hepatic veins are affected. Hematemesis due to bleeding esophageal varices is frequent in the few survivors. Death from renal failure may occur in rare cases of congenital hepatic fibrosis.

Treatment

Efforts to correct underlying causes must be undertaken promptly. Surgical removal of the occluding tumor or of the hepatic vein thrombi is possible when the large ostia are involved. Transcardiac membranotomy can be attempted when the obstruction lies in the inferior vena cava. Mesocaval and portacaval shunts and right atrial to inferior vena cava grafts have been attempted. Liver transplant should be seriously considered in refractory cases not amenable to surgical correction. Medical management with heparin, corticosteroids, and diuretics has had inconsistent results. Simple portacaval shunting is the treatment of choice in patients with congenital hepatic fibrosis and may be done prophylactically or after an esophageal bleed.

Prognosis

The mortality rate of hepatic vein obstruction is very high—95%. In veno-occlusive disease, the prognosis is better, with complete recovery possible in 50% of acute forms and 5–10% of subacute forms.

Etzioni A et al: Defective humoral and cellular immune functions associated with veno-occlusive disease of the liver. *J Pediatr* 1987;**110:**549.

Gentil-Kocher S et al: Budd-Chiari syndrome in children: Report of 22 cases. *J Pediatr* 1988;**113:**30.

Shulman HM et al: An analysis of hepatic venocclusive disease and centrilobular hepatic degeneration following bone marrow transplantation. *Gastroenterology* 1980; **79:**1178.

HEPATOMAS

Essentials of Diagnosis

- Abdominal enlargement and pain, weight loss, anemia.
- Hepatomegaly with or without a definable mass.
- Laparotomy and tissue biopsy.

General Considerations

Primary epithelial neoplasms of the liver represent 0.2–5.8% of all malignant conditions in the pediatric age group. After Wilms's tumor and neuroblastoma, it is the third most common intra-abdominal cancer. The incidence is higher in Southeast Asia, where childhood cirrhosis is more common. There are 2 basic morphologic types with certain clinical and prognostic differences. Hepatoblastoma predominates in male infants and children, with most cases appearing before age 3. Most lesions are found in the right lobe of the liver. Pathologic differentiation from hepatocarcinoma may be difficult.

Hepatocarcinoma, the other major malignant tumor of the liver, occurs more frequently after age 3. This type of neoplasm carries a poorer prognosis than hepatoblastoma and causes more abdominal discomfort. Hepatocarcinoma has been reported in chronic carriers of hepatitis B virus and in those with postnecrotic cirrhosis or biliary cirrhosis, but these are the exceptions rather than the rule. Patients with glycogen storage disease type I have an increased risk to hepatic adenoma and carcinoma. The association of hepatocarcinoma with tyrosinemia and α_1-antitrypsin deficiency cirrhosis has also been reported. The late development of hepatoma in patients treated with androgens for de Toni-Fanconi syndrome and aplastic anemia must also be kept in mind. The increased use of anabolic steroids by body-conscious adolescent patients poses a risk of hepatic neoplasia. An interesting aspect of primary epithelial neoplasms of the liver has been the increased incidence of associated anomalies and unusual conditions found in these children. Virilization has been reported as a consequence of gonadotropin activity of the tumor. Feminization with bilateral gynecomastia may occur in association with high estradiol levels in blood, the latter a consequence of increased aromatization of circulating androgens by the liver. Leydig cell hyperplasia without spermatogenesis is found on testicular biopsy. Hemihypertrophy, congenital absence of the kidney, macroglossia, and Meckel's diverticulum have been found in association with hepatocarcinoma.

Clinical Findings

A. History: Noticeable increase in abdominal girth with or without pain is the most constant feature of the history. A parent may note a "bulge" in the upper abdomen or report feeling a hard mass. Constitutional symptoms (anorexia, fatigue, fever, chills, etc) may be present. A teenage male may complain of gynecomastia.

B. Symptoms and Signs: Weight loss, pallor, and abdominal pain associated with a large abdomen are common. Physical examination reveals hepatomegaly with or without a definite tumor mass, usually to the right of the midline. Signs of chronic liver disease are usually absent. However, evidence of virilization or feminization in prepubertal children may be noted.

C. Laboratory Findings: Normal to slightly distorted liver function tests are the rule. Anemia is frequently seen, especially in cases of hepatoblastoma. Cystathioninuria has been reported. Alpha-fetoprotein levels may be elevated, especially in hepatoblastoma. Elevated estradiol levels are sometimes seen. Final tissue diagnosis is best obtained at laparotomy, though some physicians utilize skinny needle aspiration of the liver mass guided either by ultrasound or CT.

D. Imaging: Plain abdominal x-ray is at times helpful in demonstrating the tumor shadow or calcified foci in the neoplasm. Both ultrasound and CT scanning are useful for diagnosis and for following tumor response to therapy. Magnetic resonance imaging has similar capability, but experience in pediatric patients is limited. A scintigram study of bone and lung and selective angiography are generally part of the preoperative workup to evaluate metastatic disease.

Differential Diagnosis

In the absence of a palpable mass, the differential diagnosis is that of hepatomegaly with or without anemia or jaundice. Hematologic and nutritional conditions should be ruled out, as well as α_1-antitrypsin deficiency disease, lipid storage diseases, histiocytosis X, glycogen storage disease, congenital hepatic fibrosis, hepatic abscess (pyogenic or amebic), cysts, adenoma, focal nodular hyperplasia, and hemangiomas. If fever is present, hepatic abscess (pyogenic or amebic) must be considered. Veno-occlusive disease and hepatic vein thrombosis are also rare possibilities. Tumors in the left lobe may be mistaken for pancreatic pseudocysts.

Complications

Progressive enlargement of the tumor, abdominal discomfort, ascites, respiratory difficulty, and widespread metastases (especially to lungs and abdominal lymph nodes) are the rule. Rupture of the neoplastic liver and intraperitoneal hemorrhage have been reported. Progressive anemia and emaciation predispose the patient to an early septic death.

Treatment

An energetic surgical approach has brought forth the only long-term survivors. Complete resection of the lesion offers the only chance for a cure. It appears that every isolated lung metastasis should also be surgically resected. Radiotherapy and chemotherapy have been disappointing in the treatment of primary liver neoplasms, although new combinations of drugs are continually being evaluated. These modalities are also used for initial cytoreduction of tumors found unresectable at time of primary surgery. Second-look celiotomy has in some cases allowed resection of the tumor, resulting in a reduced mortality rate. Organ transplantation has been disappointing but continues to be performed in selected patients. The survival rate may be better for those patients in which the tumor is incidental to another disorder (tyrosinemia, biliary atresia, cirrhosis).

Prognosis

The survival rate if the tumor is completely removed is 60% for hepatoblastoma and 33% for hepatocellular carcinoma. Fibrolamellar oncocytic hepatocarcinoma has a more favorable prognosis. The overall survival and cure rate is less than 20%.

Ehren H, Mahour GH, Isaacs H: Benign liver tumors in infancy and childhood. *Am J Surg* 1983;**145**:325.

Giacomantonio M et al: Thirty years of experience with pediatric primary malignant liver tumors. *J Pediatr Surg* 1984;**19**:523.

Mahour GH et al: Improved survival in infants and children with primary malignant liver tumors. *Am J Surg* 1983;**146**:236.

Weinberg AG, Finegold MJ: Primary hepatic tumors of childhood. *Hum Pathol* 1983;**14**:512.

WILSON'S DISEASE
(Hepatolenticular Degeneration)

Essentials of Diagnosis

- Acute or chronic liver disease.
- Deteriorating neurologic status.
- Kayser-Fleischer rings.
- Elevated liver copper.
- Abnormalities in levels of ceruloplasmin and serum and urine copper.

General Considerations

In Wilson's disease, the increased hepatic copper may be due to an abnormal copper-binding protein or to a lysosomal defect that impairs the excretion of biliary copper. The disease should be considered in all children with evidence of liver disease or with suggestive neurologic signs. A family history is often present, and 25% of cases are identified by screening asymptomatic homozygous family members.

Clinical Findings

A. Symptoms and Signs: Hepatic involvement may be fulminant, may masquerade as chronic active liver disease, or may progress insidiously to postnecrotic cirrhosis. Findings include jaundice, hepatomegaly early in childhood, splenomegaly, Kayser-Fleischer (K-F) rings, and neurologic manifestations such as tremor, dysarthria, and drooling beginning after 10 years of age. Deterioration in school performance is often the earliest neurologic expression of disease. The K-F rings can sometimes be detected by unaided visual inspection as a brown band at the junction of the iris and cornea, but slit lamp examination is usually necessary. Absence of K-F rings does not exclude this diagnosis unless neurologic signs are present.

B. Laboratory Findings: The laboratory diagnosis is sometimes difficult. Serum ceruloplasmin levels are usually less than 20 mg/dL. (Normal values are 23–43 mg/dL.) Low values, however, are seen normally in infants under 3 months of age, and in 3–5% of homozygotes the levels may be low-normal. Serum copper levels are low, but the overlap with normal is too great for satisfactory discrimination. Urine copper excretion in children over 3 years of age is normally less than 30 μg/d; in Wilson's disease, it is greater than 100 μg/d. Finally, the tissue content of copper from a liver biopsy, normally less than 20 μg/g wet tissue, is greater than 50 μg/g in Wilson's disease.

Glycosuria, aminoaciduria, and depressed serum uric acid levels have been reported. Hemolysis and, on rare occasions, gallstones may be present; bone lesions simulating those of osteochondritis dissecans have also been found.

The coarse nodular cirrhosis and glycogen nuclei seen on liver biopsy may distinguish Wilson's disease from other types of cirrhosis. Early in the disease, vacuolation of liver cells, fatty degeneration, and lipofuscin granules can be seen, as well as Mallory bodies. The presence of the latter in a child is strongly suggestive of Wilson's disease. Stains for copper may sometimes be negative despite high copper content in the liver.

Differential Diagnosis

During the icteric phase, acute viral hepatitis, α_1-antitrypsin deficiency, chronic active hepatitis, Indian childhood cirrhosis, and drug-induced hepatitis are the unusual diagnostic possibilities. Later, other causes of cirrhosis and portal hypertension need consideration. Laboratory testing for the specific factors listed above will differentiate Wilson's disease from the others. The radiocopper ceruloplasmin incorporation test is sometimes needed to differentiate Wilson's disease with a normal ceruloplasmin level from other liver disease with increased liver and urine copper values.

Complications

Progressive liver disease and hepatic coma and death are not uncommon. Recovery from the initial episode usually results in cirrhosis of the postnecrotic type. The complications of portal hypertension (variceal hemorrhage, ascites) are poorly tolerated by these patients. Progressive degenerating central nervous system disease and terminal aspiration pneumonia are common in untreated older people. Acute hemolytic disease may result in renal impairment and profound jaundice as part of a presentation of fulminant hepatitis.

Treatment

Penicillamine, 900–1200 mg/d orally, is the drug of choice in all cases, whether symptomatic or not. It is best to begin with 250 mg/d and increase the dose weekly by 250-mg increments. The target dose is 20 mg/kg/d. Dietary restriction of copper intake is not practical. Supplementation with zinc sulfate may negate this problem. Penicillamine is continued for life, although doses may be transiently reduced at the time of surgery. Vitamin B_6 (25 mg) is given daily to prevent optic neuritis. For patients who cannot tolerate penicillamine, trientine hydrochloride is effective at a dose of 1–1.5 g/d.

General treatment measures for acute hepatitis are as outlined for infectious hepatitis. Portacaval shunting may be contraindicated in Wilson's disease. Liver transplantation is indicated for all cases of acute fulminant disease, progressive hepatic decompensation despite several months of penicillamine, and severe progressive hepatic insufficiency in patients who suddenly discontinue penicillamine therapy.

Prognosis

The prognosis of untreated Wilson's disease is poor. Without transplantation, all patients with the fulminant presentation succumb. Copper chelation reduces hepatic copper content and reverses many of the liver lesions, but it does not have a profound effect on established cirrhosis. Neurologic symptoms generally respond to therapy. All siblings should be immediately screened and homozygotes treated with copper chelation even if asymptomatic.

Perman JA et al: Laboratory measures of copper metabolism in the differentiation of chronic active hepatitis and Wilson's disease in children. *Pediatrics* 1979;**94:**564.

Saito T: Presenting symptoms and natural history of Wilson's disease. *Eur J Pediatr* 1987;**146:**261.

Scheinberg IH, Sternlieb I: *Wilson's Disease.* Saunders, 1984.

Sokol RJ et al: Orthotopic liver transplantation for acute fulminant Wilson's disease. *J Pediatr* 1985;**107:**549.

Werlin SL et al: Diagnostic dilemmas of Wilson's disease: Diagnosis and treatment. *Pediatrics* 1978;**62:**47.

REYE'S SYNDROME
(Encephalopathy With Fatty Degeneration of the Viscera; White Liver Disease)

Essentials of Diagnosis

- Prodromal upper respiratory tract infection, influenza A or B illness, or chickenpox.
- Vomiting.
- Lethargy, drowsiness progressing to semicoma.
- Elevated AST (SGOT), hyperammonemia, normal or slightly elevated bilirubin, prolonged prothrombin time.

- Variable hypoglycemia.
- Microvesicular steatosis of liver, kidneys, brain, etc.

General Considerations

The number of reported cases of Reye's syndrome is decreasing, perhaps owing to a decline in the use of salicylates among younger children, who seem to be at greater risk. Persistent attempts to implicate a single etiologic factor have failed. Varicella, influenza A and B, echovirus 2, coxsackie A virus, reovirus, and Epstein-Barr virus have been isolated from some patients. Epidemics of Reye's syndrome seem to cluster during influenza B epidemics. Toxic causes (insecticides, herbicides, aflatoxins), drugs (salicylates), and metabolic causes (defects in the urea cycle) have also been implicated. The mode of onset may lead to confusion with other causes of coma, particularly toxic encephalopathy and hepatic coma.

The mechanism is thought to be damage to mitochondria caused by salicylate metabolites or some other toxin/chemical in the milieu of a viral infection. Mitochondrial dysfunction leads to elevated short-chain fatty acids and hyperammonemia, as well as directly to cerebral edema.

Clinical Findings

A. Symptoms and Signs: Most cases give a history of chickenpox or minor upper respiratory tract illness of short duration preceding the development of vomiting, irrational behavior, progressive stupor, and coma. Restlessness and convulsions may also occur. Striking physical findings are hyperpnea, irregular respirations, and dilated, sluggishly reacting pupils. Jaundice is minimal or absent. The liver may be normal or slightly enlarged. If the prodrome has been prolonged, the liver may be small. Splenomegaly is absent. A positive Babinski sign, hyperreflexia, and decorticate and decerebrate posturing are consistent with severe cerebral edema.

B. Laboratory Findings: Cerebrospinal fluid is acellular, and cerebrospinal fluid glucose may be low in younger patients. Cerebrospinal fluid pressure is variably elevated. The serum glucose is proportionately decreased. Moderate to severe elevations of AST (SGOT), ALT (SGPT), and lactate dehydrogenase are found. Serum bilirubin and alkaline phosphatase values are normal to slightly elevated. The prothrombin time is usually prolonged, and the blood ammonia is usually elevated. A mixed respiratory alkalosis and metabolic acidosis is seen. In a few cases, the blood urea nitrogen has been elevated. Hyperaminoacidemia (glutamine, alanine, lysine) and hypocitrullinemia are present.

Histopathologic changes in Reye's syndrome are most striking in the brain, liver, and kidneys, less so in the heart and pancreas. The brain shows gross cerebral edema, occasionally with evidence of herniation.

Histologically, loss of neurons and fatty vacuolation around small vessels has been noted. The liver shows diffuse microvesicular steatosis with minimal inflammatory changes. Glycogen is virtually absent from the hepatocytes in biopsies taken before giving hypertonic glucose. Ultrastructural changes are mitochondrial.

The kidney changes include swelling and fatty degeneration of the proximal lobules.

C. Electroencephalography: The EEG shows diffuse slow-wave activity.

Differential Diagnosis

Differentiation of Reye's syndrome from acute toxic encephalopathy, hepatic coma, or fulminant hepatitis can be made on clinical and laboratory grounds. A negative history and urine screen for ingestion of poisons and drugs, absence of cells in the cerebrospinal fluid, and absence of jaundice favor a diagnosis of Reye's syndrome. The fatty acid oxidation defects (eg, medium-chain acyl-CoA dehydrogenase deficiency) and other metabolic disorders may resemble Reye's syndrome; urine organic and amino acid analysis will help differentiate them. Liver biopsy and electromicroscopy can be diagnostic, and the procedure is indicated in atypical cases.

Complications

Aspiration pneumonitis and respiratory failure are common, as with any comatose patient. Most patients die of cerebral edema rather than hepatic or renal failure. Cardiac dysrhythmias may develop, as may inappropriate vasopressin excretion, diabetes insipidus, and acute pancreatitis.

Treatment

Treatment is supportive. A nasogastric tube, Foley catheter, and arterial and central venous pressure lines should be inserted immediately. Mechanical ventilation may become necessary if the patient reaches stage III coma (Lovejoy). Intracranial pressure (ICP) should be monitored directly and kept below 15–20 mm Hg, and systemic blood pressure should be kept sufficiently high to maintain cerebral perfusion pressure above 45–50 mm Hg. Hyperventilation, mannitol infusions (0.5–1 g/kg every 4 hours), or ventricular drainage is used to lower ICP. At times, urea (1 g/kg intravenously) or glycerol (1.5 g/kg by nasogastric tube) is required. Maintenance fluids using 10% glucose should be given at a rate sufficient to produce a urine flow of 1–1.5 mL/kg/h. Careful attention to central venous pressure is needed when using hyperosmolar agents. Exchange transfusions have been used with success. Vitamin K, 3–5 mg intramuscularly, should be administered. Hypothermia (30–33 °C) and pharmacologic doses of pentobarbital (10–50 mg/kg/d) have been employed

to decrease body (brain) metabolic needs during the period of uncontrolled intracranial pressure.

Prognosis

At least 70% of these patients survive. The prognosis is related to the depth of coma and the peak ammonia level on admission. Severe neurologic residuals are not uncommon in the younger children (< 2 years) who recover from prolonged stage III-IV coma. If relapse occurs, the patient should be screened for other metabolic defect.

Arrowsmith JB et al: National patterns of aspirin use and Reye's syndrome reporting, United States, 1980 to 1985. *Pediatrics* 1987;**79**:858.

Delong GR, Glick TH: Encephalopathy of Reye's syndrome: A review of pathogenetic hypotheses. *Pediatrics* 1982;**69**:53.

Heubi JE et al: Grade I Reye's syndrome: Outcome and predictors of progression to deeper coma grades. *N Engl J Med* 1984;**311**:1539.

Hurwitz ES et al: Public Health Service study on Reye's syndrome and medications. *N Engl J Med* 1985; **313**:849.

Orlowski JP et al: A catch in the Reye. *Pediatrics* 1987; **80**:638.

Shaywitz BA, Rothstein P, Venes JL: Monitoring and management of increased intracranial pressure in Reye's syndrome: Results in 29 patients. *Pediatrics* 1980; **66**:198.

LIVER TRANSPLANTATION

Orthotopic liver transplantation is no longer considered experimental. Children with end-stage liver disease or complications from metabolic liver disorders should be considered for liver transplantation. Recent advances in immunosuppression (eg, introduction of cyclosporine), better candidate selection, improvements in surgical techniques, and experience in postoperative management have contributed to improved results.

The major indications for childhood transplantation are (1) a failed Kasai operation or decompensated cirrhosis caused by extrahepatic biliary atresia, (2) α_1-antitrypsin deficiency, (3) posthepatitic cirrhosis, (4) tyrosinemia, (5) Crigler-Najjar syndrome type I, (6) Wilson's disease, (7) acute fulminant hepatic failure when recovery is unlikely, and (8) cases in which the consequences of chronic cholestasis severely impair the patient's quality of life. Children should be referred early for transplantation evaluation, because the limiting factor for success is the small donor pool. Pared-down adult livers are being used in children in several centers. In general, 65–85% of children survive at least 1–2 years after transplantation, with long-term survival expected to be comparable. Lifetime immunosuppression therapy using combinations of cyclosporine, prednisone, or azathioprine, with its incumbent risks, is necessary to prevent rejection. Overall quality of life for children with transplanted livers appears to be excellent.

Malatack JJ et al: Choosing a pediatric recipient for orthotopic liver transplantation. *J Pediatr* 1987;**111**:479.

Shaw BW et al: Liver transplantation therapy for children. (2 parts.) *J Pediatr Gastroenterol Nutr* 1988;**7**:157, 797.

Zitelli BJ et al: Changes in life-style after liver transplantation. *Pediatrics* 1988;**82**:173.

Zitelli BJ et al: Orthotopic liver transplantation in children with hepatic-based metabolic disease. *Transplant Proc* 1983;**15**:1284.

PANCREAS

ACUTE PANCREATITIS

Most cases of acute pancreatitis are due to drugs, viral infections, systemic diseases, or accidental or nonaccidental abdominal trauma, although more than 20% are idiopathic. Other cases resulting in obstruction to pancreatic flow include stones in the ampulla hepatopancreatica, choledochal cysts, tumors of the duodenum, pancreas divisum, and ascariasis. The exact mechanism(s) by which intra-acinar or intraductal activation of pancreatic zymogens occurs remains a controversial topic. Acute pancreatitis has been seen with high-dosage corticosteroid therapy and administration of sulfasalazine, thiazides, valproic acid, azathioprine 6-mercaptopurine, L-asparaginase, and other drugs. It may also occur in cystic fibrosis, systemic lupus erythematosus, α_1-antitrypsin deficiency, diabetes, Crohn's disease, glycogen storage disease type I, hyperlipidemia types I and V and familial (hereditary) cases, hyperparathyroidism, Schönlein-Henoch purpura, Reye's syndrome, Kawasaki disease, chronic renal failure, and during rapid refeeding in cases of malnutrition. Alcohol-induced pancreatitis should be considered in the teenage patient.

Clinical Findings

A. Symptoms and Signs: An acute onset of persistent (hours to days), severe upper abdominal and midabdominal pain occasionally referred to the back, with vomiting and fever, is the common presenting picture. The abdomen is tender but not rigid, and bowel sounds are diminished, suggesting peritoneal irritation. Abdominal distention is common in infants and younger children. In cases due to trauma, an abdominal mass that is suggestive of pseudocyst may be felt. Jaundice is unusual. Ascites may be noted, and a left-sided pleural effusion is present in some. Cullen's and Grey Turner's signs indicate hemorrhagic pancreatitis.

B. Laboratory Findings: Leukocytosis and an elevated serum (greater than 1½–2 times normal) and urine amylase should be expected early, except in infants under 6 months of age who may have hypoamylasemia. Serum lipase is elevated and persists longer than serum amylase. The immunoreactive trypsinogen test may also be of value. Hyperglycemia (serum glucose > 300 mg/dL), hypocalcemia, falling hematocrit, rising blood urea nitrogen, hypoxemia, and acidosis may all occur in severe cases and impart a poor prognosis.

C. Imaging: Plain x-ray films of the abdomen may show a localized ileus (sentinel loop). Ultrasonography shows decreased echodensity of the gland in comparison to the left lobe of the liver. Pseudocyst formation can also be seen early in the course. CT scanning is better for detecting pancreatic phlegmon or abscess formation. Endoscopic retrograde pancreatography may be useful in confirming patency of the main pancreatic duct in cases of abdominal trauma or in revealing stones, strictures, pancreas divisum, etc.

Differential Diagnosis

Other causes of acute upper abdominal pain include lesions of the stomach, duodenum, liver, and biliary system; acute gastroenteritis or atypical appendicitis; pneumonia; volvulus; intussusception; and nonaccidental trauma.

Complications

Complications early in the disease include shock due to fluid and electrolyte disturbances, ileus, and hypocalcemic tetany. Impairment of oxygenation and respiratory distress (pancreatic lung) may require assisted ventilation in some patients. Hypervolemia is seen between the third and fifth days, at which time renal tubular necrosis may occur. The gastrointestinal, neurologic, musculoskeletal, hepatobiliary, dermatologic, and hematologic systems may also be involved.

Later, 5–10% of patients develop a pseudocyst heralded by recurrence of abdominal pain and rise in the serum amylase. From 15 to 25% of these will resolve spontaneously. Infection, hemorrhage, rupture, fistulization, or obstruction may occur. Phlegmon formation is frequently seen (30–50%) and may extend from the gland into the retroperitoneum or into the lesser sac. Most regress, but some require drainage. Infection in this inflammatory mass is a constant threat. Pancreatic abscess formation is fortunately rare (3–5%) and develops 2–3 weeks after the initial insult. Fever, leukocytosis, and pain occur; diagnosis is by ultrasound or CT scanning.

Chronic pancreatitis, pancreatic insufficiency, and pancreatic lithiasis are rare sequelae of acute pancreatitis.

Treatment

Medical management includes rest, gastric suction, fluids, electrolyte replacement, and blood or colloid as needed. Peritoneal lavage is still being evaluated in severe cases. Pain should be controlled with meperidine. Oxygen may be required if desaturation occurs. An H_2 blocker helps to maintain gastric neutrality at a pH greater than 4.5. Nutrition is provided by the parenteral route. Broad-spectrum antibiotic coverage is employed only in severe hemorrhagic pancreatitis. Recurrence of pain after oral feedings may be prevented by giving pancreatic enzymes with the meal.

Surgical treatment is reserved for traumatic disruption of the gland, intraductal stone, unresolved or infected pseudocysts or abscesses, and other anatomic obstructive lesions. Drugs known to produce acute pancreatitis should be discontinued.

Prognosis

In the pediatric age group, the prognosis is surprisingly good with conservative management. The mortality rate is 5–10% in patients treated by operation and 1% in those treated medically. The morbidity rate is high in the surgical group as a result of fistula formation.

Siegel MJ, Martin KW, Worthington JL: Normal and abnormal pancreas in children: US studies. *Radiology* 1987;**165**:15.

Weizman Z, Durie PR: Acute pancreatitis in childhood. *J Pediatr* 1988;**113**:24.

Ziegler DW et al: Pancreatitis in childhood. *Ann Surg* 1988;**207**:256.

CHRONIC PANCREATITIS

Two forms of chronic pancreatitis have been reported: chronic fibrosing pancreatitis and the more common familial autosomal dominant chronic relapsing pancreatitis.

The causes include stenotic lesions of the ampulla hepatopancreatica, strictures of the pancreatic ducts, intraductal stones, or persisting pseudocyst following acute pancreatitis. The role of pancreas divisum in chronic pancreatitis remains controversial. Chronic disease rarely follows acute nontraumatic pancreatitis. Choledochal and duplication cysts may give rise to episodes of pancreatitis before they are recognized as the cause of the pancreatitis. Hyperlipidemias (types I and V), hyperparathyroidism, and cystic fibrosis should be considered.

In hereditary pancreatitis, the morphologic findings are not specific. The ductus pancreaticus is dilatated but not obstructed.

Clinical Findings

The diagnosis of the hereditary form is usually not made in childhood unless there is a similar history in other family members. The diagnosis of chronic fibrosing pancreatitis is made by surgical exploration

demonstrating a normal duct system and typical histologic findings in the pancreatic biopsy.

A. Symptoms and Signs: There is usually a history of recurrent upper abdominal pain of variable severity but prolonged (1–6 days) duration. Radiation of the pain into the back is a frequent complaint. Fever and vomiting are not common in the chronic form. Abnormal stools and symptoms of diabetes may develop later in the course of this disease, and malnutrition due to failure of pancreatic exocrine secretions may also occur.

B. Laboratory Findings: The serum or urine amylase is usually elevated during the early acute attacks. Pancreatic insufficiency and reduced volume and bicarbonate response may be found at duodenal intubation after intravenous administration of synthetic cholecystokinin (0.2 μg/kg) and secretin (2 units/kg). A 3-fold increase of normal serum amylase values is considered a positive test for obstruction. An indirect screening test for pancreatic insufficiency, bentiromide, a synthetic peptide, measures urine excretion of the chymotrypsin cleaved marker *p*-aminobenzoic acid (PABA). Normal subjects excrete over 50% of the ingested dose, with some overlap occurring in normal and diseased patients who have mild pancreatic insufficiency.

Blood lipids and urinary amino acids are elevated in familial forms of the disease associated with hyperlipoproteinemia and should be studied in all cases. Elevated blood glucose levels and glycosuria are frequently found in protracted disease. Sweat chloride should be checked for cystic fibrosis and serum calcium for hyperparathyroidism.

C. Imaging: X-rays of the abdomen may show pancreatic or gallbladder calcifications. Contrast studies may demonstrate other obstructive lesions in the region of the duodenum. Endoscopic retrograde cholangiopancreatography (ERCP) is a helpful tool in the nonsurgical diagnosis. Pancreatograms show ductal dilatation, stones, strictures, or stenotic segments.

Differential Diagnosis

Other causes of recurrent abdominal pain must be considered. Specific causes such as hyperparathyroidism, systemic lupus erythematosus, infectious disease, and ductal obstruction by tumors, stones, or helminths must be excluded by appropriate tests.

Complications

Disabling abdominal pain, steatorrhea, nutritional deprivation, and diabetes are the most frequent long-term complications. Pancreatic carcinoma occurs more frequently in hereditary pancreatitis, especially in patients with calcifications within the gland.

Treatment

When the hereditary form of chronic pancreatitis is suspected or proved, medical management of acute attacks is indicated (see Acute Pancreatitis, above). If ductal obstruction is strongly suspected, surgical exploration should be undertaken if endoscopic means of therapy fail (balloon dilatation, stone removal, sphincterotomy). Pancreatography and cholangiography can also be performed at laparotomy. Sphincterotomy and biopsy are recommended even when obvious obstruction is not found. Relapses seem to occur in most patients. Orally ingested pancreatic enzymes at mealtime may reduce pain episodes in some patients. The daily injection of a somatostatin analog has shown promise in relieving pain episodes and decreasing the serum amylase of some patients. Pseudocysts may be marsupialized to the surface or drained into the stomach or into a loop of jejunum in those failing to regress spontaneously. Prophylactic total or subtotal pancreatic resection is advocated by some workers.

Prognosis

In the absence of a correctable lesion, the prognosis is not good. Disabling episodes of pain, pancreatic insufficiency, and diabetes may ensue. Narcotic addiction and suicide are risks in teenagers with disabling disease.

Ghishan FK et al: Chronic relapsing pancreatitis in childhood. *J Pediatr* 1983;**102**:514.

Niederau C, Glendell JH: Diagnosis of chronic pancreatitis. *Gastroenterology* 1985;**88**:1973.

GASTROINTESTINAL & HEPATOBILIARY MANIFESTATIONS OF CYSTIC FIBROSIS

Cystic fibrosis is a disease with protean manifestations. Although pulmonary and pancreatic involvement dominates the clinical picture for most patients (see Chapter 15), a variety of other organs can be involved. Table 21–5 lists the important gastrointestinal, pancreatic and hepatobiliary conditions that may affect cystic fibrosis patients and includes their respective clinical findings, incidence, most useful diagnostic studies, and preferred treatment.

Park RW, Grand RJ: Gastrointestinal manifestations of cystic fibrosis: A review. *Gastroenterology* 1981;**81**:1143.

Roy CC et al: Hepatobiliary disease in cystic fibrosis: A survey of current issues and concepts. *J Pediatr Gastroenterol Nutr* 1982;**1**:469.

Rubenstein S, Moss R, Lewiston N: Constipation and meconium ileus equivalent in patients with cystic fibrosis. *Pediatrics* 1986;**78**:473.

Scott RB, O'Loughlin EV, Gall DG: Gastroesophageal reflux in patients with cystic fibrosis. *J Pediatr* 1985;**106**:223.

Stern RC, Rothstein FC, Doershuk CF: Treatment and prognosis of symptomatic gallbladder disease in patients with cystic fibrosis. *J Pediatr Gastroenterol Nutr* 1986;**5**:35.

PANCREATIC EXOCRINE HYPOPLASIA & CHRONIC NEUTROPENIA (Shwachman Syndrome)

This uncommon disease, characterized by diarrhea and failure to thrive, is due to pancreatic exocrine insufficiency. Pathologically, there is widespread fatty replacement of the gland acinar tissue. This is easily recognized on abdominal CT scan. There is no fibrosis or inflammation, and the pancreatic ducts appear to be normal. The islet cells are spared. There is evidence that the disease is genetically determined.

The history of failure to thrive, diarrhea, fatty stools, and, in most cases, freedom from respiratory infections should make one suspect this entity. Important laboratory findings include normal sweat electrolytes but absent or reduced pancreatic lipase, amylase, and trypsin on duodenal intubation. Leukopenia is often present, and the thrombocyte count is sometimes depressed. Small bowel is normal on histologic examination, and studies of absorption not dependent upon pancreatic enzymes yield normal results. The bone marrow is typically hypocellular, showing a "maturation arrest" of the granulocyte series. Metaphyseal dysostosis and an elevated fetal hemoglobin may occur. Immunoglobulin deficiencies and hepatic dysfunction are also reported in some cases.

Normal sweat electrolytes and a negative history of repeated pulmonary infections differentiate this disease from cystic fibrosis. Small bowel biopsy supported by absorption tests, particularly with D-xylose, distinguishes the disorder from celiac disease. Cases of isolated lipase or enterokinase deficiency may be more difficult to distinguish by functional tests alone. The association of exocrine pancreatic insufficiency with congenital anomalies (aplastic alae nasi, aplasia cutis, deafness) needs to be recognized. Cyclic neutropenia, transient neutropenia, and pancreatic exocrine hypofunction due to viral causes must be considered.

The complications and sequelae of deficient pancreatic enzyme secretion are malnutrition, diarrhea, and growth failure. The degree of steatorrhea may lessen with age. Intragastric lipolysis mainly due to lingual lipase may be the compensatory mechanism in patients with low or absent pancreatic function. The major sequela seems to be short stature, although long-term follow-up are not available. Increased numbers of infections may be the results of chronic neutropenia. Neutrophil mobility is also impaired in many patients and perhaps contributes to their susceptibility to infections.

Pancreatic enzyme replacement therapy has been fairly successful, although some patients get along without it. The prognosis appears to be good for those able to survive the increased number of bacte-

Table 21–5. Gastrointestinal and hepatobiliary manifestations of cystic fibrosis.

Organ	Condition	Symptoms	Age of Presentation	Incidence	Diagnostic Evaluation	Management
Esophagus	Gastro-esophageal reflux, esophagitis	Pyrosis, dysphagia, epigastric pain, hematemesis.	School age and older.	10–20%	Endoscopy and biopsy, overnight pH study.	H_2 blocker, antacids, surgical antireflux procedure.
	Varices	Hematemesis, melena.	Childhood and adolescents.	3–10%	Endoscopy, barium swallow.	Endosclerosis, drugs (see p 595), portacaval shunt, liver transplant.
Stomach	Gastritis	Upper abdominal pain, vomiting, hematemesis.	School age and older.	10–25%	Endoscopy and biopsy.	H_2 blockers, antacids.
	Hiatal hernia	Reflux symptoms (see above), epigastric pain.	School age and older.	3–5%	Endoscopy, barium swallow.	As above. Surgery in some.
Intestine	Meconium ileus	Abdominal distention, bilious emesis.	Neonate.	10–15%	X-ray studies, plain abdominal films; contrast enema shows microcolon. Neonatal CF screening test (immunoreactive trypsinogen [IRT]), then sweat chloride test.	Dislodgement of obstruction with gastrografin enema. Surgery if unsuccessful or if case complicated by atresia, perforation, or volvulus.
	Meconium ileus equivalent syndrome	Abdominal pain, acute and recurrent; distention; occasional vomiting.	Any age, usually school age through adolescence.	10–15%	Palpable mass in right lower quadrant, x-ray studies.	Gastrografin enema, intestinal lavage solution, diet, bulk laxatives, adjustment of pancreatic enzyme intake.
	Intussusception	Acute, intermittent abdominal pain; distention; emesis.	Infants through adolescence.	1–3%	X-ray studies, barium enema.	Reduction by barium enema or surgery if needed, diet, bulk laxatives. Adjustment of pancreatic enzyme intake.
	Rectal prolapse	Anal discomfort, rectal bleeding.	Infants and children to age 4–5 years.	15–25%	Visual mass protruding from anus.	Manual reduction, adjustment of pancreatic enzyme dosage, reassurance as problem resolves by age 3–5 years.
	Carbohydrate intolerance	Abdominal pain, flatulence, continued diarrhea with adequate replacement therapy.	Any age.	10–25%	Intestinal mucosal biopsy and disaccharidase analysis. Breath hydrogen after lactose load.	Reduce lactose intake; reduction of gastric hyperacidity if mucosa shows partial villous atrophy. Beware concurrent celiac disease or *Giardia* infection.
Pancreas	Total exocrine insufficiency	Diarrhea, steatorrhea, malnutrition, failure to thrive. Specific fat-soluble vitamin deficiency states.	Neonate through infancy.	80–90%	Quantitative sweat chloride iontophoresis test.	Pancreatic enzyme replacement, elemental formula, fat-soluble vitamin supplements.
	Partial exocrine insufficiency	Occasional diarrhea, mild growth delay.	Any age.	5–10%	Sweat test, 72-hour fecal fat evaluation, direct pancreatic function tests.	Pancreatic enzyme replacement in selected patients. Fat-soluble vitamin supplements as indicated by biochemical evaluation.
	Pancreatitis	Recurrent abdominal pain, vomiting.	Older children through adolescence.	0.1%	Increase serum lipase and amylase, pancreatic provocative test, endoscopic pancreatogram.	Addition of pancreatic enzymes to feeds, endoscopic removal of sludge or stone(s) if present, endoscopic papillotomy.
	Diabetes	Weight loss, polyuria, polydipsia.	Older children through adolescence.	5–7%	Glucose tolerance test and insulin levels.	Diet, insulin.

Table 21–5 (cont'd). Gastrointestinal and hepatobiliary manifestations of cystic fibrosis.

Organ	Condition	Symptoms	Age of Presentation	Incidence	Diagnostic Evaluation	Management
Liver	Steatosis	Hepatomegaly.	Neonates and infants, but some cases are seen at all ages.	15–30%	Liver biopsy.	Improved nutrition, replacement of pancreatic enzymes and vitamins.
	Focal biliary cirrhosis	Hepatomegaly.	Infants and older patients.	20–25%	Liver biopsy.	As above. Taurine supplements (still experimental).
	Multilobular biliary cirrhosis	Hepatosplenomegaly, hematemesis from esophageal varices; hypersplenism, jaundice, ascites late in course.	School age through adolescence.	1–3%	Liver biopsy, endoscopy.	Improved nutrition, endosclerosis of varices, splenic embolization, liver transplantation.
	Neonatal jaundice	Cholestatic jaundice hepatomegaly; often seen with meconium ileus.	Neonates.	0.1–1%	Neonatal CF screening (IRT), sweat chloride test, liver biopsy.	Nutritional support, special formula with medium-chain triglyceride-containing oil, pancreatic enzyme replacement.
Gallbladder	Microgallbladder	None.	Congenital—present at any age.	15–20%	Ultrasound or by hepatobiliary scintigraphy.	None needed.
	Cholelithiasis	Recurrent abdominal pain, rarely jaundice.	School age through adolescence.	3–5%	Ultrasound, CT scan.	Surgery if symptomatic and low risk, trial of cholelitholytics or lithotripsy in others.
Extrahepatic Bile Ducts	Obstruction Intraluminal (sludge, stones, tumor)	Jaundice, hepatomegaly, abdominal pain.	Neonates, then older children through adolescence	Rare in neonates (< 0.01%)	Ultrasound and hepatobiliary scintigraphy, endoscopic cholangiography, surgery.	Surgery in neonates, endoscopic intervention in older patients or surgery.
	Extraluminal (intrapancreatic compression, tumor)	As above.	As above.	Rare (< 0.01%)	As above.	Surgical biliary drainage procedure or biliary stint placement endoscopically.
	Stenosis	As above.	As above.	1–40%	As above.	Endoscopic balloon dilatation, surgical drainage procedure.

rial infections early in life. However, an increased incidence of leukemia has been noted in these patients.

Aggett PJ: Shwachman's syndrome *Arch Dis Child* 1980;**55**:331.

Hill RE et al: Steatorrhea and pancreatic insufficiency in Shwachman's syndrome *Gastroenterology* 1982;**83**:22.

Woods WG et al: The occurrence of leukemia in patients with the Shwachman syndrome. *J Pediatr* 1981;**99**:425.

ISOLATED EXOCRINE PANCREATIC ENZYME DEFECT

Normal premature infants and most newborns produce little if any pancreatic amylase following meals or exogenous hormonal stimulation. This temporary physiologic insufficiency may persist for the first 3–6 months of life and be responsible for diarrhea when complex carbohydrates (cereals) are introduced into their diet.

Congenital pancreatic lipase deficiency and congenital colipase deficiency are extremely rare disorders, causing diarrhea and variable malnutrition with malabsorption of dietary fat and fat-soluble vitamins. The sweat chloride iontophoresis test is normal, and neutropenia is absent. Treatment involves use of oral replacement of pancreatic enzymes and a low-fat diet or formula containing medium-chain triglycerides.

Exocrine pancreatic insufficiency of proteolytic enzymes (trypsinogen, trypsin, chymotrypsin, etc) is in fact due to enterokinase deficiency, a duodenal mucosal enzyme required for activation of the pancreatic proenzymes. These patients present with malnutrition associated with hypoproteinemia and edema but are free of respiratory symptoms and have a normal sweat test. They respond to pancreatic enzyme replacement therapy and feeding formulas that contain a case in hydrolysate (eg, Nutramigen or Pregestimil).

Gaskin KJ et al: Colipase and lipase secretion in childhood-onset pancreatic insufficiency. *Gastroenterology* 1984;**86**:1.

Table 21–6. Pancreatic Tumors.

	Age	Major Findings	Diagnosis	Treatment	Associated Conditions
Insulinoma	After age 3–4	Hypoglycemia, seizures; high serum insulin; abdominal pain and mass infrequent	Ultrasound, CT scan	Surgery	
Adenocarcinoma	Any age	Epigastric pain, mass, weight loss, anemia, biliary obstruction	Ultrasound, CT scan	Surgery	Hereditary (calcific) pancreatitis
Gastrinoma	Over age 5–8	Male sex, gastric hypersecretion, peptic symptoms, multiple ulcers, gastrointestinal bleeding, anemia, diarrhea	Elevated fasting gastrin and postsecretin suppression test (>300 pg/mL), CT scan, MRI, laparotomy	Histamine H_2 blockers, omeprazole, surgical resection, total gastrectomy	Zollinger-Ellison syndrome, multiple endocrine neoplasia syndrome type I, neurofibromatosis
Vipoma	Any age	Secretory diarrhea, hypokalemia, weight loss	Elevated vasoactive intestinal polypeptide (VIP) levels; sometimes, elevated serum gastrin and pancreatic polypeptide	Surgery	
Glucagonoma	Older patients	Necrolytic rash, diarrhea, anemia, thrombotic events	Elevated glucagon, gastrin, VIP	Surgery	

Ghishan FK et al: Isolated congenital enterokinase deficiency. *Gastroenterology* 1983;**85**:727.

Lebenthal E: The development of pancreatic function in premature infants after milk-based and soy-based formulas. *Pediatr Res* 1981;**15**:1240.

PANCREATIC TUMORS

Pancreatic tumors, whether benign or malignant, are rare lesions. They most often arise from duct or acinar epithelium (malignant adenocarcinoma) or from islet (endocrine) components within the gland, such as the benign insulinoma (adenoma) derived from beta cells. Other pancreatic tumors also originate from these pluripotential endocrine cells (gastrinoma, vipoma, glucagonoma). These malignant lesions produce diverse symptoms, because they release biologically active polypeptides from this ectopic location. The clinical features of these tumors are summarized in Table 21–6. The differential diagnosis of these abdominal tumors includes Wilms's tumor, neuroblastoma, and malignant lymphoma.

Tersigni R et al: Pancreatic carcinoma in childhood: Case report of long survival and review of the literature. *Surgery* 1984;**96**:560.

Wolfe MM, Jensen RT: Zollinger-Ellison syndrome. *N Engl J Med* 1987;**317**:1200.

Wynick D, Williams SJ, Bloom SR: Symptomatic secondary hormone syndromes in patients with established malignant pancreatic endocrine tumors. *N Engl J Med* 1988;**319**:605.

SELECTED REFERENCES

Alagille D, Odievre M: *Liver and Biliary Tract Disease in Children.* Wiley, 1978.

Gryboski J, Walker A: *Gastrointestinal Problems in the Infant,* 2nd ed. Saunders, 1983.

Lebenthal E (editor): Pediatric gastroenterology. (2 parts.) *Pediatr Clin North Am* 1988;**35**:1, 215.

Mowat A: *Liver Disorders in Childhood.* Butterworth, 1979.

Schiff L, Schiff ER: *Diseases of the Liver,* 6th ed. Lippincott, 1987.

Silverman A, Roy CC: *Pediatric Clinical Gastroenterology,* 3rd ed. Mosby, 1983.

22

Kidney & Urinary Tract

Gary M. Lum, MD

EVALUATION OF THE KIDNEY & URINARY TRACT

HISTORY

When renal disease is suspected, a careful history should elicit the following: (1) family history of cystic disease, hereditary nephritis, deafness, dialysis, or transplantation; (2) preceding acute or chronic illnesses (eg, urinary tract infection, pharyngitis, impetigo, or endocarditis); (3) rashes or joint pains; (4) growth delay or failure to thrive; (5) polyuria, polydipsia, enuresis, frequency, or dysuria; (6) hematuria or discolored urine; (7) pain (abdominal, costovertebral angle, or flank) or trauma; (8) sudden weight gain or edema; and (9) drug or toxin exposure. In the newborn or small infant, additional information should be obtained regarding birth history, eg, prenatal ultrasonographic studies, birth asphyxia, Apgar scores, oligohydramnios, dysmorphic features, abdominal masses, voiding patterns, anomalous development, and umbilical artery catheterization.

PHYSICAL EXAMINATION

Certain aspects of the physical examination deserve emphasis. General appearance is noted, with attention to height, weight, skin lesions (café au lait or ash leaf spots), pallor, edema, or skeletal deformities. Anomalies of the ears or eye defects may be associated with renal disease, as are anomalies of the external genitalia. The blood pressure should be carefully measured in a quiet setting. The cuff should cover two-thirds of the child's upper arm, and peripheral pulses should be noted. An ultrasonic device is useful for measurements in infants. The abdomen should be palpated, with careful attention to the kidneys, abdominal masses, musculature, and the presence of ascites.

LABORATORY EVALUATION OF RENAL FUNCTION

Urinalysis

A carefully performed urinalysis is the keystone in the evaluation of possible renal disease. Commercially available dipsticks can be used to screen for the presence of blood and protein and to approximate the pH. Such detection, however, must be followed by a careful microscopic examination of the urinary sediment. The use of low illumination and a urine stain facilitates the examination. Casts should be sought at the periphery of the coverslip. Bacteria and cells are studied with the high-power objective. Crystals should be carefully described. The urine, if collected properly, can be sent for culture when indicated.

Serum Analysis

The standard indicators of renal function are serum levels of creatinine and urea nitrogen. The ratio of blood urea nitrogen to creatinine is normally about 10:1. The ratio may increase in cases where renal perfusion or urine flow is decreased, because blood urea nitrogen levels are more affected by these and other factors (eg, nitrogen intake, catabolism, use of tetracyclines) than are creatinine levels. Therefore, the most reliable, easily assessed blood indicator of glomerular function is the serum level of creatinine.

Most laboratories report a "normal" range of serum creatinine. However, the majority of small children should have serum creatinine levels well under 0.8 mg/dL, and only the larger adolescents should have levels exceeding 1 mg/dL. Thus, one must interpret with caution the "normal" creatinine levels reported because incremental increases in these lower levels of creatinine reflect significant decreases in glomerular filtration rate (GFR). For example, serum creatinine increasing from 0.5 mg/dL to 1 mg/dL represents a 50% decrease in GFR.

Less precise but nonetheless important indicators of the presence of renal disease are abnormalities of serum electrolytes, pH, calcium, phosphorus, magnesium, albumin, or serum complement.

Measurement of Glomerular Filtration Rate (GFR)

The determination of GFR is of paramount importance in the evaluation of suspected renal disease or in the serial follow-up of the child with established renal insufficiency.

An estimate of GFR may be attained by measurements of the endogenous creatinine clearance (C_{Cr})

in milliliters per minute. A 24-hour urine collection is usually obtained; however, in small children from whom collection is difficult, a 12-hour daytime specimen, collected when urine flow rate is greatest, is acceptable. The procedure for collecting a quantitative urine specimen should be carefully explained so that the parent or patient understands fully the rationale of (1) first emptying the bladder (discarding that urine) and noting the time; and (2) putting all urine subsequently voided into the collection receptacle, including the last void, 12 or 24 hours later. Reliability of the 24-hour collection can be approximated by measurement of the total 24-hour creatinine excretion in the specimen. Total daily creatinine excretion in milligrams per kilogram of the patient's weight (creatinine index) should be in the range of 14–20. If the creatinine index does not fall within this range, collections may be inadequate or excessive. Calculation by the following formula requires measurements of plasma creatinine (P_{Cr}) in milligrams per milliliter, urine creatinine (U_{Cr}) in milligrams per milliliter, and urine volume (V) expressed as milliliters per minute.

$$C_{Cr} = \frac{U_{Cr} \, V}{P_{Cr}}$$

Creatinine is a reflection of body muscle mass. Because accepted ranges of normal creatinine clearance are based on adult parameters, "correction" for size is needed to determine normal ranges in children. Clearance is "corrected" to a standard body surface area of 1.73 m², as shown in the following formula:

$$\text{"Corrected" } C_{Cr} = \frac{\text{Patient's } C_{Cr} \times 1.73 \text{ m}^2}{\text{Patient's body surface area}}$$

Although 80–125 mL/min/1.73 m² is considered a normal range for creatinine clearance, estimates in the lower end of this range may nonetheless suggest problems.

A simple and tested formula for quick approximation of creatinine clearance incorporates the use of the plasma creatinine level and the child's length in centimeters:

$$C_{Cr} \text{ (mL/min/1.73 m}^2) = \frac{0.55 \times \text{Height in cm}}{P_{Cr} \text{ in mg/dL}}$$

Note: This formula takes into consideration an expression of body surface area; thus, further correction is not necessary. Use 0.45 × length in centimeters in newborns less than 1 year old. This method of calculation is not meant to detract from the importance of clearance determinations but is of great help to the clinician who desires a quick estimate of the appropriateness of a suspect level of plasma creatinine.

Counahan R et al: Estimation of glomerular filtration rate from plasma creatinine concentration. *Arch Dis Child* 1976;**51**:875.
Schwartz GJ et al: Plasma creatinine and urea concentration in children: Normal values for age and sex. *J Pediatr* 1976;**88**:828.

Urine Concentrating Ability

Inability to concentrate urine is often the first sign of chronic renal failure and is very often a factor responsible for severe dehydration and the concomitant "prerenal" picture seen in children with chronic renal failure. A history of polyuria, polydipsia, or enuresis raises doubts concerning the ability to concentrate the urine, thus suggesting chronic renal failure. Except under unusual circumstances, a first morning void is expected to be concentrated and can be screened with a specific gravity analysis. Evaluation of other abnormalities of urinary concentration or dilution is discussed under specific disease entities.

Evaluation of Hematuria & Proteinuria

Hematuria and proteinuria deserve special emphasis because they are hallmarks of possibly significant glomerular alterations. In children with *asymptomatic* hematuria or proteinuria, the search for renal origins will yield the most results.

Initial detection of hematuria, usually by dipstick but at times by the appearance of the urine, should be followed by confirmation with careful microscopic analysis. The presence of red cell casts supports the diagnosis of glomerulonephritis, but the absence of casts does not rule out the disease.

Poststreptococcal glomerulonephritis is the most commonly suspected entity in the differential diagnosis of childhood glomerulonephritis; therefore, associated streptococcal infections should be considered and ruled out on the basis of antistreptolysin, streptozyme, and serum complement tests. However, other infections can also elicit this mechanism, thereby producing glomerulonephritis. Furthermore, asymptomatic presentations of microhematuria may also indicate the presence of other forms of glomerular disease (see Table 22–1).

Special serologic and immunologic studies, such as tests for antinuclear antibodies, anti-DNA antibodies, serum cryoglobulins, immune complexes, complement components, immunoglobulins, antiglomerular basement membrane antibodies, and hepatitis-associated antigen, are useful in diagnosing various glomerulonephritides and may be appropriate in evaluating hematuria.

The diagnosis of benign hematuria therefore becomes one of exclusion and includes the entity of benign familial hematuria. It is interesting to note that included in this group may be children who are found to have asymptomatic hypercalciuria as an explanation for their hematuria.

Table 22–1. Glomerular diseases encountered in childhood.

Entity	Clinical Course	Prognosis
Postinfection Glomerulonephritis (GN). Onset occurs 10–14 days after acute illness, commonly streptococcal. Characteristics include acute onset, tea-colored urine, mild to severe renal insufficiency (severe insufficiency is rare), edema.	Acute phase is usually over in 2 wks. There is complete resolution in 95% of cases. Severity of renal failure and hypertension varies. Microhematuria may persist to 18 months. Hypocomplementemia resolves in 1–30 days.	Excellent. Chronic disease is rare. Severe proteinuria, atypical presentation/course, or persistent hypocomplementemia suggest another entity is likely.
Membranoproliferative Glomerulonephritis. Presentation ranges from mild microhematuria to acute GN syndrome. Diagnosis is made by renal biopsy. Etiologic origin is unknown. Type I and Type II are most common. Lesion is chronic.	Course can be mild to severe (rapid deterioration in renal function). May mimic postinfection GN. Proteinuria can be severe. Complement depression is intermittent to persistent. Hypertension is usually significant.	Type I may be responsive to medication (corticosteroids e.g.). Type II (dense deposit disease) is less treatable; functions decrease immediately to as long as 15 years later in 30–50% of untreated cases.
IgA Nephropathy. Classic presentation consists of asymptomatic gross hematuria during acute unrelated illness, with microhematuria between episodes. There are occasional instances of acute GN syndrome. Etiologic origin is unknown. Diagnosis is made by biopsy.	90% of cases resolve in 1–5 years. Gross hematuric episodes resolve with recovery from acute illness. Severity of renal insufficiency and hypertension varies. Proteinuria occurs in more severe, atypical cases.	Generally good. Small percentage develops chronic renal failure. Proteinuria in the nephrotic range is a poor sign. There is no universally accepted medication. (Corticosteroids may be useful in severe cases.)
Schönlein-Henoch Purpura Glomerulonephritis. Degree of renal involvement varies. Asymptomatic microhematuria is most common, but GN syndrome can occur. Renal biopsy is recommended in severe cases; it can provide prognostic information.	Presentation varies with severity of renal lesion. In rare cases, course may progress rapidly to serious renal failure. Hypertension varies. Proteinuria in the nephrotic range and severe decline in function can occur.	Overall, prognosis is good. Cases presenting with greater than 50% reduction in function or proteinuria exceeding 1 g/24 h may develop chronic renal failure. Severity of renal biopsy picture can best guide approach in such cases. There is no universally accepted medication.
Glomerulonephritis of Systemic Lupus Erythematosus (SLE). Microhematuria and proteinuria on rare occasions are first signs of this systemic disease. Renal involvement varies. GN often causes the most concern. Histologic picture is variable.	Renal involvement is mild to severe. Clinical complexity depends on degree of renal insufficiency and other systems involved. Hypertension is significant. Manifestations of the severity of the renal lesion guide therapeutic intervention.	Renal involvement accounts for most of significant morbidity in SLE. Control of hypertension affects renal prognosis. Medication is guided by symptoms, serology, and renal lesion. End-stage renal failure can occur.
Hereditary Glomerulonephritis (eg, Alport's syndrome). Transmission is autosomal dominant/x-linked, with family history marked by end-stage renal failure, especially in young males. Deafness and eye abnormalities are associated.	There is no acute syndrome. Females are generally less affected but are carriers. Hypertension and increasing proteinuria occur with advancing renal failure. There is no known medication. Management of manifestations of renal failure is appropriate.	Progressive proteinuria and hypertension occur early, with gradual decline in renal function in those most severely affected. Disease progresses to end-stage renal failure in most males.

The association of proteinuria with hematuria is characteristic of more significant glomerular disease. Proteinuria alone, however, may indicate the presence of some benign as well as some more serious entities.

The dipstick test for proteinuria should be followed by quantitation of urinary protein excretion. The collection procedure is the same as described above for measurement of creatinine clearance. A 24-hour collection for protein excretion divided into "recumbent" and "upright" collections is needed if orthostatic proteinuria is to be ruled out; otherwise, a 12-hour timed collection could suffice.

In the 24-hour collection used to determine the presence of orthostatic proteinuria, urine formed in the recumbent position must be separated from that formed in the upright position. This is easily accomplished by having the patient complete the upright collection with a void just before going to bed. Urine voided during the night or upon awakening in the morning, when the 24-hour collection is completed, constitutes the recumbent collection. The 2 quantities can then be used to calculate total protein excretion, and the amount of protein can be compared in upright versus recumbent specimens to determine an orthostatic component. Significant quantitative proteinuria exceeds 150 mg/24 h. If the proteinuria is orthostatic in nature, an abnormal quantity will be noted in the upright specimen and an acceptable quantity will be found in the recumbent specimen. Proteinuria exceeding 1.5 g should generally not be regarded as simply orthostatic. Even when a creatinine clearance is not required from a specimen, measuring the creatinine in the specimen and calculating the creatinine index can confirm specimen reliability.

In children under 6 years of age, proteinuria may reflect anatomic abnormalities that require radiographic analysis (excretory urography or ultrasonography). The presence of proteinuria severe enough to cause hypoproteinemia (24-hour excretion usually exceeding 2 g), edema, and hyperlipidemia may represent idiopathic nephrotic syndrome of childhood (ie, "nil" disease, minimal change disease, or lipoid nephrosis), especially in the absence of any other abnormalities. The presumptive diagnosis of idiopathic nephrotic syndrome of childhood is generally "tested" by response to corticosteroid therapy (see Proteinuria and Renal Disease, below). Renal biopsy may be indicated in cases of suspected idiopathic nephrotic syndrome of childhood with numerous relapses, severe corticosteroid side effects, or a dependency on or resistance to corticosteroid therapy. In older children, there is a greater likelihood of a more serious renal lesion causing nephrotic syndrome. Typical lesions that would not be expected to respond to corticosteroid therapy are focal glomerular sclerosis and membranous nephropathy (see Proteinuria and Renal Disease, below). A renal biopsy is required to confirm the diagnosis.

Indications for diagnostic renal biopsy include atypical or clinically severe presentations of glomerulonephritis or the suspicion of acute or insidiously chronic processes that may require therapeutic intervention. Such indicators include glomerulonephritic presentations with significant proteinuria (especially in the "nephrotic range"), rapidly deteriorating renal function, evidence of systemic disease, severe or persistent hypertension, and prolonged or intermittent hypocomplementemia.

Abuelo JG: Proteinuria: Diagnostic principles and procedures. *Ann Intern Med* 1983;**98**:186.

Fairley KF et al: Hematuria: A simple method for identifying glomerular bleeding. *Kidney Int* 1982;**21**:105.

Stapleton FB et al: Hypercalciuria in children with hematuria. *N Engl J Med* 1984;**310**:1345.

West CD: Asymptomatic hematuria and proteinuria in children: Causes and appropriate diagnostic studies. *J Pediatr* 1976;**89**:173.

Special Tests of Renal Function

Measurements of urinary sodium, creatinine, and osmolality are useful in differentiating prerenal causes of renal insufficiency from renal causes when the possibility of acute tubular necrosis (ATN) is raised.

The physiologic response to decreased renal perfusion is an increase in urine concentration (osmolality usually > 800 mosm/L), a rise in urinary solutes, and a decrease in urinary sodium (usually < 20 meq/L). Therefore, when an increase in serum creatinine or blood urea nitrogen level or a decrease in urinary output suggests the possibility of renal failure, appropriate steps can be taken to assess the status of renal function by qualitative and quantitative urinalysis

The detection of some substances in urine may reflect tubular dysfunction. For example, glucose should not be present in concentrations greater than 5 mg/dL. Hyperphosphaturia is generally seen in cases of significant tubular abnormalities (eg, Fanconi's syndrome). Measurement of the phosphate concentration of a 24-hour urine specimen and evaluation of tubular reabsorption of phosphorus (TRP) will help document renal tubular diseases as well as hyperparathyroid states.

TRP (expressed as percentage of reabsorption) is calculated as follows:

$$TRP = 100 \left[1 - \frac{S_{Cr} \times U_{PO_4}}{S_{PO_4} \times U_{Cr}} \right]$$

where S_{Cr} = serum creatinine; U_{Cr} = urine creatinine; S_{PO_4} = serum phosphate; and U_{PO_4} = urine phosphate. All values for creatinine and phosphate are expressed in milligrams per deciliter for purposes of calculation. A TRP value of 80% or more is considered normal, although it depends somewhat on the S_{PO_4}.

The urinary excretion of amino acids in generalized tubular disease reflects a quantitative increase rather than a qualitative change.

The ability of the proximal tubule to reabsorb bicarbonate is affected in several disease states—including isolated renal tubular acidosis, Fanconi's syndrome (which is present in diseases such as cystinosis), and chronic renal failure—and is discussed under specific entities, below.

LABORATORY EVALUATION OF IMMUNOLOGIC FUNCTION

Much of parenchymal renal disease is mediated by immune mechanisms, many of which are not well defined or known. Examples of mechanisms in the kidney include (1) deposition of circulating antigen-antibody complexes that are themselves injurious or incite injurious responses and (2) formation of antibody directed against the glomerular basement membrane itself (rare in children).

Complete immunologic assessment of a patient requires many studies that are not routinely performed in all laboratories. Nonetheless, some basic tests are generally available. Total serum complement (and components if possible) should be measured when immune-mediated renal injury or chronic glomerulonephritis is suspected. Serum immunoglobulins should be quantitated. Abnormal serum protein levels are often associated with immune complex deposition; in such cases, tests should be performed to detect antinuclear antibodies, hepatitis-associated antigen, rheumatoid factor, and cold-precipitable proteins (cryoglobulins).

Where indicated, special studies to measure circulating immune complexes, C3 "nephritic" factor, and anti-glomerular basement membrane (anti-

GBM) antibody may be performed. Very often, the diagnosis rests on the description of renal histology.

Berger J et al: Immunochemistry of glomerulonephritis. In: *Advances in Nephrology*. Vol 1. Hamburger J, Crosnier J, Maxwell MH (editors). Year Book, 1971.

McIntosh RM et al: Cryoglobulins. 3. Further studies on the nature, incidence, clinical, diagnostic, prognostic, and immunopathologic significance of cryoproteins in renal disease. *Q J Med* 1975;**44**:285.

Wilson CB, Dixon FJ: Diagnosis of immunopathologic renal disease. *Kidney Int* 1974;**5**:389.

RADIOGRAPHIC EVALUATION

Although excretory urography remains a valuable procedure in assessing the anatomy and function of the kidney, collecting system, and bladder, renal ultrasonography is often the initial procedure in evaluation of a child's urinary tract. Such a noninvasive diagnostic method is especially helpful in evaluating small infants with renal insufficiency; abdominal masses (eg, Wilms's tumor, neuroblastoma); or renal enlargement due to obstructive uropathy, renal vein thrombosis, or cystic disease. Ultrasonography has also contributed greatly to the examination of the fetal kidneys in utero and has provided a means to demonstrate the prenatal presence of a normal urinary tract.

Radioisotope studies can provide valuable information concerning renal anatomy, blood flow, and glomerular, tubular, and collecting system function.

Evaluation of the lower urinary tract (voiding cystourethrography or cystoscopy) is indicated when vesicoureteral reflux or bladder outlet obstruction is suspected.

When clinically indicated, computed tomography or magnetic resonance imaging may be helpful if less costly studies have failed to produce desired results.

Renal arteriography or venography is rarely indicated in children, except when necessary for defining vascular abnormalities (eg, renal artery stenosis) prior to surgical intervention. Less invasive measures such as ultrasonography and doppler studies can be employed to demonstrate renal blood flow or thromboses.

The excretory urogram and voiding cystourethrogram are used in the diagnosis of ureteral reflux, bladder dysfunction, and various levels of urinary tract obstruction. However, the aforementioned noninvasive diagnostic tools can be helpful in many of these cases as well.

Except for the evaluation of patients with suspected anatomic abnormalities, cystoscopy is rarely indicated in the evaluation of asymptomatic hematuria or proteinuria in children, because the yield is minimal.

Chevalier RL, Campbell F, Brenbridge AN: Nephrosonography and renal scintigraphy in evaluation of newborns with renomegaly. *Urology* 1984;**24**:96.

Gusmano R et al: Natural history of reflux nephropathy in children. *Contrib Nephrol* 1988;**61**:200.

Lebowitz RL: Urography in children: When should it be done? 2. Conditions other than infection. *Postgrad Med* (Nov) 1978;**64**:61.

Vinocur L et al: Follow up studies of multicystic kidneys. *Radiology* 1988;**167**:311.

RENAL BIOPSY

The ultimate diagnostic procedure in children with suspected renal parenchymal disease is renal biopsy. Histologic information valuable for diagnosis, treatment, and prognosis can be obtained from a well-performed renal biopsy followed by proper tissue preparation, examination, and interpretation of findings. Satisfactory evaluation of renal tissue requires examination by light microscopy, immunofluorescence microscopy, and electron microscopy.

When a biopsy is anticipated, a pediatric nephrologist should be consulted. In children, percutaneous renal biopsy with a Vim-Silverman needle is an acceptable, low-risk procedure when performed by an experienced physician; it avoids the risks of general anesthesia. An experienced surgeon should perform the biopsy if operative exposure of the kidney is necessary, if an increased risk factor (eg, bleeding disorder) is present, or if a wedge biopsy is preferred.

CONGENITAL ANOMALIES OF THE URINARY TRACT

RENAL PARENCHYMAL ANOMALIES

Congenital anomalies of the genitourinary tract are present in about 10% of children. Severity ranges from asymptomatic abnormalities, which may never cause problems even into adult years and are often found only at autopsy, to malformations incompatible with intrauterine or extrauterine life.

Although an anomaly may be inconsequential in and of itself, there may be associated abnormalities. For example, in patients with horseshoe kidney (ie, kidneys fused in their lower poles), there is a reported higher incidence of renal calculi. Unilateral agenesis can occur and is usually accompanied by compensatory hypertrophy of the contralateral kidney and thus should be compatible with normal renal function. Supernumerary and ectopic kidneys can also occur and are usually of no significance. Nonetheless, any problems occurring during any stage of genitourinary development can result in varying degrees of renal maldevelopment and function. The most severe manifestation of such maldevelopment is, of course, complete renal agenesis.

Bilateral renal agenesis is a rare malformation resulting in early death. Oligohydramnios is present and probably is the cause of the pulmonary hypoplasia and peculiar (Potter) facies of infants with this anomaly.

Renal Hypoplasia & Dysplasia

Renal hypoplasia and dysplasia represent a spectrum of anomalies. In simple hypoplasia, which may be unilateral or bilateral, histologic findings on renal biopsy are normal, but the affected organs are smaller than normal. In the various forms of dysplasia, immature, undifferentiated renal tissue persists. In some of the dysplasias, the number of normal nephrons is insufficient to sustain life once the child reaches a critical body size. Such lack of renal tissue may not be readily discernible in the newborn period because the infant's urine production, although poor in concentration, may be adequate in volume. Often, the search for renal insufficiency is initiated only when growth failure or (unfortunately) even later manifestations of chronic renal failure are noted.

Other forms of renal dysplasia include oligomeganephronia, which is characterized by the presence of only a few large glomeruli, and the cystic dysplasias, which are a broad group of malformations in the hypoplasia-dysplasia group and are characterized by the presence of renal cysts. This group includes microcystic disease (congenital nephrosis).

Unlike the cystic dysplasias, the occurrence of a simple cyst within a kidney may lack clinical relevance because it represents no overall defect predisposing to progressive polycystic development. An entire kidney lost to multicystic development with concomitant hypertrophy and, thus, normal function of the contralateral side may also be of little clinical consequence. Nonetheless, even a simple cyst could pose problems because it may become a site for lithiasis or infection (or even symptomatic hematuria), prompting the cyst's removal.

Polycystic Kidney Disease

The autosomal recessive form of polycystic kidney disease ("infantile" PKD) is characterized by large cystic kidneys, often associated with multiple organ systems affected by cystic malformations. Some children with this type die in the newborn period, but many will develop progressive deterioration toward end-stage renal failure. When autosomal recessive PKD is diagnosed at a later age, it may be predominantly manifested by liver rather than renal involvement. Autosomal dominant PKD ("adult" form), although rarely of clinical significance (if at all) before the fourth decade, may also be detected in

the newborn period and, depending on degree of severity, could be fatal. Although renal insufficiency and hypertension usually occur late in this type, there are exceptions. Detailed discussion of this entity is beyond the scope of this text. Careful documentation (usually by ultrasonography), close monitoring and management of the complications of renal insufficiency, and strict attention to hypertension control—as well as genetic counseling—are suggested.

Medullary Cystic Disease
(Juvenile Nephronophthisis)

Medullary cystic disease is characterized by varying sizes of cysts in the medulla and is associated with tubular and interstitial nephritis. Children present with renal failure and signs of tubular dysfunction (decreased concentrating ability, Fanconi's syndrome). This lesion should not be confused with medullary sponge kidney (renal tubular ectasia), a frequently asymptomatic cystic disease usually found in adults.

Grantham JJ: Polycystic kidney disease: Hereditary and acquired. *Kidney* 1984;**17**:19.

Pretorius DH et al: Diagnosis of autosomal dominant polycystic kidney disease in utero and in the young infant. *J Ultrasound Med* 1987;**6**:249.

Steele BT, Lirenman DS, Beattie CW: Nephronophthisis. *Am J Med* 1980;**68**:531.

DISTAL URINARY TRACT ANOMALIES

Obstruction of urine flow, infection, and stone formation, alone or in combination, are the hallmarks of distal urinary tract anomalies. Many of these abnormalities may be noted upon abdominal palpation and subsequently demonstrated by ultrasonography, excretory urography, or cystourethography. Some may be managed surgically; in others, therapy is limited to supportive treatment and prompt recognition and management of infection and chronic renal failure. Early recognition of reversible lesions is of the greatest importance. However, immediate postnatal detection and intervention may not be able to reverse the detrimental intrauterine effects.

Obstruction at the ureteropelvic junction may be the result of intrinsic muscle abnormalities, aberrant vessels, or fibrous bands. The lesion can cause hydronephrosis and usually presents as an abdominal mass in the newborn. Obstruction can occur in other parts of the ureter, especially at its entrance into the bladder, with resulting proximal hydroureter and hydronephrosis. Whether impediments to normal flow of urine are intrinsic or extrinsic, immediate attention must be paid and steps toward rectifying the problem taken to minimize the adverse effects on renal parenchyma.

Severe bladder malformations such as exstrophy are clinically obvious and provide a surgical challenge. More subtle—but urgent in terms of diagnosis—is obstruction of urine flow from aberrant posterior urethral valves. This anomaly, almost invariably confined to males, usually presents as anuria or a poor voiding stream in the newborn period; with severe obstruction of urine flow, ascites may occur and the kidneys and bladder may be easily palpable. Provided that severe, irreversible damage to renal development has not occurred in utero, prompt intervention must be taken to avert further renal damage. The same can be said of many such complex genitourinary anomalies, including those of the external genitalia.

Complex Anomalies

The prune-belly syndrome is an association of urinary tract anomalies with cryptorchidism and absent abdominal musculature. Although complex anomalies, especially renal dysplasia, usually cause early death or the need for dialysis or transplantation, some patients have lived into the third decade with varying degrees of renal insufficiency. Early urinary diversion is essential to sustain renal function. At the time of this surgery, a renal biopsy can be obtained and may suggest the likelihood of adequate function in the future.

Discussion of other complex malformations, as well as such external genitalia anomalies as hypospadias, is beyond the scope of this text.

Aliabadi H et al: Management of ureteropelvic junction obstruction in infants and neonates. *Eur Urol* 1988; **15**:103.

Lennert T et al: Multicystic renal dysplasia: Nephrectomy versus conservative treatment. *Contrib Nephrol* 1988: **67**:183.

Poole CA: Congenital obstructive uropathies. *Pediatr Nephrol* 1974;**1**:231.

Rittenberg MH et al: Protective factors in posterior urethral valves. *J Urol* 1988;**140**:993.

GLOMERULAR DISEASE

POSTSTREPTOCOCCAL GLOMERULONEPHRITIS

Acute poststreptococcal glomerulonephritis is the most common form of postinfectious glomerulonephritis and the most frequently encountered in childhood. Although the cause is not certain, the condition is thought to be an immune-mediated disease. The epidemiologic relationship between certain strains of streptococci and glomerulonephritis is well

recognized. Presumably, antigen-antibody complexes induced by the infection are formed in the bloodstream and deposited in the glomeruli. These deposited complexes may cause glomerular damage through activation of the complement system, or the decrease in serum C3 levels may simply be the result of induced inflammation.

The diagnosis of poststreptococcal disease may be supported by a recent history (7–14 days previously) of group A β-hemolytic streptococcal infection. Recent streptococcal infection can be demonstrated by an elevated antistreptolysin O titer or by elevation of one or more antibody titers in the streptozyme panel.

Other infections have been shown to cause similar glomerular injury; thus, postinfection glomerulonephritis is the better term for this type of acute glomerulonephritis.

In general, the vast majority of clinical presentations of glomerulonephritis are largely asymptomatic. Gross hematuria ("coffee- or tea-colored" urine), with or without some noticeable, usually mild (eg, periorbital) edema, usually brings the problem to light. Any symptoms reported are usually nonspecific, eg, malaise; in cases of severe hypertension, there may be headache. Fever is not expected. Severe glomerular injury (which usually occurs in severe, acute presentations of the more chronic or destructive forms of glomerulonephritis) may be accompanied by massive proteinuria (nephrotic syndrome), anasarca or ascites, and severe compromise in renal function.

There is no specific treatment for the nephritis. Appropriate antibiotic therapy is indicated for streptococcal infection, if still present. The disturbances in renal function and resulting hypertension may require dietary management, diuretics, or antihypertensive drugs. In severe cases with rapidly deteriorating renal function, renal biopsy and hemodialysis or peritoneal dialysis may be necessary; corticosteroids may also be administered in an attempt to influence the course.

The acute abnormalities generally are resolved in 2–3 weeks. Serum complement may be normal as early as 3 days or as late as 30 days. Most children will recover completely, although microscopic hematuria may persist for 1–2 years. Although there are reports of significant chronic disease or abnormalities in adults, the outlook for children remains for the most part good, except in the rarest of instances. Typical resolution is expected. Nonetheless, persistent deterioration in renal function, urinary abnormalities beyond 18 months, persistent hypocomplementemia, and associated presence of nephrotic syndrome are ominous signs and are indications for renal biopsy.

Although the clinical presentations of the variety of glomerulonephritides are similar, the severity of presentation and clinical course influence differential diagnostic pursuits. The most commonly encountered entities in childhood and their clinical and histopathologic descriptions are listed in Table 22-1. Severe glomerular histopathologic and clinical entities, such as anti-glomerular basement membrane (anti-GBM) antibody disease (Goodpasture's syndrome) and idiopathic, rapidly progressive glomerulonephritis, may be considered in the differential diagnosis of acute glomerulonephritis, but these disorders are exceedingly rare in children.

Holliday MA, Barratt TM, Vernier RL: Isolated glomerular diseases. Pages 407–481 in *Pediatric Nephrology*. Williams & Wilkins, 1987.

McIntosh RM, Allen JE, Lum GM: Postviral glomerulonephritis. Chap 10, pp 263–277, in: *Clinical Immunology of the Kidney*. Zabriskie JB et al (editors). Wiley, 1983.

Southwest Pediatric Nephrology Study Group: A clinicopathologic study of crescentic glomerulonephritis in 50 children. *Kidney Int* 1985;**27**:450.

Southwest Pediatric Nephrology Study Group: Dense deposit disease in children: Prognostic value of clinical and pathologic indicators. *Am J Kidney Dis* 1985;**6**:161.

Southwest Pediatric Nephrology Study Group: A multicenter study of IgA nephropathy in children. *Kidney Int* 1982;**22**:643.

Warady BA et al: Prednisone therapy of membranoproliferative glomerulonephritis in children. *J Pediatr* 1985;**107**:702.

PROTEINURIA & RENAL DISEASE

Urine is not normally completely protein-free, but the average excretion is well below 150 mg/24 h. Although isolated asymptomatic proteinuria may be secondary to renal disease or genitourinary tract abnormalities, proteinuria is not always associated with renal disease.

Exertional proteinuria (the result of increased activity) is well recognized and may be accompanied by hematuria. Exertional proteinuria can be diagnosed by comparing urine specimens collected during or following activity with those collected at other times.

Febrile proteinuria can be seen in about 5% of febrile illnesses and is not necessarily due to the presence of underlying renal disease.

Orthostatic proteinuria is explained by hemodynamic adjustments leading to renal vein congestion. It has been suggested that lordosis may produce this proteinuria by increasing the convexity of the aorta, resulting in compression of the left renal vein. Documentation is accomplished by comparing the level of protein in urine produced in the upright position with that produced in the recumbent position (see Evaluation of Hematuria and Proteinuria, above).

CONGENITAL NEPHROSIS

Congenital nephrosis is a rare, uniformly fatal renal disorder that is often observed in more than one sibling in a family. Autosomal recessive inheritance is suggested. The kidneys are pale and large and may show microcystic dilatations (microcystic disease) of the proximal tubules and glomerular changes. The latter consist of proliferation, crescent formation, and thickening of capillary walls. The pathogenesis is not well understood.

Low birth weight (with an obstetric history of a large placenta), wide cranial sutures, delayed ossification, and mild edema are commonly noted at birth in infants with congenital nephrosis. The edema may become apparent after the first few weeks or months of life. Anasarca follows, and the abdomen can become greatly distended by ascites. Massive proteinuria associated with typically appearing nephrotic syndrome and hyperlipidemia is the rule. Hematuria is common. If the patient lives long enough, progressive renal failure occurs. Most affected infants succumb to infections at the age of a few months.

Treatment has little to offer. Supportive therapy with attention to nutrition and management of the manifestations of chronic renal failure is helpful. Timely institution of renal dialytic therapy or transplantation may be undertaken.

IDIOPATHIC NEPHROTIC SYNDROME OF CHILDHOOD ("Nil" Disease, Lipoid Nephrosis, Minimal Change Disease)

Nephrotic syndrome is characterized by proteinuria, hypoproteinemia, edema, and hyperlipidemia. It may occur as a result of any form of glomerular disease and may be associated with a variety of extrarenal conditions. In children under 5 years of age, the disease usually takes the form of idiopathic nephrotic syndrome of childhood ("nil" disease, lipoid nephrosis), which is characterized by certain clinical and laboratory findings.

Clinical Findings

Affected patients are generally under 5 years of age at the time of their first episode. Often following an influenzalike syndrome, the child is noted to have periorbital swelling and perhaps oliguria. Within a few days, increasing edema—even anasarca—becomes evident. Other than vague malaise and, occasionally, abdominal pain, complaints are few. However, with significant "third spacing" of plasma volume, some children may even present with shock. With marked edema, there may also be dyspnea due to pleural effusions.

Despite heavy proteinuria, the urine sediment is usually normal. Although microscopic hematuria may rarely be found, its presence should raise the suspicion of a glomerular lesion (such as focal glomerular sclerosis). Serum chemistries reveal hypoalbuminemia and hyperlipidemia. Abnormal immunoglobulin levels such as high IgM and low IgG have also been reported. However, no other evidence of immunologic disorder is present (eg, complement is normal, and there is no cryoglobulinemia). Some azotemia may occur but is related to intravascular volume depletion rather than to impairment of function.

Glomerular morphology is unremarkable except for fusion of foot processes of the visceral epithelium of the glomerular basement membrane. This finding, however, is nonspecific and is seen in many proteinuric states. There may be "minimal changes" in the glomerular mesangium, with unremarkable findings on immunofluorescence and electron microscopic examination.

Complications

Infectious complications (eg, peritonitis) are occasionally encountered, and pneumococci are frequently responsible for these complications. Immunization with pneumococcal vaccine is helpful. Hypercoagulability may be present, and thromboembolic phenomena are commonly reported.

Treatment and Prognosis

As soon as the diagnosis of idiopathic nephrotic syndrome is made, therapy with corticosteroids should be initiated. Prednisone, 2 mg/kg/d (maximum of 60 mg), is given daily for a maximum of 8 weeks until the dipstick test reveals trace to negative protein in the urine. The same dose is then administered on an alternate-day schedule for 1–2 months; thereafter, the dose is very gradually tapered and discontinued over an ensuing month. Lack of response—either total or partial—to treatment raises the suspicion of a true glomerular histopathologic condition that accounts for the nephrotic syndrome. If remission is achieved only to be followed by another relapse, the treatment course may be repeated. If at any time the nephrosis becomes refractory to treatment or if there are 3 relapses within a year's time, renal biopsy should be considered. If findings are consistent with the presumed diagnosis of "minimal change disease," other cytotoxic agents can be considered; however, these agents are generally most helpful when there is steroid dependence and not resistance.

Other therapeutic measures may be directed to the complications of the nephrotic syndrome itself. Unless the edema is of symptomatic proportions (eg, respiratory compromise due to ascites), diuretics should be used with extreme care: the patients are expected to have a decreased circulating volume and are also at risk for intravenous thrombosis. However, careful restoration of compromised circulating volume with intravenous albumin infusion and administration of diuretics is helpful in mobilizing edema.

Immediate attention to the development of infection (eg, acute peritonitis) is of paramount importance in reducing the morbidity of the syndrome.

The prognosis of idiopathic nephrotic syndrome is often suggested by the initial response to corticosteroids. A prompt remission lasting for 3 years is almost always permanent. Failure to respond or early relapse usually heralds a prolonged series of relapses, which may indicate the presence of more serious nephropathy. Chlorambucil or other cytotoxic drug therapy is predictably successful only in children who respond to corticosteroids. As mentioned above, renal biopsy is recommended in atypical cases.

Childhood nephrotic syndrome associated with diffuse mesangial hypercellularity: A report of the Southwest Pediatric Nephrology Study Group. *Kidney Int* 1983; **23:**87.

Kher KK, Sweet M, Makker SP: Nephrotic syndrome in children. *Curr Probl Pediatr* (April) 1988;**18:**197.

Oliver WJ, Kelsch RC: Nephrotic syndrome due to primary nephropathies. *Pediatr Rev* 1981;**2:**311.

Shulman SL et al: Predicting the response to cytotoxic therapy for childhood nephrotic syndrome: Superiority of response to corticosteroid therapy over histopathologic patterns. *J Pediatr* 1988;**113:**996.

Sibley RK et al: A clinicopathologic study of forty-eight infants with nephrotic syndrome. *Kidney Int* 1985; **27:**544.

Williams SA et al: Long-term evaluation of chlorambucil plus prednisone in the idiopathic nephrotic syndrome of childhood. *N Engl J Med* 1980;**302:**929.

FOCAL GLOMERULAR SCLEROSIS

Focal glomerular sclerosis is characterized by the presence in renal biopsy specimens of normal-appearing glomeruli as well as some partially or completely sclerosed glomeruli. At presentation, the disease is often quite similar to idiopathic nephrotic syndrome; however, in most cases the response to corticosteroid therapy is poor, and a diagnostic renal biopsy is likely. The lesion has serious prognostic implications; as many as 15–20% of cases can progress to end-stage renal failure. Clinical response to various therapies is variable. Although experience with cyclosporine treatment is limited, early results show some promise.

Arbus GS et al: Focal segmental glomerulosclerosis with idiopathic nephrotic syndrome: Three types of clinical response. *J Pediatr* 1982;**101:**40.

Kohaut EC et al: The significance of focal glomerular sclerosis in children who have nephrotic syndrome. *Am J Clin Pathol* 1976;**66:**545.

Nash MA et al: Late development of chronic renal failure in steroid-responsive nephrotic syndrome. *J Pediatr* 1982;**101:**411.

Niaudet P et al: Treatment of severe childhood nephrosis. *Adv Nephrol* 1988;**17**:151.

Tejani A et al: Cyclosporine-induced remission of relapsing nephrotic syndrome in children. *J Pediatr* 1987;**111** (Part 2):1056.

Wyszynska T et al: Evaluation of prednisolone pulse therapy in steroid-resistant nephrotic syndrome: A multicenter collaborative study. *Contrib Nephrol* 1988; **67**:183.

MEMBRANOUS NEPHROPATHY
(Membranous Glomerulonephritis)

Membranous nephropathy is occasionally seen in children and thus deserves mention. The usual presenting feature is proteinuria of variable degree. This lesion has been reported to occur in children of all ages, but the diagnosis is more frequently made in older children with "nephrotic range" proteinuria.

Although largely idiopathic in nature, this renal lesion can be found in association with diseases such as hepatitis B antigenemia, systemic lupus erythematosus, congenital and secondary syphilis, and renal vein thrombosis; with immunologic disorders such as autoimmune thyroiditis; and with administration of drugs such as penicillamine. The pathogenesis is unknown, but it is thought that the glomerular lesion is the result of prolonged deposition of circulating antigen-antibody complexes.

The onset of membranous nephropathy is often insidious, but onset may be similar to that of idiopathic nephrotic syndrome of childhood (see above). Unlike that entity, membranous nephropathy is not expected to respond dramatically (ie, exhibit decreased proteinuria or complete remission of the nephrotic state) to corticosteroid therapy. However, low-dose exposure to steroid therapy has been shown to result in long-term favorable prognosis regarding the development of chronic renal insufficiency.

A controlled study of short-term prednisone treatment in adults with membranous nephropathy: Collaborative study of the adult idiopathic nephrotic syndrome. *N Engl J Med* 1979;**301**:1302.

Gaffney EF et al: Segmental membranous glomerulonephritis. *Arch Pathol Lab Med* 1982;**106**:409.

Latham P et al: Idiopathic membranous glomerulopathy in Canadian children: A clinicopathologic study. *J Pediatr* 1982;**101**:682.

Wagoner RD et al: Renal vein thrombosis in idiopathic membranous glomerulopathy and nephrotic syndrome: Incidence and significance. *Kidney Int* 1983:**23**:368.

ACUTE INTERSTITIAL NEPHRITIS

Acute interstitial nephritis, a relatively uncommon form of nephritis, is characterized by diffuse or focal inflammation and edema of the renal interstitium and secondary involvement of the tubules but little or no secondary glomerular damage unless a combined or chronic picture is encountered. It seems to be related most often to drugs (eg, antibiotics, especially methicillin).

Fever, rigor, abdominal or flank pain, and rashes may occur in drug-associated cases. Urinalysis may reveal leukocyturia and hematuria. Hansel's staining of the urinary sediment is helpful in demonstrating the presence of eosinophils. The inflammation can be severe enough to cause rapid deterioration of renal function. Histologic demonstration of tubular and interstitial inflammation of the kidneys is helpful for diagnosis. Immediate identification and removal of the causative agent is imperative. A relentless course with progressive renal insufficiency or nephrotic syndrome may require supportive dialysis and treatment with corticosteroids.

Ellis D et al: Acute interstitial nephritis in children. *Pediatrics* 1981;**67**:862.

HEMOLYTIC-UREMIC SYNDROME

Although the glomerulonephritides as a group account for the majority of renal parenchymal causes of renal failure, the hemolytic-uremic syndrome is the most common single cause of renal failure in childhood. Because of the usual gastrointestinal prodrome, severe fluid imbalances contribute to the degree of renal insufficiency; however, direct renal glomerular injury is primarily responsible.

The cause of the hemolytic-uremic syndrome is not well established, but epidemiologic studies have suggested both a genetic and an infectious or immunologic component. The primary lesion seems to be one of the endothelium of arterioles, especially in the kidney, with formation of platelet thrombi and resulting microangiopathic hemolysis. Recent data suggest that hemolytic-uremic syndrome involves a disorder of immunoregulation and that a unique class of antiendothelial cell antibodies which may take part in the pathogenesis of the vascular injury is produced.

Clinical Findings

Hemolytic-uremic syndrome is found most often in children under 2 years of age. It usually begins with a prodromal phase characterized by gastrointestinal symptoms, including abdominal pain, diarrhea, and vomiting. Oliguria, pallor, and bleeding manifestations, principally cutaneous and gastrointestinal, occur next. Hypertension and seizures develop in some infants, especially those who develop severe renal failure and fluid overload.

The triad of anemia, thrombocytopenia, and renal failure characterizes the syndrome. Anemia is profound and is associated with findings of red blood cell fragments on smear. A high reticulocyte count confirms the hemolytic nature of the anemia. The platelet count is almost invariably below 100,000/μL. Other coagulation abnormalities are less consistent. Serum fibrin split products are often present, but fulminant disseminated intravascular coagulation is rare. Renal failure is characterized by a high blood urea nitrogen level and, usually, severe oliguria. Macroscopic hematuria is often present; proteinuria and the nephrotic syndrome may also occur. The serum complement level is normal.

Complications

The complications of hemolytic-uremic syndrome are usually those associated with acute renal failure. Neurologic problems, particularly seizures, may result from electrolyte abnormalities such as hyponatremia, hypertension, or central nervous system vascular disease. Severe bleeding and complicating infections must be anticipated.

Treatment

As with any case of acute renal failure, meticulous attention to fluid and electrolyte status is crucial. There is evidence that early dialysis improves the prognosis; the size of the patient and the bleeding tendency will usually dictate peritoneal dialysis as the technique of choice. Seizures usually respond to control of hypertension and electrolyte abnormalities. It has been suggested that the plasma in some cases lacks a prostacyclin-stimulating factor, which is a potent inhibitor of platelet aggregation. Therefore, plasma infusion or plasmapheresis has been advocated in severe cases. Platelet inhibitors have also been tried, but the results have not been impressive, especially late in the disease. Aspirin can provide the same effect but at certain doses also undesirably inhibits prostacyclin synthesis. Red cell and platelet transfusions may be necessary; although the risk of volume overload is significant, it can be minimized by use of dialysis. While there is no universally accepted therapy for patients with this syndrome, the strict control of hypertension and nutrition and the use of dialysis appear to affect the long-term outcome.

Course & Prognosis

It has been suggested that geographic factors may determine the severity of hemolytic-uremic syndrome. Most commonly, children recover from the acute episode within a week, and follow-up examination reveals no residual renal insufficiency. However, some patients who recover from the acute episode have severe and occasionally progressive renal

dysfunction. Thus, follow-up of children recovering from hemolytic-uremic syndrome should include serial determinations of renal function for 1–2 years and meticulous attention to blood pressure for 5 years. Although a very small group of patients die in the early phase from the complications of acute renal failure, most children—even those with renal failure requiring dialysis—recover completely.

Leung DYM: Lytic anti-endothelial cell antibodies in haemolytic-uraemic syndrome. *Lancet* 1988;**2**:183.

Neild G: The haemolytic uraemic syndrome: A review. *Q J Med* 1987;**63**:367.

Rizzoni G et al: Plasma infusion for hemolytic-uremic syndrome in children: Results of a multicenter controlled trial. *J Pediatr* 1988;**112**:284.

Van Damme-Lombaerts et al: Heparin plus dipyridamole in childhood hemolytic-uremic syndrome: A prospective, randomized study. *J Pediatr* 1988;**113**:913.

DISEASES OF THE RENAL VESSELS

RENAL VEIN THROMBOSIS

In the newborn period, renal vein thrombosis may suddenly complicate the course of sepsis or dehydration. It may be observed in an infant of a diabetic mother, or it may be the result of umbilical vein catheterization. In older children and adolescents, renal vein thrombosis may develop following trauma or without any apparent predisposing factors; in these cases, nephrotic syndrome may be associated with renal vein thrombosis. There may also be an underlying membranous glomerulonephropathy.

Clinical Findings

In the newborn, renal vein thrombosis generally presents with the sudden development of an abdominal mass. If the thrombosis is bilateral, oliguria may be present; urine output may be normal with a unilateral thrombus. In older children, flank pain, sometimes with a palpable mass, is a common presentation. In some children with proteinuria, however, the nephrotic syndrome may be the first sign of renal vein thrombosis.

No single laboratory test is diagnostic of renal vein thrombosis. Hematuria usually is present and occasionally is gross. Proteinuria is less constant. In the newborn, thrombocytopenia may be found; this is rare in older children. Thrombosis may be demonstrated by ultrasonography and doppler-flow studies.

Treatment

Anticoagulation with heparin is the treatment of

choice both in newborns and in older children. In the newborn, a course of heparin combined with treatment of the underlying problem is usually all that is required. Management in other cases is less straightforward. The tendency for recurrence and embolization has led some workers in this field to recommend long-term anticoagulation. If an underlying membranous glomerulonephritis is suspected, biopsy should be performed.

Course & Prognosis

The rate of deaths due to renal vein thrombosis in the newborn is usually related to the underlying cause. If the child survives the acute phase, the prognosis for adequate renal function is good. The entity is much less common in older children, but they may be expected to follow the course known to occur in adults. Renal vein thrombosis may recur in the same kidney or occur in the other kidney years after the original episode of thrombus formation. Extension into the vena cava, with fatal pulmonary emboli, is a known complication.

The nephrotic syndrome, often with membranous glomerulonephritis, is associated with renal vein thrombosis. In some cases, thrombosis may be a complication of nephrotic syndrome. There is also evidence that the thrombus itself may result in glomerulonephritis, possibly through the release of renal tubular antigens.

Mauer SM et al: Bilateral renal vein thrombosis in infancy: Report of a survivor following surgical intervention. *J Pediatr* 1971;**78**:509.

Moore HL et al: Unilateral renal vein thrombosis and the nephrotic syndrome. *Pediatrics* 1972;**50**:598.

RENAL ARTERIAL DISEASE

Children are susceptible to renovascular hypertension due to fibromuscular hyperplasia, congenital stenosis, or other renal arterial lesions. The proportion of hypertensive children with such demonstrable abnormalities, however, is quite small. Unfortunately, there are few clinical clues to underlying arterial lesions. Nonetheless, arterial lesions should be suspected in children whose hypertension is severe, beginning at 10 years of age or under, or associated with delayed visualization on excretory urogram. The diagnosis is established by renal arteriography with selective renal vein renin measurements. Some of these lesions may be repaired surgically (see Hypertension, below), but repair may be technically impossible in many small children. Although thrombosis of renal arteries is rare, it should be considered in a patient with acute onset of hypertension and hematuria in an appropriate setting (eg, in association with hyperviscosity or umbilical artery catheterization).

RENAL FAILURE

ACUTE RENAL FAILURE

Acute renal failure (ARF) is a major complication of many conditions. It can be defined as the sudden inability to excrete urine of sufficient quantity or adequate composition to maintain normal body fluid homeostasis. It may be due to impaired renal perfusion, acute renal disease, renal ischemia, renal vascular compromise, or obstructive uropathy. Prerenal, renal, and postrenal causes are shown in Table 22–2.

Clinical Findings

The hallmark of early renal failure is oliguria. The initial approach to an oliguric child should be aimed at classifying the problem in one of the categories outlined in Table 22–2. While an exact etiologic diagnosis is not necessary, accurate classification is helpful before initiating appropriate therapy.

If the cause of renal failure or oliguria is not clear, entities that can be treated (eg, volume depletion)

Table 22–2. Classification of causes of renal failure.

Prerenal
Dehydration due to gastroenteritis, malnutrition, or diarrhea
Hemorrhage, blood loss, aortic or renal vessel injury, trauma, surgery, cardiac surgery, renal arterial thrombosis
Diabetic acidosis
Pooling of interstitial fluid into local area of injury—burns, operative site, peritonitis
Hypovolemia associated with nephrotic syndrome
Shock
Heart failure
Renal
Hemolytic-uremic syndrome
Acute glomerulonephritis
Extension of prerenal hypoperfusion
Nephrotoxins
Acute tubular necrosis or vascular nephropathy
Renal (cortical) necrosis
Intravascular coagulation—septic shock, hemorrhage
Diseases of the kidney and vessels
Iatrogenic disorders
Severe infections
Drowning, especially fresh water
Treatment of neoplasms—hyperuricacidemia, hyperuricaciduria
Postrenal
Obstruction due to tumor, hematoma, or the presence of posterior urethral valves or ureteropelvic junction stricture, uretovesicle junction stricture, ureterocele
Sulfonamide crystals
Uric acid crystals
Stones
Trauma to a solitary kidney or collecting system
Renal vein thrombosis

should be considered first. After treatable problems or glomerular diseases are ruled out, a diagnosis of acute tubular necrosis (eg, vasomotor nephropathy, ischemic injury) may be entertained.

A. Postrenal Causes: Postrenal failure, which is quite rare in children, is found in newborns with anatomic abnormalities. If there is obstruction of the bladder outlet, it can be relieved by insertion of a urethral catheter; surgical correction follows. Occult postrenal obstruction must always be considered; if the diagnosis is made early enough, removal of the obstruction may prevent irreversible renal injury and the development of secondary chronic renal failure. Delayed voiding in the newborn period, anuria, or poor urinary stream usually suggests obstruction. The clinician must also consider lesions higher in the urinary system, such as ureteropelvic junctional obstruction, which usually presents as abdominal mass. Obstructive uropathy may or may not be accompanied by variable degrees of renal insufficiency.

B. Prerenal Causes: The most common reason for observed decreases in renal function in children is compromised renal perfusion. It is usually a result of problems associated with dehydration, although abnormalities of renal vasculature and poor cardiac performance may also be considered. All such concerns in given clinical settings should be addressed and, if possible, eliminated in order to determine if true renal functional disturbances are present.

C. Renal Causes: The various acute glomerulonephritides, the hemolytic-uremic syndrome, acute interstitial nephritis, and nephrotoxic injury are examples of "renal" entities that would be expected to produce varying degrees of ARF. The diagnosis of acute tubular necrosis or vasomotor nephropathy is considered in clinical situations where—with no evidence of specific renal parenchymal diseases—the elimination of any prerenal or postrenal factors produces no improvement in renal performance.

Table 22–3 lists the urinary indices that are helpful in distinguishing prerenal conditions from ARF.

Complications

Once the clinical situation becomes one of awaiting the recovery of renal function in response to therapy, whether direct or supportive, attention continues to be directed toward the management of the complications of ARF. The clinical severity of such complications depends, of course, on the degree of renal functional impairment and oliguria. Among the most commonly anticipated complications are (1) fluid overload (hypertension, congestive heart failure, pulmonary edema), (2) electrolyte disturbances (hyperkalemia), (3) metabolic acidosis, (4) hyperphosphatemia, and (5) uremia.

Treatment

An indwelling catheter should be inserted and urine output monitored hourly. If insignificant quantities of urine are produced and renal failure is established, the catheter should be removed because it then represents more of a hazard than an aid.

All prerenal or postrenal factors should be excluded or rectified. Disturbances in circulating volume should be corrected with appropriate fluids and response assessed by physical examination and observed urinary output. Measurement of central venous pressure may be indicated.

If diuresis does not occur in response to the above measures, give furosemide (Lasix), 2.5 mg/kg as an intravenous push. Allow 1 hour for a response to occur. If the urine output remains low ($< 200–250$ mL/m^2/24 h), repeat and double the dose of furosemide (5 mg/kg). If no diuresis occurs, no further administration of diuretics will be helpful.

If these maneuvers produce return of urine flow but biochemical evidence of ARF persists, the resulting "nonoliguric" ARF or acute tubular necrosis should, at the very least, be more manageable. Fluid overload and its attendant problems may then be avoided, and dialysis may be averted. However, if administration of clinically indicated medications and nutrients threatens to overwhelm the degree of urinary output, or if reduction in such medications and nutrients would result in less than optimal care, dialysis may still be considered. Therefore, institution of dialysis therapy in time to avoid the aforementioned early complications of ARF is preferred and will likely result in improved clinical management and outcome.

A. Indications for Dialysis: The need for dialysis in individual cases is determined on the basis of clinical findings. However, there are some immediate, clinical indications for dialysis: (1) severe hyperkalemia; (2) unrelenting metabolic acidosis (usually in a situation where fluid overload prevents sodium bicarbonate administration); (3) fluid overload with or without severe hypertension or congestive heart failure (a situation that would seriously compromise caloric or drug administration—a definite problem in the oliguric patient); and (4) symptoms of uremia, usually manifested in children by central nervous system depression.

The rate of rise of both blood urea nitrogen and serum creatinine levels may indicate the need for dialysis; it is generally accepted that the blood urea nitrogen level should not be allowed to exceed 100 mg/dL.

Table 22–3. Urine studies.

Prerenal Failure	Acute Tubular Necrosis
Urine osmolality 50 mosm/kg greater than plasma osmolality	Urine osmolality equal to or less than plasma osmolality
Urine sodium < 10 meq/L	Urinary sodium > 20 meq/L
Ratio of urine creatinine to plasma creatinine $> 14:1$	Ratio of urine creatinine to plasma creatinine $< 14:1$
Specific gravity > 1.020	Specific gravity 1.012–1.018

Early dialysis, when properly performed, can simplify management and reduce morbidity and mortality of ARF.

B. Methods of Dialysis: The choice between peritoneal dialysis and hemodialysis depends largely on the availability of either technique and the relative indications or contraindications of each procedure in a given patient. Peritoneal dialysis is generally preferred in children because of the ease of performance and patient tolerance. Although peritoneal dialysis is technically less efficient than hemodialysis, hemodynamic stability and metabolic control can be better sustained because this technique can be applied on a relatively continuous basis. However, hemodialysis should be considered in the following situations: (1) if rapid removal of toxins is desired; (2) if the size of the patient makes hemodialysis less technically cumbersome and hemodynamically well-tolerated; or (3) if impediments to efficient peritoneal dialysis are present (eg, ileus).

C. Complications of Dialysis: Complications of peritoneal dialysis include peritonitis, volume depletion, and technical complications such as dialysate leakage or respiratory compromise from intra-abdominal dialysate fluid. Peritonitis can be avoided by strict adherence to aseptic technique. Experienced personnel are largely responsible for minimizing the incidence of this complication. Peritoneal fluid cultures are obtained as clinically indicated. Dialysate can leak around the dialysis catheter or through tissue planes, causing dissection. However, leakage can be reduced by good catheter placement technique and appropriate intra-abdominal dialysate volumes. Any technical problems that result in abnormal flow of dialysate in and out of the peritoneal cavity require the attention of the nephrology consultant. Dialysis is useful in maintaining electrolyte balance; because potassium is absent from standard dialysate solutions, however, serum potassium levels may fluctuate significantly. Potassium may be added to the dialysate as indicated. Phosphate is also absent because hyperphosphatemia is an expected problem in renal failure. Nonetheless, in situations where nutritional impairments result in inadequate phosphate intake, care must be taken to avert hypophosphatemia when implementing dialysis. Because dextrose is used in the dialysate to produce osmotic removal of water, hyperglycemia may result, especially when the higher dextrose concentrations are used (maximum 4.25%). Using the higher concentrations of dextrose can achieve relatively rapid correction of fluid overload. Fluid removal may also be increased with more frequent exchanges of the dialysate. However, rapid osmotic transfer of water may result in hypernatremia. Careful monitoring of all these parameters must accompany the process.

Hemodialysis is expected to correct major metabolic and electrolyte disturbances, as well as volume overload, rapidly. The process itself is highly efficient, but there can be significant symptomatology

and pathophysiologic responses to the rapidity of the induced physiologic and metabolic changes. Furthermore, the specific condition of equipment and materials plays a major and variable role in individual patient tolerance. All such technical problems are minimized or avoided when experienced personnel under the direction of a nephrology consultant administer hemodialysis.

Hemodynamic instability during the procedure is a common problem but, again, can be managed. Anticoagulation is usually required for the procedure and may have clinical significance. Under appropriate conditions, the procedure may be performed with minimal exposure to heparin and its attendant risks. Again, careful monitoring of all these factors, as well as appropriate biochemical parameters, is advised. Note, however, that during or immediately following the procedure, blood sampling will produce misleading results because equilibration between extravascular compartments and the blood will not yet have been completed.

Access devices (eg, subclavian catheters) must be inspected for thrombotic or infectious complications. Such problems are greatly reduced when only experienced personnel are permitted to manipulate the various cannulas or catheters employed in the procedure.

The chronic applications of these forms of dialysis are also available for children. Continuous ambulatory peritoneal dialysis (CAPD) and continuous cycling peritoneal dialysis (CCPD) are both extremely useful for children and adults alike. These methods carry the advantages of simple application in the home setting and avoidance of the vascular access problems inherent with chronic hemodialysis. Technology that permits hemodialysis of even the small infant is available. Although eventual renal transplantation is the ultimate goal for most children with end-stage renal failure, the improvement in the techniques of dialysis has greatly enhanced the long-term management of the child in irreversible renal failure.

Course & Prognosis

The period of severe oliguria, if it occurs, usually lasts about 10 days. If oliguria lasts longer than 3 weeks or if there is complete anuria, a diagnosis of acute tubular necrosis is very unlikely; vascular injury, severe ischemia, or glomerulonephritis is more probable. The diuretic phase begins with progressive increases in urinary output, followed by the passage of large volumes of isosthenuric urine containing sodium levels of 80–150 meq/L. During the recovery phase, signs and symptoms subside rapidly, although polyuria may persist for several days or weeks. Urinary abnormalities usually disappear completely within a few months.

Dobrin RS et al: The critically ill child: Acute renal failure. *Pediatrics* 1971;**48**:286.
Ford DM et al: Unsuspected seizures during hemodialysis:

Effect of dialysate prescription. *Int J Pediatr Nephrol* 1987;**1**:597.

Kleinknecht D et al: Uremic and non-uremic complications in acute renal failure: Evaluation of early and frequent dialysis on prognosis. *Kidney Int* 1972;**1**:190.

Lum GM: Comparison of CAPD and CCPD in children. Southwest Pediatric Nephrology Study Group. In: *CAPD in Children.* Fine RN, Schurer K, Mehls O (editors). S. Karger, 1985.

Lum GM: Growth velocity of children on continuous ambulatory vs continuous cycling peritoneal dialysis. *Eur J Pediatr* 1983;**140**:204.

Lum GM: Peritonitis in infants and children on CAPD/CCPD. Pages 189–200 in: *Chronic Ambulatory Peritoneal Dialysis (CAPD) and Chronic Cycling Peritoneal Dialysis (CCPD) in Children,* Fine RN (editor). Martinus Nijhoff Publishing, 1987.

CHRONIC RENAL FAILURE

Chronic renal failure (CRF) in children most commonly results from developmental abnormalities of the kidneys or urinary tract. The kidneys may develop poorly (hypoplasia/dysplasia) or not at all (aplasia). Cystic development may result in immediate or progressive insufficiency. Abnormal development of the urinary tract may not permit normal renal development. However, depending on the degree of interference with normal renal parenchymal development, timely surgical intervention may minimize parenchymal injury and perhaps even achieve totally normal function. In older children, the chronic glomerulonephritides and nephropathies, irreversible nephrotoxic injury, or the hemolytic-uremic syndrome may also result in CRF.

In early life, when CRF is the result of an inadequate amount of normally functioning renal tissue, the clinical presentation is marked by inability to produce a concentrated urine (polyuria/polydipsia/enuresis). Depending on the degree of renal insufficiency, failure to thrive may be the chief concern. If abnormalities of the collecting system are responsible, there may be a history of urinary tract infection that had somehow missed medical attention and intervention. However, progressive deterioration of renal function may occur in the absence of infection. Usually, it is only in situations where appropriate health maintenance has not been available that such children present with overt complications of long-standing CRF, such as rickets and long-bone disfigurement.

Chronic renal failure resulting from glomerulonephritis is not expected to present with polyuria. Growth failure depends on the age of presentation and the rapidity of functional decline. Given the usually acute initial presentation of the disease, it is likely that such a child would have early intervention and follow-up by a nephrologist. However, some of the chronic glomerulonephritides (eg, membranoproliferative glomerulonephritis) can progress unnoticed if subtle abnormalities of the urinary sediment are undetected or ignored. Any child with a history of chronic glomerulonephritis or significant renal injury (eg, hemolytic-uremic syndrome with residual renal insufficiency) needs close follow-up and monitoring of renal function, as well as careful attention directed at controlling associated abnormalities that contribute to the rate of functional decline (eg, hypertension, urinary tract infection).

Complications

Despite the kidney's ability to compensate for gradual loss of functioning nephrons in most cases of CRF progression, there are resulting complications that are expected early in the course of CRF as well as those that occur toward end-stage renal disease (GFR < 15 mL/min/1.73 m^2); at this point, the compensatory capability is exhausted. In children who have developmentally reduced function but who are unable to concentrate the urine, polyuria and thus dehydration is more likely to be a problem than fluid overload. As renal homeostatic capability approaches end-stage, there may be a reduction in output; however, many such children can continue to produce generous quantities of urine (but not ''good quality'' urine), even when renal replacement therapies are initiated. Moreover, a ''salt-wasting'' state can occur. On the other hand, those children who develop CRF due to the glomerular disease will characteristically have difficulty with sodium/water retention and hypertension relatively early in the course of CRF.

Other rather early manifestations of CRF include metabolic acidosis and growth retardation. Disturbances in calcium, phosphorus, and vitamin D metabolism leading to renal osteodystrophy require prompt attention. Although renal compensation and increased parathyroid hormone can maintain a normal serum phosphate early in the course, there is a price to be paid: tertiary hyperparathyroidism with resulting skeletal abnormalities.

Overt uremic symptoms, as expected, are late manifestations of CRF, (eg, severe hyperkalemia, and pericarditis). These complications are best averted by timely renal replacement therapy, ie, dialysis or transplant. Keep in mind that if left unchecked, CRF eventually will adversely affect every organ system. The subjective symptoms of uremia (eg, anorexia, nausea, lethargy) may be somewhat ameliorated by dietary protein restriction. However, although some compromise in adequate caloric intake can result from the protein restriction, there will be considerable interference with growth in the uremic state anyway. The most difficult aspect of dietary restriction is patient compliance. A diet restricted in sodium, potassium, and phosphorus that at the same time provides adequate caloric intake is often rejected. Dietary supplementation with essential amino or keto acids is helpful, if the child will accept it. Nasogastric feeding may be necessary, especially for the infant or small child, even while the child is maintained on chronic dialysis.

A nearly constant finding in CRF is anemia. It is usually normochromic and normocytic and results from decreased production secondary to diminished renal erythropoietin synthesis as renal parenchyma atrophies. Nutritional deficiency and the uremic state also play a role. Platelet dysfunction and other abnormalities of the coagulation system may be present. Bleeding phenomena, especially gastrointestinal bleeding, may be a problem.

Central nervous system manifestations of the condition may be subtle but are usually present. Confusion, apathy, and lethargy usually occur late in the course of disease; these may be unsuspected clinically until the patient is carefully evaluated. With advancing uremia, stupor and coma may be present. Associated electrolyte abnormalities (eg, hyponatremia) may precipitate seizures (more commonly, a result of untreated hypertension).

Cardiovascular manifestations may be life-threatening. Uremic pericarditis may develop. Congestive heart failure is seen more often, and hypertension is quite common. The hypertension may relate to volume overload, excessive renin excretion, or both.

Patients with CRF tend to be more susceptible to infections. Because of their generally debilitated state, they often handle infections poorly.

Treatment

The aim of treatment in CRF is to minimize the occurrence of the aforementioned complications. However, presuming nothing more can be done for the underlying renal disease, efforts are still aimed at preserving as much renal function for as long as possible, provided that the patient tolerates the withholding of renal replacement therapies.

Controlling hypertension (see Treatment of Hypertension), hyperphosphatemia, and urinary tract infection can contribute greatly toward this endeavor. Acidosis may be treated with sodium citrate solutions, provided that the added sodium will not aggravate hypertension. Hyperphosphatemia is controlled by attempts at dietary restriction and the use of dietary phosphate binders (eg, calcium carbonate). Vitamin D should be administered to maintain normal serum calcium. When the blood urea nitrogen exceeds approximately 50 mg/dL, or if the child is lethargic or anorexic, dietary protein restriction should be initiated. Sodium restriction is advisable when hypertension is present. Potassium restriction will be necessary as the GFR falls to a level where urinary output decreases sharply. Meanwhile, the diet must continue to meet the child's specific daily requirements.

Renal function must be regularly monitored (creatinine and blood urea nitrogen), as well as serum electrolytes, calcium, phosphorus, and alkaline phosphates. Loss of the endocrine functions due to renal failure will become clinically evident at various times during the progression of chronic renal parenchymal deterioration. Problems with skeletal homeostasis, for example, are compounded by the abnormalities of vitamin D metabolism and its actions, because final hydroxylation of active vitamin D occurs in the healthy kidney. Anemia resulting from the reduction in renal erythropoietin will become symptomatic close to the time when renal replacement therapy becomes necessary. All of these areas require careful monitoring in order to minimize symptomatology while continuing to assess the success or failure of the CRF treatment regimen and the need for the institution of chronic dialysis and transplantation.

Caution must also be taken to avoid medications that (1) aggravate the uremic condition (eg, tetracyclines, which increase blood urea); (2) depend upon renal excretion (eg, compounds containing magnesium); (3) raise blood pressure (eg, over-the-counter cold preparations containing vasoconstrictive agents); or (4) contain high amounts of substances of particular concern in the management of CRF (eg, sodium, potassium, and phosphate). Successful management relies greatly upon the education of patient and family regarding such matters.

Attention must also be directed to the psychosocial needs of the patient and family during this very difficult period of adjustment to severe chronic illness and the impact of chronic dialysis and renal transplantation. Once end-stage renal replacement therapy, such as dialysis, is initiated, however, changes in management will occur. These changes will take advantage of that treatment process and may permit reduction in oral medications or dietary limitations, improve the appetite, and even alleviate anemia (or safely permit administration of blood transfusion) and bring about better control of bone disease. Moreover, growth can improve—still a primary aim in the management of the child requiring renal replacement therapy, whether dialysis or transplantation.

Dialysis & Transplantation:

The method of treatment of end-stage renal disease best tolerated by the child is a successful and uncomplicated renal transplant. Transplantation at first seems ideal; however, despite the advances that have been made in organ transplantation procedures, there are some problems. Adequate growth and well-being are directly related to acceptance of the graft, the degree of normal function, and the side effects of medications employed.

Great advances have also been made in peritoneal dialysis and hemodialysis, both in technique and in our understanding of the specialized approach required by the treatments. Hemodialysis is now performed in major centers that devote their entire effort in dialysis toward the management of pediatric patients, and it is now regarded as a reasonable long-range method of treating the child with end-stage renal disease. Treatment of terminal renal failure in children may thus consist of transplantation or dialysis, as the situation warrants. The demonstrated feasibility of chronic peritoneal dialysis in children has made this treatment most often the initial choice of dialysis therapy for children. Peritoneal dialysis via an indwelling chronic catheter is well accepted by children and can be performed in the home.

The best measure of the success of chronic dialysis in children is the level of physical and psychosocial rehabilitation achieved. Patients continue to participate in day-to-day activities and attend school; they have even recorded reasonable growth. Although catch-up growth rarely occurs, patients can grow at an acceptable rate even though they remain in the 3rd percentile. Even associated problems such as chronic anemia and bone disease are being better controlled.

Alliopoulous JC et al: Comparison of continuous cycling peritoneal dialysis with continuous ambulatory peritoneal dialysis in children. *J Pediatr* 1984;**105**:721.

Beckman et al: Measurement of erythropoietin in anephric children: A report of the Southwest Pediatric Nephrology Study Group. *Pediatr Nephrol* 1989;**3**:75.

Chesney RW et al: Increased growth after long-term oral 1 alpha, 25-vitamin D_3 in childhood renal osteodystrophy. *N Engl J Med* 1978;**298**:238.

Lum GM et al: Southwest Pediatric Nephrology Study Group: Continuous ambulatory and continuous cycling peritoneal dialysis in children. *Kidney Int* 1985;**27**:558.

Nakano M et al: Protein intake and renal function in children. *Am J Dis Child* 1989;**143**:160.

Potter DE et al: Treatment of end-stage renal disease in children: A 15 year experience. *Kidney Int* 1980;**18**:103.

Tejani et al: Strategies for optimizing growth in children with kidney transplants. *Transplantation* 1989;**47**:229.

HYPERTENSION

Hypertension in children is commonly of renal origin. It is usually encountered as an anticipated complication of known renal parenchymal disease, but it may be found on routine physical examination in an otherwise normal child. Increased understanding of the roles of water and salt retention on the one hand and overactivity of the renin-angiotensin system on the other has done much to guide therapy; it is nevertheless clear that not all forms of hypertension can be explained by these 2 mechanisms.

Hypertension in the newborn period is frequently encountered in the ill infant, usually in an intensive care setting. Etiologic origins include (1) congenital anomalies of the kidneys or renal vasculature, (2) obstruction of the urinary tract, (3) thrombosis of renal vasculature or kidneys, and (4) volume overload. There are also reported instances of apparent paradoxical elevations of blood pressure in clinical situations where chronic diuretic therapy is employed, eg, bronchopulmonary dysplasia. Asymptomatic hypertension in the newborn also elicits a search for renal, vascular, or aortic abnormalities (eg, polycystic kidneys, obstruction, renal vascular stenosis, thrombosis, neurofibromatosis, coarctation, etc), as well as some endocrine disorders.

Diagnosis

Confirmation of the diagnosis depends upon the repeated demonstration of a diastolic pressure 2 standard deviations above the mean (Table 22–4). Careful measurement of the blood pressure includes ensuring that the size of the cuff is correct and that the equipment is reliable. The cuff should be wide enough to cover two-thirds of the upper arm and should encircle the arm completely without causing an overlap in the inflatable bladder. Although an anxious child may display an elevation in blood pressure, all abnormal readings must not be too hastily attributed to this cause. Repeat measurement is helpful, especially after the child has been consoled.

Evaluation of renal hypertension in children is particularly directed toward the possibility of a unilateral lesion or other abnormality that might be susceptible to remedy by surgery. The evaluation of nonrenal possibilities suggested by the history or physical signs is detailed under these respective conditions.

Routine laboratory studies include a complete blood count, urinalysis, and urine culture and radio-

Table 22–4. Normal blood pressure for various ages (mm Hg).[1]

Ages	Mean Systolic ± 2 SD	Mean Diastolic ± 2 SD
1 month	80 ± 16	46 ± 16
6 months to 1 year	89 ± 29	60 ± 10[2]
1 year	96 ± 30	66 ± 25[2]
2 years	99 ± 25	64 ± 25[2]
3 years	100 ± 25	67 ± 23[2]
4 years	99 ± 20	65 ± 20[2]
5–6 years	94 ± 14	55 ± 9
6–7 years	100 ± 15	56 ± 8
7–8 years	102 ± 15	56 ± 8
8–9 years	105 ± 16	57 ± 9
9–10 years	107 ± 16	57 ± 9
10–11 years	111 ± 17	58 ± 10
11–12 years	113 ± 18	59 ± 10
12–13 years	115 ± 19	59 ± 10
13–14 years	118 ± 19	60 ± 10

[1]Reproduced, with permission, from Nadas A: *Pediatric Cardiology*, 2nd ed. Saunders, 1963.
[2]In this study, the point of muffling was taken as the diastolic pressure.

graphic delineation of the urinary tract. A renal biopsy (which rarely reveals the cause of hypertension unless there is clinical evidence of renal disease) should always be undertaken with special care in the hypertensive patient and preferably after pressures have been controlled by therapy. Ureteric catheterization is not used now in lateralizing lesions; instead, the appropriate information is obtained from renal size, a rapid-sequence intravenous urogram, the renal scan, aortography with renal arteriography, and differential renal vein renin levels.

Treatment

A. Treatment of Acute Emergent Hypertension:
A hypertensive emergency may be said to exist when central nervous system signs of hypertension appear, eg, papilledema or seizures. Retinal hemorrhages or exudates also indicate a need for prompt and effective control.

1. One of the most effective drugs for use in a true hypertensive emergency is diazoxide (Hyperstat IV), 5 mg/kg by a single, rapid intravenous injection.

2. Intravenous hydralazine can be effective in some cases. Dosage varies according to the severity of the hypertension and should begin at around 0.15 mg/kg.

3. Sodium nitroprusside is also effective in an intensive care setting for reducing severely elevated blood pressure. Intravenous administration of 0.5—10 μg/kg/min will reduce blood pressure in seconds, but the dose must be carefully monitored.

4. Furosemide, 1—5 mg/kg intravenously, will reduce blood volume and enhance the effectiveness of other drugs.

5. Sublingual nifedipine, a calcium channel blocker, is rapid-acting and in appropriate doses should not result in hypotensive blood pressure levels. The liquid from a 10-mg capsule can be withdrawn with a syringe, and dosage can be approximated. The exact dosage for children who weigh less than 10–30 kg is difficult to ascertain by this method, but 5 mg is a safe starting point. Because the treatment is directed at emergent levels of blood pressure, it is unlikely that the effects will be greater than desired. Larger children with malignant hypertension require 10 mg. In such cases, the capsule may simply be pierced and the medication squeezed under the patient's tongue. Whatever method is used to control emergent hypertension safely and rapidly, concomitant administration of oral medications for sustained control should also be initiated so that the effect will be maintained and the emergent measures reduced and discontinued.

Acute elevations of blood pressure not exceeding the 95th percentile for age may be approached with oral medication, and measures should be aimed at progressive improvement and control within 48 hours.

B. Treatment of Sustained Hypertension:
A large number of antihypertensive medications are available for the treatment of sustained hypertension. None of the medications has been extensively studied in children, but wide clinical experience with several allows for a choice among those that are more commonly used (Table 22–5).

The approach to the child with renal disease and hypertension includes assessing the degree of functional disturbances that result in the retention of sodium and water. When there is significant retention, the contribution of intravascular volume to the resulting elevated blood pressure supports the rational use of a diuretic. Thus, in some instances a diuretic alone may offer therapeutic benefit; however, diuretics more often are used in combination with other medications aimed at the other pathophysiologic factors that contribute to hypertension. As a single drug, the beta-blockers may be more widely applicable than diuretics and certainly lack the possible complications of electrolyte disturbances and excessive volume depletion. Nonetheless, these two classes of "first-order" medications for mild hypertension are very likely to be inadequate in the control of moderate to severe (ie, greater than the 95th percentile) hypertension.

The angiotensin-I converting enzyme (ACE) inhibitors, as well as the calcium channel blockers are being used more frequently in pediatrics, either alone or in combination with a diuretic or a beta-blocker. Of course, other drug combinations are

Table 22–5. Antihypertensive drugs for ambulatory treatment.

Drug	Oral Dose	Major Side Effects[1]
Hydrochloro-thiazide	2–4 mg/kg/24 h as single dose or in 2 individual doses	Potassium depletion, hyperuricemia.
Furosemide	1–5 mg/kg/dose, 2–3 doses per day	Potassium and volume depletion.
Hydralazine	0.75 mg/kg/24 h in 4–6 divided doses	Lupus erythematosus, tachycardia, headache.
Methyldopa	10–40 mg/kg/24 h in 3 divided doses	False-positive Coombs test, hemolytic anemia, fever, leukopenia, abnormal liver function tests.
Propranolol	0.2–5 mg/kg/dose, 2–3 doses per day	Syncope, cardiac failure, hypoglycemia.
Minoxidil	0.15 mg/kg/dose, 2–3 doses per day	Tachycardia, angina, fluid retention, hirsutism.
Captopril	0.3–2 mg/kg/dose, 2–3 doses per day	Rash, hyperkalemia, glomerulopathy.
Nifedipine	0.5–1 mg/kg/d, 3 doses per day	Flushing, tachycardia

[1]Many more side effects than those listed have been reported.

used as their therapeutic efficacy is evaluated and individualized.

The use of the vasodilator type of antihypertensive drug requires concomitant administration of a diuretic to counter the effect of vasodilation on increasing renal sodium and water retention and a beta-blocker to counter reflex tachycardia. Minoxidil, considered the most powerful of the orally administered vasodilators, can be extremely efficacious in the treatment of severe, sustained hypertension, but its effect is greatly offset by the other effects described. Hirsutism is a significant side effect; consequently, minoxidil is a troublesome drug to use in girls. Hydralazine hydrochloride may still be the most common vasodilator in pediatric use, but, again, the necessity of using 2 additional drugs for maximum benefit keeps vasodilators in reserve for those severe situations that mandate the intervention of 3 to 4 drugs.

Abman SH et al: Systemic hypertension in infants with bronchopulmonary dysplasia. *J Pediatr* 1984;**104:**928.

Flamanbaum W: Beta-blockers and hypertension. *Am J Hypertens* 1989;**2:**865.

Friedman A: Effective use of captopril (angiotensin I converting enzyme inhibitor) in severe childhood hypertension. *J Pediatr* 1980;**97:**664.

Ingelfinger JR: Investigating hypertension in children. *Nephro News Issues* (Feb) 1989;**3:**29.

Leonetti G, Terzoli L, Bragato R: Advantages and limitations of diuretic therapy in essential hypertension. *Am J Hypertens* 1989;**2:**825.

Loggie JMH et al: Hypertension in the pediatric patient: A reappraisal. *J Pediatr* 1979;**94:**688.

Parent R, Chiasson JL, Larochelle P: Hemodynamic and endocrine effects of acute and chronic administration of nifedipine. *J Clin Pharmacol* 1989;**29:**107.

Richard GA et al: A pathophysiologic basis for the diagnosis and treatment of the renal hypertensions. *Adv Pediatr* 1977;**24:**339.

INHERITED OR DEVELOPMENTAL DEFECTS OF THE URINARY TRACT

Numerous entities and syndromes involve developmental, hereditary, or metabolic abnormalities of the kidneys and collecting system. The clinical problems encountered include concerns with overall metabolic consequences, failure to thrive, nephrolithiasis, renal glomerular or tubular dysfunction, and chronic renal failure. Specific discussion of all such entities is beyond the scope of this text. However, Table 22–6 lists some of the major entities and groups them into clinically, metabolically, or anatomically related problems.

DISORDERS OF THE RENAL TUBULES

Three subtypes of renal tubular acidosis are well recognized: (1) the "classic" form, called type I or distal renal tubular acidosis; (2) the bicarbonate "wasting" form, designated as type II or proximal renal tubular acidosis; and (3) type IV, or hyperkalemic renal tubular acidosis (rare in children), which is associated with hyporeninemic hypoaldosteronism. Type I and type II and their variants are encountered most frequently in children. Thus, discussion will focus on these 2 most commonly seen problems of urinary acidification.

Primary tubular disorders in childhood, such as glycinuria, hypouricemia, or renal glycosuria, may result from a defect in a single tubular transport pathway (see Table 22–6).

Table 22–6. Inherited or developmental defects of the urinary tract.

Cystic Diseases of Genetic Origin
Polycystic disease
  Autosomal recessive form (infantile)
  Autosomal dominant form (adult)
  Other syndromes that include either form
Cortical cysts
  Several syndromes are known to have various renal cystic manifestations, including "simple" cysts; may not have significant effect on renal functional status nor be associated with progressive disease
Medullary cysts
  Medullary sponge kidney
  Medullary cystic disease (nephronophthisis)
Hereditary and familial cystic dysplasia
  Congenital nephrosis
  "Finnish" disease
Dysplastic Renal Diseases
Renal aplasia (unilateral, bilateral)
Renal hypoplasia (unilateral, bilateral, total, segmental)
Multicystic renal dysplasia (unilateral, bilateral, multilocular, postobstructive, etc)
Familial and hereditary renal dysplasias
Oligomeganephronia
Hereditary Diseases Associated With Nephritis
Hereditary nephritis with deafness and ocular defects (Alport's syndrome)
Nail-patella syndrome
Familial hyperprolinemia
Hereditary nephrotic syndrome
Hereditary osteolysis with nephropathy
Hereditary nephritis with thoracic asphyxiant dystrophy syndrome
Hereditary Diseases Associated With Intrarenal Deposition of Metabolites
Angiokeratoma corporis diffusum (Fabry's disease)
Heredopathia atactica polyneuritiformis (Refsum disease)
Various storage diseases (eg, G_{M1} monosialogangliosidosis, Hurler syndrome, Niemann-Pick disease, familial metachromatic leukodystrophy, glycogenosis type I [von Gierke's disease], glycogenosis type II [Pompe's disease])

Table 22–6 (cont'd). Inherited or developmental defects of the urinary tract.

Hereditary amyloidosis (familial Mediterranean fever; heredofamilial urticaria with deafness and neuropathy; primary familial amyloidosis with polyneuropathy)
Hereditary Renal Diseases Associated With Tubular Transport Defects
Hartnup disease
Immunoglycinuria
Fanconi's syndrome
Oculocerebrorenal syndrome of Lowe
Cystinosis (infantile, adolescent, adult types)
Wilson's disease
Galactosemia
Hereditary fructose intolerance
Renal tubular acidosis (many types)
Hereditary tyrosinemia
Renal glycosuria
Vitamin D-resistant rickets
Pseudohypoparathyroidism
Vasopressin-resistant diabetes insipidus
Hypouricemia
Hereditary Diseases Associated With Lithiasis
Hyperoxaluria
L-Glyceric aciduria
Xanthinuria
Lesch-Nyhan syndrome and variants, gout
Nephropathy due to familial hyperparathyroidism
Cystinuria (types I, II, III)
Glycinuria
Miscellaneous
Hereditary intestinal vitamin B_{12} malabsorption
Total and partial lipodystrophy
Sickle cell anemia
Bartter's syndrome

DISTAL RENAL TUBULAR ACIDOSIS (Type I)

The most common form of distal renal tubular acidosis in childhood is the hereditary form. The clinical presentation is one of failure to thrive, anorexia, vomiting, and dehydration. Hyperchloremic metabolic acidosis occurs, with hypokalemia and a urinary pH exceeding 6.5. The severity of the acidosis depends usually on the presence of a bicarbonate "leak." (This variant of distal renal tubular acidosis with bicarbonate wasting has been called type III but for clinical purposes need not be considered as a distinct entity.) Concomitant hypercalciuria may lead to rickets, nephrocalcinosis, nephrolithiasis, and renal failure.

Other situations that may be responsible for distal renal tubular acidosis are listed in Table 22–6.

The pathogenesis of distal renal tubular acidosis has not yet been clearly defined. Basically, there appears to be a defect in the distal nephron, in the tubular transport of hydrogen ion, or in the maintenance of a steep enough gradient for proper excretion of hydrogen ion. This defect can be accompanied by degrees of bicarbonate wasting, or the defect may not be severe enough to lead to frank acidosis. More studies are needed to clarify the role of a variety of abnormalities that may be associated with the distal defect.

The classic method for determining the ability to handle an acid load in suspected distal renal tubular acidosis is the administration of NH_4Cl. However, this approach has been challenged. Recent evidence has shown that during sodium bicarbonate loading, the CO_2 tension of the urine does not increase in patients with distal renal tubular acidosis as it does in normal controls; this reflects a problem with the dehydration of H_2CO_3 in these patients.

Because acid load testing can be somewhat cumbersome to perform and could produce severe acidosis, it is best to use a simplified method of bicarbonate titration (described in the next section) and alkali administration to rule out proximal (type II) renal tubular acidosis. The dose of alkali required to achieve a normal plasma HCO_3^- concentration in patients with distal renal tubular acidosis is low (seldom exceeds 2–3 meq/kg/24 h) in contrast to that required in proximal renal tubular acidosis (> 10 meq/kg/24 h). Higher doses are, however, needed if distal renal tubular acidosis is accompanied by bicarbonate wasting. Alkali therapy can result in reduced complications and improved growth.

Distal renal tubular acidosis is usually a permanent disorder, although it sometimes occurs as a secondary complication. If irreversible renal damage is prevented, the prognosis is good.

Chan CM: Renal tubular acidosis. *J Pediatr* 1982;**102**:327.
Quintanilla AP: Renal tubular acidosis. *Postgrad Med* (April) 1980;**67**:60.
Rodriguez-Soriano J et al: Natural history of primary distal renal tubular acidosis treated since infancy. *J Pediatr* 1982;**101**:669.
Roth KS, Diagnosis of renal tubular disorders: A guide for the clinician. *Clin Pediatr (Phila)* 1988;**27**:463.
Sabastian A et al: Disorders of distal nephron function. *Am J Med* 1982;**72**:289.

PROXIMAL RENAL TUBULAR ACIDOSIS (Type II)

In the proximal tubule, the dominant process in the control of acid-base balance is the exchange of tubule cell hydrogen ion for intraluminal sodium. Proximal renal tubular acidosis is characterized by an alkaline urine pH, loss of bicarbonate in the urine, and mildly reduced serum bicarbonate concentrations. About 85–90% of bicarbonate reabsorption occurs in the proximal tubules. The lesion in proximal renal tubular acidosis is a lowering of the renal bicarbonate threshold, ie, the concentration of serum bicarbonate above which bicarbonate appears in the urine. With more severe acidosis, the concentration of serum bicarbonate drops and bicarbonate disappears from the urine; this reflects normal distal tubular acidification.

The proximal type is the most common type of renal tubular acidosis encountered in children. It is often an isolated defect, and in the small or preterm infant, it can be considered to be a factor of renal immaturity. The onset in infants is accompanied by failure to thrive, hyperchloremic acidosis, hypokalemia, and, rarely, nephrocalcinosis. Secondary forms are the result of reflux or obstructive uropathy and are seen in association with other tubular disorders (see Table 22–6).

Bicarbonate titration can be used to demonstrate the lowered renal threshold for bicarbonate reabsorption in proximal renal tubular acidosis, thereby distinguishing the proximal defect from the distal defect. This procedure is rather cumbersome and requires strict adherence to a protocol of bicarbonate infusion and measurement of urine pH and bicarbonate levels. A practical differentiation can be made by oral administration of citrate or bicarbonate, gradually increasing the dose until the serum level of bicarbonate reaches 22 meq/L. Larger doses, usually exceeding 5 meq/kg/24 h, are generally required to achieve the described level of serum bicarbonate in proximal renal tubular acidosis.

The available forms of bicarbonate therapy that are somewhat more easily tolerated than sodium bicarbonate are the citrate solutions (eg, Bicitra, Polycitra). Bicitra contains 1 meq of Na^+ and citrate per milliliter. Polycitra contains 2 meq per milliliter of citrate and 1 each of Na^+ and K^+. The required daily dosage is given in 3 divided doses. Potassium supplementation may be required, because the added sodium load presenting to the distal tubule may exaggerate potassium losses.

In cases of isolated defects, especially where the problem is related to renal immaturity, the prognosis is excellent. Alkali therapy can usually be discontinued after several months to 2 years. Growth should be normal, and the gradual increase in the serum bicarbonate level to above 22 meq/L heralds the presence of a raised bicarbonate threshold in the tubules. If the defect is part of a more complex tubular abnormality, the prognosis depends on the underlying disorder or syndrome.

Buckalew VM et al: Hereditary renal tubular acidosis. *Medicine* 1974;**53**:229.

Fraser D et al: Pathogenesis of hereditary vitamin D dependent rickets. *N Engl J Med* 1973;**289**:817.

Girardin EP et al: Treatment of cystinosis with cysteamine. *J Pediatr* 1979;**94**:838.

Haussler MR, McCain TA: Basic and clinical concepts related to vitamin D metabolism and action. *N Engl J Med* 1977;**297**:974.

Matin MA, Sylvester PE: Clinicopathological studies of the oculocerebrorenal syndrome of Lowe, Terrey and MacLachlen. *J Ment Defic Res* 1980;**24**:1.

McSherry E: Renal tubular acidosis in childhood. *Kidney Int* 1981;**20**:799.

Reddy V et al: Magnesium-dependent vitamin-D-resistant rickets. *Lancet* 1974;**1**:963.

Rodriguez-Soriano J, Vallo A, Garcia-Fuentes M: Distal renal tubular acidosis in infancy: A bicarbonate wasting state. *J Pediatr* 1975;**86**:524.

Schneider JA et al: Cystinosis: A review. *Metabolism* 1977;**26**:817.

Segal S: Cystinosis and its treatment. *N Engl J Med* 1979;**300**:789.

Segal S: Disorders of renal amino acid transport. *N Engl J Med* 1976;**294**:1044.

Smolin LA et al: A comparison of the effectiveness of cysteamine and phosphacysteamine in elevating plasma cysteamine concentration and decreasing leucocyte-free cystine in nephropathic cystinosis. *Pediatr Res* 1988;**23**:616.

Vladuti A: Renal tubular acidosis: An autoimmune disease. *Lancet* 1973;**1**:265.

NEPHROGENIC DIABETES INSIPIDUS

In the normal kidney, the interstitial fluid of the papilla is hyperosmolar to the fluid in the collecting duct. The luminal cells have a specific receptor for antidiuretic hormone (ADH), which, acting via cAMP, permits water to move across the cell membrane in response to the osmotic gradient. In the common X-linked recessive form (type I) of nephrogenic diabetes insipidus, there is a disorder of the ADH:adenylate cyclase receptor, and urinary adenylate cyclase is not increased after administration of vasopressin. In the type II variety, cAMP is formed by ADH action but has no effect on water transport. There are probably many variants of this complex mechanism, which is also influenced by prostaglandin E_1 and by its inhibitor, indomethacin.

The symptoms are limited to polyuria, polydipsia, and failure to thrive. In some children, particularly if the solute intake is unrestricted, some acclimatization to an elevated serum osmolality may develop. However, these children are particularly liable to episodes of dehydration, fever, vomiting, and convulsions.

Clinically, the diagnosis can be made on the basis of a history of polydipsia and polyuria that are not sensitive to the administration of vasopressin, desmopressin acetate (DDAVP), or lypressin. It is wise to confirm this in all cases by performing a vasopressin test. Maximal water restriction, overnight if possible, does not increase the tubular reabsorption of water (T^cH_2O) to above 3 mL/min/m². If 5% dextrose is administered at the rate of 275 mL/m²/h for 2 hours and vasopressin is given after 1 hour as an intravenous bolus of 0.005 unit/kg, the urine osmolality will not change during the period of infusion. The intravenous infusion of 2.5% saline at the rate of 0.25 mL/kg/min for not more than 45 minutes will result in only a small rise in urine osmolality in comparison to control infusion periods of normal saline. Theoretically, in psychogenic diabetes insipidus, vasopressin and hypertonic saline increase urine osmolality, but constant water loading seems to diminish renal response to ADH. Urine concentrating ability is impaired in a number of conditions—sickle cell anemia, pyelonephritis, potassium depletion, hypercalcemia, cystinosis and other renal tubular disorders, and obstructive uropathy—and as a result of nephrotoxic drugs.

In infants, it is usually best to allow water as demanded and to restrict salt. Serum sodium levels should be evaluated at intervals to ensure against hyperosmolality from inadvertent water restriction. In later childhood, sodium intake should continue to be restricted to 2–2.5 meq/kg/24 h. Studies have suggested that levels of C_{H2O} are significantly decreased by use of chlorothiazide, 60 mg/m^2/24 h orally; ethacrynic acid (Edecrin), 120 mg/m^2/24 h orally; and indomethacin, 3 mg/kg/24 h. When ethacrynic acid is given, potassium chloride, 2–3 meq/kg/24 h orally, should also be given to prevent alkalosis due to excessive potassium loss.

Bell NH et al: Demonstration of a defect in the formation of 3′,5′-monophosphate in vasopressin-resistant diabetes insipidus. *Pediatr Res* 1974;**8**:223.

Schreiner RL et al: Congenital nephrogenic diabetes insipidus in a baby girl. *Arch Dis Child* 1978;**53**:906.

Usberti M et al: Renal prostaglandin E$_2$ in nephrogenic diabetes insipidus: Effects of inhibition of prostaglandin synthesis by indomethacin. *J Pediatr* 1980;**97**:476.

Verhoeven GFM, Wilson JD: The syndromes of primary hormone resistance. *Metabolism* 1979;**28**:253.

URINARY TRACT INFECTION

Predisposing Factors

Urinary tract infections occur in approximately 1% of premature infants and newborns. Most of these infections are hematogenously spread; however, outside the clinical setting of perinatal acute illness and prematurity, urinary tract infections raise the possibility of urinary tract abnormalities. Within the first year of life, males are more likely to have an anatomic basis for developing urinary tract infection; nevertheless, the initial infection in a small child should alert the physician to the possibility of abnormal anatomy regardless of the patient's sex.

Older boys with a first infection should be examined for urinary tract abnormalities, whereas a more conservative, watchful approach may be taken with older girls, especially if sexual activity or poor personal hygiene is a possible cause. Such an approach, of course, assumes there are no other clinical abnormalities present that raise the suspicion of significant urinary tract disease (eg, enuresis or short stature).

Bacteria are by far the most common cause of urinary tract infections. The most predominant organisms are *Escherichia coli, Klebsiella, Staphylococcus,* and the enteric streptococci (all present in normal rectal and perineal flora). Unless there is reason to suspect that bacteremia is responsible for the development of the urinary tract infection, bacteria usually are presumed to gain access to the urinary tract via the urethra. The problem is greatly aggravated by poor hygiene, perineal infection or infestation (eg, pinworms), sexual activity, and instrumentation. Despite the fact that voiding provides some safeguard against such contamination developing into infection, abnormalities of the collecting system contribute to clinical infection and may lead to upper tract disease and renal parenchymal damage.

Clinical Findings

A. Symptoms and Signs: Newborns may present with fever, hypothermia, poor feeding, jaundice, failure to thrive, or sepsis. Infants may have fever of unknown origin, poor feeding, failure to thrive, strong-smelling urine, and irritability. Preschool children may have abdominal pain, vomiting, strong-smelling urine, fever, enuresis, increased frequency of urination, dysuria, or urgency. School-age children may develop the "classic" signs of urinary tract infection, including enuresis, increased frequency of urination, dysuria, urgency, fever, and costovertebral angle tenderness (flank pain). Occasionally, children with bacterial urinary tract infection will present with hemorrhagic cystitis.

Not all symptoms suggestive of urinary tract infection will actually prove to be related to bacterial infection. Anatomic abnormalities producing voiding discomfort, irritation of the external genitalia, or viral hemorrhagic cystitis are examples of such problems. On the other hand, some infections may actually be relatively asymptomatic. In either case, the presence of a urinary tract infection should be documented through the performance of a urinalysis and urine culture.

B. Laboratory Tests: A properly obtained clean-catch, midstream specimen is useful for urine culture, but poor technique can result in specimen contamination and subsequent false-positive test results. The clean-catch, midstream method may be satisfactory for children who can void upon request and who can be assisted in obtaining a proper specimen or be relied upon to obtain one unassisted. A bladder catheterization or suprapubic bladder tap may be performed when necessary (eg, highly suspicious clinical picture with the inability to obtain a satisfactory clean-catch specimen). Any procedure, however, carries the risk of contamination; for this reason, the more invasive procedures demand appropriate indication as well as the proper technique.

After the specimen is obtained care must be taken to decant an aliquot for urinalysis prior to sending the specimen for culture and sensitivity. The aliquot is then spun and prepared for microscopic analysis. The presence of bacteria in the specimen is highly suggestive of a urinary tract infection, provided that the aforementioned conditions of specimen collection have been met. The presence of pyuria (> 5 white blood cells per high-power field) is also consistent with infection, but, again, specimen reliability is important because the perineal region, vagina, or external genitalia may be responsible for the presence of white or red blood cells in urine specimens. Nonetheless, such findings in the face of highly suspicious clinical symptoms should prompt the initiation of antibiotic treatment until the culture results are obtained.

The mainstay in the diagnosis of urinary tract infection is a reliably obtained culture of the urine. The presence of multiple organisms suggests specimen contamination; however, this possibility must be evaluated in light of the method used in obtaining the specimen, as well as the level of confidence in the technical performance of the procedure employed. If the child is not already receiving the appropriate antibiotic as indicated by the sensitivities, a change should be made accordingly.

Nonculture methods, such as the nitrite sticks, for early detection of the possible presence of a urinary tract infection may be useful in following the child who is being watched for recurrent infection or being treated prophylactically with antibiotic suppression therapy.

Treatment

A. Initial Treatment: Once urinary tract infection is confirmed, initial therapy should be based on the patient's history of antibiotic use, the location of the infection, and the cost of alternative antibiotics. Many drugs are available for treating urinary tract infection, but all of them will occasionally be ineffective because of inherent resistance of the organism.

For uncomplicated cases of urethritis or cystitis, a single oral antibiotic (eg, ampicillin, a sulfonamide, nitrofurantoin) that the patient has not used recently can be administered for 10 days. The choice of antibiotic therapy must be verified by prior culture and sensitivity. A patient with suspected pyelonephritis need not always be admitted to the hospital but should be treated with 2 antibiotics (ampicillin, a sulfonamide, or a cephalosporin plus gentamicin). This regimen ensures adequate coverage until the patient improves and the results of antibiotic sensitivity tests are available, allowing selection of a single effective oral antibiotic. Antibiotic dosages (depending on choice of drug) are appropriately modified in patients with acute or chronic renal failure.

Most urinary tract infections can be successfully treated with inexpensive drugs given orally. Follow-up urinalysis or use of nitrite sticks within 2–3 days can confirm therapeutic success. If symptoms persist, reexamination and repeat urine culture are necessary.

B. Treatment of Refractory Infection: Persistent bacteriuria indicates superinfection with a different organism or with the same organism due to obstruction, the presence of a foreign body, or conversion of the organism to a variant form.

Intravenous urography and voiding cystourethrography should be considered with proved infection in newborns, boys, girls with symptoms of pyelonephritis, and girls with second urinary tract infections. Renal ultrasonography is a helpful, noninvasive tool for evaluating the anatomy of the urinary tract.

Obvious structural or obstructive anomalies require referral to a urologist experienced in dealing with children. Vesicoureteral reflux is common in younger children. If not severe, it will not result in renal damage and will disappear in time if repeated infections can be prevented. The presence of mild reflux does not ordinarily necessitate urologic consultation.

In patients without structural or functional urinary tract abnormalities, possible causes of recurrent infection include infrequent or incomplete voiding, poor perineal hygiene, pinworms, constipation, and the use of bubble bath. If attempts to deal with these problems are unsuccessful, single-dose prophylaxis at bedtime with agents such as nitrofurantoin or trimethoprim-sulfamethoxazole may be useful in combination with a program of frequent voiding.

C. Follow-Up of Patients With Urinary Tract Infection: All patients with urinary tract infection should be checked for recurrence every 1–2 months until they have remained free of infection for 1 year. Use of the nitrite test for home testing of first morning concentrated urine specimens may significantly reduce the cost of follow-up without compromising accuracy.

Prognosis

As long as urinary tract infections can be confined to the lower urinary tract (bladder and below), the prognosis is excellent. Once an infectious process has entered the kidney, the prognosis becomes more guarded. Hence, every diagnostic and therapeutic effort should be made to prevent recurrences.

American Academy of Pediatrics Section on Urology: Screening school children for urologic disease. *Pediatrics* 1977;**60**:239.

Johnson CE: Renal ultrasound evaluation of UTI in children. *Pediatrics* 1986;**78**:871.

Kunin CM: *Detection, Prevention and Management of Urinary Tract Infections,* 3rd ed. Lea & Febiger, 1979.

Levitt SB: Medical versus surgical treatment of primary vesicoureteral reflux. *Pediatrics* 1981;**67**:392.

McCracken GH: Diagnosis and management of acute UTI in infants and children. *Pediatr Infect Dis J* 1987;**6**:107.

Spencer JR, Schaeffer AJ: Pediatric urinary tract infections. *Urol Clin North Am* 1986;**113**:661.

SELECTED REFERENCES

Brenner BM, Rector FC: *The Kidney.* Saunders, 1986.

Fine RN, Gruskin A: *End Stage Renal Disease.* Saunders, 1984.

Heptinstall RH: *Pathology of the Kidney,* 3rd ed. Little, Brown, 1983.

Holliday MA, Barratt TM, Vernier RL: *Pediatric Nephrology.* Williams & Wilkins, 1987.

Kelalis PP, King LR, Bellman AB: *Clinical Pediatric Urology.* Saunders, 1985.

Orthopedics

Robert E. Eilert, MD

Orthopedics is the medical discipline that deals with disorders of neuromuscular and skeletal systems. Patients with orthopedic problems usually present with pain, loss of function, or deformity. Their symptoms must be considered not only in terms of the bones and joints but also in a more general sense relating to the anatomy, particularly of the extremities, and the blood vessels, skin, nerves, tendons, and muscles. As is true of most medical and surgical disorders, the diagnosis of orthopedic disorders can often be made on the basis of a carefully taken history. However, the physical examination is the most important feature of orthopedic diagnosis and depends upon an intimate knowledge of human anatomy.

DISTURBANCES OF PRENATAL ORIGIN

CONGENITAL AMPUTATIONS

Congenital amputations may be due to teratogens (eg, drugs or viruses), amniotic bands, or metabolic diseases (eg, diabetes in the mother) or, in rare cases, may be hereditary defects. Most are spontaneous and not genetically determined. The history of the pregnancy must be carefully reviewed in a search for possible teratogenic factors. According to the currently accepted international classification, amputations are either terminal or longitudinal. In terminal amputation, all parts are missing distal to the level of involvement—eg, absence of the forearm, wrist, and hand in the case of a terminal below-the-elbow amputation. A longitudinal amputation consists of partial absence of structures in the extremity along one side or the other. In radial clubhand, the entire radius is absent, but the thumb may be either hypoplastic or completely absent—ie, the effect on structures distal to the amputation may vary. Complex tissue defects are nearly always associated with longitudinal amputations in that the associated nerves and muscles are usually not completely represented when a bone is absent. Bones within the axial skeleton likewise may be absent. Congenital absence of the sacrum is often associated with diabetes in the mother.

Terminal amputations are treated by means of a prosthesis, eg, to compensate for shortness of one leg. With longitudinal deficiencies, constructive surgery may be feasible with the objective of reducing deformity and stabilizing joints. In certain types of severe anomalies, operative treatment is indicated to remove a portion of the malformed foot so that a prosthesis can be fitted early. This applies to such anomalies as congenital absence of the fibula, which is the lower extremity bone most commonly congenitally absent. Fortunately, there is rarely a problem with tenting of the skin by relative overgrowth of bone within the stump in congenital amputations.

Lower extremity prostheses are best fitted at about the time of normal walking (12–15 months of age). Lower extremity prostheses are consistently well accepted, as they are necessary for balancing and walking. Upper extremity prostheses are not as well accepted. Fitting the child with a dummy type prosthesis as early as 6 months of age has the advantage of instilling an accustomed pattern of proper length and bimanual manipulation. Children fitted later than age 2 years nearly always reject upper extremity prostheses.

Children quickly learn how to function with their prostheses and can lead active lives, participating in sports with peers.

Scotland TR, Gallway HR: A long-term view of children with congenital and acquired upper limb deficiency. *J Bone Joint Surg[Br]* 1983;**65**:346.

Shaperman J, Surnida CT: Recent advances in research in prosthetics for children. *Clin Orthop* (May) 1980; **148**:26.

Swanson AB, Swanson GD, Tada K: A classification of congenital limb malformation. *J Hand Surg[Am]* 1983; **8**:693.

DEFORMITIES OF THE EXTREMITIES

1. METATARSUS VARUS

Metatarsus varus is characterized by adduction of the forefoot on the hindfoot, with the heel in normal position or slight valgus. The longitudinal arch is often creased vertically when the deformity is more rigid. The lateral border of the foot demonstrates sharp angulation at the level of the base of the fifth metatarsal, and this bone will be especially prominent. The deformity varies from flexible to rigid. Most flexible deformities are secondary to intrauterine posture and usually resolve spontaneously.

If the deformity is rigid and cannot be manipulated past the midline, it is worthwhile to use a plaster cast changed at weekly intervals to correct the deformity.

"Corrective" shoes do not live up to their name. Shoes are supportive, but shoe wedges have not been effective in correcting this type of deformity and are of more use for placating the parent than for any true therapeutic value. A few minutes spent explaining what can be achieved with shoes may avoid an unnecessary expense for the family. The prognosis for this common deformity of the foot is excellent, and few long-term problems are reported.

Bleck EE: Metatarsus adductus: Classification and relationship to outcomes of treatment. *J Pediatr Orthop* 1983;**3**:2.

Rushforth GF: The natural history of the hooked forefoot. *J Bone Joint Surg [Br]* 1978;**60**:530.

2. CLUBFOOT
(Talipes Equinovarus)

When foot deformity consists of the following 3 elements, the diagnosis of classic talipes equinovarus, or clubfoot, is made: (1) equinus or plantar flexion of the foot at the ankle joint, (2) varus or inversion deformity of the heel, and (3) forefoot varus. The incidence of talipes equinovarus is approximately 1:1000 live births. Any infant with a clubfoot should be examined carefully for associated anomalies, especially of the spine. Clubfoot tends to follow a hereditary pattern in some families or may be part of a generalized neuromuscular syndrome such as arthrogryposis or myelodysplasia.

Treatment consists of massage and manipulation of the foot to stretch the contracted tissues on the medial and posterior aspects, followed by splinting to hold the correction. When this treatment is instituted in the nursery shortly after birth, correction is achieved much more rapidly. When treatment is delayed, the foot tends to become more rigid within a matter of days. Treatment in the nursery by strapping and splinting is often effective. As the child gets older, casting following manipulation and stretching is necessary. The casts are applied sequentially, correcting first the forefoot adduction, then the inversion of the heel, and finally the equinus of the ankle. Treatment by means of casting requires patience and experience; if it is not done properly in sequence, iatrogenic deformities of the foot may result, such as rocker-bottom foot.

After full correction is obtained, a night brace is often prescribed for long-term maintenance of correction.

About half of children with clubfoot eventually need an operative procedure to lengthen the tightened structures about the foot.

A supple foot that is easily corrected by strapping and casting has a more favorable prognosis. If the foot is rigid and requires prolonged treatment to obtain correction, perhaps combined with surgery, the prognosis must be guarded.

Cummings RJ, Lovell WW: Operative treatment of congenital idiopathic club foot. *J Bone Joint Surg [Am]* 1988;**70**:1108.

Kite JH: Conservative treatment of the resistant recurrent clubfoot. *Clin Orthop* (May–June) 1970;**70**:93.

3. CONGENITAL DYSPLASIA OF THE HIP JOINT
(Congenital Dislocation of the Hip)

In a child with congenital dysplasia of the hip, the femoral head and the acetabulum may be in partial contact at birth. This condition is termed subluxation of the hip. A more severe defect is complete loss of contact between the femoral head and acetabulum, in which case there is frank dislocation of the hip, with the femoral head nearly always displaced laterally and superiorly due to muscle pull. At birth, there is lack of the development of both the acetabulum and the femur in cases of congenital hip dysplasia. The dysplasia becomes progressive with growth unless the dislocation is corrected. If the dislocation is corrected in the first few days or weeks of life, the dysplasia is completely reversible and a normal hip will develop. As the child becomes older and the dislocation or subluxation persists, the deformity will worsen to the point where it will not be completely reversible, especially after the walking age. For this reason, it is important to diagnose the deformity in the nursery or, at the latest, the 6-week checkup.

Clinical Findings

The diagnosis of congenital hip dislocation in the newborn depends upon demonstrating instability of the joint by placing the infant on its back and obtaining complete relaxation by feeding with a bottle if necessary. The examiner's long finger is then placed over the greater trochanter and the thumb over the inner side of the thigh. Both hips are flexed 90 degrees and then slowly abducted from the midline. With gentle pressure, an attempt is made to lift the greater trochanter forward. A feeling of slipping as the head goes into the acetabulum is a sign of instability (as first described by Ortolani). In other infants, the joint is more stable, and the deformity must be provoked by applying slight pressure with the thumb on the medial side of the thigh as the thigh is adducted, thus slipping the hip posteriorly and eliciting a jerk as the hip dislocates. This sign was first described by Barlow. The signs of instability are the most reliable criteria for diagnosing congenital dislocation of the hip in the newborn. X-rays of the pelvis are notoriously unreliable until about 6 weeks of age. Asymmetric skin folds are present in about 40% of newborns and therefore are not particularly helpful.

After the first month of life, the signs of instability as demonstrated by Ortolani's test or Barlow's test become less evident. Contractures begin to develop about the hip joint, causing limitation of abduction. Normally, the hip should abduct fully to 90 degrees on either side during the first few months of life. It is important that the pelvis be held level to detect asymmetry of abduction. When the hips and knees are flexed, the knees are at unequal heights, with the dislocated side lower (Allis's sign). After the first few weeks of life, x-ray examination becomes more valuable, with lateral displacement of the femoral head being the most reliable sign. In mild cases, the only abnormality may be increased steepness of acetabular alignment, so that the acetabular angle is greater than 35 degrees.

If congenital dislocation of the hip has not been diagnosed during the first year of life and the child begins to walk, there will be a painless limp and a lurch to the affected side, as first described by Trendelenburg. When the child stands on the affected leg, there is a dip of the pelvis on the opposite side owing to weakness of the gluteus medius muscle. This has been termed Trendelenburg's sign and accounts for the unusual swaying gait. In children with bilateral dislocations, the loss of abduction is almost symmetric and may be deceiving. Abduction, however, is never complete, and x-ray of the pelvis is indicated in children with incomplete abduction in the first few months of life. As a child with bilateral dislocation of the hips begins to walk, the gait is waddling. The perineum is widened as a result of lateral displacement of the hips, and there is flexion contracture as a result of posterior displacement of the hips. This flexion contracture contributes to marked lordosis, and the greater trochanters are easily palpable in their elevated position. Treatment is still possible in the first 2 years of life, but the results are not nearly as effective as in children treated in the nursery.

Treatment

Dislocation or dysplasia diagnosed in the first few weeks or months of life can easily be treated by splinting, with the hip maintained in flexion and abduction. Full abduction is contraindicated, as this often leads to avascular necrosis of the femoral head. The use of double or triple diapers is never indicated for medical reasons, because diapers are not adequate to obtain proper positioning of the hip. In cases of joint laxity without true dislocation, improvement will be spontaneous; diapers are excessive treatment.

Various splints to maintain flexion and abduction of the hip, such as the ones designed by Pavlik, Ilfeld, or von Rosen, are available. Treatment of children requiring splints is best supervised by an orthopedic surgeon with a special interest in the problem.

In the first 4 months of life, reduction can be obtained by simply flexing and abducting the hip; no other manipulation is usually necessary. If force is used to reduce the hip, the excessive pressure may cause avascular necrosis. In such cases, preoperative traction for 2–3 weeks is important to relax soft tissues about the hip. Following traction in which the femur is brought down opposite the acetabulum, reduction can be easily achieved without force under general anesthesia. It is then necessary to place the child in a plaster cast, which is used for approximately 6 months. The position in the cast should be carefully adjusted in order to avoid stretching of the delicate blood supply to the femoral head. The hip is flexed slightly more than 90 degrees and abducted only 45–60 degrees. Internal rotation is avoided, because this tends to "wring out" the blood vessels in the capsule of the joint. If the reduction is not stable within a reasonable range following closed reduction, open reduction, combined with plication of the lax capsule in order to maintain reduction, may be necessary.

If reduction is done at an older age, operations to correct the deformities of the acetabulum and femur may be necessary during growth.

Coleman SS: *Congenital Dysplasia and Dislocation of the Hip.* Mosby, 1978.

Hensinger RN: Congenital dislocation of the hip: Treatment in infancy to walking age. *Orthop Clin North Am* 1987;**18**:597.

Morrissy RT, Cowie GH: Congenital dislocation of the hip: Early detection and prevention of late complications. *Clin Orthop* (Sept) 1987;**222**:79.

4. TORTICOLLIS

Wryneck deformities in infancy may be due either to injury to the sternocleidomastoid muscle during delivery or to disease affecting the cervical spine. In the case of muscular deformity, the chin is rotated to the side opposite to the affected sternocleidomastoid muscle contracture, and the head is tilted toward the side of the contracture. A mass felt in the midportion of the sternocleidomastoid muscle does not represent a true tumor but fibrous transformation within the muscle.

In mild cases, passive stretching is usually effective. If the deformity has not been corrected by passive stretching within the first year of life, surgical division of the muscle will correct it. It is not necessary to excise the ''tumor'' of the sternocleidomastoid muscle, because this tends to resolve spontaneously. If the deformity is left untreated, an unsightly facial asymmetry will result.

Torticollis is occasionally associated with congenital deformities of the cervical spine, and x-rays of the spine are indicated in all cases.

Acute torticollis may follow upper respiratory infection or mild trauma in children. Rotatory subluxation of the upper cervical spine should be sought by appropriate x-ray views. Traction or a cervical collar usually results in resolution of the symptoms within 1 or 2 days.

Binder H, Eng GE, Gaiser JF: Congenital muscular torticollis: Results of conservative management with long-term follow-up in 85 cases. *Arch Phys Med Rehabil* 1987;**68**:222.

Dawson EG, Smith L: Atlantoaxial subluxation in children due to vertebral anomalies. *J Bone Joint Surg [Am]* 1979; **61**:582.

GENERALIZED AFFECTIONS OF SKELETON OR MESODERMAL TISSUES

1. ARTHROGRYPOSIS MULTIPLEX CONGENITA (Amyoplasia Congenita)

Arthrogryposis multiplex congenita consists of incomplete fibrous ankylosis (usually symmetric) of many or all of the joints of the body. There may be contractures either in flexion or extension. Upper extremity deformities usually consist of adduction of the shoulders, extension of the elbows, flexion of the wrists, and stiff, straight fingers with poor muscle control of the thumbs. In the lower extremities, common deformities are dislocation of the hips, extension of the knees, and severe clubfoot. The joints are fusiform and the joint capsules decreased in volume, producing contractures. Various investigations have attributed the basic defect to an abnormality of muscle or of the lower motor neuron. Muscular development is poor, and muscles may be represented only by fibrous bands. The joint deformities appear to be secondary to a lack of active motion during intrauterine development.

Passive mobilization of joints should be done early. Because of poor muscle control, however, joint mobility cannot be maintained by active motion. Prolonged casting for correction of deformities is contraindicated in these children because further stiffness is often produced. Use of removable splints combined with vigorous therapy is the most effective conservative treatment. Surgical release of the affected joints is often necessary. The clubfoot associated with arthrogryposis is very stiff and nearly always requires an operation. Surgery about the knees, including capsulotomy, osteotomy, and tendon lengthening, is used to correct deformity. Dynamic correction by 2-pin skeletal traction may be effective in some knee contractures when combined with therapy to maintain motion while in traction. In the young child, a single vigorous attempt at reduction of the dislocated hip is worthwhile. Multiple operative procedures about the hip are contraindicated because further stiffness may be produced with consequent impairment of motion. The dislocation of the hip that occurs in arthrogryposis is associated with severe dysplasia of the bones and does not respond to treatment as ordinary congenital hip dislocation does. Affected children are often able to walk with bilateral dislocation of the hips, and in cases of severe rigidity it is better to leave the hips out of joint. With lesser demands, the long-term disability is not as severe as it would be in a person with normal mobility and strength.

The long-term prognosis for physical and vocational independence is poor. Patients usually have normal intelligence, but they have such severe physical restrictions that gainful employment is hard to find.

Hahn G: Arthrogryposis: Pediatric review and habilitative aspects. *Clin Orthop* (April) 1985;**194**:104.

2. MARFAN'S SYNDROME

Marfan's syndrome is characterized by unusually long fingers and toes (arachnodactyly); hypermobility of the joints; subluxation of the ocular lenses; other eye abnormalities including cataract, coloboma, megalocornea, strabismus, and nystagmus; a high-arched palate; a strong tendency to scoliosis; pectus carinatum; and thoracic aneurysms due to weakness of the media of the vessels. Serum mucoproteins may be decreased and urinary excretion of hydroxyproline increased. The condition is easily confused with homocystinuria, as the phenotypic presentation is identical. The 2 diseases may be differentiated by the presence of homocystine in the urine in homocystinuria.

Treatment is usually supportive for associated problems such as flatfeet. Scoliosis may involve more vigorous treatment by bracing or spine fusion. The long-term prognosis has improved for patients as better treatment for their aortic aneurysms has been devised.

Bornstein D, Byers DH: Collagen metabolism. In: *Current Concepts.* Upjohn, 1980.

3. CLEIDOCRANIAL DYSOSTOSIS

Cleidocranial dysostosis consists of absence of part or all of the clavicle and delay in ossification of the skull. The facial bones are often underdeveloped, with absence of the sinuses, a high-arched palate, and defective teeth. The skull is enlarged, especially in the parietal and frontal regions. Coxa vara deformity of the proximal femur is sometimes present but usually is not of sufficient magnitude to require surgery. Deficiency of ossification of the symphysis pubica may persist into adult life. The clavicular deformity allows affected patients to touch their shoulders in the midline but otherwise presents no difficulty. The pelvic deformities do not prevent normal pregnancy and childbirth. The syndrome has a strong hereditary tendency.

4. CRANIOFACIAL DYSOSTOSIS (Crouzon's Disease)

Craniofacial dysostosis is a syndrome consisting of acrocephaly, hypoplastic maxilla, beaked nose, protrusion of the lower lip, exophthalmos, exotropia, and hypertelorism. It is usually familial. No orthopedic treatment is necessary. Heroic efforts have been made by neurosurgeons and plastic surgeons to correct the grotesque deformity of patients, who generally have normal intelligence. These operative procedures are complicated and hazardous, involving multiple osteotomies of the skull and facial bones.

5. KLIPPEL-FEIL SYNDROME

Klippel-Feil syndrome is characterized by fusion of some or all of the cervical vertebrae. Multiple spinal anomalies may be present, with hemivertebrae and scoliosis. The neck is short and stiff, the hairline is low, and the ears are often low-set. Common associated defects include congenital scoliosis, cervical rib, spina bifida, torticollis, web neck, high scapula, renal anomalies, and deafness. Examination of the urinary tract by urinalysis, blood urea nitrogen, and intravenous urograms is indicated as well as a hearing test.

Scoliotic deformities, if progressive, may require treatment. Occasionally, it is necessary to correct the high scapula, also called **Sprengel's deformity** (see below).

Hensinger RN et al: Klippel-Feil syndrome. *J Bone Joint Surg [Am]* 1974;**56**:1246.

6. SPRENGEL'S DEFORMITY

Sprengel's deformity is a congenital condition in which one or both scapulas are elevated and small. The child cannot raise the arm completely on the affected side, and there may be torticollis. The deformity occurs alone or may be associated with Klippel-Feil syndrome.

If the deformity is functionally limiting, the scapula may be surgically relocated lower in the thorax. Excision of the upper portion of the scapula improves cosmetic appearance but has little effect on function.

Samilson RL: Congenital and development anomalies of the shoulder girdle. *Orthop Clin North Am* 1980; **11**:219.

7. OSTEOGENESIS IMPERFECTA

Osteogenesis imperfecta is a rare, mainly dominantly inherited connective tissue disease. The severe fetal type (osteogenesis imperfecta congenita) is characterized by multiple intrauterine or perinatal fractures. Affected children continue to have fractures and are dwarfed as a result of bony deformities and growth retardation. Intelligence is not affected. The shafts of the long bones are reduced in cortical thickness, and wormian bones are present in the skull. Other features include blue scleras, thin skin, hyperextensibility of ligaments, "otosclerosis" with significant hearing loss, and hypoplastic and deformed teeth. Recurrent epistaxis, easy bruisability, mild hyperpyrexia (which may increase significantly during anesthesia), and excessive diaphoresis are common. In the tarda type, fractures begin to occur at variable times after the perinatal period, resulting in relatively fewer fractures and deformities in these cases. The patients are sometimes suspected of having suffered induced fractures, and the condition should be ruled out in any case of nonaccidental trauma.

Metabolic defects include elevated serum pyrophosphate, decreased platelet aggregation, and decreased incorporation of sulfate into acid mucopolysaccharides by skin fibroblasts. Normal parents can be counseled that the likelihood of a second affected child is negligible.

There is no effective treatment by medication. Surgical treatment involves correction of deformity of the long bones. Multiple intramedullary rods have been used to prevent deformity from poor healing of fractures.

The overall prognosis is poor, and patients are often confined to wheelchairs during adulthood.

Albright JA, Miller EA: Osteogenesis imperfecta. (Editorial.) *Clin Orthop* (Sept) 1981;**159**:2.
Bauze RJ et al: A new look at osteogenesis imperfecta: A clinical, radiological and biochemical study of 42 patients. *J Bone Joint Surg [Br]* 1975;**57**:2.

8. IDIOPATHIC JUVENILE OSTEOPOROSIS

Idiopathic juvenile osteoporosis is an acute bone disease characterized by unexplained pathologic fractures of the spine and long bones. It affects boys and girls equally in the prepubertal years, and the degree of severity is variable. There is evidence of gross enteric malabsorption of calcium, which may reflect an abnormality of 1,25-dihydroxyergocalciferol synthesis.

9. OSTEOPETROSIS (Osteitis Condensans Generalisata; Marble Bone Disease; Albers-Schönberg Disease)

The clinical manifestations of osteopetrosis, a familial and hereditary syndrome, are bony deformities due to pathologic fractures, myelophthisic anemia, splenomegaly, visual and auditory disturbances, square head, facial paralysis, pigeon breast, and dwarfing. The findings may appear at any age. On x-ray examination, the bones show increased density, transverse bands in the shafts, clubbing of ends, and vertical striations of long bones. There is thickening about the cranial foramens, and there may be heterotopic calcification of soft tissues. Treatment with corticosteroids to ameliorate the hematologic abnormalities should be tried.

Sief CA et al: Allogenic bone-marrow transplantation in infantile malignant osteopetrosis. *Lancet* 1983;**1:**437.

10. ACHONDROPLASIA (Classic Chondrodystrophy)

In achondroplasia, the arms and legs are short, with the upper arms and thighs proportionately shorter than the forearms and legs. Findings frequently include bowing of the extremities, a waddling gait, limitation of motion of major joints, relaxation of the ligaments, short stubby fingers of almost equal length, a prominent forehead, moderate hydrocephalus, depressed nasal bridge, and lumbar lordosis. Mentality and sexual function are normal. A family history is often present. X-rays demonstrate short, thick tubular bones and irregular epiphyseal plates. The ends of the bones are thick, with broadening and cupping. Epiphyseal ossification may be delayed.

Osteotomies of the long bones are occasionally necessary if deformities are severe.

The medullary canal is narrowed, so that herniated disk in adulthood may lead to acute paraplegia.

11. OSTEOCHONDRODYSTROPHY (Morquio's Disease)

Osteochondrodystrophy is characterized by shortening of the spine, kyphosis, scoliosis, moderate shortening of the extremities, pectus carinatum, protuberant abdomen, hepatosplenomegaly, and a wad-

dling gait resulting from instability of the hips and laxity of the knee joints. The skull is minimally involved. The child may appear normal at birth but begins to develop deformities between 1 and 4 years of age as a result of abnormal deposition of mucopolysaccharides. The disorder is commonly familial. Inheritance appears to be on an autosomal recessive basis.

X-rays demonstrate wedge-shaped flattened vertebrae and irregular, malformed epiphyses. The ribs are broad and have been likened to canoe paddles. The lower extremities are more severely involved than the upper ones.

There is no treatment, and the prognosis is poor. Death may occur in childhood or adolescence. Progressive clouding of the cornea leads to increasing visual impairment.

Stanescu V, Stanescu R, Maroteaux P: Pathogenic mechanisms in osteochondrodysplasias. *J Bone Joint Surg [Am]* 1984;**66:**817.

12. CHONDROECTODERMAL DYSPLASIA (Ellis-van Creveld Syndrome)

Manifestations include ectodermal dysplasia, congenital heart disease, polydactyly, syndactyly, poorly formed teeth, and mental retardation. The disease is familial and inbred in certain ethnic groups such as the Amish people of Pennsylvania.

X-ray changes include chondrodystrophy; shortening and bowing of the tibias and fibulas; hyperplastic, eccentric proximal tibial metaphyses; and fusion of the carpal bones.

No treatment is available. The long-term prognosis depends on the severity of heart involvement.

Beals RK: Orthopaedic care for patients with skeletal dysplasia. In: *AAOS Symposium on Heritable Disorders of Connective Tissue.* Akeson WH, Bornstein P, Glimcher MJ (editors). Mosby, 1982.

McKusick VA: *Heritable Disorders of Connective Tissue,* 4th ed. Mosby, 1972.

Sillence DO, Rimoin DL: Chondroosseous morphology in the skeletal dysplasias. In: *AAOS Symposium on Heritable Disorders of Connective Tissue.* Akeson WH, Bornstein P, Glimcher MJ (editors). Mosby, 1982.

GROWTH DISTURBANCES OF THE MUSCULOSKELETAL SYSTEM

SCOLIOSIS

The term scoliosis denotes lateral curvature of the spine, which is always associated with some rotation of the involved vertebrae. Scoliosis is classified by its anatomic location, in either the thoracic or lumbar spine, with rare involvement of the cervical spine. The apex of the curve is designated right or left. Thus, a left thoracic scoliosis would denote a convex leftward curve in the thoracic region, and this is the most common type of idiopathic curve. Posterior curvature of the spine (kyphosis) is normal in the thoracic area, though excessive curvature may become pathologic. Anterior curvature is called lordosis and is normal in the lumbar spine. Idiopathic scoliosis generally begins at about 8 or 10 years of age and progresses during growth. In rare instances, infantile scoliosis may be seen in children 2 years of age or less.

Idiopathic scoliosis is about 4–5 times more common in girls than in boys. The disorder is usually asymptomatic in the adolescent years, but severe curvature may lead to impairment of pulmonary function or low back pain in later years. It is important to examine the back of any adolescent coming in for an incidental physical examination in order to identify scoliosis early. The examination is performed by having the patient bend forward 90 degrees with the hands joined in the midline. An abnormal finding consists of asymmetry of the height of the ribs or paravertebral muscles on one side, indicating rotation of the trunk associated with lateral curvature.

Diseases that may be associated with scoliosis include neurofibromatosis, Marfan's syndrome, cerebral palsy, muscular dystrophy, and poliomyelitis. Neurologic examination should be performed in all children with scoliosis to determine whether these disorders are present.

Five to 7% of cases of scoliosis are due to congenital vertebral anomalies such as a hemivertebral or unilateral vertebral bridge. These curves are more rigid than the more common idiopathic curve (see below) and will often increase with growth, especially during the rapid growth spurt during adolescence.

The most common type of scoliosis is so-called idiopathic scoliosis, which may be due to asymmetry of neuromuscular development. In 30% of cases, other family members are affected also; thus, a family survey is valuable for detecting the problem in siblings if one child has been found to have scoliosis.

Idiopathic infantile scoliosis, occurring in children 2–4 years of age, is quite uncommon in the USA; it is more common in Great Britain. If the curvature is less than 30 degrees, the prognosis is excellent, as 70% resolve spontaneously. If the curvature is more than 30 degrees, there may be progression, and the prognosis is therefore guarded.

Postural compensation of the spine may lead to lateral curvature from such causes as unequal length of the lower extremities. Antalgic scoliosis may re-

sult from pressure on the spinal cord or roots by infectious processes or herniation of the nucleus pulposus; the underlying cause must be sought. The curvature will resolve as the primary problem is treated.

Clinical Findings

A. Symptoms and Signs: Scoliosis in adolescents is classically asymptomatic. It is imperative to seek the underlying cause in any case where there is pain, since in these instances the scoliosis is almost always secondary to some other disorder such as a bone or spinal cord tumor. Deformity of the rib cage and asymmetry of the waistline are evident with curvatures of 30 degrees or more. A lesser curvature may be detected by the forward bending test as described above, which is designed to detect early abnormalities of rotation that are not apparent when the patient is standing erect.

B. Imaging: The most valuable x-rays are those taken of the entire spine in the standing position in both the anteroposterior and lateral planes. Usually, there is one primary curvature with a compensatory curvature that develops to balance the body. At times there may be 2 primary curvatures, usually in the left thoracic and right lumbar regions. Any right thoracic curvature should be suspected of being secondary to neurologic or muscular disease, prompting a more meticulous neurologic examination. If the curvatures of the spine are balanced (compensated), the head is centered over the center of the pelvis and the patient is "in balance." If the spinal alignment is uncompensated, the head will be displaced to one side, which produces an unsightly deformity. Rotation of the spine may be measured by use of spirit level as described by Bunnell (1984). This rotation is associated with a marked rib hump as the lateral curvature increases in severity. Deformity of the rib cage produces a decrease in the space available for the lung and is the cause of long-term problems.

Treatment

Curvatures of less than 20 degrees usually do not require treatment unless they show progression. Bracing is indicated for curvature of 20–40 degrees in a skeletally immature child. Treatment is indicated for any curvature that demonstrates progression on serial x-ray examination. Curvatures greater than 40 degrees are resistant to treatment by bracing. Thoracic curvatures greater than 60 degrees have been correlated with a poor pulmonary prognosis in adult life. Curvatures of such severity are an indication for surgical correction of the deformity and posterior spinal fusion to maintain the correction. Curvatures between 40 and 60 degrees may also require spinal fusion if they appear to be progressive or are causing decompensation of the spine or are cosmetically unacceptable.

Surgical fusion involves decortication of the bone

over the laminas and spinous processes, with the addition of autogenous bone graft from the iliac crest. Postoperative correction is usually maintained by a Harrington or Luque rod, with activity restriction for several months until the fusion is solid.

Treatment is prolonged and difficult and is best done in centers where full support facilities are available.

Prognosis

Compensated small curvatures that do not progress may be well tolerated throughout life, with very little cosmetic concern. The patients should be counseled regarding the genetic transmission of scoliosis and cautioned that their children should be examined at regular intervals during growth. Large thoracic curvatures greater than 60 degrees are associated with shortened life span and may progress even during adult life. Large lumbar curvatures may lead to subluxation of the vertebrae and premature arthritic degeneration of the spine, producing disabling pain in adulthood. Early detection allows for simple brace treatment or surface electrical stimulation. In patients so treated, the long-term prognosis is excellent and surgery is not necessary. For this reason, school screening programs for scoliosis have gained popular support in many sections of the country.

Bunnell WP: An objective criterion for scoliosis screening. *J Bone Joint Surg [Am]* 1984;**66:**1381.

Byrd JA: Current theories on the etiology of idiopathic scoliosis. *Clin Orthop* (April) 1988;**229:**114.

Clayson D, Luz-Alterman S, Cataletto MM et al: Long-term psychological sequelae of surgically versus nonsurgically treated scoliosis. *Spine* 1987;**12:**983.

McCarthy RE: Prevention of the complications of scoliosis by early detection. *Clin Orthop* (Sept) 1987;**222:**73.

Moe JH et al: *Scoliosis and Other Spinal Deformities.* Saunders, 1978.

Weinstein SL, Favala DC, Ponseti IV: Idiopathic scoliosis: Long-term follow-up and prognosis of untreated patients. *J Bone Joint Surg [Am]* 1981;**63:**702.

EPIPHYSIOLYSIS
(Slipped Capital Femoral Epiphysis)

Epiphysiolysis is the separation of the proximal femoral epiphysis through the growth plate. The head of the femur is usually displaced medially and posteriorly relative to the neck of the femur. The condition occurs in adolescence and is more common in overweight children. Slightly over 40% of the children so affected are of the obese, hypogenital body type. The cause is not clear, although some authorities have shown experimentally that the decreased strength of the perichondral ring stabilizing the epiphyseal area is sufficiently weakened by anatomic changes in adolescent years that the simple overload by excessive body weight can produce a pathologic fracture through the growth plate. Hormonal studies in these children have not demonstrated any abnormality. Anatomic study of the area of separation demonstrates a histologic picture identical to that seen with traumatic separation, and the condition occasionally occurs as an acute episode resulting from a fall or direct trauma to the hip.

More commonly, however, there are vague symptoms over a protracted period of time in an otherwise healthy child who presents with pain and limp. The pain is often referred into the thigh or the medial side of the knee. It is important to examine the hip joint in any child complaining of knee pain, particularly in adolescents. The consistent finding on physical examination is limitation of internal rotation of the hip. There usually is also an associated hip flexion contracture as well as local tenderness about the hip. X-rays should be taken in both the anteroposterior and lateral planes. These must be carefully examined in early cases in order to show an abnormality where displacement of the femoral head occurs posteriorly, which is usually most easily seen on the lateral view.

Treatment is based on the same principles that govern treatment of fracture of the femoral neck in adults in that the head of the femur is fixed to the neck of the femur and the fracture line allowed to heal. Unfortunately, the severe complication of avascular necrosis occurs in 30% of these patients. There has been a positive correlation between forceful reduction of the slip and avascular necrosis. In cases of acute slip, as evidenced by the absence of any callus formation about the growth plate, it may be possible to reduce the hip by gentle traction. In more chronic cases, a more expeditious procedure is to pin the slip in situ and perform correctional osteotomy later in order to realign the deformity. Remodeling of the fracture site often improves the position of the hip without further surgery. The pins used to maintain reduction should be removed once healing has occurred.

The long-term prognosis is guarded because most of these patients continue to be overweight and overstress their hip joints. Follow-up studies have shown a high incidence of premature degenerative arthritis in this group of patients—even those who do not develop avascular necrosis. The development of avascular necrosis almost guarantees a poor prognosis, because new bone does not replace the femoral head at this late stage of skeletal growth.

About 30% of patients have bilateral involvement, and patients should be followed for slipping of the opposite side, which may occur as long as 1 or 2 years after the primary episode.

Crawford AH: Slipped capital femoral epiphysis: Current concepts review. *J Bone Joint Surg[Am]* 1988;**70:**1422.

Dreghorn CR et al: Slipped upper femoral epiphysis: A review of 12 years of experience in Glasgow (1972–1983). *J Pediatr Orthop* 1987;**7:**283.

Wilcox PG, Weiner DS, Leighley B: Maturation factors in slipped capital femoral epiphysis. *J Pediatr Orthop* 1988;**8**:196.

GENU VARUM & GENU VALGUM

Genu varum (bowleg) is normal from infancy through 2 years of life. The alignment then changes to genu valgum (knock-knee) until about 8 years of age, at which time adult alignment is attained. Criteria for referral to an orthopedist include persistent bowing beyond age 2, bowing that is increasing rather than decreasing, bowing of one leg only, and knock-knee associated with short stature.

Bracing may be appropriate, or, rarely, an osteotomy is necessary for a severe problem such as Blount's disease (proximal tibial epiphyseal dysplasia).

Brighton CT: Structure and function of the growth plate. *Clin Orthop* (Oct) 1978;**136**:22.
Staheli LT: Torsional deformity. *Pediatr Clin North Am* 1977;**24**:799.
Vankka E, Salenius P: Spontaneous correction of severe tibiofemoral deformity in growing children. *Acta Orthop Scand* 1982;**53**:567.

TIBIAL TORSION

The physician is often asked about "toeing in" in small children. The disorder is routinely asymptomatic. Tibial torsion is rotation of the leg between the knee and the ankle. Internal rotation amounts to about 20 degrees at birth but decreases to neutral rotation by 1 year of age. The deformity is sometimes accentuated by laxity of the knee ligaments, allowing excessive internal rotation of the leg in small children. In children who have a persistent internal rotation of the tibia beyond 1 year of age, the condition is often due to sleeping with feet turned in and can be reversed with an external rotation splint worn only at night.

FEMORAL ANTEVERSION

"Toeing in" beyond 2 or 3 years of age is usually based on femoral anteversion, which produces excessive internal rotation of the femur as compared to external rotation. This femoral alignment follows a natural history of progressive decrease toward neutral up to 8 years of age, with slower change to 16 years of age. Studies comparing the results of treatment with shoes or braces to the natural history have shown that little is gained by active treatment. Active external rotation exercises such as ballet, skating, or bicycle riding may be worthwhile. Osteotomy for rotational correction is rarely required.

Refer those who have no external rotation of hip in extension.

Fabry G, MacEwen GD, Shands AR Jr: Torsion of the femur. *J Bone Joint Surg [Am]* 1973;**55**:1726.

COMMON FOOT PROBLEMS

When a child begins to stand and walk, the long arch of the foot is flat with a medial bulge over the inner border of the foot. The forefeet are mildly pronated or rotated inward, with a slight valgus alignment of the knees. As the child grows and muscle power improves, the long arch is better supported and more normal relationships occur in the lower extremities. (See also Metatarsus Varus and Talipes Equinovarus.)

1. FLATFOOT

Flatfoot is a normal condition in infants. Children presenting for examination should be checked to determine that the heel cord is of normal length when the heel is aligned in the neutral position, allowing complete dorsiflexion and plantar flexion. As long as the foot is supple and the presence of a longitudinal arch is noted when the child is sitting in a nonweight-bearing position, the parents can be assured that a normal arch will probably develop. There is usually a familial incidence of relaxed flatfeet in children who have prolonged malalignment of the foot. In any child with a shortened heel cord or stiffness of the foot, other causes of flatfoot such as tarsal coalition or vertical talus should be ruled out by a complete orthopedic examination and x-ray.

In the child with an ordinary relaxed flatfoot, no active treatment is indicated unless there is calf or leg pain. In children who have leg pains attributable to flatfeet, an orthopedic shoe with Thomas heel may relieve discomfort. An arch insert should not be prescribed unless passive correction of the arch is easily accomplished; otherwise, there will be irritation of the skin over the medial side of the foot.

Mosier KM, Asher M: Tarsal coalitions and peroneal spastic flatfoot: A review. *J Bone Joint Surg [Am]* 1984;**66**:976.

2. TALIPES CALCANEOVALGUS

Talipes calcaneovalgus is characterized by excessive dorsiflexion at the ankle and eversion of the foot. It is often present at birth and almost always corrects spontaneously. The deformity is the reverse of classic clubfoot (talipes equinovarus) and is due to intrauterine position.

Treatment consists of passive exercises by the mother, stretching the foot into plantar flexion. In rare instances, it may be necessary to use plaster casts to help with manipulation and positioning.

Complete correction is the rule.

3. CAVUS FOOT

In cavus foot, the deformity consists of an unusually high longitudinal arch of the foot. It may be hereditary or associated with neurologic conditions such as poliomyelitis, Charcot-Marie-Tooth disease, Friedreich's ataxia, or diastematomyelia. There is usually an associated contracture of the toe extensor, producing a claw toe deformity in which the metatarsal phalangeal joints are hyperextended and the interphalangeal joints acutely flexed. Any child presenting with cavus feet should have a careful neurologic examination including x-rays of the spine.

Stretching exercises for the heel cord and arch of the foot are indicated for conservative therapy. In resistant cases that do not respond to shoe adjustments (metatarsal bars and supports), operation may be necessary to lengthen the contracted extensor and flexor tendons. Arthrodesis of the foot may be necessary later. If these feet are left untreated, they are often painful and limit walking.

The overall prognosis is much poorer than with low arch or pes planus.

4. CLAW TOES

In patients with claw toes, there is a flexion deformity of either or both interphalangeal joints, which results in the "claw." The condition is usually congenital and may be seen in association with disorders of motor weakness, such as Charcot-Marie-Tooth disease or pes cavus. Surgical correction can alleviate symptoms if the toes are painful.

5. BUNIONS (Hallux Valgus)

Girls may present in adolescence with lateral deviation of the great toe associated with a prominence over the head of the first metatarsal. This deformity is painful only with shoe wear and almost always can be relieved by fitting shoes that are wide enough. Surgery should be avoided in the adolescent age group, because the results are much less successful than in adult patients with the same condition.

Coleman SS: *Complex Foot Deformities in Children.* Lea & Febiger, 1983.

Jones BS: Flatfoot. *J Bone Joint Surg [Br]* 1975;**57**:279.

Micheli LJ, Ireland ML: Prevention and management of calcaneal apophysitis in children: An overuse syndrome. *J Pediatr Orthop* 1987;**7**:34.

EPIPHYSEAL GROWTH DISTURBANCES SECONDARY TO INFECTION OR TRAUMA

In the child under 1 year of age, there is direct vascular communication from the metaphysis to the epiphysis across the growth plate. For this reason, osteomyelitis occurring in the infant may produce permanent damage to the growth cartilage of the epiphysis with resulting angular deformity or decreased growth potential for the bone. Likewise, trauma, particularly of a compression variety, may damage part or all of the epiphysis. Once such damage occurs, deformity is progressive and may be severe, requiring osteotomy for angular deformity or epiphysiodesis for correction of leg length discrepancy.

DEGENERATIVE PROBLEMS (Arthritis, Bursitis, & Tenosynovitis)

Degenerative arthritis may follow childhood skeletal problems such as infection, slipped capital femoral epiphysis, avascular necrosis, or trauma or may occur in association with hemophilia. Early effective treatment of these disorders will prevent arthritis. Late treatment is often unsatisfactory.

Degenerative changes in the soft tissues around joints may occur as a result of overuse syndrome in adolescent athletes. Young boys throwing excessive numbers of pitches, especially curve balls, may develop "little leaguer's elbow," consisting of degenerative changes around the humeral condyles associated with pain, swelling, and limitation of motion. In order to enforce the rest necessary for healing, a plaster cast may be necessary. A more reasonable preventive measure is to limit the number of pitches thrown by children.

Acute bursitis is quite uncommon in childhood, and other causes should be ruled out before this diagnosis is accepted.

Tenosynovitis is most common in the region of the knees and feet. Children taking dancing lessons, particularly toe dancing, may have pain around the flexor tendon sheaths in the toes or ankles. Rest is effective treatment. At the knee level, there may be irritation of the patellar ligament, with associated swelling in the infrapatellar fat pad. Synovitis in this area is usually due to overuse and is also treated by rest. Corticosteroid injections are contraindicated.

Kunnamo I et al: Clinical signs and laboratory tests in the differential diagnosis of arthritis in children. *Am J Dis Child* 1987;**141**:34.

TRAUMA

SOFT TISSUE TRAUMA
(Sprains, Strains, & Contusions)

A sprain is the stretching of a ligament, and a strain is a stretch of a muscle or tendon. In either of these injuries, there may be some degree of tissue tearing. Contusions are generally due to tissue compression, with damage to blood vessels within the tissue and the formation of hematoma.

A severe sprain is one in which the ligament is completely divided, resulting in instability of the joint. A mild or moderate sprain is one in which incomplete tearing of the ligament occurs, but in which there is associated local pain and swelling.

Mild or moderate sprains are treated by rest of the affected joint, with ice and elevation to prevent prolonged symptoms. By definition, mild or moderate sprain is not associated with instability of the joint.

If there is more severe trauma resulting in tearing of a ligament, instability of the joint may be demonstrated by gross examination or by stress testing with x-ray documentation. Such deformity of the joint may cause persistent instability resulting from inaccurate apposition of the ligament ends during healing. If instability is evident, surgical repair of the torn ligament is indicated. If a muscle is torn, usually at its end, it should be repaired.

The initial treatment of any sprain consists of ice, compression, and elevation. The purpose of the treatment is to decrease local edema and residual stiffness resulting from gelling of blood proteins in the interstitial space. Splinting of the affected joint protects against further injury and relieves swelling and pain.

1. ANKLE SPRAINS

The history will indicate that the injury was by either forceful inversion or eversion. The more common inversion injury results in tearing or injury to the lateral ligaments, whereas an eversion injury will injure the medial ligaments of the ankle. The injured ligaments may be identified by means of careful palpation for point tenderness around the ankle. The joint should be supported or immobilized at a right angle, which is the functional position. Adhesive taping may be effective to maintain this position but should be applied by one skilled in the use of tape and changed frequently in order to prevent the formation of blisters and skin damage. A posterior plaster splint is more easily applied and gives good joint rest if the extremity is protected by using crutches for weight bearing. Prolonged use of a plaster cast is usually not necessary, but the sprained ankle should be rested sufficiently to allow complete healing. This may take 3–6 weeks. Because fractures usually receive more attention and adequate follow-up, the results are often better. A properly treated ankle sprain should not be the source of prolonged and repeated disability.

2. KNEE SPRAINS

Sprains of the collateral and cruciate ligaments are uncommon in children. These ligaments are so strong that it is more common to injure the epiphyseal growth plates, which are the weakest structures in the region of the knees of children. In adolescence, however, the joints and growth plates attain adult growth, and a rupture of the anterior cruciate ligament can result from a twisting injury that may avulse the anterior tibial spine. In such instances, the injury is apparent on physical examination and x-ray and requires anatomic reduction and immobilization for 6 weeks. In most instances, this means open operative correction.

Effusion of the knee after trauma deserves referral to an orthopedic specialist. The differential diagnosis includes torn ligament, torn meniscus, and osteochondral fracture. Nontraumatic effusion should be evaluated for inflammatory conditions (such as juvenile rheumatoid arthritis) or patellar malalignment.

3. INTERNAL DERANGEMENTS OF THE KNEE

Meniscal injuries are uncommon under age 12. Clicking or locking of the knee may occur in young children as a result of a discoid lateral meniscus, which is a rare type of congenital anomaly. As the child approaches adolescence, internal damage to the knee from a torsion weight-bearing injury may result in locking of the knee if tearing and displacement of the meniscus occur. Osteochondral fractures secondary to osteochondritis dissecans may also present as internal derangements of the knee in adolescence. Posttraumatic synovitis may mimic a meniscal lesion as well. In any severe injury to the knee, epiphyseal injury should be suspected; stress films will sometimes demonstrate separation of the distal femoral epiphysis in such cases. Epiphyseal injury should be suspected whenever there is tenderness on both sides of the metaphysis of the femur after injury.

Zaman M, Leonard MA: Meniscectomy in children: Results in 59 knees. *Injury* 1981;**12**:425.

4. BACK SPRAINS

Sprains of the ligaments and muscles of the back are unusual in children but may occur as a result of violent trauma from automobile accidents or athletic injuries. A child with back pain should not be presumed to have had trauma to the spine unless the history warrants that conclusion. The reason for back pain should be carefully sought by x-ray and physical examination. Inflammation, infection, and tumors are more common causes of back pain in children than sprains.

5. CONTUSIONS

Contusion of muscle with hematoma formation produces the familiar "charley horse" injury. Treatment of such injuries is by application of ice, compression, and rest. Exercise should be avoided for 5–7 days. Local heat may hasten healing once the acute phase of tenderness and swelling is past.

6. MYOSITIS OSSIFICANS

Ossification within muscle occurs when there is sufficient trauma to cause a hematoma that later heals in the manner of a fracture. The injury is usually a contusion and occurs most commonly in the quadriceps of the thigh or the triceps of the arm. When such a severe injury with hematoma is recognized, it is important to splint the extremity and avoid activity. If further activity is allowed, ossification may reach spectacular proportions and resemble an osteosarcoma.

Disability is great, with local swelling and heat and extreme pain upon the slightest motion of the adjacent joint. The limb should be rested, with the knee in extension or the elbow in 90 degrees of flexion, until the local reaction has subsided. Once local heat and tenderness have decreased, gentle active exercises may be initiated. Passive stretching exercises are not indicated, because they may stimulate the ossification reaction. It is occasionally necessary to excise excessive bony tissue if it interferes with muscle function once the reaction is mature. Surgery should not be attempted before 9 months to a year after injury, because it may restart the process and lead to an even more severe reaction.

Micheli LJ (editor): Injuries in the young athlete. *Clin Sports Med* 1988;7:459.

TRAUMATIC SUBLUXATIONS & DISLOCATIONS

Dislocation of a joint is always associated with severe damage to the ligaments and joint capsule. In contrast to fracture treatment, which may be safely postponed, dislocations must be reduced immediately. Dislocations can usually be reduced by gentle sustained traction. It often happens that no anesthetic is necessary for several hours after the injury, because of the protective anesthesia produced by the injury. Following reduction, the joint should be splinted for transportation of the patient.

The dislocated joint should be treated by immobilization for at least 3 weeks, followed by graduated active exercises through a full range of motion. Physical therapy is usually not indicated for children with injuries. As a matter of fact, vigorous manipulation of the joint by a therapist may be harmful. The child should be permitted to perform therapy alone. No stretching should be permitted.

1. SUBLUXATION OF THE RADIAL HEAD (Nursemaid's Elbow)

Infants frequently sustain subluxation of the radial head as a result of being lifted or pulled by the hand. The child appears with the elbow fully pronated and painful. The usual complaint is that the child's elbow will not bend. X-ray findings are normal, but there is point tenderness over the radial head. When the elbow is placed in full supination and slowly moved from full flexion to full extension, a click may be palpated at the level of the radial head. The relief of pain is remarkable, as the child usually stops crying immediately. The elbow may be immobilized in a sling for comfort for a day.

Pulled elbow may be a clue to battering. This should be remembered during examination especially if the problem is recurrent.

2. RECURRENT DISLOCATION OF THE PATELLA

Recurrent dislocation of the patella is more common in loose-jointed individuals, especially adolescent girls. If the patella completely dislocates, it nearly always goes laterally. Pain is severe, and the patient is brought to the doctor with the knee slightly flexed and an obvious bony mass lateral to the knee joint and a flat area over the usual location of the patella anteriorly. X-ray findings confirm the diagnosis. The patella may be reduced by extending the knee and placing slight pressure on the patella while gentle traction is exerted on the leg. In subluxation of the patella, the symptoms may be more subtle, and the patient may say that the knee "gives out" or "jumps out of place."

In the case of complete dislocation, the knee should be immobilized for 3–4 weeks, followed by a physical therapy program for strengthening the quadriceps muscle. Operation may be necessary to tighten the knee joint capsule if dislocation or subluxation is recurrent. In such instances, if the patella is not stabilized, repeated dislocation produces damage to the articular cartilage of the patellofemoral joint and premature degenerative arthritis.

EPIPHYSEAL SEPARATIONS

In children, epiphyseal separations and fractures are more common than ligamentous injuries. This finding is based on the fact that the ligaments of the joints are generally stronger than the associated growth plates. In instances where dislocation is suspected, an x-ray should be taken in order to rule out epiphyseal fracture. Films of the opposite extremity, especially around the elbow, may be valuable for comparison. Reduction of a fractured epiphysis should be done under anesthesia in order to align the growth plate with the least amount of force necessary. Fractures across the growth plate may produce bony bridges that will cause premature cessation of growth or angular deformities in the growth plate. Epiphyseal fractures around the shoulder, wrist, and fingers can usually be treated by closed reduction, but fractures of the epiphyses around the elbow often require open reduction. In the lower extremity, accurate reduction of the epiphyseal plate is necessary to prevent joint deformity if a joint surface is involved. Unfortunately, some of the most severe injuries to the epiphyseal plate occur from compression injuries, where the amount of force is not immediately apparent. If angular deformities result, corrective osteotomy may be necessary.

Mizuta T et al: Statistical analysis of the incidence of physeal injuries. *J Pediatr Orthop* 1987;**7**:518.

TORUS FRACTURES

Torus fractures consist of "buckling" of the cortex as a result of minimal angular trauma. They usually occur in the distal radius or ulna. Alignment is satisfactory, and simple immobilization for 3–5 weeks is sufficient.

GREENSTICK FRACTURES

With greenstick fractures there is frank disruption of the cortex on one side of the bone but no discernible cleavage plane on the opposite side. These fractures are angulated but not displaced, as the bone ends are not separated. Reduction is achieved by straightening the arm into normal alignment, and reduction is maintained by a snugly fitting plaster cast. It is necessary to x-ray children with greenstick fractures again in a week to 10 days to make certain that the reduction has been maintained in plaster. A slight angular deformity will be corrected by remod-

eling of the bone. The farther the fracture is from the growing end of the bone, the longer the time required for healing. The fracture can be considered healed when there are no findings of tenderness and local swelling or heat and when adequate bony callus is seen on x-ray.

FRACTURE OF THE CLAVICLE

Clavicular fractures are very common injuries in infants and children. They can be immobilized by a figure-of-8 dressing that retracts the shoulders and brings the clavicle to normal length. The healing callus will be apparent when the fracture has consolidated, but this unsightly lump will generally resolve over a period of months to a year.

SUPRACONDYLAR FRACTURES OF THE HUMERUS

Supracondylar fractures tend to occur in the age group from 3 to 6 years and are potentially dangerous because of the proximity to the brachial artery in the distal arm. They are usually associated with a significant amount of trauma, so that swelling may be severe. **Volkmann's ischemic contracture** of muscle may occur as a result of vascular embarrassment. When severe swelling is present, the safest course is to place the arm in traction and carefully observe nerve function and the vascular supply to the hand. In these cases, the children should be hospitalized and followed carefully by experienced nurses. If the blood supply is compromised, exposure of the brachial artery may be necessary, although this is rarely needed when satisfactory reduction and traction are employed. Complications associated with supracondylar fractures also include a resultant cubitus valgus secondary to poor reduction. It is often difficult to ascertain adequacy of the reduction because a flexed position is necessary to maintain normal alignment. Such a "gunstock" deformity of the elbow may be somewhat unsightly but does not usually interfere with joint function.

Landin L, Danielsson L: Elbow fractures in children: An epidemiological analysis of 589 cases. *Acta Orthop Scand* 1986;**57**:309.
Millis MB, Singer U, Hall JE: Supracondylar fracture of the humerus in children: Further experience with a study in orthopaedic decision-making. *Clin Orthop* (Sept) 1984;**188**:90.

GENERAL COMMENTS ON OTHER FRACTURES IN CHILDREN

Reduction of fractures in children is usually accomplished by simple traction and manipulation;

open reduction is rarely indicated. Remodeling of the fracture callus will usually produce an almost normal appearance of the bone over a matter of months. The younger the child, the more remodeling is possible. Angular deformities remodel with ease. Rotatory deformities do not remodel, and this produces the cubitus valgus deformity sometimes seen after supracondylar fractures.

The physician should be suspicious of child battering whenever the age of a fracture does not match the history given or when the severity of the injury is more than the alleged accident would have produced. In suspected cases of battering where no fracture is present on the initial x-ray film, a repeat film 10 days later is in order. Bleeding beneath the periosteum will be calcified by 7–10 days, and the x-ray appearance is almost diagnostic of severe closed trauma characteristic of a battered child.

Cumming WA: Neonatal skeletal fractures: Birth trauma or child abuse? *J Can Assoc Radiol* 1979;**30**:30.

Ogden JA: *Skeletal Injury in the Child.* Lea & Febiger, 1982.

Rang M: *Children's Fractures,* 2nd ed. Lippincott, 1983.

Weber BG, Brunner C, Freuler F (editors): *Treatment of Fractures in Children and Adolescents.* Springer-Verlag, 1980.

INFECTIONS OF THE BONES & JOINTS

OSTEOMYELITIS

Osteomyelitis is an infectious process that usually starts in the spongy or medullary bone and then extends to involve compact or cortical bone. It is more common in boys than in girls or in adults of either sex. The lower extremities are most often affected, and there is commonly a history of trauma. Osteomyelitis may occur as a result of direct invasion from the outside through a penetrating wound (nail) or open fracture, but hematogenous spread of infection (eg, pyoderma or upper respiratory tract infection) from other infected areas is more common. The most common infecting organism is *Staphylococcus aureus,* which seems to have a special tendency to infect the metaphyses of growing bones. Anatomically, circulation in the long bones is such that the arterial supply to the metaphysis just below the growth plate is by end arteries, which turn sharply to end in venous sinusoids, causing a relative stasis. In the infant under 1 year of age, there is direct vascular communication with the epiphysis across the growth plate, so that direct spread may occur from the metaphysis to the epiphysis and subsequently

into the joint. In the older child, the growth plate provides an effective barrier and the epiphysis is usually not involved, although the infection spreads retrograde from the metaphysis into the diaphysis and, by rupture through the cortical bone, down along the diaphysis beneath the periosteum.

1. EXOGENOUS OSTEOMYELITIS

In order to avoid osteomyelitis by direct extension, all wounds must be carefully examined and cleansed. Puncture wounds are especially liable to lead to osteomyelitis if not carefully debrided. Cultures of the wound made at the time of exploration and debridement may be useful if signs of inflammation and infection develop subsequently. Copious irrigation is necessary, and all nonviable skin, subcutaneous tissue, fascia, and muscle must be excised. In extensive or contaminated wounds, antibiotic coverage is indicated. Contaminated wounds should be left open and secondary closure performed 3–5 days later. If at the time of delayed closure further necrotic tissue is present, it should be excised. Leaving the wound open allows the infection to stay at the surface rather than extend inward to the bone.

Parenteral administration of antibiotics is satisfactory, and local irrigation is not needed. If the wound is acquired outside the hospital, penicillin is adequate for most wounds. After cultures have been read, an appropriate alternative antibiotic can be chosen if there is lingering inflammation. A tetanus toxoid booster is indicated for any questionable wound, but gas gangrene is better prevented by adequate debridement than by antitoxin.

Once exogenous osteomyelitis has become established, treatment becomes more complicated, requiring extensive surgical debridement and drainage followed by careful antibiotic management. These cases require hospitalization and the use of intravenous antibiotics.

2. HEMATOGENOUS OSTEOMYELITIS

Hematogenous osteomyelitis is usually caused by pyogenic bacteria; 85% of cases are due to staphylococci. Streptococci are rare causes of osteomyelitis today, but *Pseudomonas* organisms have often been documented in cases of nail puncture wounds. Children with sickle cell anemia are especially prone to osteomyelitis caused by salmonellae.

Clinical Findings
A. Symptoms and Signs: In infants, the manifestations of osteomyelitis may be quite subtle, presenting as irritability, diarrhea, or failure to feed properly; the temperature may be normal or slightly low; and the white blood count may be normal or

only slightly elevated. In older children, the manifestations are more striking, with severe local tenderness and pain, high fever, rapid pulse, and elevated white blood count and sedimentation rate. Osteomyelitis of a lower extremity often presents around the knee in a child 7–10 years of age. Tenderness is most marked over the metaphysis of the bone where the process has its origin.

B. Laboratory Findings: Blood cultures are often positive early. The most significant test in infancy is the aspiration of pus when suspicion arises because of lack of movement in a painful extremity. It is useful to insert a needle to the bone in the area of suspected infection and aspirate any fluid present. This fluid can be smeared and stained for organisms as well as cultured. Even edema fluid may be useful for determining the causative organism. The white blood cell count is usually elevated, as is the sedimentation rate.

C. Imaging: The first manifestation to appear on x-ray film is nonspecific local swelling. This is followed by elevation of the periosteum, with formation of new bone from the cambium layer of the periosteum occurring after 3–6 days. As the infection becomes chronic, areas of cortical bone are isolated by pus spreading down the medullary canal, causing rarefaction and demineralization of the bone. Such isolated pieces of cortex become ischemic and form sequestra (dead bone fragments). These x-ray findings are late, and osteomyelitis should be diagnosed clinically before significant x-ray findings are present. Bone scan is valuable in suspected cases before x-ray findings become positive.

Treatment

A. Specific Measures: Antibiotics should be started intravenously as soon as the diagnosis of osteomyelitis is made. Agents that cover *Staphylococcus aureus* and *Streptococcus pyogenes* (e.g., oxacillin, nafcillin, or cefazolin, all at 150 mg/kg/day) are appropriate for most cases. For possible *Pseudomonas* infection, add ceftazidime (150 mg/kg/d) or an aminoglycoside. Parenteral antibiotic therapy should be continued until all clinical signs, the white blood count and sedimentation rate are improved, usually for 5–10 days. For a reliable family an oral antibiotic may then be begun; the dosage of most antistaphylococcal drugs (dicloxacillin, cephalexin, cephradine) must be 100–150 mg/kg/d in 4 divided doses to achieve adequate serum killing powers. At least 4 weeks of therapy (with normalization of the sedimentation rate and resolution of all local signs) should be completed. Chronic infections are treated for months. Following surgical debridement, *Pseudomonas* foot infections usually respond to 1–2 weeks of treatment.

B. General Measures: Splinting of the limb minimizes pain and decreases spread of the infection by lymphatic channels through the soft tissue. The splint should be removed periodically to allow active use of adjacent joints and prevent stiffening and muscle atrophy. In chronic osteomyelitis, splinting may be necessary to guard against fracture of the weakened bone.

C. Surgical Measures: Aspiration of the metaphysis is a useful diagnostic measure in any case of suspected osteomyelitis. Osteomyelitis represents a collection of pus under pressure within the body. In the first 24–72 hours, it may be possible to abort osteomyelitis by the use of antibiotics alone. However, if frank pus is aspirated from the bone, surgical drainage is indicated. If the infection has not shown a dramatic response within 24 hours in questionable cases, surgical drainage is also indicated. It is important that all devitalized soft tissue be removed and adequate exposure of the bone obtained in order to permit free drainage. Excessive amounts of bone should not be removed when draining acute osteomyelitis, because they may not be completely replaced by the normal healing process.

In questionable cases, little damage has been done by surgical drainage, but failure to drain the pus in acute cases may lead to more severe damage.

Prognosis

When osteomyelitis is diagnosed in the early clinical stages and prompt antibiotic therapy is begun, the prognosis is excellent. If the process has been unattended for a week to 10 days, there is almost always some permanent loss of bone structure, as well as the possibility of growth abnormality.

Amir N et al: Gowers' sign in discitis in childhood. *Clin Pediatr (Phila)* 1986;**25**:459.

Jacobs RF et al: Management of *Pseudomonas* osteochondritis complicating puncture wounds of the foot. *Pediatrics* 1982;**69**:432.

LaMont RL et al: Acute hematogenous osteomyelitis in children. *J Pediatr Orthop* 1987;**7**:579.

Scoles PV, Aronoff SC: Antimicrobial therapy of childhood skeletal infections: Current concepts review. *J Bone Joint Surg [Am]* 1984;**66**:1487.

PYOGENIC ARTHRITIS

The source of pyogenic arthritis varies according to the age of the child. In the infant, pyogenic arthritis often develops by spread from adjacent osteomyelitis. In the older child, it presents as an isolated infection, usually without bony involvement. In teenagers with pyogenic arthritis, an underlying systemic disease is usually the cause, eg, an obvious generalized infection or an organism that has an affinity for joints, such as the gonococcus.

The infecting organism varies with age: group B streptococcus and *Staphylococcus aureus* in those under 4 m; *Haemophilus influenzae* and *Staphylococcus* in those 4 m to 4 y old; and *Staphylococcus* and *Streptococcus pyogenes* in older children.

The initial effusion of the joint rapidly becomes purulent. An effusion of the joint may accompany osteomyelitis in the adjacent bone. A white blood cell count exceeding 100,000/μL in the joint fluid indicates a definite purulent infection. Generally, spread of infection is from the bone into the joint, but unattended pyogenic arthritis may also affect adjacent bone. The sedimentation rate is elevated.

Clinical Findings

A. Symptoms and Signs: In older children, the signs are striking, with fever, malaise, vomiting, and restriction of motion. In infants, paralysis of the limb due to inflammatory neuritis may be evident. Infection of the hip joint in infants can be diagnosed if suspicion is aroused by decreased abduction of the hip in an infant who is irritable or feeding poorly. A history of umbilical catheter treatment in the newborn nursery should alert the physician to the possibility of pyogenic arthritis of the hip.

B. Imaging: Early distention of the joint capsule is nonspecific and difficult to measure by x-ray. In the infant with unrecognized pyogenic arthritis, dislocation of the joint may follow within a few days as a result of distention of the capsule by pus. Later changes include destruction of the joint space, resorption of epiphyseal cartilage, and erosion of the adjacent bone of the metaphysis. The bone scan shows increased flow and symmetrical increased uptake about the joint, unless there is a concomitant osteomyelitis.

Treatment

Diagnosis may be made by aspiration of the joint. In the hip joint, pyogenic arthritis is most easily treated by surgical drainage because the joint is deep and difficult to aspirate as well as being inaccessible to thorough cleaning through needle aspiration. In more superficial joints, such as the knee, aspiration of the joint at least twice daily may maintain adequate drainage. If fever and clinical symptoms do not subside within 24 hours after treatment is begun, open surgical drainage is indicated. Antibiotics can be selected based on age and smears and cultures of the aspirated pus. Reasonable empiric therapy in infants includes cefuroxime (200 mg/kg/d in 4 divided doses) or oxacillin (150 mg/kg/d) plus a third-generation cephalosporin. An antistaphylococcal alone is usually adequate for children over 5 yrs. For staphylococcal infections, 3 weeks of therapy is recommended; for other organisms, 2 weeks is usually sufficient. Oral therapy may be begun when clinical signs have markedly improved. It is not necessary to give intra-articular antibiotics, since good levels are achieved in the synovial fluid.

Prognosis

The prognosis is excellent if the joint is drained early, before damage to the articular cartilage has occurred. If infection is present for more than 24 hours, there is dissolution of the proteoglycans in the articular cartilage, with subsequent arthrosis and fibrosis of the joint. Damage to the growth plate may also occur, especially within the hip joint, where the epiphyseal plate is intracapsular.

Almquist EE: The changing epidemiology of septic arthritis in children. *Clin Orthop* (Jan–Feb) 1980;**68**:96.

Barton LL, Dunkle LM, Habib FH: Septic arthritis in childhood. A thirteen-year review. *Am J Dis Child* 1987;**141**:898.

TUBERCULOUS ARTHRITIS

Tuberculous arthritis is now a rare disease in the USA. It must be considered, however, in children with resistant infections of the joints, especially if there is a history of tuberculosis in family members. Generally, the infection may be ruled out by skin testing. The joints most commonly affected in children are the intervertebral disks, resulting in gibbus or dorsal angular deformity at the site of the involvement.

Treatment is by local drainage of the "cold abscess," followed by antituberculosis therapy with isoniazid, rifampin, and ethambutol. Prolonged immobilization in a plaster bed is necessary in order to promote healing. Spinal fusion may be required to preserve stability of the vertebral column.

TRANSIENT SYNOVITIS OF THE HIP

The most common cause of limping and pain in the hip of children in the USA is transitory synovitis, an acute inflammatory reaction that often follows an upper respiratory infection and is generally self-limited. In questionable cases, aspiration of the hip yields only yellowish fluid, ruling out pyogenic arthritis. Generally, however, toxic synovitis of the hip is not associated with elevation of the erythrocyte sedimentation rate, the white blood count or a temperature above 38.3 °C (101 °F). It classically affects children 3–10 years of age and is more common in boys. There is limitation of motion of the hip joint, particularly internal rotation, and x-ray changes are nonspecific, with some swelling apparent in the soft tissues around the joint.

Treatment consists of bed rest and the use of traction with slight flexion of the hip. Aspirin may shorten the course of the disease, although even with no treatment the disease usually is self-limited to a matter of days. It is important to maintain x-ray follow-up because toxic synovitis may be the precursor of avascular necrosis of the femoral head (see next section) in a small percentage of patients. X-ray films can be obtained at 1 month and 3 months, or earlier if there is persistent limp or pain.

Hodges DL, McGuire TJ: Hip pain in children: An anatomic approach. *Orthop Rev* 1988;**17**:251.

Kallio P, Tyoppy S, Kunnamo I: Transient synovitis and Perthes disease. Is there an aetiological connection? *J Bone Joint Surg [Br]* 1986;**68**:808.

Landin LA, Danielsson LG, Wattsgard C: Transient synovitis of the hip: Its incidence, epidemiology and relation to Perthes disease. *J Bone Joint Surg [Br]* 1987; **69**:238.

VASCULAR LESIONS & AVASCULAR NECROSIS

AVASCULAR NECROSIS OF THE PROXIMAL FEMUR
(Legg-Calvé-Perthes Disease)

The vascular supply of bone is generally precarious, and when it is interrupted, necrosis results. In contrast to other body tissues that undergo infarction, bone removes necrotic tissue and replaces it with living bone in a process called "creeping substitution." This replacement of necrotic bone may be so complete and so perfect that a completely normal bone results. Adequacy of replacement depends upon the age of the patient, the presence or absence of associated infection, congruity of the involved joint, and other physiologic and mechanical factors.

Because of their rapid growth in relation to their blood supply, the secondary ossification centers in the epiphyses are subject to avascular necrosis. The physicians who originally described the avascular lesions of the epiphyses and distinguished them from tuberculosis in the early 20th century were identified with the processes. Despite the number of different names referring to avascular necrosis of the epiphyses, the process is identical, ie, necrosis of bone followed by replacement.

Even though the pathologic and radiologic features of avascular necrosis of the epiphyses are well known, the cause is not generally agreed upon. Necrosis may follow known causes such as trauma or infection, but idiopathic lesions usually develop during periods of rapid growth of the epiphyses. Thus, the highest incidence of Legg-Calvé-Perthes disease is between 4 and 8 years of age.

Clinical Findings

A. Symptoms and Signs: Persistent pain is the most common symptom, and the patient may present with limp or limitation of motion.

B. Laboratory Findings: Laboratory findings, including studies of joint aspirates, are normal.

C. Imaging: X-ray findings correlate with the progression of the process and the extent of necrosis. The early finding is effusion of the joint associated with slight widening of the joint space and periarticular swelling. Decreased bone density in and around the joint is apparent after a few weeks. The necrotic ossification center appears more dense than the surrounding viable structures, and there is collapse or narrowing of the femoral head.

As replacement of the necrotic ossification center occurs, there is rarefaction of the bone in a patchwork fashion, producing alternating areas of rarefaction and relative density or "fragmentation" of the epiphysis.

In the hip, there may be widening of the femoral head associated with flattening, giving rise to the term **coxa plana.** If infarction has extended across the growth plate, there will be a radiolucent lesion within the metaphysis. If the growth center of the femoral head has been damaged so that normal growth does not occur, varus deformity of the femoral neck will occur as a result of overgrowth of the greater trochanteric apophysis.

Eventually, complete replacement of the epiphysis will become apparent as new bone replaces necrotic bone. The final shape of the head will depend upon the extent of the necrosis and collapse that has been allowed to occur.

Differential Diagnosis

Differential diagnosis must include inflammatory and infectious lesions of the joints or apophyses. Transient synovitis of the hip may be distinguished from Legg-Calvé-Perthes disease by serial x-rays.

Treatment

Treatment consists simply of protection of the joint. If the joint is deeply seated within the acetabulum and normal joint motion is maintained, a reasonably good result can be expected. The hip is held in abduction and internal rotation in order to fulfill this purpose. Braces are generally used. Surgery may be necessary for an uncooperative patient or one whose social or geographic circumstances do not allow use of a brace (living in a house trailer, in an unpaved rural area, etc).

Prognosis

The prognosis for complete replacement of the necrotic femoral head in a child is excellent, but the functional result will depend upon the amount of deformity that develops during the time the softened structure exists. In Legg-Calvé-Perthes disease, the prognosis depends upon the completeness of involvement of the epiphyseal center. In general, patients with metaphyseal defects, those in whom the disease develops late in childhood, and those who have more complete involvement of the femoral head have a poorer prognosis.

Osteochondrosis due to vascular lesion may affect various growth centers. Table 23–1 indicates the common sites and the typical ages at presentation.

Table 23–1. The osteochondroses.

Ossification Center	Eponym	Typical Age
Capital femoral	Legg-Calvé-Perthes disease	3–5
Tarsal navicular	Köhler's bone disease	6
Second metatarsal head	Freiberg's disease	12–14
Vertebral ring	Scheuermann's disease	13–16
Capitellum	Panner's disease	9–11
Tibial tubercle	Osgood-Schlatter disease	11–13
Calcaneus	Sever's disease	8–9

Bowen JR, Foster BK, Hartzell CR: Legg-Calvé-Perthes disease. *Clin Orthop* (May) 1984;**185**:97.

McAndrew MP, Weinstein SL: A long-term follow-up of Legg-Calvé-Perthes disease. *J Bone Joint Surg [Am]* 1984;**66**:860.

Schoenecker PL: Legg-Calvé-Perthes disease. *Orthop Rev* 1986;**15**:561.

Thompson GH, Salter RB: Legg-Calvé-Perthes disease: Current concepts and controversies. *Orthop Clin North Am* 1987;**18**:617.

OSTEOCHONDRITIS DISSECANS

In osteochondritis dissecans, there is a pie-shaped necrotic area of bone and cartilage adjacent to the articular surface. The fragment of bone may be broken off from the host bone and displaced into the joint as a loose body. If it remains attached, the necrotic fragment may be completely replaced by creeping substitution.

The pathologic process is precisely the same as that described above for avascular necrosing lesions of ossification centers. However, because these lesions are adjacent to articular cartilage, there may be joint damage.

The most common sites of these lesions are the knee (medial femoral condyle), the elbow joint (capitellum), and the talus (superior lateral dome).

Joint pain is the usual presenting complaint. However, local swelling or locking may be present, particularly if there is a fragment free in the joint. Laboratory studies are normal.

Treatment consists of protection of the involved area from mechanical damage. If there is a fragment free within the joint as a loose body, it must be surgically removed. For some marginal lesions, it may be worthwhile to drill the necrotic fragment in order to encourage more rapid vascular ingrowth and replacement. If large areas of a weight-bearing joint are involved, secondary degenerative arthritis may result.

Hughston JC, Hergenroeder PT, Courtenay BG: Osteochondritis dissecans of the femoral condyles. *J Bone Joint Surg [Am]* 1984;**66**:1340.

NEUROLOGIC DISORDERS INVOLVING THE MUSCULOSKELETAL SYSTEM

ORTHOPEDIC ASPECTS OF CEREBRAL PALSY

Early physical therapy to encourage completion of the normal developmental patterns may be of benefit in patients with cerebral palsy. The greatest gains from this type of therapy are obtained during the first few years of life, and therapy should not be continued with unrealistic goals when no improvement is apparent.

Bracing and splinting are of questionable benefit, although night splints may be useful in preventing equinus deformity of the feet or adduction contractures of the hips. Orthopedic surgery can offer procedures to weaken hyperactive spastic muscles, to transfer function of deforming spastic muscles, or to stabilize joints. In general, muscle transfers are unpredictable in cerebral palsy, and most orthopedic procedures are directed at weakening deforming forces or bony stabilization by osteotomy or arthrodesis.

Flexion and adduction of the hip due to hyperactivity of the adductors and flexors may produce a progressive paralytic dislocation of the hip. Congenital dislocation of the hip is unusual in cerebral palsy, but in more severely involved children, paralytic dislocation can lead to pain and dysfunction. Treatment of the dislocation once it has occurred is difficult and unsatisfactory. The principal preventive measure is abduction bracing, but this must often be supplemented by release of the adductors or hip flexors in order to prevent dislocation. In severe cases, osteotomy of the femur may also be necessary to correct the bony deformities of femoral anteversion and coxa valga that are invariably present.

Patients with predominantly an athetotic pattern are poor candidates for any surgical procedue or bracing. Neurosurgical procedures may be of some help.

Because it is difficult to predict the outcome of surgical procedures in cerebral palsy, the surgeon must examine patients on several occasions before any operative procedure is undertaken. Follow-up care by a physical therapist to maximize the anticipated long-term gains should be arranged before the operation.

Bleck EE: *Orthopaedic Management of Cerebral Palsy.* Mac Keith, 1987.

Harris SR: Early neuromotor predictors of cerebral palsy in low birthweight infants. *Dev Med Child Neurol* 1987;**29**:508.

Palmer FB et al: The effects of physical therapy on cerebral palsy: A controlled trial in infants with spastic diplegia. *N Engl J Med* 1988;**318**:803.

ORTHOPEDIC ASPECTS OF MYELODYSPLASIA

Patients born with spina bifida cystica (aperta) should be examined early by an orthopedic surgeon. The level of neurologic involvement determines the imbalance of muscular force that will be present and apt to produce deformity with growth. The involvement is often asymmetric and tends to change during the first 12–18 months of life. Early closure of the sac is the rule, although there has been some hesitancy to treat all of these patients because of the extremely poor prognosis associated with congenital hydrocephalus, high levels of paralysis, and associated congenital anomalies. Associated musculoskeletal problems may include clubfoot, congenital dislocation of the hip, arthrogryposis type changes of the lower extremities, and congenital scoliosis, among others. The most common lesions are at the level of L3–4 and tend to affect the hip joint, with progressive dislocation occurring during growth. Foot deformities may be in any direction and are complicated by the fact that sensation is generally absent. Spinal deformities develop in a high percentage of these children, with scoliosis being present in approximately 40%. Ambulation is impossible without braces or splints, and careful urologic follow-up must be obtained to prevent complications from incontinence. A high percentage of these children have hydrocephalus, which may be evident at birth or shortly thereafter, requiring shunting. The shunts are sources of infection and may require frequent replacement.

In children who have a reasonable likelihood of walking, operative treatment consists of reduction of the hip and alignment of the feet in the weight-bearing position as well as stabilization of the vertebral scoliosis. In children who do not have extension power of the knee, ie, those who lack active quadriceps function, the likelihood of ambulation is greatly decreased. In such patients, aggressive surgery in the hip region may result in stiffening of the joints, thus preventing sitting. Multiple foot operations are also contraindicated in these children.

The overall management of the child with spina bifida should be coordinated in a multidiscipline clinic where all doctors working in cooperation with each other can work also with therapists, social workers, and teachers to provide the best possible care.

Findley TW et al: Ambulation in the adolescent with myelomeningocele. 1. Early childhood predictors. *Arch Phys Med Rehabil* 1987;**68**:518.

Menelaus MB: *The Orthopaedic Management of Spina Bifida Cystica,* 2nd ed. Churchill Livingstone, 1980.

MISCELLANEOUS DISEASES OF BONE

FIBROUS DYSPLASIA

Dysplastic fibrous tissue replacement of the medullary canal is accompanied by the formation of metaplastic bone in fibrous dysplasia. Three forms of the disease are recognized: monostotic, polyostotic, and polyostotic with endocrine disturbances (precocious puberty in females, hyperthyroidism, and hyperadrenalism, ie, Albright's syndrome).

Clinical Findings

A. Symptoms and Signs: The lesion or lesions may be asymptomatic. Pain, if present, is probably due to pathologic fractures. In females, endocrine disturbances may be present in the polyostotic variety and associated with café-au-lait spots.

B. Laboratory Findings: Laboratory findings are normal unless endocrine disturbances are present, in which case there may be increased secretion of gonadotropic, thyroid, or adrenal hormones.

C. Imaging: The lesion begins centrally within the medullary canal, usually of a long bone, and expands slowly. Pathologic fracture may occur. If metaplastic bone predominates, the contents of the lesion will be of the density of bone. Marked deformity of the bone may result, and a shepherd's crook deformity of the upper femur is a classic feature of the disease. The disease is often asymmetric, and limb length disturbances may occur as a result of stimulation of epiphyseal cartilage growth.

Differential Diagnosis

The differential diagnosis may include other fibrous lesions of bone as well as destructive lesions such as bone cyst, eosinophilic granuloma, aneurysmal bone cyst, nonossifying fibroma, enchondroma, and chondromyxoid fibroma.

Treatment

If the lesion is small and asymptomatic, no treatment is needed. If the lesion is large and produces or threatens pathologic fracture, curettage and bone grafting are indicated.

Prognosis

Unless the lesions impair epiphyseal growth, the prognosis is good. Lesions tend to enlarge during the growth period but are stable during adult life. Malignant transformation has not been recorded.

UNICAMERAL BONE CYST

Unicameral bone cyst appears in the metaphysis of a long bone, usually in the femur or humerus. It begins within the medullary canal adjacent to the epiphyseal cartilage. It probably results from some fault in enchondral ossification. The cyst is "active" as long as it abuts onto the metaphyseal side of the epiphyseal cartilage and "inactive" when a border of normal bone exists between the cyst and the epiphyseal cartilage. The lesion is usually identified when a pathologic fracture occurs, producing pain. Laboratory findings are normal. On x-ray films, the cyst is identified centrally within the medullary canal, producing expansion of the cortex and thinning over the widest portion of the cyst.

Treatment consists of curettage of the cyst if it is producing pain. The cyst may heal after a fracture and not require treatment. Curettage should be delayed if surgery would risk damage to the adjacent growth plate. In such cases, methylprednisolone injection may be curative.

The prognosis is excellent. Many cysts will heal following pathologic fracture.

dePalma L, Santuccil A: [Treatment of bone cysts with methylprednisolone acetate.] *Int Orthop* 1987;**11**:23. [French.]

ANEURYSMAL BONE CYST

Aneurysmal bone cyst is similar to unicameral bone cyst, but it contains blood rather than clear fluid. It usually occurs in a slightly eccentric position in the long bone, expanding the cortex of the bone but not breaking the cortex, although some extraosseous mass may be produced. On x-ray films, the lesion appears somewhat larger than the width of the epiphyseal cartilage, and this feature distinguishes it from unicameral bone cyst.

The aneurysmal bone cyst is filled by large vascular lakes, and the stoma of the cyst contains fibrous tissue and areas of metaplastic ossification.

The lesion may appear quite aggressive histologically, and it is important to differentiate it from osteosarcoma or hemangioma. Treatment is by curettage and bone grafting, and the prognosis is excellent.

INFANTILE CORTICAL HYPEROSTOSIS (Caffey's Syndrome)

Infantile cortical hyperostosis is a benign disease of unknown cause that has its onset before 6 months of age and is characterized by irritability, fever, and nonsuppurating, tender, painful swellings. Swellings may involve almost any bone of the body and are frequently widespread. Classically, there are swellings of the mandible and clavicle in 50% of cases as well as of the ulna, humerus, and ribs. The disease is limited to the shafts of bones and does not involve subcutaneous tissues or joints. It is self-limited but may persist for weeks or months. Anemia, leukocytosis, an increased sedimentation rate, and elevation of the serum alkaline phosphatase are usually present. Cortical hyperostosis is demonstrable by a typical x-ray appearance and may be diagnosed on physical examination by an experienced pediatrician.

Fortunately, the disease appears to be decreasing in frequency. Corticosteroids are effective in severe cases.

The prognosis is good, and the disease usually terminates without deformity.

GANGLION

A ganglion is a smooth, small cystic mass connected by a pedicle to the joint capsule, usually on the dorsum of the wrist. It may also be seen in the tendon sheath over the flexor surfaces of the fingers. These ganglions can be excised if they interfere with function or cause persistent pain.

BAKER'S CYST

Baker's cyst is a herniation of the synovium in the knee joint into the popliteal region. In children, the diagnosis may be made by aspiration of mucinous fluid, but the cyst nearly always disappears with time. Whereas Baker's cysts may be indicative of intraarticular disease in the adult, they usually are of no clinical significance in children and rarely require excision.

Dinham JM: Popliteal cysts in children: The case against surgery. *J Bone Joint Surg [Br]* 1975;**57**:69.

24

Neurologic & Muscular Disorders

Paul G. Moe, MD, & Alan Seay, MD

NEUROLOGIC ASSESSMENT & NEURODIAGNOSTIC PROCEDURES

NEUROLOGIC HISTORY & EXAMINATION

The history is usually taken with the child and parents together. Questions can be addressed directly to the older child with further details supplemented by the parent. If time permits, a teenager should be interviewed alone. If strong psychosocial factors become evident by the end of the joint interview, the parent may leave. Sensitive issues (for example, drug use, sexual history) can then be reexplored with the older child.

A patient data form filled out by the parent in advance of the visit or in the physician's waiting room is helpful. The form should include the chief complaint, the youngster's strengths and talents, birth and family history, medical history, and school and behavioral history. A checklist of behavioral issues such as hyperactivity, depression, short attention span, etc. can bring attention to areas that need to be more carefully explored during the interview. Developmental delays suspected in the infant or older child can also be addressed in a checklist. A physician interviewing a child of the age of 5–7 can begin with neutral questions regarding age and birthday. It is often informative to see whether these children know their birthday or even year of birth.

The core of the history is the present illness. What the parent or child sees as important should be the initial focus. In recurrent conditions (for example, seizures or headaches), it is important to find out what happened during the first as well as the most recent episode. Details of recurrent episodes should be thoroughly discussed, including frequency, duration, change in character over time, and precipitating and alleviating factors. The effect of emotions, medications, and environmental manipulations such as diet change should be reviewed. The physician should ascertain, if possible, whether the disease is congenital or age-acquired and whether it is progressive.

As the interview progresses, the clinician begins to form ideas about a possible diagnosis; these can be explored with searching questions. Occasionally, the patient and parent see things from different viewpoints. The child, for instance, may consider the headaches a trivial matter that does not interfere with activity; the mother may feel quite different. It may be helpful to observe the emotional interchange between parent and child and to learn each person's views regarding the severity of disease, the degree of interference with peer group and school activities, side effects and efficacy of medications, etc.

Depending on the nature of the complaint, the past medical history may or may not be extremely detailed. For example, in a case of a teenager with headaches, the history of pregnancy and birth is of little importance. In a case of a 2-month-old with hypotonia, detailed information about those areas is essential. The family and genetic history are often important. A strong family history of migraine or a history of myotonic dystrophy in an uncle might be key to diagnosis in the cases cited. Sometimes the parents may have to do some searching with letters to relatives or hospitals to get family history details.

Available health records, roentgenograms, electroencephalograms, and school records may complement the interview. Developmental history is essential in the assessment of any infant. The Denver Developmental Screening Test (DDST) is one helpful tool for reviewing each major area of behavior in infancy, namely, gross motor, fine motor, personal/social, and language. Some developmental expectations and landmarks are listed in Table 24–1.

In the older child, the developmental history can be explored with questions concerning school progress. The clinician should inquire how the patient is getting along with the peer group, in physical activities, and in the family setting. Open-ended questions (eg, "What is she like? What is an average day in her life? What does she do?") can help the clinician assess the child's social functioning.

During examination, the infant or toddler is often held in the mother's lap. Much information can be obtained by **observing** a child in reference to spontaneous movements, curiosity, ability to understand directions, and alertness to visual and auditory cues (eg, a tinkling bell).

Part of the neurologic examination includes a brief **general physical examination** with emphasis on the

Table 24–1. Developmental landmarks.

	Birth	3 Months	6 Months	9 Months	12–15 Months	24 Months
Motor	Flexor posture, lifts head prone, hands grasped	Sits: head forward, bobbing, lifts head supine, hands open, retains briefly	Rolls both ways, begins to sit alone, supports (erect), bounces	Creeps, pulls up standing, pincer grasp, sits well	Walks with 1–2 hands held, stands alone briefly, releases on command	Walks and runs well, walks downstairs, turns pages singly
Special senses	Regards (vision), may follow 45 degrees	Looks at hands, follows 90–180 degrees	Discriminates voices, localizes sounds	Picks up raisin, "bye-bye"	Localizes noises, localizes pain	Towers 6–7 cubes, imitates scribble
Adaptive	Startles to sound, delayed nociceptive response	Smiles socially, vocalizes socially, follows vertically	Holds cube, palmar grasp, retrieves toy, transfers and rakes raisin	Bangs toys together, pat-a-cake	Assists in dressing, attempts spoon feeding, tries 2-cube tower	Asks for toilet, pulls on garments, spoon-feeds well, parallel play
Language	Throaty noises	Coos, chuckles, vocal social response	Babbles (polysyllables), "mmm-mmm"	"Ma-ma, Da-da," one other "word"	Understands simple commands, speaks 1–3 words	Speaks in phrases, names 3–5 pictures, pronouns: "I, me, you"
Reflex	Tonic neck, palmar grasp	Disappearing tonic neck, Moro reflex	Begins voluntary stepping	Parachute response		
Automatisms	Moro reflex, sucks, roots, stepping, supporting, traction: head lag	Landau response, traction: no head lag	Neck righting, blinks to threat			

skin (birth marks), spine, neck, and skull (including palpation of the fontanelle and measurement of the head circumference). Simple explanations to parent and child during the exam can reassure both the patient and the parent: "I'm checking the soft spot to be sure the headache isn't causing high pressure in the head; it feels soft. That is normal. The pressure is fine." At some point in the exam, the baby should be inspected virtually unclothed. In an older child, asking about birth marks and inspecting the spine with the shirt pulled up and the child bent over for evaluation of scoliosis may be sufficient. Again, an explanation may aid: "It is very important that I look at your spine to be sure there isn't any curvature. It looks straight. That's fine."

Developmental assessment should be included in the neurologic examination of the infant. At an appropriate age, for example 6–18 months, the physician may start with handing blocks to the baby, offering a raisin, and evaluating the child's reach and type of grasp. A younger baby often enjoys a bell, the older child a reflex hammer. Using the block and the raisin, the clinician can carry out the items on the DDST that have not been elucidated by the history.

Running around the room and retrieving a ball is a test for the child's **station and gait.** Children usually enjoy having their **reflexes** tested. Be sure reflexes are present proximally and distally, eg, knee jerk/ankle jerk, triceps/brachial radialis. Sometimes,

a subtle case of hemiparesis can be indicated by a unilateral absence of abdominal or cremasteric cutaneous reflexes. Occasionally, tapping one's finger over a hamstring or biceps reflex can show an absent reflex or asymmetry in a lumbosacral plexus or brachial plexus injury.

Infantile automatisms, their presence, absence or asymmetry, are important in examination of the newborn and very young infant (see Table 24–1).

Running around the room, squatting, jumping, etc are tests of the child's **motor function.** In infants, tone, the subjective feeling of manipulating the limb, is important. (See the section on hypotonic infant.) Occasionally, formal muscle testing is necessary, eg, abduction at the shoulder and hand grasp; rising from a squat, and dorsiflexion of the foot to test proximal and distal strength. **Sensory testing** is rarely contributory; touch, tickle, and pinprick can be used in small children.

By this time, the infant **cranial nerves** have usually been satisfactorily assessed by observation (eg, extraocular movements, vision, and hearing). If there is concern about swallowing or tongue size or function, these areas can be examined by flashlight and tongue blade. Lastly, the fundi should be assessed by having the infant look at a distant object or by having the parent get the youngster's attention with a pinwheel or bell. The physician can approach from the side to get a look at the disc before light on

Table 24–2. Mental status.

Orientation: time, place, situation, name, date, year.
Memory: recent and remote, eg, "What did you have for lunch?" "What did you do on your birthday?" Remember (for 10 minutes): "Red flag, Washington's birthday, Christmas presents."
Calculation: (depends on educational background) subtract serial 7s.
Proverbs: (interpret) "Too many cooks spoil the broth." "A rolling stone gathers no moss."
Situation: "What would you do if you saw a fire?"
Aphasia: "What's this?" (chalk). "Stick out your tongue." "Put your right finger on your left ear." Sample speech, reading and writing.

the macula causes miosis. Sometimes, mydriatics to dilate the pupil are necessary.

In the older youngster, formal examination of **mental status** is rarely necessary. Some simple assessment of cognition can be obtained by having the child obey right-and-left commands (eg, "Put your right hand on your left ear"), do simple math problems, and read paragraphs appropriate for grade level (see Table 24–2).

In the older child, the Romberg test (standing with eyes closed, feet together, and hands straight out), tandem walking, and standing and hopping on each foot are tests for **station and gait. Limb coordination** can be tested by finger pursuit, that is, having children touch the clinician's moving finger with their own. Finger-nose alternating movements and patting the palm and the back of the hand alternately on the lap are other tests of lateral coordination. In the older child, tests for sense of position, vibration, and even cortical sensory status (for example, position of the limb in space and finger writing) are occasionally important.

Because children can be uncooperative and findings uncertain, serial exams are sometimes necessary. The reasons for the follow-up exam should be explained in detail to the parent. No neurologic examination is a complete failure. The clinician has the opportunity to observe the child during the interview and during play; these observations may give a reasonable assessment of neurologic function.

Finally, it must be emphasized that a complete examination should be performed and results told to the parents in plain language, even when the complaint seems trivial.

LUMBAR PUNCTURE

The principal purpose of lumbar puncture is to obtain an aliquot of cerebrospinal fluid for the diagnosis of infectious and inflammatory conditions of the central nervous system (Table 24–3). The uses of specimens of cerebrospinal fluid in cytologic studies, bioassays of enzymes and neurotransmitters, and specific immunofluorescent staining tests for viruses are widening the clinical (and research) applicability of lumbar puncture. However, performing lumbar puncture for manometric determinations, cellular content, and protein levels in many conditions—including head injuries, brain and spinal cord tumors, and seizure disorders—has been superseded by the use of brain imaging and biochemical techniques that are far more specific.

Therapeutically, lumbar puncture may be employed for drainage of cerebrospinal fluid to reduce its hematotoxic effects in hemorrhagic conditions (eg, intraventricular hemorrhage in newborns, ruptured berry aneurysm) and to lower intracranial pressure in pseudotumor cerebri.

Lumbar puncture is usually performed with the patient in the lateral recumbent or decubitus position. Entry is at the level of the iliac crest or the L3–4 interspace, with the patient's head initially flexed and then extended. In small infants—especially premature infants and neonates in the first months of life—lumbar puncture is more safely and satisfactorily performed with the infant in the sitting position and the head only slightly flexed or supported with a pillow propped between the outstretched arms and legs resting against the infant's chest and abdomen. The wrists and ankles should be held by an assisting nurse, and the needle should be pointed slightly cephalad.

Note: Before lumbar puncture is performed, the fundi should always be checked for papilledema. Lumbar puncture is contraindicated in the presence of elevated intracranial pressure, especially when there are focal neurologic deficits, because of the risk of tentorial or tonsillar herniation. This risk is less likely when there is diffuse cerebral swelling than when elevated pressure is due to a mass lesion. Therefore, if equipment for CT brain scanning is readily available, lumbar puncture should usually be delayed until a scan can be done; it should not be delayed, however, if examination of cerebrospinal fluids is indispensable for diagnosis and vital therapeutic intervention.

Lumbar puncture must be performed promptly when a diffuse central nervous system infection (meningitis, meningoencephalitis, encephalitis, cerebritis) is suspected. Only a small-gauge needle should be used, and only enough fluid should be withdrawn to permit cell count, protein and glucose determination, and such stains and cultures (bacterial, fungal, and viral) and other studies that may be helpful. A specimen of 2–3 mL is usually adequate for microchemical determinations.

It is occasionally important to obtain opening and closing cerebrospinal fluid pressures. To obtain valid pressure readings, the head, neck, and legs should gently be brought into a straight line. Pressure in the sitting position should be measured with the level of the foramen magnum as "zero"; the length of the

Table 24—3. Characteristics of cerebrospinal fluid (CSF) in the normal child and in central nervous system infections and inflammatory conditions.

Condition	Initial Pressure (mm H₂O)	Appearance	Cells/μL	Protein (mg/dL)	Glucose (mg/dl)	Other Tests	Comments
Normal	<180	Clear	0–5 lymphocytes. First 3 months, 1–3 PMNs. Neonates, up to 30 lymphocytes, 20–50 RBCs.	15–35 (lumbar). 5–15 (ventricular). Up to 150 (lumbar) for short time after birth; to 6 months, up to 65.	50–80 (two-thirds of blood glucose). May be increased after seizure.	CSF IgG index; < 0.7 units = CSF IgG/Serum IgG CSF albumin/Serum albumin Lactate dehydrogenase (LDH), 2–27 IU/L.	CSF protein in first month may be up to 170 mg/dL. in small-for-dates or premature infants. No increase in WBCs due to seizure.
Bloody tap	Normal or low	Bloody (sometimes with clot)	One additional WBC/700 RBCs.[1] RBCs not crenated.	One additional mg/800 RBCs.[1]	Normal	RBC number should fall between first and third tube; wait 5 minutes between tubes.	Spin down fluid; supernatant will be clear and colorless.
Bacterial meningitis, acute	200–750+	Opalescent to purulent	Up to 1000s, mostly PMNs. Early, few cells	Up to 100s.	Decreased; may be none.	Smear and culture mandatory. LDH > 24 IU/L.	Very early, glucose may be normal. Immunofluorescence tests.
Bacterial meningitis, partially treated	Usually increased	Clear or opalescent	Usually increased. PMNs usually predominate.	Elevated	Normal or decreased	LDH usually > 24 IU/L.	Smear and culture often negative.
Tuberculous meningitis	150–750+	Opalescent; fibrin web or pellicle	250–500, mostly lymphocytes. Early, more PMNs.	45–500; parallels cell count.	Decreased; may be none.	Smear for acid-fast organism; CSF culture and inoculation.	**Note:** Bacterial meningitis may be superimposed.
Fungal meningitis	Increased	Variable; often clear	10–500. Early, more PMNs; then mostly lymphocytes.	Elevated and increasing.	Decreased	India ink preparations, cryptococcal antigen, culture, inoculations, immuno-fluorescence tests.	Often superimposed in patients who are debilitated or on immuno-suppressive or tumor therapy.
Aseptic meningo-encephalitides (poliomyelitis)	Normal or slightly increased	Clear unless cell count > 300	0 to few hundred, mostly lymphocytes; PMNs predominate early.	20–125	Normal; may be low in mumps.	CSF, stool, throat wash for viral cultures. LDH < 28 IU/L (90% < 24 IU/L).	Acute and convalescent antibody titers. In mumps, up to 1000 lymphocytes; serum amylase often elevated. Rarely, several thousand cells present in enteroviral infection.
Neurosyphilis	Normal to 400	Clear unless protein is very high	10–100, mostly lymphocytes.	25–150; higher in meningitis.	Normal	Positive CSF serology. CSF IgG index increased.	Blood serology positive in untreated cases; *Treponema pallidum* immobilization test positive.
Parainfectious encephalomyelitis	80–450, usually increased	Usually clear	0–50, mostly lymphocytes.	15–75	Normal	CSF IgG index may be increased. Oligoclonal bands variable.	No organisms. Fulminant cases resemble purulent bacterial meningitis.
Polyneuritis Early	Normal and occasionally increased	Normal	Normal; occasionally slight increase.	Normal	Normal	Bacterial cultures negative; gamma globulin may be elevated.	Try to find cause (viral infections, toxins, lupus, infectious mononucleosis, diabetes, etc).
Late		Xanthochromic if protein high		45–1500			
Meningeal carcinomatosis	Often elevated	Clear to opalescent	Cytologic identification of tumor cells.	Often mildly to moderately elevated.	Often depressed		Seen with leukemia, medulloblastoma, meningeal melanosis, histiocytosis X. **Note:** May mimic meningitis.
Brain abscess	Normal or increased	Usually clear	5–500 in 80%; mostly PMNs.	Usually slightly increased.	Normal; occasionally decreased.		Cell count related to proximity to meninges; findings as in purulent meningitis if abscess perforates. (See references.)

[1]Multiple articles document pitfalls in using these ratios due to WBC lysis. Clinical judgment and repeat taps may be necessary to rule out meningitis in this situation.

fluid column above that level is the pressure in millimeters of water.

Multiple other components of cerebrospinal fluid have useful clinical applications. See Table 24–4.

Anbar R: Pitfalls in interpretation of traumatic lumbar puncture formula. (Letter.) *Am J Dis Child* 1986; **140:**638.

Anderson G: Neurotransmitter precursors and metabolites in CSF of human neonates. *Dev Med Child Neurol* 1985;**27:**207.

Chow G, Schmidley JW: Lysis of erythrocytes and leukocytes in traumatic lumbar puncture. *Arch Neurol* 1984;**41:**1984.

Cutler RWP, Spertel RB: Cerebrospinal fluid: A selective review. *Ann Neurol* 1982;**11:**1.

Markowitz H, Kokmen E: Neurologic diseases and the cerebrospinal fluid immunoglobin profile. *Mayo Clin Proc* 1983;**58:**273.

Novak RW: Lack of validity of standard corrections for white blood cell counts of blood-contaminated cerebrospinal fluid in infants. *Am J Clin Pathol* 1984;**82:**95.

Phillips P et al: Cerebrospinal fluid polyamines: Biochemical markers of malignant childhood brain tumors. *Ann Neurol* 1986;**19:**360.

Portnoy J, Olson L: Normal cerebrospinal fluid values in children: Another look. *Pediatrics* 1985;**75:**484.

Ricevuti G: Meningeal leukemia diagnosed by cytocentrifuge study of cerebrospinal fluid. *Arch Neurol* 1986; **43:**466.

Rubenstein S, Yager R: What represents pleocytosis in blood-contamined ("traumatic tap") CSF in childhood? *J Pediatr* 1985;**107:**249.

Shaywitz S, Shaywitz B: Attention deficit disorder: Current perspectives. *Pediatr Neurol* 1987;**3:**129.

Snead OC: Concentration of gamma-hydroxybutyric acid in ventricular and lumbar cerebrospinal fluid. *N Engl J Med* 1987;**304:**93.

Wood J (editor): *Neurology of CSF*. Plenum Press, 1982.

ELECTROENCEPHALOGRAPHY

This widely used, noninvasive electrophysiologic method for recording cerebral activity has its most distinct clinical applicability in the study of seizure disorders. "Activation" techniques to accentuate abnormalities or disclose latent abnormalities include photic stimulation, well-sustained hyperventilation for 3 minutes, and depriving the patient of sleep from about midnight until after breakfast, at which time the EEG is recorded. The latter is an excellent though less widely employed "activation" method.

Electroencephalography is also used in the evaluation of tumors, cerebrovascular accidents, neurodegenerative diseases, and other neurologic disorders causing brain dysfunction; but, with some notable exceptions, it is nonspecific. Recordings over a 24-hour period or all-night recordings are invaluable in the diagnosis of sleep disturbances and narcolepsy. Electroencephalography with telemetry or simultaneous monitoring of behavior on videotape, although limited by cost to a relatively few laboratories, has

Table 24–4. Cerebrospinal fluid: other useful constituents.

Measurement	Examples
Cytology	Leukemia, brain tumor cells, lipomacrophages (CNS damage), iron-laden macrophages (subarachnoid hemorrhage)
Immunoglobulins IgG, IgM, IgA, IgD, IgE, oligoclonal bands	Demyelinating disease, infection, neoplasms
Polyamines (eg, putrescine)	Some childhood brain tumors (diagnosis, monitoring); neural tube defects
Neurotransmitters (metabolites, eg, homovanillic acid)	Epilepsy, febrile seizures, Lesch-Nyhan syndrome, attention deficit disorder
Lactate/pyruvate; pH	Anoxia, hemorrhage, meningitis, metabolic disease
Enzymes: LDH, CK	Newborn anoxia; infection (bacterial versus viral), CVA
Ferritin	meningitis: viral versus bacterial

great usefulness in selected cases. The EEG can be helpful in determining a possible cause or mechanism of coma and is frequently used to determine if coma is irreversible and brain death has occurred.

The limitations of electroencephalography are considerable, and results are often misinterpreted. In most cases, the duration of the actual tracing is only about 30 minutes, which is a very small fraction of the brain's overall activity. Many drugs—especially barbiturates, benzodiazepines, and most of those used in psychiatry—and "functional" disturbances have considerable effects on the EEG. About 15% of normal (nonepileptic) individuals, especially children, may show some paroxysmal activity on EEG. Electroencephalographic findings such as those seen in migraine, learning disabilities, or behavior disorders do not reflect permanent "brain damage." In fact, one of the very useful applications of the EEG is to show "normalization" as behavior disorders are relieved and certain seizure disorders are controlled by anticonvulsant drugs.

At present, use of CT scans, evoked potentials, positron emission tomography, regional cerebral blood flow studies, and magnetic resonance imaging has replaced the use of electroencephalography as a diagnostic and prognostic tool.

EVOKED POTENTIALS

Cortical auditory, visual, or somatosensory evoked potentials (evoked responses) may be recorded from the scalp surface over the temporal, occipital, or frontoparietal cortex after repetitive stimulation of the retina by light flashes, of the cochlea by sounds, or of the skin by galvanic stimuli of varying frequency and intensity, respectively. Computer averaging is used to recognize and enhance these responses while subtracting or suppressing the asynchronous background electroencephalographic activity. The presence or absence of evoked potential waves and their latencies (time from stimulus to wave peak or time between peaks) figure in the clinical interpretation.

The reproducible and quantifiable results obtained from brain stem auditory, pattern-shift visual, and short-latency somatosensory evoked potentials (see below) indicate the level of function of the relevant sensory pathway or system and indicate the site of anatomic disruption. While results of these tests alone are usually not diagnostic, the tests are noninvasive, sensitive, objective, and relatively inexpensive extensions of the clinical neurologic examination. Because the auditory and somatosensory tests and one type of visual test are totally passive, requiring only that the patient remain still, they are particularly useful in the evaluation of functions in neonates and small children as well as in patients unable to cooperate (eg, due to mental retardation, degenerative disorder, anesthesia, or coma). Knowledge of normal values and experience in testing of the applicable patient group are mandatory.

Brain Stem Auditory Evoked Potentials

A brief auditory stimulus (click) of varying intensity and frequency is delivered to the ear to activate the auditory nerve (nerve VIII) and sequentially activate the cochlear nucleus, tracts and nuclei of the lateral lemniscus, and inferior colliculus. Thus, this technique assesses hearing and function of the brain stem auditory tracts.

Hearing in the neonate or uncooperative (but sedated) patient can be objectively assessed, making the technique particularly useful in high-risk infants, especially those in intensive care nurseries, and in retarded and autistic patients. Brain stem auditory evoked potentials are used to judge brain stem dysfunction in sleep apnea and in ''near miss'' for sudden infant death syndrome. As high doses of anesthetic agents or barbiturates do not seriously affect results, the test is used to assess and monitor brain stem function of patients during surgery (in the operating room) and those in hypoxic-ischemic coma or coma following head injury. Absence of evoked potential waves beyond the first wave from the auditory nerve usually portends brain death. Brain stem auditory evoked potentials are also useful in the early evaluation of diseases affecting myelin—ie, the various leukodystrophies and multiple sclerosis (although auditory evoked potentials are less valuable than visual evoked potentials in the latter)—and in intrinsic brain stem gliomas. They are sometimes useful in evaluation of hereditary ataxias, Wilson's disease (hepatolenticular degeneration), and other degenerative disorders affecting the brain stem.

Pattern-Shift Visual Evoked Potentials

The preferred stimulus is a shift (reversal) of a checkerboard pattern, and the response is a single wave (called P100) generated in the striate and parastriate visual cortex. The absolute latency of P100 (time from stimulus to wave peak) and the difference in latency between the 2 eyes are sensitive indicators of disease. The amplitude of response is affected by any process resulting in poor fixation on the stimulus screen or affecting visual acuity. Ability to focus on a checkerboard pattern is thus necessary to evaluate visual acuity. (A bright flash visual evoked potential can be used in younger and uncooperative children, but the norms are less standardized.) Evoked potentials suggest that visual acuity may be 20/20 in infants by 6–7 months of age.

Clinical application of the test includes detection and monitoring of strabismus (ie, in amblyopia ex anopsia), optic neuritis, and lesions near the optic nerve and chiasm such as optic gliomas and craniopharyngiomas. Degenerative and immunologic diseases that affect visual transmission and may be detected early and followed by serial evaluations by this technique include adrenoleukodystrophy, Pelizaeus-Merzbacher disease, some spinocerebellar degenerations, sarcoidosis, and even multiple sclerosis. Flash visual evoked potentials are used to monitor function during surgery involving the eyes and optic nerve; to assess cortical or hysterical blindness; and to evaluate patients with photosensitive epilepsy, who may have exaggerated responses.

Short-Latency Somatosensory Evoked Potentials.

Responses are commonly produced by electrical stimulation of peripheral sensory nerves, as this evokes potentials of greatest amplitude and clarity; finger tapping and muscle stretching may also be used. The function of this test is similar to that of the auditory test in closely correlating wave forms with function of the sensory pathways and permitting localization of conduction defects.

Short-latency somatosensory evoked potentials are used in the assessment of a wide variety of lesions of the peripheral nerve, root, spinal cord, and central nervous system following trauma, neuropathies (eg, in diabetes mellitus or Landry-Guillian-Barré syndrome), myelodysplasias, cerebral palsy, and many other disorders. The test procedure is often performed on an outpatient basis. One method is to stimulate the median nerve at the wrist with small (nonpainful) electrical shocks and record responses from the brachial plexus above the clavicle, the neck (cervical cord), and the opposite scalp area overlying the sensorimotor cortex. After stimulation from the knee (peroneal nerve) or ankle (tibial nerve), impulses are recorded from the lower lumbar spinal cord, cervical cord, and sensorimotor cortex. Such potentials are used to monitor spinal cord sensory functioning during surgery for disorders including scoliosis, myelodysplasias, and tumors and other lesions of the spinal cord or blood vessels supplying the cord. The technique is also used in leukodystrophies involving peripheral nerves, in multiple sclerosis, and in hysteria and malingering (anesthetic limbs). In the diagnosis of coma and brain death, somatosensory evoked potentials supplement the results of auditory evoked potentials.

Chiappa KH, Ropper AH: Evoked potentials in clinical medicine. (2 parts). *N Engl J Med* 1982;**306**:1140, 1205. [An overall summary of the field.]

Cohen BA, Schenk VA, Sweeney DB: Meningitis-related hearing loss evaluated with evoked potentials. *Pediatr Neurol* 1988;**4**:18.

DeMeirleir LJ, Taylor MJ: Prognostic utility of SEPs in comatose children. *Pediatr Neurol* 1987;**3**:78. [Initial and serial studies of this noninvasive test can be helpful in predicting outcome.]

Fagan ER, Taylor MJ, Logan WJ: Somatosensory evoked potentials. P2. A review of the clinical applications in pediatric neurology. *Pediatr Neurol* 1987;**3**:189.

Gilmore R (editor): *Neurol Clin* 1988;**6(4).** [Entire issue; up-to-date articles.]

Goldie WD et al: Brain stem auditory evoked potentials as a tool in the clinical assessment of children with posterior fossa tumors. *J Child Neurol* 1987;**2**:272.

Hecox KE, Cone B, Blaw ME: Brain stem auditory evoked response in the diagnosis of pediatric neurologic disease. *Neurology* 1981;**31**:832. [Early applications in pediatrics.]

Kamimura N et al: Spinal somatosensory evoked potentials in infants and children with spinal cord lesions. *Brain Dev* 1988;**10**:355.

Mutoh K et al: Maturation of somatosensory evoked potentials upon posterior tibial nerve stimulation. *Pediatr Neurol* 1988;**4**:342. [Helpful normal data.]

Rotteveel JJ et al: The applications of evoked potentials in the diagnosis and follow-up of children with intracranial tumors. *Childs Nerv Syst* 1985;**1**:172.

Rowe MJ III: The brain stem auditory evoked response in neurologic disease: A review. *Ear Hear* 1981;**2**:41.

Roy M et al: Evaluation of children and young adults with tethered spinal cord syndrome. *Surg Neurol* 1986; **26**:241. [One of many helpful articles from the Kentucky group; here, a large series of rare pediatric pertinent entity.]

Sokol S: Infant visual stimulation: Visual evoked potential estimates. *Ann N Y Acad Sci* 1982;**388**:514. [Research article.]

Stockard J: Brain stem auditory evoked potentials in adult and infant sleep apnea syndrome, including sudden infant death syndrome, and near-miss for sudden infant death. *Ann N Y Acad Sci* 1982;**388**:443.

Stockard J et al: Prognostic value of brain stem auditory evoked potentials in neonates. *Arch Neurol* 1983; **40**:360.

Whyte HE et al: Prognostic utility of visual evoked potentials in term asphyxiated neonates. *Pediatr Neurol* 1986; **2**:220. An objective, noninvasive test; these are provocative early results that need confirmation.]

BRAIN ELECTRICAL ACTIVITY MAPPING (BEAM)

Brain electrical activity mapping is a relatively new technique in which electroencephalographic and evoked potential data recorded from multiple scalp electrodes are graphically displayed in color on a computer-driven video screen. Values between electrodes are obtained by interpolation. Learning-disabled, dyslexic, and epileptic children are being studied in research protocols. Expense, lack of normative data, and lack of numbers of homogenous clinical patients preclude current use of this modality in the field.

Duffy FH: The BEAM method for neurophysiological diagnosis. *Ann N Y Acad Sci* 1985;**457**:19.

Nuwer M: Quantitative EEG. 1. Techniques and problems of frequency, analysis, and topographic mapping. *Neurol Clin* 1988;**5**:1. [A careful analysis of pitfalls in this area.]

Nuwer M, Sharbrough F: American EEG Society statement on clinical use of quantitative EEG. *Neurology* 1987;**37**:28A. [An official statement of current usefulness.]

PEDIATRIC NEURORADIOLOGIC PROCEDURES

Sedation for Procedures

Radiologic procedures in infants and children are usually performed by pediatric radiologists, but sedation for these procedures remains largely the responsibility of the physician caring for the child. The choice of sedation must take into account the patient's age and physical condition, the type of neurologic disorder, the effect and duration of the procedure, and whether immediate neurosurgery is anticipated. The prescribing physician should be familiar with the agent used.

Oral or rectal chloral hydrate is safest, 30–60 mg/kg/dose. However, many radiology departments use only nonoral administration because of the risks of vomiting and aspiration. One favorite is pentobarbital, 6 mg/kg for children weighing less than 15 kg and 5 mg/kg for larger children (up to a maximum of 200 mg) given intramuscularly or rectally (at least 20 minutes before a procedure) or 2–4 mg/kg given intravenously. Training and equipment to support blood pressure and respirations must be available. This dosage usually achieves sedation for up to 2 hours. However, if sedation is inadequate 30 minutes after injection, and if the condition of the child so allows, a second dose of pentobarbital, 2 mg/kg, is given. A "cardiac cocktail," usually of intramuscularly administered meperidine hydrochloride, secobarbital, and promethazine hydrochloride or chlorpromazine, may be employed by pediatricians who are familiar with it. General anesthesia may be indicated especially if the child is to undergo surgery immediately on completion of a radiologic problem.

Computed Tomography (CT Scanning)

Computed tomography (CT) consists of a series of cross-sectional (''axial'') roentgenograms. The procedure is almost risk-free and can be performed on an outpatient basis. Radiation exposure is approximately the same as that from a skull roentgenogram series; shielded gonads receive less than 0.1 mrad. The images can be viewed on an oscilloscope as the scan is being done and later examined on printed-out films; both oscilloscope views and films record variations in tissue densities. CT scanning is of high sensitivity (88–96% of lesions larger than 1–2 cm can be seen) but low specificity (a tumor, focus of infection, or infarct may have the same appearance).

The CT scan is often repeated after intravenous injection of iodized contrast for ''enhancement,'' which reflects the vascularity of a lesion or its surrounding tissues. Precautions should be taken to ensure that the patient is not hypersensitive to iodinated dyes and that allergic reactions can be managed promptly. Sufficient information is often obtained from a nonenhanced scan; in these cases, cost and risk are minimized.

Sedation may be required for CT scanning. For positioning the head of children up to 8 years of age, a specially shaped headrest may be needed. The indications for CT scanning and the findings in specific conditions are discussed below in the sections on specific disorders.

There have been rapid advances in the application of CT techniques to further refine brain imaging, eg, with magnetic resonance imaging and positron emission tomography, which are discussed below. Coupling regional cerebral blood flow techniques with CT procedures in exploring physiologic processes is also under investigation.

Single Photon Emission Computed Tomography (SPECT)

This technique is a research tool: using an intravenous radioactive ligand (eg, iodine 123) that is lipophilic and taken up by neurons, images can be made far early in the tracer's half-life (for about 20–60 minutes). Demented patients show lessened uptake in diseased areas. Pediatric applications are pending.

Magnetic Resonance Imaging (MRI)

Magnetic or nuclear magnetic resonance (NMR) imaging is a noninvasive technique that uses the magnetic properties of certain nuclei to produce signals known as the proton spin-lattice relaxation time and the spin-spin relaxation time—signals that are based on the density of nuclei at a given point and on their immediate environment (lattice). Currently, the technique is based on detecting the response (resonance) of hydrogen proton nuclei to applied radiofrequency electromagnetic radiation; these nuclei are abundant in the body and more sensitive to magnetic resonance imaging than other nuclei. The strength of relaxation signals varies with the relationship of water to protein and the amount of lipids present. The image displayed, which is made up of a mixture of signals and is similar to the CT film, provides high-resolution contrast of soft tissues. Magnetic resonance imaging can, in fact, provide information about the histologic, physiologic, and biochemical status of tissues, in addition to gross anatomic data.

Clinically, magnetic resonance imaging has been applied chiefly to the study of lesions in the head, but it can be used in examinations of the spine, body organs, and tissues such as muscles and nerves. It has been used to delineate brain tumors, edema, ischemic and hemorrhagic lesions, hydrocephalus, vascular disorders, inflammatory and infectious lesions, and degenerative processes. Magnetic resonance imaging can be used to study myelination and demyelination and, through the demonstration of changes in relaxation time, metabolic disorders of the brain, muscles, and glands. Because bone causes no artifact in the images, the posterior fossa and its contents can be studied far better using MRI than using CT scans; even blood vessels and the cranial nerves can be imaged. On the other hand, the inability to detect calcification limits the detection of calcified lesions such as craniopharyngioma or leptomeningeal angiomatosis.

It is believed that the strong magnetic fields used in this procedure do not cause molecular or cellular damage. Work is progressing on imaging from nuclei other than hydrogen, such as phosphorus and sodium.

Cost is 2–3 times that of a contrast-enhanced CT scan. The procedure can be frightening and requires sedated sleep or light anesthesia for the child to ensure complete immobility.

Positron Emission Tomography (PET)

Positron emission tomography is an imaging technique that measures the metabolic rate at a given site by CT scanning to detect positron (proton) emission. For measurement of local cerebral metabolism, the radiolabeled substrate most frequently used has been fluorodeoxyglucose ^{18}F by injection. Gray matter and white matter are clearly distinguishable; the skull and air- or fluid-filled cavities are least active metabolically.

Positron emission tomography has been used to study the cerebral metabolism of neonates and brain activation by visual or auditory stimuli. Pathologic states that have been studied include epilepsy (during and between seizures), brain infarcts and tumors, and dementias. This functional test of brain metabolism is clinically useful in preoperative evaluation for epilepsy surgery. The "epileptogenic zone" will often be hypermetabolic during ictal events and hypoactive during the time between seizures. The information complements electrical (EEG) and imaging (MRI) findings to aid in the decision of what tissue to remove.

Other radiolabeled substances sometimes used are ^{11}C-glucose, also by injection, and [11]CO by inhalation detectable subsequently in carboxyhemoglobin.

Clinical application is limited by the cost of the procedure and the clinician's need for access to a nearby cyclotron where the radiopharmaceuticals can be prepared.

Ultrasonography

Ultrasonography offers a pictorial display (eg, echoencephalogram, echocardiogram) of the varying density of tissues in a given anatomic region or structure by recording the echoes of ultrasonic waves reflected from it. These waves, modulated by pulsations, are introduced into the tissue by means of a piezoelectric transducer. The many advantages of ultrasonography include the ability to make quick assessment of a structure and its positioning by means of portable equipment, without ionizing radiation and at about one-fourth the cost of CT scanning. Sedation is usually not necessary, and ultrasonography can be repeated as often as indicated. In brain imaging, B mode and real-time sector scanners are usually employed, permitting excellent detail to be obtained in the coronal and sagittal planes. Contiguous structures can be studied by a continuous sweep and reviewed on videotape.

Ultrasonography has been used for in utero diagnosis of hydrocephalus and other anomalies. In neonates, the thin skull and the open anterior fontanelle have facilitated imaging of the brain, and ultrasonography is now used in many nurseries to screen and follow all infants of less than 32 weeks of gestation or under 1500 g for intracranial hemorrhage. Other uses in neonates include detection of hydrocephalus, major brain and spine malformations, and even calcifications from intrauterine infection with cytomegalovirus or *Toxoplasma*.

Cerebral Angiography

Arteriography remains a very useful procedure in the diagnosis of many cerebrovascular disorders, particularly vascular malformations, and is sometimes used when a potentially operable lesion is suspected. In some instances of brain tumor, arteriography may be necessary to define the precise location or vascular bed, to differentiate among tumors, or to distinguish tumor from abscess or infarction. Noninvasive CT scanning and MRI scans are often satisfactory in cases of static or flowing blood disorders (eg, sinus thromboses). Thus, invasive arteriography

is less often being used instead of these less dangerous procedures.

Metrizamide Ventriculography

A small amount (1 or 2 mL) of metrizamide, a water-soluble contrast material, may be injected into a lateral ventricle by direct puncture or via a preexisting shunt. Imaging is then carried out by standard x-ray or CT scanning. This procedure permits visualization of the flow of cerebrospinal fluid (within the ventricle, between the ventricles, or between the ventricle and an intracerebral cyst) to determine the appropriate site of shunt placement or other surgical procedure.

Myelography

X-ray examination of the spine following injection of a dye, water-soluble contrast medium, or air into the subarachnoid space via the lumbar or, rarely, the cervical route may be indicated in cases of spinal cord tumors or various forms of spinal dysraphism and in rare instances of herniated discs in children. However, in most institutions, spin scanning (magnetic resonance imaging) or CT metrizamide myelography is now employed instead.

Altman NR, Purser RK, Post MJ: Tuberous sclerosis: Characteristics at CT and MR imaging. *Radiology* 1988; **167**:527.

Brody AS, Gooding CA: Magnetic resonance imaging: Review article. *Pediatr Rev* 1986;**8**:87.

Doyle LW et al: Regional cerebral glucose metabolism of newborn infants measured by positron emission tomography. *Dev Med Child Neurol* 1983;**25**:143.

Duchowny MS, Bonis I: Long-term cassette electroencephalogram monitoring in childhood seizures. *Ann Neurol* 1983;**14**:359.

Nowell MA et al: Magnetic resonance imaging of white matter disease in children. *AJR* 1988;**151**:359.

Powers TA et al: Central nervous system lesions in pediatric patients. *Radiology* 1988;**169**:723.

Roach E et al: Magnetic resonance imaging in pediatric neurologic disorders. *J Child Neurol* 1987;**2**:110.

Rumack CM, Johnson ML: Role of computed tomography and ultrasound in neonatal brain imaging. *J Comput Tomogr* 1983;**7**:17.

Scher MS: A developmental marker of central nervous system maturation. *Pediatr Neurol* 1988;**4**:265.

DISORDERS AFFECTING THE NERVOUS SYSTEM IN INFANTS & CHILDREN

ALTERED STATES OF CONSCIOUSNESS

Essentials of Diagnosis

- Reduction or alteration in cognitive and affective

Table 24–5. Gradation of coma.

| | "Deep Coma" | | "Light coma" | | Stupor |
	Grade 4	Grade 3	Grade 2	Grade 1	
Response to pain	0	+	Avoidance	Avoidance	Arousal unsustained
Tone/posture	Flaccid	Decerebrate			Normal
Tendon reflexes	0	+/−	+	+	+
Pupil response	0	+	+	+	+
Response to verbal stimuli	0	0	0	0	+
Other corneal reflex	0	+	+	+	+
Gag reflex	0	+	+	+	+

mental functioning and in arousability or attentiveness.

■ Acute onset.

General Considerations

Coma and other states of unconsciousness are imprecisely defined. Many terms are used to describe the continuum from full alertness and attentiveness or consciousness to complete unresponsivity and deep coma. This continuum might include clouding, obtundation, somnolence or stupor, semicoma or light coma, and deep coma. Several scales have been used to grade the depth of unconsciousness. Table 24–5 and Table 24–6 delineate some of these. Physicians should use one of these tables and further describe in their narratives what they mean. These descriptions help subsequent observers quantify unconsciousness and decide whether the patient is improving or deteriorating.

The neurologic substrate for consciousness is the reticular activating system in the brain stem, up to and including the thalamus and paraventricular hypothalamus. Large lesions of the cortex, especially of the left hemisphere, can also cause coma. "Locked-in syndrome" is a term used for patients who are conscious but have no access to motor or verbal expression because of massive loss of motor function of the brain stem. "Coma vigil" is the term used for patients who seem to be comatose but have some spontaneous motor behavior, such as eye opening or eye tracking, almost always at a reflex level. "Persistent vegetative state" refers to a chronic condition

Table 24–6. "Glasgow Coma Scale" for recording assessment of consciousness.[1,2]

| | | Date | | | | |
		Time	Time	Time	Time	etc
Best motor response	6 Obeys commands 5 Localizes pain 4 Withdraws 3 Abnormal flexing 2 Extensor response 1 None					
Best verbal response	5 Oriented 4 Confused conversation (words) 3 Inappropriate words (vocal sounds) 2 Incomprehensible sounds (cries) 1 None					
Eye opening	4 Spontaneous 3 To speech 2 To pain 1 None					
Total Score						

[1]Modified and reproduced, with permission, from Jennett B, Teasdale G: Aspects of coma after severe head injury. *Lancet* 1977;**1**:878.
[2]The scale can also be modified for infants. The sections regarding motor response and eye opening remain unchanged; items in parentheses in verbal response section are to be applied to infants. Under 6 months of age, the best verbal response is a cry (score 2) and the best motor response is usually flexion (score 3), for a total maximal score of 9. Adjusted maximal scores are as follows:

Birth–6 months:	9	2–5 years:	13
6–12 months:	11	over 5 years:	14–15
1–2 years:	12		

in which there is preservation of the sleep-waking cycle but no awareness and no recovery of mental function; this has been documented in infants.

Emergency Measures

The clinician's first response is to assure that the patient will survive the initial examination. The "ABCs" of resuscitation are pertinent. *Airway* must be kept open with positioning or even endotracheal intubation. *Breathing* and adequate air exchange can be assessed by auscultation; hand bag respiratory assistance with oxygen might be needed. *Circulation* must be assured by assessing pulse and blood pressure. An intravenous line will always be necessary. Fluids, plasma, blood, or even a dopamine drip (5–20 μg/kg/min) might be necessary in cases of hypotension. An extremely hypothermic or febrile child may require vigorous cooling or warming to save life. The assessment of vital signs may signal the diagnosis. Slow, insufficient respirations suggest poisoning by hypnotic drugs; apnea might indicate diphenoxylate hydrochloride poisoning. Rapid, deep respirations suggest acidosis, possibly metabolic, as with diabetic coma; toxic, eg, that due to aspirin; or neurogenic, as in Reye's syndrome. Hyperthermia might indicate infection or heat stroke; hypothermia might indicate cold exposure, ethanol poisoning, or hypoglycemia (especially in infancy).

The signs of impending brain herniation are another priority of the initial assessment. Bradycardia, high blood pressure, irregular breathing, increased extensor tone, and third nerve palsy with the eye and pupil deviated outward and dilatated are possible signs of impending temporal lobe or brain stem herniation. These signs suggest a need for hyperventilation, reducing cerebral edema, prompt neurosurgical consultation, and possibly, in an infant with a bulging fontanelle, subdural or ventricular tap (or both).

Initial intravenous fluids should contain glucose until further assessment disproves hypoglycemia as a cause.

A history obtained from parents or witnesses is desirable. Sometimes the only history will be obtained from ambulance attendants. An important point is whether the child is known to have a chronic illness, for example, diabetes, hemophilia, epilepsy, or cystic fibrosis. Recent acute illness raises the possibility of coma caused by Reye's syndrome, viral or bacterial meningitis, or the much rarer hemolytic-uremic syndrome. A combination of viral illness with 1–3 days of sudden and intractable vomiting invariably precedes the coma of Reye's syndrome. (The illness is usually respiratory, sometimes varicella.)

Trauma is a common cause of coma. Lack of a history of trauma, especially in infants, doesn't rule it out; nonaccidental trauma or a fall unwitnessed by caretakers may have occurred.

In coma of unknown cause, poisoning is always a possibility. Lack of a history of ingestion of a toxic substance or of medication in the home does not rule out poisoning as a cause for coma of unknown origin.

Often the history is obtained concurrent with a brief pediatric and neurologic screening examination. After the assessment of vital signs and their meaning, the general examination proceeds with an assessment for trauma. Palpation of the head and fontanelle, inspection of the ears for infection or hemorrhage, and a careful examination for neck stiffness are indicated. If circumstances suggest head or neck trauma, the head and neck must be immobilized so that any fracture or dislocation will not be aggravated. The skin must be inspected for petechiae or purpura that might suggest bacteremia, infection, bleeding disorder, or traumatic bruising. An examination of the chest, abdomen, and limbs is important to exclude enclosed hemorrhage, traumatic fractures, etc.

Neurologic examination quantifies the stimulus response and depth of coma, eg, responsiveness to verbal or painful stimuli. Examination of the eyes in reference to pupils, fundi, and eye movements is important. Are the eye movements spontaneous, or is it necessary to do the doll's-eye maneuver, ie, rotating the head rapidly to see whether the eyes follow? Motor and sensory examination assess reflex asymmetries, Babinski sign, and evidence for spontaneous posturing or posturing induced by noxious stimuli (eg, decorticate or decerebrate posturing).

If the cause of the coma is not obvious, emergency laboratory tests must be obtained. Table 24–7 and Table 24–8, respectively, list some of the causes of coma in children and mnemonics for its investigation. An immediate blood sugar (or Dextrostix), complete blood count, urine obtained by catheterization if necessary, electrolytes (including pH and bicarbonate), blood urea nitrogen, and SGOT are initial screens. Urine, blood, and even gastric contents must be saved for toxin screen if the underlying cause is not obvious. Spinal tap is often necessary to rule out central nervous system infection. Papilledema is a relative contraindication to lumbar puncture. Occasionally, blood culture is obtained, antibiotics started, and imaging study of the brain done prior to a diagnostic spinal tap. If meningitis is suspected and a tap is thought hazardous, antibiotics should be started and the diagnostic spinal puncture done later. Tests that are less readily available but helpful in obscure cases of coma include Po_2, Pco_2, ammonia levels, serum and urine osmolality, porphyrins, lead levels, and (in the newborn) urine and serum amino acids, and urine organic acids.

If there is any suspicion of head trauma or increased pressure, an emergency CT scan or MRI is necessary. Bone windows on the former study or skull x-rays can be done at the same sitting. The absence of skull fracture, of course, does not rule out

Table 24–7. Some causes of coma in childhood.[1]

Mechanism of Coma	Likely Cause	
	Newborn, Infant	Older Child

Anoxia
  Asphyxia
  Respiratory
    obstruction
  Severe anemia
	Birth asphyxia
	Meconium aspiration, infection (especially respiratory syncytial virus)
	Hydrops fetalis
		CO poisoning
		Croup, epiglottiditis
		
		Hemolysis, blood loss

Ischemia
  Cardiac
  Shock
	Shunting lesions, hypoplastic left heart
	Asphyxia (cardiac), sepsis
		Shunting lesions, aortic stenosis
		Blood loss, infection

Trauma	Birth contusion, hemorrhage, nonaccidental trauma	Falls, auto accidents
Infection	Gram-negative meningitis, herpes II encephalitis, postimmunization encephalitis	Bacterial meningitis, viral encephalitis, postinfectious encephalitis
Vascular	Intraventricular hemorrhage (premature), sinus thrombosis	Arterial, venous occlusion with congenital heart disease
Neoplasm	Rare; variety, medulloblastoma	Brainstem glioma, increased pressure with posterior fossa tumors
Drugs	Maternal sedatives, injected analgesics	"Any" drugs
Epilepsy	Constant minor motor seizures	Constant minor motor seizures, petit mal status, postictal state
Toxins	Lead	Arsenic, alcohol, drugs, pesticides
Hypoglycemia	Birth injury, diabetic progeny, toxemic progeny	Diabetes, "prediabetes," "idiopathic," hypoglycemic agents

Increased
  intracranial
  pressure
	Anoxic brain damage, hydrocephalus, unusual metabolic disorders (urea cycle; amino, organic acidurias)	Toxic encephalopathy, Reye's syndrome, head trauma, tumor of posterior fossa

Hepatic causes	Hepatitis, fulminant (rare), bile duct atresia, inborn metabolic errors in bilirubin conjugation	Acute hepatitis, chronic aggressive hepatitis
Renal causes	Hypoplastic kidneys	Nephritis, acute and chronic
Hypertensive encephalopathy		Acute nephritis, vasculitis
Hypercarbia	Congenital lung anomalies, bronchopulmonary dysplasia	Cystic fibrosis

Electrolyte abnormalities
  Hypernatremia
  Hyponatremia
 	
  Severe acidosis
  Hyperkalemia
	Iatrogenic ($NaHCO_3$ use), salt poisoning
	Inappropriate antidiuretic hormone, adrenogenital syndrome, dialysis (iatrogenic)
	Septicemia, cold injury, metabolic errors
	Renal failure, adrenogenital syndrome
		Diarrhea, dehydration
		Diarrhea, dehydration, gastroenteritis
		
		Infection, diabetic coma, poisoning (ASA, etc)
		Poisoning (ASA, etc)

Purpuric	Disseminated intravascular coagulation (many causes), hemolytic-uremic syndrome	Disseminated intravascular coagulation (many causes), leukemia, thrombotic purpura (rare)

[1]Modified and reproduced, with permission, from Lewis J, Moe PG: The unconscious child. In: *Current Diagnosis,* 5th ed. Conn H, Conn R (editors). Saunders, 1977.

coma caused by life-threatening closed head trauma; injury that results from shaking a child is one example. In a child with an open fontanelle, a real-time ultrasound may be substituted for the other, more definitive imaging studies if there is good local expertise.

Rarely, an emergency electroencephalogram aids in diagnosing the cause of coma. A nonconvulsive status epilepticus or focal finding seen with herpes encephalitis (periodic lateralized epileptiform discharges, or PLEDS) or focal slowing as seen with stroke or cerebritis are cases in which the EEG might be helpful. The EEG also may correlate with the stage of coma (for example, in Reye's syndrome) and add prognostic information. (See Table 24–9.) An improving (or deteriorating) EEG may herald clinical improvement, aid in predicting outcome, and suggest the need for more (or less) heroic therapy.

Treatment

Treatment, of course, depends on the underlying cause. Emergency measures were outlined at the beginning of this section.

A. General Measures: Vital signs must be monitored and maintained. Most emergency rooms and intensive care units have flow sheets to monitor

Table 24–8. Mnemonics for investigating
coma in children.[1]

7 Hs	5 Is
Hypoglycemia	Ictal (or postictal)
Hyperosmotic	Ingestion
Hyponatremia	Infection
Hypertensive	Injury
Hypoxia	Illness
Hemorrhage	(extracranial, intracranial)
Hepatic	
(Reye's syndrome)	

[1]Modified and reproduced, with permission, from
Lewis J, Moe PG: The unconscious child. In: *Current
Diagnosis,* 5th ed. Conn H, Conn R (editors). Saunders, 1977.

vital signs. The flow sheets provide space for repeated monitoring of the coma; one of the coma scales can be a useful tool for this purpose. The patient's response to vocal or painful stimuli and orientation to time, place, and situation when coming out of the coma are monitored. Posture and movements of the varied limbs, either spontaneous or in response to pain, is serially noted. Pupillary size, equality, and reaction to light and movement of the eyes to the doll's-eye maneuver or ice-water calorics should be on the flow sheet. Intravenous fluids can be tailored to the situation, eg, for treatment of acidosis, shock, or hypovolemia. Nasogastric suction is initially important; when the coma is prolonged, nasogastric feedings are sometimes part of treatment. The patient needs to be catheterized for monitoring urine output and for urinalysis. The child should be protected from decubiti with frequent turning and, if necessary, foam mattress. Eyes should be protected with pads and artificial tears.

B. Seizures: The doctor should order an EEG if there is a question of ongoing seizures. If there are obvious motor seizures, treatment for status epilepticus is given with intravenous drugs (see below). If there is suggestion of brain stem herniation or increased pressure, an intracranial monitor may be necessary. (This procedure is described in more detail in other sections of this book.) Initial treatment

Table 24–9. Electroencephalogram—coma
correlates.[1]

Rhythmic 4–7/sec (1–3/sec)	I	Lethargy
Dysrhythmic 1–3/sec (4–7/sec)	II	Disorientation, delirium
Disorganized 1–3/sec, low amplitude	III	Coma—decorticate
Low amplitude (< 50 microvolt), burst suppression	IV	Coma—decerebrate
Almost isoelectric	V	"Coma depasse"

[1]Modified and reproduced, with permission, from
Aoki Y, Lombroso CT: Prognostic value of electroencephalography in Reye's syndrome. *Neurology* 1973;23:333.

of this possible complication includes keeping the patient's head up (15–30 degrees) and hyperventilation. Mannitol, diuretics, steroids, and drainage of the spinal fluid are other, more heroic measures covered in detail in other sections.

Prognosis

About half of children with nontraumatic causes of coma have a good outcome. In studies of adults assessed on admission or within the first days after the onset of coma, an analysis of multiple variables was most helpful in suggesting prognosis. Abnormal neuro-ophthalmologic signs (eg, the absence of pupillary movement or of movement in response to the doll's-eye maneuver or ice-water calorics and the absence of corneal responses) were inauspicious. Delay in the return of motor responses, tone, or eye opening was also unfavorable. In children, the assessment done on admission is about as predictive as one done in succeeding days. Approximately two-thirds of outcomes can be successfully predicted at an early stage on the basis of coma severity, extraocular movements, pupillary reactions, motor patterns, blood pressure, temperature, and seizure type. Other characteristics, eg, the need for assisted respiration, the presence of increased intracranial pressure, and the duration of coma, were not significantly predictive.

Other series suggest that an anoxic (as compared to traumatic, metabolic, toxic, etc) cause of coma, eg, that caused by near drowning, has a much grimmer outlook.

BRAIN DEATH

Many medical and law associations have endorsed the following definition of death: "An individual who has sustained either (1) irreversible cessation of circulatory and respiratory functions, or (2) irreversible cessation of all functions of the entire brain, including the brain stem, is dead. A determination of death must be made in accordance with accepted medical standards." Recently, representatives from multiple pediatric and neurologic associations endorsed the Guidelines for the Determination of Brain Death in Children (see reference below). The criteria in term infants (> 38 weeks) were applicable one week after the neurologic insult. Difficulties in assessing premature infants and term infants shortly after birth were acknowledged.

Prerequisites

History is important: the physician must determine proximate causes to make sure that there are no remediable or reversible conditions. Examples of such causes are metabolic conditions, toxic agents, sedative/hypnotic drugs, surgically remediable conditions, hypothermia, and paralytic agents.

Physical Examination Criteria

These criteria are those established by the Task Force on Brain Death in Children (see reference, below).

(1) Coexistence of coma and apnea. The patient must exhibit complete loss of consciousness, vocalization, and volitional activity.

(2) Absence of brain stem function as defined by the following: (a) Midposition or fully dilated pupils that do not respond to light. Drugs may influence and invalidate pupillary assessment. (b) Absence of spontaneous eye movements and those induced by oculocephalic and caloric (oculovestibular) testing. (c) Absence of movement of bulbar musculature, including facial and oropharyngeal muscles. The corneal, gag, cough, sucking, and rooting reflexes are absent. (d) Absence of respiratory movements when the patient is off the respirator. Apnea testing using standardized methods can be performed but is done after other criteria are met.

(3) The patient must not be significantly hypothermic or hypotensive for age.

(4) Tone is flaccid, and spontaneous or induced movements, excluding spinal cord events such as reflex withdrawal or spinal myoclonus, are absent.

(5) The examination should remain consistent with brain death throughout the observation and testing period.

Confirmation

Details of apnea testing suggest documentation of a Pco_2 level reaching > 60 torr, with oxygenation maintained throughout; this level may be reached 3–15 minutes after taking the patient off the respirator. The recommended observation period to confirm brain death (repeated examinations) is 12–24 hours (longer in infancy); reversible causes *must* be ruled out.

If an irreversible cause is documented, laboratory testing is not essential. Helpful tests to support the clinical contention of brain death include the following:

(1) Electroencephalography: electrocerebral silence should persist for 30 minutes. Drug concentrations must be insufficient to suppress EEG activity.

(2) Angiography: failure of arterial intracerebral blood flow confirms brain death. Carotid arteriography and cerebral radionuclide angiogram are 2 methods. Dural sinus flow may persist and not disqualify the diagnosis of brain death.

Other laboratory studies have not been sufficiently documented to be considered definitive; cerebral evoked potentials and ultrasound blood pulsations are 2 common examples. Xenon-enhanced computer tomography is a more elaborate method.

Rarely, children have had documented preserved intracranial perfusion with EEG electrocerebral silence; the converse has also been reported. Furthermore, thoughtful clinicians have highlighted the controversy and problem regarding the definition and criteria of brain death and the special situation of brain death in the newborn. This situation includes the acknowledgement of the cessation of support in infants with nil prognosis who are not brain dead.

Ashwal S, Schneider S: Brain death in children. (2 parts.) *Pediatr Neurol* 1987;**3**:5,69.

Darby JM et al: Xenon-enhanced computed tomography in brain death. *Arch Neurol* 1987;**44**:551.

Freeman JM, Ferry PC: New brain death guidelines in children: Further confusion. *Pediatrics* 1988;**81**:301.

Goldie WD: Physiologic parameters for evaluating severe brain injury in infants and young children. *Am J EEG Technol* 1988;**28**:153.

Lewis J, Moe PG: The unconscious child. In: *Current Diagnosis*, 5th ed. Conn H, Conn R (editors). Saunders, 1977.

Mizrahi EM, Pollack MA, Kellaway P: Neocortical death in infants: Behavioral, neurologic, and electroencephalographic characteristics. *Pediatr Neurol* 1985;**1**:302.

Shewmon DA: Commentary on guidelines for the determination of brain death in children. *Ann Neurol* 1988;**24**:789.

Task Force on Brain Death in Children: Guidelines for the determination of brain death in children. *Ann Neurol* 1987;**21**:616. [Also *Arch Neurol* 1987;**44**:587. *Neurology* 1987;**37**:1077. *Pediatr Neurol* 1987;**3**:242. *Pediatrics* 1987;**80**:298.]

Teasdale G, Jennett B: Assessment of coma and impaired consciousness: A practical scale. *Lancet* 1974;**2**:81.

Toffol GJ et al: Pitfalls in diagnosing brain death in infancy. *J Child Neurol* 1987;**2**:134.

SEIZURE DISORDERS (Epilepsies)

Essentials of Diagnosis

- Recurrent nonfebrile seizures.
- Often, interictal (between seizures) EEG changes.

General Considerations

A seizure is a sudden, transient disturbance of brain function, manifested by involuntary motor, sensory, autonomic, or psychic phenomena, alone or in any combination, often accompanied by alteration or loss of consciousness. A seizure may occur after a transient metabolic, traumatic, anoxic, or infectious insult to the brain.

Repeated seizures without evident time-limited cause justify the label of epilepsy. Seizures and epilepsy occur most commonly at the extremes of life. The incidence is highest in the newborn and higher in childhood than in later life. Epilepsy in childhood often remits. Prevalence (the number of people with epilepsy in the population at any given time) flattens out after age 10–15. The chance of having a second seizure after an initial unprovoked episode is 30%. The chance of remission from epilepsy in childhood is 50%. The recurrence rate after the withdrawal of drugs is about 30%. Factors adversely influencing recurrence include (1) difficulty in getting the seizures under control (that is, the number of seizures occurring before control is achieved), (2) neurologic dysfunction or mental retardation, (3) age of onset under 2 years, and (4) abnormal EEG at the time of discontinuing medication. The type of seizures also often determines prognosis.

Seizures are caused by any factor that can disturb brain function. Seizures and epilepsy are often classified as symptomatic (the cause is strongly identified or presumed) or idiopathic (the cause is unknown, or genetic influences are strongly etiologic). The younger the infant or child, the more likely the cause can be identified. Idiopathic or genetic epilepsy most often appears from ages 4–16. A seizure disorder or epilepsy should not be considered idiopathic unless a searching history, examination, and appropriate laboratory tests have turned up no apparent cause.

Clinical Findings

A. Symptoms and Signs: The key to the diagnosis of epilepsy is, of course, the history. The initial symptom often identifies the aura to the seizure itself. A feeling of fear, numbness or tingling in the fingers, or bright lights in one visual field might be examples of an aura (really the onset of a seizure). Sometimes the patient recalls nothing; there has been no aura or warning. The parent might report that the youngster's eyes went off to one side or that extreme pallor, trismus, or overall body stiffening occurred first. Occasionally there is a prodrome to the seizure, eg, a feeling of unwellness, a feeling of something about to happen, or a recurrent thought that occurred over minutes or hours prior to the aura and seizure itself.

Minute details of the seizure can help determine the site of onset and aid in classification of the seizure. Did the patient become extremely pale before falling? Was the patient able to respond to queries during the episode? Did the patient become completely unconscious? Did the patient fall stiffly or gradually slump to the floor? Was there an injury? How long did the stiffening or jerking last? Where were the sites of jerking?

Events after the seizure can be helpful in diagnosis. Was there loss of speech? Was the patient able to respond accurately prior to going to sleep?

All these events prior to, during, and after the seizure can help to classify the seizure and, indeed, may help to determine if the event actually was a probable epileptic seizure or a pseudoseizure, ie, a nonepileptic phenomenon mimicking a seizure. Classifying the seizure type may aid in diagnosis and prognosis and suggest desirable or necessary laboratory tests and medication choices. (See Table 24–10 and Table 24–11.)

B. Status Epilepticus: Status epilepticus is a clinical or electrical seizure lasting at least 30 min-utes or a series of seizures without complete recovery over the same period of time. After 30 minutes, the brain begins to suffer from hypoxia and acidosis, with depletion of local energy stores, cerebral edema, and structural damage. Eventually, high fever, hypotension, respiratory depression, and even death may occur. Thus, status epilepticus is a relative medical emergency.

Status epilepticus is classified as (1) convulsive, ie, the common tonic-clonic, or "grand mal" status epilepticus or (2) nonconvulsive, eg, simple motor status without loss of consciousness. Other nonconvulsive types include absence status, or "spike-wave stupor," and (very rare) partial complex status epilepticus.

An EEG may be necessary to aid in diagnosing the less common variants, such as a patient with known absence who now is in a partially-in-contact, stuporous state.

Table 24–10. Clinical seizure correlation with electroencephalographic patterns.[1]

Clinical Seizure Type	EEG Ictal	EEG Interictal
Focal Simple partial ("focal") Motor Sensory	Local contralateral discharge (spike, slow wave, etc)	Same
Complex partial ("psychomotor")	Focal or bilateral frontal, temporal discharge	T-F local or asynchronous discharge
Partial seizures with generalization	Above discharges become lateralized	
Generalized Absence ("petit mal") Simple (impairment of consciousness only) Complex (with tonic, clonic, autonomic component)	3/sec spike wave	Normal
Atypical absence	Irregular 1–4/sec spike-wave	Abnormal, often slow spike-wave, asymmetric
Myoclonic seizures	Multiple spike-wave	Same
Tonic-clonic ("grand mal")	10/sec spike/ slowing, then spike/slow wave	Multiple spikes, spike-wave sharp, slow
Atonic (astatic, akinetic)	Multiple spike-wave	Same

[1]According to the International Classification of Epileptic Seizures. Some subtypes are not listed. Some age-limited syndromes occurring in childhood are not easily incorporated into this scheme.

A child with status epilepticus often has a high fever with or without intracranial infection, eg, viral encephalitis or bacterial meningitis. Status epilepticus may be the youngster's initial seizure; various studies show that one-fourth to three-fourths of children experience status epilepticus as the initial seizure. Often, it is a reflection of a remote insult (for example, anoxic or traumatic). Tumor, vascular disease (strokes), or head trauma, which are common causes of status epilepticus in adults, are uncommon causes in childhood. One-half of cases are symptomatic of acute (25%) or chronic (25%) CNS disorders. Infection or metabolic disorders are the most common symptomatic causes in children. The cause is unknown in half of cases, but many of these will be febrile.

Status epilepticus is more common in children less than one year of age, with 37% of cases occurring under that age and 85% under the age of five. Thus, the pediatrician sees status epilepticus most commonly in infants and preschoolers. For treatment, see Table 24–12.

C. Febrile Seizures: Criteria for febrile seizures are (1) age of 3 months to 5 years (most occur between the ages of 6 months and 3 years), (2) fever of 38.8 °C (102 °F), and (3) non-CNS infection. Most (greater than 90%) are generalized and brief (less than 5 minutes) and occur early in an OMPA (otitis media, pharyngitis, adenitis) illness. Febrile seizures occur in 2–3% of children. Gastroenteritis, especially due to *Shigella* or *Campylobacter,* and urinary tract infections are less common causes. Roseola infantum is a rare but classic cause. One study implicated viral causes in 86% of cases. Immunizations may be a cause.

Rarely, status epilepticus may occur: fever is a common cause of status epilepticus in early childhood. Febrile seizures rarely (2–4%) lead to epilepsy or recurrent nonfebrile seizures in later childhood and adult life. The chance of later epilepsy is higher if the febrile seizures have complex features, eg, a duration of greater than 15 minutes, more than one seizure in the same day, or focal features. Other adverse factors are an abnormal neurologic status preceding the seizures (eg, cerebral palsy or mental retardation), early onset of febrile seizure (before one year of age), and a family history of epilepsy. Even with adverse factors, the risk of epilepsy in later life is low, in the range of 15–20%.

Recurrent febrile seizures occur in 20–40% of cases but, in general, do not worsen the long-term outlook.

The child with a febrile seizure must be examined. Routine studies such as electrolytes, glucose, calcium, skull x-rays, or brain imaging studies are seldom helpful. A white count above 20,000 or with extreme left shift may correlate with bacteremia; a complete blood count and blood cultures may be appropriate studies. Serum sodium is often slightly low but not low enough to require treatment or to cause the seizure. *Meningitis must be ruled out.* Bacterial meningitis can present with a fever and seizure. Signs of meningitis (eg, bulging fontanelle, stiff neck, stupor, and irritability) may all be absent, especially in a child under 18 months.

After controlling the fever and stopping an ongoing seizure, the physician must decide whether to do a spinal tap. The fact that the child has had a previous febrile seizure does not rule out meningitis as the cause of the current episode. The younger the child, the more important the tap as the less reliable are physical findings in diagnosing meningitis. Although the yield is low, a tap should probably be done if the child is under age 2, if recovery is slow, if no other cause for the fever is found, or if close follow-up will not be possible. Occasionally, observation in the emergency room for several hours obviates the need for a tap. A negative tap does not rule out the emergence of meningitis during the same febrile illness; sometimes a second tap needs to be done.

Treatment after the seizure is problematic. Many clinicians choose to treat the child with a maintenance dosage of anticonvulsant medication during the course of that febrile illness. Diazepam (Valium), 0.5 mg/kg 2–3 times per day orally or rectally, has been used in Europe and Japan with success both for prophylaxis and for prevention of subsequent seizures. (Suppositories aren't currently available in the United States.) Phenobarbital and valproate sodium are other possible choices; however, the somnolence due to the phenobarbital load (about 5–10 mg/kilo) is often discomforting to both the doctor and parent and sometimes confuses follow-up assessments. Valproic acid has more dangers and should be avoided in a patient with vomiting or acidosis.

Most clinicians choose to follow the youngster without administering anticonvulsant medication. Measures to control fever (sponging, antipyretics, and appropriate antibiotics if a bacterial illness is suspected or found) are the major treatment. The family can be reassured that simple febrile seizures are not thought to have any long-term adverse consequences. An EEG should be ordered if the febrile seizure is complicated or unusual; in the uncomplicated febrile seizure, the EEG is most often normal. About 10% will have slowing or other occipital abnormalities. Ideally, the study should be done at least a week after the illness to avoid transient findings due to the fever or seizure itself. In older children, 3-second spike-wave discharge, suggestive of a genetic propensity to epilepsy, may occur. In the young infant, EEG findings seldom aid in predicting the chance of recurrence of febrile or nonfebrile seizures.

Prophylactic anticonvulsants are not indicated in the uncomplicated febrile seizure patient. If febrile seizures are complicated or prolonged or if medical reassurance fails to relieve family anxiety, anticon-

Table 24–11. Seizures by age at onset, pattern, and preferred treatment.

Age Group and Seizure Type	Age at Onset	Clinical Manifestations	Causative Factors	Electroencephalographic Pattern	Other Diagnostic Studies	Treatment and Comments (Anticonvulsants by Order of Choice)[2]
Neonatal Seizures	Birth to 2 weeks	Often "atypical"; sudden limpness or tonic posturing, brief apnea, and cyanosis; odd cry; eyes "rolling up"; blinking or mouthing or chewing movements; nystagmus, twitchiness or clonic movements—focal, multifocal or generalized.	Neurologic insults (hypoxia/ischemia; intracranial hemorrhage) present more in first 3 days or after eighth day; metabolic disturbances alone between third and eighth days: hypoglycemia, hypocalcemia, hypermia and hyponatremia. Drug withdrawal. Pyridoxine deficiency and other metabolic causes. CNS infections and snuctural abnormalities.	May correlate poorly with clinical seizures. Focal spikes or slow rhythms; multifocal discharges.	Lumbar puncture; serum Ca^{2+} $PO_4{}^{3-}$, glucose, Mg^{2+}, BUN, amino acid screen, blood ammonia, organic acid screen, TORCHES[1] screen. Ultrasound or CT scan for suspected intracranial hemorrhage and structural abnormalities.	Phenobarbital, IV or IM; if seizures not controlled, add phenytoin IV (loading dose 20 mg/kg each). Diazepam, approximately 0.2 mg/kg. Treat underlying disorder. Seizures due to brain damage often resistant to anticonvulsants. When cause in doubt, stop protein feedings until enzyme deficiencies of urea cycle or amino metabolism ruled out.
West's syndrome: "infantile spasms." (See also Lennox-Gastaut syndrome, below.)	3–18 months; occasionally up to 4 years	Sudden, usually symmetric adduction and flexion of limbs with concomitant flexion of head and trunk; also abduction and extensor movements like Moro reflex. Tendency for spasms to occur in clusters, on waking or falling asleep, or when fatigued, or may be noted particularly when the infant is being handled, is ill, or is otherwise irritable. Tendency for each patient to have own stereotyped pattern.	Pre- or perinatal brain damage or malformation in approximately one-third; biochemical, infectious, degenerative causes in approximately one-third; unknown in approximately one-third. With early onset, pyridoxine deficiency, amino- or organic aciduria. Tuberous sclerosis in 5–10%. Chronic inflammatory disease and toxoplasmosis. Aicardi syndrome (females with mental retardation, agenesis of corpus callosum, ocular and vertebral anomalies).	Hypsarrhythmia; chaotic highvoltage slow waves, random spikes, all leads (90%); other abnormalities in rest. Rarely "normal." EEG normalization usually correlates with reduction of seizures; not helpful prognostically regarding mental development.	Funduscopic and skin examination, trial of pyridoxine. Amino- and organic acid screen. Chronic inflammatory disease. TORCHES[1] screen. CT or MRI scan shall be done to (1) establish definite diagnosis, (2) aid in genetic counseling.	Corticotropin preferred (2–4 units/kg/d IM Acthar gel 1/d, then slow withdrawal). Some prefer oral corticosteroids. Diazepam, clonazepam, valproic acid. In resistant cases, ketogenic or medium-chain triglyceride (MCT) diet (see text). Retardation of varying degree in approximately 90% of cases.
Febrile convulsions	3 months to 5 years	Usually generalized seizures, less than 15 minutes; rarely focal in onset. May lead to status epilepticus.	Nonneurologic febrile illness (temperature rises to 102.5 °F or higher); family history frequently positive for febrile convulsions.	Normal interictal EEG, especially when obtained 8–10 days after seizure. In older infants, 3/s spikes often seen.	In infants or whenever suspicion of meningitis exists, perform lumbar puncture.	Treat underlying illness, fever. Diazepam orally or rectally as needed 0.3–0.5 mg/kg 3 times daily during illness. Prophylaxis with phenobarbital (valproic acid if phenobarbital not tolerated), with neurologic deficits, prolonged seizure, family history of epilepsy.
Myoclonic-astatic (akinetic, atonic) seizures, formerly atypical absence. With mental retardation. Lennox-Gastaut syndrome.	Any time in childhood; normally 2–7 years	Shocklike violent contractions of one or more muscle groups, singly or irregularly repetitive; may fling patient suddenly to side, forward, or backward. Usually no or only brief loss of consciousness. Half of patients or more also have generalized grand mal seizures.	Multiple causes, usually resulting in diffuse neuronal damage. History of West's syndrome; prenatal or perinatal brain damage: viral meningoencephalitides; subacute sclerosing panencephalitis; CNS degenerative disorders; lead or other encephalopathies; structural cerebral abnormalities, eg, porencephaly.	Atypical slow (1–2.5 Hz) spikewave complexes ("petit mal variant") and bursts of highvoltage generalized spikes, often with diffusely slow background frequencies. See text.	As dictated by index of suspicion. Lumbar puncture with measles antibody titer and CSF IgG index. Nerve conduction studies. Urine for lead, arylsulfatase A, etc. Skin biopsy for electron microscopy and enzyme studies. CT scan and brain biopsy may be justified.	Difficult to treat. Valproic acid, clonazepam, or ethosuximide. Imipramine as adjunct. Diazepam. Ketogenic or mediumchain triglyceride (MCT) diet. ACTH or corticosteroids as in West's syndrome. Protect head with helmet and chin padding.
Absence ("petit mal"). Also juvenile and myoclonic absence.	3–15 years	Lapses of consciousness or vacant stares, lasting about 10 seconds, often in "clusters." Automatisms of face and hands; clonic activity in 30–45%. Often confused with complex partial seizures but no aura or postictal confusion.	Unknown. Genetic component: probably an autosomal dominant gene	Three-second bilaterally synchronous, symmetric, highvoltage spikes and waves. EEG "normalization" correlates closely with control of seizures.	Hyperventilation when patient on inadequate or no medication often provokes attacks. CT scan is rarely of value.	Valproic acid or ethosuximide; with latter, add phenobarbital if EEG suggests other abnormalities (grand mal). In resistant cases, ketogenic or MCT diet. Also, in resistant cases, valproic acid and ethosuximide together.

Table 24–11 (cont'd). Seizures by age at onset, pattern, and preferred treatment.

Age Group and Seizure Type	Age at Onset	Clinical Manifestations	Causative Factors	Electroencephalographic Pattern	Other Diagnostic Studies	Treatment and Comments (Anticonvulsants by Order of Choice)[2]
Simple partial or focal seizures (motor/sensory/jacksonian). (Complex partial or psychomotor seizures, below.)	Any age	Seizure may involve any part of body; may spread in fixed pattern (jacksonian march), becoming generalized. In children, epileptogenic focus often "shifts," and epileptic manifestations may change concomitantly.	Often secondary to birth trauma, inflammatory process, vascular accidents, meningoencephalitis, etc. If seizures are coupled with new or progressive neurologic deficits, a structural lesion (eg, brain tumor) is likely.	Focal spikes or slow waves in appropriate cortical region; sometimes diffusely abnormal or even normal.	If seizures are difficult to control or progressive deficits occur, neuroradiodiagnostic studies, particularly CT brain scan, imperative (see text).	Carbamazepine, phenytoin, phenobarbital or primidone. Valproic acid useful adjunct.
Complex partial seizures (psychomotor, temporal lobe, or limbic seizures).	Any age	Aura may be a sensation of fear, epigastric discomfort, odd smell or taste (usually unpleasant), visual or auditory hallucination (either vague and "unformed" or well-formed image, words, music). Aura and seizure stereotyped for each patient. Seizure may consist of vague stare; facial tongue, or swallowing movements and throaty sounds; or various complex automatisms. Unlike absences, complex partial seizures tend not to occur in clusters but singly and to last longer (1 minute or more), followed by confusion. History of aura (or child running to adult from "vague fear") and of automatisms involving more than face and hands establishes diagnosis. About 60% also develop generalized grand mal seizures.	As above. Temporal lobes especially sensitive to hypoxia; thus, this seizure type may be sequela of birth trauma, febrile convulsions, etc. Also especially vulnerable to certain viral infections, especially herpes simplex. Remediable other causes are small cryptic tumors or vascular malformations.	As above, but occurring in temporal lobe and its connections, eg. frontotemporal, temporoparietal, temporo-occipital regions.	CT scan when structural lesions suspected. Temporal lobe biopsy when herpes simplex encephalitis suspected. Carotid amobarbital injection when lateralization of speech dominance in question.	Carbamazepine, phenytoin, phenobarbital, or primidone. More than one drug may be necessary. Valproic acid may be useful. Phenacemide in seizures difficult to control. In cases uncontrolled by drugs and where a primary epileptogenic focus is identifiable, excision of anterior third of temporal lobe. Adjunctive psychotherapy required frequently.
"Benign epilepsy of childhood" (with "centrotemporal" or "rolandic" foci).	5–16 years	Partial motor or generalized seizures. Similar seizure patterns may be observed in patients with focal cortical lesions.	Seizure history of abnormal EEG findings in relatives of 40% of affected probands and 18–20% of parents and siblings, suggesting transmission by a single autosomal dominant gene, possibly with age-dependent penetrance.	Centrotemporal spikes or sharp waves ("rolandic discharges") appearing paroxysmally against a normal EEG background.	Serum Ca^{2+} and glucose, BUN, urinalysis. Seldom need CT scan.	Carbamazepine or phenytoin. Primidone or phenobarbital.
Juvenile myoclonic epilepsy (of Janz).	Late childhood and adolescence, peaking at 13 years	Mild myoclonic jerks of neck and shoulder flexor muscles after waking up ("awakening" grand mal seizures). Intelligence usually normal.	40% of relatives have myoclonias, especially in females; 15% have the abnormal EEG pattern without clinical attacks.	Interictal EEG shows fast variety of spike-and-wave sequences or 4-to 6-Hz multi-spike-and wave complexes.	Differentiate from progressive myoclonic encephalopathy of Unverricht-Lafora and other degenerative disorders by appropriate biopsies (muscle, liver, etc).	Valproic acid.
Generalized tonic-clonic seizures (grand mal).	Any age	Loss of consciousness; tonic-clonic movements, often preceded by vague aura or cry. Bladder and bowel incontinence in approximately 15%. Postictal confusion; sleep. Often mixed with or masking other seizure patterns.	Often unknown. Genetic component. May be seen with metabolic disturbances, trauma, infection, intoxication, degenerative disorders, brain tumors, etc.	Bilaterally synchronous, symmetric multiple high-voltage spikes, spikes and waves, mixed patterns. Often normal under age 4.	As above.	Phenobarbital in first 12 months; carbamazepine or valproic acid; phenytoin; primidone. Combinations may be necessary.

[1]TORCHES is a mnemonic formula for *toxoplasmosis, rubella, cytomegalovirus, herpes simplex,* and *syphilis.*

Table 24–12. Status epilepticus treatment.

1. ABCs
   a. Airway: maintain oral airway; intubation may be necessary.
   b. Breathing: Oxygen by mouth (if available).
   c. Circulation: Assess pulse, blood pressure; support with IV fluids, drugs. Monitor vital signs.
2. Start glucose-containing IV; draw Dextrostix/blood glucose; evaluate electrolytes, HCO_3, CBC, BUN, anticonvulsant levels.
3. Arterial blood gases, pH.
4. Give 50% glucose if dextrose low (1–2 mL/kg).
5. Begin IV drug therapy; goal is to control status in 20–60 minutes.
   a. Diazepam 0.1–0.3 mg/kg over 1–5 minutes (20 mg maximum); may repeat in 5–20 minutes (short action: 20 minutes; watch for respiratory depression). *or,* lorazepam 0.05–0.2 mg/kg, less effective with repeated doses. Longer-acting than diazepam; midazolam hydrochloride; ICU use only. IM, IV; intubation desirable.
   b. Phenytoin 10–20 mg/kg over 5–20 minutes (*not* IM) (1000 mg maximum); monitor with blood pressure and ECG if available.
   c. Phenobarbital 5–20 mg/kg (sometimes higher for newborns, refractory status in intubated patients in hospital and with monitored blood levels.
6. Correct metabolic perturbations (eg, low Na acidosis).
7. Other drug approaches in refractory status:
   a. Repeat phenytoin, phenobarbital (5 mg/kg); monitor blood levels. Support respiration, BP as necessary.
   b. IV paraldehyde 4% solution or rectal paraldehyde 0.1–0.3 mL/kg diluted 1:1 in olive oil.
   c. Valproic acid suspension 50 mg/mL diluted 1:1, 30–60 mg/kg orally or rectally.
8. General anesthetic.
9. Consider underlying causes:
   a. Structural disorders or trauma (even nonaccidental trauma). Consider CT scan.
   b. Infection: Spinal tap, blood culture, antibiotics.
   c. Metabolic disorders: Lactic acidosis, toxins uremia. May need HCO_3, medication, toxin screen, judicious fluid administration.
10. Give maintenance drug (if diazepam only was sufficient to halt status epilepticus): phenytoin 10 mg/kg, phenobarbital 5–10 mg/kg, etc.

vulsant prophylaxis may be indicated and can reduce the incidence of recurrent febrile or nonfebrile seizures. One remedy is to use diazepam (Valium) at the first onset of fever for the duration of the febrile illness as noted above. Phenobarbital, 3–5 mg/kg/d as a single bedtime dose, is an inexpensive and safe option. Often, increasing the dose gradually (for example, starting with 2 mg/kg/d the first week, 3 mg/kg/d the second week, etc) decreases side effects and noncompliance. A phenobarbital level in the 15–40 μg/mL range is desirable.

Valproate sodium, the other medication that has been used with success, is more hazardous. In infants, liquid suspension is often necessary but has a short half-life and causes more gastrointestinal upset than the coated capsules used in older children. The dose is 15–60 mg/kg/d divided in 3 or 4 doses. Precautionary laboratory studies are necessary.

Diphenylhydantoin and carbamazepine have not shown effectiveness in the prophylaxis of febrile seizures.

D. Laboratory Findings and Imaging: Ordering of laboratory tests depends on the age of the child, the severity and type of the seizure, whether the child is ill or injured, and the clinician's suspicion of underlying cause. Every case of suspected seizure disorder warrants an electroencephalogram. Other studies are used selectively. Seizures in early infancy are often symptomatic. Therefore, the younger the child, the more careful the laboratory assessment (see Table 24–13).

Metabolic abnormalities are seldom found in the well child with seizures; unless there is high clinical suspicion of uremia, hyponatremia, etc, it is unnecessary to order laboratory tests. Special studies may be necessary in unusual circumstances, eg, if hemolytic-uremic syndrome or lead poisoning, is a suspected cause. CT scans are overused in patients with seizures. The youngster with a routine febrile seizure, a nonfebrile generalized seizure with normal examination and normal EEG, or an absence seizure does not need a CT scan or MRI scan. The yield in a child with normal neurologic examination and EEG is less than 5%. Conversely, in children with symptomatic epileptic syndromes, the yield of positive results is as high as 60–80%. Examples include infantile spasms, Lennox-Gastaut syndrome, or progressive myoclonic epilepsy syndromes.

In focal seizures, children with benign rolandic epilepsy do not need a CT scan; it will invariably be normal. The yield on other focal seizures is 15–30%, with most of the findings unimportant in relation to

Table 24–13. Laboratory studies in first seizure of epilepsy (nonneonatal).

Well infant: EEG. Calcium, BUN, or urinalysis, and perhaps CT or MRI (abnormal examination or focally abnormal EEG may prompt an imaging study).
Well older child: EEG. Consider CT or MRI.
Ill infant: Calcium, magnesium, CBC, BUN, electrolytes, blood culture, lumbar puncture (LP) EEG, possibly CT or MRI.
Ill older child: CBC, BUN, LP, EEG, CT, or MRI.
Generalized tonic-clonic seizure: As above.
Generalized absence: EEG only.
Atypical absence: EEG, CT, MRI: consider studies for mental retardation: serum and urine amino and organic acids, and chromosomes, including fragile X. If there is progressive worsening, consider lysosomal enzymes, LP (protein, enzymes, IgG), perhaps long-chain fatty acids, skin/conjunctival biopsies.
Infantile spasms: See atypical absence.
Myoclonic, progressive seizure with mental retardation: See atypical absence.
Focal: EEG. In cases of mental retardation, positive neurologic examination, EEG focal slow wave, or poorly controlled seizures, do CT or MRI. In refractory cases, consider surgical evaluation.

diagnosis and prognosis (eg, a mildly dilatated single ventricle, superficial atrophy, etc). Nonetheless, an imaging study eases anxiety and rules out the remote possibility of tumor or vascular malformation. Other indications for CT scan or MRI include difficulty in controlling seizures, progressive neurologic findings on serial exams, worsening focal findings on the EEG, suspicion of increased pressure, and, of course, any case in which surgery is being considered. A previous normal scan does not rule out an emerging tumor; if the course is unsatisfactory, repeating the scan may be necessary. A neoplasm or other unexpected treatable lesion is found in a small number, perhaps 2–3%, of CT scans.

E. Electroencephalography: The limitations of electroencephalography, even in epilepsy where it is most useful, are considerable. *A seizure is a clinical phenomenon;* an EEG showing epileptiform activity may confirm and even extend the clinical diagnosis, but it cannot make it.

The EEG need not be abnormal in the presence of a definite seizure disorder. Normal EEGs are seen following a first generalized seizure in one-third of children under 4 years of age; the initial EEG is normal in about 20% of older epileptic children and in around 10% of adults with epilepsy. These percentages are reduced when serial tracings are obtained but never completely eliminated. On the other hand, various grades of "dysrhythmias" are frequently observed in children; focal spikes and generalized spike-wave discharges are seen in 30% of close nonepileptic relatives of patients with centrencephalic epilepsy.

1. Diagnostic value—The greatest value of the EEG in convulsive disorders is in helping to classify seizure types and thus to select appropriate therapy (Table 24–10). Petit mal absences and partial complex or psychomotor seizures are sometimes difficult to distinguish, especially when the physician must rely on the history and cannot observe one; their differing electroencephalographic patterns will then prove most helpful. Another rather frequent illustration of the role of the EEG in guiding therapy is the finding of mixed seizure patterns in a child who clinically has only grand mal or only petit mal absences, since some anticonvulsants efficacious for one seizure type may provoke the other. The EEG may often help in diagnosing neonatal seizures with minimal and "atypical" clinical manifestations; it may show "hypsarrhythmia" in infantile spasms or the pattern associated with the Lennox-Gastaut syndrome, both expressions of diffuse brain dysfunctioning of multiple causes and generally of grave significance. The EEG may help differentiate "convulsive equivalents" from somatic complaints of psychogenic origin.

The EEG may show focal slowing that, if constant—particularly when there are corresponding focal seizure manifestations and abnormal neurologic findings—will alert the physician to the presence of a structural lesion, in which case brain imaging may establish the cause and help determine further investigation and treatment.

2. Prognostic value—A normal EEG following a first convulsion suggests (but does not guarantee) a favorable prognosis. Markedly abnormal EEGs may become normal with treatment (1) immediately following intravenous injection of 50 mg vitamin B$_6$ in pyridoxine dependency or deficiency; (2) in infantile spasms and sometimes the Lennox-Gastaut syndrome (corticotropin or corticosteroids); (3) in petit mal absences (anticonvulsants); and (4) in petit mal and other minor motor seizures, including the Lennox-Gastaut syndrome (ketogenic diet). If so, it is likely that seizure control will be achieved (although this offers no clues to the mental status of the patient).

Electroencephalography should be repeated when there is an increase in the severity and frequency of seizures despite exhaustive and adequate anticonvulsant therapy; when there is a significant change in the clinical seizure pattern; or when there are progressive neurologic deficits. Focal or diffuse slowing may indicate a progressive lesion.

The EEG may be quite helpful in determining when to discontinue anticonvulsant therapy. The presence or absence of epileptiform activity on the EEG prior to withdrawal of anticonvulsants after a seizure-free period of several years on the medications has been shown to be correlated with the degree of risk of recurrence of seizures.

Differential Diagnosis

It is extremely important that a nonepileptic condition be accurately labeled. To the lay person, epilepsy often has connotations of brain damage and limitation of activity; a person so diagnosed may be precluded from certain occupations in later life. It is often very difficult to change an inaccurate diagnosis of many years' standing.

Some of the common nonepileptic events that mimic seizure disorder are listed in Table 24–14.

Complications

Emotional disturbances—notably anxiety, depression, anger, feelings of guilt and inadequacy—often occur as a reaction to the seizures in the parents of the affected child as well as in the child old enough to understand. The seizures—and particularly the hallucinatory auras and psychomotor attacks—frequently set off in the prepubescent and adolescent youngster fantasies (and sometimes obsessive ruminations) about dying and death that may become so strong that they lead to suicidal behavior and suicidal attempts. The limitations many school systems place on epileptic children add to the problem. Commonly, the child expresses feelings by "acting out."

Table 24–14. Nonepileptic paroxysmal events.

Breath-holding Attacks: Age 6 months to 3 years. Always precipitated by trauma and fright. Cyanosis; sometimes stiffening, tonic (or jerking-clonic), convulsion (anoxic seizure). Patient may sleep following attack. Family history positive in 30%. EEG is normal. Treatment is interpretation and reassurance.

Infantile syncope (pallid breath holding): No external precipitant (perhaps internal pain, cramp, or fear?). Pallor may be followed by seizure (anoxic/ischemic). Vagally (heart-slowing) mediated, like adult syncope. EEG normal; may get cardiac slowing with vagal stimulation (eyeball pressure, cold cloth on face) during EEG.

Tics or Tourette's syndrome: Simple or complex stereotyped (the same time after time) jerks or movements, coughs, grunts, sniffs. Worse at repose or with stress. May be suppressed during physician visit. Family history often positive. EEG negative. Nonanticonvulsant drugs may benefit.

Night terrors, Sleep talking, walking, "sit-ups": Age 3–10. Usually occur in first sleep cycle (30–90 minutes after going to sleep), with crying, screaming, and "autonomic discharge" (pupils dilatated, perspiring, etc). Lasts minutes. Child goes back to sleep and has no recall of event the next day. Sleep studies (polysomnogram and EEG) are normal. Disappears with maturation. Sleep talking and walking and short "sit-ups" in bed are fragmentary arousals. If a spell is recorded, EEG shows arousal from deep sleep, but the behavior seems wakeful. The youngster needs to be protected from injury and gradually settled down and taken back to bed.

Nightmares: Nightmares or vivid dreams occur in subsequent cycles of sleep, often in the early morning hours, and generally are partially recalled the next day. The bizarre and frightening behavior may sometimes be confused with complex partial seizures. These occur during REM (rapid eye movement) sleep; epilepsy usually does not occur during that phase of sleep. In extreme or difficult cases, an all-night sleep EEG may help to differentiate seizures from nightmares.

Migraine: One variant of migraine can be associated with an acute confusional state. There may be the usual migraine prodrome with spots before the eyes, dizziness, visual field defects, and then agitated confusion. A history of other, more typical migraine with severe headache and vomiting but without confusion may aid in the diagnosis. The severe headache with vomiting as the youngster comes out of the migraine may aid in distinguishing the attack from epilepsy. Other seizure manifestations are practically never seen, eg, tonic-clonic movements, falling, and complete loss of consciousness. The EEG in migraine is usually normal and seldom has epileptiform abnormalities often seen in patients with epilepsy. Lastly, migraine and epilepsy are sometimes linked: migraine-caused ischemia on the brain surface sometimes leads to later epilepsy.

Syncope: Syncope often has a precipitant. The patient may remember feeling dizzy, lightheaded, and nauseated or ill, and sensing the room going dark. Observers will often notice extreme pallor at the onset. The fall is often but not necessarily gradual; injury may occur. Heart rate is often very slow. Patient may often have memory of beginning to fall. Occasionally, a tonic or tonic-clonic seizure due to anoxia may occur, especially if the patient is held upright and circulation to the head not restored. An EEG is invariably normal. The family history is often positive for syncope.

Shuddering: Shuddering or shivering attacks can occur in infancy and be a forerunner of essential tremor in later life. Often, the family history is positive for tremor. The shivering may be very frequent. EEG is normal. There is no clouding or loss of consciousness.

Gastroesophageal reflux: Seen more commonly in children with cerebral palsy or brain damage, reflux of acid gastric contents may cause pain that cannot be described by the child. At times, there may be unusual posturings (dystonic or other) of the head and neck or trunk, an apparent attempt to stretch the esophagus or close the opening. There is no loss of consciousness, but there may be eye rolling, apnea, occasional vomiting that may simulate a seizure. Appropriate circumstances and upper GI series, cine of swallowing, sometimes even an EEG (which is always normal) may be necessary to distinguish this from seizures.

Masturbation: Rarely in infants, repetitive rocking or rubbing motions may simulate seizures. The youngster may look out of contact, be poorly responsive to the environment, and have autonomic expressions (eg, perspiration, dilatated pupils) that may be confused with seizures. Observation by a skilled individual, sometimes even in a hospital situation, may be necessary to distinguish this from seizures. EEG is of course normal between or during attacks. Interpretation and reassurance are the only necessary treatment.

Conversion reaction/pseudoseizures: As many as 50% of patients with pseudoseizures are epileptic. The episodes may be writhing, intercourselike movements, tonic episodes, bizarre jerking and thrashing around, or even apparently sudden unresponsiveness. Often, there is ongoing psychological trauma. Often, but not invariably, the patients are developmentally delayed. The spells must often be seen or recorded on videotape in a controlled situation to distinguish them from epilepsy. A normal EEG during a spell is a key diagnostic feature. Often the spells are so bizarre that they are easily distinguished. Sometimes, pseudoseizures can be precipitated by suggestion with injection of normal saline in a controlled situation. Combativeness is common, self-injury and incontinence rare.

Temper tantrums and rage attacks: These are sometimes confused with epilepsy. The youngster is often amnesic or at least claim amnesia for events during the spell. The attacks are usually precipitated by frustration or anger and are often directed either verbally or physically and subside with behavior modification and isolation. EEGs are generally normal but unfortunately seldom obtained during an attack. Anterior temporal leads may be helpful in ruling out temporal or lateral frontal abnormalities, the latter sometimes seen in partial complex seizures. Improvement of the attacks with psychotherapy, milieu therapy, or behavioral modification helps rule out epilepsy.

Benign paroxysmal vertigo: These are brief attacks of vertigo in which the youngster often appears frightened and pale and clutches the parent. The attacks last 5–30 seconds. Sometimes, nystagmus is identified. There is no loss of consciousness. Usually, the child is well and returns to play immediately afterward. The attacks may occur in clusters, then disappear for months. Attacks are usually seen in infants and preschoolers aged 2–5. EEG is normal. If caloric tests can be obtained (often very difficult in this age group), abnormalities with hypofunction of one side are sometimes seen. Medications are usually not desirable or necessary.

Staring spells: Teachers often make referral for absence or petit mal seizures in youngsters who stare or seem preoccupied at school. Helpful in the history is the lack of these spells at home, eg, in the early morning hours prior to breakfast, as might be seen with absence seizures. A lack of other epilepsy in the child or family history often is helpful. Sometimes, these children have difficulties with school and a cognitive or learning disability. The child can generally be brought out of this spell by a firm command. An EEG is sometimes necessary to confirm that absence seizures are not occurring. A 24-hour ambulatory EEG to record attacks during the child's everyday school activities is occasionally necessary.

Pseudoretardation may occur in poorly controlled epileptic children because their seizures—or the subclinical paroxysms sustained—may interfere with their learning ability. Anticonvulsants are less likely to "slow the child down" but may do so when given in toxic amounts; phenobarbital is particularly implicated.

True mental retardation is most commonly part of the same pathologic process that causes the seizures but may occasionally occur when seizures are frequent, prolonged, and accompanied by hypoxia.

Physical injuries, especially lacerations of the forehead and chin, are frequent in astatic or akinetic seizures (drop attacks). In all other seizure disorders in childhood, injuries as a direct result of an attack are impressively rare.

Treatment

The ideal treatment of seizures is the correction of specific causes. However, even when a biochemical disorder (eg, leucine hypoglycemia), a tumor, or septic meningitis is being treated, anticonvulsant drugs are often still required.

A. Precautionary Management of Individual Brief Seizures: Protect the patient against self-injury and aspiration of vomitus. Beyond that, no specific therapy is necessary. The less done to the patient during a relatively brief seizure (up to 10 or 15 minutes), the better. Thrusting a spoon handle or tongue depressor into the clenched mouth of a convulsing patient or trying to restrain tonic-clonic movements may cause worse injuries than a bitten tongue or bruised limb. Mouth-to-mouth resuscitation is rarely (if ever) necessary.

B. General Management of the Young Epileptic:

1. Education—The patient and the parents must be helped to understand the problem of seizures and their management. Many children—some even as young as 3 years of age—are capable of cooperating with the physician in problems of seizure control.

All bottles containing antiepileptic drugs should bear a contents label. The parents should know the names and dosage of the anticonvulsants being administered.

Materials on epilepsy—including pamphlets (some in Spanish), monographs, films, and videotapes suitable for children and teenagers, parents, teachers, and medical professionals—may be purchased through the Epilepsy Foundation of America, Materials Service Center, 4351 Garden City Drive, Landover, MD 20785. The Foundation's local chapter and other community organizations are eager to provide guidance and other services. In many cities, there are support groups for older children and adolescents and for their parents and others concerned.

2. Privileges and precautions in daily life— Encourage normal living within reasonable bounds. Children should engage in physical activities appropriate to their age and social group. After seizure control is established, swimming is generally permissible with a "buddy system" or adequate lifeguard coverage. High diving and high climbing should not be permitted. Physical training and sports (other than "contact" sports) are usually to be welcomed rather than restricted. Driving is discussed below.

Loss of sleep should be avoided. Emotional disturbances may need therapy. Alcoholic intake, a serious problem usually beginning in adolescence, should be avoided, as it may precipitate seizures. Prompt attention should be given to infections. Further neurologic disturbances should be brought to the physician's attention promptly.

Although every effort should be made to control seizures, this must not interfere with a child's ability to function. Sometimes a child is better off having an occasional mild seizure than being so heavily sedated that function at home, in school, or at play is impaired. This often requires much art and fortitude on the part of the physician. Indeed, some pediatricians and pediatric neurologists, after discussion with the parents, are now *not* instituting anticonvulsant therapy after up to 3 nonfebrile convulsions in an otherwise neurologically intact child.

3. Driving—Driving becomes important to most youngsters at age 15 or 16. Restrictions vary from state to state; in most, a learner's permit or driver's license will be issued if the patient has been under a physician's care and free of seizures for at least 2 years, provided that the treatment or basic neurologic problem does not interfere with the ability to drive. A guide to this and other legal matters pertaining to persons with epilepsy is published by the Epilepsy Foundation of America, whose Legal Advocacy Department may be able to provide additional information (see reference below).

4. Pregnancy—In the pregnant teenager with epilepsy, the possibility of teratogenic effects of anticonvulsants, such as facial clefts (about 5%), must be weighed against the risks from seizures. Such malformations occur in the infants of about 2.5% of untreated epileptic mothers.

C. Principles of Anticonvulsant Therapy:

1. Treat with the drug appropriate to the clinical situation, as outlined in Table 24–15.

2. Start with one drug in conventional dosage, and increase the dosage until seizures are controlled. If seizures are not controlled on the tolerated maximal dosage of one major anticonvulsant, gradually switch over to another before adding a second anticonvulsant. The dosages and usually effective blood levels listed in Table 24–14 are guides. Individual variations must be expected. The "therapeutic range" may also vary somewhat with the method used to determine levels. *Note:* Blood levels of antiepileptic drugs are discussed below.

3. Advise the parents and the patient that the pro-

Table 24–15. Guide to pediatric anticonvulsant drug therapy.

Drug	Average Total (mg/kg/d)	in	Divided Doses	Steady State: Days	Effective Blood Levels (μg/mL)[1]	Side Effects and Precautions[2]	Usage and Remarks
Primary anticonvulsant							
Carbamazepine (Tegretol)	15–25	:	2–4	3–6	4–12 (> 15)	Thrombocytopenia, leukopenia, rash. Rare: hepatotoxicity; bone marrow depression; dystonia; inappropriate ADH secretion; bizarre behaviors; tics.	Monitor CBC, platelet count, liver functions first 6 months closely; then periodically. Blood effects usually early and transient.
Valproic acid (Depakene, Depakote)	15–60[2]	:	2–4	2–4	50–120 (> 140)	Few side effects. Occasional gastric discomfort, constipation. Rare: hepatotoxicity; hyperammonemia, leukopenia. Tremor, hair loss in 5%.	For prophylaxis in febrile convulsion, see text. Monitor CBC, platelets, liver functions first 6 months closely; then periodically. Can be given rectally (suspension: 250 mg/5 mL).
Phenytoin (Dilantin)	5–10	:	1–2	5–10	5–20 (> 25)	Gum hypertrophy, hirsutism, ataxia, nystagmus, diplopia, rash, anorexia, nausea, osteomalacia. Severe toxicity may cause pseudodementia and liver damage. Rare: macrocytic anemia, lymph node involvement, exfoliative dermatitis, peripheral neuropathy.	Generally very effective and safe effect on behavior. Good dental hygiene reduces gum hyperplasia. May aggravate absence and myoclonic seizures. Consider supplemental vitamin D. Poorly absorbed by neonatal gut. Absorption after intramuscular injection erratic. Useful in neonatal seizures and status epilepticus. **Note:** Suspension not recommended.
Phenobarbital	3–8	:	1	10–21	15–40 (> 45)	Irritability and overactivity in many children; sedative effects in others. Mild ataxia, nystagmus, skin rash. Osteomalacia. May interfere with learning.	Safest overall drug. Bitter taste. Higher blood levels sometimes required and tolerated in severe chronic epileptics. Check linear growth periodically; obtain Ca²⁺ and bone films as indicated; consider supplemental vitamin D. Useful in neonatal seizures and status epilepticus.
Primidone (Mysoline)	10–25	:	3–4	1–5	4–12 (> 15)	Drowsiness, ataxia, vertigo, anorexia, nausea, vomiting, rash.	Start slowly with 25–35% of expected maintenance dose; increase every 2 days until full dose reached. Most useful when phenobarbital not tolerated. Suspension pleasant.
Ethosuximide (Zarontin)	10–40	:	1–2	5–6	40–100 (> 150)	Nausea, gastric discomfort. Rare: Bone marrow depression; hepatotoxicity, lupus.	May aggravate generalized seizures. Combine with valproic acid in refractory absence seizures.
Clonazepam (Clonopin)	0.1–0.2	:	2–3	5–10	15–80 ng/mL (> 80)	Drowsiness (> 50%): soporific effects greatest drawback. Behavior problems (25%). Slurred speech, ataxia, salivation.	Start slowly with 10–25% of expected maintenance dose; increase every 2–3 days. Very useful with difficult to treat minor motor seizures (astatic, myoclonic, infantile spasms; absences). Tolerance often occurs after a few months, but drug may be restarted after period of withdrawal.
Adjunctive or secondary drug							
Acetazolamide (Diamox)	5–20	:	2–3	(Not known)	...	Anorexia; numbness and tingling. Increase in urinary frequency; hence, do not give in evening.	Supplement to other medications, especially in absences and complex partial seizures. Also in females 4 days prior to and in the first 2–3 days of menstrual periods.
Methsuximide (Celontin)	15–30	:	3–4	(Not known)	10–40 (nomethsuximide)	Drowsiness, ataxia, headache, diplopia. Skin rash.	Useful in complex partial and myoclonic-astatic seizures.
Clorazepate (Tranxene)	0.3–1	:	2–3	(Not known)	0.2–1.5 (> 2)	Lethargy.	May be useful adjunct in generalized tonic-clonic, partial, and astatic seizures.

Table 24–15 (cont'd.). Guide to Pediatric anticonvulsant drug therapy.

Drug	Average Total (mg/kg/d)	in	Divided Doses	Steady State: Days	Effective Blood Levels (µg/mL)[1]	Side Effects and Precautions[2]	Usage and Remarks
Mephenytoin (Mesantoin)	4–15	:	2	(Not known)	5–25 (as ethylphenylhydantoin)	Mild: Rash, drowsiness, ataxia. *Warning:* Aplastic anemia, agranulocytosis.	A good anticonvulsant, especially in difficult to control complex partial, and possibly myoclonic-astatic, seizures. Fear of bone marrow depression limits its use. Monthly CBC.
Phenacemide (Phenurone)	25–50	:	2–4	(Not known)	...	Rash, anorexia, nausea. *Warning:* Hepatitis, psychosis, blood dyscrasias.	Especially effective in complex partial seizures when all other drugs fail. Frequent CBC, liver function tests initial 3–4 months, then 2–4/yr.
Diazepam (Valium)	0.20 ± 0.05	:	3	(Not known)	...	Somnolence.	Useful in myoclonic-astatic and absence seizures and infantile spasms. Often ineffective after a few months. First choice in status epilepticus, below.
Dextroamphetamine (Dexedrine)	0.25–0.75	:	Breakfast and noon	(Not known)	...	Nervousness, palpitations, anorexia, insomnia.	To counteract sedative effect of other drugs. Narcolepsy. In behavior disorders of younger children. Growth retardation with chronic use reversible.
Trimethadione (Tridione)	20–50	:	3–4	(Not known)	470–1200 (dimethadione)	Rash, photophobia, irritability. *Warning:* Leukopenia, agranulocytosis, nephrosis. LE phenomenon.	Useful primary in absences if ethosuximide and valproic acid fail. May aggravate generalized seizures; if so, add phenobarbital. Monthly CBC, urinalysis.
Mephobarbital (Mebaral)	4–10	:	1–2	(Not known)	15–40 (phenobarbital)	As with phenobarbital.	Twice the quantity of phenobarbital required for comparable effect.

Treatment of status epilepticus

Drug	Dose					Side Effects and Precautions	Usage and Remarks
Diazepam (Valium)	0.3 mg/kg IV initially. Repeat dose 0.1–0.3					Administer slowly IV. Monitor pulse and blood pressure. May cause respiratory depression in presence of phenobarbital.	May need to be repeated every 3–4 hours. Follow with phenytoin or phenobarbital for long-range control. *Note:* Administration IM for status epilepticus ineffective.
Lorazepam	0.05–0.2 mg/kg IV. May repeat.					Mild respiratory depression.	May be more effective than diazepam. Longer-acting.
Phenobarbital	5–20 mg/kg IV initially. Repeat dose 5 mg/kg IV.					See above.	Rule out pyridoxine deficiency. In neonatal seizures, load with 15–30 mg/kg IV (IM if IV impossible).
Phenytoin (Dilantin)	10–20 mg/kg IV initially. Repeat dose every 6–8 hours 2 or 3 times.					Administer IV over a 5-minute period. IM adsorption uncertain. Monitor blood levels.	Adjunct in neonatal seizures (20 mg/kg IV) if phenobarbital alone fails.
Paraldehyde	0.1–0.15 mL/kg IV; 0.2–0.3 mL/kg rectally.					Administer slowly IV mixed in saline; rectal dose in vegetable oil 1:1. Avoid in patient with pulmonary disease or in croupette.	Avoid IM administration if possible: may cause fat necrosis. Do not use plastic syringes.
Lidocaine (Xylocaine)	2 mg/kg IV.					Administer slowly.	Useful especially when reluctant to give more diazepam, barbiturates, or paraldehyde. Effect brief (about 30 min).

General anesthesia if other measures fail.

Treatment of infantile spasms.
See text regarding use of corticotropin or corticosteroids and of ketogenic diet. Also, clonazepam, diazepam, or valproic acid, especially with recurrences.

[1]In monotherapy. (Level at which clinical toxicity usually becomes manifest.)
[2]The interaction of antiepileptic drugs is outlined in Table 24–16.

longed use of anticonvulsant drugs will not produce significant or permanent "mental slowing" (although the underlying cause of the seizures might) and that prevention of seizures for 3–4 years or so substantially reduces the chances of recurrence. Advise them also that anticonvulsants are given to prevent further seizures and that they should be taken as prescribed. Changes in medications or dosages should not be made without the physician's knowledge. Unsupervised sudden withdrawal of anticonvulsant drugs may precipitate severe seizures or even status epilepticus.

Anticonvulsants must be kept where they cannot be ingested by small children or suicidal patients.

4. Check the patient at intervals, depending on the underlying cause of the seizures, the degree of control, and the toxic properties of the anticonvulsant drug or drugs used. Blood counts, urinalyses, and liver function or other biologic tests must be obtained periodically in the case of some anticonvulsants, as indicated in Table 24–15.

Periodic neurologic reevaluation is important. CT scanning may be indicated. Repeat EEGs are not needed to achieve seizure control. Indications for repeat EEGs are discussed above.

5. Continue anticonvulsant treatment until the patient is free of seizures for 2 or more years or, in some cases, through adolescence. In about 75% of cases, seizures may not recur. Such variables as younger age at onset, normal EEG, and ease of controlling seizures carry a favorable prognosis, whereas later onset, slowing or spikes on EEG, a history of atypical febrile convulsions, and possibly an abnormal neurologic examination carry a higher risk of recurrence.

6. In general, there is no need to withdraw anticonvulsants before taking an EEG.

7. Discontinue anticonvulsants gradually. If it becomes necessary to withdraw anticonvulsants abruptly, the patient should be under close medical surveillance. If seizures recur during or after withdrawal, anticonvulsant therapy should be reinstituted and again maintained for at least 2 or more years.

D. Blood Levels of Antiepileptic Drugs:

1. General comments—Most anticonvulsants take 5–6 times the length of their half-life to reach the "steady state" indicated in Table 24–15. This must be considered when blood levels are assessed after anticonvulsants are started or dosages are changed.

Individuals vary in their metabolism and their particular pharmacokinetic characteristics. These and external factors, including, for example, food intake or illness, also affect the blood level. Thus, the level reached on a milligram per kilogram or surface area basis varies among patients.

Experience and clinical research in the determination of antiepileptic blood levels have shown that there is *some* correlation between (1) drug dose and

blood level, (2) blood level and therapeutic effect, and (3) blood level and *some* toxic effects.

2. Effective levels—The ranges given in Table 24–14 are those within which seizure control without toxicity will be achieved in most patients. The level for any given individual will vary not only with metabolic makeup (including biochemical defects) but also with the nature and severity of the seizures and their underlying cause, with other medications being taken, and other factors. Seizure control may be achieved at lower levels in some; and higher levels may be reached without toxicity in others. When control is achieved at a lower level, the dose should *not* be increased merely to get the level into the "therapeutic range." Likewise, toxic side effects will be experienced at different levels even *within* the "therapeutic range"; lowering the dose will usually resolve the problem, but sometimes the drug must be withdrawn or another added (or both). Some serious toxic effects, including allergic reactions, LE phenomenon, and bone marrow or liver toxicity, are independent of dosage; liver toxicity especially may be the effect not just of a particular drug but also of its use in a patient who is or has been on several—and often a whole gamut—of other drugs.

3. Interaction of antiepileptic drugs—Blood levels of anticonvulsants may be affected by other drugs used. Examples are shown in Table 24–16. Individual variations occur; adjustment of doses may be required.

4. Indications for blood levels—Drug blood levels should be measured in a new patient or after a

Table 24–16. Interaction of epileptic drugs.

Level of	Increased by	Decreased by	Variable or Unchanged by
Carbamazepine	Acetazolamide Erythromycin[2]	Phenobarbital[3] Phenytoin[3] Primidone[3]	Valproic acid[1,3]
Clonazepam		Carbamazepine[3]	
Ethosuximide	Valproic acid[2]	Carbamazepine[3]	
Phenobarbital (primidone similar)	Valproic acid[1]		Phenytoin
Phenytoin	High level of phenobarbital[2]	ASA[1] Low-level phenobarbital Valproic acid[1] Carbamazepine[3]	
Valproic acid[4]		Phenobarbital Carbamazepine[4] Phenytoin	

[1]May unbind from protein, causing overall lower blood level but increased *free* drug; the latter may cause toxicity despite overall normal or low total blood level.
[2]Impairs metabolism.
[3]Increases (hepatic) metabolism.
[4]Carbamazepine and valproic acid may decrease each other.

new drug is introduced and seizure control without toxicity is achieved to determine the "effective level" for that patient. Blood level monitoring is useful also when expected control on a "usual" dosage has not been achieved, either with a single drug or after adding another; when seizures recur in a previously well-controlled patient; or when control is poor in a patient on anticonvulsants seen for the first time. A low level may indicate inadequate dosage, drug interaction, or—quite frequently—noncompliance with the therapeutic regimen prescribed. A high level may indicate refractoriness, drug interaction, or a worsening neurologic process. *Note:* Brief and limited "breakthroughs" are common in children (particularly younger ones) with intercurrent infections or significant excitement or other stresses, and they do *not* necessitate blood levels.

Blood levels are mandatory when there are signs and symptoms of toxicity—particularly where there is polydrug therapy, the dosage of a drug has been raised, or another drug has been added. Blood levels may be the only means of detecting intoxication in a comatose patient or very young child. Toxic levels also occur with drug abuse or liver disease.

Finally, when the patient is well controlled (or is controlled as well as one may hope for in a patient refractory to antiepileptics or one with difficult-to-control seizures) and free of toxic signs, blood levels are desirable once or twice a year.

E. Side Effects of Antiepileptic Drugs: (See also Table 24–15.)

1. Serious allergic reactions usually necessitate discontinuance of a drug. However, not every rash in a child receiving an anticonvulsant is due to the drug. If a useful antiepileptic drug is discontinued for this reason and the rash disappears, restarting the drug in a smaller dosage is often warranted to see if the reaction recurs.

2. Signs of drug toxicity will often disappear when the daily dosage is reduced by 25–30%.

3. The sedative effect of many of the anticonvulsants is often easily counteracted by the judicious use of coffee or dextroamphetamine sulfate, 2.5–5 mg at breakfast and 2.5 mg at noon.

4. Gingival hyperplasia secondary to phenytoin is best minimized through good dental hygiene but occasionally requires gingivectomy. This condition (but not hypertrichosis) usually disappears within about 6 months after the drug is discontinued.

F. Corticotropin and Corticosteroids:

1. Indications—These drugs are indicated for infantile spasms not due to causes amenable to specific therapy and in the Lennox-Gastaut syndrome, which cannot be controlled by anticonvulsant drugs.

The duration of the therapy is guided by cessation of clinical seizures and normalization of the EEG. Corticotropins or the oral steroids are usually continued in full doses for 2 weeks and then, if seizures have ceased, tapered over one week. Others use a total treatment period of about 2 months. If seizures recur, the dosage is increased to the last effective level and repeated for 2–4 weeks, or the alternative prednisone is tried. Some clinicians maintain the patient for up to 6 months on this dosage before attempting withdrawal. There is no strong evidence, however, that longer courses of treatment are more beneficial.

2. Dosages—

a. Corticotropin gel (Acthar Gel), starting with 2–4 units/kg/d intramuscularly in a single morning dose. Parents can be taught to give injections.

b. Prednisone, starting with 2–4 mg/kg/d orally in 2–3 divided doses.

3. Precautions—Give additional potassium, guard against infections, and discuss the cushingoid appearance and its disappearance. Do not withdraw oral corticosteroids suddenly. Side effects in some series occur in up to 40% of cases, especially with higher doses than those listed here (used by some authorities).

G. Ketogenic or Medium-Chain Triglyceride Diet in Treatment of Epilepsy: A ketogenic diet should be recommended in astatic and myoclonic seizures and absence seizures not responsive to drug therapy; it is occasionally recommended for infantile spasms that do not respond to corticotropin or the corticosteroids. Ketosis is induced by a diet high in fats and very limited in carbohydrates with sufficient protein for body maintenance and growth; by the feeding of medium-chain triglycerides (MCT); or by a combination of these methods. The MCT diet induces ketosis more readily than does a high level of dietary fats and hence requires less carbohydrate restriction. The mechanism for the anticonvulsant action of the ketogenic diet is not yet understood, although various hypotheses have been put forth. However, it is the ketosis, not the acidosis, that raises the seizure threshold. It is usually most effective in young children (ie, those under the age of 8 years), but when all other measures fail, it should be tried even in adolescents.

As ketosis is achieved, a repeat EEG may be helpful; seizure control by the diet is more likely to occur if the EEG shows improvement.

The ketogenic diet is difficult and expensive, tends to be monotonous, and depends upon the ability of the mother to weigh out the foods as well as upon absolute adherence to the diet prescribed. Whether the ketosis is achieved by high fat meals or an MCT diet is often a matter of the physician's, the dietitian's, or the patient's preference. The result may also depend on which form of the diet is better tolerated. Full cooperation of *all* family members is required, including the patient if old enough. However, when seizure control is achieved by this method, the child is alert, often needs no anticonvulsants or only small amounts, and parental and patient satisfaction is most gratifying.

H. Surgery: In seizure disorders intractable to

anticonvulsant therapy and primarily of focal origin, neurosurgery should be considered. Useful procedures, depending on the lesion, include corticectomy, hemispherectomy, anterior temporal lobectomy (for complex partial seizures), callosotomy (or commissurotomy), and stereotactic ablation.

Aicardi J, Chevrie JJ: Convulsive status epilepticus in infants and children: A study of 239 cases. *Epilepsia* 1970;**11**:187.

Annegars J: Factors prognostic of unprovoked seizures after febrile convulsions. *N Engl J Med* 1987;**316**:493.

Camfield PR et al: Epilepsy after a first unprovoked seizure in childhood. *Neurology* 1985;**35**:1657.

Committee on Drugs, American Academy of Pediatrics: Behavioral and cognitive effects of anticonvulsant therapy. *Pediatrics* 1985;**76**:644.

Crawford TO et al: Lorazepam in childhood status epilepticus and serial seizures. *Neurology* 1987;**37**:190.

Crawford TO et al: Very high dose phenobarbital for refractory status epilepticus in children. *Neurology* 1988;**38**:1035.

Delgado-Escueta AV, Treiman DM, Walsh GO: Medical progress: The treatable epilepsies. (2 parts.) *N Engl J Med* 1983;**308**:1508, 1576.

Dreifuss FE: Proposal for revised and clinical and EEG classification of epilepsy. *Epilepsia* 1981;**22**:489.

Holmes GL: *Diagnosis and Management of Seizures in Childhood.* Saunders, 1987.

Huttenlocher PR: Ketonemia and seizures: Metabolic and anticonvulsant effects of two ketogenic diets in childhood epilepsy. *Pediatr Res* 1976;**10**:536.

Lowenstein OH et al: Barbiturate anesthesia in the treatment of status epilepticus. *Neurol* 1988;**38**:395.

Maytal, J: Low Morbidity and Mortality of Status Epilepticus in Children. *Pediatrics* 1989;**83**:323.

Newton RW, McKinley I: Subsequent management of children with febrile convulsions. *Dev Med Child Neurol* 1988;**30**:391.

Phillips S, Shanohan R: Etiology and morbidity of status epilepticus in children. *Ann Neurol* 1989;**46**:74.

Reitter B, Walther B (editors): Proceedings of the symposium on infantile spasms, Mainz, Germany. *Brain Dev* 1987;**9**:345.

Riikonen R: Infantile spasms: Modern practical aspects. *Acta Paediatr Scand* 1984;**73**:1.

Shinnar S et al: Discontinuing antiepileptic medication in children with epilepsy after two years without seizures: A prospective study. *N Engl J Med* 1985;**313**:976.

Taylor DC, McKinlay I: When not to treat epilepsy with drugs: Annotations. *Dev Med Child Neurol* 1984; **26**:822.

Vian F et al: Infantile febrile status epilepticus: Risk factors and outcome. *Dev Med Child Neurol* 1987;**29**:495.

HEADACHES

Headache is not usually a psychosomatic symptom in very young children, whereas this is more often the case in older children and adolescents. Headaches occur in 37% and migraine in 2.7% of children by 7 years of age; by 14 years, the rates are 69% and 10.9%, respectively. A careful description of the headaches, associated circumstances, and other neurologic and systemic symptoms should be obtained. The family history and emotional problems should be discussed in detail. Systemic and neurologic examination, including blood pressure, ophthalmoscopic examination, and station and gait, will usually distinguish organic from psychogenic headaches. Differential features are given in Table 24–17.

If there is evidence of a specific intracranial cause or systemic disorder (eg, renal disease), diagnosis and treatment should be directed at the primary disorder.

Migraine attacks are usually paroxysmal, throbbing, pulsating, or pounding in character (initial vasoconstriction of intracranial vessels followed by vasodilatation of extracranial vessels). The pain in children is as often bilateral as unilateral, frontal or retroorbital as hemicranial. Between attacks, the child is asymptomatic. Migraine in children is associated (in order of frequency) with nausea, gastric discomfort, or vomiting; dizziness or vertigo; photophobia, visual auras, and, less frequently, visual loss; sensory and motor disturbances, especially involving face and arm; speech disturbances; and, occasionally, hemiplegia (sometimes alternating), acute confusional states, or impairment of space, time, and body image perceptions (termed the "Alice-in-Wonderland syndrome"). The child frequently seeks rest in a dark, quiet room.

Migraine of varying severity may occur in up to 6.6% of children between 7 and 14 years of age. Onset by age 4 is not uncommon. After 10 years of age, it is twice as common in girls as in boys. The family history is positive for migraine in up to 75% of patients and not infrequently also for epilepsy. School stresses (headache often occurs after school) and foods occasionally precipitate migraine. Head trauma may precipitate onset. In most instances, the migraine attack is brief (hours, not days), and sleep gives relief. Motion sickness is an associated feature in 45% of cases.

EEG may be abnormally slow to mildly or moderately dysrhythmic in up to 80% of patients soon after an attack of complicated migraine (emphasizing the relationship between migraine and epilepsy). Neuroradiologic studies, such as CT scanning, are usually not warranted unless there are definite neurologic or progressive abnormalities.

Acetaminophen is often effective in children. The patient should be allowed to remain quiet in a darkened room. In children over 12 years of age, severe migraine may often be controlled by Fiorinal,[1] Lanorinal,[1] or Fioricet,[2] 1 capsule every 4 hours. If

---

[1]One capsule of Fiorinal or Lanorinal contains butalbital, 50 mg; aspirin, 325 mg; and caffeine, 40 mg.

[2]One capsule of Fioricet contains butalbital, 50 mg; acetaminophen, 325 mg; and caffeine, 40 mg.

Table 24–17. Differential features of headaches in children.

	Muscule Contraction (Tension/Psychogenic)	Vascular (Migraine)	Traction and Inflammatory (Increased Intracranial Pressure)
Time course	Chronic, recurrent.	Acute, paroxysmal, recurrent.	Chronic or intermittent but increasingly frequent; *progressive severity.*
Prodromes	No.	Yes.	No.
Description	Diffuse, bandlike, tight.	Intense, pulsatile, unilateral in older child (70%).	Diffuse; more occipital with infratentorial mass, more frontal with supratentorial mass.
Characteristic findings	Feelings of inadequacy, depression, or anxiety.	Neurologic symptoms and signs usually transient.	Positive neurologic signs, especially papilledema.
Predisposing factors	Problems at home or school or socially (sexually).	Positive family history (75%); head trauma.	No.

these measures are ineffective, especially in the older child, and when anxiety and nausea are prominent symptoms, Cafergot P-B,[3] ½–1 tablet at the first sign of an attack and ½–1 additional tablet every 30 minutes for a total of 2–4 tablets, is often useful. Cafergot P-B suppositories may be used when vomiting precludes oral medication.

In the prevention of severe, frequent, and disabling migraine—especially in children too young to alert an adult to their symptoms or to follow the above regimen—prophylaxis is recommended as follows: propranolol (Inderal), 10–40 mg 3 times daily depending on weight (contraindications are respiratory and cardiac disorders); cyproheptadine (Periactin), 0.2–0.4 mg/kg/d in 2–3 divided doses; or calcium channel blockers may be used (varying forms and doses; they may have anticonvulsant action as well). Antidepressants such as imipramine (Tofranil) or amitriptyline (Elavil) may be useful (25–50 mg at bedtime). In children, methysergide maleate (Sansert) is not recommended.

Cho C, Pruitt AW: Therapeutic uses of calcium channel blocking drugs in the young. *Am J Dis Child* 1986; **140**:360.

Diamond S, Millstein E: Current concepts of migraine therapy. *J Clin Pharmacol* 1988;**28**:193.

Fenichel GM: Migraine in children. *Neurol Clin* 1985;**3**:77.

Gascon GG: Chronic and recurrent headaches in children and adolescents. *Pediatr Clin North Am* 1984;**31**:1027.

Larson B et al: Therapist-assisted self-help relaxation treatment of chronic headaches in adolescents: A school-based intervention. *J Child Psychol Psychiatry* 1987; **28**:127.

SLEEP DISORDERS

Sleep Apnea Syndrome in Older Children

Sleep apnea syndrome should be considered if there is a history of restless sleep with snoring or respiratory noise during sleep and frequent awakenings from sleep in an older child who shows poor school performance associated with excessive daytime sleepiness or irritability and hyperactivity. Children with these problems frequently have hypertrophied tonsils or adenoids, causing partial airway obstruction; occasionally, they have facial dysmorphism, neuromuscular disorders with muscle hypotonia and poor pharyngeal muscle control, and hyperplastic tissues, as seen in myxedema, Hodgkin's disease, or pickwickian syndrome. Evaluation includes soft tissue x-rays of the lateral neck; chest x-ray; electrocardiography to rule out cardiomegaly, sinus dysrhythmias, and incipient or actual right-sided heart failure; arterial blood gas determinations while awake and during sleep; and polysomnography. Therapy is generally surgical, ranging from tonsillectomy and adenoidectomy when appropriate to tracheostomy when medical measures fail.

Narcolepsy

Narcolepsy, a primary disorder of sleep and wakefulness, is characterized by chronic, excessive daytime sleeping that occurs regardless of activity or surroundings and is not relieved by increased sleep at night. Onset occurs as early as 3 years of age and has been reported before 10 years of age in about 18% of patients and between puberty and the late teens in 60%. Narcolepsy usually interferes severely with normal living. Often months to years after onset, there may also be cataplexy (transient partial or total loss of muscle tone, often triggered by laughter, anger, or other emotional upsurge), hypnagogic hallucinations (visual or auditory), and the sensation of paralysis on falling asleep. Studies have shown that rapid eye movement (REM) sleep, with loss of muscle tone and an electroencephalographic low-amplitude mixed frequency pattern, occurs within 15 minutes of sleep onset in patients with narcolepsy, whereas normal subjects experience 80–100 minutes or longer of non-REM (NREM) sleep before the initial REM period.

Narcolepsy is treated with a central nervous system stimulant (dextroamphetamine or long-acting

---

[3]Cafergot P-B contains ergotamine tartrate, 1 mg; caffeine, 100 mg; Bellafoline (alkaloids of belladonna, as malates), 0.125 mg; and pentobarbital sodium, 30 mg.

methylphenidate is preferred); occasionally, a tricyclic antidepressant, in low dosages titrated to the need of the patient, is added to the treatment regimen. The condition persists throughout life.

Somnambulism

Somnambulism has been assigned to a group of sleep disturbances known as disorders of arousal. It is characterized by abrupt onset early in the night of an episode of veiled consciousness and coordinated activity (eg, walking, sometimes moving objects without seeming purpose). The episode is of relatively brief duration and ceases spontaneously. There is poor recall of the event on waking in the morning. Somnambulism may be related to mental activities occurring in stages 3 and 4 of NREM sleep. The incidence has been estimated at only 2–3%, but up to 15% of cases are reported in children 6–16 years of age, with boys affected more often than girls and many youngsters having recurrent episodes. No psychopathologic features can usually be demonstrated, but a strong association (30%) between childhood migraine and somnambulism has been noted, and episodes of somnambulism may be triggered in predisposed children by stresses, including febrile illnesses.

No treatment of somnambulism is required, and it is not necessary to seek psychiatric counsel.

Night Terrors

Night terrors (pavor nocturnus) is a disorder of arousal from NREM sleep. It usually occurs in children 3–8 years of age and rarely occurs after adolescence. The disorder is characterized by sudden (but only partial) waking, with the severely frightened child unable to be fully roused or comforted. Concomitant autonomic symptoms include rapid breathing, tachycardia, and perspiring. The next morning, the child has no recall of any nightmare. Psychopathologic mechanisms are unclear, but falling asleep after watching scenes of violence on television or hearing frightening stories may play a role. Elimination of such causes and administration of a mild antianxiety agent such as chlordiazepoxide (Librium) may be helpful. It is important to differentiate these episodes from complex partial (psychomotor) seizures.

Barabas G, Ferrari M, Matthews WS: Childhood migraine and somnambulism. *Neurology* 1983;**33**:948.

Douglas AB et al: Monozygotic twins concordant for the narcoleptic syndrome. *Neurology* 1989;**39**:140.

Guilleminault C: Obstructive sleep apnea syndrome and its treatment in children. *Pediatr Pulmonol* 1987;**3**:429.

Guilleminault C: *Sleep and Its Disorders in Children.* Raven Press, 1987.

Klackenberg G: Somnambulism in childhood: Prevalence, course and behavioral correlations. *Acta Paediatr Scand* 1982;**71**:495.

Regestein QR, Reich P, Mufson MJ: Narcolepsy: An initial clinical approach. *J Clin Psychiatry* 1983;**44**:166.

HEAD INJURIES

General Considerations

Serious accidental injury constitutes one of the most common causes of childhood hospitalization and death in the United States.

Injury of the brain can result from sudden acceleration-deceleration movements or from sudden rotational or torsional movements of the head. Direct impact of the brain against the inner table of the skull, together with blood vessel rupture and dural tears, leads to parenchymal damage.

''Closed head injury'' includes those injuries in which the skull remains intact or in which there is only a small linear fracture. ''Open head injury'' consists of those injuries involving major scalp lacerations and compound or depressed skull fractures. Brain parenchymal injury can occur in either ''closed'' or ''open'' head injuries but is more frequent and often more severe with open head injury.

The clinical severity of head injury is classified as mild, moderate, or severe, depending on the type and extent of brain damage, the presence of brain edema, and presence or absence of intracranial hemorrhage. Intracranial hemorrhages can occupy a variety of potential spaces within the cranial vault, including epidural, subdural, and subarachnoid spaces. Cerebral contusions consist of a localized region of petechial hemorrhage and edema. Intraparenchymal hemorrhages can be small, or they can be massive, rapidly expanding to produce markedly elevated intracranial pressure and cerebral herniation.

Clinical Findings

A. Symptoms and Signs: In mild head injuries, loss of consciousness may not occur or may be only momentary. Frequently, patients experience mild to moderate headache, nausea, vomiting, vertigo, and light-headedness. Although tachycardia may be present, blood pressure and other vital signs are normal. There is rapid resolution of all symptoms. Occasionally, a brief, generalized clonic seizure may occur shortly after the head injury, but posttraumatic epilepsy is rare.

Moderately severe head injuries are associated with loss of consciousness for several minutes to one hour. Headache may be severe, and the patient may experience severe irritability, drowsiness, emotional lability, and signs of mild to moderate delirium. Nausea and vomiting can be prominent. Vertigo, tinnitus, and light-headedness can be moderately severe for a short period. Symptoms resolve in 1–2 days, although vertigo and some alteration in behavior, mood, and concentration persist for several days. Some children also experience relatively protracted problems regarding attention, concentration, and school performance after seemingly mild or moderate head injury.

Severe head injury is associated with prolonged

loss of consciousness, usually greater than one hour. Headache, nausea, vomiting, and tinnitus are severe and at times incapacitating. Marked behavioral changes and seizures can develop immediately after the head injury, and posttraumatic epilepsy occurs in approximately 10 percent of children. Symptoms usually persist for several days or weeks, in some patients for months.

When intracranial hemorrhages occur, symptoms of progressively increasing intracranial pressure may develop. Patients have progressive loss of consciousness and severe nausea and vomiting. Seizures occur in about 50–70% of children with subdural hematomas. Fever and nuchal rigidity are often present with subdural hematomas, and meningitis may be suspected. Epidural and acute subdural hematomas may be acute and require emergency surgical drainage. These forms of intracranial hemorrhage can rapidly lead to death, particularly if they occur in the posterior fossa. Subarachnoid hemorrhages are unusual in childhood unless they are associated with an underlying cerebrovascular malformation. Intracerebral hematomas, particularly in the frontal and temporal regions, can occur after either a closed or open head injury. When intracerebral hemorrhages occur, underlying bleeding diathesis should be excluded by appropriate laboratory testing.

B. Physical Examination: Initial assessment of patients who have suffered head injury includes frequent monitoring of heart rate, blood pressure, and temperature. Sudden changes in blood pressure, particularly hypotension, may be an indication of intrathoracic, intra-abdominal, or other systemic injury associated with bleeding.

Head circumference should be measured in infants after head injury, and the fontanelle size and tension should be carefully documented. Evaluation of the head and neck region is important in the search for signs of cerebrospinal fluid leakage from the ear and nose. Care should be taken to move the head as little as possible because injury to the spinal cord and cervical vertebrae may not be initially apparent. The patient should be examined thoroughly for signs of injury to extremities, abdomen, back, and chest. Skin should also be carefully examined for evidence of recent or remote injury. The possibility of nonaccidental trauma should be suspected when multiple sites of injury or injuries of different ages are present.

Neurologic examination includes assessment of the pupillary size, symmetry, and light reflexes. Evidence of ocular and orbital injury may be associated with basilar skull fracture. Funduscopic examination may disclose retinal, flame-shaped hemorrhages that can be indicative of subdural or subarachnoid hemorrhages. Increased intracranial pressure related to intracranial hemorrhages or cerebral edema may result in dilatated, nonpulsating retinal veins and swelling of the optic disc. Assessment of muscle tone, strength, and reflexes may provide evidence of focal or lateralized neurologic dysfunction.

C. Laboratory Studies and Imaging: A sudden or progressive decrease in hematocrit may suggest rapidly evolving acute subdural hematoma. Injury may result in fluid and electrolyte abnormalities as a consequence of inappropriate antidiuretic hormone (ADH) or diabetes insipidus.

Radiographic studies, particularly CT scanning, should be carried out to search for skull fracture, intracranial hemorrhage, and intracranial foreign bodies. Skull films in general are not as helpful as CT scanning; however, in certain situations when CT scanning is not available, skull films may demonstrate clinically significant depressed or comminuted skull fractures. In addition, plain radiographs of the neck, chest, abdomen, and extremities are important in searching for more generalized evidence of injury. X-ray films of the neck should be obtained on all patients with head injury because unsuspected spinal injury can be present and require immediate stabilization. Magnetic resonance imaging can also demonstrate intracranial hemorrhage and some types of foreign bodies. However, MRI is not as helpful as CT scanning at defining bony abnormalities. Cerebral angiography may be required at times when major vascular damage is suspected or when the patient develops clinical signs suggesting arterial dissection.

Lumbar puncture is rarely needed in the evaluation of patients with head injury and in most instances is contraindicated. Infants with tense fontanelles and fever may be suspected initially of having bacterial meningitis, and in this situation lumbar puncture may be necessary.

Subdural tap is an important immediate diagnostic as well as therapeutic maneuver in acute and rapidly progressing subdural or epidural hematomas. When an acute subdural hematoma is clinically suspected and the patient is deteriorating rapidly, a subdural tap should be performed as an emergency procedure. The tap should not be delayed in order to obtain a CT scan. With posterior fossa subdural and epidural hematomas, a cisternal tap can also be life-saving.

EEGs after acute head injury are frequently abnormal but nonspecific, and their role is quite limited in the initial evaluation and management of head injury. EEGs may be useful in monitoring seizure activity and can complement serial neurologic examinations and assessments of a patient's progress after head injury.

Differential Diagnosis

Whenever the cause for the head injury is not readily apparent, nonaccidental trauma should be suspected. Intracranial hemorrhage may occur with relatively minor injuries in patients with bleeding diathesis. Some metabolic disorders, such as scurvy, rickets, and Menkes' disease, may predispose the patient to pathologic fractures and intracranial hemorrhage.

Complications

Seizures, either focal or generalized, have been reported in 5–15% of children with head injury. Usually the seizures are brief, but a few patients experience status epilepticus. Chronic posttraumatic epilepsy develops in 10% of children who have suffered brain lacerations or who have experienced prolonged loss of consciousness immediately after head injury. When posttraumatic seizures develop, approximately 50% will occur in the first 6 months after the injury, and 80% will have developed within 2 years. Antiepileptic medications may be started when patients have one or more immediate posttraumatic seizures and continued for up to 6 months. If seizures develop later, chronic antiepileptic medication is continued for 2–4 years.

Massive cerebral swelling, cerebral edema, and intracranial hematomas may lead to herniation of the temporal lobe through the tentorial notch with subsequent brain stem compression and rapid deterioration of the patient's mental status and neurologic function. Cerebellar tonsillar herniation results from posterior fossa hematomas and leads to clinical evidence of lower brain stem dysfunction, progressive loss of consciousness, and impaired cardiorespiratory functions.

CSF leakage through basilar skull fractures predisposes the patient to chronic, recurrent bacterial meningitis with organisms that normally inhabit the upper airway, such as *Streptococcus pneumoniae* and *Haemophilus influenzae*. Most CSF leaks stop spontaneously, but chronic leaks require surgical closure. If the patient develops signs of fever, nuchal rigidity, or other evidence of possible meningitis, antibiotics are necessary.

Hydrocephalus can develop after head injury, particularly when subarachnoid hemorrhage leads to basilar arachnoiditis or impairment of the CSF absorption through the arachnoid villi.

Some patients develop pseudotumor cerebri shortly after head injury, but the mechanism is not clear.

Patients with diastatic linear fractures develop leptomeningeal cysts. This cyst develops when a tear in the dura and arachnoid is followed by entrapment of the arachnoid between the margins of the diastatic fracture. Spinal fluid accumulates within the cyst and produces a progressively enlarging, fluid-filled mass over the fracture line. Removal of the cyst and closure of the dural tear requires surgical repair.

Postconcussion syndrome is seen in children, adolescents, and adults, but its pathogenesis is not clear. Principal manifestations are changes in behavior, personality, and sleep pattern, headache, vertigo, tinnitus, and various head and neck pains. School or job performance deteriorates, and the ability to concentrate is impaired. Hyperactivity can impair the child's normal daily function. Treatment is symptomatic, and postconcussion syndrome usually abates gradually over a period of days to weeks.

Treatment

Immediate treatment of a patient with serious head injury consists of securing the airway and supporting the cardiovascular system. Seizures, particularly status epilepticus, may require acute anticonvulsant medication. As described above, subdural or cisternal taps are required if the patient is rapidly deteriorating because of an acute subdural or epidural hematoma.

After the initial assessment, the patient must be observed carefully for several hours after head injury, whether in the emergency room, in an ambulatory clinic setting, or at home. The patient's arousability, pupillary light reflexes, extraocular movements, and extremity movements must be serially documented. Hospitalization of patients after head injury is necessary when the patient has focal or asymmetric neurologic deficits that do not rapidly resolve or when loss of consciousness is prolonged. It is important to admit and monitor carefully patients who show signs of deterioration and to initiate rapid treatment to relieve intracranial pressure.

Severe headache, nausea, vomiting, and restlessness can usually be treated symptomatically. Tetanus prophylaxis (0.5 mL tetanus toxoid) should be given to patients with scalp lacerations or open head injuries. Most patients do not require prophylactic antibiotics. However, patients with CSF leakage from the nose or ears should be monitored carefully and antibiotics started if meningitis is suspected. Cerebral edema may be treated with diuretics, osmotic agents, or glucocorticoids or by lowering the patient's P_{CO_2}. If acute obstructive hydrocephalus occurs, a ventricular drain aids in controlling increased intracranial pressure.

Patients with depressed or displaced fractures, epidural hematomas, progressive acute subdural hematomas, and some chronic subdural hematomas require surgical intervention. Evacuation of intracerebral hematomas is usually not indicated, although superficial intracerebral hematomas occasionally may be evacuated in an attempt to relieve severe and rapidly increasing mass affect.

Prognosis

Ninety percent or more of children who suffer from mild to moderate head injuries become free of symptoms and do not develop serious, long-term complications. Severe head injury is associated with a mortality rate of 5–10%. From 3 to 5% of children with severe head injury have severe, long-term neurologic deficits, and another 5–6% have moderate long-term deficits. Over 80% of children with severe head injury, however, enjoy good functional recovery.

PERINATAL HEAD INJURY

Injury to the scalp and skull occurs during the perinatal period in association with prolonged pressure on the infant's skull, breech presentation, shoulder dystocia, or malpositioned forceps. Several types of head and scalp injury may be visibly apparent at the time of birth. Caput succedaneum is characterized by hemorrhagic edema of the scalp skin and muscles. Cephalohematoma is a localized subperiosteal hemorrhage; this type of hemorrhage is limited in extent by the periosteum that attaches at suture margins. Caput and cephalohematomas resolve spontaneously and do not require specific treatment. Cephalohematomas occasionally prolong neonatal jaundice, and approximately 25% of them overlie linear skull fractures. Subgaleal hemorrhage represents the most dangerous and serious extracranial hemorrhage in the neonate. The blood of this hemorrhage dissects underneath the fascia of muscles of the head and neck. Blood may dissect and extend into the face, down the neck, and over the chest and back. Massive blood loss can take place, and subgaleal hemorrhage can result in exsanguination. Subgaleal hemorrhage usually occurs in association with an underlying bleeding-coagulation disorder or after severe head trauma that results in tears of the dura that form the dural sinuses.

Skull fractures in the perinatal period involving the skull base and occipital region can be associated with dural tears and massive intracranial hemorrhage. Hemorrhage secondary to dural tear often results in catastrophic, rapid clinical deterioration and death.

Intracranial hemorrhage is the most serious consequence of head injury during the perinatal period. Epidural hematomas are usually associated with depressed skull fractures. Emergency surgical removal is mandatory. Subarachnoid hemorrhage is relatively frequent in the perinatal period and is often asymptomatic. However, hydrocephalus may develop after subarachnoid hemorrhage and require ventriculoperitoneal shunting. Subdural hematomas are occasionally seen in the perinatal period and are often associated with cerebral laceration or contusion. Acute subdural hematomas may progress rapidly, and the patient may require emergency surgery for evacuation of the hematoma. Chronic subdural hematomas are manifested by increasing head circumference and the gradual appearance of neurologic deficits, anemia, poor weight gain, irritability, and somnolence.

Intracerebral hematomas usually indicate severe head trauma in the perinatal period and are frequently associated with dural lacerations or with bleeding-coagulation disorder.

Intracranial Hemorrhage in the Premature

Approximately 25–40% of all newborns weighing less than 2000 g develop periventricular-interventricular hemorrhage. This type of hemorrhage originates in the germinal matrix and is related to immature blood vessel structure, poor blood vessel support by the germinal matrix, and the unusual tortuous course of veins in the region of the germinal matrix in the premature brain. Germinal matrix hemorrhages are classified as grade I, II, or III. Grade I indicates a hemorrhage limited to the subependymal, germinal matrix region with little or no intraventricular extension. Grade II represents the germinal matrix hemorrhage with moderate extension into the ventricular system. Grade III represents germinal matrix hemorrhage with massive intraventricular extension and usually ventriculomegaly. Furthermore, intraventricular hemorrhage may be associated with hemorrhagic infarction of the white matter dorsal and lateral to the anterior lateral ventricle.

Clinical symptoms of intraventricular-periventricular hemorrhage are related to the size of the hemorrhage and its degree of extension into the ventricular system. In addition, clinical symptoms are modified by the degree of the infant's systemic illness. Small grade I hemorrhages limited to the germinal matrix can be asymptomatic and are often diagnosed by ultrasound but not suspected clinically. Some patients develop a waxing and waning course with a gradual, stuttering evolution of neurologic deficits. The most dramatic presentation of intraventricular-periventricular hemorrhage, however, is the sudden catastrophic onset of seizures, anemia, and cardiovascular instability. Acute grade III hemorrhages combined with periventricular hemorrhagic infarction are associated with a mortality rate of greater than 60% (see Table 24–18).

Laboratory evaluation of infants with periventricular-intraventricular hemorrhage includes assessment of the hematocrit, electrolytes, calcium, magnesium, blood glucose concentration, coagulation system, and acid-base status. Examination of spinal

Table 24–18. Prognosis of periventricular-intraventricular hemorrhage in premature infants.

	Acute		Long-Term
	Mortality (%)	**Hydrocephalus (%)**	**Neurologic Impairment (%)**
Grade I	15	5	15
Grade II	20	25	30
Grade III	40	55	40
IVH & periventricular hemorrhagic infarction	> 60	80	90

fluid after intraventricular hemorrhage is usually not necessary, but reveals grossly bloody spinal fluid with elevated protein and decreased glucose concentration.

The primary diagnostic test in neonates suspected of having periventricular-intraventricular hemorrhage is cranial ultrasonography. This test is excellent for displaying germinal matrix hemorrhage with or without intraventricular extension and can be used for serial monitoring of ventricular size. However, ultrasonography is not an adequate method for evaluating cerebral hemispheres or structures of the posterior fossa. CT or MRI scanning is necessary for full evaluation of the cerebral parenchyma, the posterior fossa, and the subarachnoid, subdural, and epidural spaces.

Treatment

Treatment of infants with periventricular-intraventricular hemorrhage is directed at stabilizing and supporting the cardiovascular system. Abnormalities of the cardiovascular, renal, gastrointestinal, and other organ systems require specific monitoring and management. Fluid, electrolyte, and acid-base disturbances should be identified and corrected. Secondary infections and seizures should be treated with antibiotics and anticonvulsant medications. Any underlying bleeding diathesis should be corrected, and vitamin K_1 should be given to infants to ensure that a bleeding diathesis secondary to Vitamin K deficiency does not contribute to the patient's problems.

For patients with progressive ventriculomegaly and hydrocephalus, ventricular drains and subsequent ventriculoperitoneal shunting is often required. The value of serial lumbar punctures is controversial but can be useful in some patients if ventriculostomy is not readily available to relieve acute posthemorrhagic ventriculomegaly.

Prognosis

The outcome of intracranial hemorrhage is related to the extent of underlying brain injury. Brain laceration and contusions predispose the patient to the development of posttraumatic epilepsy and focal or multifocal areas of cerebral atrophy.

The outcome of neonatal intraventricular-periventricular hemorrhage is related to the size and extent of the hemorrhage and associated factors such as the presence of hemorrhagic infarction and systemic complications secondary to cardiovascular, renal, gastrointestinal, and other systemic abnormalities. Table 24–18 displays the overall mortality rates and morbidity rates with regard to neurologic deficits and hydrocephalus.

Bruce DA et al: Pathophysiology, treatment and outcome following severe head injury in children. *Childs Brain* 1979;**5**:174.

Hennes H et al: Clinical predictors of severe head trauma in children. *Am J Dis Child* 1988;**142**:1045.

Ivan LP, Choo SH, Ventureyra ECG: Head injuries in childhood: A 2-year survey. *Can Med Assoc J* 1983; **128**:281.

Jenkins A et al: Brain lesions detected by magnetic resonance imaging in mild and severe head injuries. *Lancet* 1986;**2**:445.

Jennett B, Teasdale G: *Management of Head Injuries*. FA Davis, 1981.

Kraus JF et al: Incidence, severity, and external causes of pediatric brain injury. *Am J Dis Child* 1986;**140**:687.

Sneed RC, Stover SL: Undiagnosed spinal cord injuries in brain-injured children. *Am J Dis Child* 1988;**142**:965.

NEOPLASMS OF THE CENTRAL NERVOUS SYSTEM

1. INTRACRANIAL TUMORS

Neoplasms of the central nervous system account for approximately 20% of all malignant neoplasms of childhood and are second only to leukemia in frequency. The incidence of primary CNS tumors in people less than 20 years old is 20–25 per million per year, or about one-third to one-half of the incidence of childhood leukemia. The incidence of CNS tumors in children under age 2 is approximately one-tenth of that in older children, or approximately 2–2.5 per million per year. Approximately 1500 new cases of brain tumor occur each year in the United States, including 150–200 cases in children under 2 years old. The peak incidence of brain tumors occurs between the ages of 5 and 10 years, and the male-to-female ratio for brain tumors is approximately 1.2:1. Primary brain tumors can be classified generally by their cell of origin (see Table 24–19). In children over the age of 2, approximately 65% of brain tumors are infratentorial and 35% supratentorial. Secondary involvement of the nervous system is com-

Table 24–19. Classification of primary brain tumors of childhood.

Tumor Type	Incidence (%)	Common Examples
Glial cell tumors	50–60	Astrocytoma Optic nerve glioma Brainstem glioma Ependymoma
Neuroectodermal tumors	25–35	Medulloblastoma Pinealoblastoma
Craniopharyngioma	5–10	
Germ cell tumors	< 10	Teratoma Dermoid Germinoma
Meningeal tumors	< 5	Meningioma Meningeal sarcoma
Lymphoma (non-Hodgkins)	< 1	

mon in the early stages of acute leukemia, and the brain may be invaded directly by tumors that involve extraneural tissue in the head and neck region. Hematogenous metastatic spread from solid malignant tumors outside the nervous system is rare in childhood, but the true incidence of this phenomenon is unknown. Some highly aggressive and malignant intracranial tumors in childhood, such as medulloblastoma, commonly spread throughout the subarachnoid spaces within the central nervous system. Rarely, primary CNS tumors may metastasize to extraneural sites such as bone marrow, lung, and viscera. The cause and pathogenesis of brain tumors is unknown.

Clinical Manifestations

Manifestations of intracranial tumors consist of nonspecific signs due to increased intracranial pressure (see Table 24–20). Infratentorial tumors, regardless of histologic type, frequently present with gait disturbance, incoordination, multiple and often asymmetric cranial nerve deficits, and nystagmus. The patient may tilt the head in an attempt to relieve discomfort at the base of the skull due to cerebellar tonsillar herniation, or head tilt may be a compensatory adjustment to correct double vision.

Specific neurologic manifestations of supratentorial tumors are dictated by the location of the tumor. Focal motor and sensory abnormalities and focal seizures occur frequently in the more common types of hemispheral tumors. Abnormalities of eye movements and vision are also common. Endocrine and autonomic disturbances may indicate the presence of a hypothalamic or thalamic tumor.

Diagnosis

When the clinical history and the findings of physical examination suggest the presence of an intracranial mass, a CT scan or MRI scan of the head should be obtained to define the precise anatomic site and extent of the tumor. Skull x-rays may show scalloping of the inner table of the skull, truncation of the

Table 24–20. Signs of increased intracranial pressure.

Acute
Macrocephaly
Excessive rate of head growth
Altered behavior
Decreased level of consciousness
Vomiting
Blurred vision
Double vision
Optic disk swelling
Abducens nerve paresis
Chronic
Macrocephaly
Growth impairment
Developmental delay
Optic atrophy
Visual field loss

sella turcica, or widening of the suture lines as evidence of increased intracranial pressure. EEG findings in brain tumors are nonspecific, and EEGs are rarely necessary in the initial diagnostic evaluation of brain tumor. However, EEGs done on patients who have focal or generalized seizures as a manifestation of their tumor may show localized epileptiform discharges. An EEG done before initiation of treatment for the brain tumor may provide a useful baseline assessment of electrocerebral activity for future reference. Examination of cerebrospinal fluid is usually not necessary in the diagnosis of localized mass lesions within the nervous system. However, examination of spinal fluid, particularly cytopathologic examination, may be helpful when tumors are disseminated throughout the subarachnoid space.

Treatment

Some tumors, such as cerebellar astrocytomas, may be completely removed by surgery and require no additional treatment. However, most primary CNS tumors are currently treated by a combination of surgery, radiation, and chemotherapy. Surgery is frequently used to reduce the mass of tumor and is followed by localized radiation to the tumor bed. Some tumors with a propensity for subarachnoid seeding and spread (eg, medulloblastoma) are also treated with prophylactic total craniocerebral radiation. Chemotherapeutic agents currently being used for treatment of childhood brain tumors include prednisone, vincristine sulfate, VP = 16 = 213 (etoposide), methotrexate, carmustine, cisplatin and thiotepa. These drugs are often used in combinations over a period of several weeks. Current recommendations are that children with brain tumors be enrolled in multicenter protocols that use combinations of surgery, radiation, and chemotherapy.

2. PSEUDOTUMOR CEREBRI

Pseudotumor cerebri is a condition characterized by increased intracranial pressure in the absence of an identifiable intracranial mass or hydrocephalus. Clinical manifestations of pseudotumor cerebri are those of increased intracranial pressure as outlined in Table 24–20. The precise cause is usually not known, but pseudotumor cerebri has been described in association with a variety of inflammatory, metabolic, toxic, and connective tissue disorders (Table 24–21). The diagnosis of pseudotumor cerebri is one of exclusion. CT scans or MRI scans of the head are needed to exclude hydrocephalus and intracranial masses; these studies demonstrate ventricles of small or normal size but no other structural abnormalities. Lumbar puncture should be performed to document elevated cerebrospinal fluid pressure. Examination of cerebrospinal fluid reveals a normal cell count, a normal glucose concentration, and a normal or low

Table 24–21. Conditions associated with pseudotumor cerebri.

Metabolic-toxic disorders
  Hypervitaminosis A
  Hypovitaminosis A
  Prolonged steroid therapy
  Steroid withdrawal
  Tetracycline therapy
  Nalidixic acid therapy
  Iron deficiency
  Plumbism
  Hypocalcemia
  Hyperparathyroidism
  Adrenal insufficiency
  Lupus erythematosus
  Chronic CO_2 retention
Infectious and parainfectious disorders
  Chronic otitis media
  Poliomyelitis
  Guillain-Barré syndrome
Dural sinus thrombosis
Minor head injury

protein concentration. In some inflammatory and connective tissue diseases, however, the CSF protein may be increased.

Specific treatment of pseudotumor cerebri is aimed at correcting any identifiable underlying predisposing condition. In addition, some patients may benefit from the use of furosemide or acetazolamide to decrease the volume and pressure of cerebrospinal fluid within the central nervous system. These drugs may be used in combination with repeated lumbar punctures to remove cerebrospinal fluid. If a program of repeated spinal fluid removal and medical management is not successful or if visual field loss is detected despite these measures, lumboperitoneal shunt or another surgical decompression procedure may be necessary to prevent irreparable visual loss and damage to the optic nerves.

3. SPINAL CORD TUMORS

The incidence of tumors within the spinal canal is one-fifth to one-sixth that of tumors within the intracranial compartment. The peak age of occurrence is approximately 4 years. Spinal tumors can be classified as intradural and extradural. Intradural tumors within the substance of the spinal cord are referred to as intramedullary, and those outside the substance of the spinal cord are referred to as extramedullary. Recent reports suggest that approximately one-third of intraspinal tumors are intramedullary, approximately one-third are intradural extramedullary, and approximately one-third are extradural. Approximately 10% of intraspinal tumors arise in the sacral region, and the remaining 90% are distributed equally in the cervical, thoracic, and lumbar regions. Neurofibromas, meningiomas, dermoid cysts, teratomas, and metastatic tumors constitute the most frequent tumors that are extradural or intradural extramedullary. Astrocytomas and ependymomas are the most common intramedullary tumors.

Clinical manifestations of spinal cord tumors result from direct invasion of the tumor into neural tissue, as well as from compression of neural tissue. Symptoms of gait disturbance, pain, and bowel and bladder dysfunction occur in association with abnormal muscle stretch reflexes, weakness, and sensory loss. The specific pattern of neurologic deficits are determined by the location and size of tumor mass.

When the clinical course and physical examination suggest the presence of an intraspinal mass, neuroimaging procedures are required. Spinal CT scan, metrizamide myelography and spinal MRI scans are currently the methods by which a tumor can be defined. The use of gadolinium with MRI scanning enhances the definition of tumors within the spinal cord and within the spinal subarachnoid and extradural spaces. Although examination of cerebrospinal fluid may demonstrate the presence of neoplastic cells and markedly elevated protein concentrations, this test is not required for the diagnosis of intraspinal tumors and is contraindicated when significant cord compression is suspected clinically.

Primary intraspinal tumors may be totally removed by surgery, but many intramedullary tumors require a combination of surgery, radiation, and chemotherapy similar to the treatment of intracranial tumors discussed in the preceding section.

In addition to primary intraspinal tumors, the spinal cord and intraspinal compartment may be the site of direct invasion or hematogenous metastatic spread of tumors that arise outside the nervous system. Important examples include spinal neuroblastoma that may be an extension of paraspinous, retroperitoneal neuroblastoma. Lymphoma, sarcoma, and leukemia may involve paraspinous tissue and spread to the intraspinal compartment through neural foramina. Treatment of these secondary neoplasms usually requires some combination of surgical excision, radiation, and chemotherapy.

Allen JC: Childhood brain tumors: Current status of clinical trials in newly diagnosed and recurrent disease. *Pediatr Clin North Am* 1985;**32**:633.

Baker RS, Baumann RJ, Buncic JR: Idiopathic intracranial hypertension (pseudotumor cerebri) in pediatric patients. *Pediatr Neurol* 1989;**5**:5.

Cohen ME, Duffner PK: *Brain Tumors in Children: Principles of Diagnosis and Treatment.* Raven Press, 1984.

Donaldson JO: Pathogenesis of pseudotumor cerebri syndromes. *Neurology* 1981;**31**:877.

Haft H, Ransohoff J, Carter S: Spinal cord tumors in children. *Pediatrics* 1959;**23**:1152.

Kadota RP et al: Brain tumors in children. *J Pediatr* 1989;**114**:511.

Rush JA: Pseudotumor cerebri: Clinical profile and visual outcome in 63 patients. *Mayo Clin Proc* 1980;**55**:541.

Simpson DA, Carter RF, Ducrou W: Intracranial tumors in infancy. *Dev Med Child Neurol* 1968;**10**:190.

Weisberg LA, Chutorian AM: Pseudotumor cerebri of childhood. *Am J Dis Child* 1977;**131**:1243.

CEREBROVASCULAR DISEASE

Cerebrovascular disease, or stroke, occurs with an incidence of approximately 2.5 per 100,000 per year. Although stroke occurs most frequently between the ages of 1 and 5 years, it may occur at any age during infancy and childhood. Congenital cyanotic heart disease is the most common underlying systemic disorder predisposing to stroke.

The initial approach to the patient should take into account the patient's age and any underlying systemic or neurologic illness. A systematic search for evidence of cardiac disease, vascular disease, hematologic disease, and intracranial disorders should be undertaken (Table 24–22).

Clinical Findings

A. Symptoms and Signs: The clinical manifestations of stroke in childhood vary according to the vascular distribution to the brain that is involved. Because many conditions leading to childhood stroke result in emboli, multifocal neurologic involvement is common. Children may present with an acute hemiplegia similar to stroke in adults. Symptoms of unilateral weakness, sensory disturbance, dysarthria, and dysphasia may develop over a period of minutes, but at times progressive worsening of symptoms may evolve over several hours. Bilateral hemispheral involvement may lead to a depressed level of consciousness. The patient may also demonstrate disturbances of mood and behavior and experience focal or multifocal seizures. Physical examination of the patient is aimed not only at identifying the specific deficits related to impaired cerebral blood flow but also at seeking evidence for any predisposing disorder. Retinal hemorrhages, splinter hemorrhages in the nailbeds, cardiac murmurs, and signs of trauma are especially important findings.

When stroke is ushered in by a focal hemiconvulsion followed by hemiplegia, a chronic epilepsy syndrome may persist for years in association with hemiplegia. This combination of hemiconvulsion, hemiplegia, and chronic epilepsy has been referred to as the "HHE syndrome."

B. Laboratory Findings: Laboratory investigation can be carried out systemically, with particular attention to disorders involving the heart, blood vessels, platelets, red cells, and coagulation protein. Additional laboratory tests for systemic disorders such as systemic lupus erythematosus and polyarteritis nodosa are usually indicated.

Examination of spinal fluid is indicated in patients with fever, nuchal rigidity, or marked obtundation when the diagnosis of intracranial infection requires

Table 24–22. Etiologic risk factors for stroke in children.

Cardiac disorders
  Cyanotic heart disease
  Valvular disease
    Rheumatic
    Infection (SBE)
  Cardiomyopathy
  Cardiac dysrhythmia
Vascular occlusive disorders
  Arterial trauma (carotid dissections)
  Homocystinuria
  Vasculitis
    Meningitis
    Polyarteritis nodosa
    Systemic lupus erythematosus
    Drug abuse (amphetamines)
  Fibromuscular dysplasia
  Diabetes
  Nephrotic syndrome
  Systemic hypertension
  Dural sinus and cerebral venous thrombosis
    Meningitis
    Hyperviscosity
    Hypovolemia
  Cortical venous thrombosis
  Carotid-cavernous fistula
Hematologic disorders
  Polycythemia
  Thrombotic thrombocytopenia
  Thrombocytopenic purpura
  Thrombocythemia
  Hemoglobinopathies
    Sickle cell disease
    S-C disease
  Coagulation defects
    Hemophilia
    Vitamin K deficiency
  Hypercoagulable states
    Pregnancy
    Use of oral contraceptives
    Antithrombin III deficiency
    Protein C and S deficiencies
  Leukemia
Intracranial vascular anomalies
  Arteriovenous malformation
  Arterial aneurysm
  Carotid-cavernous fistula

exclusion. The lumbar puncture, however, may be deferred until a neuroimage excluding brain abscess or a space-occupying lesion that might contraindicate lumbar puncture has been obtained. In the absence of infection and frank intracranial subarachnoid hemorrhage, the spinal fluid examination is rarely helpful in defining the cause of the cerebrovascular disorder.

C. Imaging: CT scans of the brain and magnetic resonance images are often helpful in defining the extent of cerebral involvement with ischemia or hemorrhage. CT scans, however, may be normal within the first few hours of an ischemic stroke and, therefore, may need to be repeated several hours later. A CT scan early after the onset of neurologic deficits is valuable in excluding significant intracranial hemorrhage. This information may be helpful in the early stages of the patient's management and the decision to treat with anticoagulants.

Cerebral angiography is usually not urgently needed in the evaluation. However, cerebral angiography may be needed to confirm such disorders as fibromuscular dysplasia and cerebral arteritis. If angiography is done, all major vessels should be studied. If evidence of fibromuscular dysplasia is present in the intracranial or extracranial vessels, renal arteriography is indicated.

When seizures are prominent, an EEG may be used as an adjunct in the patient's evaluation. An EEG and sequential electroencephalographic monitoring may help in the evaluation of patients with severely depressed levels of consciousness.

Electrocardiography and echocardiography are useful both in the diagnostic approach to the patient and in ongoing monitoring and management, particularly when hypotension or cardiac irregularities complicate the clinical course.

Differential Diagnosis

Patients with an acute onset of neurologic deficits must be evaluated not only for cerebrovascular disease but also for other disorders that can cause focal neurologic deficits. Hypoglycemia, prolonged focal seizures, a prolonged postictal paresis (Todd's paralysis), meningitis, encephalitis, and brain abscess should all be considered. Migraine with focal neurologic deficits may be initially difficult to differentiate from ischemic stroke. Occasionally, the onset of a neurodegenerative disorder (eg, adrenoleukodystrophy) may begin with the abrupt onset of seizures and focal neurologic deficits. Drug abuse, particularly cocaine, and other toxin exposures must be sought for diligently.

Treatment

The initial management of children with stroke is aimed at providing support for their pulmonary, cardiovascular, and renal function. Appropriate fluid and electrolyte infusions should be started, and careful monitoring of heart rate and rhythm and blood pressure are required. Specific treatment of stroke depends in part upon the underlying pathogenesis and the specific predisposing disorder. In some situations, heparinization for emboli and consumption coagulopathies is indicated. In other disorders, such as fibromuscular dysplasia, treatment aimed at decreasing platelet adhesiveness may be an acceptable alternative to anticoagulation.

Long-term management requires intensive rehabilitation efforts, anticonvulsant treatment, and therapy aimed at improving the child's language, educational, and psychologic performance.

Prognosis

The outcome of stroke in infants and children is variable. Underlying predisposing conditions and the vascular territory involved all play a role in dictating the outcome for an individual patient. When the stroke involves extremely large portions of one hemisphere or large portions of both hemispheres and cerebral edema develops, the patient's level of consciousness may deteriorate rapidly, and death may occur within the first few days. Some patients may achieve almost complete recovery of neurologic function within several days if the cerebral territory is small. Seizures, either focal or generalized, may occur in 30–50% of patients at some point in the course of their cerebrovascular disorder. Chronic problems with learning, behavior, and activity are seen in many patients.

Gold AJ et al: Report of joint committee for stroke facilities. 9. Strokes in children (2 parts.) *Stroke* 1973;**4**:835, 1009.

Golden GS: Stroke syndromes in childhood. *Neurol Clin* 1985;**3**:59.

Roach ES, Riela AR: *Pediatric Cerebrovascular Disorders.* Futura, 1988.

Schoenberg BS, Mellinger JF, Schoenberg DG: Cerebrovascular disease in infants and children: A study of incidence, clinical features, and survival. *Neurology* 1978;**28**:763.

CONGENITAL MALFORMATIONS OF THE NERVOUS SYSTEM

Malformations of the nervous system occur in 1–3% of living neonates and are present in 40% of infants who die. Developmental anomalies of the central nervous system may result from a variety of causes, including infectious, toxic, metabolic, and vascular insults that affect the fetus. The specific type of malformation that results from such insults, however, may depend more upon the gestational period in which the insult occurs than on the specific cause. The period of induction, 0–28 days of gestation, is the period during which the neural plate appears and the neural tube forms and closes. Insults during this phase can result in a major absence of neural structures, such as anencephaly, or in a defect of neural tube closure, such as spina bifida, meningomyelocele, or encephalocele. Cellular proliferation and migration characterize neural development that occurs after 28 days of gestation. Lissencephaly, pachygyria, agyria, and agenesis of the corpus callosum represent disorders caused by insults that occur during the period of cellular proliferation and migration.

1. ABNORMALITIES OF NEURAL TUBE CLOSURE

Defects of neural tube closure constitute some of the most common forms of congenital malformations affecting the nervous system. Spina bifida with associated meningomyelocele or meningocele is commonly found in the lumbosacral region. Depending on the extent and severity of the involvement of the spinal cord and peripheral nerves, clinical findings include lower extremity weakness, bowel and bladder dysfunction, and hip dislocation. Surgical intervention to close meningoceles and meningomyeloceles is usually indicated. Additional treatment is necessary to manage chronic abnormalities of the urinary tract, orthopedic abnormalities such as kyphosis and scoliosis, and paresis of the lower extremities. Hydrocephalus commonly associated with meningomyelocele usually requires ventriculoperitoneal shunting.

Arnold-Chiari Malformations

Arnold-Chiari malformation type I consists of elongation and displacement of the caudal end of the brain stem into the spinal canal with protrusion of the cerebellar tonsils through the foramen magnum. In association with this hind brain malformation, there are often minor to moderate abnormalities of the base of the skull, including basilar impression (platybasia) and small foramen magnum. Arnold-Chiari malformation type I may remain asymptomatic for years, but in older children and young adults it may cause progressive ataxia, paresis of the lower cranial nerves, and progressive vertigo. Posterior cervical laminectomy may be necessary to provide relief from cervical cord compression. Ventriculoperitoneal shunting is required for hydrocephalus.

Arnold-Chiari malformation type II consists of the malformations found in Arnold-Chiari type I plus an associated lumbosacral meningomyelocele. Hydrocephalus is present in approximately 90% of children with Arnold-Chiari type II. These patients may also have aquaductal stenosis, hydromyelia, or syringomyelia. The clinical manifestations of Arnold-Chiari type II are most commonly caused by the associated hydrocephalus and meningomyelocele. In addition, dysfunction of the lower cranial nerves may be present.

Arnold-Chiari malformation type III is characterized by occipital encephalocele, a closure defect of the rostral end of the neural tube. Hydrocephalus is extremely common with this malformation.

In general, the diagnosis of neural tube defects is obvious at the time of birth. Diagnosis may be strongly suspected prenatally on the basis of ultrasonographic findings and the presence of elevated alpha-fetoprotein in the amniotic fluid.

2. DISORDERS OF CELLULAR PROLIFERATION AND MIGRATION

Lissencephaly

Lissencephaly is a sever malformation of brain characterized by an extremely smooth cortical surface with minimal sulcal and gyral development. Such a smooth surface is characteristic of fetal brain at the end of the first trimester. In addition, many brains with lissencephaly have a primitive cytoarchitectural construction with a 4-layered cerebral mantle instead of the mature 6-layered cerebral mantle. Pachygyria and agyria are closely associated with lissencephaly but represent more restricted forms of migrational abnormalities. Patients with lissencephaly usually suffer from severe neurodevelopmental delay, microcephaly, and seizures (including infantile spasms) and frequently have additional associated malformations and dysmorphic features. The Walker-Warburg syndrome or Miller-Dieker syndrome can often be identified in some of these patients. It is particularly important to identify these syndromes because of their genetic importance; Walker-Warburg syndrome is an autosomal recessive disorder, and Miller-Dieker syndrome is associated with defects of chromosome 17. In addition to these 2 syndromes, lissencephaly may be a component of Zellweger syndrome, a metabolic peroxisomal abnormality. Zellweger syndrome is diagnosed by the presence of elevated concentrations of very long chain fatty acids in plasma. A peroxisomal defect in fatty acid degradation in cultured skin fibroblasts confirms the diagnosis. No specific treatment for lissencephaly is available. Seizures may be controlled by the use of phenobarbital, phenytoin, or clonazepam.

Agenesis of the Corpus Callosum

Agenesis of the corpus callosum, once thought to be a relatively rare cerebral malformation, has been seen frequently with modern neuroimaging techniques such as CT and MRI. The cause of this malformation is unknown. Occasionally, it appears to be inherited in an autosomal dominant or autosomal recessive pattern. X-linked recessive patterns have also been described. Agenesis of the corpus callosum has been found in some patients with pyruvate dehydrogenase deficiency and in others with nonketotic hyperglycinemia. Most cases, however, are sporadic. Maldevelopment of the corpus callosum may be partial or complete. No specific clinical syndrome is typical of agenesis of the corpus callosum, although many patients have seizures, developmental delay, microcephaly, or mental retardation. Neurologic abnormalities may be related to microscopic cytoarchitectural abnormalities of the brain that occur in association with the agenesis of the corpus callosum. The malformation may be found coincidentally by neuroimaging studies in otherwise normal patients and has been described as a coincidental finding at autopsy in neurologically normal individuals. A special form of agenesis of the corpus callosum occurs in Aicardi's syndrome. In this X-linked disorder, agenesis of the corpus callosum is associated with infantile spasms, mental retardation, lacunar choreoretinopathy, and vertebral body abnormalities.

Dandy-Walker Malformation

Dandy-Walker malformation is characterized by vermian aplasia, cystic enlargement of the fourth ventricle, rostral displacement of the tentorium, and absence or atresia of the foramina of Magendie and Luschka. Although hydrocephalus is usually not present congenitally, it develops within the first few months of life, and 90% of those patients who develop hydrocephalus do so by the age of one year. On physical examination, there is often a rounded protuberance or exaggeration of the occiput of the cranium. In the absence of hydrocephalus and increased intracranial pressure, there may be few physical findings to suggest neurologic dysfunction. An ataxic syndrome occurs in fewer than 20% of patients and is usually late in appearing. Many long-term neurologic deficits result directly from hydrocephalus. Diagnosis of Dandy-Walker malformation is confirmed by CT or MRI scanning of the head. Treatment is directed at the management of hydrocephalus.

3. CRANIOSYNOSTOSIS

Craniosynostosis, or premature closure of cranial sutures, is usually sporadic and idiopathic. However, some patients have hereditary disorders, such as Apert syndrome and Crouzon's disease, that are associated with abnormalities of the digits, extremities, and heart. Occasionally, craniosynostosis may be associated with an underlying metabolic disturbance such as hyperthyroidism and hypophosphotasia. The most common form of craniosynostosis involves the sagittal suture and results in scaphocephaly, an elongation of the head in the anterior to posterior direction. Premature closure of the coronal sutures causes brachycephaly, an increase in cranial diameter from left to right. Unless many or all cranial sutures close prematurely, intracranial volume will not be compromised, and the brain's growth will not be impaired. Closure of only one or a few sutures will not cause impaired brain growth or neurologic dysfunction. Management of craniosynostosis is directed at preserving normal skull shape and consists of excising the fused suture and applying material to the edge of the craniectomy to prevent reossification of the bone edges. The best cosmetic effect on the skull is achieved when surgery is done during the first 6 months of life.

4. HYDROCEPHALUS

Hydrocephalus is characterized by an increased volume of cerebrospinal fluid in association with progressive ventricular dilatation. In communicating hydrocephalus, cerebrospinal fluid can circulate through the ventricular system and into the subarachnoid space without obstruction. In noncommunicating hydrocephalus, an obstruction blocks the flow of spinal fluid within the ventricular system or blocks the egress of spinal fluid from the ventricular system into the subarachnoid space. A wide variety of disorders, such as hemorrhage, infection, tumors, and congenital malformations, may play an etiologic role in development of hydrocephalus.

Clinical features of hydrocephalus include macrocephaly, an excessive rate of head growth, irritability, vomiting, loss of appetite, impaired up gaze, impaired extraocular movements, hypertonia of the lower extremities, and generalized hyperreflexia. Without treatment, optic atrophy may occur. In infants, papilledema may not be present, whereas older children with closed cranial sutures can eventually develop swelling of the optic disk.

Hydrocephalus can be diagnosed on the basis of the clinical course, physical examination findings, and CT scan or MRI findings. Radionuclide scans also demonstrate impaired CSF circulation through the ventricular and subarachnoid systems but are rarely needed for clinical diagnosis or management.

Treatment of hydrocephalus is directed at providing an alternative outlet for CSF from the intracranial compartment. The most common method is ventriculoperitoneal shunting. Other treatment should be directed, if possible, at the underlying cause of the hydrocephalus.

Barth PG: Disorders of neuronal migration. *Can J Neurol Sci* 1987;**14:**1.

Dobyns WB: Agenesis of the corpus callosum and gyral malformations are frequent manifestations of nonketotic hyperglycenemia. *Neurology* 1989;**39:**817.

Dobyns WB: The neurogenetics of lissencephaly. *Neurol Clin* 1989;**7:**89.

Hirsch JF et al: The Dandy-Walker malformation. *J Neurosurg* 1984;**61:**515.

Hoffman HJ, Epstein F (editors): *Disorders of the Developing Nervous System: Diagnosis and Treatment.* Blackwell, 1986.

Holmes LB, Driscoll SG, Atkins L: Etiologic heterogenicity of neural-tube defects. *N Engl J Med* 1976;**294:**365.

Parrish ML, Roessmann U, Levinsohn MW: Agenesis of the corpus callosum: A study of the frequency of associated malformations. *Ann Neurol* 1979;**6:**349.

Sarnat HB: Disturbances of late neuronal migrations in the perinatal period. *Am J Dis Child* 1987;**141:**969.

ABNORMAL HEAD SIZE

Head size reflects brain growth. Many variables govern head growth. The average head circumference of males is about 1 cm larger than that of females from term birth on, except during girls' earlier pubertal spurt. Generally, taller and heavier people have larger heads, and parental head sizes influence the child's head size. Worldwide, significantly undernourished populations show head circumference curves as much as 1 SD below those in well-fed populations. Within the range of normal, head size and degree of intelligence cannot be correlated. Furthermore, most children with head sizes between 2 and 3 SD from the mean will be normal, especially if the head circumference correlates with body size.

Head circumference should be measured at each well-child visit and more often in certain cases, eg, when the child—or even the adolescent—is seen for a possible disorder of growth and development or for a neurologic problem or when the head circumference falls 2 SD below or above the mean or crosses percentiles.

A thin, flexible, nonexpandable measuring tape should be used and the maximal occipitofrontal circumference checked at least twice. Variances of 0.5 cm in measurement are common and are about equal to the difference between a full or close-cut hair style. The measurement should then be plotted on a graph of standard head circumference based on sex.

1. MICROCEPHALY

A head circumference 3 SD or more below the mean for age and sex or one that increases too slowly or not at all denotes microcephaly. A head circumference of nearly 2 SD below the mean and falling off is equally significant.

Etiology

The causes of microcephaly resulting in irreparable interference to brain development are listed in Table 24–23.

Advanced maternal age may suggest a risk for trisomy. A careful history may uncover gestational maternal alcohol abuse, radiation exposure, or primary herpes infection at term. Perinatal insults as a cause are usually obvious. The placenta should be examined.

A head size small at birth proves intrauterine onset; a baby suffering insult at birth will have normal newborn head size with later dramatic fall-off and failure of head growth.

A family history of small heads and measuring those of close relatives may aid in diagnosing (rare) autosomal dominant microcephaly.

Clinical Findings

A. Symptoms and Signs: Microcephaly may be suspected in the full-term newborn and in infants up to 6 months of age whose chest circumference exceeds the head circumference (unless the child is very obese). Microcephaly may be discovered when the child is examined because of delayed developmental milestones or neurologic problems, such as

Table 24–23. Microcephaly.

Causes	Examples
Prenatal chromosomal	Trisomy 13, 18, 21
Malformation	Lissencephaly, schizencephaly
Syndromes	Rubenstein-Taybi, Cornelia de Lange
Toxins	alcohol, anticonvulsants (?), maternal phenylketonuria
Infections (intrauterine)	TORCHES[1]
Radiation	Maternal pelvis, 1st and 2nd trimester
Placental insufficiency	Toxemia, infection
Familial	Autosomal dominant, autosomal recessive
Perinatal hypoxia, trauma	Birth asphyxia, injury
Infections (perinatal)	Bacterial meningitis (especially group B streptococci) Viral encephalitis (coxsackie B, herpes II)
Metabolic	Hypoglycemia, phenylketonuria, maple syrup urine disease
Postnatal sequela from earlier insult	As above
Degenerative disease	Tay-Sachs, Krabbe's

[1]A mnemonic formula for *t*oxoplasmosis, *r*ubella, *c*ytomegalovirus, *h*erpes simplex, and *s*yphilis.

seizures or spasticity. There may be a marked backward slope of the forehead (as in familial microcephaly) with narrowing of the bitemporal diameter, and there may be occipital flattening that is not positional. The fontanelle may close earlier than expected; sutures may be unexpectedly prominent.

B. Laboratory Findings: These vary with the cause. Abdominal dermatoglyphics may be present when the injury occurred before the 19th week of gestation. If clinical factors warrant, titers for TORCHES (*t*oxoplasmosis, *r*ubella, *c*ytomegalovirus, *h*erpes simplex, *s*yphilis) then must be assessed. Elevated IgM titer, if obtained at birth, is most helpful; comparison to maternal titers, passive transfer to the infant, and rising titer postnatally are all important factors to analyze. Amino and organic acid screens on the baby are occasionally diagnostic. The mother may need to be screened for phenylketonuria. Karyotyping, including fragile X, should be considered.

C. Imaging: Skull films are indicated if there is suspicion of craniosynostosis. Sometimes microcephaly causes secondary acquired craniosynostosis. The head is usually "small normal" in congenital acquired craniostenosis; the head shape, however, is almost invariably abnormal. CT or MRI may aid in diagnosis (eg, of intracranial calcification, malformations, atrophy) and prognosis. Genetic counseling should be done in any infant with significant microcephaly. The radiologist may see typical findings of early intrauterine malformations. Examples include single ventricle of holoprosencephaly, periventricular calcifications of cytomegalovirus or other intrauterine TORCHES infection, or multiloculated encephalomalacia of birth asphyxia.

Differential Diagnosis

Congenital craniosynostosis involving multiple sutures is easily differentiated by inspection (head shape), history, identification of syndromes, hereditary pattern, and sometimes signs and symptoms of increased intracranial pressure. Treatable undergrowth of the brain due to hypopituitarism or severe protein-calorie undernutrition is recognized by the history and clinical findings.

Treatment & Prognosis

Except for the treatable disorders noted above, treatment is usually supportive and directed at the multiple neurologic and sensory deficits and any endocrine disturbances (eg, diabetes insipidus) encountered. Many children with head circumferences more than 2 SD below the mean show variable degrees of mental retardation (as in premature infants). The notable exceptions are found in cases of hypopituitarism (rare) or familial autosomal dominant microcephaly. However, one population study (926 children) showed that only one of 6 microcephalic children followed to age 15 achieved poorly in school.

Ahlfors K et al: Microcephaly and congenital cytomegalovirus infection: Prospective and retrospective study. *Pediatrics* 1986;**78:**1058. [Circumspection required re TORCHES titer and cytomegalovirus urine cultures.]

Ishihara T et al: Growth and achievement of large and small headed children in a normal population. *Brain Dev* 1988;**10:**295. [Population study of microcephaly.]

Jaffe M et al: The dilemma in prenatal diagnosis of idiopathic microcephaly. *Dev Med Child Neurol* 1987; **29:**187. [Diagnosis of idiopathic microcephaly in utero isn't practical until it is too late for therapeutic abortion.]

Jawarski M et al: Computed tomography of the head in evaluation of microcephaly. *Pediatrics* 1986;**78:**1064.

Rossi L et al: Autosomal dominant microcephaly without mental retardation. *Am J Dis Child* 1987;**141:**655. [Rare.]

2. MACROCEPHALY (Megalencephaly)

A head circumference more than 3 SD above the mean for age and sex or one that increases too rapidly denotes macrocephaly and suggests an abnormally large brain (megalencephaly). A head circumference of 2 SD above the mean, followed by accelerating growth, is equally significant but may not be pathologic.

Clinical Findings

Clinical and laboratory findings vary with the underlying process. In infants, transillumination of the skull with an intensely bright flashlight or "Chun's gun" in a completely darkened room may disclose chronic subdural effusions, hydrocephalus, hydranencephaly, and large cystic defects.

A surgically or medically treatable condition must be ruled out; thus, the first major decision is whether and when to perform an imaging study.

A. Imaging Study Deferred:

1. "Catch-up growth," as in the thriving, neurologically intact premature infant whose rapid head enlargement is most marked in the first weeks of life, or the infant in the early phase of recovery from deprivation dwarfism. As the expected "normal" is reached, head circumference growth slows down, then follows the percentile curve normal for the child. If the fontanelle is open, the less expensive (noninvasive) cranial ultrasound can assess ventricles and reassure that hydrocephalus is not occurring.

2. Familial macrocephaly, where another family member may have an unusually large head and there are no signs or symptoms referable to such disorders as neurocutaneous dysplasias (especially neurofibromatosis) or cerebral gigantism (Sotos' syndrome) nor significant mental or neurologic abnormalities in the child.

3. The older infant or child who is either so relatively intact or so profoundly neurologically damaged that serial head circumference measurements about 2–4 weeks apart for a few weeks or months, with equally close attention to neurologic status, may obviate the need for a CT scan.

B. Brain Scan Indicated: CT or magnetic resonance brain imaging—or ultrasonography, if the anterior fontanelle is open—is used to define any structural cause of macrocephaly and to determine an operable disorder. Even when the condition is not treatable (or benign), the information gained may permit more accurate diagnosis and prognosis, guide management and genetic counseling, and serve as a basis for comparison should future abnormal cranial growth or neurologic changes necessitate a repeat study. An imaging study is necessary if there are any signs or symptoms of increased intracranial pressure (see Table 24–20).

Classification

Macrocephaly with increased intracranial pressure requires diagnosis; aggressive hydrocephalus is the most common cause. Mild, nonprogressive hydrocephalus—mildly dilatated ventricles that do not serially enlarge or that are not causing any adverse symptoms or signs—can be followed without medical or surgical therapy. The same principal is true for intracranial cysts or effusions. Details regarding types of hydrocephalus and therapies are discussed in that section.

There is some nosologic confusion regarding the third subdivision of macrocephaly. Alvarez et al blend benign familial macrocephaly and idiopathic external hydrocephalus. This syndrome is that of an infant with large head, large subarachnoid space (especially frontally), and, often, mild ventriculomegaly. Motor development may be delayed. There is a positive family history in most cases. Measurements of parents, especially the father, are important (as is an imaging study) in establishing the diagnosis. Progressive hydrocephalus rarely develops. Eventual motor and speech development, even if initially delayed, is usually normal. Invasive studies are not needed; observation is all that is necessary. Familial macrocephaly is a benign, self-limited condition that resolves without active treatment.

In summary, familial macrocephaly is a relatively common cause of a large head. Serial imaging studies show dilatated subarachnoid spaces and, sometimes, dilatated ventricles that do not progressively enlarge. The head of at least one parent is often large. Serial examinations to make sure the child has normal development and serial imaging studies establish the diagnosis.

Megalencephaly, or large brain, is most often a normal variant. The most frequent pathologic cause is a neurocutaneous disorder such as neurofibromatosis or tuberous sclerosis. Rarely, a large brain and sometimes mildly dilatated ventricles are associated with Sotos' syndrome of cerebral gigantism. Occasionally, patients with dwarfism syndromes such as achondroplasia have a large head, sometimes even hydrocephalus, usually nonprogressive. After identification of this syndrome, the head size needs to be followed, and sometimes serial imaging studies are necessary. A rare cause of a large brain is storage of brain lipids due to lack of catabolic enzyme. Patients with Hurler syndrome or mucopolysaccharidosis may have large brains from stored gangliosides and obstructed subarachnoid spaces from mucopolysaccharides.

Another possible cause of macrocephaly is a thick skull. Table 24–24 provides some examples.

In sporadic megalencephaly, the child is normal, and no other family member is of unusually large size or has an unusually large head size. The child may be excessively tall. In some of these cases, CT ventricular measurements (bifrontal and bicaudate distances) may be slightly enlarged. These children should be followed with serial measurements of head circumference and neurologic examinations.

Alvarez L et al: Idiopathic external hydrocephalus: Natural history and relationship to benign familial macrocephaly. *Pediatrics* 1986;**77**:901.

Bosnjak V: Cranial ultrasonography in the evaluation of macrocrania in infancy. *Dev Med Child Neurol* 1989; **31**:66.

Table 24–24. Macrocephaly.

Causes	Examples
"Pseudomacrocephaly," "pseudohydrocephalus," "catch-up growth" crossing percentiles	Premature "grower," cystic fibrosis treatment, congenital heart disease recovery. Parenteral alimentation.
Increased intracranial pressure With dilatated ventricles With other mass	Progressive hydrocephalus Subdural effusion Arachnoid, porencephalic cyst Tumor
Benign familial macrocephaly: idiopathic external hydrocephalus	"External hydrocephalus" "Benign enlargement of the subarachnoid spaces" "Congenital communicating Hydrocephalus" "Benign subdural collections of infancy"
Megalencephaly (large brain) With neurocutaneous disorder	Benign familial (see above) Neurofibromatosis Tuberous Sclerosis, etc
With gigantism	Sotos' syndrome
With dwarfism	Achondroplasia
Metabolic Lysosomal	Mucopolysaccharidoses Metachromatic leukodystrophy
Other leukodystrophy	Canavan's spongy degeneration
Thickened skull	Fibrous dysplasia (bone) Hemolytic anemia (marrow) (sicklemia, thalassemia)

Bray PF et al: Occipitofrontal head circumference: An accurate measure of intracranial volume. *J Pediatr* 1986; **75**:303.

DeMeyer W: Megalencephaly: Types, clinical syndromes, and management. *Pediatr Neurol* 1986;**2**:321.

Dodge PR, Holmes SJ, Sotos JF: Cerebral gigantism. *Dev Med Child Neurol* 1983;**25**:248.

Gooskens RHJM et al: Megalencephaly: Definition and classification. *Brain Dev* 1988;**10**:1.

Lorber J, Priestley BL: Children with large heads: A practical approach to diagnosis in 557 children with special reference to 109 children with megalencephaly. *Dev Med Child Neurol* 1981;**23**:494.

Nellhaus G: Head circumference from birth to eighteen years: Practical composite international and interracial graphs. *Pediatrics* 1968;**41**:106.

Nickle RE, Gallenstein JS: Developmental prognosis for infants with benign enlargement of the subarachnoid spaces. *Dev Med Child Neurol* 1987;**29**:181.

NEUROCUTANEOUS DYSPLASIAS

Neurocutaneous dysplasias are diseases of the neuroectoderm and sometimes involve endoderm and mesoderm. Birth marks and skin growths appearing later often suggest a need to look for brain, spinal cord, and eye disease. Hamartomas (histologically normal tissue growing abnormally rapidly or in aberrant sites) are common. The most common dysplasias are genetically dominantly inherited. Benign and even malignant tumors may develop.

1. NEUROFIBROMATOSIS (Recklinghausen's Disease)

Essentials of Diagnosis

- More than 6 café au lait spots 5 mm in greatest diameter in prepubertal individuals and over 15 mm of greatest diameter in postpubertal individuals.
- 2 or more neurofibromas of any type or one plexiform neurofibroma.
- Freckling in the axillary or inguinal regions.
- Optic glioma.
- 2 or more Lisch nodules (iris hamartomas).
- Distinctive osseous lesions, such as sphenoid dysplasia or thinning of long bone with or without pseudarthroses.
- First-degree relative (parent, sibling, offspring) with neurofibromatosis type I by above criteria.

Clinical Findings

A. Symptoms and Signs: The most common presenting symptoms are cognitive or psychomotor problems, eg, school difficulties; 40% of patients have learning disabilities, and mental retardation is seen in 8%. Family history is important in identifying dominant gene manifestations in parents; they should be examined in detail. The history should focus on lumps or masses causing disfigurement, functional problems, or pain. The clinician should ask about visual problems; strabismus or amblyopia dictate a search for optic glioma, a common tumor in this disease. Any progressive neurologic deficit might indicate studies for a tumor of the spinal cord or central nervous system. Tumors of the eighth nerve virtually are not seen in the common neurofibromatosis type I.

The physician should check blood pressure and examine the spine for scoliosis and the limbs for pseudarthroses. Head measurement often shows macrocephaly. Hearing and vision need to be assessed. The eye examination should include a check for proptosis and iris Lisch nodules; the optic disk should be examined for atrophy or papilledema. Short stature or precocious puberty are occasional findings. An examination for neurologic manifestations of tumors (eg, asymmetric reflexes, spasticity) is important.

B. Laboratory Findings: Laboratory tests are not likely to be of any value in asymptomatic patients. Selected patients require brain MRI or CT with special cuts through the optic nerves to rule out optic glioma. Hypertension necessitates a look at renal arteries for dysplasia and stenosis as a cause. Cognitive and school achievement testing may be indicated. Scoliosis or limb abnormalities should be studied by appropriate roentgenograms, even an MRI scan of the spinal cord and roots.

Differential Diagnosis

Patients with Albright's syndrome often have larger café au lait spots with precocious puberty. Many normal individuals have one or 2 café au lait spots.

Treatment

Genetic counseling is important. The risk to siblings is up to 50%. The disease may be progressive, with serious complications rarely seen. Sometimes patients worsen during puberty or pregnancy. Family members need to be evaluated for presence of the gene. Annual or semiannual visits are important in the early detection of school problems or bony or neurologic abnormalities.

Multidisciplinary clinics are being established at medical centers around the United States and are often an excellent resource. Prenatal diagnosis is likely on the horizon, but the variability of manifestations (trivial to severe) will make therapeutic abortion an unlikely option.

Information for lay people and physicians is available from the National Neurofibromatosis Foundation, Inc, 70 West 40th Street, New York, NY 10018.

Gomez MR (editor): *Neurocutaneous Diseases*. Butterworth, 1987.

National Institutes of Health Consensus Statement: Neurofibromatosis. Vol 6, No. 12, 1987.

Riccardi VM: The multiple forms of neurofibromatosis. *Pediatr Rev* 1982;**3**:293.

2. TUBEROUS SCLEROSIS (Bourneville's Disease)

Essentials of Diagnosis

- Facial angiofibromas or subungual fibromas.
- Often hypomelanotic macules, gingival fibromas.
- Retinal hamartomas.
- Cortical tubers or subependymal glial nodules often calcified.
- Renal angiomyolipomas.

General Considerations

Tuberous sclerosis, a disease of unknown cause, is of autosomal dominant inheritance. The classic triad of seizures, mental retardation, and adenoma sebaceum are seen in only one-third of patients. The disease, thought to have a high rate of mutation, as a result of more sophisticated techniques such as MRI, parents formerly thought not to harbor the gene are now being diagnosed as asymptomatic carriers.

Like neurofibromatosis, tuberous sclerosis may present with a wide variety of symptoms. The patient may be asymptomatic but for skin findings or may be devastated by severe infantile spasms in early infancy, continuing epilepsy, and mental retardation. Seizures in early infancy correlate with later mental retardation.

Clinical Findings

A. Symptoms and Signs:

1. Dermatologic features—Skin findings bring most cases to the physician's attention. Ninety-six percent have one or more hypomelanotic macules, facial angiofibromas, ungual fibromas, or shagreen patches. Adenoma sebaceum or the facial skin hamartomas may first appear in early childhood, often on the cheek, chin, and dry sites of the skin where acne is not usually seen. They often have a reddish hue. The off-white hypomelanotic macules are more easily seen in tanned or dark-skinned individuals. They often are oval or "ash leaf" in shape and follow dermatomes. A Wood's lamp or ultraviolet light shows the macules more clearly—a great help in the light-skinned patient. In the scalp, poliosis, or whitened hair, is the equivalent. In infancy, the presence of these macules accompanied by seizures is virtually diagnostic of the disease. Subungual or periungual fibromas are more common in the toes. Leathery, orange peel-like shagreen patches support the diagnosis. Café au lait spots can occasionally be seen. Fibrous or raised plaques may resemble coalescent angiofibromas.

2. Neurologic features—Seizures are the most common presenting symptom. Five percent of infantile spasms (a malign epileptic syndrome) occur in patients with tuberous sclerosis. Thus, any patient presenting with infantile spasms (and the parents as well) should be carefully examined for this disorder. An imaging study of the central nervous system, such as a CT scan, may show calcified subependymal nodules; an MRI scan may show dysmyelinating white matter lesions or cortical tubers. Virtually any kind of symptomatic seizure, eg, atypical absence, partial complex, and generalized tonic-clonic seizures, may occur.

3. Mental retardation—Mental retardation is seen in up to 50% of patients referred to centers; the incidence is likely much lower in randomly selected patients. Patients with seizures are more prone to retardation or learning disabilities.

4. Renal lesions—Renal cysts or angiomyolipomas may be asymptomatic. Sometimes, hematuria or obstruction of urine flow occurs; the latter requires an operation. An ultrasound of the kidneys should be done in any patient suspected of tuberous sclerosis, both to aid in diagnosis if lesions are found and to rule out renal obstructive disease.

5. Cardiopulmonary involvement—Rarely, cystic lung disease may occur. Rhabdomyomas of the heart may be asymptomatic but can lead to outflow obstruction, conduction difficulties, and death. Chest x-rays and echocardiograms can detect these rare manifestations.

6. Eye involvement—Retinal hamartomas are often near the disk; if distant from the disk, they are more "diagnostic" for this syndrome.

7. Skeletal involvement—Findings sometimes helpful in diagnosis are cystic rarefactions of the bones of the fingers or toes.

B. Diagnostic Studies: Plain radiographs may detect areas of thickening within the skull, spine, and pelvis and cystic lesions in the hands and feet. Chest x-rays may show lung honeycombing. More helpful is CT scanning, which can show the virtually pathognomonic subependymal nodular calcifications and sometimes widened gyri or tubers and brain tumors. Contrast material may show the often classically located tumors near the foramen interventriculare. Hypomyelinated lesions may be seen with magnetic resonance imaging.

The EEG is helpful in delineating the presence of seizure discharges.

Treatment

Therapy is as indicated by underlying disease, eg, seizures and tumors of the brain, kidney, and heart. Skin lesions on the face may need dermabrasion or other removal. Genetic counseling emphasizes identification of the carrier. There is a 50% risk for appearance in offspring if the parent is a carrier. The patient should be seen annually for counseling and reexamination in childhood. Identification of the chromosome on a DNA marker link may in the future make intrauterine diagnosis possible.

Hunt A, Dennis J: Psychiatric disorder among children with tuberous sclerosis. *Dev Med Child Neurol* 1987; **29:**191.

Oppenheimer EY et al: Late appearance of hypopigmented maculae in tuberous sclerosis. *Am J Dis Child* 1985; **139:**408.

Roche ES et al: Magnetic resonance imaging in tuberous sclerosis. *Arch Neurol* 1987;**44:**301.

Sugita K et al: Tuberous sclerosis: Report of two cases studied by computer assisted cranial tomography within one week after birth. *Brain Dev* 1985;**7:**438.

3. ENCEPHALOFACIAL ANGIOMATOSIS (Sturge-Weber Disease)

Sturge-Weber disease consists of a facial port wine nevus involving the upper part of the face (in the first division of the fifth nerve), a venous angioma of the meninges in the occipitoparietal regions, and choroidal angioma. The syndrome has been described without the facial nevus.

Clinical Findings

In infancy, the eye may show congenital glaucoma, or buphthalmos, with a cloudy, enlarged cornea. In early stages, the facial nevus may be the only indication, with no findings in the brain, even on radiologic studies. The characteristic atrophy and calcifications of the cortex and meningoangiomatosis may appear with time, solidifying the diagnosis.

Physical examination may show focal seizures or hemiparesis on the side opposite the cerebral lesion. The facial nevus may be much more extensive than just the first division of the fifth nerve; for example, it can involve the lower face, mouth, lip, neck, and even torso. Hemiatrophy of the opposite limbs may occur. Mental handicap may result from poorly controlled seizures. Late-appearing glaucoma and, rarely, central nervous system hemorrhage occur.

Radiologic studies may show calcification of the cortex; CT scanning may show this much earlier than plain film studies. MRI scans often show underlying brain involvement.

The EEG often shows depression of voltage over the involved area in early stages; later, epileptiform abnormalities may be present focally.

Treatment

The disease is sporadic. Early control of seizures is important to avoid consequent developmental setback. If seizures do not occur, normal development is expected. Careful examination of the newborn, with ophthalmologic assessment to detect early buphthalmos, is indicated. Rarely, surgical removal of the involved meninges and the involved portion of the brain may be indicated, even hemispherectomy.

Taly AB et al: Sturge-Weber-Dimitri disease without facial nevus. *Neurology* 1987;**37**:1063.

4. VON HIPPEL-LINDAU DISEASE (Retinocerebellar Angiomatosis)

Von Hippel-Lindau disease is a rare, dominantly inherited condition with retinal and cerebellar hemangioblastomas, cysts of the kidneys, pancreas, and epididymis, and sometimes renal cancers. The patient may present with ataxia, slurred speech, and nystagmus due to a hemangioblastoma of the cerebellum or with a medullary spinal cord cystic hemangioblastoma. Retinal detachment may occur from hemorrhage or exudate in the retinal vascular malformation. Rarely, a pancreatic cyst or renal tumor may be the presenting symptom.

The diagnostic criteria for the disease are a retinal or cerebellar hemangioblastoma with or without positive family history, intra-abdominal cyst, or renal cancer.

Coulam CM et al: Hippel-Lindau syndrome. *Semin Roentgenol* 1976;**11**:61.

CENTRAL NERVOUS SYSTEM DEGENERATIVE DISORDERS OF INFANCY & CHILDHOOD

Essentials of Diagnosis

■ Arrest of psychomotor development.

■ Loss, usually progressive but at variable rates, of mental and motor functioning and often vision.

■ Seizures are common in some disorders.

■ Symptoms and signs vary with age at onset and primary sites of involvement of specific types.

General Considerations

The central nervous system degenerative disorders of infancy and childhood are fortunately rare. An early clinical pattern of decline often follows normal early development. Referral for sophisticated biochemical testing is usually necessary before definitive diagnosis can be made. (See Table 24–25 and Table 24–26.)

Kimura S, Goebel H: Light and electron microscopy study of juvenile neuronal ceroid-lipofuscinosis lymphocytes. *Pediatr Neurol* 1988;**4**:148.

Mehler M, Rabinowich L: Inflammatory myeloclastic diffuse sclerosis. *Ann Neurol* 1988;**23**:413.

Menkes J: Huntington disease: Finding the gene and after. *Pediatr Neurol* 1988;**4**:73.

Naidu S et al: Phenotypic and genotypic variability of generalized peroxisomal disorders. *Pediatr Neurol* 1988;**4**:5.

ATAXIAS OF CHILDHOOD

1. ACUTE CEREBELLAR ATAXIA

Acute cerebellar ataxia occurs most commonly in children 2–6 years of age. The onset is abrupt, and the evolution of symptoms is rapid. In about half of cases, there is a prodromal illness with fever, respiratory or gastrointestinal symptoms, or an exanthem within 3 weeks of onset. Associated viral infections include varicella, rubeola, mumps, rubella, echovirus infections, poliomyelitis, infectious mononucleosis, and influenza. Bacterial infections such as scarlet fever and salmonellosis have also been incriminated.

Clinical Findings

A. Symptoms and Signs: Ataxia of the trunk and extremities may be severe, so that the child exhibits a staggering, reeling gait and inability to sit without support or to reach for objects; or there may be only mild unsteadiness. Hypotonia, tremor of the extremities, and horizontal nystagmus may be present. Speech may be slurred. The child frequently is irritable, and vomiting may occur.

There are no clinical signs of increased intracranial pressure. Sensory and reflex testing usually shows no abnormalities.

B. Laboratory Findings: Cerebrospinal fluid pressure and protein and glucose levels are normal; slight lymphocytosis (up to about 30/μL) may be present. Attempts should be made to identify the eti-

Table 24–25. Central nervous system degenerative disorders of infancy.

Disease	Enzyme Defect and Genetics	Onset	Early Manifestations	Vision and Hearing	Somatic Findings	Motor System	Seizures	Laboratory and Tissue Studies	Course
WHITE MATTER									
Globoid (Krabbe's) leukodystrophy	Recessive. Galactocerebrosidase and lactosylceramidase 1 deficiency.	First 6 months; "late-onset forms."	Feeding difficulties. Shrill cry. Irritability. Arching of back.	Optic atrophy, mid-course to late. Hyperacusis occasionally.	Head often small. Often underweight.	Early spasticity, occasionally preceded by hypotonia. Prolonged nerve conduction.	Early. Myoclonic and generalized.	CSF protein elevated; usually normal in late-onset forms. Sural nerve: nonspecific myelin breakdown. Enzyme deficiency in leukocytes, cultured skin fibroblasts.	Rapid. Death usually by 1½–2 years. Late-onset cases may live 5–10 years.
Metachromatic leukodystrophy	Recessive. Arylsulfatase A deficiency.	Second year. Less often, later in childhood.	Incoordination, especially gait disturbance; then general regression. Reverse in juveniles.	Optic atrophy, usually late. Hearing normal.	Head enlarged late. None in juvenile form.	Combined upper and lower motor neuron signs. Ataxia. Prolonged nerve conduction.	Infrequent, usually late and generalized.	Metachromatic cells in urine: negative sulfatase A test. CSF protein elevated; occasionally normal early. Sural nerve biopsy: metachromasia. Enzyme deficiency in leukocytes, cultured skin fibroblasts.	Moderately slow. Death in infantile form by 3–8 years, in "juvenile" form by 10–15 years.
Adrenoleukodystrophy and variants	X-linked recessive. Neonatal form recessive.	5–10 years New-born.	Impaired intellect, behavioral problems.	"Cortical blindness and deafness."		Ataxia, spasticity. Motor deficits may be asymmetric, or one-sided initially.	Occasionally.	Hyperpigmentation and adrenocortical insufficiency.[1] ACTH elevated. Accumulation of very long chain fatty acids. Plasma test available.	Fairly rapid, death usually within 2–3 years after onset.
Pelizaeus-Merzbacher disease	X-linked recessive; rare female.	(?) Birth to 2 years.	"Eye rolling" often shortly after birth. Head bobbing. Slow loss of intellect.	Slowly developing optic atrophy. Hearing normal.	Head and body normal.	Cerebellar signs early, hyperactive deep reflexes. Spasticity usually only very late.	Usually only late.	None specific. Brain biopsy: extensive demyelination with small perivascular islands of intact myelin.	Exceedingly slow, often seemingly stationary. Many survive well into adult life.
DIFFUSE, BUT PRIMARILY GRAY MATTER									
Poliodystrophy (Alpers' disease)	Occasionally familial, recessive. Possibly viral. Metabolic forms.	Infancy to adolescence.	Variable: loss of intellect, seizures, incoordination.	"Cortical blindness and deafness."	Head normal initially; may fail to grow.	Variable: incoordination, spasticity.	Often initial manifestation: myoclonic, akinetic, and generalized.	Non specific. CSF protein normal or slightly elevated. Extensive neuronal loss in cortex: may ocur very late. Citric acid cycle defects. Increased serum pyruvate, lactate.	Usually rapid, with death within 1–3 years after onset.
Tay-Sachs disease and G_{M2} gangliosidosis variants: Sandhoff disease; juvenile; chronic-adult.	Recessive. Hexosaminidase deficiencies. Tay-Sachs 93% East European Jewish; hexosaminidase A and S. Others panethnic. Sandhoff hexosaminidase A and B.	Tay-Sachs, Sandhoff similar: 3–6 months. Others 2–6 years or later. Juvenile: partial hexosaminidase A.	Variable: shrill cry, loss of vision, infantile spasms, arrest of development. In juvenile and chronic forms: motor difficulties; later, mental difficulties.	Cherry-red macula, early blindness. Hyperacusis early. Strabismus in juvenile form, blindness late.	Head enlarged late. Liver occasionally enlarged. None in juvenile or chronic forms.	Initially floppy. Eventual decerebrate rigidity. In juvenile and chronic forms: dysarthria, ataxia, spasticity.	Frequent, in mid-course and late. Infantile spasms and generalized.	Blood smears: vacuolated lymphocytes; basophilic hypergranulation. Enzyme deficienceis in serum, leukocytes, cultured skin fibroblasts.	Moderately rapid. Death usually by 2–5 years. In juvenile form, 5–15 years.
Niemann-Pick disease and variants	50% Jewish. Recessive. Sphingomyelinase deficiency. In variants, enzyme defects unknown.	First 6 months. In variants, later onset; often non-Jewish.	Slow development. Protruding belly.	Cherry-red macula in 35–50%. Blindness late. Deafness occasionally.	Head usually normal. Spleen enlarged more than liver. Occasional xanthomas of skin.	Initially floppy. Eventually spastic. Occasionally extrapyramidal signs.	Rare and late.	Blood: vacuolated lymphocytes; increased lipids. X-rays: "mottled" lungs, decalcified bones. "Foam cells" in bone marrow, spleen, lymph nodes; lipid analysis of nodes.	Moderately slow. Death usually by 3–5 years.

Table 24–25 (cont'd.). Central nervous system degenerative disorders of infancy.

Disease	Enzyme Defect and Genetics	Onset	Early Manifestations	Vision and Hearing	Somatic Findings	Motor System	Seizures	Laboratory and Tissue Studies	Course
Infantile Gaucher's disease (glucosyl ceramide lipidosis)	Recessive. Glucocerebrosidase deficiency	First 6 months; rarely, late infancy.	Stridor or hoarse cry. Retraction. Feeding difficulties.	Occasional cherry-red macula. Convergent squint. Deafness occasionally.	Head usually normal. Liver and spleen equally enlarged.	Opisthotonos early, followed rapidly by decerebrate rigidity.	Rare and late.	Anemia. Increased acid phosphatase. X-rays: thinned cortex, trabeculation of bones. "Gaucher cells" in bone marrow, spleen. Enzyme deficiency in leukocytes or cultured skin fibroblasts.	Very rapid.
Lipogranulomatosis (Farber's disease)	Ceramidase deficiency.	Early in infancy.	Hoarseness, irritability, restricted joint movements.	Usually normal.	Painful nodular swelling of joints; subcutaneous nodules.	Psychomotor retardation and progressive paralysis.	Usually none.	Chest x-rays may show pulmonary infiltrates. Nodules: granulomatous lesions, resembling those in reticuloendotheliosis.	Rapid; death usually in 1–2 years.
Generalized gangliosidosis and juvenile type (G_{M1} gangliosidoses)	Recessive. Beta-galactosidase deficiency.	First year; less often, second year.	Arrest of development. Protruding belly. Coarse facies in infantile (generalized) form.	50% "cherry-red spot." Hearing usually normal. In juvenile type, occasionally retinitis pigmentosa.	Head enlarged early. Liver enlarged more than spleen.	Initially floppy, eventually spastic.	Usually late.	Blood: vacuolated lymphocytes. X-rays: dorsolumbar kyphosis, "beaking" of vertebrae. "Foam cells" similar to those in Niemann-Pick disease.	Very rapid. Death within a few years. Slower in juvenile type.
Subacute necrotizing encephalomyelopathy (Leigh's disease)	Recessive Variable: thiamine triphosphate "inhibitor." Also deficiency of pyruvate carboxylase, pyruvate dehydrogenase.	Infancy to late childhood.	Difficulties in feeding. Feeble or absent cry. Floppiness.	Optic atrophy, often early. Roving eye movements.	Head usually normal, occasionally small. Cardiac and renal tubular dysfunction occasionally.	Flaccid and immobile; may become spastic. Spinocerebellar forms.	Rare and late.	Increased blood lactate and pyruvate. CSF, urine for "inhibitor." "Inhibitor" in brain, liver, heart, skeletal muscle.	Usually rapid in infants, but may be slow with death after several years. Central hypoventilation a frequent cause of death.
"Steel wool," or "kinky hair," disease (Menkes')	X-linked recessive. Defect in copper absorption.	Infancy.	Peculiar facies. Secondary hair white, twisted, split. Hypothermia.	May show optic disk pallor and microcysts of pigment epithelium.	Normal to small.	Variable: floppy to spastic.	Myoclonic, infantile spasms, status epilepticus.	Defective adsorption of copper. Cerebralangiography shows elongated arteries. Hair shows pili torti, split shafts. CT scan may show diffuse multifocal areas of low density.	Moderately rapid. Death usually by 3–4 years.
Huntington's disease	Dominant. Genetic marker on chromosome 4.	10% childhood onset.	Rigidity, dementia.	Ophthalmoplegia late.	None.	Rigidity. Chorea frequently absent in children.	50% with major motor seizures.	CT scan may show "butterfly" atrophy of caudate and putamen.	Moderately rapid with death in 5–15 years.
Bassen-Kornzweig disease	Recessive. Primary defect unknown.	Early childhood.	Diarrhea in infancy.	Retinitis pigmentosa; late ophthalmoplegia.	None.	Ataxia, late extrapyramidal movement disorder.	None.	Abetalipoproteinemia; acanthocytosis, low serum vitamin E.	Progression arrested with vitamin E.

[1] CSF gamma globulin (IgG) is considered elevated in children when above 9% of total protein (possibly even > 8.3%); definitely elevated when > 14%.

Table 24–26. Central nervous system degenerative disorders of childhood.[1]

Disease	Enzyme Defect and Genetics	Onset	Early Manifestations	Vision and Hearing	Motor System	Seizures	Laboratory and Tissue Studies	Course
Neuroaxonal degeneration (Seitelberger's disease). Same as, or resembling, Hallervorden-Spatz disease	Familial, (?) recessive. Girls more frequent than boys. Defect unknown.	1–3 years.	Arrest of development and dementia. Loss of motor functions. Occasionally hypesthesia over trunk and legs.	Nystagmus frequent; optic atrophy, hearing impairment.	Combined upper and lower motor neuron lesions. Early, may lie in "frog" position.	Variable, but usually not a prominent feature.	Denervation on EMG; elevated serum LDH and transaminase. Increased iron uptake in region of basal ganglia by scintillation counter probes over the temples. Brain and sural nerve: axonal swellings or "spheroids." Iron deposition in globus pallidus.	Very slowly progressive, with death early in second decade or earlier.
Neuronal ceroid lipofuscinosis (cerebromacular degenerations): Late infantile cerebral sphingolipidosis (Bielschowsky-Jansky disease)	Recessive. Defect unknown.	2–4 years.	Ataxia. Visual difficulties. Arrested intellectual development.	Pigmentary degeneration of macula. Optic atrophy. Hearing may be impaired.	Ataxia, spasticity progressing to decerebrate rigidity.	Often early: myoclonic and later generalized; difficult to control.	Blood: vacuolated lymphocytes, azurophilic dispersed hypergranulation of polymorphonuclear cells. Electroretinography helpful. Bone marrow: sea-blue histiocytes. In skin, skeletal muscle, peripheral nerves, brain: "curvilinear bodies" and "fingerprint profiles"; autofluorescent lipopigments.	Moderately slow. Death in 3–8 years.
Subacute sclerosing panencephalitis (Dawson's disease, SSPE)	None. Relatively common. Measles "slow virus" infection. Also reported as result of rubella.	3–22 years. Rarely earlier or later.	Impaired intellect, emotional lability, incoordination.	Occasionally chorioretinitis or optic atrophy. Hearing normal.	Ataxia, slurred speech, occasionally involuntary movements, spasticity progressing to decerebrate rigidity.	Myoclonic and akinetic seizures relatively early; later, focal and generalized.	CSF protein normal to moderately elevated. High CSF gamma globulin;[2] oligoclonal bands. Elevated CSF and serum measles (or rubella) antibody titers. Characteristic EEG. Brain biopsy: inclusion body encephalitis; culturing of measles virus, possibly rubella virus.	Variable, from death in months to years. Remissions of variable duration may occur. Isoprinosine produces long-term remissions.
Multiple sclerosis (See also Transverse Myelitis and Neuromyelitis Optica, Table 24–31).	None. Diagnosis difficult in childhood. Defect unknown. ?Slow virus infection.	2 years on.	Highly variable: may strike one or more sites of CNS. Paresthesias common.	Optic neuritis; diplopia, nystagmus at some time. Vestibulocochlear nerves occasionally affected.	Motor weakness, spasticity, ataxia, sphincter disturbances, slurred speech, mental difficulties.	Rare: focal or generalized.	CSF may show slight pleocytosis, elevation of protein and gamma globulin;[2] oligoclonal bands present. CT scan may show areas of demyelination. Auditory, visual, and somatosensory evoked responses often show lesions in respective pathways. Changes in T cell subsets.	Variable: complete remission possible. Recurrent attacks and involvement of multiple sites are prerequisites for diagnosis.
Cerebrotendinous xanthomatosis	?Recessive. Abnormal accumulation of cholesterol.	Late childhood to adolescence.	Xanthomas in tendons. Mental deterioration.	Cataracts; xanthelasma.	Cerebellar deficits. Late: bulbar paralysis.	Myoclonus.	Xanthomas may appear in lungs. Xanthomas in tendons (especially Achilles).	Very slowly progressive into middle life. Replace deficient bile acid.
Wilson's disease (hepatolenticular degeneration)	Recessive. Accumulation of copper.	Adolescence.	Ataxia, dysarthria, mental changes.	Normal. Kayser-Fleischer rings.	Spasticity and incoordination.	Rare.	Liver copper, 24-hour urine copper increased.	Reversed with chelators.
Refsum's disease	Recessive. Phytanic acid oxidase deficiency.	5–10 years.	Ataxia, ichthyosis, cardiomyopathy.	Retinitis pigmentosa.	Ataxia	None.	Serum phytanic acid elevated; slow nerve conduction velocity, elevated CSF protein. Peroxisomal disease.	Treat with low phytanic acid diet.

[1] For late infantile metachromatic leukodystrophy, Pelizaeus-Merzbacher disease, poliodystrophy, Gaucher's disease of later onset, and subacute necrotizing encephalomyelopathy, see Table 24–25.

[2] CSF gamma globulin (IgG) is considered elevated in children when > 9% of total protein (possibly even > 8.3%); definitively elevated when > 14%.

ologic viral agent by appropriate studies of spinal fluid, stool, throat washings, and paired sera.

C. Imaging: CT scans and x-rays of long bones are normal. The EEG may be normal or may show nonspecific slowing.

Differential Diagnosis

Acute cerebellar ataxia must be differentiated from acute cerebellar syndromes due to phenytoin, phenobarbital, primidone, or lead intoxication. For phenytoin, the toxic level in serum is usually above 25 μg/mL; for phenobarbital, above 50 μg/mL; for primidone, above 14 μg/mL. (See Seizure Disorders.) With lead intoxication, papilledema, anemia, basophilic stippling of erythrocytes, proteinuria, typical x-rays, and elevated cerebrospinal fluid protein are clinical clues, confirmed by serum, urine, or hair lead levels. An occult neuroblastoma, usually seen with the polymyoclonia-opsoclonus syndrome (see below) that once was included in acute cerebellar ataxia, must also be ruled out.

In rare cases, acute cerebellar ataxia may be the presenting sign of acute bacterial meningitis or may be mimicked by corticosteroid withdrawal, vasculitides such as in polyarteritis nodosa, trauma, the first attack of ataxia in a metabolic disorder such as Hartnup disease, or the onset of acute disseminated encephalomyelitis or of multiple sclerosis. The history and physical findings may differentiate these disturbances, but appropriate laboratory studies are often necessary. For ataxias with more chronic onset and course, see the sections on spinocerebellar degeneration (below) and the other degenerative disorders.

Treatment & Prognosis

Treatment is supportive. The use of corticosteroids has no rational justification.

Between 80 and 90% of children with acute cerebellar ataxia not secondary to drugs recover without sequelae within 6–8 weeks. In the remainder, neurologic disturbances, including disorders of behavior and of learning, ataxia, abnormal eye movements, and speech impairment, may persist for months or years, and recovery may remain incomplete.

French JH, Familusi JB: Cerebellar disorders in childhood. *Pediatr Ann* 1983;**12**:825.

2. POLYMYOCLONIA-OPSOCLONUS SYNDROME OF CHILDHOOD (Infantile Myoclonic Encephalopathy, "Dancing Eyes-Dancing Feet" Syndrome)

The symptoms and signs of this syndrome are at first similar to those of "acute cerebellar ataxia."

Often of sudden onset, the disorder is characterized by severe incoordination of the trunk and extremities with lightninglike jerking or flinging movements of a group of muscles, causing the child to be in constant motion while awake. Extraocular muscle involvement results in sudden irregular eye movements (opsoclonus). Irritability and vomiting are present often, but there is no depression of level of consciousness. This syndrome occurs in association with viral infections, tumors of neural crest origin, and many other disorders. Immunologic mechanisms have been postulated to be responsible. There are usually no signs of increased intracranial pressure. Cerebrospinal fluid may show normal or mildly increased protein levels. Special techniques show increased cerebrospinal fluid levels of plasmocytes and abnormal immunoglobulins. The EEG may be slightly slow, but when performed together with electromyography, it shows no evidence of association between cortical discharges and the muscle movements. An assiduous search must be made to rule out tumor of neural crest origin by x-rays of the chest and CT scan or ultrasound (or both) of the adrenal area as well as by assays of urinary catecholamine metabolites (vanilmandelic acid, etc) and cystathionine.

The symptoms respond (often dramatically) to large doses of corticotropin. Otherwise, treatment is as for specific entities. When a neural crest (or possibly other) tumor is found, surgical excision should be followed by irradiation and chemotherapy. Life span is determined by the biologic behavior of the tumor.

The syndrome is usually self-limited but may be characterized by exacerbations and remissions. However, even after removal of a neural crest tumor and without other evidence of its recurrence, symptoms may reappear. A high incidence of mild mental retardation has also been recorded.

Boltshauser E, Deonna TH, Hirt HR: Myoclonic encephalopathy of infants or "dancing eyes syndrome": Report of 7 cases with long-term follow-up and review of the literature (cases with and without neuroblastoma). *Helv Paediatr Acta* 1979;**34**:119.

Rivner MH et al: Opsoclonus in *Hemophilus influenzae* meningitis. *Neurology* 1982;**32**:661.

3. SPINOCEREBELLAR DEGENERATION DISORDERS

Spinocerebellar degeneration disorders may be hereditary or may occur in sporadic distribution. Hereditary disorders include Friedreich's ataxia, dominant hereditary ataxia, and a group of miscellaneous diseases.

Friedreich's Ataxia

This is a recessive disorder characterized by onset of gait ataxia or scoliosis before puberty, becoming progressively worse in the first 2 years and later. Reflexes, light touch, and position sensation are reduced. Dysarthria becomes progressively more severe. Cardiomyopathy usually develops, and diabetes mellitus is found in 40% of patients, with half of these requiring insulin. Pes cavus typically is found.

Patients with Friedreich's ataxia have a deficiency of the mitochondrial malic enzyme in fibroblasts and muscle. However, it may not be the primary defect, or there may be more than one gene coding for the subunits of this enzyme.

Treatment includes surgery for scoliosis and intervention as needed for cardiac disease and diabetes. Patients are usually confined to a wheelchair after age 20 years. Death occurs, usually from heart failure or dysrhythmias, in the third or fourth decade; some patients survive longer.

Dominant Ataxia

This disease (also known as olivopontocerebellar atrophy, Holmes's ataxia, Marie's ataxia, etc) occurs with varying manifestations, even among members of the same family. Ataxia occurs at onset, and progression continues with ophthalmoplegias, extrapyramidal tract and motor neuron degeneration, and later dementia. Levodopa may ameliorate rigidity and bradykinesia, but no other therapy is available. Only 10% have onset in childhood, and their course is often more rapid.

Miscellaneous Hereditary Ataxias

Associated findings permit identification of these recessive disorders. These include ataxia-telangiectasia (telangiectasia, immune defects; see below), Wilson's disease (Kayser-Fleischer rings), Refsum disease (ichthyosis, cardiomyopathy, retinitis pigmentosa, large nerves), Rett's syndrome (regression to autism at 7–18 months in girls, loss of use of hands, progressive failure of brain growth), and abetalipoproteinemia (infantile diarrhea, acanthocytosis, retinitis pigmentosa). Patients with juvenile and chronic gangliosidoses and some hemolytic anemias and long-term survivors of Chédiak-Higashi disease may develop a spinocerebellar degeneration. Idiopathic familial ataxia is called Behr's syndrome. Neuropathies such as Charcot-Marie-Tooth disease produce ataxia.

Haas R, Rapin I, Moser H: Rett syndrome and autism. *J Child Neurol* 1988;**3(Suppl):** 52.

Sheu KFR et al: Mitochondrial enzymes in hereditary ataxias. *Metab Brain Dis* 1988;**3:**151.

Stumpf DA: The inherited ataxias. *Neurol Clin* 1985;**3:**47.

ATAXIA-TELANGIECTASIA (Louis-Bar Syndrome)

Ataxia-telangiectasia is a multisystemic disorder, inherited as an autosomal recessive trait. It is characterized by progressive ataxia; telangiectasia of the bulbar conjunctiva, external ears, nares, and (later) other body surfaces, appearing in the third to sixth year; and recurrent respiratory, sinus, and ear infections. Ocular dyspraxia, slurred speech, choreoathetosis, hypotonia and areflexia, and psychomotor and growth retardation may be present. Endocrinopathies are common. Nerve conduction velocities may be reduced. The entire nervous system may be affected in late stages of the disease. A spectrum of involvement may be seen in the same family. Immunodeficiencies of IgA and IgE are common (see Chapter 18), and the incidence of certain cancers is high.

Ataxia-telangiectasia: A multisystem hereditary disease with immunodeficiency, impaired organ maturation, x-ray hypersensitivity, and a high incidence of neoplasia. (NIH Conference.) *Ann Intern Med* 1983;**99:**367.

EXTRAPYRAMIDAL DISORDERS

Extrapyramidal disorders are characterized by the presence in the waking state of one or more of the following features: dyskinesias, athetosis, ballismus, tremors, rigidity, and dystonias.

For the most part, precise pathologic and anatomic localization is not completely understood. Motor pathways synapsing in the striatum (putamen and caudate nucleus), globus pallidus, red nucleus, substantia nigra, and the body of Luys are involved; this "system" is modulated by pathways originating in the thalamus, cerebellum, and reticular formation.

1. SYDENHAM'S POSTRHEUMATIC CHOREA

Sydenham's chorea is characterized by an acute onset of choreiform movements and variable degrees of psychologic disturbance. It is frequently associated with endocarditis and arthritis. Although the disorder follows infections with β-hemolytic streptococci, the interval between infection and chorea may be greatly delayed; throat cultures and antistreptolysin O (ASO) titers may therefore be negative. Psychic predisposition may also play a role. Chorea has also been associated with hypocalcemia, with vascular lupus erythematosus, and with toxic, viral, infectious and parainfectious, and degenerative encephalopathies.

Clinical Findings

A. Symptoms and Signs: Chorea, or rapid, involuntary movements of the limbs and face, is the hallmark physical finding. In addition to the jerky incoordinate movements, the following are noted: emotional lability, waxing and waning ("milkmaid's") grip, darting tongue, "spooning" of the extended hands and their tendency to pronate, and knee jerks slow to return from the extended to their prestimulus position ("hung up"). Seizures, while uncommon, may be masked by choreic jerks.

B. Laboratory Findings: Anemia, leukocytosis, and an increased erythrocyte sedimentation rate may be present. The ASO titer may be elevated and C-reactive protein present. Throat culture is sometimes positive for β-hemolytic streptococci.

Elecrocardiography may occasionally show cardiac involvement. Electroencephalography may show nonspecific slowing or seizure activity.

Differential Diagnosis

The diagnosis is usually not difficult. Tics, drug-induced extrapyramidal syndromes, Huntington's chorea, and hepatolenticular degeneration (Wilson's disease), as well as other rare movement disorders, can usually be ruled out on historical and clinical grounds.

Treatment

There is no specific treatment. Sodium valproate in a dosage of 20 mg plus 5 mg/kg may suppress the involuntary movements in a few days, or one of the following may be used for sedation: (1) chlorpromazine (Thorazine), 15–25 mg 3 times daily initially and increased slowly until the involuntary movements are markedly reduced or cease or until the patient is overly drowsy; or (2) phenobarbital, 2–3 mg/kg orally 3 times daily. Corticosteroids have also been used.

All patients should be given antistreptococcal prophylaxis with penicillin G (200,000 units twice daily) or sulfonamide drugs.

Prognosis

Sydenham's chorea is a self-limiting disease that may last from a few weeks to about 2 years. Two-thirds of patients relapse one or more times, but the ultimate outcome does not appear to be worse in those with recurrences. Valvular heart disease occurs in about one-third of patients, particularly if other rheumatic manifestations appear. Psychoneurotic disturbances, if not already present at the onset of illness, occur in a significant percentage of patients.

Dhanaraj M et al: Sodium valproate in Sydenham's chorea. *Neurology* 1985;**35**:114.

Nausieda PA et al: Sydenham chorea: An update. *Neurology* 1980;**30**:331.

Peters ACB et al: ECHO 25 focal encephalitis and subacute hemichorea. *Neurology* 1979;**29**:676.

2. TICS (Habit Spasms)

Tics, or habit spasms, are quick repetitive but irregular movements, often stereotyped, and briefly suppressible. Coordination and muscle tone are not affected. A psychogenic basis is seldom discernible.

Transient tics of childhood (12–24% incidence in school-age children) last from 1 month to 1 year and seldom need treatment. Many children with tics have a history of encephalopathic past events, "soft signs" on neurologic examination, and school problems.

Facial tics such as grimaces, twitches, and blinking predominate, but the trunk and extremities are often involved and there are twisting or flinging movements. Vocal tics are less common.

Gilles de la Tourette's syndrome is a chronic disorder of multiple fluctuating motor tics and involuntary vocalizations. Tics evolve slowly, new ones being added to or replacing old ones. Coprolalia and echolalia are relatively infrequent. Partial forms are common. The usual age at onset is 2–15 years, and familial incidence is 35–50%; the disorder is now reported in almost all ethnic groups. Gilles de la Tourette's syndrome may be triggered by stimulants or other chemical agents; one of the authors has observed similar findings in 2 retardates receiving long-term neuroleptic drug therapy for aggressivity. Thus, the syndrome may have multiple causes. An imbalance of neurotransmitters, especially dopamine and serotonin, has been hypothesized.

In relatively mild cases, tics are self-limited and, when disregarded, disappear. When attention is paid to one tic, it may disappear only to be replaced by another that is often worse. If the tic and its underlying anxiety or compulsive neurosis are severe, psychiatric evaluation and treatment are needed. Drug therapy has little place in the treatment of tics except in Gilles de la Tourette's syndrome, for which haloperidol (Haldol), 1–5 mg/d, is the best-established treatment, benefiting 80% of patients. Because of side effects, including tardive dyskinesia, its usefulness may be limited. Use of clonidine, 0.125–0.3 mg/d, results in significant improvement in at least half of cases, without serious side effects or the development of tolerance to the drug. Attention to speech, academic, and behavior problems is at least as important as medication.

Barbas G (editor): Multiple articles on Tourette syndrome. *Psychiatr Ann* (July) 1988;**18**:393–425.

Caine ED: Gilles de la Tourette's syndrome: A review of clinical and research studies and consideration of future directions for investigation. *Arch Neurol* 1985;**42**:393.

Harlan R et al: Sensory tics in Tourette's syndrome. *Neurology* 1989;**39**:731.

Harlan R et al: Transient tic disorder and the spectrum of Tourette syndrome. *Arch Neurol* 1988;**45**:1200.

INFECTIOUS & INFLAMMATORY DISORDERS OF THE CENTRAL NERVOUS SYSTEM

Infections of the central nervous system (CNS) are some of the most common neurologic disorders encountered by the pediatrician. While infections are among the CNS disorders most amenable to treatment, they are also among the disorders that have the highest potential for causing catastrophic destruction of the nervous system. It is imperative for the clinician to recognize infections early and to identify those disorders that are treatable with antimicrobial agents. Appropriate therapy must be started as early as possible in order to prevent massive tissue destruction.

Clinical Manifestations

Patients with CNS infections, whether the infections are caused by bacteria, viruses, or other microorganisms, present with similar manifestations. Often, the patient has systemic signs of infection, including fever, generalized malaise, or impaired heart, lung, liver, or kidney functions. General features suggesting CNS infection consist of headache, stiff neck, fever or hypothermia, changes in mental status (including hyperirritability evolving into lethargy and coma), seizures, and focal sensory and motor deficits. On examination, meningeal irritation is manifest by the presence of Kernig's and Brudzinski's signs. In very young infants, signs of meningeal irritation may be absent, and temperature instability and hypothermia are often more prominent than fever. In young infants, a bulging fontanelle and an increased head circumference are common. Papilledema may eventually develop, particularly in older children and adolescents. Cranial nerve palsies may develop acutely or gradually during the course of neurologic infections. No specific clinical sign or symptom is reliable in distinguishing bacterial infections from infections caused by other microbes.

During the initial clinical assessment, conditions that predispose the patient to infection of the CNS should be sought. Infections involving the sinuses or other structures in the head and neck region can result in direct extension of infection into the intracranial compartment. Open head injuries, recent neurosurgical procedures, immunodeficiencies, and the presence of a mechanical shunt may provide strong evidence regarding the nature of the underlying illness.

Laboratory Investigation

When CNS infections are suspected, blood should be obtained for a complete blood count, general chemistry panel, and culture. Most important, however, is obtaining cerebrospinal fluid. In the absence of focal neurologic deficits or signs of increased intracranial pressure, spinal fluid should be obtained immediately from any patient in whom serious CNS infection is suspected. When papilledema or focal motor signs are present, a lumbar puncture may be delayed until a neuroimaging procedure has been done to exclude brain abscess or other space-occupying lesion. It is generally safe to obtain spinal fluid from infants with nonfocal neurologic examination, even if the fontanelle is full. Once spinal fluid is obtained, it should be examined for the presence of red and white blood cells, protein concentration, glucose concentration, bacteria, and other microorganisms, and a sample should be cultured. In addition, serologic and immunologic tests may be performed on the spinal fluid in an attempt to identify the specific organism. Special studies such as IgG-albumin ratios may be helpful in distinguishing primary infections from parainfectious, inflammatory disorders. As a general rule, spinal fluid that contains a high proportion of polymorphonuclear leukocytes, a high protein concentration, and a low glucose concentration strongly suggests bacterial infection. Spinal fluid containing predominantly lymphocytes, a high protein concentration, and low glucose concentration suggests an infection with mycobacteria, fungi, uncommon bacteria, and some viruses such as lymphocytic choriomeningitis virus, herpes simplex virus, mumps virus, and arboviruses. Cerebrospinal fluid that contains a high proportion of lymphocytes, normal or only slightly elevated protein concentration, and a normal glucose concentration is most suggestive of viral infections, although partially treated bacterial meningitis and parameningeal infections may also result in this type of CSF formula. Typical CSF findings in a variety of infectious and inflammatory disorders are shown in Table 24–3.

Neuroimaging procedures such as CT and MRI may be helpful in demonstrating the presence of brain abscess, meningeal inflammation, or secondary problems such as venous and arterial infarctions, hemorrhages, and subdural effusions. In addition, these neuroimaging procedures may identify sinus infections or other focal infections in the head or neck region that are related to the CNS infection. CT scanning may demonstrate bony abnormalities, such as basilar fractures, that are etiologically important to the CNS infection.

EEGs may be helpful in the assessment of patients who have had seizures at the time of presentation. The changes are often nonspecific and characterized by generalized slowing. In some instances, such as herpes simplex virus infection, focal electronegative activity may be seen early in the course and may be one of the earliest laboratory abnormalities to suggest the diagnosis. EEGs may also show focal slowing over regions of abscesses. Unusual, characteristic electroencephalographic patterns are seen in some patients with subacute sclerosing panencephalitis (SSPE).

In some cases, brain biopsy may be needed to identify the presence of specific organisms and clarify the diagnosis. Herpes simplex virus infections are confirmed by culturing brain tissue. Brain biopsy is often needed to distinguish herpes simplex encephalitis from parasitic infections, brain tumors, and other structural abnormalities.

BACTERIAL MENINGITIS

Clinical Findings

Bacterial infections of the central nervous system may present acutely (symptoms evolving rapidly over 1–24 hours), subacutely (symptoms evolving over 1–7 days), or chronically (symptoms evolving over more than one week). Diffuse bacterial infections involve the leptomeninges, superficial cortical structures, and blood vessels. Although the term "meningitis" is used to describe these infections, it should not be forgotten that the brain parenchyma is also inflamed and that blood vessel walls may also be infiltrated by inflammatory cells that result in endothelial cell injury, vessel stenosis, and secondary ischemia and infarction.

Symptoms and findings of bacterial meningitis are described above. No specific features reliably distinguish infections caused by bacteria from infections caused by viruses, fungi, parasites, or other microbes.

Pathologically, the inflammatory process involves all intracranial structures to some degree. Acutely, this inflammatory process may result in cerebral edema or impaired CSF flow through and out of the ventricular system resulting in hydrocephalus. Many bacterial infections are characterized by early and extensive involvement of blood vessels, both arteries and veins, resulting in ischemia, ischemic infarction, or hemorrhagic infarction.

Treatment

A. Specific: (See also Chapter 28, *Haemophilus influenzae* type B infections, and Chapter 38.) Children less than 3 months of age are treated initially with cefotaxime (or ceftriaxone if over 1 month of age) and ampicillin; the latter agent is used to treat *Listeria* and enterococcus, agents that rarely affect older children. Children older than 3 months are treated with ceftriaxone; cefotaxime; or ampicillin plus chloramphenicol. Therapy may be narrowed if organism sensitivity allows. Duration of therapy is 7

days for meningococcal infections; 10 days for *H influenzae* or pneumococcal infection; and 14–21 days for other organisms. Slow clinical response or the occurrence of complications may prolong duration. Although therapy duration of 7 days has proved successful in many children with *Haemophilus* infection, it cannot be recommended if steroids are also used (see below) without further study.

B. General: Children with bacterial meningitis are often systemically ill. The following complications should be looked for and treated aggressively: hypovolemia, hypoglycemia, hyponatremia, acidosis, septic shock, increased intracranial pressure, seizures, disseminated intravascular coagulation, and metastatic infection (eg, pericarditis, arthritis, and pneumonia). Children should initially be monitored closely (cardiorespiratory monitor, strict fluid balance and frequent urine specific gravity assessment, daily weights, neurologic assessment every few hours), not fed until neurologically very stable, isolated until the organism is known, rehydrated with isotonic solutions until euvolemic, and then given intravenous fluids containing dextrose and sodium at no more than maintenance rate (assuming no unusual losses occur).

Complications

Abnormalities of water and electrolyte balance result from either excessive or insufficient production of antidiuretic hormone and require careful monitoring and appropriate adjustments in fluid administration. Monitoring serum sodium every 8–12 hours during the first 1 or 2 days—and urine sodium if the inappropriate secretion of antidiuretic hormone is suspected—usually detects significant problems.

Seizures occur in up to 30% of children with bacterial meningitis. Seizures tend to be most frequent in neonates and less common in older children. Persistent focal seizures or focal seizures associated with focal neurologic deficits strongly suggest a subdural effusion, abscess, or vascular lesions, such as arterial infarct, cortical venous infarcts, or dural sinus thrombosis. Because generalized seizures in a metabolically compromised child may have severe sequelae, early recognition and therapy are critical; some practitioners prefer phenytoin for acute management because it is less sedating than phenobarbital.

Subdural effusions occur in as many as 50% of young children with *H influenzae* meningitis. Subdural effusions are often seen on CT scans of the head during the course of meningitis. They do not require treatment unless they are producing increased intracranial pressure or progressive mass affect. Although subdural effusions may be detected in children with persistent fever, such effusions do not usually have to be sampled or drained if the infecting organism is *Haemophilus,* meningococcus, or pneumococcus. These are usually sterilized with the standard treatment duration, and slowly waning fever during an otherwise uncomplicated recovery may be followed clinically. Under any other circumstance, however, aspiration of the fluid for documentation of sterilization or relief of pressure should be considered.

Cerebral edema can participate in the production of increased intracranial pressure, requiring treatment with dexamethasone, osmotic agents, diuretics, or hyperventilation; continuous pressure monitoring may be needed.

Long-term sequelae of meningitis result from direct inflammatory destruction of brain cells, vascular injuries, or secondary gliosis. Focal motor and sensory deficits, visual impairment, hearing loss, seizures, hydrocephalus, and a variety of cranial nerve deficits can result from meningitis. Sensorineural hearing loss in *H influenzae* meningitis occurs in approximately 5–10% of cases during long-term follow-up. Recent studies have suggested that the early addition of dexamethasone to the antibiotic regimen may modestly decrease the risk of hearing loss in some children with *H influenzae* meningitis (see Chapter 28).

In addition to the variety of disorders mentioned above, some patients with meningitis suffer from mental retardation and severe behavioral disorders that limit their function at school and later performance in life. Table 24–27 lists the overall mortality and morbidity figures for the most common organisms associated with acute bacterial meningitis in childhood.

BRAIN ABSCESS

Patients with brain abscess often appear to have systemic illness similar to patients with bacterial meningitis, but in addition, they show signs of focal neurologic deficits, papilledema, and other evidence of increased intracranial pressure or evidence of a mass lesion. Symptoms may be present for a week or more; children with bacterial meningitis usually present within a few days. Conditions predisposing to development of brain abscess include penetrating head trauma; chronic infection of middle ear, mastoid, or sinuses (especially the frontal sinus); cardiovascular lesions allowing right-to-left shunting of blood (including arteriovenous malformations); endocarditis; and meningeal infection, especially with necrotizing organisms such as enterics or staphylococci.

When brain abscess is strongly suspected, a neuroimaging procedure such as CT or MRI should be done prior to lumbar puncture. If a brain abscess is identified, lumbar puncture may be dangerous and rarely alters choice of antibiotic or clinical management since the spinal fluid abnormalities usually reflect only parameningeal inflammation. Table 24–28 lists organisms most often recovered from brain abscesses in children. Unfortunately, cultures from a large number of brain abscesses remain negative and the organisms responsible unknown.

The diagnosis of brain abscess is based primarily on strong clinical suspicion and confirmed by a neuroimaging procedure. As mentioned earlier, electroencephalographic changes are nonspecific but frequently demonstrate focal slowing in the region of brain abscess. Treatment includes antibiotic management (as outlined in Table 24–28), neurologic consultation, and anticonvulsant and edema therapy if necessary. In their early stages, brain abscesses are areas of focal cerebritis and can be "cured" with antibiotic treatment alone, without surgical intervention. Well-developed abscesses require surgical drainage.

Differential diagnosis of brain abscess includes any condition that produces focal neurologic deficits and increased intracranial pressure, such as neoplasms, subdural effusions, cerebral infarctions, and cerebral edema.

The surgical mortality in the treatment of brain abscess is less than 5%. Untreated cerebral abscesses lead to irreversible tissue destruction and may rupture into the ventricle, producing catastrophic deterioration in neurologic function and death. Because brain abscesses are often associated with systemic illness and systemic infections, the death rate is frequently high in these patients.

Table 24–27. Outcome of acute bacterial meningitis by organism.

Organism	Mortality (%)	Motor Handicap (%)		Intellect (%)	
		None	Severe	Normal	Severe Mental Retardation
Escherichia coli gram-negative organisms	20–50	62	25	75	25
Haemophilus influenzae	5–10	87	3	82	5
Streptococcus pneumoniae	10–30	96	0	83	0
Neisseria meningitidis	5–10	100	0	93	0
Group B streptococci	20				
Overall total	10–25	85	5	82	6

Table 24–28. Initial antibiotic coverage for organisms commonly found in brain abscesses.

Suspected Organism	Drug
Staphylococcus aureus	Nafcillin or methicillin
β-hemolytic streptococcus	Penicillin G
Streptococcus viridans	Penicillin G
Gram-negative bacteria	Cefotaxime, ceftriaxone, or chloramphenicol
Anaerobic bacteria	Penicillin G and chloramphenicol or metronidazole
Unknown—cultures pending	Nafcillin or methicillin combined with chloramphenicol

VIRAL INFECTIONS

Viral infections of the central nervous system can involve primarily meninges (meningitis) (see Chapter 27) or cerebral parenchyma (encephalitis). All patients, however, have some degree of involvement of both the meninges and cerebral parenchyma (meningoencephalitis). Many viral infections are generalized and diffuse, but some viruses, notably herpes simplex and some arboviruses, characteristically cause prominent focal disease. Focal cerebral involvement is clearly evident on neuroimaging procedures. Some viruses have an affinity for specific CNS cell populations. Poliovirus and other enteroviruses can selectively infect anterior horn cells (poliomyelitis) and some intracranial motor neurons.

Although most viral infections of the nervous system present with an acute or subacute course in childhood, chronic infections can occur. Subacute sclerosing panencephalitis, for example, represents a chronic indolent infection caused by measles virus and is characterized clinically by progressive neurodegeneration and seizures.

Inflammatory reactions within the nervous system may occur during the convalescent stage of systemic viral infections. Parainfectious or postinfectious inflammation of the central nervous system results in several well-recognized disorders: acute disseminated encephalomyelitis, transverse myelitis, optic neuritis, polyneuritis, and Guillain-Barré-Strohl syndrome.

Congenital viral infections can also affect the central nervous system. Cytomegalovirus, herpes simplex virus and rubella virus are the most notable causes of viral brain injury in utero.

Treatment of viral infections of the nervous system is usually limited to symptomatic and supportive measures. In recent years, however, antiviral agents effective against herpes simplex virus have been constructed. Acyclovir is considered the treatment of choice in suspected or proved cases of herpes simplex virus encephalitis. Acyclovir may also be useful in some patients with varicella-zoster virus infections of the CNS.

Encephalopathy of HIV infection. In the past several years, there has been an increased number of patients with acquired immunodeficiency syndrome caused by human immunodeficiency virus (HIV). Neurologic abnormalities are seen in many patients with HIV infection (Table 24–29). Neurologic syndromes associated directly with HIV infection include subacute encephalitis, meningitis, myelopathy, polyneuropathy, and myositis. In addition, secondary opportunistic infections of the central nervous system occur in patients with HIV-induced immunosuppression; toxoplasmal and cytomegaloviral infections have been particularly common. Progressive multifocal leukoencephalopathy, a secondary papovavirus infection, and herpes simplex virus and herpes zoster virus infections also occur frequently in patients with HIV infection. A variety of other fungal, mycobacterial, and bacterial infections have been described. Neurologic abnormalities in these patients can also be the result of noninfectious, neoplastic disorders. Primary CNS lymphoma and metastatic lymphoma to the nervous system are the most frequent neoplasms involving the nervous system in these patients. See Chapters 18 and 27 for the diagnosis and management of HIV infection.

OTHER INFECTIONS

A wide variety of other microorganisms, including toxoplasma, mycobacteria, spirochetes, rickettsia, ameba, and mycoplasma, can cause CNS infections. CNS involvement in these infections is usually secondary to systemic infection or other predisposing factors. Appropriate cultures and serologic testing is required to confirm infections by these organisms. Parenteral antimicrobial treatment for these infections is discussed elsewhere in this text.

NONINFECTIOUS, INFLAMMATORY DISORDERS OF THE CENTRAL NERVOUS SYSTEM

In the differential diagnosis of bacterial, viral, and other microbial infections of the central nervous system are disorders that cause inflammation but for which no specific etiologic organism has been identified. Sarcoidosis, Behçet's syndrome, systemic lupus erythematosus, other collagen-vascular disorders, and Kawasaki disease represent examples of these disorders. In these disorders, CNS inflammation in general occurs in association with characteristic systemic manifestations that allow proper diagnosis. Management of CNS involvement in these disorders is the same as the treatment of the systemic illness.

Table 24–29. Neurologic aspects of HIV infection.

Direct HIV effects
  Encephalopathy
  Meningitis
  Myelopathy
  Neuropathy-Neuritis
  Myositis
Secondary infections
  Toxoplasma meningoencephalitis
  Cytomegalovirus infections
  Herpes simplex virus infections
  Papovavirus infection (progressive multifocal leukoencephalopathy)
  Fungal infections
  Mycobacterial infections
Neoplasms
  Primary CNS lymphoma
  Metastatic lymphoma

OTHER PARAINFECTIOUS ENCEPHALOPATHIES

In association with systemic infections or other illnesses, CNS dysfunction may occur in the absence of direct CNS inflammation or infection. Reye's syndrome is a prominent example of this type of encephalopathy that often occurs in association with varicella virus or other respiratory or systemic viral infections. In Reye's syndrome, cerebral edema and cerebral dysfunction occur, but there is no evidence of any direct involvement of the nervous system by the associated microorganism or inflammation. Cerebral edema in Reye's syndrome is accompanied by liver dysfunction and fatty infiltration of the liver. Perhaps as a result of recent efforts to discourage use of aspirin in childhood febrile illnesses, there has been a marked decrease in the number of patients with Reye's syndrome. The precise relationship, however, between aspirin and Reye's syndrome is not clear.

Falloon J et al: Human immunodeficiency virus infection in children. *J Pediatr* 1989;**114**:1.

Johnson RT: *Viral Infections of the Nervous System.* Raven Press, 1982.

Klein JO, Feigin RD, McCracken GH: Report of the task force on diagnosis and management of meningitis. *Pediatrics* 1986;**78(Suppl)**:959.

Kohl S: Herpes simplex virus encephalitis in children. *Pediatr Clin North Am* 1988;**35**:465.

Lebel MH et al: Dexamethasone therapy for bacterial meningitis. *N Engl J Med* 1988;**319**:964.

Patrick CC, Kaplan SL: Current concepts in the pathogenesis and management of brain abscesses in children. *Pediatr Clin North Am* 1988;**35**:625.

Plotkin SA et al: Treatment of bacterial meningitis. *Pediatrics* 1988;**81**:904.

Seay AR: Bacterial meningitis: Future directions. *J Child Neurol* 1988;**3**:80.

Sever JL Gibbs CJ (editors): Retroviruses in the nervous system. *Ann Neurol* 1988;**23(Suppl)**:S4.

Swartz MN: "Chronic meningitis": Many causes to consider. *N Engl J Med* 1987;**317**:957.

SYNDROMES PRESENTING AS ACUTE FLACCID PARALYSIS

General Considerations

Flaccid paralysis evolving over hours or a few days suggests involvement of the lower motor neuron complex (see Floppy Infant Syndrome). **Anterior horn cells** (spinal cord) may be involved by viral infection (paralytic poliomyelitis) or paraviral or postviral immunologically mediated disease (acute transverse myelitis). The **nerve trunks** (polyneuritis) may be diseased as in Landry-Guillain-Barré syndrome or affected by toxins (diphtheria, porphyria). The **neuromuscular junction** may be blocked by tick toxin or botulinum toxin. The paralysis rarely will be due to metabolic (periodic paralysis) or inflammatory muscle disease (myositis). *A lesion compressing the spinal cord must be ruled out.*

Clinical Findings

A. Symptoms and Signs: The features that aid in diagnosis are age, a history of preceding or waning illness, the presence (at time of paralysis) of fever, rapidity of progression, cranial nerve findings, and sensory findings. The examination may show "long tract" findings (pyramidal tract), causing increased reflexes and positive Babinski sign. The spinothalamic tract may be interrupted, causing loss of pain and temperature. Back pain, even tenderness to percussion, may occur. Bowel and bladder dysfunction (incontinence) may occur. Often, the paralysis is ascending, symmetric, and painful (muscle tenderness or myalgia). Table 24–30 details many of these points. Laboratory findings occasionally are diagnostic.

B. Laboratory Findings: The examination of spinal fluid is most helpful (see Table 24–30). Imaging studies of the spinal column (plain films) and spinal cord (MRI, myelogram) are occasionally essential. Viral cultures (CSF, throat, stool) and titers aid in diagnosing polio. A high sedimentation rate may suggest tumor or abscess; antinuclear antibody (ANA) may suggest lupus arteritis.

Electromyography and nerve conduction velocity can be helpful in diagnosing polyneuropathy. Nerve conduction is usually slowed after 7–10 days. Findings in botulism and tick-bite paralysis can be specific and diagnostic. Rarely, elevation of muscle enzymes, even myoglobinuria, may aid in diagnosis of myopathic paralysis. Porphyrin urine studies and heavy metal assays (arsenic, thallium, lead) can reveal those rare toxic causes of polyneuropathic paralysis.

Table 24–30. Acute flaccid paralysis in children.

	Poliomyelitis (Paralytic, Spinal, and Bulbar), With or Without Encephalitis	Landry-Guillain-Barré Syndrome ("Acute Idiopathic Polyneuritis")	Botulism	Tick-Bite Paralysis	Transverse Myelitis and Neuromyelitis Optica
Etiology	Poliovirus types I, II, and III; Other enteroviruses; Immunization virus (rare).	Likely delayed hypersensitivity-immunologic. Mycoplasmal and viral infections (including infectious mononucleosis) and various systemic or toxic disorders may be underlying cause.	*Clostridium botulinum* toxin. Block at neuromusclar junction. Under age one, toxin forms in bowel from ingested dust or honey in formula. At older ages, contamined food (preformed toxin). Rarely from wound infection.	Probable interference with transmission of nerve impulse caused by toxin in tick saliva.	Usually unknown; immunodeficiency state (?)
History	None, or inadequate polio immunization. Upper respiratory or gastrointestinal symptoms followed by brief respite. Bulbar paralysis more frequent after tonsillectomy. Often in epidemics, in summer and early fall.	Nonspecific respiratory or gastrointestinal symptoms in preceding 5–14 days common. Any season, though slightly lower incidence in summer. *Campylobacter.* Hepatitis.	Infancy: dusty environment (eg, construction area), suburbs; honey. Older: "food poisoning." Multiple cases hours to days after ingesting contaminated food.	Exposure to ticks (dog tick in eastern USA; wood ticks). Irritability 12–24 hours before onset of a rapidly progressive ascending paralysis.	Occasionally, symptoms compatible with multiple sclerosis or optic neuritis. Progression from onset to paraplegia very rapid, usually without a history of bacterial infection.
Presenting complaints	Febrile at time of paralysis. Meningeal signs, muscle tenderness, and spasm. Asymmetric weakness widespread or segmental (cervical, thoracic, lumbar). Bulbar symptoms early or before extremity weakness. Anxiety. Delirium.	Symmetric weakness of lower extremities, which may ascend rapidly to arms, trunk, and face. Verbal child may complain of paresthesias. Fever uncommon. Facial weakness early. Miller-Fisher variant presents as ataxia and ophthalmoplegia.	Infancy: constipation, poor suck and cry. "Floppy." Apnea. Lethargy. Choking (cause of SIDS?). Older: Blurred vision, diplopia, ptosis, choking, weakness.	Rapid onset and progression of ascending flaccid paralysis; often accompanied by pain and paresthesias. Paralysis of upper extremities usually occurs on second day after onset.	Root and back pain in about one-third to one-half of cases. Sensory loss below level of lesion accompanying rapidly developing paralysis. Sphincter difficulties common.
Findings	Flaccid weakness, usually asymmetric. Lumbar: legs, lower abdomen. Cervical: shoulder, arm, neck, diaphragm. Thoracic: intercostals, spine, upper abdomen. Bulbar: respiratory, lower cranial nerves. Fever in first days.	Flaccid weakness, symmetric, usually greater proximally, but may be more distal or equal in distribution. Facial diplegia in about 85%, then IX–X, XI, III–VI. Bulbar involvement may occur. Slight distal impairment of position, vibration, touch; difficult to assess in young children.	Infants: flaccid weakness. Alert. Eye, pupil, facial weakness. Deep tendon reflexes (DTR) decreased to 0? Absent suck, gag. Constipation. Older: Paralysis accommodation, eye movements. Weak swallow. Respiratory paralysis.	Flaccid, symmetric paralysis. Cranial nerve and bulbar (respiratory) paralysis, ataxia, sphincter disturbances, and sensory deficits may occur. Some fever. Diagnosis rests on finding tick, which is especially likely to be on occipital scalp.	Paraplegia with areflexia below level of lesion early; later, may have hyperreflexia. Sensory loss below and hyperesthesia or normal sensation above level of lesion. Paralysis of bladder and rectum. Optic atrophy or neuritis may be present.
CSF	Pleocytosis (20–500+ cells) with PMN predominance in first few days, followed by rapid decrease and monocytic preponderance. Glucose normal. Protein frequently elevated (50–150 mg/dL).	Cytoalbuminologic dissociation; 10 or fewer mononuclear cells with high protein after first week. Normal glucose. Gamma globulin may be elevated.	Normal.	Normal.	Usually no manometric block; CSF may show increased protein, pleocytosis with predominantly mononuclear cells, increased gamma globulin.
EMG	Denervation after 10–21 days. Nerve conduction normal.	Nerve conduction velocities markedly decreased, may be normal early.	EMG distinctive: BSAP ("brief small abundant potentials").	Nerve conduction slowed; returns rapidly to normal after removal of tick.	Normal early. Denervation at level of lesion after 10–21 days.
Other studies	Initially, leukocytosis. Virus in stool and throat. Serologic titers.	Search for specific cause such as infection, intoxication, metabolic or endocrine disease, allergic phenomena, neoplasm. Lymphocyte transformation demonstrated. *Mycoplasma pneumoniae* implicated.	Infancy: stool culture, toxin. Rare serum toxin +. Older: Serum (or wound) toxin.	Leukocytosis, often with moderate eosinophilia.	Normal spine x-rays do not exclude spinal epidural abscess. MRI has largely replaced myelography to rule out cord-compressive lesions. Cord may be swelled in myelitis.

Table 24–30 (cont'd). Acute flaccid paralysis in children.

	Poliomyelitis (Para-lytic, Spinal, and Bul-bar), With or Without Encephalitis	Landry-Guillain-Barré Syndrome ("Acute Idiopathic Polyneuritis")	Botulism	Tick-Bite Paralysis	Transverse Myelitis and Neuromyelitis Optica
Course and prognosis	Paralysis usually maximal 3–5 days after onset. Transient bladder paralysis may occur. Outlook varies with extent and severity of involvement. *Note:* Threat greatest from respiratory failure and superinfection. Early muscle atrophy common.	Course progressive over a few days to about 2 weeks. Transient bladder paralysis may occur. *Note:* Threat greatest from respiratory failure, autonomic crises (eg, BP, arrhythmia) and superinfection. Majority recover completely. Plasmapheresis may have a role.	Infancy: Supportive. Penicillin ? Purge stool ? Antitoxin unnecessary. Respiratory support (prolonged often), gavage feeding. Avoid aminoglycosides. Older: Penicillin, antitoxin, prolonged respiratory support. Prognosis: excellent with good quality intensive care. Fatality 3%.	Total removal of tick is followed by rapid improvement and recovery. Otherwise, mortality rate due to respiratory paralysis is very high.	Large degree of functional recovery possible. Corticosteroids are of controversial benefit in shortening duration of acute attack but not in preventing recurrences or altering the overall course.

Differential Diagnosis

The child who is "well" and becomes paralyzed often has polyneuritis. Sometimes, acute transverse myelitis (ATM) occurs in an afebrile child. The child who is ill and febrile at the time of paralysis often has ATM (or polio); *acute* epidural spinal cord abscess (or other compressive lesion) must be ruled out. Poliomyelitis is very rare in our immunized population. Paralysis due to tick bites occurs seasonally (spring and summer). The tick is usually found in the occipital hair. Removal is curative.

Paralysis due to botulism occurs most commonly under age one; food-borne and wound botulism are very rare. An investigative history and laboratory studies are diagnostic. Intravenous drug abuse can lead to myelitis and paralysis. Furthermore, *chronic* myelopathy is emerging as a result of 2 human immunodeficiency viruses, HTLV-I and HTLV-III.

Complications

A. Respiratory Paralysis: Early and careful attention to oxygenation is essential; administration of oxygen, intubation, mechanical respiratory assistance, and careful suctioning of secretions may be required. Increasing anxiety and a rise in diastolic and systolic blood pressures are early signs of hypoxia. Cyanosis is a late sign. Deteriorating spirometric findings (forced expiratory volume in one second [FEV_1] and total vital capacity) may indicate the need for controlled intubation and respiratory support.

B. Infections: Pneumonia is common, especially in cases of respiratory paralysis. Prophylactic antibiotic administration is generally contraindicated. Antibiotic therapy is best guided by results of cultures. Bladder infections occur most commonly when an indwelling catheter is required because of bladder paralysis. Recovery from myelitis may be delayed by urinary tract infection.

C. Autonomic Crisis: This may be a cause of death in Guillain-Barré syndrome; strict attention to vital signs to detect and treat hypotension or hypertension and cardiac arrhythmias in an intensive care setting is advisable, at least early in the course in severely ill patients.

Treatment

There is no specific treatment in most of these syndromes; however, ticks causing paralysis must be removed. Other therapies include the use of erythromycin in *Mycoplasma* infections and botulism equine antitoxin in wound botulism. Recognized associated disorders (eg, endocrine, neoplastic, toxic) should be treated by appropriate means. Supportive care also involves "pulmonary toilet," adequate fluids and nutrition, bladder and bowel care, prevention of decubiti, and often, psychiatric support.

A. Corticosteroids: These agents are believed by most to be of no benefit in Landry-Guillain-Barré syndrome. Autonomic symptoms (eg, hypertension) in polyneuritis may require treatment.

B. Plasmapheresis: Plasma exchange has been beneficial in severe cases of Landry-Guillain-Barré syndrome.

C. Physical Therapy: Rehabilitative measures are best instituted when acute symptoms have subsided and the patient is stable.

Prognosis

The prognosis varies greatly with the extent of involvement, duration of the inflammatory process, complications, and other factors.

Briscoe DM et al: Prognosis in Guillain-Barré syndrome. *Arch Dis Child* 1987;**62**:733.

Dunne K et al: Acute transverse myelopathy in childhood. *Dev Med Child Neurol* 1986;**28**:198.

Freeman JM: Diagnosis and evaluation of acute paraplegia. *Pediatr Rev* 1983;**4**:328.

Johnson RT, McArthur J: Myelopathic and retrovirus infections. *Ann Neurol* 1987;**21**:113.

Keller MA et al: Wound botulism in pediatrics. *Am J Dis Child* 1982;**136**:320.

Kleyweg RP et al: Treatment of Guillain-Barré syndrome with high dose gammaglobulin. *Neurology* 1988; **38**:1639.

McKhahn G, Griffin JW: Plasmapheresis and GB syndrome. (Editorial.) *Ann Neurol* 1987;**22**:762.

Novak RW, Jones G, Chi'ien LT: Acute transverse myelopathy in childhood: A study of four cases. *Clin Pediatr* 1978;**17**:894.

Packer RJ et al: Magnetic resonance imaging of spinal cord disease in childhood. *Pediatrics* 1986;**78**:251.

Yoshioka M, Kuroki S, Mizue H: Plasmapheresis in the treatment of Guillain-Barré syndrome in childhood. *Pediatr Neurol* 1985;**1**:329.

DISORDERS OF CHILDHOOD AFFECTING MUSCLES

This section is concerned with specific muscle and neuromuscular disorders, including the muscular dystrophies, myasthenia gravis, and miscellaneous congenital neuromuscular disorders. (See Table 24–31.)

Certain studies that are commonly used in the diagnosis of muscle diseases merit special consideration.

Serum Enzymes

Among muscle enzymes—creatine kinase (CK), aldolase, glutamic-oxaloacetic transaminase (GOT), and lactic dehydrogenase—helpful in diagnosing and following the course of some muscle disorders, usually only CK is now followed. CK (or CPK) reflects muscle damage or "leak" from muscle into plasma; the other enzymes are less available (aldolase) or also have liver origin. Normal CK values may vary by laboratory. Blood should be drawn before electromyography (EMG) or muscle biopsy, which may lead to release of the enzyme. Corticosteroids may suppress levels despite very active muscle disease.

Muscle Imaging

Ultrasonography, CT scanning, and MRI are employed in a research situation to aid in the diagnosis and assessment of muscular dystrophies, congenital myopathies and myotonias, spinal muscular atrophies, and some neuropathies.

Electromyography (EMG)

Electromyography is often helpful in grossly differentiating "myopathic" from "neurogenic" processes. Fibrillations occur in both. In the myopa-
thies, very low spikes are more typical, and the motor unit action potentials seen during contraction characteristically are of short duration, polyphasic, and increased in number for the strength of the contraction (increased interference pattern). "Neurogenic" findings include decreased numbers of motor units, which may be polyphasic, larger than normal, or both. The interference pattern is decreased.

In myotonic dystrophy, the EMG is characterized by prolonged discharge of electrical activity on movement of the probing needle ("dive bomber" sound), although these discharges may be found to a lesser degree in other conditions. During attempted relaxation after a contraction, electrical activity persists parallel with the protracted relaxation of muscle.

Muscle Biopsy

Properly executed (by "open" biopsy or by using the Bergstrom muscle biopsy needle), this procedure is usually most helpful. Histochemical techniques, histogram analysis of muscle fiber types, and electron microscopy are offering new classifications of the myopathies. Findings common to the myopathies include variation in the size and shape of muscle fibers, increase in connective tissue, interstitial infiltration of fatty tissue, degenerative changes in muscle fibers, and central location of nuclei.

Findings more characteristic of certain myopathies include the sarcoplasmic masses and striking chains of central nuclei in myotonic dystrophy; the cysts in trichinosis and toxoplasmosis; the vacuoles in the periodic paralyses, thyrotoxicosis, chloroquine myopathy, and lupus erythematosus; the patterns of special stains in central core disease and nemaline myopathy; and the electron microscopic findings in giant mitochondrial myopathy.

Genetic Testing & Carrier Detection

To date, detection of carriers for Duchenne's dystrophy (mothers and sisters of involved boys) has rested on CK enzyme elevations (two-thirds will have this), physical findings of mild dystrophy (large calves, muscle weakness), abnormal muscle EMG, or biopsy results. All are unreliable for diagnostic purposes.

DNA probes are now available for carrier detection and prenatal diagnosis of Duchenne's and Becker's dystrophy. Deletions are often found on the short arm of the X chromosome; it is postulated that all patients and most mothers will show deletions when sufficient probes are developed to search the whole Duchenne genome (perhaps 4000 kilo bases in length).

Another more laborious method is to use recombinant DNA linkage analysis of nearby genes to chromosome band Xp21. Restriction fragment length polymorphisms (RFLPs) have no functional significance but may be inherited together with the nearby deleted Xp21 Duchenne genes and enable carrier detection.

Dystrophin is a normal intracellular plasma membrane protein in muscle, the "gene product" missing in Duchenne's (and Becker's) dystrophy. Assays in muscle biopsies have shown very low levels or absent dystrophin in severe Duchenne's dystrophy, low concentrations in "intermediate" forms (eg, manifesting female carrier), and qualitatively abnormal dystrophin at intermediate levels in Becker's dystrophy.

Arahata K: Mosaic expression of dystrophin in symptomatic carriers of Duchenne's muscular dystrophy. *N Engl J Med* 1989;**320**:138.

Bartlett RJ: Duchenne muscular dystrophy: High frequency of deletions. *Neurology* 1989;**38**:1.

Brooke MH: *A Clinician's View of Neuromuscular Diseases*, 2nd ed. Williams & Wilkins, 1985.

Hejtmancik JF: Carrier diagnosis of Duchenne muscular dystrophy using restriction fragment length polymorphisms. *Neurology* 1986;**36**:1553.

Hoffman EP: Characterization of dystrophin in muscle biopsy specimens from patients with Duchenne's or Becker's muscular dystrophy. *N Engl J Med* 1988;**318**:1363.

Lanzi G et al: Myotonic dystrophy in childhood. *Acta Neurol Belg* 1982;**82**:150.

Martinez BA: Childhood nemaline myopathy: A review. *Dev Med Child Neurol* 1987;**29**:815.

McMenamin JB, Becker LE, Murphy EG: Congenital muscular dystrophy: A clinicopathologic report of 24 cases. *J Pediatr* 1982;**100**:692.

Roses A: Mutants in Duchenne's muscular dystrophy. *Arch Neurol* 1988;**45**:84.

Schmalbruch H: Early fatal nemaline myopathy: Case review. *Dev Med Child Neurol* 1987;**29**:784.

Stanley CA: New genetic defects in mitochondrial fatty acid oxidation and carnitine deficiency. *Adv Pediatr* 1987;**34**:59.

BENIGN ACUTE CHILDHOOD MYOSITIS

Benign acute childhood myositis (myalgia cruris epidemica) is characterized by transient severe muscle pain and weakness affecting mainly the calves and occurring 1–2 days following an upper respiratory tract infection. Though symptoms involve mainly the gastrocnemius muscles, all skeletal muscles appear to be invaded directly by virus; recurrent episodes are due to different viral types. By demonstration of seroconversion or by isolation of the virus, acute myositis has been shown to be largely due to influenza types B and A and occasionally due to parainfluenza and adenovirus.

Ruff RL, Secrist D: Viral studies in benign acute childhood myositis. *Arch Neurol* 1982;**39**:261.

THE PERIODIC PARALYSES

Hypokalemic Periodic Paralysis

This rare condition is inherited as a dominant trait, with decreased occurrence in females, but it may appear sporadically. Onset occurs during childhood. The proximal muscles are affected first. Cranial and respiratory muscles are spared. Attacks of weakness may be precipitated by rest after exercise, exposure to cold, emotional stress, and high dietary intake of carbohydrate and sodium.

Attacks usually last for hours but may last for days and may be shortened by rest. The disease may progress to permanent weakness and atrophy.

The serum potassium level is low during an attack. Provocative tests that induce weakness and thus confirm the diagnosis include (1) exercise and (2) giving insulin 0.25 unit/kg subcutaneously, simultaneously with glucose 0.8 g/kg orally.

Hyperthyroidism, particularly in Japanese persons, may produce similar periodic weakness.

Acetazolamide, 5–30 mg/kg/d orally, is usually effective in preventing attacks. Alternative treatment consists of giving potassium chloride, 2–10 g orally to terminate an attack and 2–10 g at bedtime between attacks. The patient should be encouraged to eat a low-carbohydrate, low-sodium diet. Thiamine may abort the effects of carbohydrates. Unnecessary exposure to cold should be avoided.

The disorder is consistent with a normal life span. There are rare hyperkalemic and normokalemic variants.

Hyperkalemic Periodic Paralysis

This form of periodic paralysis has its onset in the first decade of life and is usually detected in infancy because of "staring" eyes (myotonic form of lid lag) or a very feeble cry (especially on waking). It is inherited as an autosomal dominant. Pseudohypertrophy of the calves is often present. There is an increased incidence of diabetes mellitus. The attacks are relatively short, lasting 30 minutes to 2 hours, and may be precipitated by rest after exercise, cold, and fatigue. Attacks usually occur in children of school age and then abate, although permanent muscle weakness may develop.

The serum potassium level rises during attacks. The EMG may show myotonia of the external ocular and facial muscles.

Treatment is with hydrochlorothiazide, 50 mg/d orally, or acetazolamide, 250 mg/d orally. Dichlorphenamide (Daranide), 50 mg/d orally, has also been recommended. The dose must be adjusted for each case. The disorder is consistent with a normal life span.

Normokalemic Periodic Paralysis

The onset of this disorder occurs in the first decade of life. The disorder is inherited as an autosomal

Table 24–31. Muscular dystrophies and myotonias of childhood.

Disease	Genetic Pattern	Age at Onset	Early Manifestations	Involved Muscles	Reflexes
Muscular dystrophies Duchenne's muscular dystrophy (pseudohypertrophic infantile)	X-linked recessive; autosomal recessive unusual. Thirty to 50% have no family history.	2–6 years; rarer in infancy.	Clumsiness, easy fatigability on walking, running, and climbing stairs. Walking on toes; waddling gait. Lordosis. (Climbing up on legs rising from supine position—Gower's maneuver.)	Axial and proximal before distal. Pelvic girdle; pseudohypertrophy of gastrocnemius (90%), triceps brachii, and vastus lateralis. Shoulder girdle usually later, also articulation difficulties. Eventually cardiomyopathy (50%).	Knee jerks ± or 0; ankle jerks + to + +.
Becker's Muscular Dystrophy (late onset)	X-linked recessive.	Childhood (usually later than in Duchenne's).	Similar to Duchenne's.	Similar to Duchenne's.	Similar to Duchenne's.
Limb-girdle muscular dystrophy A. Pelvifemoral (Leyden-Möbius) B. Scapulohumeral (Erb's juvenile)	Autosomal recessive in 60%; high sporadic incidence. A. Relatively common. B. Rare.	Variable; early childhood to adulthood.	Weakness, with distribution according to type. Waddling gait, difficulty climbing stairs. Lordosis.	A. Pelvic girdle usually involved first and to greater extent. B. Shoulder girdle often asymmetric. Quadriceps and hamstrings may be weakest. Pseudohypertrophy of calves uncommon.	Usually present.
Facioscapulohumeral muscular dystrophy (Landouzy-Déjérine) Scapuloperoneal variant	Autosomal dominant; sporadic cases not uncommon.	Usually late in childhood and adolescence; rare in infancy; not uncommon in twenties.	Diminished facial movements with inability to close eyes, smile, or whistle. Face may be flat, unlined. Difficulty in raising arms over head. Lordosis. Tripping in scapuloperoneal type.	Facial muscles followed by shoulder girdle, with occasional spread to hips or distal legs (scapuloperoneal variant).	Present.
Spinal muscular atrophy (SMA) Infantile SMA (Werdnig-Hoffman disease)	Autosomal recessive.	0–2 years.	Floppy infant	Big muscles: shoulder, hip. Tongue. Intercostals. Fingers-toes spared.	0 or nearly so.
Juvenile SMA (Kugelburg-Welander disease)	Autosomal recessive.	Onset after age 2 usually (Age 5–15 typical).	Weakness. "Fasciculations" 50%. Rarely a cause of "floppy infant."	Same.	Same.
Metabolic myopathies Carnitine deficiency (lipid storage myopathy) Primary (rare) Secondary: multiple forms	Genetics variable.	Infancy to adolescence.	Fasting hypoglycemia and coma; less ketosis than expected. Myopathy. Cardiomyopathy. Fatty liver. Don't confuse with Reye's, SIDS.	Weakness variable; may be precipitated by exercise (with resultant myoglobulinuria) or fasting.	Normal to decreased.
"Oculocraniosomatic syndrome" (ophthalmoplegia and "ragged reds"; progressive external ophthalmoloplegia)	(?) Acquired; 80% female; other hereditary neurologic disorders may be found in patient or family.	Variable; from infancy to adult life; most at about 10 years of age.	Ptosis and limitation of eye movements; hearing and visual loss (retinitis pigmentosa); intellectual loss; cerebellular disturbance (ataxia).	Extraocular muscles, often asymmetric. Variable involvement of axial muscles; cardiac muscles, with conduction defect.	Depressed to ± or 0.
Myasthenia gravis Transient neonatal	Variable.	At birth.	Difficulty sucking, swallowing; trouble with secretions.	Somatic and cranial muscles.	Normal to decreased.
Persistent neonatal	Variable.	Variable: birth, neonatal, infancy.	Same.	Same.	Same.
Congenital myopathies Myotonic dystrophy	Autosomal dominant.	At birth.	Same as myasthenia. Ptosis. Facial diplegia. Arthrogyposis, club feet, thin ribs.	Cranial and somatic, pharyngeal.	Decreased to 0.
"Other" Central core Nemaline (rod body) Myotubular (centronuclear) Congenital fiber type disproportion	Variable, often autosomal recessive.	Severe variants present at birth; milder variants (more common) infancy, childhood.	Severe variant, as in myasthenia, myotonic dystrophy. Later presentation—facial weakness, mild to moderate weakness, even "toe walking" only.	Similar to myotonic dystrophy.	Decreased to 0.
Congenital muscular dystrophy (Fukayama)	? Genetic. ? Infectious.	Birth.	Hypotonia. Facial weakness, joint contractures, mental retardation.	Heterogenous. Facial (cranial) and somatic. Contracture common.	Variable.
Congenital muscular dystrophy ("occidental")	Unknown. Usually not familial.	Birth (or early infancy).	As above. Normal IQ.	Same.	Same.
Benign congenital hypotonia (Oppenheim)	Variable.	Variable.	Hypotonia only. Deep tendon reflexes +. Laboratory tests, biopsy normal.	Somatic muscles (respiratory muscles spared).	Normal to decreased.
Myotonias Myotonia congenita (Thomsen)	Autosomal dominant (autosomal recessive cases reported).	Early infancy to late childhood.	Difficulty in relaxing muscles after contracting them, especially after sleep; aggravated by cold, excitement.	Hands especially; muscles may be diffusely enlarged, giving patient Herculean appearance.	Normal.
Myotonic dystrophy (Steinert) (Childhood and adult form)	Autosomal dominant.	Late childhood to adolescence; neonatal and infantile forms increasingly recognized (see above).	Myotonia of grasp, tongue; worsened by cold, emotions. "Hatchet-face." Nasal voice. Weakness and easy fatigability. Mild to moderate mental retardation noted.	Wasting and weakness of facial muscles, including muscles of mastication; sternocleidomastoids, hands. Myotonic phenomena: "bunching up" of muscles of tongue, thenar eminence, finger extensors after tapping with percussion hammer.	In infantile form, marked hyporeflexia.

Table 24–31 (cont.). Muscular dystrophies and myotonias of childhood.

Muscle Biopsy Findings	Other Diagnostic Tests	Treatment	Prognosis
Degeneration and variation in fiber size; proliferation of connective tissue. Basophilia, phagocytosis. Poor differentiation of fiber types on ATPase reaction; deficiency of type 2B fibers.	EMG myopathic. CK (4000–5000 IU) very high with decrease toward normal over the years. ECG. Chest x-ray. Cloned dystrophin cDNA probes.	Physical therapy, braces, wheelchair eventually, weight control.	Ten percent show nonprogressive mental retardation. Death from pneumonia 10–15 years after diagnosis with 75% of patients dead by age 20.
Similar to above, except type 2B fibers present.	Similar to above, although muscle enzymes may not be as elevated.	As above. Wheelchair in late childhood or early adult life.	Slower progression than Duchenne's, with death usually in adulthood.
Variation in muscle fiber size with many very large fibers. Fiber splitting and internal nuclei common. Many "moth-eaten" whorled fibers.	EMG myopathic. CK variable; often normal but may be elevated. ECG.	Physical therapy, weight control.	Mildly progressive: spread from lower to upper limbs may take 15–20 years. Life expectancy mid to late adulthood.
Predominantly large fibers with scattered tiny atrophic fibers, "moth-eaten" and whorled fibers. Inflammatory response. Little or no fiber splitting, fibrosis or type 1 fiber predominance.	EMG myopathic. Muscle enzymes usually normal.	Physical therapy where indicated. Wheelchair in old age. ? steroids in inflammatory infant variant.	Very slowly progressive, often with plateaus, except in infantile form where there may be difficulties in walking by adolescence. Usually normal life span.
Small, group atrophy. Twin peak fiber size. Fiber type grouping. Minimal fibrosis.	EMG "neuropathic." Nerve conduction, CSF, muscle enzymes normal.	Supportive: respiratory care, positioning, secretion management. Genetic counseling.	80–95% of patients 0–4 years die of pneumonia and respiratory failure.
Same.	Same. CK ("enzymnes") may be mildly elevated.	Physical therapy, wheelchair positioning to avoid scoliosis. May walk, usually later lose this.	Fairly normal life expectancy. 4–40+ years.
Normal or lipid droplets ("Ragged red" fibers with lipid stain, eg, oil red O).	Muscle biochemistry (carnitine, CPT enzyme) Urine organic acids (at time of illness). Plasma carnitine. WBC, Fibroblast enzyme studies.	Avoid fasting and mitochondrial toxins, eg, ASA, valproic acid. Carbohydrate. Treat acidosis. Carnitine orally.	Variable: occasionally fatal in infants. Progressive weakness, developmental delay, cardiomyopathy may occur.
Mitrochondrial abnormalities. "Ragged red" fibers. Changes in fiber size, usually due to type 2 fiber atrophy.	CK usually normal. ECG with conduction block. CSF protein elevated. Nerve conduction slowed. CT, brain scan, and brain stem auditory evoked response may be abnormal.	Plastic retraction of eyelids. Cardiac support. Anticipate diabetes mellitus. CoEnzyme Q?	Dysphagia may develop (50%) as well as generalized muscle weakness. Prognosis fair if disease is confined to ocular muscles. In severe cases, spongy vacuolization of brain and brain stem.
Unnecessary	Edrophonium or neostigmine tests. Acetylcholine receptor (AChR) antibodies. Repetitive nerve stimulation, EMG.	Supportive. Anticholinergic drugs.	Usually transient (< 2 months).
Sophisticated end plate, nerve terminal ultrastructural studies may be necessary.	May be similar to above. AChR antibodies negative.	May not respond to ACh-ase drugs, steroids or immunosuppressants.	Variable, may have long-term severe course.
Generalized fiber hypertrophy, delay in maturation. Type I atrophy. Internal nuclei	EMG "myotonic" in some (waning amplitude and pitch). Test mother. CK often normal.	Supportive, even respiratory support. Genetic counseling.	Severely involved infant may improve dramatically over months; expect mental retardation.
Distinctive diagnostic histochemistry, eg. "central cores," "nemaline rods."	Myopathic EMG.	Supportive. Genetic counseling.	Variable. May shorten life. Death in infancy or severe handicap. Scoliosis prominent.
"Dystrophic" changes. Fibrosis. Necrotic fibers. Internal nuclei. ? regenerative fibers.	Myopathic EMG, CK increased or normal. Positive CT, MRI scans: white matter low density, polymicrogyria, lissencephaly, etc.	Supportive.	Physical and mental handicap lifelong.
Same.	As above, CT, MRI variably low density.		May improve, walk. Scoliosis.
Normal with sophisticated studies (histochemistry, electron microscopy, even metabolic studies.)	Use of this diagnosis is shrinking with increasingly sophisticated biochemical (eg, cytochrome oxidase) studies.	Supportive.	Good (by definition). (Few documented long-term studies.)
Nonspecific and minor changes; type 2B fibers may be absent.	EMG "myotonic."	Usually none. Phenytoin, especially in cold weather, may improve muscle functioning.	Normal life expectancy, with only mild disability.
Type I fiber atrophy, type 2 hypertrophy, sarcoplasmic masses, internal nuclei, phagocytosis, fibrosis and cellular reaction.	EMG markedly "myotonic." Glucose tolerance test, thyroid tests. ECG. Chest x-ray and pulmonary function tests. Immunoglobulins.	Procainamide, 250 mg 3 times daily orally, increased to tolerance; phenytoin 5–7 mg/kg/d orally. (Drugs usually little role.)	Frontal baldness, cataracts (85%), gonadal atrophy (85% of males), thyroid dysfunction, diabetes mellitus (20%). Cardiac conduction defects; impaired pulmonary function. Low IgG. Life expectancy decreased.

dominant. Attacks come on during rest after exercise, with cold, following ingestion of foods high in potassium (eg, many fruit juices), and following ingestion of alcohol. The attacks may last for days.

In normokalemic paralysis, serum electrolyte levels do not change during attacks. Muscle biopsy may show vacuolar myopathy.

Treatment consists of increasing salt intake; acetazolamide, 250 mg/d orally, with dosage adjusted for each case; and fludrocortisone, 0.1 mg/d orally. The prognosis is good.

Bendheim P et al: Beta adrenergic treatment of hyperkalemic periodic paralysis. *Neurology* 1985;**35**:746.

Pearson CM: The periodic paralyses: Differential features and pathological observations in permanent myopathic weakness. *Brain* 1964;**87**:341.

MYASTHENIA GRAVIS

Essentials of Diagnosis

- Weakness, chiefly of muscles innervated by the brain stem, usually coming on or increasing with use (fatigue).
- Positive response to neostigmine and edrophonium.
- Acetylcholine receptor antibodies in serum (except in congenital form).

General Considerations

Myasthenia gravis is characterized by easy fatigability of muscles, particularly the extraocular muscles and those of mastication, swallowing, and respiration. However, in the neonatal period or in early infancy, the weakness may be so constant and general that an affected infant may present nonspecifically as a "floppy infant." Girls are affected more frequently than boys. The age at onset is over 10 years in 75% of cases, often shortly after menarche. If diagnosed before age 10, congenital myasthenia should be considered in retrospect. Thyrotoxicosis is found in almost 10% of affected female patients. The essential abnormality is a circulating antibody that binds to the acetylcholine receptor protein and thus reduces the number of motor end plates for binding by acetylcholine.

Clinical Findings

A. Symptoms and Signs:

1. Neonatal (transient) myasthenia gravis— This occurs in 12% of infants born to myasthenic mothers. The condition is due to maternal acetylcholine receptor antibody transferred across the placenta; a thymic factor in the infant may also be involved. A sibling may have died in the neonatal period with similar symptoms and nondiagnostic autopsy.

2. Congenital (persistent) myasthenia gravis— In this form of the disease, the mothers of the

affected infants rarely have myasthenia gravis, but other relatives may. Sex distribution is equal. Symptoms are often subtle and not recognized initially. Differential diagnosis includes many other causes of the "floppy infant" syndrome, such as infant botulism, ocular myopathy, congenital ptosis, and Möbius' syndrome (facial nuclear aplasia and other anomalies). This condition is not caused by receptor antibodies and often responds poorly to therapy. It may result from a genetic abnormality of the acetylcholine receptor protein or other neurotransmitter vagaries.

3. Juvenile myasthenia gravis— In this autoimmune form, the symptoms and signs are like those in adults. Receptor antibodies are usually present. The patient may be first seen by an otolaryngologist or psychiatrist. The more prominent signs are difficulty in chewing, dysphagia, a nasal voice, ptosis, and ophthalmoplegia. Pathologic fatigability of limbs, chiefly involving the proximal limb and neck muscles, may be more prominent than the bulbar signs and may lead to an initial diagnosis of conversion hysteria, muscular dystrophy, or polymyositis. Weakness may be limited to ocular muscles only. Associated disorders include autoimmune conditions, especially thyroid disease.

An acute fulminant form of myasthenia gravis has been reported in children of age 2–10 years and presents with rapidly progressive respiratory difficulties. Bulbar paralysis may evolve within 24 hours. There is no history of myasthenia. The differential diagnosis includes Landry-Guillain-Barré syndrome and bulbar poliomyelitis. Administration of anticholinesterase agents establishes the diagnosis and is lifesaving.

B. Laboratory Findings:

1. Neostigmine test— In newborns and very young infants, the neostigmine (Prostigmin) test may be preferable to the edrophonium (Tensilon) test because the longer duration of its response permits better observation, especially of sucking and swallowing movements. The test dose of neostigmine is 0.02 mg/kg subcutaneously, usually given with atropine, 0.01 mg/kg subcutaneously. There is a delay of about 10 minutes before the effect may be manifest. The physician should be prepared to suction secretions.

2. Edrophonium test— Testing with edrophonium is used in older children who are capable of cooperating in certain tasks, such as raising and lowering their eyelids and squeezing a sphygmomanometer bulb or the examiner's hands. The test dose is 0.1–1 mL intravenously, depending on the size of the child. Maximum improvement occurs within 2 minutes.

3. Other laboratory tests— Serum acetylcholine receptor antibodies are often found in the neonatal and juvenile forms. Ophthalmologic tests of ocular motility with edrophonium are often positive in patients able to cooperate. In juveniles, thyroid studies are appropriate.

C. Electrical Studies of Muscle: Repetitive stimulation of a motor nerve at slow rates (3/s) with recording over the appropriate muscle reveals a progressive fall in amplitude of the muscle potential in myasthenic patients. A maximal stimulus must be given. At higher rates of stimulation (50/s), there may be a transient repair of this defect before the progressive decline is seen.

If this study is negative, single fiber electromyography is now employed to determine if ''mean jitter'' exceeds normal.

D. Imaging: Chest x-ray and laminagraphy in older children may disclose benign thymus enlargement. Thymus tumors are rare in children.

Treatment

A. General and Supportive Care: In the newborn or in a child in myasthenic or cholinergic crisis (see below), suctioning of secretions is essential. Respiratory assistance may be required.

Treatment should be carried out by physicians with experience in this disorder.

B. Anticholinesterase Drug Therapy:

1. Pyridostigmine bromide (Mestinon)—The dose must be adjusted for each patient. A frequent starting dose is 15–30 mg orally every 6 hours.

2. Neostigmine (Prostigmin)—Fifteen milligrams of neostigmine are roughly equivalent to 60 mg of pyridostigmine bromide. Neostigmine often causes gastric hypermobility with diarrhea, but it is the drug of choice in newborns, in whom prompt treatment may be lifesaving. It may be given parenterally.

3. Atropine—Atropine may be added on a maintenance basis to control mild cholinergic side effects such as hypersecretion, abdominal cramps, and nausea and vomiting.

4. Immunologic intervention—This is primarily by use of prednisone. Plasmapheresis is effective in removing acetylcholine receptor antibody in severely affected patients.

5. Myasthenic crisis—Relatively sudden difficulties in swallowing and respiration may be observed in myasthenic patients. Edrophonium results in dramatic but brief improvement; this may make evaluation of the condition of the small child difficult. Suctioning, tracheostomy, respiratory assistance, and fluid and electrolyte maintenance may be required.

6. Cholinergic crisis—Cholinergic crisis may result from overdosage of anticholinesterase drugs. The resulting weakness may be similar to that of myasthenia, and the muscarinic effects (diarrhea, sweating, lacrimation, miosis, bradycardia, hypotension) are often absent or difficult to evaluate. The edrophonium test may help to determine whether the patient is receiving too little of the drug or is manifesting toxic symptoms due to overdosage. Improvement after the drugs are withdrawn suggests cholinergic crisis. Respirator facilities should be available. The patient may require atropine and tracheostomy.

C. Surgical Measures: Early thymectomy is beneficial in many patients whose disease is not confined to ocular symptoms; the effects may be delayed. Experienced surgical and postsurgical care are prerequisites.

Prognosis

Neonatal (transient) myasthenia presents a great threat to life, primarily due to aspiration of secretions. With proper treatment, the symptoms usually begin to disappear within a few days to 2–3 weeks, after which the child usually requires no further treatment.

In the congenital (persistent) form, the symptoms may initially be as acute as in the transient variety; more commonly, however, they are relatively benign and constant, with gradual worsening as the child grows older. Fatal cases occur.

In the juvenile form, patients may become resistant or unresponsive to anticholinesterase compounds and require corticosteroids or treatment in a hospital, where respiratory assistance can be given as needed. The overall prognosis for survival, for remission, and for improvement after therapy with prednisone and thymectomy is favorable.

Death in myasthenic or cholinergic crisis may occur unless prompt treatment is given.

Engel AG: Myasthenia gravis and myasthenic syndromes: Neurologic progress. *Ann Neurol* 1984;**16:**519.

Gordon N: Congenital myasthenia. *Dev Med Child Neurol* 1986;**28:**810.

Lefvert AK, Osterman PO: Newborn infants to myasthenic mothers: A clinical study and investigation of acetylcholine receptor antibodies in 17 children. *Neurology* 1983;**33:**133.

Morel E et al: Neonatal myasthenia gravis: A new clinical and immunologic appraisal in 30 cases. *Neurology* 1988;**38:**138.

Pascuzzi RM, Coslett HB, Johns TR: Long-term corticosteroid treatment of myasthenia gravis: Report of 116 patients. *Ann Neurol* 1984;**15:**291.

Rodriguez M et al: Myasthenia gravis in children: Long-term follow-up. *Ann Neurol* 1983;**13:**504.

Snead OC et al: Juvenile myasthenia gravis. *Neurology* 1980;**30:**732.

CONGENITAL ABSENCE OF MUSCLES*

Congenital absence (sometimes only partial) of one or more muscles, usually unilateral, and particularly of the pectoralis (sternal portion), trapezius,

---

*Arthrogryposis multiplex, or contractures and fixation about multiple joints, is discussed briefly in a later section on the floppy infant. Clubfoot, Sprengel's deformity, and torticollis are discussed in Chapter 22.

serratus anterior, quadratus femoris, or omohyoid, is not unusual. Heredofamilial cases have been reported. Other deformities, eg, syndactyly, microdactyly, and muscular dystrophy, may be present. Absence of muscles of the abdominal wall (prune belly) may be associated with anomalies of the gastrointestinal tract, urinary tract (Eagle's syndrome), or extremities or with cryptorchidism. Treatment is determined by the specific abnormalities present.

PERIPHERAL NERVE PALSIES

1. FACIAL WEAKNESS

Facial asymmetry may be present at birth or develop later, either suddenly or gradually, unilaterally or bilaterally. Nuclear or peripheral involvement of the facial nerves results in sagging or drooping of the mouth and inability to close one or both eyes, particularly when newborns and infants cry. Inability to wrinkle the forehead may be demonstrated in infants and young children by getting them to follow an object (light) moved vertically above the forehead. Loss of taste of the anterior two-thirds of the tongue on the involved side may be demonstrated in intelligent, cooperative children by age 4 or 5; playing with a younger child and the judicious use of a tongue blade may enable the physician to note whether the child's face puckers up when something sour (eg, lemon juice) is applied with a swab to the anterior tongue. Ability to wrinkle the forehead is preserved, owing to bilateral innervation, in supranuclear or central facial paralysis.

Injuries to the facial nerve at birth occur in 0.25–6.5% of consecutive live births. Forceps delivery is the cause in some cases; in others, the side of the face affected may have abutted in utero against the sacral prominence. Often, no cause can be established.

Facial asymmetry due to hypoplasia of one side of the cranium associated with contralateral hemiatrophy and spastic hemiparesis (due, in most instances, to an intrauterine cerebrovascular accident affecting one hemisphere) is usually differentiated easily, as is the hemiatrophy of one side of the body seen in Silver's syndrome.

Acquired peripheral facial weakness (Bell's palsy) of sudden onset and unknown cause is common in children. It often follows a viral illness (postinfectious) or physical trauma (eg, cold). It may be a presenting sign of a disorder such as tumor, hypertension, infectious mononucleosis, or Landry-Guillain-Barré syndrome, usually diagnosable by the history, physical examination, and appropriate laboratory tests.

Bilateral facial weakness in early life may be due to agenesis of the affected muscles or to nuclear causes (part of Möbius' syndrome) or may even be familial. Myasthenia gravis, polyneuritis, and myotonic dystrophy must be considered.

"Asymmetric crying facies," in which one side of the lower lip depresses with crying (this is the *normal* side) and the other does not, is a common innocent congenital malformation inherited as an autosomal dominant. The defect in the parent (the asymmetry often improves with age) may be almost inapparent. Electromyography suggests congenital absence of the depressor anguli oris muscle of the lower lip. Forceps pressure is often indicted as a cause of this innocent congenital anomaly. Occasionally, other major (eg, cardiac septal) congenital defects accompany the palsy.

In the vast majority of cases of isolated peripheral facial palsy—both those present at birth and those acquired later—improvement begins within 1–2 weeks, and near or total recovery of function is observed within 2 months. Methylcellulose drops, 1%, should be instilled into the eyes to protect the cornea during the day; at night, the lid should be taped down with cellophane tape. Upward massage of the face for 5–10 minutes 3–4 times a day may help maintain muscle tone. Prednisone therapy reduces the pain of Bell's palsy and promotes recovery of facial strength and reduction of motor synkinesis ("crocodile tears").

Faradic or galvanic stimulation of facial muscles is not advised.

In the few children with permanent and cosmetically disfiguring facial weakness, plastic surgical intervention at 6 years of age or older may be of benefit. New procedures, such as attachment of facial muscles to the temporal muscle or transplantation of cranial XI, are being developed.

2. BRACHIAL PLEXUS INJURIES
(Erb's Palsy, Klumpke's Paralysis)

Traction injuries of the brachial plexus are most common in newborns, occurring in 0.1% of spontaneous, 1.2% of breech, 1.3% of forceps, and 0.25% of all deliveries. The complexity of the brachial plexus precludes any absolute classification, but injuries are usually divided into those affecting the upper plexus (Erb's palsy) and those affecting the lower plexus (Klumpke's paralysis).

Erb's palsy, involving chiefly the fifth and sixth cervical roots, is seen in 99% of cases. It is usually associated with difficult breech delivery, forceps delivery (especially in brow and face presentations), or misapplication of the vacuum extractor. The arm is maintained in adduction and internal rotation at the shoulder, with the lower arm pronated, assuming the "waiter's tip" position. Loss of sensation may be difficult to assess in newborns.

In Klumpke's paralysis, involving chiefly the

lower brachial plexus (eighth cervical and first thoracic roots), the small muscles of the hand and wrist flexors are affected, causing a "claw hand." Horner's syndrome may also be present. The injury, usually caused by manipulation during delivery, results from hyperabduction of the arm at the shoulder.

Swinging a child by one arm or jerking the arm may also cause lower plexus injuries ("nursemaid's palsy").

The palsies observed are usually due to avulsion of the plexus, with contusion, edema, and some hemorrhage. X-ray studies of the shoulder will rule out fractures of the clavicle or cervical spine as well as dislocations.

In most instances, recovery occurs spontaneously within a few days or weeks. However, contractures of the shoulder and especially the elbow joints and atrophy of the affected muscles may occur; positioning in the so-called Statue of Liberty or airplane wing position, formerly advised, has been said to contribute to these problems. Passive range-of-motion exercises, which can be taught to the parents, are most helpful in preventing contractures. Electromyography and CT metrizamide myelography can delineate the extent of injury and aid in prognosis, as well as determine the patients in whom surgical exploration and reparative procedures may be justified.

Adour KK: Current concepts in neurology: Diagnosis and management of facial paralysis. *N Engl J Med* 1982; **307:**348.

Greenwald AG, Schute PC, Shiveley JL: Brachial plexus at birth palsy: A 10-year report on the incidence and prognosis. *J Pediatr Orthop* 1984;**4:**689.

Hunt D: Surgical management of brachial plexus injuries at birth. *Dev Med Child Neurol* 1988;**30:**824.

Miller M, Hall J: Familial asymmetric crying facies. *Am J Dis Child* 1979;**133:**743.

Painter ML, Bergman I: Obstetrical trauma to the neonatal central and peripheral nervous system. *Semin Perinatol* 1982;**6:**89.

Reroque H et al: Möbius' syndrome and transposition of the great vessels. *Neurology* 1988;**38:**1894.

Sudarshan A, Goldie WD: The spectrum of congenital facial diplegia (Moebius syndrome). *Pediatr Neurol* 1985; **1:**180.

CHRONIC POLYNEUROPATHY

Polyneuropathy, usually insidious in onset and slowly progressive, occurs in children of any age. The presenting complaints are chiefly disturbances of gait and easy fatigability in walking or running and, slightly less often, weakness or clumsiness of the hands. Pain, tenderness, or paresthesias are less frequently mentioned. Neurologic examination discloses muscular weakness, greatest in the distal portions of the extremities, with steppage gait and depressed or absent deep tendon reflexes. Cranial

nerves are sometimes affected. Sensory deficits (difficult to demonstrate in fearful children or those under 5 years of age) occur in a stocking and glove distribution. The muscles may be tender, and trophic changes such as glassy or "parchment" skin and absent sweating may occur. Thickening of the ulnar and peroneal nerves may be felt. Pure sensory neuropathies show up as chronic trauma, ie, the patient does not feel minor trauma and burns to the fingers and toes.

Known causes include (1) toxins, eg, lead, arsenic, mercurials, vincristine, and benzene; (2) systemic disorders, eg, diabetes mellitus, chronic uremia, recurrent hypoglycemia, porphyria, polyarteritis nodosa, and lupus erythematosus; (3) "inflammatory" states, eg, chronic or recurrent Landry-Guillain-Barré syndrome and neuritis associated with mumps or diphtheria; (4) hereditary, often degenerative conditions, which in some classifications include certain storage diseases, leukodystrophies, spinocerebellar degenerations with neurogenic components, and Bassen-Kornzweig syndrome (Table 24–32); and (5) the hereditary sensory or combined motor and sensory neuropathies. Polyneuropathies associated with carcinomas, beriberi or other vitamin deficiencies, or excessive vitamin B_6 intake are not reported or are exceedingly rare in children.

The most common chronic neuropathy of insidious onset often has no identifiable cause. This "chronic idiopathic neuropathy" is assumed to be immunologically mediated and may have a relapsing course. Sometimes there is facial weakness. Spinal fluid protein is elevated. Nerve conduction is slowed, and nerve biopsies are abnormal. Immunologic abnormalities are seldom demonstrated, although nerve biopsies may show round cell infiltration. Steroids and other immunosuppressants may give long-term benefit.

Of the 4 defined hereditary sensory neuropathies, the prototype is familial dysautonomia, also called

Table 24–32. Hereditary neuropathies with known metabolic error.[1]

Disorder	Characteristics
Amyloidosis	Rarely seen in children.
Acute intermittent porphyria (AD)	Abdominal pain, emotional disease.
Krabbe's disease and metachromatic leukodystrophy (AR)	Onset usually in infancy. Dementia. WBC enzyme to diagnose.
Adrenoleukodystrophy (XLR) and myeloneuropathy (AR)	Peroxisomal disease. Long-chain fatty acid to diagnose either one.
Abetalipoproteinemia (AR), Fabry's disease (XLR), Tangier disease (AR), Refsum dis ease (AR)	Disordered lipid metabolism in these 4 diseases.

[1]AD = autosomal dominant; AR = autosomal recessive; XLR = sex-linked recessive.

Riley-Day syndrome and hereditary sensory neuropathy type III. Transmitted as an autosomal recessive trait and seen mostly in Jewish children, this disorder has its onset in infancy. It is characterized by vomiting and difficulties in feeding that are due to abnormal esophageal motility; pulmonary infections; decreased or absent tearing; indifference to pain; diminished or absent tendon reflexes; absence of fungiform papillae of the tongue; emotional lability; abnormal temperature control with excessive sweating; labile blood pressure; abnormal intradermal histamine responses; and other evidences of autonomic dysfunction. Mental retardation may be present. Neurologic findings include a marked decrease in unmyelinated fibers of cutaneous nerves and decreased myelinization in dorsal root fibers and the posterior columns of the spinal cord.

A careful genetic history (pedigree) and examination and electrical testing (motor and sensory nerve conduction, electromyography) of relatives are keys to diagnosis of hereditary neuropathy.

Other hereditary neuropathies may have ataxia as a prominent finding often overshadowing the neuropathy. Examples are Friedreich's ataxia, dominant cerebellar ataxia, and Marinesco-Sjögren's syndrome. Finally, some hereditary neuropathics have identifiable and occasionally treatable metabolic errors (see Table 24–33). Other sections (eg, CNS Degenerative Disorders of Infancy & Childhood) describe these in more detail.

Laboratory diagnosis of chronic polyneuropathy is made by measurement of motor and sensory nerve conduction velocities; electromyography may show a neurogenic polyphasic pattern. Cerebrospinal protein levels are often elevated, with an IgG index sometimes increased as well. Nerve biopsy, with teasing of the fibers as well as staining for metachromasia, is advised to demonstrate loss of myelin and (to a lesser degree) loss of axons and increased connective tissue or concentric lamellas ("onion skin appearance") around the nerve fiber. Muscle biopsy may show the pattern associated with denervation. Other laboratory studies, directed toward specific causes mentioned above, include screening for heavy metals and for metabolic, renal, or vascular disorders. Chronic lead intoxication, which rarely causes neuropathy in childhood, may escape detection until the child is given edentate calcium disodium (EDTA) and lead levels are determined in timed urines. Three- and 4-fold rises are then diagnostic.

Table 24–33. Hereditary motor and sensory neuropathies; metabolic error unknown.

Name	Prototype Unknown	Inheritance	Clinical Features	Nerve Biopsy
Sensory and autonomic neuropathy	(1) Familial dysautonomia (2) other	Autosomal recessive (AR) AR, ? autosomal dominant (AD)	See text Rare (see references)	(1) Decreased unmyelin fibers posterior column and cord (2) Variable (see references)
HMSN I (Hereditary motor and sensory neuropathy I) (If tremor is present, Roussy-Lévy syndrome)	"Classic" Charcot-Marie-Tooth disease	AD	Onset 0–15 y. Weakness, atrophy of feet, calves (pes cavus, "stork legs"), hands. Sensory loss 0 or variable. Deep tendon reflexes (DTR) 0. Motor nerve conduction velocities (MNCV) slowed. Often hypertrophic (palpable) nerves. Linked to Duffy blood group.	Segmental
HMSN II	Neuronal/axonal Charcot-Marie-Tooth disease	AD	Less severe; onset 10–20. Leg cramps, numbness, MNCV normal or slightly slow. CSF protein often normal.	Axonal loss, secondary demyelination
HMSN III	Hypertrophic Charcot-Marie-Tooth disease; Dejerine-Sottas disease	AR	Onset in infancy. Severe. CSF protein increased. Very slow MNCV. Slowly progressive.	Hypertrophic ("onion bulb") interstitial changes
HMSN IV	Refsum disease		Severe sensory, mild motor. Thick nerves. CSF protein elevated. Ichthyosis, retinitis pigmentosa, ataxia, deafness. Urine phytanic acid.	See HMSN III
HSMN V	Charcot-Marie-Tooth disease with spastic paraparesis		Abnormal pyramidal tract findings. Rule out adrenomyelopathy.	Defined in pedigrees
HMSN VI, VII	Optic atrophy, retinitis pigmentosa, etc.		Poorly defined. Multiple-systems involved.	See HMSN V

Therapy is directed at specific disorders whenever possible. Occasionally, the weakness is profound and involves bulbar nerves, in which case tracheostomy and respiratory assistance are required. Corticosteroid therapy may be of considerable benefit in cases where the cause is unknown or neuropathy is considered to be due to "chronic inflammation" (this is not the case in acute Landry-Guillain-Barré syndrome). Prednisone, 1–2.5 mg/kg/d orally, with tapering to the least effective dose—discontinued if the process seems to be arresting and reinstituted when symptoms recur—is recommended. Prednisone should probably not be used for treatment of peroneal muscular atrophy. In all cases considered for corticosteroid therapy, the risks and benefits should be carefully weighed. When treatable, symptoms regress and may disappear altogether over a period of months.

Long-term prognosis varies with the cause and the ability to offer specific therapy. In the "corticosteroid-dependent" group, residual deficits and deaths within a few years are more frequent.

Axelrod FB, Pearson J: Congenital sensory neuropathies: Diagnostic distinction from familial dysautonomia. *Am J Dis Child* 1984;**138**:947.

Chatorian, AM: Chronic polyneuropathy in childhood. *Int Pediatr* 1988;**3**:125.

Dyck PJ et al: *Peripheral Neuropathy*, 2nd ed. Saunders, 1988.

Dyck PJ et al: Prednisone improves chronic inflammatory demyelinating polyradiculoneuropathy more than no treatment. *Ann Neurol* 1982;**11**:136.

Dyck PJ et al: Prednisone-responsive hereditary motor and sensory neuropathy. *Mayo Clin Proc* 1982;**57**:239.

Evans OB: Polyneuropathy in childhood. *Pediatrics* 1979;**64**:96.

Hagberg B, Westerberg B: The nosology of genetic peripheral neuropathies in Swedish children. *Dev Med Child Neurol* 1983;**25**:3.

Prensky AL, Dodson WE: The steroid treatment of hereditary motor and sensory neuropathy. *Neuropediatrics* 1984;**15**:203.

MISCELLANEOUS NEUROMUSCULAR DISORDERS

FLOPPY INFANT SYNDROME

Essentials of Diagnosis

- In early infancy, decreased muscular activity, both spontaneous and in response to postural reflex testing and to passive motion.
- In young infants, "frog posture" or other unusual positions at rest.
- In older infants, delay in motor milestones.

General Considerations

In the young infant, ventral suspension, ie, supporting the infant with a hand under the chest, normally results in the infant's holding its head slightly up (45 degrees or less), the back straight or nearly so, the arms flexed at the elbows and slightly abducted, and the knees partly flexed. The floppy infant droops over the hand like an inverted U. Even the normal newborn attempts to keep the head in the same plane as the body when pulled up from supine to sitting by the hands ("traction response"). Marked head lag is characteristic of the floppy infant. Hyperextensibility of the joints is not a dependable criterion.

The usual reasons for seeking medical evaluation in older infants are delays in walking, running, or climbing stairs or difficulties and lack of endurance in motor activities.

Hypotonia or decreased motor activity is a frequent presenting complaint in neuromuscular disorders but may also accompany a variety of systemic conditions or may be due to certain disorders of connective tissue.

Clinical Types

A. Paralytic Group: There is significant lack of movement against gravity (eg, failure to kick the legs, hold up the arms, or attempt to stand when held) or in response to stimuli such as tickling or slight pain.

B. Nonparalytic Group: There is floppiness without significant paralysis.

Note: Deep tendon reflexes may be depressed or absent in the nonparalytic group also. Brisk reflexes with hypotonia point to suprasegmental or general cerebral dysfunction.

1. PARALYTIC GROUP

The hypotonic infant who is weak ("paralyzed") usually has a lesion of the lower motor neuron complex. (See Table 24–34.) Infantile progressive spinal muscular atrophy (Werdnig-Hoffman disease) is the most common cause. Neuropathy is rare. Botulism and myasthenia gravis (rare) are neuromuscular junction causes. Myotonic dystrophy and rare myopathies (eg, central core myopathy) are muscle disease entities.

In anterior horn cell or muscle disease, weakness is proximal, eg, shoulder and hips; finger movement is preserved. Tendon reflexes are absent or depressed; strength (to noxious stimuli) is decreased ("paralytic"). Intelligence is preserved. Fine motor, personal/social, and language milestones are normal, for example, on a Denver Developmental Screening Test (DDST).

Table 24–34. Floppy infant: paralytic causes.

Disease	Genetic	Early Manifestations
IPSMA (Infantile Progressive Spinal Muscular Atrophy) "Malignant" form	Autosomal recessive (AR)	In utero movements decreased by one-third. Gradual weakness, delay in gross motor milestones. Weak cry. Abdominal breathing. Poor limb motion ("no kicking"). Deep tendon reflexes (DTR)—0. Fasciculations of tongue. Normal personal-social behavior.
"Intermediate" form	AR	Onset under age 1 usual. *Progression slower:* may be impossible to predict early course of IPSMA. Hand tremors common.
Infantile botulism	Acquired under age 1 (mostly under 6 months); botulism spore in stool makes toxin	Poor feeding. Constipation. Weak cry. Failure to thrive. Lethargy. Facial weakness, ptosis, ocular muscle palsy. Inability to suck, swallow. Apnea. Source: soil dust (outdoor construction workers may bring it home on clothes), honey.
Myasthenia gravis Neonatal transient	12% of infants born from a myasthenia mother	Floppiness. Poor sucking and feeding; choking. Respiratory distress. Weak cry.
Congenital persistent	Mother normal. Rare AR (AD)	As above; may improve and later exacerbate.
Myotonic dystrophy	Autosomal dominant (AD) (almost always *mother* transmits gene in neonatal/ infant severe form)	Polyhydramnios; failure of suck, respirations. Facial diplegia. Ptosis. Arthrogryposis. Thin ribs. Later, developmental delay.
Neonatal "rare myopathy," severe variant Nemaline central core "minimal change" myotubular (centronuclear) reducing body	AR, AD	Virtually all of the rare myopathies may have a severe (even fatal) neonatal or early infant form. Clinical features similar in infancy to infantile myotonic dystrophy.
Congenital muscular dystrophy Fukayama	? Genetic ? Infectious	Early onset. Facial weakness. Joint contractures. Severe mental retardation. Ill-defined.
Other		Severe or benign (improve). No mental retardation.
Essential hypotonia ("benign congenital hypotonia")	Unknown cause	Diagnosis of exclusion. Family history variable. Mild to moderate hypotonia with weakness.

Myopathies

The congenital, relatively nonprogressive myopathies, muscular dystrophy, myotonic dystrophy, polymyositis, and periodic paralysis are discussed elsewhere. Most cases of congenital or early infantile muscular dystrophy reported in the past probably represented congenital myopathies (Table 24–31). Congenital muscular dystrophy, diagnosed by muscle biopsy, occurs in 2 forms: (1) a benign form, with gradual improvement in strength; and (2) a severe form, in which there is either rapid progression of weakness and death in the first months or year of life or severe disability with little or no progression but lifelong marked limitation of activity.

Glycogenosis With Muscle Involvement

Glycogen storage diseases are described in Chapter 33. Patients with type II (Pompe's disease, due to a deficiency of acid maltase) are most likely to present as floppy infants. The weakness in type III (limit dextrinosis) is less marked than in type II, while the rare instances of type IV (amylopectinosis) are severely hypotonic. Muscle cramps on exertion or easy fatigability, rather than floppiness in infancy, is the presenting complaint in type V (McArdle's phosphorylase deficiency) or the glycogenosis due to phosphofructokinase deficiency or phosphohexose isomerase inhibition.

Myasthenia Gravis

Neonatal transient and congenital persistent myasthenia gravis, presenting as "paralytic" floppy infants, is described elsewhere in this chapter.

Arthrogryposis Multiplex (Congenital Deformities About Multiple Joints)

This symptom complex, sometimes associated with hypotonia, may be of "neurogenic" or "myopathic" origin (or both) and may be associated with a wide variety of other anomalies. Orthopedic aspects are discussed in Chapter 23.

Spinal Cord Lesions

Severe limpness in newborns following breech extraction with stretching or actual tearing of the lower cervical to upper thoracic spinal cord is rarely seen today, owing to improved obstetric delivery. Klumpke's lower brachial plexus paralysis may be present; the abdomen is usually exceedingly soft, and the lower extremities are flaccid. Urinary retention is present initially; later, the bladder may function autonomously. Myelography or MRI scanning may define the lesion. After a few weeks, spasticity of the lower limbs becomes obvious. Treatment is symptomatic and consists of bladder and skin care and eventual mobilization on crutches or in a wheelchair.

2. NONPARALYTIC GROUP

The nonparalytic group often has "brain damage." (See Table 24–35.) Intrauterine or perinatal insults to brain or spinal cord, while sometimes difficult to document, are major causes. (Occasionally, severe congenital myopathies presenting in the newborn period cause confusion.) Persisting severe hypotonia is ominous. Tone will often vary. Spasticity and other forms of cerebral palsy may emerge; hypertonia and hypotonia may occur at varying times in the same infant. Choreoathetoid or ataxic movements and developmental delay can clarify the diagnosis. Reflexes are often increased; pathologic reflexes (Babinski, tonic neck) may persist or worsen.

Creatine kinase and electromyogram are usually normal. Prolonged nerve conduction velocities point to polyneuritis or leukodystrophy. Muscle biopsies, utilizing special stains and histographic analysis, often show a remarkable reduction in size of type II fibers associated with decreased voluntary motor activity.

Limpness in the neonatal period and early infancy and subsequent delay in achieving motor milestones are the presenting features in a large number of children with a variety of central nervous system disorders, including mental retardation, as in trisomy 21. In many such cases, no specific diagnosis can be made. Close observation and scoring of motor patterns and adaptive behavior, as by the Denver Developmental Screening Test, are most helpful.

Brooke MH: *A Clinician's View of Neuromuscular Disease.* Williams & Wilkins, 1986.

Dubowitz V: *The Floppy Infant,* 2nd ed. No. 76 of: *Clinics in Developmental Medicine.* Heinemann, 1980.

Gamstorp I, Sarnat HG (editors): *Progressive Spinal Muscular Atrophies.* Raven Press, 1984.

Greenberg F et al: X-linked infantile spinal muscular atrophy. *Am J Dis Child* 1988;**142**:217.

Long SS: Botulism in infancy. *Pediatr Infect Dis J* 1984; **3**:266.

Zellweger H: The floppy infant: A practical approach. *Helv Paediatr Acta* 1984;**38**:301.

Table 24–35. Floppy infant: nonparalytic causes.

	Causes	Manifestations
Central nervous system disorders Atonic diplegia ("prespastic diplegia")	Intrauterine, perinatal asphyxia, cord injury	Limpness, stupor; poor suck, cry, Moro reflex, grasp; later, irritability, increased tone and reflexes
Choreoathetosis	As above; kernicterus	Hypotonic early; movement disorder emerges later (6–18 months)
Ataxic cerebral palsy	Same	Same
Syndromes with hypotonia (CNS origin) Trisomy 21	Genetic	100% have hypotonia early
Prader-Willi syndrome	Genetic ?	Hypotonia, hypomentia, hypogonadism, obesity
Marfan syndrome	Autosomal dominant (AD)	Arachnodactyly
Dysautonomia	Autosomal recessive (AR)	Respiratory, corneal anesthesia
Degenerative disorders Tay-Sachs	AR	Macular cherry-red spot
Metachromatic leukodystrophy	AR	Deep tendon reflexes (DTR) increased early, polyneuropathy late; mental retardation
Systemic diseases Malnutrition	Deprivation, cystic fibrosis, celiac disease	See underlying disease elsewhere in text
Chronic illness	Congenital heart disease; chronic pulmonary disease (eg, bronchopulmonary dysplasia); uremic, renal acidosis	
Metabolic	Hypercalcemia, Lowe's disease	
Endocrine	Hypothyroid, Turner's syndrome	

CEREBRAL PALSY

Essentials of Diagnosis

- Impairment of movement and posture since birth or early infancy.
- Nonprogressive and nonhereditary.

General Considerations

Cerebral palsy is a term of clinical convenience for disorders of impaired motor functioning and posture with onset before or at birth or during the first year of life, basically nonprogressive, and varying widely in their causes, manifestations, and prognosis. The most obvious manifestation is impaired ability of voluntary muscles. In the USA, cerebral palsy affects about 0.2% of neonatal survivors.

Classification

Classification is commonly based on the predominant motor deficit.

A. Spastic Forms: About 75% of cases. Often associated with other forms.

1. Quadriplegia (tetraplegia)—The 4 extremities may be involved about equally, or upper limbs may show more severe involvement. The main lesion is in the cerebral white matter. Quadriplegia due to perinatal damage often shows symptoms earlier than that due to fetal undernutrition or prematurity. Nearly 90% of patients are profoundly retarded.

2. Diplegia—Legs involved more than arms.

3. Hemiplegia—One side involved primarily.

4. Paraplegia—Legs only involved.

5. Monoplegia—One extremity only involved.

6. Triplegia—Three extremities involved.

B. Ataxia: About 15% of cases. Pure and in combination with other forms.

C. Dyskinesia (Choreoathetosis): About 5% of cases. Often associated with rigidity or spastic quadri- or diplegia.

D. Hypotonic Form: Fewer than 1% of cases. Persistent hypotonia with variable degrees of weakness.

Etiology

The cause is often obscure or multiple. No definite etiologic diagnosis is possible in over one-third of cases. The incidence is high among infants small for gestational age. Intrauterine hypoxia is a frequent cause. Other known causes are intrauterine bleeding, infections, toxins, congenital malformations, obstetric complications (including birth hypoxia), neonatal infections, kernicterus, neonatal hypoglycemia, acidosis, and a small number of genetic syndromes (about 2%).

Associated Deficits

A. Seizures: Seizures afflict about 50% of all children with cerebral palsy and are more prevalent in those with severe involvement.

B. Mental Retardation: Mild to moderate retardation is seen in 26% of patients and profound retardation in 27%. The incidence highly correlates with the severity of cerebral palsy.

C. Sensory and Speech Deficits: Impairment of speech, vision, hearing, and perceptual functions is found often in varying degrees and combinations.

Clinical Findings

A. Symptoms and Signs: The typical spastic child exhibits muscular hypertonicity of the clasp knife type that may eventually end in contractures. In the limb or limbs involved, tendon reflexes, if sufficient muscle relaxation can be achieved, are hyperactive; clonus may be present, and the plantar responses are often extensor. While voluntary control, especially of fine movements, is decreased, there is spread or overflow of associated movements. In extreme cases, the child may lie with elbows flexed and fists clenched (straphanger's posture) and legs crossed or scissored. In early infancy, the child may appear floppy, although tendon jerks are abnormally increased (hypotonic, atonic, or prespastic diplegia). Rigidity often accompanies cerebral palsy.

Ataxia may be difficult to delineate in the presence of spasticity or hyperkinetic movements.

Microcephaly (head circumference < 2 SD below the mean for age and sex and decreasing) is present in about 25% of spastic quadri- and diplegics.

Partial atrophy of the cranium on the involved side or of involved extremities is observed frequently, but dependable statistics are not available.

A smaller hand or foot, when coupled with mild weakness on muscle testing or hyperreflexia, often justifies a diagnosis of mild cerebral palsy of which the patient or the family may not even have been aware.

B. Laboratory and Other Findings: No routine workup can be outlined. The clinical findings, the presence or absence of seizures, and the overall outlook for the child—particularly with respect to intelligence and the ability to carry on activities of daily living—determine what studies, if any, should be performed. Hip films in abduction are indicated to rule out dislocations secondary to spasticity. Electroencephalography is indicated when seizures are present or suspected. In some cases, CT scanning may aid in determining the prognosis.

Urine screening tests for aminoacidurias (and in choreoathetosis with self-abuse, serum uric acid determinations) should be considered to rule out Lesch-Nyhan syndrome.

Differential Diagnosis

The diagnosis is usually not difficult. Progressive deterioration in the first 3 months is more likely to denote a metabolic disorder; subsequently, it denotes one of the central nervous system degenerative disorders (Tables 24–25 and 24–26). In the ataxic form, cerebellar dysgenesis (sometimes familial) or a spinocerebellar degeneration may have to be ruled out.

Prevention

Obstetric advances involving late third-trimester management and delivery have resulted in significant gains. Much more needs to be done in prenatal care, especially during the second and early third trimester. The number of cases in which cerebral palsy is associated with aggressive efforts to salvage premature infants has decreased as a result of advances in neonatal care.

Treatment

Realistically, a child with cerebral palsy should be helped to achieve maximum potential rather than "normality." Special educational programming depends on the physical and mental potential of the child. The degree of improvement with physical therapy correlates positively with better intelligence. Treat seizures as in other children. The orthopedic aspects of cerebral palsy are discussed in Chapter 23.

Spasticity occasionally is reduced by diazepam (Valium), dantrolene (Dantrium), or baclofen (Lioresal). Optimal doses vary with degree of spasticity, size and age of the child, and other medications taken. Surgical amelioration of moderate to severe spasticity in cerebral palsy has been attempted by various procedures over many years; dorsal rhizotomy is the newest procedure.

Management of "hyperactivity" is dealt with below in connection with attention deficit disorder.

Psychologic counseling and support of the child and family are of paramount importance.

Prognosis

In patients with severe cerebral palsy, especially spastics with profound retardation and seizures that are difficult to control, death due to intercurrent infections is not uncommon; nearly half die by 10 years of age. In nearly 30% of patients, chiefly in those with mild involvement, motor deficits resolve by the seventh birthday. Many children with cerebral palsy and average or near-average intelligence lead fairly normal, satisfying, and productive lives.

Freeman JM, Nelson BL: Intrapartum asphyxia and cerebral palsy. *Pediatrics* 1988;**82**:240.

Nelson KB: What proportion of cerebral palsy is related to birth asphyxia? (Editorial.) *J Pediatr* 1988;**112**:572.

Neville BGR: Selective dorsal rhizotomy for spastic cerebral palsy. (Annotation.) *Dev Med Child Neurol* 1988; **30**:395.

Palmer FB et al: The effects of physical therapy on cerebral palsy: A controlled trial in infants with spastic diplegia. *N Engl J Med* 1988;**318**:803.

Physical therapy for spastic diplegia. *Lancet* (Editorial.) 1988;**2**:201.

What causes cerebral palsy? *Lancet* 1988;**2**:142.

ATTENTION DEFICIT DISORDER (ADD)

Essentials of Diagnosis

■ Developmentally inappropriate attention and impulsivity (ADD).

■ Hyperactivity a frequent, but not invariable, component (ADD-H).

General Considerations As defined by the American Psychiatric Association's *Diagnostic and Statistical Manual of Mental Disorders* (DSM-III-Revised), the criteria for ADD-H are as follows:

(1) A period of 6 months or more during which at least 8 of the following behaviors are present:

(a) Has difficulty remaining seated when required to do so.

(b) Often fidgets with hands or feet or squirms in seat.

(c) Has difficulty playing quietly.

(d) Often talks excessively.

(e) Often shifts from one uncompleted activity to another.

(f) Has difficulty sustaining attention to tasks or play activities.

(g) Has difficulty following through on instructions from others (not due to oppositional behavior or failure of comprehension), eg, fails to finish chores.

(h) Is easily distracted by extraneous stimuli.

(i) Often interrupts or intrudes on others, eg, butts into other children's games.

(j) Often blurts out answers to questions before they have been completed.

(k) Has difficulty waiting for a turn in games or group situations.

(l) Often engages in physically dangerous activities for the purpose of thrill seeking, eg, runs into street without looking.

(m) Is often extremely messy or sloppy.

(n) Often loses things necessary for tasks or activities at school or at home (eg, toys, pencils, books, assignments).

(o) Often does not seem to listen to what is being said to him or her.

(2) Onset before 7 years of age.

(3) Occurrence not only during the course of autistic disorder.

The absence of hyperactivity characterizes another subtype of the disorder. A third subtype, known as residual, refers to children who previously had the whole syndrome with hyperactivity but are no longer hyperactive.

The terminology in the past has been quite confused. Minimal brain dysfunction, hyperactive child, hyperkinetic reaction of childhood, and learning disability are terms that have been used interchangeably with poor precision. In Great Britain, conduct disorder is emphasized as a cardinal finding. In psychiatry, the associated problems of depression and family imbalance are often emphasized as needing careful treatment.

Etiology

The cause of attention deficit disorder is usually multifactorial. Genetic influences are important, a fact confirmed by studies of families and twins and of children raised in foster or adoptive homes. It is possible that deficiencies of amino monoaminergic brain neurotransmitters are an inherited biochemical lesion in some patients. Most recent studies have shown reduced concentrations of homovanillic acid (HVA), the principle metabolite of dopamine in cerebrospinal fluid of children with ADD. The principle metabolite of brain norepinephrine, 3-methoxy-4-hydroxyphenylglycol (MHPG), may also be reduced. Other studies have shown brain insults, often perinatally, in children with this syndrome; this is especially true in the subgroup with hyperactivity.

Because premature infants and those who are small for gestational age are more likely to have this malady, it is thought that perinatal leukoencephalopathy may be the underlying disease in some cases. Virtually any significant insult to the brain—traumatic, infectious, or other—at an early age may lead to this syndrome in a school-aged child.

Can food additives cause or aggravate the syndrome? Most careful blind studies have shown such an effect in only a small minority of cases. At this writing, there is no uniform biochemical or neuropathologic substrate for these children.

Clinical Findings

A. Symptoms and Signs: The diagnostic criteria listed above summarize many of the findings. Core terms are inattention and impulsivity with or without hyperactivity. Other descriptions used are distractibility, inconsistency, impaired selectivity, and disinhibition. Symptoms are especially noticeable in group situations, eg, in the classroom or group activities in the home. The child may not appear inattentive or hyperactive in the physician's office.

Rating assessments are useful. The Conners scale and teacher and parent questionnaires are widely used to assess behavior features such as increased mood lability, inability to get along with others, destructiveness, mendacity, impudence, etc. Peer relationships may be characterized by rejection and poor acceptance. Clumsiness, delay in achievement of motor milestones, a history of erratic feeding and sleeping habits in infancy, and, often, delayed language development or ongoing articulation problems are present. The neurologic examination is often abnormal, especially in "soft" or fine motor tasks, such as abnormal finger sequential movements and dysdiadochokinesia (abnormal alternating movements, such as turning the hand over rapidly from front to back). There may be difficulties in hopping, mixed dominance, or choreiform movements. Mirror movements are in excess of that expected for age. Eye-following movements and visual pursuit may be erratic and incoordinate. Catching a bounced ball, tandem gait, and oral-buccal movements (for example, placing the tongue in various positions) may be abnormal. Learning disability may be evident during the examination. The child may read below grade level and have difficulties in writing and in verbal expression.

Minor somatic abnormalities are more common in these children. Rarely, the physician identifies an underlying neurologic syndrome, eg, neurofibromatosis, arrested hydrocephalus, microcephaly, or macrocephaly.

The diagnosis is made on the basis of the history obtained from the parents and teachers. The Conners questionnaires are often helpful. Reports of psychologic testing at school or through a referral source

can be helpful, especially if the psychologist comments on inattentiveness or hyperactivity during the testing.

There are several structured neurologic examinations that might aid in quantifying the standard neurologic examination. The patients often perform poorly in visual perception, visual sequential memory, auditory association, or reading and writing tests on formal psychologic examinations.

B. Electroencephalography, Imaging, and Other Studies: Electroencephalographic and radiologic imaging studies are frequently abnormal; they are not helpful, however, in making the diagnosis or excluding it. An EEG should be done if seizures are suspected. Thus, some cases of attention deficit are thought to be caused by absence seizures. This possibility is generally easily ruled out with an EEG. In rare circumstances, 24-hour ambulatory monitoring can be carried out during the child's normal activities (for example, in the schoolroom) in an attempt to prove that the inattention is not due to complex partial seizures, absence epilepsy, etc.

The most helpful laboratory tests are an extensive neuropsychologic battery, either done through the school system or referral source. Children differ from controls most commonly in the measures listed above. In the Wechsler Intelligence Scale for Children, a profile for attention deficit shows arithmetic, digit span, and coding scores to be low relative to other subtest scores. Especially useful in some cases are such instruments as the Luria-Nebraska Children's Battery or the Halstead-Reitan Neuropsychological Test Batteries for Children.

At this time, evoked potential studies and brain electrical activity mapping (BEAM) are research tools and are not useful in diagnosis or therapy.

Treatment (Table 24–36)

A. General and Supportive Care: One of the major responsibilities of the physician is to be sure that there is no underlying medical condition needing further assessment, interpretation, or treatment. As noted above, it is rare for a disorder of vision or hearing or some medical syndrome to underlie problems with attention and hyperactivity, but a thorough medical history and physical examination must rule out these possibilities. Formal vision and hearing

Table 24–36. Therapies for attention deficit disorder-hyperactivity.

Pediatric counseling: interpretation, advocacy, advice, goals.
Mental health counseling: family therapy, school counseling, behavior therapy, cognition therapy, "stop, look, listen."
Educational intervention: milieu changes, tutors, realistic goals, special education.
Pharmacotherapy: stimulant drugs, antidepressants.
Avoiding therapies of unproved benefit: optometric training, Feingold diet, megavitamins, etc.

testing may need to be done to supplement screening tests done in the school system. The physician should ascertain who is complaining. Is this a difficulty mainly in the classroom or in the home?

The physician must be an advocate for the child and family and order testing through the school system or through community or hospital resources by psychologists, speech and language experts, etc. Evaluation for perceptual learning disabilities includes psychometric tests, school achievement tests, and projective personality tests and interviews. The physician can gather the results of these tests and interpret them to the parents, helping to clarify difficult terminology.

Physicians can help interpret labels. They may choose to explain the symptoms as a maturation phenomenon expected to improve with treatment and time. Therapy in the home might include behavior modification, strict routines, and rewards for sustained attention to home jobs, studying, etc. Psychotherapy for the child or family therapy (or both) may be helpful where the home situation is in disorder, eg, if there is alcoholism or depression in family members. Formal therapy may be needed for a youngster with a conduct disorder or depression. In the adolescent with attention deficit, antisocial behavior and substance abuse can be anticipated.

In school, the child with learning disabilities may need special class placement or even tutors. A small, self-contained classroom, even a resource room, may be necessary; a large, noisy, open classroom is often detrimental.

The physician's role includes interpreting to the parents therapies of questionable aid. Special diets, such as the Feingold diet, are of little scientific validity. Vision training by optometrists and patterning as popularized by Doman and Delacato have not been shown in scientific studies to be of benefit.

B. Drug Therapy: Drug therapy often plays a role in improving attention, vigilance, and reaction time and in reducing impulsivity. Relative contraindications include motor tics, Tourette's syndrome, anorexia nervosa, growth failure, cardiac arrhythmias, and hypertension. The effects may be mediated through central monoaminergic neurotransmitters (see Etiology, above). CNS stimulants do not increase overall IQ but sometimes cause improvements on performance items of the Wechsler Intelligence Scale. Some studies show response rates as high as 60–80%. Children with attention deficit disorder alone or with hyperactivity improve.

The 2 most commonly used drugs are methylphenidate and dextroamphetamine. Both need to be given 2 or 3 times a day. Sustained-release methylphenidate, 20 mg, is available, (Ritalin SR) but whether it is effective as a single dose or must be given twice daily is controversial. The usual dose is 0.3–1 mg/kg of methylphenidate; that for dextroamphetamine (Dexedrine) is 2.5–10 mg morning and noon. For both drugs, the medication is generally concentrated during school hours (hence, the morning and noon doses). Sometimes, hyperactive behavior at home in the evening requires a third dose.

Magnesium pemoline (Cylert) has a slower onset and more sustained action, with a dosage range of 18.75 mg/d orally at first to a maximum of 75 mg daily. The most common side effects (sometimes necessitating discontinuation of the medication) are changes in mood or personality, including tearfulness and even depression. Anorexia, poor weight gain, and a lag in growth are other possible side effects. The youngster's height and weight should be monitored carefully. There is often catch-up growth once the medication is stopped, such as during the summer holidays. Other, less common side effects are tachycardia or hypertension, tics, headaches, and stomach aches. Disturbance of sleep and insomnia are other possible concerns.

Medications are not contraindicated in a youngster who has seizures; the drugs may even have a beneficial effect of counteracting some of the soporific affects of anticonvulsive medications. Other drugs used with success for target symptoms are antidepressants such as imipramine, hydrochloride (Tofranil) and desmethylimipramine (DMI).

All of the medications may be used into adolescence, if necessary. The drugs are not thought to have addiction or abuse potential. Of course, it is important not to look upon the drugs as a panacea; the other therapy issues addressed above must be included in any treatment protocols.

Prognosis

Follow-up studies have suggested that two-thirds of children improve. Difficulties with school achievement often continue to be a major problem in adolescence; children with aggression seem to fare worse. Antisocial behavior and substance abuse are threats in adolescents. The children often need help with social skills. Academic and social problems are the most common sequelae in adolescents.

Some studies have shown that 30% are diagnosed with psychiatric disorders as adults. On the other hand, many studies have shown normal or good work performance in adults who suffered from attention deficit disorder in childhood.

American Psychiatric Association: *Diagnostic and Statistical Manual of Mental Disorders,* 3rd rev ed. American Psychiatric Association, 1987.

Berry CA, Shaywitz SE, Shaywitz BA: Girls with attention deficit disorder: A silent minority? A report on behavioral and cognitive characteristics. *Pediatrics* 1985; **76**:801.

Coleman WM, LeVine M: Attention deficit disorder in adolescence: Description, evaluation and management. *Pediatr Rev* 1988;**9**:287.

Frank Y, Ben-Nun Y: Toward a clinical subgrouping of hyperactive and nonhyperactive attention deficit disorder. *Am J Dis Child* 1988;**142:**153.

Kelly PC et al: Self-esteem in children medically managed for attention deficit disorder. *Pediatrics* 1989;**83:**211.

Klein RG: Prognosis of attention deficit disorder and its management in adolescence. *Pediatr Rev* 1987;**8:**216.

Pelham WE et al: Sustained release and standard methylphenidate effects on cognition and social behavior in children with attention deficit disorder. *Pediatrics* 1987;**80:**491.

Shaywitz S, Shaywitz B: Attention deficit disorder: Current perspectives. *Pediatr Neurol* 1987;**3:**129.

SELECTED REFERENCES

Illingworth RS: *The Development of the Infant and Young Child: Normal and Abnormal,* 8th ed. Churchill Livingstone, 1984.

Menkes JH: *Textbook of Child Neurology,* 3rd ed. Lea & Febiger, 1985.

Plum F, Posner J: *The Diagnosis of Stupor and Coma,* 3rd ed. F. A. Davis, 1980.

Swaiman KF, Wright FS (editors): *The Practice of Pediatric Neurology,* 3rd ed. Mosby, 1989.

Volpe JJ: *Neurology of the Newborn.* Saunders, 1987.

Psychosocial Aspects of Pediatrics & Psychiatric Disorders

25

R. Barkley Clark, MD

HIGHLIGHTS OF CHILD & FAMILY DEVELOPMENT

DEVELOPMENTAL STAGES

Anyone who provides for the medical or emotional needs of children understands that children change dramatically throughout the process of growing up. Each period of development presents children and parents its own characteristic set of challenges and problems. Likewise, the manifestations of stress and of disease change as the child changes over time. The planning of interventions by health care providers must therefore be in tune with the developmental level of the child and the corresponding needs of the parents. For these reasons, the chapter begins with a review of some of the highlights of child development that relate particularly to the psychosocial care of children. The struggles that caretakers face in providing a nurturing environment for their children are also noted. (See also Table 25–1.)

The Infant

The central developmental challenge of infancy is the development of specific emotional attachments, or bonds, between infant and caretakers. Those attachment bonds, in turn, form the basis for all meaningful and rewarding human relationships throughout the life span.

This period of forming emotional attachments is now recognized as a time of great reciprocal interaction between the child and the caretakers, with the child being an active participant in the attachment process. Shortly after birth, the child begins to display a powerful attachment behavior—the innate capacity to smile, particularly in response to the visual presentation of the human face. By the age of 2 or 3 months, the child is already beginning to smile preferentially in response to the face and voice of the primary caretakers, and by 6 months of age, a substantial bond has already been formed.

In assessing the process of attachment, one can learn much from observing the reciprocally reinforc-ing smiling that occurs between the 3- to 6-month-old infant and the primary attachment figure (typically, but not necessarily, the mother). If this process is progressing normally, the infant and the mother experience an obvious mutual pleasure in the interaction of smiling and "talking softly" to one another. In fact, the mutual pleasure in the interaction encourages further smiling and talking, which in turn further strengthens the emotional attachment bonds. Infants aged 3–4 months who do not smile interactively in response to the slow approach of a smiling, nodding, and cooing human face should be considered at risk for a primary disorder of attachment (for example, a pervasive developmental disorder). Likewise, infants at 4–6 months of age who do not smile preferentially and enthusiastically at their primary caretaker's smiling and nodding face should be considered at risk for a reactive attachment disorder (for example, maternal deprivation or disabilities in mothering).

By 6–8 months of age, the infant can clearly differentiate the primary attachment figure from other individuals. This ability is manifest even before 6 months in the wariness of infants around "strangers" (even fathers), and by 6–8 months of age, overt distress in the presence of strangers is usually apparent. This developmental landmark of stranger distress heralds the onset of the infant's capacity to recognize and remember the mother's face in contrast to the faces of other human beings. At the same time, beginning at 8–10 months of age, the inability of the infant to evoke a memory of the mother relates to the separation anxiety that is seen with the threatened absence of the mother.

An understanding of these developmental landmarks can assist in the clinical assessment of the attachment process; the physician can use information about a child's distress at strangers and the onset of separation anxiety as early as 7–8 months of age. The infant who is normally attached is at ease and smiling while on the mother's lap and while looking at her face. As the physician approaches the infant and mother, and as the baby notices the physician, the face sobers; the infant then turns to face the mother. The child may cry vigorously when taken off the mother's lap for examination. The child's

Table 25–1. Highlights of child and family development.

Stage (Age)	Developmental Tasks	Developmental Landmarks	Developmental Concerns	Pitfalls for Caregivers
Infancy (birth–1 y)	Emotional attachment	2–3 mo: responsive social smile; 7–9 mo: distress in the presence of "strangers."	Temperamental variations (including colic).	Exhaustion; lack of emotional support; unexpected temperament; unfulfilled expectations and fantasies.
Toddler (1–3 y)	Beginning of the separation-individuation process	8–24 mo: separation anxiety; 12 mo: locomotion; 15 mo: "no"; 24–36 mos: bowel training.	Sleep disturbances (separation or overstimulation); breath holding and temper tantrums; "terrible two's," ie, oppositional behavior; accident proneness.	Exhaustion; autonomous strivings of child seen as rejection or adversarial relationship; need for parents to set limits seen as parental failure; "permissiveness" seen as good parent-child interaction.
Preschooler (3–6 y)	Taming of the internal world of fantasy	Symbolic play.	Childhood fears: bedtime, darkness, ghosts and monsters.	Competitive strivings of child seen as personal challenge; egocentricity of child seen as selfishness.
School age (6–11 y)	Skills development	7 y: logical thought processes (cause-and-effect thinking); games and organizations with rules.	Continued childhood fears; school phobia; learning disabilities; primary nocturnal enuresis.	Parental discomfort with separation from child; high expectations for child's performance; child's performance experienced as parents' own self-esteem.
Adolescence (11–20 y)	Continuation of the separation-individuation process: identity formation ("Who am I?"); gaining independence.			
Early adolescence (11–15 y)		Puberty; "best friends" of same sex; self-absorption; painful concerns about appearance.	Adolescent "turmoil."	Child's attachment to peer group seen as rejection; self-absorption seen as irresponsible disregard for others; exasperation with the child's changing moods.
Middle adolescence (15–17 y)		Heterosexual interests; beginning of a truce with parents.	Adolescent sexuality.	Prudish indignation; sexual stimulation in the parent; envy and anger at child's youthful energy and appearance; rivalry and competition with suitors.
Late adolescence (17–20 y)		Orientation toward future; pursuit of an adult, work-role identity.	Will the young adult make it?	"Empty nest syndrome"; sense of loss and grief.

distress at seeing a strange face approaching and further distress when separated from the mother are signs that the attachment process is proceeding satisfactorily.

By 12 months of age, strong attachment bonds are firmly in place with primary caretakers and, to a somewhat lesser degree, with other prominent persons involved in caring for the child. By 12 months, prolonged separation from attachment figures, particularly in the context of unfamiliar surroundings, such as a hospital, can lead to a predictable series of reactions (described by John Bowlby) involving stages of protest, despair, and, ultimately, emotional detachment.

Bowlby J: Childhood mourning and its implications for psychiatry. *Am J Psychiatry* 1961;**118**:481.
Metcalf AW: Child and adolescent development. Pages 58–61 in: *Review of General Psychiatry*. Goldman, HH (editor). Appleton & Lange, 1988.
Scharfman MA: The infant. Pages 165–181 in: *Under-*

standing Human Behavior in Health and Illness. Simons RC (editor). Williams & Wilkins, 1985.

The Toddlers

The toddler stage of development begins at about 1 year of age with the onset of locomotion and the use of a pincer grasp. These 2 developmental milestones allow children first to begin to move away from their caretakers to explore the world and second to begin to provide for themselves by self-feeding. These landmarks herald the onset of the child's innate thrust toward independence that will unfold more completely during childhood, adolescence, and early adult life. This beginning process of developing independence during the toddler years is referred to as separation-individuation, a term adopted from the now famous work of Margaret Mahler.

The developmental challenge of the separation-individuation phase is the child's development of a sense of personal mastery and autonomy, particularly in relation to a sense of control over the child's own body. This stage of development provides children with a deep sense of pride in the experience of their own activities and accomplishments and, finally, in the achievement of bowel control.

Mahler describes the young toddler as having a love affair with the world. Children at this age are enamored of their own activities and excited by all that they find in the world around them. At the same time, the children are encouraged and reinforced by the delight that they perceive in the expressions of caretakers regarding those wonderful, newly found skills.

It is important at this point to stress the development of good self-esteem. A central concept is "mirroring," namely, the information that children learn, over time, about themselves from the expressions on the faces of those around them and, in particular, those people to whom they are emotionally attached. The earliest underpinnings of good self-esteem arise in the reciprocal and interactive smiling that occurs between the infant and the caretakers and then continue in the delight that the caretakers feel in their toddler's emerging skills of independence. The personal pleasure that the caretaker experiences in being with the child and observing the child's newly found skills of independence is reflected, or mirrored, back to the child as information about the self. Over many years, the facial expressions of caretakers become internalized within children as deep-seated feelings and convictions about their own positive self-worth. In short, children learn much about themselves by what the world mirrors back.

While the toddler is in the midst of a love affair with the world (in the form of physical activity, exploration, and beginning independence), the developmental process is complicated, at least for caretakers, by 3 conflicting developmental problems: willfulness, poor judgment, and separation anxiety. Regarding willfulness, Rene Spitz pointed out the importance of the child's acquisition and use of the word "no." After "Mama" and "Dada," "no" is frequently the first word in a child's vocabulary. Children's use of "no," either in verbal expression or in action through behavioral opposition, signifies the powerful wish on their part to be in control of themselves. This drive for self-control and self-determination is strong and should ultimately result in responsible, self-directed behavior in the future, but in the meantime it is responsible for the temper tantrums, the breath holding, and the oppositional behavior that characterize many toddlers. Because this strong-mindedness (and in particular the use of "no") this period is often called "the terrible two's."

One of the biggest problems regarding children's exuberance and powerful wish for self-determination is that their judgment is poor at this time. For exam-

ple, running into the street, thrusting objects into electrical outlets, and getting into medicine cabinets are clear and distinct dangers for the toddler. These impulses elicit in caretakers a sense of duty to limit their child's behavior—ie, the parents must say "no" themselves, figuratively and literally. The first noticeable conflict between caretaker and child now surfaces, and that state of conflict, although absolutely necessary, is experienced as unpleasant by both child and caretaker. It marks the beginning of many disagreements to come in the future, and it places caretakers in the sometimes difficult position of feeling like "the heavy." An important key to child rearing (in relation to the child's innate thrust toward functioning independently) is to strike a balance: autonomous behavior is enthusiastically rewarded and supported, while dangerous, destructive, or disruptive behavior is consistently and calmly limited.

The child's delight with activity and exploration is further complicated by the presence of separation anxiety. Separation anxiety begins as early as 8–10 months of age, generally peaks during the middle of the second year of life, and then gradually subsides in the latter part of the second and the beginning of the third year of life. Separation anxiety becomes manifest when the toddler perceives the threatened loss of the support of the primary attachment figures. Signs typically include a distressed expression, with or without crying, and active behavioral attempts on the part of the toddler to become reunited with the parenting figures. Separation anxiety is thought by Bowlby to represent a genetically determined adaptive mechanism that promotes the safety of young children by increasing physical proximity with caretakers. Margaret Mahler refers to the need of toddlers to be "emotionally refueled" by intermittent contact with their primary attachment figures during times of exploration of the environment. Depending on the intensity of the separation anxiety, the toddler may need only brief visual contact with the parent, or the child may need physical contact and even comfort from that parent. Although remnants of separation anxiety can be seen in young school-age children, particularly in times of stress such as the start of school, the intensity and frequency of separation anxiety are thought to wane in the third year of life as the children become able to calm themselves by evoking the image of their attachment figures or, at least, the feelings of safety associated with them.

In addition, the array of factors that come to play in the important achievement of bowel control must be mentioned. The development of bowel control can be viewed as a prototype for the development of self-control in a more general sense. First, adults need to remind themselves that bowel movement, in and of itself, is not inherently unpleasant or disgusting to young toddlers. Toddlers play happily while soiled or even with feces. In fact, 2- and 3-year-olds often express pleasure in the "wonderful" bowel movement that they have produced. The importance of this concept lies in the fact that the child must accept and take on the caretaker's view that a bowel movement is something that belongs only in certain places (ie, in the potty) and does not belong in public (eg, in one's pants).

To incorporate the caretakers' point of view about bowel movement, the child must have the desire to please them. This desire implies a strong and positive attachment to caretakers, and it implies that the child's needs, eg, appropriate care, emotional responsiveness, and positive mirroring responses from the parents, are being met. In short, the relationship between the child and caretaker is not tinged with the anger that exhausted and disillusioned caretakers feel when dealing with demanding and frustrated children.

Finally, the wish to please the responsive parent must then be reconciled with the toddlers' powerful wish to be in control of themselves. If the child's wish for self-determination is not adequately respected nor the playful explorations encouraged, the child then feels overly controlled or coerced by too many "no's" from caretakers. The child can then develop an attitude that reflects in effect, this view: "One thing that you cannot control is where I put my bowel movement." And, in this case, the child is correct.

If, however, the child's developmental thrust toward exploration and independence has not been thwarted by too many stifling parental "no's," and if the parent-child relationship is such that the child wishes to please those parents, the child will then internalize the parent's attitude about where to put bowel movements (ie, how to behave); such children experience the personal pleasure and pride associated with *their* own correct use of the potty. In the end, children who voluntarily elect to use the toilet not only experience the positive reinforcement from their caretakers but also at the same time feel a sense of personal pride in their own accomplishment. An important step toward socially appropriate autonomous functioning has been taken.

Bowlby J: Childhood mourning and its implications for psychiatry. *Am J Psychiatry* 1961;**118**:481.

Mahler MS et al: *The Psychological Birth of the Human Infant.* Basic Books, 1975.

Metcalf AW: Child and adolescent development. Pages 61–63 in: *Review of General Psychiatry.* Goldman HH (editor). Appleton and Lange, 1988.

Scharfman MA: The toddler. Pages 182–196 in: *Understanding Human Behavior in Health and Illness.* Simons RC (editor). Williams & Wilkins, 1985.

The Preschool Child

By the time children reach 3 years of age, a prominent developmental shift is already occurring: the child no longer behaves simply in relation to caretak-

ers. The focus turns to the mental world of thoughts and feelings within the child. This shift was described by Piaget as a movement from a plane of action (the sensory-motor stage of cognitive development) to the plane of thought (the preoperational stage of cognitive development). While the behavior of the infant is directed primarily toward facilitating and maintaining attachment with primary caretakers and that of the toddler toward expressing the beginning of independence from the parents, the preschool child is mentally aware of thoughts and feelings regarding the caretakers. The 3- and 4-year-old child can begin to think (albeit very illogically), and with that developmental achievement a tremendous new world of thought, fantasy, and worry opens for the child.

The central developmental task of the preschool child is essentially the sorting out of the wondrous and sometimes frightening world that comes with thought. This new cognizance includes awareness of such exciting issues as the perception of differences between the sexes and the ensuing curiosity and worry about those differences. It includes the boastful wish to be big and powerful and the fantasy of being on a par with one's parents and even being able to displace them from their perceived position of power and privilege.

Because preschoolers perceive themselves as being at the center of the universe, they come to believe that everyone around them must be also aware of their thoughts and motives. This perceived exposure makes the mental world of the preschool child filled with unspeakable dangers, leading to worries about caretakers' withdrawal of their love and admiration, and even angry and physical retaliation against the child. Preschool children are caught between exciting and wondrous fantasies on the one hand and prohibitions, dangers, and worries on the other.

The outward behavioral manifestations of this wondrous world of thought and fantasy include "showing off" behaviors, exhibiting the "private parts," sexual curiosity (exploration and comparison between children), and competitive struggles for favored status with parents. At the same time, children display the content of their mental worlds in symbolic play. The little girl may act out coming home to favored status with daddy, and the little boy may portray superboy slaying a dangerous dragon.

The frightening and worrisome aspects of the child's mental world become manifest in fears (particularly at night) about ghosts, monsters, dangerous animals, and the dark. In addition, children may even develop transient phobic symptoms that represent the displacement of internal worries onto objects in the outside world. Finally, preschool children are usually greatly concerned about bodily injury; thus, everyday "ouchies" need special care, and trips to the doctor for shots, stitches, and throat cultures are associated with considerable anxiety.

The preschool stage of mental development comes to a close as the child learns to moderate, and in a sense give up, the wild fantasies of power and privilege by identifying with the rules and the self-control represented by the child's own loved ones. The internalization of parental rules and values means that children no longer have to worry so intensely about angering people they love and depend on. Furthermore, despite all the emotional turmoil, the child remains the apple of the parent's eye. Recognizing this fact ultimately leaves the child in a calmer mental state. Generally, the child clearly identifies with an adult model of the same sex and is now ready to focus mental energies on adapting to the challenges at school and in the social community beyond home.

Farley GK: Cognitive development Pages 249–254 in: *Understanding Human Behavior in Health and Illness* Simons RC (editor). Williams & Wilkins, 1985.

Scharfman MA: The preschool child. Pages 213–226 in: *Understanding Human Behavior in Health and Illness.* Simons RC (editor). Williams & Wilkins, 1985.

Sours JA: The Oedipal and latency years. Pages 197–216 in: *Handbook of Clinical Assessment of Children and Adolescents.* Kestenbaum CH, Williams DT (editors). New York Univ Press, 1988.

The School-Aged Child

Although the child of gradeschool age may still show residual evidence of earlier developmental challenges in the form of stress-induced separation anxiety (for example, with the start of school) and persistent nighttime fears, the child at this age should generally be prepared to devote mental energies to learning and to expanding social interactions beyond the family. The developmental challenge of this age is the development of confidence in mastering skills, whether athletic, academic, or social.

By the age of 7–8 years, the school-age child has developed the more logical and coherent thought processes that are necessary for more formal academic learning (Piaget's stage of concrete mental operations, during which logical relationships of cause and effect begin to exist). At the same time, the school-age child becomes more and more involved with organized peer group activities (for example, clubs and teams), during which the rules of the game and acceptable codes of conduct become very important. The child begins to devote considerable time, focused energy, and practice on the development of skills, whether on the athletic field, in hobbies, or in schoolwork. Girls at this age are frequently more developmentally advanced than boys, particularly in the academic work of the classroom. Kindergarten and first-grade boys are much more apt to be "developmentally immature" (ie, lacking in impulse control) than are girls of the same age.

Children of this age also begin to experience pleasure in their ability to organize and catagorize information. One may see the development of collections (for example, stamps, baseball cards, and dolls) and, at the same time, the exclusion of other children from activities because they are in some way perceived as different from the rest of the peer group.

During the school-age years, children should develop a sense of confidence about their abilities. The development of skills (whether athletic, academic, or social) is an important source of enhancement to self-esteem. Children with learning disorders, developmental disabilities, or temperamental variations, including problems with attention or self-control, are at risk for developing deficiencies in self-esteem. Likewise, families that place unrealistically high expectations of performance on their children may in fact emotionally burden them; these children feel they must excel to remain in parental favor.

Scharfman MA: The grade school child. Pages 240–248 in: *Understanding Human Behavior in Health and Illness.* Simons RC (editor). Williams & Wilkins, 1985.

Sours JA: The Oedipal and latency years. Pages 197–216 in: *Handbook of Clinical Assessment of Children and Adolescents.* Kestenbaum CH, Williams DT (editors). New York Univ Press. 1988.

The Adolescent

Adolescence is a stage of transition between childhood, where more emotional and physical dependence on caretakers is the rule, and adulthood, where independent and autonomous functioning is sustained without the continuous support of the family of origin. The stage of adolescence is relatively long in Western society, lasting from the onset of puberty (roughly, 11 years of age) to the early period beyond the high school years (roughly, age 18–20), when the young person makes plans toward an adult identity in the working world. Theoreticians refer to this developmental period as the second period of separation and individuation (a reliving of aspects of the "terrible two's"). For parents, it can be a dreaded period of turmoil and rebellion in their children. In fact, the developmental tasks of adolescence are quite noble: developing a unique identity (answering the question, "Who am I?") and letting go the dependent childhood attachments to primary caretakers. It is more the *form* of the journey that stirs concern among those responsible for the care of adolescents.

The extended period of adolescence can be divided into early, middle, and late adolescence. For most parents, early adolescence (roughly, ages 11–15) is the most difficult. Young people clearly turn their interests outside the family toward strengthening attachments with peers of the same sex. That shift to an emotional investment outside the family may be coupled with an active distancing and pushing away from the family, a transition that is frequently painful to parents. In addition, early adolescents are notoriously inconsistent and somewhat volatile in their frequently anxious moods. They are egocentrically self-absorbed and painfully concerned about outward appearances, and they frequently question parental authority. In all, early adolescence represents a large shift away from the relatively compliant and family-oriented school-age child.

Middle adolescence (roughly, ages 15–17) tends to be a less difficult time for parents. Although young people begin to focus their attention more earnestly on relationships with members of the opposite sex (certainly a source of concern for most parents), middle adolescents have typically become less emotionally labile, less anxious about physical appearance, and less desperate in their need to fit in with their peer group. The result is a relative truce with parents and an overall increasing sense of calm in the adolescent's daily life. In addition, by middle adolescence, 30–50% of teens have achieved the developmental capacity for the abstract thought processes associated with Piaget's stage of formal mental operations. For this reason, the adolescent now takes a more thoughtful approach to situations that previously elicited more impulsive action.

In late adolescence (roughly, age 17–20), the young person is more aware of and focused on the future. This shift in focus coincides with high school graduation and plans for leaving home. The young person begins to assume patterns of behavior that are strikingly similar to those of the parents. The young person is, in effect, coming full circle from the initial rejection of parental values in early adolescence to a partial internalization of those values by late adolescence. As late adolescence closes, the young person begins to plan future work goals that are realistically designed to support independence from the family of origin.

Goldings HJ: Development from ten to thirteen years. Pages 199–204 in: *Basic Handbook of Child Psychiatry*. Vol 1. Noshpitz JD et al (editors). Basic Books, 1979.

Hamburg BA, Wortman RN: Adolescent development and psychopathology. Pages 21–36 in: *Child Psychiatry*. Vol 6. Solnit AJ et al (editors). Basic Books, 1986.

Malmquist CP: Development from thirteen to sixteen years. Pages 205–212 in: *Basic Handbook of Child Psychiatry*. Vol 1. Noshpitz JD et al (editors). Basic Books, 1979.

Metcalf AW: Child and adolescent development. Pages 66–69 in: *Review of General Psychiatry*. Goldman HH (editor). Appleton and Lange, 1988.

Peterson AC, Offer D: Adolescent development: Sixteen to nineteen years. Pages 213–232 in: *Basic Handbook of Child Psychiatry*. Vol 1. Noshpitz JD et al (editors). Basic Books, 1979.

TEMPERAMENTAL VARIATION

Each child has an innate characteristic pattern of behavioral expression. This concept of an individual behavior style was put forth by Thomas and Chess in their description of the concept of temperament. According to Thomas and Chess, temperament is not what the child does or why the child is motivated to behave in a certain fashion; rather, temperament describes how behavior is manifest.

In this study, a child's particular temperament could be identified and studied from early infancy through childhood. Thomas and Chess proposed that a child's temperament was primarily the result of constitutional factors that act on the environment to modify caretakers' reactions to the child. They observed temperamental differences in children interacting with their environments and noted that a child's temperamental style needed to mesh with, or "fit," the expectations of caretakers in order for development to proceed smoothly. For example, if a parent expected an infant to be calm and quiet, and instead the child tended to be intense and active, fertile ground for conflict between the child and caretakers was then created.

Thomas and Chess identified 9 categories of temperament:

(1) Activity level—general motoric activity level.
(2) Regularity—rythmicity in biologic functions such as sleep-wake cycles and hunger and feeding patterns.
(3) Approach or withdrawal in new situations—the initial response to a new stimulus.
(4) Adaptability—ease of accommodation to new situations.
(5) Sensory threshold—intensity level of sensory stimulation required to evoke a response.
(6) Intensity of reaction—energy level in responsiveness.
(7) Quality of mood—the predominant or basic mood of the child.
(8) Distractibility—ability of extraneous environmental stimuli to interfere with concentration.
(9) Persistence—the ability to remain engaged in activity.

In addition to the 9 categories of temperament, Thomas and Chess found that over 60% of the children in their study displayed patterns, or constellations, of temperamental traits that related to the child's general adaptability to life's challenges and to the quality of "fit" between caretaker and child. Approximately 40% of the sample displayed characteristics of an "easy child," and approximately 10–15% displayed the temperamental characteristics of a "difficult child." The characteristics of those temperamental constellations are described in Table 25–2.

The clinical importance of understanding a child's temperament lies in 2 areas: first, in helping parents individualize expectations and approaches toward their children and, second, in associating difficult, temperamental constellations with behavior problems in childhood. Regarding the former, the concept of "fit" between child and caretaker is important. This concept refers to how a child's behavior matches with environmental and caretaker expectations about childhood behavior. A good fit optimizes development, because the child behaves in harmony with parental expectations. A poor fit, by contrast, creates dissonance in the relationship that can promote parental dissatisfaction, conflict between child and parent, and poor self-esteem in the child.

If parents can understand that their child has a temperamental style that is different from parental hope or expectation, the change in perspective about the child can led to (1) less parental dissatisfaction and, therefore, less guilt about their feelings of frustration with the child and (2) a more effective dealings with the child.

A number of authors have reported a significant association between difficult temperamental constellations and behavior problems in childhood. Most notable is the finding that the "difficult child" temperament is associated with a significant increase in behavior problems at home and at school, as well as an increased frequency of psychiatric referrals. In Thomas and Chess's study, 70% of children found to have "difficult temperament" in the first 3 years of life developed clinically evident behavior problems during later childhood. Knowledge of this predictive

association between difficult temperament and behavior disorders can allow a physician to monitor the "fit" between child and environment more closely and to maximize opportunities to improve the "fit" in the relationship. An excellent resource for physicians and parents is Turecki and Tonner's book on difficult temperamental styles.

Table 25–2 can be used to help parents "diagnose" their child's temperamental characteristics. Knowledge of a child's individual variation in 1 or 2 categories of temperament (even if the child does not fit completely within a temperamental constellation) can help parents better understand their child's individual characteristics and needs.

Hertz ME, Snow ME: The assessment of temperament. Pages 133–153 in: *Handbook of Clinical Assessment of Children and Adolescents*. Kestenbaum CH, Williams DT (editors). New York Univ Press, 1988.

Thomas AA, Chess S: *Temperament and Development*. Bruner/Mazel, 1977.

Turecki S, Tonner L: *The Difficult Child*. Bantam Books, 1985.

FAMILY LIFE

Family Functions

The structure of families has changed in recent years with the increase in the number of single-

Table 25–2. Temperamental variations.[1]

Temperamental Category	Assessment in Infancy (6 mo ± 2)	Assessment in Childhood	Characteristics of the "Easy Child"	Characteristics of the "Difficult Child"
Activity level	Activity during diaper changes and dressing	Preference for physical or quiet activities; reaction to sitting quietly (eg, school, car trips)	Lower	Higher
Regularity	Regularity of patterns in sleeping, awakening	Regularity of patterns of sleepiness, hunger, bowel habits	Regular patterns	Irregular patterns
Approach/ withdrawal	Reactions to new foods, clothing, caretakers	Reactions to newness (new friends, clothes, classroom)	Initial approach	Initial withdrawal
Adaptability	Speed with which child becomes accustomed to new situations	Ability to go along with changes in routine and with the preferences of other children	More rapid adjustment to change	Slow adjustment to change
Sensory threshold	Sensitivity to sound, light and textures	Any unusual sensitivities to sound, light, touch	Higher	Lower
Intensity of reaction	Strength of reactions when hungry or frustrated	Responses to disappointment and pleasure	Lower	Higher
Quality of mood	Fussy or pleasant disposition	Is the child's predominant mood contented or distressed?	Positive mood	Negative mood
Distractability	Ease of distraction while feeding	Tendency to get easily sidetracked	Lower	Higher
Persistence	Does the infant become engrossed with toys and mobiles?	Ability to "stick to" difficult tasks	Higher	Lower

[1]Source: Thomas AA, Chess S: *Temperament and Development*. Bruner/Mazel, 1977.

parent homes and reconstituted families and the decline in the involvement with and dependence on extended families. Despite these changes, the nuclear family unit continues to play a vital role in meeting the needs of society and of the individual family members. The family serves the following functions: (1) the rearing of offspring to become autonomous adults, and eventually competent parents, within the context of societal expectations and (2) meeting the needs of individual family members for nurturance, protection, feedback, recognition (mirroring), promoting adaptive behaviors, and emotional closeness and support.

The Parental Subsystem

The cornerstone of family functioning is the parental subsystem or the parental unit. Whether this parental unit consists of a marriage relationship, single parent, or other family members, it must stand alone as the source of leadership and power in the family. The parental unit must meet the emotional and physical needs of other, more dependent family members, while at the same time defining the norms of behavior that will lead to adaptive, independent functioning in the future. In short, the ways in which the parental unit exercises its leadership roles determine in large part the health or sickness of the family and its individual members.

Parenthood, as defined above, is emotionally and physically draining. In order for the parental unit to fulfill its vital role as provider and setter of limits for the family, the members of the parental unit must have their own source of adult support and nurturance so that they can reenergize themselves. In the case of a healthy marriage, the marital partners provide the emotional support, the respite, the problem-solving advice, and the source of adult companionship that is necessary to refuel the parental unit emotionally. Finding this support is more difficult for single parents, who have no "built-in" source of adult support within the immediate family unit; in such cases, unfortunately, the child is at risk of becoming a pseudoadult companion to the single parent.

The lack of a solid marital relationship can be an important factor in virtually any child-centered problem. To function successfully as a parental unit, the couple must find the marriage mutually satisfying in the following ways: (1) the couple nurtures and affirms one another; (2) the couple has trust and respect for one another; (3) the couple is able to recognize and resolve conflict within the marriage; and (4) the couple's needs for intimacy and sexuality are met satisfactorily within the marriage.

When the parental subsystem is weakened by marital dissatisfaction or by persistent marital conflict, children are at risk of becoming the focus of parental conflict. In effect, the child becomes the focus of parental attention and concern, thus "detouring" the conflict within the marriage unit onto the child. The parental concern about the child distracts the parents from their own marital problems, and the child ends up functioning as a buffer between the parents. Questions designed to screen the quality of the marital and parental relationship are outlined in the section on screening for psychosocial problems and disorders.

Barker P: Healthy families and their development. Pages 19–32 in: *Basic Family Therapy*. Oxford Univ Press, 1986.

Gurwitt A, Muir RC: Family development. Pages 37–48 in: *Child Psychiatry*. Vol 6. Solnit AJ et al (editors). Basic Books, 1986.

Malone CA: Family therapy and childhood disorders. Pages 228–241 in: *Psychiatry Update*. Vol 2. Grinspoon L (editor). American Psychiatric Press, 1983.

Issues in Parenthood

In rearing children, parents face a potentially rewarding but at the same time tiring and frequently frustrating task. In general, the greatest pitfalls in parenting involve (1) physical and emotional exhaustion and (2) unfulfilled expectations about having children.

Meeting the caretaking needs of children is tiring work. The physical and emotional energy that is expended in caring for a child must be replenished by rest, time to meet one's personal needs, and the emotional support of others. All of these can be provided in part by a mate who shares in the parenting responsibilities. In this regard, the "woman's movement" has helped men broaden their parental roles and personal identities to include more nurturing activities. At the same time, single parents are at a relative disadvantage regarding the availability of a built-in support system.

In addition to the physical and emotional support derived from a mate or "significant other" (for example, a relative, a roommate, or an adult child-care provider), primary caretakers are partly replenished emotionally by the feedback that they receive in their child's responsiveness to them (in the form of smiles and excitement in the presence of the parent), as well as the dim but powerful memories of having been warmly and consistently cared for by their own parents. Children who are developmentally disabled or temperamentally difficult not only require greater amounts of parental energy but also may not be as emotionally responsive and rewarding to the parent. In addition, the caretaker who experienced deficiencies in parental care as a child has fewer positive feelings and memories from the past to call on to replenish depleting energy stores.

Parental exhaustion can "endanger" the child's development: it decreases the parent's emotional and physical responsiveness toward the child and brings about a state of anger and frustration inherent to feeling exhausted and depleted. Both factors adversely affect the ensuing interaction between the parent and child. A mild consequence may be a state of tension—a more extreme one, child abuse and neglect.

The second major pitfall in parenting involves the disappointment brought about by the unfulfilled fantasies and expectations that inevitably come with parenthood. Most parents consciously hope, and to some degree expect, that their offspring will be healthy, competent, and happy. In addition, they hope that they will be reasonably able to meet the needs of their growing child and that in doing so they will feel a sense of accomplishment and emotional closeness that will lead to a greater sense of fulfillment within their own lives.

In addition to those conscious hopes, parents also develop less conscious and more unrealistic fantasies about their children. These fantasies frequently serve to fill a void created by their own unmet needs for admiration, prowess, and respect. As a result, fantasies about their children frequently include basking in the glow of a child with exceptional abilities in skill development and social interaction. Parents may fantasize that their children will thank them for all of their hard work in parenting, and they may even hope that they will feel loved by their children in ways that will relieve the pain and loneliness that they feel in their own lives.

Parents who have children with illness, disabilities, and temperamental difficulties have to adjust their expectations about their children so that they can realistically meet the special needs of that child. That adjustment involves the painful grieving of the loss of the child that was hoped for or expected.

For parents whose hope was to relieve their own personal unhappiness and sense of incompleteness through parenthood, raising children can become an emotional exercise in futility and a source of emotional burden to their children, who sense their own inability to meet the needs of the parent.

Although emotional and physical exhaustion and unfulfilled parental expectations are issues that parents must struggle with throughout their child's development, each new phase of development presents the parent with a unique set of challenges. In infancy, the irregularity of the child's sleep-wake cycles and the child's need for constant care become physically exhausting, especially to a parent functioning alone without the support of a mate or "significant other." The physical demands are then made even more draining if the child is not easily soothed and does not develop rythmicity of states.

During the toddler years, the child's striving for autonomy and independence can be misunderstood. To parents, the behavioral opposition and verbal "no's" of toddlers can seem like a rejection of parental caretaking. The resulting pain and anger can manifest itself either in irritation with the child or in attempts to smooth the relationship by giving in to the child's demands. In the former case, the child's autonomous strivings are met with parental displeasure; in the latter, the child becomes a tyrant.

In the later preschool years, parents are faced with competitive rivalrous challenges from their children. A sense of humor and perspective, combined with a solid marital relationship, allows parents to balance respect for the child's wishes to be "big" with the ability to set firm limits that maintain boundaries between the private lives of the parents (for example, the parents' bedroom) and their children.

During the elementary school years, parents must come to grips with allowing their children to experience the challenges that await outside the home and family. Parental support of skill development must be balanced with realistic definitions of success. Persistent separation anxiety on the part of parents and unrealistic standards of performance can contribute to the child's development of anxiety during school years.

Adolescence presents a number of challenges to parents. The early adolescent presents unpredictable changes of mood, intense attachment to peers, and a self-centered point of view, all of which deprive parents of the positive feedback that they once enjoyed from the child who wanted to please the parents. Not since infancy and the toddler years have parents received so little gratitude for their efforts. And, as in toddler years, parents must remind themselves that what may seem to be a rebuff is in fact a further step along the child's road to independence. Again, like parents of toddlers, the parents of young adolescents need to support autonomy while preventing tyranny and disaster.

The sexual interests of the middle adolescent can elicit a variety of parental reactions related to parents' own concerns about sexuality. The parental reactions range from pride to fear to rivalrous envy to sexual stimulation.

Finally, as the late adolescent prepares to leave home, parents face the sense of loss and grief associated with the launching of offspring into the world. Parents need to mourn the loss and, at the same time, begin to recommit to the primary importance of the marriage once the offspring leave the nest.

PSYCHOSOCIAL ASSESSMENT OF CHILDREN & FAMILIES

Recent epidemiologic data suggest that 5–15% of children in the USA are affected by psychiatric disorders, and nearly 50% of pediatric office visits are related to psychosocial or developmental problems. These statistics underscore the importance of being able to screen for and recognize psychosocial problems in children and their families.

SCREENING FOR PSYCHOSOCIAL PROBLEMS & PSYCHIATRIC DISORDERS WITHIN THE CONTEXT OF HEALTH MAINTENANCE

Although important information about psychosocial problems is obtained by interviewing children and observing the interaction of parents and their children, most authorities agree that the most efficient indicator in screening for psychosocial problems is the history provided by caretakers. Psychosocial screening with a focus on the caretaker can lead to information from 3 sources of data found in the pediatric office: checklists of specific symptoms completed by caretakers, general questioning of parents about psychosocial functioning, and physician-parent discussions of normal and expected child behavior at different developmental levels.

Murphy and Jellinek have recently devised a pediatric symptom checklist designed to screen school-age children (ie, 6–12 years of age) for psychosocial dysfunction. The 35-item checklist is to be completed in the waiting room by a parent or caretaker. (See Table 25–3.) Each item is rated by the parents

Table 25–3. Pediatric symptom checklist.[1]

	Never	Sometimes	Often
1. Complains of aches or pains			
2. Spends more time alone			
3. Tires easily, little energy			
4. Fidgets, is unable to sit still			
5. Has trouble with a teacher			
6. Is less interested in school			
7. Acts as if driven by a motor			
8. Daydreams too much			
9. Is distracted easily			
10. Is afraid of new situations			
11. Feels sad, unhappy			
12. Is irritable, angry			
13. Feels hopeless			
14. Has trouble concentrating			
15. Has less interest in friends			
16. Fights with other children			
17. Is absent from school			
18. Experiences a drop in school grades			
19. Is down on himself or herself			
20. Visits doctor, with doctor finding nothing wrong			
21. Has trouble with sleeping			
22. Worries a lot			
23. Wants to be with you more than before			
24. Feels he or she is bad			
25. Takes unnecessary risks			
26. Gets hurt frequently			
27. Seems to be having less fun			
28. Acts younger than children the same age			
29. Does not listen to rules			
30. Does not show feelings			
31. Does not understand other people's feelings			
32. Teases others			
33. Blames others for his or her troubles			
34. Takes things that belong to others			
35. Refuses to share			

Parents are asked to indicate which category—Never, Sometimes, or Often—best fits their child, with 0, 1, or 2 points assigned to each answer, respectively. For the interpretation of scores, see text.
[1]Modified and reproduced, with permission, from Murphy JM, Jellinek M: Screening for psychosocial dysfunction in economically disadvantaged and minority children: Further validation of the pediatric symptom checklist. *Am J Orthopsychiatry* 1988;**58**:450. Copyright 1988 by the American Orthopsychiatric Association, Inc.

as "often," "sometimes," or "never" present, with 2, 1, or 0 points assigned to each answer, respectively. The information obtained can be used in 2 ways: first, as a psychosocial review of symptoms and a point of departure for the discussion of problems that "often" or "sometimes" occur; and, second, as a general screening device, with a total score of 28 or greater indicating a need for more in-depth psychosocial evaluation of the child.

Jellinek has also suggested 5 general screening questions to be addressed to parents during an office consultation that will provide the opportunity for uncovering areas of parental concern. These same questions can be slightly rephrased and then directed to children as well:

(1) How are things going with you and your child? (Assessing parent-child interaction)
(2) How are things going in school? (Academically and behaviorally)
(3) How are things with peers and with play?
(4) How is the child's mood? (Comfortable and happy versus tense and unhappy)
(5) How are things going within the family? (Including siblings, marriage, and parents as individuals)

Finally, within the context of anticipatory guidance, age-appropriate, expected behavior is brought forth for review and for parental reaction. Parental concern about infant attachment, "the terrible two's," childhood fears, school problems, and adolescent problems can be brought out in the open for further discussion (see Table 25–1).

ASSESSMENT OF PSYCHOSOCIAL SIGNS & SYMPTOMS

General Comments

When an emotional or behavioral sign or symptom is presented for evaluation, a more thorough psychosocial evaluation is indicated. Data will need to be collected from caretakers, from the child, and (when available) from school personnel and "significant others." When beginning the assessment, it is important to schedule enough time at least to get a picture of the presenting problem (generally, at least 30 minutes).

Whenever possible, it is advantageous to see parents and child together, the parents alone, and the school-age and adolescent child alone. Doing so allows the physician to view interactions among family members, as well as to give both the parents and the child the opportunity to speak confidentially regarding concerns and problems. When assessing psychosocial problems, it is important to remember that parents and child frequently experience shame and guilt about a personal inadequacy that they perceive to be the cause of the presenting problem. The

physician can ease the family's burden and at the same time facilitate the assessment by remembering that the family is doing its best to cope with its problems, that no one is morally to blame for the difficulty, and that the task of the assessment is to identify where the family's efforts could be better refocused in support of the family's emotional needs. An attitude of nonjudgmental inquiry can be captured in supportive statements to the family, eg, "Let's see if we can figure out what might be happening."

Obtaining Data

The psychosocial information obtained from the parents, the child, and "significant others" can be organized into the format that follows. That format should be used as a framework for gathering information, not as a "cookbook" to be followed in rigid sequence. The appropriate interviewing technique allows for a blending of individual descriptions of concerns, supplemented by specific questions designed to glean information about important areas of psychosocial functioning. By the end of the assessment, whether it is completed in one or more appointments, the physician should have obtained relevant information in the different areas that follow:

A. History of the Presenting Problem: First, the physician should obtain a detailed description of the problem. When did it start? Were there changes or stresses at the time that it began? How is the problem affecting the child's life and the family's functioning? What does the child say about the problem? What attempts have been made alleviate the problems? Are there any theories about the cause of the problem?

B. Review of other Psychosocial Symptoms: The techniques used in screening for psychosocial problems that were described above can be used as a guide.

C. Developmental History:
1. Review the landmarks of psychosocial development (see Table 25–1).
2. Profile the child's temperamental traits (see Table 25–2).
3. Review stressful life events and the child's reactions to them—
   a. Separations.
   b. Losses.
   c. Marital conflict.
   d. Illnesses, injuries, and hospitalizations.
4. Obtain details of any past mental health treatment.

D. Family History:
1. Marital history—
a. Overall satisfaction with the marriage.
b. Conflicts or disagreements within the relationship.
c. Quantity and quality of time together away from children.

d. Whether the child comes between or causes a conflict between parents.

e. Marital history prior to having children.

2. Parenting history—

a. Feelings about parenthood.

b. Whether parents feel together/united in dealing with the child.

c. "Division of labor" in parenting.

d. Parental energy or stress level.

e. Sleeping arrangements.

f. Privacy practices.

g. Attitudes about discipline.

h. Interferences with discipline from outside the family (eg ex-spouses and grandparents).

3. Stresses on the family—

a. Problems with employment?

b. Financial problems?

c. Moves?

d. Illnesses/injuries/deaths?

4. Family history of mental health problems—

a. Depression? Who?

b. Suicide attempts? Who?

c. Psychiatric hospitalizations? Who?

d. Nervous breakdowns? Who?

e. Substance abuse problems? Who?

f. Nervousness or anxiety? Who?

D. Observation of Parents:

1. Do they agree on the existence of the problem or concern?

2. Are they uncooperative or antagonistic about the evaluation?

3. Does the parent appear depressed or overwhelmed?

4. Can the parents present a coherent picture of the problem and their family life?

5. Do the parents assume some sense of responsibility for the child's problems, or do they blame forces outside the family and beyond their control?

6. Do they appear burdened with guilt about the child's problem?

E. Observation of the Child:

1. Can the child acknowledge the existence of a problem or concern?

2. Does the child want help?

3. Is the child uncooperative or antagonistic about the assessment?

4. What is the child's predominant mood or attitude?

5. What does the child wish could be different in his life (for example, "3 wishes")?

6. Does the child display unusual behavior (activity level, mannerisms, or fearfulness)?

7. What is the estimate of the child's cognitive level?

F. Observation of Parent-Child Interaction:

1. Do the parents show concern about and sensitivity toward the child's feelings?

2. Does the child control or disrupt the joint interview?

3. Does the child respond to parental limits and control?

4. Do the parents inappropriately answer questions addressed to the child?

5. Is there obvious tension between family members?

6. Data from Other Sources:

1. Waiting room observations by office staff.

2. School (teacher, nurse, social worker, counselor).

3. Department of social services.

THE CHILD INTERVIEW

Interviewing the Preschool Child

Because preschool children frequently experience significant distress when separated from their parents in a physician's office and because they lack the cognitive capacity to describe their problems in much detail, the physician can frequently gather more information by interviewing parents and child together. As the parents discuss their concerns, the physician can look for the following behaviors:

(1) Does the child use the parent as a source of security and support appropriately?

(2) Does the 2- to 5-year-old warm up to the strange environment and begin to explore the room and even interact with the physician from a distance?

(3) How does the child relate to toys that are offered?

(4) What is the child's activity level?

(5) Does the child display unusual mannerisms (eg, intense clinging, stereotypic motor behaviors)?

(6) Does the child disrupt or control the interview session?

(7) Does the parent attempt to place appropriate limits on behavior? How does the child respond?

It is helpful to have in the office toy figures with which the child can portray emotional states and interpersonal interactions. After hearing the history from the parents and after observing the child's activities, play, and affect, the physician may question the 3- to 5-year-old child about toy figures who appear to be feeling sad, worried, angry, or bossy. Children aged 3–5 are frequently able to confirm important interpersonal relationships and attitudes in their symbolic play activities.

Interviewing The School-Aged Child

Most school-age children have mastered separation anxiety sufficiently to tolerate at least a brief interview with the physician. In addition, they have important information to share about their own worries, concerns, and problems.

The individual interview of the school-age child should be preceded by an explanation from the parents or the physician (or both) that the doctor wishes to talk only to the child today about how he or she is feeling. School-age children understand and even appreciate parental concern about unhappiness, worries, and difficulty in getting along with people, and they are usually willing to discuss their own perceptions of these problems.

In the beginning, it is good to restate the purpose of the interview, ie, to discuss and understand the child's view of certain issues raised by the parents. This helps to set the stage and break the ice for the meeting. Rapport can be enhanced by asking if the child has ever talked with anyone before about how he or she feels. If so, the child may explain more about what he or she liked or did not like about that discussion. If the child has never before talked about personal feelings with a professional, that focus can help to reassure the child that the physician understands that it is not easy to speak with someone about a difficult topic.

The next step in the interview involves ascertaining whether the child agrees about the existence of a problem (for example, unhappiness, worry, or not getting along). If so, the physician should try to discover what the child can tell the physician about the magnitude of the problem, how it affects the child and the family, and what seems to bring the problem about.

It is important to try to understand something of how children perceive the world around them. Asking directly about how mom and dad get along can yield surprising information about parental conflicts. A kinetic family drawing ("Draw your family and have everyone doing and saying something") can sometimes give important clues to how the child fits into the family and how members of the family interact with one another. Likewise, questions about school can yield information about life outside the home and with peers.

It is also important to try to understand something of the child's inner world of emotions and fantasy. Asking about worries, unhappy feelings, and getting angry can be very informative. Asking "3 wishes" (ie, "Let's pretend you could have anything or change anything. What would you wish for and why?") can help to uncover important concerns that may not have been apparent from the history of overt problems or symptoms.

At the end of the child interview, it is important to share or reiterate the salient points derived from the interview and to state that the next step is to talk further with the parents about trying to find some ways to make things better for the child. At that time, it is good to discuss any concerns or misgivings that the child might have about sharing information with parents so that the child's right to privacy is not arbitrarily violated. Most children want and appreciate help to make things better and, therefore, will allow the physician to share appropriate concerns with their parents.

Interviewing the Adolescent

Because the developmental task of adolescence is to develop an identity separate from that of the parents, the physician who interviews an adolescent needs to make a point of conveying respect for the young person's point of view. That process begins with including the adolescent from the outset in deciding on an initial format for the evaluation. The need for the adolescent to have a say in the consultation should be expressed to the parents, and then the adolescent is informed of his parents' expressed concern and the physician's wish to be helpful to the family in determining whether a problem does in fact exist. The physician might ask if the adolescent was aware of the parental concern and if the adolescent would feel most comfortable in beginning the process by meeting alone with the physician, together with the parents, or after the physician has talked further with the parents.

When meeting with the adolescent, it is important to clarify the issue of confidentiality. A good policy is to say to the adolescent, "What we talk about today is between you and me, unless we decide someone should know or unless it appears to me that you might be in some danger."

The interview might then start with a restatement of parental concern. Adolescents are then encouraged to describe the situation in their own words, being sure to explain their point of view. In developing a working relationship with the adolescent, it can be helpful to sum up the salient elements in the adolescent's recounting of the story. Doing so confirms that the physician has been listening and understands the young person's perspective.

The physician should then ask questions designed to obtain information about the following areas of concern:

(1) Predominant mood state.
(2) Nature of relationships with family members.
(3) Level of satisfaction with school and peer relationships.
(4) Plans for the future.
(5) Drug and alcohol use.
(6) Worries or concerns.
(7) Biggest "stumbling block" in the adolescent's life.
(8) What the adolescent would like to be different about himself or herself and also about the family.

In closing the interview, it is important that the physician review the salient points with the adolescent and discuss a plan either for further evaluation or for developing a plan to address the problems that have been identified.

Murphy JM, Jellinek M: Screening for psychosocial dysfunction in economically disadvantaged and minority children: Further validation of the pediatric symptom checklist. *Am J Orthopsychiatry* 1988;**58**:450.

Simmons JE: *Psychiatric Examination of the Child.* Lea & Febiger, 1987.

DIAGNOSTIC FORMULATION & INTERPRETATION OF FINDINGS

Whenever behavioral or emotional symptoms are presented for evaluation, those symptoms must be explained in some fashion. The diagnostic process starts with a thorough description of the presenting problem. Those presenting problems or symptoms are then understood in the context of the child's age, developmental needs and tasks, temperament, the stresses and strains on the child and the family, and the functioning of the family system. The physician develops a diagnostic hypothesis, and when all is considered, the presenting problem is understood from one or more of the following perspectives:

(1) The presenting behavior is within the range of normal, given the child's developmental level.
(2) The presenting behavior is a reflection of temperamental variation.
(3) The presenting behavior is the result of dysfunction of the nervous system.
(4) The presenting behavior represents the child's expected reaction to exposure to stressful circumstances, (eg, medical illness, change in family structure, loss of a loved one).
(5) The presenting problems are primarily a reflection of dysfunction or inbalance within the family system.
(6) The presenting problem is a manisfestation of a psychiatric disorder in the child.
(7) Some combination of the above.

The physician's interpretation of the findings are then presented to the family; the interpretive process includes the following components: (1) An explanation of how the presenting problem or symptom is a reflection of a hypothesized cause (For example, children frequently display a disturbance in conduct in the wake of stressful circumstances or become bossy or demanding when parent and child roles are not defined clearly enough); (2) a suggested plan of interaction that is based on the hypothesized etiologic mechanism.

A plan is then developed in conjunction with the parents and child to address the developmental needs of the child in light of the family structure and cur-

rent stresses. If a plan cannot be reasonably developed, the question of referral to a mental health practitioner should be considered.

DEVELOPMENTAL DISTURBANCES & CONCERNS

Developmental disturbances represent variations in normal development; they are associated with symptoms in children that cause distress or concern on the part of their adult caretakers. As a result, parents frequently contact their health care providers with questions about fussiness in infancy, the "terrible two's," childhood fears and anxieties, and finally adolescent rebellion. In these circumstances, the health care provider is faced with making the correct diagnosis, educating the concerned parents about normal developmental variations, and then (when needed) finding strategies to help the distressed parents facilitate normal parent-child interaction.

COLIC & FUSSINESS

In addition to the important temperamental variations among children described earlier, most infants display at least some unexplained fussiness (not related to feeding) in the first 3 months of life. This fussiness takes the form of crying that typically begins at about 2–3 weeks of age and declines toward the end of the third month of life. The fussiness tends to be most prominent in the afternoon and evening hours. In approximately one-fourth of babies, it is extreme enough to be referred to as infantile colic.

Infantile fussiness can be a source of considerable distress to parents for a number of reasons. First, although the baby sounds distressed, no known painful stimulus can be found in the vast majority of babies, and hunger does not appear to be motivating this type of crying. In addition, attempts at soothing a fussy baby are not predictably successful. This situation can result in tired parents who feel they must be doing something wrong; in fact, infantile fussiness is largely independent of caretaking functions.

The cause of infantile fussiness is unknown. However, some have speculated that immaturity of the central nervous system mechanisms regulating states of being in infants may be responsible for the problem. Another hypothesis is that prior to the emergence of the social smile at about 2–3 months of age, the infant's crying may serve as an adaptive function to promote caretaker-infant proximity.

In helping parents cope with the fussy or colicky baby, 2 issues need to be stressed. First, the parents need to understand that this is a normal variant and also that it is time-limited. It is helpful for parents to know that if they can survive for 3 to 4 months, the fussiness will invariably diminish considerably. Second, the parents need permission to have a break away from the fussy baby by sharing caretaking responsibilities and taking time away from the crying child.

Efforts focused on decreasing the fussiness meet with variable success. Many babies tend to be quiet and alert when held snugly to the shoulder. Some babies quiet with movement, such as walking or rocking in an infant seat. For others, rhythmic sounds and pacifiers can be of some help. The real key to intervention is helping the parents to survive the first 3 to 4 months of life.

Emde RN, Robinson J: The first 2 months: Recent research on developmental psychobiology and the changing view of the newborn. Page 91 in: *Basic Handbook of Child Psychiatry*. Vol 1. Noshpitz JD et al (editors). Basic Books, 1979.

Green M: Psychogenic pain disorders. Page 248 in: *Ambulatory Pediatrics*. Green M, Haggerty R (editors). Saunders, 1984.

THE PUSHY PRESCHOOLER

The push for independence and autonomy that begins in the second year of life can pose problems for parents who are uncertain or insecure about their own role as parents when faced with setting limits on their child's behavior. Preschool children typically want their way, no matter what, even when it poses a danger or violates the appropriate intergenerational boundaries between parents and child. Many children at this age express the desire and even the intent to decide when and what the family eats, what time they go to bed, and who sleeps in what bed. In short, preschool children can be quite demanding, pushy, and bossy, all as part of their rudimentary push to become independent.

The formidable task for parents and caretaking adults is to respect the child's wish for self-determination while limiting and guiding the child's exuberance so that the child does not become tyrannical or out of control. Parents who are having difficulty in placing limits on their child's behavior will present with one of the following types of complaints:

(1) "Discipline won't work with this child."
(2) "I can't get her to do what I ask without getting mad."
(3) "He says, 'I don't have to do it if I don't want to.'"
(4) "She won't sleep in her own bed."
(5) "Children his age don't like him because he always wants his way."
(6) "Is this child hyperactive?"

Parents who have difficulty saying "no" calmly and yet firmly and convincingly frequently have one of two problems in parenting: (1) They are emotionally drained and don't have the energy to say "no" effectively, or (2) they have the unspoken belief that conflicts and disagreements are to be avoided in interpersonal relationships. In the former case, parental depression or emotional exhaustion from working and single parenthood is common. In the latter case, the parent typically overidentifies with the child's distress when faced with frustration and is then reminded of painful conflicts or unhappiness in the parent's own life. Keeping the child "happy," ie, avoiding conflict, keeps the parent from feeling distressed and unhappy.

In planning interventions, the physician must educate the parents about the sometimes pushy nature of children who are "feeling their oats" of independence. With that explanation comes the need for external limits, because a child's judgment and self-control are as yet underdeveloped. Parents need to know that a child's disappointment and frustration with limits does not mean poor parenting or an unhappy child.

Parents who are emotionally depleted or depressed need to be cared for themselves, either through rest, emotional support, and assistance with parenting or through professional care for their depression.

In the case of a parent who avoids conflict, the physician should suggest addressing one or two discipline problems. For example, if toys are not picked up after a reminder, they are put away for some period of time. Likewise, if the meal is not eaten within a reasonable and specific time limit, the meal is disposed of, and there are no snacks until the next meal. Once the parent begins to feel more comfortably in control, the child's behavior typically becomes less oppositional; at this point, the parent should use positive reinforcement, eg, "I like the way you picked up your toys; let's read a story together."

Green M: Toddler out-of-control behavior. Pages 289–291 in: *Ambulatory Pediatrics*. Green M, Haggerty R (editors). Saunders, 1984.

CHILDHOOD FEARS & ANXIETIES

The mental world of the child is filled with magical wonders and, at the same time, threatening dangers. The result is that childhood is a time of both excitement and worry, the latter of which is manifest by fears and anxieties.

In a study of nearly 500 randomly selected families, mothers reported that some 43% of their children had displayed at least 7 fears or worries between 6 and 12 years of age. The vast majority of childhood fears are not associated with psychologic disorders; in fact, the fearful stimuli tend to evolve and change with age in a developmental sequence (see Table 25–4).

Although the manifestations of many developmental anxieties, such as separation distress and fear of the dark, may wax and wane over many months and even years, most specific childhood fears are transient (days to weeks in duration) and are not associated with significant interferences in day-to-day life. In most cases, all that is needed is to reassure the parents about the developmental nature of fears; the parents, in turn, are able to reassure the children that they will be fine even though they feel frightened at times. Fears become a source of greater concern to health care providers when they appear outside the normal developmental sequence of fears, when they are persistent, when they cause much subjective distress in the child, or when they are severe enough to be associated with impairments in adaptive functioning, such as poor attendance at school or avoiding peer relationships. Approximately 2–3% of children have fears significant enough to require specific mental health treatment interventions.

Campbell SB: Developmental issues in childhood anxiety. Pages 24–57 in: *Anxiety Disorders in Children*. Gittelman R (editor). Gilford Press, 1986.

Childhood fears and anxieties. *The Harvard Medical School Mental Health Letter* (Aug) 1988;**5**:1.

Lapouse R, Monk MA: Fears and worries in a representative sample of children. *Am J Orthopsychiatry* 1959; **29**:803.

ADOLESCENT REBELLION & TURMOIL

Large surveys of adolescent populations confirm that adolescence is not the turbulent state that is depicted in individual clinical case studies. Previously, general theoretic impressions and sampling bias have tended to exaggerate the turmoil of normal adolescence.

Table 25–4. Sequence of developmental anxieties.

Age of Appearance	Fearful Stimuli
Young infants	Sudden loud noises, unpredictable stimuli, loss of postural support, heights
1 year	Strangers, novel situations and objects, beginning of separation distress
2–6 years of age	Animals, darkness, imaginary creatures (ghosts and monsters)
School age	Bodily injury, physical danger, fear of the loss of a loved one
Teens and adults	Fear of failure (test anxiety), concerns about social acceptance, loss of a loved one, physical danger, natural disasters

Daniel Offer's longitudinal study of a sample of normal, suburban, middle-class boys through their high school years identified only 21% as experiencing tumultuous unrest. On closer inspection, this population was found to be distinguished from the remainder of the sample by lower socioeconomic status, more overt marital conflicts in the family, and a greater than normal incidence of mental illness in the family. Overall, approximately 20% of normal adolescents have a stormy course; another 20% progress continuously and smoothly through adolescence; and the remainder show normal overall adjustment but have had temporary, noticeable difficulty during times of stress. In total, 80% of adolescents adjust successfully and do not display signs and symptoms of emotional disturbances unless confronted with clear socioenvironmental stressors.

When behavioral deviance or a clearly psychopathologic disorder is identified in adolescence, those problems tend not to remit with time. In short, adolescents with significant problems tend not to outgrow them with time. A continuity does therefore seem to exist between adolescent and adult psychopathology.

Hamburg BA, Wortman RN: Adolescent development and psychopathology. Pages 28–30 in: *Child Psychiatry*. Vol 6. Solnit AJ et al (editors). Basic Books, 1986.

Offer D: *The Psychological World of the Teenager*. Basic Books, 1969.

Rutter M et al: Adolescent turmoil: Fact or fiction. *J Child Psychol Psychiatry* 1976;**17**:35.

PSYCHIATRIC DISORDERS

Since the publication of the third edition of the American Psychiatric Association's *Diagnostic and Statistical Manual of Mental Disorders* in 1980, psychiatric disturbances have been classified on the basis of descriptive and phenomenologic data rather than on the basis of presumed or hypothesized etiologic mechanisms for the disorders. That trend was maintained in the revised third edition of the manual, which was published in 1987.

In this current psychiatric nomenclature, a psychiatric disorder is defined as a cluster of symptoms (ie, emotions, behaviors, psychologic states) that occur together with statistical frequency within the population; furthermore, the cluster of symptoms is associated with subjective distress or maladaptive behavior within the affected individual. This definition presumes that the individual's symptoms are of such intensity, persistence, and duration that the ability to adapt to life's challenges is compromised by the disorder.

A number of reports suggest that approximately 10% of children and adolescents are personally affected by psychiatric disorders. As a general rule, these affected children will benefit most from treatment by professionals experienced in the treatment of psychiatric disturbances.

American Psychiatric Association: *Diagnostic and Statistical Manual of Mental Disorders,* 3rd rev ed. American Psychiatric Press, 1987.

Child Psychiatry: A Plan for the Coming Decades. American Academy of Child and Adolescent Psychiatry, 1983.

DISTURBANCES IN PARENT-INFANT INTERACTION

1. PRIMARY CARETAKER DYSFUNCTION

Essentials of Diagnosis

■ Inability of primary caretaker(s) to meet the physical, emotional, or developmental needs of the child.

General Considerations

Primary caretaker dysfunction can be defined as a failure in providing parenting functions (usually, but not necessarily, by the mother) because of parental vulnerability or disability, with the result that the parent is unable to meet the caretaking or developmental needs of the child. Although these parents have no single psychiatric diagnosis (in fact, they may not be formally diagnosable at all), they can manifest anxiety, distress, exhaustion, anger, or indifference in relation to the tasks of child care. Caretaker dysfunction can result in a number of symptoms that are presented to the health care provider, usually within the first 6 months of life (see Table 25–5).

These parents frequently have difficult psychosocial histories, find themselves currently without emotional or physical support, and have many unmet personal needs of their own (see Table 25–6). Likewise, characteristics of the child may also contribute

Table 25–5. Signs and symptoms suggesting primary caretaker dysfunction.

Failure to thrive
Feeding problems
Delays in development
Signs of abuse
Frequent physician visits, especially for nonspecific concerns
Excessive parental worry about illness in the child
Inadequate physical care
Child perceived as "difficult to deal with"
Sleep problems

Table 25–6. Parental risk factors contributing to primary caretaker dysfunction.

Personal history of inadequate relations with own mothering figure
Isolation from an adult support system (eg, single parenthood)
Psychiatric disorders (particularly acute or chronic depression)
Chronic psychosocial or cognitive dysfunctions (eg, unstable relationships, school problems, legal problems, employment problems)
Unresolved grief over past losses
Marital discord
Poverty/financial problems
Personal or family illnesses
Unwanted or difficult pregnancy
Current life stresses (eg, loss of a relationship, recent illness, job loss)

to the parent's failure to "tune in and turn on" to the child's needs. These characteristics frequently define the child as different, defective, or disappointing in the parent's eyes (see Table 25–7).

Clinical Findings

The diagnosis of caretaker dysfunction lies primarily in interviewing the parent(s) and in observing the interaction between parent and child. In addition, the child should be evaluated for organic disorders that could explain the presenting symptoms.

History regarding specific parental risk factors should be obtained directly from the parent (see Table 25–6), with particular reference to feelings of stress or being overwhelmed by the caretaking needs of the child or by the demands of daily life. Particular attention should be paid to the parents' description of the child and to parental symptoms of anxiety or depression manifest by tenseness, irritability, fatigability, tearfulness, sleep disturbance, and a wish to avoid or withdraw from daily activities.

In observing the parent-child interaction, the physician should look for the presence of reciprocity and mutual enthusiasm and enjoyment in the relationship, as opposed to pathologic signs of tension, irritability, or apathy on either side of the relationship.

Differential Diagnosis

Physical disorders that may explain the presenting symptoms must be ruled out, but it should also be

Table 25–7. Characteristics of the child contributing to primary caretaker dysfunction.

Prematurity
Perinatal complications
Illness in the newborn
Birth defects
Multiple births
Difficult temperament (eg, unresponsive, irritable, difficult to soothe)

noted that caretaker dysfunction and organic disease not infrequently coexist.

Complications

Unrecognized parental dysfunction can result in nonorganic failure to thrive, child abuse, later behavior problems in the child, and another generation of children who will themselves likely display caretaker dysfunction as parents.

Treatment

Treatment is focused primarily on supporting and educating the parental unit of the family. First, the physician should empathize with the parent, explaining that being a parent is difficult and tiring work and that it requires health, energy, and emotional support. The task is to help the parent feel well physically and emotionally and then to facilitate the development of appropriate child-care skills. Any underlying medical or psychiatric disorder in the parent should be treated, and a social support system for the parent should be identified. Parenting skills are taught and positively reinforced over time.

Prognosis

Prognosis depends greatly on the ability of the parent to view professional support and education as helpful rather than critical or indifferent.

Green M: Mothering disabilities. Pages 240–243 in: *Ambulatory Pediatrics.* Green M, Haggerty R (editors). Saunders, 1984.
Pruitt KD: Disorders of the parent/child relationship. Pages 367–373 in: *Child Psychiatry.* Vol 6. Solnit AJ et al (editors). Basic Books, 1986.

2. NONORGANIC FAILURE TO THRIVE

Essentials of Diagnosis

- Failure to thrive, not caused primarily by an organic disorder or by inadvertent inadequate caloric intake.
- Deficiency in caretaker-child interaction that results in inadequate child care.

General Considerations

Failure to thrive is a clinical syndrome that accounts for 1–5% of general pediatric hospital admissions. Failure to thrive is classified into 2 major etiologic subgroups: (1) failure to thrive caused by organic disease or deficiency and (2) nonorganic failure to thrive caused by a defect in parent-child interaction. Nonorganic failure to thrive accounts for approximately 50% of all cases of failure to thrive, and perhaps an additional 20–25% are cases where organic disease and parent-child dysfunction combine to result in failure to thrive. Primary caretaker dysfunction is seen as a major etiologic factor in nonorganic failure to thrive.

Clinical Findings

Two clinical patterns of nonorganic failure to thrive have been described. A pattern of early onset of failure to thrive, where a disorder of attachment is presumed primary, and a pattern of later onset of failure to thrive, where a disorder of separation and individuation is presumed to be the cause. The characteristics of these 2 patterns are outlined in Table 25–8.

The diagnosis of nonorganic failure to thrive is based on interviewing the parent/caretaker, observing parent-child interaction, and evaluation of the child. History should be obtained directly from the parent regarding parental risk factors, including current emotional state (ie, mood, energy level, and level of frustration), perceptions of the child, view of the tasks of parenting, nature of a parental support system, a history of losses, and a history of childhood parenting experiences.

The interaction between parent and child should

Table 25–8. Patterns of nonorganic failure to thrive.

	Disorder of Attachment	**Disorder of Separation**
Age at onset	First 6 months	6–24 months
Characteristics of child	Exhibits developmental delays, listlessness, apathy; has a diminished ability to relate socially.	Shows no developmental delays; exhibits oppositional behavior; is socially interactive.
Characteristics of mothering figure	Is young, unsupported; has a history of childhood deprivation or abuse; feels emotionally overwhelmed by the child's needs.	Feels overly anxious about eating behaviors.
Pathogenic mechanisms	Inconsistent care and parent-child interaction (ie, *deprivation*).	Oppositional food *refusal* in response to anxious or coercive feeding.
Parental risk factors	Isolation during pregnancy; lack of emotional support; recent loss; chronic depression; view of child as damaged or disappointing.	Medical disorder in child that causes parental anxiety; feeding disorder; lack of support by marriage partner.
Treatment interventions	Identify a parental support system; supply positive reinforcement of caretaking behaviors; treat maternal depression.	Ignore refusals; limit feedings to a specified time period (ie, "If you don't eat now, you'll have to wait until the next meal."); keep play time separate from meal time.

be viewed both during feedings and during play. Is feeding successful, interactive, and mutually pleasing? During play, is there reciprocity of interaction between parent and child, and is there mutual enjoyment and enthusiasm in the interaction?

Finally, the child must be evaluated for the presence of organic disorders and for the adequacy of caloric intake. In addition, an estimate of the child's temperamental characteristics should be made, along with an assessment of the child's ability to be emotionally responsive and reinforcing to the parent.

Differential Diagnosis

Although medical disorders causing failure to thrive must be ruled out, a significant minority of cases of failure to thrive (perhaps 20–25%) have mixed organic and nonorganic etiologic origins.

Complications

Nonorganic failure to thrive and its associated parental dysfunction can result in all of the complications associated with unrecognized and untreated primary caretaker dysfunction. In addition, developmental handicaps and death can be the outcome of severe nonorganic failure to thrive.

Treatment

The treatment of nonorganic failure to thrive must include meeting the caretaking needs of the child, meeting the emotional needs of the parent, and facilitating more adequate parent-child involvement and interaction.

Initial hospitalization of the child should be considered when the diagnosis is uncertain (the baby will typically begin to thrive with adequate nursing care in the hospital), when the baby's physical health is in jeopardy, or when the parents appear difficult to engage in addressing the problem. During hospitalization, social workers and nursing staff can begin to build a treatment alliance around assessing the parent's own needs and beginning to teach more adequate caretaking skills. Ideally, the parents begin to develop some sense of trust and support from their health care providers and begin to feel some confidence in their own ability.

The backbone of treatment for the parents is the development of a social and parenting support system for them (for example, family, friends, church, social services), the ongoing teaching and positive reinforcement of parenting skills, and the treatment of any underlying psychiatric disorder in the parent.

The child's growth and development are carefully monitored medically. The child should not only gain and grow but also become more appropriately socially responsive.

Prognosis

As in cases of primary caretaker dysfunction, prognosis depends greatly on the ability of the parents to view professional care, support, and education as desirable and helpful, rather than viewing these efforts as critical intrusions into private family affairs.

Chatoor I et al: Pediatric assessment of nonorganic failure to thrive. *Pediatr Ann* (Nov) 1984;**13**:844.

Egan J et al: Clinical evaluation of nonorganic failure to thrive. Pages 831–841 in: *Handbook of Clinical Assessment of Children and Adolescents.* Kestenbaum CJ, Williams DT (editors). New York Univ Press, 1988.

PERVASIVE DEVELOPMENTAL DISORDERS & SCHIZOPHRENIA

Pervasive developmental disorders and childhood schizophrenia are a group of early-onset, severe neuropsychiatric disorders that were once referred to as childhood psychoses. Today, pervasive developmental disorders (including autism) are categorized separately from childhood schizophrenia on the basis of clinical differences and family histories. *Pervasive developmental disorder* is a term that actually refers to a spectrum of disorders, the most severe of which is autistic disorder and the mildest language-related disorders.

1. AUTISTIC DISORDER

Essentials of Diagnosis

- Profound deficits in social responsiveness and interpersonal relatedness.
- Abnormal speech and language development.
- Behavioral peculiarities.
- Onset in infancy or early childhood.

General Considerations

Autism is an infrequent disorder having an incidence of approximately 4–5 per 10,000 school-age children. More boys than girls are affected, at a rate of 3–4:1.

Although the cause of autism remains unknown, central nervous system dysfunction is suggested by the increased incidence of autism in populations affected by perinatal problems, rubella, phenylketonuria, tuberous sclerosis, infantile spasms, encephalitis, and the fragile X syndrome. In addition, studies of twins reveal greater than 90% concordance for autism in monozygotic twins, compared to a 24% concordance in dizygotic twins. There is no consistent psychopathologic pattern seen in the parents of autistic youngsters, although 25% of families with an autistic child have other family members with language-related disorders.

Clinical Findings

Profound deficits in reciprocal social interaction, eg, delayed or absent social smile, failure to anticipate interaction with caretakers, and a lack of attention to a primary caretakers' face, are often evident even in the first year of life. In toddlers, findings include deficiencies in imitative play and a relative lack of interest in interpersonal interactions. Language development is often quite delayed. In fact, children are often first referred for evaluation because they appear to lack responsiveness to spoken language and are presumed to be hearing-impaired. When speech does begin to develop, it frequently is not used for meaningful symbolic communication but is instead echolalic and nonsensical.

Autistic children often display peculiar interests, bizarre responses to sensory stimuli, repetitive, stereotypic motor behaviors (eg, twirling and hand flapping), odd posturing, self-injurious behavior, abnormal patterns of eating and sleeping, and unpredictable mood changes. In addition, some 75% have an IQ of less than 70.

Differential Diagnosis

Although autism and mental retardation often coexist, the vast majority of mentally retarded children do not show the essential characteristics of autism. A hearing or visual impairment must be ruled out with appropriate screening. Children with developmental speech and language disorders typically show an interest in interpersonal interaction that is not seen in autistic children. Youngsters should be investigated for metabolic disorders and for the fragile X syndrome.

Complications

Approximately 25% of autistic individuals eventually develop a seizure disorder. Some autistic adolescents who have higher cognitive skills become depressed as they become partially aware of their deficits.

Treatment

Behaviorally oriented special education or day treatment programs are vital in helping the autistic child acquire more appropriate social, linguistic, self-care, and cognitive skills. The goal is to normalize the child's behavior and adaptive social skills.

Antipsychotic medications (particularly haloperidol in doses of 0.5–4 mg/d) can modify a variety of disruptive symptoms, including hyperactivity, aggressiveness, and negativism, thus making the child more amenable to learning. Fenfluramine hydrochloride may be helpful for a few autistic children, but stimulants can sometimes make the symptoms of autism more severe.

Parents and families need tremendous support and education in coping with their child's chronic disability.

Prognosis

Autism is a lifelong disorder with an overall poor prognosis. Approximately one-sixth of autistics become gainfully employed, and another one-sixth can function in sheltered workshops and halfway houses. Two-thirds need ongoing supervision and support. The best prognosis is seen in children who have normal, testable intelligence and who have developed significant symbolic language skills by the age of 5 years.

Perry R et al: Long-term efficacy of haloperidol in autistic children: Continuous vs. discontinuous drug administration. *J Am Acad Child Adolesc Psychiatry* 1989;**28**:87.

Ritvo ER et al: Concordance for the syndrome of autism in 40 pairs of afflicted twins. *Am J Psychiatry* 1985;**142**:74.

Volkmar FR, Cohen DJ: Pervasive developmental disorders. Pages 201–210 in: *Child Psychiatry*. Vol 6. Solnit AJ et al (editors). Basic Books, 1986.

2. LESS SEVERE PERVASIVE DEVELOPMENTAL DISORDERS

Essentials of Diagnosis

- Pattern of social impairment, delayed language development, and some behavioral peculiarities.
- Children much less severely affected than autistic children.
- Onset of symptoms by early childhood.

General Considerations

At the less severe end of the spectrum of pervasive developmental disorders are children who display a wide range of deficits in social and language skills but who are not so severely affected that they are identified as autistic. In the past, many of these youngsters would have been classed in the group manifesting "atypical development." Children with less severe forms of pervasive developmental disorders probably outnumber autistic children by as much as 2–3:1.

Clinical Findings

Despite having traits reminiscent of autism, these children are generally much less severely affected and therefore have a greater ability to develop more appropriate social relationships, although they may be viewed by their peers as odd or eccentric. They frequently have delays in speech and language, particularly in understanding the nuances of communication. They generally tend to be concrete, rote thinkers. Many are able to control their behavioral peculiarities and are therefore seen as more socially appropriate.

Differential Diagnosis

Specific developmental speech and language disorders should be distinguished diagnostically. Hearing impairments should be ruled out with appropriate screening.

Complications

Complications are uncertain.

Treatment

The backbone of treatment is special education services designed to develop more appropriate social and language skills. Parental and family education and support are important in the process of dealing with these disabled youngsters over time.

Some children may benefit from mental health treatment for depression as they become more aware of their own deficiencies. Psychoactive medications may occasionally be helpful for specific target symptoms.

Prognosis

The prognosis is variable, depending on the severity of social and language deficits.

American Psychiatric Association: Pervasive developmental disorders. Pages 33–39 in: *Diagnostic and Statistical Manual of Mental Disorders,* 3rd rev ed. American Psychiatric Press, 1987.
Rutter M: Infantile autism and other pervasive developmental disorders. Pages 545–566 in: *Child and Adolescent Psychiatry,* 2nd ed. Rutter M, Hersov L (editors). Blackwell, 1985.

3. CHILDHOOD SCHIZOPHRENIA

Essentials of Diagnosis

- Rambling or illogical speech patterns.
- Bizarre thought content.
- Patient out of tune with environmental reality.

General Considerations

Childhood schizophrenia probably represents a more severe form of the spectrum of schizophrenic disorders. It is rare, affecting only 1 or 2 children in every 10,000 of the general population under 15 years of age. The onset is usually after 5 years of age, and approximately equal numbers of males and females are affected. Childhood schizophrenia appears to be genetically related to the adult type of schizophrenia.

Clinical Findings

Affected children display many of the same clinical symptoms that adult schizophrenics do. Bizarre and morbid thought content, or rambling, illogical speech (or both) are the hallmarks of the disorder. Many children have hallucinations or delusions, especially when they have reached 8 years of age or older. They tend to withdraw into an internal world of fantasy and then may react by behaving as though the fantasy were in fact external reality. These children generally have difficulty with schoolwork and with peer relationships.

Differential Diagnosis

Psychotic symptoms in young children (less than 8 years of age) must be differentiated from the normal vivid fantasy life. Rambling speech and bizarreness of thought content can be helpful distinguishing factors. Associated learning disabilities should also be identified.

Treatment

The treatment of childhood schizophrenia focuses on 4 main areas: (1) ameliorating active psychotic symptoms, (2) teaching appropriate social and cognitive skills, (3) reducing the risk of relapse of psychotic symptoms, and (4) providing support and education to parents and family members. Antipsychotic medications and a supportive, reality-oriented focus in relationships can help in reducing hallucinations, delusions, frightening thoughts, and social withdrawal. Teaching appropriate life skills is probably best accomplished in a special education program or a day treatment setting. Support for the family emphasizes the importance of clear, focused communication and an emotionally calm climate in preventing recurrences of overtly psychotic symptoms in schizophrenic individuals.

Prognosis

Childhood schizophrenia is generally considered a chronic disorder with exacerbations and remissions in active psychotic symptoms. The onset of symptoms in children less than 10 years of age is a relatively poor pronostic sign. When the onset of the disorder occurs after age 10, approximately 20% do well and 30–40% improve to some significant degree, leaving approximately 40–50% who have a more chronic course with only modest amelioration of symptoms.

Beichtman JH: Childhood schizophrenia: A review and comparison with adult onset schizophrenia. *Psychiatr Clin North Am* 1985;**8**:793.
Tanguay PE, Cantor SL: Childhood schizophrenia: Introduction. *J Am Acad Child Adolesc Psychiatry* 1986;**25**:591.

MOOD DISORDERS

1. DEPRESSION IN CHILDREN & ADOLESCENTS

Essentials of Diagnosis

- Unhappy, dysphoric mood or depressed appearance (or both), persisting days to weeks at a time.

General Considerations

The term *depression* can refer to an emotional state, a symptom, or a clinical syndrome. All 3 are now well-recognized entities occuring in children and adolescents.

The clinical syndrome of depression probably occurs approximately as frequently among boys as girls. Estimates of the incidence of depression within the general population of school-age children range from 1.9% to as high as 9%. In one study, 10% of parents of 10- and 11-year-old children characterized their children as unhappy. The incidence of depression in children is significantly higher when other family members have been affected by depressive disorders.

Clinical Findings

Clinical depression can be defined as an intense, persistent state of unhappiness and misery that interferes with the child's enjoyment or productivity. The signs and symptoms of depression are surprisingly constant across the age range from early childhood to adolescence and adulthood. (See Table 25–9.) Various combinations of these signs and symptoms are seen in individual children and adults with depression.

Typically, a child or adolescent with depression begins to look unhappy and may make comments such as, "I have no friends; life is boring; there is nothing I can do to make things better; I wish I were dead." There is usually a change in behavior patterns that includes social isolation, deterioration in schoolwork, loss of interest in usual activities, and flashes of intense anger and irritability. Sleep and appetite patterns frequently change, and the child may complain of tiredness and somatic pain.

Differential Diagnosis

Youngsters with clinical depression can be identified by actively questioning them about depressive symptoms. When symptoms are many, persistent, and intense, a diagnosis of major depressive disorder is most appropriate. When symptoms are fewer and of less intensity but have persisted over a number of months, a diagnosis of dysthymic disorder is made. When depressive symptoms are milder and of relatively short duration and clearly follow some stressful life event, a diagnosis of adjustment disorder with depressed mood is made.

Children with attention deficit disorders, conduct disorders, and developmental disabilities can become quite "demoralized" or "reactively depressed" by their chronic difficulties in life. Medically ill patients also have an increased incidence of depression.

Complications

Because the emotional pain associated with severe depression can be intensely distressing, suicide can become an option to the depressed person. In addition, adolescents have a particular propensity to try to escape the pain of depression through substance abuse or excitement-seeking behaviors (for example, "partying," negativism and defiance, and reckless behavior).

Treatment

The treatment of depression focuses on 2 issues: (1) helping those in the environment to respond more effectively to the child's emotional needs and (2) diminishing the child's depressive symptoms. Within the context of the family, efforts are made to resolve conflicts between family members and to increase the opportunity for mutually enjoyable time together. Attitudes, expectations, and disciplinary methods are evaluated. The child is encouraged to become involved in activities and to pursue opportunities for maximizing skills and talents.

Individual psychotherapy with the child or adolescent can increase a sense of caring, concern, and interest from adults. It also helps the young person to identify, label, and verbalize feelings and misperceptions.

When the symptoms of depression are severe, persistent, and disabling, tricyclic antidepressants can be of considerable help, especially when there is a positive family history of depressive disorder that has responded favorably to antidepressants.

Prognosis

Although follow-up studies on depressed children are few, evidence to date suggests that clinical depression tends to be a chronically recurring disorder in children. That possibility must certainly be kept in mind when monitoring previously depressed children over time.

Carlson GA: Phenomenology of major depression childhood through adulthood: Analysis of 3 studies. *Am J Psychiatry* 1988;**145:**1222.

Table 25–9. Clinical manifestations of depression in children and adolescents.

Depressive Symptom	Clinical Manifestations
Dysphoric mood	Tearfulness; sad, downturned expression; unhappiness; slumped posture; quick temper; irritability; anger.
Anhedonia	Loss of interest and enthusiasm in play, socializing, school, and usual activities; boredom; loss of pleasure.
Fatigability	Lethargy and tiredness; no play after school
Morbid ideation	Self-deprecating thoughts, statements; thoughts of disaster, abandonment, death, suicide, or hopelessness.
Somatic symptoms	Changes in sleep or appetite patterns; difficulty in concentrating; bodily complaints, particularly headache and stomachache.

Jellinek MS, Herzog DB: The child. Pages 619–622 in: *The New Harvard Guide to Psychiatry.* Nicholi AM (editor). Belknap Press, 1988.

Poznanski EO: Affective disorders. Pages 231–239 in: *Child Psychiatry.* Vol 6. Solnit AJ et al (editors). Basic Books, 1986.

Clayton PJ: Bipolar illness. Pages 39–59 in: *The Medical Basis of Psychiatry.* Winokur G, Clayton P (editors). Saunders, 1986.

Weller RA et al: Pre-pubertal mania: Has it been under-diagnosed? *J Affective Dis* 1986;**11**:151.

2. BIPOLAR DISORDER

Essentials of Diagnosis

- A distinct period (days in duration) of abnormally and persistently elevated, expansive, or irritable mood.
- Not due to substance abuse.

General Considerations

Bipolar disorder (previously referred to as manic-depressive disease) is an episodic mood disorder that includes patients who have both manic and depressive episodes or, less commonly, manic episodes alone. Some 20% of patients experience the onset of symptoms before the age of 20 years. The onset of bipolar disorder before puberty is thought to be infrequent.

Clinical Findings

In perhaps 70% of patients, the first episode presents as depression. In perhaps 30% of patients, the onset is a manic or hypomanic episode. Manic patients present a variable pattern of elevated, expansive, or irritable mood, along with more rapid speech, higher energy levels, some difficulty sustaining concentration, and a decreased need for sleep. Many times, patients do not perceive any problem with their mood or behavior. The symptom picture can be quite severe and dramatic, with florid psychotic symptoms of delusions and hallucinations (a full-blown manic psychosis) or may be manifest more subtly in changes in mood or behavior (hypomania). The episode clearly represents a change from usual patterns of emotional responsiveness and behavior.

Differential Diagnosis

Diagnostic considerations must include an acute organic process, particularly substance abuse disorder. Hyperthyroidism should be ruled out.

Complications

The poor judgment associated with manic episodes predisposes the patient to dangerous, impulsive, and (sometimes) illegal activities. Affective disorders are associated with a 30 times greater incidence of completed suicide.

Treatment & Prognosis

The majority of bipolar patients respond favorably to treatment with lithium carbonate and supportive psychotherapy.

DISRUPTIVE BEHAVIOR DISORDERS

1. ATTENTION-DEFICIT HYPERACTIVITY DISORDER

Essentials of Diagnosis

- Pattern of behaviors related to the following: excessive motoric activity, impulsivity, distractibility.
- Developmentally excessive and inappropriate behaviors.
- Behaviors that are persistent over time and are not primarily reactive to life stressors.

General Considerations

The history of attention-deficit hyperactivity disorder is reflected in the many names it has taken over the years: minimal brain damage, minimal brain dysfunction, hyperkinetic syndrome, and attention deficit disorder. When careful diagnostic criteria are applied, the incidence of the disorder is found to be approximately 3% of school age children, with males far outnumbering females by a ratio of 5–9:1. Although the behavioral syndrome has been statistically associated with perinatal problems, brain injury and dysfunction, and a family history of learning disability and behavior disorders, no etiologic or structural abnormality can be identified in the affected child in the vast majority of cases. A recent review of research suggested the importance of noradrenergic-mediated inhibitory processes in the pathogenesis of the disorder. At the same time, the syndrome is viewed by some as reflective of an extreme in the temperamental characteristics of "the difficult child."

Clinical Findings

There are 2 common clinical presentations for attention-deficit hyperactivity disorder. In the first, the "difficult child," the history of a fussy, hard to soothe, overactive, behaviorally impulsive child goes as far back as the family can remember. The child is frequently described as having been "a handful" since day one of life.

The second common clinical presentation is that of the "immature child" whose silliness, distractibility, and motoric restlessness and clumsiness become apparent at the time of entry into school, when behavioral self-control, the focusing of attention, and relating to peers are emphasized. In either case, with time, these children have difficulty completing schoolwork because of their distractibility and short attention span; they also have difficulty with interpersonal relationships because of their intrusiveness, excitability, and motoric restlessness.

The diagnosis is a clinical one, based largely on the history of a persistent behavioral pattern that interferes both with the development of relationships and with academic performance commensurate with the child's intellectual capacity. These children are almost always academic underachievers, and in perhaps 40% of cases, a specific learning disability is associated with the attention deficit disorder.

Differential Diagnosis

The differential diagnosis includes reactive behavioral disorders, in which a precipitating stressful event is associated with the onset of behavioral symptoms that represent a change in usual behavior patterns. In addition, children from chaotic, disorganized home environments may display behavioral dyscontrol. The symptoms of attention-deficit hyperactivity disorder can also be seen early in the course of children with Tourette's disorder, with the symptoms of attention deficit disorder frequently preceding the onset of tics. Symptoms of attention deficit disorder are also associated with mental retardation and pervasive developmental disorders. On occasion, mood disorders can present with psychomotor agitation in childhood. Vision and hearing abnormalities should be ruled out as a cause of social and academic dysfunction.

Complications

Many children with attention-deficit hyperactivity disorder develop depressed mood states and a significant syndrome of ''demoralization'' due to the difficulties they experience in getting along socially and functioning satisfactorily in academic settings. Perhaps 25% of these children go on to develop disorders of conduct.

Treatment
(See also Chapter 3.)

Attention-deficit hyperactivity disorder is a chronic disorder that requires a comprehensive, multimodel approach over many years. In school, children with attention-deficit hyperactivity disorder do best in small, quiet, structured classrooms with teachers who are nonjudgmental yet have firm and consistent behavioral expectations. Extra tutoring assistance in small group settings can be helpful; occasionally, a self-contained special education classroom may be necessary for the very distractible and impulsive child.

Positive reinforcement programs that reward the child for socially appropriate behavior and for on task performance can be helpful both at school and at home. Cognitive and behavioral training programs such as Think Aloud can diminish symptoms of impulsivity. When specific learning disabilities are present, additional educational assistance is indicated.

The families of children with attention-deficit hyperactivity disorder need to understand the nature of their child's problem, and they need support in structuring discipline at home so that the disciplinary techniques do not become overly harsh and filled with conflict.

Individual psychotherapy can be helpful when depression or disorders of conduct (or both) coexist with the attention deficit disorder.

Finally, the psychostimulants (dextroamphetamine [Dexedrine], methylphenidate hydrochloride, and sodium pemoline) and the tricyclic antidepressants are helpful in symptomatic control in perhaps 70% of cases. Psychoactive medications alone are never sufficient treatment.

Prognosis

In past years, physicians believed that youngsters with attention-deficit hyperactivity disorder would outgrow their problems once they reached puberty. There is now a growing body of literature to suggest that just the opposite is true: at least 50–60% of these youngsters have problems with short attention span, impulsivity, and emotional immaturity into adolescence and even adult life. In addition, significant numbers are chronically unhappy, repeat grades, drop out of school, and develop conduct disorders that bring them into conflict with the legal authorities. Although attention-deficit hyperactivity disorder is clearly not a benign disorder, comprehensive treatment does lead to better social skills, higher self-esteem, and less difficulty in dealing with aggression.

Barkley RA: *Hyperactive Children.* Gilford Press, 1981.

Camp BW, Bash MS: *Think Aloud.* Research Press, 1981.

Weiss G, Hechtman LT: *Hyperactive Children Grown Up.* Gilford Press, 1986.

Wender PH: *The Hyperactive Child, Adolescent, and Adult.* Oxford Univ Press, 1987.

Zametkin AJ, Rapoport JL: Neurobiology of ADHD: Where have we come in 50 years? *J Am Acad Child Adolesc Psychiatry* 1987;**26:**676.

2. CONDUCT DISORDERS

Essentials of Diagnosis

A persistent pattern of behavior that includes the following:

- Defiance of authority.
- Violating the rights of others or society's norms.
- Aggressive behavior towards others.

General Considerations

Disorders of conduct affect approximately 9% of males and 2% of females under the age of 18 years.

This is a very heterogeneous population, with significant overlap among attention-deficit hyperactivity disorder, learning disabilities, and family dysfunction. Many of these youngsters have "difficult temperaments" and come from broken homes where domestic violence, child abuse, drug abuse, shifting parental figures, and poverty are frequent.

Clinical Findings

The typical child with conduct disorder is a boy with rampant social and academic difficulties. Defiance of authority, fighting, tantrums, running away, school failure, and destruction of property are frequent symptoms. Occasionally, fire setting and cruelty to animals are seen. Later in childhood and in adolescence, truancy, antisocial acts, and substance abuse may be seen.

Differential Diagnosis

Young people with conduct disorders, especially those with more violent histories, have been found to have an increased incidence of neurologic signs and symptoms, psychomotor seizures, psychotic symptomatology, mood disorders, attention-deficit hyperactivity disorder, and learning disabilities. Efforts should be made to identify any of these associated disorders.

Treatment

The treatment of conduct disorders is notoriously difficult and not terribly effective. Efforts should be made to stabilize the youngster's environment and to improve functioning within the home. Any associated neurologic, psychiatric, or educational disorders should be treated specifically. In severe cases, residential treatment may be needed.

Prognosis

The prognosis for children with conduct disorders is not good, particularly for those children who present with early onset and who are aggressive and academically unsuccessful. Nearly half of those youngsters become antisocial adults. In one study, 37% of a population of children with conduct disorders seen in a child guidance setting suffered from a variety of psychiatric symptoms as adults.

American Psychiatric Association: Conduct disorder. Pages 53–56 in: *Diagnostic and Statistical Manual of Mental Disorders*, 3rd rev. ed. American Psychiatric Press, 1987.

Lewis DO: Conduct disorder. Pages 275–284 in: *Child Psychiatry*. Vol 6. Solnit AJ et al (editors). Basic Books, 1986.

Lewis DO et al: Neuropsychiatric, psychoeducational, and family characteristics of 14 juveniles condemned to death in the United States. *Am J Psychiatry* 1988; **145**:584.

ANXIETY DISORDERS

1. SCHOOL REFUSAL

Essentials of Diagnosis

- A persistent pattern of school avoidance related to a morbid dread of leaving home.
- Prominent somatic symptoms of anxiety on school mornings, with the symptoms resolving if the child is allowed to remain at home.
- No organic medical disorder that accounts for the child's symptoms.

General Considerations

School refusal, or school phobia, is a clinical syndrome rather than a diagnostic entity. It refers to a pattern of school nonattendance due to anxiety about being away from home, rather than a true fear or phobia of some aspect of the school environment. In many cases, it represents a prototype of persistent, developmentally inappropriate separation anxiety. It affects boys and girls with approximately equal frequency, and there appear to be peaks in the incidence at the ages of 6 and 7 years, again at 10 to 11 years of age, and finally in early adolescence.

Clinical Findings

In preadolescent children, school refusal often begins after some clear precipitating stress, such as an illness in the child, the birth of a sibling, or parental illness. The child's anxiety is then manifest either in somatic symptoms or in the displacement of the child's anxiety onto some aspect of the school environment that the child perceives as frightening.

The child's physical symptoms are often somatic manifestations of anxiety, such as dizziness, nausea, and stomach distress. Characteristically, the somatic symptoms become more prominent as the time to leave for school approaches then remit if the child is allowed to remain at home for the day. In older children, the onset of school refusal is more insidious and is often associated with prominent symptoms of social withdrawal and depression. The parents of children with school refusal are themselves quite anxious about any distress in their children and in themselves. There is an increased incidence of both anxiety and mood disorders in these families.

Differential Diagnosis

A medical disorder that causes the child's somatic symptoms must be ruled out. Other causes of school refusal that need to be considered include the appropriate avoidance of school, eg, a case of a youngster who is being threatened or intimidated by either bullying students or an abusive teacher. Children with learning disabilities may also wish to avoid the sense of failure that they experience at school. Normal children may also have very transient episodes of wanting to stay at home while they struggle with some internal conflict. Finally, truants are to be differentiated on the basis of their chronic noncompliance with adult authority and their preference to be with peers rather than at home.

Complications

The longer a child remains out of school, the more difficult it is to return and the more strained the relationship between child and parent becomes. Many parents of nonattending children feel tyrannized by their defiant, clinging child.

Treatment

The cornerstone of treatment is helping the child to confront the anxiety and overcome it by returning to school. This requires the development of a strong alliance between the parents and the care provider that is built on trust. The parent must understand and believe that no underlying medical disorder exists, that the child's symptoms are a manifestation of anxiety, and that the basic problem is a recrudescence of old developmental anxieties that must be faced to be overcome. Parents must understand and must be reminded that in this case being good parents means helping the children to face their own distress. Children are also reassured that these are predictable symptoms of "worry" they will overcome once they return to school.

A plan for returning the child to school is then developed with parents and school personnel. The child is then brought to school by someone least likely to waver in the face of the child's distress. This person might be the father or perhaps even an older sibling. If the child develops significant symptoms at school, the child is checked by the school nurse and then returned to class after a brief rest. The parents are reassured that school staff will handle the situation at school and that the school can reach the child's primary health care provider if any questions arise.

In cases where parents are unable to enter into such a treatment contract, more in-depth mental health assistance in supporting autonomy in family members must be provided. For children with symptoms of panic anxiety disorder or major depression (or both), tricyclic antidepressants may be an important adjunct to treatment.

Prognosis

Although the vast majority of preadolescent children can be effectively returned to school, the long-term prognosis is more questionable. Recent studies suggest that a history of school refusal is significantly more frequent in adults with "neuroticism," panic anxiety, and agoraphobia than in the general population. Thus, there may be some correlation between symptoms of school refusal in childhood and the development of psychiatric disorders in adulthood.

Bernstein GA, Garfinkel BD: Pedigrees, functioning, and psychopathology in families of school phobic children. *Am J Psychiatry* 1988;**145:**70.

Gittelman R: Anxiety disorders: Correlates and outcome. Pages 116–121 in: *Anxiety Disorders in Childhood.* Gittelman R (editor). Gilford Press, 1986.

Green M: School refusal (avoidance). Pages 254–256 in: *Ambulatory Pediatrics.* Green M, Haggerty R (editors). Saunders, 1984.

Mansdorf IJ, Lukens E: Cognitive-behavioral psychotherapy for separation anxious children exhibiting school phobia. *J Am Acad Child Adolesc Psychiatry* 1987; **26:**222.

2. THE OVERLY ANXIOUS CHILD

Transient developmental fears are common in early childhood. Therefore, the person evaluating the clinical significance of anxiety symptoms in children must consider the age of the child, the developmental fears typical of that age, the form of the symptoms, the degree to which the symptoms disrupt the child's life, and the duration and persistence of those symptoms.

Clinical anxiety can be manifest either directly in psychologic, psychomotor, or psychophysiologic symptoms or indirectly through problems related to the presence of anxiety (see Table 25–10). The characteristics of the anxiety disorders that are evident in childhood are listed in Table 25–11.

The treatment of the overanxious child frequently involves interventions on a number of levels. First

Table 25–10. Signs and symptoms of clinical anxiety in children.

Direct Manifestations of Anxiety
Psychologic manifestations:
  Fears and worries
  Uneasiness and apprehension
  Frightening themes in play and fantasy
Psychomotor manifestations:
  Motoric restlessness and hyperactivity
  Sleep disturbances
  Decreased concentration
Psychophysiologic manifestations:
  Autonomic hyperarousal—
    Dizziness and lightheadedness
    Palpitations
    Shortness of breath
    Flushing, sweating, dry mouth
    Nausea and vomiting
    Panic
  Headaches and stomachaches
Indirect Manifestations of Anxiety
Increased dependence on home and parents
Avoidance of social interaction outside the family
Avoidance of anxiety-producing stimuli
Decreased school performance
Increased self-doubt and irritability
Ritualistic behaviors (eg, washing and counting)

...

Table 25–11. Anxiety disorders evident in childhood.

Disorder	Major Clinical Manifestations
Separation anxiety disorder	Intense, developmentally inappropriate separation anxiety; morbid worries of threats to family integrity; homesickness.
Avoidant disorder	Abnormal shyness in the child.
Overanxious disorder	Worry about everything.
Phobic disorders	Anxiety focused on specific stimuli.
Obsessive-compulsive disorder	Intrusive thoughts suggesting danger; urge to perform meaningless rituals such as washing, counting, or checking.

and foremost, the child's environment (ie, the family and school environment) should be evaluated for anxiety-producing circumstances, eg, marital discord, family violence, harsh or inappropriate disciplinary methods, or emotional overstimulation. The child's experience of anxiety and its relationships to life events are explored, and the child is taught specific cognitive and behavioral techniques to deal with the anxiety. Finally, when panic anxiety appears to play a prominent role in the child's anxiety disorder or when the child has persistent obsessive-compulsive disorder, tricyclic antidepressants can be helpful. The long-term prognosis for these disorders is largely unknown.

Gittelman R: *The Anxiety Disorders of Childhood.* Gilford Press, 1986.
McDermott JF: Anxiety disorders. Pages 293–302 in: *Child Psychiatry.* Vol 6. Solnit AJ et al (editors). Basic Books, 1986.
Rapoport JL: The new biology of obsessive compulsive disorder. *The Harvard Medical School Mental Health Letter* (Jan) 1989;**5**:4.

3. POSTTRAUMATIC STRESS DISORDER

Essentials of Diagnosis

- Signs and symptoms of autonomic hyperarousal.
- Avoidant behaviors.
- Flashbacks of a traumatic event.
- All of the above following the occurrence of a traumatic event.

General Considerations

Interest in posttraumatic stress disorder in children really began in 1979 with Lenor Terr's now classic study of the children of Chowchilla. Since then, the field has mushroomed; at present, great interest is focused on the developing body of knowledge connecting child physical and sexual abuse with symptoms of posttraumatic stress disorder.

Clinical Findings

Children who have been psychically traumatized show persistent evidence of fear and anxiety. They are hypervigilant to the possibility of a recurrence of a traumatic event. In addition, they regress developmentally and experience fears of strangers, of the dark, and of being alone. They avoid reminders of the traumatic event.

In addition, children frequently reexperience elements of the traumatic events in frightening dreams and intrusive daytime flashbacks. In their symbolic play, one can often notice a monotonous repetition of some aspect of the traumatic event.

Treatment

The cornerstone of treatment for posttraumatic stress disorder is the intense education of the child and family regarding the nature of posttraumatic stress disorder so that the child's emotional reactions and regressive behavior are not mistakenly viewed as "crazy" or "manipulative." Support, reassurance, repeated explanations, and understanding are all intensely needed. "Tincture of time" and behavioral desensitization are helpful to combat specific fears. The presence of a supportive relationship with a caretaking adult is enormously helpful to children with posttraumatic stress disorders.

Prognosis

Children who have experienced psychic trauma are often left with significant emotional scars. At 4- to 5-year follow-ups, children continue to have vivid, frightening memories, a more pessimistic view of the future, and posttraumatic dreams.

Eth S, Pynoos RS: *Post Traumatic Disorder in Children.* American Psychiatric Press, 1985.
McLeer SV et al: Post traumatic stress disorder in sexually abused children. *J Am Acad Child Adolesc Psychiatry* 1988;**27**:650.
Terr LC: Children at acute risk: Psychic trauma. Pages 104–120 in: *Psychiatry Update.* Vol 3. Grinspoon L (editor). American Psychiatric Press, 1984.
Terr LC: The children of Chowchilla. *Psychoanal Study Child* 1979;**34**:52.

CONVERSION DISORDER

Essentials of Diagnosis

- The appearance of a symptom suggesting physical dysfunction.
- No known physical disorder accounting for the symptom.
- A psychosocially stressful event associated in time with the onset of the symptom.

Clinical Findings

Conversion symptoms most frequently occur in school-age children and adolescents. Their exact incidence is unclear, but they are probably much more frequently seen in pediatric practice as transient symptoms rather than as chronic disorders requiring the treatment of mental health practitioners. The appearance of the conversion symptom is thought to represent the surfacing of underlying psychologic conflict or stress that is being expressed through the symptom. Although children with conversion disorder can present with a variety of clinical symptoms, many presentations initially suggest a disorder of neurologic or sensory origin. Symptoms include unusual sensory phenomena, paralysis, and movement or seizurelike disorders.

In the classic case, the child's symptom complex and examination are not consistent with the clinical manifestations of any organic disease process. In addition, the symptoms frequently begin as an intercurrent illness within the context of a family experiencing significant stress, eg, serious illness, a death, or family discord. On closer examination, the child's symptoms are often found to resemble symptoms present in other significant family members. Children with conversion symptoms often but not always have some secondary gain associated with their symptoms.

A number of recent reports have also pointed to the increased association of conversion symptoms with sexual overstimulation or sexual abuse. Health care providers should always keep that possibility in mind.

Differential Diagnosis

In some cases, it is not possible to be sure that the symptoms are not due to an underlying disease process. In those cases, particular care should be taken to follow up to see whether further symptoms evolve.

Somatic symptoms can certainly be prominent in children with anxiety and depressive disorders. The child's mood state and associated symptoms of avoidance are helpful indicators in determining whether such disorders are present. Occasionally, psychotic children present with somatic preoccupations and even somatic delusions.

Treatment

In most cases, conversion symptoms resolve quickly when the child and family are reassured that the symptom is a way of reacting to identifiable stresses in the child's life. The child is encouraged to go about daily life as normally as possible, knowing that the symptom will resolve when the stress is resolved.

If identifiable stresses are not clearly understood or if the symptom does not resolve with reassurance, the physician should assume that the underlying stress must be further explored by a mental health professional. In such cases, in-depth exploration of

the child's inner conflicts may be helpful in elucidating the meaning of the conversion symptom.

Futterman EH: Somatoform disorders in children and adolescents. Pages 337–343 in: *Child Psychiatry*. Vol 6. Solnit AJ et al (editors). Basic Books, 1986.

Kriechman AM: Siblings with somatoform disorders in childhood and adolescence. *J Am Acad Child Adolesc Psychiatry* 1987;**26**:222.

Volkmar FR et al: Conversion reactions in children and adolescents. *J Am Acad Child Adolesc Psychiatry* 1984; **23**:424.

EATING DISORDERS

1. ANOREXIA NERVOSA (See also Chapter 10.)

Essentials of Diagnosis

- Intense fear of becoming fat.
- Distorted view of self as overweight.
- Refusal to keep weight at a reasonable minimum.
- Amenorrhea.
- No known physical illness causing weight loss.

General Considerations

Anorexia nervosa is a disorder characterized by the relentless pursuit of thinness. It affects 0.5–1% of females between the ages of 12 and 18 years. Females account for 90–95% of all cases. The incidence of the disorder has increased significantly in recent years, presumably related in part to the high premium that society places on the thin female figure. The disorder is found more frequently in families with histories of eating disorders or affective disorders.

Clinical Findings

There is a bimodal distribution to the onset of symptoms in anorexia nervosa at ages 13–14 and again at ages 17–18. Typically, the disorder begins in an overly compliant and highly achievement-oriented girl who perceives herself as overweight and therefore begins a diet. Over a period of weeks to months, the diet evolves into an obsessive preoccupation with being thin. This pathologic pursuit of thinness is manifest primarily in the restriction of caloric intake but may also include excessive exercising and purging behaviors (ie, vomiting and the use of laxatives and diuretics). Some 40–50% of anorectics also have a history of binge eating. Although amenorrhea typically follows the onset of weight loss, the cessation of menses precedes significant weight loss in about 20% of cases.

As the disorder progresses, most anorectics curtail their social relationships and become anxious, irritable, or depressed. Their thoughts increasingly focus on food and weight loss; all the while, anorectics deny that any problems exist. Physical and psychologic symptoms of starvation then ensue. In some cases, the pursuit of thinness runs a constant course toward emaciation; in others, the disorder runs a more episodic course, with exacerbations and partial remissions.

Differential Diagnosis

The diagnosis rests in the characteristic findings of fear of fatness and the distorted perception of self as overweight. In bulimia, weight loss is not as pronounced as in anorexia nervosa. Other psychiatric disorders associated with weight loss or bizarre behaviors include depressive disorders, food phobias, and psychotic disorders, but these do not present with the same fear of fatness that is characteristic of patients with eating disorders.

Physical disorders to be ruled out include tumors of the hypothalamus or third ventricle, hyperthyroidism, diabetes mellitus, panhypopituitarism, inflammatory bowel disease, and peptic ulcer disease.

Complications

The complications of anorexia nervosa are frequent and numerous. The most frequent complications reflect the effects of starvation (see Table 25–12). In fact, the physical and psychologic effects of starvation are thought to be prominent in perpetuating many symptoms associated with anorexia nervosa.

Dehydration, hypokalemia (particularly in patients who purge), cardiac irregularity, and gastric fullness secondary to delayed gastric emptying are not uncommon.

As many as 50% of anorectics have an associated major depressive syndrome.

Mortality rates for anorexia nervosa range from 5–10%, with 2–5% of chronic anorectics eventually committing suicide.

Table 25–12. Effects of starvation states.

Physical Effects
  Dry skin
  Hair loss
  Lanugo
  Paresthesias
  Sensitivity to noise
  Hypothermia
  Cold intolerance
Psychologic Effects
  Anxiety states
  Depressed mood
  Labile moods
  Irritability and anger
  Fatigue
  Loss of motivation
  Feelings of inadequacy
  Decreased concentration
  Social withdrawal
  Intense hunger, even after eating
  Preoccupation with food, including food fads

Treatment

The treatment of anorectic patients is at best difficult. A multidimensional approach to treatment is needed. Three major areas need attention: (1) the management of medical dangers, including metabolic problems (particularly hypokalemia), cardiac irregularities, hypotension, and dehydration; (2) the restoration of normal nutrition and eating patterns; and (3) the psychiatric treatment needs of the patient and the family. Because anorectics usually deny their illness, it is important to be direct and firm in addressing their serious problem. Treatment often begins with an open acknowledgment to the patient and the family that although the striving for thinness and control is obviously very important to the patient, it has serious, inherent dangers, including physical illness, psychologic morbidity, and even death. It is helpful to relate the patients' weight to norms for their age and to relate the effects of starvation to many of their symptoms. It is helpful to state that the purpose of treatment is both to restore physical and nutritional health and to help them find more effective ways to feel good about themselves and to feel in control of their lives.

In approximately 50% of cases, treatment is begun in the hospital. Indications for hospitalization include the following: (1) Rapid weight loss—equal to or greater than 30% of body weight loss within 3 months; (2) Medical complications—heart rate equal to or less than 40; body temperature less than 36° C; systolic blood pressure less than 70; serum K less than 2.5 meq/L; (3) Unwavering denial of the illness; (4) Failure to agree to or comply with a contract for weight gain and ongoing treatment; (5) Severe depression, particularly with risk of suicide; and (6) Severe binging and purging.

Treatment focuses on identifying a target weight to be achieved. Small, frequent meals are eaten to attain weekly weight increments of 2–3 pounds. The nutritionist can often be of great help in planning such a program.

The psychiatric treatment of the child and family goes hand in hand with the nutritional rehabilitation. Individual treatment is based on the assumption that the preoccupation with food and weight is a smokescreen for underlying problems of inadequacy and self-doubt. The patients are therefore encouraged to express their feelings and needs, to get to know themselves, and to feel more comfortable with the range of feelings that they are so desperately trying to control and deny. The core cognitive distortion in anorexia nervosa is the anorectics' belief that the only way to feel good about their own competence is to be in rigid control of their weight. In the course of psychiatric treatment, many issues surface: the need to behave perfectly; self-doubt; the perception that self-worth depends on the approval of others; and fear of the turbulent emotions so characteristic of a normal adolescent's inner life.

Because most families of anorectic patients have

dysfunctional structures, family treatment often must accompany individual psychiatric care. Here, the focus is often on strengthening intergenerational boundaries between parents and children, decreasing parental overprotectiveness, and freeing the anorectic child from the role of peacemaker between silently warring parents.

Finally, attention must be paid to the major depression that is present in up to 50% of anorectic patients. Antidepressant medications can be of help in medically stable anorectics.

Prognosis

The course and outcome of anorexia nervosa are highly variable. In general, the younger the age of onset, the better the prognosis. At 5-year follow-up, approximately 40% of anorectics are asymptomatic, 30% are significantly improved, 25% are actively symptomatic, and 5% have died. More than 50% of those patients whose weight returns to normal continue to experience depression, anxiety, social maladjustment, pathologic eating patterns, or difficult relationships with family members.

Herzog DB: Eating disorders. Pages 434–445 in: *The New Harvard Guide to Psychiatry*. Nicholi AM (editor). Belknap Press, 1988.

Hsu LKG: The treatment of anorexia nervosa. *Am J Psychiatry* 1986;**143:**573.

Yager J: Section on eating disorders. Pages 438–516 in: *American Psychiatric Association Annual Review*. Vol 4. Hales RE, Frances AJ (editors). American Psychiatric Press, 1985.

2. BULIMIA

Essentials of Diagnosis

- Recurrent episodes of binge eating.
- Feeling a lack of control of eating during a binge.
- Efforts to prevent weight gain.
- Overconcern with body weight and shape.

General Considerations

Binge eating is defined as the rapid consumption of large amounts of food in a brief period. Binge eating is quite common, particularly among college-age females. Up to 50% of college-age students admit to some binge eating at some time, and some 5–10% of females of high school and college age admit to binging weekly. When clinical bulimia is defined as binging at least 2 times per week with active attempts to prevent weight gain, 1–4% of college females meet diagnostic criteria. As is the case with anorexia nervosa, over 95% of bulimics are female.

Clinical Findings

Bulimia is an episodic eating disorder that typically begins in later adolescence and frequently persists for years before it comes to medical attention. During an episode of binge eating, bulimics frequently consume from 5000 to 20,000 kcal of high-carbohydrate foods. About 50–60% practice binge eating daily. The binging is followed by attempts to control weight gain by means of strict dietary measures, excessive exercising, or purging by self-induced vomiting or the use of laxatives or diuretics. These patients know that their eating behavior is abnormal, and they feel ashamed and uncomfortable about being out of control. Episodes of binging are frequently associated with stressful life events, and depression, guilt, and self-deprecation frequently follow an episode of binge eating. Most commonly, bulimics are of normal weight, but bulimia is also associated with anorexia nervosa and even with being overweight.

Differential Diagnosis

The major diagnostic question is whether the binge-eating behavior and the resultant attempts to control weight are also associated with the severe weight loss and denial of symptoms found in anorexia nervosa. Very rarely, tumors of the central nervous system or seizurelike states can result in binge eating.

Complications

Serious medical complications can result from the purging behaviors so commonly seen in bulimics. The complications include the following: hypokalemia, metabolic alkalosis, dehydration, cardiac arrythmias, dental erosion, esophageal tears, esophagitis, gastric rupture, abraded knuckles, parotid hypertrophy, and myocardial dysfunction secondary to ipecac poisoning.

The psychiatric complications of bulimia are likewise frequent. Major depression is found in up to 80% of cases, and impulse control disorders, such as substance abuse and sexual promiscuity, are not uncommon.

Treatment

After medical safety is ensured, treatment often focuses on improving the patient's self-monitoring techniques (including an understanding of precipitating life stressors, alternative strategies in dealing with the urge to eat, and relaxation training) and on working with the bulimic's distorted self-image. This type of psychotherapeutic work lends itself very well to a group therapy model.

In addition, antidepressant medications not only are helpful for the frequently associated depressive symptoms but also have been shown to decrease the frequency of binges in some 70% of bulimic patients.

Prognosis

Although long-term prognosis is uncertain, bulimics of normal weight generally do much better than patients with anorexia nervosa. One 20-month follow-up study found that 43% of bulimics of normal weight had improved, regardless of the treatment they had received. Many probably continue to have episodes of bulimic behavior associated with stressful life events.

Brownell KD, Foreyt JP: *Handbook of Eating Disorders.* Basic Books, 1986.

Mitchell JE et al: Bulimia. Pages 464–480 in: *American Psychiatric Association Annual Review.* Vol 4. Hales RE, Frances AJ (editors). American Psychiatric Press, 1985.

Yager J et al: A 20-month follow-up study of 623 women with eating disorders: Course and severity. *Am J Psychiatry* 1987;**144:**1172.

ADJUSTMENT REACTIONS

Essentials of Diagnosis

- A change in behavior or emotional reaction in response to the occurrence of a psychosocial stressor.

Clinical Findings

Children's lives are filled with stresses and changes, many of which are personally upsetting and not of their choosing. The list of these is endless, but the most frequent and most disturbing for children and adolescents include marital discord or dissolution, family illness, the loss of a loved one, or a family move.

When faced with stress, children can manifest many different symptoms, including changes in mood state, changes in behavior, and physical complaints. Key findings include the following: (1) the precipitating event or circumstance is identifiable; (2) the symptoms have appeared since the occurrence of the stressful event; (3) the intensity of the child's reaction is not severe and disabling; and (4) the reaction does not persist beyond a few months. The range of symptoms of patients with adjustment disorders are listed in Table 25–13.

Differential Diagnosis

When symptoms are clearly a reaction to an identifiable stressor but are severe, persistent, or disabling in nature, depressive, anxiety, and conduct disorders must be considered.

Treatment

The mainstay of treatment is a supportive state-

Table 25–13. Signs and symptoms of adjustment reactions.

Irritable, angry mood
Anxious, worried mood
Unhappy, depressed mood
Angry resistance to authority
Fatigue
Aches and pains
Decreased school performance
Social withdrawal
Any combination of the above

ment that the emotional or behavioral change is a rather predictable consequence of the stressful events. Such a statement serves both to validate the child's reaction and to encourage the child to talk about the feelings associated with the stressful occurrence and its aftermath. Parents are asked to understand the child's reaction and encourage the appropriate verbal expression of feelings but, at the same time, to spell out clear boundaries for behavior that prevent the child from feeling out of control.

Prognosis

The duration of symptoms in adjustment reactions depends on the severity of the stress, the child's personal sensitivity to stress, and the support system available to the child. The prognosis is generally good when these children feel understood by someone to whom they can verbally express their feelings. Nonetheless, the loss of a parent or the breakup of a marriage can lead to years of intermittent distress in normal children.

American Psychiatric Association: *Diagnostic and Statistical Manual of Mental Disorders,* 3rd rev ed. American Psychiatric Press, pp 329–331, Section on Adjustment Disorders, 1987.

Herman SP: Adjustment disorders in children and adolescents. Pages 375–580 in: *Child Psychiatry.* Vol 6. Solnit AJ (editor). Basic Books, 1986.

ELIMINATION DISORDERS

1. ENURESIS

Essentials of Diagnosis

- Involuntary urinary incontinence in a child 5 years of age or older.
- No physical abnormality causing the urinary incontinence.

General Considerations

Enuresis refers to the involuntary passage of urine into bedclothes or undergarments. At least 90% of enuretics have primary nocturnal enuresis: that is, they wet only at night during sleep, and they have never had a sustained period of dryness. Diurnal enuresis (daytime wetting) is much less common, as is secondary enuresis, which develops after a child has had a sustained period of bladder control. The latter 2 varieties of enuresis are much more frequently associated with emotional stress, anxiety, and psychiatric disorders. Primary nocturnal enuresis is generally viewed as a developmental disorder or maturational lag that is only infrequently associated with a significant psychopathologic disorder.

Clinical Findings

Primary nocturnal enuresis is a very common

symptom in childhood. (See Table 25–14.) The incidence is 3 times higher in boys than in girls. With each year that passes, approximately 15–20% of nighttime wetters stop wetting without any form of treatment. The family history of these children frequently reveals other family members, particularly fathers, who have had prolonged nighttime bed wetting.

Although the cause of primary nocturnal enuresis is not established, it does appear to be related to a maturational delay either of sleep and arousal mechanisms or of the development of increased functional bladder capacity.

Daytime wetting most often occurs in timid and shy children or in children with temperamental differences characteristic of attention deficit disorders. It occurs with about equal frequency in boys and girls, and 60–80% of daytime wetters also wet at night.

Secondary enuresis typically follows a stressful event, such as the birth of a sibling, a significant loss, or discord within the family. The enuretic symptom can be seen as a nonspecific regression in the face of stress or as a more symbolic expression of the child's feelings.

Differential Diagnosis

The differential diagnosis includes neurologic abnormalities, seizure disorders, diabetes mellitus, and abnormalities of the urinary tract. Obtaining a urinalysis and urine culture and observing the child's urine stream can essentially rule out the vast majority of organic causes of enuresis. Some children with daytime wetting can have ''difficult'' temperamental variations or overt depression.

Complications

The most common complication of enuresis is the development of poor self-esteem from harsh criticism by caretakers and the resultant shame experienced by the child.

Treatment

The most important aspect of treatment for children with primary nocturnal enuresis is reassuring the family and child that the symptom is a developmental lag and not indicative of emotional problems

Table 25–14. Incidence of enuresis in children.

Age (Years)	Incidence of Primary Nocturnal Enuresis (%)	Incidence of Occasional Daytime Enuresis (%)
5	15	8
7–8	7	—
10	3–5	—
12	2–3	1
14	1	—

or ''badness.'' Treatment then can be pursued if this largely ''cosmetic'' problem is a source of concern and distress to the child. If the child chooses to pursue treatment, the positive motivation of the child is an important aspect of any successful intervention.

Treatment can begin with a program of bladder exercises that include holding urine as long as possible during the day and then starting and stopping the urine stream during micturition. In addition, the child is instructed to practice getting up from bed and going to the bathroom at bedtime. The youngster lies down, counts to 50, gets up, goes to the bathroom, and tries to urinate. The child repeats this procedure 10–20 times each night before retiring. The combination of these procedures is helpful in perhaps 30–40% of children with nighttime wetting. For the remainder, an alert buzzer that sounds early in the bedwetting process is helpful to about 70% of children. The child is instructed to get up and go to the bathroom and finish emptying the bladder if the alarm goes off.

For others, a trial of imipramine hydrochloride is worthwhile at dosages of 25–50 mg at bedtime for children less than 12 years of age and 50–75 mg at bedtime for children over 12 years of age. Imipramine generally provides satisfactory results in about 70% of children. Unfortunately, many relapse once the drug is stopped; thus, its primary use is for camp or overnight visits, where a temporary period of dryness is important to the child. Scharf et al have described an even more elaborate training program for children with primary nocturnal enuresis.

Mental health treatment is more often needed for children with daytime wetting or secondary enuresis. The focus is on the verbal expression of feelings that may be associated with the perpetuation of the symptom.

Shaffer D: Enuresis. Pages 465–481 in: *Child and Adolescent Psychiatry.* Rutter M, Hersov L (editors). Blackwell, 1985.

Scharf MB et al: Childhood enuresis: A comprehensive treatment program. *Psychiatr Clin North Am* 1987; **10:**655.

2. FUNCTIONAL ENCOPRESIS

Essentials of Diagnosis

- Fecal incontinence in a child 4 years of age or older.
- No physical abnormality causing the fecal incontinence.

General Considerations

Functional encopresis is defined as the repeated, usually involuntary passage of feces into inappropriate places in a child at least 4 years of age. It affects approximately 1–1.5% of school-age children, and boys are affected 4 times as often as girls. Functional fecal incontinence is rare in adolescence.

Clinical Findings

Functional encopresis can be divided into 4 subgroups: retentive, continuous, discontinuous, and "toilet phobia."

In the retentive type of encopresis, also known as psychogenic megacolon, the child withholds bowel movement, leading to the development of constipation, a fecal impaction, and the seepage of soft or liquid bowel movement into the child's underclothing. Marked constipation and painful defecation are often factors that contribute to a vicious cycle of withholding, leading to larger impaction, leading to further seepage. These children often have a history of crossing their legs to resist the urge to defecate and of infrequent but large bowel movements that can plug the toilet, and they are found on examination to have large fecal masses in their rectal vaults. Most of these children are distressed by their symptom of soiling.

The continuous encopretics have never gained primary control of bowel function. Usually, the bowel movement is randomly deposited in underclothing without regard to social norms. Typically, family structure does not encourage organization and skill training, and therefore the youngster has never had adequate, consistent bowel training. These children and their parents are more apt to be socially or intellectually limited.

The discontinuous encopretics have a clear history of having attained an extended period of normal bowel control prior to their "breakdown" in fecal continence. That "breakdown" often occurs in the face of a stressful event, such as the birth of a sibling, a separation, family illness, or discord within the family. Encopretic children then begin to "place" normal bowel movement in "irritating places" as an expression of anger or as an expression of their wish to be seen as younger children. Typically, these children display relative indifference to their symptoms.

In the infrequent case of "toilet phobia," a relatively young child views the toilet as a frightening structure to be avoided. These children may view the bowel movement as an extension of themselves, which is then swept away in a frightening manner. They may have the thought that they too may be swept away by the toilet.

Differential Diagnosis

The main differential diagnosis involves the medical causes of constipation and retentive encopresis. Hirschsprung's disease can be reasonably ruled out by the history of passing large-caliber bowel movements in the past. Neurologic disorders, hypothyroidism, hypercalcemia, and diseases of smooth muscle must be considered as well. The child should be examined for anal fissures, which tend to encourage the withholding of bowel movement.

In addition, fecal soiling can be a presenting symptom in childhood depression and is sometimes a concomitant finding in children with attention-deficit hyperactivity disorder.

Treatment

Identifying the type of encopresis is important in treatment planning. Another important variable is the child's own concern and level of distress about the symptom. Children who display denial or indifference about their symptoms are much harder to treat.

With the most common type of encopresis, the retentive type, efforts are made to soften stool so that constipation and painful defecation do not continue to perpetuate the child's withholding. These children are then instructed in how *they* can begin to overcome *their* problem by developing a regular schedule of postprandial visits to the toilet to defecate. A system of positive reinforcement can be added, in which the child is rewarded for each day with no soiled underclothes. The youngsters are given the responsibility for rinsing their own soiled undergarments and then placing them in the appropriate receptacle. In the case of continuous fecal soiling, the family is encouraged and taught to train their youngster. For children with fears of the toilet, a gradual series of steps with rewards is designed to increase their familiarity with the toilet and in turn to desensitize them to the toilet.

Children with discontinuous soiling that persists over a number of weeks often need psychotherapeutic assistance in recognizing and expressing their anger and wish to be dependent verbally rather than through their symptoms of soiling.

Prognosis

The ultimate prognosis for the disappearance of symptoms of fecal soiling is excellent. The natural history of soiling is that it resolves by adolescence in all but the most severely disturbed teenagers.

Hersov L: Fecal soiling. Pages 484–489 in: *Child and Adolescent Psychiatry*. Rutter M, Hersov L (editors). Blackwell, 1985.

Levine MD: Encopresis: Its potentiation, evaluation, and alleviation. *Pediatr Clin North Am* 1982;**29**:315.

SPECIAL PROBLEMS

SUICIDE IN CHILDREN & ADOLESCENTS

General Considerations

Suicide has become the second leading cause of death among youth 15–24 years of age. From 1960 to 1984, the suicide rate among youths rose from approximately 5 per 100,000 to 12.5 per 100,000, a 2½-fold increase. For children 14 years of age and younger, the rate of completed suicide is low (0.7 per 100,000), but even that rate has doubled over the same time period.

Adolescent females make 3–4 times the number of suicide attempts made by their male counterparts. On the other hand, suicide attempts of adolescent males are more lethal—the number of completed suicides is 3–4 times greater in males than in females. Firearms are the most frequent method in successful suicides, accounting for 40–60% of cases; hanging, carbon monoxide poisoning, and drug overdoses each account for approximately 10–15% of completed suicides. Among youth, there are perhaps 50–100 suicide attempts for every completed suicide.

Suicide is associated with psychopathologic disorder and should not be viewed as a philosophic choice about life or death. Over 50% of suicides occur in youths who are sad, despairing, or depressed; another 20% are described as angry, with the suicide attempt occurring rather impulsively. Substance abuse is implicated in at least 20% of suicides.

The vast majority of youths who commit suicide give some clue to their distress or tentative plans for suicide. Most show signs of depression, such as social withdrawal, loss of interest in activities, and an irritable or depressed mood. Over 60% make comments such as, "I wish I were dead" or "I just can't continue to deal with this any longer" within the last 24 hours prior to their death. In one study, nearly 70% of youths experienced a crisis event, such as a loss, a failure, or an arrest prior to their completed suicide.

Assessment of Suicide Risk

The best assessment of suicide risk comes from a high index of suspicion and a direct interview with the patient and "significant others" such as family members, peers, and teachers. A format for the interview for the adolescent is provided in Table 25–15.

The highest risk of suicide is associated with older white males who express an intent to die, especially when they are away from their family members. Previous suicide attempts, a written note, and a viable plan for suicide with the availability of lethal means are high risk factors. Likewise, signs and symptoms of major depression, a family history of suicide, a recent death in the family, and a view of death as a relief from the pain in their lives are also further risk factors. Persons who have little or no family support, are facing a crisis in their lives at work or school, or refuse to agree not to commit suicide are also at high risk.

Principles of Intervention

Intervention in cases of potential teen suicide must

Table 25–15. Clinical interview to assess suicide risk.

1. An observation or change has been noted.
2. How have you been feeling (inside/emotionally)?
3. Have you had periods of feeling down or discouraged?
   a. How often?
   b. How long?
   c. How severe?
4. Do they interfere with your life?
   a. Daily activities?
   b. School/work?
   c. Sleep or appetite (or both)?
   d. Family life?
5. Do you have feelings of
   a. Self-criticism/worthlessness?
   b. Helplessness?
   c. Hopelessness?
   d. Wanting to give up?
6. Are the feelings ever so strong that life does not seem worth living? Have you had thoughts of suicide?
   a. Are you having thoughts of suicide now?
   b. How persistent are they?
   c. How much effort does it take to resist?
   d. Can you tolerate the pain you are feeling?
7. Have you made any plans to carry out suicide?
   a. What are the plans?
   b. Have you taken any tentative action (eg, obtaining a gun or rope; stockpiling pills)?
   c. As you have thought about suicide, how have you viewed the idea of death?
8. What deters you from trying suicide?
9. If the suicidal feelings are subsiding, could you resist the feelings if they returned?
10. Is there someone you can turn to for help at those times? Who?
11. Has the idea of suicide come up in the past?
    a. How often?
    b. When and under what circumstances?
    c. What has happened at those times?
12. Can you tolerate the pain that you are feeling right now?

follow certain principles. The health care provider must (1) consider any suicide attempt a serious matter; (2) not allow the patient to be left alone; (3) make an effort to understand the young person's pain and to convey the desire to help; (4) meet with the patient and the family, both alone and together, and listen carefully to their problems and perceptions; and (5) let these young persons know that their pain and feelings of hopelessness are understood. At the same time, the health care provider should express the firm conviction that with the assistance of mental health professionals, solutions can in fact be found once the young person is no longer quite as tired and discouraged.

These adolescents should be hospitalized if there appears to be a high potential for suicide, if they are severely depressed or intoxicated, if the family does not appear appropriately concerned, or if there are practical limitations to providing supervision, support, or safety to the young person. If there is any doubt, do hospitalize the patient!

Any decision to send the patient home should be made only after consultation with an appropriate mental health expert. The decision should rest on a decrease in the risk of suicide and the ability of the family to provide for the 24-hour supervision of the patient. The patient's home must be "sterilized" of guns, pills, knives, and razor blades, and the young person should be restricted from driving for at least the first 24 hours. The focus is on supporting the youth, easing the emotional strain, and meeting the young person's needs so that the young person can regain strength. Phone contact must be available, and the family must commit to follow through with appropriate mental health treatment.

Finally, examining physicians should be aware of their own emotional reactions to dealing with potentially suicidal adolescents and their families. Because the assessment takes a considerable period of time and a considerable amount of energy, the physician should be aware of becoming tired, irritable, or angry over the suicide attempt. The physician should also be wary of blaming parents for this problem. The physician need not fear precipitating suicide by direct, open, and frank discussions of suicide risk.

Hoberman HM, Garfinkel BD: Completed suicide in children and adolescents. *J Am Acad Child Adolesc Psychiatry* 1988;**27**:689.

Peck ML et al: *Youth Suicide.* Springer-Verlag, 1985.

Pfeffer CR: Suicidal behavior among children and adolescents: Risk identification and intervention. Pages 386–402 in: *American Psychiatric Association Annual Review of Psychiatry.* Vol 7. Frances AJ, Hales RE (editors). American Psychiatric Press, 1988.

SUBSTANCE ABUSE
(See Chapter 10.)

General Considerations

Illegal drug use in adolescents has been a major public health concern since the early 1960s. From 1960 through the early 1980s, the incidence of drug abuse was largely on the rise, but fortunately the 1980s appear to be a decade in which public education is beginning to turn the tide toward lowered rates of substance abuse. (See Table 25–16.) The one exception for which good statistical data are not available is "crack," a highly addictive and relatively inexpensive form of cocaine. "Crack" use is exploding, especially within socioeconomically disadvantaged populations that are influenced by street gang activities.

Patterns of Drug Use

Macdonald has described a predictable sequence in the evolution of serious substance abuse in adolescence (see Table 25–17). That progression begins with occasional recreational use under the influence of the peer group, proceeds to experimental use not limited to social settings then to the regular use of

Table 25–16. Trends in drug use among high school seniors.[1]

	Incidence (%)			
	1975	1981	1985	1987
Alcohol				
Used in past month	68	71	66	66.4
Daily use	6	6	5	4.8
Marihuana				
Used in past year	40	46	41	36.3
Used in past month	27	32	26	21.0
Daily use	6	7	5	3.3
Cocaine				
Ever used	9	17	17	15.2
Used in past month	2	6	7	4.3
Stimulants				
Ever used	22	32	26	21.6
Used in past month	9	16	7	5.2
Illicit drugs				
Ever used	55	66	60.6	56.6
Used in past year	45	52	46.3	41.7

[1]Modified and reproduced, with permission, from Macdonald DI: Substance abuse. *Pediatr Rev* 1988;**10**:89.

drugs as in integral part of daily life, and finally ends in serious, compulsive addiction. Throughout this evolutionary course, alcohol and marihuana are used regularly and act as "gateway substances" to the use of other illicit drugs. A problem with alcohol use is considered a sign of seriously progressing substance abuse and predicts the future use of other illicit drugs.

Factors Associated with Increased Risk of Substance Abuse in Adolescence

A number of factors have been associated with the development of substance abuse disorders in adolescence. Factors within the family include "permissive attitudes" about substance use, parental marihuana use, and a father absent from the household. In addition, adolescents are more likely to use the substances that they believe have been used by their parents.

It is clear that genetic factors are influential in the development of substance abuse disorders. Adoption studies reveal a 4-fold increase in the risk of alcoholism in the adopted sons of alcoholics when compared to the risk of alcoholism in the adopted sons of nonalcoholics.

Individual characteristics of the adolescents prior to drug use are influential factors and predictive as well. Early and persistent drug use is predicted by life patterns of aggressive behavior, antisocial behavior, poor school performance, resistance to au-

Table 25–17. Stages in the evolution of adolescent drug use.[1]

Stage 1: Occasional recreational use
Adolescent engages in experimentation and social use.
Alcohol precedes marihuana use ("gateway substances").
Clinical signs and symptoms are not present.

Stage 2: Experimental use
User seeks drugs to deal with stress.
Drugs are used in nonsocial settings.
User buys and maintains a "supply."
Adolescent tries drugs other than alcohol and marihuana.
User dresses in "drug culture" garb.
School performance slips.
Family conflict increases.
User exhibits irritable and moody behavior.
Adolescent associates more and more with drug-using peers.

Stage 3: Regular use (drugs as an integral part of life)
Adolescent uses several drugs, but primary drugs remain alcohol and marihuana.
User experiences clear problems with family, school, and even law enforcement.
Money is needed to support use.
Major focus is trying to get high and feel better.
User often avoids eye contact, or eyes look lost or empty.

Stage 4: Compulsive use
Physical signs and symptoms are frequently present: cough, sore throat, malaise, weight loss, fatigue.
User drops out of school or loses job.
Crime becomes a way of life.
User has no family life.

[1]Source: Macdonald DI: Substance abuse. *Pediatr Rev* 1988;**10:**89.

thority, "hyperactivity," lowered self-esteem, and depressed mood.

In addition, the onset of drug use before the age of 20 predicts more sustained use over time. From 70 to 90% of males and 50–60% of females who abused drugs in adolescence continue to do so in adult life. In addition, drug abuse in teen years is associated with an increased risk of criminality, pregnancy before the age of 20 years, lower socioeconomic status, and mental health referrals.

Principles of Treatment

Physicians who treat adolescents with substance abuse must assess not only their current level of functioning within the family, within the peer group, and in school but also their functioning prior to the onset of the substance abuse disorder. This assessment can give some indication of the presence of underlying psychiatric disorders such as depression, anxiety, attention-deficit hyperactivity disorder, and learning disabilities, which need attention in addition to the substance abuse problem.

In all cases, the patients' first step in treatment is to acknowledge the disorder and its impact on their lives so that the goal of abstinence can be reasonably pursued. But many adolescents deny or minimize their drug use, even in the face of evidence of their deteriorating psychosocial functioning. Biochemical drug screening during and immediately after weekends can be helpful in confronting the denial and in promoting abstinence.

Many times, an initial, short-term hospitalization is helpful in removing the teen from peer group in-

fluence, in initiating abstinence, and in providing for an honest, critical appraisal of drug use.

Therapeutic peer group confrontation, either in the hospital or in an outpatient setting, can be very important in helping the teens to address and accept their problem. A commitment to abstinence is made, which is then supported by the family, the therapy group, and ongoing drug screening. Emphasis is then placed on the development of the social skills, positive self-esteem, and academic and work skills that are needed in order to remain abstinent from substances. The family is helped to understand the nature of substance abuse and to find patterns of behavior that facilitate abstinence.

Hendren RL: Adolescent alcoholism and substance abuse. Pages 468–479 in: *American Psychiatric Association Annual Review of Psychiatry*. Vol 5. Frances AJ, Hales RE (editors). American Psychiatric Press, 1986.
Macdonald DI: Substance abuse. *Pediatr Rev* 1988;**10:**89.
Sbriglio R et al: Drug and alcohol abuse in children and adolescents. Pages 915–937 in: *Handbook of Clinical Assessment of Children and Adolescents*. Kestenbaum CJ, Williams DT (editors). New York Univ Press, 1988.

THE CHRONICALLY ILL CHILD

Reactions to Chronic Illness or Disability

From 5 to 10% of children experience a prolonged illness or disability during childhood, and the psychosocial effects of that illness are often profound for the children and their families. Although the specific impact of illness on children and their families depends on the characteristics of the illness, the age of the child, and premorbid functioning, it can be expected that both child and parents will go through predictable stages toward the eventual acceptance of the disease state. Shock and disbelief at the time of diagnosis give way in time to anger and to mourning the loss of the normal, healthy child. Finally, after many months, the family reaches a level of realistic acceptance of the disease, at which time the family is better able to cope effectively with the demands and stresses created by the child's illness and at the same time carry on as normal a life as possible. These stages are, in fact, the stages of grief that one goes through with the loss of a loved one. When the stages are mastered successfully, the illness (ie, the loss of the healthy child) is painfully accepted, and life proceeds with a new set of ground rules that take accurately into account the needs of the sick child and the other members of the family. On the other hand, when anxiety and guilt remain prominent within the family, a pattern of overprotection can evolve. Likewise, when the illness is not accepted as a reality to be dealt with, a pattern of denial may become prominent. The clinical manifestations of these patterns of behavior are put forth in Table 25–18.

Assistance from Health Care Providers

Health care providers can do much to promote more effective coping in families struggling with chronic illness:

A. Educating the Patient and Family: Children and their families should repeatedly be given information regarding the illness, its course, and its treatment. Truthful, open discussions minimize the anxieties that are created by family secrets about the illness. The explanation should be comprehensible to all, and there should be plenty of time set aside for questions and answers. The setting can be created with the statement, "Let's take some time to review again the situation together."

B. Preparing the Child for Changes and Procedures: The physician should carefully explain what can be expected with a new turn in the illness or with upcoming medical procedures. This explanation enables the child to anticipate and in turn to master the new development and promotes trust between the patient and the caregivers.

C. Encouraging the Normalization of Activities: The child should attend school and play with peers as much as the illness allows. At the same time, parents should be encouraged to apply the same rules of discipline and behavior to the ill child as are applied to normal siblings.

D. Encouraging Compensatory Activities, Interests, and Skill Development: For example, a child whose athletic ability has been limited might pursue the development of computer skills.

E. Promoting Self-Reliance: The health care provider should guide and encourage parents in helping ill children assume appropriate responsibility for their own medical care.

F. Periodically Reviewing Family Coping: From time to time, the physician should ask, "How is everyone doing with this?" The feelings of the patient, the parents, and the siblings are explored, as well as concerns about finances and the state of the marriage. Inevitable feelings of fear, guilt, anger, and grief should be watched for and accepted as normal reactions to very difficult circumstances.

G. Recommending Support Groups: Patient and parent lay support groups are to be encouraged.

Long-Term Coping

The process of coping with a chronic illness is an ongoing one. Each change in the course of the illness and each new developmental stage for the child bring new challenges for readjustment. With each step comes the need for new and painful acceptance of the disease and its limitations.

Mattsson A: Long-term physical illness in childhood: A challenge to psychosocial adaptations. *Pediatrics* 1972; **50:**801.

Rae-Grant Q: Psychological problems of the medically ill child. *Psychiatr Clin North Am* 1985;**8:**653.

Schowalter JE: The chronically ill child. Pages 432–436 in: *The Basic Handbook of Child Psychiatry.* Vol 1. Nospitz JD et al (editors). Basic Books, 1979.

THE TERMINALLY ILL CHILD

The diagnosis of fatal illness in a child is a severe blow, even to suspecting families. Most parents face the news of a fatal illness as the worst thing that they have ever experienced, and although parents want and need to know the truth, they are best told in piecemeal fashion beginning with phrases such as the following: "The news is not good; it's a life threatening illness." The parents' reactions and

Table 25–18. Patterns of coping with chronic illness.

Overprotection	Effective Coping	Denial
Persistent anxiety or guilt (or both)	Realistic acceptance of limits imposed by the illness	Lack of acceptance of the illness
Few friends and peer activities	Normalization of daily activities with peers, play, and school	Poor medical compliance
Poor school attendance		Risk-taking behaviors
Overconcern with somatic symptoms		Lack of parental follow-through with medical instruction
Secondary gain from the illness		General pattern of acting-out behaviors

questions can then be followed as a guide to how much they want to know at any one point in time. Parental reactions to the child with a fatal illness then follow a sequence of grief, including initial shock and disbelief lasting days to weeks, followed by anger, despair, and guilt.

Although children probably don't fully understand the permanent and irreversible nature of death until approximately 8 years of age, most ill children experience a sense of danger and doom that is associated with death before that age. Even so, the question of telling children about the fatal nature of their disease is to be answered in the affirmative in most cases, unless there is parental objection. The refusal of the adults to tell the child, especially when the adults themselves are very sad, leads to a "conspiracy of silence" that increases fear of the unknown in the child and leads to feelings of loneliness and isolation at the time of the child's greatest need. In fact, children who are able to discuss their illness with family members are less depressed, have fewer behavior problems, have higher self-esteem, feel closer to their families, and adapt better to the rigors of their disease and its treatment.

Children are very observant and intuitive when it comes to understanding their illness and its general prognosis. At the same time, their primary concerns are the effects of the illness on day-to-day life, feeling ill, and the limitations on normal activities. Children are also keenly aware of their families' reactions and are reluctant to bring up issues that they know are upsetting to their parents. Whenever possible, parents should be encouraged to discuss the child's illness and to answer questions openly and honestly, including discussion about the child's fears and fantasies. Such discussions promote proximity between child and parents and decrease the sense of aloneness that is so common in fatally ill individuals. Even with these active attempts to promote effective sharing between the child and the family, ill children frequently experience fear and anxiety, irritability and anger over their illness, and guilt over causing family distress. Sleep disturbances, tears, and clingy, dependent behavior are not infrequent or abnormal.

The siblings of dying children are also significantly affected by the stress on the family. Siblings feel relatively neglected and deprived because of the time that their parents must spend with the fatally ill child. They feel anger and jealousy and then guilt over having such "bad" feelings about their sick sibling.

Finally, after the death of the ill child, the family's period of bereavement may extend up to 3 years, with considerable emotional pain and dysfunction. Many times, family members will need outside assistance in dealing with their intense grief.

Gardner GG: The dying child and adolescent: Ethical perspectives. Pages 299–302 in: *Understanding Human Behavior in Health and Illness.* Simons RS (editor). Williams & Wilkins, 1985.

Thunberg U: The dying child and adolescent: Clinical perspectives. Pages 302–314 in: *Understanding Human Behavior in Health and Illness.* Simons RC (editor). Williams & Wilkins, 1985.

VanDongen-Melman JEWM, Sanders-Woudstra JAR: The fatally ill child and his family. Pages 541–551 in: *Child Psychiatry.* Vol 6. Solnit AJ et al (editors). Basic Books, 1986.

EFFECTS OF DIVORCE

General Considerations

As of the mid 1980s, statistics indicate that some 40% of families experience divorce. 75% of divorced parents remarry, and then another 50% divorce again. In addition, approximately 90% of single parents are mothers, and some 50% of their children have little or no contact with their noncustodial parent.

Clinical Effects of Divorce

The adverse emotional effects of divorce are far-reaching for both adults and children. Many adult women who have been through divorce report that it takes 3 years for a sense of order and stability to return to their lives. As a result, there are significant effects on the parent-child relationship. First, there is a decrease in the parenting capacity, which is manifest in irregularity of daily schedules, flares of parental temper, decreased emotional sensitivity and support of the child, inconsistent discipline, and decreased pleasure in the parent-child relationship. In addition, a tendency exists for the divorced parent to look to the child as a source of emotional support. Younger children become inappropriately close to their parents by acting as "proud little helpers" and parental advisors. Adolescents, on the other hand, may rebel in order to distance themselves from the emotional needs of their distressed parents.

The effects of divorce on children are most dramatically seen in the first 2 years following the divorce period. Very few children experience the dissolution of even unhappy marriages as a relief, because the breakup of the nuclear family is perceived by the children as a loss of the structure that provides for their safety and support. Children would rarely choose divorce for their parents.

The effects of divorce on children vary with the child's age and developmental level. Most preschoolers display a behavioral regression, experiencing fears of separation at night and when they are with babysitters. In addition, sleep disturbances and irritability toward parents, peers, and siblings are common. In children aged 5–8, grief, sadness, and tears predominate. These children are heartbroken and wish for the reconciliation of their parents. Approximately 50% experience a decrease in school performance. In children aged 9–12, anger is the predominant affect, with the child blaming one or another parent and taking sides. At the same time, children of this age are most at risk for becoming "little parental helpers." In adolescence, anger and depression go hand in hand. In addition, teenagers are at risk of developing a sense of pessimism about their own future involvement in intimate relationships because of what they have been through in their own families.

Outcome

The most favorable outcome of divorce is seen when the divorced parents are able to put aside old conflicts and anger and return to meaningful caretaking relationships with their children. Younger children actually fare the best, particularly when they have a support network (for example, siblings or grandparents) during the period that parents are self-absorbed in their own emotional pain. When the parents have their own adult support network, the children are not so apt to be burdened with the responsibility of caring for their own parents.

At 5-year follow-up, nearly 33% of children of divorces are moderately depressed.

Wallestein JS: Children of divorce: The dilemma of a decade. Pages 144–158 in: *Psychiatry Update*. Vol 3. Grinspoon L (editor). American Psychiatric Press, 1984.

Wolkind S, Rutter M: Separation and loss in Family Relationships. Pages 43–47 in: *Child and Adolescent Psychiatry*. Rutter M, Hersov L (editor). 1985.

OVERVIEW OF CHILDHOOD PSYCHOPHARMACOLOGY

In recent years, psychopharmacologic agents have established a clearer role in the treatment of psychiatric disorders in children and adolescents. The greater specificity of diagnostic criteria has allowed for more precise treatment planning based on diagnostic classification rather than on vague clinical impression. Despite the therapeutic optimism that has evolved, one must remember that psychopharmacologic agents are never the only treatment indicated for any psychiatric disorder.

A few rules of thumb apply to the use of psychoactive medications in children. First, identify target symptoms that can be followed to evaluate the efficacy of the treatment. When initiating treatment, start with low doses and increase slowly, monitoring the side effects along with effects of the medication on the target symptoms. Divided daily doses are the rule in children.

Table 25–19 represents a basic overview of the major indications for psychopharmacologic agents in children and adolescents, as well as a limited number of the more frequently used psychoactive medications. The most common side effects are noted as well.

Campbell M, Spencer EK: Psychopharmacology in child and adolescent psychiatry: A review of the last 5 years. *J Am Acad Child Adolesc Psychiatry* 1988;**27**:269.

Popper CW: Child and adolescent psychopharmacology. Pages 417–439 in: *Child Psychiatry*. Vol 6. Solnit AJ et al (editors). Basic Books, 1986.

Wiener JM (editor): *Diagnosis and Psychopharmacology of Childhood and Adolescent Disorders*. Wiley and Sons, 1985.

CHILD ABUSE & NEGLECT*

In the USA, over 80% of cases of abuse and neglect causing physical or developmental trauma in children and adolescents are the result of harmful actions of parents or other caretakers, with the vast majority attributable to the parents themselves. At least 10% of major injuries in children under 4 years of age are due to nonaccidental trauma. The number of sexual abuse cases that are reported is increasing rapidly, probably because of increased professional and public awareness and detection of the problem. Survey studies indicate that as many as 40% of women and 20% of men have been sexually molested at some time and that only a small percentage of these incidents had been reported. Currently, almost 16% of reports of child abuse fall into the category of sexual abuse, but in light of the above survey statistics, it appears that this figure is not an accurate reflection of the number of cases that actually occur. The offender in sexual abuse cases is usually a relative (the parent or stepparent in 50% of cases), neighbor, baby-sitter, or trusted family friend. Occasionally, several members of a family are involved in an incestuous relationship.

Physicians and nurses (and other specified classes of child care professionals) are legally required to report suspected child abuse or neglect. Remaining alert to the possibility of abuse or neglect in children with injuries, developmental and emotional problems, and vague symptoms of illness will help make the diagnosis in more subtle cases.

Classification

A. Physical Abuse: This category includes injuries caused by undue physical punishment, violence, or poisoning.

B. Neglect: Neglect is the primary diagnosis in over 45% of cases of child maltreatment and is a concomitant of many other forms of abuse. Neglect is not always willful; lack of knowledge, financial hardship, and other factors may prevent parents from providing adequately for their children. Types of neglect include (1) lack of nurturance, leading to growth failure (often called nonorganic failure to thrive), attachment difficulties and other psychologic

---

*Contributed by Ruth S. Kempe, MD.

Table 25–19. Overview of childhood psychopharmacology.

Drug Class	Drug (Trade) Name	Daily Dose Range	Clinical Indications	Side Effects
Psychostimulants	Methylphenidate hydrochloride (Ritalin) Dextroamphetamine (Dexedrine) Magnesium pemoline (Cylert)	0.2–0.5 mg/kg/dose (5–20 mg/dose) at AM, noon, and about 4:00 PM 2.5–10 mg/dose at AM, noon, and about 4:00 PM 37.5–112.5 mg/d in single AM dose	Attention-deficit hyperactivity disorder.	Trouble falling asleep; diminished appetite; increase in pulse and blood pressure; growth retardation; dysphoria and tearfulness; headache and stomachache; lethargy; emergence of tics; interdose rebound.
Antidepressants	Imipramine hydrochloride (Tofranil) Desipramine hydrochloride (Norpramin) Nortriptyline hydrochloride (Aventyl)	1–3 mg/kg/d (higher doses with ECG monitoring) One-third of the daily dose of imipramine and desipramine (Except when the drug is prescribed for enuresis, daily dosage is divided in 2 or 3 doses.)	Major depression; attention-deficit hyperactivity disorder; enuresis; panic anxiety.	Sedation; dry mouth; stuffy nose; orthostatic hypotension; tachycardia and mild hypertension; risk of cardiac conduction abnormalities in doses greater than 3 mg/kg/d; irritability.
Neuroleptics	Haloperidol (Haldol) Thioridazine hydrochloride (Mellaril)	0.5–4 mg/d 20–200 mg/d (Daily dosage is frequently divided in 2 or 3 doses.)	Autistic disorder; childhood schizophrenia; Gilles de la Tourette's syndrome; psychotic disorders; temporary control of agitation.	Sedation; weight gain; photosensitivity; dry mouth; stuffy nose; orthostatic hypotension; acute dystonias; akathisia, parkinsonian tremor; tardive dyskinesias.
Mood stabilizer	Lithium carbonate	Serum lithium 0.6–1.2 meq/L	Bipolar disorder.	Gastrointestinal upset; tremor; polyuria and polydipsia; acne; goiter; possible renal damage.

disturbances, and developmental delays associated with failure to respond appropriately to the needs of a developing infant or child; (2) lack of supervision, which exposes the child to increased risks of injury and emotional trauma; (3) medical neglect, including failure to provide for well child care (eg, immunizations) and failure to seek medical attention for illness, which may result in exacerbation of an easily treated problem (eg, untreated recurrent otitis media resulting in hearing loss); and (4) educational neglect, including failure to teach the child moral values or the minimal information necessary to cope with his or her environment and failure to send the school-age child to school on a regular schedule.

C. Emotional Abuse: This is usually manifested as verbal criticism and demeaning and overt rejection of the child. It may progress to ignoring the child completely, isolating him or her from all social contact, or scapegoating of one child in the family. Emotional abuse almost always accompanies other forms of neglect and abuse.

D. Sexual Abuse: Sexual abuse may be confined to fondling or may involve seduction with oral, anal, and vaginal intercourse or rape. Children of any age may be sexually abused, but the offender is usually at least 5 years older than the victim. At least one-third of sexually abused children are physically abused or neglected as well.

E. "Munchausen-by-Proxy" Syndrome: Munchausen's syndrome involves seeking medical help for fictitious illnesses and providing a false history to support the claims. In the "by-proxy" form of the syndrome, the parent or caretaker (usually the mother) reports fictitious illnesses in the child or even induces illness (eg, by giving the child drugs or noxious substances) to obtain medical attention. The disturbed adult is very persistent and usually goes from one doctor to the next to obtain medical and surgical care and is sometimes successful in having the child hospitalized repeatedly.

Diagnosis

A multidisciplinary approach to diagnosis and treatment of child abuse and neglect involves physicians, nurses, social workers, and other medical and community professionals, often forming a special child protection team in larger communities or hospitals. Expertise is directed toward protecting the abused child and siblings but also preventing wrongful accusations of parents or caretakers by investigating whether injuries could have been accidental or self-inflicted.

A. History and Physical Examination:

1. Physical abuse—Details of the circumstances leading to injury should be elicited, and the child's medical history should be taken as described elsewhere in the text. Findings should be carefully recorded and photographs taken if appropriate.

In cases due to violence or excessive punishment, there may be obvious signs of injury, such as bruises, swelling, abrasions, lacerations, or cuts; marks made by slapping, tying, choking, or striking with a belt and belt buckle; or stocking and glove burns on an extremity, often due to immersion in hot water. With dislocations or fractures, commonly of the long bones and ribs, there may be tenderness or pain and resistance to movement. Skull fractures may be present even if there are no signs of intracranial injury. Retinal hemorrhages, an early sign of subdural hematoma, usually appear within 2 hours of injury. Subdural hematoma may be caused by direct trauma or shaking of an infant. Alterations in mental status may be due to head injury, drug ingestion, or poisoning.

2. Neglect—Signs of neglect include malnutrition, cradle cap (in infants) or dental caries (in children), evidence of chronic lack of personal cleanliness, and inadequate or dirty clothing. The parents may show lack of concern and support for the child, and the child may exhibit poor attachment to the parents, delayed development, and inappropriate social responses to parents and others.

3. Sexual abuse—Specific or generalized fears, social withdrawal, psychosomatic symptoms, school failure, or sexual preoccupation (often evidenced in overt masturbation or sexually seductive behavior with adults or other children) may alert teachers, parents, or physicians to the possibility of recent or past sexual abuse in a child or adolescent. In most cases, however, the diagnosis usually depends on the ability of the child to tell someone who will respond by enlisting medical or social service help.

The adequacy of the initial interview of the child is particularly important, and law enforcement personnel and the medical specialist may wish to arrange for a joint meeting or a videotaped interview performed by someone skilled in the field of interviewing children who are sexually abused. The child's comfort in the interviewing situation is of primary importance. The child should be encouraged to talk freely and provide details about who was involved and where, how, when, and how often the sexual encounters occurred. Questions should be nonleading, specific, and appropriate to the child's developmental age, so that there is confidence in the reliability of the child's report. Children under 3 years of age may only be able to indicate who was involved and how they were handled. Observing the young child's behavior in a play situation or the child's ability to demonstrate sexual experience by use of dolls may be helpful if these techniques are accompanied by appropriate questioning.

Perineal examination, performed in the presence of another person, should be done only after a good relationship has been established with the child so that there is a minimum of anxiety. The sex of the examiner may depend on the sex and age of the child and of the sex offender. Inspection of the genitalia may reveal hymenal tears or scars, or there may be irritation and redness of the vaginal or anal area. Some investigators believe that a vaginal opening exceeding 4 mm in a prepubertal girl is indicative of sexual abuse, but this requires further studies. The absence of specific findings on perineal examination does not rule out sexual abuse.

B. Laboratory, Radiologic, and Other Studies:

1. Physical abuse or neglect—If caretakers attribute bruises and similar marks to the child's easy bruisability, a bleeding screen (see Chapter 17) should be performed. If poisoning or ingestion of drugs or other noxious substances (eg, salt added to an infant formula) is suspected, a blood and urine screen and determination of electrolyte values should be performed. Ultrasonography can be useful in diagnosing some visceral injuries. X-ray films should be taken in cases in which physical abuse is suspected in infants under 3 years of age and in older children with physical findings or with siblings who have been abused. Fractures in different stages of healing are usually diagnostic of nonaccidental trauma unless there is documented bone disease. Radionuclide bone scanning may be especially useful in detecting recent fractures, and CT scanning or magnetic resonance imaging (MRI) is helpful in the diagnosis of intracranial injuries.

In cases in which sudden death occurs in a child and abuse or neglect is suspected, a thorough postmortem examination should be performed to detect signs of bone or visceral injury, poisoning, and other indications of abuse, especially if the child is over the usual age for sudden infant death syndrome (see Chapter 15).

2. Sexual abuse—Rape kits for collecting appropriate specimens should be available for those who treat sexual abuse regularly. A serologic test for syphilis should be performed, and specimens from oral, anal, and vaginal orifices should be cultured for gonococci. Swabs should also be analyzed for prostatic acid phosphatase, spermatozoa, and ABO antigen if sexual abuse has occurred within 48 hours; however, only about 20–30% of these will yield positive results. Rape kits also include equipment to collect and analyze pubic hair.

C. Psychosocial Evaluation: An evaluation of the family should be undertaken if any form of abuse (physical, sexual, emotional, etc) or neglect is suspected. This should include a thorough evaluation of (1) the family's current environmental and socioeconomic status, including housing and financial problems; (2) the parents' marital situation, including the quality and status of the marriage (discord, stress, separation); (3) psychologic support systems (help from relatives and friends, isolation of the family, inability to trust or use outside support) and family responses to crises; (4) health problems of the parents, eg, physical illness, mental retardation, emotional problems, psychiatric disorders, or drug or alcohol abuse; (5) social problems of the parents, eg, history of violence or law breaking; (6) parent-child interactions, including attachment, ability to perceive and respond to the needs of the child, expectations of the child (realistic or unrealistic), and specific methods of discipline and how frequently they are employed; (7) the parents' perceptions of their child's behavior and, if perceived as unacceptable, examples of this; and (8) the parents' own experience during childhood. The majority of abusive and neglectful parents were themselves abused and neglected during childhood.

Management

A. Acute Medical Care: The acute medical needs of the child are addressed while the diagnostic process is under way. Treatment and follow-up for fractures, malnutrition, and other injuries and disorders are discussed elsewhere in the text. In cases of sexual abuse, the reader should consult Chapter 10 for discussions of sexually transmitted disease and pregnancy. Studies indicate that the risk of pregnancy is low, with incidence rates varying from 1 to 10% in several reports.

B. Immediate Protection of the Child: Hospitalization is often indicated because of the child's medical condition. In other cases, hospitalization or placement in a crisis care facility may be indicated for the child's protection while the home environment is evaluated.

High-risk factors that mitigate against an early return to the home include any injury in a young infant, because injuries tend to escalate in severity in cases of recurrent abuse; present serious or life-threatening injuries; a history of repeated injuries requiring treatment in the child or a sibling; fatal injury in a sibling; injuries resulting from sadistic behavior; abuse or neglect of a child who is particularly vulnerable, eg, physically handicapped, mentally retarded, or suffering from a severe behavior disorder; and cases in which a parent is mentally retarded, violent, emotionally disturbed, or addicted to drugs or alcohol. In the latter category, psychiatric evaluation of the parent is indicated to determine if parenting skills are adequate, and careful follow-up is needed to ensure that the parent is functioning well.

C. Long-Term Planning for the Family: Planning for protection of the child and treatment of the parents and child may require the expertise of various medical, social, and law enforcement personnel. In about 25% of substantiated reports of child abuse

or neglect, the courts become involved in determining placement of the child.

While foster care placement is sometimes indicated, it should be considered a temporary measure to ensure the child's safety during the early stages of treatment for the parents and child.

1. Services to aid the parents—One or more of the following may be recommended: individual psychotherapy or individual counseling; self-help groups, such as Parents Anonymous; parenting classes or parent-child interaction sessions with a developmental specialist; respite care (ie, use of day-care centers, crisis nurseries, or voluntary temporary placement at times of major stress); and family or marriage counseling. The latter is considered most effective in coping with incest but should be considered in all cases of abuse or neglect when the family is to be reunited. In some cases, drug dependency programs or job training or rehabilitation services may be indicated.

2. Services to aid the child—For young children with developmental delays or emotional disturbances, therapeutic or specialized day-care services or preschool sessions may be indicated. Issues to be addressed in individual or group therapy for older children who show emotional disturbances subsequent to abuse or neglect include difficulties with relationships, expressed by lack of basic trust and by feelings of deprivation, dependency, sadness, and anger; behavioral difficulties, such as poor control of impulses and poor socialization skills; and negative self-image, with lack of self-confidence and poorly developed sense of identity. A few children will require psychiatric hospitalization or residential treatment because of the extensive nature of their emotional difficulties (eg, severe depression with suicidal tendencies, severe behavior disorders). Chapter 10 discusses treatment of problems that may develop or reach serious proportions in adolescence (eg, school truancy or failure, drug or alcohol abuse, depression, and suicidal behavior).

Prognosis & Prevention

Early diagnosis and treatment in cases of child abuse and neglect are essential to prevent future episodes of maltreatment and reduce the severity of physical, developmental, and psychologic effects on the victimized children. Parents who have themselves been severely neglected or abused in childhood are often the offenders in these cases and may respond slowly to counseling or therapy, whereas the children usually respond quickly to a safe and supportive environment. This poses the dilemma of how much time to allow parents to change their behavior while the child is without a permanent home (eg, in a foster home). If it appears that the parents will never achieve adequate parenting skills (as occurs in about 10% of those in treatment), it may be advantageous to the child to seek early court involvement to terminate parental rights and place the child in a permanent home.

Because of the generational repetition of abuse and neglect, as well as the difficulties in treating parents quickly, prevention of this problem is an urgent and major social concern. Measures to heighten social awareness and prevent abuse and neglect could include incorporation of concepts of human development (both physical and psychologic) into the school curriculum at all levels, educational programs for future parents, and support programs for all new parents.

Bross DC et al (editors): *The New Child Protection Team Handbook*. Garland, 1988.

Finkelhor D: *Child Sexual Abuse: New Theory and Research*. Free Press, 1984.

Fraiberg S: *Clinical Studies in Infant Mental Health*. Basic Books, 1980.

Helfer RE, Kempe RS: *The Battered Child*. Chicago Univ Press, 1986.

Mrazek PB, Kempe CH (editors): *Sexually Abused Children and Their Families*. Pergamon Press, 1981.

Summit RC: The child sexual abuse accommodation syndrome. *Child Abuse Negl* 1983;**7**:177.

26

Endocrine Disorders

Ronald W. Gotlin, MD, & Georgeanna J. Klingensmith, MD

In the health care of children and adolescents, a knowledge of the endocrine system is essential in order to differentiate disturbances in hormonal secretion and action from normal variations in the timing and pattern of development (ie, "constitutional" deviations from the average). In the pediatric age group, longitudinal changes in physical features invariably provide the basis for diagnosis and treatment.

DISTURBANCES OF GROWTH & SEXUAL DEVELOPMENT

Disturbances of growth and development are the most common presenting complaints in the pediatric endocrine clinic. It is estimated that over 1 million children in the USA have abnormal short stature and that there are at least 10 million children whose growth is potentially abnormal.

Failure to thrive is a term usually reserved for infants who fail to gain weight and is most often due to undernutrition (see below).

Tall stature is currently an unusual presenting complaint in our society. Because of the preference for tallness in both males and females, the number of young people evaluated and treated for tall stature has decreased.

SHORT STATURE

Short stature, in most instances, is due to a normal variation of the usual pattern of growth. Influencing factors include sex, race, size of parents and other family members, nutrition, intrauterine growth pattern, timing of puberty, dysmorphia, the presence of systemic or chronic diseases, and psychosocial status; all must be considered in the total assessment of the child.

The causes of unusually short stature are listed in Table 26–1. The causes can generally be differentiated on the basis of the history, the physical examination, and the stage of skeletal maturation as assessed by radiography.

1. CONSTITUTIONAL SHORT STATURE

Many children have a constitutional delay in growth and skeletal maturation. In all other respects, they appear entirely normal. In children with constitutional short stature, birth weight and length are not affected, but typically the rate of growth is decreased during infancy. There is often a history of a similar pattern of growth in one of the parents or in other members of the family. Puberty is delayed ("late bloomer"), and these children characteristically reach normal adult height at a later than average age.

Treatment with anabolic agents or low dose-estrogen (girls) or testosterone (boys) may be useful in hastening the timing of puberty, but adult height is not enhanced. The future role (if any) of a growth hormone for these normal children is unknown; ethical, economic, and social concerns have all appropriately been voiced.

2. GROWTH HORMONE & GROWTH HORMONE DEFICIENCY

Human growth hormone (hGH) is a 191-amino-acid peptide with 2 intramolecular disulfide bridges. The hGH gene is present on chromosome 17 in association with genes for human chorionic sommatomammotropin. Human growth hormone has been synthesized recently in bacterial and mouse-cell lines, an accomplishment that has provided unlimited quantities of hGH for study and treatment in humans.

The recent biosynthesis of hGH employing recombinant DNA methods has made sufficient hormone available to treat all children with a deficiency state. Moreover, children with severe short stature and normal growth hormone secretion who may benefit from hGH in large doses can be evaluated in clinical trials. When rigid diagnostic criteria are employed, instances of hGH deficiency are found in approximately one in 4000 children. About two-thirds of the cases are idiopathic (rarely familial): a deficiency or impairment in the hypothalamic secretion of hGH-

Table 26–1. Causes of short stature.

Familial, racial, or genetic	**Inborn errors of metabolism (cont'd)**
	Sphingolipidoses (eg, Tay-Sachs disease, Niemann-Pick disease, Gaucher's disease)
Constitutional short stature and delayed adolescence	Miscellaneous (eg, cystinosis)
	Aminoacidemias and aminoacidurias
Endocrine disturbances	Epithelial transport disorders (eg, renal tubular acidosis, cystic fibrosis, Bartter's syndrome, vasopressin-resistant diabetes insipidus, pseudohypoparathyroidism)
Growth hormone deficiency	
Hereditary—gene deletion	
Idiopathic—deficiency of growth hormone or growth hormone releasing hormone (or both) with and without associated abnormalities of midline structures of the central nervous system	Organic acidemias and acidurias (eg, methylmalonic aciduria, orotic aciduria, maple syrup urine disease, isovaleric acidemia)
Acquired	Metabolic anemias (eg, sickle cell disease, thalassemia, pyruvate kinase deficiency)
Transient—eg, psychosocial short stature	Disorders of mineral metabolism (eg, Wilson's disease, magnesium malabsorption syndrome)
Organic—tumor, irradiation of the central nervous system, infection, or trauma	Body defense disorders (eg, Bruton's agammaglobulinemia, thymic aplasia, chronic granulomatous disease)
Hypothyroidism	
Adrenal insufficiency	**Constitutional (intrinsic) diseases of bone**
Cushing's disease and Cushing's syndrome (including iatrogenic causes)	Defects of growth of tubular bones or spine (eg, achondroplasia, metatropic dwarfism, diastrophic dwarfism, metaphyseal chondrodysplasia)
Sexual precocity (androgen or estrogen excess)	Disorganized development of cartilage and fibrous components of the skeleton (eg, multiple cartilaginous exostoses, fibrous dysplasia with skin pigmentation, precocious puberty of McCune-Albright)
Diabetes mellitus (poorly controlled)	
Diabetes insipidus	
Hyperaldosteronism	Abnormalities of density of cortical diaphyseal structure or metaphyseal modeling (eg, osteogenesis imperfecta congenita, osteopetrosis, tubular stenosis)
Primordial short stature	
Intrauterine growth retardation	**Short stature associated with chromosomal defects**
Placental insufficiency	Autosomal (eg, Down's syndrome, cri du chat syndrome, trisomy 18)
Intrauterine infection	Sex chromosomal (eg, Turner's syndrome-XO, penta X, XXXY)
Primordial dwarfism with premature aging	
Progeria (Hutchinson-Gilford syndrome)	
Progeroid syndrome	**Chronic systemic diseases, congenital defects, and cancers** (eg, chronic infection and infestation, inflammatory bowel disease, hepatic disease, cardiovascular disease, hematologic disease, central nervous system disease, pulmonary disease, renal disease, malnutrition, cancers, collagen vascular disease)
Werner's syndrome	
Cachectic (Cockayne's syndrome)	
Short stature without dysmorphism	
Short stature with dysmorphism (eg, Seckel's bird-headed dwarfism, leprechaunism, Silver's syndrome, Bloom's syndrome, Cornelia de Lange syndrome, Hallerman-Streiff syndrome)	
	Psychosocial short stature (deprivation dwarfism)
Inborn errors of metabolism	**Miscellaneous syndromes** (eg, arthrogryposis multiplex congenita, cerebrohepatorenal syndrome, Noonan's syndrome, Prader-Willi syndrome, Riley-Day syndrome)
Altered metabolism of calcium or phosphorus (eg, hypophosphatemic rickets, hypophosphatasia, infantile hypercalcemia, pseudohypoparathyroidism)	
Storage diseases	
Mucopolysaccharidoses (eg, Hurler's syndrome, Hunter's syndrome)	
Mucolipidoses (eg, generalized gangliosidosis, fucosidosis, mannosidosis)	

releasing hormone is suspected. The remainder are secondary to pituitary or hypothalmic disease, infection, trauma, reticuloendotheliosis, and craniopharyngioma or other tumors (eg, gliomas). The deficiency of hGH may be an isolated defect or may occur in combination with other pituitary hormone deficiencies. Idiopathic hGH deficiency affects both sexes equally.

At birth, affected children are of normal weight, but length may be reduced. The most characteristic clinical feature of the child with hGH deficiency is a linear growth rate as little as one-half that of the normal child. Growth retardation may begin during infancy or may be delayed until later childhood. Other findings include infantile fat distribution, youthful facial features, midfacial hypoplasia, and

delayed sexual maturation. Epiphyseal maturation ("bone age") is delayed. Headaches, visual field defects, polyuria, and polydipsia may precede or accompany the onset of growth failure in cases resulting from central nervous system disease. Abnormal skull radiographs, CT scans, or MRIs are common in organic hypopituitarism.

The deficiency of hGH is generally associated with low levels of hGH in the serum and with the failure of hGH levels to increase appreciably during normal physiologic sleep, after exercise, or in response to arginine, glucagon, levodopa, clonidine, or insulin induced hypoglycemia. It is important to assess thyroid function and correct deficiency states prior to testing. Spontaneous hypoglycemia, augmented insulin sensitivity, and additional clinical features due to other pituitary hormone deficiencies may be present.

When results of growth hormone testing are equivocal, a trial of hGH treatment may be useful in determining whether an abnormally short child will benefit from growth hormone. Currently, the treatment of choice is synthetic hGH alone or in combination with other hormones. The dose of hGH is 0.05–0.1 mg/kg administered subcutaneously 3 times weekly; preferably, one-seventh of the total weekly dose is given daily. Results of clinical trials with hGH-releasing hormone (somatotropin-releasing hormone) have been encouraging, and this agent may be employed in the future in patients with hypothalamic hGH-releasing hormone deficiency. Protein anabolic agents may be effective in promoting linear growth but may cause undue acceleration of epiphyseal closure, with a resultant lessening of adult height. Anabolic agents should ideally be used at the time of puberty and in combination with hGH.

The efficacy of hGH treatment for conditions associated with severe short stature and normal hGH secretion (eg, intrauterine growth retardation, dysmorphism) is currently under clinical investigation. In Turner's syndrome (see below) results over a 5-year study have been encouraging. Similarly adults with hGH deficiency may benefit from continued therapy. The use of hGH in conditions other than definite deficiency states prompts scientific, social, and ethical questions. The greatest controversy surrounding hGH therapy is its role, if any, in a normal, short child and the elderly.

Physiologically, hGH is released from the anterior pituitary in response to a delicate interplay of hypothalamic releasing and inhibitory factors. Moreover, a variety of stimuli, including adrenergic and serotoninergic agents, arginine, glucagon, and insulin-induced hypoglycemia, have been employed clinically to provoke hGH secretion. Physiologically, serum levels of hGH vary considerably; episodic surges occur in relation to nutrients, to activity, and particularly to natural sleep. The latter typically is associated with significant sustained elevation of hGH during the first 2 hours after the onset of sleep. Electroencephalographic monitoring during this interval reflects slow-wave or "deep" sleep, suggesting a role for specific neurotransmitter influence.

Following secretion, hGH exerts its biologic effects following binding to specific receptors in a large variety of tissues. Actions are divided into direct and indirect. The latter division is used to designate actions, hormonal and panacrine, resulting from the activity of the somatomedin family (insulin-like growth factors; IGFs) in response to hGH.

3. HYPOTHYROIDISM

Hypothyroidism in childhood (discussed in a subsequent section) is invariably associated with poor growth and delayed osseous maturation. In occasional cases, short stature may be the principal finding.

4. INTRAUTERINE GROWTH RETARDATION (Primordial Short Stature)

Intrauterine growth retardation may occur in a number of disorders, including craniofacial disproportion (eg, Seckel's dwarfism), Silver's syndrome noonan syndrome, some cases of progeria (eg, Hutchinson-Gilford syndrome), and cachectic dwarfism, or may occur in individuals with no accompanying significant dysmorphism. Children with these conditions are small at birth; both birth weight and length are below normal for gestational age. They grow parallel to but below the 5th percentile. Plasma hGH levels are usually normal but may be elevated. In most instances, skeletal maturation ("bone age") corresponds to chronologic age or is only mildly delayed, in contrast to the striking delay often present in children with hGH and thyroid deficiency.

There is no satisfactory long-term treatment for primordial short stature, although growth hormone in large doses may be efficacious and is being evaluated in clinical trials.

5. SHORT STATURE DUE TO EMOTIONAL FACTORS (Psychosocial Short Stature, Deprivation Dwarfism)

Psychologic deprivation with disturbances in motor and personality development may be associated with short stature. Although the growth retardation in some affected individuals is the result of undernutrition, in others undernutrition does not seem to be the major factor. In some instances, the child may have increased (often voracious) appetite; polydipsia and polyuria are sometimes present. These children are of normal size at birth and grow normally for a variable period of time before growth slows. A history of feeding problems in early infancy is common. Sleep is often restless. Emotional disturbances in the family are the rule. Skeletal maturation is delayed and plasma hGH levels during sleep or in response to pharmacologic stimulation may be diminished.

Foster home placement or a change in the psychologic and emotional environment at home usually results in significantly improved growth (return of normal hGH secretion), normalization of, personality, appetite and dietary intake.

DIFFERENTIAL DIAGNOSIS OF SHORT STATURE

Short stature may accompany or be caused by a large number of conditions (Table 26–1). When the etiologic diagnosis is not apparent from the history and physical examination, the following laboratory studies, in addition to bone age, are useful in detecting or categorizing the common causes of short stature:

(1) Complete blood count (to detect chronic anemia, infection, cancer).

(2) Erythrocyte sedimentation rate (often elevated in collagen-vascular disease, cancer, chronic infection, inflammatory bowel disease).

(3) Urinalysis and microscopic examination (occult pyelonephritis, glomerulonephritis, renal tubular disease, etc).

(4) Stool examination for occult blood, parasites, and parasite ova (inflammatory bowel disease, overwhelming parasitism).

(5) Serum electrolytes and phosphorus (mild adrenal insufficiency, renal tubular diseases, parathyroid disease, rickets, etc); antigliadin antibody (for celiac disease).

(6) Blood urea nitrogen and creatinine (occult renal insufficiency).

(7) Karyotyping (should be performed in all short girls with delayed sexual maturation with or without phenotypic features of Turner's syndrome).

(8) Thyroid function assessment: thyroxine (T_4), free T_4, and thyroid-stimulating hormone (TSH) assay (short stature may be the only sign of hypothyroidism).

(9) Currently, considerable controversy concerning the diagnostic determination of hGH deficiency remains. The authors prefer a combination of physiologic assessments: hGH levels obtained during natural sleep and following the administration of the provocative agent clonidine. Other provocative choices include arginine, insulin, and levodopa, administered after priming with sex steroids (in children with bone ages greater than 8 years).

Cuttler L: Evaluation of growth disorders in children. *Pediatrician* 1987;**14:**109.

Grumbach MM: Growth hormone therapy and the short end of the stick. (Editorial.) *N Engl J Med* 1988; **319:**238.

Miller WL, Eberhardt NL: Structure and evolution of the growth hormone gene family. *Endocr Rev* 1983;**4:**97.

Thorner MO et al: Acceleration of growth rate in growth hormone-deficient children treated with human growth hormone releasing hormone. *Pediatr Res* 1988;**24:**145.

Wilson DM, Rosenfeld RG: Treatment of short stature and delayed adolescence. *Pediatr Clin North Am* 1987; **34:**865.

FAILURE TO THRIVE

Failure to thrive is present when there is a perceptible declination of growth from an established pattern or when the patient's height and weight plot consistently below the 3rd percentile. (The term is optimally reserved for infants who for various reasons fail to gain weight.) Head circumference may also be affected; when this occurs, the underlying condition is generally more severe. There are many reasons for failure to thrive (see below and Table 26–1). Inadequate caloric intake is the most important cause of failure to thrive.

Classification & Etiologic Diagnosis

The diagnosis of failure to thrive is usually apparent on the basis of the history and physical examination. When it is not, it is helpful to compare the patient's chronologic age with the height age (median age for the patient's height), weight age, and head circumference. On the basis of these measurements, 3 principal patterns can be defined that provide a starting point in the diagnostic approach.

Group 1. (Most common type.) Normal head circumference; weight reduced out of proportion to height: In the majority of cases of failure to thrive, malnutrition is present as a result of either deficient caloric intake or malabsorption.

Group 2. Normal or increased head circumference; weight only moderately reduced, usually in proportion to height: Structural dystrophies, constitutional dwarfism, endocrinopathies.

Group 3. Subnormal head circumference; weight reduced in proportion to height: Primary central nervous system deficit; intrauterine growth retardation.

An initial period of observed nutritional rehabilitation, usually in a hospital setting, is often helpful in the diagnosis. The child should be placed on a regular diet for age, and intake and weight should be carefully plotted for 1–2 weeks. If stools are abnormal, evaluate for carbohydrate intolerance and malabsorption. Caloric intake should be increased if weight gain does not occur but intake is well tolerated. The following 3 patterns are often noted during rehabilitation.

Pattern 1. (Most common type.) Intake adequate; weight gain satisfactory: Feeding technique or amount at fault. Disturbed infant-mother relationship leading to decreased caloric intake.

Pattern 2. Intake adequate; no weight gain: If weight gain is unsatisfactory after increasing the calories to an adequate level (based on the infant's ideal weight for height), malabsorption is the most likely diagnosis. A diencephalic tumor may also cause this pattern, with or without associated microcephaly or ocular abnormalities.

If malabsorption is present, it is usually necessary to differentiate pancreatic exocrine insufficiency (cystic fibrosis, Shwachman syndrome) from abnormalities of intestinal mucosa (eg, celiac disease). In cystic fibrosis, growth velocity commonly declines from the time of birth, and appetite usually is voracious. In celiac disease, growth velocity is usually not reduced until 6–12 months of age, and inadequate caloric intake may be a prominent feature.

Pattern 3. Intake inadequate:

(1) Sucking or swallowing difficulties: Central nervous system or neuromuscular disease; esophageal or oropharyngeal malformations.

(2) Inability to eat large amounts is common in patients with cardiopulmonary disease or in anorexic children suffering from chronic infections, systemic diseases, inflammatory bowel disease, and endocrine problems (eg, hypothyroidism). Patients with celiac disease often have inadequate caloric intake in addition to malabsorption. Zinc deficiency may cause anorexia and resultant poor weight gain.

(3) Vomiting, spitting up, or rumination: Upper intestinal obstruction (eg, pyloric stenosis, hiatal hernia, chalasia), chronic metabolic aberrations and acidosis (eg, renal insufficiency, diabetes mellitus and insipidus, organic acidemias), aldosterone insufficiency, increased intracranial pressure, psychosocial abnormalities.

Laboratory Aids to Diagnosis

The laboratory may provide helpful diagnostic information:

A. Inital: Initial laboratory investigations at the time of admission might be limited to the following:

1. Blood—Complete blood count, sedimentation rate antigliadin antibody.

2. Urine—Urinalysis (including microscopic examination of sediment) and culture.

3. Stool (if abnormal)—Culture, pH, reducing substances, examination for occult blood, fat, and parasites.

4. Other tests only if clinically indicated.

B. Definitive: The following laboratory investigations are recommended after the period of nutritional rehabilitation, when the patient has been classified in one of the 3 categories listed above.

1. Pattern 1—No further laboratory tests are indicated. Maternal (and family) social and psychologic evaluation may be indicated.

2. Pattern 2—

a. Evaluate for malabsorption (see Chapter 20) if stools are abnormal.

b. If stools are normal or malabsorption excluded, consider cerebral imaging for diencephalic tumor.

3. Pattern 3—

a. With vomiting—

(1) Serum electrolytes, pH, glucose, creatinine, zinc, ammonia, and lactate/pyruvate; serum and urine osmolarities; serum and urine organic and amino acids.

(2) Upper gastrointestinal series and cineesophageography.

(3) Cerebral imaging for causes of increased intracranial pressure, (eg, subdural hematoma, hydrocephalus, tumor) or central vomiting.

b. Without vomiting—

(1) Sigmoidoscopy, rectal biopsy (ulcerative or granulomatous colitis).

(2) Barium enema (ulcerative colitis or Hirschsprung's disease).

(3) Upper gastrointestinal series and follow-through (regional enteritis, malrotations).

(4) Thyroid function tests.

C. Other Tests: Further testing (adrenal function tests, intravenous urograms, etc) may be indicated.

Treatment & Prognosis

Treatment varies according to the underlying disorder. Most patients will gain weight and thrive on an adequate caloric intake. Maternal counseling and support placement may be required.

The outcome is dependent on the underlying disorder. In general, infants whose length and, particularly, head circumference are affected along with weight have a less favorable prognosis.

TALL STATURE

Currently, tall stature is usually of concern only to adolescent and preadolescent girls. The upper limit of acceptable height of both sexes appears to be increasing, but there are occasions when the patient and her parents may wish to influence the pattern of growth. On the basis of family history, previous pattern of growth, stage of physiologic development, assessment of epiphyseal development (''bone age''), and standard growth data, the physician should make a tentative estimate of the patient's eventual height. Although there are several conditions (Table 26–2) that may produce tall stature, by

Table 26–2. Causes of tall stature.

Constitutional (familial)

Endocrine causes
  Somatotropin excess (pituitary gigantism)
  Androgen excess (tall as children, short as adults)
    True sexual precocity
    Pseudosexual precocity
  Androgen deficiency (normal height as children, tall as adults)
    Klinefelter's syndrome
    Anorchia (infection, trauma, idiopathic)
  Hyperthyroidism

Genetic causes
  Klinefelter's syndrome
  Syndromes of XYY, XXYY (tall as adults)

Miscellaneous syndromes and entities
  Marfan's syndrome
  Cerebral gigantism (Sotos' syndrome)
  Total lipodystrophy
  Diencephalic syndrome
  Homocystinuria

far the most common cause is a constitutional or familial variation from the average.

Reassurance, counseling, and education are generally all that is required. If the predicted height appears to be excessive, hormonal therapy with estrogen (eg, ethinyl estradiol, 0.2–0.3 mg daily), cycled with a progestational agent for 7 out of 28 days, may be effective. Estrogens are of less value when the physiologic age (as determined by stage of sexual maturity and epiphyseal development) has reached the 12-year-old level and may be of little value even when administered at earlier ages. Estrogens act to accelerate epiphyseal closure and may be continued until fusion occurs. In the male, a course of testosterone may be effective.

Wettenhall HNB, Cahill C, Roche AF: Tall girls: A survey of 15 years of management and treatment. *J Pediatr* 1975;**86**:602.

Whitehead EM et al: Pituitary gigantism: A disabling condition. *Clin Endocrinol (Oxf)* 1982;**17**:2271.

THE POSTERIOR PITUITARY GLAND

The posterior pituitary (neurohypophysis) is an extension of the ventral hypothalamus. The 2 principal neurohormones of the posterior pituitary, oxytocin and vasopressin, are synthesized in the supraoptic and paraventricular nuclei. After synthesis, these neurohormones are packaged in granules with specific neurophysins and transported via the axons to their storage site in the neurohypophysis. Oxytocin is primarily important during parturition and breast-feeding and is not discussed further.

ANTIDIURETIC HORMONE (Vasopressin)

Antidiuretic hormone (ADH) release is controlled by a complex system that under physiologic conditions modulates the effective osmotic pressure of plasma. Osmoreceptors in the anterolateral hypothalamus and baroreceptors in the cardiac atria respond to changes in osmolality and blood volume and pressure, respectively. Moreover, a large number of putative chemical mediators within the central nervous system, as well as nausea, vomiting, and a variety of drugs and hormones, influences the release of vasopressin. In the text, 3 important conditions involving abnormalities of ADH secretion and action are addressed: (1) central neurogenic diabetes insipidus (below), (2) nephrogenic diabetes insipidus (Chapter 22), and (3) syndrome of inappropriate antidiuretic hormone (SIADH) (Chapter 36).

DIABETES INSIPIDUS

Essentials of Diagnosis

■ Polydipsia and polyuria (4–40 L/d).
■ Urine specific gravity < 1.010; osmolality < 280 mosm/kg.
■ Inability to concentrate urine on fluid restriction.
■ Hyperosmolality of plasma.
■ Subnormal plasma ADH concentration.
■ Vasopressin responsiveness.

General Considerations

Hypofunction of the hypothalamus or posterior pituitary with deficiency of ADH (neurogenic diabetes insipidus) is usually due to loss of neurosecretory neurons in the neurohypophysis. The condition may be idiopathic or may be associated with lesions of the posterior pituitary or hypothalamus (trauma, infections, suprasellar cysts, tumors, reticuloendotheliosis, or some developmental abnormality). Familial ADH deficiency may be transmitted as an autosomal dominant or X-linked recessive trait. When no specific cause of neurogenic diabetes insipidus can be determined, the search for an underlying lesion should be continued for many years.

In nephrogenic diabetes insipidus, the renal tubules fail to respond to physiologic or pharmacologic doses of vasopressin, and no lesion of the pituitary or hypothalamus can be demonstrated; this disease is believed to be X-linked with variable degrees of penetrance, with a milder variant present in carrier females (see Chapter 22).

Clinical Findings

The onset is often sudden, with polyuria, intense thirst, constipation, fever, and dehydration, particularly in infants. A desire for very cold beverages is a common historical notation. The child who awakens at night to urinate is very thirsty and drinks copiously is a typical presentation of this unusual condition. In young infants on an ordinary feeding regimen, polyuria may not be recognized as abnormal and the infant may present with severe dehydration manifested by a high fever, circulatory collapse, and convulsions. In long-standing cases, growth retardation, lack of sexual maturation, and central nervous system damage may occur. The inability to concentrate urine is reflected by serum osmolalities that may be elevated to 300 mosm/kg or greater; urine osmolality remains below this level (usually < 280 mosm/kg). Familial diabetes insipidus may have a more insidious onset and a progressive course.

In cases of ADH deficiency and associated damage to the hypothalamic thirst center or hypothalamic-pituitary centers controlling corticotropin (ACTH) production, the clinical features may be "masked," and polydipsia may not occur. The administration of ACTH or adrenocorticosteroids in the latter condition may "unmask" the ADH deficiency by increasing the glomerular filtration rate and enhancing distal tubule perfusion (site of ADH action).

Differential Diagnosis

Diabetes insipidus may be differentiated from psychogenic polydipsia (compulsive water drinking, potomania) and polyuria by limiting the usual excessive intake of fluid for 2–3 days and then withholding water for 7 hours. The test should be terminated if distress is clinically notable or associated with a weight loss exceeding 3% of body weight. Patients with long-standing psychogenic polydipsia may be unable to concentrate urine initially, and the test may have to be repeated after several days of limited fluid intake monitored carefully. In these patients, dehydration eventually increases urine osmolality well above plasma osmolality. Normal children and those with psychogenic polydipsia respond to dehydration with urinary osmolality above 450 mosm/kg (specific gravity 1.020). With neurogenic and nephrogenic diabetes insipidus, the urine osmolality usually does not increase above 280 mosm/kg (specific gravity 1.010), even after the period of dehydration. The vasopressin (Pitressin) and hypertonic saline tests may be employed to distinguish between the various forms and degrees of diabetes insipidus.

Decreased ability to concentrate urine may also occur with hypokalemia (eg, hyperaldosteronism) and with various forms of hypercalcemia (including hypervitaminosis D) and renal tubular abnormalities (eg, Fanconi's syndrome).

Treatment

A. Medical Treatment: The treatment of choice for partial and total diabetes insipidus is desmopressin acetate (1-deamino-8-D-arginine vasopressin; DDAVP) administered intrasally. The dosage must be adjusted, but the duration of action is generally at least 12 hours and lessens or eliminates the inconvenience of nocturia.

Chlorpropamide has been found to have an antidiuretic action through its potentiation of endogenous ADH effect; hypotension and hypoglycemia are, however, uncommon side effects limiting its use.

B. Other Therapy: X-ray therapy, surgery, antitumor chemotherapy, or a combination of these is, of course, indicated in the treatment of known causative diseases (eg, reticuloendotheliosis).

Prognosis

In absence of central nervous system damage in infancy resulting from severe dehydration and in the absence of associated defects, life expectancy should be normal. Hydronephrosis and hydroureter are not uncommon sequelae of prolonged polyuria; patients should also be observed carefully for urinary tract infection.

Anderson RJ et al: Hyponatremia: A prospective analysis of its epidemiology and the pathogenetic role of vasopressin. *Ann Intern Med* 1985;**102**:164.

THE PINEAL GLAND

The pineal gland is made up of parenchymal cells (pinealocytes) and is often assigned an endocrine function (eg, regulation of somatic growth, sexual maturation, body pigmentation, blood glucose regulation, and a day/night-sensitive neuroendocrine regulatory function). Pineal tumors are rarely associated with sexual precocity in the male. Cases of gonadotropin-secreting choriocarcinomas of the pineal with secondary Leydig cell activation and resultant sexual precocity have been reported.

Preslock JP: The pineal gland: Basic implications and clinical correlations. *Endocr Rev* 1984;**5**:282.

THE THYROID GLAND

FETAL DEVELOPMENT OF THE THYROID

By the seventh week of intrauterine development, the thyroid gland has migrated to its definitive location, and the thyroglossal duct has atrophied. Cell differentiation and function progress over the next 7 weeks, and by the fourteenth week the thyroid is capable of hormone synthesis. At this stage, thyroid-stimulating hormone (TSH) is detectable in the fetal serum and pituitary gland.

Under normal conditions, neither TSH nor thyroid hormones cross the placenta in appreciable amounts, and the fetal pituitary-thyroid axis functions independently of the maternal pituitary-thyroid axis. Antithyroid drugs, including radioactive iodine, freely cross the placenta, and goitrous hypothyroid newborns may be born to hyperthyroid mothers who undergo treatment during pregnancy.

Although maternal TSH does not reach the fetus, pregnant hyperthyroid or previously hyperthyroid mothers may transmit human-specific thyroid stimulator immunoglobulin (HTSI) transplacentally, resulting in thyrotoxic newborns who may develop goiter and exophthalmos. Because HTSI may be present in the serum of "controlled," previously hyperthyroid mothers, the possible transmission of HTSI should be considered in all mothers in whom hyperthyroidism is or has been present.

Physiology

Under the stimulation of pituitary TSH, the thyroid gland traps, concentrates, and organifies iodine, synthesizes and couples mono- and diiodotyrosine, and releases active thyroid hormones into the circulation.

The quantity released is proportionate to the needs of the organism and is maintained by a negative feedback mechanism involving pituitary TSH and ''free'' thyroid hormone (Fig 26–1).

Active hormone produced in excess of physiologic needs is stored within the thyroid follicles as colloid. Upon release into circulation, T_4 and T_3 are bound to thyroid hormone-binding globulin (TBG), albumin, and prealbumin. The binding affinity of TBG for T_4 is approximately 20 times greater than that for T_3. A small percentage (1%) of T_3 and T_4 is not bound but is ''free'' and exists in equilibrium with the ''bound'' form. In the peripheral tissues, T_4 is deiodinated to either T_3 (active) or reverse T_3 (inactive), and the physiologic activity of thyroid hormone depends primarily on the amount of free T_3 presented to the cells. In the fetus, the majority of T_4 is converted to reverse T_3.

Causes of Thyroid Disturbances

Physiologic disturbances of the thyroid gland may be due to the following causes, of which only the first is common:

(1) Decreased thyroid tissue: Hypofunction may result from congenital aplasia or hypoplasia, destruction due to inflammatory disease (thyroiditis), neoplasm, thyroidectomy, or irradiation.

(2) Inborn errors in the synthesis of thyroid hormone: Defects may occur in any of the metabolic steps outlined above, as well as the binding and release of T_4 and T_3 from thyroglobulin.

(3) Iodine deficiency.

(4) Inhibition of thyroidal iodide uptake and concentration by drugs (eg, thiocyanates, perchlorates, lithium nitrates).

(5) Interference with thyroid enzyme activity by antithyroid compounds. Antithyroid compounds include thiourea, thiouracil and its derivatives, cobalt, large doses of iodides, and certain foods such as cabbage, turnips, and soybeans. Iodides also interfere with the release of thyroid hormone.

(6) Disorders of the hypothalamus and pituitary gland that result in impairment of either thyrotropin-releasing hormone (TRH) or thyrotropin secretion.

(7) Defects in the peripheral tissue conversion of T_4 to T_3.

(8) Absence or alteration in tissue receptor(s) for thyroid hormones.

Synthesis, Release, Binding, & Transport of Thyroid Hormone & Its Function

The principal functions of the thyroid gland are to synthesize and store T_4 and T_3 and to release them in response to bodily need. A number of chemical reactions are involved in thyroid hormone formation. The thyroid gland is regulated and stimulated by TSH; HTSI is important only in hyperthyroid states. TSH production may be inhibited by either endogenous or exogenous thyroid hormone. At birth, the T_4 approximates that of the mother. There is a rapid increase of T_4 during the second to fifth days of life in response to a TSH surge resulting from umbilical cord clamping and then a gradual decrease over several weeks or months.

The total T_4 is low in various forms of hypothyroidism and may be reduced in premature infants (particularly those with sepsis or respiratory distress), subacute and chronic thyroiditis, hypopituitarism, nephrosis, cirrhosis, hypoproteinemia, malnutrition, and following therapy with T_3. Prolonged administration of high doses of adrenocorticosteroids, as well as sulfonamides, testosterone, phenytoin, and salicylates, may also produce a decrease in total T_4. TSH and ''free'' T_4 levels remain in the normal range. The total T_3 and T_4 are high in hyperthyroidism and may be elevated in the acute forms of thyroiditis and acute hepatitis; in some types of inborn errors in the synthesis, release, or binding of thyroid hormone; following the administration of estrogens or clofibrate or during pregnancy; and following the administration of various iodine-containing globulins.

TBG is increased in pregnancy, after estrogen therapy (including oral contraceptives), occasionally as a genetic variation, in certain hepatic disorders, following administration of phenothiazines, and occasionally from an unknown cause. TBG is decreased in familial TBG deficiency; following the administration of glucocorticoids, androgens, or an-

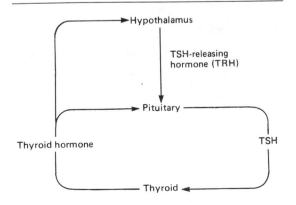

Figure 26–1. Pituitary-thyroid control.

abolic steroids; in nephrotic syndrome with marked hypoproteinemia; in some forms of hepatic disease; in patients receiving phenytoin; and as an idiopathic finding. T_3, which appears to be the active thyroid hormone, acts fairly rapidly and has a shorter duration of action. Receptors for T_3 are present in the cell membrane, mitochondria, and nucleus and within the cytosol; the physiologic action of thyroid hormone is complex.

HYPOTHYROIDISM (Congenital & Acquired Hypothyroidism)

Essentials of Diagnosis

- Growth retardation, diminished physical activity, sluggish circulation, constipation, thick tongue, poor muscle tone, hoarseness, anemia; intellectual retardation if hypothyroid in infancy.
- Delayed dental and skeletal maturation. Rarely, "stippling" of epiphyses.
- Thyroid function studies low (T_4, FT_4 and T_3 resin uptake); TSH levels elevated in primary hypothyroidism.

General Considerations

Thyroid hormone deficiency may be either congenital (with or without the physical features of cretinism) or acquired (juvenile hypothyroidism) and may be due to many causes. In the majority of these cases in childhood, particularly in the presence of a history of goiter, hypothyroidism is the result of chronic lymphocytic thyroiditis (see Thyroiditis, below).

Various types of enzymatic defects have been described (Table 26–3) that result from inborn errors of metabolism. With the exception of the defects associated with congenital nerve deafness (Pendred's syndrome), there are no distinguishing clinical features among the various types. In children who have enzymatic defects, thyroid enlargement may not be present in the newborn period but generally occurs within the first 2 decades of life. Enzymatic defects have a familial autosomal recessive inheritance pattern. Although thyroid function tests (including radioactive iodide uptake studies) may be helpful in diagnosis, final clarification of the defect generally requires chromatographic fractionation of iodinated compounds in the serum, urine, and thyroid tissue.

Several drugs and goitrogens taken during pregnancy (eg, cabbage, soybeans, aminosalicyclic acid, thiourea derivatives, resorcinol, phenylbutazone, cobalt, and iodides in therapeutic doses for asthma— particularly in individuals who have also received adrenocortical steroids) have been reported to cause goiter and, in some instances, hypothyroidism. Because many of these agents cross the placenta freely, they should be used with great caution during pregnancy. If these agents are taken by pregnant women, the goiter and decreased thyroid function that are produced in the newborn are generally transient and seldom a problem.

Clinical Findings

The severity of the findings in cases of thyroid

Table 26–3. Causes of hypothyroidism.

A. Congenital (Cretinism):
1. Aplasia, hypoplasia, or associated with maldescent of thyroid—
   a. Embryonic defect of development.
   b. Autoimmune disease (?).
2. Familial iodine-induced goiter secondary to metabolic inborn errors—
   a. Iodide transport defect (defect 1).
   b. Organification defect (defect 2)—
      (1) Lack of iodine peroxidase.
      (2) Lack of iodine transferase; Pendred's syndrome, associated with congenital nerve deafness.
   c. Coupling defect (defect 3).
   d. Iodotyrosine deiodinase defect (defect 4).
   e. Abnormal iodinated polypeptide (defects 5a and 5b)—
      (1) Resulting from defect in intrathyroidal proteolysis of thyroglobulin.
      (2) Abnormal plasma binding preventing use of T_4 by peripheral cells.
   f. Inability of tissues to convert T_4 to T_3.
3. Maternal ingestion of medications during pregnancy—
   a. Maternal radioiodine.
   b. Goitrogens (propylthiouracil, methimazole).
   c. Iodides.

4. Iodide deficiency (endemic cretinism).
5. Idiopathic.

B. Acquired (Juvenile Hypothyroidism):
1. Thyroidectomy or radioiodine therapy for—
   a. Thyrotoxicosis.
   b. Cancer.
   c. Lingual thyroid.
   d. Isolated midline thyroid.
2. Destruction by x-ray.
3. Thyrotropin deficiency—
   a. Isolated.
   b. Associated with other pituitary tropic hormone deficiencies.
4. TRH deficiency due to hypothalamic injury or disease.
5. Autoimmune disease (lymphocytic thyroiditis).
6. Chronic infections.
7. Medications—
   a. Iodides—
      (1) Prolonged, excessive ingestion.
      (2) Deficiency.
   b. Cobalt.
8. Idiopathic.

deficiency depends on the age at onset and the degree of deficiency of production of thyroid hormone.

A. Symptoms and Signs:

1. Functional changes—Even with congenital absence of the thyroid gland, the first finding may not appear for several days or weeks. Findings include physical and mental sluggishness; pale, gray, cool, or mottled skin; nonpitting myxedema; decreased intestinal activity (constipation); large tongue; poor muscle tone, giving rise to a protuberant abdomen, umbilical hernia, and lumbar lordosis; hypothermia; bradycardia; diminished sweating (variable); decreased pulse pressure; hoarse voice or cry; delayed transient deafness; and a low relaxation component of deep tendon reflexes (best appreciated in the ankles). Nasal obstruction and discharge and persistent jaundice may be present in the neonatal period.

The skin may be dry, thick, scaly, and coarse, with a yellowish tinge due to excessive deposition of carotene. The hair is dry, coarse, and brittle (variable) and may be excessive. Lateral thinning of the eyebrows may occur. The axillary and supraclavicular fat pads may be prominent in infants. Muscular hypertrophy (Kocher-Debré-Sémélaigne syndrome) is an unusual poorly understood presentation.

2. Retardation of growth and development—Findings include shortness of stature; infantile skeletal proportions with relatively short extremities; infantile naso-orbital configuration (bridge of nose flat, broad, and underdeveloped; eyes seem to be widely spaced); delayed osseous development; delayed closure of fontanelles; and retarded dental eruption. Treatment of acquired hypothyroidism may not result in the predicted final adult target height. In hypothyroidism resulting from enzymatic defects, ingestion of goitrogens, or chronic lymphocytic thyroiditis, the thyroid gland may be enlarged. Thyroid enlargement in children is usually symmetric, and the gland is moderately firm without nodularity. In chronic lymphocytic thyroiditis, however, a cobblestone surface frequently is present; size and shape are apparent on inspection in children. Slowing of mental responsiveness and retardation of development of the brain may occur in neonates and infants and in many cases a coincidental congenital malformation of the brain is present also.

3. Alterations in sexual development (usually retardation, sometimes precocity)—Menometrorrhagia may be seen in older girls; galactorrhea has been reported.

B. Laboratory Findings: T_4 and FT_4 are is decreased. Radioiodine uptake is below 10% (normal: 10–50%).* (Both may be normal or elevated in goitrous cretinism and in some cases of thyroiditis.) The binding of T_3 by erythrocytes or resin in vitro (T_3 RU test) is lowered. With primary hypothyroidism, the plasma TSH is elevated. A normocytic anemia is common, but microcytic or macrocytic anemia may occur because of decreased iron, folate, and cobalamin absorbtion. Serum cholesterol and carotene are usually elevated in childhood but may be low or normal in infants. Cessation of therapy in previously treated hypothyroid patients produces a marked rise in serum cholesterol levels in 6–8 weeks. Urinary creatine excretion is decreased, and urinary hydroxyproline is low. Serum alkaline phosphatase is occasionally reduced. Circulating autoantibodies to thyroid constituents may be present. Erythrocyte glucose 6-phosphate dehydrogenase activity is decreased. Plasma growth hormone may be decreased, with subnormal response to insulin-induced hypoglycemia and arginine stimulation.

C. Imaging: Epiphyseal development ("bone age") is delayed. Centers of ossification, especially of the hip, may show multiple small centers or a single, stippled, porous, or fragmented center (epiphyseal dysgenesis). Vertebrae may show anterior beaking. Cardiomegly is common. Coxa vara and coxa plana may occur.

Screening Programs for Neonatal Hypothyroidism

Congenital hypothyroidism may be clinically recognized during the first month of life but may be so mild that it remains unrecognized clinically for months. Every effort should be made to establish the diagnosis of hypothyroidism as early as possible, because untreated hypothyroidism may be associated with irreversible damage to the central nervous system. Adequate treatment initiated prior to the second or third month of life is associated with a favorable prognosis. Mandatory screening programs for newborn infants facilitate prompt diagnosis (within 30–60 days after birth) and therapy of congenital hypothyroidism. Screening programs utilize either T_4 or TSH or both.

Differential Diagnosis

The various causes of primary hypothyroidism due to intrinsic defects of the thyroid gland must be differentiated from pituitary and hypothalamic failure with secondary thyroid insufficiency. TSH measurements before and after TSH administration and, in certain circumstances, radioactive iodide uptake studies before and after exogenous TSH administration (5–10 units daily for 3 days) are useful in differentiation. Practically, TSH and free T_4 levels are the most useful and are usually sufficient in directing treatment or the need for further investigations.

Down's syndrome, chondrodystrophy, generalized gangliosidosis, I-cell disease, Hurler's and Hunter's syndromes, and certain other causes of short stature

---

*The presence of iodides in bread has resulted in a significant decrease in previous values of radioiodine uptake. The normal levels for any particular age group and area should be ascertained.

and coarse features can all be readily distinguished by the clinical manifestations and by appropriate laboratory studies. Although other individual findings of the hypothyroid child may suggest exogenous obesity, congenital heart disease, or some type of anemia as the primary diagnosis, a careful appraisal of the entire clinical and laboratory picture should permit establishment of the proper diagnosis.

Treatment

Levothyroxine is the drug of choice in a dose of 100 $\mu g/m^2$ once daily. In newborns and infants, a dose of 10–12 $\mu g/kg$ is employed; a dose of 0.025 mg (25 μg) of levothyroxine is used initially and subsequently increased to the final dose in 1–2 weeks. Serum T_4 or free T_4 and TSH levels should be used as a guide to adequate therapy.

The hypothyroid patient may be quite responsive to thyroid and may be sensitive to slight excesses of thyroid hormone. After therapy is started, improvement in 7–21 days can be anticipated.

Triiodothyronine may be employed when a more rapid and short-lived effect is desired (eg, in the TSH suppression test) but probably is not as effective for maintenance therapy as levothyroxine. In the treatment of neonatal goiter with or without hypothyroidism resulting from drugs and goitrogens taken by the pregnant woman, temporary use of levothyroxine may be helpful in decreasing the size of the goiter.

Glorieux J et al: Useful parameters to predict the eventual mental outcome of hypothyroid children. *Pediatr Res* 1988;**24**:6.

Rivkees SA, Bode HH, Crawford JD: Long-term growth in juvenile acquired hypothyroidism: The failure to achieve normal adult stature. *N Engl J Med* 1988; **318**:599. [A familial clinical observation is documented in a formal study.]

Roti E, Gnudi A, Braverman LE: The placental transport, synthesis and metabolism of hormones and drugs which affect thyroid function. *Endocr Rev* 1983;**4**:131.

Sklar CA, Oazi R, David R: Juvenile autoimmune thyroiditis: Hormonal status at presentation after long-term follow-up. *Am J Dis Child* 1986;**140**:877.

Tachman ML, Guthrie GP Jr: Hypothyroidism: Diversity of presentation. *Endocr Rev* 1984;**5**:456.

THYROIDITIS

With the exception of chronic lymphocytic thyroiditis (Hashimoto's disease), the forms of thyroiditis listed in Table 26–4 are uncommon in childhood. In contrast, Hashimoto's disease is perhaps the most common endocrine condition in pediatric patients, particularly in adolescent females.

1. ACUTE SUPPURATIVE THYROIDITIS

Acute thyroiditis is rare and generally is thought to result from seeding of oropharyngeal organisms via

Table 26–4. Causes of thyroiditis.

I. Thyroiditis due to infectious agents.
   A. Acute bacterial thyroiditis (acute suppurative thyroiditis).
   B. Subacute viral thyroiditis (nonsuppurative, or De Quervain's, thyroiditis).
   C. Chronic or recurring thyroiditis.
II. Thyroiditis due to autoimmunity (chronic lymphocytic, or Hashimoto's, thyroiditis).
III. Thyroiditis due to physical agents.
   A. Radiation.
   B. Trauma.
IV. Thyroiditis of unknown etiology.
   A. Riedel's thyroiditis.

a patent foramen cecum and thyroglossal duct track. As a result, the most common pathogens are streptococci, pneumococci, staphylococci, and anaerobic agents. The patient is invariably toxic, and the thyroid gland is exquisitely tender. There may be radiation of pain to the ear or chest. There is usually no consistently associated endocrine disturbance. Specific antibiotic therapy should be administered.

2. SUBACUTE NONSUPPURATIVE THYROIDITIS

Subacute thyroiditis (de Quervain's thyroiditis) is rare in the USA. In most cases, the cause is a virus (mumps, influenza, echovirus, coxsackievirus, Epstein-Barr, or adenovirus). Presenting features are similar to those of acute thyroiditis: fever, malaise, sore throat, dysphagia, pain in the thyroid gland that may radiate to the ears, and mild and transient manifestations of hypermetabolism. In contrast to acute thyroiditis, the onset is generally insidious. The thyroid gland is firm, and the enlargement may be confined to one lobe. Radioiodine uptake is usually reduced, but thyroid hormone levels in the blood are normal or elevated.

3. CHRONIC LYMPHOCYTIC THYROIDITIS (Chronic Autoimmune Thyroiditis, Hashimoto's Thyroiditis, Lymphadenoid Goiter)

Essentials of Diagnosis

- Firm, freely movable, nontender, and diffusely enlarged goiter.
- T_4 generally normal but may be elevated or decreased, depending on stage of the disease.

General Considerations

Chronic lymphocytic thyroiditis is being seen with increasing frequency in all age groups and currently is the most common cause of goiter and hypothyroidism in childhood. In children and adolescents, the incidence peaks between the age of 8 and 15 years and occurs most commonly in females (4:1 ratio). The disease is the result of a defect in immunoregulation (probably involving suppressor T cells) that permits a cell-mediated immune response (autoimmunity) to occur in the thyroid gland. The defect is probably inherited and may be associated with other autoimmune disorders (eg, type I diabetes mellitus, Graves' disease, Addison's disease, hypoparathyroidism, pernicious anemia). The defect can be located on histocompatibility loci of chromosome 6, most frequently at HLA-Dw3.

Clinical Findings
A. Symptoms and Signs: The goiter is characteristically firm, freely movable, nontender, ''pebbly'' in consistency, and diffusely enlarged, although it may be asymmetric. In long-standing cases, nodules and, rarely, malignant changes have been described. The onset is usually insidious. Most cases occur without clinical manifestations and are completely painless. Occasionally, a sensation of tracheal compression or fullness, hoarseness, and dysphagia are described by the patient. There are no local signs of inflammation and no evidence of systemic infection.

B. Laboratory Findings: Laboratory findings are variable. Levels of T_4, free T_4 and T_3 resin uptake are usually normal but may be elevated or depressed. TSH levels may be slightly elevated. Thyroid antibodies are usually present, though sometimes at low levels. A variety of abnormalities in radioactive iodide uptake studies have been described; thyroid scans usually show a diffuse or patchy pattern, and cold nodules have been reported. Thyroid scans and uptake studies add little to the diagnosis. Surgical or needle biopsy is diagnostic but seldom indicated.

Treatment
The treatment of choice for autoimmune thyroiditis is thyroid hormone in full therapeutic doses (levothyroxine, 100 µg/m²). Approximately two-thirds of patients will have some decrease in the size of the goiter within 3 months. Hypothyroidism is believed to be a common end result of autoimmune thyroiditis in the second to third decade of life.

4. RIEDEL'S STRUMA (Chronic Fibrous Thyroiditis, Woody Thyroiditis, Invasive Thyroiditis)

Riedel's struma is an extremely rare condition in the USA, particularly in children. The disease is characterized by marked and invasive fibrosis that extends beyond the thyroid gland to involve the trachea, esophagus, blood vessels, nerves, and muscles of the neck, so that the gland becomes fixed to these tissues. Surgery is necessary to ascertain that carcinoma is not the cause and to relieve fibrotic obstruction or constriction of neighboring structures.

Mäenpää J et al: Natural course of juvenile autoimmune thyroiditis. *J Pediatr* 1985;**10**:898.

Reiter EO et al: Childhood thyromegaly: Recent developments. *J Pediatr* 1981;**99**:507.

Weetman AP, McGregor AM: Autoimmune thyroid disease: Developments in our understanding. *Endocr Rev* 1984;**5**:309.

HYPERTHYROIDISM

Essentials of Diagnosis
- Nervousness, irritability, emotional lability, tremor, excessive appetite, weight loss, smooth and warm skin, increased perspiration, and heat intolerance.
- Goiter, exophthalmos, tachycardia, increased pulse pressure.
- Thyroid function studies elevated (eg, T_4, FT_4 T_3, radioiodine uptake). TSH level suppressed.

General Considerations
The cause of hyperthyroidism has not been precisely determined; abnormalities in the immune system are operative in the pathophysiology. The association of hyperthyroidism and certain additional diseases that have an autoimmune basis and a familial pattern with a predilection for females supports the supposition of a heritable and autoimmune basis. In addition, psychic trauma, psychologic maladjustments, disturbances in pituitary function, and infectious diseases may play a part in triggering the thyrotoxic state. Human-specific thyroid stimulator immunoglobulin (HTSI), an IgG antibody to thyroid receptors that stimulates thyroid hormone production, has been identified. Since HTSI is an IgG, it may cross the placenta from a thyrotoxic mother and affect the fetus and neonate. Transient congenital hyperthyroidism may occur in infants of thyrotoxic mothers. Hyperthyroidism may be associated with chronic thyroiditis, tumors of the thyroid, other tumors producing thyrotropinlike substances, and exogenous thyroid hormone excess.

Clinical Findings
A. Symptoms and Signs: With the exception of neonatal hypothyroidism (sex ratio 1:1), hyperthyroidism is 5 times as common in females as in males. The disease is most likely to appear in childhood at age 12–14 years: only 20% of cases present before 10 years of age. The course of hyperthyroidism tends to be cyclic, with spontaneous remissions and exacerbations. A deterioration in school performance is a common presenting feature. Findings include weakness, dyspnea, dysphagia emotional instability, ''nervousness'', marked variability

in mood, personality disturbances, tremors and movements that may simulate chorea. The skin is warm and moist, the face is flushed. Palpitation, tachycardia, systolic hypertension with increased pulse pressure, are common. Proptosis and exophthalmos are common in hyperthyroid children. Goiter is present in more than 90% of cases and is characteristically diffuse and usually firm. A bruit and thrill may be present. Variable degrees of accelerated growth and development occur, and loss of weight is common despite polyphagia. (An occasional adolescent may gain weight.) Amenorrhea may occur in adolescent girls. In neonatal hyperthyroidism, hepatosplenomegaly and thrombo cytopenia with antiplatelet antibodies is common.

B. Laboratory Findings: The T_4, T_3 uptake, and free T_4 are elevated, except in rare cases in which only the blood T_3 level is elevated ("T_3 thyrotoxicosis"). Radioiodine uptake is above 35–40% at 24 hours and suppressed less than 40% after administration of T_3 (25 μg 3–4 times daily for 7 days). The basal metabolic rate is elevated, but testing for this is frequently unreliable and is seldom used. Serum cholesterol is low; glycosuria may occur. Agglutinating antibodies of thyroglobulin are found in most patients. Circulating TSH is usually depressed, and HTSI is often present in plasma. Erythrocyte glucose 6-phosphate dehydrogenase activity, urinary hydroxyproline and creatine are increased.

C. Imaging: Skeletal maturation assessed radiographically is advanced in younger children. In newborns, accelerated bony maturation may be associated with subsequent premature closure of the cranial sutures.

Differential Diagnosis

Although the well-established case of hyperthyroidism seldom presents a problem in diagnosis, the findings in the early stages of the disease may be confused with chorea or, more commonly, with euthyroid goiter. Typically, the patient is an adolescent with a decrease in school performance, nervousness, emotional lability, and increased perspiration. Careful and sometimes repeated clinical and laboratory evaluation may be required before a definitive diagnosis is established. Various disease states associated with hypermetabolism (severe anemia, leukemia, chronic infections, pheochromocytoma, as well as muscle-wasting disease) may occasionally be confused with hyperthyroidism, but differentiation is readily made by the appropriate laboratory studies.

Treatment

The course of hyperthyroidism may exhibit fluctuations of improvement and remission. In some mild cases, therapy may not be required.

Both surgical and medical methods are available for treating the manifestations of hyperthyroidism.

A. General Measures: Bed rest is advisable only in severe cases, in preparation for surgery, or at the beginning of a medical regimen. The diet should be high in calories, carbohydrates, and vitamins (particularly vitamin B_1).

B. Medical Treatment: With medical treatment, clinical response may be noted in 2–3 weeks, and adequate control may be achieved in 2–3 months. The thyroid frequently increases in size after initiation of treatment but usually decreases in size within several months.

1. Propranolol—This β-adrenergic blocking agent may be useful in controlling symptoms of nervous instability and tachycardia. In mild cases, propranolol without other antithyroid treatment may be adequate. Propranolol may also be helpful in controlling life-threatening cardiac complications that may occur in thyroid storm (severe thyrotoxicosis, fever, and altered consciousness). In large doses, propranolol decreases the peripheral conversion of T_4 to T_3.

2. Propylthiouracil—This drug interferes with the intrathyroidal hormonogenesis and in large doses the peripheral conversion of T_4 to T_3. The correct dose must always be individually assessed. Propylthiouracil is frequently used in the initial treatment of children with hyperthyroidism. Short-term therapy is occasionally successful, but treatment usually must be continued for at least 2–3 years with the smallest drug dosage that will produce a euthyroid state. If T_4 levels rise rapidly with reduction in drug dosage after 18–24 months of therapy, continued or alternative therapy will be necessary; relapses occur in 10–30% of cases, and severe cases may not respond. The safety of prolonged treatment has not been evaluated.

a. Initial dosage—Give 75–300 mg/d in 3–4 divided doses 6–8 hours apart until tests of thyroid function are normal and all signs and symptoms have subsided. Larger doses are frequently necessary.

b. Maintenance—Give 50–100 mg/d in 2–3 divided doses. Some authors recommend continuing the drug at higher levels until the euthyroid state is approached or reached and then, as the TSH level rises, adding thyroid hormone. If goiter develops or persists after 2–3 months with propylthiouracil therapy, T_4 and TSH levels should be obtained to determine whether the patient is becoming hypothyroid; thyroid hormone is added when indicated.

c. Toxicity—Granulocytopenia, fever, rash, and arthralgia may occur. The drug must be discontinued, and antibiotics and a short course of one of the adrenocorticosteroids should be prescribed if indicated.

2. Methimazole—This drug may be used in one-fifteenth to one-tenth the dosage of propylthiouracil and may be effective with a bid dosage schedule. However, toxic reactions may be more common with methimazole than with propylthiouracil.

3. Iodide—Medical treatment with continuous iodide administration alone usually produces a rapid but brief response. Because the efficacy of iodide is short-lived, it is generally recommended only for acute management. A progressive increase in dosage is often required for satisfactory control, and toxic reactions to iodide are not uncommon.

C. Radiation Therapy: Radioactive iodide (^{131}I) is currently being used as alternative therapy for children and adolescents. Reports do not support the fear of an increased incidence of thyroid cancer, particularly when an ablative dose of ^{131}I is employed. Therapy with thyroid hormone is necessary after thyroid ablation.

D. Surgical Measures: Subtotal thyroidectomy is considered by many to be the treatment of choice, especially when a close follow-up of the patient is difficult or impossible. In childhood, surgery should be employed in patients when medical treatment is impossible or has been unsuccessful. The patient should be prepared first with bed rest, diet, and propranolol (as above) and with iodide and propylthiouracil as follows: Propylthiouracil (as above) should be given for 2–4 weeks. Iodide (as saturated solution of potassium iodide) is added 10–21 days before surgery is scheduled. Iodides act by blocking the effect of TSH on the thyroid, with a resultant decrease in iodine trapping and reduction of vascularity, and by inhibiting the release of hormone, thus reducing the possibility of thyroid storm. Give 1–10 drops daily for 10–21 days. Continue the drug for 1 week after surgery.

E. Course & Prognosis: Improvement may occur without therapy in as many as one-third of cases, but partial remissions and exacerbations may continue for several years. With medical treatment alone, prolonged remissions may be expected in one-half to two-thirds of cases. Surgical therapy yields similar results. Postoperative hypothyroidism is not uncommon, and hypoparathyroidism and other complications may occur. Because of the comparatively high incidence of carcinoma in nodular goiters of childhood, such glands should be removed routinely once the thyrotoxicosis is in remission. Progressive exophthalmos following surgery is uncommon in childhood.

F. Management of Congenital (Transient) Hyperthyroidism: Congenital hyperthyroidism has a significant death rate in the neonatal period, but the eventual prognosis in surviving infants is excellent. Temporary treatment of congenital hyperthyroidism may be necessary, in which case iodides appear to be the drug of choice. Reserpine or propranolol may be necessary to control cardiac arrthymias. Transection of an enlarged thyroid isthmus may be of value if respiratory distress due to tracheal compression is present.

Becker DV: Choice of therapy for Graves' hyperthyroidism. (Editorial.) *N Engl J Med* 1984;**311**:464.

Buckingham BA et al: Hyperthyroidism in children: A reevaluation of treatment. *Am J Dis Child* 1981;**135**:112.

Burros GN: Hyperthyroidism During Pregnancy. *N Engl J Med* 1978;**298**:150.

Collen RJ et al: Remission rates of children and adolescents with thyrotoxicosis treated with antithyroid drugs. *Pediatrics* 1980;**65**:550.

Fisher DA, Klein AH: Thyroid development and disorders of thyroid function in the newborn. *N Engl J Med* 1981; **304**:702.

Hamburger JI: Management of hyperthyroidism in children and adolescents. *J Clin Endocrinol Metab* 1985; **60**:1019.

CARCINOMA OF THE THYROID

Carcinoma of the thyroid is uncommon in childhood. The presentation is usually asymptomatic, asymmetric thyroid enlargement. Neck discomfort, dysphagia, voice changes, and respiratory difficulty are unusual but may be noted. Fifty percent of children have metastatic disease at the time of presentation, usually to regional lymph nodes. Pulmonary metastasis occurs in 5% of cases.

Thyroid function tests are normal. Thyroid carcinoma may elaborate thyroglobulin; if present, it is a useful tumor marker. A technetium or iodine scan of the thyroid shows a "cold" nodule and is the most definitive diagnostic test. Pulmonary metastases should be excluded by a CT scan of the chest.

Papillary carcinoma is the most common form in childhood, and the prognosis with treatment is relatively good, with a survival rate greater than 80% after 10–20 years. The treatment of choice is surgical extirpation of the entire gland and removal of all involved lymph nodes. Radical neck dissection is usually not indicated. If metastatic disease is not identified at surgery, replacement thyroid hormone is generally the only further therapy required. Follow-up thyroid scans every 2–5 years are recommended.

Other, less common malignant tumors of the thyroid include follicular, medullary, and undifferentiated carcinomas, lymphomas, and sarcomas. Medullary carcinoma of the thyroid may be familial (autosomal dominant), usually occurs as a component of type II multiple endocrine neoplasia. Thus this condition may be associated with excessive elaboration of gastrin and calcitonin, with pheochromocytoma, parathyroid hyperplasia, "marfanoid habitus," and mucosal neuromas. The treatment and prognosis depend upon the cell type present but the outcome is generally less favorable.

Panza N et al:[131] I total body scan and serum thyroglobulin assay in the follow-up of surgically treated patients affected by differentiated thyroid carcinoma. *J Nucl Med Allied Sci* 1984;**28**:9.

Schmike RN: Genetic aspects of multiple endocrine neoplasia. *Annu Rev Med* 1984;**35**:25.

DISORDERS OF CALCIUM HOMEOSTASIS

Parathyroid hormone (PTH) and vitamin D are the principal hormonal factors in the human that maintain calcium homeostasis. These agents exert their action primarily in bone, small intestine, and kidney. The integrated action of PTH and vitamin D maintains the serum calcium level within a narrow normal range and contributes to normal bone mineralization. Deficiencies and excesses of these agents—as well as abnormalities in their receptors or in the metabolic transformation of vitamin D—lead to the clinical disturbances described below and shown in Tables 26–5 and 26–6. Less important calciotropic factors (eg, calcitonin, magnesium, and phosphorus) also influence calcium homeostasis.

HYPOPARATHYROIDISM

Essentials of Diagnosis

- Tetany with numbness, tingling, cramps, spontaneous muscle contractures, carpopedal spasm, positive Trousseau and Chvostek signs, loss of consciousness, convulsions.
- Diarrhea, photophobia, prolongation of electrical systole (QT interval) and laryngospasm.
- Candidal infections, defective nails and teeth, cataracts, and calcific bodies in the subcutaneous tissues and basal ganglia.
- Serum and urine calcium normal or low; serum phosphorus high; urine phosphorus low; alkaline phosphatase normal or low; azotemia absent. Inappropriately low parathyroid hormone:ionized calcium ratio.

General Considerations

Bone and kidney are the target organs of PTH, and most of the hormonal effects are mediated by interaction with a plasma membrane-bound receptor and activation of the adenylate cyclase complex—a complex consisting of at least 3 distinct proteins. Manifestations of PTH deficiency (Table 26–5) result either from an absolute deficiency in the hormone or from "resistant states" related to abnormalities of the receptor complex of the PTH molecule. Hypoparathyroidism may be idiopathic result from an autoimmune phenomenon or from parathyroidectomy. Hypoparathyroidism may develop from thyroidectomy, with either acute or insidious onset, and may be transient or permanent. Parathyroid deficiency has been reported following irradiation of the neck or the administration of therapeutic doses of radioactive iodine for carcinoma of the thyroid. Two types of transient hypoparathyroidism may be present in the newborn, both of which are due to a relative deficiency of PTH or hormone action. An early form occurs within the first 2 weeks of life in newborns with a history of birth asphyxia or those born to mothers with diabetes mellitus or hyperparathyroidism. Hypomagnesemia may also be seen in the early form and augments the severity of hypocalcemia. The more common later form occurs almost exclusively in infants fed a milk formula with a high phosphate:calcium ratio. In this group, episodes of tetany are often precipitated by febrile illnesses.

Autoimmune hypoparathyroidism with demonstrable antibodies to parathyroid tissue may be associated with candidal infection, Addison's disease, diabetes mellitus, pernicious anemia, alopecia, thyroiditis, hypogonadism, steatorrhea and malabsorption. This form of hypoparathyroidism is often familial (autosomal recessive) and is associated with certain human leukocyte antigen (HLA) types. Infections resulting from lack of immune reaction to *Candida* (in spite of normal generalized T cell function) may lead to severe intractable cutaneous and gastrointestinal candidiasis. Because of the frequent association of adrenocortical insufficiency with parathyroid insufficiency, adrenocortical function should be tested repeatedly.

Congenital absence of the parathyroids may occur in association with congenital absence of the thymus (with resultant thymic-dependent immunologic deficiency) and cardiovascular (DiGeorge syndrome), cerebral, and ocular defects.

Clinical Findings

A. Symptoms and Signs: Prolonged hypocalcemia causes tetany (see below), photophobia, blepharospasm, and diarrhea. It may be associated with chronic conjunctivitis, cataracts, numbness of the extremities, poor dentition, skin rashes, alopecia, ectodermal dysplasias, candidal infections, "idiopathic" epilepsy, or symmetric punctate calcifications of basal ganglia. In early infancy, respiratory distress may be the presenting finding.

Tetany (hyperexcitability of the central and peripheral nervous system) is manifested by numbness, cramps, and twitchings of the extremities; carpopedal spasm and laryngospasm; a positive Chvostek sign (tapping of the face in front of the ear produces spasm of the facial muscles); a positive Trousseau sign (compression of the upper arm with a blood pressure cuff inflated to a pressure above systole for 2–4 minutes produces carpopedal spasm); unexplained bizarre behavior; irritability; loss of consciousness; convulsions; and retarded physical and mental development. Headache, vomiting, diarrhea, photophobia, increased intracranial pressure, papilledema, and pseudopapilledema may occur.

B. Laboratory Findings: (Table 26–5) Serum calcium is decreased, serum phosphorus increased, and serum alkaline phosphatase is usually low nor-

Table 26–5. Parathyroid deficiency states.

Disease or Condition	Synonym	Inheritance Pattern	Major Clinical Features	Serum Concentration Ca²⁺	P	Alk Ptase	PTH	Urinary Excretion Basal Conditions Ca²⁺	P	Response to Parathyroid Hormone[3] P	Cyclic AMP
"Idiopathic" (spontaneous), surgical, or "autoimmune" hypoparathyroidism	Autoimmune polyendocrinopathy. Thyroiditis and hypoparathyroidism (Schmidt's syndrome). Absence of parathyroid glands and thymic aplasia (DiGeorge's syndrome)	X-linked or autosomal recessive in autoimmune type	Tetany, seizures, photophobia, diarrhea, positive Chvostek and Trousseau signs, candidiasis. In autoimmune type, other autoimmune diseases (eg, adrenal insufficiency, thyroiditis, pernicious anemia, diabetes mellitus).	↓ (N)	↑	↓ (N)	↓	↓ (N)	↓	N	N
Pseudohypoparathyroidism and pseudopseudohypoparathyroidism	Albright's syndrome	X-linked dominant	Brachymetacarpal and metatarsal short stature; mental subnormality; ectopic calcification of lenses, basal ganglia, and subcutaneous tissue.	↓ (N)	↑ (N)	↓ ↑ (N)	↑	↓ (N)	↓	↓	↓
Pseudohypoparathyroidism type II	PTH unresponsiveness	Unknown	Seizures. Phenotype normal.	↓	↑		↑	↓	↓	↓	N
Pseudohypohyperparathyroidism with osteitis fibrosa[1]	Renal resistance to parathyroid hormone with osteitis fibrosa	Probably familial	Clinical features of hypocalcemia. Phenotype normal.	↓	↑	↑	↑	N (↑)	↓ (N)	↓	↓
Pseudoidiopathic hypoparathyroidism[2]			Clinical features of hypoparathyroidism. Phenotype normal.	↓	↑		↑↑	↓	↑	N	N

[1]The opposite (ie, skeletal unresponsiveness to PTH with normal renal responsiveness) has been described.
[2]Structural anomaly of PTH molecule has been proposed.
[3]Parathyroid hormone is not commercially available for testing.

Table 26–6. Rickets and disorders of calcium metabolism.[1]

Disease or Condition	Synonym	Inheritance Pattern	Clinical Features	Serum Concentration				Urinary Excretion		Treatment
				Ca²⁺	P	Alk Ptase	PTH	Ca²⁺	P	
Hypoparathyroid states	See Table 26–5.									Vitamin D and calcium
Transient tetany of the newborn			Tetany, focal seizures. More common in prematures and infants of diabetic mothers. Rarely described in association with maternal hyperparathyroidism.	↓	↓(N)	↓(N)	↓(N)	↓(N)	↑(N)	Diet high in calcium, low in phosphate. Vitamin D may be necessary.
Malabsorption syndrome	Disease entities associated with malabsorption include cystic fibrosis, celiac disease, sprue, Shwachman syndrome; hypoplasia of cartilage and hair.	Generally familial with mode of inheritance related to specific disease	Steatorrhea, failure to thrive. Some forms associated with neutropenia, skeletal anomalies, immunologic deficiencies, and abnormalities of cartilage and hair.	↓(N)	(N)↓	↑(N)	↑(N)	↓	N(↑↓)	Vitamin D, calcium, and magnesium (hypomagnesemic states)
Chronic renal insufficiency			Growth failure, undernutrition, skeletal changes.	↓(N)	↑	↑(N)	↑	↓(N)	↓	Diet high in calcium, low in phosphorus; vitamin D
Vitamin D-deficient rickets	Infantile rickets		Rickets.	↓(N)	↓	↑	↑	↑	↑	Vitamin D and calcium
Familial hypophosphatemic vitamin D-resistant rickets[2]	(1) Hereditary vitamin D-resistant rickets (2) Phosphate diabetes (3) X-linked hypophosphatemia	X-linked dominant (occasionally autosomal dominant or sporadic)	Skeletal deformities, growth retardation.	N(↓)	↓	N	N(↑)	N	↑	Oral phosphate and vitamin D
Hereditary vitamin D-refractory rickets[3] Type I Type II	(1) Hypophosphatemic vitamin D-refractory rickets (2) Pseudo-vitamin D-deficiency rickets	Autosomal recessive	Severe rachitic bone changes; generalized aminoaciduria.	↓	↓(N)	↑	↑	↓	↑	Vitamin D (calciferol) in large doses or approximately physiologic doses of 1,25-dihydroxycholecalciferol

[1]Normal tubular reabsorption of phosphate (TRP) is 83–98%; the lower values are associated with higher serum levels of phosphorus. In hypoparathroidism, TRP varies from 40 to 70%. Low values for TRP are also found in some forms of inherited renal tubular disease, eg, vitamin D-resistant rickets.

[2]A variety of diseases (cystinosis, galactosemia, tyrosinosis, Wilson's disease, hereditary fructose intolerance) are associated with renal tubular defects and should be considered in the differential diagnosis.

[3]Type I has been shown to be the result of defective renal 1α-hydroxylation of 25-hydroxycholecalciferol; type II is due to tissue unresponsiveness to normal levels of 1,25-dihydroxycholecalciferol; in this type, the vitamin D receptor complex fails to bind to DNA.

mal. Urinary excretion of calcium and phosphorus is decreased. Renal clearance of phosphorus is decreased, and the maximum tubular reabsorption of phosphate falls by 12–30%. PTH levels are inappropriately reduced for the ionized calcium concentration.

C. Imaging: Soft tissue and basal ganglia calcification may occur in idiopathic hypoparathyroidism but is less common than in pseudohypoparathyroidism.

Differential Diagnosis

The differential diagnosis of hypoparathyroid states is outlined in Table 26–5. Convulsions suggest epilepsy and other chronic disorders of the central nervous system. The group of findings referable to the central nervous system (headache, vomiting, increased intracranial pressure, and convulsions) may make differentiation from brain tumor difficult.

Treatment

The objective of treatment is to maintain the serum calcium and phosphate at an approximately normal level.

A. Acute or Severe Tetany: Correct hypocalcemia immediately with calcium intravenously and orally. Thiazide diuretics (eg, chlorthalidone) are also useful in acute management.

Calcium lactate or carbonate is the treatment of choice for prolonged oral therapy for both the raising of calcium and lowering of phosphate in the serum.

B. Maintenance Management of Hypoparathyroidism and Chronic Hypocalcemia:

1. Drugs—Give ergocalciferol, dihydrotachysterol, or calcitriol. Ergocalciferol may not reach its peak effect for 3–7 days, but activity of all vitamin D preparations persists for weeks or months. Careful control of dosage with frequent determinations of serum and urine calcium and of the ability to concentrate urine is essential to avoid hypercalcemia and the resultant nephrocalcinosis and potential renal damage.

2. Diet—Give a low-phosphate, high-calcium diet, with added calcium lactate or carbonate. The dose is 300–1200 mg of calcium lactate or carbonate 3–4 times daily with meals. Because calcium is efficiently absorbed, large doses of vitamin D are rarely necessary.

Course & Prognosis

Abnormal mineral concentrations in extracellular fluid are easily corrected and most signs and symptoms can be ameliorated with conventional dietary and drug treatments. Central nervous system manifestations are usually reversible, and the prognosis for intellectual development is excellent. A major goal of therapy is avoidance of hypercalcemia and resultant renal damage; therefore, high doses of long-acting vitamin D preparations must be carefully monitored. Difficult therapeutic problems arise when manifestations are referable to other autoimmune diseases or when the immune defect gives rise to overgrowth of *Candida.*

Canalis E: The hormonal and local regulation of bone formation. *Endocr Rev* 1983;**4**:62.

Norman AW, Roth J, Orci L: The vitamin D endocrine system: Steroid metabolism, hormone receptors, and biological response (calcium binding proteins). *Endocr Rev* 1982;**3**:331.

PSEUDOHYPOPARATHYROIDISM (Albright's Syndrome & Pseudopseudohypoparathyroidism)

Pseudohypoparathyroidism is a familial hereditary X-linked disease with a female to male ratio of approximately 2:1. It is characterized by the adequacy of parathyroid hormone but a failure of response of the end-organ (the renal tubule, bone, or both) to the hormone. The failure of response is the result of an abnormality in the adenylate cyclase complex, a complex consisting of at least 3 distinct proteins; specifically, there is a quantitative diminution in one of these units (the G unit), which is also low in other tissues. Hence, resistance to other hormones acting through the adenylate cyclase complex has been described in pseudohypoparathyroidism.

Patients with pseudohypoparathyroidism may have the same signs and symptoms seen in hypocalcemia and the same chemical findings seen in idiopathic hypoparathyroidism (Table 26–5). In addition, these patients have round, full faces; irregularly shortened hands (with the index and third metatarsal often longer than the first, fourth, and fifth metatarsals); a short, thickset body; delayed and defective dentition; and mental retardation. The hair is dry and coarse, and nails and skin are thickened. Candidiasis has not been reported. X-ray films may show thickness of the long bones with limitation of growth at the metaphyseal ends. There may be chondrodysplastic changes in the bones of the hands, demineralization of the bones, thickening of the cortices, and exostoses. Ectopic calcification of the basal ganglia and subcutaneous tissues may occur with or without abnormal serum calcium levels. Corneal and lenticular opacities may be present.

Treatment is the same as that for hypoparathyroidism.

Similar phenotypic findings may be found in **pseudopseudohypoparathyroidism,** a variant of pseudohypoparathyroidism in which the blood chemistry findings are normal. No treatment is necessary.

In both pseudo- and pseudopseudohypoparathyroidism, the parathyroid glands are hyperplastic, serum levels of PTH are elevated, and the kidneys are relatively unresponsive to PTH. Elevated calcitonin concentration is the consequence rather than the cause of hypocalcemia.

HYPERPARATHYROIDISM & HYPERCALCEMIC STATES

Essentials of Diagnosis

- Elevated blood levels of PTH.
- Serum (and urine) ionized calcium elevated; urine phosphate high with low or normal serum phosphate; alkaline phosphatase normal or elevated.
- Abdominal pain, polyuria, polydipsia, hypertension, nephrocalcinosis, renal stones, intractable peptic ulcer, constipation, uremia, and pancreatitis.
- Bone pain and, rarely, pathologic fractures. X-ray film shows subperiosteal resorption, loss of the lamina dura of the teeth, renal parenchymal calcification or stones, and bone cysts or "brown tumors."
- Unusual (often bizarre) behavior and mood swings.

General Considerations

Hyperparathyroidism is rare in childhood and may be primary or secondary (Table 26–7). The most common cause of primary hyperparathyroidism is adenoma of the gland. Diffuse parathyroid hyperplasia or multiple adenoma has also been described in families. The most common causes of the secondary form are chronic renal disease (glomerulonephritis, pyelonephritis), congenital anomalies of the genitourinary tract rickets. Rarely, hyperparathyroidism may be found in osteogenesis imperfecta and cancers with bony metastases. Familial hyperparathyroidism

Table 26–7. Hypercalcemic states.

I. Primary hyperparathyroidism:
  A. Hyperplasia.
  B. Adenoma.
  C. Familial, including multiple endocrine neoplasia types I and II.
  D. Ectopic parathyroid hormone secretion.
II. Hypercalcemic states other than primary hyperparathyroidism associated with increased intestinal or renal absorption of calcium:
  A. Hypervitaminosis D (including idiopathic hypercalcemia of infancy).
  B. Familial hypercalciuric hypercalcemia.
  C. Lithium therapy.
  D. Sarcoidosis.
  E. Phosphate depletion.
  F. Aluminum intoxication.
III. Hypercalcemic states other than hyperparathyroidism associated with increased immobilization of bone mineral: A. Hyperthyroidism.
  B. Immobilization.
  C. Thiazides.
  D. Vitamin A intoxication.
  E. Malignant neoplasims.
    1. Ectopic parathyroid hormone secretion:
    2. Prostaglandin-secreting tumor and perhaps prostaglandin release from subcutaneous fat necrosis.
    3. Tumors metastatic to bone.
    4. Myeloma.

---

may be an isolated disease or may be associated with other endocrine adenomas of type I and, less commonly, type II multiple endocrine neoplasia (MEN) syndromes.

Clinical Findings

A. Symptoms and Signs:

1. Due to hypercalcemia—Findings include hypotonicity and weakness of muscles; apathy, mood swings, and bizarre behavior; nausea, vomiting, abdominal pain, constipation, and loss of weight; hyperextensibility of joints; and hypertension, cardiac irregularities, bradycardia, and shortening of the QT interval. Calcium deposits may occur in the cornea or conjunctiva ("band keratopathy"). Detection of this important finding may require slit lamp examination of the eye. Coma occurs rarely. Intractable peptic ulcer and pancreatitis occur in adults and rarely in children.

2. Due to increased calcium and phosphorus excretion—Findings include loss of renal concentrating ability, polyuria, polydipsia, precipitation of calcium phosphate in the renal parenchyma or as urinary calculi, and progressive renal damage.

3. Related to changes in the skeleton—There may be bone pain, osteitis fibrosa, subperiosteal absorption of phalanges, absence of lamina dura around the teeth, spontaneous fractures, and a "moth-eaten" appearance of the skull.

B. Imaging: Bone changes may be subtle in children, even when radiography shows nephrocalcinosis. When bone changes occur, the distal clavicle and middle phalanges are initially affected. Later, there is a generalized demineralization with a predilection for subperiosteal cortical bone.

Treatment

Treatment consists of complete removal of the tumor or subtotal removal of hyperplastic parathyroid glands. Preoperatively, intake of dietary calcium should be restricted and hypercalcemia controlled with normal saline infusion and nonthiazide diuretics. Postoperatively, observe carefully for evidence of hypocalcemic tetany; this may occur with total serum calcium within normal limits if a precipitous drop in calcium has occurred. The diet should be high in calcium and vitamin D.

Treatment of secondary hyperparathyroidism is directed at the underlying disease. Diminution in the absorption of phosphate with aluminum hydroxide orally is helpful. The hypocalcemia of severe renal disease (creatinine clearance < 15 mL/min) results from impaired renal activation of vitamin D. Treatment with calcitriol has been useful in this disorder.

Course & Prognosis

The prognosis following removal of a single adenoma is excellent. The prognosis following subtotal parathyroidectomy and removal of multiple adenomas and diffuse hyperplasia or removal of an adenoma is usually good and depends on correction of the underlying defect. In patients with multiple sites of parathyroid adenoma or hyperplasia, the possibility of a familial disease (eg, multiple endocrine neoplasia) must be considered. Because this may be either a sporadic or autosomal dominant condition, other family members may be at risk, and genetic counseling is indicated.

Scholz DA et al: Primary hyperparathyroidism with multiple parathyroid gland enlargement: Review of 53 cases. *Mayo Clin Proc* 1978;**53**:792.

HYPERVITAMINOSIS D

Exposure to sunlight and ingestion of vitamin D in a normal diet do not result in hypervitaminosis D and hypercalcemia, except possibly in sarcoidosis. Vitamin D intoxication is the result of ingestion of excessive amounts of vitamin D, some forms of which may be stored for months in adipose tissue.

Signs and symptoms of vitamin D-induced hypercalcemia are the same as those in other hypercalcemic states and include abdominal, renal, central nervous system, and bone findings. Renal insufficiency may be irreversible and is the result of renovascular effects of hypercalcemia and precipitation of calcium phosphate in the renal interstitial tissue. Ectopic calcification can occur in many other tissues, including the cornea and the gastric mucosa.

Treatment depends on the stage of hypercalcemic toxicity. Because of adipose tissue storage of vitamin D, several months of treatment may be necessary. Dietary intake of foods fortified with vitamin D (eg, milk) and calcium should be reduced or eliminated, if possible. Hypercalcemia can be treated with intravenous fluids and nonthiazide diuretics. Adrenocorticosteroids, salmon calcitonin, and the antineoplastic agent plicamycin have also been employed with some success.

The central nervous system manifestations may be dramatic, and deaths have occurred during acute crises. Chronic brain damage in young infants has been reported. The insidious occult nature of the renal insult may result in renal insufficiency and failure by the time diagnosis is established.

IDIOPATHIC HYPERCALCEMIA OF INFANCY

Idiopathic hypercalcemia (Williams syndrome) is an uncommon disorder characterized in its severe form by peculiar (''elfin'') facies (receding mandible, depressed bridge of nose, relatively large mouth, prominent eyes, occasional esotropia, and hypertelorism), failure to thrive, mental and motor retardation, irritability, purposeless movements, constipation, hypotonia, polyuria, polydipsia, hyper-

tension, and cardiac defects (ie, supravavular aortic stenosis or peripheral pulmonic stenosis). Generalized osteosclerosis is common, and there may be premature craniosynostosis and nephrocalcinosis with evidence of urinary tract disease. In addition to the hypercalcemia, there may be hypophosphatemia, hypercholesterolemia, azotemia, and elevation of serum carotene and vitamin A.

Clinical manifestations may not appear for several months. Serum concentration of 1,25-dihyroxycholecalciferol is frequently elevated. This disease may be due to the increased intake of vitamin D during pregnancy, a defect in the metabolism of or responsiveness to vitamin D, abnormal sterol synthesis, or some as yet undefined mechanism.

Treatment consists of rigid restriction of dietary calcium and vitamin D and, in severe, unresponsive conditions, moderate doses of glucocorticoids.

IMMOBILIZATION HYPERCALCEMIA

Abrupt immobilization of a rapidly growing adolescent following an injury may lead to a rapid decrease in bone deposition with continued bone resorption, calcium mobilization, and hypercalcemia. For reasons that are not completely understood, immobilization may be associated with elevated parathyroid hormone levels in spite of elevated levels of ionized calcium.

HYPOPHOSPHATASIA

Hypophosphatasia is an uncommon inherited (autosomal recessive) condition characterized by a specific deficiency of alkaline phosphatase activity in serum, bone, and tissues. Radiographically, there is inadequate mineralization of epiphyseal cartilage and osteoid, with localized areas of radiolucency. The disease is radiographically and histologically similar to rickets, but the lesions are not more severe in sites of rapid growth. The earlier the age at onset, the more severe the condition. Failure to thrive, feeding problems, dwarfing, hyperpyrexia, delayed dentition, or premature loss of teeth, widening of the sutures, bulging fontanelles, convulsions, bony deformities indistinguishable from rickets, hyperpigmentation, conjunctival calcification, band keratopathy, and renal lesions have been reported in some cases. Premature closure of cranial sutures may occur. Calcium and phosphate concentrations in the extracellular fluid are usually normal; calcium levels, however, may be elevated. In the latter case, signs and symptoms may be similar to those of idiopathic hypercalcemia; late features include osteoporosis, osteopenia, and pseudofractures. The plasma and urine of patients and heterozygote carriers contain phosphoethanolamine in excessive amounts. In some cases, marked metaphyseal irregularities may occur. A condition known as

pseudohypophosphatasia has been described in which the clinical features of hypophosphatasia are seen in association with normal levels of alkaline phosphatase.

No specific treatment is available, but adrenocorticosteroids may be of value. The mortality rate is high in infancy. Adults are usually asymptomatic.

THE GONADS (Ovaries & Testes)

DEVELOPMENT & PHYSIOLOGY

The gonads develop from a bipotential anlage in the genital ridge of the coelomic cavity. The primordial germ cells, which will become the oocytes and spermatocytes, arise in the yolk sac and migrate to the genital ridge by the fourth week after conception, when the gonad is identifiable. Between the fourth and eighth weeks of gestation, differentiation into an ovary or testis occurs; by 7–9 weeks, the fetal testis begins to produce androgens, and granulosa cells can be identified in the ovary. Testicular androgen production at this time occurs in response to placental human chorionic gonadotropin (hCG) and is necessary for male sexual differentiation. Between 9 and 12 weeks of gestational age, the fetal pituitary starts to produce luteinizing hormone (LH) and follicle-stimulating hormone (FSH); these fetal pituitary hormones are important for gonadal development. In response to fetal gonadotropins, ovarian follicular stage. In the testes, Leydig cell production of testosterone continues until several months after birth.

Throughout childhood, pulsatile secretion of FSH and LH occurs at 60- to 90-minute intervals and affects the output of gonadal hormones (Fig 26–2). As puberty approaches, the amplitude of the peaks increases, initially at night during sleep. As the basal

LH levels rise, estrogen production from the ovaries or testosterone production from the testes increases toward adult levels.

SEXUAL DIFFERENTIATION

Normal Sexual Differentiation

For normal sexual differentiation to occur, a specific sequence of events must take place. The bipotential gonad requires at least two X chromosomes to develop into an ovary; in the absence of a second X chromosome, a fibrous streak develops along the genital ridge. If a Y chromosome is present, a testis develops. Between the seventh and fourteenth weeks of gestation, testosterone (produced by the fetal testis in response to placental hCG) acts locally to induce the formation and growth of the internal male accessory sex structures and acts peripherally to induce masculinization of the external genitalia (eg, fusion of the labioscrotal folds and formation of a penile urethra). Growth of the penis occurs mainly in the late second and third trimesters, requiring stimulation of the testis by fetal pituitary gonadotropins. In the absence of androgens, the external genitalia feminize and a vagina is formed. Müllerian duct inhibiting factor, a glycoprotein produced by the testis, causes regression of the internal female duct structures; in the absence of this factor, the uterus and uterine (fallopian) tubes develop and mature.

Abnormal Sexual Differentiation

Abnormalities of sexual differentiation frequently result in ambiguous external genitalia. The causes for abnormal sexual differentiation may be divided into 4 major categories:

A. Abnormalities in Normal Gonadal Differentiation: These usually result from an unidentifiable abnormality of the sex chromosomes. Klinefelter's syndrome (see Chapter 34) with an XXY karyotype usually is associated with a male phenotype. Turner's syndrome (see Chapter 34) is usually associated with a female phenotype. Mosaic forms of gonadal dysgenesis that contain a Y-bearing cell line have an ambiguous phenotype and variable external phenotype. Idiopathic testicular failure prior to completion of sexual differentiation results in ambiguous genitalia. True hermaphroditism, with the presence of both spermatocytes and oocytes, is rare and produces external genitalia that range in type from fully masculine to almost completely feminine.

B. Abnormalities in Testosterone Synthesis or Action: These disorders cause male pseudohermaphroditism, frequently with ambiguous genitalia. Enzyme defects in testosterone synthesis may affect only testosterone synthesis, or they may also affect the synthesis of cortisol, as in variants of the adrenogenital syndrome. Defects in testosterone action result from either absent or defective end-organ recep-

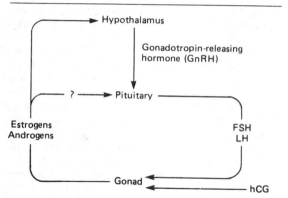

Figure 26–2. Hormonal regulation of gonadal function.

tors or a defect in peripheral testosterone metabolism to dihydrotestosterone due to 5α-reductase deficiency. The androgen receptor defect may be complete (testicular feminization) or incomplete (Reifenstein's syndrome and its variants).

C. Presence of Excessive Androgens in a Female Fetus: These disorders cause female pseudohermaphroditism and usually result in ambiguous genitalia. Excessive adrenal androgen production secondary to an adrenal enzyme defect in cortisol synthesis (ie, adrenal hyperplasia) is the cause of 95% of cases of XX patients with female pseudohermaphroditism and approximately half of all cases of patients with ambiguous genitalia. Occasionally, maternally derived androgens may cause masculinization of the female fetus.

D. Miscellaneous Syndromes: These are usually associated with multiple congenital anomalies, especially of the urinary tract and intestine. Occasionally, teratogenic agents may result in anomalous sexual development.

Saengen P: Abnormal sexual differentiation. *J Pediatr* 1984;**104**:1.

ABNORMALITIES IN OVARIAN FUNCTION

The ovary is composed of follicles (germ cells surrounded by granulosa cells), theca cells immediately surrounding the follicle, as stromal or supporting tissue. The ovary produces several types of hormones, the most important of which are estrogens and progesterone. At least 3 natural estrogens have been identified; estrone, 17β-estradiol (the most potent), and estriol. Production of the major ovarian estrogen, estradiol, is stimulated by pituitary LH secretion (Fig 26–2). Significant quantities of estrogen are not produced until the onset of puberty. Estrogens stimulate the growth of the uterus, vagina, and breasts. They also appear to be essential for the adolescent growth spurt occurring in girls.

Most patients with significant ovarian abnormalities in childhood exhibit precocious puberty, delayed puberty (primary amenorrhea), or secondary amenorrhea.

1. PRECOCIOUS PUBERTY IN GIRLS

General Considerations

Puberty is considered precocious if the onset of secondary sexual characteristics occurs prior to 8 years of age. Precocious puberty is 9 times more common in girls than in boys. The onset may occur at any age. True (complete) precocious puberty refers to sexual maturation in which hypothalamic-pituitary maturation initiates the sexual development;

in pseudoprecocity, the process is initiated elsewhere (eg, adrenal or gonadal tumor, exogenous hormones). True precocious puberty is always isosexual and may progress to the production of mature ova. In pseudoprecocity, sexual characteristics may be isosexual or heterosexual; secondary sexual characteristics develop, but the hypothalamic-pituitary-gonadal axis (Fig 26–2) does not mature, and oocyte maturation does not occur.

Clinical Findings

A. Symptoms and Signs: Although the first sign of sexual development in girls is usually breast development, followed by pubic hair growth and vaginal bleeding, the pattern of development may be variable. The interval between breast development and menstruation (normally about 2 years) may be less than 1 year or more than 6 years. On careful abdominal examination of girls with ovarian or adrenal tumors, a mass may be palpated and then confirmed by an ultrasonography. A growth spurt may precede or accompany the development of secondary sexual characteristics. A history of excessive mood changes and emotional lability frequently is obtained. Children with precocious puberty have accelerated growth and may be tall during childhood; because osseous maturation (bone age) advances at a more rapid rate than linear growth (particularly in the female), adult short stature may occur.

B. Laboratory Findings: In true precocious puberty, radioimmunoassays generally reveal that levels of serum or plasma gonadotropins are in the pubertal range. Early in the course of the disorder, random gonadotropin determinations may be within the prepubertal range. In these cases, further evaluation of serum LH and FSH levels during sleep and after stimulation with gonadotropin-releasing hormone (GnRH) is necessary (levels are obtained 30 and 60 minutes after intravenous stimulation with 100 μg of GnRH).

C. Imaging: A determination of bone age at the onset and every 6–12 months is helpful in predicting the effect of the precocity on adult height.

Abdominal and pelvic ultrasonography performed by a skilled radiologist can usually identify an ovarian mass, demonstrate an adrenal mass greater than 5 cm, and reveal presence of follicular ovarian cysts. Serial examinations are useful in demonstrating significant changes. A cranial CT scan or MRI with special attention to the hypothalamic and pituitary regions will identify mass lesions and other structural abnormalities of the central nervous system. Some cases of precocious puberty are due to organic brain lesions and other structural abnormalities of the central nervous system. Some cases of precocious puberty due to organic brain lesions may produce no clinical manifestations for prolonged periods. When these conditions are suspected, examinations for central nervous system lesions should be performed periodically.

Differential Diagnosis

The causes of true precocious and pseudoprecocious puberty are outlined in Table 26–8. Precocious and pseudoprecocious puberty should be differentiated from premature thelarche and premature adrenarche, which are both benign. Initially, differentiation of true precocious and pseudoprecocious puberty is important. Laboratory and x-ray findings helpful in differentiating these are discussed above. Most girls (80–90%) with precocious puberty have true precocious puberty. Prior to the advent of sophisticated CT scanners, 75–95% of these cases were considered idiopathic. CT scanning and MRI now demonstrate that many of them are due to static (presumably congenital) mass lesions in the hypothalamus.

Treatment

Treatment of the underlying cause of pseudoprecocious puberty (removal of the tumor or correction of the adrenal enzyme disorder) usually results in cessation of abnormal pubertal development. Successful medical intervention in true precocious puberty is effective, but long-term safety has not been established. The most successful therapy employs analogues of gonadotropin-releasing hormone (GnRH agonists). The analogues given in sustained doses either by daily injection or depot sustained-release preparations, interrupt the physiologic pulsatile state described above. "Down regulation" occurs, resulting in a block in pituitary LH synthesis and release and in the return of estrogen levels to prepubertal values. In most cases, menses cease, secondary sexual development stabilizes or re-

gresses, and linear growth and bone maturation slow to prepubertal rates.

In patients with McCune-Albright syndrome, analogues of gonadotropin-releasing hormone are not initially helpful. Therapy with antiandrogens, agents that block steroid synthesis (eg, ketoconazole), or both may be effective.

Regardless of the cause of precocious puberty or the medical therapy selected, the psychologic management of the patient and family is essential.

Fleischer AC, Shawker TH: The role of sonography in pediatric gynecology. *Clin Obstet Gynecol* 1987;**30**:35. [Review article; 28 references.]

Manasco PK et al: Resumption of puberty after long term luteinizing hormone-releasing hormone agonist treatment of central precocious puberty. *J Clin Endocr Metab* 1988;**67**:368.

Pescovitz OH et al: Premature thelarche and central precocious puberty: The relationship between clinical presentation and the gonadotropin response to luteinizing hormone-releasing hormone. *J Clin Endocr Metab* 1988; **67**:474.

Rudd BT: Precocious and delayed sexual development in children. *Acta Endocrinol Suppl (Copenh)* 1988;**288**:66 [Review article; 65 references.]

Temeck JW et al: Genetic defects of steroidogenesis in premature pubarche. *J Clin Endocr Metab* 1987;**64**:609.

2. AMENORRHEA

Amenorrhea is the absence of menstruation in a female 14 years of age or older or in a female of any age who is over 2½–3 years postpubarche. Secondary amenorrhea is cessation of menses after an inter-

Table 26–8. Causes of isosexual precocious development.

True (complete) gonadotropin dependent precocious puberty Constitutional (functional, idiopathic) Tumors producing destruction of the pineal (principally in males) Hypothalamic lesions (hamartomas, hyperplasia, congenital malformations, tumors) Tumors in vicinity of the third ventricle Internal hydrocephalus Cerebral and meningocerebral infections (postencephalitis, postmeningitis) Degenerative, possibly congenital encephalopathy Tuberous sclerosis Recklinghausen's disease Cystic arachnoiditis Therapeutic administration of gonadotropin Exogenous obesity **Pseudoprecocious (incomplete) puberty** Polyostotic fibrous dysplasia (McCune-Albright syndrome) (principally in females; often incomplete; usually infertile) Adrenal abnormalities Adrenocortical hyperplasia (males) Adrenocortical tumors Hyperplastic ectopic adrenal tissue Cushing's syndrome (males)	Gonadal tumors Tumors of the ovary—Granulosa cell tumor (most common), theca cell tumor, teratoma, choriocarcinoma, dysgerminoma, luteoma Tumors of the testes—Interstitial (Leydig) cell tumor, teratoma Premature pubarche (premature adrenarche) (both sexes) Without cerebral disease (constitutional?) With cerebral disease Premature thelarche (premature gynarche) (females) Without cerebral disease (constitutional?) With cerebral disease Drug-induced **Unclassified causes** With elevated gonadotropins Associated with hypothyroidism Presacral teratoma Primary liver cell tumors (hepatoma) (males only) Choriocarcinoma and seminoma of the testes Others Hyperinsulinism Primordial dwarfism Silver's syndrome (short stature, congenital asymmetry, and variations in the pattern of sexual development) Thyrotropin-releasing hormone excess

val of time equal to at least 6 months postmenarche or 3 menstrual cycles. A history and physical examination (including pelvic examination) often determines possible causes of amenorrhea (Table 26–9).

Primary Amenorrhea

Common causes of primary amenorrhea include physiologic or constitutional delay. Turner's syndrome, chronic illness, and severe undernutrition or strenuous exercise are also common.

Pseudoamenorrhea is a term employed when the patient is menstruating but has a genital tract obstruction that prevents release of menstrual blood. Sexual development is usually at Tanner stage IV or V, and cyclic abdominal pain without menstruation

Table 26–9. Causes of secondary amenorrhea.[1]

With Normal Ovarian Function
A. Congenital
    1. Cryptomenorrhea
    2. Absence of uterus
    3. Mayer Rokitarsky Küsten Hausen Syndrome
B. Acquired
    1. Intrauterine synechia (Asherman's syndrome)
    2. Hysterectomy
    3. After abortion, infection, or cesarean section
With Decreased Ovarian Secretion of Estrogen, Progestogen, or Androgen
A. With high gonadotropins (primary ovarian failure)
    1. Congenital
       a. Ovarian agenesis
       b. Gonadal dysgenesis
       c. Gonadotropin-resistant ovary syndrome
    2. Acquired
       a. Premature menopause
       b. Surgical oophorectomy
       c. Radiation castration
       d. Ovarian destruction by infection (rarely)
       e. Following chemotherapy (cyclophosphamide [Cytoxan])
B. With low or normal gonadotropins (secondary ovarian failure)
    1. Feminizing ovarian tumor
    2. Hypothalamic-pituitary dysfunction
       a. Congenital deficiency of gonadotropin secretion
       b. Acquired
          i. Organic CNS disease
          ii. Functional aberration of hypothalamic-pituitary axis
            Psychogenic
            Starvation (eg, anorexia nervosa)
            Physical exertion (eg, marathon runners, ballet dancers)
            Chronic systemic disease
            Extragenital endocrine disorders
            Pharmacologic (eg, with tranquilizers or after prolonged use of antifertility hormones)
            Unknown
With Increased Ovarian Androgen Secretion
A. Masculinizing ovarian tumor
B. Continuous estrus syndrome (polycystic ovary syndrome)

[1]Modified and reproduced, with permission, from Ross G. Vande Wiele R: Ovaries. In: *Textbook of Endocrinology*, 6th ed. Williams RH (editor). Saunders, 1981.

is noted. Pelvic examination may reveal an imperforate hymen, transverse vaginal ridge, or other obstruction. Treatment is surgical.

Turner's syndrome (XO syndrome, gonadal dysgenesis) should be considered in patients with short stature and sexual infantilism or pubarche without normal pubertal progression. This is a form of hypergonadotropic hypogonadism in which the estrogen level is low (or absent), FSH and LH levels are elevated, bone maturation is usually delayed, buccal smear is sometimes chromatin-negative, and karyotype is abnormal. The phenotypic features of Turner's syndrome (described in Chapter 34) may be absent in 40–50% of girls with the syndrome. Current treatment for the short stature includes human growth hormone, anabolic steroids, and low doses of estrogens separately or in combination. At the time of adolescence, a combination of estrogen and progesterone in physiologic doses is indicated.

Mayer-Rokitansky-Küster-Hauser syndrome is characterized by congenital müllerian agenesis with normal ovaries, normal ovarian function, and normal breast development. Pelvic examination reveals an absent vagina and various uterine abnormalities with or without additional renal and skeletal anomalies. Full evaluation is necessary, including karyotyping, intravenous pyelography, and laparoscopy. Therapy for this syndrome is surgical vaginoplasty.

Secondary Amenorrhea

Common causes of secondary amenorrhea include stress, pregnancy, major weight loss, polycystic ovary syndrome, and prolactin excess. Stress-induced amenorrhea is often noted in teenagers, but it should be diagnosed only after a careful evaluation. Pregnancy and its complications are the most frequent causes of secondary amenorrhea in sexually active teenagers.

Irregular menses (oligomenorrhea) or amenorrhea may result from severe weight loss secondary to dieting, vigorous exercise (eg, in marathon runners), depression, anorexia nervosa, or chronic illness. In the normal ovulating female, it is believed that a major source of estrogen is aromatization of androgens in peripheral adipose tissue. When the proportion of body weight as fat falls below a critical level (15–25%), estrogen production is decreased. This hypothesis has been advanced to explain amenorrhea in athletes and patients with anorexia nervosa.

In polycystic ovary syndrome (Stein-Leventhal syndrome), secondary amenorrhea is the result of chronic anovulation. Occasionally, dysfunctional uterine bleeding is the only finding; the full syndrome consists of obesity, hirsutism, secondary amenorrhea, bilaterally enlarged ovaries, and, in some cases, clitoromegaly. The results of tests of endocrine function reveal normal FSH concentrations, elevated LH levels, and borderline to elevated adrenal or ovarian androgen levels. The ratio of estrone:estradiol is often increased. Polycystic ovary syndrome may be idiopathic or secondary to adrenocortical hyperplasia or an adrenocortical neoplasm. Laparoscopy, ovarian biopsy, endometrial biopsy, or a combination of these procedures may be necessary for final diagnosis. Treatment consists of correction of the estrogen:androgen ratio and induction of ovulation in patients who wish to become pregnant. Agents with antiandrogen activity (eg, spironolactone) may be helpful in controlling the hirsutism.

Other causes of amenorrhea are shown in Table 26–9. Chronic illness and central nervous system disorders should always be considered. When galactorrhea and amenorrhea occur together, hyperprolactinemia, drug ingestion, hypothyroidism, stress, and hypothalamic injury should be considered.

Hall JG et al: Turner's syndrome. *West J Med* 1982; **137**:32.

Hurley DM et al: Induction of ovulation and fertility in amenorrheic women by pulsatile low-dose gonadotropin-releasing hormone. *N Engl J Med* 1984; **310**:1069.

Patton ML, Woolf PD: Hyperprolactinemia and delayed puberty: A report of three cases and their response to therapy. *Pediatrics* 1983;**71**:572.

Soules, MR: Adolescent amenorrhea. *Pediatr Clin North Am* 1987;**34**:1083.

OVARIAN TUMORS

Ovarian tumors are not rare in children. They may occur at any age and are usually large, benign, and unilateral. They may be estrogen-producing; ovarian tumors account for approximately 1% of cases of female sexual precocity. The most common estrogen-producing tumor is the granulosa cell tumor, but thecomas, luteomas, mixed types, and theca-lutein and follicular cysts have all been described in association with sexual precocity. In most instances, an ovarian tumor is palpable abdominally or rectally by the time sexual development has occurred.

Other ovarian tumors (teratomas, choriocarcinomas, and dysgerminomas) have been reported in association with sexual precocity.

Treatment is surgical removal. Recurrences are uncommon.

Grosfeld JL, Billmire DF: Teratomas in infancy and childhood. *Curr Probl Cancer* 1984;**2**:53.

ABNORMALITIES IN TESTICULAR FUNCTION

The major testicular hormone, testosterone, is produced by the Leydig (interstitial) cells. Production of testicular androgens is stimulated by LH secretion (Fig 26–2). Appreciable amounts of androgen usu-

ally begin to appear in boys at 12 years of age and are responsible, wholly or in part, for growth of internal and external genitalia and development of secondary sexual characteristics, including pubic, axillary, and facial hair. Androgens induce nitrogen retention, accelerate bone growth, and determine the closure of bony epiphyseal growth centers.

The seminiferous tubules are composed of germinal epithelium and Sertoli's cells. Testicular androgens in combination with pituitary FSH stimulate the development and maturation of the germinal epithelium and thus promote spermatogenesis. The Sertoli cells provide mechanical support for the germinal epithelium.

Patients with abnormalities in testicular function may present with delayed or precocious sexual development, cryptorchidism, or gynecomastia.

1. PRECOCIOUS PUBERTY IN BOYS

General Considerations

Puberty is considered precocious in boys if secondary sexual characteristics appear prior to 9 years of age. Precocious puberty is much less common in boys than in girls. In boys presenting with sexual precocity, pseudoprecocious puberty is as common as true precocious puberty. In addition, boys with true precocious puberty are more likely to have an identifiable pathologic process (eg, tumor) rather than idiopathic precocious puberty.

Descriptions of gonadotropin-independent precocious puberty have suggested that this may be the cause of familial male precocious puberty. In affected males, testicular production of testosterone is apparently independent of gonadotropin.

Clinical Findings

A. Symptoms and Signs: In precocious development, increases in somatic growth and growth of pubic hair are the common presenting complaints. Testicular size may differentiate true precocity, in which the testicles usually enlarge, from pseudoprecocity (most commonly due to andrenocortical hyperplasia), in which the testicles usually remain small. There are some exceptions: in advanced cases of pseudoprecocity, for example, some testicular enlargement may occur, because seminiferous tubule elements may be stimulated by prolonged elevated testosterone levels. In the very young child with early true precocity, minimal increases of testosterone may result in dramatic increases in penis size and pubic hair growth, with very little testicular enlargement. Tumors of the testis present with asymmetric testicular enlargement.

B. Laboratory Findings: LH and FSH levels are elevated in boys with true sexual precocity. Sexual precocity caused by the adrenogenital syndrome is associated with abnormal levels of plasma dehydroepiandosterone, androstenedione, 17α-hydroxyprogesterone, plasma 11-deoxycortisol, urinary 17-ketosteroids, or a combination of these steroids. The level of serum or plasma testosterone aids in the differentiation of true precocity and pseudoprecocity. Obtaining hCG levels to determine the presence of hepatoma may be necessary in boys with true sexual precocity.

C. Imaging: Diagnostic studies are similar to those used to evaluate sexual precocity in girls (see above). Ultrasonography may be useful in detection of hepatic, presacral, and testicular tumors.

Differential Diagnosis

The causes of sexual precocity are outlined in Table 26–8. In boys, it is particularly important to differentiate pseudoprecocity from true sexual precocity.

Treatment

Specific therapy should be used in cases in which the cause is known and amenable to therapy. Treatment of idiopathic true precocious puberty in boys is similar to that in girls (see above).

Treatment of gonadotropin-independent precocious puberty (testitoxicosis) with agents that block steroid synthesis (eg, ketoconazole), antiandrogens (eg, spironolactone), or with a combination of both has been successful.

2. SEXUAL INFANTILISM (Primary & Secondary Testicular Failure)

General Considerations

Lack of development of secondary sexual characteristics after the age of 17 years suggests abnormal testicular maturation. While delay of puberty until 17 years of age may be physiologically normal, it is generally of concern to a boy if pubertal changes do not occur by 14–15 years of age, and evaluation should be initiated at that time.

Sexual infantilism may be difficult to differentiate from constitutionally delayed adolescence. Although the latter may be associated with a delay in testicular function, normal puberty occurs at a later date.

The differentiation of primary and secondary testicular failure is based on the cause of the disorder. In general, primary failure results from absence, malfunction, or destruction of testicular tissue; secondary failure results from pituitary or hypothalamic insufficiency.

Primary testicular failure may be due to anorchia, surgical castration, Klinefelter's syndrome or other sex chromosomal abnormalities, a genetic defect in testosterone synthesis or action, inflammation and destruction of the testes following infection or toxic agents (mumps, irradiation, autoimmune disorders, syphilis, gonorrhea), trauma, or tumor.

Causes of secondary testicular failure resulting from central nervous system or hypothalamic-pituitary dysfunction include panhypopituitarism, empty sella syndrome, Kallmann's syndrome, isolated LH deficiency, and isolated FSH deficiency. Destructive lesions in or near the anterior pituitary, especially craniopharyngiomas and gliomas, may result in hypothalamic or pituitary dysfunction as can infection. These tumors may require irradiation to the central nervous system employing greater than 3500 rad. Prader-Willi syndrome and Laurence-Moon syndrome (Bardet-Biedl syndrome, Biemond syndrome II) are frequently associated with LH and FSH deficiency secondary to deficiency of hypothalamic gonadotropin-releasing hormone. Miscellaneous causes include chronic debilitating disease and hypothyroidism.

Clinical Findings

A. Symptoms and Signs: Physical examination may not be helpful in differentiating primary from secondary gonadal insufficiency. While cryptorchidism suggests primary testicular failure, hypothalamic or pituitary insufficiency as well as anatomic abnormalities may lead to failure of testicular descent.

B. Laboratory Findings: In primary testicular failure, the serum testosterone level is low, whereas LH and FSH values are elevated into the castrate range. In secondary testicular failure, levels of all 3 hormones are below the normal adult range. To establish the presence of the testes and their ability to respond to stimulation, the clinician may administer hCG; a dose of 2000 units/m^2 given intramuscularly every other day for 2–3 doses should result in a rise in the serum testosterone level to above 200 mg/dL 48 h. after the final dose. Determination of LH and FSH responses to exogenous GnRH may be useful.

Chromosomal karyotype should be determined in primary testicular failure of unknown cause.

C. Imaging: Skeletal maturation is usually delayed. A cranial CT scan or MRI should be performed in cases of secondary testicular failure.

Treatment

Specific therapy is indicated when the cause of testicular failure is known. Treatment with depot testosterone (eg enanthate) 200 mg every 3–4 weeks intramuscularly, may be given until sexual maturity is reached. In patients with primary testicular failure, replacement therapy with testosterone, 300–400 mg every 3–4 weeks, may be continued indefinitely. Specific therapy (GnRH pulsations) may result in fertility in patients with hypothalamic-pituitary insufficiency.

Bourguignon JP et al: Hypopituitarism and idiopathic delayed puberty: A longitudinal study in an attempt to diagnose gonadotropin deficiency before puberty. *J Clin Endocrinol Metab* 1982;**54**:733.

Hoffman AR et al: Induction of puberty in men by long-term pulsatile administration of low-dose gonadotropin-releasing hormone. *N Engl J Med* 1982;**307**:1237.

Reiter EO, Grumbach MM: Neuroendocrine control mechanisms and the onset of puberty. *Annu Rev Physiol* 1982;**44**:595.

Swerdlott RS, Overstreet JW, Sokal RS: Infertility in the male. *Ann Intern Med* 1985;**103**:901.

Winters SJ, Troen P: Reexamination of pulsatile luteinizing hormone secretion in primary testicular failure. *J Clin Endocrinol Metab* 1983;**57**:432.

3. CRYPTORCHIDISM

General Considerations

Cryptorchidism (undescended testes) is a common disorder in children. It may be unilateral or bilateral and may be classified as ectopic cryptorchidism or true cryptorchidism.

Approximately 3% of term male newborns and 30% of premature males have undescended testes at birth. In over half of these cases, the testes descend by the second month; by the age of 1 year, 80% of all undescended testes are in the scrotum. Further descent may occur through puberty, the latter perhaps stimulated by endogenous gonadotropin. If cryptorchidism persists into adult life, failure of spermatogenesis occurs, but testicular androgen production usually remains intact. The incidence of malignant neoplasm (usually seminoma) is appreciably greater in those testes which remain in the abdomen after puberty.

Ectopic testes are presumed to develop normally but are diverted as they descend through the inguinal canal. They are subclassified on the basis of their location; surgery is indicated once the diagnosis is established.

True cryptorchidism in most cases is thought to be the result of an abnormality in testicular development (dysgenesis). Cryptorchid testes frequently have a short spermatic artery, poor blood supply, or both. Although early scrotal positioning of these testes will obviate further damage related to intra-abdominal location, the testes generally remain abnormal, spermatogenesis is rare, and the risk of malignant neoplasm is increased. These testes should probably be removed if spermatogenesis does not occur after a reasonable period of observation.

Bilateral cryptorchidism is a common feature in prepubertal castrate syndrome (the vanishing testes syndrome), Noonan's syndrome, and disorders of androgen synthesis or action; it is seen less commonly with Klinefelter's syndrome, Sertoli-cell-only syndrome, and hypogonadotropin states.

Clinical Findings

Testosterone levels may be obtained after hCG stimulation to confirm the presence or absence of abdominal testes. The child with bilaterally unde-scended testes should be evaluated for sex chromosome abnormalities; genetic sex should be determined by buccal smear or chromosome analysis in the newborn period.

Differential Diagnosis

In palpating for the testes, the cremasteric reflex may be elicited, with a resultant ascent of the testes into the inguinal canal or abdomen (pseudocryptorchidism). To prevent this, the fingers first should be placed across the upper portion of the inguinal canal, obstructing ascent. Examination while the child is in the squatting position or a warm bath is also helpful. No treatment is necessary, and the prognosis for testicular descent and competence is excellent.

Treatment

The best age for medical or surgical treatment has not been determined, but there is a trend toward operation in infancy or early childhood. Surgical repair is indicated for cryptorchidism persisting beyond puberty.

Gonadotropin therapy (chorionic gonadotropin, 4000–5000 units intramuscularly 3–5 times a week for 2–3 weeks) is generally ineffective unless the child has retractile testes (pseudocryptorchidism) rather than cryptorchidism.

Androgen treatment (eg, depot testosterone enanthate) is indicated as replacement therapy in the male beyond the normal age of puberty who has been shown to lack functional testes.

Rajfer J et al: Hormonal therapy of cryptorchidism: A randomized, double-blind study comparing human chorionic gonadotropin and gonadotropin-releasing hormone. *N Engl J Med* 1986;**314**:466.

4. GYNECOMASTIA

See Chapter 10.

TESTICULAR TUMORS

The primary malignant tumors of the testis are seminomas and teratomas. Seminomas are rare in childhood; they may be hormone-producing. The major hormone-producing tumor of the testis is the Leydig cell tumor. It is frequently associated with sexual precocity. Other testicular tumors (choriocarcinomas and dysgerminomas) have been reported in association with sexual precocity.

Treatment of testicular tumors is surgical removal. The prognosis in patients with Leydig cell tumors is generally good.

Murphy CP: Testicular cancer. *CA* 1983;**33**:100.

ADRENAL CORTEX

The adrenal cortex develops from the dorsal coelomic mesothelium between the fourth and sixth weeks of fetal life. By 8–9 weeks of gestation, the fetal adrenal cortex contains the enzymes necessary to produce cortisol from progesterone. At 7–9 weeks of gestation, the fetal pituitary seems capable of producing and releasing adrenocorticotropic hormone (ACTH) to provide regulation of adrenal hormone production.

The adult adrenal cortex is composed of 3 distinct zones. The glomerulosa is the outermost zone and seems to be the exclusive source of aldosterone, the major mineralocorticoid in humans. The zona fasciculata is the largest cortical zone and is the source of cortisol, the major glucocorticoid, as well as small amounts of mineralocorticoids. The zona reticularis is the innermost zone (adjacent to the adrenal medulla) and appears to produce mainly adrenal androgens and estrogens.

During fetal life, these zones comprise only a minor portion of the adrenal cortex. The predominant portion is the fetal zone, or provisional cortex, which is capable of producing glucocorticoids, mineralocorticoids, androgens, and estrogens but is relatively deficient in production of 3β-hydroxydehydrogenase and $\Delta^5 = \Delta^4$ isomerase (Fig 26–3). Therefore, placentally produced progesterone serves as the major precursor for fetal adrenal production of cortisol and aldosterone.

The adrenal cortex produces cortisol under the control of pituitary ACTH. The quantity of cortisol produced is regulated by a negative-feedback mechanism involving the pituitary and hypothalamus (Fig 26–4). This negative-feedback control is superimposed in a diurnal pattern of ACTH release. ACTH release is greatest during early morning hours and least around midnight.

The actions of glucocorticoids are myriad and incompletely understood. Glucocorticoids are catabolic and antianabolic; ie, they promote the release of amino acids from muscle and increase gluconeogenesis while decreasing incorporation of amino acids into muscle protein. They also antagonize insulin action and permit lipogenesis. Glucocorticoids influence blood pressure through their "permissive effect" (norepinephrine enhancing peripheral vascular tone) and by affecting sodium and water retention.

Mineralocorticoids (primarily aldosterone in humans) promote sodium retention and permit potassium excretion. While ACTH can affect aldosterone production, the predominant regulators of aldosterone secretion are mediated via the renin-aldosterone system in response to changes in intravascular volume and serum sodium concentrations. Serum potassium concentrations also directly influence aldosterone release.

The zona reticularis of the adrenal cortex produces androgens (eg, dehydroepiandrosterone and androstenedione). In normal subjects, adrenal androgen production is insignificant; at pubarche, androgen production increases and may be an important factor in the initiation of puberty. The adrenal gland is the major source of androgen in the pubertal and adult female.

ADRENOCORTICAL INSUFFICIENCY
(Adrenal Crisis, Addison's Disease)

Essentials of Diagnosis

Acute form (adrenal crisis):
- Vomiting, dehydration, hypotension, circulatory collapse.
- Low serum sodium, high serum potassium, low glucose; eosinophilia.
- Low blood and urine adrenocorticosteroids.
- Weakness, fatigue, pallor; episodes of nausea, vomiting, and diarrhea; increased craving for salt.
- Increased pigmentation, hypotension; small heart.

General Considerations

Adrenocortical hypofunction may be due to congenital absence or atrophy (toxic factors, autoimmune phenomena) of the adrenal glands; an enzymatic defect leading to decreased production of cortisol; infection (eg, tuberculosis); or destruction of the gland by tumor, calcification, or hemorrhage (Waterhouse-Friderichsen syndrome). Rarely, adrenal insufficiency is the result of corticotropin (ACTH) or corticotropin releasing hormone (CRH) deficiency due to anterior pituitary or hypothalamic disease. In the latter condition, hyperpigmentation does not occur. Any acute illness, surgery, trauma, or exposure to excessive heat may precipitate an adrenal crisis. A temporary salt-losing disorder due to partial mineralocorticoid deficiency or renal subresponsiveness may occur during infancy.

Fractional types of adrenocortical insufficiency (relative or absolute deficiency of a single group [glucocorticoids] with normal production of other hormones of the adrenal glands) have been described.

Clinical Findings
A. Symptoms and Signs:
1. Acute form (adrenal crisis)—Manifestations include nausea and vomiting, diarrhea, abdominal pain, dehydration, fever (which may be followed by hypothermia), hypotension, circulatory collapse, and confusion or coma.

2. Chronic form (Addison's disease)—The leading causes of adrenal insufficiency today are hereditary enzymatic defects with congenital adrenal

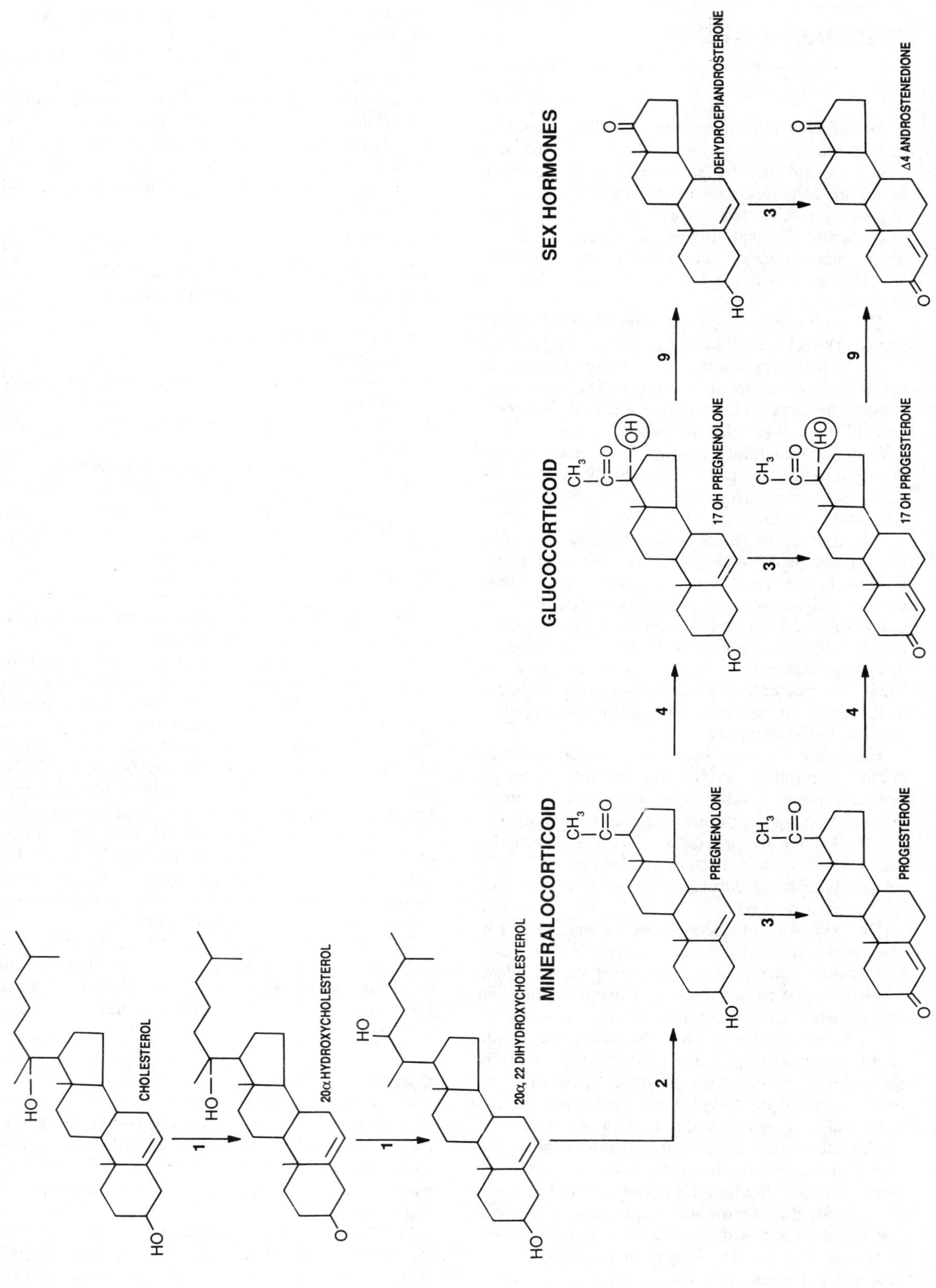
CHOLESTEROL
20α HYDROXYCHOLESTEROL
20α, 22 DIHYDROXYCHOLESTEROL
MINERALOCORTICOID
GLUCOCORTICOID
SEX HORMONES
PREGNENOLONE
17 OH PREGNENOLONE
DEHYDROEPIANDROSTERONE
PROGESTERONE
17 OH PROGESTERONE
Δ4 ANDROSTENEDIONE

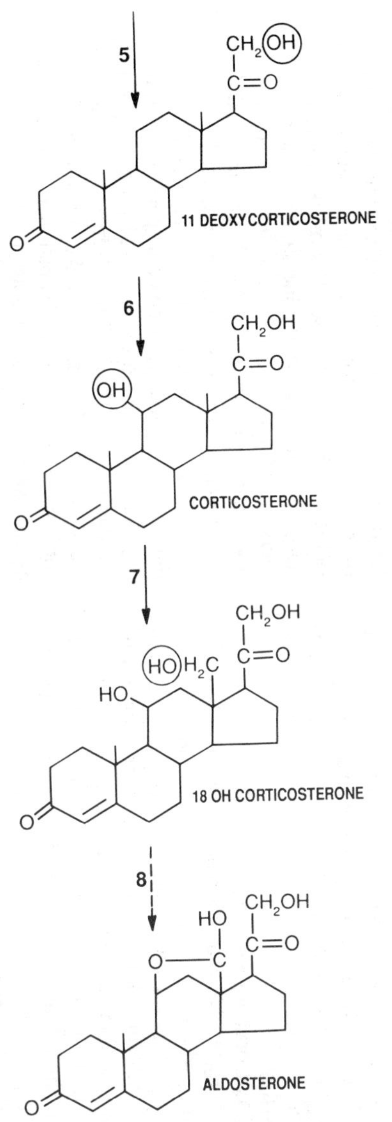

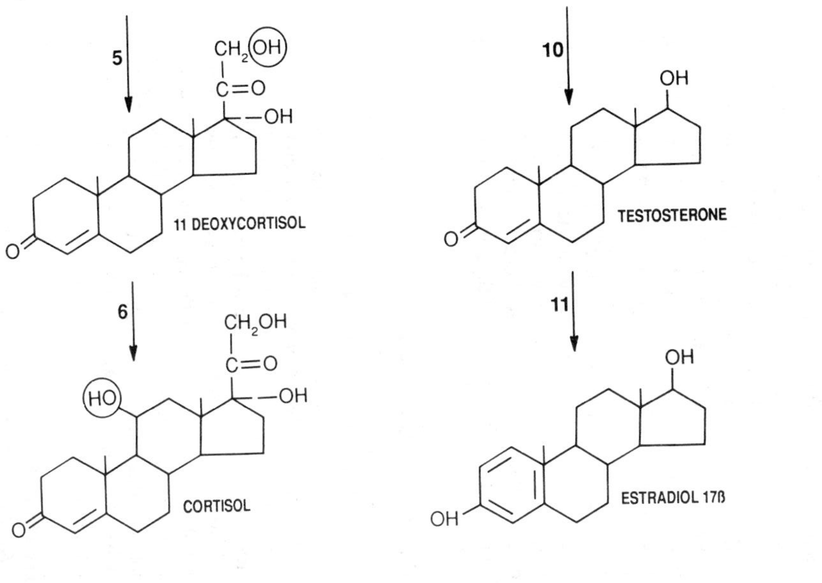

Figure 26-3. Adrenal steroid pathways.

TRADITIONAL

1. 20α Hydroxylase
2. 20,22-Desmolase
3. 3β-Hydroxydehydrogenase; Δ⁵–Δ⁴ isomerase*
4. 17-Hydroxylase
5. 21-Hydroxylase
6. 11-Hydroxylase
7. 18-Hydroxylase
8. 18-Hydroxydehydrogenase
9. 17, 20-lyase
10. 17-Keto-reductase
11. Aromatase

REVISED	GENE LOCATION
P 450 SCC	15
P 450 C17	10
P 450 C21	6 p
P 450 C11	8 q
P 450 ARO	15 q

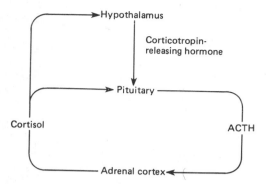

Figure 26–4. Pituitary-adrenal cortex control.

hyperplasia and idiopathic loss of adrenal function, the latter thought to be due to autoimmune mechanisms. Adrenal destruction may also occur secondary to infectious processes (eg, tuberculosis or fungal infection) and neoplasms. A rare form of familial Addison's disease may be seen in association with cerebral sclerosis and spastic paraplegia. Idiopathic Addison's disease may be familial and has been described in association with hypoparathyroidism, candidiasis, hypothyroidism, pernicious anemia, hypogonadism, and diabetes mellitus. The finding of circulating antibodies to adrenal tissue and other tissues involved in these conditions suggests that an autoimmune mechanism, probably related to a defect in immunoregulation involving suppressor T cell function, is the cause.

Signs and symptoms include fatigue, hypotension, weakness, failure to gain weight or loss of weight, increased appetite for salt, diarrhea, vomiting (which may become forceful and sometimes projectile), and dehydration. Diffuse tanning with increased pigmentation over pressure points, scars, and mucous membranes may be present. A small heart may be seen on x-ray film.

B. Laboratory Findings:
1. Suggestive of adrenal insufficiency— Serum sodium, chloride, and bicarbonate, P_{CO_2}, blood pH, and blood volume are decreased. Serum potassium and blood urea nitrogen are increased. Urinary sodium is elevated, and the sodium:potassium ratio is high despite low serum sodium. Eosinophilia* and moderate neutropenia may be present.

2. Confirmatory tests—The following tests measure the functional capacity of the adrenal cortex:

a. The corticotropin (ACTH) stimulation test is the most definitive test. (For details of ACTH stimulation test, see Adrenocorticosteroids and Corticotropin: Treatment for Nonendocrine Diseases.)

---

*A normal number of eosinophils during stress (eg, the day after operation or in the presence of a severe infection) is also suggestive of insufficiency.

b. Plasma ACTH levels are elevated, whereas cortisol is low and fails to rise with ACTH stimulation.

c. Urinary free cortisol and 17-hydroxycorticosteroid excretion are decreased.

d. Urinary 17-ketosteroid output is lower except in cases due to congenital adrenal hyperplasia or adrenal cortex tumor. (This test is of little value in younger children, who normally excrete less than 1 mg/d.)

e. The metyrapone test is useful in demonstrating normal pituitary function and in the diagnosis of adrenal insufficiency secondary to pituitary insufficiency. This test may provoke acute adrenal insufficiency in an individual with compromised adrenal function.

Differential Diagnosis

Acute adrenal insufficiency must be differentiated from severe acute infections, diabetic coma, various disturbances of the central nervous system, and acute poisoning. In the neonatal period, adrenal insufficiency may be clinically indistinguishable from respiratory distress, intracranial hemorrhage, or sepsis.

Chronic adrenocortical insufficiency must be differentiated from anorexia nervosa, certain muscular disorders (myasthenia gravis, etc), salt-losing nephritis, and chronic debilitating infections (tuberculosis, etc) and must be considered in cases of recurrent spontaneous hypoglycemia.

Treatment
A. Acute Form (Adrenal Crisis);
1. Replacement therapy—
a. Hydrocortisone sodium succinate, 2 mg/kg diluted in 2–10 mL of water intravenously, is given over 2–5 minutes, followed by an infusion of normal saline and 5–10% glucose, 100 mL/kg/24 h intravenously. Then, hydrocortisone sodium succinate, 1.5 mg/kg in infants or 12.5 mg/m² in older children, is given intravenously every 4–6 hours until stabilization is achieved and oral therapy tolerated.

b. Desoxycorticosterone acetate (DOCA), 1–2 mg/d intramuscularly, is given as part of initial therapy. This is repeated every 12–24 hours, depending on the state of hydration, electrolyte status, and blood pressure. When oral intake is tolerated, fludrocortisone, 0.1 mg daily, is substituted and continued as necessary every 12–24 hours.

c. Ten percent glucose in normal saline, 20 mL/kg intravenously in the first 2 hours, may be of value, particularly in infants with adrenal crisis who have congenital adrenal hyperplasia. Overtreatment must be avoided.

2. Hypotension—Specific treatment includes volume expansion (eg, normal saline solution, albumin) and hydrocortisone sodium succinate. Rarely, inotropic agents such as dopamine or dobutamine are needed.

3. Infections—Infections are treated with large

doses of appropriate antibiotic or chemotherapeutic agents.

4. Waterhouse-Friderichsen syndrome with fulminant infections—The use of adrenocorticosteroids and norepinphrine in the treatment or "prophylaxis" of fulminant infections is still controversial; steroids may augment the generalized Shwartzman reaction in fatal cases of meningococcemia. However, corticosteroids should always be considered in the presence of adrenal insufficiency, particularly with hypotension and circulatory collapse.

5. Fluids and electrolytes— Ten percent glucose in saline, 20 mL/kg intravenously, is given. *Caution:* Overtreatment must be avoided. Total parenteral fluid in the first 8 hours should not exceed the maintenance fluid requirement of the normal child (see Chapter 36).

B. Maintenance Therapy of Chronic Form (Addison's Disease): Following initial stabilization, the most effective substitution therapy is hydrocortisone given with fludrocortisone. Overtreatment should be avoided, because it may result in obesity, growth retardation, and other cushingoid features.

Additional hydrocortisone, desoxycorticosterone, or sodium chloride, singly or in combination, may be necessary with acute illness, surgery, trauma, or other stress reactions.

Supportive adrenocortical therapy should be given whenever surgical operations are performed in patients who have at some time received prolonged therapy with adrenocorticosteroids. (See below.)

1. Glucocorticoids (hydrocortisone or equivalent)—The dosage of all glucocorticoids is increased to 2–4 times the usual dosage during intercurrent illness or times of stress.

a. Hydrocortisone—A dosage of 10–20 mg/m²/d is given orally in 3–4 divided doses. For adrenal enzyme defects with excess ACTH, 25% of the dose is given in the morning and afternoon and 50% at night. For all other causes of adrenocortical insufficiency, 50% of the daily dose is given in the morning.

b. Prednisone—A dosage of 5–6 mg/m²/d is given orally in 2–3 divided doses. Its potency may preclude necessary minor modulations in dosage.

2. Mineralocorticoids (desoxycorticosterone acetate [DOCA] and related drugs)—The dosage should gradually be increased or decreased to maintain normal serum sodium levels and blood volume; avoid hypertension. Increases with stress are not necessary.

a. Fludrocortisone—A dose of 0.05–0.2 mg is given orally once a day or in 2 divided doses.

b. DOCA in oil—A dose of 1 mg/d is given intramuscularly.

3. Salt—The child should be given ready access to table salt. Frequent blood pressure determinations in the recumbent position should be made to ensure that hypertension is avoided.

C. Corticosteroids in Patients With Adreno-cortical Insufficiency Who Undergo Surgery: Hydrocortisone sodium succinate, 30 mg/m² intramuscularly or intravenously, is given 1 hour before surgery.

2. During operation—Hydrocortisone sodium succinate, 25–100 mg intravenously is administered with 5–10% glucose in saline throughout surgery.

3. During recovery—Hydrocortisone sodium succinate, 12.5 mg/m² intravenously, is given every 4–6 hours until oral doses are tolerated. The oral dose of 3–5 times the maintenance dose is gradually tapered to the maintenance dose as the patient recovers.

Course & Prognosis

A. Acute: The course of acute adrenal insufficiency is rapid, and death may occur within a few hours, particularly in infants, unless adequate treatment is given. Spontaneous recovery is unlikely. Patients who have received long-term treatment with adrenocorticosteroids may exhibit adrenal collapse if they undergo surgery or other acute stress. Pharmacologic doses of glucocorticoids during these episodes may be needed throughout life.

In all forms of acute adrenal insufficiency, the patient should be observed carefully once the crisis has passed and evaluated with laboratory tests to assess the degree of permanent adrenal insufficiency.

B. Chronic: Adequately treated chronic adrenocortical insufficiency is consistent with a relatively normal life. Patients on maintenance doses of glucocorticoids may require increases (2- to 3-fold) during severe illnesses and operations.

CONGENITAL ADRENAL HYPERPLASIA (Adrenogenital Syndrome)

Essentials of Diagnosis

- Pseudohermaphroditism in females, with urogenital sinus, enlargement of clitoris, and other evidence of virilization.
- Isosexual precocity in males with infantile testes.
- Increased linear growth in young children; advancement of skeletal maturation.
- Urinary and plasma androgen elevation; plasma 17α-hydroxyprogesterone and urinary pregnanetriol concentrations increased in the common form.
- May be associated with electrolyte and water disturbances, particularly in the newborn period.

General Considerations

The adrenogenital syndrome occurs when adrenal androgens or estrogens or both are produced in excessive amounts for the age of the child, resulting in precocious and sometimes heterosexual development of the genitalia. The most common form of this syndrome is the congenital familial (autosomal recessive) form, also known as congenital adrenal hyperplasia. This form, which affects males and females equally, is due to an inborn error of metabolism that has traditionally been equated to a deficiency in one of a number of distinct enzymes involved in adrenal steroidogenesis or sex hormone synthesis. Recent studies employing tools in molecular biology and protein chemistry have yielded evidence that has altered this view. It appears that the P-450 group of oxidases are the operative enzymes, and 4 distinct multipurpose enzymes within the cytochrome P-450 enzyme group are believed to be responsible for adrenal steroidogenesis. Within the text material and Table 26–10, the traditional terminology is retained to avoid confusion. In Fig 26–3, the new terminology is provided with the traditional terminology, and together the presumed gene location for the enzymes is indicated.

Over 80% of cases are caused by a 21-hydroxylase enzyme deficiency, approximately 10% by an 11-hydroxylase enzyme deficiency, and the remainder by deficiencies of the other 5 enzymes (Fig 26–3). In some forms, the infant may appear normal at birth, with symptoms occurring later. In all forms except 17,20-desmolase deficiency, diminished secretion of cortisol results in excessive secretion of ACTH. ACTH excess results in adrenal hyperplasia with increased production of various adrenal hormone precursors and increased urinary excretion of their metabolites. Increased pigmentation, especially of the scrotum, labia majora, and nipples, frequently results from excessive ACTH secretion.

Studies in patients with 21-hydroxylase deficiency indicate that the clinical type (salt-wasting versus nonsalt-wasting) is usually consistent within a family and that there is a close genetic linkage of the 21-hydroxylase gene to the HLA complex on chromosome 6. The latter finding has allowed more precise heterozygote detection and prenatal diagnosis. Population studies indicate that the defective gene is present in one of 50–100 people and that the incidence of the disorder is one per 5000–15,000. Hormonal evaluation of unaffected family members following ACTH stimulation allows detection of the heterozygote with a certainty of 80–90%, and a combination of hormonal and HLA studies can increase the number of cases detected. HLA typing in combination with the measurement of 17α-hydroxyprogesterone and androstenedione in amniotic fluid has been used in the prenatal diagnosis of 21-hydroxylase deficiency. The potential for mass screening with a microfilter paper technique to evaluate 17α-hydroxyprogesterone is in progress in some centers.

Nonclassic presentations of 21-hydroxylase deficiency have been reported with increasing frequency. Affected individuals have a normal phenotype at birth and develop evidence of virilization during later childhood, adolescence, or early adulthood. In these cases, previously referred to as late-onset or acquired enzyme deficiencies, results of hormonal studies are characteristic of 21-hydroxylase deficiency. An asymptomatic form has also been identified, in which individuals have none of the phenotypic features of the disorder but have hormonal study results identical to those in patients with nonclassic 21-hydroxylase deficiency. The nonclassic form appears to be less severe than the classic form. Because members of the same family may have classic, nonclassic, and asymptomatic forms, the disorders may be due to allelic variations of the same enzyme.

Pseudohermaphroditism can be caused by factors other than enzyme deficiencies. In females, these include virilizing maternal tumors or androgens or related hormones taken by the mother during the first trimester of pregnancy. In these cases, the condition does not progress after birth, and cortisol efficiency with abnormal steroidogenesis is not present. Pseudohermaphroditism occurs rarely with gonadal dysgenesis.

Adrenogenital syndrome may also result from tumors of the adrenal gland, ovary, or testis or from idiopathic adrenal hyperplasia later in life. Symptoms begin after birth and progress until treated.

Clinical Findings

A. Symptoms and Signs:

1. Adrenogenital syndrome in females—In females with potentially normal ovaries and uterus, masculinization occurs, and sexual development is along heterosexual lines.

a. Congenital bilateral hyperplasia of the adrenal cortex secondary to enzyme deficiency (pseudohermaphroditism)—The abnormality of the external genitalia may vary from mild enlargement of the clitoris to complete fusion of the labioscrotal folds, forming a penile urethra, and enlargement of the clitoris to form a normal-sized phallus. When the defect is incomplete, signs of adrenal insufficiency may not occur; signs and symptoms of virilization predominate. In the complete form left untreated, growth in height and skeletal maturation are excessive, and patients become muscular. Pubic hair appears early (often before the second birthday); acne may be excessive; and the voice may deepen. Excessive pigmentation may develop. Dentition is normal or only slightly advanced for the chronologic age. Similar abnormalities may be present in siblings and cousins. Signs of associated adrenal insufficiency may be present during the first days of life (typically in the first or second week). In some cases, adrenal insufficiency does not occur for months or years.

b. Postnatal adrenogenital syndrome (virilism)—This disorder may be due to adrenal hyperplasia or tumor or to arrhenoblastoma (extremely rare). Enlargement of the clitoris occurs, but other changes of the genitalia are not found. The family history is negative for similar abnormalities. If a tumor is present, it may be palpably enlarged. Other findings are similar to those of pseudohermaphroditism.

2. Adrenogenital syndrome in males (macrogenitosomia precox)—In males, sexual development proceeds along isosexual lines.

a. Congenital bilateral hyperplasia of the adrenal cortex due to enzyme deficiency—The infant may appear normal at birth, but during the first few months of life enlargement of the penis will be noted. There may be increased pigmentation resulting from excessive secretion of β-lipotropin and ACTH. Other symptoms and signs are similar to those of the congenital form in females. The testes are soft and not enlarged, except in the rare male in whom aberrant adrenal cells are present in the testes and produce unilateral or bilateral symmetric or asymmetric enlargement.

b. Tumor—The findings may be identical with those of congenital bilateral hyperplasia of the adrenal cortex, except that they appear at a later age. The tumor may be palpably enlarged. Rarely, an adrenal tumor in a male may produce feminization with gynecomastia.

B. Laboratory Findings:

1. Blood and urine—Hormonal studies are essential for accurate diagnosis. Findings characteristic of the enzyme deficiencies are shown in Table 26–10. With adrenal tumor, production and excretion of dehydroepiandrosterone are greatly elevated.

2. Genetic studies—When available, rapid chromosomal diagnosis should be obtained.

3. Dexamethasone suppression test—If dexamethasone, 2–4 mg/d in 4 divided doses for 7 days,

reduces 17-ketosteroids to normal, hyperplasia rather than adenoma is the probable diagnosis.

C. Imaging: Adrenal ultrasonography, CT scanning, and MRI may be useful in defining pelvic anatomy or enlarged adrenals or in localizing an adrenal tumor. Vaginograms using contrast material may indicate the presence of a urogenital sinus and cervix. Calcification in the area of the adrenal with displacement of the kidney may be seen on x-ray films of patients with tumors. Bone age is advanced with 21- and 11-hydroxylase defects but may not be evident in the first year.

Treatment
A. Congenital Hyperplasia of the Adrenal Cortex:

1. Initially, hydrocortisone given in a dosage of 25–30 mg/m^2/d orally suppresses abnormal adrenal steroidogenesis within 2 weeks. The maintenance dose is the same as that in Addison's disease. In congenital hyperplasia, 50% of the daily dose should be given in the late evening to suppress the early morning ACTH rise. Dosage is regulated to maintain a normal growth rate and a normal rate of osseous maturation; in cases of 21-hydroxylase deficiency, the plasma 17-hydroxyprogesterone and dehydroepiandrosterone sulfate levels should also be kept within the normal range. In adolescent females, menses are a sensitive index of the adequacy of therapy. Therapy should be continued throughout life in both males and females because of the possibility of malignant degeneration of the hyperplastic adrenal gland.

2. Other aspects of treatment are as for Addison's disease (eg, mineralocorticoid therapy and glucocorticoid increases with stress; see p 801. Occasionally, inadequate mineralocorticoid therapy leads to increased renin levels and elevated 17α-

Table 26–10. Laboratory and clinical findings in adrenal enzyme defects resulting in adrenogenital syndrome.

Enzyme Deficiency[1]	Urinary 17-Ketosteroids	Elevated Plasma Metabolite	Plasma Androgens	Aldosterone	Hypertension/ Salt Loss	External Genitalia[2]
20,22-Desmolase (1)	↓↓↓		↓↓↓	↓↓↓	−/+	M: feminized F: normal
3β-Hydroxydehydrogenase (2)	↑↑(DHEA)	Pregnenolone	↑(DHEA)	↓↓↓	−/+	M: feminized F: masculinized
17-Hydroxylase (3)	↓↓↓	Progesterone	↓↓	↓↓(↑ Deoxycorticosterone)	+/−	M: feminized F: normal
21-Hydroxylase (simple) (4)	↑↑↑	17α-Hydroxyprogesterone	↑↑	↑	−/−	M:normal F:masculinized
21-Hydroxylase (salt-wasting) (4)	↑↑↑	17α-Hydroxyprogesterone	↑↑	↓↓	−/+	M: normal F: masculinized
11-Hydroxylase (5)	↑↑	11-Deoxycortisol	↑↑	↓↓(↑ Deoxycorticosterone)	+/−	M: normal F: masculinized
17,20-Desmolase (7)	↓↓↓		↓↓	Normal	−/−	M: feminized F: normal

[1]The numbers refer to the position of enzyme action as shown in Fig 26–3.
[2]M = male, F = female.

hydroxyprogesterone production in the face of adequate or excessive glucocorticoid therapy.

3. Clitororecession is often indicated in the first year of life. Vaginoplasty for labial fusion should be performed in early childhood; it may be necessary during infancy if vaginal-urinary reflux and genitourinary tract infections occur. Partial clitorectomy is occasionally indicated if the clitoris is abnormally large or sensitive.

B. Tumor: Because the malignant and benign lesions cannot be distinguished clinically, surgical removal is indicated whenever a tumor has been diagnosed. Preoperative and postoperative treatment is as for Cushing's syndrome due to tumor.

Course & Prognosis

When therapy is initiated in early infancy, abnormal metabolic effects are not observed, and masculinization does not progress. Unless adequately controlled, adrenal hyperplasia results in sexual precocity and masculinization throughout childhood. Affected individuals will be tall as children but short as adults. Treatment with the corticosteroids permits normal growth, development, and sexual maturation. If treatment is delayed until somatic development is over 12–14 years (as determined by bone age), true sexual precocity may occur in males and females.

Patient education stressing lifelong therapy is important to ensure compliance in adolescence and later life.

Female pseudohermaphrodites mistakenly raised as males for more than 3 years may have serious psychologic disturbances if their sex is "changed" after that time. Extensive psychologic evaluation is mandatory in determining the optimal course of action.

When adrenogenital syndrome is caused by a tumor, the progression of signs and symptoms ceases after surgical removal; however, evidence of masculinization, particularly deepening of the voice, may persist.

ADRENOCORTICAL HYPERFUNCTION (Cushing's Disease, Cushing's Syndrome)

Essentials of Diagnosis

- "Truncal type" adiposity with thin extremities, moon face, muscle wasting, weakness, plethora, easy bruisability, purplish striae, growth retardation.
- Hypertension, osteoporosis, glycosuria.
- Elevated serum and urine adrenocorticosteroids; low postassium; eosinopenia.

General Considerations

The principal findings in Cushing's syndrome in childhood result from excessive secretion of glucocorticoids and androgens. Depletion of body protein is typical. There may also be lesser degrees of overproduction of the mineralocorticoids. It has been suggested that in Cushing's syndrome with bilateral adrenal hyperplasia there is decreased responsiveness of the hypothalamic-pituitary "feedback" mechanism that regulates the release or production of ACTH. This may then result in a constant but only slightly excessive elevation in the secretion of ACTH or lead to qualitative or quantitative change in the diurnal variation.

Cushing's syndrome is more common in females. In children under 12, it is usually iatrogenic (secondary to therapeutic doses of corticotropin or one of the corticosteroids). It may rarely be due to an adrenal tumor or to adrenocortical hyperplasia, or associated with basophilic adenoma of the pituitary gland or, rarely, with an extrapituitary ACTH-producing tumor.

Clinical Findings

A. Symptoms and Signs:

1. Due to excessive secretion of the glucocorticoid hormones—Findings include "buffalo type" adiposity, most marked on the face, neck, and trunk (a fat pad in the interscapular area is characteristic); easy fatigability and weakness; plethoric facies; purplish striae; easy bruisability; ecchymoses; hirsutism; osteoporosis; hypertension; diabetes mellitus (usually latent), pain in the back; muscle wasting and weakness; and marked retardation of growth.

2. Due to excessive secretion of mineralocorticoids—Hypernatremia, increased blood volume, edema, and hypertension may be found.

3. Due to excessive secretion of androgens—Manifestations include hirsutism, acne, and varying degrees of excessive masculinization. Menstrual irregularities occur during puberty in older girls.

B. Laboratory Findings:

1. Blood—

a. Serum cortisol levels are elevated. There may be a loss of the normal diurnal variation.

b. Serum chloride and potassium may be lowered. Serum sodium and HCO_3^- content may be elevated (metabolic alkalosis).

c. Plasma ACTH concentrations are slightly elevated with adrenal hyperplasia; decreased in cases of adrenal tumor; and greatly increased with ACTH-producing pituitary or extrapituitary tumors.

d. The leukocyte count shows polymorphonuclear leukocytosis with lymphopenia, and the eosinophil count is low ($< 50/\mu L$). The erythrocyte count may be elevated.

2. Urine—

a. Urinary free cortisol excretion is elevated. This is the most useful diagnostic test.

b. Urinary 17-hydroxycorticosteroid levels are elevated.

c. Urinary 17-ketosteroids may be normal but usually elevated in association with adrenal tumor.

d. Glycosuria may be present.

3. Response to corticotropin (ACTH) and corticosteroids—The response to corticotropin (ACTH) stimulation is excessive in patients with adrenal hyperplasia; a poor response is usually found in those with tumor. There is a diminished adrenal response to small doses (0.5 mg) of dexamethasone in the dexamethasone suppression test; larger doses cause suppression of adrenal activity when the disease is due to adrenal hyperplasia. Adenomas and adrenal carcinomas may rarely be suppressed by large doses of dexamethasone (4–16 mg/d in 4 divided doses).

C. Imaging: Pituitary imaging may demonstrate a pituitary adenoma. Adrenal imaging demonstrates adenoma and may demonstrate bilateral hyperplasia. Radionuclide studies of the adrenals may be useful in complete cases. Urograms may be abnormal. Adrenal calcification may be present. Osteoporosis (evident first in the spine and pelvis) with compression fractures may be seen in advanced cases.

Differential Diagnosis

Children with obesity, particularly in the presence of striae and hypertension, are frequently suspected of having Cushing's syndrome. The growth rate is helpful in differentiating the two. Children with Cushing's syndrome have a poor growth rate, whereas those with exogenous obesity usually have a normal or slightly increased growth rate. In addition, the color of the striae (purplish in Cushing's syndrome, pink in obesity) and the distribution of the obesity assist in the differentiation. The urinary free cortisol excretion is alway normal in obesity.

Treatment

In all cases of primary hyperfunction due to tumor, surgical removal, if possible, is indicated. Corticotropin (ACTH) should be given preoperatively and postoperatively to stimulate the nontumorous adrenal cortex, which is generally atrophied. Adrenocorticosteroids should be administered during and after surgery until the patient is stable. Supplemental potassium, salt, and mineralocorticoids may be necessary. (See above outline of corticosteroid administration in surgical patients.)

Adrenal hyperplasia resulting from a pituitary microadenoma may respond to pituitary surgery irradiation, or partial adrenalectomy. In some cases, total adrenalectomy is necessary. Substitution therapy is usually necessary after these measures.

The use of mitotane, a DDT derivative toxic to the adrenal cortex, and aminoglutethimide, an inhibitor of steroid synthesis, have been suggested, but the efficacy of these agents in children with adrenal tumors has not been determined.

Prognosis

If the tumor is malignant, the prognosis is poor; if benign, cure is to be expected following proper preparation and surgery.

Pituitary enlargement has been reported in some cases of Cushing's syndrome following both partial and complete adrenalectomy.

Cushing's syndrome (perhaps due to pituitary adenoma) may occasionally undergo spontaneous remission.

Although most of the changes resulting from adrenocorticosteroid excess disappear, hypertension, diabetes mellitus, and osteoporosis may persist, and the rate of growth may continue to be poor.

Aron DC et al: Cushing's syndrome: Problems in management. *Endocr Rev* 1982;**3**:229.

Drucker A, New M: Disorders of adrenal steroidogenesis. *Pediatr Clin North Am* 1987;**34**:1055.

Homoki J, Solyom J, Teller WM: Detection of late onset steroid 21-hydroxylase deficiency by capillary gas chromatographic profiling of urinary steroids in children and adolescents. *Eur J Pediatr* Apr, 1988:147(3):257.

Killean AA et al: Diagnosis of classical steroid 21-hydroxylase deficiency using an HLA-B locus-specific DNA-probe. *Am J Med Genet* 1988;**29**:703.

Krieger DT: Physiopathology of Cushing's disease. *Endocr Rev* 1983;**4**:22.

Miller WL, Levine LS: Molecular and clinical advances in congenital adrenal hyperplasia. *J Pediatr J*, 1987;**111**:1.

Streeten DH et al: Normal and abnormal function of the hypothalamic-pituitary-adrenocortical system in man. *Endocr Rev* 1984;**5**:371.

White PC, New MI, Dupont B: Congenital adrenal hyperplasia. (2 Parts.) *N Engl J Med* 1987;**316**:1519, 1580.

PRIMARY HYPERALDOSTERONISM

Primary hyperaldosteronism may be caused by a benign adrenal tumor or by adrenal hyperplasia. It is characterized by paresthesias, tetany, weakness, polyuria (nocturnal enunesis is common in young children), periodic ''paralysis,'' low serum potassium, elevated serum sodium, hypertension, metabolic alkalosis, and production of a large volume of alkaline urine with a low fixed specific gravity; the latter does not respond to vasopressin. Edema is rare. The glucose tolerance test is frequently abnormal. Plasma and urinary aldosterone are elevated, but other steroid levels are variable. Plasma renin levels are decreased (in contrast to increased levels in secondary hyperaldosteronism, eg, that due to renal vascular disease and Bartter's syndrome). In patients with tumor, the administration of ACTH may further increase the excretion of aldosterone. Marked decrease of aldosterone-induced hypokalemia, alkalosis, hypochloremia, or hypernatremia after the administration of a glucocorticoid or an aldosterone antagonist such a spironolactone, which blocks the action of aldosterone upon the renal tubule, may be of diagnostic value.

Treatment is glucocorticoid administration, subtotal or total adrenalectomy for hyperplasia, and surgical removal of the tumor.

Findling JW, Adams AH, Raff H: Selective hypoaldosteronism due to an endogenous impairment in angiotensin II production. *N Engl J Med* 1987;**316:**1632.

ADRENOCORTICOSTEROIDS & CORTICOTROPIN (ACTH): TREATMENT FOR NONENDOCRINE DISEASES

The adrenocorticosteroids and corticotropin are commonly employed for their anti-inflammatory and immunosuppressive properties in a variety of conditions in childhood. Pharmacologic doses are necessary to achieve these actions effects, and side effects are, unfortunately, common. Numerous synthetic preparations possessing variable ratios of glucocorticoid to mineralocorticoid activity are available (Table 26–11).

Actions

The adrenocorticosteroids exert a direct or permissive effect on virtually every tissue of the body; major known effects include the following:

(1) Gluconeogenesis and glycogen synthesis in the liver.

(2) Stimulation of fat synthesis and redistribution of body fat.

(3) Catabolism of protein with an increase in nitrogen and phosphorus excretion.

(4) Decrease in lymphoid and thymic tissue, resulting in a decreased cellular response to inflammation and hypersensitivity.

(5) Alteration of central nervous system excitation.

(6) Retardation of connective tissue mitosis and migration, decreasing wound healing.

(7) Improved capillary tone and increased vascular compartment volume and pressure.

(8) In the case of mineralocorticoids, control of cation flux across membranes, with sodium retention and potassium excretion.

Uses

The adrenocorticosteroids and corticotropin are commonly employed in the following nonendocrine deficiency states in childhood:

(1) Adrenogenital syndrome, adrenal insufficiency. (Corticotropin is not effective in these disorders.)

(2) Nephrotic syndrome.

(3) Ulcerative colitis and ileitis.

(4) Allergic disorders: Bronchial asthma (including status asthmaticus), intractable hay fever (pollinosis), urticaria, angioneurotic edema, serum sickness, atopic dermatitis, atopic eczema, exfoliative dermatitis.

Table 26–11. Adrenocorticosteroids.

	Trade Names	Potency/mg Compared to Cortisol[1] (Glucocorticoid Effect)	Potency/mg Compared to Cortisol (Sodium-Retaining Effect)
Glucocorticoids			
Hydrocortisone (cortisol)	Cortef, Cortril, Hydrocortone, Solu-Cortef	1	1
Cortisone	Cortone	4/5	1
Prednisone	Deltasone, Meticorten	4–5	2/5
Methylpredinisolone	Medrol	5–6	Minimal effect
Triamcinolone	Aristocort, Kenacort, Kenalog	5–6	Minimal effect
Paramethasone	Haldrone	10–12	
Dexamethasone	Decadron, Hexadrol	25–30	Minimal effect
Betamethasone	Celestone	25	
Mineralocorticoids			
Fludrocortisone (9α-fluorocortisol)	Florinef	15–20	300–400
Desoxycorticosterone acetate	DOCA, Percorten Acetate	No effect	15
Desoxycorticosterone pivalate (trimethylacetate)	Percorten Pivalate	No effect	
Aldosterone	Not available commercially	30	500

[1]To convert hydrocortisone dosage to equivalent dosage in any of the other preparations listed in this table, divide by the potency factors shown.

(5) Inflammatory eye disease: Uveitis, chorioretinitis, sympathetic ophthalmia, iritis, iridocyclitis, retinitis centralis, herpes zoster (not herpes simplex) ophthalmicus, optic neuritis, retrobulbar neuritis.

(6) Collagen vascular diseases: Rheumatoid arthritis, acute rheumatic fever, disseminated lupus erythematosus, scleroderma, dermatomyositis.

(7) Neoplastic diseases (temporary remission): Pulmonary granulomatosis, lymphoma, Hodgkin's disease, acute leukemia.

(8) Blood dyscrasias: Idiopathic thrombocytopenic purpura, allergic purpura, aplastic anemia, acquired hemolytic anemia.

(9) Miscellaneous conditions: Idiopathic hypoglycemia, infantile cortical hyperostosis, reticuloendotheliosis, thymic enlargement, sarcoidosis, pulmonary fibrosis, transfusion reactions, contact dermatitis (including poison oak), drug reactions, neurodermatitis.

Contraindications

A. Absolute: Use is contraindicated in active, questionably healed, or suspected tuberculosis.

B. Relative: These drugs should be used with extreme caution in the presence of herpes simplex of the eye, osteoporosis, peptic ulcer, active infections, emotional instability, and thrombophlebitis.

Side Effects of Therapy

When pharmacologic doses or prolonged use of adrenocorticosteroids are necessary clinical manifestations of Cushing's syndrome are common. Side effects may result either from the use of synthetic exogenous agents by any route, including inhalation and topical administration (inflamed skin), or from the use of corticotropin (ACTH), which stimulates excessive production of endogenous adrenocorticosteroids. Use of a large, single dose of glucocorticoids given once every 48 hours (alternate-day therapy) lessens the incidence and severity of some of the side effects.

A. Endocrine Disorders:

1. Hyperglycemia and glycosuria (of particular significance in early chemical diabetes).

2. Cushing's syndrome.

3. Persistent suppression of pituitary-adrenal responsiveness to stress with resultant hypoadrenocorticism.

B. Electrolyte and Mineral Disorders:

1. Marked retention of sodium and water, producing edema, increased blood volume, and hypertension (more common in endogenous hyperadrenal states).

2. Potassium loss with symptoms of hypokalemia.

3. Hypocalcemia, tetany.

C. Protein and Skeletal Disorders:

1. Negative nitrogen balance, with loss of body protein and bone protein, resulting in osteoporosis, pathologic fractures, and aseptic bone necrosis.

2. Suppression of growth, retarded skeletal maturation.

3. Muscular weakness and wasting.

D. Effect on Gastrointestinal Tract:

1. Excessive appetite and intake of food.

2. Activation or production of peptic ulcer.

3. Gastrointestinal bleeding from ulceration or from unknown cause (particularly in children with hepatic disease).

4. Fatty liver with embolism, pancreatitis, nodular panniculitis.

E. Lowering of Resistance to Infectious Agents; Silent Infection; Decreased Inflammatory Reaction:

1. Susceptibility to acute pulmonary or disseminated fungal infections; intestinal parasitic infections.

2. Activation of tuberculosis; false-negative tuberculin reaction.

3. Stimulation of activity of herpes simplex virus.

F. Neuropsychiatric Disorders:

1. Euphoria, excitability, psychotic behavior, and status epilepticus with electroencephalographic changes.

2. Increased intracranial pressure with "pseudotumor cerebri" syndrome.

G. Hemorrhagic Disorders:

1. Bleeding into the skin as a result of increased capillary fragility.

2. Thrombosis, thrombophlebitis, cerebral hemorrhage.

H. Miscellaneous:

1. Myocarditis, pleuritis, and arteritis following abrupt cessation of therapy.

2. Cardiomegaly.

3. Nephrosclerosis, proteinuria.

4. Acne (in older children), hirsutism, amenorrhea or irregular menses.

5. Posterior subcapsular cataracts; glaucoma.

Tapering of Pharmacologic Doses of Steroids

Prolonged use of pharmacologic doses of glucocorticoids may result in suppression of ACTH and consequent adrenal atrophy; discontinuation of glucocorticoids may result in clinical adrenal insufficiency. A gradual reduction in the steroid dose may allow resumption of ACTH stimulation of the adrenal gland, thereby lessening the risk of adrenal insufficiency. ACTH elaboration will generally not occur until the administered steroid is given in subphysiologic doses. If glucocorticoid therapy is not considered necessary for more than 2 weeks, the drug can be discontinued abruptly because adrenal suppression is unlikely. Thus, pharmacologic doses of glucocorticoid employed for 2 weeks or less may be tapered and withdrawn as rapidly as the condition for which the glucocorticoid is prescribed allows. As a rule of thumb, a reduction of 25–50% every 2–7 days is sufficiently rapid to permit observation of clinical symptomatology. Moreover, withdrawal through use of an alternate-day schedule (eg, a single dose given every 48 hours) may allow for a 50% decrease in the total dosage while providing the desired pharmacologic effect.

Once a physiologic equivalent is achieved, the dose may be reduced by 25% every 5–7 days until a subphysiologic level is reached. At this point, assessment of endogenous adrenal activity is estimated by obtaining fasting plasma cortisol levels drawn prior to the morning steroid dose. When an alternate-day schedule is followed, a plasma cortisol level is drawn the morning prior to treatment. A cortisol level within the physiologic range (8–15 µg/dL) demonstrates return of basal physiologic adrenal function; exogenous steroids may then be discontinued. Once basal physiologic adrenal function returns, the adrenal reserve or capacity to respond to stress and infection is estimated by the ACTH stimulation test, in which 250 µg of synthetic ACTH is administered intravenously. Cortisol levels are obtained prior to and at 0, 30, and 60 minutes after infusion. A cortisol level above 20 µg/dL at 30 or 60 minutes indicates a satisfactory adrenal reserve. The ACTH test should be performed in all patients who have received pharmacologic doses of steroids for more than 2 weeks. Even if the results of the test are normal, however, patients who have received prolonged treatment with adrenocorticosteroids may exhibit signs and symptoms of adrenal insufficiency during acute stress, infection, or surgery for months to years after glucocorticoids have been withdrawn. Careful monitoring and (when necessary), the use of pharmacologic doses of glucocorticoids should be considered during severe illnesses and surgery for life.

Axelrod L: Corticosteroid therapy. Chapter 79 in: *Principles and Practice of Endocrinology and Metabolism.* Becker, KL (editor). Lippincott, 1990.

Byyny RC: Withdrawal from glucocorticoid therapy. *N Engl J Med* 1976;**295**:30.

Chamberlain P, Meyer WJ: Management of pituitary-adrenal suppression secondary to corticosteroid therapy. *Pediatrics* 1981;**67**:245.

Messer J et al: Association of adrenocorticosteroid therapy and peptic ulcer disease. *N Engl J Med* 1983;**309**:21.

ADRENAL MEDULLA

PHEOCHROMOCYTOMA
(Chromaffinoma)

Pheochromocytoma is an uncommon tumor. Approximately 10% of the total number of cases occur in childhood. The tumor may be located wherever there is any chromaffin tissue (adrenal medulla, sympathetic ganglia, carotid body, etc). It may be multiple, familial (autosomal dominant, in which case a high prevalence of multiple endocrine neoplasia exists), recurrent, and (sometimes) malignant.

Although clinical manifestation of pheochromocytoma may result from physical expansion of lesions into surrounding tissue (eg, spinal cord), manifestations are generally due to excessive secretion of epinephrine or norepinephrine. Attacks of anxiety, unexplained perspiration, and headaches should arouse suspicion. Other findings are palpitation and tachycardia, dizziness, weakness, nausea and vomiting, diarrhea, dilated pupils with blurring of vision, abdominal and precordial pain, hypertension (usually persistent), postural hypotension, discomfort from heat, and vasomotor instability. The symptoms may be sustained, producing all of the above findings plus papilledema, retinopathy, and enlargement of the heart. There is an increased incidence of pheochromocytomas in patients and families with pheochromatoses, neurofibromatosis, and type II multiple endocrine neoplasia (see Carcinoma of the Thyroid). Neuroblastomas, neurogangliomas, and other neural tumors may cause increased secretion of pressor amines and occasionally simulate the findings of a pheochromocytoma. Carcinoid tumors may produce cardiovascular changes similar to those associated with pheochromocytoma.

Laboratory diagnosis is possible in over 90% of cases. Serum catecholamines are elevated, particularly while the patient is symptomatic, and urinary excretion of catecholamines parallels this elevation. Elevated levels are characteristically high enough to be diagnostic but may be limited to the period of a paroxysm. The 24-hour urine collection shows increased excretion of metanephrines and vanillylmandelic acid (VMA, 4-hydroxy-3-methoxymandelic acid). Provocative tests employing histamine, tyramine, or glucagon and the phentolamine tests may be abnormal; the former are dangerous, however, and these agents are rarely necessary for diagnosis. Displacement of the kidney may be shown by routine x-ray and the tumor identified by CT scanning or MRI. Angiocatheterization and measurement of blood levels of catecholamines may be helpful in localizing the tumor prior to surgery.

Surgical removal of the tumor is the treatment of choice; this is a dangerous procedure and may produce sudden death. Oral phenoxybenzamine or intravenous phentolamine is used preoperatively. Profound hypotension may occur as the tumor is removed but may be controlled with an infusion of norepinephrine, which may have to be continued for 1–2 days.

Complete relief of symptoms is to be expected after recovery from removal of the nonmalignant tumor unless irreversible secondary vascular changes have occurred. If the disorder remains untreated, severe cardiac, renal, and cerebral damage may result.

Bravo EB, Gifford RW Jr: Pheochromocytoma: Diagnosis, localization and management. *N Engl J Med* 1984; **311:**1298.

Cryer PE: Physiology and pathophysiology of the human sympathoadrenal neuroendocrine system. *N Engl J Med* 1980;**303:**436.

DIABETES MELLITUS

Essentials of Diagnosis

- Weight loss, polyuria, polydipsia, and abdominal or leg cramps.
- Hyperglycemia and glycosuria with or without ketonuria.
- Enuresis, loss of appetite, emotional disturbances, and lassitude may occur.
- Fewer than 5% of cases present in coma or precoma.

General Considerations

In individuals under 18 years of age, the incidence of diabetes mellitus is between 1 and 3.5 per 1000, depending on the population surveyed. Genetic susceptibility is associated with markers on chromosome 6 within the HLA region. The risk in DR3 heterozygotes compared to the population at large is 3.7; in DR4 heterozygotes, 9.7; and in DR3/DR4 mixed heterozygotes, 45.8.

Insulin-dependent diabetes mellitus (IDDM), or type I diabetes, occurs when an inflammatory insult of the islet cells results in destruction of beta cells and insulin deficiency. In most cases of type I diabetes, the pathologic process is thought to have been taking place for several months or years before evidence of clinical deficiency occurs. The actual trigger of the inflammatory response in genetically susceptible individuals is unknown. With the progressive destruction of islet cells, insulin is no longer available to stimulate protein synthesis at the ribosomal level or to bind heterokinase to the electron transport chain on the mitochondrial surface. The latter leads to diminished availability of oxaloacetate. Diminished energy sources from glucose are replaced by an increased breakdown of fat and protein to acetylcoenzyme A. Peripheral utilization of fatty acids and amino acids, however, is impaired, and both are converted to ketone bodies in the liver.

Recently, it has been learned that some siblings of patients with IDDM have circulating anti islet cell cytoplasmic antibodies and that the presence of these antibodies is associated with a progressive impairment of insulin secretion in response to an intravenous glucose infusion. These findings may seem to represent the earliest stages of IDDM, and treatment studies have been designed to evaluate the possibility that immunosuppressive agents at this early stage may prevent or delay the onset of clinical IDDM.

Clinical Findings

A. Symptoms and Signs:

1. Moderate to severe acidosis—In most affected children, clinical diabetes is first recognized when insulin production falls below physiologic needs: Five to 10% of patients present in severe metabolic ketoacidosis; in this group, the symptoms of weight loss, polyuria, and polydipsia are recognized only in retrospect. Dehydration, increased respiratory effort, mental confusion, and lethargy (which are characteristic of acidosis) are common in this category.

2. Mild or absent acidosis at time of presentation—Ten to 20% of patients have mild to moderate metabolic derangement at the time of diagnosis and clinically present with enuresis, failure to grow or gain weight, or a decreased endurance. A few children are detected by routine urinalysis before overt symptoms appear. Rare presenting manifestations include a delayed insulin release following a glucose load; postprandial hypoglycemia; or nonketotic (hyperosmolar) coma (see below).

3. Maturity-onset diabetes in youth (MODY)—This condition, occasionally diagnosed in an obese teenager, may be more common than realized. The condition can usually be managed effectively by diet restriction.

4. Pseudodiabetes—Pseudodiabetes is a transient hyperglycemia state occurring in the newborn or, occasionally, in a young child with an infection. It is probably the result of increased concentrations of counterregulatory hormones (eg, epinephrine and glucagon) and rarely requires a short course of treatment with regular insulin.

5. Hyperosmolar nonketotic coma—This condition, primarily seen in adults, is characterized by severe hyperglycemia, hyperosmolality, and dehydration without ketoacidosis. The condition is thought to be the result of a mild insulinopenia in the splanchnic (portal) circulation and moderate insulinopenia in the peripheral circulations. Cautious restoration of extracellular water with isotonic fluids is a primary goal of treatment.

B. Laboratory Findings:

1. Glycosuria—Glycosuria may be identified by glucose oxidase tapes.

2. Hyperglycemia—A fasting blood glucose value exceeding 120 mg/dL or a random blood sugar value in excess of 180 mg/dL is usually the result of diabetes mellitus.

3. Oral glucose tolerance tests—The oral glucose tolerance test (Fig 26–5) is not usually necessary for diagnosis of type I diabetes mellitus.

4. Serum insulin levels—Serum insulin concen-

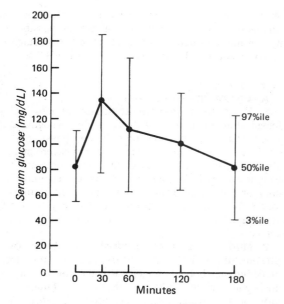

Figure 26–5. Serum glucose percentile levels after administration of glucose, 1.75 g/kg orally.

trations are rarely helpful at the onset of juvenile diabetes; they may be low, normal, or moderately elevated.

5. Other laboratory measurements—Stable hemoglobin A_{1c} or total glycosylated hemoglobin measurements are used to evaluate long-term glucose control. Levels of 10–25% are seen at the time of diagnosis. Stable hemoglobin A_{1c} levels are 6.3% +2% in normal children and are 10% + 2%, of total hemoglobin in children with reasonably well controlled diabetes. Abnormal hemoglobins can falsely affect the stable hemoglobin A_{1c} levels but do not affect total glycosolated hemoglobin. Fasting plasma cholesterol and HDL levels should be monitored during long-term management.

Cytoplasmic islet cell antibodies and complement-fixing islet cell antibodies are usually present in the serum many months before the disease is clinically overt and may presist for 6–24 months after diagnosis. Moreover, at the onset of type I diabetes, there is an increase in activated T cells reflecting immunologic activity.

Differential Diagnosis

The combination of glycosuria, hyperglycemia, and ketoacidosis is diagnostic of diabetes mellitus. Abnormal glucose tolerance tests with glycosuria may be encountered in a variety of conditions in which there is an excess of counterregulatory hormones (eg, glucagon, glucocorticoids, or catecholamines). These include certain exogenous hypothalamic and pituitary tumors, adrenal tumor or hyperplasia, exogenous pharmacologic doses of glu-

cocorticoids, and pheochomocytomas. Because the hyperglycemia in these states is a reflection of increased glyconeogenesis and glucogenolysis and not of insulin insufficiency, there is no ketosis unless there is a concomittant decrease in insulin reserve.

Renal glucosuria (see Chapter 22) is not associated with hyperglycemia.

Treatment

A. Management of Moderate to Severe Ketoacidosis:

1. General management—The treatment of severe diabetic acidosis is based on fundamental principles. Extracellular fluid volume must be restored to compensate for losses due to vomiting and to the osmotic diuresis accompanying glucosuria. Insulin is given to restore normal carbohydrate utilization and synthesis of triglycerides and protein. Serum hyperosmolality must be gradually normalized, intracellular stores of potassium must be replenished, and disturbances in acid-base balance must be corrected. Moderate to severe diabetic ketoacidosis, except as an initial presentation, is generally due to poor compliance with treatment.

2. Initial laboratory studies—The acid-base status should be estimated by measuring blood pH, serum bicarbonate, and anion gap. Baseline serum (or plasma) ketones, glucose, sodium, potassium, and chloride levels should be recorded, as well as blood urea nitrogen, serum calcium and phosphate, and, in severe cases, serum osmolality.

Additional laboratory measurements usually include a complete blood count; examination of the urine for blood cells, protein, ketone bodies, glucose, and bacteria; appropriate cultures should be obtained in cases of suspected infection.

3. Initial management—The following protocol is employed for children with newly diagnosed diabetic ketoacidosis, severe ketoacidosis, central nervous system symptoms, and repeated vomiting; for patients unable to tolerate oral fluids; or for those who have not responded to home or outpatient management. Ketoacidosis generally resolves in 6–8 hours, but the severely acidotic patient may require 12–48 hours for complete correction.

a. Clinical assessment—

(1) Medical history and a physical examination are obtained, with special attention to possible precipitating causes, such as emotional stress, failure to take insulin, or infection. The degree of shock and the need for volume expanders are assessed and corrective measures initiated promptly. Because of the risk of cardiac failure and cerebral edema, plasma volume expansion with colloid should be used with caution in the child whose lean body mass has been depleted. Correction is indirectly *but more safely* achieved by replacement of extracellular fluid losses with near isotonic fluids.

(2) A flow sheet for fluids, insulin, and other

medications and laboratory data is initiated. All intake and output must be meticuously recorded.

(3) An electrocardiogram is obtained in severely ill children for quick assessment of the effect of potassium or calcium abnormalities on conduction; cardiac monitoring is continued.

(4) If there is vomiting, abdominal distention, or the risk of aspiration due to coma or precoma, a continuous gastric suction should be started.

(5) A urinary catheter is placed in severely ill children for acurate fluid loss measurement.

b. Laboratory management—Following the initial laboratory studies above, blood glucose, HCO_3^- or pH, and K+ should be measured hourly until the HCO_3^- is greater than 10 meq/L or the pH is greater than 7.25. These indices can then be assessed every 2–3 hours until normalized. Bedside blood glucose monitoring is useful in management.

c. Fluid and electrolyte management—

(1) Initial volume expansion—If the patient is severely dehydrated, a physiologic solution (isotonic saline or lactated Ringer's injection) is given as rapidly as needed to normalize perfusion and blood pressure. If the patient is severely acidotic or has not voided, the addition of potassium must be delayed until after the initial fluid volume reexpansion has been given.

(2) Twenty-four-hour fluid replacement—

(a) Fluids—A convenient rule is to give normal saline in a dosage of 600 mL/m^2 for the first 1–2 hours. Insulin is added as soon as the blood glucose level is known; potassium and bicarbonate may be added as detailed below. Depending on the hydration needs, intravenous fluids can be slowed to twice the maintenance dose (see Table 36–3) after 2–3 hours.

(b) Glucose—Hydration fluids should be changed to 5–10% dextrose in 0.45 normal saline with added potassium when the glucose reaches 250–300 mg/dL. The percentage of dextrose in the solution should be selected to maintain the serum glucose between 200 and 300 mg/dL.

(c) Potassium—The maintainance of normal serum potassium concentration is a special problem. In the presence of insulinopenia and acidosis, potassium moves from the intracellular to the extracellular compartment, and high urinary and, occasionally, gastric losses occur. As acidosis is corrected, it is not unusual for serum potassium levels to fall in spite of large potassium replacements. Once voiding is established, therefore, all intravenous fluids should contain 20–40 meq of K+ per liter. Electrocardiographic monitoring (lead II) may provide an additional estimate of total body potassium deficit or change. Supplements may be in the form of potassium chloride or acetate. Additional oral potassium supplements of 1 meq/kg every 2–4 hours may be necessary to maintain a potassium concentration at the desired levels of greater than 3.5 meq/L.

(d) Acid-base management—Specific acid-base correction with alkali is usually not necessary unless the blood pH is under 7.1. The acidosis appears to be of 2 types: low and high renal perfusion states. In the low renal perfusion state, ketoacids cannot be excreted. In the less common normal renal perfusion state, the urine contains large amounts of sodium salts of ketoacids. As a consequence, distal luminal acidosis exists; There is impaired distal excretion of the hydrogen ion in spite of the acidosis, resulting in a hyperchloremic acidosis. Hyperchloremic acidosis resolves more slowly; bicarbonate therapy may be useful in this instance.

(e) Osmolarity—Measurement of serum osmolarity may be helpful in severely acidotic patients. If the serum osmolarity is markedly elevated (greater than 350 mmol/L), the danger of cerebral edema is increased, and blood glucose and dehydration should be corrected less rapidly.

d. Insulin management—No insulin should be given until the baseline serum glucose level has been determined. Insulin is then given by continuous intravenous infusion (0.1 unit/kg/hour) until the acidosis resolves. This dosage achieves a relatively constant serum insulin level with a smooth and predictable fall in serum glucose.

If the serum glucose falls below 250 mg/dL and acidosis is still present, the intravenous insulin regime should be continued, and glucose should be administered intravenously with an electrolyte solution. In the interval between the resolution of the acidosis and the initiation of daily long-acting doses of insulin, the intravenous insulin, 0.025–0.05 unit/kg/h, can be continued with intravenous dextros. Alternatively, one or more doses of regular insulin, 0.1–0.2 unit/kg/dose, can be given subcutaneously.

The first dose of long-acting insulin should be given the morning after admission, provided that vomiting has ceased (see Long-Term Management of All Patients).

4. Complications of diabetic ketoacidosis—

a. Cerebral edema is an unusual complication in the treatment of ketoacidosis but is often fatal. The pathophysiology is unclear, but edema generally occurs in patients less than 18 years of age who present with moderate to severe dehydration and are treated with large volumes of fluid rapidly administered. Meticulous monitoring of fluid and electrolyte replacement in this type of setting is mandatory. When cerebral edema occurs, treatment should be initiated promptly (see Chapter 36).

b. Hypokalemia and hypoglycemia, the other common serious risks of ketoacidosis therapy, can be easily prevented by frequent monitoring.

B. Management of Mild Ketoacidosis: When children with previously known diabetes develop mild diabetic ketoacidosis, they can be treated at home with additional regular insulin and fluids such as diet drinks and fruit juice; more serious cases can often be managed in an outpatient setting with a few hours of fluid therapy. The insulin dosage is 0.2 to 0.5 unit per kilogram per day and may gradually be increased until hyperglycemia and glycosuria are controlled. In the newly diagnosed juvenile diabetic without severe ketoacidosis, both treatment and education can often be conducted in an outpatient setting if the family and physician can devote sufficient time. Subsequently, the patient should be encouraged to return to full activity and diet, while the insulin dose is adjusted on the basis of blood glucose levels.

C. Long-Term Management of All Patients: The objective of long-term management is to achieve "control." In children, this can be defined as a high level of physical and emotional health, continuing normal growth, freedom from hypoglycemic reactions, absence of polyuria, and absence of acetones in the urine. Employing home glucose monitoring, blood glucose levels should be maintained between 80 and 180 mg/dL. The glycosylated hemoglobin concentration, depending on methodology, should be less than 10%. The following are important in achieving these goals:

1. Patient education and follow-up—This is the cornerstone of satisfactory patient care. Initially, regular weekly (or more frequent) encounters are necessary; telephone contact is encouraged. Education begins immediately after diagnosis and includes the keeping of a record diary, the techniques of giving insulin, testing the urine for acetone, and home monitoring of blood glucose. The constant renewal and augmentation of the patient's and the family's understanding of diabetes is particularly important in the early months. Many families need emotional support and counseling. As the family becomes more familiar with diabetes management, visits can be extended to every 3 months. This may be particularly important to the adolescent diabetic.

2. Insulin—(See Table 26–12). Human or pork insulin is recommended; little difference can be demonstrated in vitro between human and purified pork insulins. Human insulin is more rapidly absorbed than pork insulin, and the duration of action of human NPH may be shorter than that of pork NPH. Beef/pork or pure beef insulins are not recommended because of high antigenicity of beef insulin.

In established diabetes, the total dose of insulin is usually 0.8–1 unit/kg/d. During adolescence, relative insulin resistance may develop. A requirement of 1.2 unit/kg/d is not unusual and may reach 1.8 unit/kg/d. Nevertheless, insulin overdose must always be considered, (ie, Somogyi effect) whenever insulin requirements exceed 1 unit/kg/d. While it is always worthwhile to try to achieve satisfactory control with one injection per day, most patients require both a morning and an evening dose; a 3-dose regimen may improve glycemic control in a small number of patients. The daily insulin dose is usually divided at approximately 12 hour intervals, with two-thirds of the dose given in the morning before breakfast and one-third given in the evening before supper. For most individuals, regular insulin constitutes one-third of the morning dose and one-half of the evening dose; the remainder is either NPH or Lente. This pattern is then adjusted to the needs of the individual patient.

When 3 doses per day appear necessary, the following 2 regimens are often effective: (1) regular and NPH insulin in the morning, regular insulin at supper, and NPH at bedtime (10:00–11:00 PM); (2) regular and ultralente before breakfast and supper and regular insulin before lunch. Both of these schedules provide more flexibility for meals and activities.

The insulin dosage should be readjusted from time to time on the basis of routine home blood glucose determinations. Parents and patients should be encouraged to acquire confidence in making small adjustments in insulin dosage in response to gradual changes (growth) and short-term changes (physical activity, illness, or diet).

Insulin can also be administered by external computerized minipumps. This technology can offer excellent control. However, they are cumbersome and do not offer significantly improved control over injections given 3 times daily. At the present time, these pumps do not have glucose sensors and must be used only in conjunction with frequent capillary blood glucose determinations.

3. Diet—Instructions concerning the diet should be given by a dietitian or nutritionist. A balanced diet providing adequate nutrition for normal growth and development is pivotal. The diabetic child should eat the same kinds of food at the same time and in the same amounts each day. Snacks in the mid morning, afternoon, and evening avert hypoglycemia and spread the carbohydrate load throughout the day. Weighing of the food is seldom necessary, but an understanding of basic nutrition is important. In small children, good dietary discipline should not be pressed to the point of causing emotional problems; in the child of school age and the adolescent, however, every effort should be made to obtain compliance in the interest of good control and a diminished prospect of complications. Daily caloric intake

Table 26–12. Duration of action of various insulins.

Insulin	Duration of Maximum Effect (hours)	End of Effect (hours)
Human regular	1–3	5
Pure pork regular	2–4	7
Human NPH	4–6	12
Pork NPH	6–8	16
Pork Lente	7–15	22
Ultralente	10–24	36

for growth in childhood is estimated at 100 calories multiplied by the age in years, plus 1000. Ten to 15% of the calories should be derived from protein sources, 30–35% from fat, and 45–60% from carbohydrates. Understanding the dietary exchange system may be helpful in achieving control. This system is outlined in the pamphlet *Exchange Lists for Meal Planning,* published by the American Diabetes Association, 600 Fifth Avenue, New York, NY 10020.

If at all possible, foods that are not good for the diabetic child should be excluded from the home. Special dietetic foods, with the exception of artificial sweeteners, should not be encouraged for young diabetics. Providing 2 menus within the home differentiates the affected child from the remainder of the family and may contribute to the development of emotional problems.

The use of alternative sweeteners such as saccharin and aspartame makes life easier for the child with diabetes. Sorbitol and fructose are sugars that can be metabolized without forming glucose; sufficient insulin is still required.

A high-fiber, low-fat diet in which carbohydrates are given in the form of complex carbohydrates may be helpful and is being investigated at the present time; these foods are considered by many to be unpalatable. Obesity in a young diabetic requires the same attention as in the nondiabetic. When insulin resistance develops, however, more frequent glucose monitoring and insulin adjustments may be necessary.

Alcohol and drug intake can be a considerable problem in teenagers with diabetes. The use of alcoholic beverages usually results in an initial increase in blood glucose levels. Later, low blood glucose levels will be more likely secondary to a reduction in gluconeogenesis; missed snacks and meals can also contribute to the hypoglycemia.

4. Exercise—Patients should be encouraged to participate in a variety of activities. Exercise often reduces the amount of insulin required as a result of increased insulin-independent glucose utilization. Adjustments in snack times and the content of snacks may also be necessary to cover increases in exercise and avoid hypoglycemia.

Vigorous exercise in the late afternoon or evening may cause an increase in hypoglycemia for 6–12 hours after the event. This fact should always be considered when the bedtime snack is selected; in such cases, protein or fat is substituted for carbohydrate.

5. Avoiding hypoglycemia—Education of the patient concerning the physiology of insulin absorption and action, the importance of regular meal timing and content, and the effect of exercise on glucose utilization is the most important factor in avoiding hypoglycemia. The patient is taught to recognize the signs and symptoms of hypoglycemia and is instructed to carry a glucose source for treatment of hypoglycemia. Medications that may mask symptoms of hypoglycemia (eg, beta-blockers) should be avoided. Parents are also instructed in the use of glucagon when the child is unable to eat (eg, vomiting and coma). Recent studies have suggested that nocturnal hypoglycemia is likely to be associated with a late-evening glucose level of less than 100 mg/dL and may be avoided by appropriate adjustment in the bedtime snack.

6. Blood glucose estimations—Home monitoring of blood glucose, with testing 2–4 times per day, has become the standard for assessing control and for optimal blood glucose regulation. Isolated and occasional blood glucose estimations are of little value except during acute illness or when the child is symptomatic. These tests should be done in the morning before breakfast, in the mid afternoon, before dinner, and before bed. During illness, more frequent testing is helpful. If patients keep careful records of blood glucose levels, it is usually possible to identify situations in which small alternations in insulin dosages, food choices, or exercise will aid in maintaining appropriate glucose levels.

7. Urine testing—Because of the variability in the renal clearance of glucose, routine urine testing for glucose in type I diabetes has been replaced by home blood glucose monitoring. Monitoring of urine ketones during episodes of acute illness remains helpful in certain instances.

8. Recent advances—Continued improvement in home blood glucose monitors has decreased user error. These monitors now have memory capability to store results of recent blood tests; computer assisted analysis of blood sugar records may aid in improved adjustments of insulin dosage.

Increased knowledge of the immunologic nature of the primary lesion of diabetes is leading to transplantation and equivocally successful trials of immunosuppresive therapy in the early stages of diabetes.

Complications

Complications during the course of childhood diabetes include ketoacidosis, fatal cerebral edema, and hypoglycemia with resultant brain damage. Peripheral neuritis renal compromise and exudative retinopathy may occur but are infrequent. Poorly controlled diabetes in young children over a long period may lead to a syndrome of hepatomegaly, delayed puberty, and dwarfism (Mauriac syndrome). Limited joint mobility occurs in poorly controlled diabetes and seems to be an index of later degenerative vascular disease. Vaginal candidiasis is seen occasionally. Both atrophy and hypertrophy of subcutaneous fat occur around injection sites but are much less common with the use of purified insulins. These frequently occur as a result of localized injections of insulin over an extended interval. Occult hypoglycemia, followed by counterregulatory hormone-induced hyperglycemia, presumably occurs when the resultant hyperglycemia is incorrectly interpreted as the result of insufficient insulin. Misinterpretation that has led an increase in insulin dosage should be corrected with a reduction of the insulin dosage.

Emotional disturbances are common, especially in the early teen years. During these years, adherence to the recommended routine of blood testing, insulin injections, and dietary restrictions is frequently impossible. Every attempt should be made to allow the adolescent to express his or her frustrations and to identify an adult who can perform some of the required management tasks. Inability to follow the recommended treatment plan is the most common cause of poor control during the adolescent period.

Prognosis

Parents will want to know in what ways the overall life expectancy for their diabetic children may be altered. In this respect, there is currently a mean interval of 20 years after the onset of disease before the onset of major complications. It is possible that the prepubertal years may not be included in the 20-year interval. Improved metabolic control achieved with more precise home monitoring of blood glucose offers the hope of decreasing the risk of microvascular complications.

Chase HP et al: Diagnosis of pre-type 1 diabetes. *J Pediatr* 1987;**111**:807.

Friberg TR et al: The effect of long-term near normal glycemic control on mild diabetic retinopathy. *Ophthalmology* 1985;**92**:1051.

Krane EJ: Diabetic ketoacidosis. Biochemistry, physiology, treatment, and prevention. *Pediatr Clin North Am* 1987;**34**:935.

Krolewaki AS et al: Epidemiologic approach to the etiology of type 1 diabetes mellitus and its complications. *N Engl J Med* 1987;**317**:1390.

Morris LR, Murphy MB, Kitabchi AE: Bicarbonate therapy in severe diabetic ketoacidosis. *Ann Intern Med* 1986;**105**:836.

Nelson RL: Oral glucose tolerance test: Indications and limitations. *Mayo Clin Proc* 1988;**63**:263.

Perriello G et al: The effect of symptomatic nocturnal hypoglycemia on glycemic control in diabetes mellitus. *N Engl J Med* 1988;**319**:1233.

Rizza RA: Treatment options for insulin-predependent diabetes mellitus: A comparison of the artificial endocrine pancreas, continuous subcutaneous insulin infusion, and multiple daily insulin injections. *Mayo Clin Proc* 1986;**61**:796.

Whincup G, Milner RDG: Prediction and management of nocturnal hypoglycemia in diabetes. *Arch Dis Child* 1987;**62**:333.

SELECTED REFERENCES

Alsever RN, Gotlin RW: *Handbook of Endocrine Tests in Adults and Children,* 2nd ed. Year Book, 1978.

DeGroot LJ et al (editors): *Endocrinology,* 2nd ed. 3 vols. Saunders, 1989.

Felig P et al: *Endocrinology and Metabolism,* 2nd ed. McGraw-Hill, 1987.

Greenspan FS, Forsham PH: *Basic and Clinical Endocrinology,* 2nd ed. Lange, 1986.

Hung W, August GP, Glasgow AM: *Pediatric Endocrinology.* Medical Examination Publishing, 1983.

Travis LB, Bronhard BH, Schreiner BJ: *Diabetes Mellitus in Children and Adolescents,* Saunders, 1987.

Infections: Viral & Rickettsial

27

John W. Paisley, MD, & Myron J. Levin, MD

I. VIRAL INFECTIONS

Viruses cause most pediatric infections. Although immunizations have made some viral infections rare, new viruses have been discovered. Familiarity with the clinical syndromes and complications of common viral illnesses is mandatory. Mixed viral or viral-bacterial infections of the respiratory and intestinal tracts are rather common, as is prolonged, asymptomatic shedding of some viruses in childhood. Thus the detection of a virus is not always a definitive indication that it is the cause of that illness.

Diagnosis of many viral illnesses is now possible through antigen detection techniques. These are more rapid than the more sensitive method of isolation in tissue culture. Electron microscopy, nucleic acid hybridization, and enzyme amplification of viral genome permit recognition of previously undetectable infections. This will change many basic concepts about viral disease and make viral diagnosis an increasingly complex and commercialized field. Only reputable laboratories with excellent quality controls should be used, and results of new tests must be interpreted cautiously. The availability of specific antiviral agents increases the need for early diagnosis in some serious viral infections. Table 27–1 lists some viral agents causing common clinical signs, and Table 27–2 lists some diagnostic tests.

The local viral diagnostic laboratory should be contacted for details regarding specimen collection, handling, and shipping.

MYXOVIRUSES

INFLUENZA

Because children have little prior experience with influenza, infection is common. Upper respiratory infection is typical. More severe disease may be seen at any age, but lower respiratory tract symptoms are more common in children under the age of 5, especially with primary influenza infection. Spread is respiratory. Neonates are partially protected by maternal antibody.

Although only three main types (A/H1N1, A/H3N2, B) have been prevalent recently, antigenic shift and drift ensure the supply of susceptible hosts of all ages.

Clinical Findings

A. History: Prior exposure to a respiratory infection is common but not specific unless the contact had classic influenza symptoms during an epidemic. The incubation period is 2–7 days, similar to that of other respiratory viruses but shorter than that of *Mycoplasma pneumoniae* (10–20 d).

B. Symptoms and Signs: Classic influenza in older children and adults is characterized by sudden onset of high fever, severe myalgia, headache, and chills. These overshadow the associated coryza, pharyngitis, and cough. Usually absent are rash, marked conjunctivitis, adenopathy, exudative pharyngitis, arthritis, jaundice, and dehydrating enteritis. Diarrhea and vomiting are common in infants. Unusual clinical findings or variants include the following: croup (a severe form due to type A may occur), myositis (especially calf muscles), abdominal pain, myocarditis, parotitis, encephalopathy (distinct from Reye's syndrome); nephritis, and a transient maculopapular rash.

Acute illness lasts 2–5 days. Cough and fatigue last several weeks.

C. Laboratory Findings: Leukocyte counts are normal to low with variable shift. The virus may be found in respiratory mucosal cells by rapid fluorescent antibody (FA) staining or enzyme immunoassay (EIA). It can also be cultured within 3–5 days from pharyngeal swabs or throat washings. Other body fluids or tissue (except lung) rarely yield the virus. Diagnosis may also be made with paired serology, using hemagglutination inhibition.

D. Imaging: The chest x-ray film is nonspecific; it may show hyperaeration, peribronchial thickening, diffuse interstitial infiltrates, or bronchopneumonia in severe cases. Pneumothorax may occur. Hilar nodes are not enlarged. Pleural effusion is rare in uncomplicated influenza.

Table 27–1. Viral Causes of common clinical syndromes.

Rash	**Pneumonia**
Enterovirus	RSV[7]
Adenovirus	Adenovirus
Measles	Parainfluenza
Rubella	Measles
HHV-6[1]	Varicella[8]
Varicella	Rhinovirus[7]
Parvovirus B19[2]	CMV[7,8]
EBV	**Enteritis**
Dengue	Rotavirus
Fever	Enteric adenovirus
Enterovirus	Hepatitis A[9]
Adenovirus	Enterovirus
EBV	Norwalk agent
HHV-6[1]	Calicivirus
Arbovirus	**Hepatitis**
Colorado tick fever	Hepatitis A, B[9],C
CMV	Hepatitis non-A, non-B,
Influenza	(other)
Many others	EBV
Conjunctivitis	CMV
Adenovirus	Adenovirus
Enterovirus 70	Yellow fever
Influenza	**Arthritis**
Measles	Parvovirus B19
Herpes simplex[3]	Rubella
Parotitis	Arbovirus
Mumps	**Congenital Infection**
Parainfluenza	CMV
Enterovirus	Rubella
Influenza	HIV
CMV	Parvovirus B19
EBV	Enterovirus
HIV	Varicella
Pharyngitis	HSV
Adenovirus	**Meningoencephalitis**
Enterovirus	Enterovirus
EBV	Mumps
HSV[4]	Arbovirus
Influenza	HSV
Adenopathy	CMV
EBV	Lymphocytic choriomeningi-
CMV	tis virus
Rubella[5]	Measles
HIV	Varicella
Croup	Rabies
Parainfluenza	Adenovirus
Influenza	HIV
Adenovirus	EBV
Measles	
Bronchiolitis	
RSV[6]	
Adenovirus	
Parainfluenza	
Influenza	

CMV = cytomegalovirus; EBV = Epstein-Barr virus; HIV = human immunodeficiency virus; HHV-6 = human herpes virus type 6; HSV = herpes simplex virus.
[1]Roseola agent.
[2]Erythema infectiosum agent.
[3]Conjunctivitis rare, only in primary infections; keratitis in older patients.
[4]May cause isolated phayngeal vesicles at any age.
[5]May cause adenopathy without rash.
[6]Over 90% of cases.
[7]Usually only in young infants.
[8]Immunosuppressed, pregnant (varicella only), rarely other adults.
[9]Anicteric cases more common in children; these may resemble viral gastritis.

Differential Diagnosis

The following may be considered: all other respiratory viruses, *M pneumoniae* or *c pneumoniae* (longer incubation period, prolonged illness), streptococcal pharyngitis (pharyngeal exudate or petechiae, adenitis, no cough), bacterial sepsis (petechial or purpuric rash may occur), meningitis, toxic shock syndrome (rash, hypotension), arboviral infections (fewer respiratory symptoms, summer onset), and rickettsial infections (rash, different season, insect exposure).

Complications & Sequelae

Secondary bacterial infections (especially staphylococcal) of the middle ear, sinuses, or lungs are most common. Of the viral infections that precede Reye's syndrome, varicella and influenza (usually type B) are the most notable. During an influenza outbreak, ill children who develop protracted vomiting or altered behavior should be evaluated for Reye's syndrome (see Chapter 21). Influenza can also cause a viral or postviral encephalitis with symptoms much more prominent than those of the accompanying respiratory infection.

Children with underlying cardiopulmonary disease may develop severe viral pneumonia.

Prevention

Influenza vaccine is moderately protective in older children (see Chapter 6). Type A infections may be prevented by amantadine (3 mg/kg/dose orally, 2 times a day, max 200 mg/d). The physician should consider administering amantadine during an epidemic to high-risk children who cannot be immunized or who have not yet developed immunity (about 6 weeks after primary vaccination or 2 weeks after a booster dose).

Therapy & Prognosis

Therapy consists of general support and management of pulmonary complications, especially bacterial superinfections. Ribavirin is active in vitro. The efficacy of aerosolized ribavirin in humans is controversial, but it may be tried in severe infections or compromised hosts. Amantidine (same dose as above) is of some benefit if begun within 48 hours of onset.

Recovery is usually complete unless severe cardiopulmonary or neurologic damage has occurred.

Glezen WP et al: Acute respiratory disease associated with influenza epidemics in Houston, 1981–1983. *J Infect Dis* 1987;**155**:1119.

Liou Y et al: Children hospitalized with influenza B infection. *Pediatr Inf Dis* 1987;**6**:541. [Clinical review. All children less than 3 years of age.]

PARAINFLUENZA

Parainfluenza virus (types 1–4) is most notable as a cause of croup. Most infants are infected with type

Table 27–2. Diagnostic tests for viral infections

Agent	Rapid Antigen Detection (Specimen)	Tissue Culture (Days to Positive; Mean, Range)	Serology Acute	Serology Paired	Comments
Adenovirus	–	+10(1–21)	–	+	"Enteric" strains detected by electron microscopy of stool or culture on special cell line
Arboviruses	–	–	+	+	Acute serum may diagnose Eastern equine; mouse inoculation possible
Colorado tick fever	–	–	–	+	Mouse inoculation may be used; antigen may be detected in red blood cells
Cytomegalovirus	+(Ur, T, Rs)	+(1–28)	–*	+	Use culture followed by antigen detection (EIA):
Enterovirus	–	+4(2–15)	–	+	No serology available for many coxsackie A viruses, echoviruses
Epstein-Barr virus	–	–	+	+	Single serologic panel defines infection status; heterophil titer less specific
Hepatitis A	–	–	+	+	Usually diagnosed by presence of IgM antibody
Hepatitis B	+(B)	–	+	+	Infection diagnosed by presence of surface antigen or anti-core IgM antibody
Herpes simplex	+(Sk, Rs, CSF, T)	+2(1–5)	–	+	Serology rarely used for herpes simplex. Tzanck preparation of vesicle easy, 50% sensitive
Human herpes-6	–	–	–	–	Roseola agent
Human immunodeficiency virus	+(B)	+10(5–28)	+	+	Antibody proves infection unless passively acquired (age 15 m), culture not widely available
Influenza	+(Rs)	+3(2–7)	–	+	Antigen detection 50% sensitive
Measles	–(Rs)	+(5–14)	+	+	Difficult to grow; IgM serology available
Mumps	–(Rs CSF)	+(>5)	+	+	Complement fixation titers may allow single specimen diagnosis
Parvovirus B19	–	–	–	–	Erythema infectiosum agent; serologic tests being studied
Parainfluenza	+(Rs)	+5(2–10)	–	+	
Rabies	+(Sk, T)	–	–	+	Usually diagnosed by antigen detection in cornea, skin
Respiratory syncytial virus	+(Rs)	+5(3–14)	–	+	Rapid antigen detection reliable
Rhinovirus	–	+4(2–7)	–	–	Too many types to diagnose serologically
Rotavirus	+(Fe)	–	–	–	Usually detected by electron microscopy or antigen detection
Rubella	–	+(>10)	–*	+	Recommended that paired sera be tested simultaneously
Varicella-zoster	+(Sk, T)	+7(3–14)	–	+	Tzanck preparation useful

[1]Ur = urine; T = tissue biopsy; B = blood; Sk = skin; Rs = respiratory secretions; CSF = cerebrospinal fluid; Fe = feces; + = Commercially or widely available; – = Not available commercially; –* = Specific antibody titers available by arrangement with individual research laboratories or the Centers for Disease Control, Atlanta, Georgia. Results from some commercial laboratories are unreliable.

3 in the first 2 years of life; all types may cause outbreaks. The season and extent vary by location and prior immunity. In many areas, extensive outbreaks occur every other fall.

Clinical diseases include febrile upper respiratory infection, laryngitis, croup, and bronchiolitis (second most common cause after respiratory syncytial virus); pneumonia occurs in infants and immunodeficient children.

There is no specific therapy or vaccine. Croup management is discussed in Chapter 15. Ribavirin is active in vitro and has been used in immunocompromised children, but it is still experimental.

Glezen WP et al: Parainfluenza virus type 3: Seasonality and risk of infection and reinfection in young children. *J Infect Dis* 1984;**150**:851. [Excellent epidemiologic study.]

Welliver R et al: Natural history of parainfluenza virus infection in childhood. *J Pediatr* 1982;**101**:180.

Welliver RC et al: Parainfluenza virus bronchiolitis. *Am J Dis Child* 1986;**140**:34.

MUMPS

Essentials of Diagnosis

- No prior mumps vaccine; exposure 14–21 days previously.
- Parotid gland swelling.
- Aseptic meningitis with or without parotitis.
- Orchitis, pancreatitis, or oophoritis.

General Considerations

Mumps is one of the classic childhood infections; the virus attacks almost all unimmunized children (asymptomatically in 30–40% of cases) and produces lifelong immunity. The vaccine is so efficacious that clinical disease is rare in immunized children. Due to the many subclinical infections, 95% of adults with no history of mumps are seropositive.

Clinical Findings

A. History: A history of exposure to a child with parotitis is not proof of mumps exposure. In an adequately immunized individual, parotitis is usually due to another virus.

B. Symptoms and Signs:

1. Salivary Gland Disease—Tender swelling of one or more glands, variable fever, and facial lymphedema are typical. Parotid involvement is most common. The ear is displaced upward and outward; the mandibular angle is obliterated. Systemic toxicity is usually absent. Parotid stimulation with sour foods may be quite painful. Stensen's duct may be red and swollen; yellow secretions may be expressed, but pus is absent.

2. Meningoencephalitis—Prior to widespread immunization, mumps was the most common cause of aseptic meningitis, which would occur in up to 50% of cases, usually manifested by mild headache or asymptomatic pleocytosis. Cerebral symptoms have no direct relation to the parotid symptoms. Although neck stiffness, nausea, and vomiting can occur, encephalitic symptoms are rare; recovery in 3–10 days is the rule.

3. Pancreatitis—Abdominal pain associated with parotitis may represent transient pancreatitis. Because salivary disease may elevate serum amylase, specific markers of pancreatic function (lipase, amylase isoenzymes) need to be assayed.

4. Orchitis, Oophoritis—Involvement of these glands is associated with fever and local tenderness and swelling. Orchitis is unusual in children but occurs in up to a third of affected postpubertal males. Usually it is unilateral and resolves in 1–2 weeks. Although a third of infected testes atrophy, bilateral involvement and total sterility are rare. Atrophic testes may become malignant.

5. Other—Thyroiditis, mastitis, arthritis, and presternal edema (occasionally with dysphagia or hoarseness) may be seen.

C. Laboratory Findings: Leukocyte counts are usually normal. Up to 1000 leukocytes (predominantly lymphocytes) may be present in the spinal fluid, with mildly elevated protein and normal to slightly decreased glucose. Viral culture of saliva, throat, urine, or spinal fluid may be positive. Paired sera assayed by enzyme immuno assay is currently used for diagnosis. Complement-fixing antibody to the soluble antigen disappears in several months; its presence in a single specimen thus indicates recent infection.

Differential Diagnosis

Mumps parotitis may resemble the following: cervical adenitis (the jaw angle may be obliterated, but the ear does not usually protrude; Stensen's duct is normal; leukocytosis and neutrophilia are observed), bacterial parotitis (pus in Stensen's duct, toxicity, exquisite tenderness); recurrent parotitis (idiopathic or associated with calculi), tumors, and tooth infections. Many viruses, including parainfluenza, enteroviruses, Epstein-Barr virus, cytomegalovirus, human immunodeficiency virus, and influenza, can cause parotitis.

Unless parotitis is also present, mumps meningitis resembles that caused by enteroviruses or early bacterial infection. An elevated amylase is a useful clue in this situation. Isolated pancreatitis is not distinguishable from many other causes of epigastric pain and vomiting. Mumps is a classic cause of orchitis, but torsion, epididymitis, hematomas, hernias, and tumors must also be considered.

Complications

The major neurologic complication is nerve deafness (usually unilateral), which may be transient, usually results in inability to hear high tones, and may occur without meningitis. Permanent damage is rare, occurring in less than 0.1% of cases of mumps. Aqueductal stenosis and hydrocephalus (especially following congenital infection), myocarditis, transverse myelitis, and facial paralysis are other rare complications.

Treatment & Prognosis

Treatment is supportive and includes provision of fluids, analgesics, and scrotal support for orchitis. Systemic steroids have been used for orchitis; surgery is not recommended.

Brunell PA:Mumps. Page 1628 in: *Textbook of Pediatric Infectious Diseases.* Feigin RD, Cherry JD (editors). Saunders, 1987. [Recent review of all aspects.]

Koskiniemi M et al: Clinical appearance and outcome in mumps encephalitis in children. *Acta Paediatr Scand* 1983;**72**:603.

RESPIRATORY SYNCYTIAL VIRUS (RSV) DISEASE

Essentials of Diagnosis
- Diffuse wheezing, tachypnea following upper respiratory symptoms in an infant (bronchiolitis).
- Hyperinflation on chest x-ray film.

General Considerations
RSV is the most important cause of lower respiratory tract illness in young children, accounting for over 90% of cases of bronchiolitis and many cases of pneumonia. Yearly winter outbreaks are seen, and attack rates are high; most children are infected in the first year of life. Despite the presence of serum antibody, reinfection is common. No vaccine is available.

Clinical Findings
A. History: Initial symptoms are those of an upper respiratory infection. Fever is common.

B. Symptoms and Signs: The classic disease is bronchiolitis, characterized by diffuse wheezing, variable fever, cough, tachypnea, difficulty feeding, and cyanosis if severe. Hyperinflation ("barrel chest" appearance), rales, rhonchi, wheezing, and retractions are present. Rash and conjunctivitis are unusual. The liver and spleen may be palpable because of lung hyperinflation, but are not enlarged. The disease usually lasts 3–7 days.

Apnea may be the presenting manifestation, especially in premature infants in the first few months of life; it usually resolves in the first day or 2 of illness, often being replaced by more obvious signs of bronchiolitis. No specific etiology for the apnea has been found, and it may occur with other respiratory infections as well.

C. Laboratory Findings: Routine tests are nonspecific. A markedly elevated leukocyte count should suggest bacterial superinfection (neutrophilia) or pertussis (lymphocytosis). Rapid detection of RSV antigen in nasal or pulmonary secretions by immunofluorescent staining or enzyme immunoassay is over 90% sensitive and specific compared to culture. Routine culture takes 3–7 days to turn positive.

D. Imaging: Diffuse hyperinflation and peribronchiolar thickening are most common; atelectasis and patchy infiltrates also occur in uncomplicated infection, but not consolidation or pleural effusion.

Differential Diagnosis
Although almost all cases of bronchiolitis are due to RSV during an epidemic, other viruses cannot be excluded. Mixed infections are not uncommon. Wheezing may be due to asthma, a foreign body, or other airway obstruction. RSV may closely resemble *Chlamydia* pneumonitis when fine rales are present and fever and wheezing are not prominent. The two may also coexist. Cystic fibrosis may resemble RSV; a positive family history or failure to thrive associated with hyponatremia or hypoalbuminemia should prompt a sweat chloride test. Pertussis should also be considered in this age group, especially if cough is prominent.

Complications
Secondary bacterial infection of middle ear or lung (usually due to pneumococcus or *Haemophilus influenzae*) is the most common complication. Sudden onset of fever and leukocytosis should suggest bacterial infection. Respiratory failure or apnea may require mechanical ventilation. Cardiac failure may occur due to pulmonary disease or myocarditis. RSV, as well as parainfluenza and influenza, can cause acute exacerbations of asthma.

Treatment
Children who are very hypoxic or cannot feed due to respiratory distress must be hospitalized and given humidified oxygen and tube or intravenous feedings. Antibiotics, decongestants, expectorants, and steroids are of no value in routine infections. The child should be in respiratory isolation.

Often a trial of brochodilator therapy is given to determine if bronchospasm coexists. Terbutaline (0.01/mg/kg; up to 0.25 mg) or epinephrine (0.01 mL of 1:1000 solution/kg up to 0.3 mL) may be administered subcutaneously or bronchodilator inhalation therapy may be used. Discontinue these if there is no improvement. If they do help, nebulized treatments (every 2–6 h, as needed) or intravenous or oral theophylline may be continued (see Chapter 15). Toxic levels of theophylline are easily reached in infants less than a year of age, and the level needs close monitoring for this reason.

Ribavirin is the only antiviral proved active against RSV in humans. It is given by continuous aerosolization (6 g in a 300 mL vial of water) by a special nebulizer (Small Particle Aerosol Generator, ICN Pharmaceuticals) for 12–18 h/d for 3–7 days. This agent has minimal effect on viral shedding and a measurable, but very modest, effect on disease severity. It is very expensive (about $250 per daily dose, wholesale cost). It is teratogenic in animals, but this is of unknown significance in humans. It should be used in a negative-pressure room preferably with additional respiratory care equipment capable of preventing contamination of the room air. Caregivers should wear masks, and pregnant women should not care for children receiving ribavirin. Bronchospasm may be exacerbated by this drug. It should be used with extreme caution in ventilated patients and only by therapists expert in pediatric ventilator management. In general, it should be considered for use only for children with underlying cardiopulmonary or immunologic diseases predisposing them to severe or fatal infections.

Prognosis

Although mild bronchiolitis does not produce long-term problems, 30–40% of patients hospitalized with this infection will wheeze later in childhood. Chronic restrictive lung disease and bronchiolitis obliterans are rare sequelae.

Hall CB et al: Long-term prospective study in children after respiratory syncytial virus infection. *J Pediatr* 1984;**105**:358.

Hall CB et al: Ribavirin treatment of respiratory syncytial viral infection in infants with underlying cardiopulmonary disease. *JAMA* 1985;**254**:3047.

Janai HK et al: Ribavirin: Adverse drug reactions, 1986 to 1988. *Pediatr Infect Dis J* 1990;**9**:209.

Krasinski K: Severe respiratory syncytial virus infection: Clinical features, nosocomial acquisition and outcome. *Pediatr Infect Dis J* 1985;**4**:250.

McConnochie KM, Roghman KJ: Bronciolitis as a possible cause of wheezing in childhood: New evidence. *Pediatrics* 1984;**74**:1.

Wohl MEB, Chernick V: Bronciolitis. *Amer Rev Respir Dis* 1978;**118**:759. [An excellent review with photos of pathologic and radiographic findings.]

MEASLES

Essentials of Diagnosis

- Exposure to measles 9–14 days previously.
- Prodrome of fever, cough, conjunctivitis, and coryza.
- Koplik's spots (few to countless small white papules on a diffusely red base on the buccal mucosa) 1–2 days prior to and after rash onset.
- Maculopapular rash spreading down from the face and hairline over 3 days and later becoming confluent.
- Leukopenia.

General Considerations

Until 1989 this classic childhood exanthem had greatly decreased in incidence in the USA because of vaccination against it (see Chapter 6). The recent increase in cases may be a result of no or improper immunization or of vaccine failure. The recommendation has been changed to include revaccination of all children upon entrance to primary or secondary school. The attack rate in susceptibles is extremely high; spread is respiratory. Morbidity and mortality in the developing world are substantial due to underlying malnutrition and secondary infections. Immunity following natural disease is lifelong.

Clinical Findings

A. History: A history of contact with a suspected case is often obtainable during an epidemic. Many suspected cases at other times are misdiagnoses of other viral infections. Since airborne spread is effi-

cient and patients are very contagious during the prodrome, no contact history may be obtained.

B. Symptoms and Signs: High fever and lethargy begin 8–14 days after exposure. Sneezing, eyelid edema, tearing, copious coryza, photophobia, and harsh cough ensue and worsen. Koplik's spots are almost pathognomonic for rubeola. They have rarely been described with rubella and enteroviral infection and may be absent in measles.

The discrete maculopapular rash spreads quickly over the face and trunk, coalescing to a bright red. As it involves the extremities, it fades from the face and is completely gone within 6 days; fine desquamation may occur. Fever usually falls 2–3 days after the onset of the rash.

The use of killed-virus vaccine until 1967 resulted in partial immunity; upon exposure to wild virus, some vaccinees develop a severe atypical measles characterized by peripheral rash, pneumonia, headache, high fever, and abdominal pain. Koplik's spots are absent. Many adults who were not reimmunized with live-virus vaccines are still at risk for this atypical disease. Mild cases of measles may be seen in infants with residual maternal antibody or in those given immune globulin.

C. Laboratory Findings: Total leukocyte counts may fall to $1500/\mu L$. An experienced cytologist may see multinucleated giant cells (Warthin-Finkeldey cells) in oral mucosal scrapings and in nasal secretions, but diagnosis is usually made by detection of IgM antibody in serum drawn at least 2 days after the onset of rash or by detection of a significant rise in antibody. Tissue culture may also be used, but it takes longer and is less sensitive in many laboratories. Direct detection of measles antigen by fluorescent staining of nasopharyngeal cell is promising.

D. Imaging: Chest radiographs often show perihilar infiltrates or parenchymal patchy densities. Secondary bacterial infection produces consolidation or effusion.

Differential Diagnosis

Table 27–3 lists other illnesses that may resemble measles and some distinguishing features.

Complications & Sequelae

A. Respiratory Complications: These occur in up to 15% of cases. Bacterial superinfection of lung, middle ear, sinus, and cervical nodes are most common. Bronchospasm, severe croup, and progressive viral pneumonia or bronchiolitis (in infants) also occur. Immunosuppressed patients are at much greater risk of fatal pneumonia.

B. Cerebral Complications: Encephalitis occurs in 1 in 1000 cases. Onset is usually within a week of rash appearance. Symptoms include combativeness, ataxia, vomiting, seizures, and coma. Lymphocytic pleocytosis and a mildly elevated protein level are usual findings of spinal fluid tests; spi-

Table 27-3. Red rashes in children

Disease	Incubation Period (Days)	Prodrome	Rash	Laboratory Tests	Comments, Other Diagnostic Features
Measles	9–14	Cough, rhinitis, conjunctivitis	Maculopapular; face to extremities; lasts 7–10 d; Koplik's spots	Leukopenia	Toxic. Bright red rash becomes confluent, may desquamate.
Rubella	14–21	Usually none	Mild maculopapular; rapid spread face to extremities; gone by day 4	Normal or leukopenia	Postauricular, occipital adenopathy common. Polyarthralgia in some older girls. Mild clinical illness.
Roseola (exanthem subitum)	10–14	Fever (3–4 d)	Pink, macular rash occurs at end of illness; transient	Normal	Fever often high, and disappears when rash develops; child appears well. Usually occurs in children 6 m–2 y of age.
Erythema infectiosum	13–18	None	Erythematous "slapped" cheeks; then reticular rash on extremities, trunk	Normal; (reticulocytopenia)	Fifth disease. Rash may reappear over weeks, especially with exposure to heat, sunlight. May cause arthralgia/arthritis, usually in older children or adults. Red cell maturation arrest in children with chronic hemolysis can cause aplastic crisis.
Enterovirus	2–7	Variable fever, chills, myalgia, sore throat	Usually macular, maculopapular on trunk or palms, soles; vesicles, petechiae also seen	Variable	Varied rashes may resemble those of many other infections. Pharyngeal or hand-foot-mouth vesicles with certain coxsackie A types.
Streptococcal scarlet fever	1–7	Fever, abdominal pain, headache, sore throat	Diffuse erythema, "sandpaper" texture; neck, axillae, inguinal areas; spreads to rest of body; desquamates 7–14 d	Leukocytosis; positive group A streptococcus culture of throat or wound	Strawberry tongue, red pharynx with or without exudate. Eyes, perioral area, palms, and soles spared. Pastia's lines. Brief prodrome. Mild variant, scarlatina. Usually occurs in children 2–10 y of age.
Staphylococcal scarlet fever	1–7	Variable fever	Diffuse erythroderma; resembles streptococcal scarlet fever except eyes may be hyperemic, no coated "strawberry" tongue, pharynx spared	Variable leukocytosis if infected	Focal *Staphylococcus aureus* infection may be present.
Staph scalded skin	Variable	Irritability, absent to low fever	Painful erythroderma, followed in 1–2 d by dry cracking around eyes, mouth; bullae form with friction (Nikolsky's sign)	Normal if colonized only by staph; leukocytosis and sometimes bacteremia if infected	Normal pharynx. Look for focal staph infection. Usually occurs in infants.
Toxic shock syndrome	Variable	Fever, myalgia, headache, diarrhea, vomiting	Nontender erythroderma; red eyes, palms, soles, pharynx, lips	Leukocytosis; abnormal liver enzymes, coagulation tests; proteinuria	*S aureus* infection (especially vaginal during menses), multiorgan involvement. Swollen hands, feet. Hypotension or shock.
Erythema multiforme	—	Usually none or related to underlying cause	Discrete, red maculopapular lesions; symmetric, distal, palms and soles; target lesions classic	Normal or eosinophilia	Reaction to drugs (especially sulfas), or infectious agents. Uriticaria, arthralgia also seen.
Stevens-Johnson syndrome	—	Pharyngitis, conjunctivitis, fever, malaise	Bullous erythema multiforme; may slough in large areas; hemorrhagic lips; purulent conjunctivitis	Leukocytosis	Classic precipitants are drugs (especially sulfas), *Mycoplasma pneumoniae* infections. Pneumonitis and urethritis also seen.
Drug allergy	—	No fever or fever, myalgia, pruritus	Macular, maculopapular, urticarial, or erythroderma	Leukopenia, eosinophilia	Rash variable. Severe reactions may resemble measles, scarlet fever; adenopathy, hepatosplenomegaly, marked toxicity possible.
Kawaski syndrome	Unknown	Fever, cervical adenopathy, irritability	Polymorphous (may be erythroderma) on trunk and extremities; red palms and soles, lips, tongue, pharynx	Leukocytosis, thrombocytosis, elevated ESR; negative cultures and streptococcal serology	Swollen hands, feet; prolonged illness; bulbar hyperemia; uveitis; no response to antibiotics. Vasculitis and aneurysms of coronary and other arteries occur.
Leptospirosis	4–19	Fever, myalgia, chills	Variable erythroderma	Leukocytosis; hematuria, proteinuria; hyperbilirubinemia	Conjunctivitis; toxic. Hepatitis, aseptic meningitis may be seen. Rodent, dog contact.

nal fluid may be normal. Fifty percent die or are severely damaged.

Subacute sclerosing panencephalitis occurs years later in about 1 in 100,000 previously infected children. This progressive cerebral deterioration with myoclonic jerks is fatal in 6–12 months. It may occur following administration of vaccine, with an estimated incidence of 1 in 1,000,000. High titers of measles antibody are present in serum and spinal fluid. Virus has been cultured from brain using special techniques, supporting the hypothesis that this paneuchephalitis is a latent measles infection.

C. Other Complications: These include hemorrhagic or "black" measles (severe disease with multiorgan bleeding, fever, cerebral symptoms), thrombocytopenia, appendicitis, keratitis, myocarditis, optic neuritis, reactivation or progression of tuberculosis (including transient cutaneous anergy), and premature delivery or stillbirth.

Treatment, Prognosis, & Prevention

Recovery generally occurs 7 to 10 days after onset of symptoms. Therapy is supportive: eye care, cough relief (avoid narcotic suppressants in infants), and fever reduction (acetaminophen, lukewarm baths; avoid salicylates). Secondary bacterial infections should be treated promptly; antimicrobial prophylaxis is not indicated. Ribavirin is active in vitro and being studied in human infections.

Vaccination prevents the disease in susceptible contacts if given within 72 hours (see Chapter 6). Suspected cases should be diagnosed promptly and reported to the local health department.

Aaby P et al: High measles mortality in infancy related to intensity of exposure. *J Pediatr* 1986;**109**:40.

Kipps A, Dick G, Moodie JW: Measles and the central nervous system. *Lancet* 1983;**2**:1406.

Markowitz LE et al: Patterns of transmission in measles outbreaks in the United States, 1985–1986. *N Engl J Med* 1989;**320**:75.

Narain JP et al: Imported measles outbreak in a university. *Am J Public Health* 1985;**75**:397.

PICORNAVIRUSES

The picornaviruses are small RNA viruses that include the enteroviruses (poliovirus, 3 types; echovirus, 32 types; and coxsackievirus, 24 type A, 6 type B), rhinoviruses (more than 100 types), and hepatitis A.

ENTEROVIRAL INFECTIONS

Enteroviruses are a major cause of illness in children. They are physically and biochemically similar and may produce identical syndromes. The multiple types make vaccine development impractical and have hindered development of antigen-detection and serologic tests. Recent discovery of common RNA fragments and group antigens should improve future diagnostic capability. Tissue culture is the best diagnostic method for echoviruses, polioviruses, and coxsackie B viruses. Many coxsackie A viruses fail to grow.

Transmission is fecal-oral. Multiple enteroviruses circulate in the community at any one time; although summer–fall outbreaks are common, illness is seen year round. After poliovirus, coxsackie B virus is most virulent, followed by echovirus. Neurologic, cardiac, and overwhelming neonatal infections are the severest forms of illness.

1. ACUTE FEBRILE ILLNESS

Accompanied by nonspecific upper respiratory or enteric symptoms, sudden onset of fever and irritability in young infants is often enteroviral in origin. Occasionally, a petechial rash is seen; more often, a diffuse maculopapular eruption (often prominent on palms and soles) occurs on the second to fourth day of fever. Rapid recovery is the rule. Leukocyte counts are usually normal. Many types of coxsackievirus and echovirus may cause this presentation, which often prompts an evaluation for bacteremia or meningitis.

2. RESPIRATORY TRACT ILLNESSES

A. Nonspecific, Febrile Upper Respiratory Infection with Pharyngitis: This infection is most common. Pneumonia or wheezing is unusual.

B. Herpangina: This syndrome is characterized by acute onset of fever and posterior pharyngeal ulcers, often linearly arranged on the anterior fauces. Single "kissing" faucial ulcers may also be seen. Dysphagia, vomiting, and anorexia also occur and rarely parotitis or vaginal ulcers. Symptoms disappear in a week. The epidemic form is due to a variety of coxsackie A viruses; coxsackie B viruses and echoviruses cause sporadic cases.

The differential diagnosis includes primary herpes simplex gingivostomatitis (ulcers are more prominent anteriorly and gingivitis is present); aphthous stomatitis (fever absent, recurrent episodes, anterior lesions); trauma; burns (usually not discrete); hand-foot-and-mouth disease (see below); Vincent's angina (spreading painful ulcer from the gum line, underlying dental disease).

C. Acute Lymphonodular Pharyngitis: Coxsackievirus A10 has been associated with a febrile pharyngitis characterized by nonulcerating yellow-white posterior pharyngeal papules. The duration is 1–2 weeks; therapy is supportive.

D. Pleurodynia (Bornholm Disease, Devil's Grip): Caused by coxsackie B virus (epidemic form) or many nonpolio enteroviruses (sporadic form), pleurodynia presents with abrupt onset of unilateral pleuritic pain of variable intensity. Symptoms are episodic; relapses are seen. Associated symptoms include headache, fever, vomiting, and abdominal and neck pain. Physical findings include fever, chest muscle tenderness, decreased thoracic excursion, and occasionally a friction rub. The chest x-ray film is normal. Hematologic tests are nondiagnostic.

Differential diagnosis includes bacterial pneumonia, empyema, tuberculosis, and coccidioidomycosis (all excluded radiographically), costochondritis (no fever or other symptoms), and a variety of abdominal problems, especially those causing diaphragmatic irritation.

There is no specific therapy. Potent analgesic agents and chest splinting alleviate the pain.

3. RASHES

The rash may be macular, maculopapular, urticarial, scarlatiniform, petechial, or vesicular. One of the most characteristic is that of hand-foot-and-mouth disease (caused by coxsackievirus, especially types A5, A10, and A16), in which vesicles or red papules are found on the tongue, oral mucosa, hands, and feet. Associated fever and malaise are mild. The rash may appear when fever abates, simulating roseola.

4. CARDIAC INVOLVEMENT

Myocarditis and pericarditis may be caused by a number of nonpolio enteroviruses, particularly type B coxsackieviruses; disease may be mild or fatal. In infants, other organs may be involved at the same time; in older patients, cardiac disease is usually isolated (see Chapter 16 for therapy).

5. SEVERE NEONATAL INFECTION

Sporadic and nosocomial nursery cases of severe systemic enteroviral disease occur. Clinical manifestations include combinations of fever, rash, pneumonitis, encephalitis, hepatitis, gastroenteritis, myocarditis, pancreatitis, and myositis. The differential diagnosis includes bacterial and herpes infections, necrotizing enterocolitis, other causes of heart or liver failure, and metabolic diseases. Diagnosis is suggested by the finding of pleocytosis and confirmed by the isolation of virus from urine, stool, cerebrospinal fluid, or pharynx. Strict isolation is needed; therapy is supportive. The role of intravenous immunoglobulin is not defined.

6. CENTRAL NERVOUS SYSTEM ILLNESSES

Poliomyelitis
A. Essentials of Diagnosis:
- Usually no prior immunization.
- Headache, fever, nausea, vomiting, muscle weakness.
- Asymptomatic, flaccid paralysis; muscle tenderness; intact sensation; late atrophy.
- Aseptic meningitis.

B. General Considerations: Poliovirus infection is subclinical in 90–95% of cases, causes nonspecific febrile illness in about 5%, and causes aseptic meningitis or paralytic disease in only 1–3%. In endemic areas, most older children and adults are immune because of prior inapparent infections. Most cases in the USA occur in patients who have traveled to foreign countries or who are immunodeficient. Severe poliovirus infections can rarely follow oral poliovirus vaccination, as a result of reversion of the vaccine virus. The incidence varies from 1 in 3–10 million doses, depending on virus type and age of the vaccinee.

C. Clinical Findings:

1. Symptoms and Signs—The initial symptoms are fever, myalgia, sore throat, and headache for 2–6 days. Several symptom-free days are followed by signs of aseptic meningitis—recurrent fever, headache, stiff neck, spinal rigidity, and nausea. Mild cases resolve completely. High fever, severe myalgia, and anxiety usually portend progression to loss of reflexes and subsequent flaccid paralysis. Sensation remains intact. The disease progression is variable, especially in infants.

Paralysis is usually asymmetric. Bulbar involvement affects swallowing, speech, and cardiorespiratory function and accounts for most deaths. Paralysis is usually complete by the time the temperature normalizes. Weakness usually resolves completely. Most improvement of paralysis occurs within 6 months; the remainder, during the next 18 months.

2. Laboratory Findings—In patients with meningeal symptoms, the cerebrospinal fluid has up to several hundred leukocytes (mostly lymphocytes); glucose level is normal, and protein concentration is mildly elevated. Poliovirus is relatively easy to grow in cell culture and can be readily differentiated from other enteroviruses. It may be isolated from spinal fluid for 3–5 days after meningitis is appreciated or from throat and stool for several weeks following infection. Paired serology is also diagnostic. Differentiation of wild from live attenuated vaccine strains requires expertise. Paired serology is also helpful in this differentiation.

D. Differential Diagnosis: Aseptic meningitis due to poliovirus is indistinguishable from that due to other viruses. Paralytic disease may be due to nonpolio enteroviruses. Polio may resemble Guillain-Barré syndrome (variable sensory loss, symmetric loss of function, minimal pleocytosis, high protein concentration in spinal fluid), polyneuritis (sensory loss), pseudoparalysis due to bone or joint problems (eg, trauma, infection), botulism, or tick paralysis.

E. Complications & Sequelae: Complications are the result of the acute and permanent effects of paralysis. Respiratory, pharyngeal, bladder, and bowel malfunction are most critical. Assisted ventilation, tracheostomy, and enteral feeding may be needed. Deaths are usually due to complications arising from respiratory dysfunction.

F. Treatment & Prognosis: Therapy is supportive. Bed rest, fever and pain control (heat therapy is helpful), and careful attention to progression of weakness (particularly of respiratory muscles) are important. Intubation or tracheostomy for secretion control and catheter drainage of the bladder may be needed. Paralysis is mild in about 30%, permanent in 15%, and results in death in 5–10%. Disease is worse in adults and pregnant women than in children.

Hovi T et al: Outbreak of paralytic poliomyelitis in Finland: Widespread circulation of antigenically altered poliovirus type 3 in a vaccinated population. *Lancet* 1986; **1:**1427.

Moore LM et al: Poliomyelitis in the United States 1969–1981. *J Infect Dis* 1982;**146:**558.

Nikowane BM et al: Vaccine associated paralytic poliomyelitis. *JAMA* 1987;**257:**1335.

Aseptic Meningitis

A. General Considerations: Nonpolio enteroviruses cause over 80% of cases of aseptic meningitis at all ages. In the summer and fall, multiple cases may be seen associated with circulation of neurotropic strains. Nosocomial outbreaks also occur; severe disease and death may occur in neonates. Spread is fecal-oral.

B. Clinical Findings:

1. History—The usual enteroviral incubation period is 4–6 days. Since enteroviral infections may be subclinical, a history of contact with a patient with meningitis is unusual. Neonates may acquire infection from maternal blood, vaginal secretions or feces at birth; occasionally, the mother has had a febrile illness just prior to delivery.

2. Symptoms and Signs—Onset is usually acute with variable fever—up to 40.5°C (105°F)—marked irritability, and lethargy in infants. Older children also describe frontal headache, photophobia, and myalgia. Abdominal pain, diarrhea, and vomiting may occur. The incidence of rash varies with the infecting strain. If rash occurs, it is usually seen after several days of illness and is diffuse, macular or maculopapular, occasionally petechial, but not purpuric. Oropharyngeal vesicles and rash on the palms and soles suggest an enteroviral etiology. The anterior fontanelle may be full. In older children, it is easier to demonstrate neck stiffness, Kernig's sign, and Brudzinski's sign. Seizures are unusual, and focal neurologic findings so rare that they suggest another agent or diagnosis. Frank encephalitis is rare at all ages, although more common in neonates.

3. Laboratory Findings—Leukocyte counts are nonspecific and often within the normal range. The spinal fluid contains 50–500 leukocytes/μL. Early in the illness, polymorphonuclear cells predominate; a shift to mononuclear cells occurs later. In about 95% of cases, spinal fluid parameters include total leukocyte count <3000/μL, protein <80 mg/dL, and glucose >40% of serum values. Marked deviation from any of these values should prompt consideration of another diagnosis (see below). Cerebral imaging is not often indicated; if done, it is usually normal; subdural effusions, infarcts, edema, or focal abnormalities seen in bacterial meningitis are absent. The syndrome of inappropriate secretion antidiuretic hormone may occur but is rarely clinically significant.

Culture of cerebrospinal fluid may yield an enterovirus within a few days; virus may be found in acellular spinal fluids. Isolation of an enterovirus from throat or stool suggests but does not prove enteroviral meningitis. Vaccine poliovirus may be present in feces in infants being evaluated for aseptic meningitis; it does not cause the illness.

C. Differential Diagnosis: In the prevaccine era, mumps and polio were leading causes of aseptic meningitis. Other viral agents include arbovirus and herpes simplex. In adolescents, herpesvirus type 2 may cause concomitant aseptic meningitis and genital infection. In neonates, early herpesvirus meningoencephalitis may mimic enteroviral disease (see the section on herpesviruses, below). Other entities that may resemble enteroviral infection include partially treated bacterial meningitis (recent antibiotic treatment, spinal fluid parameters resembling those seen in bacterial disease, bacterial antigen possibly detected in cerebrospinal fluid); parameningeal focus of bacterial infection such as brain abscess, subdural empyema, mastoiditis (predisposing factors, glucose level in cerebrospinal fluid possibly lower, focal neurologic signs); tumors or cysts (malignant cells possibly detected by cytologic exam, longer history of neurologic symptoms, higher protein concentration or lower glucose level in cerebrospinal fluid); trauma (presence, without exception, of red blood cells, which are often assumed due to traumatic lumbar puncture but are crenated and fail to clear); vasculitis (other systemic or neurologic signs; older children); tuberculous or fungal meningitis (see Chapter 28); cysticercosis; parainfectious encephalopathies (*Mycoplasma pneumoniae*, respiratory viruses); Lyme disease; and leptospirosis.

D. Treatment & Prevention: There is no specific therapy. Infants are usually hospitalized, isolated, and treated with fluids and antipyretics. If they are moderately to severely ill, infants are given antibiotics for bacterial pathogens (including ampicillin for infants less than 3 months old for the possibility of *Listeria monocytogenes*) until cultures are negative for 48–72 hours. If patients, especially older children, are mildly ill, antibiotics may be withheld and a repeat lumbar puncture done in 8–12 hours; with viral infection, the Gram's stain is again negative, the cell count does not rise substantially, and there is a further shift to mononuclear cells. In these cases, children who are clinically stable may be closely observed in the hospital or at home. Pain relief may be needed. With clinical deterioration, repeat lumbar puncture, cerebral imaging, neurologic consultation, and more aggressive diagnostic tests (eg, viral cultures, brain biopsy) should be considered. Herpesvirus encephalitis is of graver concern in such cases, particularly in infants 1 month of age or younger.

Measures to prevent enteroviral infection include good hygiene, scrupulous hand washing, and proper isolation in the hospital.

Prognosis: In general, enteroviral meningitis has no significant sequelae; mild developmental delay may follow infection in the first few months of life. Unlike mumps, enteroviruses rarely cause hearing loss. Frank encephalitis may cause diffuse brain damage.

Cherry JD: Aseptic meningitis and viral meningitis. Page 478 in: *Textbook of Pediatric Infectious Disease.* Feigin RD, Cherry JD (editors). Saunders, 1987.

Sumaya CV, Corman LI: Enteroviral meningitis in early infancy: Significance in community outbreaks. *Pediatr Infect Dis J* 1982;**1**:151.

Wilfert CM, Lehrman SN, Katz SL: Enteroviruses and meningitis. *Pediatr Infect Dis J* 1983;**2**:333.

RHINOVIRAL INFECTIONS

The many serotypes of this virus are best known as agents of the common cold. Profuse rhinorrhea, sneezing, cough, mild pharyngitis, and mild fever are typical. They have been isolated from the lower respiratory tract in normal infants and children and in immunosuppressed patients. Therapy is supportive.

HERPESVIRUSES

HERPES SIMPLEX

Essentials of Diagnosis

- Grouped vesicles on an erythematous base.
- Recurrent episodes in many patients.
- Tender regional adenopathy, especially with primary infection.

General Considerations

There are two types of herpes simplex viruses (HSV). Type 1 causes most oral, skin, and cerebral disease. Type 2 causes most genital and congenital infections. Latent infection in sensory ganglia routinely follows primary infection. Recurrences may be spontaneous, induced by external events (eg, fever, menstruation, or trauma) or immunosuppression. Transmission is by direct contact with infected secretions. Herpes simplex is the virus most susceptible to antiviral drugs.

Primary infection usually occurs early in childhood, although many adults (20%–50%) have never been infected. Primary infection with type 1 HSV is asymptomatic in 90% of cases and causes gingivostomatitis in the remainder. Type 2 HSV is mainly sexually transmitted. Infection with one type usually precludes infection with other strains of that type. Recurrent episodes are due to reactivation of latent virus.

Clinical Findings

A. History: The source of primary infection is often an asymptomatic excretor; at any one time, 1–2% of normal seropositive adults excrete type 1 HSV in the saliva. Prior infection and subclinical disease are so common that the history is of little diagnostic value.

B. Symptoms and Signs

1. Gingivostomatitis—High fever, irritability, and drooling are seen in infants. Multiple oral ulcers are seen on the tongue and buccal and gingival mucosa, occasionally extending to the pharynx. Pharyngeal ulcers may be predominate in older children. Diffusely swollen, red gums that are friable and bleed easily are typical. Cervical nodes are swollen and tender. Duration is 7–14 days. Herpangina, aphthous stomatitis, thrush, and Vincent's angina should be excluded.

2. Vulvovaginitis or Urethritis—Genital herpes in a prepubertal child should suggest sexual abuse. Vesicles or ulcers on the vulva, vagina, or penis and tender adenopathy are seen. Painful urination may cause retention. Primary infections last 7–14 days. Lesions may resemble folliculitis, trauma, syphilis, or chancroid in the adolescent, and bullous impetigo, trauma, severe chemical irritation, and burns in younger children.

3. Cutaneous Infections—Direct inoculation onto cuts (eg, herpetic whitlow on a thumb) or abrasions may produce localized or extensive vesicles or ulcers. A whitlow may be mistaken for a bacterial felon or paronychia; surgical drainage is of no value and contraindicated. HSV infection of eczematous skin may result in extensive areas of vesicles and shallow ulcers (eczema herpeticum), which may be mistaken for impetigo or varicella.

4. Recurrent Cutaneous Infection—Recurrent intra-oral herpes is usually asymptomatic. Perioral recurrences often begin with a prodrome of tingling or burning limited to the vermilion border, followed by vesiculation, scabbing, and crusting around the lips over the next few days. Rarely, intraoral lesions recur. Fever, adenopathy, and other symptoms are absent. Recurrent cutaneous herpes most closely resembles impetigo; the latter is often outside the perinasal and perioral region, responds to antibiotics, and yields *Streptococcus pyogenes* or *Staphylococcus aureus* on culture.

5. Keratoconjunctivitis—Caused by reactivation of virus latent in the ciliary ganglion, keratoconjunctivitis produces photophobia, pain, conjunctival irritation, and a dendritic corneal ulcer demonstrable with fluorescein staining. Stromal invasion may occur. Steroids should never be used without opthalmologic consultation. Conjunctivitis may be seen in neonates, but eye disease is not common in older children despite presumed frequent inoculation via infected secretions. Other causes of these symptoms include trauma and bacterial and viral (especially adenovirus) infection.

6. Encephalitis—Although unusual in infants outside the neonatal period, encephalitis may occur at any age and usually without cutaneous herpes lesions. HSV is probably the most common cause of sporadic severe encephalitis. Fever, headache, behavioral changes, and focal seizures (as a result of the typical temporal lobe involvement) occur. Early in infection, all studies may be normal. Later, mild mononuclear pleocytosis (often with erythrocytes) is present along with elevated protein concentration, which continues to rise on repeat lumbar punctures. Hypodense areas with a temporal lobe predilection are seen on cerebral images, and periodic focal epileptiform discharges (PLEDS) are seen on electroencephalograms. Viral cultures of spinal fluid are usually negative; a brain biopsy should be considered for specific diagnosis. Without early antiviral therapy, prognosis is very poor. Differential diagnosis includes mumps, arbovirus encephalitis, rabies, parainfectious encephalopathy, Reye's syndrome, acute demyelinating syndromes, and bacterial meningoencephalitis.

7. Neonatal Infections—The infection is acquired by ascending spread (5–10% of cases) prior to delivery or at the time of a vaginal delivery of a mother with genital infection. A history of genital herpes in the parents is usually absent. Within a few days to weeks, skin vesicles (especially at sites of trauma, such as the sites where scalp monitors were placed) appear in about half of infected infants. Some infants are acutely ill, presenting with jaundice, shock, bleeding or respiratory distress. Others appear well initially, but dissemination to brain or other organs usually occurs over the next week if the infection is untreated. Other infants present with only neurologic symptoms: apnea, lethargy, fever, poor feeding, or overt seizures. The skin lesions

may resemble impetigo, bacterial scalp abscesses, trauma, or miliaria. The systemic signs may be due to many other causes.

C. Laboratory Findings: Routine tests are nonspecific. A finding of lymphocytic pleocytosis is the rule in aseptic meningitis or encephalitis. Virus may be cultured from infected epithelial sites (vesicles, ulcers, or corneal scrapings) and from infected tissue (skin, brain) obtained by biopsy. Cultures of spinal fluid are seldom positive in older children, but often so (50%) in infants. Isolation from throat, eye, urine, or stool of a newborn is diagnostic. Vaginal culture of the mother may offer circumstantial evidence for the diagnosis.

HSV is a somewhat labile virus, and survival in transport media is impaired by prolonged contact with calcium alginate swabs. HSV tolerates heat and drying poorly. It often grows within 2–3 days in tissue culture. The value of serologic tests in older individuals is limited by the presence of antibody in all patients with latent infections, the lack of serologic rise during most reactivations, and cross reactivity between type 1 and 2 antibody. A negative convalescent titer, however, excludes HSV infection.

Rapid diagnostic tests include cytology of scrapings from the base of vesicles or ulcers using chemical stains (Tzanck test) to look for characteristic multinucleated giant cells or immunofluorescent stains to detect viral antigen.

Complications, Sequelae, & Prognosis

Gingivostomatitis may result in dehydration due to dysphagia; severe chronic oral disease and esophageal involvement may occur in immunosuppressed patients.

Severe primary vulvovaginitis may be associated with aseptic meningitis, paresthesias, autonomic dysfunction due to neuritis (urinary retention, constipation), and secondary candidal infection. The social implications and frequent recurrences may cause significant depression.

Extensive cutaneous disease (as in eczema) may be associated with dissemination, bacterial superinfection, and death.

Keratitis may result in blindness or perforation.

Untreated encephalitis is fatal in 70% of patients and causes severe damage in most of the remainder. When acyclovir treatment is instituted early, 20% die and 40% are normal.

Disseminated neonatal infection is often fatal in spite of therapy.

Treatment

A. Specific Measures: HSV is very sensitive to antiviral therapy. Topical antivirals are most effective for corneal disease and include 1% trifluridine, 3% acyclovir, and 3% vidarabine. Trifluridine appears superior; cure rates over 95% are reported. The dose is one drop every 2 hours while the patient is awake until the ulcer heals, then one drop every 4 hours for 7 more days. Vidarabine ointment requires fewer treatments and may be more practical for young children.

Moderate cutaneous HSV infections respond to oral administration of acyclovir. The main indication is severe genital HSV in adolescents; acyclovir (200 mg orally 5 times a day for 5–10 d) is beneficial for primary disease. Recurrent disease rarely requires therapy. Frequent recurrences may be suppressed by oral administration of acyclovir (200 mg) 3 times a day, but this regimen should be used sparingly. Other forms of severe cutaneous disease, such as eczema herpeticum and HSV infections in immunocompromised children, also respond. The safety and efficacy of acyclovir in prepubertal children are not known, and there are currently no specific indications for its use.

The only two parenteral drugs of value are acyclovir and vidarabine. Although they are equally effective in neonatal disease, acyclovir requires less free water administration, a potential advantage in patients with encephalitis. In encephalitis, acyclovir is superior; the dosage is 10 mg/kg every 8 hours intravenously for 14 days. The same dose is given to affected neonates for 14–21 days. Severe mucocutaneous disease, even in immunocompromised patients, is treated with 5 mg/kg every 8 hours.

No controlled studies support the administration of immune globulin for herpes infections.

Antiviral therapy does not alter the incidence or severity of recurrences of genital infection. Development of resistance to acyclovir is rare after standard courses but is increasingly reported in immunocompromised patients after prolonged therapy.

B. General Measures:

1. Gingivostomatitis — Gingivostomatitis is treated with pain relief and temperature control. Maintaining hydration is important due to the long duration (7–14 d). Nonacidic, cool fluids are best. Topical anesthetic agents (such as viscous lidocaine or an equal mixture of Kaopectate, diphenhydramine, and viscous lidocaine) may be used as a mouthwash for older children who won't swallow it; ingested xylocaine may be toxic to infants, however. Antiviral therapy is not generally indicated in normal hosts, although it could be considered for those with severe disease. Antibiotics are not helpful.

2. Genital Infections—Genital infections require pain relief, assistance with voiding (warm baths, topical anesthetics, rarely catheterization), and psychologic support. Lesions should be kept clean; drying decreases the potential for spread and may shorten the duration. Sexual contact should be avoided between the prodrome and crusting stages.

3. Cutaneous Lesions—Skin lesions should be kept clean, dry, and covered if possible to prevent spread. Systemic analgesics may be helpful. Second-

ary bacterial infection is uncommon in patients with lesions on mucosa or involving small areas. Secondary infection should be considered and treated if necessary (usually with an antistaphylococcal agent) in patients with more extensive lesions. *Candida* superinfection occurs in 10% of women with primary genital infections.

4. Recurrent Cutaneous Disease—Recurrent disease is usually milder than primary infection. Sun block lip balm helps prevent labial recurrences. There is no evidence that the many popular topical or vitamin therapies are efficacious.

5. Keratoconjunctivitis—An ophthalmologist should be consulted regarding the use of cycloplegics, antiinflammatory agents, local debridement, and other therapies.

6. Encephalitis—See Chapter 24.

7. Neonatal Infection—The affected infant should be isolated from other neonates or immunocompromised children. Therapy is supportive. A cesarian section is indicated if there are obvious maternal lesions, especially if these represent primary infection. In women with a prior history of genital HSV, vaginal delivery with peripartum cultures of maternal cervix and infant (conjuctiva, throat, skin) and meticulous clinical follow-up are recommended. Repeated cervical cultures during pregnancy are not recommended.

Steroids may exacerbate HSV infections not concomitantly treated with antivirals; their use in conjunction with antiviral therapy is discouraged (except in certain forms of ocular disease) due to lack of proved benefit and potential for impairing the immune response.

Arvin AM: Oral therapy with acyclovir in infants and children. *Pediatr Infect Dis J* 1987;**6**:56.

Arvin AM, Johnson RT, Whitley RJ, et al: Consensus management of the patient with herpes simplex encephalitis. *Pediatr Infect Dis J* 1987;**6**:2.

Brown ZA, Berry S, Vontver LA: Genital herpes simplex infection complicating pregnancy: Natural history and peripartum management. *J Reprod Med* 1986;**31(Suppl 5)**:420.

Bryson YJ: The use of acyclovir in children. *Pediatr Infect Dis J* 1984;**3**:345.

Corey L, Spear PG: Infections with herpes simplex viruses (parts 1 and 2). *N Engl J Med* 1986;**314**:686, 749.

Koskiniemi M et al: Neonatal herpes simples virus infection: A report of 43 patients. *Pediatr Infect Dis* 1989;**8**:30.

Whitley RJ: Neonatal herpes simplex infections: Presentation and management: *J Reprod Med* 1986;**31**:426.

VARICELLA (Chickenpox) & HERPES ZOSTER (Shingles)

Essentials of Diagnosis

Varicella:

■ Exposure to varicella or herpes zoster 10–20 days previously; no prior history of varicella.

- Widely scattered macules and papules rapidly progressing over 5–6 days to small, clear vesicles, then crusting. Different forms present at any one time. Variable fever and nonspecific systemic symptoms.

Herpes zoster:
- History of varicella.
- Local paresthesias and pain prior to eruption (more common in older children).
- Dermatomal distribution of grouped vesicles on erythematous base.
- Multinucleated giant cells on cytologic stain (Tzanck test) of scraping from vesicle base strongly suggestive of infection by herpes zoster or herpes simplex.

General Considerations

Primary infection results in varicella, which almost always confers lifelong immunity; the virus remains latent in sensory ganglia and reappears in 10–15% of individuals as shingles. The incidence of reactivation is increased in immunosuppressed patients. Spread from a contact with varicella during primary infection is respiratory with a > 95% infection rate in susceptibles. Infection may also be caused by direct contact with vesicles. Herpes zoster is about one third as infectious. Over 95% of young adults with a prior history of varicella are immune, as are 90% of native-born Americans who are unaware of having had varicella. Humans are the only reservoir.

Clinical Findings

A. History: Usually exposure to varicella has occurred 14–16 days previously (range 10–20 days). Contact with a patient with herpes zoster or mild varicella may go unrecognized. Although varicella is the most distinctive childhood exanthem, inexperienced observers may mistake other diseases for varicella. A 1–3 day prodrome of fever and respiratory symptoms may be seen in patients with varicella, especially older children. The preeruptive pain of shingles may last several days and resemble that of other illnesses.

B. Symptoms and Signs

1. Varicella—The usual case consists of mild systemic symptoms followed by crops of red macules that rapidly become tiny vesicles with surrounding erythema (''dew drop on a rose petal''), form pustules, become crusted and then scabbed over, and leave no scar. The rash appears predominantly on the trunk and face. Lesions occur in the scalp, nose, mouth (where they are nonspecific ulcers), and intestine (usually asymptomatic). Systemic symptoms usually parallel skin involvement. Up to 5 crops of lesions may be seen. New ones usually stop forming after 5–7 days. A zosterlike cluster of lesions may occur. If varicella occurs in the first few months of life, it is often mild due to persisting maternal anti-

body. Once crusting begins, the patient is no longer contagious.

2. Herpes zoster—The eruption of shingles involves a single dermatome, usually truncal or cranial. The rash does not cross the midline. Ophthalmic zoster may be associated with corneal involvement. The closely grouped vesicles often coalesce. The duration is 7–10 days before crusting. Postherpetic neuralgia is rare in children. A few vesicles are occasionally seen outside the involved dermatome.

C. Laboratory Findings: Leukocyte counts are normal or low. Leukocytosis suggests secondary bacterial infection. Tzanck tests must be carefully interpreted. Although cultures may be done, they take 7–21 days to turn positive and are thus of limited clinical value. Diagnosis may also be made with paired serology. Serum transaminase levels may be modestly elevated during normal varicella.

D. Imaging: Varicella pneumonia classically produces numerous bilateral nodular densities and hyperinflation. Abnormal chest x-ray films are not uncommon in young adults but do not necessarily portend a poor outcome.

Differential Diagnosis

Varicella is usually distinctive. Similar rashes include those of coxsackievirus infection (fewer lesions, lack of crusting), impetigo (fewer lesions, no classic vesicles, response to antimicrobial agents, perioral or peripheral lesions), papular urticaria (insect bite history, nonvesicular rash), scabies (burrows, no typical vesicles), parapsoriasis (rare in children under 10 years of age, chronic or recurrent, often a history of prior varicella), rickettsialpox (eschar at mite bite site, smaller lesions, no crusting), dermatitis herpetiformis (chronic, urticaria, residual pigmentation), and folliculitis.

Complications & Sequelae

Secondary bacterial infection with *Staphylococcus* spp or group A streptococcus is most common, presenting as impetigo, cellulitis, abscesses, scarlet fever, toxic shock syndrome, or sepsis.

Protracted vomiting or a change in sensorium suggests Reye's syndrome or encephalitis. In one study, subclinical, histologic Reye's syndrome was common in patients with varicella, vomiting, and minimal neurologic changes. Since Reye's syndrome usually occurs with salicylate use, this drug should be especially avoided in patients with varicella. Encephalitis occurs in less than 0.1% of cases, usually in the first week of illness. It is often limited to cerebellitis with ataxia and resolves completely. Diffuse encephalitis may result in some mortality (5%).

Varicella pneumonia is usually seen in immunocompromised or pregnant patients and may be fatal. Cough, dyspnea, tachypnea, rales, and cyanosis are seen several days after rash onset.

Hemorrhagic varicella lesions may be seen without other complications. Usually due to autoimmune thrombocytopenia, hemorrhagic lesions can represent disseminated intravascular coagulation or purpura fulminans.

Varicella may be life-threatening in immunosuppressed patients (especially those with leukemia or lymphoma or those receiving high doses of steroids). Their disease is complicated by severe pneumonitis, hepatitis, and encephalitis. Varicella exposure in such patients must be evaluated immediately (see Chapter 6).

Neonates born to mothers who develop varicella from 6 days before to 2 days after delivery are at high risk for severe or fatal (in 5%) disease and must be given varicella-zoster immune globulin and followed closely (see Chapter 6).

Unusual complications of varicella include optic neuritis, transverse myelitis, orchitis, and arthritis.

Complications of herpes zoster include prolonged pain, secondary bacterial infection, motor or cranial nerve paralysis, encephalitis, keratitis, and dissemination in immunosuppressed patients.

Treatment

A. General: Supportive measures include maintenance of hydration, administration of acetaminophen for discomfort, cool soaks or antipruritics for itching (diphenhydramine, 1.25 mg/kg/dose q6h; or hydroxyzine, 0.5 mg/kg/dose q6h), and observance of general hygiene measures (keep nails trimmed and clean, skin clean). Topical or systemic antistaphylococcal antibiotics may be needed.

B. Specific: Although acyclovir is more active against herpes simplex, it is the preferred drug for varicella and herpes zoster infections. Topical therapy is reserved for ocular infections. Recommended parenteral acyclovir dosage for severe disease is 30–50 mg/kg/d intravenously in 3 divided doses, infused over 1 hour. Parenteral therapy should be started early in immunosuppressed patients or high-risk, infected neonates. Varicella-zoster immune globulin is of no proved therapeutic value. The effect of oral acyclovir on the course of varicella in normal children is being evaluated. In one study, doses of 40–80 mg/kg/d were modestly beneficial and non-toxic.

Prevention

See Chapter 6 for a discussion of the live attenuated vaccine and the use of varicella-zoster immune globulin for prevention of varicella.

Prognosis

Except for secondary bacterial infections, serious complications are rare and recovery complete in normal hosts.

Balfour HH et al: Acyclovir treatment of varicella in otherwise healthy children. *J Pediatr* 1990;**116**:633.

Fleischer G et al: Life-threatening complications of varicella. *Am J Dis Child* 1981;**135**:896.
Preblud S et al: Varicella: Clinical manifestations, epidemiology and health impact in children. *Pediatr Infect Dis J* 1984;**3**:505.
Shepp DH: Treatment of varicella-zoster virus infections in severely immunocompromised patients. *N Engl J Med* 1986;**314**:208.

ROSEOLA INFANTUM
(Exanthema Subitum)

Roseola infantum is a benign illness probably caused by a newly discovered human herpesvirus (human herpesvirus 6; HHV-6), which can be isolated from circulating T cells during the early course of the illness. The significance of this common disease is its ability to mimic more serious causes of high fever and its role in inciting febrile seizures.

Clinical Findings

A. History: Most prominent is the abrupt onset of fever, reaching 38.9–40.6 °C (102–105 °F) and continuing for 3–5 days in an otherwise mildly ill child. The fever then ceases abruptly, and the characteristic rash appears. Roseola occurs predominantly in children 6 months to 4 years old, with 90% of cases occurring before the second year. It is the most common recognized cause of exanthem in this age group.

B. Symptoms and Signs: Mild lethargy and irritability may be present, but generally there is a dissociation between systemic symptoms and the febrile course. The pharynx, tonsils, and tympanic membranes may be injected. Conjunctivitis, coryza, cough, and pharyngeal exudate are notably absent. Adenopathy of the head and neck often occurs. The most notable feature is the rash—upon cessation of fever—which begins on the trunk and spreads to the face, neck, and extremities. Rose-pink macules or maculopapules, 2–3 mm in diameter, are nonpruritic and disappear in 1–2 days without pigmentation or desquamation.

C. Laboratory Findings: An early leukocytosis gives way to leukopenia, a relative lymphocytosis, and atypical lymphocytes before the rash appears.

Differential Diagnosis

The initial high fever may suggest serious bacterial infection. However, the relative well-being of most children, and the typical course and rash soon clarify the diagnosis. If the child has a febrile seizure, it is important to exclude bacterial meningitis. The cerebrospinal fluid is normal in children with roseola. In children who receive antibiotics or other medication at the beginning of the fever, the rash may be incorrectly attributed to a drug allergy.

Complications & Sequelae

Febrile seizures occur, but no more commonly than with other self-limited infections.

Treatment & Prognosis

Fever is readily managed with acetaminophen and sponge baths. Fever control should be a major consideration in children with a history of febrile seizures. Roseola infantum is otherwise entirely benign.

Veda K et al: Exanthem subitum and antibody to human herpesvirus-6. *J Infect Dis* 1989;**159**:750.

Yoshiyama H et al: Role of human herpesvirus-6 infection in infants with exanthem subitum. *Pediatr Infect Dis J* 1990;**9**:71.

CYTOMEGALOVIRUS INFECTIONS

Cytomegalovirus (CMV) is a ubiquitous human herpesvirus transmitted by many routes. It can be acquired following maternal viremia or from birth canal secretions and maternal milk. Young children are infected by the saliva of playmates; older individuals are infected by sexual partners (saliva, vaginal secretions, and semen). Transfused blood products and transplanted organs can be a source of CMV infection. Clinical illness is largely determined by the immune competence of the patient. Normal individuals usually develop a mild, self-limited illness, whereas immunocompromised children are likely to develop severe, progressive, often multiorgan disease. In addition, in utero infection can be teratogenic.

1. IN UTERO CMV INFECTION

Clinical Findings

A. History: Approximately 0.5–1.5% of children are born with CMV infections acquired during maternal viremia. Over 95% of them are asymptomatic and are usually born to mothers with reactivation of latent CMV infection during the pregnancy. Symptomatic infants are born to mothers with primary CMV infection. Even after primary maternal CMV infection, less than 50% of fetuses are infected, and only 10% of those infected are symptomatic at birth. Primary infection in the first half of pregnancy poses the greatest risk for severe fetal damage.

B. Symptoms and Signs: Severely affected infants are born ill; they are often small for gestational age, floppy, and lethargic. They feed poorly and have poor temperature control. Hepatosplenomegaly, jaundice, petechiae, seizures, and microcephaly are often present. Characteristic signs are a distinctive chorioretinitis and periventricular calcification.

A purpuric ("blueberry muffin") rash similar to that seen with congenital rubella may be present. The mortality rate is 20–30%. Survivors usually have significant sequelae. Less severely ill children are born with one or more of the above findings. Isolated hepatosplenomegaly or thrombocytopenia may occur. Even mildly affected children may subsequently manifest mental retardation and psychomotor delay. Most infected infants (90%) have no clinical manifestations at birth. Of these, 10–15% develop sensorineural hearing loss, which is often bilateral.

C. Laboratory Findings: Anemia, thrombocytopenia, hyperbilirubinemia, and elevated transaminase levels are common. Lymphocytosis is occasionally seen. Pleocytosis and an elevated protein content are found on examination of cerebrospinal fluid. The diagnosis is readily confirmed by isolation of CMV from urine, saliva, cerebrospinal fluid, and stool. Urine isolates can often be obtained in 7 days using tissue culture alone and in 1 or 2 days combining culture with enzyme immunoassay. The presence in the infant of IgM-specific CMV antibodies suggests the diagnosis, but currently available reagents are associated with 25% false-negative and false-positive tests.

D. Imaging: Skull films show microcephaly and periventricular calcification. Long bone films show the "celery stalk" pattern characteristic of congenital viral infections. Interstitial pneumonia may be present.

Differential Diagnosis

CMV infection should be considered in any newborn who is seriously ill shortly after birth, especially once bacterial sepsis, metabolic disease, intracranial bleeding, and cardiac disease have been excluded. Other congenital infections to be considered in the differential diagnosis include: toxoplasmosis (serology, more diffuse calcification of the central nervous system, specific type of retinitis, macrocephaly), rubella (serology, specific type of retinitis, cardiac lesions, eye abnormalities); enteroviral infections (isolation, time of the year, maternal illness), syphilis (serology for both infant and mother, skin lesions, bone involvement).

Treatment & Prevention

Support is rarely required for anemia and thrombocytopenia. The antiviral drug, ganciclovir, may be of value in severely ill children, but this is not an approved use of the drug, which in addition frequently produces neutropenia. Possibly the late sequelae of CMV infection—including abnormalities occurring in initially asymptomatic infants—may be ameliorated by ganciclovir use. Delayed development and hearing loss should be discovered and treated as soon as possible.

2. PERINATAL CMV INFECTION

Clinical Findings

A. History: CMV infection can be acquired from birth canal secretions or shortly after birth from maternal milk. In some socioeconomic groups, 10–20% of infants are infected at birth and excrete CMV for many months. Infection can also be acquired in the postnatal period from transfused blood products.

B. Symptoms and Signs: Ninety percent of normal infants infected by their mothers at birth develop subclinical illness (ie, virus excretion only) or a minor illness within 1–3 months. The remainder develop an illness lasting several weeks and characterized by hepatosplenomegaly, lymphadenopathy, and interstitial pneumonitis in various combinations. The severity of the pneumonitis may be increased by the simultaneous presence of *Chlamydia trachomatis*. Infants who receive blood products are often premature and immunologically impaired. If they are born to CMV-negative mothers and subsequently receive CMV-containing blood, they frequently develop severe infection and pneumonia after a 2–6 week incubation period.

C. Laboratory Findings: Lymphocytosis, atypical lymphocytes, anemia, and thrombocytopenia may be present, especially in premature infants. Liver function is abnormal. CMV can be isolated from urine and saliva. Secretions obtained at bronchoscopy contain CMV and epithelial cells bearing CMV antigens. Serum levels of CMV antibody rise significantly.

D. Imaging: Chest films show a diffuse, interstitial pneumonitis.

Differential Diagnosis

CMV should be considered as a cause of any prolonged illness in early infancy, especially if hepatosplenomegaly, lymphadenopathy, or atypical lymphocytosis is present. This must be distinguished from granulomatous or malignant diseases and from congenital infections (syphilis, toxoplasmosis, hepatitis B) not previously appreciated. Other viruses (Epstein-Barr virus, human immunodeficiency virus, adenovirus) can cause this syndrome. CMV is a recognized cause of viral pneumonia in this age group. However, since asymptomatic CMV excretion is common in early infancy, care must be taken to establish the diagnosis and to rule out concomitant copathogens such as *Chlamydia* and respiratory syncytial virus.

Treatment & Prevention

The self-limited disease of normal infants requires no therapy. Severe pneumonitis in premature infants requires oxygen administration and often intubation. Very ill infants may benefit from ganciclovir (currently obtainable on a compassionate basis from Syntex Corporation). CMV infection acquired by transfusion can be prevented by excluding CMV-seropositive blood donors. Alternatively, washed deglycerolized frozen red blood cells can be used. Milk donors should also be screened for prior CMV infection. It is likely that high-risk infants receiving large doses of intravenous gamma globulin for other reasons will be protected against severe CMV disease.

3. CMV ACQUIRED IN CHILDHOOD AND ADOLESCENCE

Clinical Findings

A. History: Young children are readily infected by playmates, especially since CMV continues to be excreted in saliva and urine for many months after infection. The annual incidence of CMV excretion by children in day care centers exceeds 75%. In fact, young children in a family are often the source of primary CMV infection of the mother during subsequent pregnancies. An additional peak of CMV infection occurs in sexually active individuals. Blood transfusion represents another source of CMV infection.

B. Symptoms and Signs: The large majority of young children acquiring CMV are asymptomatic or have a minor febrile illness, occasionally with adenopathy. They provide the reservoir of virus shedders that facilitate spread of CMV. Occasionally a child may have a prolonged fever with hepatosplenomegaly and adenopathy. Older children and adults are more likely to be symptomatic in this fashion and can present with a syndrome that mimics the infectious mononucleosis syndrome following infection by Epstein-Barr virus (1–2 weeks of fever, malaise, anorexia, splenomegaly, and some adenopathy). This syndrome can also occur 2–4 weeks after transfusion of CMV-infected blood.

C. Laboratory Findings: In the CMV mononucleosis syndrome, lymphocytosis and atypical lymphocytes are common, as is a mild rise in transaminase levels. CMV is present in saliva and urine, and diagnosis is made as for the other syndromes.

Differential Diagnosis

In older children, CMV should be included as a possible cause of fever of unknown origin, especially when lymphocytosis and atypical lymphocytes are present. CMV is distinguished from Epstein-Barr virus infection by the absence of pharyngitis, the relatively minor adenopathy, and the absence of serologic evidence of acute Epstein-Barr virus infection. Other mononucleosis syndromes are caused by *Toxoplasma gondii*, rubella, adenovirus, hepatitis A and, infection by the human immunodeficiency virus.

Treatment & Prevention

Screening of transfused blood would prevent cases related to this source.

4. CMV IN IMMUNOCOMPROMISED CHILDREN

Clinical Findings

A. History: CMV in this setting is usually acquired from infused blood products or transplanted tissue. In addition, reactivation of latent CMV can cause symptomatic disease. This is clearly seen in children with AIDS or congenital immunodeficiencies. However, in most other immunocompromised patients, primary infection is much more likely to cause severe symptoms than is reactivation disease. The severity of the resulting disease is generally proportional to the degree of immunosuppression.

B. Symptoms and Signs: A mild febrile illness with myalgia, malaise, and arthralgia may occur, especially with reactivation disease. Severe disease often includes subacute onset of dyspnea and cyanosis as manifestations of an interstitial pneumonitis. Auscultation reveals only coarse breath sounds and scattered rales. Rapid respiratory rate may precede the clinical or x-ray evidence of pneumonia. Hepatitis, without jaundice and hepatomegaly, is common. Diarrhea, which can be impressive in degree, occurs with CMV colitis, and CMV can cause esophagitis with symptoms of odynophagia or dysphagia. These enteropathies are most common in AIDS, as is the presence of a retinitis that often progresses to blindness.

C. Laboratory Findings: Neutropenia and thrombocytopenia are common. Atypical lymphocytosis is not a frequent occurrence. Serum transaminase levels are often elevated. The stools may contain occult blood if enteropathy is present. CMV is readily isolated from saliva, urine, buffy coat, and bronchial secretions. The technique of centrifugation of the specimen onto tissue culture and subsequent immunoassay will show the presence of CMV within 48 hours.

D. Imaging: Bilateral interstitial pneumonitis is present on chest film.

Differential Diagnosis

The initial febrile illness must be distinguished from intrapulmonary hemorrhage, drug-induced or radiation pneumonitis, pulmonary edema, and bacterial, fungal, and parasitic infection in this population. However, systemic CMV infection is not usually accompanied by much toxicity. Similarly, the pulmonary disease must be distinguished from treatable bacterial and fungal infections. In this regard, it is noteworthy that CMV is bilateral and interstitial on x-ray films of the chest, cough is nonproductive, and chest pain is absent. *Pneumocystis carinii* may present in a very similar manner. Polymicrobial disease may be present in these patients. It is suspected that bacterial and fungal infections are enhanced by the neutropenia that can accompany CMV infection. Infection of the gastrointestinal tract is diagnosed by endoscopy, mainly to exclude candidal and herpes simplex etiologies.

Treatment & Prognosis

Blood donors should be screened for prior CMV infection. Ideally, seronegative transplant recipients should receive organs from seronegative donors. Severe symptoms, most commonly pneumonitis, sometimes respond to early therapy with intravenous ganciclovir (2.5 mg/kg every 6–8 hours for 10–14 days). Neutropenia is a frequent side effect of this therapy.

Jordan CJ et al: Spontaneous cytomegalovirus mononucleosis. *Ann Intern Med* 1973;**79**:153.

Kumar ML et al: Postnatally acquired cytomegalovirus infections in infants of CMV-excreting mothers. *J Pediatr* 1984;**104**:669.

Pass RF et al: Outcome of symptomatic congenital cytomegalovirus infection: Results of long-term longitudinal follow-up. *Pediatrics* 1980;**66**:758.

Stagno S, Whitley RJ: Herpesvirus infections of pregnancy. Part 1. Cytomegalovvirus and Epstein-Barr virus infections. *N Engl J Med* 1985;**313**:1270.

Stagno S et al: Infant pneumonitis associated with cytomegalovirus, *Chlamydia, Pneumocystis,* and *Ureaplasma:* A prospective study. *Pediatrics* 1981;**68**:322.

Yeager AS et al: Prevention of transfusion-acquired cytomegalovirus infections in newborn infants. *J Pediatr* 1981;**98**:281.

INFECTIOUS MONONUCLEOSIS

General Considerations

Mononucleosis in the most characteristic syndrome produced by infection with the Epstein-Barr virus (EBV). Its elements are fever, pharyngitis, lymphadenopathy, splenomegaly, atypical lymphocytosis, and the production of heterophil antibodies. Young children infected with EBV have either no symptoms or a mild nonspecific febrile illness. As the age of the host increases, EBV infection is likely to be followed by the mononucleosis syndrome, occurring in 20–25% of infected adolescents. EBV is readily acquired from asymptomatic carriers (15–20% of whom excrete the virus on any given day) and from recently ill patients, who excrete virus for many months. Young children are infected from the saliva of playmates and family members. Adolescents may be infected through sexual activity. EBV can also be transmitted by blood transfusion and transplantation.

Clinical Findings

A. Symptoms and Signs: After an incubation period of 1–2 months, a 2–3 day prodrome of malaise and anorexia yields, abruptly or insidiously, to a febrile illness with temperatures exceeding 38.8°C (102°F). The major complaint is pharyngitis, which is often (50%) exudative. Lymph nodes are enlarged, firm, and mildly tender. Any area may be affected, but posterior and anterior cervical nodes are almost always enlarged. Splenomegaly is present in 50 to 75% of patients. Hepatomegaly is uncommon (10%), but the liver is frequently tender. Five percent of patients have a rash, which can be macular, scarlatiniform, or urticarial. Rash is almost universal in patients taking penicillin or ampicillin.

B. Laboratory Findings:

1. Peripheral Blood—Leukopenia may occur early, but an atypical lymphocytosis (comprising over 10% of the total leukocytes at some time in the illness) is most notable. Hematologic changes may not be seen until the third week of illness and may be entirely absent in some EBV syndromes, eg, neurologic ones.

2. Heterophil Antibodies—These nonspecific antibodies appear in over 90% of older patients with mononucleosis but in fewer than 50% of children under age 5. They may not be detectable until the second week of illness and may persist for up to 12 months after recovery. Rapid screening tests (slide agglutination) are usually positive if the titer is significant; a positive result strongly suggests but does not prove EBV infection.

3. Anti-EBV Antibodies—It may be necessary to measure specific antibody titers when heterophil antibodies fail to appear, as in young children. EBV infection is established by detecting IgM antibody to the viral capsid antigen (VCA); by detecting a rise over several weeks of IgG antibody to VCA; or by detecting IgG-VCA antibody in the absence of antibody to the Epstein-Barr nuclear antigen (EBNA), which appears late in the illness. Seroconversion of antibody to EBNA confirms the above indicators.

4. Transaminase, GGT, and Bilirubin Levels—Transaminase and gammaglutamyltransferase (GGT) levels are mildly elevated in 80% of patients; **bilirubin** is mildly elevated in 25%.

Differential Diagnosis

Severe pharyngitis may suggest group A streptococcal infection. The presence of anterior cervical adenopathy only, neutrophilic leukocytosis, and the absence of splenomegaly suggest bacterial infection. Although a child with a positive throat culture usually requires therapy, up to 10% of children with mononucleosis are asymptomatic carriers. In this group, penicillin therapy is unnecessary and often causes a rash. Severe primary herpes simplex pharyngitis, which is common in adolescence, may also mimic infectious mononucleosis. In this pharyngitis, some anterior mouth ulcerations should suggest the correct diagnosis. EBV infection should be considered in the differential diagnosis of any perplexing prolonged febrile illness. Some similar illnesses that produce atypical lymphocytosis include rubella (pharyngitis not prominent, shorter illness, less ade-

nopathy and splenomegaly), adenovirus (upper respiratory infection symptom and cough, conjunctivitis, less adenopathy, fewer atypical lymphocytes), hepatitis (more severe liver function abnormalities, no pharyngitis or splenomegaly), and toxoplasmosis (negative heterophil test and less pharyngitis). Serum sickness–like drug reactions and leukemia (smear morphology is important) may be confused with infectious mononucleosis. Cytomegalovirus mononucleosis is a close mimic except for minimal pharyngitis and less adenopathy; it is much less common. The serology for EBV and cytomegalovirus is important for correct diagnosis.

Complications

Splenic rupture is a very rare complication, which usually follows significant trauma. Hematologic complications, including hemolytic anemia, thrombocytopenia, or neutropenia, are more common. Neurologic involvement can include aseptic meningitis, encephalitis, isolated neuropathy such as Bell's palsy, and Guillain-Barré syndrome. Any of these may appear prior to or in the absence of the more typical signs and symptoms of infectious mononucleosis. Rare complications include myocarditis, pericarditis, and atypical pneumonia. Very rarely, EBV infection becomes a progressive lymphoproliferative disorder characterized by persistent fever, multiple organ involvement, neutropenia or pancytopenia, and agammaglobulinemia. Hemocytophagia is often present in the bone marrow. An X-linked genetic defect in immune response has been inferred for some patients (Duncan's syndrome, X-linked lymphoproliferative disorder). Children with other congenital immunodeficiencies, or chemotherapy-induced immunosuppression, can also develop progressive EBV infection or EBV-induced lymphomas.

Treatment & Prognosis

Bed rest may be necessary for severe cases. Acetaminophen controls high fever. Potential airway obstruction due to swollen pharyngeal lymphoid tissue responds rapidly to systemic steroids. Steroids may also be given for hematologic and neurologic complications, although no controlled trials have proved their efficacy in these conditions. Fever and pharyngitis disappear by 10 to 14 days. Adenopathy and splenomegaly can persist several weeks longer. Some patients complain of fatigue, malaise, or lack of well-being for several months. Although chronic EBV infection has been suggested as a cause of the chronic fatigue syndrome, this must be considered completely speculative. Although steroids may shorten the duration of fatigue and malaise, their long-term effects on this potentially oncogenic viral infection are unknown, and indiscriminant use is discouraged. Patients with splenic enlargement should avoid contact sports for 6 to 8 weeks.

Alpert G, Fleisher GR: Complications of infection with Epstein-Barr virus during childhood: A study of children admitted to the hospital. *Pediatr Infect Dis* 1984;**3**:304.

Andiman WA: Epstein-Barr virus associated syndromes: A critical reexamination. *Pediatr Infect Dis J* 1984;**3**:198.

Sumaya CV: Epstein-Barr virus serologic testing: Diagnostic indications and interpretations. *Pediatr Infect Dis J* 1986;**5**:337.

Sumaya CV, Ench Y: Epstein-Barr virus infectious mononucleosis in children. 1. Clinical and general laboratory findings. *Pediatrics* 1985;**75**:1003.

ARBOVIRUSES
See Table 27–4 for the common arboviral diseases in children.

Bell WE, McCormick WF: Viral encephalitis and aseptic meningitis. Chapter 13 in: *Neurologic Infections in Children*. Major Problems in Clinical Pediatrics (monographs). Vol 12. 1981.

Goodpasture HC et al: Colorado tick fever: Clinical, epidemiologic, and laboratory aspects of 228 cases in Colorado in 1973–74. *Ann Intern Med* 1978;**88**:303.

Malinson MD, Waterman SH: Dengue fever in the United States. *JAMA* 1983;**249**:496.

ADENOVIRUSES

There are over 40 types of adenoviruses, which account for 2–10% of all respiratory illnesses. In addition, enteric adenoviruses are an important cause of childhood diarrhea. Adenoviral infections are common early in life. Because of latent infection in lymphoid tissue, asymptomatic shedding from the respiratory or intestinal tract is more common than with other respiratory viruses.

Specific clinical syndromes include the following:

(1) Pharyngoconjunctival fever: Fever, follicular conjunctivitis, and pharyngitis (sometimes exudative) are present.

(2) Follicular conjunctivitis: This form of conjunctivitis may be prolonged and associated with preauricular adenopathy and corneal damage.

(3) Epidemic keratoconjunctivitis: Severe conjunctivitis with punctate keratitis and occasionally visual impairment occurs.

(4) Pneumonia: Severe, sometimes fatal pneumonia may occur at all ages. Epidemics in adults are seen.

(5) Rash: A diffuse morbilliform (rarely petechial) rash resembling measles, rubella, or roseola may occur.

(6) Other: Immunosuppressed patients, including neonates, may develop severe or fatal pulmonary or gastrointestinal infections. Other rare complications include hemorrhagic cystitis, mesenteric adenitis, encephalitis, hepatitis, and myocarditis. Although adenovirus may be isolated in cases of pertussis syndrome, *Bordetella pertussis* is usually also present.

Diagnosis is by culture of conjunctival, respiratory, or rectal specimens (several days to weeks are required for growth) or paired serology; rapid antigen detection tests for respiratory specimens are being evaluated.

Therapy is supportive.

MISCELLANEOUS VIRUSES

ERYTHEMA INFECTIOSUM

This benign exanthematous illness of school-aged children is caused by a human parvovirus designated B19. The incubation period is about 2 weeks (4–20 days). Springtime outbreaks are typical. It is mildly contagious; only about half of susceptible household contacts are infected.

Approximately one-half of infected individuals have a subclinical illness. Most cases (70%) occur in children between the ages of 5 and 15, with an additional 20% occurring later in life. One-half of adults are seronegative. Rare complications of parvovirus infection include aplastic crises in children with chronic hemolytic anemia and occasionally hydrops fetalis when susceptible pregnant women are infected.

Clinical Findings

A. History: Due to the nonspecific nature of the exanthem and the many subclinical cases, a contact history is often absent or unreliable. Recognition of the illness is easier during outbreaks.

B. Symptoms and Signs: Typically the first sign of illness is the rash, which begins as raised maculopapular lesions on the cheeks that coalesce to give a "slapped cheek" appearance. The lesions are warm, nontender, and sometimes pruritic. They may be scattered on the forehead, chin, and postauricular areas, but the circumoral region is spared. Within 1 to 2 days, similar lesions appear on the proximal extensor surfaces of the extremities and spread distally in a symmetric fashion. The trunk, neck, and buttocks are also commonly involved. Central clearing of confluent lesions produces a characteristic lacelike pattern. The rash fades in several days to several weeks, but frequently reappears in response

Table 27–4. Arboviral diseases

Disease[1]	Natural Reservoir, (Vector)	Geographic Distribution	Incubation Period	Clinical Disease	Laboratory Findings	Complications, Sequelae	Diagnosis, Therapy, Comments[2]
St. Louis encephalitis	Birds (*Culex* mosquitos)	Mid- and South-Central USA; Central, South America	2–5 d (up to 3 weeks)	Abrupt onset fever, chills, headache, nausea, vomiting; may develop generalized weakness, seizures, coma, paralysis	Modest leukocytosis, neutrophilia; CSF: 100–200 WBC/μL (PMNs predominate early)	Mortality 2–5% in children; neurologic sequelae in 1–20%	Most important arbovirus in USA; 20–500 cases/yr; < 2% of infections are symptomatic. Worse in elderly. Horses infected, not ill. Therapy: supportive. Diagnosis: serology. Specific antibody often present within 5 d.
California encephalitis (LaCrosse, Jamestown Canyon, 3 others)	Chipmunks (*Aedes* mosquitos)	North and Mid-Central USA	2–5 d	Similar to St. Louis encephalitis; focal neurologic signs in up to 25%	Variable WBC counts; CSF: 30-100 (up to 600) WBC/μL; variable PMN %.	Mortality <1%	About 50–150 cases/yr in USA, 5% of infections are symptomatic. Therapy: supportive. Diagnosis: serology. Up to 90% have specific IgM antibody in first week; 25% of population in endemic area has IgG antibody.
Western equine encephalitis	Birds (*Culex* mosquitos)	Canada, USA and Mexico west of Mississippi River longitude; South America	2–5 d	Similar to St. Louis encephalitis	Variable WBC counts; CSF: 10-300 WBC/μL	Permanent brain damage 10% overall; 30% in <1 y old	About 10–100 cases/year in USA. Worse in infants. Equine illness precedes human outbreaks. Therapy: supportive. Diagnosis: serology. Often positive in first week; specific IgM or CF antibody testing preferred.
Eastern equine encephalitis	Birds (*Culex, Aedes* mosquitos)	Eastern US Seaboard; Caribbean; South America	2–5 d	Similar to St. Louis encephalitis but more severe; progresses rapidly	Leukocytosis with neutrophilia; CSF: 500–2000 WBC/μL; PMNs predominate early	Mortality 20–70%; neurologic sequelae in over 50% of children	Most severe arboviral encephalitis in USA, <20 cases/year. Only 3–10% of cases are symptomatic. Therapy: supportive. Diagnosis: serology. Background seropositivity very low. Titers often positive in first week.
Colorado tick fever	(*Dermacentor andersoni*, or wood tick)	Rocky Mountain region	3–4 d (range 1–14 d)	Fever, myalgia, conjunctivitis, headache, retroorbital pain; rash in <10%; no respiratory symptoms; biphasic in 50%	Leukopenia (maximum at 4–6 d); mild thrombocytopenia	Rare encephalitis, coagulopathy	Patient may have no known tick bite. Acute illness lasts 7 d; prolonged fatigue in adults. Therapy: supportive. Diagnosis: serology.
Dengue (4 types)	*Aedes* mosquitos	Asia, Africa, Central and South America, Caribbean; rarely in southern USA	2–7 d	Fever, headache, myalgia, retroocular pain, pharyngitis, cough; maculopapular or petechial rash in 20%; adenopathy	Leukopenia, thrombocytopenia	Hemorrhagic fever, shock syndrome, prolonged weakness	High infection rate. Biphasic course may occur. Therapy: supportive. Diagnosis: serology.
Yellow fever	(*Aedes* mosquitos) Humans	Africa	3–7 d (up to 13 d)	Abrupt onset fever, headache, vomiting; may progress to jaundice, GI bleeding, hepatitis, death	Leukopenia; abnormal liver functions; proteinuria creatinine	Severe in 10–20% with 50% mortality in this group; milder in children	May be biphasic. Liver biopsy: characteristic midzonal necrosis, eosinophilic inclusions. Therapy: supportive. Diagnosis: paired serology; mouse inoculation with blood, liver tissue.

CSF = cerebrospinal fluid; WBC = white blood cells (leukocytes); PMN = polymorphonuclear leukocytes.
[1]Viral agent has same name as disease unless noted.
[2]Vaccine available only for yellow fever.

to local irritation, heat (bathing), sunlight, and stress. Almost one-half of infected children have some rash remaining (or recurring) for 10 days. Fine desquamation may be present.

Mild systemic symptoms occur in up to 50% of children during outbreaks. These include low-grade fever (38–38.5°C [100.4–101.3°F]) mild malaise, sore throat, and coryza.

C. Laboratory Findings: A mild leukopenia occurs early in some patients, followed by leukocytosis and lymphocytosis. Blood tests for antigen and antibody are being developed.

Differential Diagnosis

The characteristic rash and the mild nature of the illness distinguish erythema infectiosum from other childhood exanthems. It lacks the prodromal symptoms of measles and the lymphadenopathy of rubella. Systemic symptoms and pharyngitis are more prominent with enteroviral infections and scarlet fever.

Complications & Sequelae

A. Arthritis: This occurs in older patients, beginning with late adolescence. Pain and stiffness occur symmetrically in the peripheral joints. Arthritis usually follows the rash and may persist for 2–4 weeks but resolves without permanent damage.

B. Aplastic Crisis: Parvovirus B19 replicates primarily in erythroid progenitor cells. Consequently, reticulocytopenia occurs for approximately one week during the illness. This goes unnoticed in normal individuals but results in severe anemia in patients with chronic hemolytic anemia. The rash of erythema infectiosum is usually absent in these patients.

C. In Utero Infections: Infection of susceptible pregnant women may produce fetal infection with hydrops fetalis; fetal death occurs in about 10%. The risk of fetal infection is not known. There is no obvious relationship between the outcome of such infections and the age of the fetus at the time of infection. Congenital anomalies have not been associated with parvovirus B19 infection during pregnancy.

Treatment & Prognosis

Erythema infectiosum is a benign and inconsequential illness for normal individuals. Patients with aplastic crisis may require blood transfusions. It is unlikely that this complication can be prevented by quarantine measures, since acute parvovirus infection in contacts is often unrecognized and most contagious prior to the rash. Pregnant women who are exposed to erythema infectiosum or who work in a setting where an epidemic occurs should be tested for evidence of prior infection, if a reliable serologic test is available. Susceptible pregnant women should then be followed for evidence of parvovirus infection. If maternal infection occurs, the fetus should be followed for evidence of hydrops and distress. In utero transfusion or early delivery may salvage some fetuses. Pregnancies should not be terminated because of parvovirus infection.

Anand A et al: Human parvovirus infection, pregnancy and hydrops fetalis. *N Engl J Med* 1987;**316**:183.

Centers for Disease Control, USA: Risks associated with human parvovirus B19 infection. *MMWR* 1989;**38**:83.

Ware R: Human parvovirus infections. *J Pediatr* 1989;**114**:343.

HUMAN IMMUNODEFICIENCY VIRUS (HIV) INFECTIONS (Acquired Immune Deficiency Syndrome, AIDS)

Essentials of Diagnosis

Children older than 15 months:
- Presence of HIV in blood or tissue determined by culture or antigen detection method.

or

- Presence of HIV antibody determined by repeated screening tests and confirmatory test.

or

- Symptoms of AIDS (multiple infections, opportunistic infections, lymphoid interstitial pneumonitis, encephalopathy, Kaposi's sarcoma, other; see Centers for Disease Control case definition, MMWR 1987;**36**:25).

Children younger than 15 months:
- HIV in blood or tissue as above.

or

- Symptoms of AIDS.

or

- HIV antibody as above and evidence of cellular and humoral immunodeficiency (without an obvious cause) and nonspecific symptoms compatible with immunodeficiency, eg, weight loss, hepatosplenomegaly, generalized adenopathy, chronic thrush, diarrhea, lymphoid interstitial pneumonitis, progressive developmental delay, unexplained fevers, or opportunistic infections.

General Considerations

HIV is the most common cause of acquired immunodeficiency in children. AIDS is caused by a retrovirus that infects helper T cells, monocytes/macrophages, neural cells, and many other types of cell. The destruction of helper T cells profoundly affects B cells, suppressor T cells, and cell-mediated immunity and results in progressive generalized immune incompetence. Venereal and contaminated-needle spread account for most infections after puberty; younger children are infected perinatally (transplacentally or at birth) or by blood transfusion. Of hemophiliacs who received blood products prior to 1985, when screening began, 65–90% are infected.

About 80% of infected women are of childbearing age. About half are intravenous drug abusers, and most of the remainder are sexual partners of infected men. The number of women who are unknowingly exposed by heterosexual contact is increasing, however. About 30–50% of infants born to infected mothers will be infected.

The incubation period for primary infection is about 2–4 weeks. Primary infection is nonspecific (a "flu" or mild mononucleosislike illness) and often subclinical. The latent period before AIDS is diagnosed is a median of 9 months for congenital infection and 17 months for transfusion-acquired infection. Sexually acquired infections may not be clinically manifest for years. Current evidence suggests that eventually everyone infected with HIV will develop symptomatic immunodeficiency.

Clinical Findings

A. History: Risk factors for HIV infection include exposure to blood products from 1978 to the spring of 1985, a history of parenteral illicit drug use, multiple heterosexual or homosexual contacts, heterosexual partner, or mother with one of the above risk factors.

Casual, classroom, or household contact with an HIV-infected person poses no risk.

History of frequent illness may include recurrent otitis media, poor weight gain, chronic cough, chronic diarrhea or candidal infection, developmental delay, or unexplained fevers.

B. Symptoms and Signs: See Table 27–5.

1. Nonspecific—See above. These are the most common and earliest findings and may be present for years in an otherwise well child.

2. Infections—Recurrent or severe infections include sepsis, pneumonia, abscesses, meningitis, and cellulitis. Organisms include *Haemophilus influenzae,* pneumococcus, *Staphylococcus aureus, Salmonella,* and opportunistic pathogens.

3. Pulmonary—Chronic lymphoid interstitial pneumonitis, perhaps related to EBV infection, is seen in about half of children with AIDS; it may be

asymptomatic or associated with dry cough, hypoxemia, and dyspnea on exertion. *Pneumocystis carinii* pneumonia is also common, but it is a more acute illness preseating with fever and abnormal findings on auscultation.

4. Encephalopathy—This is rather common as a late sequela and consists of acquired microcephaly, retardation, weakness, ataxia, pseudobulbar palsy, and failure to attain (or loss of previously attained) developmental milestones. The course is variable, but it is usually not acute; seizures are uncommon.

5. Other—Chronic parotid enlargement, thrombocytopenia, hepatitis, cardiomyopathy, nephritis, pancreatitis, and Bell's palsy have all been described.

C. Laboratory Findings: Routine tests are often nonspecific and reflect inflammation in the affected organs. In children, the leukocyte counts and lymphocyte counts are often normal until late in the disease, when lymphopenia often occurs. With progression of disease, the helper T cells are reduced and helper/suppressor T cell ratios reversed. The sedimentation rate is often elevated. Anemia and thrombocytopenia may occur. Hypergammaglobulinemia is characteristic: Some children fail to make specific antibody to antigens (eg, tetanus, *Haemophilus influenzae* type b, pneumococcus). This failure may play a role in subsequent infections. With brain involvement, the protein level in cerebrospinal fluid may be elevated, and a mononuclear pleocytosis may be present. Serum lactate dehydrogenase levels are high in children with *P carinii* infection.

HIV antibody should be positive, both by the enzyme immunoassay and confirmatory blot test. Maternal antibody may persist up to 15 months in uninfected infants. No reliable IgM antibody test is available, and diagnosis of infection in infants requires culture of the virus (usually from blood; not widely available), demonstration of antigen in blood or tissue (less sensitive than culture), or evidence of immunodeficiency with no other etiology in a child with signs of AIDS. Infants who are antibody positive after 15 months are probably infected even if clinically well.

D. Imaging: Chest x-ray films of children with lymphoid interstitial pneumonitis show a diffuse interstitial reticulonodular infiltrate, occasionally with hilar adenopathy. Cerebral images demonstrate atrophy and calcification in the basal ganglia and frontal lobes in patients with brain infection. Infection with all other opportunistic pathogens usually results in x-ray findings typical of each agent: The more severe the immunodeficiency, however, the more atypical these presentations can be.

Differential Diagnosis

In children older than 15 months the diagnosis of infection can be quickly made by serology. In younger children, a negative result rules out under-

Table 27–5. Clinical characteristics of AIDS in children and adults

	Infants and Children Under 13 Years	Adolescents/ Adults
Disorders		
Infections Bacterial	Very common	Occurs
Opportunistic	Very common	Very common
Failure to thrive or weight loss	Very common (95%)	Common
Hepatosplenomegaly, adenopathy	Very common (95%)	Common
Lymphoid interstitial pneumonitis	Very common (50%)	Unusual
CNS disorders	Very common (50%)	Very common
Malignances	Unusual (4%)	Very common
Parotitis	Occurs (10%)	Rare
Laboratory findings		
Hypergammaglobulinemia	Very common	Common
Lymphopenia	Unusual	Very common
Decreased T-helper cells	Occurs	Very common

lying HIV infection, but a positive result must be followed by careful confirmatory testing. In these children, other congenital immunodeficiencies, congenital infections (CMV, toxoplasmosis, syphilis), and many other illnesses may cause similar presenting clinical signs.

Complications & Sequelae

These result from direct viral invasion (brain, lung, heart, kidney), secondary malignancies (less common than in adults; Kaposi's sarcoma has been seen in children, as have lymphomas and polyclonal B cell lymphoproliferative syndromes), and infections with a multitude of agents (eg, *P carinii, Candida albicans,* herpes simplex, CMV, measles, *Toxoplasma gondii Cryptosporidium* spp, *Mycobacterium avium -intracellulare, Cryptococcus neoformans, Nocardia* spp, and *Histoplasma capsulatum*).

Prevention

Awareness of modes of transmission is crucial for prevention. Caregivers should encourage AIDS education for children entering puberty. Heterosexual spread may be the primary problem in the future. Although condom use may not be fully preventive, it is highly recommended.

All medical equipment that can penetrate skin should be sterile. Infected blood and secretions should be handled according to the recommendations made by the Centers for Disease Control (see below).

There is currently no way to prevent perinatal transmission; cesarian section is not effective. It is recommended that HIV-infected mothers not become pregnant. Since breast milk can carry the virus, breast-feeding by HIV-positive mothers is contraindicated.

Therapy

A. Specific Measures: The only specific antiviral available currently is azidothymidine (AZT), an orally absorbed nucleoside analog that prevents viral DNA synthesis and secondarily inhibits replication. Being virostatic, it must be taken for life. In adults, it has improved survival and immune function in patients with AIDS or those with very low helper T cell counts. The major toxicities are anemia, neutropenia, headache, myalgia, and insomnia. Preliminary studies in children have been promising; a suspension has been approved by the FDA for use in children. Whenever possible, children should be enrolled in collaborative treatment studies. Recommendations for therapy change rapidly; consultation must be obtained.

B. General Measures:

1. Immunizations—Combined diphtheria-tetanus-pertussis (DTP), conjugated *Haemophilus influenzae* type b (Hib), pneumococcal, and influenza vaccines should be given at the recommended times. Due to the possibility of vaccine-associated polio developing in the patient or immunodeficient contacts after oral polio vaccine, the inactivated polio vaccine is recommended both for patients and well children in households with HIV-infected patients (see Chapter 6). The risk of wild measles is considered greater than the potential risk of the vaccine in asymptomatic children; thus, measles-mumps-rubella vaccine should be given at the usual time. It is not recommended for symptomatic children. Varicella or measles may be fatal; prophylaxis with immune serum globulin or varicella-zoster immune globulin should be given after each exposure to all unimmunized HIV-infected children and to symptomatic immunized children.

2. Infections—Bacterial infections should be diagnosed and treated aggressively. Antibiotic prophylaxis is not recommended unless the patient has had *P carinii* pneumonia, in which case therapy is often continued indefinitely. Adverse reactions to some agents (eg, sulfonamides) limit this approach in many patients. Unusual infections may require invasive diagnostic techniques such as biopsy or brochoscopy. Agents such as *Mycombacterium avium-itracellulare,* CMV, and *cryptosporidium* spp are often impossible to eradicate due to the lack of immune response.

Prevention of infection and immune enhancement using periodic intravenous immune globulin therapy is being evaluated.

3. Lymphoid Interstitial Pneumonitis—This may respond to steroid therapy. The long-term toxicity of steroids in patients with HIV infection is unknown.

4. General Support—Careful attention to psychosocial needs and nutrition is important. Ideally, care should be coordinated by a team of caregivers familiar with this disease, the newest therapies, and all community support systems available. Transfusions may be needed; CMV seronegative blood is preferred.

Prognosis

Poor prognosis is associated with perinatal infection, encephalopathy, infection with *P carinii,* and early development of AIDS. Some children, especially those infected by blood products, may live many years. The presence of lymphoid interstitial pneumonitis is a relatively good indicator (median survival over 7 years). Due to the great variability in individual response to infection and treatment, definite statements regarding the prognosis for duration or quality of life should not be made.

Public Health Issues

In general, the toilet-trained child who is well enough to attend school should be educated as any other child. Although health-care providers and the teacher and nurse need to be aware of the underlying diagnosis, it is otherwise confidential. The social consequences of HIV infection often overshadow the medical problems.

Secretions are not considered contagious in routine living situations. The virus in blood or serum is easily neutralized by a variety of agents, including household bleach (1:10 dilution), some commercial disinfectants (eg, Lysol), or 70% isopropyl alcohol.

Centers for Disease Control, USA: Classification system for human immunodeficiency virus (HIV) infection in children under 13 years of age. *MMWR* 1987;**36**:225.

Centers for Disease Control, USA: Immunization of children infected with human immunodeficiency virus: Supplemental ACIP statement. *MMWR* 1988;**37**:181.

Falloon J et al: Human immunodeficiency virus infection in children. *J Pediatr* 1989;**114**:1. [A comprehensive review and bibliography from the National Institutes of Health.]

McKinney RE et al: Safety and tolerance of intermittent intravenous and oral zidovudine therapy in human immunodeficiency virus-infected pediatric patients. *J Pediatr* 1990;**116**:640.

Scott GB et al: Survival in children with perinatally acquired human immunodeficiency virus type 1 infection. *N Engl J Med* 1989;**321**:1791.

Yarchoan R et al: Clinical and basic advances in the antiretroviral therapy of human immunodeficiency virus infection. *Am J Med* 1989;**87**:191.

MOLLUSCUM CONTAGIOSUM

This virus causes small pink to flesh-colored asymptomatic umbilicated papular lesions on the face, back, buttocks, and arms. Transmission by close contact is presumed, with a 6–8 week incubation period. School outbreaks have been described. Sexual transmission occurs. Diagnosis is usually visual; rarely is biopsy required. Therapeutic measures include 0.9% cantharidin (rapid and nonpainful), curettage, topical liquid nitrogen, podophyllin, or silver nitrate. Although molluscum is usually benign and self-limited, autoinoculation may produce many lesions.

RABIES

Essentials of Diagnosis

- History of animal bite 10 days to 1 year previously.
- Paresthesias or hyperesthesia in bite area.
- Irritability followed by fever, confusion, combativeness, muscle spasms (especially pharyngeal with swallowing).
- Progressive symptoms, death.
- Rabies antigen detected in corneal scrapings or tissue obtained by brain or skin biopsy; Negri bodies seen in brain tissue.

General Considerations

Rabies remains a serious public health problem wherever animal immunization is not widely prac-

ticed. Although infection does not always follow a bite by a rabid animal (about 40% infection rate following rabid dog bites), infection is fatal. Although any warm-blooded animal may be infected, susceptibility and transmissibility vary with species. Bats may be well yet carry and excrete the virus in saliva or feces for prolonged periods. Dogs and cats are usually clinically ill within 10 days of becoming contagious (the standard quarantine period for well animals). Valid quarantine periods or signs of illness are not fully known for many species. Rodents rarely transmit infection. Animal vaccines are only partially immunogenic; a single inoculation may fail to produce immunity in up to 20% of dogs.

Clinical Findings

A. History: The risk is assessed according to the type of animal (bats always considered rabid), the animal's behavior (unprovoked bite or unusual behavior), wound extent and location (infection more common after head or arm bites, or if wounds have extensive salivary contamination or are not quickly and thoroughly cleaned), geographic area (urban rabies rare to nonexistent in many US cities; rural rabies always possible, especially outside USA), and animal vaccination history (risk low if documented). Due partially to the long incubation period, a bite history is not always obtained. Rarely, aerosolized virus in caves inhabited by bats causes infection.

B. Symptoms and Signs: Paresthesias at the bite site are usually the first symptom. Nonspecific anxiety and excitability follow; then muscle spasms, drooling, hydrophobia, delirium, and lethargy. Swallowing or even the sensation of air blown on the face may cause pharyngeal spasms. Seizures, fever, coma, and death follow within a week of onset.

C. Laboratory Findings: Leukocytosis is common. The spinal fluid may be normal or show elevation of protein and mononuclear cells. Cerebral imaging and electroencephalography are not diagnostic.

Infection in an animal may be determined by use of the fluorescent antibody test to examine brain tissue for antigen.

Rabies virus is excreted in the saliva of infected humans, but the diagnosis is usually made by antigen detection in scrapings or tissue samples of richly innervated epithelium (the site of early viral migration), eg, the cornea or hairline of the neck. Classic Negri cytoplasmic inclusion bodies in brain tissue are not always present.

Seroconversion occurs after 7–10 days.

Differential Diagnosis

Failure to elicit the bite history in areas where rabies is rare may delay diagnosis. Other disorders to be considered include pseudorabies (hysterical belief that one has the disease); parainfectious encephalopathy; encephalitis due to herpes simplex, arboviruses, enteroviruses, and lymphocytic choriomeningitis virus; and Guillain-Barré syndrome.

Prevention

See Chapter 6 for information regarding vaccination and postexposure prophylaxis. The development of human immune globulin and diploid cell vaccine has made prophylaxis more effective and minimally toxic. Since rabies is almost always fatal, the decision to use vaccine and immune globulin must be carefully made.

Treatment & Prognosis

Survival is rare but has been reported in patients receiving meticulous, intensive care. No antiviral preparations are of proved benefit.

Anderson LJ et al: Human rabies in the United States 1960–1979. *Ann Intern Med* 1984;**100:**728.
Mann JM: Systematic decision-making in rabies prophylaxis. *Pediatr Infect Dis* 1983;**2:**162.
Shah U, Jaswal GS: Victims of a rabid wolf in India: Effect of severity and location of bites on development of rabies. *J Infect Dis* 1976;**134:**25.

RUBELLA

Essentials of Diagnosis

"Typical case":
- History of rubella vaccination usually absent.
- Prodromal nonspecific respiratory symptoms and adenopathy (postauricular and occipital).
- Maculopapular rash beginning on face, rapidly spreading to entire body, and disappearing by fourth day.
- Few systemic symptoms.

Congenital infection:
- Retarded growth, development.
- Cataracts, retinopathy.
- Purpuric "blueberry muffin" rash at birth, jaundice, thrombocytopenia.
- Deafness.
- Congenital heart defect.

General Considerations

If it were not teratogenic, rubella would be of little clinical importance. Clinical diagnosis is difficult in some cases due to its variable expression. In one study, over 80% of infections were subclinical. Because of inadequate vaccination, many outbreaks now occur in adolescents or adults.

Clinical Findings

A. History: The incubation period is 14–21 days. The nondistinctive signs may make exposure history unreliable. A history of immunization makes rubella very unlikely.

Congenital rubella usually follows maternal infection in the first trimester.

B. Symptoms and Signs:
1. Infection in Children—Young children may present with the rash. Older patients often have a nonspecific prodrome of low-grade fever, ocular pain, sore throat, and myalgia. Postauricular and suboccipital adenopathy (sometimes generalized) is characteristic. This often precedes and may occur without the rash. The rash consists of discrete maculopapules beginning on the face. A "slapped cheek" appearance or pruritus may occur. The rash spreads to the trunk and extremities quickly after it fades from the face, it is gone by the fourth day. Exanthem is usually absent or consists of nonspecific erythema or a few macules or petechiae.

2. Congenital Infection—Over 80% of women infected in the first 4 months of gestation deliver affected infants, only 5–10% of those infected later in pregnancy do so. Later infections also result in more isolated defects, eg, deafness. The main manifestations are the following:

a. Growth retardation: 50–85% small at birth and remain so.

b. Cardiac anomalies: Pulmonary artery stenosis, patent ductus, ventricular septal defect.

c. Ocular anomalies: Cataracts, microphthalmia, glaucoma, retinitis.

d. Deafness.

e. Cerebral disorders: Chronic encephalitis.

f. Hematologic disorders: Thrombocytopenia, dermal nests of extramedullary hematopoiesis or purpura ("blueberry muffin" spots), lymphopenia.

g. Other: Hepatitis, osteomyelitis, immune disorders, malabsorption, diabetes.

C. Laboratory Findings: Leukopenia is common, and platelet counts may be low. Congenital infection is associated with low platelet counts, abnormal liver function tests, hemolytic anemia, pleocytosis, and very high rubella IgM antibody titers. Total serum IgM is elevated, and IgA and IgG levels may be depressed.

D. Imaging: Pneumonitis and bone metaphyseal longitudinal lucencies may be present in films of children with congenital infection.

Diagnosis

Virus may be isolated from throat or urine from 1 week prior to 2 weeks after rash onset. Children with congenital infection are infectious for months. The virus laboratory must be notified that rubella is suspected. Serologic diagnosis is best made by demonstrating a 2-dilution rise in antibody titer between specimens drawn 1–2 weeks apart. The first should be drawn promptly, since titers increase rapidly after rash onset. For the sake of accuracy, it is recommended that both specimens be tested simultaneously by a single laboratory. Specific IgM titers are not reliable for diagnosing disease outside the neonatal period. Because the decision to terminate a pregnancy is usually based on serologic results, testing must be done carefully.

Differential Diagnosis

Rubella may resemble infections due to enterovirus, adenovirus, measles, Epstein-Barr virus, roseola, parvovirus (erythema infectiosum), and *Toxoplasma gondii*. Because public health implications are great, sporadic suspected cases should be serologically or virologically confirmed.

Congenital rubella must be differentiated from congenital CMV, toxoplasmosis, and syphilis.

Complications & Sequelae

A. Arthralgia/Arthritis: Both occur more often in older females. Polyarticular involvement (fingers, knees, wrists), lasting a few days to weeks, is typical. Frank arthritis occurs in a few percent. It may resemble acute rheumatoid arthritis.

B. Encephalitis: With an incidence of about 1 in 6000, this is a nonspecific parainfectious encephalitis associated with a low mortality rate. A syndrome resembling subacute sclerosing panencephalitis (see rubeola) has also been described in congenital rubella.

C. Rubella in Pregnancy: Infection in the mother is self-limited and not unusually severe (see above for sequelae).

Prevention

See Chapter 6 for the indications for and efficacy of rubella vaccine. Standard prenatal care in many areas includes rubella antibody testing. Seropositive mothers are at no risk; seronegative mothers are vaccinated after delivery.

A pregnant woman possibly exposed to rubella should be tested immediately; if seropositive, she is immune and need not worry. If she is seronegative, a second specimen should be drawn and both specimens should be tested simultaneously in 4–6 weeks. Seroconversion suggests high fetal risk; such women require counseling regarding therapeutic abortion.

When pregnancy termination is not an option, some experts recommend intramuscular administration of 20 mL of standard immune serum globulin within 72 hours of exposure in an attempt to prevent infection. (This negates the value of subsequent antibody testing.) The efficacy of this is unknown.

Therapy & Prognosis

Symptomatic therapy is sufficient. Arthritis may improve with administration of anti-inflammatory agents. Prognosis is excellent in those with acquired disease but poor in congenitally infected infants, in whom most defects are irreversible or progressive.

Chantler JK et al: Persistent rubella virus infection associated with chronic arthritis in children. *N Engl J Med* 1985;**313**:1117.

Desmond MM et al: The longitudinal course of congenital rubella encephalitis in non-retarded children. *J Pediatr* 1978;**93**:584.

Herrman KL: Available rubella serologic tests. *Rev Infect Dis* 1985;**7** (**Suppl**):108.

Miller E et al: Consequences of confirmed maternal rubella at successive stages of pregnancy. *Lancet* 1982;**2**:781.

II. RICKETTSIAL INFECTIONS

These pleomorphic, gram-negative coccobacilli are obligate intracellular parasites. They are often in the differential diagnosis of febrile rashes, although they may cause a variety of other illnesses not characterized by rash. The endothelium is the primary target tissue, and the ensuing vasculitis is responsible for severe illness.

All except Q fever are transmitted by cutaneous arthropod contact, either by bite or fecal contamination of skin breaks. Evidence of such contact by history or physical exam may be completely lacking, especially in young children. The geographic distribution of the vector is often the primary determinant for suspicion of these infections.

Diagnosis is serologic; elevation of antibodies to *Proteus* strains (OX19, OX2, OX K, the classic Weil-Felix test) is easily measured but less specific than many other tests now available. Therapy must often be empirical. Most new broad-spectrum antimicrobials are inactive against these cell wall–deficient organisms; chloramphenicol and tetracycline are usually effective.

EHRLICHIA CANIS INFECTION

Ehrlichia spp are known to cause febrile pancytopenia in dogs (*E canis*) and other animals and a mononucleosis-like syndrome in humans in Japan (*E sennetsu*). Recent evidence suggests that human infection with *E. canis* is underrecognized; in one study 10% of adults suspected of having Rocky Mountain spotted fever had serologic evidence of *E canis* infection. Canines serve as the reservoir, and ticks are the vectors. Most cases in the United States have been diagnosed in the South, in the spring.

The clinical presentation consists of fever, headache, myalgia, and anorexia; nausea and vomiting may occur. A nondiagnostic rash has also been described, occasionally suggesting Kawasaki disease. The physical examination is usually normal; although mild cervical adenopathy and organomegaly have been described, their absence is more typical. Characteristic laboratory abnormalities include mild leukopenia and thrombocytopenia and elevated transaminase levels.

Diagnosis is made serologically; characteristic intracytoplasmic inclusions in leukocytes may be present. Although the disease may last several weeks, it is usually self-limited. Tetracycline therapy is beneficial; chloramphenicol may also be effective. The differential diagnosis includes other rickettsial infections, leptospirosis, Epstein-Barr virus infection, cytomegalovirus infection, hepatitis, other viral infections, lupus, and leukemia.

Barton LL, Foy TM: *Ehrlichia canis* infection in a child. *Pediatrics* 1989;**4**:580.
Fishbein DB et al: Human ehrlichiosis: Prospective active surveillance in febrile hospitalized patients. *J Infect Dis* 1989;**160**:803.

RICKETTSIALPOX

Rickettsia akari is transmitted by mites on infected house mice. Infection is rarely diagnosed; most cases have occurred in Northeastern cities, particularly New York. The bite site becomes a papule, then a pustule; it ulcerates and then scabs at about the time fever develops, at 9–14 days. Local adenopathy is the rule. Headache, myalgia, and photophobia are followed in 2–4 days by a generalized, central, and discrete papular rash. Vesicles develop on the papules and form crusts. The fever lasts about a week.

The differential diagnosis includes varicella, enteroviral infections, the other rickettsial spotted fevers, meningococcemia, and gonococcemia. Mild cases require no therapy. The Weil-Felix test is negative.

Brettman LK et al: Rickettsialpox: Report of an outbreak and contemporary review. *South Afr Med J* 1981; **60**:363.

ROCKY MOUNTAIN SPOTTED FEVER

Rickettsia rickettsii infection causes one of many similar tick-borne illnesses characterized by fever and a rash. Most are named for their geographic area—Siberian, Queensland, Kenyan, etc. In all except Rocky Mountain spotted fever, there is a characteristic eschar at the bite site, the "tache noire." Dogs and rodents are reservoirs of the *R rickettsii*.

Rocky Mountain spotted fever is the most severe of these infections and most important in the USA. It occurs predominantly in the South and Southeast, rarely in the West. Most cases are in children exposed in rural areas in the spring and summer. Since tick attachment lasting 4 hours or longer is needed, frequent tick removal is a preventive measure.

After the incubation period of 2–8 days, there is high fever (over 40°C [104°F], often hectic) of abrupt onset, myalgia, severe and persistent headache (less obvious in infants), general toxicity, vomiting, and diarrhea. The characteristic rash occurs in over 95% of patients and appears 2–6 days after fever onset as macules on the palms, soles, and extremities, becoming petechial and spreading centrally. Conjunctivitis, splenomegaly, muscle tenderness, edema, and meningismus may be seen.

Laboratory findings are nonspecific and reflect diffuse vasculitis: thrombocytopenia, hyponatremia, early mild leukopenia, proteinuria, and hematuria. Elevated *Proteus* OX 19 and OX 2 titers are found in the second week.

Complications and death result from severe vasculitis, especially in the brain, heart, and lung. The mortality rate is 5–7%. To be effective therapy must be early and is often based on a presumptive diagnosis in endemic areas prior to rash onset. Chloramphenicol is the agent of choice for children less than 8 years of age; a tetracycline may be used for older children.

The differential diagnosis includes meningococcemia, measles, meningitis, staphylococcal sepsis, enteroviral infection, leptospirosis, Colorado tick fever or infection by other arboviruses, and streptococcal pharyngitis.

Bernard K et al: Surveillance of Rocky Mountain spotted fever in the United States, 1978–1980. *J Infect Dis* 1982;**146**:297.
Helmick CG, Bernard KW, D'Angelo LJ: Rocky Mountain spotted fever: Clinical, laboratory and epidemiological features of 262 cases. *J Infect Dis* 1984;**150**:480.
Linnemann CC, Janson PJ: The clinical presentations of Rocky Mountain spotted fever. *Clin Pediatr* 1978; **17**:683.
Woodward TE: Rocky Mountain spotted fever: Epidemiology and early clinical signs are keys to treatment and reduced mortality. *J Infect Dis* 1984;**150**:465.

ENDEMIC TYPHUS (Murine Typhus)

Endemic typhus is present in the USA, mainly in Southern Texas. The disease is transmitted by fleas on infected rodents. There is no eschar at the bite, which may go unnoticed. The incubation period is 6–14 days. Headache, myalgia, and chills slowly worsen. Fever may last 10–14 days. After 3–8 days a rash appears. Truncal macules spread to the extremities but spare the palms and soles; the rash may become petechial. Intestinal and respiratory symptoms may occur. The illness is self-limited and milder than epidemic typhus. Therapy is not usually needed. Diagnosis is serologic.

SELECTED REFERENCES

Feigin RD, Cherry JD (editors): *Textbook of Pediatric Infectious Diseases,* 2nd ed. Saunders, 1987. [The most useful and comprehensive text for all pediatric infections.]

Galasso GH, Merigan TC, Buchanan RA (editors): *Antiviral Agents and Viral Diseases of Man,* 2nd ed. Raven, 1984.

Hanshaw JB, Dudgeon JA, Marshall WC: *Viral Diseases of the Fetus and Newborn.* Vol 17 of: *Major Problems in Clinical Pediatrics.* Saunders, 1985.

Moffett HL: *Pediatric Infectious Diseases,* 3rd ed. Lippincott, 1989. [This very current reference by a single author takes a problem-oriented approach useful for a basic understanding of many infections.]

Zuckerman AJ, Banatvala JE, Pattison JR: *Principles and Practice of Clinical Virology.* Wiley, 1987.

28

Infections: Bacterial & Spirochetal

Brian A. Lauer, MD, Mary P. Glodé, MD, & John W. Ogle, MD

BACTERIAL INFECTIONS

GROUP A STREPTOCOCCAL INFECTIONS

Essentials of Diagnosis

Streptococcal pharyngitis:
- Clinical diagnosis based entirely on symptoms; signs and physical examination unreliable.
- Throat culture yielding group A streptococci is essential.

Impetigo:
- Rapidly spreading, highly infectious skin rash.
- Erythematous denuded areas and honey-colored crusts.
- On culture, group A streptococci are grown in most (not all) cases.

General Considerations

Group A streptococci are common gram-positive bacteria capable of producing a wide variety of clinical illnesses. Prominent among these are acute pharyngitis; impetigo; cellulitis; and scarlet fever, the generalized illness caused by strains that elaborate erythrogenic toxin. Group A streptococci can also cause pneumonia, septic arthritis, osteomyelitis, meningitis, and numerous other less common infections. Group A streptococcal infections may also produce nonsuppurative sequelae (rheumatic fever or acute glomerulonephritis).

The cell walls of streptococci contain both carbohydrate and protein antigens. The C-carbohydrate antigen determines the *group,* and the M- or T-protein antigens determine the specific *type.* In most strains, the M protein appears to confer virulence, and antibodies developed against the M protein are protective against reinfection with that type.

Group A streptococci are almost all β-hemolytic. These organisms may be carried asymptomatically on the skin and in the pharynx, rectum, and vagina. Ten to 15% of school children in some studies are asymptomatic pharyngeal carriers of group A streptococci. Streptococcal carriers are asymptomatic individuals who do not mount an immune response to

the organism and are therefore believed to be at low risk for nonsuppurative sequelae. Unfortunately, there are no accepted criteria for identification of streptococcal carriers.

All group A streptococci are sensitive to penicillin. A small percentage have become resistant to erythromycin, the other mainstay of treatment.

Clinical Findings

A. Symptoms and Signs:

1. Respiratory infections—

a. Infancy and early types (under 3 years of age)—The onset of infection is insidious, with mild symptoms, eg, low-grade fever, serous nasal discharge, and pallor. Otitis media is common. Pharyngitis with exudate and cervical adenitis are uncommon in this age group.

b. Childhood type—Onset is sudden, with fever and marked malaise and often with repeated vomiting. The pharynx is sore and edematous, and the tonsillar area generally shows exudate. Anterior cervical lymph nodes are tender and enlarged. Small petechiae are frequently seen on the soft palate. Fine discrete petechiae on the upper abdomen and trunk occasionally also appear. In scarlet fever, the skin is diffusely erythematous and appears sunburned and roughened (sandpaper rash). The rash is most intense in the axillas and groin and on the abdomen and trunk. It blanches on pressure except in the skin folds, which do not blanch and are pigmented (Pastia's sign). The rash usually appears 24 hours after the onset of fever and rapidly spreads over the next 1–2 days. Desquamation begins on the face at the end of the first week and becomes generalized by the third week. Early, the surface of the tongue is coated white, with the papillae enlarged and bright red ("white strawberry tongue"). Subsequently, desquamation occurs, and the tongue appears beefy red ("red strawberry tongue"). The face generally shows circumoral pallor. Petechiae may be seen on all mucosal surfaces.

c. Adult type—The adult type is characterized by exudative or nonexudative tonsillitis with fewer systemic manifestations, lower fever, and no vomiting. Scarlet fever is uncommon in this age group.

2. Impetigo—Streptococcal impetigo begins as a papule that vesiculates and then breaks, leaving a denuded area covered by a honey-colored crust. Both *Staphylococcus aureus* and group A streptococci are isolated in some cases. The lesions spread readily and diffusely. Local lymph nodes may become swollen and inflamed. Although the affected child often lacks systemic symptoms, occasionally a high fever and toxicity are present. If flaccid bullae are present, the disease is called bullous impetigo and it is caused by an epidermolytic toxin-producing strain of *S. aureus*.

3. Cellulitis—The portal of entry is often an insect bite or superficial abrasion on an extremity. There is a diffuse and rapidly spreading cellulitis that involves the subcutaneous tissues and extends along the lymphatic pathways with only minimal local suppuration. Local acute lymphadenitis occurs. The child is usually acutely ill, with fever and malaise. In classic erysipelas, the involved area is bright red, swollen, warm, and very tender. The infection may extend rapidly from the lymphatics to the bloodstream.

Streptococcal perianal cellulitis is an entity peculiar to young children. Pain with defecation often leads to constipation, which may be the presenting complaint. The child is afebrile and otherwise well. Perianal erythema and tenderness and painful rectal examination are the only abnormal physical findings. Culture of a perianal swab specimen usually yields a heavy growth of group A streptococcus. Any of the antimicrobial regimens for streptococcal infection is usually effective. A variant of this syndrome is streptococcal vaginitis in prepubertal girls. Symptoms are dysuria and pain; marked erythema and tenderness of the introitus and blood-tinged discharge are seen.

4. Necrotizing fasciitis—Formerly called streptococcal gangrene, this is an uncommon but dangerous entity. Only 20–40% of cases are due to group A streptococci. About 30–40% are due to *S. aureus* and the rest to mixed bacterial infections. The disease is characterized by extensive necrosis of superficial fasciae, with undermining of surrounding tissue and extreme systemic toxicity. Initially, the skin overlying the infection is pale red without distinct borders, resembling subcutaneous cellulitis. Blisters or bullae may appear. The color deepens to a distinct purple. The involved area may develop mild to massive edema. Early recognition and aggressive debridement of necrotic tissue are essential.

5. Group A streptococcal infections in newborn nurseries—Group A streptococcal epidemics still occasionally occur in nurseries. The organism may be introduced into the nursery from the vaginal tract of a mother or from the throat or nose of a mother or member of the staff. The organism then spreads from infant to infant. The umbilical stump is colonized while the infant is in the nursery. As is true also in staphylococcal infections, there may be no or few clinical manifestations while infants are still in the nursery; most often, a colonized infant develops a chronic, oozing omphalitis days later at home. The organism may spread from the infant to other family members. More serious and even fatal infections may develop, including sepsis, meningitis, empyema, septic arthritis, and peritonitis.

B. Laboratory Findings: Leukocytosis with a marked shift to the left is seen early. Eosinophilia regularly appears during convalescence. β-hemolytic streptococci are cultured with ease from the throat. The organism may be cultured from the skin and by needle aspiration from subcutaneous tissues and other involved sites, such as infected nodes. Occasionally, blood cultures are positive. Group A streptococci may be identified most easily by demonstrable sensitivity to bacitracin. Grouping by immunofluorescence or coagglutination studies correlates best with the original precipitin reactions described by Lancefield. Typing is not routinely done and is dependent upon the presence of specific M and T antigens in the cell wall.

Rapid antigen detection tests are 60–95% sensitive and over 95% specific for detecting group A streptococci in throat swabs. The predictive value of negative tests is about 80%, meaning that 1 in 5 patients with a positive throat culture will have a negative rapid antigen test. Rapid tests may be useful when early antibiotic therapy is considered, but because the currently available tests lack sensitivity, a standard culture should be done on specimens testing negative.

Antistreptolysin O (ASO) titers rise about 150 units within 2 weeks after an acute infection. Elevated ASO and anti-DNase B titers are useful in documenting prior throat infections in cases of acute rheumatic fever. However, elevated anti-DNase B and antihyaluronidase titers are most useful in associating pyoderma and acute glomerulonephritis. The streptozyme test is a useful 2-minute slide test that detects antibodies to streptolysin O, hyaluronidase, streptokinase, DNase B, and NADase. It is somewhat more sensitive than the measurement of ASO titers.

Proteinuria, cylindruria, and minimal hematuria may be seen early in children with streptococcal infection. More commonly, true poststreptococcal glomerulonephritis is seen 1–4 weeks after the respiratory infection.

Differential Diagnosis

Streptococcosis of the early childhood type must be differentiated from adenovirus and other respiratory virus infections.

Adenoviruses, coxsackieviruses (both A and B), echoviruses, Epstein-Barr virus (infectious mononucleosis), and many other respiratory viruses can produce pharyngitis. The pharyngitis in herpangina (coxsackie A viruses) is vesicular or ulcerative. Herpes simplex also causes ulcerative lesions, which most commonly involve the anterior pharynx, tongue, and gums. With other viruses (coxsackie viruses and echoviruses), rashes are common. In infectious mononucleosis, the pharyngitis is often exudative, but generalized lymphadenopathy is also present, and laboratory findings are often diagnostic (atypical lymphocytes, elevated liver enzymes, and a positive heterophil or other serologic test for mononucleosis). Uncomplicated streptococcal pharyngitis improves within 24–48 hours on penicillin therapy, and by 72–96 hours without antimicrobials.

In diphtheria, systemic symptoms, vomiting, and fever are less marked; the pseudomembrane is confluent and adherent; the throat is less red; and cervical adenopathy is prominent.

Pharyngeal tularemia causes white rather than yellow exudate. There is little erythema, and cultures for β-hemolytic streptococci are negative. A history of exposure to rabbits and a failure to respond to antimicrobials may suggest a diagnosis of tularemia. Response to specific antibiotic therapy is prompt.

Leukemia and agranulocytosis may present with pharyngitis and are diagnosed by bone marrow examination.

Scarlet fever must be differentiated from other exanthematous diseases, principally rubella. Erythema due to sunburn, drug reactions, fever, Kawasaki disease, toxic shock syndrome, and staphylococcal scalded skin syndrome must at times be considered.

Complications

The most common suppurative complications of group A streptococcal infections are purulent or serous rhinitis, sinusitis, otitis, mastoiditis, cervical lymphadenitis, pneumonia, empyema, septic arthritis, and meningitis. Spread of streptococcal infection from the throat to other sites, principally the skin (impetigo) and vagina, is common also and should be considered in every instance of chronic vaginal discharge or chronic skin infection, such as that complicating childhood eczema.

Both acute rheumatic fever and acute glomerulonephritis are nonsuppurative complications of group A streptococcal infections.

A. Acute Rheumatic Fever: See Chapter 16.

B. Acute Glomerulonephritis: Acute nephritis can follow streptococcal infections of either the pharynx or the skin, in contrast to rheumatic fever, which follows pharyngeal infection only. Glomerulonephritis may occur at any age, including infancy. In most reported series of acute glomerulonephritis, males predominate by a ratio of 2:1, whereas acute rheumatic fever occurs with equal frequency in both sexes.

Certain M types are strongly associated with poststreptococcal glomerulonephritis (''nephritogenic types''). Moreover, the serotypes resident on or producing disease on the skin often differ from those found in the pharynx. Pharyngeal infections leading to glomerulonephritis include M types 1, 4, 12, and

18, with limited evidence for 3, 6, and 25. Skin M types leading to nephritis include 2, 31, 49, 52–55, 57, and 60.

The incidence of acute glomerulonephritis after streptococcal infection is variable and has ranged from 0 to 28%. Several outbreaks of acute glomerulonephritis in families have involved 50–75% of siblings of affected patients in 1- to 7-week periods. Second attacks of glomerulonephritis are rare. The median latent period between infection and the development of glomerulonephritis is 10 days. This contrasts with acute rheumatic fever, which occurs after a median latent period of 18 days.

Treatment

A. Specific Measures: Treatment is directed not only toward eradication of acute infection but also toward the prevention of rheumatic fever. In patients with pharyngitis, antibiotics should be started early to relieve symptoms and should be continued for 10 days to prevent rheumatic fever. Although early therapy has not been shown to prevent glomerulonephritis, it seems advisable to promptly treat impetigo in sibling contacts of patients with poststreptococcal nephritis. Neither sulfonamides nor trimethoprim-sulfamethoxazole is effective in the treatment of streptococcal infections.

Although topical therapy for impetigo with antimicrobial ointments (eg, bacitracin, mupiricin) is as effective as systemic therapy, it does not eradicate pharyngeal carriage and is less practical for extensive disease.

1. Penicillin—A single dose of benzathine penicillin G (Bicillin) given intramuscularly (0.6 million units for children weighing less than 60 pounds and 1.2 million units for children weighing more than 60 pounds) is preferred for treatment of pharyngitis and impetigo. Phenoxymethyl penicillin (penicillin V) 250 mg administered orally 3 or 4 times daily between meals for 10 days is successful in about 90% of cases. Giving penicillin V (250 mg) twice daily is as effective as more frequent oral administration or intramuscular therapy, but a single daily dose results in a higher failure rate. Parenteral therapy is indicated if there is vomiting or sepsis. Mild cellulitis may be similarly treated. Cellulitis requiring hospitalization should be treated with aqueous penicillin G, (150,000 units/kg/d intravenously in 4–6 divided doses) or procaine penicillin (50,000 units/kg intramuscularly once or twice a day) until there is marked improvement. Penicillin V, 125–250 mg every 6 hours, may then be given orally to complete a 10-day course. Acute cervical lymphadenitis may require incision and drainage. Treatment of necrotizing fasciitis requires emergency surgical debridement followed by high-dose parenteral antibiotics appropriate to the organisms cultured.

2. Other antibiotics—For pharyngitis or impetigo, erythromycin estolate (20–40 mg/kg per day in 2 to 4 divided doses) should be given for 10 days. Erythromycin ethyl succinate (40–50 mg/kg per day) is best tolerated if given in 4 divided doses. Both erythromycin preparations are best absorbed and tolerated when taken with food. Clindamycin, cephalexin, cephradine and cefadroxil are also effective oral antimicrobials. The dosage of clindamycin is 10–20 mg/kg/d in 4 divided doses. Each of these drugs should be given for 10 days. Many strains are resistant to tetracycline. For serious or life-threatening infections in patients with known penicillin allergy, cephalothin (100–200 mg/kg/d intravenously in 4 divided doses) or cefazolin (100–150 mg/kg/d intravenously or intramuscularly in 3 divided doses) should be given.

3. Treatment failure—Reculture after cessation of therapy is indicated only in the patient with pharyngitis who has a personal or family history of rheumatic fever. Even when compliance is perfect, organisms will be found at this time in 5–15% of children with infections. Retreatment at least once with benzathine penicillin G or a different oral antibiotic is indicated.

4. Prevention of recurrences in rheumatic individuals—The preferred prophylaxis for rheumatic individuals is benzathine penicillin G, 1.2 million units given intramuscularly once every 3 weeks. One of the following alternative oral prophylactic regimens may be used: sulfadiazine, 0.5–1 g daily; penicillin G, 200,000 units twice daily; or erythromycin, 250 mg twice daily. Most authorities feel that lifelong prophylaxis is indicated, particularly in the presence of rheumatic heart disease. A similar approach to the prevention of recurrences of glomerulonephritis is debatable but may be indicated during childhood when there is a suspicion that repeated streptococcal infections coincide with flare-ups of acute glomerulonephritis.

B. General Measures: Analgesic lozenges or gargles with 30% glucose or warm saline solution may be used for relief of sore throat. A soft, bland diet that includes noncarbonated high-glucose drinks (such as apple, grape, and pear juice) and iced milk or sherbet is helpful. Acetaminophen is useful for pain or fever.

With impetigo, local treatment may promote earlier healing. Crusts should first be soaked off; areas beneath the crusts should then be washed with soap daily.

C. Treatment of Complications: Acute complications are best treated with penicillin. Rheumatic fever is best prevented by early adequate penicillin treatment of the streptococcal infection (see above).

D. Treatment of Carriers: Identification and management of group A streptococcal carriers is difficult. There are no established clinical or serologic criteria for differentiating carriers from the truly infected. Some children receive multiple courses of antimicrobials, with persistence of group A strepto-

cocci in the throat, leading to a "streptococcal neurosis" on the part of families.

Clindamycin (20 mg/kg/d in 4 divided doses) given orally or a combination of rifampin (20 mg/kg/d for 4 days) given orally and penicillin in standard dosage given orally has been used to improve bacteriologic cure rates after streptococcal pharyngitis and may be useful in selected streptococcal carriers.

Prognosis

Death is rare except in infants or young children with sepsis or pneumonia. The febrile course is shortened and complications eliminated by early and adequate treatment with penicillin.

Chaudhary S et al: Penicillin V and rifampin for the treatment of group A streptococcal pharyngitis: A randomized trial of 10 days penicillin vs 10 days penicillin with rifampin during the final 4 days of therapy. *J Pediatr* 1985;**106**:481.

Christie CDC, Havens PL, Shapiro ED: Bacteremia with group A streptococci in childhood. *Am J Dis Child* 1988; **142**:559.

Gerber MA: Diagnosis of group A β-hemolytic streptococcal pharyngitis. Use of antigen detection tests. *Diagn Microbiol Infect Dis* 1986;**4(Suppl)**:5.

Gerber MA, Randolph MF, Mayo DR: The group A streptococcal carrier state. *Am J Dis Child* 1988;**142**:562.

Gerber MA et al: Failure of once-daily penicillin V therapy for streptococcal pharyngitis. *Am J Dis Child* 1989; **143**:153.

Kaplan EL: The group A streptococcal upper respiratory tract carrier state: An enigma. *J Pediatr* 1980;**97**:337.

Randolph MF et al: Effect of antibiotic therapy on the clinical course of streptococcal pharyngitis. *J Pediatr* 1985; **106**:870.

Todd JK: Special series: Infectious diseases and the office laboratory. *J Infect Dis* 1982;**4**:265.

GROUP B STREPTOCOCCAL INFECTIONS

Essentials of Diagnosis

Early-onset neonatal sepsis or meningitis:
■ Newborn infant, age birth to 5 days, with rapidly progressing overwhelming sepsis, with or without meningitis.
■ Pneumonia with respiratory failure frequently present; chest x-ray resembles that seen in hyaline membrane disease.
■ Leukopenia with a shift to the left.
■ Blood or spinal fluid cultures growing group B streptococci.

Late-onset neonatal sepsis or meningitis:
■ Meningitis in a child 1–16 weeks old with spinal fluid or blood cultures growing group B streptococci.

General Considerations

Most patients with group B streptococcal disease are infants under 3 months of age. However, serious infection has been reported in women with puerperal sepsis, in immunocompromised patients, in patients with cirrhosis and spontaneous peritonitis, and in diabetics with cellulitis. Group B streptococcal infections occur as frequently as gram-negative infections in the newborn period. Two distinct clinical syndromes distinguished by differing perinatal events, age at onset, and serotype of the infecting strain have been described in these infants.

Clinical Findings

The first syndrome, early-onset illness, is observed in the newborn less than 5 days old. The onset of symptoms in the majority of these infants occurs in the first 48 hours of life. Apnea is often the first sign. There is high incidence of associated maternal obstetric complications, especially premature labor and prolonged rupture of the membranes. Newborns with early-onset disease are severely ill at the time of diagnosis, and the mortality rate is more than 50%. Although the majority of infants with early-onset infections have low birth weights, term infants may also develop fatal infection. Newborns with early-onset infection acquire the group B streptococcal organism from the maternal genital tract in utero or during passage through the birth canal. When early-onset infection is complicated by meningitis, as occurs in approximately 30% of cases, more than 80% of the bacterial isolates belong to serotype III. Postmortem examination of infants with early-onset disease almost always reveals pulmonary inflammatory infiltrates and hyaline membranes containing large numbers of group B streptococci.

Late-onset infection occurs in infants between 10 days and 4 months of age; the median age at onset is about 4 weeks. Maternal obstetric complications are infrequently associated with late-onset infection. These infants are usually not as severely ill at the time of diagnosis as those with early-onset disease, and the mortality rate is significantly lower (approximately 20%). However, up to 50% of infants with late-onset disease have meningitis. Other clinical manifestations, eg, septic arthritis and osteomyelitis, "occult" bacteremia, otitis media, ethmoiditis, conjunctivitis, cellulitis (particularly of the face or submandibular area), lymphadenitis, breast abscess, empyema, and impetigo, have been described. Strains of group B streptococci possessing the capsular type III polysaccharide antigen are isolated from more than 95% of infants with late-onset disease, regardless of clinical manifestations. The exact mode of transmission of the organisms is not well defined.

Prevention

Many women of childbearing age possess circulating antibody to the polysaccharide antigen of type III group B streptococci. This antibody is transferred to the newborn via the placental circulation. Carriers delivering healthy infants have significant serum levels of IgG antibody to this antigen. In contrast, women delivering infants who develop type III group B streptococcal disease of either the early- or late-onset type rarely have detectable antibody in their sera. Similar findings have recently been described for type Ia infections.

A vaccine prepared with type III polysaccharide has been evaluated in pregnant women. Although the vaccine is not optimally immunogenic, 63% of mothers produced IgG antibody.

Recent studies of the use of prophylactic penicillin in newborns to prevent early-onset group B streptococcal disease have produced conflicting results. Many infants with early-onset disease are bacteremic at birth, and use of penicillin in this group fails to control infection. Intrapartum ampicillin prophylaxis of mothers with positive cultures prevents early-onset disease.

Treatment

Penicillin G is the drug of choice. Group B streptococci are less susceptible than other streptococci to penicillin, and high doses are recommended, especially for meningitis (at least 250,000 units/kg/d, given in 3 doses per day to infants less than 1 week old and in 4 doses per day to older infants). Aminoglycosides act synergistically with penicillin in vitro; for this reason, some experts use both penicillin and gentamicin for meningitis and other serious infections. Penicillin dosage for nonmeningeal infections is 50,000 units/kg/d (q. 12 h doses) for infants less than 1 week old and 75,000–100,000 units/kg/d (q. 8 h doses) for older infants. Duration of therapy is 3 weeks for meningitis, at least 4 weeks for osteomyelitis or endocarditis, and 10–14 days for other infections. Therapy does not eradicate carriage of the organism.

Ablow RC et al: A comparison of early-onset group B streptococcal neonatal infection and the respiratory-distress syndrome of the newborn. *N Engl J Med* 1976; **294:**65.

Baker CJ: Prevention of neonatal group B streptococcal disease. *Pediatr Infect Dis J* 1983;**2:**1.

Baker CJ et al: Immunization of pregnant women with a polysaccharide vaccine of group B streptococcus. *N Engl J Med* 1988;**319:**1180.

Edwards MS et al: Long-term sequelae of group B streptococcal meningitis in infants. *J Pediatr* 1985;**106:**717.

Fischer GW: Immunoglobulin therapy of neonatal group B streptococcal infections: An overview. *Pediatr Infect Dis J* 1988;**7(Suppl):**13.

Paredes A et al: Nosocomial transmission of group B streptococci in a newborn nursery. *Pediatrics* 1977;**59:**679.

Pyati SP et al: Penicillin in infants weighing two kilograms or less with early-onset group B streptococcal disease. *N Engl J Med* 1983;**308:**1383.

Siegel JD et al: Single-dose penicillin prophylaxis of neonatal group B streptococcal disease. *Lancet* 1982;**1:**426.

STREPTOCOCCAL INFECTIONS WITH ORGANISMS OTHER THAN GROUP A OR B

General Considerations

Streptococci of groups other than A and B are part of the normal flora of humans and can cause disease. Group C or G organisms occasionally produce pharyngitis (with an ASO rise) but without risk of subsequent rheumatic fever, although acute glomerulonephritis may occasionally occur. Group D streptococci and enterococci are normal inhabitants of the gastrointestinal tract and may produce urinary tract infections, meningitis and sepsis in the newborn, and endocarditis. Nosocomial infections caused by enterococci are frequent in neonatal and oncology units. Nonhemolytic aerobic streptococci and α-hemolytic streptococci are normal flora of the mouth. They are involved in the production of dental plaque and probably dental caries and are the most common cause of subacute bacterial endocarditis. Finally, there are numerous anaerobic and microaerophilic streptococci, normal flora of the mouth, skin, and gastrointestinal tract, which alone or in combination with other bacteria may cause sinusitis, dental abscesses, brain abscesses, and intra-abdominal or lung abscesses.

Treatment

A. Enterococcal Infections: Urinary tract infections can be treated with oral ampicillin alone. Sepsis or meningitis in the newborn should be treated intravenously with a combination of ampicillin (100–200 mg/kg/d in 3 divided doses) and gentamicin (7.5 mg/kg/d in 3 divided doses). Endocarditis requires 6 weeks of intravenous treatment. Usually, penicillin G (250,000 units/kg/d in 6–8 divided doses), plus streptomycin (30 mg/kg/d) or gentamicin (6–7.5 mg/kg/d in 3 divided doses) is used. Third-generation cephalosporins are not useful. Ampicillin-resistant enterococci are susceptible to vancomycin (40–60 mg/kg/d in 4 divided doses). Careful monitoring of aminoglycoside levels is required, both to avoid toxicity and to ensure therapeutic levels.

Whenever endocarditis is being treated, peak and trough serum killing powers should be obtained. A bactericidal level of 1:8 or greater immediately before the next penicillin dose should be maintained.

B. Viridans Streptococcal Infections (Subacute Bacterial Endocarditis): It is important to determine the penicillin sensitivity of the infecting strain as early as possible in the treatment of viridans streptococcal endocarditis. Resistant organisms are most commonly seen in patients receiving chronic penicillin prophylaxis for rheumatic heart disease. Strains sensitive to penicillin G (minimum inhibitory concentrations, MIC, less than 0.1 μg/mL) may be treated for 4 weeks with penicillin, 150,000–200,000 units/kg/d IV, with streptomycin or gentamicin added during the first 2 weeks. If the MIC is 0.5 μg/mL or higher, longer therapy (at least 4 weeks) and higher doses of penicillin G must be used (200,000–300,000 units/kg/d IV in combination with streptomycin or gentamicin for 4–6 weeks). If the MIC is 0.1–0.5 μg/mL, penicillin G at the higher dose for a minimum of 4 weeks is recommended with gentamicin added for the first 2 weeks. Vancomycin 40 mg/kg/d is usually preferred for resistant strains and patients allergic to penicillin.

Bisno AL et al: Antimicrobial treatment of infective endocarditis due to viridans streptococci, enterococci, and staphylococci. *JAMA* 1989;**261:**1471.

Luginbuhl LM et al: Neonatal enterococcal sepsis: Case-control study and description of an outbreak. *Pediatr Infect Dis J* 1987;**11:**1022.

PNEUMOCOCCAL INFECTIONS

Essentials of Diagnosis

Bacteremia:
- High fever (≥ 39.4 °C [102.9 °F]).
- Leukocytosis (≥ 15,000/μL).
- Age 6–24 months.

Pneumonia:
- Fever, leukocytosis, and cough.
- Localized chest pain.
- Localized or diffuse rales. Chest x-ray may show lobar infiltrate (with effusion).

Meningitis:
- Fever, leukocytosis.
- Bulging fontanelle, neck stiffness.
- Irritability and lethargy.

All types:
- Diagnoses confirmed by cultures of blood, spinal fluid, pleural fluid, or other body fluid or by detection of pneumococcal antigen in urine or spinal fluid.

General Considerations

Pneumococcal sepsis, sinusitis, otitis media, pneumonitis, meningitis, osteomyelitis, cellulitis, arthritis, vaginitis, and peritonitis are all part of a spectrum of pneumococcal infection. Clinical findings that correlate with occult bacteremia in ambulatory patients include age (6–24 months), degree of temperature elevation (≥ 39.4 °C [102.9 °F]), and leukocytosis (≥ 15,000/μL). Although each of these findings is in itself nonspecific, a combination of them should arouse suspicion. This constellation of findings in a child who has no focus of infection may be an indication for blood cultures and antibiotic therapy. The cause of two-thirds of such bacteremic episodes is pneumococci. *Haemophilus influenzae* type b is the second most frequent cause.

Streptococcus pneumonae is the most common cause of acute purulent otitis media.

Pneumococci are the organisms responsible for most cases of acute bacterial pneumonia in children. The disease is indistinguishable on clinical grounds from other bacterial pneumonias. Effusions are common, although frank empyema is less common. Abscesses also occasionally occur.

Pneumococcal meningitis is much less common than *H influenzae* type b meningitis in children under age 5, but it is more common in older children. Pneumococcal meningitis, sometimes recurrent, may complicate serious head trauma, particularly if there is persistent leakage of cerebrospinal fluid. This has prompted some physicians to recommend the prophylactic administration of penicillin or other antimicrobials in such cases.

Children with sickle cell disease, other hemoglobinopathies, congenital or acquired asplenia, and some immunoglobulin and complement deficiencies are unusually susceptible to overwhelming pneumococcal sepsis and meningitis. These children often have a catastrophic illness with shock and disseminated intravascular coagulation. Even with excellent supportive care, the mortality rate is 20–50%. The spleen is important in the control of pneumococcal infection by clearing organisms from the blood and producing an opsonin that enhances phagocytosis. Autosplenectomy may explain why children with sickle cell disease are at increased risk for developing serious pneumococcal infections.

For more than 30 years, penicillin has been the agent of choice for pneumococcal infections. The majority of strains are still highly susceptible to penicillin; however, during the last 10 years, there have been increasing reports of pneumococci with moderately increased resistance to penicillin and reports of treatment failure, particularly in meningitis. The prevalence of these relatively penicillin-resistant strains in North America is about 3–15%. An outbreak of infections due to markedly penicillin-resistant pneumococci has been reported from South Africa. Pneumococci from normally sterile body fluids should be screened routinely for penicillin susceptibility. Pneumococci may also be resistant to chloramphenicol, erythromycin, and other antimicrobials.

Pneumococci have been classified into 83 serotypes based on capsular polysaccharide antigens. Serotypes 6, 14, 18, 19, and 23 cause most pneumococcal infections in children. The frequency distribution of serotypes varies at different times, in different geographic areas, and with different sites of infection. The most recently developed polyvalent pneumococcal vaccine contains capsular polysaccharides of 23 serotypes and is discussed in Chapter 6. Specific antibody induced by the vaccine protects only against the serotypes included in the vaccine. Children under age 18–24 months generally do not have a good antibody response to this vaccine, and the protective efficacy of the vaccine in older children is controversial. Despite these limitations, the vaccine is recommended for high-risk children over 2 years of age.

Clinical Findings

A. Symptoms and Signs: In pneumococcal sepsis, fever usually appears abruptly, often accompanied by chills. There may be no respiratory symptoms. In pneumococcal sinusitis, mucopurulent nasal discharge may occur. In infants and young children with pneumonia, cough and diffuse rales are found more often than the lobar distribution characteristic of adult forms of pneumococcal pneumonia. Respiratory distress is manifest by flaring of the alae nasi, chest retractions, and tachypnea. Abdominal pain is common. In older children, the adult form of pneumococcal pneumonia with signs of lobar consolidation may be found, but sputum is rarely bloody. Thoracic pain resulting from pleural involvement is sometimes present, but less often in children than in adults. With involvement of the right hemidiaphragm, pain may be referred to the right lower quadrant, suggesting appendicitis. Vomiting is common at onset but seldom persists. Convulsions are relatively common at onset in infants.

Meningitis is characterized by fever, irritability, convulsions, and neck stiffness. The most important sign in very young infants is a tense, bulging anterior fontanelle. In older children, fever, chills, headache, and vomiting are common symptoms. Classic signs are nuchal rigidity associated with positive Brudzinski and Kernig signs. With progression of untreated disease, the child may develop opisthotonos, stupor, and coma.

B. Laboratory Findings: Leukocytosis is often pronounced $(20,000–45,000/\mu L)$, with 80–90% polymorphonuclear neutrophils. Neutropenia may be seen early in very serious infections. The presence of pneumococci in the nasopharynx is not a helpful finding, because up to 40% of normal children carry pneumococci in the upper respiratory tract. Large numbers of organisms seen on gram-stained smears of endotracheal aspirate are seen with pneumonia. Needle aspiration of the lung rarely is indicated. In meningitis, cerebrospinal fluid usually shows an elevated white cell count of several thousand, chiefly polymorphonuclear neutrophils, with decreased glucose and elevated protein levels. Grampositive diplococci are seen on stained smears of cerebrospinal fluid sediment in 70–90% of cases. Detection of pneumococcal antigen allows rapid diagnosis and is most valuable when a child has been partially treated with antibiotics prior to lumbar puncture and the gram-stained smear and culture of spinal fluid are negative. Antigen detection in pleural fluid, serum, or joint fluid may also be helpful in selected cases. Testing urine for pneumococcal antigen is generally not helpful; this test lacks sensitivity, presumably because the antigen is degraded and only small molecular-size fragments are found in the urine.

Differential Diagnosis

There are many causes of high fever and leukocytosis in young infants; 80–90% of children presenting with these signs have a disease other than pneumococcal bacteremia, such as enteroviral or other viral infection, urinary tract infection, unrecognized focal infection elsewhere in the body, roseola infantum, or early acute shigellosis (diarrhea will appear later).

Infants with upper respiratory tract infection who subsequently develop signs of lower respiratory disease are most likely to be infected with a respiratory virus. Hoarseness or wheezing is often present. X-ray of the chest typically shows perihilar infiltrates and increased bronchovascular markings. It must be remembered, however, that viral respiratory infection often precedes pneumococcal pneumonia and that the clinical picture may be mixed.

Staphylococcal pneumonia frequently causes cavity formation and empyema, but it may be indistinguishable early in the course from pneumococcal pneumonia. It is most common in infants.

In primary pulmonary tuberculosis, children are not toxic, and x-rays show a primary focus associated with hilar adenopathy and often with signs of pleurisy. Miliary tuberculosis presents a classic x-ray appearance.

Pneumonia caused by *Mycoplasma pneumoniae* is most common in children 5 years of age and older. Onset is insidious, with infrequent chills, low-grade fever, prominent headache and malaise, cough, and, often, striking x-ray changes. Marked leukocytosis (eg, > 18,000/μL) is unusual.

Pneumococcal meningitis is diagnosed by lumbar puncture. Without a gram-stained smear and culture of spinal fluid, it is not distinguishable from other types of acute bacterial meningitis.

Complications

Complications of sepsis include meningitis and osteomyelitis; complications of pneumonia include empyema, parapneumonic effusion, and, rarely, lung abscess. Mastoiditis and meningitis may follow untreated pneumococcal otitis media. Both pneumococcal meningitis and peritonitis are more likely to occur independently without coexisting pneumonia. Shock, disseminated intravascular coagulation, and Waterhouse-Friderichsen syndrome resembling meningococcemia are occasionally seen in pneumococcal sepsis, particularly in asplenic patients.

Treatment

A. Specific Measures: Penicillin is the drug of choice, but erythromycin and cephalosporins are also effective.

1. Sepsis—All children with blood cultures that grow pneumococci must be reexamined as soon as possible. The child who has a focal infection such as pneumonia or meningitis or who appears septic should be admitted to the hospital and should receive parenteral penicillin G. Only if the child is afebrile and appears well should management on an ambulatory basis be considered. If the physician is assured of close follow-up, a second blood culture is performed (lumbar puncture is not mandatory); penicillin V (50–100 mg/kg/d orally for 10 days), is prescribed, and the initial dose is given at once. Some children may be intermittently afebrile yet still progress to meningitis.

2. Pneumonia—For infants, severely ill patients, and immunocompromised hosts, aqueous penicillin G (150,000–200,000 units/kg/d intravenously in 4–6 divided doses) is given. Mild pneumonia may be treated with phenoxymethyl penicillin (50 mg/kg/d orally in 4 divided doses for 7–10 days). Erythromycin (40–50 mg/kg/d orally in 4 divided doses) is given to patients allergic to penicillin. Oral cephalosporins may be used.

3. Otitis media—Treat with oral ampicillin, amoxicillin, trimethoprim-sulfamethoxazole, or erythromycin for 10 days.

4. Meningitis—Until bacteriologic confirmation, ampicillin plus chloramphenicol, cefotaxime, or ceftriaxone should be given intravenously. After bacteriologic confirmation, aqueous penicillin G (300,000 units/kg/d intravenously in 6 divided doses for 10–14 days) should be given. Meningitis due to organisms that are resistant or relatively resistant to penicillin should be treated with chloramphenicol, a third generation cephalosporin, or vancomycin (also see H influenzae, meningitis).

B. General Measures: Supportive and symptomatic care is required.

Prognosis

In children, case fatality rates of less than 1% should be achieved except in meningitis, in which rates of 5–20% still prevail. The presence of large numbers of organisms without a prominent cerebrospinal fluid inflammatory response or of meningitis due to a penicillin-resistant strain indicates a poor prognosis. Serious neurologic sequelae, particularly hearing loss, are more frequent following pneumococcal meningitis than following meningococcal or *H influenzae* type b meningitis.

Burman LA, Norrby R, Trollfors B: Invasive pneumococcal infections: Incidence, predisposing factors, and prognosis. *Rev Infect Dis* 1985;**7**:133.

Davies AJ, Kumaratne DS: The continuing problem of pneumococcal infection. *J Antimicrob Chemother* 1988;**21(4)**:387.

Gorensek MJ, Lebel MH, Nelson JD: Peritonitis in children with nephrotic syndrome. *Pediatrics* 1988;**81**:849.

Gray BM, Dillon HC Jr: Epidemiological studies of *Streptococcus pneumoniae* in infants: Antibody to types 3, 6, 14, and 23 in the first two years of life. *J Infect Dis* 1988;**158**:948.

Jackson MA et al: Relatively penicillin-resistant pneumococcal infections in pediatric patients. *Pediatr Infect Dis* 1984;**3**:129.

Klein JO: Bacteremia in ambulatory children. *Pediatr Infect Dis* 1984:**3(Suppl):**S5.

STAPHYLOCOCCAL INFECTIONS

Staphylococcal infections are common and important in childhood. Staphylococcal skin infections range from minor furuncles to the varied syndromes now collected under the encompassing term "scalded skin syndrome." Staphylococci are the major cause of osteomyelitis and, in older children, of septic arthritis. They are an uncommon but important cause of bacterial pneumonia. A toxin produced by certain strains causes staphylococcal food poisoning. Staphylococci are now responsible for most infections of artificial heart valves. They cause toxic shock syndrome (see below). Finally, they are found in infections at all ages and in multiple sites, particularly when infection is introduced from the skin or upper respiratory tract or when closed compartments become infected (pericarditis, sinusitis, cervical adenitis, surgical wounds, abscesses in the liver or brain, and abscesses elsewhere in the body).

Staphylococcus aureus and *Staphylococcus epidermidis* are normal flora of the skin and respiratory tract. The latter rarely causes disease except in compromised hosts, the newborn, or patients with a plastic prosthesis in place.

Many strains of *S aureus* elaborate a β-lactamase that confers penicillin resistance. This can be overcome in clinical practice by the use of a nonpenicillin antibiotic, a cephalosporin, or a penicillinase-resistant penicillin such as methicillin, oxacillin, nafcillin, cloxacillin, or dicloxacillin. Methicillin-resistant strains are found worldwide and are now common in certain hospitals and areas in the USA. Most of these strains retain β-lactamase production, and many are resistant to other antibiotics as well. Methicillin-resistant strains are also resistant in vivo to cephalosporins.

S aureus produces a variety of exotoxins, most of which are of uncertain importance. Two toxins are recognized as playing a central role in specific diseases: exfoliatin and staphylococcal enterotoxin. The former is largely responsible for the various clinical presentations of the scalded skin syndrome. Most strains that elaborate exfoliatin are of phage group II. The latter toxin causes staphylococcal food poisoning. The exoprotein toxin most commonly associated with toxic shock syndrome has been termed TSST-1. However, *S aureus* strains isolated from patients with toxic shock syndrome who have focal infections do not produce detectable TSST-1. Their organisms have been found to produce enterotoxins B or C, suggesting that the syndrome may be caused by more than one *S aureus* exoprotein.

Clinical Findings

A. Symptoms and Signs:

1. Staphylococcal skin diseases—Dermal infection with *S aureus* causes furuncles or cellulitis. More superficial infections are often found along with streptococci in impetigo. If the strains produce exfoliatin, localized lesions become bullous (bullous impetigo).

Generalized exfoliative disease (scalded skin syndrome) occurs as a result of more generalized involvement with exfoliatin-producing strains. The infection may begin at any site but appears to be introduced through the respiratory tract in most cases. There is a prodromal phase of erythema, often beginning around the mouth, accompanied by fever and irritability. The involved skin becomes tender, and a sick infant will cry when picked up or touched. A day or so later, exfoliation begins, usually around the mouth. The inside of the mouth is red, and a peeling rash is present around the lips, often in a radial pattern resembling rhagades. Generalized, painful peeling may follow, involving the limbs and trunk but often sparing the feet. More commonly, peeling is confined to areas around body orifices. If erythematous but unpeeled skin is rubbed sideways, superficial epidermal layers separate from deeper ones and a blister appears (Nikolsky's sign). In the newborn, the disease is termed **Ritter's disease** and may be fulminating. If there is tender erythema but not exfoliation, the disease is termed nonstreptococcal scarlet fever. The scarlatiniform rash is sandpaperlike, but strawberry tongue is not seen, and cultures grow *S aureus* rather than streptococci.

2. Osteomyelitis and septic arthritis—See Chapter 23.

3. Staphylococcal pneumonia—Staphylococcal pneumonia in infancy is characterized by abdominal distention, high fever, respiratory distress, and toxemia. It often occurs without predisposing factors or after minor skin infections. The organism is necrotizing, producing bronchoalveolar destruction. Pneumatoceles, pyopneumothorax, and empyema are frequently encountered. Rapid progression of disease is characteristic. Frequent chest x-rays to monitor the progress of disease are indicated and may be lifesaving. Presenting symptoms may be typical of paralytic ileus, suggestive of an abdominal catastrophe. When this is suspected, the abdominal films should always be accompanied by a chest film to rule out staphylococcal pneumonitis.

Staphylococcal pneumonia usually is peribronchial and diffuse and begins with a focal infiltrative lesion progressing to patchy consolidation. Most often only one lung is involved (80%), more often the right. Purulent pericarditis occurs by direct extension in about 10% of cases, with or without empyema.

4. Staphylococcal food poisoning—Staphylococcal food poisoning is produced by enterotoxin. The most common source is poorly refrigerated and contaminated food. The disease is characterized by vomiting, prostration, and diarrhea occurring 2–6 hours after ingestion of contaminated foods.

5. Staphylococcal endocarditis—*S aureus* may produce infection of normal heart valves, of valves or endocardium in children with congenital or rheumatic heart disease, or of artificial valves. In large recent series, about 25% of all cases of endocarditis are due to *S aureus*. The great majority of artificial heart valve infections involve either *S aureus* or *S epidermidis*. Infection usually begins in an extracardiac focus, often the skin. Involvement of the endocardium must be suspected in every case of *S aureus* bacteremia regardless of the presence of signs. Suspicion must be highest in the presence of congenital heart disease, particularly ventricular septal defects with aortic insufficiency but also simple ventricular septal defect, patent ductus arteriosus, and tetralogy of Fallot.

Clinical presentation in staphylococcal endocarditis is with fever, weight loss, weakness, muscle pain or diffuse skeletal pain, poor feeding, pallor, and cardiac decompensation. Signs include splenomegaly, cardiomegaly, petechiae, hematuria, and a new or changing murmur. The course of *S aureus* endocarditis is commonly rapid, although subacute disease is occasionally seen. Peripheral septic embolization and uncontrollable cardiac failure are not uncommon, even when optimal antibiotic therapy is administered, and may be indications for surgical intervention (see below).

6. Nursery Infections—*S aureus* colonizes the umbilicus and respiratory tract of a highly variable proportion of newborn infants (10–90%) during their nursery stay. The source of colonization is the skin and anterior nares of those handling the infants. Under normal circumstances, such colonization is harmless, since the bacterial strains involved are of low virulence. However, if a virulent strain is introduced (usually from an infected lesion), the proportion of sick to colonized infants can rise from less than 1% to over 50%. Such outbreaks may begin insidiously, since infants usually do not develop symptoms (furuncles, omphalitis, mastitis, impetigo, with occasional more serious disease) until after discharge. Thus, the occurrence of even a single case of staphylococcal disease in a nursery is an indication for epidemiologic surveillance of infants recently resident in that nursery, with possible subsequent institution of control measures.

7. Toxic shock syndrome—In 1978, Todd et al described a new syndrome of fever, blanching erythroderma, diarrhea, vomiting, myalgia, prostration, hypotension, and multiple organ involvement associated with cultures of *S aureus*. In that series, infection occurred equally in male and female children, with apparent heavy mucosal colonization (particularly in the female genital tract) or with clinically evident infection. Bacteremia did not occur.

Subsequently, large numbers of cases have been described in menstruating adolescents and young women using vaginal tampons. Toxic shock syndrome has also been seen in both male and female patients with focal staphylococcal infections as well as in individuals with postoperative wound infections due to *S aureus*. The epidemiologic connection with *S aureus* in this group has remained strong. Additional clinical features include sudden onset; conjunctival suffusion; mucosal hyperemia; desquamation of skin on the palms, soles, fingers, and toes during convalescence; disseminated intravascular coagulation in severe cases; renal and hepatic functional abnormalities; and evidence of myolysis. The mortality rate is now about 2%. Recurrences were seen during subsequent menstrual periods in as many as 60% of untreated women who continued to use tampons. Recurrences were reported in up to 15% of those who were treated with antistaphylococcal antibiotics and stopped using tampons. The disease is probably due to a toxin resembling one of the staphylococcal enterotoxins and elaborated by certain strains of *S aureus*.

8. S epidermidis infections—Localized and systemic *S epidermidis* infections occur primarily in immunocompromised patients, high-risk newborns, and patients with plastic prostheses or catheters. In one survey, *S epidermidis* was the fourth most common organism isolated from cases of septicemia in children with leukemia; in this group, there was a 10% mortality rate with a high incidence of antibiotic resistance. In low birth weight infants, *S epidermidis* has emerged as the commonest nosocomial pathogen in nurseries in the USA. In patients with an artificial heart valve, Dacron patch, ventriculoperitoneal shunt for hydrocephalus, or a Hickman or Broviac vascular catheter, *S epidermidis* is one of the very common causes of sepsis or catheter infection, often necessitating removal of the foreign material and prolonged antibiotic therapy. Because blood cultures are frequently contaminated by this organism, diagnosis of genuine localized or systemic infection is often difficult and sometimes uncertain.

B. Laboratory Findings: Moderate leukocytosis (15,000–20,000/μL) with a shift to the left is occasionally found, although normal counts are common, particularly in infants. The sedimentation rate is elevated. Blood cultures are frequently positive in systemic staphylococcal disease and should always be obtained when it is suspected. Similarly, pus from sites of infection should always be aspirated or obtained surgically, examined with Gram's stain, and cultured both aerobically and anaerobically.

Bacteriophage typing may be useful for epidemiologic studies but is rarely of value in individual cases. There are at present no useful serologic tests for staphylococcal disease.

Differential Diagnosis

Staphylococcal skin disease has many morphologic forms and therefore many differential diagnoses. Bullous impetigo must be differentiated from chemical or thermal burns, from drug reactions, and, in the very young, from the various congenital epidermolytic syndromes or even herpes simplex infections. Staphylococcal scalded skin syndrome resembles scarlet fever in some instances and in others appears similar to Kawasaki disease, Stevens-Johnson syndrome, erythema multiforme, and other drug reactions. A skin biopsy may be critical in establishing the correct diagnosis. The skin lesions of varicella may become superinfected with exfoliatin-producing staphylococci and produce a combination of the 2 diseases (bullous varicella).

Osteomyelitis of the long bones and septic arthritis must often be differentiated (see Chapter 23).

Severe, rapidly progressing pneumonia, even including ileus, may occasionally be produced by pneumococci. Abscesses and pneumatoceles may be seen in pneumonia due to pneumococci, *Haemophilus influenzae*, and group A streptococci. Empyema formation occurs with all bacterial pneumonias.

Staphylococcal food poisoning is often epidemic. It is differentiated from other common-source gastroenteritis syndromes (*Salmonella, Clostridium perfringens, Vibrio parahaemolyticus*) by the short incubation period (2–6 hours), the prominence of vomiting (as opposed to diarrhea), and the general absence of fever.

Endocarditis must be suspected in any instance of *S aureus* bacteremia, particularly when there is a significant heart murmur or preexisting cardiac disease (see Chapter 16).

Newborn infections with *S aureus* can resemble infections with streptococci and a variety of gram-negative organisms. Umbilical and respiratory tract colonization occurs with a variety of pathogenic organisms (group B streptococci, *Escherichia coli, Klebsiella*), and both skin and systemic infections occur with virtually all of these.

Toxic shock syndrome must be differentiated from Rocky Mountain spotted fever, leptospirosis, Kawasaki disease, drug reactions, and measles.

Treatment

A. Specific Measures: Since 85% of *S aureus* strains are penicillin-resistant, it is important to use a β-lactamase-resistant penicillin as the first drug in treatment. In serious systemic disease, in osteomyelitis, and in the treatment of large abscesses, intravenous therapy is indicated initially (oxacillin or nafcillin, 100–200 mg/kg/d in 4 divided doses, or methicillin, 200–300 mg/kg/d in 4 divided doses). When high doses over a long period are required, it is preferable not to use methicillin, because of the frequency with which interstitial nephritis is seen. In life-threatening illness, an aminoglycoside antibiotic (kanamycin or gentamicin) may be used in addition for its possible synergistic action.

In those instances where *S aureus* is penicillin-sensitive, penicillin G should be used for treatment.

When children with established penicillin sensitivity are treated, cephalosporins may be used (cephalothin, 100–200 mg/kg/d intravenously in 4 divided doses; cefazolin, 100–150 mg/kg/d intravenously in 3 divided doses; or cephalexin, 50–100 mg/kg/d orally in 4 divided doses). The newer cephalosporins should not generally be used for staphylococcal infections.

For methicillin-resistant infections, vancomycin (40 mg/kg/d intravenously in 3–4 divided doses) should be used. Although such strains are often sensitive to cephalosporins in vitro, resistance emerges rapidly in vivo. Combinations including rifampin may be either synergistic or antagonistic.

1. Skin Infections—See Chapter 11.

2. Osteomyelitis and septic arthritis—Treatment should be begun intravenously, with antibiotics selected to cover the most likely organisms (staphylococci in hematogenous osteomyelitis; *H influenzae*, meningococci, pneumococci, staphylococci in arthritic children under the age of 3 years; staphylococci and gonococci in arthritis in older children). Antibiotic levels should be kept high at all times, with monitoring by serum killing powers at least once and at suitable intervals if dosage or route of administration is changed.

In osteomyelitis, clinical studies support the use of intravenous treatment until local symptoms and signs have subsided—at least 1 week—followed by oral therapy (dicloxacillin, 100 mg/kg/d in 4 divided doses, or cephalexin, 100 mg/kg/d in 4 divided doses) for at least 3 additional weeks. Longer treatment may be required, particularly when x-rays show extensive involvement. In arthritis, where drug diffusion into synovial fluid is good, intravenous therapy need be given only for a few days, followed by adequate oral therapy for at least 3 weeks. In all instances, oral therapy should be administered under careful supervision, either in the hospital or, in some instances, at home with frequent support and reinforcement from physicians or visiting nurses.

Surgical drainage of osteomyelitis or septic arthritis is often required (see Chapter 23).

3. Staphylococcal pneumonia—Antibiotic therapy should consist of a parenteral penicillinase-resistant penicillin with or without an aminoglycoside. Empyema or pyopneumothorax require chest tube drainage. The tube should be removed as soon as drainage has become clinically insignificant.

If staphylococcal pneumonia is promptly treated

and empyema promptly drained, resolution in children is almost always complete—in spite of evidence of widespread parenchymal destruction and the persistence of bullae, blebs, and even pockets of empyema or abscess fluid well into convalescence. Surgical decortication or segmental resection is very rarely required.

4. Staphylococcal food poisoning—Therapy is supportive and usually not required except in severe cases or for small infants with marked dehydration.

5. Staphylococcal endocarditis—As outlined above, high-dose, prolonged, parenteral treatment with oxacillin, nafcillin, or methicillin plus kanamycin or gentamicin is indicated. In penicillin-allergic patients, vancomycin should be used. With penicillin-sensitive organisms, penicillin G is the drug of choice. Therapy lasts in all instances for at least 6 weeks.

In some patients, medical treatment may fail. Signs of this are (1) recurrent fever without apparent treatable other cause (eg, thrombophlebitis, incidental respiratory or urinary tract infection, drug fever), (2) persistently positive blood cultures, (3) intractable and progressive congestive heart failure, and (4) recurrent (septic) embolization. In such circumstances—particularly (2), (3), and (4)—valve replacement becomes necessary as part of good management of a difficult situation. Antibiotics are continued for at least another 4 weeks. Persistent or recurrent infection may require a second surgical procedure.

6. Nursery Infections—(See also Chapter 4.) Methods available to stop a nursery epidemic include the following:

a. Emphasis and reemphasis on the first principle of infection control: thorough washing of hands with soap, an iodophore, or other antiseptic agent between handling of infants.

b. Prompt and adequate management of known infections.

c. Prevention of colonization of newborns with epidemic strains by the following means:

(1) Treatment of the umbilical cord with triple dye immediately after birth.

(2) Removal and treatment of personnel carrying the epidemic strain.

(3) Segregation of infants according to age; discharge as soon as medically safe.

(4) Cohorting of nursing personnel.

(5) Restriction of visitors to the nursery area.

(6) Complete cleansing and disinfection of nurseries after discharge of colonized and infected infants.

7. Toxic shock syndrome—Treatment is first with volume expansion and inotropic agents and later with oxacillin, nafcillin, or cephalosporins. If a tampon is in place, it should be removed. All focal staphylococcal infections should be drained aggressively. Some experts feel that corticosteroid therapy may be effective if given to patients with severe illness early in the course of their disease. Antibiotic treatment reduces risk of recurrence.

8. *S epidermidis* infections—*S epidermidis* infections are usually treated with vancomycin (see Chapter 38 for dosing); clindamycin and occasionally trimethoprim-sulfamethoxazole are alternative agents.

B. General Measures: Localized pus should be drained. Oxygen, intravenous fluids, and other supportive care are indicated in staphylococcal pneumonia and other systemic infections. Blood transfusion may be indicated if the patient is severely anemic.

Prognosis

Septicemia, endocarditis, and widespread pneumonitis in infancy all have a serious prognosis. Infants and children who recover from serious staphylococcal pneumonia have a good long-term prognosis without development of chronic respiratory disease. Osteomyelitis is now never fatal if promptly treated.

Baumgart S et al: Sepsis with coagulase-negative staphylococci in critically ill newborns. *Am J Dis Child* 1983; **137**:461.

Friedman LE et al: *Staphylococcus epidermidis* septicemia in children with leukemia and lymphoma. *Am J Dis Child* 1984;**138**:715.

Hieber JP, Nelson AJ, McCracken GH: Acute disseminated staphylococcal disease in childhood. *Am J Dis Child* 1977;**131**:181.

MacDonald KL, Osterholm MT, Hedberg CW, et al: Toxic shock syndrome: A newly recognized complication of influenza and influenza-like illness. *JAMA* 1987; **257**:1053.

Melish ME, Glasgow LA: The staphylococcal scalded skin syndrome: The expanded clinical syndrome. *J Pediatr* 1971;**78**:958.

Shulman ST, Ayoub EM: Severe staphylococcal sepsis in adolescents. *Pediatrics* 1976;**58**:59.

Todd J et al: Toxic-shock syndrome associated with phage group I staphylococci. *Lancet* 1978;**2**:1116.

Todd JKT: Toxic shock syndrome. *Clin Microbiol Rev* 1988;**1**:432.

MENINGOCOCCAL INFECTIONS

Essentials of Diagnosis

- Fever, headache, vomiting, convulsions, shock (meningitis).
- Fever, shock, petechial or purpuric skin rash (meningococcemia).
- Diagnosis confirmed by culture or detection of meningococcal antigen in normally sterile body fluids.

General Considerations

Meningococci may be carried asymptomatically for many months in the upper respiratory tract. Fewer than 1% of carriers develop disease. Meningitis and sepsis are the 2 commonest forms of illness, but septic arthritis, pericarditis, pneumonia, chronic meningococcemia, otitis media, conjunctivitis, and vaginitis also occur. The highest attack rate for meningococcal meningitis is in the first year of life. The incidence in the USA is about 1.2 cases per 100,000 people.

Meningococci are classified serologically into groups A, B, C, D, X, Y, Z, 29-E, and W-135. The serologic groups serve as specific markers for studying outbreaks and transmission of disease. Major epidemics of meningococcal disease in the USA prior to 1950 were caused by group A strains. In recent years, however, group A organisms have accounted for only about 2% of meningococcal isolates. Group B, the most common serogroup, accounts for about 40%; group C, for 30%; and group Y, for 20%. Sulfonamide resistance is common in non-group A strains. Few isolates are resistant to rifampin. Pathogenic strains differ in their virulence and in their potential for epidemic spread. Serogroup A meningococci have the greatest propensity to cause widespread outbreaks.

Children develop immunity from asymptomatic carriage of meningococci (usually nontypeable, nonpathogenic strains) or other cross-reacting bacteria. Patients deficient in one of the late components of complement (C6, C7, or C8) are uniquely susceptible to meningococcal infection.

Meningococci are gram-negative organisms containing endotoxin in their cell walls. Endotoxins may damage the walls of blood vessels and may also cause disseminated intravascular coagulation. Myocarditis is a significant factor in the fatal outcome of acute meningococcal infections.

Vaccines prepared from purified meningococcal polysaccharides (A, C, Y, and W-135) are available for controlling outbreaks and preventing spread in special high-risk groups such as household contacts and military recruits. Unfortunately, the vaccines, except for the A component, are ineffective in children under 2 years of age (see Chapter 6).

Clinical Findings

A. Symptoms and Signs: Many children with clinical meningococcemia also have meningitis, and some may have other foci of infection. All children with suspected meningococcemia should have a lumbar puncture.

1. Meningococcemia—A prodrome of upper respiratory infection is followed by high fever, headache, nausea, marked toxicity, and hypotension. Purpura, petechiae, and occasionally bright pink, tender macules or papules over the extremities and trunk are seen. The rash usually progresses rapidly.

Fulminant meningococcemia (Waterhouse-Friderichsen syndrome) progresses rapidly and is characterized by disseminated intravascular coagulation, massive skin and mucosal hemorrhages, and shock. This syndrome also may be due to *Haemophilus influenzae*, *Streptococcus pneumoniae* or other bacteria.

Chronic meningococcemia is characterized by periodic bouts of fever, arthralgia or arthritis, and recurrent petechiae. Splenomegaly is often present. The patient may be free of symptoms between bouts. Chronic meningococcemia occurs primarily in adults and mimics Henoch-Schönlein purpura.

2. Meningitis—In many children, meningococcemia is followed within a few hours by symptoms and signs of acute purulent meningitis, with severe headache, stiff neck, nausea, vomiting, and stupor. Children with meningitis and meningococcemia generally fare better than children with meningococcemia alone.

B. Laboratory Findings: The peripheral white blood cell count may be either low or elevated. Thrombocytopenia may be present with or without disseminated intravascular coagulation (see Chapter 17). If petechial or hemorrhagic lesions are present, meningococci can sometimes be demonstrated on smear by puncturing the lesions and expressing a drop of tissue fluid. The spinal fluid is generally cloudy and contains more than 1000 white cells per microliter, with many polymorphonuclear cells and gram-negative intracellular diplococci.

Meningococcal polysaccharide antigen of some types may be detected in body fluids, but the available tests are much less sensitive than tests for other bacterial antigens. They are most useful when prior antibiotic therapy makes culture results unreliable.

With recurrent disease, a total hemolytic complement assay may reveal absence of late components as an underlying cause.

Differential Diagnosis

The lesions of meningococcemia may be mistaken for those seen in sepsis, infections due to *H influenzae* or pneumococci, enterovirus infection, endocarditis, leptospirosis, Rocky Mountain spotted fever, other rickettsial diseases, Henoch-Schönlein purpura, and blood dyscrasias. Other causes of sepsis and meningitis are distinguished by appropriate Gram's stain and cultures.

Complications

Meningitis may lead to permanent central nervous system damage, with deafness, convulsions, paralysis, or impairment of intellectual function. Subdural collections of fluid and hydrocephalus are important complications, but they usually resolve spontaneously. Extensive skin necrosis, loss of digits or extremities, intestinal hemorrhage, and late adrenal insufficiency may complicate fulminant meningococcemia.

Prevention

Household contacts, day-care center contacts, and hospital personnel directly exposed to the respiratory secretions of patients are at increased risk of developing meningococcal infection and should be given chemoprophylaxis with rifampin. The secondary attack rate among household members is 1–5% during epidemics and less than 1% in nonepidemic situations. Children 3 months to 2 years of age are at the greatest risk, presumably because they lack protective antibodies. Secondary cases reported in day-care centers are not uncommon, but school classroom outbreaks are rare. Hospital personnel are not at increased risk unless they have had contact with a patient's oral secretions, eg, during mouth-to-mouth resuscitation, intubation, or suctioning procedures. Approximately 50% of secondary cases in households have their onset within 24 hours of identification of the index case. Exposed children should be examined promptly. If they are febrile, they should be fully evaluated and treated with high doses of penicillin pending the results of blood cultures.

All intimate contacts should be given chemoprophylaxis with rifampin given orally in the following dosages twice daily for 2 days: 600 mg for adults, 10 mg/kg for children 1 month–12 years of age, and 5 mg/kg for infants under 1 month of age. An alternate dosing schedule for rifampin, which is also effective chemoprophylaxis for H influenzae type b, is 20 mg/kg/day (maximum adult dose 600 mg/day) once daily for 4 days. If the organism is sensitive to sulfonamides, sulfadiazine may be used. Penicillin and most other antibiotics (even with parenteral administration) are not effective chemoprophylactic agents, since they do not eradicate upper respiratory tract carriage of meningococci. In some situations, meningococcal polysaccharide vaccine should be given to contacts in addition to chemoprophylaxis. Throat cultures to identify carriers are not useful.

Treatment

Blood cultures should be obtained for all children with fever and purpura or other signs of meningococcemia, and antibiotics should be administered immediately as an emergency procedure. There is a good correlation between survival rates and initiation of prompt antibiotic therapy. Purpura and fever should be considered a medical emergency.

Children with meningococcemia or meningococcal meningitis should be managed as though shock were imminent even if their vital signs are stable when they are first seen. If hypotension already is present, supportive measures should be aggressive, because the prognosis is grave in such situations. It is optimal to initiate treatment in an intensive care setting. To minimize the risk of nosocomial transmission, patients should be placed in respiratory isolation for the first 24 hours of antibiotic treatment.

A. Specific Measures: Antibiotics should be begun promptly. Since other bacteria, especially H influenzae, can cause identical syndromes in young children, initial therapy should be effective against that organism until the diagnosis is made. Cefotaxime, ceftriaxone, or ampicillin and chloramphenicol are alternatives (see Chapter 38 for dosages). When the diagnosis is made, penicillin G (250,000 units/kg/d in 6 doses) is the drug of choice.

B. General Measures:

1. Cardiovascular—See Chapter 8 for management of septic shock. Recent evidence suggests that corticosteroids are not beneficial.

2. Hematologic—Since hypercoagulability is frequently present in patients with meningococcemia, administration of heparin is recommended for patients who exhibit either hypotension or other evidence of shock. A loading dose of 100 units/kg is followed by 15 units/kg/h as a continuous drip for 48 hours. The patient is monitored by following the partial thromboplastin time. See Chapter 17 for the management of disseminated intravascular coagulation.

Prognosis

Unfavorable prognostic features include shock, disseminated intravascular coagulation, and extensive skin lesions. The case fatality rate in fulminant meningococcemia is very high—over 50%. In uncomplicated meningococcal meningitis, the fatality rate is much lower—generally 10–20%.

Band JD et al: Trends in meningococcal disease in the United States, 1975–1980. *J Infect Dis* 1983;**148:**754.

Dashefsky B, Teele DW, Klein JO: Unsuspected meningococcemia. *J Pediatr* 1983;**102:**69.

Edwards MS, Baker CJ: Complications and sequelae of meningococcal infections in children. *J Pediatr* 1981;**99:**540.

Griffiss JM et al: Immune response of infants and children to disseminated infections with *Neisseria meningitidis. J Infect Dis* 1984;**150:**71.

Jacobson JA et al: The risk of meningitis among classroom contacts during an epidemic of meningococcal disease. *Am J Epidemiol* 1976;**104:**552.

Leggiadro RJ, Winkelstein JA: Prevalence of complement deficiencies in children with systemic meningococcal infections. *Pediatr Infect Dis J* 1987;**6:**75.

Nguyen QV, Nguyen EA, Weiner LB: Incidence of invasive bacterial disease in children with fever and petechiae. *Pediatrics* 1984;**74:**77.

Van-Esso D et al: *Neisseria meningitidis* strains with decreased susceptibility to penicillin. *Pediatr Infect Dis J* 1987;**6:**438.

Waage A, Halstensen A, Espevik T: Association between tumor necrosis factor in serum and fatal outcome in patients with meningococcal disease. *Lancet* 1987; **1:**355.

GONOCOCCAL INFECTIONS

Essentials of Diagnosis

- Purulent urethral discharge showing intracellular gram-negative diplococci on smear in male patient (usually adolescent).
- Purulent, edematous, sometimes hemorrhagic conjunctivitis showing intracellular gram-negative diplococci on smear in infant 2–4 days of age.
- Fever, arthritis (often polyarticular) or tenosynovitis, and maculopapular peripheral rash that may be vesiculopustular or hemorrhagic.
- Positive culture of blood or pharyngeal or genital secretions.

General Considerations

Gonorrhea is the most commonly reported communicable disease. *Neisseria gonorrhoeae* is a gram-negative diplococcus. Although morphologically similar to other neisseriae, it differs in its ability to grow on selective media and to ferment only glucose. The cell wall of *N gonorrhoeae* contains endotoxin, which is liberated when the organism dies and is responsible for the production of a cellular exudate. The incubation period is short, usually 2–5 days.

Gonococci that elaborate penicillinase and are highly resistant to penicillin are now being encountered. Resistance to penicillin has also been recognized in isolates that do not produce β-lactamase but have a chromosomally mediated resistance. A high level of resistance to tetracycline has also been identified.

Gonococcal disease in children may be transmitted sexually or nonsexually. Prepubertal girls usually manifest gonococcal vulvovaginitis because of the neutral-alkaline pH of the vagina and thin vaginal mucosa.

Prepubertal gonococcal infection outside the neonatal period should be considered presumptive evidence of sexual play or child abuse. In the adolescent or adult, the workup of every case of gonorrhea should include a careful and accurate inquiry into sexual practices, since pharyngeal infection must be detected if present and may be difficult to eradicate. In addition, efforts should be made to identify and treat all sexual contacts. When prepubertal children are infected, all family members should be cultured, and epidemiologic investigation should be thorough.

Clinical Findings
A. Symptoms and Signs:

1. Asymptomatic gonorrhea—The ratio of asymptomatic to symptomatic gonorrheal infections in adolescents and adults is probably 3–4:1 in women and 0.5–1:1 in men. Asymptomatic infections are considered as infectious as symptomatic ones.

2. Uncomplicated genital gonorrhea—
a. Male with urethritis—Urethral discharge is sometimes painful and bloody and may be white, yellow, or green. There may be associated dysuria. The patient is usually afebrile.

b. Prepubertal female with vaginitis—The only clinical findings initially may be dysuria and polymorphonuclear neutrophils in the urine. Vulvitis characterized by erythema, edema, and excoriation accompanied by a purulent discharge may follow.

c. Postpubertal female with cervicitis— Symptomatic disease is characterized by a purulent discharge, dysuria, and, occasionally, dyspareunia. Lower abdominal pain is absent. Physical examination reveals an afebrile patient with a yellow, foul-smelling discharge. The cervix is frequently hyperemic and tender when touched by the examining finger. This tenderness is not worsened by moving the cervix, nor are the adnexa tender to palpation.

d. Rectal gonorrhea—Rectal gonorrhea is often asymptomatic. There may be purulent discharge, edema, and pain during evacuation.

3. Pharyngeal gonorrhea—Pharyngeal involvement is usually asymptomatic. There may be some sore throat and, rarely, acute exudative tonsillitis with bilateral cervical lymphadenopathy and fever.

4. Conjunctivitis and iridocyclitis—In the adolescent or adult eye, infection probably is spread from infected genital secretions by the fingers.*

5. Pelvic inflammatory disease (salpingitis)—The interval between initiation of genital infection and its ascent to the uterine tubes is variable and may range from days to months, with menses frequently the initiating factor. With the onset of a menstrual period, gonococci invade the endometrium, causing transient endometritis. Subsequently, salpingitis may occur, resulting in pyosalpinx or hydrosalpinx; rarely, it leads to peritonitis or perihepatitis. Gonococcal salpingitis occurs in an acute, subacute, or chronic form. All 3 forms have in common tenderness on gentle movement of the cervix and bilateral tubal tenderness during pelvic examination.

Not all pelvic inflammatory disease is due to gonococci. In many instances, gonococci may be an initial cause of infection, but the predominant intrapelvic organisms may be enteric bacilli, *Bacteroides fragilis,* or other anaerobes. In other cases, *Chlamydia trachomatis* may be the triggering or sole cause. Nongonococcal salpingitis is sometimes seen in girls or women with intrauterine devices.

6. Gonococcal perihepatitis (Fitz-Hugh-Curtis syndrome)—In the typical clinical pattern, there is right upper quadrant tenderness in association with signs of acute or subacute salpingitis. Pain may be

---

*Gonococcal ophthalmia neonatorum is discussed in Chapter 12. Infants may also develop anogenital colonization during birth, with subsequent gonococcal sepsis and arthritis.

pleuritic and referred to the shoulder. Hepatic friction rub is a valuable but inconstant sign.

7. Disseminated gonorrhea—Dissemination follows asymptomatic more often than symptomatic genital infection and often results from gonococcal pharyngitis or anorectal gonorrhea. The most common form of disseminated gonorrhea is polyarthritis or polytenosynovitis, with or without dermatitis. Monarticular arthritis is less common, and gonococcal endocarditis and meningitis are fortunately rare.

a. Polyarthritis—Disease usually begins with the simultaneous onset of low-grade fever, polyarthralgia, and general malaise. After a day or so, the joint symptoms become acute, and swelling, redness, and acute tenderness occur, frequently over the wrists, ankles, and knees but also in the fingers, feet, and other peripheral joints. Skin lesions may be noted at the same time: individual, tender, evolving 5- to 8-mm maculopapular lesions that may become vesicular, pustular, and then hemorrhagic. They are noted on the fingers, palms, feet, and other distal surfaces and may be single or multiple.

In patients with this form of the disease, blood cultures are often positive, but joint fluids rarely yield organisms. Skin lesions often are positive by Gram's stain but rarely by culture. Genital, rectal, and pharyngeal cultures must always be performed.

b. Monarticular arthritis—In this somewhat less common form of disseminated gonorrhea, fever is often absent. Arthritis evolves in a single joint. Dermatitis usually does not occur. Systemic symptoms are minimal. Blood cultures are negative, but joint aspirates may yield gonococci on smear and culture. Genital, rectal, and pharyngeal cultures must always be performed.

B. Laboratory Findings: Demonstration of gram-negative, kidney bean-shaped diplococci on smears of urethral exudate in males is presumptive evidence of gonorrhea. Positive culture confirms the diagnosis. Negative smears do not rule out gonorrhea. Gram-stained smears of cervical or vaginal discharge in girls are more difficult to interpret because of normal gram-negative flora, but they may be useful when technical personnel are experienced. In girls with suspected gonorrhea, both the cervical os and the anus should be cultured. Gonococcal pharyngitis requires culture to substantiate the etiologic diagnosis.

Cultures for *N gonorrhoeae* are plated on a selective chocolate agar containing antibiotics (eg, Thayer-Martin agar) to suppress normal flora. If bacteriologic diagnosis is critical, suspected material should be cultured on chocolate agar as well. Since gonococci are labile, swabs should be inoculated immediately and agar plates placed without delay in an atmosphere containing CO_2 (candle jar). When transportation is necessary, material should be directly inoculated into Transgrow medium prior to shipment to an appropriate laboratory. In cases of possible sexual molestation, notify the laboratory that definite speciation is needed, since nongonococcal *Neisseria* spp can grow on the selective media.

All children or adolescents with a suspected or established diagnosis of gonorrhea should have a serologic test for syphilis.

Differential Diagnosis

Urethritis in the male may be gonococcal or ''nonspecific.'' The latter is a syndrome characterized by discharge (rarely painful), mild dysuria, and a subacute course. The discharge is usually scant or moderate in amount but may be profuse. The responsible microorganisms cannot all be identified, but about half of cases are probably due to *C trachomatis*. The remainder are probably due to *Ureaplasma*, trichomonads, or other as yet unknown agents. Most cases respond to tetracycline therapy (500 mg orally 4 times a day for 7 days in adolescents). *C trachomatis* has been shown to cause epididymitis in males and salpingitis in females.

Vulvovaginitis in a prepubertal female may be due to infection caused by miscellaneous bacteria, *Candida,* and herpesvirus; discharges may be caused by trichomonads, *Enterobius vermicularis* (pin-worm), or foreign bodies. Symptom-free discharge (leukorrhea) normally accompanies rising estrogen levels.

Cervicitis in a postpubertal female, alone or in association with urethritis and involvement of Skene's and Bartholin's glands, may be due to infection caused by *Candida,* herpesvirus, *Trichomonas,* or discharge resulting from inflammation caused by foreign bodies (usually some form of contraceptive device). Leukorrhea may be associated with birth control pills.

Salpingitis may be due to infection with other organisms. The symptoms must be differentiated from those of appendicitis, urinary tract infection, ectopic pregnancy, endometriosis, or ovarian cysts or torsion.

Disseminated gonorrhea presents a wide differential diagnosis that must include meningococcemia, acute rheumatic fever, Henoch-Schönlein purpura, juvenile rheumatoid arthritis, lupus erythematosus, leptospirosis, secondary syphilis, certain viral infections (particularly rubella, but also enteroviruses), serum sickness, type B hepatitis (in the prodromal phase), infective endocarditis, and even acute leukemia and other types of cancer. The fully evolved skin lesions of disseminated gonorrhea are remarkably specific, and genital, rectal, or pharyngeal cultures, plus cultures of blood and joint fluid, usually yield gonococci from at least one source.

Prevention

Prevention of gonorrhea is principally a problem of sex education and treatment of contacts.

Treatment

A. Uncomplicated Urethral, Endocervical, or Rectal Gonococcal Infections in Adolescents:
Due to increasing penicillin resistance, current recommended therapy is ceftriaxone (250 mg intramuscularly once) plus, for concurrent *Chlamydia trachomatis* infection, doxycycline (100 mg orally 2 times daily for 7 days). Erythromycin base (500 mg orally 4 times daily for 7 days) should be substituted for the doxycycline in pregnant patients. An alternative regimen is spectinomycin (2 g intramuscularly once) plus the same doxycycline regimen. If the contact's infecting strain was proved susceptible to penicillin, the patient may be treated orally with amoxicillin, 3 g, and probenecid, 0.5 g, taken together as a single dose. A "test of cure" culture is not necessary after the ceftriaxone/doxycycline regimen; repeat screening in 1–2 months is preferable.

B. Pharyngeal Gonococcal Infection:
Ceftriaxone (250 mg intramuscularly once) should be used; ciprofloxacin (0.5 g orally once) is an alternative. Neither spectinomycin nor amoxicillin is recommended. A repeat culture is recommended 4–7 days after therapy.

C. Disseminated Gonorrhea:
Recommended regimens include ceftriaxone (1 g intramuscularly or intravenously once daily) or cefotaxime (1 g intravenously every 8 hours). Proved penicillin-sensitive organisms may be treated with ampicillin (1 g intravenously every 6 hours) or an equivalent penicillin regimen. Oral therapy may follow parenteral therapy after clinical resolution. Recommended regimens include cefuroxime axetil, (0.5 g 2 times daily), amoxicillin (0.5 g plus clavulanic acid 3 times daily), or ciprofloxacin (0.5 g 2 times daily; not used for pregnant patients). If concurrent infection with *Chlamydia* is present or has not been excluded, a course of doxycycline or erythromycin should also be prescribed.

Total duration of therapy is 7 days for disseminated infections.

D. Prepubertal Gonococcal Infections:

1. Uncomplicated genitourinary, rectal, or pharnygeal infections—These infections may be treated with ceftriaxone (125 mg intramuscularly once). Children over 8 years of age should also be treated with doxycycline (100 mg orally 2 times daily for 7 days). The physician should evaluate all children for evidence of sexual abuse and coinfection with syphilis and *Chlamydia*.

2. Disseminated gonorrhea—This should be treated with ceftriaxone (25–50 mg/kg once daily parenterally) or cefotaxime (25 mg/kg 2 times daily parenterally).

Alexander ER: Misidentification of sexually transmitted organisms in children: Medicolegal implications. *Pediatr Infect Dis J* 1988;**7:**1.

Centers for Disease Control: Sexually transmitted diseases: Treatment guidelines 1989;**38(Suppl):**8.

Hammerschlag MR, Cummings C, Roblin PM, et al: Efficacy of neonatal ocular prophylaxis for the prevention of chlamydial and gonococcal conjunctivitis. *N Engl J Med* 1989;**320:**769.

Ingram D et al: Sexual contact in children with gonorrhea. *Am J Dis Child* 1982;**136:**994.

Whittington WL, Knapp JS: Trends in resistance of *Neisseria gonorrheae* to antimicrobial agents in the United States. *Sex Transm Dis* 1988;**15:**202.

Whittington WL et al: Incorrect identification of *Neisseria gonorrheae* from infants and children. *Pediatr Infect Dis J* 1988;**7:**3.

BOTULISM

Essentials of Diagnosis
- Dry mucous membranes.
- Nausea and vomiting.
- Diplopia; dilated, unreactive pupils.
- Descending paralysis.
- Difficulty in swallowing and speech occurring within 12–36 hours after ingestion of toxin contaminated home-canned food.
- Multiple cases in a family or group.
- Hypotonia and constipation in infants.
- Diagnosis by clinical findings and identification of toxin in blood, stool, or implicated food.

General Considerations
Botulism is a paralytic disease caused by *Clostridium botulinum,* an anaerobic, gram-positive, spore-forming bacillus normally found in soil. The organism produces an extremely potent neurotoxin. Of the 7 types of toxin (A–G), types A, B, and E cause most human disease, and types C and D cause outbreaks of botulism in birds and mammals. The toxin, a polypeptide, is so potent that 0.1 μg is lethal for humans.

Food-borne botulism usually results from ingestion of toxin-containing food. Preformed toxin is absorbed from the gut and produces paralysis by preventing acetylcholine release from cholinergic fibers at myoneural junctions.

In Japan, a raw fish and vegetable dish that is allowed to ferment for 4 weeks is responsible for most botulism outbreaks. In Germany, smoked sausage is often implicated. In the USA, home-canned vegetables are usually the cause. Commercially canned foods rarely are responsible. Virtually any food will support the growth of *C botulinum* spores into vegetative toxin-producing bacilli if an anaerobic, nonacid environment is provided. The food may not appear or taste spoiled. The toxin is heat-labile, but the spores are heat-resistant. Inadequate heating during processing (temperature < 115 °C) allows the spores to survive and later resume toxin production. Boiling of foods for 10 minutes or heating at 80 °C (176 °F) for 30 minutes before eating will destroy the toxin.

Infant botulism is a newly recognized form of the disease seen in infants less than 6 months of age. It usually presents as constipation and severe hypotonia. The toxin appears to be produced by *C botulinum* organisms residing in the gastrointestinal tract. In some instances, honey has been the source of spores. Clinical findings include constipation, weak suck and cry, pooled oral secretions, cranial nerve deficits, generalized weakness, and, on occasion, sudden apnea. A characteristic electromyographic pattern termed "brief, small, abundant motor-unit action potentials" (BSAP) is observed. Infant botulism may be responsible for some cases of sudden infant death syndrome (SIDS). In the USA, 60–80 cases are reported annually. Studies are under way to determine the full clinical spectrum, incidence, and public health importance of this form of botulism.

Clinical Findings

A. Symptoms and Signs: The incubation period for food-borne botulism is 8–36 hours. Initially, there is lassitude or fatigue, generally with headache. This is followed by double vision, dilated pupils, ptosis, and, within a few hours, difficulty in swallowing and in speech. Pharyngeal paralysis occurs in some cases, and food may be regurgitated. The mucous membranes often are very dry. Descending skeletal muscle paralysis may be seen. The sensorium is clear, and the temperature normal. Death usually results from respiratory failure.

B. Laboratory Findings: Feces, vomitus, serum, and suspect food should be examined for the presence of toxin by injection into mice. The organism also may be cultured from feces or the suspect food. Laboratory findings, including cerebrospinal fluid examination, are usually normal. With the use of electrophysiologic techniques, the characteristic electrical abnormalities can be found.

Differential Diagnosis

Staphylococcal food poisoning, chemical food poisoning, carbon monoxide poisoning, and Guillain-Barré syndrome are commonly misdiagnosed as botulism. Staphylococcal food poisoning is characterized by nausea, vomiting, and diarrhea; paralysis is not a feature of the illness. Chemical food poisonings generally are characterized by nausea and vomiting beginning minutes after ingestion of contaminated food.

Carbon monoxide poisoning causes unconsciousness without cranial nerve paralysis, and carboxyhemoglobin can be detected in blood. Guillain-Barré syndrome is characterized by ascending paralysis, sensory deficits, and elevated cerebrospinal fluid protein without pleocytosis.

Other illnesses that should be considered include poliomyelitis, postdiphtheritic polyneuritis, certain chemical intoxications, tick paralysis, and myasthenia gravis. The history and elevated cerebrospinal fluid protein characterize postdiphtheritic polyneuritis.

Poisoning with methyl alcohol, organic phosphorus compounds, methyl chloride, sodium fluoride, or atropine may have to be ruled out.

Tick paralysis is characterized by a flaccid ascending motor paralysis that begins in the legs. An attached tick should be sought.

Myasthenia gravis usually occurs in adolescent girls. It is characterized by ocular and bulbar symptoms, with normal pupils, fluctuating weakness, the absence of other neurologic signs, and clinical response to cholinesterase inhibitors.

Complications

Difficulty in swallowing leads to aspiration pneumonia. Serious respiratory paralysis may be fatal despite assisted ventilation and modern intensive supportive measures.

Prevention

Proper sterilization of foods during canning requires a temperature of 115°C to destroy the spores of *C botulinum;* this temperature can be reached in a pressure cooker but not by open boiling. Heating food at 80°C for 30 minutes or allowing it to boil energetically for 10 minutes before it is served will prevent the disease by destroying any toxin produced during storage. Foods that look or smell abnormal, cans with bulging lids, and jars with leaking rings should be destroyed.

Prophylactic use of botulism equine antitoxin (available from the Centers for Disease Control) may be given to asymptomatic persons within 72 hours of ingesting an incriminated food, but because of frequent hypersensitivity reactions (20%), this decision should not be made lightly. Vomiting should be induced, and purgatives and high enemas should be administered.

Treatment

A. Specific Measures: Equine botulism antitoxin is of probable value in the treatment of botulism. Trivalent antitoxin (types A, B, and E) should be given intramuscularly as soon as the diagnosis is made after skin testing for horse serum sensitivity. The antitoxin, 24-hour diagnostic consultation, epidemic assistance, and laboratory testing services are available from the Centers for Disease Control. Guanidine hydrochloride, 15–35 mg/kg/d orally in 3 doses, may reverse the neuromuscular block, but its efficacy is questionable.

B. General Measures: General and supportive therapy consists of bed rest, ventilatory support (if necessary), fluid therapy, and administration of purgatives and high enemas. In cases of infant botulism, some authorities recommend penicillin to eliminate organisms continuing to produce toxin within the gastrointestinal tract.

Prognosis

The mortality rate is about 25% and is lower in children than adults. In nonfatal cases, symptoms subside over 2–3 months and recovery is eventually complete. The availability of antitoxin and modern respiratory support affects the prognosis.

Cherington M: Electrophysiologic methods as an aid in diagnosis of botulism: A review. *Muscle Nerve* 1982; **5(Suppl 9):**S28.

Dowell VR Jr.: Botulism and tetanus: Selected epidemiologic and microbiologic aspects. *Rev Infect Dis* 1984; **6(Suppl 1):**S202.

Long SS: Botulism in infancy. *Pediatr Infect Dis* 1984; **3:**266.

Mills DC, Arnon SS: The large intestine as the site of *Clostridium botulinum* colonization in human infant botulism. *J Infect Dis* 1987;**156:**997.

Wainwright RB et al: Food-borne botulism in Alaska, 1947–1985: Epidemiology and clinical findings. *J Infect Dis* 1988;**157:**158.

Wilcox P et al: Long-term follow-up of symptoms, pulmonary function, respiratory muscle strength, and exercise performance after botulism. *Am Rev Respir Dis* 1989; **139:**157.

TETANUS

Essentials of Diagnosis

- Unimmunized or partially immunized patient.
- History of skin wound.
- Spasms of jaw muscles (trismus).
- Stiffness of neck, back, and abdominal muscles, with hyperirritability and hyperreflexia.
- Episodic, generalized muscle contractions.
- Diagnosis is based on clinical findings and the immunization history.

General Considerations

Tetanus is caused by *Clostridium tetani*, an anaerobic, gram-positive bacillus that produces a potent neurotoxin, tetanospasmin. In unimmunized or incompletely immunized individuals, infection follows contamination of a wound by soil containing clostridial spores from animal manure. The toxin reaches the central nervous system by retrograde axon transport, is bound to cerebral gangliosides, and is thought to increase reflex excitability in neurons of the spinal cord by blocking function of inhibitory synapses. Intense muscle spasms result. Two-thirds of cases in the USA follow minor puncture wounds of the hands or feet. In many cases, no history of a wound can be obtained. In the newborn, infection usually results from contamination of the umbilical cord. The incubation period typically is 4–14 days but may be longer.

In the USA, there is an increased incidence of tetanus in the lower Mississippi Valley and in the Southeast. Over the past 25 years, the overall incidence of tetanus in the USA has been declining. Tetanus is much more prevalent in developing countries, where immunization is not always available. There are an estimated 500,000 deaths yearly from tetanus worldwide. The World Health Organization estimates that about 1% of newborns in developing countries die of tetanus.

Clinical Findings

A. Symptoms and Signs: In children and adults, the first symptom is often minimal pain at the site of inoculation, followed by hypertonicity and spasm of the regional muscles. Characteristically, difficulty in opening the mouth (trismus) is evident within 48 hours. In newborns, the first signs are irritability and inability to suck at the breast. The disease may then progress to stiffness of the jaw and neck, increasing dysphagia, and generalized hyperreflexia with extreme rigidity and spasms of all muscles of the abdomen and back (opisthotonos). The facial distortion resembles a grimace (risus sardonicus). Difficulty in swallowing and convulsions triggered by minimal stimuli such as sound, light, or movement may occur. Individual spasms may last seconds or minutes. Recurrent spasms are seen several times each hour, or they may be almost continuous. In most cases, the temperature is normal or only mildly elevated. A high or subnormal temperature is a bad prognostic sign. Patients are fully conscious and lucid. A profound circulatory disturbance associated with sympathetic overactivity may occur on the second to fourth day, which may contribute to the mortality. This is characterized by elevated blood pressure, increased cardiac output, tachycardia (> 120 beats/min), and dysrhythmia.

B. Laboratory Findings: The diagnosis is made on clinical grounds. There may be a mild polymorphonuclear leukocytosis. The cerebrospinal fluid is normal with the exception of some elevation of pressure. Serum muscle enzymes may be elevated. Transient electrocardiographic and electroencephalographic abnormalities may occur. Anaerobic culture and microscopic examination of pus from the wound can be helpful, but *C tetani* is difficult to grow, and the drumstick-shaped gram-positive bacilli often cannot be found.

Differential Diagnosis

In areas where tetanus is rarely seen, physicians may not recognize the infection until classic findings are present. Poliomyelitis is characterized by asymmetric paralysis in an incompletely immunized child. The history of an animal bite, absence of trismus, and pleocytosis suggest rabies. Local infections of the throat and jaw should be easily recognized. In strychnine poisoning, spasms of the jaw muscles are not common, and periods of complete relaxation between spasms are more obvious. Bacterial meningitis, phenothiazine reactions, decerebrate posturing, narcotic withdrawal, spondylitis, and hypocalcemic tetany may be confused with tetanus.

Complications

Complications include malnutrition, pneumonitis, asphyxial spasms, nosocomial infections, decubitus ulcers, and fractures of the spine due to intense contractions. They can be prevented in part by skilled supportive care.

Prevention

A. Tetanus Toxoid: Active immunization with tetanus toxoid is the cornerstone of prevention of tetanus (see Chapter 6). A serum antitoxin level of 0.01 unit/mL indicates a protective level and almost always is achieved after the third dose of vaccine. A booster at the time of injury is needed if none has been given in the past 10 years—or within 5 years in case of a heavily contaminated wound. Nearly all cases of tetanus (99%) in the USA are in unimmunized or incompletely immunized individuals. Because an attack of tetanus does not confer immunity, every patient who recovers should be immunized.

B. Tetanus Antitoxin: Horse serum antitoxin was formerly used in nonimmunized individuals with soil-contaminated wounds. Human tetanus immune globulin (TIG) should now be employed instead. For children who have had no or one tetanus toxoid immunization, 250–500 units should be given intramuscularly. Tetanus toxoid and TIG should be administered concurrently at different sites using different syringes; there is no evidence of significant interference with the immune response to tetanus toxoid by concomitantly administered TIG.

C. Treatment of Wounds: Proper surgical cleansing and debridement of contaminated wounds will decrease the risk of tetanus.

D. Prophylactic Antimicrobials: Prophylactic antimicrobials are useful if the child is unimmunized and TIG is not available.

Treatment

A. Specific Measures: Serotherapy lowers the mortality rate from tetanus, but not dramatically. TIG, 500 units intramuscularly for newborns and 3000–6000 units intramuscularly for children and adults, is preferred to horse serum. Surgical debridement of wounds is indicated, but more extensive surgery or amputation to eliminate the site of infection is not necessary. Penicillin G is given in a dosage of 150,000 units/kg/d intravenously for 10–14 days. Cephalosporins may be substituted in penicillin-sensitive children.

B. General Measures: The patient is kept in a quiet room with minimal stimulation. Control of spasms and prevention of hypoxic episodes are crucial. Sedatives such as diazepam are useful. Diazepam dosage is 0.6–1.2 mg/kg/d intravenously in 6 divided doses. In the newborn, 2 or 3 divided doses

should be given. Large doses (up to 25 mg/kg/d) may be required for older children. Diazepam is given intravenously until muscular spasms become infrequent and the generalized muscular rigidity much less prominent. The drug may then be given orally and the dose reduced as the child improves. Barbiturates, chlorpromazine, and paraldehyde may also be useful.

Mechanical ventilation and muscle paralysis are necessary in severe cases.

Prognosis

The fatality rate in newborns and heroin addicts is high (70–90%). The overall mortality rate in the USA is 65%. The fatality rate depends primarily on the quality of supportive care. Many deaths are due to pneumonia or respiratory failure. If the patient survives 1 week, recovery is likely.

Mortality rates tend to be high when (1) the incubation time is short, (2) the site of infection is less accessible, (3) there is no immunity, (4) spasms are frequent and severe and are associated with apnea, and (5) the temperature is under 36.7 °C (98 °F) or over 38.9 °C (102 °F).

Bowen V et al: Tetanus—a continuing problem in minor injuries. *Can J Surg* 1988;**31:**7.

Farquhar I, Hutchinson A, Curran J: Dantrolene in severe tetanus. *Intensive Care Med* 1988;**14:**249.

Gultekin A et al: Double-blind trial of intramuscular and intramuscular plus intrathecal human tetanus immunoglobulin and intramuscular equine tetanus antitoxin in the treatment of tetanus neonatorum. *Turk J Pediatr* 1988;**30:**9.

Stanfield JP, Galazka A: Neonatal tetanus in the world today. *Bull WHO* 1984;**62:**647.

GAS GANGRENE

Essentials of Diagnosis

- Contamination of a wound with soil or feces.
- Massive edema, skin discoloration, bleb formation, and pain in an area of trauma.
- Serosanguineous exudate from wound.
- Crepitation of subcutaneous tissue.
- Rapid progression of signs and symptoms.
- Clostridia cultured or seen on stained smears.

General Considerations

Gas gangrene (clostridial myonecrosis) is a necrotizing infection that follows trauma or surgery and is caused by several anaerobic, gram-positive, spore-forming bacilli of the genus *Clostridium*. These are soil, genital tract (female), and fecal organisms. In devitalized tissue, the spores germinate into vegetative bacilli that proliferate and produce toxins causing thrombosis, hemolysis, and tissue necrosis. *Clostridium perfringens,* the species causing approximately 80% of cases of gas gangrene, produces at least 8 such toxins. These toxins, together with tissue distention caused by interference with blood supply and by gas formation, favor the spread of gangrene. The areas involved most often are the extremities, abdomen, and uterus. Nonclostridial infections with gas formation can mimic clostridial infections and are more common.

Clinical Findings

A. Symptoms and Signs: The onset is sudden, usually 1–20 days (mean 3–4 days) after trauma or surgery. The skin around the wound becomes discolored, with hemorrhagic bullae, serosanguineous exudate, and crepitation in the subcutaneous tissues. Pain and swelling are usually intense. Systemic illness appears early and progresses rapidly to intravascular hemolysis, jaundice, shock, toxic delirium, and renal failure. Toxic delirium may precede any obvious signs of wound infection.

B. Laboratory Findings: Isolation of the organism requires anaerobic culture. Gram-stained smears may demonstrate many gram-positive rods and few inflammatory cells.

C. Imaging: X-ray films may demonstrate gas in tissues, but this is a late finding and is also seen in infections with other gas-forming organisms or may be due to air introduced into tissues during trauma or surgery.

D. Surgical Findings: Direct visualization of the muscle at surgery may be necessary to diagnose gas gangrene. Early, the muscle is pale and edematous and does not contract normally; later, the muscle may be frankly gangrenous.

Differential Diagnosis

Gangrene and cellulitis caused by other organisms and clostridial cellulitis (not myonecrosis) must be distinguished. Necrotizing fasciitis may resemble gas gangrene.

Prevention

Gas gangrene can be prevented by the adequate cleansing and debridement of all wounds. It is essential that foreign bodies and dead tissue be removed. A clean wound does not provide a suitable anaerobic environment for the growth of clostridial species.

Treatment

A. Specific Measures: Penicillin G (300,000–400,000 units/kg/d intravenously in 6 divided doses) should be given. The use of polyvalent gas gangrene antitoxin is controversial because of adverse reactions to horse serum and because its effectiveness is questionable.

B. Surgical Measures: Surgery should be prompt and extensive, with removal of all necrotic tissue.

C. Hyperbaric Oxygen: Hyperbaric oxygen therapy has been shown to be effective, but it is not a substitute for surgery. A patient may be exposed to 2–3 atmospheres in pure oxygen for 1- to 2-hour periods for as many sessions as necessary until there is clinical remission.

Prognosis

Clostridial myonecrosis is fatal if untreated. With early diagnosis, antibiotics, and surgery, the mortality rate is about 20–60%. Involvement of the abdominal wall, leukopenia, intravascular hemolysis, renal failure, and shock are ominous prognostic findings.

Bessman AN, Wagner W: Nonclostridial gas gangrene: Report of 48 cases and review of the literature. *JAMA* 1975;**233:**958.

Hart GB et al: Gas gangrene. *J Trauma* 1983;**23:**991.

Hirn M, Niinikoski J: Hyperbaric oxygen in the treatment of clostridial gas gangrene. *Ann Chir Gynaecol* 1988;**77:**37.

Stevens DL et al: Comparison of clindamycin, rifampin, tetracycline, metronidazole, and penicillin for efficacy in prevention of experimental gas gangrene due to *Clostridium perfringens. J Infect Dis* 1987;**155:**220.

DIPHTHERIA

Essentials of Diagnosis

- A gray, adherent pseudomembrane, most often in the pharynx but also in the nasopharynx or trachea.
- Sore throat, serosanguineous nasal discharge, hoarseness, and fever in a nonimmunized child.
- Peripheral neuritis or myocarditis.
- Positive culture.
- Treatment should *not* be withheld pending culture results.

General Considerations

Diphtheria is an acute infection of the upper respiratory tract or skin caused by toxin-producing *Corynebacterium diphtheriae.* Five or fewer cases per year are reported in the USA, but significant numbers of elderly adults and unimmunized children are susceptible to infection. Corynebacteria are gram-positive club-shaped rods with a beaded appearance on Gram's stain.

The capacity to produce exotoxin is conferred by a lysogenic bacteriophage and is not present in all strains of *C diphtheriae.* In immunized communities, infection probably occurs through spread of the phage among carriers of susceptible bacteria rather than through spread of phage-containing bacteria themselves. Diphtheria toxin kills susceptible cells by irreversible inhibition of protein synthesis.

The toxin is absorbed into the mucous membranes and causes destruction of epithelium and a superficial inflammatory response. The necrotic epithelium becomes embedded in exuding fibrin and red and white cells, forming a grayish "pseudomembrane" commonly present over the tonsils, pharynx, or larynx. Any attempt to remove the membrane exposes and tears the capillaries, resulting in bleeding. The diphtheria bacilli within the membrane continue to produce toxin, which is absorbed and may result in toxic injury to heart muscle, liver, kidneys, and adrenals, and is sometimes accompanied by hemorrhage. The toxin also produces neuritis, resulting in paralysis of the soft palate, eye muscles, or extremities. Death may occur as a result of respiratory obstruction or acute toxemia and circulatory collapse. The patient may succumb after a somewhat longer time as a result of cardiac damage. The incubation period is 1–6 days.

Clinical Findings

A. Symptoms and Signs:

1. Pharyngeal diphtheria—Early manifestations of diphtheritic pharyngitis are mild sore throat, moderate fever, and malaise, followed fairly rapidly by severe prostration and circulatory collapse. The pulse is more rapid than the fever would seem to justify. A pharyngeal membrane forms and may spread into the nasopharynx or the trachea, producing respiratory obstruction. The membrane is tenacious and gray and is surrounded by a narrow zone of erythema and a broader zone of edema. The cervical lymph nodes become swollen, and swelling is associated with brawny edema of the neck (''bull neck'').

2. Laryngeal diphtheria—In about 25% of cases, the larynx is invaded. Occasionally, it may be the only manifestation of the disease. Stridor is apparent. Progressive laryngeal obstruction can lead to cyanosis and suffocation.

3. Other forms—Cutaneous, vaginal diphtheria and wound diphtheria currently account for as many as 33% of cases and are characterized by ulcerative lesions with membrane formation.

B. Laboratory Findings: Diagnosis is clinical. Direct smears are unreliable. Material is first obtained from the nose and throat and from skin lesions, if present, for culture on Loffler's and tellurite agar. Sixteen to 48 hours are required before identification of the organism is possible. A toxigenicity test is then performed. Cultures may be negative in individuals who have received antibiotics. The white blood cell count is usually normal, but there may be a slight leukocytosis. The red blood cell count may show evidence of rapid destruction of erythrocytes. Thrombocytopenia due to peripheral destruction is frequent.

Differential Diagnosis

Pharyngeal diphtheria resembles acute streptococcal pharyngitis, mononucleosis, and occasionally, other viral pharyngitis. Nasal diphtheria may be mimicked by a foreign body or purulent sinusitis. Other causes of laryngeal obstruction are epiglottitis

and viral croup. Neuropathy may be a manifestation of Guillain-Barré syndrome, poliomyelitis, or acute poisoning.

Complications

A. Myocarditis: Diphtheritic myocarditis is characterized by a rapid, thready pulse; indistinct heart sounds, ST–T wave changes, conduction abnormalities, dysrhythmias, or cardiac failure; hepatomegaly; and fluid retention. Myocardial dysfunction may occur from 2 to 40 days after the onset of pharyngitis, most commonly during the second week.

B. Polyneuritis: Neuritis of the nerves innervating the palate and pharyngeal muscles occurs during the first or second week. Nasal speech and regurgitation of food through the nose are seen. Diplopia and strabismus occur during the third week or later. Neuritis may also involve peripheral motor nerves supplying the intercostal muscles and diaphragm and other muscle groups. Generalized paresis usually occurs after the fourth week.

C. Bronchopneumonia: Secondary pneumonia is common in fatal cases.

Prevention

A. Immunization: Immunization with diphtheria toxoid combined with pertussis and tetanus toxoids (DTP) should be used routinely for infants and children (see Chapter 6).

B. Care of Exposed Susceptibles: Children exposed to diphtheria should be examined, and nose and throat cultures obtained. If signs and symptoms of early diphtheria are found, treatment should be as for diphtheria. Immunized asymptomatic individuals should receive diphtheria toxoid if a booster has not been received within 5 years. Unimmunized close contacts should receive either erythromycin orally (40 mg/kg/d in 4 divided doses) for 7 days or benzathine penicillin G intramuscularly (25,000 units/kg), active immunization with diphtheria toxoid and be observed daily.

Treatment

A. Specific Measures:

1. Antitoxin—Diphtheria antitoxin should be administered within 48 hours to be effective (see Chapter 6).

2. Antibiotics—Procaine penicillin G (250,000 units/kg/d twice daily intramuscularly) or penicillin G (150,000 units/kg/d intravenously) should be given for 10 days. For the patient allergic to penicillin, erythromycin, 40 mg/kg/d, is given orally for 10 days.

3. Other—Therapy with corticosteroids did not reduce the occurrence of electrocardiographic abnormalities or neuritis in a recent controlled trial. In one study, oral administration of carnitine appeared to prevent cardiac damage.

B. General Measures: Bed rest in the hospital for 10–14 days is usually required. All patients must be strictly isolated from other persons until antibiotic treatment has made respiratory secretions noninfectious (1–7 days). Isolation may be discontinued when 3 successive nose and throat cultures at 24-hour intervals are negative. These cultures should not be taken until at least 48 hours have elapsed since the cessation of antibiotic treatment.

C. Treatment of Carriers: All carriers should be treated. Erythromycin (40 mg/kg/d orally in 3 or 4 divided doses), penicillin VK (50/mg/kg/d for 10 days), or benzathine penicillin G (600,000–1,200,000 units intramuscularly) should be given. All carriers must be confined at home. Before they can be released, carriers must have 3 negative cultures of both the nose and the throat taken 24 hours apart and obtained at least 24 hours after the cessation of antibiotic therapy.

Prognosis

Mortality rates vary from 3 to 25% and are particularly high in the presence of early myocarditis. Neuritis is reversible; it is fatal only if an intact airway and adequate respiration cannot be maintained. Permanent damage due to myocarditis occurs rarely.

Chen RT et al: Diphtheria in the United States, 1971–1981. *Am J Pub Health* 1985;**75**:1393.

English PC: Diphtheria and theories of infectious disease: Centennial appreciation of the critical role of diphtheria in the history of medicine. *Pediatrics* 1985;**76**:1.

Pappenheimer AM Jr, Murphy JR: Studies on the molecular epidemiology of diphtheria. *Lancet* 1983;**2**:923.

Thisyakorn USA, Wongvanich J, Kumpeng V: Failure of corticosteroid therapy to prevent diphtheritic myocarditis or neuritis. *Pediatr Infect Dis J* 1984;**3**:126.

INFECTIONS DUE TO *ENTEROBACTERIACEAE*

Essentials of Diagnosis

- Diarrhea by several different mechanisms due to *Escherichia coli*.
- Neonatal sepsis or meningitis.
- Urinary tract infection.
- Opportunistic infections.
- Diagnosis confirmed by culture.

General Considerations

Enterobacteriaceae is a family of gram-negative bacilli that are part of the normal flora of the gastrointestinal tract and are also found in water and soil. They cause gastroenteritis, urinary tract infections, neonatal sepsis and meningitis, opportunistic infections, and, occasionally, other infections. *Escherichia coli* is the organism in this family that most commonly causes infection in children, but

Klebsiella, Morganella, Enterobacter, Serratia, Proteus, and other genera are also important, particularly in the compromised host. *Shigella* and *Salmonella* are discussed in separate sections.

E coli strains capable of causing diarrhea were originally termed enteropathogenic and were recognized by serotype. It is now known that *E coli* may cause diarrhea by several distinct mechanisms. The mechanism(s) responsible for diarrhea in the originally described EPEC strains are not known. Enterotoxigenic *E coli* cause a secretory, watery diarrhea. ETEC adhere to enterocytes and secrete one or more plasmid-encoded enterotoxins. One of these toxins resembles cholera toxin in structure, function, and mechanism of action. Enteroinvasive *E coli* are very similar to *Shigella* in pathogenetic mechanism. *E coli* serotype 0157:H7 was recently reported to cause hemorrhagic colitis and hemolytic-uremic syndrome. This strain and several others are termed enterohemorrhagic and elaborate toxins very similar to Shiga toxin.

Eighty percent of *E coli* strains causing neonatal meningitis possess specific capsular polysaccharide (K1 antigen), which, alone or in association with specific somatic antigens, confers virulence. K1 antigen is also present on approximately 40% of strains causing neonatal septicemia. The *E coli* K1 organisms do not appear to cause gastrointestinal disease.

Approximately 90% of urinary tract infections in children are caused by *E coli*. *E coli* bind to the uroepithelium by P-fimbria, which are present in greater than 90% of *E coli* that cause pyelonephritis. Other bacterial cell-surface structures, such as O and K antigens, and host factors are also important in the pathogenesis of urinary tract infections.

Klebsiella, Enterobacter, Serratia, and *Morganella* are normally found in the gastrointestinal tract and in soil and water. *Klebsiella* may cause a bronchopneumonia with cavity formation. *Klebsiella, Enterobacter,* and *Serratia* are often opportunists associated with antibiotic usage, debilitating states, and chronic respiratory conditions. They frequently cause urinary tract infection or sepsis. In many newborn nurseries, nosocomial outbreaks caused by aminoglycoside-resistant *Klebsiella pneumoniae* are a major problem.

Many of these infections are difficult to treat because of antibiotic resistance. Antibiotic susceptibility tests are necessary. Parenteral third-generation cephalosporins are usually more active than ampicillin, but resistance due to depressed chromosomal cephalosporinase may occur. Aminoglycoside antibiotics (gentamicin, tobramycin, amikacin) are usually effective.

Clinical Findings

A. Symptoms and Signs:

1. *E coli* gastroenteritis—*E coli* may cause diarrhea of varying type and severity. Enterotoxigenic

E coli usually produce mild, self-limiting illness without significant fever or systemic toxicity, often known as traveler's diarrhea. However, diarrhea may be severe in newborns and infants, and occasionally an older child or adult will have a cholera-like syndrome. Enteroinvasive strains cause a shigella-like illness characterized by fever, systemic symptoms, blood and mucus in the stool, and leukocytosis, but currently are uncommon in the USA. Enterohemorrhagic strains cause bloody diarrhea, abdominal cramps, nausea, and vomiting, often without fever.

2. Neonatal sepsis—Findings include jaundice, hepatosplenomegaly, fever, temperature lability, apneic spells, irritability, and failure to suck vigorously. Meningitis is associated with sepsis in 25–40% of cases. Other metastatic foci of infection may be present, including pneumonia and pyelonephritis. Sepsis may lead to severe metabolic acidosis, shock, disseminated intravascular coagulation, and death.

3. Neonatal meningitis—Findings include high fever, full fontanelles, vomiting, coma, convulsions, pareses or paralyses, poor or absent Moro reflex, opisthotonos, and, occasionally, hyper- or hypotonia. Sepsis coexists or precedes meningitis in most cases. Thus, signs of sepsis often accompany those of meningitis. Cerebrospinal fluid usually shows a cell count of over $1000/\mu L$, mostly polymorphonuclear neutrophils, and bacteria on Gram's stain. Cerebrospinal fluid glucose concentration is low (usually less than half that of blood), and the protein is elevated above the levels normally seen in newborns and premature infants (> 150 mg/dL).

4. Acute urinary tract infection—Symptoms include dysuria, increased urinary frequency, and fever in the older child. Nonspecific symptoms such as anorexia, vomiting, irritability, failure to thrive, and unexplained fever are seen in children under 2 years of age. Young infants may present with jaundice. As many as 1% of girls of school age and 0.05% of boys have asymptomatic bacteriuria.

B. Laboratory Findings: Serotyping, tests for enterotoxin production or invasiveness, and tests for P-fimbria are performed in research laboratories, but these tests are not available in most laboratories. Blood cultures are positive in neonatal sepsis. Cultures of cerebrospinal fluid and urine should also be obtained. The diagnosis of urinary tract infections is discussed in Chapter 22.

Differential Diagnosis

The clinical picture of enteropathogenic *E coli* infection may resemble that of salmonellosis, shigellosis, or viral gastroenteritis.

Neonatal sepsis and meningitis caused by *E coli* can be differentiated from other causes of neonatal infection only by blood and cerebrospinal fluid culture.

Treatment
A. Specific Measures:

1. *E coli* gastroenteritis—*E coli* gastroenteritis seldom requires antimicrobial treatment. In nursery outbreaks, infants have been treated with neomycin (100/mg/kg/d orally in 3 divided doses for 5 days) or colistin (10–15 mg/kg/d orally in 3 divided doses for 5 days). Clinical efficacy is not established. Trimethoprim-sulfamethoxazole may be used in older children.

2. *E coli* sepsis, pneumonia, or pyelonephritis—The drugs of choice are ampicillin (150–200 mg/kg/d intravenously or intramuscularly in divided doses every 4–6 hours) or gentamicin (5–7.5 mg/kg/d intramuscularly or intravenously in divided doses every 8 hours). Treatment is for 10–14 days. Amikacin or tobramycin may be used instead of gentamicin if the strain is susceptible. Third-generation cephalosporins are often an attractive alternative as single-drug therapy and do not require monitoring for toxicity.

3. *E coli* meningitis—Ampicillin (200–300 mg/kg/d intravenously in 4–6 divided doses) and gentamicin (5–7.5 mg/kg/d intramuscularly or intravenously in 3 divided doses) are given for a minimum of 3 weeks. Third-generation cephalosporins such as cefotaxime (200 mg/kg/d intravenously in 4 divided doses) are also effective. Treatment with intrathecal and intraventricular aminoglycosides does not improve outcome. Newborns treated with aminoglycosides or chloramphenicol must have serum levels monitored.

4. Acute urinary tract infection—See Chapter 22.

Prognosis

Death due to gastroenteritis can be prevented by early fluid and electrolyte therapy. Neonatal sepsis with meningitis is still associated with a mortality rate of over 50%. Most children with recurrent urinary tract infections do well if they have no serious underlying anatomic defects. The mortality rate in opportunistic infections usually depends on the severity of infection and the underlying condition.

Durbin WA, Peter G: Management of urinary tract infections in infants and children. *Pediatr Infect Dis* 1984; **3**:564.

Levine MM: *Escherichia coli* that cause diarrhea: Enterotoxigenic, enteropathogenic, enteroinvasive, enterohemorrhagic, and enteroadherent. *J Infect Dis* 1987; **155**:377.

McCracken GH: Diagnosis and management of acute urinary tract infections in infants and children. *Pediatr Infect Dis J* 1987;**6**:107.

McCracken GH et al: Moxalactam therapy for neonatal meningitis due to gram-negative enteric bacilli. *JAMA* 1984;**252**:1427.

MacDonald KL et al: *Escherichia coli* 0157:H7, an emerging gastrointestinal pathogen. *JAMA* 1988;**259**:3567.

Travelers' Diarrhea—Consensus Conference, *JAMA* 1985; **253**:2700.

PSEUDOMONAS INFECTIONS

Essentials of Diagnosis

- Opportunistic infection.
- Confirmed by cultures.

General Considerations

Pseudomonas aeruginosa is an important cause of infection in children with cystic fibrosis, neoplastic disease, neutropenia, or extensive burns and in those receiving antibiotic therapy. Infections of the urinary and respiratory tracts, ears, mastoids, paranasal sinuses, eyes, skin, meninges, and bones are seen. *Pseudomonas* pneumonia is a common nosocomial infection in patients receiving assisted ventilation. *P aeruginosa* sepsis may be accompanied by characteristic peripheral lesions called ecthyma gangrenosum. *P aeruginosa* osteomyelitis sometimes complicates puncture wounds of the feet. *P aeruginosa* is a frequent cause of malignant external otitis media. Outbreaks of vesiculopustular skin rash have been associated with exposure to contaminated water in whirlpool baths and hot tubs.

P aeruginosa is a aerobic gram-negative rod with versatile metabolic requirements. *P aeruginosa* may grow in distilled water and in commonly used disinfectants, complicating the problem of infection control. *P aeruginosa* is both invasive and destructive to tissue, and toxigenic due to secreted exotoxins, which contribute to virulence. Other *Pseudomonas* species occasionally cause nosocomial infections. *Xanthomonas maltophilia* (previously *P maltophilia*) and *P cepacia* are the most frequent.

P aeruginosa infects the tracheobronchial tree of nearly all patients with cystic fibrosis. Mucoid exopolysaccharide, an exuberant capsule, is characteristically overproduced by isolates from patients with cystic fibrosis. Although bacteremia seldom occurs, patients with cystic fibrosis ultimately succumb to chronic lung infection with *P aeruginosa*. *P cepacia* has been increasingly a problem in some cystic fibrosis centers.

Clinical Findings

The clinical findings depend on the site of infection and the patient's underlying disease. Sepsis with these organisms resembles gram-negative sepsis with other organisms. The diagnosis is made by culture. *Pseudomonas* infection should be suspected in neutropenic patients with clinical sepsis.

Prevention

A. Infections in Debilitated Patients: Colonization of extensive second- and third-degree burns by *Pseudomonas* can lead to fatal septicemia. Aggressive debridement and topical treatment with 0.5% silver nitrate solution, 10% mafenide (Sulfamylon) cream, or gentamicin ointment will greatly inhibit *Pseudomonas* contamination of burns. (See Chapter 8 for a discussion of burn wound infections and prevention.)

B. Nosocomial Infections: Faucet aerators, communal soap dispensers, disinfectants, improperly cleaned inhalation therapy equipment, infant incubators, and back rub lotions have all been associated with *Pseudomonas* epidemics. Infant-to-infant transmission by nursery personnel carrying *Pseudomonas* on the hands is frequent in neonatal units. Careful maintenance of equipment and enforcement of infection control procedures are essential to minimize nosocomial transmission.

C. Patients with Cystic Fibrosis: Chronic infection of the lower respiratory tract occurs in nearly all patients with cystic fibrosis. The infecting organism is seldom cleared from the respiratory tract, even with intensive antimicrobial therapy, and the resultant injury to the lung eventually leads to pulmonary insufficiency. Treatment is aimed at controlling signs and symptoms of the infection.

Treatment

P aeruginosa is inherently resistant to many antimicrobials and may develop resistance during therapy. Mortality rates in hospitalized patients exceed 50%, due both to the severity of underlying illnesses in patients predisposed to *Pseudomonas* infection and to the limitations of therapy. Aminoglycoside antimicrobials; expanded-spectrum cephalosporins, such as ceftazidime; imipenem; and the fluoroquinolones are active against most *P aeruginosa* strains, as well as other enteric gram-negative rods. However, antimicrobial susceptibility patterns vary from area to area, and resistance tends to appear as new drugs become popular. Treatment of infections is best guided by clinical response and susceptibility tests.

Use of gentamicin (5–7.5 mg/kg/d intramuscularly or intravenously in 3 divided doses) in combination with ticarcillin (200–300 mg/kg/d intravenously in 6 divided doses) or with another anti-*Pseudomonas* β-lactam antibiotic is recommended for treatment of serious *Pseudomonas* infections. Treatment should be continued for 10–14 days. Treatment with 2 active drugs is recommended for all serious infections.

Pseudomonas osteomyelitis requires surgical debridement and antimicrobial therapy for 2 weeks.

Prognosis

Because debilitated patients are most frequently affected, the mortality rate is high. These infections may have a protracted course, and eradication of the organisms may be difficult.

Bodey GP et al: Infections caused by *Pseudomonas aeruginosa*. *Rev Infect Dis* 1983;**5**:279.

Chusid MJ, Hillmann SM: Community-acquired *Pseudomonas* sepsis in previously healthy infants. *Pediatr Infect Dis J* 1987;**6**:681.

Gustafson TL et al: *Pseudomonas* folliculitis: An outbreak and review. *Rev Infect Dis* 1983;**5**:1.

Jackson MA, Wong KY, Lampkin B: *Pseudomonas aeruginosa* septicemia in childhood cancer patients. *Pediatr Infect Dis J* 1982;**1**:239.

Pier GB: Pulmonary disease associated with *Pseudomonas aeruginosa* in cystic fibrosis: Current status of the host-bacterium interaction. *J Infect Dis* 1985;**151**:575.

Ruvalo C, Bauer CR: Intrauterinely acquired *Pseudomonas* infection in the neonate. *Clin Pediatr* 1982;**21**:664.

SALMONELLA GASTROENTERITIS

Essentials of Diagnosis

- Nausea, vomiting, headache, meningismus.
- Fever, diarrhea, abdominal pain.
- Culture or organism from stool, blood, or other specimens.

General Considerations

Salmonellae are gram-negative rods that frequently cause food-borne gastroenteritis and occasionally bacteremic infection of bone, meninges, and other foci. Three species—*Salmonella typhi, Salmonella choleraesuis,* and *Salmonella enteritidis*—and approximately 1700 serotypes are recognized. *S typhimurium* is the most frequently isolated serotype in most parts of the world. Approximately 50,000 cases of salmonellosis are reported annually in the USA, but many cases are either not reported or not recognized.

Salmonellae are able to penetrate the mucin layer of the small bowel and attach to epithelial cells. Organisms penetrate beneath the epithelial surface and multiply there. Infection results in fever, vomiting, watery diarrhea, and occasionally, mucus with some polymorphonuclear leukocytes in the stool. Although the small intestine is generally regarded as the principal site of infection, colitis also occurs. *S typhimurium* frequently involves the large bowel.

Salmonella infections in childhood occur in 2 major forms: (1) gastroenteritis (including food poisoning), which may be complicated by sepsis and focal suppurative complications; and (2) enteric fever (typhoid fever and paratyphoid fever). (See next section.) Although the incidence of typhoid fever has decreased in the USA, the incidence of *Salmonella* gastroenteritis has greatly increased in the past 15–20 years. The highest attack rates occur in children under 6 years of age, with a peak in the age group from 6 months to 2 years old.

Salmonellae are widespread in nature, infecting domestic and wild animals. Fowl and reptiles have a particularly high carriage rate. Contaminated egg powder and frozen whole egg preparations used to make ice cream, custards, fresh eggs, and mayonnaise are responsible for outbreaks. Transmission results primarily from ingestion of contaminated food.

Transmission from human to human occurs by the fecal-oral route via contaminated food, water, and fomites.

Most cases of *Salmonella* meningitis (80%) and bacteremia occur in infancy. Newborns may acquire the infection from their mothers during delivery and may precipitate outbreaks in nurseries. Newborns are at special risk of developing meningitis.

Clinical Findings

A. Symptoms and Signs: Infants usually develop fever, vomiting, and diarrhea. The older child may also complain of headache, nausea, and abdominal pain. Stools are often watery or may contain mucus and, in some instances, blood, suggesting shigellosis. Drowsiness and disorientation may be associated with meningismus. Convulsions occur less frequently than with shigellosis. Splenomegaly is occasionally noted. In the usual case, diarrhea is moderate and subsides after 4–5 days, but it may be protracted.

B. Laboratory Findings: Diagnosis is made by isolation of the organism from stool, blood, or, in some cases, from urine, cerebrospinal fluid, or pus from a suppurative lesion. The white blood cell count usually shows a polymorphonuclear leukocytosis but may show leukopenia. Typing of isolates is done with specific antisera. *Salmonella* isolates should be reported to public health authorities for epidemiologic purposes.

Differential Diagnosis

In staphylococcal food poisoning, the incubation period is shorter (2–4 hours) than in *Salmonella* food poisoning (12–24 hours). Fever is absent, and vomiting rather than diarrhea is the main symptom. In shigellosis, many pus cells are likely to be seen on a stained smear of stool, and there is more likely to be a marked shift to the left in the peripheral white count, although some cases of salmonellosis are indistinguishable from shigellosis. *Campylobacter* gastroenteritis commonly resembles shigellosis clinically. *Arizona* organisms are closely related to the salmonellae and cause a similar illness. Culture of the stools will establish the diagnosis.

Complications

Unlike most types of infectious diarrhea, salmonellosis is frequently accompanied by bacteremia, especially in newborns and infants. Septicemia with extraintestinal infection is seen, most commonly with *S choleraesuis* but also with *S enteritidis, S typhimurium,* and *S paratyphi* B and C. The organism may localize in any tissue and may cause arthritis, osteomyelitis, cholecystitis, endocarditis, meningitis, pericarditis, pneumonia, or pyelonephritis. In patients with sickle cell anemia or other hemoglobinopathies, there is an unusual predilection for osteomyelitis to develop. Severe dehydration and shock are more likely to occur with shigellosis but may occur with *Salmonella* gastroenteritis.

Prevention

Measures for the prevention of *Salmonella* infections include thorough cooking of foodstuffs derived from potentially infected sources; proper refrigeration during storage; and recognition and control of infection among domestic animals, combined with proper meat and poultry inspections. Adults with salmonellosis who are food handlers or who have occupations involving care of young children should have 3 negative stool cultures before resuming work.

Treatment

A. Specific Measures: In uncomplicated *Salmonella* gastroenteritis antibiotic treatment does not shorten the course of the clinical illness and may prolong convalescent carriage of the organism.

However, to prevent sepsis and focal disease, antibiotic treatment is recommended for newborns, for severely ill children, and for children with sickle cell disease, liver disease, recent gastrointestinal surgery, cancer, depressed immunity, and chronic renal or cardiac disease. Ampicillin (150–200 mg/kg/d intravenously in 4 divided doses for 5–10 days), amoxicillin (50 mg/kg/d orally in 3 divided doses), or trimethoprim-sulfamethoxazole is recommended. Patients developing bacteremia during the course of gastroenteritis should receive parenteral treatment initially, and a careful search should be made for additional foci of infection. After signs and symptoms subside, they should receive oral medication. Parenteral and oral treatment should last a total of 7–10 days. Longer treatment is indicated for specific complications. If susceptibility tests indicate resistance to ampicillin, chloramphenicol or trimethoprim-sulfamethoxazole should be given. Clinical experience with third-generation cephalosporins is limited, and some failures are reported despite the excellent in vitro activity of these antimicrobials.

Salmonella meningitis is best treated with a combination of chloramphenicol (100 mg/kg/d intravenously in 4 divided doses) and ampicillin (200–300 mg/kg/d intravenously in 4–6 divided doses) for 3 weeks or a third-generation cephalosporin (cefotaxime, ceftriaxone) for 3 weeks. If the child improves rapidly and the cerebrospinal fluid is sterile, treatment may be completed with a single drug, the choice guided by results of susceptibility tests.

Outbreaks on pediatric wards are difficult to control. Strict hand washing, cohorting of patients and personnel, and ultimate closure of the unit may be necessary.

B. Treatment of the Carrier States: About half of patients are still infectious after 4 weeks. Infants tend to remain convalescent carriers for up to a year. Antibiotic treatment of carriers is not effective.

C. General Measures: Careful attention must be given to maintaining fluid and electrolyte balance, especially in infants.

Prognosis

In gastroenteritis, the prognosis is good. In sepsis with focal suppurative complications, the prognosis is more guarded.

The case fatality rate of *Salmonella* meningitis is high in infants. There is a strong tendency to relapse if treatment is not prolonged.

Blaser MJ, Newman LS: A review of human salmonellosis: I. Infective dose. *Rev Infect Dis* 1982;**4:**1096.

Buchwald DS, Balser MJ: A review of human salmonellosis: II. Duration of excretion following infection with nontyphi *Salmonella. Rev Infect Dis* 1984;**6:**345.

Chalker RB, Blaser MJ: A review of human salmonellosis: III. Magnitude of *Salmonella* infection in the United States. *Rev Infect Dis* 1988;**10:**111.

Rennels MB, Leving MM: Classical bacterial diarrhea: Perspectives and update—*Salmonella, Shigella, Escherichia coli, Aeromonas* and *Plesiomonas. Pediatr Infect Dis J* 1986;**5(Suppl):**21.

Ryan CA et al: Massive outbreak of antimicrobial-resistant salmonellosis traced to pasteurized milk. *JAMA* 1987; **258:**3269.

St Geme JW III et al: Consensus: management of *Salmonella* infection in the first year of life. *Pediatr Infect Dis J* 1988;**7:**615.

TYPHOID FEVER & PARATYPHOID FEVER

Essentials of Diagnosis

- Insidious or acute onset of headache, anorexia, vomiting, constipation or diarrhea, ileus, and high fever.
- Meningismus, splenomegaly, and rose spots.
- Leukopenia; positive blood, stool, bone marrow, and urine cultures.

General Considerations

Typhoid fever is caused by the gram-negative bacillus *Salmonella typhi;* paratyphoid fevers, which are usually milder but may be clinically indistinguishable, are caused by *Salmonella paratyphi* A, *Salmonella schottmeulleri,* or *Salmonella hirschfeldi* (formerly *Salmonella paratyphi* A, B, and C.) Children have a shorter incubation period than do adults (usually 5–8 days instead of 8–14 days). The organism enters the body through the walls of the intestinal tract and, following a transient bacteremia, multiplies in the reticuloendothelial cells of the liver and spleen. Persistent bacteremia and symptoms then follow. Reinfection of the intestine occurs as organisms are excreted in the bile. Bacterial emboli produce the characteristic skin lesions (rose spots). Symptoms in children may be mild or severe, but in general, except for the very young, the disease is milder than in adults.

Chloramphenicol-resistant typhoid fever has been reported in Southeast Asia, India, and South America, and ampicillin- and chloramphenicol-resistant strains are seen in Latin America and elsewhere.

Typhoid fever is transmitted by the fecal-oral route and by contamination of food or water. Unlike other *Salmonella* species, there are no animal reservoirs of *S typhi;* each case is the result of direct or indirect contact with the organism or with an individual who is actively infected or a chronic carrier. Laboratory-acquired infections are common.

About 500 cases per year are reported in the USA, 60% of which are acquired during foreign travel.

Clinical Findings

A. Symptoms and Signs: In children, the onset is apt to be sudden rather than insidious, with malaise, headache, crampy abdominal pains and distention, and sometimes constipation followed within 48 hours by diarrhea, high fever, and toxemia. An encephalopathy may be seen with irritability, confusion, delirium, and stupor. Vomiting and meningismus may be prominent in the young. The classic prolonged 3-stage disease seen in adult patients is often shortened in children. The prodrome may be only 2–4 days; the toxic stage may last only 2–3 days; and the defervescence stage may last 1–2 weeks.

During the prodromal stage, physical findings may be absent, or there may merely be some abdominal distension and tenderness, meningismus, mild hepatomegaly, and minimal splenomegaly. The typical typhoidal rash (rose spots) is present in 10–15% of children. It appears during the second week of the disease and may erupt in crops for the succeeding 10–14 days. Rose spots are erythematous maculopapular lesions 2–3 mm in diameter that fade on pressure. They are found principally on the trunk and chest, and they generally disappear within 3–4 days. The lesions usually number less than 20.

B. Laboratory Findings: Typhoid bacilli can be isolated from many sites, including blood, stool, urine, and bone marrow. Blood cultures are positive in 50–80% of cases during the first week and less often later in the illness. Stool cultures are positive in about 50% of cases after the first week. Urine and bone marrow cultures are also valuable. Most patients will have negative cultures (including stool) by the end of a 6-week period. Serologic tests (Widal reaction) are not as useful as cultures because both false-positive and false-negative results occur. A 4-fold rise in titer of O (somatic) agglutinins is suggestive but not diagnostic of infection.

Leukopenia is common in the second week of the disease, but in the first week, leukocytosis may be seen. Proteinuria, mild elevation of liver enzymes, thrombocytopenia, and disseminated intravascular coagulation are common.

Differential Diagnosis

Typhoid and paratyphoid fevers must be distinguished from other serious prolonged fevers. These include typhus, brucellosis, tularemia, miliary tuberculosis, psittacosis, vasculitis, lymphoma, mononucleosis, and Kawasaki disease.

The diagnosis of typhoid fever if often made clinically in developing countries. In developed countries, where typhoid fever is uncommon and physicians are unfamiliar with the clinical picture, the diagnosis is often not suspected until late. Positive cultures confirm the diagnosis.

Complications

The most important complications of typhoid fever are gastrointestinal hemorrhage (2–10%) and perforation (1–3%). They occur toward the end of the second week or during the third week of the disease.

Intestinal perforation is one of the principal causes of death. The site of perforation generally is the terminal ileum or cecum. The clinical manifestations are indistinguishable from those of acute appendicitis, with pain, tenderness, and rigidity in the right lower quadrant. The x-ray finding of free air in the peritoneal cavity is diagnostic.

Bacterial pneumonia, meningitis, septic arthritis, abscesses, and osteomyelitis are uncommon complications, particularly if specific treatment is given promptly. Shock and electrolyte disturbances may lead to death.

About 1–3% of patients become chronic carriers of *S typhi*. Chronic carriage is defined as excretion of typhoid bacilli for more than a year, but carriage is often lifelong. Adults with underlying biliary or urinary tract disease are much more likely than children to become chronic carriers.

Prevention

Although vaccine is available, routine typhoid immunization is not recommended in the USA (see Chapter 6).

Treatment

A. Specific Measures: Equally effective regimens for susceptible strains include the following: chloramphenicol (50–100 mg/kg/d orally or intravenously in 4 doses), trimethoprim-sulfamethoxazole (10 mg/kg trimethoprim and 50 mg/kg sulfamethoxazole per day orally in 2–3 divided doses), amoxicillin (100 mg/kg/d orally in 4 divided doses), and ampicillin (100–200 mg/kg/d intravenously in 4 divided doses). Aminoglycosides and first- and second-generation cephalosporins are clinically ineffective regardless of in vitro susceptibility results. Limited data suggest that ceftriaxone and cefotaxime are effective; one of these should be used initially in infections caused by strains with proved or suspected resistance to the more standard agents.

Treatment duration is 14–21 days. Patients remain febrile for 3–5 days even on appropriate therapy.

B. General Measures: General support of the patient is exceedingly important and includes rest, good nutrition, and careful observation, with particular regard to evidence of intestinal bleeding or perforation. Blood transfusions may be needed even in the absence of frank hemorrhage.

Prognosis

A prolonged convalescent carrier stage in children often continues 3–6 months. This does not require retreatment with antibiotics or exclusion from school or other activities.

With early antibiotic therapy, the prognosis is excellent. With early treatment, the mortality rate is less than 1%. Relapse occurs 1–3 weeks later in 10–20% of cases despite appropriate antibiotic treatment.

Bitar R, Tarpley J: Intestinal perforation in typhoid fever: A historical and state-of-the-art review. *Rev Infect Dis* 1985;**7**:257.

Hoffman SL et al: Reduction of mortality in chloramphenicol-treated severe typhoid fever by high-dose dexamethasone. *N Engl J Med* 1984;**310**:82.

Hornick RB: Selective primary health care: Strategies for control of disease in the developing world. 20. Typhoid fever. *Rev Infect Dis* 1985;**7**:537.

Meloni T et al: Ceftriaxone treatment of *Salmonella* enteric fever. *Pediatr Infect Dis J* 1988;**7**:734.

Scully RE, Mark EJ, McNeely BU: Case records of the Massachusetts General Hospital. *N Engl J Med* 1983; **309**:600.

Thisyakorn U, Mansuwan P, Taylor DN: Typhoid and paratyphoid fever in 192 hospitalized children in Thailand. *Am J Dis Child* 1987;**141**:862.

SHIGELLOSIS
(Bacillary Dysentery)

Essentials of Diagnosis

- Cramps and bloody diarrhea.
- High fever, malaise, convulsions.
- Pus and blood in diarrheal stools examined microscopically.
- Diagnosis confirmed by stool culture.

General Considerations

Shigellae are nonmotile gram-negative rods of the family *Enterobacteriaceae* and are closely related to *Escherichia coli*. The genus *Shigella* is divided into 4 major groups, A–D: *Shigella dysenteriae, Shigella flexneri, Shigella boydii,* and *Shigella sonnei.* Approximately 20,000 cases of shigellosis are reported each year in the USA. *S sonnei* followed by *S flex-*

neri are the most common isolates. *S dysenteriae,* which causes the most severe diarrhea of all species and the greatest number of extraintestinal complications, accounts for fewer than 1% of all *Shigella* infections in the USA.

Shigellosis is often a serious disease, particularly in children under 2 years of age, and without supportive treatment there is an appreciable mortality rate. In older children and adults, the disease tends to be self-limited and milder. Shigellosis is unusual in infants under 3 months of age, although rarely, shigellae may be transmitted from the mother to the newborn infant during delivery. Diarrhea and refusal to take feedings are the most common symptoms in neonatal shigellosis, and bloody diarrhea and fever occur less frequently. Vomiting, convulsions, or high fever is almost never encountered.

Shigella is usually transmitted by the fecal-oral route. Food- and water-borne outbreaks occur but are less important overall than person-to-person transmission. The disease is very communicable; as few as 200 bacteria can produce illness in an adult. The secondary attack rate in families is high, and shigellosis is a serious problem in day-care centers and custodial institutions. *Shigella* organisms produce disease by invading the colonic mucosa, causing mucosal ulcerations and microabscesses. A plasmid-encoded gene is required for enterotoxin production, chromosomal genes are required for invasiveness, and smooth lipopolysaccharide are required for virulence.

Clinical Findings

A. Symptoms and Signs: The incubation period usually is 2–4 days. Onset is abrupt, with abdominal cramps, urgency, tenesmus, chills, fever, malaise, and diarrhea. In severe forms, blood and mucus are seen in small volume in the watery stool (dysentery), and meningismus and convulsions may occur. In older children, the disease may be mild, and the diagnosis therefore missed. In young children, a fever of 39.4–40° C (103–104° F) is common. Rarely, there is rectal prolapse. Symptoms generally last 3–7 days.

B. Laboratory Findings: The total white blood cell count varies, but often there is a marked shift to the left. The stool may contain gross blood and mucus, and many neutrophils are seen if mucus from the stool is examined microscopically. Stool cultures usually are positive; however, they may be negative because the organism is somewhat fragile and present in small numbers late in the disease, and because laboratory techniques are suboptimal for the recovery of shigellae.

Differential Diagnosis

Diarrhea due to rotavirus infection is a winter rather than a summer disease, usually children are not as febrile or toxic, and stool does not contain gross blood or neutrophils. Intestinal infections caused by *Salmonella* or *Campylobacter* are differentiated by culture. Amebic dysentery is diagnosed by microscopic examination of fresh stools; intussusception is characterized by an abdominal mass, "currant jelly" stools without leukocytes, and absence of fever. Mild shigellosis is not distinguishable clinically from other forms of infectious diarrhea.

Complications

Dehydration, acidosis, shock, and renal failure are the major complications. In some cases, a chronic form of dysentery occurs, characterized by mucoid stools and poor nutrition. Bacteremia and metastatic infections are rare. Febrile seizures are common. Fulminating fatal dysentery (Ikari syndrome) and hemolytic-uremic syndrome occur rarely.

Treatment

A. Specific Measures: Trimethoprim-sulfamethoxazole (10 mg/kg/d trimethoprim and 50 mg/kg/d sulfamethoxazole, in 2 divided doses orally for 5 days) is the treatment of choice. Amoxicillin is not effective. Ampicillin (100 mg/kg/d in 4 divided doses) is also efficacious if the strain is sensitive. Successful treatment results in reduced duration of fever, cramping, and diarrhea and in termination of fecal excretion of *Shigella*. Strains resistant to ampicillin and trimethoprim-sulfamethoxazole are common in Mexico, underdeveloped countries, and increasingly in the USA. Tetracycline and chloramphenicol are also effective, but resistance may be seen. Third-generation cephalosporins and quinolones are active in vitro against resistant strains, but clinical experience is limited.

B. General Measures: In severe cases, immediate rehydration is critical. A mild form of chronic malabsorption syndrome may supervene and require prolonged dietary control.

Prognosis

The prognosis is excellent if vascular collapse is treated promptly by adequate fluid therapy. The mortality rate is high in very young, malnourished infants who do not receive fluid and electrolyte therapy. Convalescent fecal excretion of *Shigella* lasts 1–4 weeks in patients not receiving antimicrobial therapy. Long-term carriers are rare.

Ashkenazi S et al: Convulsions in shigellosis: Evaluation of possible risk factors. *Am J Dis Child* 1983;**137**:985.

Blaser MJ et al: *Shigella* infections in the United States, 1974–1980. *J Infect Dis* 1983;**147**:771.

DeWitt TG, Humphrey KF, McParthy P: Clinical predictors of acute bacterial diarrhea in young children. *Pediatrics* 1985;**76**:551.

Dupont HL, Nornick RB: Adverse effects of Lomotil therapy in shigellosis. *J Am Med Assoc* 1973;**226**:1525.

Ling J et al: Susceptibilities of Hong Kong isolates of multiply resistant *Shigella* spp to 25 antimicrobial agents, including ampicillin plus sulbactam and new 4-quinolones. *Antimicrob Agents Chemother* 1988;**32**:20.

Martin T, Habbick BF, Nyssen J: Shigellosis with bacteremia: A report of two cases and a review of the literature. *Pediatr Infect Dis* 1983;**2**:21.

O'Brien AD, Holmes RK: Shiga and Shiga-like toxins. *Microbiol Rev* 1987;**51**:206.

Tacket CO, Cohen ML: Shigellosis in day-care centers: Use of plasmid analysis to assess control measures. *Pediatr Infect Dis* 1983;**2**:127.

CHOLERA

Essentials of Diagnosis

- Sudden onset of severe watery diarrhea.
- Persistent vomiting without nausea or fever.
- Extreme and rapid dehydration and electrolyte loss, with rapid development of vascular collapse.
- Contact with a case of cholera, with shellfish, or the presence of cholera in the community.
- Diagnosis confirmed by stool culture.

General Considerations

Cholera is an acute diarrheal disease caused by the gram-negative organism *Vibrio cholerae*. It is transmitted by contaminated water or food, especially contaminated shellfish. The disease is generally so dramatic that in endemic areas the diagnosis is obvious. Individuals with mild illness and young children may play an important role in transmission of the infection.

Asymptomatic infection is far more common than clinical disease. In endemic areas, rising titers of vibriocidal antibody are seen with increasing age; infection occurs in individuals with low titers. The age-specific attack rate is highest in children under 5 years and declines with age. Cholera is unusual in infancy.

Cholera toxin is a protein enterotoxin that is primarily responsible for symptoms. Cholera toxin binds to a regulatory subunit of adenylcyclase in enterocytes, causing increased cyclic adenosine monophosphate and an outpouring of NaCl and water into the lumen of the small bowel.

Nutritional status is an important factor determining the severity of the diarrhea. Duration of diarrhea is prolonged in adults and children suffering from severe malnutrition.

Cholera is endemic in India and South and Southeast Asia. Seven major pandemics have occurred since 1817. The most recent pandemic, caused by the El Tor biotype of *Vibrio cholerae* 01, began in 1961 in Indonesia. In 1982, 37 countries were affected, and 54,000 cases reported. Outbreaks of cholera occurred in Spain in 1972, in Italy in 1973, and in Guam in 1975. Although no cases of cholera occurred in the USA between 1911 and 1973; an endemic focus of *V cholerae* of a unique phage type exists along the Gulf Coast. Cholera is increasingly recognized to be associated with consumption of shellfish. Interstate shipments of oysters have resulted in cholera in several inland states.

Several recent studies provide evidence that *V cholerae* is a natural inhabitant of estuarine environments. Seasonal multiplication of *V cholerae* may provide a source for outbreaks in endemic areas. Chronic cholera carriers are rare. The incubation period is short, usually 1–3 days.

Clinical Findings

A. Symptoms and Signs: There is sudden onset of massive, frequent, watery stools, generally light gray in color (''rice water'') and containing some mucus but no pus. Vomiting may be projectile and is not accompanied by nausea. Within 2–3 hours, the tremendous loss of fluids results in severe and life-threatening dehydration, hypochloremia, and hypokalemia, with marked weakness and collapse. Renal failure with uremia and irreversible peripheral vascular collapse will occur if fluid therapy is not administered. The illness lasts 1–7 days and is shortened by appropriate therapy.

B. Laboratory Findings: Markedly elevated hemoglobin (20 g/dL), marked acidosis, hypochloremia, and hyponatremia are seen.

A presumptive diagnosis can be made rapidly by fluorescence microscopy or the vibrio-immobilization test (immobilization by specific antisera of the highly motile cholera vibrios). Cultural confirmation using thiosulfate-citrate-bile-salt-sucrose (TCBS) agar takes 16–18 hours for a presumptive diagnosis and 36–48 hours for a definitive bacteriologic diagnosis.

Prevention

Cholera vaccine dosages are discussed in Chapter 6. The vaccine offers only partial protection (50%) for 3–6 months and is ineffective in controlling outbreaks. Experimental subunit vaccines and attenuated live-bacteria oral vaccines appear to be more efficacious. In endemic areas, all water and milk must be boiled, food protected from flies, and sanitary precautions observed. Thorough cooking of shellfish prevents transmission. All patients with cholera should be isolated.

Chemoprophylaxis is indicated for household and other close contacts of cholera patients. It should be initiated as soon as possible after the onset of the disease in the index patient. Tetracycline (500 mg daily for 5 days) is effective in preventing infection. Trimethoprim-sulfamethoxazole may be substituted in children.

Tourists visiting endemic areas are at little risk if they exercise common sense in what they eat and drink and maintain good personal hygiene.

Treatment

Physiologic saline must be administered in large amounts to restore blood volume and urine output and to prevent irreversible shock. Potassium supplements are required. Sodium bicarbonate, given intravenously, may also be needed initially to overcome profound acidosis. Moderate dehydration and acidosis can be corrected in 3–6 hours by oral therapy alone, because the active glucose transport system of the small bowel is normally functional. The composition of the solution (in meq/L) is as follows: Na^+, 120; HCO_3-, 48; Cl^-, 97; and K^+, 25—together with glucose, 110 mmol/L (2% dextrose). Intravenous fluids should be given initially in severe cases.

Treatment of children with tetracycline (50 mg/kg/d orally in 4 divided doses for 2–5 days) modifies the clinical course of the disease and prevents clinical relapse but is not as important as fluid and electrolyte therapy. Trimethoprim-sulfamethoxazole should be used in children less than 9 years of age.

Prognosis

With early and rapid replacement of fluids and electrolytes, the case fatality rate is 1–2% in children. If significant symptoms appear and no treatment is given, the mortality rate is over 50%.

Finkelstein RA et al: Epitopes of the cholera family of enterotoxins. *Rev Infect Dis* 1987;**9**:544.

Johnston JM et al: Cholera on a Gulf Coast oil rig. *N Engl J Med* 1983;**309**:523.

Kaper JB et al: Molecular epidemiology of *Vibrio cholerae* in the U.S. Gulf Coast. *J Clin Microbiol* 1982;**16**:129.

Kelly MT: Cholera: A worldwide perspective. *Pediatr Infect Dis* 1986;**5(Suppl)**:101.

Morris JG Jr, Black RE: Cholera and other vibrioses in the United States. *N Engl J Med* 1985;**312**:343.

CAMPYLOBACTER INFECTION

Essentials of Diagnosis

- Fever, vomiting, abdominal pain, diarrhea.
- Blood, mucus, pus in stools (dysentery).
- Presumptive diagnosis by darkfield or phase contrast microscopy of stool wet mount or modified Gram's stain.
- Definitive diagnosis by stool culture.

General Considerations

Campylobacter species (formerly grouped with vibrios and known as *Vibrio fetus*) are small, gram-negative, curved or spiral bacilli that are commensals or pathogens in many animals. *Campylobacter jejuni* frequently causes acute enteritis in humans, and *Campylobacter fetus* causes bacteremia and meningitis in immunocompromised patients. *Helicobacter pylori* (previously named *Campylobacter pylori*) has been associated with gastritis and peptic ulcer disease in both adults and children (see Chapter 20).

In the past decade, *C jejuni* has been responsible for 3–11% of cases of acute gastroenteritis in North America and Europe; in many areas, enteritis due to *C jejuni* is more common than that due to *Salmonella* or *Shigella*.

Campylobacter colonizes domestic and wild animals, especially poultry. Numerous cases have been associated with sick puppies or other animal contacts. Contaminated food and person-to-person spread by the fecal-oral route are important in transmission. Outbreaks associated with day-care centers, contaminated water supplies, and raw milk have been reported. Newborns may acquire the organism from their mothers at delivery.

Clinical Findings

A. Symptoms and Signs: *C jejuni* enteritis can be mild or severe. In tropical countries, asymptomatic stool carriage is common. The disease usually begins with sudden onset of high fever, malaise, headache, abdominal cramps, nausea, and vomiting. Diarrhea follows and may be watery or bile-stained, mucoid, and bloody. Passage of up to 20 stools per day is not uncommon. The illness is self-limiting, lasting 2–7 days, but relapses occur in 15–25% of cases. Without antimicrobial treatment, the organism remains in the stool for 1–6 weeks.

B. Laboratory Findings: The peripheral white blood cell count generally is elevated, with many band forms. Microscopic examination of stool reveals erythrocytes and pus cells, and darkfield or phase contrast microscopic examination of wet mounts may reveal darting bacilli characteristic of *Campylobacter*. Other bacteria, particularly *Vibrio* species, may exhibit similar motility, but in areas where cholera and *Vibrio parahaemolyticus* diarrhea are rare, a positive darkfield examination has a predictive value of about 90%. Isolation of *C jejuni* from stool is not difficult but requires selective agar, incubation at 42 °C, rather than 35 °C, and incubation in an atmosphere of about 5% oxygen and 5% CO_2 (candle jar is satisfactory).

Differential Diagnosis

Campylobacter enteritis may resemble viral gastroenteritis, salmonellosis, shigellosis, amebiasis, or other infectious diarrheas. Because it also mimics ulcerative colitis, Crohn's disease, intussusception, and appendicitis, mistaken diagnosis can lead to unnecessary surgery.

Complications

The most important complications are dehydration and inappropriate treatment due to misdiagnosis as inflammatory bowel disease. Other complications are uncommon but include erythema nodosum, convulsions, reactive arthritis, bacteremia, urinary tract infection, and cholecystitis.

Prevention

No vaccine is yet available. Hand washing and adherence to basic food sanitation practices help prevent disease.

Treatment

Treatment of fluid and electrolyte disturbances is most important. Antimicrobial treatment with erythromycin in children (30–50 mg/kg/d orally in 4 divided doses for 5 days) or with tetracycline in adults terminates fecal excretion and may prevent relapses, but antimicrobial treatment does not shorten or modify the illness unless given early in the disease. Antimicrobials used for shigellosis, such as trimethoprim-sulfamethoxazole and ampicillin, are inactive against *Campylobacter*. Supportive therapy is sufficient in most cases.

Prognosis

The outlook is excellent if dehydration is corrected and misdiagnosis does not lead to inappropriate diagnostic or surgical procedures.

Anders BJ et al: Double-blind placebo controlled trial of erythromycin for treatment of *Campylobacter* enteritis. *Lancet* 1982;**1**:131.

Blaser MJ, Reller LB: *Campylobacter* enteritis. *N Engl J Med* 1981;**305**:1444.

Paisley JW et al: Dark-field microscopy of human feces for presumptive diagnosis of *Campylobacter fetus* subsp *jejuni* enteritis. *J Clin Microbiol* 1982;**15**:61.

Schwartz RH et al: Experience with the microbiologic diagnosis of *Campylobacter* enteritis in an office laboratory. *Pediatr Infect Dis* 1983;**2**:298.

TULAREMIA

Essentials of Diagnosis

- A cutaneous or mucous membrane lesion at the site of inoculation and regional lymph node enlargement.
- Sudden onset of fever, chills, and prostration.
- History of contact with infected animals, principally wild rabbits, or history of tick exposure.
- Positive culture or immunofluorescence of mucocutaneous ulcer or regional lymph nodes.
- High serum antibody titer.

General Considerations

Tularemia is caused by *Francisella tularensis*, a gram-negative organism usually acquired from infected animals, principally wild rabbits; by contamination of the skin or mucous membranes with infected blood or tissues; by inhalation of infected material; by bites of ticks, fleas, or deerflies that have been in contact with infected animals; or by ingestion of contaminated meat or water. Strains of high virulence for humans (Jellison type A) are usually associated with tick-borne tularemia of rabbits; those of lowered virulence (Jellison type B) are linked with the water-borne disease of rodents. The incubation period is short, usually 3–7 days, but may vary from 2 to 25 days.

Rabbits are the classic vectors of tularemia. It is important to seek a history of rabbit hunting, skinning, or food preparation in any patient who has a febrile illness with tender lymphadenopathy, often in the region of a draining skin ulcer. However, a history of exposure to other wild game or ticks may also be helpful in diagnosis.

Clinical Findings

A. Symptoms and Signs: Several clinical types are seen in children. Most infections are of the ulceroglandular form and start as a reddened papule that may be pruritic, quickly ulcerates, and is not very painful. Shortly thereafter, the regional lymph nodes become large and tender. Fluctuance quickly follows. At the same time, there may be marked systemic manifestations, including high fever, chills, weakness, and vomiting. Pneumonitis occasionally accompanies the ulceroglandular form or may be seen as the sole manifestation of infection (pneumonic form). A detectable skin lesion is occasionally absent, and localized lymphoid enlargement exists alone (glandular form). Oculoglandular and oropharyngeal forms also occur in children. The latter is characterized by tonsillitis, often with membrane formation, cervical adenopathy, and high fever. In the absence of any primary ulcer or localized lymphadenitis, a prolonged febrile disease reminiscent of typhoid fever can be seen (typhoidal form). Splenomegaly is common in all forms.

B. Laboratory Findings: F tularensis can be recovered from ulcers, regional lymph nodes, and sputum of patients with the pneumonic form. However, the organism grows only on an enriched medium (blood-cystine-glucose agar), and laboratory handling is dangerous. Another method of organism detection is immunofluorescence of biopsied material or aspiration of involved lymph nodes. Gram's stain is not useful.

The white blood cell count is not remarkable. Agglutinins are present after the second week of illness, and in the absence of a positive culture their development confirms the diagnosis. An agglutination titer of 1:160 or higher is considered positive.

Differential Diagnosis

The typhoidal form of tularemia may mimic typhoid, brucellosis, miliary tuberculosis, Rocky Mountain spotted fever, and infectious mononucleosis. Pneumonic tularemia resembles atypical and mycotic pneumonitis. The ulceroglandular type of tularemia resembles pyoderma caused by staphylococci

or streptococci, rat-bite fever, plague, anthrax, and cat-scratch fever. The oropharyngeal type must be distinguished from streptococcal or diphtheritic pharyngitis, infectious mononucleosis, herpangina, or other viral pharyngitides.

Prevention

Reasonable attempts should be made to protect children from bites of insects, principally ticks, fleas, and deerflies, by the use of proper clothing and repellents. Since rabbits are the source of most human infections, the dressing and handling of such game should be performed with great care. If contact occurs, thorough washing with soap and water is indicated.

Treatment

A. Specific Measures: Streptomycin (30 mg/kg/d intramuscularly in 2 divided doses for 8–10 days) is the drug of choice. The maximum daily dose is 1 g. Other aminoglycoside antibiotics have been used in individual cases and are probably effective. The tetracyclines and chloramphenicol are also effective, but the organism is not eradicated, and relapses occur.

B. General Measures: Antipyretics and analgesics may be given as necessary. Skin lesions are best left open. Glandular lesions occasionally require incision and drainage.

Prognosis

The prognosis is excellent in patients receiving streptomycin.

Evans ME et al: Tularemia: A 30-year experience with 88 cases. *Medicine* 1985;**64**:251.

Jacobs RF, Condrey YM, Yamauchi T: Tularemia in adults and children: A changing presentation. *Pediatrics* 1985;**76**:818.

Markowitz LE et al: Tick-borne tularemia. *JAMA* 1985;**254**:292. [Emphasizes a more benign, often unrecognized form of illness in children with fever and cervical adenopathy.]

Uhari M, Syrjälä H, Salminen A: Tularemia in children caused by *Francisella tularensis* biovar palaearctica *Pediatr Infect Dis J* 1990;**9**:80.

PLAGUE

Essentials of Diagnosis

- Sudden onset of fever, chills, and prostration.
- Regional lymph node tender; lymphadenitis with suppuration of nodes (bubonic form).
- Hemorrhages into skin and mucous membranes and shock (septicemia).
- Cough, dyspnea, cyanosis, and hemoptysis (pneumonia).
- History of exposure to infected animals.

General Considerations

Plague is an extremely serious, acute infection caused by a gram-negative bacillus, *Yersinia pestis*. It is a disease of rodents that is transmitted to humans by the bites of fleas. Rodent plague in animals of the field and forest is called sylvatic plague; plague in rodents associated with humans is called murine plague. Plague bacilli have been isolated from rodents in 15 of the western states in the USA. Cases associated with wild rodents occur sporadically. Ten to 20 cases of plague in humans have occurred annually in the USA since 1974. In the western part of the USA, the disease almost always occurs during the period from June through September.

Human plague in the USA appears to occur in cycles that reflect comparable cycles in wild animal reservoirs of infection.

Clinical Findings

A. Symptoms and Signs: The disease assumes several different clinical forms, the 2 most common being bubonic and septicemic. Pneumonic plague, the form that occurs when organisms enter the body through the respiratory tract, is now very uncommon.

1. Bubonic plague—Bubonic plague begins after an incubation period of 2–6 days with a sudden onset of high fever, chills, headache, vomiting, and marked delirium or clouding of consciousness. A less severe form also exists, with a less precipitous onset but with progression over several days to severe symptoms. Although the flea bite is rarely seen, the regional lymph node, usually inguinal and unilateral, is painful and tender, 1–5 cm in diameter. The node usually suppurates and drains spontaneously after 1 week. The plague bacillus is known to produce an endotoxin that causes vascular necrosis. Bacilli may overwhelm regional lymph nodes and enter the circulation to produce septicemia. Severe vascular necrosis results in widely disseminated hemorrhages in skin, mucous membranes, liver, and spleen. Myocarditis and circulatory collapse may result from damage by the endotoxin.

A septicemic form of bubonic plague also exists that begins with fever, delirium, and bacteremia, with regional lymphadenopathy and bubo formation occurring after 3–5 days.

Plague meningitis or pneumonia may occur secondarily following bacteremic spread from an infected lymph node.

2. Septicemic plague—The septicemic form is defined as any case of plague without evidence of lymphadenopathy. This form is less common than bubonic plague but carries a worse prognosis, largely because it is less likely to be recognized and treated early. It is frequently complicated by pneumonia.

B. Laboratory Findings: Aspiration of a bubo leads to visualization of bacilli on a stained smear. Pus, sputum, and blood all yield the organism, although laboratory infections are common enough to make isolation dangerous. A buffy coat Gram's stain may reveal the organism, and blood-agar cultures yield positive results in 48 hours. The white blood cell count is markedly elevated, with a shift to the left.

Sera obtained during disease and convalescence should be collected and stored for use in confirming the diagnosis in cases where the organism may not be recovered.

Differential Diagnosis

The septic phase of the disease may be confused with such illnesses as meningococcemia, sepsis, and rickettsioses. The bubonic form resembles tularemia, anthrax, cat-scratch fever, streptococcal adenitis, and cellulitis. Primary gastroenteritis and appendicitis may have to be distinguished.

Prevention

Proper disposal of household and commercial wastes and chemical control of rats are basic for control of the murine plague reservoir. Flea control is instituted and maintained with the liberal use of insecticides. Children vacationing in remote camping areas should be warned not to handle dead or dying animals. Travelers to wild areas in the enzootic western states are at low risk of infection, and immunization of visitors to these areas is not recommended.

Vaccination is recommended for those traveling or living in areas of high incidence. (See Chapter 6.)

Treatment

A. Specific Measures: Streptomycin and tetracyclines should both be used. The dose of streptomycin is 20–40 mg/kg intramuscularly in 3 divided doses for 5 days, followed by one of the tetracyclines, 50 mg/kg/d intramuscularly or orally in 3 divided doses. Treatment should be continued until the patient has been afebrile for 4 or 5 days. Chloramphenicol (75–100 mg/kg/d intravenously or orally in 4 divided doses) may be substituted for tetracycline.

In septicemia and pneumonic plague, treatment must be started in the first 15–24 hours of the disease if survival is to be expected. Treatment with streptomycin started 36–48 hours after onset of the disease may result in death due to liberation of plague toxin. The mechanism may be analogous to the Jarisch-Herxheimer reaction, with release of toxin from dead plague bacilli.

Bubonic plague is not highly contagious. Every effort is made to effect resolution of buboes without resorting to surgery. Pus from draining lymph nodes should be handled with rubber gloves.

B. General Measures: Pneumonic plague is highly infectious, and rigid isolation is required. All contacts should receive prophylaxis with sulfadiazine (100–200 mg/kg/d orally in 4 divided doses for 7 days) or tetracycline (30 mg/kg/d in 4 divided doses for 7 days).

Prognosis

The mortality rate in untreated bubonic plague is about 50%; it is 90% in the septicemic form and nearly 100% in the pneumonic form. Recent mortality rates in New Mexico were 3% for bubonic plague and 71% for the septicemic form.

Centers for Disease Control: Human plague—United States, 1988. *MMWR* 1988;**37**:653.

Eidson M et al: Feline plague in New Mexico: Risk factors and transmission to humans. *Am J Public Health* 1988; **78**:1333–1335.

Hull HF, Montes JM, Mann JM: Septicemic plague in New Mexico. *J Infect Dis* 1987;**155(1)**:113–118.

Mann JM, Shandler L, Cushing AH: Pediatric plague. *Pediatrics* 1982;**69**:762.

HAEMOPHILUS INFLUENZAE TYPE b INFECTIONS

Essentials of Diagnosis

- Purulent meningitis in children under age 4 years with direct smears of cerebrospinal fluid showing gram-negative pleomorphic rods.
- Acute epiglottitis: High fever, drooling, dysphagia, aphonia, and croup. White blood cell count over 20,000/µL.
- Septic arthritis: Fever, local redness, swelling, heat, and pain with active or passive motion of the involved joint in a child 4 months to 4 years of age.
- Cellulitis: Sudden onset of fever and distinctive cellulitis in an infant, often involving the cheek or periorbital area, and starting as a mild swelling with central erythema that rapidly progresses to a lesion without a distinct border with central reddish discoloration, surrounded by and merging into purplish areas that fade peripherally.
- In all cases, a positive culture from the blood, cerebrospinal fluid, or aspirated pus confirm the diagnosis.

General Considerations

Haemophilus influenzae type b (Hib) is perhaps the most important bacterial pathogen in childhood. It causes meningitis, epiglottitis (supraglottic croup), septic arthritis, periorbital and facial cellulitis, pneumonia, and pericarditis. Hib infections occur most frequently in the age group from 4 months to 4 years (epiglottitis: 2–5 years). This organism is the leading bacterial cause of all the above infections, with the exception of pneumonia and pericarditis, in this age range.

Ninety percent of blood samples from newborns show bactericidal antibody, reflecting passive transfer of antibody from protected mothers. The age distribution of infection is explained by the loss of passive protection by 4–6 months of age, the progressive infection of susceptible individuals, and acquisition of protective antibodies in early childhood. The chief virulence factor for Hib organisms appears to be the polyribose phosphate (PRP) capsule, which is antiphagocytic, and anti-PRP antibody is protective. Many children 4 months to 3 years of age have low or nondetectable levels of anticapsular antibodies. In the period from 3½–8 years of age, anticapsular antibodies appear in the serum and reach adult levels. Although many infants and children are colonized early with *H influenzae* species, most of the strains are nonencapsulated. The very low nasopharyngeal colonization rate (1–2%) of Hib in infants and children suggests that the homologous organism is not the usual stimulus for the development of anticapsular antibodies. The type b capsule is immunologically cross-reactive with the capsules of certain species of bacilli, diphtheroids, lactobacilli, *Staphylococcus aureus*, *Staphylococcus epidermidis*, streptococci, *Escherichia coli*, and *Pseudomonas*. Thus, it appears that natural immunity is acquired from encapsulated bacteria that share antigenic determinants with Hib PRP.

In the past 3 decades, the incidence of Hib infections serious enough to require hospitalization has been increasing. There is no clear explanation for this increase. Recently, reports of systemic disease in newborns and adults have increased. However, the number of systemic infections has increased in all age groups, and the highest age-specific attack rate still occurs in children from 4 months to 4 years of age.

In 1974, the first 2 cases of illnesses due to ampicillin-resistant Hib were reported. The mechanism of resistance was the elaboration of β-lactamase (penicillinase) by the resistant organisms. Ampicillin-resistant strains currently account for 10–40% of all type b strains isolated in certain regions of the USA. Associated clinical illnesses have included meningitis, pneumonia, epiglottitis, sepsis, and otitis media. Hib resistant to chloramphenicol and rare strains resistant to both drugs have been observed.

Tympanocentesis performed in children with acute otitis media has demonstrated that a pneumococcus can be isolated from about 35% of cases and *H influenzae* from about 25%. However, most of the *H influenzae* strains are nonencapsulated and nontypeable. Type b accounts for about 10% of the *H influenzae* strains. Ampicillin-resistant *H influenzae* should be suspected in situations where ampicillin therapy of otitis media is unsuccessful.

Acutely ill children 4–36 months of age, with temperatures higher than 39 °C (102.2 °F) and nonspecific symptoms associated with an elevated white blood cell count, may have Hib bacteremia. This syndrome is associated most frequently with pneumococcal bacteremia and next most frequently with Hib bacteremia.

Both ampicillin and chloramphenicol or a third-generation cephalosporin (cefotaxime or ceftriaxone) should be used as initial therapy for infants and children over 30 days of age with disease thought to be due to Hib. This includes all bacterial meningitis and epiglottitis, and, in infants under 4 years of age, facial cellulitis and septic arthritis. Ampicillin alone is adequate initial therapy for otitis, sinusitis, and most cases of suspected bacterial pneumonia. If Hib is cultured, sensitivities to ampicillin, chloramphenicol, and third-generation cephalosporins should be determined and therapy continued with the single most appropriate drug. If no organism is cultured and Hib is a likely cause (as with meningitis or typical cellulitis), chloramphenicol alone or a third-generation cephalosporin should be used.

Clinical Findings

A. Symptoms and Signs:

1. Meningitis—In the USA, Hib is responsible for about 80% of cases of bacterial meningitis in children after the neonatal period. In many other countries, this percentage is lower. Infants usually present with fever, irritability, lethargy, poor feeding with or without vomiting, and a high-pitched cry. Signs of localized disease elsewhere should be looked for carefully, including otitis, cellulitis, arthritis, and pneumonia. (See Chapter 24 for further details.)

2. Acute epiglottitis—The most useful clinical finding in the early diagnosis of Hib epiglottitis is evidence of dysphagia characterized by a refusal to eat or swallow saliva and by drooling. This finding, plus the presence of a high fever in a "toxic" child—even in the absence of cherry-red epiglottis on direct examination of the epiglottis—should strongly suggest the diagnosis and lead to prompt intubation. Stridor is a late sign. (See Chapter 15 for details.)

3. Septic arthritis—Hib is the most common cause of bacterial septic arthritis in children under 4 years of age in the USA. Disease may involve multiple joints and is complicated by osteomyelitis in about 20% of cases. The child is febrile and refuses to move the involved joint and limb because of pain. Examination reveals swelling, warmth, redness, tenderness on palpation, and severe pain on attempted movement of the joint.

4. Cellulitis—Cellulitis due to Hib occurs almost exclusively in the 3-month to 4-year age group. The presentation is typical. The child often gives a history of coryza or otitis media. Fever persists at the same time the cellulitis develops. The cheek or periorbital (preseptal) area is usually involved. There is mild swelling with central erythema, rapidly progressing to a lesion without a distinct border that exhibits central reddish discoloration surrounded by a purplish area. Superficial trauma is characteristically absent. Bacteremia is frequent.

Periorbital cellulitis due to Hib must be distinguished from 2 other similar entities. The first is periorbital (preseptal) cellulitis caused by other bacteria. This frequently presents with evidence of a primary local infection nearby (conjunctivitis, sinusitis) or trauma to the skin. Staphylococci, streptococci, or a combination of the 2 is usually involved. Bacteremia is rare. The second is true orbital cellulitis. This disease is rare and occurs primarily in older children with ethmoid or sphenoid sinusitis. Hib is usually not involved.

5. Pneumonia—Pneumonia due to Hib usually presents clinically in much the same fashion as pneumonia due to the pneumococcus. Disease is most common in the 3-month to 4-year age group, just as it is with *H influenzae* meningitis. Most cases are segmental or lobar in distribution, but diffuse bronchopneumonia or interstitial involvement is occasionally seen. Both empyema and lung abscesses occur. Hib involvement of other organs (meningitis, epiglottitis, otitis media) is not uncommon.

The true incidence of Hib pneumonia is not known. It is likely, however, that it varies according to geographic area. In the USA, Hib is probably second only to the pneumococcus as a cause of bacterial pneumonia in young children.

B. Laboratory Findings: The white blood cell count in Hib infections may be high or normal with a shift to the left. Blood culture is frequently positive. Positive culture of aspirated pus or fluid from the involved site or nearby proves the diagnosis.

In meningitis (before treatment), spinal fluid smear may show the characteristic pleomorphic gram-negative rods.

The diagnosis of Hib pneumonia depends on isolation of the organism from blood, lung tissue, or empyema fluid. A positive culture from the upper respiratory tract is not diagnostic. Detection of antigen in body fluids, including urine, may be helpful. Counterimmunoelectrophoresis or latex agglutination can be used to detect polyribose phosphate (PRP), the capsular antigen of Hib in cerebrospinal fluid, joint fluid, urine, sputum, and serum. The test is particularly useful in the diagnosis of patients with meningitis or arthritis who have received antibiotic therapy and have negative cultures. Antigenemia may last from days to weeks in certain infants and occurs transiently following Hib immunization.

C. Imaging: A lateral view of the neck in suspected acute epiglottitis may be helpful but should not delay intubation. Haziness of maxillary and ethmoid sinuses occurs with orbital cellulitis.

Differential Diagnosis

A. Meningitis: Meningitis must be differentiated from head injury, brain abscess, tumor, lead encephalopathy, and other forms of meningoencephalitis, including tuberculous meningitis, due to viral, fungal, and bacterial agents.

B. Acute Epiglottitis: In croup caused by viral agents (parainfluenza 1, 2, and 3, respiratory syncytial virus, influenza A, adenovirus), the child has more definite upper respiratory symptoms, cough, hoarseness, slower progression of obstructive signs, and only low-grade fever. Spasmodic croup occurs typically at night in a child with a history of previous attacks; these attacks may be of allergic origin. A history of sudden onset of choking and paroxysmal coughing suggests aspiration of a foreign body. Occasionally, retropharyngeal abscess or laryngeal diphtheria may have to be differentiated from epiglottitis.

C. Septic Arthritis: Differential diagnosis includes acute osteomyelitis, prepatellar bursitis, cellulitis, rheumatic fever, and fractures and sprains.

D. Cellulitis: Erysipelas, streptococcal cellulitis, insect bites, and trauma (including Popsicle panniculitis) may occur. Periorbital cellulitis must be differentiated from paranasal sinus disease without cellulitis, allergic inflammatory disease of the lids, conjunctivitis, and herpes zoster infection.

E. Pneumonia: See Chapter 15.

Complications

A. Meningitis: See Chapter 24.

B. Acute Epiglottitis: Mediastinal emphysema and pneumothorax may occur.

C. Septic Arthritis: Septic arthritis may result in rapid destruction of cartilage and ankylosis if diagnosis and treatment are delayed. Even with early treatment, the incidence of residual damage and disability after septic arthritis in weight-bearing joints may be as high as 25%.

D. Cellulitis: Bacteremia may lead to metastatic meningitis or pyarthrosis.

E. Pneumonia: Complications include empyema and, rarely, pneumotocele and pneumothorax.

Prevention

In Finland, field trials of a purified PRP vaccine for Hib showed greater than 90% protection of infants immunized at 2 years of age and older. This vaccine was licensed in the USA in 1985 and was recommended for routine use in children at 2 years of age (see Chapter 6 for discussion of use in older children). If ongoing trials demonstrate good immunogenicity and efficacy of these conjugate vaccines, it is likely that they will soon be recommended for use in younger children. In the past several years, three other more immunogenic vaccines containing PRP conjugated with diphtheria toxoid or other pro-

teins have been licensed for use in children 15 months of age and older.

Careful epidemiologic studies have demonstrated that families and close contacts of patients with Hib infections are at increased risk of acquiring infection. This has led to the following recommendation: The index case and all family members should be given rifampin 20 mg/kg/d (maximum adult dose 600 mg/d) orally for 4 successive days. There is controversy regarding a recommendation for chemoprophylaxis for day-care-center contacts. Some authorities recommend rifampin chemoprophylaxis for young contacts (especially children age 2 or less) of a case who regularly attended a day-care center. Other authorities believe that the risk to day-care-center contacts is low and do not recommend prophylaxis unless 2 cases of systemic Hib disease have occurred in children in the day-care center within a 60-day period. Rifampin, if used, should be given to children in the same classroom as the index case and to adults working in that classroom.

Treatment

For comments regarding the problem of ampicillin-resistant strains of Hib, see General Considerations (above). All bacteremic or potentially bacteremic Hib diseases require hospitalization for treatment. The drugs of choice in hospitalized cases are a third-generation cephalosporin (cefotaxime or ceftriaxone) or intravenous ampicillin and chloramphenicol, in combination until the sensitivity of the organism is known.

Most second-generation cephalosporins (cefamandole, cefoxitin, and cefaclor) should not be used for any Hib infection in which meningitis is a possibility, since these drugs do not reach cerebrospinal fluid in concentrations adequate to treat or prevent infection. Cefuroxime is effective for nonmeningeal infections but third-generation agents (ceftriaxone, cefotaxime) are preferred for meningitis because of more rapid and reliable sterilization of cerebrospinal fluid.

Oral therapy with amoxicillin is preferred for susceptible strains. Several agents may be used for ampicillin-resistant strains or for those of unknown susceptibility. These include trimethoprim-sulfamethoxazole, erythromycin-sulfonamide combinations, cefaclor, amoxicillin-clavulanic acid, and cefixime. Penicillin, erythromycin alone, and first-generation cephalosporins are not reliable. Oral chloramphenicol is very effective but usually reserved for children who were already exposed to it parenterally, since there are many other oral agents that do not pose the hematologic risk.

A. Meningitis: Therapy is begun as soon as bacterial meningitis has been identified and cerebrospinal fluid, blood, and other appropriate cultures have been obtained. Therapy is begun with cefotaxime (50 mg/kg intravenously every 8 hours) or ceftriaxone (50 mg/kg intravenously every 12 hours). Intravenous ampicillin (50 mg/kg every 6 hours) plus chloramphenicol (20 mg/kg every 6 hours for infants 3–6 months old, and 25 mg/kg every 6 hours for older children) may also be used. If the organism is sensitive to ampicillin, it is the drug of choice. Therapy should preferably be given intravenously for the entire course; chloramphenicol may be given orally when tolerated if it is used (levels must be monitored), and ceftriaxone may be given intramuscularly if venous access becomes difficult.

Duration of therapy is 10 days. Although a 7-day regimen appears effective in most uncomplicated cases, it has not been studied in children who have also been treated with steroids to prevent hearing loss (see below). Longer treatment is reserved for those children who respond slowly or in whom septic complications have occurred. Antibiotics can be discontinued after 10 days in a febrile child if the clinical response was rapid and satisfactory, but the source of prolonged or recurrent fevers must always be sought with great care. The most common causes for recurrence of fever or persistence of fever beyond 6 days are the following: phlebitis, hospital-acquired viral or bacterial superinfection, metastatic disease requiring drainage (eg, subdural empyema, septic pericarditis, arthritis), drug fever, and subdural effusions.

Repeated lumbar taps are usually not necessary in Hib meningitis. They should be obtained in the following circumstances: unsatisfactory or questionable clinical response, seizure occurring after several days of therapy, and prolonged (7 days) or recurrent fever. Routine lumbar tap at the end of therapy is not recommended. (See Chapter 24 for additional information.)

Supportive therapy with intravenous fluids and oxygen, should be given as required. Patients should be observed carefully for development of the syndrome of inappropriate ADH secretion (SIADH). In addition, a preliminary study has suggested that dexamethasone given immediately after diagnosis and continued for a period of 4 days may reduce the incidence of hearing loss in children with Hib meningitis. Additional studies are now under way to confirm or refute this preliminary finding. In the published study, dexamethasone at a dose of 0.6 mg/kg/d given in 4 divided doses was used for a period of 4 days. In animal models, it is important to give the dexamethasone prior to beginning antimicrobials; this maximally blocks formation of inflammatory mediators (interleukin-1-beta and tumor necrosis factor) thought responsible for eighth nerve damage.

B. Acute Epiglottitis: See Chapter 15.

C. Septic Arthritis: If the isolate is sensitive to ampicillin, it is given in a dosage of 200–300 mg/kg/d intravenously in 4 divided doses until there is marked improvement (usually 4–7 days). This may be followed by oral amoxicillin (75–100 mg/kg/d in 4 divided doses every 6 hours) administered under careful supervision to complete a 2-week course. Chloramphenicol or a third-generation cephalosporin should be used for ampicillin-resistant organisms. Oral agents for ampicillin-resistant organisms include chloramphenicol, cefaclor, trimethoprim-sulfamethoxazole, amoxicillin-clavulanic acid, and cefixime. Ideally, susceptibility to these agents should be proved prior to use. Drainage of infected joint fluid is an essential part of treatment. In joints other than the hip, this can often be accomplished by one or more needle aspirations. In hip infections—and in arthritis of other joints where treatment is delayed or clinical response is slow—open surgical drainage is advised. Local instillation of antibiotics is not necessary and may be injurious.

The joint should be immobilized. Antipyretics and analgesics are given as required, and adequate hydration is maintained.

D. Cellulitis and Orbital Cellulitis: Depending on results of susceptibility testing, ampicillin chloramphenicol, or a third-generation cephalosporin is given parenterally for 3–7 days, followed by oral treatment as for septic arthritis, and supportive and symptomatic treatment as required. There is usually marked improvement after 72 hours of treatment. Antibiotics should be given for 10–14 days.

E. Pneumonia: Ampicillin (200–300 mg/kg/d intravenously in 4 divided doses) chloramphenicol, or a third-generation cephalosporin is given, as well as oxygen, intravenous fluids, and other supportive care as required. Treatment lasts 3 weeks. Empyema should be treated by placement of one or more chest tubes into the pleural space. When possible, a chest tube should be removed after 4 or 5 days.

Prognosis

The case fatality rate for Hib meningitis is less than 5%. Young infants have the highest mortality rate. Neurologic sequelae should be watched for but are appreciably reduced with prompt antibiotic treatment. One of the most common neurologic sequelae, which develops in approximately 5–10% of patients with Hib meningitis, is significant sensory neural hearing loss. All patients with Hib meningitis should have their hearing checked at some time during the course of the illness or shortly after recovery.

The case fatality rate in acute epiglottitis is 2–5%; deaths are associated with bacteremia and the rapid development of airway obstruction.

The prognosis for the other diseases requiring hospitalization is good with the institution of early and adequate antibiotic therapy.

Asman BI et al: *Haemophilus influenzae* type b pneumonia in 43 children. *J Pediatr* 1978;**93**:389.

Claesson B et al: Incidence and prognosis of *Haemophilus influenzae* meningitis in children in a Swedish region. *Pediatr Infect Dis J* 1984;**3**:35.

Jacobs NM, Harris VJ: Acute *Haemophilus* pneumonia in childhood. *Am J Dis Child* 1979;**133**:603.

Lebel MH, Freij BJ, Syrogiannopoulos GA: Dexamethasone therapy for bacterial meningitis: Results of two double-blind, placebo-controlled trials. *N Engl J Med* 1988;**319**:964.

Letson GW et al: Comparison of active and combined passive/active immunization of Navajo children against *Haemophilus influenzae* type B. *Pediatr Infect Dis J* 1988;**7**:747.

Li KI, Wald ER: Use of rifampin in *Haemophilus influenzae* type b infections. *Am J Dis Child* 1986; **140**:381.

Makintubee S, Istre GR, Ward JI: Transmission of invasive *Haemophilus influenzae* type b disease in day care settings. *J Pediatr* 1987;**111**:180.

Mendelman PM, Smith AL: *Haemophilus influenzae* Chapter 28 in Feigin RD, Cherry JD (editors). *Textbook of Pediatric Infectious Disease,* (2nd ed) Saunders, 1987.

Molteni RA: Epiglottitis. Incidence of extraepiglottic infection: Report of 72 cases and review of the literature. *Pediatrics* 1976;**58**:526.

Rotbart HA, Glode MP: *Haemophilus influenzae* type b septic arthritis in children; Report of 23 cases. *Pediatrics* 1985;**75**:254.

Weinberg GA, Granoff DM: Polysaccharide-protein conjugate vaccines for the prevention of *Haemophilus influenzae* type B disease. *J Pediatr* 1988;**113**:621.

PERTUSSIS (Whooping Cough)

Essentials of Diagnosis

- Prodromal catarrhal stage (1–3 weeks) characterized by mild cough, coryza, and fever.
- Persistent staccato, paroxysmal cough ending with a high-pitched inspiratory "whoop."
- Leukocytosis with absolute lymphocytosis.
- Diagnosis confirmed by fluorescent stain or culture of nasopharyngeal secretions.

General Considerations

Pertussis is an acute, highly communicable infection of the respiratory tract caused by *Bordetella pertussis* and characterized by severe bronchitis. Children usually acquire the disease from symptomatic family contacts. Adults who have mild respiratory illness, not recognized as pertussis, frequently are the source of infection. Asymptomatic carriage of *B pertussis* is not documented. Infectivity is greatest during the catarrhal and early paroxysmal cough stage (for about 4 weeks after onset).

The disease is most common and most severe in early infancy. Of 5500 reported cases in the USA in 1984 and 1985, 48% were in children less than one year of age, and 37% were in children less than 6 months of age. Seventy-four percent of infants aged 6 months or less were hospitalized; 20% had pneumonia, 2.6% had seizures, 0.8% had encephalopathy, and 1% died.

Active immunity follows natural pertussis. Reinfections occur years to decades later but are usually mild. Immunity following immunization wanes in 5–10 years. The majority of young adults in the USA are susceptible to pertussis infection.

Bordetella parapertussis causes a similar but milder syndrome and is reported frequently in central Europe.

B pertussis organisms attach to the ciliated respiratory epithelium and multiply there; deeper invasion does not occur. Disease is due to several bacterial toxins; the most potent is pertussis toxin, which is responsible for lymphocytosis and many of the symptoms of pertussis.

Clinical Findings

A. Symptoms and Signs: The onset of pertussis is insidious, with catarrhal upper respiratory tract symptoms (rhinitis, sneezing, and an irritating cough). Slight fever may be present; temperature greater than 38.3 °C (101 °F) suggests bacterial superinfection or another cause of respiratory tract infection. After about 2 weeks, cough becomes paroxysmal, characterized by 10–30 forceful coughs ending with a loud inspiration (the "whoop"). Infants and adults with otherwise typical, severe pertussis often lack characteristic whooping. Vomiting commonly follows a paroxysm. Coughing is accompanied by cyanosis, sweating, prostration, and exhaustion. This stage lasts for 2–4 weeks, with gradual improvement. Cough suggestive of chronic bronchitis lasts for another 2–3 weeks. Paroxysmal coughing may continue for some months in the absence of any infection and may worsen with intercurrent viral respiratory infection. In adults, older children, and partially immunized individuals, symptoms may consist only of low-grade fever and irritating cough lasting 1–2 weeks. In the younger unimmunized child, symptoms of pertussis last about 8 weeks or longer.

B. Laboratory Findings: White blood cell counts of 20,000–30,000/μL with 70–80% lymphocytes typically appear near the end of the catarrhal stage. Many older children and adults with mild infections never demonstrate lymphocytosis. The blood picture may resemble lymphocytic leukemia or leukemoid reactions. Identification of *B pertussis* by culture from nasopharyngeal swabs proves the diagnosis. Cough plates are inferior to nasopharyngeal swabs or nasal wash specimens. The organism may be found in the respiratory tract in diminishing numbers beginning in the catarrhal stage and ending about 2 weeks after the beginning of the paroxysmal stage. After 4–5 weeks of symptoms, cultures and fluorescent antibody tests are almost always negative. Fresh Bordet-Gengou agar or a charcoal agar containing an antimicrobial should be inoculated as soon as possible; *B pertussis* does not tolerate drying nor prolonged transport. Serum agglutinins appear late in the infection and are of little value in diagnosis. Enzyme-linked immunosorbent assays for detection of antibody to pertussis toxin or filamentous hemagglutinin may be useful for diagnosis but are currently not widely available. The chest x-ray reveals thickened bronchi and sometimes shows a ''shaggy'' heart border, indicating bronchopneumonia and patchy atelectasis.

Differential Diagnosis

The differential diagnosis of pertussis includes bacterial, tuberculous, chlamydial, and viral pneumonia. Cystic fibrosis and foreign body aspiration may be considerations.

Adenoviruses and respiratory syncytial virus may cause paroxysmal coughing with an associated elevation of lymphocytes in the peripheral blood, mimicking pertussis. Coinfection with pertussis and respiratory viruses may cause symptoms indistinguishable from pertussis alone.

Complications

Bronchopneumonia due to superinfection is the most common serious complication. It is characterized by abrupt clinical deterioration during the paroxysmal stage, accompanied by high fever and sometimes a striking leukemoid reaction with a shift to predominantly polymorphonuclear leukocytes. Atelectasis is a second common pulmonary complication. Atelectasis may be patchy or extensive and may shift rapidly to involve different areas of lung. Intercurrent viral respiratory infection is also a common complication and may provoke worsening or recurrence of paroxysmal coughing. Otitis media is common. Residual chronic bronchiectasis is infrequent despite the severity of the illness. Apnea and sudden death may occur during a particularly severe paroxysm. A diffuse encephalopathy of uncertain cause may complicate severe cases and frequently is fatal. It is unclear whether anoxic brain damage, cerebral hemorrhage, or pertussis neurotoxins are to blame, but anoxia is most likely the cause. Epistaxis and subconjunctival hemorrhages are common.

Prevention

Active immunization (see Chapter 6) with pertussis vaccine in combination with diphtheria and tetanus toxoids (DTP) should be given in early infancy.

Chemoprophylaxis with erythromycin should be given to exposed family and hospital contacts, particularly those under age 2 years, for 14 days. Hospitalized children with pertussis should be isolated because of the great risk of transmission to patients and staff. Several large hospital outbreaks have been reported in the last decade.

Treatment

A. Specific Measures: Antibiotics may ameliorate early infections but not those in the paroxysmal stage. Erythromycin is the drug of choice since it promptly terminates respiratory tract carriage of *B pertussis*. Patients should be treated with erythromycin (40–50 mg/kg/24 h in 4 divided doses for 14 days). Although ampicillin is effective against *B pertussis* in vitro, it is ineffective in vivo. Steroids were efficacious in reducing number and severity of paroxysms in one controlled study.

B. General Measures: Nutritional support during the paroxysmal phase is very important. Frequent small feedings, tube feeding, or parenteral fluid supplementation may be needed. Minimizing stimuli that trigger paroxysms is probably the best way of controlling cough. In general, cough suppressants are of little benefit.

C. Treatment of Complications: Respiratory insufficiency due to pneumonia or other pulmonary complications should be treated with oxygen and assisted ventilation if necessary. Convulsions are treated with oxygen and anticonvulsants. Bacterial pneumonia or otitis media may require additional antibiotics.

Prognosis

The prognosis for patients with pertussis has improved in recent years because of adequate nursing care, treatment of complications, nutrition, and modern intensive care. However, the disease is still very serious in infants under 1 year of age; most deaths occur in this age group. Children with encephalopathy have a poor prognosis.

Mertsola J et al: Intrafamilial spread of pertussis. *J Pediatr* 1983;**103**:359.

Nkowane BM et al: Pertussis epidemic in Oklahoma. *Am J Dis Child* 1986;**140**:433.

Noble GR et al: Acellular and whole-cell pertussis vaccines in Japan. *JAMA* 1987;**257**:1351.

Placebo-controlled trial of two acellular pertussis vaccines in Sweden: Protective efficacy and adverse events. *Lancet* 1988;**1**:954.

Report of the Task Force on Pertussus and Pertussis Immunization—1988. *Pediatrics* 1988;**81**.

LISTERIOSIS

Essentials of Diagnosis

Early-onset of neonatal disease:

■ Signs of sepsis a few hours after birth in an infant born with fetal distress; hepatosplenomegaly. Maternal fever.

Late-onset neonatal disease:

■ Meningitis, sometimes with monocytes in the cerebrospinal fluid and peripheral blood. Onset at 9–30 days of age.

General Considerations

Listeria monocytogenes is a gram-positive, non-spore-forming aerobic rod distributed widely in the animal kingdom and in food, dust, and soil. It causes systemic infections in newborn infants and immunosuppressed older children. In pregnant women, infection is relatively mild, with fever, aches, and chills, but it is accompanied by bacteremia and sometimes results in intrauterine or perinatal infection with grave consequences for the fetus or newborn. Disease due to *Listeria* is uncommon even though the organism is widespread and occurs as normal fecal flora in at least 1% of the population. Persons in contact with animals seem to be at particular risk. Recent large food-borne outbreaks have been traced to contaminated cabbage in coleslaw, and contaminated soft cheese.

Like group B streptococcal infections, *Listeria* infections in the newborn can be divided into early and late forms. Early infections are more common and are frequently severe and generalized, sometimes leading to granulomatosis infantiseptica, a severe congenital form of infection. Later infections are often characterized by meningitis.

Clinical Findings

A. Symptoms and Signs: In the early neonatal form, symptoms usually appear on the first day of life and always by the third day. Infants are frequently premature and have signs of fetal distress. Respiratory distress, diarrhea, and fever occur. On examination, hepatosplenomegaly and a papular rash are found. A history of maternal fever is common. Meningitis may accompany the septic course.

The late neonatal form usually occurs after 9 days of age and can occur as late as 5 weeks. Meningitis is common, characterized by irritability, fever, and poor feeding.

Listeria infections occur rarely in older children, usually in those with animal contact or those who are immunosuppressed. Signs and symptoms are those of meningitis, usually with insidious onset.

B. Laboratory Findings: In all patients except those receiving white cell depressant drugs, the white blood cell count is elevated, with 10–20% monocytes. When meningitis is found, the characteristic cell count is high (> 500/uL) with a predominance of polymorphonuclear leukocytes in 70% of cases; monocytes predominate in up to 30%. The chief pathologic feature in severe neonatal sepsis is miliary granulomatosis with microabscesses in liver, spleen, central nervous system, lung, and bowel.

In meningitis, gram-stained smears of cerebrospinal fluid often show short gram-positive rods.

Cultures are frequently positive from multiple sites, including blood in the infant and the mother. The organisms form small, weakly hemolytic colonies on blood agar and may be mistaken for streptococci.

Differential Diagnosis

Early-onset neonatal disease resembles hemolytic disease of the newborn, group B streptococcal sepsis or severe cytomegalovirus infection, rubella, or toxoplasmosis. Late-onset disease must be differentiated from meningitis due to echovirus and coxsackievirus, group B streptococci, and gram-negative enteric bacteria.

Treatment

Ampicillin (150–300 mg/kg/d every 6 hours intravenously) is the drug of choice in most cases. Gentamicin (2.5 mg/kg every 8 hours intravenously) is added in severe illnesses by most experts, since it has a synergistic effect with ampicillin in vitro. If ampicillin cannot be used, trimethoprim-sulfamethoxazole is also effective. Cephalosporins are not effective. Treatment of severe disease should continue for at least 2 weeks.

Prognosis

In a recent outbreak of early-onset neonatal disease, the mortality rate was 27% despite aggressive and appropriate management. Meningitis in older infants has quite a good prognosis. In immunosuppressed children, prognosis depends to a great extent on that of the underlying illness.

Lennon D et al: Epidemic perinatal listeriosis. *Pediatr Infect Dis J* 1984;**3**:30.

Linnan MJ et al: Epidemic Listeriosis associated with mexican-style cheese. *N Engl J Med* 1988;**319**:823.

Schlech WF III et al: Epidemic listeriosis: Evidence for transmission by food. *N Engl J Med* 1983;**308**:203.

Visintine AM, Oleske JM, Nahmias AJ: *Listeria monocytogenes*. Infection in infants and children. *Am J Dis Child* 1977;**131**:393.

TUBERCULOSIS

Essentials of Diagnosis

- All types: Positive tuberculin test in patient or members of household, suspicious chest x-ray, history of contact, and demonstration of organism by stain and culture.
- Pulmonary: Fatigue, irritability, and undernutrition, with or without fever and cough.
- Glandular: Chronic cervical adenitis.
- Miliary: Classic "snowstorm" appearance of chest x-ray; choroidal tubercles.
- Meningitis: Fever and manifestations of meningeal irritation and increased intracranial pressure. Characteristic cerebrospinal fluid.

General Considerations

Tuberculosis is a granulomatous disease caused by *Mycobacterium tuberculosis*. It remains a leading cause of death throughout the world. Children under 3 years of age are most susceptible, and lymphohematogenous dissemination through the lungs and spread to extrapulmonary sites, including the brain and meninges, eyes, bones and joints, lymph nodes, kidneys, intestines, larynx, and skin, are more likely to occur in infants. Increased susceptibility occurs again in adolescence, particularly in girls within 2 years of menarche. Prolonged household contact with an active adult case usually leads to infection of infants and children. Tuberculosis is a particularly serious problem among crowded urban populations refugees from Southeast Asia, and AIDS patients. The case rate and death rate in nonwhite children are 2–5 times those in white children. The primary complex in infancy and childhood consists of a small parenchymal lesion in any area of the lung with caseation of regional nodes and calcification. Postprimary tuberculosis in adolescents and adults occurs in the apexes of the lungs and is likely to cause chronic, progressive cavitary pulmonary disease with less tendency for hematogenous dissemination.

Clinical Findings

A. Symptoms and Signs:

1. Pulmonary—See Chapter 15.

2. Military—Diagnosis is made on the basis of a classic snowstorm appearance of lung fields on x-ray, although early in the course of disseminated tuberculosis, the chest x-ray may show no or only subtle abnormalities. The majority also have a fresh primary complex and pleural effusion. Choroidal tubercles are sometimes seen on funduscopic examination. Other lesions may be present and produce osteomyelitis, arthritis, meningitis, tuberculomas of the brain, enteritis, or infection of the kidneys and liver.

3. Meningitis—Symptoms include fever, vomiting, headache, lethargy, and irritability, with signs of meningeal irritation and increased intracranial pressure, including cranial nerve palsies, convulsions, and coma. Choroidal tubercles are pathognomonic when associated with these signs and symptoms. Otorrhea or acute otitis media may be seen.

4. Glandular—The primary complex may be associated with a skin lesion drained by regional nodes or chronic cervical node enlargement and infection of the tonsils. Involved nodes may become fixed to the overlying skin and suppurative, and they may drain.

B. Laboratory Findings: The Mantoux text (0.1 mL of intermediate strength PPD, [5 TU] inoculated intradermally is read as positive at 48–72 hours if there is significant induration (Table 28–1). False-negative results are seen in malnourished patients, those with overwhelming disease, and in a few percent of children with isolated pulmonary disease. Temporary suppression of tuberculin reactivity may also be seen with viral infections (eg, measles, influenza, varicella, mumps), after live virus immunization, and when corticosteroids or other immunosuppressive drugs are present. For this reason, every Mantoux test should be accompanied by intradermal injection of control antigens (such as *Candida albicans* or tetanus toxoid) that are usually positive in persons with normal immune response. When tuberculosis is suspected and the child is anergic, household members and adult contacts (eg, teachers) should also be tested immediately.

The erythrocyte sedimentation rate is usually elevated. Cultures of pooled early morning gastric aspirates from 3 successive days are often valuable in children in whom tuberculosis is suspected. The cerebrospinal fluid in tuberculous meningitis shows slight to moderate pleocytosis (50–300 white blood cells, predominantly lymphocytes), decreased glucose, and increased protein.

The direct detection of mycobacteria in body fluids or discharges is best done by staining specimens with auramine O and examining them with blue-light fluorescence microscopy; this is superior to the Ziehl-Neelsen method.

C. Imaging: Chest x-ray should be obtained in all children with suspicion of tuberculosis at any site or with a positive skin test. Segmental consolidation with some volume loss and hilar adenopathy are common findings in children. Pleural effusion also occurs with primary infection. Cavities and apical disease are unusual.

Differential Diagnosis

Pulmonary tuberculosis must be differentiated from sarcoidosis; fungal, parasitic, mycoplasmal, and bacterial pneumonias; lung abscess; foreign body aspiration; lipoid pneumonia; and mediastinal cancer. Cervical lymphadenitis is most apt to be due to streptococcal or staphylococcal infections. Cat-scratch fever and infection with atypical mycobacteria may need to be distinguished from tuberculosis also. Viral meningoencephalitis, head trauma (battered child), lead poisoning, brain abscess, acute bacterial meningitis, brain tumor, and disseminated

Table 28–1. Interpretation of tuberculin skin test reactions[1].

Risk	Risk Factors	Positive Reaction
High	Recent close contact with case of active tuberculosis, Chest radiograph compatible with tuberculosis, Immunocompromise	> 5 mm induration
Medium	Current or previous residence in high prevalence area (Asia, Africa, Latin America) Intravenous drug use Homelessness, or residence in correctional institution Recent weight loss or malnutrition Leukemia, Hodgkin's disease, diabetes mellitus	> 10 mm induration
Low	All others	> 15 mm induration

[1]Standard intradermal Mantoux test, 5 test units.

fungal infections must be excluded in tuberculous meningitis. The skin test in the patient or family contacts is frequently valuable in differentiation of these conditions from tuberculosis.

Prevention

A. BCG Vaccine: Although this is often routinely given to infants and children in countries with a high prevalence of tuberculosis, protective efficacy varies greatly with vaccine potency and method of delivery. In the USA, BCG vaccination is considered only for tuberculin-negative children and neonates in high-risk situations who are unlikely to receive isoniazid (INH) prophylaxis or close follow-up (see Chapter 6).

B. Isoniazid (INH) Chemoprophylaxis: Daily administration of isoniazid (10 mg/kg/d orally; maximum 300 mg) is advised for children who cannot avoid intimate household contact with adolescents or adults with active disease. Isoniazid is given until 3 months after last contact. At the end of this time, a Mantoux test should be done, and therapy should be continued for 9–12 months if it is positive. BCG is not recommended during the period of isoniazid chemoprophylaxis.

C. Other Measures: The source contact (index case) should be identified, isolated, and treated to prevent other secondary cases. Exposed tuberculin-negative children should be skin tested every 2 months for 6 months after contact has been terminated. Routine tuberculin skin testing is advised at 12 months of age. Routine testing of school children is recommended only in certain populations.

Treatment

A. Specific Measures: Most children in the USA are hospitalized initially. If the infecting organism has not been isolated for susceptibility testing from the presumed contact, reasonable attempts should be made to obtain it from the child using gastric aspirates, sputum induction, bronchoscopy, thoracentesis, etc. Cooperation with outpatient therapy must be assured.

All children with positive skin tests (see Table 28-1) without overt disease should receive 6–12 months of isoniazid (10 mg/kg/d orally, maximum 300 mg) therapy. In children with overt pulmonary disease, therapy for 9 months using isoniazid (10 mg/kg/d), rifampin (15 mg/kg/d), and pyrazinamide (25–30 mg/kg/d) in a single daily oral dose for 2 months, followed by isoniazid plus rifampin (either in a daily or twice-weekly regimen) for 7 months appears effective for isoniazid-susceptible organisms. For more severe disease, such as miliary or central nervous system infection, duration is increased to 12 months or more, and a fourth drug (streptomycin or ethambutol) is added initially until susceptibility is known.

1. Isoniazid—The hepatotoxicity seen in adults and some adolescents is rare in children. Transient transaminitis (up to 3 times normal) may be seen at 6–12 weeks, but therapy is continued unless clinical illness occurs. Peripheral neuropathy associated with pyridoxine deficiency is rare in children, and it is not necessary to add pyridoxine unless significant malnutrition coexists.

2. Rifampin—Although an excellent bactericidal agent, rifampin is never used alone due to rapid development of resistance. Hepatotoxicity may be seen but rarely with recommended doses. The orange discoloration of secretions is benign.

3. Pyrazinamide—This excellent sterilizing agent has most effect during the first 2 months of therapy; with the recommended duration and dosing, it is well tolerated. Although it elevates the uric acid level, it rarely causes symptoms of hyperuricemia in children. Use of this drug is now common for tuberculous disease in children; resistance is almost unknown. Oral acceptance and central nervous system penetration are good.

4. Ethambutol—Since color blindness and optic neuritis are the major side effects, ethambutol is usually given only to children who can be reliably vision tested every 2 months. This complication occurs in a few percent of patients, usually those receiving more than the recommended dosage of 15 mg/kg/d.

5. Streptomycin, kanamycin, and capreomycin—One of these agents (usually streptomycin, 20–30 mg/kg/d, intramuscularly in 1–2 doses a day) may be given in severe disease, especially if resistance to other agents is likely. Hearing should be tested periodically during use.

B. Chemotherapy for Drug-Resistant Tuberculosis: The incidence of drug resistance in previously untreated patients with tuberculosis is still relatively low in the USA and Canada. However, when the organism is acquired from foreign-born adults, the incidence of resistance to isoniazid may reach 15%. If primary drug resistance is expected because of epidemiologic considerations, children should be treated with isoniazid and at least 2 other drugs (rifampin and ethambutol or pyrazinamide) to which the organisms are likely to be susceptible. Therapy should continue for 12 months or longer.

C. General Measures:

1. Corticosteroids—These drugs may be used for suppressing inflammatory reactions in meningeal, pleural, and pericardial tuberculosis and for the relief of bronchial obstruction due to hilar adenopathy. Prednisone is given orally, 1 mg/kg/d for 6–8 weeks, with gradual withdrawal at the end of that time.

2. Bed rest—Rest in bed is indicated only while the child feels ill. Isolation is necessary only for children with draining lesions or renal disease and those with chronic pulmonary tuberculosis. Most children with tuberculosis are noninfectious and can attend school while being treated.

Prognosis

If bacteria are sensitive and treatment is completed, most patients make lasting recovery. Retreatment is more difficult and less successful. With antituberculosis chemotherapy (especially isoniazid), there should now be nearly 100% recovery in miliary tuberculosis. Without treatment, the mortality rate in both miliary tuberculosis and tuberculous meningitis is almost 100%. In the latter form, about two-thirds of treated patients survive. There may be a high incidence of neurologic abnormalities among survivors if treatment is started late.

Biddulph J, Kokoha V, Sharma S: Short course chemotherapy in childhood tuberculosis. *J Trop Pediatr* 1988; **34**:20.

Grossman M et al: Consensus: Management of tuberculin-positive children without evidence of disease. *Pediatr Infect Dis J* 1988;**7**:243.

Nemir RL, Krasinski K: Tuberculosis in children and adolescents in the 1980's. *Pediatr Infect Dis J* 1988;**7**:375.

Snider DE Jr et al: Tuberculosis in children. *Pediatr Infect Dis J* 1988;**7**:271.

Starke JR: Modern approach to the diagnosis and treatment of tuberculosis in children. *Pediatr Clin North Am* 1988;**35**:441.

Visudhiphan P, Chiemchanya S: Tuberculous meningitis in children: Treatment with isoniazid and rifampicin for twelve months. *J Pediatr* 1989;**114**:875.

INFECTIONS WITH ATYPICAL MYCOBACTERIA

Essentials of Diagnosis

- Chronic unilateral cervical lymphadenitis.
- Granulomas of the skin.
- Chronic bone lesion with draining sinus (chronic osteomyelitis).
- Reaction to PPD-S (standard) of 5–8 mm, negative chest x-ray, and negative history of contact with tuberculosis.
- Positive skin reaction to a specific atypical antigen.
- Diagnosis by positive acid-fast stain or culture.

General Considerations

Various species of acid-fast mycobacteria other than *Mycobacterium tuberculosis* may cause subclinical infections and, occasionally, clinical disease closely simulating tuberculosis. Strain cross-reactivity with *M tuberculosis* can be demonstrated by simultaneous skin testing (Mantoux) with PPD-S (standard) and PPD prepared from one of the atypical antigens (available from the CDC). The larger skin reaction suggests infection with the homologous strain.

The Runyon classification of mycobacteria includes the following:

Group I—Photochromogens (PPD-Y): Yellow color develops upon exposure to light in previously white colony grown 2–4 weeks in the dark. Group 1 includes *Mycobacterium kansasii* and *Mycobacterium marinum.*

Group II—Scotochromogens (PPD-G): Colonies are definitely yellow-orange after incubation in the dark. Organisms may be found in small numbers in the normal flora of some human saliva and gastric contents. Subclinical infection is widespread in the USA, but clinical disease appears rarely. Group II includes *Mycobacterium scrofulaceum.*

Group III—Nonphotochromogens (PPD-B): "Battey-avian-swine group" grows as small white colonies after incubation in the dark, with no significant development of pigment upon exposure to light. Infection with *Mycobacterium intracellulare* ("Battey bacillus") is prevalent on the east coast of the USA, particularly the Southeast. Infection with avian strains is prevalent in Great Britain.

Group IV—"Rapid growers": *Mycobacterium fortuitum* and *Mycobacterium chelonei* are the recognized pathogens. Within 1 week after inoculation, they form colonies closely resembling *M tuberculosis* morphologically.

Clinical Findings

A. Symptoms and Signs:

1. Lymphadenitis—In children, the commonest form of infection due to mycobacteria other than tuberculosis is cervical lymphadenitis. *M scrofulaceum* or *M intracellulare* is almost always the cause. A submandibular node swells slowly and is firm and usually nontender. Over time, the node suppurates and may drain chronically. Nodes in other areas of the head and neck and elsewhere are sometimes involved. There is no fever or toxicity.

2. Pulmonary disease—In the western USA, this is usually due to *M kansasii;* in the eastern USA, it may be due to *M intracellulare.* In other countries, disease is usually caused by *M intracellulare* or *avium.* In adults, there is usually underlying chronic pulmonary disease, but in children, this is often not the case. Immunologic deficiency may be present. Presentation is clinically indistinguishable from that of tuberculosis.

3. Swimming pool granuloma—This is due to *M marinum.* A solitary chronic granulomatous lesion, frequently on the elbow, develops after minor trauma in infected swimming pools.

4. Chronic osteomyelitis—Osteomyelitis is caused by *M kansasii, M scrofulaceum,* or "rapid growers." Findings include swelling and pain over a distal extremity, radiolucent defects in bone, fever, and clinical and x-ray evidence of bronchopneumonia. Such cases are rare.

5. Meningitis—Disease is due to *M kansasii* and may be indistinguishable from tuberculous meningitis.

6. Disseminated infection—Rarely, a clinical

syndrome resembling that of acute hematopoietic cancer has been reported in association with isolation of *M kansasii*, scotochromogens, *M fortuitum*, or *M intracellulare* from bone marrow, lymph nodes, or liver. Chest x-rays are usually normal. *M intracellulare* is now recognized as an important cause of disseminated infection in individuals with HIV infection.

B. Laboratory Findings: In most cases, there is a small reaction (< 10 mm) when Mantoux testing is done with PPD-S. Larger reactions may be seen. The chest x-ray is negative, and there is no history of contact with tuberculosis. Needle aspiration of the node excludes bacterial infection and may yield acid-fast bacilli on stain or culture. Fistulization should not be a problem because total excision follows if the infection is due to atypical mycobacteria. If other organisms are found, formal excision may be avoided. Excision is usually required if aspiration is nondiagnostic and the clinical findings support the diagnosis. If performed, simultaneous tuberculin testing with the infecting atypical antigen (PPD-Y,-G, or -B) will usually give a reaction greater than the reaction to PPD-S.

Differential Diagnosis

See section on differential diagnosis in the discussion of tuberculosis above and in Chapter 15.

Treatment

A. Specific Measures The usual treatment of lymphadenitis is complete surgical excision. Chemotherapy is neither necessary nor sufficient for cure. Occasionally, resolution of the adenopathy is under way when the diagnosis is made. In these cases, careful follow-up is adequate.

Response of extensive adenopathy or other forms of infection varies according to the infecting species and susceptibility. Recent data suggest that isoniazid, rifampin, and streptomycin with or without ethambutol (depending on sensitivity to isoniazid) will result in a favorable response in almost all patients with *M kansasii* infection. Chemotherapeutic treatment of *M intracellulare* is much less satisfactory. Most authors favor surgical excision of involved tissue if possible and treatment with at least 3 drugs to which the organism has been shown to be sensitive. Effective drugs may include ethionamide, capreomycin, and pyrazinamide as well as the more familiar antituberculous agents. *M fortuitum* and *M chelonei* are usually susceptible to amikacin plus erythromycin or doxycycline and may be successfully treated with such combinations. Swimming pool granuloma due to *M marinum* is usually self-limited but may be treated either with drugs or by surgical excision, with good results.

B. General Measures: Isolation of the patient is usually not necessary. General supportive care is indicated for the child with disseminated disease.

Prognosis

The prognosis is good for localized disease, though fatalities occur in immunocompromised children with disseminated disease.

Benjamin DR: Granulomatous lymphadenitis in children. *Arch Pathol Lab Med* 1987;**111:**750.

Contreras MA, Cheung OT, Sanders DE, et al: Pulmonary infection with nontuberculous mycobacteria. *Am Rev Respir Dis* 1988;**137:**149.

Gill MJ, Fanning EA, Chomyc S: Childhood lymphadenitis in a harsh northern climate due to atypical mycobacteria. *Scand J Infect Dis* 1987;**19:**77.

Margileth AM: Management of nontuberculous (atypical) mycobacterial infections in children and adolescents. *Pediatr Infect Dis J* 1985;**4:**119.

Woods GL, Washington JA: Mycobacteria other than *Mycobacterium tuberculosis:* Review of microbiologic and clinical aspects. *Rev Infect Dis J* 1987;**9:**275.

LEGIONELLA INFECTION

Essentials of Diagnosis

- Severe progressive pneumonia in a child with compromised immunity.
- Diarrhea and neurologic signs are common.
- Positive culture requires buffered charcoal yeast extract media and proves infection.

General Considerations

Legionella pneumophila is an ubiquitous gram-negative bacillus that causes two distinct clinical syndromes: legionnaires' disease and Pontiac fever. Legionnaires' disease is an acute, severe pneumonia that is frequently fatal in immunocompromised patients. Pontiac fever is a mild, nonpneumonic, flulike illness characterized by fever, headache, myalgia, and arthralgia. The disease is self-limited and is described in outbreaks in otherwise healthy adults.

Twenty-two different species of *Legionella* have been discovered. *Legionella* is present in many natural water sources as well as domestic water supplies (faucets, showers). Contaminated cooling towers and heat exchangers have been implicated in several large institutional outbreaks. Sporadic, community-acquired cases also occur, and the source of infection is not usually clear. Person-to-person transmission has not been documented.

Few cases of legionnaires' disease have been reported in children. Most have been children with compromised cellular immunity or children receiving steroids. In adults, risk factors include smoking, underlying cardiopulmonary or renal disease, alcoholism, and diabetes.

L pneumophila is thought to be acquired by inhalation of a contaminated aerosol. The bacteria are phagocytosed but proliferate within macrophages. Cell-mediated immunity is necessary to activate macrophages to kill intracellular bacteria.

Clinical Findings

A. Signs and Symptoms: Onset of fever, chills, anorexia, and headache is abrupt. Pulmonary symptoms occur within 2–3 days but progress rapidly. The cough is nonproductive early on. Purulent sputum occurs late. Hemoptysis, diarrhea, and neurologic signs (including lethargy, irritability, tremors, and delirium) are seen.

B. Laboratory Findings: White blood count is usually elevated. Chest radiographs show rapidly progressive, patchy consolidation. Cavitation and large pleural effusions are uncommon. Cultures from sputum, tracheal aspirates, or broncoscopic specimens, when grown on buffered yeast charcoal extract media, are positive in 50–70% of patients at 3 to 7 days. Direct fluorescent antibody (DFA) staining of sputum or other respiratory specimens is only 70–75% sensitive but 95% specific. As such, a negative culture or DFA of sputum or tracheal secretions does not rule out legionnaires' disease. Serologic tests are available and aid in diagnosis, but a maximum rise in titer may require 6 to 8 weeks.

Differential diagnosis

Legionnaires' disease is usually a rapidly progressive pneumonia in a patient who appears very ill with unremitting fevers. Other bacterial pneumonias, viral pneumonias, *Mycoplasma* pneumonia, and fungal disease are all possibilities and may be difficult to differentiate in an immunocompromised patient.

Complications

In sporadic untreated cases, mortality rates are 5–25%. In untreated immunocompromised patients, mortality approaches 80%. Hematogenous dissemination may result in extrapulmonary foci of infection, including pericardium, myocardium, and renal involvement. *Legionella* may present as "culture-negative" endocarditis.

Prevention

No vaccine is available. Hyperchlorination and periodic superheating of water supplies in hospitals have been shown to reduce the number of organisms and the frequency of cases.

Treatment

Erythromycin (40–50 mg/kg/d in 4 divided doses, orally or intravenously) results in clinical improvement in 48–72 hours. Rifampin (20 mg/kg/d divided in 2 doses) is very active in vitro and is also given to gravely ill patients. Therapy is continued for 21 days to reduce the likelihood of relapse.

Prognosis

Mortality is frequent if legionnaires' disease is not recognized and appropriately treated. Malaise, problems with memory, and fatigue are common problems in patients after recovery.

Esposito AL, Gantz NM: Legionnaires' disease: The distance travelled since Philadelphia. *Pediatr Infect Dis J* 1986;**5**:163.

Helms CM et al: Legionnaires' disease associated with a hospital water system. *JAMA* 1988;**259**:2423.

Hervas JA, Alomar P: Multiple organ system failure in an infant with *Legionella* infection. *Pediatr Infect Dis J* 1988;**7**:671.

Kovatch AL et al: Legionellosis in children with leukemia in relapse. Pediatrks 1984;**73**:811.

Meyer RD: *Legionella* infections: A review of five years of research. *Rev Infect Dis* 1983;**5**:258.

Orenstein WA et al: The frequency of *Legionella* infection prospectively determined in children hospitalized with pneumonia. *J Pediatr* 1981;**99**:403.

Tompkins LS: Legionella prosthetic-valve endocarditis. *N Engl J Med* 1988;**318**:530.

PSITTACOSIS (Ornithosis) & *CHLAMYDIA PNEUMONIAE* INFECTION

Essentials of Diagnosis

- Fever, cough, malaise, chills, headache.
- Diffuse rales; no consolidation.
- Long-lasting x-ray findings of bronchopneumonia.
- Isolation of the organism or rising titer of complement-fixing antibodies.
- Exposure to infected birds.

General Considerations

Psittacosis is caused by *Chlamydia psittaci*. When the agent is transmitted to humans from psittacine birds (parrots, parakeets, cockatoos, and budgerigars), the disease is often called psittacosis or parrot fever. However, other avian genera (pigeons, turkeys) are common sources of infection in the USA, and the general term *ornithosis* is often used. The agent is an obligatory intracellular parasite. Human-to-human spread occurs rarely. The incubation period is 7–15 days. The bird from whom the disease was contracted may not be clinically ill.

Recently, a new strain of *Chlamydia*, designated the TWAR agent or *C pneumoniae*, has been found to cause an atypical pneumonia in previously well individuals. Transmission is by respiratory spread. Infection appears to become prevalent during the second decade; half of surveyed adults are seropositive. The disease may be more common than atypical pneumonia due to *M pneumoniae*. The role of this organism in pediatric infection is unknown.

Clinical Findings

A. Symptoms and Signs:

1. *C psittaci*—The disease is extremely variable but tends to be mild in children. The onset is rapid or insidious, with fever, chills, headache, backache, malaise, myalgia, and dry cough. Signs include those of pneumonitis, alteration of percussion note and breath sounds, and rales. Pulmonary findings may be absent early. Splenomegaly, epistaxis, prostration, and meningismus are occasionally seen. Delirium, constipation or diarrhea, and abdominal distress may occur. Dyspnea and cyanosis may occur later.

2. C pneumoniae—Clinically, *C pneumoniae* infection is very similar to *M pneumoniae* infection, with fever, sore throat (perhaps more severe with *C pneumoniae*), cough, and bilateral pulmonary findings and infiltrates. Prolonged symptoms in some patients suggest that therapy with erythromycin or tetracycline may have to be more prolonged than that usually given for *Mycoplasma*.

B. Laboratory Findings: In psittacosis, the white blood cell count is normal or decreased, often with a shift to the left. Proteinuria is frequently present. *C. psittaci* is present in the blood and sputum during the first 2 weeks of illness and can be isolated by inoculation of clinical specimens into mice or embryonated hens' eggs. Complement-fixing antibodies appear during or after the second week. The rise in titer may be minimized or delayed by early chemotherapy. Serologic tests for *C. pneumoniae* are now available.

C. Imaging: The x-ray findings in psittacosis are those of central pneumonia, which later becomes widespread or migratory. Psittacosis is indistinguishable from viral pneumonias by x-ray. Signs of pneumonitis may appear by x-ray in the absence of clinical suspicion of pulmonary involvement.

Differential Diagnosis

Psittacosis can be differentiated from acute viral pneumonias only by the history of contact with potentially infected birds. In severe or prolonged cases with extrapulmonary involvement, the differential diagnosis includes a wide spectrum of diseases such as typhoid fever, brucellosis, rheumatic fever, etc.

Complications

Complications of psittacosis include myocarditis, endocarditis, hepatitis, pancreatitis, and secondary bacterial pneumonia. *C. pneumoniae* infection may be prolonged or recur.

Treatment

For psittacosis, tetracyclines in full doses should be given for 14 days. Supportive oxygen may be needed. The patient should be kept in isolation. *C. pneumoniae* responds to either erythromycin or tetracycline.

Byrom NP, Wells J, Mair HJ: Fulminant psittacosis. *Lancet* 1979;**1**:353.

Durfee PT: Psittacosis in humans in the United States, 1974. *J Infect Dis* 1975;**132**:604.

Grayson JT et al: A new *Chlamydia psittaci* strain, TWAR, isolated in acute respiratory tract infections. *N Engl J Med* 1986;**315**:161.

CAT-SCRATCH DISEASE

Essentials of Diagnosis

- History of a cat scratch or cat contact.
- Primary lesion (papule, pustule, conjunctivitis) at site of inoculation.
- Acute or subacute regional lymphadenopathy.
- Positive cat-scratch skin test.
- Aspiration of sterile pus from a node.
- Laboratory studies excluding other causes.
- Biopsy of node or papule showing histopathologic findings consistent with cat-scratch disease and occasionally characteristic bacilli on Warthin-Starry stain.

General Considerations

Cat-scratch disease is a benign, self-limiting form of lymphadenitis. Patients often report a cat scratch (67%) or contact with a cat or kitten (90%). The cat almost invariably is healthy. The clinical picture is that of a regional lymphadenitis associated with an erythematous papular skin lesion without intervening lymphangitis. The disease occurs worldwide and is more common in the fall and winter. The most common systemic complication is encephalitis.

An infectious agent is now considered responsible; short, thin bacilli have been seen by Warthin-Starry stain in tissue obtained early in the infection and a fastidious gram-negative bacillus has been isolated on artificial media.

Clinical Findings

A. Symptoms and Signs: About 50% of patients develop a primary lesion at the site of inoculation, although some authors report a much higher percentage. The lesion usually is a papule or pustule and is located most often on the arm or hand (50%), head or leg (30%), or trunk or neck (10%). The lesion may be conjunctival (10%). Regional lymphadenopathy appears 10–30 days later and may be accompanied by mild malaise, lassitude, headache, and fever. Multiple sites are seen in about 10% of cases. Involved nodes may be hard or soft and 1–6 cm in diameter. They are usually tender, and about 25% of them suppurate. The overlying skin may or may not be inflamed. Lymphadenopathy usually resolves in about 2 months, but it may persist for up to 8 months.

Unusual manifestations include nonpruritic maculopapular rash, erythema multiforme or nodosum, purpura, conjunctivitis (Parinaud's oculoglandular fever), parotid swelling, pneumonia, chronic sinus drainage, osteolytic lesions, mesenteric and mediastinal adenitis, peripheral neuritis, hepatosplenomegaly, and encephalitis.

B. Laboratory Findings: Antigens prepared from pus aspirated from nodes of infected individuals have been used for skin testing. Because they are poorly standardized antigens and are not available commercially, their use is discouraged. The skin test is positive in more than 90% of patients thought to have cat-scratch disease and 5% of normal controls.

Histopathologic examination of involved nodes shows characteristic changes that are nondiagnostic unless the organism is demonstrated. The lymph node architecture is distorted by multiple areas of central necrosis with acidophilic staining. These areas are surrounded by foci of epithelioid cells and scattered giant cells of the Langhans type. There is usually some elevation in the sedimentation rate. In cases with central nervous system involvement, the cerebrospinal fluid is usually normal but may show a slight pleocytosis and modest elevation of protein. All routine cultures, including anaerobic, fungal, and mycobacterial culture, are negative.

Differential Diagnosis

Cat-scratch disease must be distinguished from pyogenic adenitis, tuberculosis (typical and atypical), tularemia, plague, brucellosis, Hodgkin's disease, lymphoma, rat-bite fever, acquired toxoplasmosis, infectious mononucleosis, lymphogranuloma venereum, and fungal infections.

Treatment

The best therapy is reassurance that the adenopathy is benign and will subside spontaneously within 4–8 weeks in most cases. In cases of suppuration, node aspiration under local anesthesia with an 18- to 19-gauge needle relieves the pain. Excision of the involved node is indicated in cases of chronic adenitis. Antimicrobial therapy has not been proved to alter the course of illness; gentamicin has been useful anecdotally in a few severe infections and is active in vitro in preliminary studies.

Prognosis

The prognosis is good if complications do not occur.

Carithers HA: Cat-scratch disease: An overview based on a study of 1200 patients. *Am J Dis Child* 1985; **139:**1124.

English CK et al: Cat-scratch disease: Isolation and culture of the bacterial agent. *JAMA* 1988;**259:**1347.

Margileth AM, Wear DJ, English CK: Systemic cat scratch disease: Report of 23 patients with prolonged or recurrent severe bacterial infection. *J Infect Dis* 1987; **155:**390.

Margileth AW et al: Cat-scratch disease: Bacteria in skin at the primary inoculation site. *JAMA* 1984;**252:**928.

Wear DJ et al: Cat-scratch disease: A bacterial infection. *Science* 1983;**221:**1403.

SPIROCHETAL INFECTIONS

SYPHILIS

Essentials of Diagnosis

Congenital:

- All types: History of untreated maternal syphilis, a positive serologic test, and a positive darkfield examination.
- Newborn: Hepatosplenomegaly, characteristic x-ray bone changes, anemia, increased nucleated red cells, thrombocytopenia, abnormal spinal fluid, jaundice, edema.
- Young infant (3–12 weeks): Snuffles, maculopapular skin rash, mucocutaneous lesions, pseudoparalysis (in addition to x-ray bone changes).
- Children: Stigmas of early congenital syphilis (saddle nose, Hutchinson's teeth, etc), interstitial keratitis, saber shins, gummas of nose and palate.

Acquired:

- Chancre of genitals, lip, or anus in child or adolescent. History of sexual contact.

General Considerations

Syphilis is a chronic, generalized infectious disease caused by a slender spirochete, *Treponema pallidum.* In the acquired form, the disease is transmitted by sexual contact. Primary syphilis is characterized by the presence of an indurated painless chancre, which heals in 7–10 days. A secondary eruption involving the skin and mucous membranes appears in 4–6 weeks. After a long latency period, late lesions of tertiary syphilis involve the eyes, skin, bones, viscera, central nervous system, and cardiovascular system.

Congenital syphilis results from transplacental infection. Characteristic disease occurs after the fourth month of gestation and may result in stillbirth or manifest illness in the newborn, in early infancy, or later in childhood. First-trimester fetal infection has been found in the products of conception in therapeutic abortions. Syphilis occurring in the newborn and young infant is comparable to secondary disease in the adult but is more severe and life-threatening. Late congenital syphilis (developing in childhood) is comparable to tertiary disease.

Congenital syphilis is increasing in the USA due to increasing primary and secondary syphilis in women of childbearing age, and perhaps due to inadequate diagnosis and treatment of syphilis in prenatal care programs.

Clinical Findings

A. Symptoms and Signs:

1. Congenital syphilis—

a. Newborns—Most newborns with congenital syphilis are well, disease not usually becoming manifest for several weeks. When clinical signs are present, they usually consist of jaundice, anemia with or without thrombocytopenia, increase in nucleated red blood cells, hepatosplenomegaly, and edema. There may be overt signs of meningitis (bulging fontanelle, opisthotonos), but subclinical infection with cerebrospinal fluid abnormalities is more likely. The majority of affected newborns show x-ray changes in the long bones.

b. Young infants (3–12 weeks)—The infant may appear normal for the first few weeks of life only to develop ''snuffles,'' a syphilitic skin eruption, mucocutaneous lesions, and pseudoparalysis of the arms or legs. Shotty lymphadenopathy may sometimes be felt in addition to hepatosplenomegaly. Other signs of disease seen in the newborn may be present. Anemia has been reported as the only presenting manifestation of congenital syphilis in this age group. ''Snuffles'' (rhinitis) almost always appears and is characterized by a profuse mucopurulent discharge that excoriates the upper lip. A syphilitic rash is common on the palms and soles but may occur anywhere on the body; it consists of bright red, raised maculopapular lesions that gradually fade. Moist lesions occur at the mucocutaneous junctions (nose, mouth, anus, genitals) and lead to fissuring and bleeding.

Syphilis in the young infant may lead to stigmas recognizable in later childhood, such as rhagades (scars) around the mouth or nose, a ''saddle'' nose, and a high forehead (secondary to mild hydrocephalus associated with low-grade meningitis and frontal periostitis). The permanent upper central incisors may be peg-shaped with a central notch (Hutchinson's teeth), and the cusps of the sixth-year molars may have a lobulated mulberry appearance.

c. Children—Bilateral interstitial keratitis (at 6–12 years) is characterized by photophobia, increased lacrimation, and vascularization of the cornea associated with exudation. Chorioretinitis and optic atrophy may also be seen. Meningovascular syphilis (at 2–10 years) is usually slowly progressive, with mental retardation, spasticity, abnormal pupil response, speech defects, and abnormal spinal fluid. Deafness sometimes occurs. Thickening of the periosteum of the anterior tibias produces saber shins. A bilateral effusion into the knee joints (Clutton's joints) may occur but is not associated with sequelae. Gummas may develop in the nasal septum, palate, long bones, and subcutaneous tissues.

2. Acquired syphilis—The primary chancre of the genitals, mouth, or anus may occur as a result of intimate sexual contact. If the chancre is missed, signs of secondary syphilis may be the first manifestation of the disease.

B. Laboratory Findings:

1. Darkfield microscopy—Treponemes can be seen in scrapings from a chancre and from moist lesions.

2. Serologic tests for syphilis (STS)—There are 2 general types of serologic tests for syphilis: treponemal and nontreponemal. The latter (Venereal Disease Research Laboratory, or VDRL) is useful both for screening and for follow-up of known cases. A rapid test (the rapid plasma reagin, or RPR) is useful for screening, but positive sera should be further examined by quantitative nontreponemal and treponemal tests. The most useful treponemal test is the fluorescent treponemal antibody absorption, or FTA-ABS, test. This test is seldom falsely positive.

One or 2 weeks after the onset of primary syphilis (chancre), the FTA-ABS test becomes positive. The VDRL or a similar nontreponemal test usually turns positive a few days later. By the time the secondary stage has arrived, virtually all patients show both positive FTA-ABS and positive nontreponemal tests. During latent and tertiary syphilis, the VDRL may become negative, but the FTA-ABS test usually remains positive. The quantitative VDRL or a similar nontreponemal test should be used to follow treated cases (see below).

Positive serologic tests in cord sera may represent passively transferred antibody rather than congenital infection and therefore must be supplemented by a combination of clinical and laboratory data. Elevated total cord IgM is a helpful but nonspecific finding. A specific IgM-FTA-ABS was developed, but it lacks sensitivity and specificity and is not widely available. Demonstration of characteristic treponemes by darkfield examination of material from a moist lesion (skin, nasal or other mucous membranes) is definitive. Serial measurement of quantitative VDRL is also very useful, since passively transferred antibody in the absence of active infection should decay with a normal half-life of about 18 days.

In one study, 15% of infants with congenital syphilis had negative cord blood serology, presumably due to maternal infection late in pregnancy.

C. Imaging: Osteochondritis and periostitis involve the long bones. Occasionally, the phalanges and metatarsals are involved. Periostitis of the skull is seen. Bilateral symmetric osteomyelitis with pathologic fractures of the medial tibial metaphyses (Wimberger's sign) is almost pathognomonic.

Differential Diagnosis

A. Congenital Syphilis:

1. Newborns—Sepsis, congestive heart failure, congenital rubella, toxoplasmosis, disseminated herpes simplex, cytomegalovirus infection, and hemolytic disease of the newborn have to be differentiated. Positive Coombs test and blood group incompatibility distinguish hemolytic disease.

2. Young infants—Pseudoparalysis (a flaccid paralysis) occurs in poliomyelitis. Signs of scurvy do not appear until the latter half of the first year of life. Injury to the brachial plexus, acute osteomyelitis, and septic arthritis must be differentiated from pseudoparalysis. Coryza due to viral infection will often respond to symptomatic treatment. Rash (ammoniacal diaper rash) and scabies may be confused with a syphilitic eruption.

3. Children—Interstitial keratitis and bone lesions of tuberculosis are distinguished by positive tuberculin reaction and chest x-ray. Arthritis associated with syphilis is unaccompanied by systemic signs, and joints are not tender. Mental retardation, spasticity, and hyperactivity are shown to be of syphilitic origin by strongly positive serologic tests.

B. Acquired Syphilis: Herpes genitalis, traumatic lesions, and other venereal diseases must be differentiated.

Prevention

A serologic test for syphilis should be performed at the initiation of prenatal care and repeated once during pregnancy. In mothers at high risk of syphilis, repeated tests may be necessary. Adequate treatment of mothers with secondary syphilis before the last month of pregnancy reduces the incidence of congenital syphilis from 90% to less than 2%. Examination and serology of sexual partners and siblings should also be done.

Treatment

A. Specific Measures: Penicillin is the drug of choice for *T pallidum*. If the patient is allergic to penicillin, erythromycin or one of the tetracyclines may be used.

1. Congenital syphilis—Prompt treatment of the infant with penicillin is indicated if there is clinical or x-ray evidence of disease, if the cord blood serology is positive and the mother has not been adequately treated, if the mother was treated with drugs other than penicillin, or if follow-up is not ensured. With equivocal findings, the infant may be followed at monthly intervals with quantitative serologic tests and physical examinations if follow-up is ensured. Rising titers or clinical signs usually occur within 4 months in infants with infection. Infants with suspected congenital syphilis should have roentenography of the long bones and a cerebrospinal fluid examination.

Infants with proved or suspected congenital syphilis should receive either of the following: (1) aqueous crystalline penicillin G (50,000 units/kg/d intramuscularly or intravenously in 2 divided doses for a minimum of 10 days) or (2) aqueous procaine penicillin G (50,000 units/kg/d intramuscularly for a minimum of 10 days). Because treatment failure in early congenital syphilis may be due to low levels of benzathine penicillin in the cerebrospinal fluid and the eye, and because cerebrospinal fluid serology may fail to detect central nervous system infection, benzathine penicillin is no longer recommended for proved or strongly suspected congenital syphilis. Asymptomatic seropositive infants with normal cerebrospinal fluid may be given benzathine penicillin G (50,000 units/kg intramuscularly in a single dose) with follow-up serologic examinations as below. Penicillin dosages for congenital syphilis after the neonatal period should be the same as dosages recommended for neonatal congenital syphilis. For larger children, the total dose of penicillin need not exceed the dosage used in adult syphilis of more than 1 year's duration.

Follow-up quantitative VDRL tests should be performed at 1, 2, 4, 6, 9, and 12 months, or until they become nonreactive. In those infants treated for late infection, follow-up should be longer to demonstrate whether the child, though adequately treated, is "serofast" (ie, seropositive for life). A repeat CSF examination at 6 months is indicated for infants with a positive CSF VDRL. If it is still positive, retreatment is indicated.

2. Acquired syphilis—Benzathine penicillin G (1.2 million units) is given intramuscularly in each buttock (total dose of 2.4 million units) to adolescents with primary, secondary, or latent disease less than 1 year's duration.

B. General Measures: Care should be given to the maintenance of adequate nutrition.

Penicillin treatment of early congenital or secondary syphilis may result in a febrile Jarisch-Herxheimer reaction. Treatment is symptomatic, with careful follow-up and aspirin or acetaminophen, although transfusion may be necessary in infants with severe hemolytic anemia.

Prognosis

Severe disease, if unexpected, may be fatal in the newborn. Complete cure can be expected if the young infant is treated with penicillin. Serologic reversal usually occurs within 1 year. Treatment of primary syphilis with penicillin is curative. Permanent neurologic sequelae may be seen with meningovascular syphilis.

Beck-Sague C, Alexander ER: Failure of benzathine penicillin G treatment in early congenital syphilis. *Pediatr Infect Dis J* 1987;**6:**1061.

Centers for Disease Control: Current trends: Continuing increase in infectious syphilis—United States. *MMWR* 1988;**37:**35.

Dobson SRM, Taber LH, Baughn RE: Characterization of the components in circulating immune complexes from infants with congenital syphilis. *J Infect Dis* 1988;**158:**940.

Ginsburg CM: Acquired syphilis in prepubertal children. *Pediatr Infect Dis J* 1983;**2:**232.

Interview with Larry H. Taber: Evaluation and management of syphilis in pregnant women and newborn infants. *Pediatr Infect Dis J* 1982;**1:**224.

Johns DR, Tierney M, Felsenstein D: Alteration in the natural history of neurosyphilis by concurrent infection with the human immunodeficiency virus. *N Engl J Med* 1987;**316:**1569.

Mascola L et al: Congenital syphilis revisited. *Am J Dis Child* 1985;**139**:575.

Mascola L et al: Congenital syphilis: Why is it still occurring? *JAMA* 1984;**252**:1719.

RELAPSING FEVER

Essentials of Diagnosis

- Episodes of fever, chills, malaise.
- Occasional rash, arthritis, cough, hepatosplenomegaly, conjunctivitis.
- Diagnosis confirmed by direct microscopic identification of spirochetes in smears of peripheral blood.

General Considerations

Relapsing fever is a vector-borne disease caused by spirochetes of the genus *Borrelia*. Epidemic relapsing fever is transmitted to humans by body lice (*Pediculus humanus*) and endemic relapsing fever by soft-bodied ticks (genus *Ornithodoros*).

Tick-borne relapsing fever is endemic in the western USA. Transmission usually takes place during the warm months, when ticks are active and recreation or work brings people into contact with *Ornithodoros* ticks. Mountain camping areas and cabins are sites where infection often is acquired. The ticks are nocturnal feeders and remain attached for only 5–20 minutes. Consequently, the patient seldom remembers a tick bite.

Rarely, neonatal relapsing fever results from transplacental transmission of *Borrelia*.

Clinical Findings

A. Symptoms and Signs: The disease is characterized by relapses lasting 3–5 days, occurring at intervals of 1–2 weeks, with interim asymptomatic periods. The relapses duplicate the initial attack but become progressively less severe. In louse-borne relapsing fever, there is usually a single relapse; in tick-borne infection, there are 2–6 relapses.

The incubation period is 5–11 days. The attack is sudden, with high fever, chills, tachycardia, nausea and vomiting, headache, myalgia, arthralgia, bronchitis, and a dry, nonproductive cough. Hepatomegaly and splenomegaly appear later. An erythematous rash may be seen over the trunk and extremities, and petechiae may be present. After 3–10 days, the fever falls by crisis. Jaundice, iritis, conjunctivitis, cranial nerve palsies, and hemorrhage are more common during relapses.

B. Laboratory Findings: During febrile episodes, the urine contains protein, casts, and, occasionally, erythrocytes; there is a marked polymorphonuclear leukocytosis and, in about one-fourth of cases, a false-positive serologic test for syphilis. Spirochetes can be found in the peripheral blood by direct microscopy in approximately 70% of cases by darkfield examination or by Wright, Giemsa, or acri-

dine orange staining of thick and thin smears. They are not found during afebrile periods. The blood may be injected into young mice and the spirochetes found 1–14 days later in the tail blood. OXK agglutinin titers in serum may be positive.

Differential Diagnosis

Relapsing fever may be confused with malaria, leptospirosis, dengue, yellow fever, typhus, rat-bite fever, Colorado tick fever, Rocky Mountain spotted fever, collagen vascular disease, or any fever of unknown origin.

Complications

Complications include facial paralysis, iridocyclitis, optic atrophy, hypochromic anemia, pneumonia, nephritis, myocarditis, endocarditis, and seizures. Central nervous system involvement is seen in 10–30% of cases.

Treatment

For children under 7 years of age with tick-borne relapsing fever, erythromycin (40–50 mg/kg/d orally in divided doses every 6 hours for 10 days) should be given. Older children may be given tetracycline instead. Penicillin and chloramphenicol are also efficacious.

In louse-borne relapsing fever, a single dose of tetracycline or erythromycin has been effective.

Severely ill patients should be hospitalized. Antibiotic treatment should be started after the fever has dropped; this will lessen the risk of severe or even fatal Jarisch-Herxheimer reaction. Isolation precautions are not necessary.

Prognosis

The mortality rate in treated cases is very low, except in debilitated or very young children. With treatment, the initial attack is shortened and relapses prevented. The response to antimicrobial therapy is dramatic.

Le CT: Tick-borne relapsing fever in children. *Pediatrics* 1980;**66**:963.

Perine PL, Teklu B: Antibiotic treatment of louse-borne relapsing fever in Ethiopia: A report of 377 cases. *Am J Trop Med Hyg* 1983;**32**:1096.

Relapsing fever: New lessons about antibiotic action. (Editorial.) *Ann Intern Med* 1985;**102**:397.

Sciotto CG et al: Detection of *Borrelia* in acridine orange–stained blood smears by fluorescence microscopy. *Arch Pathol Lab Med* 1983;**107**:384.

LEPTOSPIROSIS

Essentials of Diagnosis

- Biphasic course lasting 2 or 3 weeks.
- Initial phase: high fever, headache, myalgia, and conjunctivitis.

- Apparent recovery for 2–3 days.
- Return of fever associated with meningitis.
- Jaundice, hemorrhages, and renal insufficiency (severe cases).
- Culture of organism from blood and cerebrospinal fluid (early) and from urine (later), or direct microscopy of urine or cerebrospinal fluid.
- Positive leptospiral agglutination test.

General Considerations

Leptospirosis is a zoonosis caused by many antigenically distinct but morphologically similar spirochetes. The organism enters through the skin or respiratory tract. Classically, the severe form—Weil's disease, with jaundice and a high mortality rate—was associated with infection with *Leptospira icterohaemorrhagiae* following immersion in water contaminated with rat urine. It is now known that a variety of animals (dogs, rats, cattle, etc) may serve as reservoirs for pathogenic *Leptospira,* that a given serogroup may have multiple animal species as hosts, and that severe disease may be caused by many different serogroups other than *L icterohaemorrhagiae.*

In the USA, leptospirosis occurs more commonly from avocational activities (70% of cases) in children, students, and housewives than from occupational exposure. Urban and suburban cases are more common than rural cases. Cases acquired from contact with dogs are more than twice as frequent as those acquired from cattle, swine, or rodents. Sewer workers, farmers, abattoir workers, animal handlers, and soldiers have occupational exposure. Outbreaks have resulted from swimming in contaminated streams and harvesting field crops.

In the USA, about 100 cases are reported yearly, and about one-third are in children. Approximately 50% of cases occur in the summer or early fall.

Clinical Findings

A. Symptoms and Signs:

1. Initial phase—The incubation period is 4–19 days, with a mean of 10 days. Chills, fever, headache, myalgia, conjunctivitis (episcleral injection), photophobia, cervical lymphadenopathy, and pharyngitis occur commonly. This leptospiremic phase lasts for 3–7 days.

2. Phase of apparent recovery—Symptoms typically (but not always) subside for 2–3 days.

3. Systemic phase—Fever reappears and is associated with headache, muscular pain and tenderness in the abdomen and back, and nausea and vomiting. Lung, heart, and joint involvement occasionally occurs. These manifestations are due to extensive vasculitis.

a. Central nervous system involvement—The central nervous system is involved in 50–90% of cases. Severe headache and mild nuchal rigidity are usual, but delirium, coma, and focal neurologic signs may be seen.

b. Renal and hepatic involvement—In about 50% of cases, the kidney or liver or both are affected. Gross hematuria and oliguria or anuria are sometimes seen. Jaundice may be associated with an enlarged and tender liver.

c. Gallbladder involvement—Leptospirosis may cause acalculous cholecystitis in children. An abdominal ultrasound study may reveal a dilated, nonfunctioning gallbladder. Pancreatitis is unusual.

d. Hemorrhage—Petechiae, ecchymoses, and gastrointestinal bleeding may be severe.

e. Rash—A rash is seen in 10–30% of cases. It may be maculopapular and generalized or may be petechial or purpuric. Occasionally, erythema nodosum is seen. Peripheral desquamation of the rash may occur. Gangrenous areas are sometimes noted over the distal extremities. In such cases, skin biopsy demonstrates the presence of severe vasculitis involving both the arterial and the venous circulations.

B. Laboratory Findings: Leptospires may be seen by direct darkfield or phase contrast microscopy or immunofluorescence techniques, but they do not stain by Gram, Wright, or Giemsa methods. They appear in the blood and cerebrospinal fluid only during the first 10 days of illness. They appear in the urine during the second week, where they may persist for 30 days or longer. The organism can be isolated from blood inoculated into Fletcher's semisolid medium or EMJH semisolid medium, but culture techniques are slow (7–10 days), difficult, and not generally available.

The white blood cell count often is elevated, especially when there is liver involvement. Serum bilirubin levels usually remain below 20 mg/dL. Other liver function tests may be abnormal, although the AST (SGOT) usually shows only slight elevation. An elevated serum creatinine phosphokinase is frequently found. Cerebrospinal fluid shows moderate pleocytosis (< 500/μL), increased protein (50–100 mg/dL), and normal glucose. Urine often shows microscopic pyuria, hematuria, and, less often, proteinuria (+ + or greater). The erythrocyte sedimentation rate is markedly elevated. Chest x-ray may show pneumonitis.

The serologic test of choice is a microscopic agglutination test using live organisms (performed at the Centers for Disease Control, Atlanta, GA 30333). Leptospiral agglutinins generally reach peak levels by the third to fourth week. A 1:100 titer is considered suspicious; a 4-fold or greater rise is diagnostic.

Differential Diagnosis

Fever and myalgia associated with the characteristic conjunctival (episcleral) injection should suggest leptospirosis. During the prodrome, malaria, typhoid fever, typhus, rheumatoid arthritis, brucellosis, and influenza may be suspected. Later, depending on the organ systems involved, a variety of other diseases need to be distinguished, including encephalitis, viral or tuberculous meningitis, viral hepatitis, glomerulonephritis, viral or bacterial pneumonia, rheumatic fever, subacute bacterial endocarditis, acute surgical abdomen, and Kawasaki disease (see Table 27–3).

Prevention

Preventive measures include the avoidance of contaminated water and soil, the use of rodent control, immunization of dogs and other domestic animals, and good sanitation. Immunization or antimicrobial prophylaxis with doxycycline may be of value to certain high-risk occupational groups.

Treatment

A. Specific Measures: Treatment within the first 4 days of illness may reduce the severity of the disease but has little effect if started later. Aqueous penicillin G (150,000 units/kg/d in 4–6 divided doses intravenously for 7–10 days) should be given. A Jarisch-Herxheimer reaction may be seen. Tetracycline (40–50 mg/kg/d) also may be used.

B. General Measures: Symptomatic and supportive care is indicated, particularly for renal and hepatic failure and hemorrhage.

Prognosis

Leptospirosis generally is anicteric and self-limiting. The disease usually lasts 1–3 weeks but may be more prolonged. Relapse may occur.

There are usually no permanent sequelae associated with central nervous system infection. The mortality rate in reported cases in the USA is 5%, usually from renal failure. The mortality rate may reach 20% or more in elderly patients who have severe kidney and hepatic involvement.

Lecour H et al: Human leptospirosis: A review of 50 cases. *Infection* 1989;**17**:8.

Peter G: Leptospirosis: A zoonosis of protean manifestations. *Pediatr Infect Dis* 1982;**1**:282.

Takafuji ET et al: An efficacy trial of doxycycline chemoprophylaxis against leptospirosis. *N Engl J Med* 1984;**310**:497.

Watt G et al: Placebo-controlled trial of intravenous penicillin for severe and late leptospirosis. *Lancet* 1988;**1**:433.

Wong ML et al: Leptospirosis: A childhood disease. *J Pediatr* 1977;**90**:532.

LYME DISEASE
(Lyme Arthritis)

Essentials of Diagnosis

- Presence of skin lesion (erythema migrans) 3–30 days after tick bite.

- Arthritis, usually pauciarticular, occurring about 4 weeks after appearance of skin lesion. Headache, chills, and fever.
- Residence or travel in an endemic area during the late spring, summer, or early fall.

General Considerations

Lyme disease is a subacute or chronic spirochetal infection caused by *Borrelia burgdorferi* and transmitted by the bite of an infected deer tick (*Ixodes* spp.). The disease was known in Europe for many years as tick-borne encephalomyelitis, often associated with a characteristic rash (erythema migrans). Discovery of the agent and vector followed investigation of an outbreak of pauciarticular arthritis in Lyme, Connecticut in 1977.

Although cases are reported from many countries and states, endemic areas include the Northeast, upper Midwest, and West Coast in the US and the northern European countries. The disease is increasingly recognized and appears to be spreading due to increased infection in and distribution of the tick vector. Most cases with rash are recognized in spring and summer, when most tick bites occur. Since the incubation period for joint and neurologic disease may be months, however, cases may present at any time. Ixodes ticks are very small and the infecting bite is often unrecognized.

Clinical Findings

A. Symptoms and Signs: Erythema migrans is the most characteristic feature of the disease and develops in 60–80% of patients. Three to 30 days after the bite, a ring of erythema develops at the site and spreads over days. It may attain a diameter of 20 cm. The center of the lesion may clear (resembling tinea corporis), remain red, or become raised (suggesting a chemical or infectious cellulitis). Many patients are otherwise asymptomatic; some have fever (usually low-grade), headache, and myalgias. Multiple satellite skin lesions, urticaria or diffuse erythema may occur. Untreated, the rash lasts days to weeks and eventually disappears.

In up to 50% of patients, arthritis develops several weeks to months after the bite. Recurrent attacks of migratory, mono- or pauciarticular arthritis involving the knees and other large joints are seen. Each attack lasts for days to a few weeks. Children are not usually highly febrile nor toxic. Complete resolution between attacks is typical. Chronic arthritis develops in less than 10%, more often in those with the DR4 haplotype.

Neurologic manifestations develop in up to 20% of cases and usually consist of Bell's palsy, aseptic meningitis (which may be indistinguishable from viral meningitis), or polyradiculitis. Peripheral neuritis, Guillain-Barre syndrome, encephalitis, ataxia, chorea and other cranial neuropathies are less common. Seizures suggest another diagnosis. Untreated, the neurologic symptoms are usually self-limited but may be chronic or permanent. Although the fatigue and non-specific neurologic symptoms may be prolonged in a few patients, Lyme disease is not usually proved as a cause of the chronic fatigue syndrome.

Self-limited heart-block or myocardial dysfunction occur in about 5% of patients.

B. Laboratory Findings: Most patients with only rash have no abnormal laboratory tests. Children with arthritis may have moderately elevated sedimentation rates and white blood cell counts; the ANA and rheumatoid factor are negative or non-specific; streptoccocal antibodies are not usually elevated. Circulating IgM cryoglobulins may be present. Joint fluid may show up to 100,000 cells with a polymorphonuclear predominance, normal glucose, elevated protein and immune complexes; the Gram stain and culture are negative. In patients with central nervous system involvement, the spinal fluid may show lymphocytic pleocytosis and elevated protein; the glucose and all cultures and stains are normal or negative. Abnormal nerve conduction may be present with peripheral neuropathy.

Diagnosis

The organism can neither be seen in nor cultured easily from clinical specimens. The diagnosis is either presumptive, as in patients with the characteristic rash who are usually seronegative, or made by positive serology in the presence of a compatible clinical syndrome. Antibody titers should be measured in experienced laboratories; the enzyme immunoassay is currently the most accurate test, and confirmation of positives by Western blot testing should be considered, especially with unusual clinical syndromes. Diagnosis of central nervous system infection requires both positive serology and objective abnormalities of the neurologic exam, laboratory or radiographic tests.

Differential Diagnosis

Aside from the disorders already mentioned, the rash may resemble pityriasis, erythema multiforme, a drug eruption, or erythema nodosum. Erythema migrans is non-scaly, minimally or non-tender, and persists longer in the same place than many of the more common childhood erythematous rashes. The arthritis may resemble juvenile rheumatoid arthritis, reactive arthritis, septic arthritis, reactive effusion from a contiguous osteomyelitis, rheumatic fever, leukemic arthritis, lupus, and Henoch-Schoenlein purpura. Spontaneous resolution in a few days to weeks helps differentiate it from JRA. The neurologic signs may suggest idiopathic Bell's palsy, viral or parainfectious meningitis or meningoencephalitis, lead poisoning, psychosomatic illness, and many other conditions.

Treatment

Although antimicrobial therapy is beneficial in most cases, it is most effective if started early; prolonged treatment is important for all forms. Relapses are seen with all regimens in some patients.

Rash, other early infections: Use amoxicillin (40 mg/kg/d) orally in 3 divided doses; some experts add probenecid, 10 mg/kg/dose) for 2–3 weeks. Use erythromycin (30 mg/kg/d) in penicillin-allergic children. Doxycycline (100 mg orally twice a day) may be used in children over age 8.

Arthritis: Use the amoxicillin or doxycycline regimen (same dosage as above), but treat for 4 weeks. Parenteral ceftriaxone or penicillin in high doses for 2–3 weeks may also be used.

Bell's palsy: The same oral drug regimens may be used for 4 weeks.

Neurologic disease, other, or cardiac disease: Parenteral therapy for two weeks is recommended with either ceftriaxone, 50 mg/kg/d in one daily dose, or penicillin, G, 3–400,000 units/kg/d in 4 divided doses.

Prevention: Avoidance of endemic areas, long sleeves and pants, frequent "tick checks" and tick repellents may help. Repellents containing high concentrations of DEET may be neurotoxic and should be used cautiously and washed off when tick exposure ends. Prophylactic antibiotics cannot be currently recommended.

Dammin GJ: Erythema migrans: A chronicle. *Rev Infect Dis* 1989;**11**:142.

Dattwyler RJ et al: Treatment of late Lyme borreliosis: Randomized comparison of ceftriaxone and penicillin. *Lancet* 1988;**1**:1191.

Eichenfield AH, Athreye BH: Lyme disease: Of ticks and titers. *J Pediatr* 1989;**114**:328.

Treatment of Lyme disease. *Med Lett Drugs Ther* 1989;**31**:57.

Williams CL et al: Lyme disease in childhood: Clinical and epidemiologic features of 90 cases. *Pediatr Infect Dis J* 1990;**9**:10.

SELECTED REFERENCES

Committee on Infectious Diseases: *Report,* 21st ed. American Academy of Pediatrics, 1988.

Feigin RD, Cherry JD (editors): *Textbook of Pediatric Infectious Disease,* 2nd ed. Saunders, 1987.

Krugman S, Katz S, Gershon A, Wilfert K: *Infectious Diseases of Children,* 8th ed. Mosby, 1985.

Schaechter M, Medoff G, Schlessinger D: *Mechanisms of Microbial Disease,* Williams & Wilkins, 1989.

Infections: Parasitic & Mycotic

John W. Paisley, MD

I. INFECTIONS: PARASITIC

Parasitic diseases are common and present in a variety of ways (Table 29–1). Although travel to endemic areas suggests particular infestations, many are acquired from contact with human carriers and can occur anywhere in the country. The most common infections acquired abroad are giardiasis and malaria—at home, giardiasis, toxoplasmosis, and cryptosporidiosis. A list of antiparasitic agents is shown in Table 29–2.

PROTOZOAN INFECTIONS

MALARIA

Essentials of Diagnosis

- Residence in or travel to an endemic area.
- High fever, chills, headache, icterus, vomiting, diarrhea.
- Splenomegaly, anemia.
- Seizures, coma.
- Malaria parasites in blood smear.

General Considerations

Malaria kills a million children each year and is resurging in areas previously controlled. The female anopheline mosquito transmits the parasites—*Plasmodium vivax* (most common), *Plasmodium falciparum* (most virulent), *Plasmodium ovale* (similar to *P vivax*), and *Plasmodium malariae*. The gametocytes ingested from an infected human form sporozoites in the mosquito; when inoculated into a susceptible host, these sporozoites infect hepatocytes. Antibody, but not drugs, decreases the sporozoite infectivity. The preerythrocytic phase is about 2 weeks for all but *P malariae* infection (3–5 weeks), but the initial symptoms may be delayed for up to a year in *P falciparum*, 4 years in *P vivax,* and decades in *P malariae* infections. Merozoites released from hepatocytes infect red cells (young cells

by *P vivax,* old cells by *P malariae,* and all cells by *P falciparum*) and begin the synchronous erythrocytic cycles—rupturing the infected cells at intervals of 48 hours for all but *P malariae,* which has a 72-hour cycle. Asynchronous cycles causing daily fevers are not uncommon. Survival is associated with a progressive decrease in intensity of cycles; relapses years later may occur due to hepatic infection, which persists in all but *P falciparum* infections. Infection acquired congenitally or from transfusions or needle sticks does not result in a hepatic phase.

Susceptibility varies genetically; certain red cell phenotypes are partially resistant to infection (hemoglobin S, hemoglobin F, thalassemia, G6PD deficiency). Recurrent infections result in some natural species-specific immunity; this does not prevent sporozoite infection but does decrease parasitemia and symptoms. Maternal immunity protects the neonate, despite the placental infection seen in active infection in pregnancy.

Clinical Findings

A. Symptoms and Signs: Clinical manifestations vary according to species, strain, and host immunity. The child presents with recurrent bouts of fever, irritability, poor feeding, vomiting, jaundice, and splenomegaly. Enanthem, rash, cough, and significant dehydration are usually absent in malaria and help distinguish it from many viral infections with similar symptoms. Symptoms are similar in older children, with headache, backache, chills, myalgia, and fatigue more easily elicited. Fever may be periodic (every other day for all but *P malariae* infection, in which it occurs every third day) or daily. Between attacks, patients may look completely well. If the disease is untreated, relapses cease within a year in *P falciparum* and within several years in *P vivax* infections but may recur decades later in *P malariae* infection. Infection during pregnancy often causes intrauterine growth retardation or premature delivery but rarely true fetal infection.

Physical examination may be normal or show mild jaundice or hepatosplenomegaly.

B. Laboratory Findings: Most cases in the USA are diagnosed by a Wright stain of thin blood smears, occasionally in the course of another investigation. To exclude malaria completely, multiple thick smears must be properly made and examined

Table 29–1. Symptoms of parasitic infection.

Sign	Agent	Comments*
Abdominal pain	*Ascaris*	Heavy infection; may obstruct bowel, biliary tract.
	Clonorchis	Heavy, early infection. Hepatomegaly later.
	Entamoeba histolytica	Hematochezia, variable fever, diarrhea.
	Fasciola hepatica	Sheep liver fluke. Diarrhea, vomiting.
	Hookworm	Heavy infection. Iron deficiency anemia.
	Strongyloides	Eosinophilia, pruritus. May resemble peptic disease.
	Trichinella	Myalgia, periorbital edema, eosinophilia.
	Trichuris	Heavy infection; diarrhea, dysentery.
Cough	*Ascaris*	Wheezing, eosinophilia. During migration phase.
	Paragonimus westermani	Hemoptysis; chronic. May mimic tuberculosis.
	Strongyloides	Wheezing, pruritus, eosinophilia during migration or dissemination.
	Toxocara	Affects ages 1–5; hepatosplenomegaly; eosinophilia.
	Tropical eosinophilia	Pulmonary infiltrates, eosinophilia.
Diarrhea	*Cryptosporidium*	Watery; prolonged in normals, chronic in immunosuppressed.
	Dientamoeba fragilis	Heavy infection.
	Entamoeba histolytica	Hematochezia, variable fever; no eosinophilia.
	Giardia	Afebrile, chronic; anorexia; no hematochezia or eosinophilia.
	Schistosoma	Chronic; hepatosplenomegaly.
	Strongyloides	Abdominal pain; eosinophilia.
	Trichinella	Myalgia, periorbital edema, eosinophilia.
	Trichuris	Heavy infection.
	Blastocystis	Possibly with heavy infection in immunosuppressed or normal individuals.
Dysentery	*Balantidium coli*	Swine contact.
	Entamoeba histolytica	Few to no leukocytes in stool; fever; hematochezia
	Schistosoma	During acute infections.
	Trichuris	Heavy infection.
Dysuria	*Enterobius*	Usually girls with worms in urethra, bladder; nocturnal, perianal pruritus.
	Schistosoma	Hematuria. Exclude bacteruria, stones.
Headache (and other cerebral symptoms)	*Angiostrongylus*	Eosinophilic meningitis.
	Naegleria	Fresh-water swimming; rapidly progressive meningoencephalitis.
	Plasmodium	Fever, chills, jaundice, splenomegaly. Cerebral ischemia (with *P falciparum*).
	Taenia solium	Cysticercosis. Focal seizures, deficits; hydrocephalus, aseptic meningitis.
	Toxoplasma	Meningoencephalitis (especially in the immunosuppressed); hydrocephalus in infants.
	Trypanosoma	African forms. Chronic lethargy (sleeping sickness).
Pruritus	*Ancylostoma braziliense*	Creeping eruption; dermal serpiginous burrow.
	Enterobius	Perianal, nocturnal.
	Filaria	Variable; seen in many filarial diseases.
	Hookworm	Local at penetration site in heavy exposure.
	Strongyloides	Diffuse with migration; may be recurrent.
	Trypanosoma	African forms; one of many nonspecific symptoms.
Fever	*Entamoeba histolytica*	With acute dysentery or liver abscess.
	Leishmania donovani	Hepatosplenomegaly, anemia, leukopenia.
	Plasmodium	Chills, headache, jaundice; periodic.
	Toxocara	Cough, hepatosplenomegaly, eosinophilia.
	Toxoplasma	Generalized adenopathy; splenomegaly.
	Trichinella	Myalgia, periorbital edema, eosinophilia.
	Trypanosoma	Early stage, African forms; lymphadenopathy.
Anemia	*Diphyllobothrium*	Megaloblastic due to B_{12} deficiency; rare.
	Hookworm	Iron deficiency.
	Leishmania donovani	Fever, hepatosplenomegaly, leukopenia (kala-azar).
	Plasmodium	Hemolysis.
	Trichuris	Heavy infection, due to iron loss.

Table 29–1 (cont'd.). Symptoms of parasitic infection.

Sign	Agent	Comments*
Eosinophilia	*Angiostrongylus*	Eosinophilic meningitis.
	Fasciola	Abdominal pain.
	Filaria	Microfilariae in blood. Lymphadenopathy.
	Onchocerca	Nodules, keratitis.
	Schistosoma	Chronic; intestinal or genitourinary symptoms.
	Strongyloides	Abdominal pain, diarrhea.
	Toxocara	Hepatosplenomegaly, cough; affects ages 1–5.
	Trichinosis	Myalgia, periorbital edema.
	Tropical eosinophilia	Unknown filarial agent. Cough.
Hematuria	*Schistosoma*	*S haematobium*. Bladder, urethral granulomas. Exclude stones, bacteriuria.
Hemoptysis	*Paragonimus westermani*	Lung fluke. Variable chest pain; chronic.
Hepatomegaly	*Clonorchis*	Heavy infection. Tenderness early; cirrhosis late.
	Echinococcus	Chronic; cysts.
	Entamoeba histloytica	Toxic hepatitis or abscess. No eosinophilia.
	Leishmania donovani	Kala-azar. Splenomegaly, fever, anemia.
	Schistosoma	Chronic; cirrhosis, splenomegaly.
	Toxocara	Splenomegaly, eosinophilia, cough.
Splenomegaly	*Leishmania donovani*	Kala-azar. Hepatomegaly, fever, anemia.
	Plasmodium	Fever, chills, jaundice, headache.
	Schistosoma	Hepatomegaly.
	Toxocara	Eosinophilia, hepatomegaly.
	Toxoplasma	Lymphadenopathy, other symptoms.
Lymphadenopathy	*Filaria*	Inguinal typical; chronic.
	Leishmania donovani	Hepatosplenomegaly, leukopenia, anemia, fever (kala-azar).
	Toxoplasma	Generalized; splenomegaly.
	Trypanosoma	Localized near bite (Chagas' disease); generalized (especially posterior cervical) in African forms.

*Symptoms usually related to degree of infestation. Infestation with small numbers of organisms are often asymptomatic.

Table 29–2. Antiparasitic drugs (brand names; manufacturer).

Albendazole (Zentel; Parke-Davis)[1]
Amphotericin B (Fungizone; Squibb)
Antimony potassium tartrate (tartar emetic)
Antimony sodium gluconate (stibogluconate sodium; Pentostam; Burroughs Wellcome)[2]
Bithionol (Bitin; Tanabe) (Lorothidol; Winthrop)[2]
Chloroquine phosphate or sulfate (Aralen, others)
Dehydroemetine dihydrochloride (Hoffman-La Roche)[2]
Diethylcarbamazine citrate (Hetrazan; Lederle)[3]
Diloxanide furoate (Furamide; Boots)[2]
Furazolidone (Furoxone; Norwich Eaton)
Iodoquinol (Yodoxin; Glenwood)[5]
Ivermectin (Merck)[1]
Mebendazole (Vermox; Janssen)
Melarsoprol (Arsobal; Rhone-Poulenc)[2]
Metrifonate (Bilarcil; Bayer)[1]
Metronidazole (Flagyl; Searle) (others)
Niclosamide (Yomesan; Bayer) (Niclocide; Miles)[4]
Nifurtimox (Lampit; Bayer)[2]
Niridazole (Ambilhar; Ciba-Geigy)[1]
Oxamniquine (Vansil; Pfipharmecs)
Paromomycin (Humatin; Parke-Davis)
Pentamidine isethionate (Pentam 300; Lyphomed)
Piperazine citrate (Antepar; Burroughs Wellcome)
Praziquantel (Biltricide; Miles)[4]

Primaquine phosphate (Winthrop-Breon)
Proguanil hydrochloride (Paludrine; Rhone-Poulenc)[1]
Pyrantel pamoate (Antiminth; Pfipharmecs)
Pyrimethamine-sulfadoxine (Fansidar; Roche) (Falcidar)
Pyrvinium pamoate (Povan; Parke-Davis)
Quinacrine hydrochloride (Atabrine; Winthrop-Breon)
Quinine dihydrochloride[2] and quinine sulfate
Spiramycin (Rovamycin; Poulenc)[6]
Suramin (Germanin; Bayer)[2]
Tetrachloroethylene (veterinary; Parke-Davis)
Thiabendazole (Mintezol; Merck)
Tinidazole (Fasigyn; Pfizer)[1]
Tryparsamide (Tryparsone, others)[1]

---

[1]Not available in the USA.
[2]Available in USA only through Parasitic Disease Drug Service, Centers for Disease Control, Atlanta, GA 30333, Telephone: (404)639-3670 (evenings, weekends, and holidays [404] 639-2888).
[3]Available from Lederle Laboratories, (914)735-5000, x3644.
[4]Available from Miles Inc, Pharmaceutical Division (800)243-4153.
[5]Available from Glenwood, Inc (201)569-0050.
[6]Available from FDA, Anti-infective Drugs Office (301)443-7580.

by experienced personnel. Giemsa stain is preferable for the correct identification of species, which is critical in the selection of therapy. Improper therapy of misdiagnosed chloroquine-resistant falciparum infection may be fatal. Multiple infections should also be searched for carefully, because each type may require different drugs; fortunately, if *P falciparum* is present, it is usually the predominant form seen. Rarely, blood drawn immediately after synchronous merozoite rupture is not diagnostic; resampling several hours later may demonstrate the organism.

Finding only young trophozoites (ring forms) may make exact species identification difficult; a predominance of larger trophozoites usually reassures that the infection is not due to *P falciparum* (in which only the ring forms and gametocytes are seen in peripheral blood) and is thus sensitive to chloroquine. Gametocytes may persist for days following adequate therapy.

Laboratory findings include a normocytic, normochromic anemia, leukopenia or leukocytosis, normal to low platelet count, reticulocytosis, elevation of direct and indirect bilirubin, mild transaminase elevation, low C3 level, and hyperglobulinemia; occasionally, a positive rheumatoid factor and falsely elevated syphilis, antinuclear, and heterophile titers are present.

Differential Diagnosis

Relapsing fever may be seen with borreliosis, brucellosis, sequential common infections, Hodgkin's disease, juvenile rheumatoid arthritis, rat-bite fever, or one of the idiopathic periodic fevers. Other common causes of high fever and headache include influenza, *Mycoplasma pneumoniae* or enteroviral infection, sinusitis, meningitis, enteric fever, tuberculosis, juvenile rheumatoid arthritis, occult pneumonia, or bacteremia. Malaria may also coexist with other diseases.

Complications & Sequelae

Severe complications are usually limited to *P falciparum* infections. Chronic infections result in anemia, debilitation, and massive splenomegaly (with potential rupture). Erythrocytes infected with *P falciparum* stick to capillary endothelium, causing microthrombosis and ischemia of any organ; involvement of the intestinal tract (bleeding, enteritis), lung (pneumonitis), and brain (diffuse edema, seizures, encephalopathy) are most common. Severe hemolysis with hemoglobinuria (blackwater fever) is an unusual complication of *P falciparum* infection. Erythrocyte destruction is greatest in *P falciparum* infection, because cells of all ages may be infected. Chronic infection with *P malariae,* but not other species, has been associated with the development of the nephrotic syndrome. The immune response to *Plasmodium* plays a role in the renal and hematologic complications.

Prevention

Prophylaxis is recommended for nonimmune children traveling to or residing in endemic areas. Pregnant women should avoid exposure; chloroquine may be safely used prophylactically in pregnancy, but other agents are contraindicated.

Sporozoites are resistant to drugs; thus, prophylaxis only suppresses schizogony and symptoms.

Chloroquine-resistant *P falciparum* is present in all areas except Central America west of the Panama canal, Haiti, the Dominican Republic, Egypt, and the Middle East. In resistance-free areas, chloroquine alone is recommended for prophylaxis (5 mg/kg of the base, max of 300 mg, once a week). In all other areas, mefloquine alone is recommended (one 250 mg tablet once a week for adults; lower doses for children based on weight). Mefloquine is not recommended for children under 15 kg, however; they may be given chloroquine prophylaxis and closely observed and treated for possible resistant *P falciparum* infection if it occurs. Proguanil may also be given to young children, although it is not available in the USA. Chloroquine prophylaxis is begun one week before travel and continued for four weeks after return; consult the recent CDC recommendations for the appropriate mefloquine schedule. Some experts recommend two weeks of primaquine at the end of prophylaxis to eradicate any hepatic malarial infection.

For the most current details of prophylaxis, a 24 hour telephone information service is available through the Centers for Disease Control (404-332-4555).

Diethyltoluamide-containing insect repellents and mosquito netting at night are important preventive measures.

Treatment

Malaria should always be excluded in children with fever or unexplained coma who have traveled to an endemic area. Blood transfusion and illicit intravenous drug use also put them at risk.

A. Specific Measures: Chloroquine phosphate is the drug of choice for nonresistant falciparum infections and for infections due to other species. Three days of therapy completely eradicates the erythrocytic phase (see Table 29–3).

Although mefloquine is also effective therapy for established malaria, it is not recommended. It is equally or less effective than the quinine-containing regimens and disturbing neuropsychiatric side-effects have been seen in some patients on therapeutic doses.

B. General Measures:

1. For uncomplicated malaria, hydration and fever control are emphasized. Blood and needle precautions are indicated. Hospitalization should be considered if the patient is vomiting, severely ill, or nonimmune and infected with *P falciparum*. Tests for

Table 29–3. Malaria treatment.

Indication	Drug	Dosage
All *Plasmodium* infections except chloroquine-resistant *P falciparum*	Oral: Chloroquine	10 mg base/kg (maximum 600 mg base), then 5 mg/kg 6 h, 24 h, and 48 h later.
	Parenteral: Quinine dihydrochloride	8 mg/kg/dose, given in normal saline intravenously over 2–4 h every 8 h until oral therapy tolerated (maximum 1800 mg).
Chloroquine-resistant *P falciparum*	Oral: Quinine sulfate	8 mg/kg/dose every 8 h for 3 days (maximum 1800 mg/d).
	Plus pyrimethamine	< 10 kg (6.25 mg/d for 3 days). 10–20 kg (12.5 mg/d for 3 days). 20–40 kg (25 mg/d for 3 days). > 40 kg (25 mg twice a day for 3 days).
	Plus sulfadiazine or Quinine sulfate Plus tetracycline	100–200 mg/kg/d in 4 doses for 5 days (maximum 2 g/d). (Same as above.) 5 mg/kg 4 times a day for 7 days (in children > 8 years old).
	Parenteral: Quinine dihydrochloride or Quinidine gluconate	(Same as above.)
Prevention of *P vivax* or *P ovale* relapses	Primaquine phosphate	0.3 mg base/kg/d (maximum 15 mg) for 14 days (screen for G6PD deficiency first).

incidental hepatitis B carrier states are indicated in high-risk groups (illicit drug users, native Orientals). Iron and folate levels may be low due to preexisting deficiency and exacerbated by hemolysis.

2. For suspected cerebral malaria, other causes must be ruled out; anticonvulsants and management appropriate for ischemic cerebral edema are needed. Corticosteroids have been shown to be detrimental and should not be used.

3. For blackwater fever, parasitemia must be treated and renal failure managed.

Cook GC: Prevention and treatment of malaria. *Lancet* 1988;**1**:32.

Krogstad DJ, Herwaldt BL, Schlesinger PH: Antimalarial agents: Specific treatment regimens. *Antimicrob Agents Chemother* 1988;**32**:957.

Randall G, Seidel JS: Malaria. *Pediatr Clin North Am* 1985;**32**:893.

WHO Malaria Action Programme: Severe and complicated malaria. *Trans R Soc Trop Med Hyg* 1986;**80 (Suppl)**:1

Recommendations for the prevention of malaria among travelers. *MMWR* 1990;**39**:1.

AMEBIASIS

Essentials of Diagnosis

- Acute dysentery: Evidence of colitis (diarrhea with blood and mucus, pain, tenderness).
- Chronic dysentery: Recurrent diarrhea and abdominal pain.
- Hepatic amebiasis: Tender hepatomegaly.
- Amebas or cysts in stools or abscesses.

General Considerations

Amebiasis is a common problem in endemic areas of poor hygiene. It should be suspected in cases with a history of travel to such areas or of contact with individuals from endemic areas who may be asymptomatic carriers. In the USA, amebiasis may be seen in homes for the retarded or handicapped, where poor hygiene fosters the spread of enteric pathogens. Individuals of any age may be infected. Transmission is usually fecal-oral, often from asymptomatic carriers who pass cysts. Trophozoites are killed by stomach acid and are not infectious. *Entamoeba coli* is a nonpathogenic commensal, as is *Entamoeba hartmanni* (previously known as "smallrace" *Entamoeba histolytica*). Only 10–20% of *E histolytica* infections result in symptoms.

Clinical Findings

A. Symptoms and Signs: Clinical symptoms may be unrelated to the presence of stool cysts. A response to specific therapy and a positive serology support a causative association.

The incubation period varies from days to months. Severity, acuteness of onset, degree of fever or abdominal pain (usually present over the cecum or sigmoid), and degree of dehydration are also quite variable. Stools usually contain blood and mucus. Chronic or recurrent symptoms may occur, an atypical finding in most bacterial enteritides.

B. Laboratory Findings: In colitis, a freshly passed stool specimen should be examined immediately for trophozoites and preserved in polyvinyl alcohol. Trophozoite motility, an important diagnostic characteristic, is rapidly lost with cooling or staining. Expert technologic help is mandatory: mistaking leukocytes (usually absent in amebiasis) for trophozoites has resulted in many false diagnoses. Sigmoidoscopy allows visualization of the classic "buttonhole" ulcers and procurement of excellent material for histology.

In chronic infections, several stools collected over

a period of days should be examined for the characteristic tetranucleated cysts; because cysts are stable at room temperature, special handling is not needed. Cysts only 10 μm in diameter are classified as the nonpathogenic *E hartmanni*. Oral cathartics, barium, and antibiotics may temporarily stop shedding. Routine laboratory tests are nondiagnostic. Leukocytosis may be present acutely. Eosinophilia is absent.

A barium enema may demonstrate colitis but is not diagnostic for amebiasis.

Serology is positive in 95% of patients with amebic dysentery or abscess but only in 10% of asymptomatic carriers or normal individuals.

Differential Diagnosis

Bacterial dysentery is usually more acute in onset. Very high fever, seizure, encephalopathy, and leukopenia with many immature neutrophils are characteristic of shigellosis but unusual in amebiasis. Fecal leukocytes suggest bacterial or inflammatory colitis; colitis can also be associated with antibiotics, allergies, hemolytic-uremic syndrome, ulcerative colitis, Crohn's disease, and *Balantidium coli* infection. Other intestinal parasites do not cause dysentery. The differential diagnosis for chronic amebiasis is even longer (see Chapter 21).

Complications & Sequelae

Intestinal complications include perforation, peritonitis, granulomatous proliferation (producing a mass or ameboma, which is rare in children), hemorrhage, intussusception, fistulization to bladder or skin, and late colonic strictures. Hepatic complications include hepatitis and abscess. The former is associated with dysentery and is characterized by tender hepatomegaly and mildly abnormal liver function tests without abscess formation. It is considered a form of toxic hepatitis and resolves with therapy. The diagnosis and management of amebic liver abscess is presented in Chapter 21.

Treatment

A. Specific Measures: Although several drugs are available, none are always curative.

1. Asymptomatic intestinal infection is best eradicated with diloxanide furoate (7 mg/kg 3 times daily for 10 days) or iodoquinol (10 mg/kg 3 times daily for 20 days). Paromomycin (8 mg/kg 3 times daily for 7 days) is an alternative.

2. Mild to moderate intestinal disease is treated with metronidazole (15 mg/kg, maximum of 750 mg, 3 times daily for 10 days), followed by a luminal amebicide (because metronidazole may fail to eradicate cysts).

3. Severe intestinal disease and liver abscess is treated with oral metronidazole (see above regimen) or intravenous metronidazole. An alternative regimen is dehydroemetine (0.5 mg/kg 2 times daily intramuscularly for 5 days, maximum of 90 mg/d).

Chloroquine is effective for abscesses but not intestinal disease. Dehydroemetine is cardiotoxic. Luminal amebicides should also be given when tolerated.

B. General Measures: Enteric isolation is advised. Adequate hydration and repeated evaluations should be done to detect complications. For follow-up (particularly in cases where diloxanide has not been given), examination of 3 stool specimens on alternate days determines whether the infection has been eradicated.

Adams ED, MacLeod IN: Invasive amebiasis. 1. Amebic dysentery and its complications. *Medicine* 1977;**56**:315. [A classic review from South Africa.]

Merritt RJ et al: Spectrum of amebiasis in children. *Am J Dis Child* 1982;**136**:785. [Emphasizes the nondysenteric presentations.]

Thompson JE Jr, Forlenza S, Verma R: Amebic liver abscess: A therapeutic approach. *Rev Infect Dis* 1985; **7**:171. [Excellent discussion of the management controversies.]

Wolfe MS: Treatment of intestinal protozoan infections. *Med Clin North Am* 1982;**66**:707.

DIARRHEA ASSOCIATED WITH *BLASTOCYSTIS HOMINIS*

The role of this protozoan in causing enteritis is controversial. Although it may be found in asymptomatic children, many investigators believe that it can cause acute enteritis in normal individuals and acute or chronic diarrhea in immunocompromised children. The clinical presentation is nonspecific. The organism is usually detected by routine examination of feces for the presence of ova and parasites; it is reported if present in large numbers. There are no characteristic laboratory findings or serologic diagnostic tests. If therapy seems necessary due to the severity of the disease and the lack of another cause, either metronidazole (15 mg/kg by mouth 3 times a day for 10 days) or iodoquinol (10 mg/kg by mouth 3 times a day for 20 days) may be effective.

Miller RA, Minshew BH: *Blastocystis hominis:* An organism in search of a disease. *Rev Infect Dis* 1988;**10**:930.

Doyle PW et al: Epidemiology and pathogenicity of *Blastocystis hominis*. *J Clin Microbiol* 1990;**28**:116

DIARRHEA ASSOCIATED WITH *DIENTAMOEBA FRAGILIS*

The pathogenicity of *Dientamoeba fragilis* is controversial, and even a presumptive diagnosis requires exclusion of other enteric pathogens. Purported symptoms include abdominal pain, diarrhea, nausea, anorexia, vomiting, and fatigue. Iodoquinol, 30 mg/kg/day in 3 divided doses for 21 days, has been used with success. Efficacy of other amebicides is unknown. Given the potential toxicity of therapy, the usual mild nature of symptoms, and questionable pathogenicity, *D fragilis* should not be treated routinely.

Spencer MJ, Garcia LS, Chapin MR: *Dientamoeba fragilis:* An intestinal pathogen in children? *Am J Dis Child* 1979;**133**:390.
Turner JA: Giardiasis and infections with *Dientamoeba fragilis. Pediatr Clin North Am* 1985;**32**:865.

FREE-LIVING AMEBAS: PRIMARY AMEBIC MENINGOENCEPHALITIS & AMEBIC KERATOCONJUNCTIVITIS

Essentials of Diagnosis:
Naegleria:
- Incidence usually in young, previously well individuals who swam in warm, fresh water lakes several days prior to onset of disease.
- Upper respiratory syndrome followed by rapidly progressive, purulent nonbacterial meningoencephalitis.
- Motile amebas in the spinal fluid.

Hartmannella-Acanthamoeba:
- Preexisting immunosuppression or debilitation.
- Variable clinical presentation; multiple organ involvement.
- Insidious onset of meningoencephalitis.
- Keratitis in wearers of soft contact lenses.

General Considerations
Two genera of amebas are capable of causing fatal meningoencephalitis. *Naegleria* inhabits fresh water. Infection presumably occurs by nasal colonization with subsequent penetration of the cribriform plate into the brain. The other genus, *Acanthamoeba,* causes systemic disease only in immunosuppressed individuals but may cause local corneal infection in normal individuals. Trauma to the skin, mucous membranes, or cornea may provide an entry site. Granulomas in multiple organs often precede involvement of the central nervous system.

Clinical Findings
A. Symptoms and Signs: *Naegleria* infection is usually fatal. The early symptoms of upper respiratory infection, occasionally with an altered sense of smell or taste, are followed by high fever, headache, vomiting, seizures, and coma. Systemic *Acanthamoeba* infections present more subacutely; cutaneous granulomas and nodules and renal, adrenal, pancreatic, and cerebral involvement (hydrocephalus, abscesses) occur. Recently, a severe and sometimes blinding form of keratitis has been seen in wearers of soft contact lenses due to contamination of the lens-cleaning solution by *Acanthamoeba.*
B. Laboratory Findings: Identification can be made by direct wet mounts of cerebrospinal fluid,

nasal smears, or conjunctival scrapings, by immunofluorescent staining of fixed tissue or cerebrospinal fluid, by Wright's stain of the sediment from centrifuged cerebrospinal fluid, or by cultures on special media. Rapid examination of a warm fluid is important so that motility, which helps differentiate amebas from leukocytes, can be observed.

Differential Diagnosis
Primary amebic meningoencephalitis due to *Naegleria* resembles acute bacterial meningitis. *Acanthamoeba* infection more closely resembles chronic mycotic disease.

Prevention
Cases are rare and usually sporadic, although clusters have been reported. Swimming and diving in warm, stagnant water is discouraged.

Treatment
Therapy of *Naegleria* should be instituted as early as possible. Amphotericin B should be given intravenously (1 mg/kg/d) and perhaps intraventricularly or intrathecally (0.1 mg every other day) if improvement does not occur in 48 hours. Oral rifampin and intraventricular miconazole have also been used. Intravenous sulfadiazine is the drug of choice for *Acanthamoeba.* Both regimens are indicated if the species is unknown. The prognosis is generally poor, perhaps relating to delay in diagnosis. The true efficacy of the treatment regimens is not known because too few patients are treated early in the course. *Acanthamoeba* keratitis requires debridement; it may respond to topical miconazole, propamidine, and antibiotics.

Seidel JS et al: Successful treatment of primary amebic meningoencephalitis. *N Engl J Med* 1982;**306**:346.
Simon MW, Wilson HD: The amebic meningoencephalitides. *Pediatr Infect Dis J* 1986;**5**:562.
Stehr-Green JK et al: Acanthamoeba keratitis in soft contact lens wearers. *JAMA* 1987;**258**:57.

GIARDIASIS

Essentials of Diagnosis
- Chronic or relapsing diarrhea, flatulence, bloating, anorexia, poor weight gain.
- Absence of fever and hematochezia.
- Presence of trophozoites in loose stools or duodenal contents; cysts in formed stools.

General Considerations
Giardiasis is the most common intestinal protozoan infection in children in most areas. Endemic worldwide, it is classically associated with drinking contaminated water, either in rural areas or in areas with faulty purification systems. Because even ostensibly clean urban water supplies can be intermit-

tently contaminated, giardiasis can be acquired by almost any traveler. Recently, day-care centers have been recognized as major sources, with an incidence of up to 50% reported in some centers. Asymptomatic infections are the rule and allow spread to household contacts.

Although rare in neonates, infection occurs at any age.

Clinical Findings

A. Symptoms and Signs: Following cyst ingestion, liberated trophozoites live noninvasively in the small bowel. Symptoms develop in 1–3 weeks in some patients, particularly those with hypogammaglobulinemia. Diarrheal, soft, or steatorrheal stools with mucus, but no blood or leukocytes, are passed. Abdominal cramps, vomiting, anorexia, and weight loss may occur. Rash and fever are absent. The illness may last days to months and may relapse.

B. Laboratory Findings: Routine blood tests are normal; there is no eosinophilia. Examination of several stool specimens usually reveals the pear-shaped trophozoites (2–15 μm) (in fresh loose stools) or the oval cysts. Immediate fixation of loose stools with subsequent trichrome staining to look for trophozoites is recommended. If results are negative, samples should be taken directly from the duodenum by aspiration, biopsy, or the string test (Entero-Test). Because only trophozoites are present there, rapid processing is necessary. Cyst shedding is intermittent, and multiple stools may be negative in infected patients. Tests for *Giardia* antigen in stools are promising and could prove more cost-effective than multiple stool examinations.

Differential Diagnosis

Many other causes of steatorrhea and chronic diarrhea should be considered, including cryptosporidiosis and chronic amebiasis. (See Chapter 21.)

Prevention

Spread is fecal-oral. Untreated water or potentially contaminated foods (fresh fruit, vegetables) should be avoided; personal hygiene is important. Pets are not considered a source. Identifying and treating asymptomatic human carriers may be needed.

Treatment

Ideally, the diagnosis is made prior to treatment, although many clinicians use a single empiric course of therapy prior to invasive diagnostic tests.

Failures and reinfections occur with all regimens and can frustrate attempts at eradication. Symptomatic children in day-care centers and their contacts should be evaluated and treated if infected. Asymptomatic children should probably not be tested unless there are multiple or recurrent cases. Eradicating every cyst from a large group of infants is a monumental task.

The only stable suspension active against *Giardia* available is furazolidone (50 mg/15 mL); the dosage is 2 mg/kg 4 times daily for 7–10 days. Children able to take tablets may be treated with quinacrine hydrochloride, 2 mg/kg 3 times daily for 5–10 days. Gastrointestinal upset and yellow skin may be seen. Metronidazole, 5 mg/kg 3 times daily for 5–10 days may also be used. A single dose of tinidazole (50 mg/kg, maximum of 2 g) is also highly effective but is not available in the USA.

Giardia excretion is self-limited; if symptoms resolve with therapy, repeated stool examinations may not be necessary.

Secondary lactase deficiency may also occur; a secondary invasion of giardiasis should be considered in patients with cystic fibrosis, chronic pancreatitis, or achlorhydria. In hypogammaglobulinemic patients, relapses are common.

Dupont JL, Sullivan PS: Giardiasis: The clinical spectrum, diagnosis and therapy. *Pediatr Infect Dis J* 1986; **5(Suppl):**131.

Kavousi S: Giardiasis in infancy and childhood: A prospective study of 160 cases with comparison of quinacrine (Atabrine) and metronidazole (Flagyl). *Am J Trop Med Hyg* 1979;**28:**19.

Ranch AM et al: Longitudinal study of *Giardia lamblia* infection in a day care center population. *Pediatr Infect Dis J* 1990;**9:**186.

Smith PD: Pathophysiology and immunology of giardiasis. *Annu Rev Med* 1985;**36:**295.

CRYPTOSPORIDIOSIS

The protozoan *Cryptosporidium* belongs to the same family as *Toxoplasma* and *Isospora*. It is distributed worldwide. The parasite lines the villi of the small bowel and is noninvasive; it has been found in the biliary and respiratory tracts as well, but its role there is undefined. *Cryptosporidium* is found in many animals and is a prominent cause of diarrhea in calves; intractable, watery diarrhea and inanition may occur in immunocompromised patients, particularly those with HIV infection. A similar but self-limited (up to several weeks) diarrheal illness may occur in normal individuals of all ages. Other symptoms include vomiting, fever, and cramps; stools may be positive for occult blood but are usually free of leukocytes. Outbreaks in day-care centers and cases in travelers and handlers of large animals are noteworthy. Diagnosis is by intestinal biopsy or fecal examination for the characteristic 3-μm, round cysts. Optimal detection requires an additional laboratory procedure, such as a modified acid-fast stain, which may not be part of the routine parasitologic examination. No specific therapy is effective.

Casemore DP, Sands RL, Curry A: *Cryptosporidium* species: A "new" human pathogen. *J Clin Pathol* 1985; **38:**1321.

Isaacs D et al: Cryptosporidiosis in immunocompetent children. *J Clin Pathol* 1985;**38:**76.

Janoff EN, Reller LB: *Cryptosporidium* species: A protean protozoan. *J Clin Microbiol* 1987;**25:**967.

TRICHOMONAS

The nonpathogenic flagellates *Trichomonas hominis* and *Trichomonas tenax* are commensals in the mouth and intestinal tract, respectively. *Trichomonas vaginalis* may cause vaginitis, usually in sexually active girls and, rarely, secondary to sexual abuse in prepubertal children. Nonsexual transmission to prepubertal children may also occur, although molestation must always be excluded. Findings include pruritus, dysuria, frothy leukorrhea, vaginal erythema, and edema. Male urethritis also occurs. Diagnosis by wet prep examination is usually sufficient. Other genital pathogens may coexist. Metronidazole is often used (a single oral dose of 2 g for teenagers is usually effective; 5 mg/kg 3 times daily for 7 days is an alternative). Sexual partners should be treated concomitantly. Intravaginal clotrimazole is a less effective choice.

TOXOPLASMOSIS

Essentials of Diagnosis

- Congenital toxoplasmosis: Rash, hepatosplenomegaly, chorioretinitis, hydrocephalus or microcephaly, and mental retardation.
- Acquired toxoplasmosis: Fever, rash, lymphadenopathy, chorioretinitis, encephalitis, and myocarditis.
- Demonstration of *Toxoplasma gondii* in tissue or serologic evidence of infection is required for confirmation.

General Considerations

Toxoplasma gondii is a protozoan parasite of humans and some animals. The tachyzoite is crescentic, 4–7 μm long, and has a single nucleus. True cysts containing large numbers of bradyzoites form in various tissues but are particularly common in the brain. Affected individuals are usually asymptomatic. Reactivation and symptomatic infection may occur years later, especially with immunosuppression. Ingestion of tissue cysts (eg, cats eating mice with infected brains; humans eating infected meat) is one form of transmission.

Congenital toxoplasmosis is acquired in utero during a primary maternal infection. Reactivation of prior infection is probably never a cause of neonatal infection.

Acquired infection may be due to handling and eating raw or undercooked red meat or to contact with infected cat feces in litter boxes and soil. Felines are the definitive hosts and pass infective oocysts in the feces, especially during pregnancy. Oocyst survival is decreased by drying; this fact may explain the low incidence of infection in dry climates.

Clinical Findings

A. Symptoms and Signs:

1. Congenital toxoplasmosis—This occurs in about 2 per 1000 live births. Clinical abnormalities are more common following infection in early gestation. Hepatosplenomegaly, jaundice, rash, thrombocytopenia, a characteristic chorioretinitis, and encephalitis with calcifications, hydrocephalus, microcephaly, and mental retardation may be seen. Cardiac, pulmonary, bone, or lens abnormalities are not common; their presence suggests cytomegalovirus, rubella, or syphilis.

2. Acquired toxoplasmosis—This occurs at any age and is usually asymptomatic. Fever, adenopathy (usually cervical), hepatomegaly, myalgias, maculopapular rash, encephalitis, myocarditis, retinitis, and pneumonia are possible. Less than 1% of mononucleosislike syndromes are due to toxoplasmosis. The retinitis is thought to represent a late manifestation of congenital infection.

3. Immunocompromised hosts—Patients with lymphoma, leukemia, and HIV infection are especially prone to reactivated toxoplasmosis with severe involvement of brain, eye, heart, or lung.

B. Laboratory Findings:

Visualization of organisms in spinal fluid or biopsy material is diagnostic. Serologic tests, usually an indirect fluorescent antibody (IFA) test, should be performed by reference laboratories and interpreted carefully; commercial kits may be very inaccurate. An acute IFA titer over 1:1000, a positive IgM titer, or a 2-dilution rise suggests acute infection. Other laboratory tests are nonspecific. The retinal abnormalities are very characteristic, as are the cranial CT findings, in congenital infection. The cerebral findings in acquired disease may closely resemble bacterial abscess or tumor. The histologic findings of toxoplasma lymph node infection may closely resemble lymphoma.

Differential Diagnosis

Congenital infection may resemble that due to cytomegalovirus, syphilis, herpes, or other agents. Acquired infection mimics a number of viral or lymphoproliferative diseases.

Prevention

Pregnant women should wash hands thoroughly after handling raw meat, cook meat to 66 °C or greater, wash fruits and vegetables before consumption, and avoid contact with cat feces.

Treatment

Pyrimethamine (0.5 mg/kg twice daily for infants, 1 mg/kg twice daily for older children) and either sulfadiazine or trisulfapyrimidines (25 mg/kg 4 times a day orally) for 3–4 weeks in suspected or proved cases is recommended. Gastrointestinal upset and rash are side effects.

Pyrimethamine may cause leukopenia, thrombocytopenia, and, rarely, agranulocytosis; frequent blood counts should be performed and the drug stopped if the counts fall very low. Folinic acid, 1–3 mg intramuscularly once a week, may be given to decrease the drug toxicity.

Therapy does not alter the congenital neurologic damage. Because acquired infection is usually self-limited, the potentially toxic therapy should be prescribed with discretion, usually only if the illness is complicated.

In chorioretinitis, especially in the acquired form, a course of corticosteroids (eg, prednisone, 1 mg/kg orally initially and then tapered over 3–4 weeks) should be given along with the antimicrobial agents. Antimicrobial therapy is continued until the eye disease has improved or stabilized. For recurrence of retinitis, steroids may be given alone.

Therapy of primary infection in pregnancy decreases infection in the infant by about 50%. Spiramycin is recommended and may be obtained in the USA through the Federal Drug Administration Anti-infective Drug Office (telephone (301)443-7580); a sulfonamide and pyrimethamine are used if spiramycin is not available.

Frenkel JK: Toxoplasmosis. *Pediatr Clin North Am* 1985; **32**:917.

Hohlfeld P et al: Fetal toxoplasmosis outcome of pregnancy and infant follow-up after in utero treatment. *J Pediatr* 1989;**115**:765.

McCabe RE et al: Clinical spectrum in 107 cases of toxoplasmic lymphadenopathy. *Rev Infect Dis* 1987;**9**:754.

LEISHMANIASIS

1. VISCERAL LEISHMANIASIS (Kala-Azar)

Essentials of Diagnosis

- Fever, hepatosplenomegaly, adenopathy, anemia, leukopenia, and wasting.
- Demonstration of *Leishmania donovani* in bone marrow, spleen, liver, or lymph node.
- Positive serology.

General Considerations

Leishmania donovani is a protozoan transmitted by the sandfly from human to human (India), from dogs to humans (Mediterranean region) or from carnivores or rodents to humans (Sudan). Infantile kala-azar is common in the Mediterranean area; in India,

older children are more susceptible; and in other parts of the world, it is primarily an adult disease.

The parasites infect and multiply in reticuloendothelial cells, existing as oval bodies 2–4 μm long. A kinetoplast separate from the nucleus helps distinguish this organism from *Histoplasma* or *Toxoplasma*. Tissue touch-preparation smears stained with Giemsa or Leishman's stain demonstrate the organisms well.

Clinical Findings

A. Symptoms and Signs: High fever, intestinal symptoms, rapid splenic enlargement, hepatic enlargement, and adenopathy are common in young children. Older children have a more subacute course with progressive anemia. Posttreatment nodular cutaneous lesions containing many organisms may be seen as well.

B. Laboratory Findings: Leukopenia, thrombocytopenia, anemia, and hypergammaglobulinemia are common. Organisms may be seen in blood smears, but tissue demonstration is usually required. Serology may also help.

Differential Diagnosis

Brucellosis, typhoid fever, lymphoproliferative diseases, histiocytosis, endocarditis, schistosomiasis, trypanosomiasis, and malaria should be considered.

Treatment

Specific therapy is an antimony compound, such as stibogluconate sodium or antimony sodium gluconate, given parenterally daily for 6 days (10 mg/kg/dose slowly intravenously or intramuscularly once a day). Vomiting, diarrhea, or cramps may occur. Pentamidine (3 mg/kg intramuscularly daily for 10 days) has also been used. Nodular cutaneous leishmaniasis also requires antimony.

Indian kala-azar responds better to these drugs than the African variety.

Nonspecific therapy for secondary bacterial infections and nutritional deficiency is also needed.

2. CUTANEOUS LEISHMANIASIS (Oriental Sore)

This worldwide form of skin disease, also transmitted by sandflies, is due to *Leishmania tropica*. Although most cases come from Asia, India, and North Africa, some have been reported in Texas.

After an incubation period of weeks to months, pruritic papules develop at the bite site and develop into slowly spreading granulomatous ulcers. The face and limbs are usually affected. Healing and scar formation occur over months.

Organisms may be found in fluid or tissue obtained from the ulcer margin. The leishmanin skin test is usually positive.

Therapy for secondary bacterial infection usually suffices, allowing spontaneous healing and development of immunity. For severe infections, a 10-day course of antimony may be used. Early therapy reduces ultimate scar formation.

3. MUCOCUTANEOUS LEISHMANIASIS

This more severe form is prevalent in South America and caused by several species, including *Leishmania braziliensis* (espundia), *Leishmania mexicana* (chiclero ulcer), and *Leishmania peruviana*. Although lesions may resemble Oriental sore, disfiguring naso-oral lesions are also seen. The skin test and biopsy are both positive. Prolonged antimony therapy is needed.

Al-Taqi M, Behbehani K: Cutaneous leishmaniasis in Kuwait. *Ann Trop Med Parasitol* 1980;**74:**495.
Evans T et al: American visceral leishmaniasis (kala-azar). *West J Med* 1985;**142:**777.
Rees PG et al: The treatment of kala-azar: A review with comments drawn from experience in Kenya. *Trop Geogr Med* 1985;**37:**37.

AFRICAN TRYPANOSOMIASIS
(Sleeping Sickness)

Essentials of Diagnosis
- Chancre and red, painful nodule at the site of a bite of the tsetse fly (*Glossina*).
- Fever, progressive anemia and weakness, splenomegaly, lymphadenitis, skin rash.
- Personality disturbance, apathy, somnolence, involuntary movements, and coma.
- Trypanosomes present in peripheral blood (Rhodesian variety) and in lymph node aspirates (Gambian variety).

General Considerations
Trypanosomiasis occurs in parts of tropical Africa. The more serious form caused by *Trypanosoma brucei rhodesiense* occurs mainly in East Africa; that caused by *T brucei gambiense* is more widespread and more common in children.

Clinical Findings
A. Symptoms and Signs:
1. Rhodesian trypanosomiasis—The primary bite-site nodule develops in some patients in a week and usually resolves within days. Variable fever follows, accompanied by headache, myalgia, and transient rashes. Splenomegaly, generalized adenopathy, and hepatomegaly may occur. The neurologic changes begin within months and are rapidly fatal.

2. Gambian trypanosomiasis—The initial stages are similar to those of the Rhodesian form, but the progression is slower. Lymphadenitis is more prominent, especially of the posterior cervical glands (Winterbottom's sign). After months to years, the child becomes lethargic and sleeps most of the time. Severe emaciation and edema are common prior to death.

B. Laboratory Findings: The characteristic spindle-shaped organisms should be searched for in wet or thick blood smears; bone marrow or lymph node aspirate (early stages); or spun cerebrospinal fluid (later stages). Spinal fluid pleocytosis and protein elevation may precede clinical symptoms. Anemia, an elevation in the erythrocyte sedimentation rate and serum gamma globulins, and hypoproteinemia may also occur.

Differential Diagnosis
Kala-azar, lymphoreticular disorders, HIV infection, tuberculosis, fungal meningitis, or brain tumors may resemble stages of trypanosomiasis.

Treatment
A. Specific Measures: Suramin sodium is the drug of choice for both forms in the absence of cerebral disease. Pentamidine may also be used, although it is less effective for the Rhodesian form. With any cerebral involvement, melarsoprol, tryparsamide, or difluoromethylornithine are available.

B. General Measures: If possible, the patient should be hospitalized; superinfection and malnutrition must be treated.

Prognosis
Spontaneous recovery may occur in early cases. Therapy is very effective for early and intermediate disease. The outcome is worse for cerebral disease. Untreated, the Rhodesian form is usually fatal within a year and the Gambian form in 10 years.

Haller L et al: Clinical and pathological aspects of human African trypanosomiasis (*Trypanosoma brucei gambiense*) with particular reference to reactive arsenical encephalopathy. *Am J Trop Med Hyg* 1986;**35:**94.

AMERICAN TRYPANOSOMIASIS
(Chagas' Disease)

Essentials of Diagnosis
- Development of a red, painful nodule at the site of the bite (the chagoma).
- Conjunctivitis; lid and facial edema (Romaña's sign).
- Fever, lymphadenitis, myocarditis, or encephalitis.
- Megaesophagus, megacolon.

- *Trypanosoma cruzi* in the blood, marrow, lymph node, or spleen.

General Considerations

Present in South and Central America (especially Brazil and Argentina), Chagas' disease is caused by *Trypanosoma cruzi,* which is transmitted when reduviid bug feces contaminate conjunctivas or skin abrasions. Cases resulting from blood transfusion are common, and congenital infection with pneumonia also occurs. Organisms invade locally and systemically.

Clinical Findings

A. Symptoms and Signs: At the site of inoculation, a painful red nodule usually appears, accompanied by local adenitis and fever. Eye inoculation results in conjunctivitis, facial edema, and lid edema. Systemic spread may cause hepatosplenomegaly, myocarditis, and encephalitis. The main organs involved in late stages of disease are the heart (congestive failure) and esophagus and colon (dilatation due to involvement of the nerve plexuses).

B. Laboratory Findings: In acute Chagas' disease, the organisms may be found in peripheral blood examined by wet prep or after Giemsa staining. If results are negative, aspirates from bone marrow, lymph node, or spleen should be obtained. Cultures of clinical specimens on special media (NNN medium) or in animals may also be done. Serology is also available. A mononuclear leukocytosis may be present in the acute stage.

Differential Diagnosis

Bacterial infections, trichinosis, and kala-azar may resemble Chagas' disease. In endemic areas, non-pathogenic trypanosomes (eg, *Trypanosoma rangeli*) may also be found in humans.

Treatment

There is no specific therapy available, although a derivative of nitrofurantoin, nifurtimox, is somewhat beneficial in acute disease. Chronic disease does not respond.

Blood for transfusion is rendered noninfectious by 48 hours of contact with amphotericin B.

Prognosis

Mortality is highest with encephalitis or in very young children. Chronic damage to the heart or intestinal tract is irreparable.

Apt W: Treatment of Chagas' disease. *Rev Med Chil* 1985; **113**:162.

Schipper H et al: Tropical diseases encountered in Canada. 1. Chagas' disease. *Can Med Assoc J* 1980;**122**:165.

METAZOAN INFECTIONS

NEMATODE INFECTIONS

1. ENTEROBIASIS (Pinworms)

Essentials of Diagnosis

- Nocturnal anal pruritus.
- Worms in the stool or eggs on perianal skin.

General Considerations

This worldwide infection is caused by *Enterobius vermicularis*. The adult worms live in the colon; females deposit eggs on the perianal area, primarily at night, causing intense pruritus. Scratching contaminates the fingers and allows transmission back to the host (autoinfection) or to contacts.

Clinical Findings

A. Symptoms and Signs: Although blamed for a myriad of symptoms, pinworms are definitely associated only with local itching. They can be found within the bowel wall, in the lumen of the appendix (usually an incidental finding by the pathologist), and (in girls) in the urethra, bladder, and even the peritoneal cavity. The granulomatous reaction that may be present around these ectopic worms is usually asymptomatic. Worm eradication may correspond with the cure of recurrent urinary tract infections in some young girls.

B. Laboratory Findings: The usual diagnostic test consists of placing a piece of transparent tape over the child's anus in the morning prior to bathing. Placing the tape on a drop of xylene on a slide and examining it microscopically usually demonstrates the ova. Occasionally, eggs or adult worms are seen in fecal specimens.

Differential Diagnosis

Nonspecific irritation or vaginitis, streptococcal perianal cellulitis (usually painful), and vaginal or urinary bacterial infections may at times resemble pinworm infestation, although the symptoms of pinworms are often so suggestive that a therapeutic trial is justified without a confirmed diagnosis.

Treatment

A. Specific Measures: Treat all household members at the same time to prevent reinfections. Since the drugs are not active against the eggs, therapy should be repeated after two weeks to kill the recently hatched adults.

1. Pyrantel pamoate—This drug is given as a single dose (11 mg/kg, maximum of 1 g); it is safe and very effective.

2. Mebendazole—Mebendazole is also highly effective for this infection as well as for most of the other common nematodes. A single oral dose of 100 mg is used for all ages. It should not be given to pregnant women, nor has it been well studied in children under 2.

3. Pyrvinium pamoate—This drug is available as a syrup; nausea, vomiting, and red stools are side effects. A single dose of 5 mg/kg (up to 250 mg) is used.

4. Piperazine compounds—Piperazine compounds are available in syrup form and not very toxic but must be given nightly for 7 days (50 mg/kg, up to 2 g).

B. General Measures: Personal hygiene must be emphasized. Nails should be kept short and clean. Children should wear undergarments to bed to diminish contamination of fingers; bedclothes should be laundered frequently. Although eggs may be widely dispersed in the house and multiple family members infected, the disease is mild and treatable. Avoid creating "pinworm psychosis" in the parents.

2. ASCARIASIS

Essentials of Diagnosis
- Abdominal cramps and discomfort.
- Large, white, round worms or ova in the feces.

General Considerations
Ascaris lumbricoides is a worldwide human parasite. Ova passed by carriers may remain viable for months under the proper soil conditions. The ova contaminate food or fingers and are subsequently ingested by a new host. The larvae hatch, penetrate the intestinal wall, enter the venous system, reach the alveoli, are coughed up, and return to the small intestine, where they mature. The female lays thousands of eggs daily.

Clinical Findings
A. Symptoms and Signs: Infections usually remain asymptomatic; severe cases, however, can cause pain, weight loss, anorexia, diarrhea, or vomiting. Adult worms may be seen in feces or vomitus. Rarely, they perforate or obstruct the small bowel, biliary system, or appendix.

Large numbers of larvae migrating through the lungs may cause an acute, transient eosinophilic pneumonia (Löffler's syndrome).

B. Laboratory Findings: The diagnosis is made by observing the large, round worms in the stool or by microscopic detection of the ova.

Treatment
Because the adults live less than a year, asymptomatic infection need not be treated. Mebendazole (100 mg 2 times daily for 3 days for children over 2 years old) or pyrantel pamoate (a single dose of 11 mg/kg, maximum of 1 g) is the drug of choice. If there are large numbers of worms, intestinal obstruction may result from the mass of paralyzed parasites. Surgical removal is sometimes needed.

Crompton EWT, Nesheim MC, Pawloski ZS (editors): *Ascariasis and Its Public Health Significance.* Taylor and Francis, 1985.
Pawlowski ZS: Ascariasis: Host-pathogen biology. *Rev Infect Dis* 1982;**4**:802.

3. TRICHURIASIS (Whipworm)

Trichuris trichiura is a widespread human and animal parasite common in poor children living in warm, humid areas conducive to survival of the ova. The adult worms live in the cecum and colon; the ova are passed and become infectious after several weeks in the soil. Ingested infective eggs hatch in the upper small intestine. Usually, no symptoms are present unless the infection is severe, in which case it can cause pain, diarrhea, and mild distention. Massive infections may also cause rectal prolapse and dysentery. Detecting the characteristic barrel-shaped ova in the feces makes the diagnosis. Adult worms may be seen in the prolapsed rectum or at proctoscopy; their thin heads are buried in the mucosa, and the thicker posterior portions extrude. Mild to moderate eosinophilia may be present.

Mebendazole is the drug of choice (100 mg orally 2 times daily for 3 days for children over 2 years).

Gilman RH et al: The adverse consequences of heavy *Trichuris* infection. *Trans R Soc Trop Med Hyg* 1983; **32**:118.
Rossignol JF, Maisonneuve H: Benzimidazoles in the treatment of trichuriasis: A review. *Ann Trop Med Parasitol* 1984;**78**:135.

4. HOOKWORM

Essentials of Diagnosis
- Iron deficiency anemia.
- Hematochezia.
- Abdominal discomfort, weight loss.
- Ova in the feces.

General Considerations
The common human hookworms are *Ancylostoma duodenale* and *Necator americanus*. Both are widespread in the tropics and subtropics. The larger

Ancylostoma is more pathogenic because it consumes more blood, up to 0.5 mL per worm per day.

The adults live in the jejunum. Eggs are passed in the feces and develop and hatch in warm, damp soil within 2 weeks into infective larvae. The larvae penetrate human skin on contact, enter the blood, reach the alveoli, are coughed up and swallowed, and develop into adults in the intestine. Infection rates reach 90% in areas without sanitation.

A separate species, *Ancylostoma braziliense* (the dog or cat hookworm), causes creeping eruption (cutaneous larva migrans). This disease is seen mainly on the warm-water American coasts.

Clinical Findings

A. Symptoms and Signs: The larvae usually penetrate the skin of the feet and cause intense local itching (''ground itch''). In the cutaneous form of the disease, the larvae migrate blindly in the skin before dying, creating serpiginous burrows.

Mild infections produce no symptoms. Severe infections may cause pain, loose stools, and iron deficiency anemia.

B. Laboratory Findings: The species of the large ova are identical, and both are present in feces. Microcytic anemia, folate deficiency, hypoalbuminemia, eosinophilia, and hematochezia are seen in severe cases.

Prevention

Fecal contamination of soil should be prevented; skin contact with potentially contaminated soil should also be avoided.

Treatment

A. Specific Measures: Mebendazole (100 mg orally 2 times daily for 3 days) is the drug of choice. It is also active against a number of other nematodes that may coexist with hookworm. Pyrantel pamoate (11 mg/kg, maximum of 1 g, daily for 3 days) is an alternative.

B. General Measures: Iron therapy may be more important than worm eradication. Parenteral iron or transfusions may be needed in severe cases.

Prognosis

The outcome is usually excellent.

Gilles HM: Selective primary health care: Strategies for control of diseases in the developing world. 17. Hookworm infections and anemia. *Rev Infect Dis* 1985; 7:111.

5. STRONGYLOIDIASIS

Essentials of Diagnosis
- Cough and hemoptysis.
- Abdominal pain, diarrhea.
- Eosinophilia, malnutrition.
- Larvae in stools and duodenal aspirates.

General Considerations

The responsible parasite, *Strongyloides stercoralis,* is unique in having both parasitic and free-living forms; the latter can survive in the soil for several generations. The parasite is found in most tropical and subtropical regions of the world. The adults live in the submucosal tissue of the duodenum and occasionally in the whole intestine. Eggs deposited in the mucosa hatch rapidly; the first-stage (rhabditiform) larvae, therefore, are the predominant form found in duodenal aspirates and feces. The larvae rapidly mature to the tissue-penetrating filariform stage and initiate internal autoinfection. The filariform larvae also inhabit the soil and can penetrate the skin of another host, subsequently migrating into veins and alveoli and reaching the intestine when coughed up and swallowed.

Older children and adults are more often infected than young children. Infestations due to poor sanitation and hygiene in homes for the retarded are noteworthy. Immunosuppressed patients may develop fatal disseminated strongyloidiasis.

Clinical Findings

A. Symptoms and Signs: At the site of the skin penetration, there may be a pruritic rash. Large numbers of migrating larvae can cause wheezing, cough, and hemoptysis. The most common symptoms, if any occur, are abdominal pain, distention, diarrhea, and (sometimes) vomiting. Because the upper bowel is involved, a high obstruction or peptic disease may be simulated.

B. Laboratory Findings: Finding larvae in the feces or in duodenal aspirates makes the diagnosis. Because even multiple stools may be negative, duodenal aspirates or use of the string test (Entero-Test) should be considered.

C. Imaging: Patchy pulmonary infiltrates may be seen during the migration phase; later, inflammation or narrowing of the duodenum on a barium study is typical.

Differential Diagnosis

Strongyloidiasis should be differentiated from peptic disease, celiac disease, regional or tuberculous enteritis, hookworm infection, and other causes of malabsorption. The pulmonary phase may mimic asthma or bronchopneumonia. Severe infection can present as an acute abdomen.

Complications & Sequelae

Chronic diarrhea and malabsorption can lead to malnutrition. Overwhelming strongyloidiasis is an opportunistic infection in heavily immunosuppressed patients from endemic areas. Suspect the diagnosis if bilateral pulmonary infiltrates and paralytic ileus are seen on radiographs. *Strongyloides* larvae are usually easily found in many body fluids, including cerebrospinal fluid.

Treatment

A. Specific Measures: Thiabendazole (25 mg/kg orally 2 times daily for 2 days, maximum of 3 g/d) is the drug of choice. Relapses are common.

B. General Measures: Fluid and nutritional support are needed.

Davidson RA, Fletcher RH, Chapman LE: Risk factors for strongyloidiasis: A case control study. *Arch Intern Med* 1984;**144**:321.

Milder JE et al: Clinical features of *Strongyloides stercoralis* infection in an endemic area of the United States. *Gastroenterology* 1981;**80**:1481.

Neva FA: Biology and immunology of human strongyloidiasis. *J Infect Dis* 1986;**153**:397.

6. VISCERAL LARVA MIGRANS (Toxocariasis)

Essentials of Diagnosis

- Hepatosplenomegaly and marked eosinophilia in young children with pica.
- Hyperglobulinemia; elevated isohemagglutin titers.
- Demonstration of larvae on liver biopsy or positive serology.

General Considerations

Visceral larva migrans is a worldwide disease. The agent is the cosmopolitan intestinal ascarid of dogs and cats, *Toxocara canis* or *Toxocara cati*. The eggs passed by infected animals contaminate parks and other areas that young children frequent. After an incubation period, the organisms become infectious when inadvertently ingested. Children with pica are more at risk. Even urban areas may be contaminated; up to 30% of playground soils may contain eggs. Ingested eggs hatch and penetrate the intestinal wall, then migrate to the liver, lungs, and other organs, where they die and incite a granulomatous inflammatory reaction. The rodent whipworm, *Capillaria hepatica,* can cause a similar syndrome.

Clinical Findings

A. Symptoms and Signs: Presenting symptoms include anorexia, fever, pallor, and, occasionally, abdominal distention and cough. Hepatomegaly is common, and splenomegaly is not unusual. Adenopathy is absent. Seizures and blindness are unusual manifestations.

B. Laboratory Findings: Marked leukocytosis (with 30–90% eosinophils) is the rule. Anemia, hypergammaglobulinemia, and elevated isohemagglutinins are common. The diagnosis is confirmed by finding larvae in the liver, granulomatous lesions, muscle, or brain. Positive serology and the exclusion of other causes of hypereosinophilia allow a presumptive diagnosis to be made in typical cases.

Differential Diagnosis

Diseases with hypereosinophilia must be considered. These include trichinosis (large liver and spleen not usually seen), eosinophilic leukemia (rare in children; eosinophils are abnormal in appearance), collagen-vascular disease (those associated with eosinophilia are rare in young children), strongyloidiasis (no organomegaly; enteric symptoms are common), early ascariasis, and tropical eosinophilia (seen mainly in India).

Complications & Sequelae

Myocarditis, retinitis, and encephalitis occur. A retinal mass resembling a retinoblastoma may be the only manifestation in some children.

Treatment

A. Specific Measures: Thiabendazole is the best drug (25 mg/kg, maximum of 3 g/d, orally twice a day for 5–7 days). Diethylcarbamezine may also be used (2–4 mg/kg 3 times a day orally for 7–10 days). Significant lung involvement is one indication for therapy.

B. General Measures: Because the disease is usually self-limited, therapy is supportive and emphasizes prevention of reinfection. Treating any cause of pica, such as iron deficiency, is important. Corticosteroids are used for marked inflammation of lung, eye, or other organs.

Other children in the household may be infected. Mild eosinophilia and positive serologies may be the only clue to their infection. Therapy is not necessary for these patients.

Bejhti A: Mebendazole in toxocariasis. *Ann Intern Med* 1984;**100**:463.

Shields JA: Ocular toxocariasis: A review. *Surv Ophthalmol* 1984;**28**:361.

Zinkham WH: Visceral larva migrans: A review and reassessment indicating two forms of clinical expression: Visceral and ocular. *Am J Dis Child* 1978;**132**:627.

7. TRICHINOSIS

Essentials of Diagnosis

- Vomiting, diarrhea, and pain within 48 hours of eating infected meat.
- Fever, periorbital edema, myalgia, and marked eosinophilia.
- *Trichinella spiralis* larvae in muscle biopsy.

General Considerations

Trichinella spiralis is a small roundworm. The

adults inhabit the intestines of hogs and several other meat-eating animals. The cycle begins when the larvae in the muscle of hogs, bear, walrus, and other animals are ingested and enter the bowel mucosa, develop into adults, reemerge into the intestine, mate, and reenter the mucosa. The hundreds of larvae produced by each female over the next weeks enter the bloodstream and encyst in the striated muscle. Their migration causes marked inflammation. Humans are usually infected by eating undercooked pork. Smoking, salting, or drying the meat does not kill the larvae. Machines used to grind infected pork may contaminate other meat, such as beef.

Clinical Findings

A. Symptoms and Signs: The initial bowel penetration may cause nausea, vomiting, diarrhea, and cramps. Most patients have mild or no symptoms. In some cases, larval migration produces fever, edema (primarily of the face and eyelids), and myalgias. Many organs may be infected by the migrating larvae—diaphragm, heart, lungs, kidneys, spleen, skin, and brain. Severe cerebral involvement may be fatal. Symptoms may last months.

B. Laboratory Findings: Marked eosinophilia is the rule.

Differential Diagnosis

The classic symptoms are quite pathognomonic if one is aware of this disease. It sometimes mimics typhoid fever.

Prevention

Because a microscopic exam must be done, meat in the USA is not inspected for trichinosis. Although all states require the cooking of hog swill, hog-to-hog or hog-to-rat cycles may continue. All pork and sylvatic meat (such as bear or walrus) should be heated to at least 65 °C (149 °F). Freezing meat to at least −15 °C (5 °F) for 3 weeks may also prevent transmission.

Animals used for food should not be fed or allowed access to raw meat.

Treatment

No specific therapy is available. Thiabendazole (25 mg/kg orally twice a day for 5 days) is helpful in the intestinal phase; mebendazole and albendazole may be effective for tissue larvae. Corticosteroids are used for symptomatic therapy but may allow the mature female to produce more larvae. There is not enough data to make specific recommendations for children under 2 or for pregnant women. If exposure is recognized immediately, catharsis may eliminate some larvae before they penetrate the gut.

Prognosis

Death may occur within the first weeks, but most infections are self-limited.

Campbell WC (editor): *Trichinella and Trichinosis.* Plenum Press, 1983.

Levin ML: Treatment of trichinosis with mebendazole. *Am J Trop Med Hyg* 1983;**32**:980.

8. DRACUNCULIASIS (Guinea Worm Infection)

Dracunculus medinensis infection is common in India, Africa, and Southwest Asia. Ingestion of water containing larva-bearing small crustaceans (*Cyclops*) initiates infection. Larvae penetrate the intestinal mucosa, mature in the abdominal cavity, and migrate to the subcutaneous tissues of the lower extremities. A skin blister develops in the host over the female worm and periodically ruptures, allowing passage of eggs into warm water. Symptoms relate primarily to the local ulcer at the site of the worm, which may be visible and mechanically removed (slowly, to avoid rupture). Niridazole may decrease local inflammation and hasten worm death and removal. Metronidazole is an alternative drug.

Muller R: Guinea worm disease: Epidemiology, control, and treatment. *Bull WHO* 1979;**57**:683.

9. ONCHOCERCIASIS

Essentials of Diagnosis

- Subcutaneous nodules.
- Keratitis.
- Eosinophilia.
- *Onchocerca volvulus* on biopsy.

General Considerations

Onchocerca volvulus is a filarial nematode found in central Africa, Central America, and southern Mexico. Transmitted by the bite of the black fly (*Simulium*), the larvae develop slowly in the subcutaneous tissue. A tumor enclosing the adult worms is formed. Scalp nodules are common in the Americas, truncal nodules in Africa. Microfilariae may migrate further in subcutaneous tissue and into the eyes but do not enter the bloodstream, as do other filariae.

Clinical Findings

A. Symptoms and Signs: Pruritic, chronically pigmented nodules over bony prominences are seen in about half of patients. Migrating microfilariae in the eye cause punctate keratitis, secondary iridocyclitis, and possibly glaucoma, cataracts, and blindness.

B. Laboratory Findings Marked eosinophilia is common. Microfilariae may be present in aspirates of nodules and skin or in conjunctival snips or shavings. Adult worms are found in excised nodules.

Treatment

A. Medical Measures: Diethylcarbamazine citrate cures about 40% of cases in one course and the remainder after repeated courses. Ivermectin (150 μg/kg as a single oral dose) is also highly active against microfilariae and results in fewer side effects; it is considered the treatment of choice.

B. Surgical Measures: Excision of nodules, especially those near the eye, removes many adult worms.

Prognosis

Prognosis is excellent unless there is advanced ocular disease.

Connor DH, George GH, Gibson DW: Pathologic changes in human onchocerciasis: Implications for future research. *Trv Infect Dis* 1985;**7**:809.

Greene BM et al: Comparison of ivermectin and diethylcarbamazine in the treatment of onchocerciasis. *N Engl J Med* 1985;**313**:133.

10. FILARIASIS

Essentials of Diagnosis

- Lymphedema and inflammation of the legs and genitalia.
- Microfilariae in the blood.
- Leukocytosis and marked eosinophilia.
- Positive serology.

General Considerations

The filarial worms that cause this infection invade the bloodstream and lymphatics. Circulating microfilariae are produced. The human pathogens, *Wuchereria bancrofti* and *Brugia malayi*, are transmitted by mosquitoes. *Wuchereria* is widespread in the tropics and subtropics; *Brugia* is mainly found in India and Southeast Asia. Microfilariae deposited on human skin by mosquitoes enter the bite site and then lymphatics mature into adults, and release circulating microfilariae. Adults cause chronic lymphatic obstruction of the extremities and genitalia. *Wuchereria* usually circulate only at night; *Brugia* may be found in the daytime as well.

Nonpathogenic filariae that may be present in peripheral blood smears include *Dipetalonema perstans* (Africa and South America), *Mansonella ozzardi* (West Indies, Central and South America) and *Dirofilaria* (Florida and southern USA). The common dog heartworm, *D immitis,* is included in the latter genus and occasionally produces an asymptomatic pulmonary nodule that creates a diagnostic dilemma.

Clinical Findings

A. Symptoms and Signs: Asymptomatic infection and parasitemia may be seen with both species. By age 6, most children from endemic areas will be infected. Lymphadenopathy, usually inguinal, is common. When the adult worms die, the microfilariae disappear.

Inflammation due to adult worms causes localized areas of leg lymphangitis and episodes of epididymitis and orchitis. Fever, chills, vomiting, and malaise may persist for weeks. The chronic inflammation may result in an abscess or scarring with lymphatic obstruction; although this is the cause of the serious sequelae, it occurs in a minority of patients. Disfiguring elephantiasis results from scarring of the majority of the draining lymphatics.

B. Laboratory Findings: Early in the disease, eosinophilia occurs in up to 25% of cases. Microfilariae may be present in night blood specimens, but they decrease in number as the disease becomes chronic. A filtration technique is recommended for optimal detection of microfilariae in the blood. Differentiating the species of the filariae requires experience. A biopsy can show the adult worms but should be done carefully to avoid tissue damage. Serology is also available.

Differential Diagnosis

In endemic areas (or if the patient has traveled to such areas), fever, adenitis, or adenitis associated with eosinophilia should suggest filariasis. Other genital inflammations should be considered, such as mumps orchitis, epididymitis, or gonorrhea. Elephantiasis may resemble a hernia, hydrocele, thrombosis, or dependent edema of any cause (eg, nephrotic syndrome).

Prevention

Mosquito control and therapy of human cases is needed.

Treatment

A. Specific Measures: Single-dose ivermectin therapy rapidly eradicates microfilariae and may replace the standard diethylcarbamazine regimen of 2–3 weeks (1 mg/kg on day 1; 1 mg/kg 3 times on day 2; 2 mg/kg 3 times a day subsequently for 21 days). Neither drug reliably kills adult worms. Retreatment is often needed. Obstructive disease is not benefited by drugs; it may be surgically approached.

B. General Measures: Rest, treatment of secondary infections, and scrotal support (if needed) are recommended.

Prognosis

The prognosis is good in children with asymptomatic disease. Surgery is needed for severe elephantiasis; genital involvement may be helped more than extremity involvement.

Grove DI: Selective primary health care: Strategies for the control of disease in the developing world. 7. Filariasis. *Rev Infect Dis* 1983;**5**:933.

Kumaraswami V et al: Ivermectin for the treatment of *Wuchereria bancrofti* filariasis. *JAMA* 1988;**259**:3150.

Weller PF et al: Endemic filariasis on a Pacific island. 1. Clinical, epidemiologic, and parasitologic aspects. *Am J Trop Med Hyg* 1982;**31**:942.

11. TROPICAL EOSINOPHILIA

Symptoms of chronic cough, wheezing, and exertional dyspnea associated with generalized adenitis and splenomegaly characterize this condition. There are no specific diagnostic tests; absolute eosinophil counts over 4000/μL are usually required to support the clinical diagnosis. Chest radiographs show interstitial or nodular infiltrates.

The disease is thought to be due to an uncharacterized species of filaria, because microfilariae can be found in biopsies of nodes or other tissues. They are not found in peripheral blood. Endemic areas include southern Asia, northwest and central Africa, some parts of South America, and certain Pacific islands. Although the disorder is unusual in very young infants, all other ages may be affected. Diethylcarbamazine is often curative (2 mg/kg orally 3 times daily for 7–10 days). A longer course may be needed.

12. ANGIOSTRONGYLIASIS (Eosinophilic Meningitis, Intestinal Eosinophilic Granuloma)

Angiostrongylus cantonensis is the rat lungworm. It has an intermediate host in amphibious snails and giant land snails (found in gardens and fresh waters in the Pacific islands and in southeastern Asia). When the raw snails are ingested (usually inadvertently by young children), the larvae migrate through the liver and lung and enter the central nervous system. Eosinophilic meningitis occurs 1–4 weeks after exposure. Ocular involvement may also occur. Any age may be affected; disease severity ranges from mild to fatal.

Intestinal eosinophilic granuloma is due to infection with *Morerastrongylus (Angiostrongylus) costaricensis*. Most cases have occurred in Costa Rica. Humans inadvertently ingest the infected snails or slugs and develop abdominal pain, fever, eosinophilia, and an inflammatory intestinal mass, which is often diagnosed at laporotomy for suspected appendicitis. No medical therapy is available for either parasite.

Kuberski T, Wallace GD: Clinical manifestations of eosinophilic meningitis due to *Angiostrongylus cantonensis*. *Neurology* 1979;**29**:1566.

Loria-Cortes R, Lobo-Sanahuja JF: Clinical abdominal angiostrongylosis: A study of 116 children with intestinal eosinophilic granuloma caused by *Angiostrongylus costaricensis*. *Am J Trop Med Hyg* 1980;**29**:538.

CESTODE INFECTIONS (Flukes)

1. TAENIASIS & CYSTICERCOSIS

Essentials of Diagnosis

- Abdominal discomfort, diarrhea (taeniasis).
- Focal seizures, headaches (neurocysticercosis).
- Passage of worm segments (proglottids) and eggs in feces.
- Cysticerci present in biopsy specimens, on plain films (as calcified masses), or on CT or MRI.

General Considerations

Both the beef tapeworm (*Taenia saginata*) and the pork (*Taenia solium*) tapeworm cause taeniasis. The adults live in the intestines of humans; the egg-laden distal segments, or proglottids, break off and are passed in feces, disintegrating and releasing the ova in the soil. After ingestion in food or water by cattle or pigs, the eggs hatch and the larvae migrate to and encyst in skeletal muscle. When ingested by humans, these larvae mature into adults.

Humans can be an intermediate host for *T solium* (but not *T saginata*), and the larvae released from ingested eggs encyst in a variety of tissues, especially muscle and brain. Full larval maturation occurs in 2 months, but the cysts cause little inflammation until they die months to years later. Inflammatory edema ensues with calcification or disappearance of the cyst. A slowly expanding mass of sterile cysts at the base of the brain may cause obstructive hydrocephalus (racemose cysticercosis).

Both parasites are distributed worldwide. Contamination of foods by eggs from human feces allows infection without exposure to meat or travel to endemic areas. Asymptomatic cases are common, but neurocysticercosis is a leading cause of seizures in endemic areas.

Clinical Findings
A. Symptoms and Signs:

1. Taeniasis—In most tapeworm infections, the only clinical manifestation is the passage of fecal proglottids—white, motile bodies 1 by 2 cm. in size. They occasionally crawl out onto the skin and down the leg, especially the larger *T saginata*.

Children may harbor the adult worm for years and complain of abdominal pain, anorexia, and diarrhea. A more severe infestation may be associated with more symptoms.

2. Cysticercosis—Most cases are asymptomatic. Subcutaneous nodules of 1–2 cm may be the only sign. After several years, the cysticerci calcify and appear as radiographic opacities. Brain cysts may remain silent or cause seizures, headache, hydrocephalus, and basilar meningitis. Rarely, the spinal cord is involved. Neurocysticercosis becomes manifest an average of 5 years after exposure but may cause symptoms in the first year of life. In the eye, cysts cause bleeding, retinal detachment, and uveitis. Definitive diagnosis requires histologic demonstration of larvae or cyst membrane. Presumptive diagnosis is often made by the characteristics of the cysts seen on CT or MRI studies; the differential diagnosis may include tuberculoma, brain abscess, arachnoid cyst, and tumor. The presence of *T solium* eggs in feces is uncommon but supports the diagnosis.

B. Laboratory Findings Eggs or proglottids may be found in feces or on the perianal skin (using the tape method employed for pinworms). Eggs of both *Taenia* species are identical. The species are identified by examination of proglottids; more than 18 lateral uterine branches are present in *T saginata*, less than 12 in *T solium*.

Peripheral eosinophilia is minimal or absent. Spinal fluid eosinophilia is seen in 10–75% of cases of neurocysticercosis; its presence supports an otherwise presumptive diagnosis.

Enzyme immunoassay (EIA) titers are eventually positive in up to 98% of serum specimens and over 75% of CSF specimens in neurocysticercosis.

Treatment

A. Taeniasis: Niclosamide is relatively nontoxic and the drug of choice for all tapeworm infections. It is given as a single dose of 1 g (2 tablets) for children 11–34 kg and 1.5 gm for heavier children. The adult dose is 2 g. Tablets should be crushed or chewed well before swallowing. Paromomycin in alternative agent (11 mg/kg every 15 minutes for 4 doses). Feces free of segments or ova for 3 months suggest cure.

B. Cysticercosis: Although cysts may be removed surgically, praziquantel and albendazole have been shown to cause disappearance of noninflamed cysts. The recommended dose of praziquantel is 50 mg/kg per day in 3 divided doses for 2 weeks; that for albendazole is 15 mg/kg once daily for a month. Larval death may result in clinical worsening due to inflammatory edema. A short course of dexamethasone may decrease these symptoms, but it should not be used prophylactically because it may lower serum praziquantel levels. Once cyst inflammation is demonstrated by imaging (ring enhancement), resolution usually occurs, and therapy may not be of further benefit. The racemose cysts contain no viable larvae and do not respond to medical therapy. Follow-up scans every several months help assess the response to therapy.

Prevention

The incidence in the USA is low, because beef and pork are inspected for taeniasis. Prevention requires proper cooking of meat, careful washing of raw vegetables and fruits, treatment of intestinal carriers, avoiding the use of human excrement for fertilizer, and providing proper sanitary facilities.

Prognosis

The prognosis is good in intestinal taeniasis. Symptoms associated with a few cerebral cysts may disappear in a few months; heavy infections may cause death or chronic neurologic impairment.

Brown WJ, Voge M: Cysticercosis: A modern plague. *Pediatr Clin North Am* 1985;**32**:953.

Escobedo F et al: Albendazole therapy for neurocysticercosis. *Arch Intern Med* 1987;**147**:738.

Mitchell WG, Crawford TO: Intraparenchymal cerebral cysticercosis in children: Diagnosis and treatment. *Pediatrics* 1988;**82**:76.

Sotelo J et al: Therapy of parenchymal brain cysticercosis with praziquantel. *N Engl J Med* 1984;**310**:1001.

2. HYMENOLEPIASIS

Hymenolepis nana, the cosmopolitan human tapeworm, is a common parasite of children; *Hymenolepis diminuta*, the rat tapeworm, is rare. The former is capable of causing autoinfection, because the entire life cycle may take place in the human intestine. The larvae hatched from the ingested eggs penetrate the intestinal wall and then reenter the lumen to mature into adults. Their eggs are immediately infectious for the same or a new host. The adult is only a few centimeters long. Finding the characteristic eggs in feces is diagnostic.

H diminuta has an intermediate stage in rat fleas and other insects; children are infected when they ingest these insects.

Light infections with either tapeworm are usually asymptomatic; heavy infection can cause diarrhea and abdominal pain. The therapy is niclosamide in the same dosage as for *Taenia* infection. Paromomycin may also be used. Both drugs are given for 5–7 days, however, to allow destruction of all adults emerging from the intestinal wall.

Jones WE: Niclosamide as a treatment for *Hymenolepsis diminuta* and *Dipylidium caninum* infection in man. *Am J Trop Med Hyg* 1979;**28**:300.

Most H et al: Yomesan (niclosamide) therapy of *Hymenolepsis nana* infections. *Am J Trop Med Hyg* 1971;**20**:206.

3. DIPHYLLOBOTHRIASIS

Infection with the broad fish tapeworm, *Diphyllo-*

bothrium latum, occurs in the Scandinavian, Baltic, and Mediterranean regions; Japan, Chile, and Argentina; and in Alaska and the Great Lakes region of the USA and Canada. The adult worms attach to human intestinal mucosa. Occasionally, pain, vomiting, and diarrhea accompany the infection. Ova passed into fresh water infect copepod crustaceans (*Diaptomus*), which release larvae when eaten by a variety of fish (pike, salmon, trout, turbot, and whitefish). These first-stage larvae develop into infective forms in the muscles and connective tissue of the fish. A number of carnivores can be definitive hosts, including dogs, cats, beavers, foxes, seals, and humans. Ingestion of raw or inadequately cooked fish allows infection. Smoking or kippering does not destroy the larvae.

Rarely, progressive megaloblastic anemia occurs. as a result of vitamin B_{12} deficiency; this usually resolves after worm expulsion but may require parenteral B_{12} injections. Therapy is single-dose niclosamide (see Taeniasis). Paromomycin is an alternative.

4. ECHINOCOCCOSIS

Essentials of Diagnosis

- Cystic tumors of liver, lung, kidney, bone, brain, and other organs.
- Eosinophilia.
- Urticaria and pruritus if cysts rupture.
- Protoscoleces or daughter cysts in the primary cyst.
- Positive serology.

General Considerations

Dogs, cats, and other carnivores are the hosts for *Echinococcus granulosus.* The adult tapeworm lives in the intestine, and eggs are passed in the animal's feces. When ingested by a child, the eggs hatch, and the larvae penetrate the intestinal mucosa and disseminate in the bloodstream. The larvae produce cysts; the primary sites of involvement are the liver (60–70%) and the lungs (20–25%). A unilocular cyst is most common. Over years, it may reach 25 cm in diameter, although most are much smaller. The cysts of *Echinococcus multilocularis* are multilocular and demonstrate more rapid growth.

Clinical Findings

A. Symptoms and Signs: Clinical disease is due to pressure from the enlarging cysts, vessel erosion, and sensitization to cyst or worm antigens. Liver cysts present as slowly expanding tumors that may cause biliary obstruction. Most are in the right lobe and extend inferiorly; one-fourth are on the upper surface and may be asymptomatic for years. Omental torsion or hemorrhage from vessel erosion may occur.

Rupture of a pulmonary cyst causes coughing, dyspnea, wheezing, urticaria, chest pain, and hemoptysis; cyst and worm remnants are found in sputum. Brain cysts may cause focal neurologic signs and convulsions; renal cysts cause pain and hematuria; bone cysts cause pain.

B. Laboratory Findings: Presumptive diagnosis is made by a combination of radiographic, cytologic, and serologic findings. The appropriate body fluid (tracheal aspirate, ascitic or pleural fluid, spinal fluid, or urine, depending on the site of the cyst) should be examined for protoscoleces. Passing a large amount of fluid through a 5-μm filter and then looking for protoscoleces with an acid-fast stain or other stain has been found to be a sensitive method.

Eosinophilia is variable and may be absent. Serologic tests are useful for diagnosis and follow-up of therapy.

Diagnostic titers vary among laboratories. The bentonite flocculation test is positive at a titer of 1:5, and the indirect hemagglutination test is positive at 1:128 (Centers for Disease Control, Atlanta, GA 30333). Titers are much higher in secondary echinococcosis (due to cyst rupture). Titers remain high at least a year after surgery. They are usually negative by 10 years. Persistently elevated titers suggest persistent infection.

The skin test for echinococcosis (Casoni test) should not be used. It has never been standardized, and many false-positive results are seen.

C. Imaging: Pulmonary or bone cysts may be visible on plain films. Other imaging techniques are preferred for cysts in other organs. Visualization of daughter cysts is highly suggestive of echinococcosis.

Differential Diagnosis

Tumors, bacterial or amebic abscess, and tuberculosis (pulmonary) must be considered.

Complications

Sudden cyst rupture with anaphylaxis and death is the worst complication. If the patient survives, secondary infections from seeding of daughter cysts may occur. Segmental lung collapse, secondary bacterial infections, effects of increased intracranial pressure, and severe renal damage due to renal cysts are other potential complications.

Treatment

Definitive therapy requires meticulous surgical removal of the cysts, preceded by careful injection of the cyst with formalin or an iodine solution to sterilize infectious protoscoleces. Freezing the cyst wall and injecting silver nitrate prior to removal is another technique. A surgeon familiar with this disease should be consulted.

If the cyst leaks or ruptures, the allergic symptoms

must be managed immediately. Drug therapy for the disease may be tried in inoperable cases or when leakage of cyst fluid occurs. Both mebendazole (50 mg/kg/d) or albendazole (10 mg/kg/d) have been effective. The former has been used for 6 months, and the latter for 1 month; optimal duration of therapy has not been defined.

Prognosis

Large liver cysts may be asymptomatic for years. Surgery is often curative for lung and liver cysts but not always for cysts in other locations. Secondary disease has a much worse prognosis; about 15% of patients with this disease die.

Kammerer WS, Schantz PM: Long term follow-up of human hydatid disease (*Echinococcus granulosus*) treated with a high-dose mebendazole regimen. *Am J Trop Med Hyg* 1984;**33**:132.

Katz R, Murphy S, Kosloske A: Pulmonary echinococcosis: A pediatric disease of the Southwestern United States. *Pediatrics* 1980;**65**:1003.

Morris DL et al: Albendazole: Objective evidence of response in human hydatid disease. *JAMA* 1985;**253**:2053.

TREMATODE INFECTIONS

1. PARAGONIMIASIS, CLONORCHIASIS, FASCIOLIASIS, & FASCIOLOPSIASIS

Paragonimiasis is caused by the lung fluke *Paragonimus westermani* and occurs in Asia, South America, and parts of Africa. Carnivores acquire the infection by eating raw crabs and other crustaceans, which are the intermediate hosts carrying the encysted larvae.

The Oriental liver fluke (*Clonorchis sinensis*) and the sheep liver fluke (*Fasciola hepatica*) cause clonorchiasis and fascioliasis. *Clonorchis* encysts on fish, *Fasciola* on water plants such as watercress. Ingestion of these without cooking results in infection. *Clonorchis* is found in Asia; *Fasciola* is present throughout the world and is the only fluke found in temperate climates.

Fasciolopsis buski, the largest fluke (2–5 cm long) is also acquired by ingestion of contaminated water plants such as water chestnuts and bamboo; it causes upper intestinal infection in humans in East and Southeast Asia.

Clinical Findings

A. Paragonimiasis: The larval flukes migrate to the lungs, where they form thick-walled cysts, develop into adults, and lay eggs, inducing further inflammation. The most common symptoms are cough and hemoptysis, similar to tuberculosis. Rarely, the adult worms migrate to the brain or abdominal organs, producing seizures, paralysis, or various abdominal complaints. Although radiographic findings may suggest pulmonary disease, the diagnosis is confirmed by the presence of ova in sputum specimens (concentration improves the yield) or in stool.

B. Clonorchiasis: Once hatched in the intestine, *Clonorchis* migrates up the bile ducts; mild infections are asymptomatic, but severe infections can cause chronic obstruction. Thus, fever, tender hepatomegaly, jaundice, urticaria, and eosinophilia may be seen. Cholecystitis, stones, cirrhosis, and biliary carcinoma are serious late complications.

C. Fascioliasis: The hatched larvae penetrate the intestinal wall, enter the peritoneal cavity, and penetrate and live in the liver.

D. Fasciolopsiasis: The adults live in the upper intestine and cause pain and diarrhea. These can lead to inanition, ascites, and death. Ova of all these flukes are found in feces.

Treatment

Praziquantel (25 mg/kg 3 times daily) is given for 2 days for *Paragonimus* and *Clonorchis* and for 1 day for *Fasciolopsis*. Bithionol (30–50 mg/kg every other day for 10–15 doses) is used for *Fasciola*, which may not respond to praziquantel.

2. SCHISTOSOMIASIS

Essentials of Diagnosis

- Transient pruritic rash after exposure to fresh water.
- Fever, urticaria, arthralgias, cough, lymphadenitis, and eosinophilia.
- Weight loss, anorexia, diarrhea.
- Hematuria, dysuria.
- Eggs in stool, urine, or rectal biopsy specimens.

General Considerations

One of the most common serious parasitic diseases, schistomiasis is caused by several species of *Schistosoma* flukes; *Schistosoma japonicum*, *Schistosoma mekongi*, and *Schistosoma mansoni* involve the intestines, and *Schistosoma haematobium* the urinary tract. The first 2 are found in East and Southeast Asia; *S mansoni* in tropical Africa, the Caribbean, and parts of South America; and *S haematobium* in northern Africa.

Infection is caused by free-swimming larvae (cercariae), which emerge from the intermediate hosts, certain species of fresh-water snails. The cercariae penetrate human skin, migrate to the liver, and mature into adults, which then migrate through the portal vein to lodge in the bladder veins (*S japonicum*), superior mesenteric veins (*S mekongi, S japonicum*), or inferior mesenteric veins (*S mansoni*). Clinical disease results primarily from the inflammation caused by the many eggs that are laid in the perivascular tissues or embolize to the liver. Escape of ova into bowel or bladder lumen allows microscopic visualization and diagnosis from stool or urine specimens, as well as contamination of fresh water and infection of the snail hosts that ingest them.

Clinical Findings

Much of the population in endemic areas is infected but asymptomatic. Only heavy infections produce symptoms.

A. Symptoms and Signs: The cercarial penetration may cause a pruritic rash; larval migration may cause fever, urticaria, and cough; the maturation phase may cause tender hepatosplenomegaly followed by days to weeks of fever and malaise as the worms migrate to their final destination. Bladder infection results in dysuria, hematuria, reflux, stones, and incontinence. Secondary pyelonephritis and ureteral obstruction may occur. Intestinal infection causes pain, diarrhea (often with blood), and, finally, cirrhosis, splenomegaly, and ascites due to the chronic inflammation caused by the thousands of eggs embolized to the liver.

B. Laboratory Findings: The diagnosis is made by finding the species-specific eggs in feces (*S japonicum, S mekongi, S mansoni,* and occasionally *S haematobium*), urine (*S haematobium,* occasionally *S mansoni*). A rectal biopsy may reveal *S mansoni* and should be done if other specimens are negative. Peripheral eosinophilia is common, and eosinophils may be seen in urine.

Complications & Sequelae

The chronic inflammation in the urinary tract associated with *S haematobium* infections may result in obstructive uropathy, stones, infection, bladder cancer, fistulas, and anemia due to chronic hematuria. Spinal cord granulomas and paraplegia due to egg embolization into Batsen's plexus have been seen.

The intestinal schistosomes cause cirrhosis. Intestinal perforation and stricture are uncommon.

Prevention

The best prevention is to avoid contact with contaminated fresh water in endemic areas. Efforts to destroy the snail hosts have not been successful.

Treatment

A. Specific Measures: Praziquantel is the drug of choice for schistosomiasis. A single dose of 40 mg/kg (*S mansoni* or *S haematobium*) or 30 mg/kg twice in one day (*S japonicum* or *S mekongi*) is very effective and nontoxic. To decrease the mild enteric side effects of one dose, 20 mg/kg may be given 3 times in one day (all types).

Alternative drugs include oxamniquine (*S mansoni*), metrifonate (*S haematobium*), niridazole (*S japonicum, S mansoni,* or *S haematobium*), and antimony compounds (*S japonicum* and *S mekongi*).

B. General Measures: Medical therapy of nutritional deficiency or secondary bacterial infections may be needed. The urinary tract should be carefully evaluated in *S haematobium* infections; reconstructive surgery may be needed. Cirrhosis is treated supportively and with portal shunting if needed.

Prognosis

Medical therapy decreases the worm infestation and liver size, despite continued exposure in endemic areas. Early disease responds well to therapy, but once significant scarring or severe inflammation has occurred, eradication of the parasites is of little benefit.

II. INFECTIONS: MYCOTIC

The 3 main types of fungal infections are shown in Table 29–4. The primary pathogens, *Coccidioides, Histoplasma,* and *Blastomyces,* are restricted to certain geographic areas; prior residence in or travel to these areas, even for a brief time, is a prerequisite for inclusion in a differential diagnosis. Of these 3, *Histoplasma* is the one that may relapse years later in patients who are immunosuppressed.

Immunosuppression, foreign bodies (eg, central catheters), and broad-spectrum antimicrobial therapy are major risk factors for opportunistic fungal disease. They usually are present at least 1–2 weeks before fungal superinfections occur.

Laboratory diagnosis may be difficult because of the small number of fungi present in some lesions, the slow growth of the organism, and the lack of correlation of mucosal fungal cultures with clinical disease. A tissue biopsy with fungal stains and culture is the best method for diagnosing systemic disease. Repeated blood cultures may be negative even in the presence of intravascular infections. Positive antibody titers or skin tests suggest prior infection but rarely diagnose current disease. Tests for antibody and antigen are too insensitive to diagnose most systemic infections.

Few drugs are available for parenteral therapy. The risk of empiric treatment is greater for fungal than bacterial infections because of the toxicity of antifungals, the frequent need for prolonged parenteral administration, and the limited data available for choosing the best dose or regimen. Delay in treating systemic disease, however, may prove fatal. Susceptibility testing of fungi is not well standardized, and marked interlaboratory variation in results may be seen. Relation of in vitro susceptibility of fungi to clinical response is not well defined.

Table 29-4. Pediatric fungal infections.

Type	Host	Agents	Incidence	Diagnosis	Diagnostic Tests	Therapy	Prognosis
Superficial	Normal	*Candida* *Dermatophytes* *Sporothrix* *Malassezia*	Very common	Simple, accurate[2]	KOH prep	Topical[2]	Good
Systemic	Normal	*Coccidioides* *Histoplasma* *Blastomyces*	Common; regional	Often presumptive	Chest x-ray Skin tests Serology Culture	None or systemic	Good
Systemic	Abnormal	*Candida* *Pneumocystis*[1] *Aspergillus* *Nocardia* *Malassezia* *Zygomycetes* *Cryptococcus*	Uncommon	Difficult[3]	Tissue— biopsy, culture	Systemic, prolonged	Poor if therapy delayed

[1] Now considered a yeast. May infect many normal individuals.
[2] Sporotrichosis may require biopsy for diagnosis and systemic therapy.
[3] Except cryptococcosis which is often diagnosed by antigen detection.

Several unusual fungal infections, including actinomycosis, are presented in Table 29–5.

NORTH AMERICAN BLASTOMYCOSIS

The causative fungus, *Blastomyces dermatitidis* is a soil organism found primarily in the Mississippi and Ohio river valleys, although infections also occur in Central America. Transmission is presumably by inhalation of spores. Outbreaks associated with construction have occured.

Primary infection may be pulmonary or cutaneous. Acute symptoms include cough, chest pain, headache, weight loss, and fever occuring several weeks to months after inoculation. They are usually self-limited in normal patients. Progressive pulmonary disease may occur. Radiographic consolidation is typical; effusions, nodules, hilar nodes, and cavities are less common.

Cutaneous lesions usually represent disseminated disease, although local primary inoculation is possible. Slowly progressive ulcerating nodules are typical. Verrucous lesions may be seen. Bone disease resembles other forms of chronic osteomyelitis. Skull lesions in children and spinal involvement in adults are typical.

The genitourinary tract involvement characteristic of dissemination in adults is rare in prepubertal children. Lymph nodes, brain, and kidneys may be involved.

Diagnosis requires isolation or visualization of the fungus. Pulmonary specimens (sputum, tracheal aspirates, lung biopsy, etc) may be positive. Microscopically, the budding yeasts are large and very distinctive. The blastomycin skin test is neither sensitive nor specific. Antibody titers measured by enzyme immunoassay appear much more sensitive for detecting infection than those measured by complement fixation or immunodiffusion.

Recommended therapy is amphotericin B (30 mg/kg total dose; see Chapter 38). Hydroxystilbamidine isethionate is effective for cutaneous disease (5–8 mg/kg/d, intravenously for 30 days, maximum of 8 g).

Klein BS et al: Isolation of *Blastomyces dermatitidis* in soil associated with a large outbreak of blastomycosis in Wisconsin. *N Engl J Med* 1986;**314**:529.

Laskey WK, Serosi GA: Blastomycosis in children. *Pediatrics* 1980;**65**:111.

Steele RW, Abernathy RS: Systemic blastomycosis in children. *Pediatr Infect Dis J* 1983;**2**:304.

CANDIDIASIS

Essentials of Diagnosis

- Superficial infections in normal or immunosuppressed individuals: Oral thrush or ulcerations; vulvovaginitis; erythematous intertriginous rash with satellite lesions.
- Systemic infection in the immunosuppressed: Renal, pulmonary, or cerebral abscesses; "cotton-wool" retinal lesions; cutaneous nodules.
- Budding yeast and pseudohyphae seen in biopsy specimens, fluid, or scrapings of lesions; positive culture.

General Considerations

Disease due to *Candida* is usually caused by *Candida albicans;* similar systemic infection may be due to *Candida tropicalis,* other *Candida* species, or the closely related *Torulopsis.* In tissue, pseudohyphae are seen as well as the budding yeast phase. *Candida* grows on routine media more slowly than bacteria; growth is usually evident on agar after 2–3 days and in blood culture media in 2–7 days.

Table 29–5. Unusual fungal infections in children.

Organism	Predisposing Factors	Route of Infection	Clinical Disease	Diagnostic Tests	Therapy, Comments
Actinomyces[1] species	Dental disease, mucosal breaks, aspiration	Local invasion from colonized mucosa	Cervicofacial: chronic adenitis, sinus tracts. Thoracic: weight loss, fever, cough; effusion, sinus tracts. Abdominal: fever, pain, mass.	"Sulfur granules" (masses of branching gram-positive rods) in pus. Culture (anaerobic media).	Parenteral penicillin, 4–6 wks; then oral, 3–12 m total. Surgical drainage.
Aspergillus species	Immunosuppression	Inhalation of spores	Allergic bronchopulmonary aspergillosis: wheezing, migratory infiltrates. Progressive pulmonary: consolidation, nodules, abscesses. Disseminated: usually lung, brain; occasionally intestine, kidney, heart, bone.	Organisms in sputum; positive skin test; specific IgE antibody. Demonstrate organisms in tissues by stain or culture.	Hypersensitivity to fungal antigens, use steroids; no antifungals needed. Amphotericin B, 4–6 wks.
		Cutaneous inoculation	Focal cutaneous: pustules, hemorrhagic ulcers.	Organisms in tissue by stain or culture.	Amphotericin B (if severe).
Malassezia furfur, pachydermatis	Central venous catheter, lipid infusion (usually neonates)	Line infection from skin colonization	Sepsis; pneumonitis, thrombocytopenia.	Culture of catheter tip or catheter blood specimen on lipid-enriched media. (for M Furfur; M. pachydermatis does not need lipid)	Discontinuation of lipid may be sufficient. Remove catheter; amphotericin B. Organism ubiquitous on normal skin; requires long-chain fatty acids for growth.
Nocardia asteroides[2]	Immunosuppression or none	Inhalation(?) or from colonized mucosa	Pulmonary (pneumonia, abscess). Disseminated: lung, brain, liver, spleen, bone.	Culture; Gram and partial acid-fast stains of pus or tissue (gram-positive, partially acid-fast aerobic rods, usually branching).	Antimicrobials for weeks; drainage. Sulfonamides, trimethoprim-sulfamethoxazole. Amikacin sulfate, gentamicin adjunctive therapy for difficult cases.
N brasilienis	Minor trauma	Cutaneous	Abscess, local adenitis (resembles sporotrichosis); mycetoma.		Drainage; antimicrobials for weeks (see above).
Pseudallescheria boydii	Immunosuppression	Inhalation	Disseminated abscesses (lung, brain, liver, spleen, other).	Culture of pus or tissue.	Surgical drainage; resistant to most antifungals. Poor prognosis.
	Minor trauma	Cutaneous	Mycetoma (most common).	Yellow-white granules in pus. Culture.	Aggressive surgery; amputation may be needed.
Sporothrix schenckii	Minor trauma (thorns, splinters)	Cutaneous	Chronic skin ulcers, subcutaneous nodules along lymphatics. Pneumonia, osteomyelitis, or arthritis.	Gram or fungal stain of pus or tissue may show "hockey stick" organisms. Culture of pus, tissue.	1. Potassium iodide (oral). 2. Amphotericin B, drainage, debridement.
Zygomycetes (*Mucor, Rhizopus*)	Immunosuppression, diabetic acidosis	Inhalation, mucosal colonization, invasion of vessels or tissue	Rhinocerebral: sinus, nose, necrotizing vasculitis; central nervous system spread. Disseminated: any organ.	Broad, aseptate hyphae on tissue stains. Culture: rapidly growing, fluffy fungus.	Amphotericin B, surgical debridement. Poor prognosis.

[1]An anaerobic bacterium; *Actinomyces israelii* most common.
[2]*Nocardia* is an aerobic actinomycete.
[3]In this table, always given parenterally.

C albicans is ubiquitous and often present in small numbers on skin, mucous membranes, or in the intestinal tract. Normal bacterial flora, intact epithelial barriers, and normal lymphocyte function (manifested by skin test reactivity) prevent invasion. Disseminated infection is almost always preceded by prolonged broad-spectrum antibiotic therapy, instrumentation, or immunosuppression. Patients with diabetes mellitus are especially prone to *Candida* infection; thrush and vaginitis are most common.

Clinical Findings

A. Symptoms and Signs:

1. Oral candidiasis (thrush)—Adherent white plaques with mucosal ulceration are seen. Lesions may be few and asymptomatic, or they may be extensive, extending into the esophagus and causing pain, dysphagia, and anorexia. Thrush is very common in otherwise normal infants in the first weeks of life; it may last weeks despite topical therapy. Spontaneous thrush in older children is unusual unless they have recently received antimicrobials. Steroid inhalation for asthma greatly predisposes the patient to this problem. Infection with human immunodeficiency virus should be considered if there is no other reason.

2. Skin infection—

a. Diaper dermatitis is often due entirely or partly to *Candida*. Pronounced erythema with a sharply defined margin and satellite lesions is typical. Pustules, vesicles, papules, or scales may be seen. Any moist area, such as axillae or neck folds, may be involved.

b. Congenital skin lesions may be seen in infants born to women with *Candida* amnionitis. A red maculopapular or pustular rash is seen. Dissemination may occur.

c. Vulvovaginitis is seen in sexually active girls or diabetics. Thick, cheesy discharge with intense pruritus is typical.

d. Scattered red papules or nodules may represent cutaneous dissemination.

e. Chronic mucocutaneous candidiasis may be associated with a specific lack of T cell response to *Candida*.

f. Paronychia and onychomycosis are occasionally seen with hypoparathyroidism, adrenal insufficiency, pernicious anemia, and steatorrhea.

3. Enteric infection—Esophageal involvement in immunosuppressed patients is most common. Stomach or intestinal ulcers are also seen. A syndrome of mild diarrhea in normal individuals who have predominant *Candida* on stool culture has also been described, although *Candida* is not considered a true enteric pathogen. Its presence more often reflects recent antimicrobial therapy.

4. Pulmonary infection—Although the organism is occasionally found in respiratory secretions, demonstration of tissue invasion is needed to diagnose true *Candida* pneumonia or tracheitis. The infection may cause fever, cough, abscesses, and effusion but is rare and seen almost only in immunosuppressed patients.

5. Renal infection—Candiduria (of any quantity) may be the only manifestation of disseminated disease. More often, it is associated with instrumentation or anatomic abnormality of the urinary tract. Localized infections respond to brief local or systemic therapy. Renal abscesses and dissemination require prolonged therapy.

6. Other infections—Endocarditis, myocarditis, meningitis, and osteomyelitis are usually only seen in compromised patients.

7. Disseminated candidiasis—The clinical setting for this has been described. Mucosal colonization precedes but does not predict dissemination. Too often, dissemination mimics bacterial sepsis but fails to repond to antimicrobials. A careful search for lesions highly suggestive of disseminated *Candida* (retinal "cotton-wool" spots or dermal abscesses) should be carried out. If these findings are absent, diagnosis is often presumptively based on finding a compatible disease in a compromised patient whose symptoms have no other obvious cause, on lack of response to antimicrobials, and often on *Candida* colonization of mucosal surfaces.

B. Laboratory Findings: Budding yeast cells are easily seen in scrapings or other samples. The presence of pseudohyphae is suggestive of tissue invasion. Culture is definitive. Blood cultures may take days to yield positive results, or they may remain negative, even with disseminated disease or endocarditis. *Candida* should never be considered a contaminant in cultures from normally sterile sites. *Candida* in any number in the urine may represent true infection.

Candida antigen tests are neither sensitive nor specific. Antibody tests are not useful.

A positive skin test is common in older normal children and adults but is not diagnostic of infection. A negative skin test may be seen in normal individuals especially infants, or in compromised patients who may be infected.

Differential Diagnosis

Thrush may resemble formula, other types of ulcers, or burns. Skin lesions may resemble contact, allergic, chemical, or bacterial dermatitis, miliaria, folliculitis, or eczema. Deeper infection may resemble that due to bacteria, Herpes simplex, cytomegalovirus, toxoplasmosis, and other fungi.

Complications

Failure to recognize disseminated disease while it is still treatable is the greatest complication. Osteoarthritis and meningitis occur more often in neonates than older children. Blindness from retinitis, massive emboli from endocarditis, intestinal perforation, and abscesses in any organ are the other complications; the greater the length or degree of immunosuppression, the more complications are seen.

Treatment

A. Oral Candidiasis: In infants, oral nystatin suspension (100,000 units, 4 times a day until resolution) usually suffices. It must come in contact with the lesions because it is not systemically absorbed. Older children may use it as a mouthwash, although it is poorly tolerated due to taste. Clotrimazole troches are better tolerated. Prolonged therapy and more frequent dosing may be needed. Larger doses (up to 15 million units/d) may be needed in older children with resistant disease. Painting the lesions with a cotton swab dipped in gentian violet is visually dramatic and messy but may help refractory cases. Eradication of *Candida* from pacifiers, bottle nipples, toys, or the mother's breasts (if the infant is breast-feeding and there is monilia of the nipples) may be helpful in difficult cases.

Discontinuation of antibiotics or steroids is advised.

B. Skin Infection: Cutaneous infection usually responds to a cream containing nystatin or an imidazole. Associated inflammation, such as severe diaper dermatitis, is also helped by concurrent use of a topical mild corticosteroid cream, such as 1% hydrocortisone. The steroid should not be used alone. Keeping the area dry also helps (corn starch is a yeast nutrient and should not be used as a drying agent), as does control of secondary bacterial infection or other inciting factors. Vaginal infection is treated with clotrimazole or other antifungal suppositories or creams, usually applied once nightly for 7–14 days.

C. Renal Infection: Local candiduria may be treated with amphotericin B bladder irrigation, a short course of oral flucytosine, or fluconazole or 5–10 days of parenteral amphotericin B.

D. Systemic Infection: Systemic infection is more dangerous and resistant to therapy. Surgical drainage of abscesses or removal of infected tissue (such as a heart valve) is recommended. The clinician should administer systemic amphotericin B, beginning with 0.25 mg/kg/d and advancing by 0.25 mg/kg/d to 0.5–1 mg/kg/d. It is continued for at least 4 weeks, depending on disease response. Correcting predisposing factors is important (eg, discontinuing antibiotics and immunosuppressives, and improving control of diabetes). Addition of flucytosine (50–200 mg/kg/d orally in 4 doses; keep serum levels below 100 μg/mL) may help. Unlike amphotericin B, it penetrates tissue well; it is also synergistic with amphotericin B against many organisms. It should not be used as a single agent in serious infections because resistance develops rapidly. Leukopenia, thrombocytopenia, elevated transaminases, and enteric upset are common side effects.

Oral imidazoles, especially fluconazole, are well absorbed, reasonably nontoxic, and effective for a variety of *Candida* infections. It is the drug of choice if amphotericin is not tolerated. The dosage is 1–8 mg/kg/d in a single dose, depending on severity of infection. Experience in children and systemic infections is currently limited.

Occasionally, specific immune defects may be treatable (eg, transfer factor for chronic cutaneous candidiasis), and this treatment secondarily improves the *Candida* infection.

Prognosis

Superficial disease in normal hosts has a good prognosis; in abnormal hosts, it may be quite refractory to therapy. Early therapy of systemic disease is often curative if the underlying immune response is adequate. Prognosis is poor when therapy is delayed or when host response is poor.

Buchs S: Candida meningitis: A growing threat to premature and full term infants. *Pediatr Infect Dis J* 1985; **4**:122.

Epstein JB, Truelove EL, Izutzu KT: Oral candidiasis: Pathogenesis and host defense. *Rev Infect Dis* 1984; **6**:96.

Fisher JF et al: Urinary tract infection due to *Candida albicans*. *Rev Infect Dis* 1982;**4**:1107.

Hughes WT: Systemic candidiasis: A study of 109 fatal cases. *Pediatr Infect Dis J* 1982;**1**:11.

Robinson PA, Knirsch AK, Joseph JA: Fluconazole for life-threatening fungal infections in patients who cannot be treated with conventional antifungal agents. *Rev Infect Dis* 1990;**12**:5349.

Turner RB, Donowitz LG, Hendley JO: Consequences of candidemia for pediatric patients. *Am J Dis Child* 1985; **139**:178.

COCCIDIOIDOMYCOSIS

Essentials of Diagnosis

- Travel to an endemic area.
- Primary pulmonary form: Fever, chest pain, cough, anorexia, weight loss, and occasionally a macular rash or erythema nodosum or multiforme.
- Extrapulmonary form: Trauma followed in 1–3 weeks by an ulcer and regional adenopathy.
- Spherules seen in pus, sputum, cerebrospinal fluid, etc; positive culture.
- Positive coccidioidin skin test.
- Development of precipitating and complement-fixing antibodies.

General Considerations

This disease is caused by the dimorphic fungus *Coccidioides immitis*, which is endemic in the Southwestern USA, Mexico, and South America. Infection results from inhalation or inoculation of arthrospores (highly contagious and readily airborne in the dry climate). Rodents are naturally infected. Even brief travel in or through an endemic area may allow infection. Human-to-human transmission does not occur. Infection from accidental exposure in laboratories also occurs. About half of all infections are asymptomatic. Dissemination occurs in less than 1% of cases; the risk is much higher in Filipinos or blacks, especially in older males.

Clinical Findings
A. Symptoms and Signs:
1. Primary disease—The incubation period is 7–28 days. Symptoms vary from those of a mild

cold to severe influenzalike illness with high fever, pleurlisy, myalgias, arthralgias, headache, and anorexia. Weight loss may occur. Signs vary from none to rash, rales, pleural rubs, and signs of pulmonary consolidation.

2. Skin disease—Up to 10% of children develop erythema nodosum or multiforme. These imply a favorable host response to the organism. Primary skin inoculation sites develop indurated ulcers with local adenopathy. Contiguous involvement of skin from deep infection in nodes or bone also occurs.

3. Chronic pulmonary disease—This may be asymptomatic or associated with chronic cough (occasionally with hemoptysis), weight loss, pulmonary consolidation, effusion, cavitation, or pneumothorax.

4. Disseminated disease—This is less common in children than adults; one or more organs may be involved. The most common sites involved are bone or joint (subacute or chronic swelling, pain, redness), node, brain (slowly progressive meningeal signs, ataxia, vomiting, headache, cranial neuropathies), and kidney (dysuria, urinary frequency). As with most fungal diseases, the evolution of the illness is usually slow.

B. Laboratory Findings: Direct examination of respiratory secretions, pus, spinal fluid, or tissue may reveal the large spherules (30–60 μm). Phase-contrast microscopy is useful for demonstrating these refractile bodies; Gram or methylene blue stains are not helpful, but fungal stains are. The spherules contain many smaller endospores that can resemble yeast or other fungi if found alone in the specimen. Negative stains do not exclude the diagnosis.

The fluffy, gray-white colonies grow within 2–5 days on routine fungal or other media. They are highly infectious.

Routine laboratory tests are nonspecific. The sedimentation rate is usually elevated. Eosinophilia may occur, particularly prior to dissemination. Meningitis causes a mononuclear pleocytosis with elevated protein and mild hypoglycorrhacia.

Within 2–21 days, most patients develop a delayed hypersensitivity reaction to the skin test antigen (coccidioidin or spherulin, 0.1 mL intradermally, should produce 5 mm induration). Erythema nodosum suggests strong reactivity; the antigen should be diluted 10–100 times before use. The skin test may be negative in compromised patients or with disseminated disease. Positive reactions may remain for years and do not prove active infection.

Antibodies consist of precipitins (usually measurable by 1–3 weeks and gone by 6 weeks) and complement-fixing antibodies (elevated by several weeks and gone by 8 months, unless dissemination occurs, in which case persistent high titers may be seen). Immunodiffusion may also be used. The presence of antibody in spinal fluid diagnoses cerebral infection.

C. Imaging: Pulmonary consolidation, hilar adenopathy, effusion, thin-walled cavities, or solitary granulomas (coin lesions) may be seen. Unlike in reactivation tuberculosis, apical disease is not prominent. Bone infection causes osteolysis that enhances with technetium. Cerebral imaging may show hydrocephalus and meningitis; abscesses and calcifications are unusual. Radiographic evolution of all lesions is slow.

Differential Diagnosis

Primary pulmonary infection resembles acute viral, bacterial, or mycoplasmal infections or psittacosis; subacute presentation mimics tuberculosis, histoplasmosis and blastomycosis. Chronic pulmonary or disseminated disease must be differentiated from cancer, tuberculosis, or other fungal infections.

Complications

Dissemination of primary pulmonary disease is associated with prolonged fever (> 1 month), a negative skin test, and marked hilar adenopathy. Local pulmonary complications include effusion, empyema, and pneumothorax. Cerebral infection can cause noncommunicating hydrocephalus due to aqueductal obstruction.

Treatment

A. Specific Measures: Mild pulmonary infections require no therapy. Amphotericin B is the drug of choice for severe pulmonary disease or any form of disseminated disease. Because meningitis may be incurable, some recommend prophylactic intraventricular therapy even for disseminated disease with no documented brain involvement (see Chapter 38 for dosage).

Meningitis may best be treated with high-dose oral ketoconazole (see Chapter 38 for dosage) and intraventricular miconazole (3–5 mg daily) using a reservoir or ventricular shunt. Parenteral amphotericin B is more effective in adults. Prolonged intrathecal or intraventricular amphotericin B therapy carries a risk of adhesive arachnoiditis.

Duration of therapy is based on clinical response, normalization of laboratory values, sterilization of cultures, and antibody titer decline (in serum and cerebrospinal fluid). Outpatient therapy with parenteral amphotericin B and intraventricular therapy once or twice weekly may have to be continued for months.

Although immune stimulators such as transfer factor have been used to bolster host response, their value is not defined.

B. General Measures: Most pulmonary infections require only symptomatic therapy, self-limited activity, and good nutrition. They are not contagious. Secondary bacterial infection is unusual.

C. Surgical Measures: Excision of pulmonary cavities or abscesses may be needed. Infected nodes, sinus tracts, and bone are other operable lesions. Amphotericin B should be given prior to surgery to prevent dissemination; it is continued for 4 weeks arbitrarily or until other criteria for cure are met.

Prognosis

Most patients recover. Even with amphotericin B, however, disseminated disease may be fatal, especially in those racially predisposed to severe disease. Reversion of the skin test to negative or a rising complement-fixing antibody titer is an ominous sign. Meningitis may require lifetime therapy to prevent progression or relapse.

Ampel NM et al: Fungemia due to *Coccidioides immitis:* An analysis of 16 episodes in 15 patients and a review of the literature. *Medicine* 1986;**65:**312.

Harrison ER et al: Amphotericin B and imidazole therapy for coccidioidal meningitis. *Pediatr Infect Dis J* 1983; **2:**216.

Kafka JA, Catanzaro A: Disseminated coccidioidomycosis in children. *J Pediatr* 1981;**98:**355.

CRYPTOCOCCOSIS

Cryptococcus neoformans is a ubiquitous soil yeast. It appears to have a survival advantage in soil contaminated with bird excrement, especially that of pigeons, although most human cases do not have a history of significant contact with birds. Inhalation is the presumed route of inoculation. Infections in children are quite rare, even in heavily immunocompromised patients such as those with HIV infection. It is much more common in compromised adults. Normal individuals can also be infected. Asymptomatic carriage is not seen.

The most common clinical disease is meningitis. Symptoms of headache, vomiting, and fever occur over days to months. Cranial nerve palsies and seizures may occur. The spinal fluid usually has a lymphocytic pleocytosis; it may be completely normal in immunosuppressed patients yet grow *Cryptococcus.*

Pulmonary infection is the next most common infection and may coexist with cerebral involvement. Symptoms are nonspecific and subacute—cough, weight loss, and fatigue. Radiographic findings are usually lower lobe infiltrates or nodular densities, less often effusions, and rarely cavitation, hilar adenopathy, or calcification.

Cutaneous forms are usually secondary to dissemination. Papules, pustules, and ulcerating nodules are typical. Bones (rarely joints) may be infected; osteolytic areas are seen, and the process may resemble osteosarcoma. Many other organs can be involved with dissemination.

Laboratory findings are not specific for cryptococcosis. Direct microscopy may reveal organisms in sputum, spinal fluid, or other specimens. The india ink stain demonstrates the capsules nicely, but it is insensitive; artifacts and yeast contaminants in the ink may give false-positive results. The capsular antigen can be detected by a commercial latex agglutination test, which is both sensitive and specific. Serum, spinal fluid, and urine may be tested. False-negative cerebrospinal fluid tests have occurred. The organism grows well after several days on many routine media; for optimal culture yield, collecting and concentrating a large amount of spinal fluid (up to 10 mL) is recommended, because the number of organisms may be low.

Amphotericin B and flucytosine (150 mg/kg/d in 4 divided doses orally) are used for most systemic infections. The combination is synergistic and allows lower doses of amphotericin B to be used (final dose of 0.3 mg/kg/d). Therapy is usually 6 weeks for cerebral infections (or for 1 month after sterilization) and 8 weeks for osteomyelitis. Ketoconazole is being studied. Relapses occur in up to 25% of meningitis cases, especially with continued immunosuppression. Antigen levels should be followed every few weeks to assess the response. Disappearance is reassuring. Intraventricular therapy may be needed if response is poor.

Bennett HE et al: A comparison of amphotericin B alone and combined with flucytosine in the treatment of cryptococcal meningitis. *N Engl J Med* 1979;**301:**126.

Eng RH et al: Cryptococcal infections in patients with acquired immunodeficiency syndrome. *Am J Med* 1985; **81:**19.

Hammerschlag MR et al: Cryptococcal osteomyelitis. *Clin Pediatr (Phila)* 1982;**21:**109.

HISTOPLASMOSIS

Essentials of Diagnosis

- Residence in or travel to endemic areas.
- Pulmonary calcification.
- Hepatosplenomegaly, anemia, leukopenia.
- Positive skin test.
- Detection of the organism in smears or tissue or by culture.

General Considerations

The dimorphic fungus, *Histoplasma capsulatum,* is found in the central and eastern USA. The small yeast form (2–4 μm) is seen in tissue, especially within macrophages; the mycelial form is a slow growing, infectious, fluffy, gray-white fungus. Endemic infections are very common at all ages and are usually asymptomatic. Over two-thirds of children are infected in endemic areas. Reactivation is very rare in children; it may occur years later, usually due to significant immunosuppression. Infection is acquired by the respiratory route. Soil contamination is enhanced by the presence of bat feces or chicken or other bird feces.

Clinical Findings

Because human-to-human transmission does not occur, infection requires exposure to the endemic area—usually within the past weeks or months. Congenital infection is not seen.

A. Symptoms and Signs:

1. Asymptomatic infection—This is usually diagnosed by the presence of scattered calcifications in lungs or spleen and a positive skin test. The calcification may resemble that due to tuberculosis but may be more extensive than the usual Ghon complex.

2. Pneumonia—Acute pulmonary disease may resemble influenza, with fever, myalgia, arthralgia, and cough; the subacute form resembles infections such as tuberculosis, with weight loss, night sweats, and pleurisy. Chronic disease is unusual in children. Physical examination may be normal, or rales may be heard. Mediastinal nodes may be greatly enlarged. Effusion is uncommon. The usual duration of the disease is less than 2 weeks with complete resolution. Symptoms may last several months and still resolve without antifungal therapy.

3. Disseminated infection—Fungemia during primary infection is probably common; transient hepatosplenomegaly may occur, but resolution is the rule in normal individuals. Heavy infection, severe pulmonary disease, and immunosuppression may be followed by progressive reticuloendothelial cell infection, with anemia, fever, weight loss, organomegaly, bone marrow involvement, and death. Dissemination may occur in otherwise normal children; usually they are less than 2 years of age.

4. Other—Ocular involvement consists of multifocal choroiditis. This is usually seen in normal adults with other evidence of disseminated disease. Brain, heart valve, adrenal glands, intestine, and skin (oral ulcers, nodules) are other involved sites.

B. Laboratory Findings: Routine tests are normal or nonspecific in the benign forms. Pancytopenia is present in many cases of dissemination. Definitive diagnosis usually requires demonstration of the organism by histology or culture. Tissue yeast forms are small and may be mistaken for artifact. They are usually found in macrophages, occasionally in peripheral blood leukocytes in severe disease, but rarely in sputum, urine, or spinal fluid. Cultures of infected fluids or tissues may yield the organism after 1–6 weeks of incubation on fungal media. Mouse inoculation is also a sensitive method of isolation.

Antibodies may be detected by immunodiffusion, complement fixation, and precipitation; the latter 2 rise in the first few weeks of illness and fall unless dissemination occurs. A positive skin test (greater than 5 mm induration to histoplasmin, 0.1 mL intradermally) does not diagnose active infection; a negative skin test does not rule out infection. The skin test may itself cause seroconversion in a noninfected patient.

C. Imaging: Scattered pulmonary calcifications in a well child is typical of past infection. Bronchopneumonia occurs with acute disease, often with hilar adenopathy, occasionally with nodules, but seldom with effusion or cavity formation.

Differential Diagnosis

Pulmonary disease resembles viral infection, tuberculosis, coccidioidomycosis, and blastomycosis. Systemic disease resembles disseminated fungal or mycobacterial infection or leukemia, histiocytosis, or cancer.

Treatment

Mild infections do not require therapy. Disseminated disease in infants may respond to as little as 10 days of amphotericin B, the drug of choice, although 4–6 weeks (or 30 mg/kg total dose) is usually recommended for this and other severe forms of infection. Surgical excision of local pulmonary disease may be useful.

Prognosis

Mild infections do well. With early diagnosis and treatment, infants with disseminated disease usually recover; the prognosis worsens if immune response is poor.

Hughes WT: Hematogenous histoplasmosis in the immunocompromised child. *J Pediatr* 1984;**105**:569.

Leggiadro RJ, Barrett FF, Hughes WT: Disseminated histoplasmosis of infancy. *Pediatr Infect Dis J* 1988;**7**:799.

Weinberg GA et al: Unusual manifestations of histoplasmosis in childhood. *Pediatrics* 1983;**72**:99.

PNEUMOCYSTIS CARINII INFECTION

Recent studies have shown that this organism is a yeast, not a protozoan. The infection occurs in immunocompromised hosts, malnourished or premature infants, and occasionally in normal infants as a self-limited disease resembling viral or chlamydial pneumonitis. It presents with fever, tachypnea, cough, dyspnea, and hypoxemia. Fever and hypoxemia may precede all other findings. Bilateral, lower lobe, interstitial infiltrates without consolidation, effusion, or hilar adenopathy are the typical radiographic findings; many patterns may be seen in severely immunocompromised patients, such as those with HIV infection. Other lab tests are nonspecific, although the serum lactate dehydrogenase is markedly elevated in adult patients with HIV infection. Diffuse pulmonary uptake of gallium is also highly suggestive.

Diagnosis is based on demonstrating the round (6–8 μm) cysts in lung biopsy, bronchial brushings or washings, sputum or tracheal aspirates, or gastric aspirates. The latter 3 specimens are less sensitive but more easily obtained. Several rapid stains, as well as standard methenamine silver, are useful; all require competent laboratory evaluation because few organisms may be present.

Trimethoprim-sulfamethoxazole is the drug of choice (20 mg/kg/d of the trimethoprim plus 100 mg/ kg/d of the sulfamethoxazole in 3–4 divided oral doses for 14–21 days; the parenteral form may also be used).

Adverse reactions, especially erythema multiforme and Stevens-Johnson syndrome, are common in patients with HIV infection. Intravenous pentamidine (4 mg/kg/d) is also effective but more toxic. Combined therapy may be harmful and should not be used. A number of regimens using intermittent trimethoprim-sulfamethoxazole (eg, one-quarter of the above dose daily) are effective for prophylaxis in heavily immunosuppressed patients. For those intolerant of sulfonamides, aerosolized pentamidine once every four weeks may be used.

Respiratory isolation is recommended because spread to other immunocompromised hosts has occurred.

Davey RT, Masur H: Recent advances in the diagnosis, treatment and prevention of *Pneumocystis Carinii* pneumonia. *Antimicrob Agents Chemother* 1990; **34**:499.

Hughes WT: *Pneumocystis carinii* pneumonitis. *Chest* 1984;**85**:810.

Pearson RD, Hewlett EL: Pentamidine in the treatment of *Pneumocystis carinii* pneumonia and other protozoal diseases. *Ann Intern Med* 1985;**103**:782.

Peters SG, Prakash UB: *Pneumocystis carinii* pneumonia: Review of 53 cases. *Am J Med* 1987;**82**:73.

SELECTED REFERENCES

Parasitology

Abramowicz M (editor): Drugs for parasitic infections. *Med Lett Drugs Ther* 1988;**30**:15.

Balows A et al (editors): *Laboratory Diagnosis of Infectious Diseases: Principles and Practice.* Springer-Verlag, 1988.

Binford CH, Connor DH (editors): *Pathology of Tropical and Extraordinary Diseases.* Vols 1 and 2. Armed Forces Institute of Pathology, 1976.

James DM, Gilles HM (editors): *Human Antiparasitic Drugs: Pharmacology and Usage.* Wiley, 1985.

MacLeod CL (editor): *Parasitic Infections in Pregnancy and the Newborn.* Oxford Univ. Press, 1988.

Warren KS, Mahmoud AAF (editors): *Tropical and Geographic Medicine.* McGraw-Hill, 1989.

Mycology

Abramowicz M (editor): Drugs for the treatment of systemic fungal infections. *Med Lett Drugs Ther* 1986; **30**:15.

Bodey GP, Fainstein V (editors): *Candidiasis.* Raven Press, 1985.

Kass EH, Platt R (editors): *Current Therapy in Infectious Disease-2.* Decker, 1986.

Rippon JW: *Medical Mycology,* 3rd ed. Saunders, 1988.

Roberts SOB, Hay RJ, Mackenzie DWP: *A Clinician's Guide to Fungal Disease.* Marcel Dekker, 1984.

30

Poisoning

David G. Spoerke, MS, RPh, & Barry H. Rumack, MD

Poisonings, the fourth most common cause of death in children, result from the complex interaction of the agent, the child, and the family environment. The peak incidence is at age 2 years, and most of these episodes are not actual poisonings but ingestions that do not produce toxicity. Accidents occur most often in children under 5 years of age as a result of insecure storage of drugs, household chemicals, etc. Twenty-five percent of children will have a second episode of ingestion of a toxic substance within a year following the first one. However, repeated poisonings may be a sign of a family problem requiring intervention on the child's behalf. Accidental poisonings are unusual after age 5 years. "Poisonings" in older children and adolescents usually represent manipulative or genuine suicide attempts. Toxicity may also result in this group following the use of drugs or chemicals for their mind-altering effects.

PHARMACOLOGIC PRINCIPLES OF TOXIOCOLOGY

In the evaluation of the poisoned patient, it is important to compare the anticipated pharmacologic or toxic effects with the clinical presentation of the patient. If the history, for example, is that the patient ingested phenobarbital 30 minutes ago but the clinical examination reveals dilated pupils, tachycardia, dry mouth, absent bowel sounds, and active hallucinations, then clearly the major toxicity is anticholinergic, and therapy should be given accordingly.

Knowledge of the pharmacokinetics of the toxic agent will help the physician to plan a rational approach to definitive care after necessary life-supporting measures have been instituted.

LD50, MLD

Many health professionals, when confronted with an episode of ingestion of a potentially poisonous agent, are eager to look up the LD50 or the MLD (minimum lethal dose) because they think this information will help them decide whether or not the child is going to be ill. Unfortunately, such information is seldom of significant value, since it is usually impossible to tell how much the child has ingested,

how much has been absorbed, the metabolic status of the patient, or where the patient's response to the agent will fall in the normal distribution curve. Furthermore, these values are often not valid in humans even if the history is accurate.

Half-Life ($t_{1/2}$)

Knowledge of the $t_{1/2}$ of an agent can be confusing in the overdose situation. For example, one cannot rely upon the published $t_{1/2}$ for salicylate (2 hours) to assume rapid elimination of the drug with a concomitant short toxic course. In salicylate overdose (> 100 mg/kg), the $t_{1/2}$ is prolonged to 24–30 hours. Most published $t_{1/2}$ values are for therapeutic dosages. The $t_{1/2}$ may increase as the quantity of the ingested substance increases for many common intoxicants such as barbiturates, salicylates, and phenytoin.

Volume of Distribution (V_d)

The volume of distribution (V_d) of a drug represents the percentage of the body mass in which a drug is distributed. It is obtained by dividing the amount of drug absorbed by the blood level. With theophylline, for example, this is roughly equivalent to the body water volume and can be expressed as 0.46 L/kg body weight, or 32 L in an adult. Ethchlorvynol, a lipophilic drug, on the other hand, distributes well beyond total body water. Because the calculation produces a volume above body weight (300 L in an adult, 500% of body weight in children), this figure is frequently referred to as an **apparent volume of distribution,** a designation shared by many drugs (Table 30–1).

When a drug is differentially concentrated in body lipids or is heavily tissue- or protein-bound and has a high volume of distribution, only a small proportion of the ingested drug will be in the blood and thereby accessible to diuresis, dialysis, or exchange transfusion. On the other hand, a drug that is water-soluble and has a low volume of distribution may cross the dialysis membrane well and also respond to diuresis. The V_d can be useful in predicting which drugs will be removed by dialysis or exchange transfusion. In general, agents with a V_d greater than 1 L/kg are not significantly removable by these maneuvers.

Table 30–1. Some examples of pK_a and V_d.[1]

Drug	pK_a	Diuresis	Dialysis	Apparent V_d
Amobarbital	7.9	No	No	200–300% body weight
Amphetamine	9.8	No	Yes	60% body weight
Aspirin	3.5	Alkaline	Yes	15–40% body weight
Chlorpromazine	9.3	No	No	40–50 L/kg (2800–3500% body weight)
Codeine	8.2	No	No	5–10 L/kg (350–700% body weight)
Desipramine	10.2	No	No	30–40 L/kg (2100–2800% body weight)
Ethchlorvynol	8.7	No	No	5–10 L/kg (350–700% body weight)
Glutethimide	4.5	No	No	10–20 L/kg (700–1400% body weight)
Isoniazid	3.5	Alkaline	Yes	61% body weight
Methadone	8.3	No	No	5–10 L/kg (350–700% body weight)
Methicillin	2.8	No	Yes	60% body weight
Phenobarbital	7.4	Alkaline	Yes	75% body weight
Phenytoin	8.3	No	No	60–80% body weight
Tetracycline	7.7	No	No	200–300% body weight

[1]See Table 37–2 for additional V_d values.

Metabolism & Excretion

The route of detoxification of an agent—correlated with other information—will help in making therapeutic decisions. Methanol, for example, is metabolized to a toxic product. This metabolic step may be blocked by the administration of ethanol. Long-acting barbiturates are primarily metabolized in the liver but are also partially excreted in the urine; which means that forced diuresis will be an effective therapeutic measure. Secobarbital, a short-acting barbiturate, is poorly excreted in the urine and has a larger V_d, and forced diuresis is therefore ineffective.

Blood Levels

Care of the poisoned patient should never be guided solely by the results of laboratory measurements. Treatment should be directed first against the clinical signs and symptoms, followed by more specific therapy based on laboratory determinations. The laboratory pathologist should be given whatever information is needed regarding the history and the class of the suspected toxic agent (sedative-hypnotic, opiate, amphetamine, etc), so that the specific agent can be identified as rapidly as possible. The laboratory should know its own normal levels of therapeutic ranges so that interpretation can be rational.

Handling of Specimens

A. Vomitus and Gastric Lavage Fluid: Collect and send to the laboratory initial material produced in separate containers plus an aliquot of the remainder. Include any material that appears to be pill fragments.

B. Blood: Ask the laboratory pathologist specifically what type of container and anticoagulant are desired before drawing the sample. Inform the pathologist of the history and current physical findings.

C. Urine: Collect an initial sample—if possible, 100 mL—for analysis and then begin a timed 6- to 12-hour collection, which may be useful in determining the rate of excretion of the agent.

GENERAL TREATMENT OF POISONING

The first contact in the case of possible poisoning by ingestion involving a child under age 5 will usually be over the telephone. Proper handling of the situation by phone can significantly reduce morbidity and prevent unwarranted or excessive treatment.

After initial telephone advice has been given, a decision is made about whether the child should be seen. The decision depends upon the ingested agent, the age of the child, the time of day, the reliability of the parent, and whether child neglect is suspected.

Initial Telephone Contact

Evaluate the urgency of the situation and decide whether immediate emergency transportation to a health facility is indicated. Transportation of seriously poisoned patients should be by competent emergency rescue personnel who have suction, oxygen, and other equipment available to provide or continue emergency procedures. Determine whether the patient is in immediate danger, potential danger, or no danger.

Basic information that should be *written down* at the first telephone contact includes the patient's name, age, weight, address and telephone number, the agent and amount of agent ingested, and the time elapsed since ingestion or other exposure.

Type of Ingestion

This information is usually given by the parent in the first few words of the call. (***Example:*** "My little boy just swallowed the vitamin pills!") After a decision is made about whether the ingestion is a dangerous one and basic information has been obtained, the physician should develop more details about the suspected toxic agent. It may be difficult to obtain an accurate history. For example, an empty bottle of iron tablets may have rolled out of sight under the couch, and the parent may then assume that the empty vitamin bottle means that only the vitamin capsules have been swallowed. Obtain names of drugs or ingredients, manufacturers, prescription numbers, names and phone numbers of prescribing physician and pharmacy, etc. Find out whether the substance was shared among several children, whether it had been recently purchased, who had last used it, how full it was, and how much was spilled if any.

PREVENTING CHILDHOOD POISONINGS

Each year, thousands of children are accidentally poisoned by medicines, polishes, insecticides, drain cleaners, bleaches, household chemicals, and garage products. It is the responsibility of adults to make sure that children are not exposed to potentially toxic substances.

Here are some suggestions:

(1) Insist on packages with safety closures and learn how to use them properly.
(2) Keep household cleaning supplies, medicines, garage products, and insecticides out of the reach and sight of your child. Lock them up whenever possible. Remember the child's area of investigation and "reach."
(3) Never store food and cleaning products together. Store medicine and chemicals in original containers and never in food or beverage containers.
(4) Avoid taking medicine in your child's presence. Children love to imitate. Always call medicine by its proper name. Never suggest that medicine is "candy"—especially aspirin and children's vitamins.
(5) Read the label on all products and heed warnings and cautions. Never use medicine from an unlabeled or unreadable container. Never pour medicine in a darkened area where the label cannot be clearly seen.
(6) If you are interrupted while using a product, take it with you. It only takes a few seconds for your child to get into it.
(7) Know what your child can do physically. For example, if you have a crawling infant, keep household products stored above floor level, not beneath the kitchen sink.
(8) Keep the phone number of your doctor, poison center, hospital, police department, and fire department or paramedic emergency rescue squad near the phone.

FIRST AID FOR POISONING (Advice for Parents)

Always keep syrup of ipecac and Epsom salt (magnesium sulfate) in your home. Determine whether activated charcoal for home use is available in your area, and store it with the ipecac if obtainable. The ipecac is used to induce vomiting, and the activated charcoal is used to adsorb poisons, and Epsom salt may be used as a laxative. These drugs are used sometimes when poisons are swallowed. Use them only as instructed by your poison center or doctor, and *follow their directions for use.*

Inhaled Poisons

If smoke, gas, or fumes have been inhaled, immediately drag or carry the patient to fresh air. Then call the poison center or your doctor.

Poisons on the Skin

If the poison has been spilled on the skin or clothing, remove the clothing and flood the involved parts with water. Then wash with soapy water and rinse thoroughly. Then call the poison center or your doctor.

Swallowed Poisons

If the substance swallowed is a medicine, give nothing. If the substance is a household product or other chemical, give one glass of water or milk. Then call the poison center or your doctor. *CAUTION:* antidote labels on products may be incorrect. Do not give salt, vinegar, or lemon juice. Call before doing anything else.

Poisons in the Eye

Flush the eye with lukewarm water poured from a pitcher held 3–4 inches from the eye. Continue this flushing for 15 minutes. Call the poison center or your doctor.

DOCTOR _____
POISON CENTER _____
AMBULANCE _____
POLICE _____
FIRE DEPARTMENT _____
HOSPITAL _____

(This section may be reproduced and used for purposes of education in poison prevention. Courtesy of Rocky Mountain Poison Center, Denver, Colorado.)

Bring the Poison to the Hospital

If the patient is to be seen in the emergency department, everything in the vicinity of the patient that may be a cause of poisoning should be brought along.

Initial Therapy Over the Phone

Treatment at home should include external and internal decontamination if appropriate.

A. External:

1. Skin—If the patient has been exposed to an insecticide or has spilled a caustic agent on the skin, the area should be immediately flooded with water and washed well with soap and a soft washcloth or sponge.

2. Eye—Irrigation of the eye with plain water should begin *before* the patient arrives at the emergency room. Use plain tap water—do not try to neutralize acids or alkalies. Have the head held back over the sink and direct a gentle stream of water into the eye from the tap, or pour water into the eye from a drinking glass or pitcher. Irrigation should be continued for 15–20 minutes. Then transport the patient to the hospital for ophthalmologic examination.

B. Internal: Milk or water should be immediately administered to any patient who has ingested a strongly acid or alkaline agent. Do not give more than 15 mL/kg (250 mL maximum in a child weighing 16 kg or more). Do not induce vomiting in patients who are comatose or convulsing or who have lost the gag reflex. If vomiting occurs, the vomitus should be retained for further analysis. If emesis is induced on the way to the hospital, syrup of ipecac should be administered as described in the section on prevention of absorption (see p 932).

Poison Information

Up-to-date data on ingredients of commercial products and medications can usually be obtained from the regional poison information center. *POISINDEX® Information System* is a quarterly computerized publication that offers current data about toxic ingredients based on computer contact with over 8000 manufacturers. It is important to have the actual container at hand when calling the manufacturer so that information about serial numbers, label colors, etc, can be conveyed. In some cases, the experience of the company physician may be of value in management. *Caution:* Antidote information on labels of commercial products may be incorrect and may contain bad advice such as administration of an acidic agent like vinegar to a child who has ingested a caustic substance.

Follow-Up

In over 95% of cases of ingestion of potentially toxic substances by children, a trip to the hospital is not required. If it is decided that an ingestion is not toxic or that vomiting induced at home is the only treatment required, it is important to call the parent at 1 and 4 hours after an ingestion. If the child has actually ingested an additional unknown agent and is gradually becoming comatose or developing other symptoms, a change in management may be instituted, including transportation to the hospital. An additional call should be made 24 hours after the ingestion to begin the process of poison prevention.

Poison Prevention Over the Telephone

This may be instituted with a few simple questions about storage of hazardous substances in unsafe locations. The following is a partial list of potentially poisonous substances that must be stored safely if there are small children in the home: drain-cleaning crystals or liquid, dishwasher soap and cleaning supplies, paints and paint thinners, medicines, garden spray and other insecticide materials, automobile products, and all medications.

If it seems that there are problems that may lead to further episodes of poisoning, it will be useful to arrange an appointment with the parent to discuss the problems or to send a public health nurse to the home to examine storage practices and make suitable changes.

PREVENTION OF POISONING

A major goal of pediatricians is to reduce the number of accidental ingestions in the high-risk age group under 5 years of age. A systematic poison education effort should be part of the routine care of every patient. Parents of very young children should be encouraged to search the house and identify all hazardous substances that should be removed from the home or locked up.

The section entitled "Preventing Childhood Poisonings," reproduced on p 930, may be copied from this book and given to parents along with a bottle of syrup of ipecac at the 6-month checkup.* Reinforcement should occur at the 1-year checkup to make certain that adequate poison-proofing measures have been instituted and maintained.

INITIAL EMERGENCY ROOM CONTACT

If the decision has been made to see the child in the hospital, or if the patient has bypassed the initial phone call and is brought to the hospital emergency room—as in the case of many severe ingestions or adolescent overdoses—the following steps should be followed:

Make Certain the Patient Is Breathing

This is sometimes overlooked in the emergency room frenzy of getting intravenous lines started and searching for treatment protocols. The adequacy of

---

*No request for permission to reproduce the chart is necessary provided it is done without modification.

tidal volume should be checked, normal being 10–15 mL/kg.

Treat Shock

Initial therapy of the hypotensive patient should consist of laying the patient flat and administering colloids, blood, or isotonic solutions. Because of potential interaction and toxicity, vasopressors should be reserved for poisoned patients in shock who do not respond to these standard measures.

Treat Burns

Burns may occur following exposure to strong acid or strong alkaline agents or petroleum distillates. Burned areas should be cleaned and debrided (if extensive) and fully decontaminated by flooding with sterile saline solution or water. Skin decontamination should be performed in a patient with cutaneous exposure. Emergency department personnel in contact with a critically ill patient who has been contaminated with (for example) an organophosphate insecticide should themselves be decontaminated if their skin or clothing has been exposed to the agent. So-called barbiturate burns require treatment as for any other kind of burn. These bullous lesions, usually on the fingers, may occur following exposure to one of a wide variety of sedating agents.

Take a Pertinent History

The history should be taken from family or friends or from the patient if old enough and sufficiently alert to give useful answers to questions. It may be crucial to determine all of the kinds of toxicants in the home. These may include toxic drugs used by ill family members, chemicals associated with hobbies, occupations of family members, or purity of the water supply. Unusual eating or medication habits or other clues to the possible cause of poisoning should also be investigated.

Assess Coma, Hyperactivity, & Withdrawal

It is useful to determine the level of coma, degree of hyperactivity, or severity of withdrawal symptoms as a means of assessing the efficacy of treatment.

A. Determine the Level of Coma: Coma is graded on a scale of 0–4:

0 Asleep but can be aroused and can answer questions.

1 Comatose; withdraws from painful stimuli; reflexes intact.

2 Comatose; does *not* withdraw from painful stimuli; most reflexes intact; no respiratory or circulatory depression.

3 Comatose; most or all reflexes absent; no depression of respiration or circulation.

4 Comatose; reflexes absent; respiratory depression with cyanosis, circulatory failure, or shock.

B. Determine the Degree of Hyperactivity:

1 + Restlessness, irritability, insomnia, tremor, hyperreflexia, sweating, mydriasis, flushing.

2 + Confusion, hyperactivity, hypertension, tachypnea, tachycardia, extrasystoles, sweating, mydriasis, flushing, mild hyperpyrexia.

3 + Delirium, mania, self-injury, marked hypertension, tachycardia, cardiac arrhythmias, hyperpyrexia.

4 + The above symptoms and signs plus convulsions, coma, circulatory collapse.

C. Determine the Severity of Narcotic Withdrawal Symptoms: Score the following findings on a scale of 0–2:

Diarrhea	Insomnia
Dilated pupils	Lacrimation
Gooseflesh	Muscle cramps
Hyperactive bowel sounds	Restlessness
	Tachycardia
Hypertension	Yawning

A score of 1–5 represents mild, 6–10 moderate, and 11–15 severe withdrawal symptoms.

Seizures, which are unusual in narcotic withdrawal, indicate severe withdrawal problems.

DEFINITIVE THERAPY OF POISONING

Antidotes

There are few specific antidotes. Many of these agents are discussed in the section on treatment of specific agents. A few poisons that may require immediate antidotal therapy are listed here:

Poison	Antidote
Carbon monoxide	Oxygen
Cyanide	Sodium nitrite (pediatric dosage), sodium thiosulfate
Nitrites and nitrates	Treat methemoglobinemia with methylene blue
Organophosphate insecticides	Atropine, pralidoxime (2-PAM)
Anticholinergics	Physostigmine
Narcotics	Naloxone
Methanol, ethylene glycol	Ethanol

Prevention of Absorption

A. Emesis: Induced vomiting is *contraindicated* in patients who are comatose or convulsing, who have lost the gag reflex, or who have ingested strong acids, strong bases, or some hydrocarbons. However, in the case of hydrocarbons, vomiting should be induced if more than 1 mL/kg has been ingested, if they contain heavy metals, or if the solvent is a central nervous system depressant.

1. Ipecac method—Adult dose, 30 mL; pediatric

dose, 15 mL. Give orally and repeat once only in 20 minutes if necessary. The procedure is as follows:

a. Give ipecac orally.

b. Follow with up to 6 ounces of water or whatever fluid the child will drink (ipecac on an empty stomach is "like squeezing an empty balloon").

c. Keep the patient ambulatory.

d. After 15 minutes, stimulate the patient's throat, if necessary, to induce vomiting.

2. Other emetics—The only approved oral emetic agent is syrup of ipecac. Use of sodium chloride may lead to lethal hypernatremia. Apomorphine should not be used because its depressant effect outlasts the duration of reversal by naloxone. Other emetic agents, such as mustard and soap, are not as effective as syrup of ipecac and should be avoided.

B. Lavage: If the patient is or is becoming unconscious, is convulsing, or has lost the gag reflex, gastric lavage following endotracheal or nasotracheal intubation should be performed rather than induction of vomiting. Lavage is less effective than emesis if a small (8–16F) tube is utilized but not if the recommended 28–36F Ewald tube is used. The tube should be inserted orally, and lavage should be with warm saline solution in a small child to avoid hyponatremia or hypothermia. Save the initial aspirate for laboratory determination and lavage until the returns have been clear for 1 liter. Monitor the amount of fluid given. The amount instilled should approximate the amount removed.

Emesis and lavage recover an average of about 30% of the stomach contents. While these procedures may be helpful in reducing the amount of toxin available for absorption, approximately 70% of an ingested dose will remain. Additional measures such as charcoal and cathartics should be instituted to prevent further absorption.

C. Charcoal: Thirty grams of charcoal should be made into a slurry with a minimum of 240 mL of diluent. Give 1–2 g/kg (maximum of 100 g) per dose. The charcoal may be in an aqueous slurry or mixed with a saline cathartic or sorbitol.

In some poisonings, it may be advantageous to administer more than one dose of activated charcoal. Repeating the dose is particularly useful for those agents that undergo enterohepatic circulation or those that may slow passage through the gastrointestinal tract. When multiple doses of activated charcoal are given, repeated doses of sorbitol or saline cathartics should *not* be given. Repeated doses of cathartics may cause electrolyte imbalances and fluid loss. A few drops of anise may be added to the charcoal to improve its flavor; too much flavoring, however, can significantly reduce the adsorptive capability of charcoal. Charcoal dosing is repeated every 2–6 hours until charcoal is passed per rectum.

The patient may regurgitate some of the charcoal, but 70% is usually retained. Charcoal has been shown to reduce the half-life of an agent even when it is given after the intravenous administration of phenobarbital or theophylline.

D. Catharsis: *Caution:* Do not give cathartics containing magnesium to patients in renal failure. Pneumonitis may occur following aspiration of oil-based cathartics.

Acceptable cathartics include the following: magnesium sulfate or sodium sulfate (250 mg/kg/dose orally, maximum of 30 g); Fleet's Phospho-Soda (15–30 mL, diluted 1 to 4; give the entire amount to adolescents and about one-fourth to children); magnesium citrate (4 mL/kg/dose, maximum of 300 mL); and sorbitol (1.0–1.5 g/kg/dose, of a 35% solution, for children over 1 year of age; maximum of 50 g/dose). Sorbitol should probably be administered in a health care facility so that fluid and electrolyte status can be monitored, especially in children.

Enhancement of Urinary Excretion

Urinary excretion of certain toxins can be hastened by forced alkaline diuresis or by dialysis (hemodialysis or peritoneal dialysis).

A. Diuresis: Forced diuresis is often useful in serious poisonings (eg, salicylates, phenobarbital, and rosary peas) if the drug is excreted in the urine in active form. The technique should not be used unless it is specifically indicated because it may increase the likelihood of cerebral edema, a common cause of death in poisonings.

Hypertonic or pharmacologic diuretics should be given along with adequate fluids to increase urine flow to 3–6 mL/kg/h. Alkaline diuresis should be chosen on the basis of the toxin's pK_a, so that ionized drug will be trapped in the tubular lumen and not reabsorbed. (See Table 30–1.) Thus, if the pK_a is less than 7.5, alkaline diuresis is appropriate; if it is over 8.0, this technique will not usually be beneficial. The pK_a is usually supplied with general drug information. Osmotic load is also important, and the diuretic should be given at intervals. Proximal reabsorption will occur if adequate osmotic load is not maintained in the tubule.

1. Alkaline diuresis—Alkaline diuresis can usually be accomplished with bicarbonate. It is well to observe for potassium depletion, in which case administration of potassium citrate, which has both potassium and considerable alkalinizing ability, may be used. Potassium citrate is also available orally as K-Lyte "fizzies," which are a quite palatable form. Follow serum K^+ and observe for electrocardiographic evidence of K^+ deficiency.

2. Acid diuresis—Acid diuresis has been abandoned owing to renal complications in the face of rhabdomyolysis or myoglobinuria associated with some poisons.

B. Dialysis: Hemodialysis (or peritoneal dialysis if hemodialysis is unavailable) is useful in the poisonings listed below. Dialysis should be considered part of supportive care if the patient satisfies any of the following criteria:

1. Clinical criteria—

a. Stage 3 or 4 coma or hyperactivity that is caused by a dialyzable drug and cannot be treated by conservative means.

b. Hypotension threatening renal or hepatic function that cannot be corrected by adjusting circulating volume.

c. Apnea in a patient who cannot be ventilated.

d. Marked hyperosmolality that is not due to easily corrected fluid problems.

e. Severe acid-base disturbance not responding to therapy.

f. Severe electrolyte disturbance not responding to therapy.

g. Marked hypothermia or hyperthermia.

2. Immediate dialysis—Immediate dialysis may be considered in ethylene glycol and methanol poisoning only if acidosis is refractory and blood levels of ethanol of 100 mg/dL are consistently maintained during dialysis.

3. Dialysis indicated on basis of condition of patient—(In general, dialyze if patient is in coma deeper than level 3.)

Alcohols	Bromides	Paraldehyde
Ammonia	Calcium	Potassium
Amphetamines	Chloral hydrate	Quinidine
Anilines	Fluorides	Quinine
Antibiotics	Iodides	Salicylates
Barbiturates	Isoniazid	Strychnine
(long-acting)	Meprobamate	Thiocyanates
Boric acid		

(Other drugs may be dialyzable, but the information should be verified prior to institution of dialysis therapy.)

4. Dialysis not indicated except for support—Therapy consists of intensive care.

Antidepressants (cyclics and MAO inhibitors also)	Heroin and other opiates
Antihistamines	Methaqualone
Barbiturates (short-acting)	Methyprylon
	Oxazepam
Chlordiazepoxide	Phenothiazines
Diazepam	Phenytoin
Digitalis and related drugs	Synthetic anticholinergics and belladonna compounds
Diphenoxylate with atropine	

While the long-acting barbiturates (cleared by the kidneys) are more readily dialyzable than the short-acting ones (cleared by the liver), dialysis may be helpful if the patient satisfies the criteria for supportive dialysis needs as outlined above.

Salicylates generally respond very well to intensive alkaline diuretic therapy, but if complications such as renal failure or pulmonary edema develop, hemodialysis alone or with hemoperfusion may be helpful.

Peritoneal dialysis and **exchange transfusion** may be more useful in small children than hemodialysis, as much for fluid and electrolyte homeostasis as for poison removal.

Dialysis should *not* be performed as initial therapy but only when the criteria listed above are met.

Hemoperfusion

Perfusion of blood through charcoal- or resin-filled devices is gradually becoming more widely available in many centers. These techniques will probably allow rapid removal of many substances previously considered dialyzable but will not be likely to remove large quantities of agents with large V_ds.

MANAGEMENT OF SPECIFIC COMMON POISONS

Unless otherwise contraindicated, syrup of ipecac should be given to all conscious patients poisoned by the substances listed in the following section. Whenever possible, patients should be evaluated regarding the need for emesis, which depends on the severity of the exposure. Gastric lavage is usually indicated for comatose patients after an endotracheal tube is inserted. Apomorphine should not be used, because of the high incidence of complications.

ACETAMINOPHEN

Acetaminophen is an analgesic antipyretic contained in numerous preparations often accessible to children. In prescribed doses, the drug is a safe and effective agent for relief of fever and pain. In overdosage, acetaminophen can cause severe hepatotoxicity. The incidence of hepatotoxicity in adults and adolescents has been reported to be 10 times higher than in young children; in the latter group, only 3 of 417 patients under the age of 5 years developed transient hepatotoxicity.

Acetaminophen is normally metabolized in the liver. A small percentage of the drug goes through a pathway leading to a toxic metabolite. Normally, this nucleophilic reactant is removed harmlessly by conjugation with glutathione. In overdosage, the supply of gluthathione becomes exhausted, and the metabolite may bind covalently to hepatic macromolecules to produce necrosis.

Treatment

Treatment is to supply a surrogate glutathione by giving acetylcysteine. In the USA, it may only be given orally. Investigation protocols are available for intravenous use. Consultation may be obtained from the Rocky Mountain Poison Center (telephone number: [800] 525-6115). Blood levels should be obtained as soon as possible after 4 hours and plotted on Fig 30–1. Acetylcysteine is the drug of choice if given within 16 hours after ingestion. It is administered to patients whose acetaminophen levels plot in the toxic range on the nomogram (Fig 30–1).

The dose is 140 mg/kg orally, diluted to a 5% solution in sweet fruit juice or carbonated soft drink. The primary problems associated with administration are nausea and vomiting. After this loading dose, 70 mg/kg should be administered orally every 4 hours for 3 days. AST (SGOT), ALT (SGPT), serum bilirubin, and plasma prothrombin time should be followed closely; if the patient develops hepatic encephalopathy, supportive measures should be provided and acetylcysteine withdrawn.

Peterson RG, Rumack BH: Pharmacokinetics of acetaminophen in children. *Pediatrics* 1978;**62**:877.

Rumack BH: Acetaminophen overdose in young children. *Am J Dis Child* 1984;**138**:428.

Rumack BH et al: Acetaminophen overdose. *Arch Intern Med* 1981;**141**:380.

Smilkstein M et al: Efficacy of oral *N*-acetylcysteine in the treatment of acetaminophen overdose. *N Engl J Med* 1988;**319**:1557.

ALCOHOL, ETHYL
(Ethanol)

Alcoholic beverages, tinctures, cosmetics, and rubbing alcohol are common sources of poisoning in children. Concomitant exposure to other depressant drugs increases the seriousness of the intoxication. (Blood levels cited are for adults; comparable figures for children are not available. In most states, alcohol levels of 50–80 mg/dL are considered compatible with impaired faculties, and levels of 80–150 mg/dL are considered evidence of intoxication.)

50–150 mg/dL: Incoordination, slow reaction time, and blurred vision.

150–300 mg/dL: Visual impairment, staggering, and slurred speech. Marked hypoglycemia may be present.

300–500 mg/dL: Marked incoordination, stupor, hypoglycemia, and convulsions.

> 500 mg/dL: Coma and death, except in individuals who have developed tolerance.

Complete absorption of alcohol requires 30 minutes to 6 hours, depending upon the volume, the presence of food, the time spent in consuming the alcohol, etc. The rate of metabolic degradation is constant (about 10 mL of 50% alcohol per hour in an adult). Less than 10% is excreted in the urine. Absolute ethanol, 1 mL/kg, results in a peak blood level of about 100 mg/dL in 1 hour after ingestion. Acute intoxication and chronic alcoholism increases the risk of subarachnoid hemorrhage.

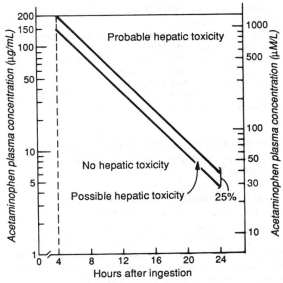

Cautions for use of this chart:
1. The time coordinates refer to time of ingestion
2. Serum levels drawn before 4 hours may not represent peak levels.
3. The graph should be used only in relation to a single acute ingestion.
4. The lower solid line 25% below the standard nomogram is included to allow for possible errors in acetaminophen plasma assays and estimated time from ingestion of an overdose.

Figure 30–1. Semilogarithmic plot of plasma acetaminophen levels versus time. (Modified and reproduced, with permission, from Rumack BH, Matthew H: Acetaminophen poisoning and toxicity. *Pediatrics* 1975; **55**:871.)

Treatment

Supportive treatment, including aggressive management of hypoglycemia and acidosis, is usually the only measure required. Glucagon does not correct the hypoglycemia, because hepatic glycogen stores are reduced. If the patient is conscious, vomiting may be induced with syrup of ipecac; however, ethanol is absorbed fairly rapidly. Monitoring of blood gases and oxygen administration are indicated in serious overdoses because death is usually caused by respiratory failure. In severe cases, cerebral edema should be treated with dexamethasone, 0.1 mg/kg intravenously every 4–6 hours. Peritoneal dialysis and hemodialysis are indicated in life-threatening intoxication.

Hammond K, Rumack B, Rodgerson D: Blood ethanol. *JAMA* 1973;**226**:63.

Leung AKC: Ethyl alcohol ingestions in children. *Clin Pediatr (Phila)* 1986;**25**:617.

Scherger DL et al: Ethyl alcohol (ethanol)-containing cologne, perfume, and aftershave ingestions in children. *Am J Dis Child* 1988;**142**:630.

Sellers EM, Kalant H: Alcohol intoxication and withdrawal. *N Engl J Med* 1976;**294**:757.

AMPHETAMINES & RELATED DRUGS (Methamphetamine, Phenmetrazine [Preludin])

Acute poisoning. Amphetamine poisoning is common because of the widespread availability of "diet pills" and the use of "speed," "crank," "crystal," and "ice" by adolescents. (Care must be taken in the interpretation of slang terms because they have multiple meanings.) Symptoms include central nervous system stimulation, anxiety, hyperactivity, hyperpyrexia, hypertension, abdominal cramps, nausea and vomiting, and inability to void urine. A toxic psychosis indistinguishable from paranoid schizophrenia may occur.

Chronic toxicity. Amphetamines are common causes of dependency and addiction. Chronic users develop such a high tolerance that more than 1500 mg of intravenous methamphetamine can be used daily. Hyperactivity, disorganization, and euphoria are followed by exhaustion, depression, and coma lasting 2–3 days. Upon awakening, the patient is ravenously hungry. Heavy users, taking more than 100 mg/d, have restlessness, incoordination of thought, insomnia, nervousness, irritability, and visual hallucinations. Psychosis may be precipitated by the chronic administration of high doses. Depression, weakness, tremors, gastrointestinal complaints, and suicidal thoughts occur frequently.

Treatment

The treatment of choice is diazepam. If this fails to reduce hyperactivity, chlorpromazine (0.5–1.0 mg/kg intravenously may repeat in 30 minutes. Maximum daily dose of 2.5–6 mg/kg.) may be used. Chlorpromazine may produce hypotension. In case of extreme agitation or hallucinations, droperidol (0.1 mg/kg/dose) or haloperidol (up to 0.1 mg/kg) parenterally has been used. When combinations of amphetamines and barbiturates (diet pills) are used, the action of the amphetamines begins first, followed by a rebound depression caused by the barbiturates. In these cases, treatment with additional barbiturates is contraindicated because of the risk of respiratory failure. Emesis or lavage, charcoal, and cathartics should be used in all cases.

Chronic users may be withdrawn rapidly from amphetamines. On the other hand, if amphetamine-barbiturate combination tablets have been used, the barbiturates must be withdrawn gradually to prevent withdrawal seizures. Psychiatric treatment should be considered.

Catravas JD et al: Haloperidol for acute amphetamine poisoning: A study in dogs. *JAMA* 1975;**231**:1340.

Cohen S: Amphetamine abuse. *JAMA* 1975;**231**:414.

Espelin DE, Done AK: Amphetamine poisoning: Effectiveness of chlorpromazine. *N Engl J Med* 1968;**278**:1361.

Gary NE, Saidi P: Methamphetamine intoxication. *Am J Med* 1978;**64**:537.

ANESTHETICS, LOCAL

Intoxication from local anesthetics may be associated with central nervous system stimulation, acidosis, delirium, shock, convulsions, and death. Methemoglobinuria has been reported following local dental analgesia.

Local anesthetics used in obstetrics cross the placental barrier and are not efficiently metabolized by the fetal liver. Mepivacaine, lidocaine, and bupivacaine can cause fetal bradycardia, neonatal depression, and death. Prilocaine causes methemoglobinemia, which should be treated if levels in the blood exceed 40% or if the patient is symptomatic.

Accidental injection of mepivacaine into the unborn infant's head during paracervical anesthesia has caused neonatal asphyxia, cyanosis, acidosis, bradycardia, convulsions, and death.

Treatment

If the anesthetic has been ingested, induced vomiting should be followed by activated charcoal. Any contaminated mucous membranes should be carefully cleansed. Oxygen administration, with assisted ventilation if necessary, is indicated. Methemoglobinemia is treated with methylene blue, 1%, 0.2 mL/kg (1 to 2 mg/kg/dose) intravenously over 5–10 minutes; this should dramatically relieve the cyanosis. Acidosis may be treated with sodium bicarbonate, seizures with diazepam. Therapeutic levels of mepivacaine, lidocaine, and procaine are less than 5 μg/mL.

Rothstein P, Dornbusch J, Shaywitz BA: Prolonged seizures associated with the use of viscous lidocaine. *J Pediatr* 1982;**101**:461.

ANTIHISTAMINES

Although antihistamines typically cause central nervous system depression, children often react paradoxically with excitement, hallucinations, delirium, tremors, and convulsions followed by central nervous system depression, respiratory failure, or cardiovascular collapse. Anticholinergic effects such as dry mouth, fixed dilated pupils, flushed face, and fever may be prominent.

Antihistamines are widely available in allergy, cold, and antiemetic preparations, and many are supplied in sustained-release forms, which increases the likelihood of dangerous overdoses. They are absorbed rapidly and metabolized by the liver, lungs, and kidneys. A potentially toxic dose of most antihistamines is 10–50 mg/kg of the most commonly used antihistamines.

Treatment

Activated charcoal should be used to delay drug absorption. Emetics may be ineffective if the antihistamine is structurally related to phenothiazines. A cathartic is indicated for sustained-release preparations. Physostigmine, 0.5–2 mg slowly intravenously, dramatically reverses the central and peripheral anticholinergic effects of antihistamines but should be used only when the anticholinergic effects are serious. Diazepam 0.1–0.2 mg/kg intravenously, can be used to control seizures. Forced diuresis is not helpful. Exchange transfusion should be considered in very severe intoxications, because most antihistamines are highly protein-bound and are concentrated in the serum.

Freedberg RS et al: Cardiogenic shock due to antihistamine overdose: Reversal with intra-aortic balloon counterpulsation. *JAMA* 1987;**257**:660.

Nigro SA: Toxic psychosis due to diphenhydramine hydrochloride. *JAMA* 1968;**203**:301.

Rumack BH et al: Ornade and anticholinergic toxicity, hypertension, hallucinations and arrhythmia. *Clin Toxicol* 1974;**7**:573.

Wallace AR, Allen E: Recovery after massive overdose of diphenhydramine and methaqualone. *Lancet* 1968; **2**:1241.

ARSENIC

Acute poisoning. Abdominal pain, vomiting, watery and bloody diarrhea, cardiovascular collapse, paresthesias, neck pain, garlic odor on breath, difficulty in walking, and exfoliative dermatitis occur. Convulsions, coma, and anuria are later signs. Inhalation may cause pulmonary edema. Death is the result of cardiovascular collapse.

Chronic toxicity. Anorexia, generalized weakness, giddiness, colic, abdominal pain, polyneuritis, dermatitis, nail changes, alopecia, and anemia often develop.

Arsenic is commonly used in insecticides (fruit tree or tobacco sprays), rodenticides, weed killers, and wallpaper. It is well absorbed primarily through the gastrointestinal and respiratory tracts, but skin absorption may occur. Arsenic can be found in the urine, hair, and nails by laboratory testing.

Poisoning with arsenic trioxide, an insoluble precursor of most arsenicals, is associated with a 12%

mortality rate. Highly toxic soluble derivatives of this compound, such as sodium arsenite, are frequently found in liquid preparations and can cause death in as many as 65% of victims. The alkyl methanearsonates found in "persistent" or "preemergence" type weed killers are relatively less soluble and do not cause deaths. Poisonings with a liquid arsenical preparation that does not contain alkyl methanearsonate compounds should be considered potentially lethal. Patients with any clinical signs other than minor gastrointestinal irritation should be treated until laboratory tests indicate that treatment is no longer necessary.

Treatment

In acute poisoning, induce vomiting and put activated charcoal into the stomach. Then immediately give dimercaprol (BAL), 2.5 mg/kg intramuscularly, and follow with 2 mg/kg intramuscularly every 4 hours. The dimercaprol-arsenic complex is dialyzable. Penicillamine 100 mg/kg orally to a maximum of 1 g/d in 4 divided doses, should be used instead of BAL after the first day or even immediately if the patient is not acutely ill. N-acetylcysteine and 2,3-dimercaptosuccinic acid (DMSA) have also been used but are not yet standard care. Dimercaprol is not effective in the treatment of arsine gas intoxication, which should be treated by exchange transfusion when the plasma hemoglobin is 1.5 g/dL or more and then by hemodialysis if there is renal damage.

Chronic arsenic intoxication should be treated with penicillamine. Collect a 24-hour baseline urine specimen and then begin chelation. If the 24-hour urine arsenic level is greater than 50 μg, continue chelation for 5 days. After 10 days, repeat the 5-day cycle once or twice depending on how soon the urine arsenic level falls below 50 μg/24 h.

Done AK: . . . and old lace. *Emergency Med* 1973;**5**:246.

Peterson RG, Rumack BH: Arsenic poisoning treated with D-penicillamine. *J Pediatr* 1977;**91**:661.

BARBITURATES

A patient who has ingested barbiturates in toxic amounts can present with a variety of findings, including confusion, poor coordination, coma, miotic or fixed dilated pupils, and increased or (more commonly) decreased respiratory effort. Respiratory acidosis is commonly associated with pulmonary atelectasis, and hypotension frequently occurs in severely poisoned patients. Ingestion of more than 6 mg of long-acting or 3 mg of short-acting barbiturates per kilogram is usually toxic; however, chronic users of barbiturates can tolerate blood levels up to 25 mg/dL.

Treatment

If the patient is awake, vomiting should be induced and activated charcoal should be given. Careful, conservative management with emphasis on maintaining a clear airway, adequate ventilation, and control of hypotension is critical. Forced alkaline diuresis is useful and often eliminates the need for dialysis. If the patient develops increasing respiratory acidosis after initial improvement during forced alkaline diuresis, pulmonary edema ("shock lung") is suggested and may require dialysis or hemoperfusion if the blood level is high. Forced alkaline diuresis or hemodialysis is not of significant help in the treatment of poisoning with short-acting barbiturates.

Analeptics are contraindicated.

Berg MJ et al: Acceleration of the body clearance of phenobarbital by oral activated charcoal. *N Engl J Med* 1982;**307**:642.

Gröschel D, Gerstein A, Rosenbaum J: Skin lesions as a diagnostic aid in barbiturate poisoning. *N Engl J Med* 1970;**283**:409.

Matthew H: Barbiturates. *Clin Toxicol* 1975;**8**:495.

BELLADONNA ALKALOIDS
(Atropine, Jimsonweed, Potato Leaves, Scopolamine, Stramonium)

Patients with atropinism have been characterized as "red as a beet, dry as a bone, and mad as a hatter." Common complaints include dry mouth; thirst; decreased sweating with hot, dry, red skin; high fever; and tachycardia that may be preceded by bradycardia. The pupils are dilated, and vision is blurred. Speech and swallowing may be impaired. Hallucinations, delirium, and coma are common. Leukocytosis may occur, confusing the diagnosis.

The onset of symptoms is quite rapid, but symptoms usually last only 3–4 hours unless large overdoses have been taken. Atropinism has been caused by normal doses of atropine or homatropine eye drops, especially in children with Down's syndrome. Many common plants and over-the-counter sleeping medications contain belladonna alkaloids.

Treatment

Emesis or lavage should be followed by activated charcoal and cathartics. Physostigmine, 0.5–2 mg slowly intravenously (can be repeated every 30 minutes as needed), dramatically reverses the central and peripheral signs of atropinism but should be used only when the anticholinergic effects are serious. Neostigmine is ineffective because it does not enter the central nervous system. High fever must be controlled. Catheterization may be needed if the patient cannot void.

Beech M, Hell C, Nightingale P: Central anticholinergic syndrome. *Lancet* 1987;**1**:1089.

Table 30–2. Clinical symptoms of carbon monoxide poisoning.

Saturation of Blood	Symptoms
0–10%	None.
10–20%	Tightness across forehead; slight headache; dilatation of cutaneous vessels.
20–30%	Headache; throbbing in temples.
30–40%	Severe headache; weakness and dizziness; dimness of vision; nausea and vomiting; collapse and syncope; increased pulse and respiratory rate.
40–50%	As above, plus increased tendency to collapse and syncope; increased pulse and respiratory rate.
50–60%	Increased pulse and respiratory rate; syncope; Cheyne-Stokes respiration; coma with intermittent convulsions.
60–70%	Coma with intermittent convulsions; depressed heart action and respiration; death possible.
70–80%	Weak pulse; depressed respiration; respiratory failure and death.

Rumack BH: Anticholinergic poisoning: Treatment with physostigmine. *Pediatrics* 1973;**52**:449.

CARBON MONOXIDE

The degree of toxicity correlates well with the carboxyhemoglobin level. Symptoms are more severe if the patient lives at a high altitude, has a high respiratory rate (ie, infants), is pregnant, or has myocardial insufficiency or lung disease. Normal blood may contain up to 5% carboxyhemoglobin.

The most prominent early clinical effect is headache. Other symptoms occur in relation to levels as shown in Table 30–2.

Proteinuria, glycosuria, elevated serum transaminase levels, or electrocardiographic changes (including ST segment and T wave abnormalities, atrial fibrillation, and interventricular block) may be present in the acute phase. Myocardial infarction most commonly occurs about a week after an acute serious exposure. Permanent cardiac, liver, renal, or central nervous system damage occasionally occurs. Even in extremely severe poisoning, central nervous system damage may be completely reversible, although months may be required for total recovery. The incidence of delayed neurologic effects is directly correlated to the initial level of consciousness.

Treatment

The biologic half-life of carbon monoxide on room air is approximately 200–300 minutes; on 100% oxygen, it is 40–90 minutes. After the level has been reduced to near zero, therapy is aimed at the nonspecific sequelae of anoxia. The addition of CO_2 is more hazardous than beneficial. A hyperbaric chamber (if readily available) at 2–2.5 atmospheres of oxygen is the ideal treatment. Hypothermia appears to be a useful adjunct to therapy. Dexamethasone, 0.1 mg/kg intravenously or intramuscularly every 4–6 hours, should be started to combat cerebral edema.

The patient should be closely observed for at least a week following severe acute poisoning, because myocardial infarction, pulmonary edema, neurologic sequelae, and myoglobinuria may occur during convalescence.

Gore I: Treatment of carbon-monoxide poisoning. *Lancet* 1970;**1**:468.

Norkool DM, Kirkpatrick JN: Treatment of acute carbon monoxide poisoning with hyperbaric oxygen: A review of 115 cases. *Ann Emerg Med* 1985;**14**:1168.

Smith JS, Brandon S: Morbidity from acute carbon monoxide poisoning at three-year follow-up. *Br Med J* 1973;**1**:318.

CAUSTICS

1. ACIDS
(Hydrochloric, Nitric, & Sulfuric Acids; Sodium Bisulfate)

Strong acids are commonly found in metal and toilet bowl cleaners, batteries, etc. Sulfuric acid is the most toxic and hydrochloric acid the least toxic of these 3 substances. However, even a few drops can be fatal if aspirated into the trachea.

Painful swallowing, mucous membrane burns, bloody emesis, abdominal pain, respiratory distress due to edema of the epiglottis, thirst, shock, and renal failure can occur. Coma and convulsions sometimes are seen terminally. Residual lesions include esophageal, gastric, and pyloric strictures as well as scars of the cornea, skin, and oropharnyx.

Treatment

Emetics and lavage are contraindicated. Water or milk (less than 15 mL/kg) is the ideal substance to dilute the ingestant, because a heat-producing chemical reaction does not occur. Take care not to induce emesis by excessive fluid administration. Alkalies should not be used. The use of gas-forming carbonates is contraindicated because they increase the likelihood of perforating already weakened tissue. Burned areas of the skin, mucous membranes, or eyes should be washed with copious amounts of warm water. Opiates for pain and antibiotics may be needed. Treatment of shock is often necessary. An endotracheal tube may be required to alleviate laryngeal edema. Esophagoscopy should be performed if the patient has significant burns or difficulty in swallowing. Acids are likely to produce gastric burns or esophageal burns. Corticosteroids may be of use.

2. BASES
(Clinitest Tablets, Clorox, Drano, Liquid-Plumr, Purex, Sani-Clor)

Alkalies produce more severe injuries than acids do. Some substances, such as Clinitest Tablets or Drano, are quite toxic, whereas the chlorinated bleaches (3–6% solutions of sodium hypochlorite) are not as toxic as formerly thought. When sodium hypochlorite comes in contact with the acid pH of the stomach, hypochlorous acid, which is very irritating to the mucous membrane and skin, is formed. However, the rapid inactivation of this substance prevents systemic toxicity from developing. If chlorinated bleach is mixed with a strong acid such as a toilet bowl cleaner or with ammonia, chlorine or chloramine is produced. Both are very irritating to the eyes and respiratory tract.

Alkalies can cause burns of the skin, mucous membranes, and eyes. Respiratory distress may be due to edema of the epiglottis, pulmonary edema resulting from inhalation of fumes, or pneumonia. Mediastinitis or other intercurrent infections or shock can occur. Perforation of the esophagus or stomach is rare.

Treatment

The skin and mucous membranes should be cleansed with copious amounts of water. A local anesthetic can be instilled in the eye if necessary to alleviate blepharospasm. The eye should be irrigated for at least 20–30 minutes. Ingestions should be treated with water or milk as a diluent. Routine esophagoscopy is no longer indicated to rule out burns of the esophagus due to chlorinated bleaches, unless an unusually large amount has been ingested or the patient is symptomatic. The absence of oral lesions does not rule out the possibility of laryngeal or esophageal burns following granular alkali ingestion. A 3-week course of corticosteroids in high doses (dexamethasone, 10 mg initially, then 1 mg every 4 hours) is indicated for the treatment of esophageal burns. Bougienage may be helpful in selected cases. Antibiotics may be needed if mediastinitis is likely, but they should not be used prophylactically.

Cello JP, Fogel RP, Boland CR: Liquid caustic ingestion: Spectrum of injury. *Arch Intern Med* 1980;**140**:501.

Gaudreault P et al: Predictability of esophageal injury from signs and symptoms: A study of caustic ingestion in 378 children. *Pediatrics* 1983;**71**:767.

Rumack BH, Burrington JP: Antidotal therapy of caustic reactions. *Clin Toxicol* 1977;**11**:27.

COCAINE

Cocaine use has become so pervasive that the pediatrician may encounter both accidental overdose and intentional misuse. Street names may include free-base, crack, rock, baseball, speedball, coke, snow, gold dust, bernice, lady, nose-candy, champagne, Dama Blanca, and rich man's drug. Freebase is prepared by treating cocaine hydrochloride with a basic solution, such as sodium hydroxide. The precipitated alkaloid is filtered, dried, and smoked. Crack is prepared by mixing the cocaine hydrochloride with baking soda and water, then heating to form a "rock," which is then smoked. Most street cocaine is adulterated. Cocaine is absorbed intranasally or via inhalation or ingestion. Effects are noted almost immediately when the drug is taken intravenously or smoked. Peak effects are delayed for about an hour when the drug is taken orally or nasally. Cocaine prevents the reuptake of endogenous catecholamines, thereby causing an initial sympathetic discharge, followed by catechol depletion after chronic abuse.

Clinical Findings

A local anesthetic and vasoconstrictor, cocaine is also a potent stimulant to both the central nervous system and the cardiovascular system. Often the initial tachycardia, hyperpnea, hypertension, and stimulation of the central nervous system are followed by coma, seizures, hypotension, and respiratory depression. In severe cases of poisoning, various arrhythmias may be seen, including sinus tachycardia, atrial arrhymias, premature ventricular contractions, bigeminy, and ventricular fibrillation. If large doses are taken intravenously, cardiac failure, arrhythmias, or hyperthermia may result in death.

Treatment

Testing for cocaine levels in blood or plasma is generally not clinically useful, but a qualitative analysis of the urine may aid in confirming the diagnosis. For severe cases, an ECG is indicated. When a teenager is suspected of being a "body packer," x-rays of the gastrointestinal tract may be warranted. Cocaine is usually smoked or taken intranasally or intravenously; for this reason, decontamination is seldom possible. When an oral dose is taken, emesis or lavage may be indicated, depending on the potential for seizures or loss of gag reflex. Activated charcoal may also be indicated. Seizures may be treated with intravenous diazepam (0.25–0.4 mg/kg to a maximum of 5 mg in children aged 1 month to 5 years and 10 mg in older children) or intravenous phenytoin (loading dose 10–15 mg/kg, maintenance 4–7 mg/kg/24h). Hypotension may be treated with standard agents. However, because cocaine abuse may deplete norepinephrine, an indirect agent such as dopamine may be less effective than a direct agent such as norepinephrine. Propranolol (0.1–0.15 mg/kg/dose, by slow intravenous administration) has

been recommended for symptomatic or life-threatening supraventricular or ventricular arrhythmias.

CONTRACEPTIVE PILLS

The only known toxic effects following acute ingestion of oral contraceptive agents are nausea, vomiting, and vaginal bleeding in girls.

COSMETICS & RELATED PRODUCTS

The relative toxicities of commonly ingested products in this group are listed in Table 30–3.

Permanent wave neutralizers may contain bromates, peroxides, or perborates. Bromates have been removed from most products because they can cause nausea, vomiting, abdominal pain, shock, hemolysis, renal failure, and convulsions. Four grams of bromate salts is potentially lethal. Poisoning is treated by induced emesis or gastric lavage with 1% sodium thiosulfate followed by demulcents to relieve gastric irritation. Sodium bicarbonate, 2%, in the lavage may reduce hydrobromic acid formation. Sodium thiosulfate, 1%, 100–500 mL, can be given intravenously, but methylene blue should not be used to treat methemoglobinemia in this situation, because it increases the toxicity of bromates. Dialysis is indicated in renal failure but does not enhance renal excretion of bromate. Perborate can cause boric acid poisoning.

Fingernail polish removers used to contain toluene or aliphatic acetates, which produce central nervous system irritation and depression. They now usually have an acetone base, which does not require specific treatment other than monitoring central nervous system status.

Cobalt, copper, cadmium, iron, lead, nickel, silver, bismuth, and tin are sometimes found in metallic hair dyes. In large amounts, they can cause skin

Table 30–3. Relative toxicities of cosmetics and similar products.

High toxicity	Low toxicity
Permanent wave	Perfume
neutralizers	Hair removers
	Deodorants
Moderate toxicity	Bath salts
Fingernail polish	
Fingernail polish remover	**No toxicity**
Metallic hair dyes	Liquid makeup
Home permanent wave	Vegetable hair dye
lotion	Cleansing cream
Bath oil	Hair dressing
Shaving lotion	(nonalcoholic)
Hair tonic (alcoholic)	Hand lotion or cream
Cologne, toilet water	Lipstick

sensitization, urticaria, dermatitis, eye damage, vertigo, hypertension, asthma, methemoglobinemia, tremors, convulsions, and coma. Treatment for ingestions is to administer demulcents and the appropriate antidote for the heavy metal involved.

Home permanent wave lotions, hair straighteners, and hair removers usually contain thioglycolic acid salts, which cause alkaline irritation and perhaps central nervous system depression.

Shaving lotion, hair tonic, hair straighteners, cologne, and toilet water contain denatured alcohol, which can cause central nervous system depression and hypoglycemia.

Deodorants usually consist of an antibacterial agent in a cream base. Antiperspirants are aluminum salts, which frequently cause skin sensitization. Zirconium oxide can cause granulomas in the axilla.

Chronic inhalation of hair sprays containing synthetic and natural resins has reportedly caused thesaurosis (hilar lymphadenopathy and diffuse pulmonary infiltration) as well as ocular irritation and keratitis.

Arena JM & Drew RH: *Poisoning: Toxicology, Symptoms, Treatments,* 5th ed. Thomas Springfield, 1986.

CYCLIC ANTIDEPRESSANTS

Cyclic antidepressants (amitriptyline, imipramine, etc) are utilized by adolescents and adults as antidepressants. Unfortunately, these drugs have a very low toxic:therapeutic ratio, and in a young child even a moderate overdose can have a disastrous effect. The 5 features of cyclic antidepressant overdosage that make it more of a problem than other drugs with anticholinergic properties are arrhythmias, coma, convulsions, hypertension (and, later, hypotension), and hallucinations. These may be life-threatening and require rapid intervention. One agent, amoxapine, differs in that it has a lower incidence of cardiovascular complications, and seizures may be associated with normal QRS complexes.

If the patient has symptoms—dry mouth, tachycardia, etc—an ECG should be taken. If there is any arrhythmias, the patient should be admitted and monitored until free of irregularity for 24 hours. Another indication for monitoring is tachycardia of more than 110 beats/min plus additional findings of anticholinergic toxicity. The onset of arrhythmias is rare beyond 24 hours after ingestion.

Treatment

Phenytoin or lidocaine may be used primarily for treatment of arrhythmias, and physostigmine for tachyarrhythmia. Alkalinization with sodium bicarbonate, 0.5 mEq/kg intravenously, or hyperventilation may dramatically reverse *ventricular* arrhythmias. Sodium bicarbonate should be administered to all patients with significant arrhythmias to achieve a plasma pH of 7.5–7.6. Forced diuresis is contraindicated. A QRS interval greater than 100 ms specifically identifies patients with major cyclic antidepressant overdosage. Diazepam should be given for convulsions.

Physostigmine is antidotal, but it is a dangerous drug that must be given slowly to avoid iatrogenic convulsions. It is contraindicated in asthma, vascular gangrene, or urinary tract obstruction. The dosage is as follows: (1) For children under 12 years of age, give 0.5 mg intravenously over 60 seconds. If there is no effect, the dose may be repeated at 5-minute intervals to a maximum of 2 mg. Repeat as necessary only for life-threatening situations. (2) For adolescents and adults, give 2 mg intravenously over 60 seconds. If there is no effect, repeat in 10 minutes to a maximum dose of 4 mg. Repeat for *life-threatening* situations.

Hypotension is a major problem. Cyclic antidepressants block the reuptake of catecholamines, thereby producing a rebound hypotension following initial hypertension. Treatment with physostigmine is not effective. Infusion of sodium bicarbonate helps avert hypotension. Vasopressors are generally ineffective, and the mortality rate is 60% in patients with hypotension who prove unresponsive to initial fluids. Orogastric charcoal, 1–2 g/kg every 2–6 hours during the first 24 hours following ingestion, appears to interrupt an enterohepatic recirculation of cyclic antidepressants and shorten the plasma $t_{1/2}$.

Callahan M et al: Epidemiology of fatal tricyclic antidepressant ingestion. *Ann Emerg Med* 1985;**14**:1.
Kulig K et al: Amoxapine overdose: Coma and seizures without cardiotoxic effects. *JAMA* 1982;**248**:1092.
Swartz CM et al: The treatment of tricyclic antidepressant overdose with repeated charcoal. *J Clin Psychopharmacol* 1984;**4**:336.

DIGITALIS & OTHER CARDIAC GLYCOSIDES

Manifestations include nausea, vomiting, diarrhea, headache, delirium, confusion, and, occasionally, coma. Cardiac irregularities such as atrial fibrillation, paroxysmal atrial tachycardia, and atrial flutter often occur. Death usually is the result of ventricular fibrillation.

Transplacental intoxication by digitalis has been reported. An accurate radioimmunoassay for digitalis is now available.

Treatment

If vomiting has not occurred, induce emesis or provide lavage followed by charcoal and cathartics.

Potassium should not be given in acute overdosage unless there is laboratory evidence of hypokalemia. In acute overdosage, hyperkalemia is more common.

The patient must be monitored carefully for electrocardiographic changes. The correction of acidosis better demonstrates the degree of potassium deficiency present. In some cases, phenytoin, a β-adrenergic blocking agent such as propranolol, or procainamide is necessary to correct arrhythmias. A pacemaker may be needed.

Clinical investigations using digoxin antibody fragments (Fab), supplied by Burroughs Wellcome Company, indicate that this is the most effective agent for treatment of cardiac glycoside poisoning and should be considered in those who are severely poisoned and fail to respond to other therapy. Specific indications for use of fab fragments are available in product literature.

Rumack BH et al: Phenytoin (diphenylhydantoin) treatment of massive digoxin overdose. *Br Heart J* 1974; **36**:405.

Wenger TL et al: Treatment of 63 severely digitalis-toxic patients with digoxin-specific antibody fragments. *J Am Coll Cardiol* 1985;**5**:118A.

DIPHENOXYLATE HYDROCHLORIDE (Lomotil)

Lomotil is a combination of diphenoxylate hydrochloride, a synthetic narcotic, and atropine sulfate. Early signs of Lomotil intoxication are due to its anticholinergic effect and consist of fever, facial flush, tachypnea, and lethargy. However, the miotic effect of the narcotic predominates. Later, hypothermia, increasing central nervous system depression, and loss of the facial flush occur. Seizures are probably secondary to hypoxia. Small amounts of Lomotil are potentially lethal when ingested by children; it is contraindicated in children under age 2 years.

Treatment

After an adequate airway has been established with an endotracheal tube, gastric lavage may be useful because of the prolonged delay in gastric emptying time. Activated charcoal may be of use. Naloxone hydrochloride (0.4–2.0 mg intravenously in children and adults) should be given.

A transient improvement in respiratory status may be followed by respiratory depression, because the duration of action of diphenoxylate is considerably longer than that of the antagonists. Repeated doses may be required. The anticholinergic effects do not usually require treatment but in severe cases can be reversed temporarily by the use of physostigmine, 0.5–2 mg slowly intravenously.

Rumack BH, Temple AR: Lomotil poisoning. *Pediatrics* 1974;**53**:495.

DISINFECTANTS & DEODORIZERS

1. NAPHTHALENE

Naphthalene is commonly found in mothballs, disinfectants, and deodorizers.

Naphthalene's toxicity is often not fully appreciated. It is absorbed not only when ingested but also through the skin and lungs. Naphthalene is very soluble in oil and relatively insoluble in water. It is potentially hazardous to store baby clothes in naphthalene because baby oil is an excellent solvent that may increase absorption of the drug through the skin.

Metabolic products of naphthalene cause a severe hemolytic anemia, similar to that due to primaquine toxicity, 2–7 days after ingestion. Other physical findings include vomiting, diarrhea, jaundice, oliguria, anuria, coma, and convulsions. The urine may contain hemoglobin, protein, and casts.

Treatment

Induced vomiting should be followed by activated charcoal and a cathartic. Forced alkaline diuresis prevents blocking of the renal tubules by acid hematin crystals. Repeated small blood transfusions may be necessary to bring the hemoglobin level up to 60–80% of normal. Corticosteroids may be useful in minimizing naphthalene hemolysis. Anuria may persist for 1–2 weeks and still be completely reversible.

2. p-DICHLOROBENZENE, PHENOLIC ACIDS, & OTHERS

Disinfectants and deodorizers containing p-dichlorobenzene or sodium sulfate are much less toxic than those containing naphthalene. Disinfectants containing phenolic acids are highly toxic, especially if they contain a borate ion. Phenol precipitates tissue proteins and causes respiratory alkalosis followed by metabolic acidosis. Some phenols cause methemoglobinemia.

Local gangrene occurs after prolonged contact with tissue. Phenol is readily absorbed from the gastrointestinal tract, causing diffuse capillary damage and, in some cases, methemoglobinemia. Pentachlorophenol, which has been used in terminal rinsing of diapers, has caused infant fatalities.

The toxicity of alkalies, quaternary ammonium compounds, pine oil, and halogenated disinfectants varies with the concentration of active ingredients. Wick deodorizers are usually of moderate toxicity. Iodophor disinfectants are the safest. Spray deodorizers are not usually toxic, because a child is not likely to swallow a very large dose.

Manifestations of acute quaternary ammonium compound ingestion include diaphoresis, strong irritation, thirst, vomiting, diarrhea, cyanosis, hyperactivity, coma, convulsions, hypotension, abdominal pain, and pulmonary edema. Acute liver or renal failure may develop later.

Treatment

Activated charcoal may be used prior to gastric lavage. Castor oil dissolves phenol and may retard its absorption. This property of castor oil, however, has not been proved clinically. Mineral oil and alcohol are contraindicated because they increase the gastric absorption of phenol. A cathartic may be useful. The metabolic acidosis must be carefully managed. Anticonvulsants or measures to treat shock may be needed.

Because phenols are absorbed through the skin, exposed areas should be irrigated copiously with water. Undiluted polyethylene glycol may be a useful solvent as well.

Pegg SP, Campbell DC: Children's burns due to cresol. *Burns* 1985;**11**:294.

DISK BATTERY

Small, flat, smooth disk-shaped batteries are used in watches, calculators, hearing aids, games, etc. They measure between 10 and 25 mm in diameter. In the past, treatment for disk battery ingestion was the same as for other smooth foreign bodies such as coins. It is now known that batteries are associated with different hazards and may represent a major emergency.

Batteries impacted in the esophagus may, like any other foreign body, cause presenting symptoms of refusal to take food, increased salivation, vomiting with or without blood, and pain or discomfort. Aspiration into the trachea may also occur. Fatalities have been reported in association with esophageal perforation.

When a history of disk battery ingestion is obtained, x-rays of the entire respiratory tract and gastrointestinal tract should be taken so that the battery can be located and the proper therapy determined. Generally, batteries less than 15.6 mm in diameter do not lodge in the esophagus.

Treatment

If the disk battery is located in the esophagus, it must be removed immediately. If ingestion occurred within the previous 24-hour period, the battery may be removed by the balloon catheter technique. The patient is placed in the steep head-down, prone-oblique position. The catheter is placed beyond the object; the balloon is inflated with barium; and the catheter is withdrawn. If the battery has been in the esophagus for more than 24 hours, the risk of caustic burn is greater, and removal by endoscopic means may be necessary.

Location of the disk battery below the esophagus has been associated with erosion, tissue damage, and colored residue in the stomach and bowel, but the course has been benign in most cases. Perforated Meckel's diverticulum has been the major complication. It may take as long as 7 days for spontaneous passage to occur, and lack of movement in the gastrointestinal tract may not be a reason for removal in an asymptomatic patient. Some have suggested repeated x-rays and surgical intervention if passage of the battery pauses, but this approach may be excessive. Batteries that have opened in the gastrointestinal tract have been associated with some toxicity due to mercury, but the patients have recovered.

Emesis is ineffective in removal of the battery from the stomach. Asymptomatic patients may simply be observed and stools examined for passage of the battery. If the battery has not passed within 7 days or if the patient becomes symptomatic, x-rays should be repeated. If the battery has come apart or appears not to be moving, a purgative, enema, or nonabsorbable intestinal lavage solution should be administered. If these methods are not successful, surgical intervention may be required. Levels of heavy metals (mainly of mercury) should be measured in patients in whom the battery has opened or symptoms have developed.

Kulig K et al: Elevated mercury levels after ingestion of a disk battery. *JAMA* 1983;**249**:2502.
Litovitz TL: Button battery ingestions. *JAMA* 1983;**249**:2495.
Rumack BH, Rumack CM: Disk battery ingestion. *JAMA* 1983;**249**:2509.
Votteler TP, Nash JC, Rutledge JC: The hazard of ingested alkaline disk batteries in children. *JAMA* 1983;**249**:2504.

HYDROCARBONS
(Benzene, Charcoal Lighter Fluid, Gasoline, Kerosene, Petroleum Distillates, Turpentine)

Ingestion causes irritation of mucous membranes, vomiting, blood-tinged diarrhea, respiratory distress, cyanosis, tachycardia, and fever. Although a small amount of certain hydrocarbons (10 mL) is potentially fatal, patients have survived ingestion of several ounces of other petroleum distillates. The more aromatic a hydrocarbon and the lower its viscosity rating, the more potentially toxic it is. Benzene, gasoline, kerosene, and red seal oil furniture polish are the most dangerous. A dose exceeding 1 mL/kg is likely to cause central nervous system depression. A history of coughing or choking, as well as vomiting, suggests aspiration with resulting hydrocarbon pneumonia. This is an acute hemorrhagic necrotizing disease that usually develops within 24 hours of the ingestion and resolves without sequelae in 3–5 days.

However, several weeks may be required for full resolution of a hydrocarbon pneumonia. Pneumonia may be caused by the aspiration of a few drops of petroleum distillate into the lung or by absorption from the circulatory system. Pulmonary edema and hemorrhage, cardiac dilatation and, arrhythmias hepatosplenomegaly, proteinuria, and hematuria can occur following large overdoses. Hypoglycemia is occasionally present. A chest film may reveal pneumonia shortly after the ingestion. An abnormal urinalysis in a child with a previously normal urinary tract suggests a large overdose.

Treatment

Both emetics and lavage should be avoided when only a small amount has been ingested. It is impossible to do a "cautious gastric lavage" unless a cuffed endotracheal tube is inserted. Under these circumstances, gastric lavage may be done using saline. Following lavage, magnesium or sodium sulfate should be left in the stomach. (Mineral oil should not be given, because it is capable of causing a low-grade lipoid pneumonia.)

Emetics are probably preferable to gastric lavage if massive ingestion has occurred. Epinephrine should not be used with halogenated hydrocarbons because it may affect an already sensitized myocardium. Analeptic drugs are contraindicated. The usefulness of corticosteroids is debated, and antibiotics should be reserved for patients with infections. Oxygen and mist are helpful.

Anas N, Namasonthi V, Ginsburg C: Criteria for hospitalizing children who have ingested products containing hydrocarbons. *JAMA* 1981;**246**:840.

Brown J et al: Experimental kerosene pneumonia. *J Pediatr* 1984;**84**:396.

Kulig K, Rumack BH: Hydrocarbon ingestion. *Curr Top Emerg Med* 1981;**3**:1.

IBUPROFEN

Ibuprofen is an anti-inflammatory and analgesic agent that has become very popular since it was made available as an over-the-counter drug. Most exposures in children do not produce symptoms (see Fig 30–2); in one study, for example, children ingesting up to 2.4 g remained asymptomatic. When symptoms do occur, the most common are abdominal pain, vomiting, drowsiness, and lethargy. In more unusual manifestations symptomatology include apnea (especially in young children), seizures, metabolic acidosis, and central nervous system depression leading to coma.

Treatment

If a child has ingested less than 100 mg/kg, dilution with water or milk may be all that is necessary to minimize the gastrointestinal upset, which occurs

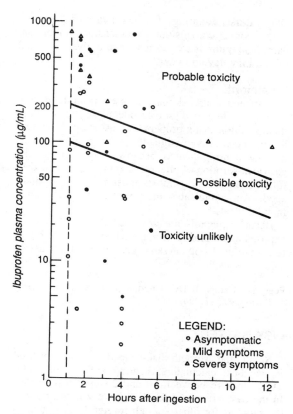

Figure 30–2. Nomogram relating ibuprofen plasma concentration and expected severity of intoxication at varying intervals following ingestion of ibuprofen. (Modified and reproduced, with permission, from Hall AH et al: Ibuprofen overdose: 126 cases. *Ann Emerg Med* 1986; **15**:1308.

even with therapeutic amounts. In children, the volume of liquid used for dilution should be less than 4 ounces. When the ingested amount is more than 500 mg/kg, there is a potential for seizures or central nervous system depression; therefore, gastric lavage may be preferred to emesis. If the ingested amount is between 100 and 400 mg/kg, emesis may be of equal value. Activated charcoal and a cathartic may also be of some value. Multiple doses of activated charcoal have also been suggested because of the possibility of enterohepatic circulation. There is no specific antidote; other treatment consists of good supportive care, eg, monitoring for hypotension, seizures, acidosis, and gastrointestinal bleeding. Neither alkalinization of the urine nor hemodialysis has been proved helpful.

Hall AH, Rumack BH: Treatment of patients with ibuprofen overdose. *Ann Emerg Med* 1988;**17**:185.

Hall AH et al: Ibuprofen overdose: 126 cases. *Ann Emerg Med* 1986;**15**:1308.

Hall AH et al: Ibuprofen overdose: A prospective study. *West J Med* 1988;**148**:653.

Perry SJ, Streete PJ, Volans GN: Ibuprofen overdose: The first 2 years of over-the-counter sales. *Hum Toxicol* 1987;**6**:173.

INSECT STINGS
(Bee, Wasp, & Hornet)

Insect stings are painful but not usually dangerous; however, these insects cause more deaths in the USA than snakes do. Deaths from insect stings are usually due to severe allergic reactions. Bee venom, for example, has hemolytic, neurotoxic, and histaminelike activities that can on rare occasions cause hemoglobinuria and severe anaphylactoid reactions.

Treatment

The physician should remove the stinger, taking care not to squeeze the attached venom sac. For allergic reactions, epinephrine 1:1000 solution, 0.01 mL/kg, should be administered intravenously or subcutaneously above the site of the sting. Three to 4 whiffs from an isoproterenol aerosol inhaler may be given at 3- to 4-minute intervals as needed. Corticosteroids (hydrocortisone), 100 mg intravenously, and diphenhydramine, 1.5 mg/kg intravenously, are useful ancillary drugs but have no immediate effect. Ephedrine or antihistamines may be used for 2 or 3 days to prevent recurrence of symptoms.

A patient who has had a potentially life-threatening insect sting should be desensitized against the Hymenoptera group, because the honey bee, wasp, hornet, and yellow jacket have common antigens in their venom.

For the more usual stings, cold compresses, aspirin, and diphenhydramine 1 mg/kg orally, are useful.

Russell F et al: Insect and scorpion bites and stings. *JAMA* 1973;**224**:131.

Yunginger JW: Advances in the diagnosis and treatment of stinging insect allergy. *Pediatrics* 1981;**67**:325.

INSECTICIDES

The petroleum distillates or other organic solvents used in these products are often as toxic as the pesticide. Unless otherwise indicated, induced vomiting or gastric lavage is warranted after insertion of an endotracheal tube.

DePalma AE, Kwalich DS, Zukerberg N: Pesticide poisoning in children. *JAMA* 1970;**211**:1979.

Rumack BH, Spoerke DG (editors): *POISINDEX ® Information System.* Micromedex, Inc., Denver, Colorado. [Published quarterly.]

1. CHLORINATED HYDROCARBONS (Aldrin, Carbinol, Chlordane, DDT, Dieldrin, Endrin, Heptachlor, Lindane, Toxaphene, Etc)

Signs of intoxication include salivation, gastrointestinal irritability, abdominal pain, nausea, vomiting, diarrhea, central nervous system depression, and convulsions. Inhalation exposure causes irritation of the eyes, nose, and throat; blurred vision; cough; and pulmonary edema.

Chlorinated hydrocarbons are absorbed through the skin, respiratory tract, and gastrointestinal tract. These compounds or their metabolic products are chronically stored in fat. Decontamination of skin (tincture of green soap) and evacuation of the stomach contents are critical. All contaminated clothing should be removed. Castor oil, milk, and other substances containing fats or oils should not be left in the stomach because they increase absorption of the chlorinated hydrocarbons. Convulsions should be treated with diazepam, 0.1–0.3 mg/kg intravenously. Epinephrine should not be used because it may cause cardiac arrhythmias.

2. ORGANOPHOSPHATE (CHOLINESTERASE-INHIBITING) INSECTICIDES (Chlorthion, Co-Ral, DFP, Diazinon, Malathion, Paraoxon, Parathion, Phosdrin, TEPP, Thio-TEPP, Etc)

Dizziness, headache, blurred vision, miosis, tearing, salivation, nausea, vomiting, diarrhea, hyperglycemia, cyanosis, sense of constriction of the chest, dyspnea, sweating, weakness, muscular twitching, convulsions, loss of reflexes and sphincter control, and coma can occur.

The clinical findings are the result of cholinesterase inhibition, which causes an accumulation of large amounts of acetylcholine. The onset of symptoms occurs within 12 hours of the exposure. Red cell cholinesterase levels should be measured as soon as possible. (Some normal individuals have a low serum cholinesterase level.) Normal values vary in different laboratories. A screening test apparatus for cholinesterase levels should be available in every hospital emergency room. In general, a decrease of red cell cholinesterase to below 25% of normal indicates significant exposure to organophosphate insecticides and is an indication for treatment with pralidoxime in addition to atropine.

Repeated low-grade exposure may result in sudden, acute toxic reactions. This syndrome usually occurs after repeated household spraying rather than agricultural exposure.

Although all organophosphates act by inhibiting

cholinesterase activity, they vary greatly in their toxicity. Parathion, for example, is 100 times more toxic than malathion. The toxicity is influenced by the specific compound, the type of formulation (liquid or solid), the vehicle, and the route of absorption (lungs, skin, or gastrointestinal tract).

Treatment

Atropine plus a cholinesterase reactivator, pralidoxime, is a chemical antidote for organophosphate insecticide poisoning. After establishing a clear airway and eliminating any cyanosis, large doses of atropine should be given and repeated every few minutes until signs of atropinism are present. An appropriate starting dose of atropine is 2–4 mg intravenously in an adult and 0.05 mg/kg in a child. The patient should receive enough atropine to stop secretions (approximately 10 times the normal dose). As much as 1 g of atropine per 24 hours may be needed in an adult.

Because atropine antagonizes the parasympathetic effects of the organophosphates but does not alter the muscular weakness, pralidoxime should also be given immediately in more severe cases and repeated every 8–12 hours as needed (25–50 mg/kg diluted to 5% and infused over 5–30 minutes at a rate of no more than 500 mg/min). Pralidoxime should be used in addition to—not in place of—atropine if red cell cholinesterase is less than 25% of normal. Pralidoxime is probably not useful later than 48 hours after the exposure. Morphine, theophylline, aminophylline, succinylcholine, and tranquilizers of the reserpine and phenothiazine types are contraindicated. Hyperglycemia is common in severe poisonings.

Decontamination of the skin (including nails and hair) and clothing with soapy water is extremely important. Decontamination of the skin must be done carefully to avoid abrasions, which increase organophosphate absorption significantly.

Bardin PG, Van Eeden SF, Joubert JR: Intensive care management of acute organophosphate poisoning: A 7-year experience in the western cape. *S Afr Med J* 1987;**72**:593.

Borowitz SM: Prolonged organophosphate toxicity in a 26-month-old child. *J Pediatr* 1988;**112**:302.

Melby TH: Prevention and management of organophosphate poisoning. *JAMA* 1971;**216**:2131.

3. CARBAMATES
(Carbaryl, Sevin, Zectran, Etc)

Carbamate insecticides are reversible inhibitors of cholinesterase. The usual laboratory procedures used to determine red cell cholinesterase will not show a depression after carbamate exposure. The reversal is often so rapid that measurements of blood cholinesterases are near normal, whereas β-naphthol, a metabolite, is present in significant amounts. The signs and symptoms of intoxication are similar to those associated with organophosphate poisoning but are generally less severe. Atropine in large doses is sufficient treatment. Pralidoxime should not be used with carbaryl poisoning but is of value with other carbamates. In combined exposures to organophosphates, give atropine but reserve pralidoxime for cases in which the red cell cholinesterase is depressed below 25% of normal.

4. BOTANICAL INSECTICIDES
(Black Flag Bug Killer, Black Leaf CPR Insect Killer, Flit Aerosol House & Garden Insect Killer, French's Flea Powder, Raid, Etc)

Allergic reactions, asthmalike symptoms, coma, and convulsions have been seen. Pyrethrins, allethrin, ryania, and rotenone do not commonly cause signs of toxicity. Antihistamines, short-acting barbiturates, and atropine are helpful when needed.

IRON

Five stages of intoxication occur following iron intoxication: (1) Hemorrhagic gastroenteritis, which occurs 30–60 minutes after ingestion and may be associated with shock, acidosis, coagulation defects, and coma. This phase usually lasts 4–6 hours and is commonly followed by a 6- to 24-hour asymptomatic period. (2) Phase of improvement, lasting 2–12 hours, during which patient looks better. (3) Delayed shock, which may occur 12–48 hours after ingestion and is usually associated with a serum iron level greater than 500 μg/dL. Metabolic acidosis, fever, leukocytosis, and coma may also be present. (4) Liver damage with hepatic failure. (5) Residual pyloric stenosis, which usually develops at least 4 weeks after the ingestion.

Diarrhea, vomiting, leukocytosis (> 15,000/μL), hyperglycemia, and a positive abdominal x-ray have been shown to correlate positively with serum iron levels exceeding 300 μg/dL. If any of these signs are present, chelation with deferoxamine should be initiated and further serum iron levels obtained.

Once iron is absorbed from the gastrointestinal tract, it is not normally eliminated in feces but may be partially excreted in the urine, giving it a red color prior to chelation. A reddish discoloration of the urine suggests a serum iron level greater than 350 μg/dL.

Treatment

Shock must be treated in the usual manner. After inducing vomiting, leave sodium bicarbonate or Fleet's Phospho-Soda (15–30 mL diluted 1:2 with water) in the stomach to form the insoluble phosphate or carbonate. Deferoxamine, a specific chelating agent for iron, is a useful adjunct in the treatment of severe iron poisoning. When given parenterally, it forms a soluble complex that is excreted in the urine. It is contraindicated in patients with renal failure unless dialysis can be used.

Deferoxamine should not be delayed in serious cases of poisoning until serum iron levels are available. Intravenous administration is indicated if the patient is in shock, in which case it should be given at a rate not to exceed 15 mg/kg/h for 8 hours. Rapid intravenous administration causes hypotension, facial flushing, urticaria, tachycardia, and shock. The dose may be repeated every 8 hours if clinically indicated. Deferoxamine, 90 mg/kg intramuscularly every 8 hours, may be given if clinically indicated. Blood levels of deferoxamine given intramuscularly and intravenously are about equal in 15 minutes if the patient is not in shock. The drug should not be given orally for chelate-absorbed iron.

Hemodialysis, peritoneal dialysis, or exchange transfusion can be used to increase the excretion of the dialyzable complex, if necessary. Urine output should be monitored and urine sediment examined for evidence of renal tubular damage. Initial laboratory studies should include blood typing and cross-matching; total protein; total iron-binding capacity; serum iron, sodium, potassium, and chloride; CO_2; pH; and liver function tests. Serum iron levels fall rapidly even if deferoxamine is not given.

After the acute episode, liver function studies and an upper gastrointestinal series are indicated to rule out residual damage.

Lacouture PG et al: Emergency assessment of severity in iron overdose by clinical and laboratory methods. *J Pediatr* 1981;**99**:89.

Propper RD, Shurin SB, Nathan DG: Reassessment of the use of desferrioxamine B in iron overload. *N Engl J Med* 1976;**294**:1421.

Robotham JL, Lietman PS: Acute iron poisoning: A review. *Am J Dis Child* 1980;**134**:875.

LEAD

Lead poisoning causes weakness, irritability, weight loss, vomiting, personality changes, ataxia, constipation, headache, transient abdominal pain, opaque flakes in the gastrointestinal tract, and a "lead line" on the gums and in many bones at the metaphyseal area. Late manifestations consist of retarded development, convulsions, and coma associated with increased intracranial pressure. The latter is a medical emergency.

Plumbism usually occurs insidiously in children under 5 years of age. The most likely sources of lead include flaking leaded paint, artist's paints, fruit tree sprays, solder, brass alloys, home-glazed pottery, and fumes from burning batteries. Only paint containing less than 1% lead is safe for interior use (furniture, toys, etc). Tetraethyl lead poisoning from gasoline sniffing is manifested by pyramidal and cerebellar dysfunction and encephalopathy. Repetitive ingestions of small amounts of lead are far more serious than a single massive exposure.

Toxic reactions are likely to occur if more than 0.5 mg of lead per day is absorbed. Only uncombined lead is removed by deleading agents. Children under 2 years of age have a poor prognosis, whereas children who develop peripheral neuritis without evidence of mental retardation or encephalitis usually recover completely.

Laboratory tests are necessary to establish a diagnosis of plumbism. Urinary coproporphyrins or, preferably, red cell δ-aminolevulinic acid dehydratase or free erythrocyte protoporphyrin (FEP) levels are satisfactory screening tests. Urine lead levels are the definitive test. The 24-hour urinary lead level exceeds 80 μg/d without treatment and should increase to greater than 1.5 mg/d on any one of the first 3 days on calcium disodium edetate (EDTA) or penicillamine therapy (or both). Dehydration and acidosis may falsely lower urinary lead levels. Glycosuria, proteinuria, hematuria, and aminoaciduria occur frequently. Blood lead levels usually exceed 80 μg/dL in symptomatic patients. Blood lead levels exceeding 40 μg/dL on 2 occasions warrant further investigation. Abnormal blood and urinary lead levels should be repeated in asymptomatic patients to rule out laboratory error. Specimens must be meticulously obtained in acid-washed containers. A normocytic, slightly hypochromic anemia with basophilic stippling of the red cells and reticulocytosis is usually present in plumbism. Stippling of red blood cells is absent in cases of sudden massive ingestion.

The cerebrospinal fluid protein is elevated, and the white cell count is usually less than 100 cells per milliliter. Cerebrospinal fluid pressure is usually elevated. Lumbar punctures must be performed cautiously to prevent herniation in patients with encephalopathy.

Treatment

Induced vomiting followed by a saline cathartic is indicated in acute cases. Combination therapy with dimercaprol (BAL), 4 mg/kg per dose every 4 hours intramuscularly, and calcium disodium edetate, 12.5 mg/kg per dose (maximum dose, 75 mg/kg/d) intravenously or intramuscularly starting with the second dose of dimercaprol, should reduce the mortality rate of acute lead encephalopathy to less than 5%. Penicillamine, 100 mg/kg/d (maximum of 1 g), should be added as soon as the patient can take oral medication. This treatment is indicated for a symptomatic patient or one with a blood lead level of 100 μg/dL. It should be started as soon as urine flow is initiated. If urine flow is delayed over 4 hours, simultaneous hemodialysis must be started. Unless the patient is severely affected, a lower dose (50 mg/kg/d) of calcium disodium edetate is adequate and is less likely to damage the kidneys or cause hypercalcemia. Elevated lead levels will usually return to normal in 3–5 days when the combination method is used; this is rarely true when calcium disodium edetate is used alone. After a 2-day pause, another course of treatment can be given if desired, again including oral penicillamine. Dimercaprol can be used with complete renal shutdown but not in patients with severe hepatic insufficiency. Dimercaprol (but not calcium disodium edetate) increases the fecal excretion of lead. The development of lacrimation, blepharospasm, paresthesias, nausea, tachycardia, and hypertension suggests a toxic reaction to dimercaprol. Iron should not be given to patients being treated for plumbism, because it forms a toxic substance with dimercaprol.

If the blood lead level is 80–100 μg/dL, one of the following regimens can be used: calcium disodium edetate and dimercaprol given for 2 days and then replaced with penicillamine orally for 5 days if there is no lead in the gut; calcium disodium edetate given alone for 5 days; or dimercaprol and calcium disodium edetate given concomitantly for 3 days.

A brief course of calcium disodium edetate or a longer course of penicillamine is indicated for lead levels of 60–80 μg/dL. Chelation therapy is not indicated for lead levels below 60 μg/dL unless there is additional evidence of toxicity.

Anticonvulsants may be needed. Mannitol or corticosteroids are indicated in patients with encephalopathy. Fluid intake should be restricted. One expert investigator feels that surgical decompression is contraindicated, but others disagree. Hypothermia and corticosteroid therapy have not altered mortality rates significantly. A high-calcium, high-phosphorus diet and large doses of vitamin D remove lead from the blood by depositing it in the bones.

Urinalysis should be done daily; serum calcium and phosphorus and blood urea nitrogen every 2 days. Calcium gluconate given intravenously as a 10% solution is helpful in controlling the colic that sometimes occurs.

A public health team should evaluate the source of the lead. Necessary corrections should be completed before the child is returned home.

Boeckx RL, Postl B, Coodin FJ: Gasoline sniffing and tetraethyl lead poisoning in children. *Pediatrics* 1977; **60**:140.

Chisholm J et al: Recognition and management of children with increased lead absorption. *Arch Dis Child* 1979; **54**:249.

Houk VN: Preventing lead poisoning in young children: A statement by the Center for Disease Control. *J Pediatr* 1978;**93**:709.

Lin-Fu J: Lead exposure among children: A reassessment. *N Engl J Med* 1979;**300**:731.

MUSHROOMS

Many toxic species of mushrooms are difficult to distinguish from edible varieties. Symptoms vary with the species ingested, the time of year, the stage of maturity, the quantity eaten, the method of preparation, and the interval since ingestion. A mushroom that is toxic to one individual may not be toxic for another. Drinking alcohol and eating certain mushrooms may cause a reaction similar to that seen with disulfiram and alcohol. Cooking destroys some toxins but not the deadly one produced by *Amanita phalloides,* which is responsible for 90% of deaths due to mushroom poisoning. Mushrooms toxins are absorbed relatively slowly. Onset of symptoms within 2 hours of ingestion suggests muscarinic toxin, whereas a delay of symptoms for 6–48 hours after ingestion strongly suggests *Amanita* poisoning. Patients who have ingested *A phalloides* may relapse and die of hepatic or renal failure following initial improvement.

Mushroom poisoning may be manifested by muscarinic symptoms (salivation, vomiting, diarrhea, cramping abdominal pain, tenesmus, miosis, and dyspnea), coma, convulsions, hallucinations, hemolysis, and hepatic and renal failure.

Treatment

Induce vomiting and follow with activated charcoal and a saline cathartic. If the patient has muscarinic signs, give atropine, 0.05 mg/kg intramuscularly (0.02 mg/kg in toddlers), and repeat as needed (usually every 30 minutes) to keep the patient atropinized. Atropine, however, is only used when there are cholinergic effects and not for all mushrooms. Hypoglycemia is most likely to occur in patients with delayed onset of symptoms. It is important, if at all possible, to identify the mushroom specifically if the patient is symptomatic. Local botanical gardens, university departments of botany, and societies of mycologists may be able to help. Supportive care is usually all that is needed except in the case of *A phalloides,* where penicillin, silibinin, or hemodialysis may be indicated.

Lampe KF, McCann MA: Differential diagnosis of poisoning by North American mushrooms, with particular emphasis on *Amanita phalloides*-like intoxication. *Ann Emerg Med* 1987;**16**:956.

Rumack BH, Salzman E: *Mushroom Poisoning, Diagnosis and Treatment.* CRC Press, 1978.

NARCOTICS & SYNTHETIC CONGENERS* (Codeine, Heroin, Methadone, Morphine, Propoxyphene)

Physicians may be called upon to treat various

---

*See p 942 for diphenoxylate poisoning.

narcotic problems, including drug addiction, withdrawal in a newborn infant, and accidental overdoses. Accidental ingestions of propoxyphene and diphenoxylate are frequent.

Unlike other narcotics, methadone is readily absorbed from the gastrointestinal tract. Drug abusers often use the intravenous route of administration. Most narcotics, including heroin, methadone, meperidine, morphine, and codeine, are excreted in the urine within 24 hours and can be readily detected.

Adolescent narcotic addicts often have other medical problems, including cellulitis, abscesses, thrombophlebitis, tetanus, infective endocarditis, HIV infection, tuberculosis, hepatitis, malaria, foreign body emboli, thrombosis of pulmonary arterioles, diabetes mellitus, obstetric complications, nephropathy, and peptic ulcer.

Treatment of Overdosage

Children receiving an overdose of opiates can develop respiratory depression, stridor, coma, increased oropharyngeal secretions, sinus bradycardia, and urinary retention. Pulmonary edema rarely occurs in children; deaths usually result from respiratory arrest and cerebral edema. Convulsions may occur with propoxyphene overdosage.

While suggested doses for naloxone hydrochloride range from 0.01 to 0.1 mg/kg, it is generally unnecessary to calculate the dosage on this basis. This extremely safe antidote should be given in sufficient quantity to reverse opiate binding sites. For children under 1 year of age, 1 ampule (0.4 mg) should be given initially; if there is no response, give 5 more ampules (2 mg) rapidly. Older children should be given 1–2 ampules, followed by 5–10 more ampules if there is no response. An improvement in respiratory status may be followed by respiratory depression, because the depressant action of narcotics may last 24–48 hours but the antagonist's duration of action is only 2–3 hours. Neonates poisoned in utero may require 10–30 μg/kg to reverse the effect.

Withdrawal in the Addict

The severity of withdrawal signs should be evaluated as explained on p 951.

Diazepam, 10 mg every 6 hours orally, has been recommended for the treatment of mild narcotic withdrawal in ambulatory adolescents. Ambulatory or hospitalized patients with moderate or severe withdrawal signs can be given the same dose of diazepam intramuscularly. Diazepam is recommended because it is nonhepatotoxic and nonmutagenic, does not affect the fetus when given to pregnant women, and is a good anticonvulsant. Diazepam therapy can be discontinued when the withdrawal score falls below 2. Diphenoxylate with atropine (Lomotil) is used to treat severe diarrhea and abdominal cramps. Chloral hydrate is the drug of choice for insomnia.

The abrupt discontinuation of narcotics (cold turkey method) is not recommended and may cause severe physical withdrawal signs.

Withdrawal in the Newborn

A newborn infant in narcotic withdrawal is small for gestational age and demonstrates yawning, sneezing, decreased Moro reflex, hunger but uncoordinated sucking action, jitteriness, tremor, constant movement, a shrill protracted cry, increased tendon reflexes, convulsions, vomiting, fever, watery diarrhea, cyanosis, dehydration, vasomotor instability, and collapse. The onset of symptoms commonly begins in the first 48 hours but may be delayed as long as 8 days depending upon the timing of the mother's last fix and her predelivery medication. The diagnosis can be easily confirmed by identifying the narcotic in the urine of the mother and baby.

Several methods of treatment have been suggested for narcotic withdrawal in the newborn. Phenobarbital, 8 mg/kg/d intramuscularly or orally in 4 doses for 4 days and then reduced by one-third every 2 days as signs decrease, may be continued for as long as 3 weeks. Methadone may be necessary in those infants with congenital methadone addiction who are not controlled in their withdrawal by large doses of phenobarbital. Dosage should be 0.5 mg/kg/d in 2 divided doses but can be gradually increased as needed. Slow tapering off may be necessary over 4 weeks for methadone addiction.

It is not clear whether prophylactic treatment with these drugs decreases the complication rate. The mortality rate of untreated narcotic withdrawal in the newborn may be as high as 45%.

Bradberry JC, Raebel MA: Continuous infusion of naloxone in the treatment of narcotic overdose. *Drug Intell Clin Pharm* 1981;**15**:945.
Lovejoy FH Jr, Mitchell AA, Goldman P: The management of propoxyphene poisoning. *J Pediatr* 1974;**85**:98.
Martin WR: Naloxone. *Ann Intern Med* 1978;**85**:765.
Reddy AM, Harper RG, Stern G: Observations on heroin and methadone withdrawal in newborn. *Pediatrics* 1971;**48**:353.

NITRITES, NITRATES, ANILINE, PENTACHLOROPHENOL, & DINITROPHENOL

Nausea, vertigo, vomiting, cyanosis (methemoglobinemia), cramping abdominal pain, tachycardia, cardiovascular collapse, tachypnea, coma, shock, convulsions, and death are possible manifestations of nitrite or nitrate poisoning.

Nitrite and nitrate compounds found in the home include amyl nitrite, butyl nitrates, isobutyl nitrates, nitroglycerin, pentaerythritol tetranitrate, sodium nitrite, nitrobenzene, and phenazopyridine. Pentachlorophenol and dinitrophenol, which are found in wood preservatives, produce methemoglobinemia and high fever because of uncoupling of oxidative phosphorylation. Headache, dizziness, and bradycardia have been reported. High concentrations of nitrites in water or spinach have been the most common cause of nitrite-induced methemoglobinemia. Symptoms do not usually occur until 40–50% of the hemoglobin has been converted to methemoglobin. A rapid test is to compare a drop of normal blood with the patient's blood on a dry filter paper. Brown discoloration of the patient's blood indicates a methemoglobin level of more than 15%.

Treatment

After inducing administer activated charcoal, vomiting and follow with a cathartic. Decontaminate any affected skin with soap and water. Oxygen and artificial respiration may be needed. If the blood methemoglobin level exceeds 40% or if levels cannot be obtained and the patient is symptomatic, give a 1% solution of methylene blue, 0.2 mL/kg intravenously over 5–10 minutes. Avoid perivascular infiltration, because it causes necrosis of the skin and subcutaneous tissues. A dramatic change in the degree of cyanosis should occur. Transfusion is occasionally necessary. Epinephrine and other vasoconstrictors are contraindicated. If reflex bradycardia occurs, atropine can be used to block it.

Bogart L, Bonsignore J, Carvalho A: Massive hemolysis following inhalation of volatile nitrites. *Am J Hematol* 1986;**22**:327.
Comly HH: Cyanosis in infants caused by nitrates in well water. *JAMA* 1987;**257**:2788.

PHENOTHIAZINES
(Chlorpromazine, Prochlorperazine, Trifluoperazine)

Extrapyramidal crisis. Episodes characterized by torticollis, stiffening of the body, spasticity, poor speech, catatonia, and inability to communicate although conscious are typical manifestations. These episodes usually last a few seconds to a few minutes but have rarely caused death. Extrapyramidal crises may represent idiosyncratic reactions and are aggravated by dehydration. The signs and symptoms occur most often in children who have received prochlorperazine. They are commonly mistaken for psychotic episodes.

Overdose. Lethargy and deep prolonged coma commonly occur. Promazine, chlorpromazine, and prochlorperazine are the drugs most likely to cause respiratory depression and precipitous drops in blood pressure. Occasionally, paradoxic hyperactivity and extrapyramidal signs as well as hyperglycemia and acetonemia are present. Seizures are uncommon.

Phenothiazines are rapidly absorbed from the gastrointestinal tract and bound to tissue. They are principally conjugated with glucuronic acid and excreted in the urine.

Treatment

Extrapyramidal signs are alleviated within minutes by the slow intravenous administration of diphenhydramine, 1–5 mg/kg, or benztropine mesylate, 1–2 mg intravenously (1 mg/min). No other treatment is usually indicated. Dialysis is ineffective.

Patients with overdoses should be treated conservatively. An attempt should be made to induce vomiting with ipecac followed by administration of activated charcoal. Charcoal adsorbs chlorpromazine and probably other phenothiazines very well. Emetics are often unsuccessful in this situation because phenothiazines are potent antiemetics; gastric lavage, therefore, may be the only practical way to remove gastric contents. A large amount of intravenous fluid without vasopressor agents is the preferred method of treating tranquilizer-induced neurogenic hypotension. If a pressor agent is required, norepinephrine (levarterenol) should be used. Epinephrine should *not* be used, because phenothiazines reverse epinephrine's effects.

Barry D, Meyskens FL Jr, Becker CE: Phenothiazine poisoning: A review of 48 cases. *Calif Med* (Jan) 1973; **118**:1.

PLANTS

Many common ornamental, garden, and wild plants are potentially toxic. Small amounts of a plant may cause severe illness or death. These effects usually involve the cardiovascular, gastrointestinal, and central nervous systems and the skin. Table 30–4 lists the most toxic plants, symptoms and signs of poisoning, and treatment.

Frohne D, Pfander HJ: *A Colour Atlas of Poisonous Plants.* Wolfe Publishing, 1984.
Lampe KF, McCann MA: *AMA Handbook of Poisonous and Injurious Plants.* American Medical Association, 1985.

PSYCHOTROPIC DRUGS

Psychotropic drugs consist of 4 general classes: stimulants (amphetamines, cocaine), depressants (narcotics, barbiturates, etc), antidepressants and tranquilizers, and hallucinogens (LSD, PCP, etc).

The following clinical findings are commonly seen in patients abusing drugs:

Stimulants. Agitation, euphoria, grandiose feelings, tachycardia, fever, abdominal cramps, visual and auditory hallucinations, mydriasis, coma, convulsions, and respiratory depression.

Depressants. Emotional lability, ataxia, diplopia,

Table 30–4. Poisoning due to plants.[1]

	Symptoms and Signs	Treatment
Arum family: *Caladium, Dieffenbachia,* calla lily, dumb cane (oxalic acid)	Burning of mucous membranes and airway obstruction secondary to edema caused by calcium oxalate crystals.	Accessible areas should be thoroughly washed. Corticosteroids relieve airway obstruction. Apply cold packs to affected mucous membranes.
Castor bean plant (ricin—a toxalbumin) Jequirity bean (abrin—a toxalbumin)	Mucous membrane irritation, nausea, vomiting, bloody diarrhea, blurred vision, circulatory collapse, acute hemolytic anemia, convulsions, uremia.	Fluid and electrolyte monitoring. Saline cathartic. Forced alkaline diuresis will prevent complications due to hemagglutination and hemolysis.
Foxglove, lily of the valley, and oleander[2]	Nausea, diarrhea, visual disturbances, and cardiac irregularities (eg, heart block).	See treatment for digitalis drugs in text (p 941).
Jimsonweed: See Belladonna Alkaloids, p 938	Mydriasis, dry mouth, tachycardia, and hallucinations.	Atropine.
Larkspur (ajacine, *Delphinium,* delphinoidine)	Nausea and vomiting, irritability, muscular paralysis, and CNS depression.	Symptomatic. Atropine may be helpful.
Monkshood (aconite)	Numbness of mucous membranes, visual disturbances, tingling, dizziness, tinnitus, hypotension, bradycardia, and convulsions.	Activated charcoal, oxygen. Atropine is probably helpful.
Poison hemlock (coniine)	Mydriasis, trembling, dizziness, bradycardia, CNS depression, muscular paralysis, and convulsions. Death is due to respiratory paralysis.	Symptomatic. Oxygen and cardiac monitoring equipment are desirable. Assisted respiration is often necessary. Give anticonvulsants if needed.
Rhododendron (grayanotoxin)	Abdominal cramps, vomiting, severe diarrhea, muscular paralysis, CNS and circulatory depression. Hypertension with very large doses.	Atropine can prevent bradycardia. Epinephrine is contraindicated. Antihypertensives may be needed.
Yellow jessamine (active ingredient, gelsemine, is related to strychnine)	Restlessness, convulsions, muscular paralysis, and respiratory depression.	Symptomatic. Because of the relation to strychnine, activated charcoal and diazepam for seizures is worth trying.

[1]Many other plants cause minor irritation but are not likely to cause serious problems unless large amounts are ingested. See Lampe KF, McCann MA: *AMA Handbook of Poisonous and Injurious Plants.* American Medical Association, 1985. See also Rumack BH, Spoerke DG (editors): *POISINDEX® Information System.* Micromedex, IAC, Denver, Colorado. [Published quarterly.]
[2]Done AK: Ornamental and deadly. *Emerg Med* (April) 1973;**5**:255.

nystagmus, vertigo, poor accommodation, respiratory depression, coma, apnea, and convulsions. Dilatation of conjunctival blood vessels suggests marijuana ingestion. Narcotics cause miotic pupils and, occasionally, pulmonary edema.

Antidepressants and tranquilizers. Hypotension, lethargy, respiratory depression, coma, and extrapyramidal reactions.

Hallucinogens and psychoactive drugs. Belladonna alkaloids cause mydriasis, dry mouth, nausea, vomiting, urinary retention, confusion, disorientation, paranoid delusions, hallucinations, fever, hypotension, aggressive behavior, convulsions, and coma. **Psychoactive drugs** such as LSD cause mydriasis, unexplained bizarre behavior, hallucinations, and generalized undifferentiated psychotic behavior.

See also other entries discussed in alphabetic sequence in this chapter.

Management of the Patient Who Abuses Drugs

Only a small percentage of the persons using drugs come to the attention of physicians; those who do are usually suffering from adverse reactions such as panic states, drug psychoses, homicidal or suicidal thoughts, and respiratory depression that could not be satisfactorily managed by friends.

Even with cooperative patients, an accurate history is difficult to obtain. The user often does not really know what drug has been taken or how much. "Street drugs" are almost always adulterated with one or more other compounds. Multiple drugs are often taken together, making it impossible to clinically define the type of drug. Friends may be a useful source of information. A drug history is most easily obtained in a quiet spot by a gentle, nonthreatening, honest examiner.

The general appearance, skin, lymphatics, cardiorespiratory status, gastrointestinal tract, and central nervous system should be stressed during the physical examination, because they often provide clues suggesting drug abuse. A drug history should not be taken from an adolescent in the parents' presence.

Although it is desirable to know the specific drug taken, it is often impossible to obtain this information. Hallucinogens are not life-threatening unless the patient is frankly homicidal or suicidal. A specific diagnosis is usually not necessary for management; instead, the presenting signs and symptoms are treated. Does the patient appear intoxicated? In withdrawal? "Flashing back?" Is some illness or injury (eg, head trauma) being masked by a drug effect? (Remember that a known drug user may still have hallucinations from meningoencephalitis.)

The signs and symptoms in a given patient are a function of not only the drug and the dose but also the level of acquired tolerance, the "setting," the patient's physical condition and personality traits, the potentiating effects of other drugs, and many other factors.

A common drug problem in hospital emergency rooms is the "bad trip," which is usually a panic reaction. This is best managed by "talking the patient down" and minimizing auditory and visual stimuli. Sitting with a friend while the drug effect dissipates may be the best treatment that can be offered. This may take 8 hours or more. The physician's job is not to terminate the drug effect but to help the patient over the bad experience.

Drugs are often unnecessary and may complicate the clinical course of a patient with a panic reaction. Although phenothiazines have been commonly used to treat "bad trips," they should be avoided if the specific drug is not known, because they may enhance toxicity or produce unwanted side effects that makes management difficult. Diazepam, 20 mg orally every 30 minutes as necessary, is the drug of choice if a sedative effect is required. Physical restraints are rarely if ever indicated and usually increase the patient's panic reaction.

For treatment of life-threatening drug abuse, consult the section on the specific drug elsewhere in this chapter and the section on general management at the beginning of the chapter.

After the acute episode, the physician must decide whether psychiatric referral is indicated; in general, patients who have made suicidal gestures or attempts and adolescents who are not communicating with their families should be referred. On the other hand, adolescents who are "experimenting" with drugs often do not need psychiatric referral.

Cohen S: The "angel dust" states: Phencyclidine. *Pediatr Rev* 1979;**1:**17.

Consroe PF: Treatment of acute hallucinogenic drug toxicity: Specific pharmacological intervention. *Am J Hosp Pharm* 1973;**30:**80.

Smith D et al: PCP problems and prevention. *J Psychedelic Drugs* 1980;**12:**181.

Teitelbaum DT: Poisoning with psychoactive drugs. *Pediatr Clin North Am* 1970;**17:**557.

SALICYLATES

The use of childproof containers and publicity regarding accidental poisoning have reduced the incidence of acute salicylate poisoning. Nevertheless,

serious intoxication still occurs and must be regarded as an emergency.

Salicylates uncouple oxidative phosphorylation, leading to increased heat production, excessive sweating, and dehydration. They also interfere with glucose metabolism and may cause hypoglycemia or hyperglycemia. Respiratory center stimulation occurs early.

Patients usually have signs of hyperventilation, sweating, dehydration, and fever. Vomiting and diarrhea sometimes occur. In severe cases, disorientation, convulsions, and coma are often present.

The severity of acute intoxication can in some measure be judged by serum salicylate levels (Fig 30–3). High levels are always dangerous irrespective of clinical signs, and low levels may be misleading in chronic cases. Other laboratory values usually indicate metabolic acidosis despite hyperventilation; low serum K^+ values; and, often, abnormal serum glucose levels.

Salicylate poisoning is classified as mild when plasma pH is greater than 7.4 and urine pH is greater than 6.0; as moderate when plasma pH is greater than 7.4 and urine pH is less than 6.0; and as severe when plasma pH is less than 7.4 and urine pH is less than 6.0.

In mild poisoning, stimulation of the respiratory

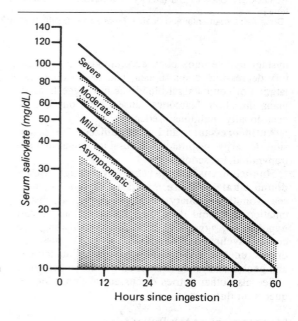

Figure 30–3. Nomogram relating serum salicylate concentration and expected severity of intoxication at varying intervals following ingestion of a single dose of salicylate. (Redrawn and reproduced, with permission, from Done AK: Salicylate intoxication. *Pediatrics* 1960; **26:**800.)

center produces respiratory alkalosis. The kidney responds by producing alkali.

In moderate poisoning, the respiratory center is still stimulated and produces respiratory alkalosis. The kidney becomes less able to excrete alkali owing to depletion of K^+. Consequently, the kidney exchanges K^+ for H^+, and a relatively acidic urine is seen.

In severe intoxication (seen in severe acute ingestion with high salicylate levels and in chronic toxicity with lower levels), respiratory response is unable to overcome the metabolic overdose.

Once the urine becomes acidic, progressively smaller amounts of salicylate are excreted. Until this process is reversed, the half-life will remain extended, because metabolism contributes little to the removal of these substances.

Chronic severe poisoning may be seen as early as 3 days after a regimen of salicylate is begun. Findings usually include vomiting, diarrhea, and dehydration due to accumulation of salicylates in the body.

Treatment

Salicylates can be recovered from the body in substantial amounts for as long as 20 hours following accidental or intentional ingestion. Charcoal binds salicylates well and, after emesis or lavage, should be given on a cyclic basis every 4 hours until charcoal appears in stool.

Mild poisoning may require only the administration of oral fluids and confirmation that the salicylate level is falling.

Moderate ingestion is reflected by moderate dehydration and depletion of renal potassium. Fluids must be administered at a rate sufficient to correct dehydration and produce urine with a pH of greater than 7.0 at a rate of flow of 2–3 mL/kg/hr. Initial hydrating solutions should be isotonic, with sodium bicarbonate constituting half the electrolyte content. Once the patient is rehydrated, the solution can contain more free water and approximately 40 mEq of potassium per liter.

Severe ingestion is marked by major dehydration in cases of chronic poisoning with a delay in diagnosis. Symptoms may be confused with those of Reye's syndrome, encephalopathy, and metabolic acidosis. Salicylate levels may even be in the "therapeutic range." Major fluid correction of dehydration is required. Once this has been accomplished, hypokalemia must be corrected and sodium bicarbonate given. Urine pH will not become alkaline until adequate potassium has been provided. Usual requirements are sodium bicarbonate, 1–2 mEq/kg/hr over the first 6–8 hours, and K^+, 20–40 mEq/L. A urine flow of 2–3 mL/kg/hr should be established.

Vitamin K should be administered, although hemorrhaging is rare except in severely poisoned patients. Renal failure or pulmonary edema is an indication for dialysis. Hemodialysis is most effective and peritoneal dialysis relatively ineffective. Acetazolamide should not be used.

Hill JB: Salicylate intoxication. *N Engl J Med* 1973;**288**:1110.

Snodgrass W et al: Salicylate toxicity following therapeutic doses in young children. *Clin Toxicol* 1981;**18**:247.

SCORPION BITES

Scorpion bites are common in arid areas of the southwestern USA. Scorpion venom is more toxic than most snake venoms, but only minute amounts are injected. Although neurologic manifestations of the bite may last a week, most clinical signs subside within 24–48 hours.

Bites by less toxic scorpion species cause local pain, redness, and swelling. Bites by more toxic species cause tingling or burning paresthesias that begin at the site of the bite and tend to progress up the extremity; other findings include throat spasm, a feeling of a thickening of the tongue, restlessness, muscular fibrillation, abdominal cramps, convulsions, urinary incontinence, and respiratory failure.

Treatment

Calcium gluconate (0.1 mg/kg of a 10% solution given intravenously), relieves muscular cramps. Hot compresses of sodium bicarbonate will soothe the bitten area. Sedation and corticosteroids may be indicated. Patients may require treatment for seizures, hypertension, or tachycardia.

The prognosis for life is good except in infants and young children.

Bartholomew C: Acute scorpion pancreatitis in Trinidad. *Br Med J* 1970;**1**:666.

Gueron M et al: Cardiovascular manifestations of severe scorpion sting: Clinicopathologic correlations. *Chest* 1970;**57**:156.

Zlotkin E et al: Recent studies on the mode of action of scorpion neurotoxins: A review. *Toxicon* 1969;**7**:217.

SNAKEBITE

Despite the lethal potential of venomous snakes, human morbidity and mortality rates are surprisingly low. The outcome depends on the size of the child, the site of the bite, the degree of envenomation, and the effectiveness of treatment.

Poisonous snakebites are most common and most severe in the early spring. Children in snake-infested areas should wear boots and long trousers, should not walk barefoot, and should be cautioned not to explore under ledges or in holes where a snake might be hiding.

Ninety-eight percent of poisonous snakebites in the USA are caused by pit vipers (rattlesnakes, water moccasins, and copperheads). A few are caused by elapids (coral snakes), and occasional bites occur from cobras and other nonindigenous exotic snakes kept as pets. Snake venom is a complex mixture of enzymes, peptides, and proteins that may have predominantly cytotoxic, neurotoxic, hemotoxic, or cardiotoxic effects but other effects as well. The snake seldom uses all its venom in a single bite. Up to 70% of bites by pit vipers do not result in venom injection.

Pit viper venom is predominantly cytotoxic and hemotoxic, causing a severe local reaction with pain, discoloration, and edema, as well as hemorrhagic effects. Peripheral and central neurologic abnormalities can also occur. Convulsions are common in children.

Swelling and pain occur soon after rattlesnake bite and are a certain indication that envenomation has occurred. During the first few hours, swelling and ecchymosis extend proximally from the bite. The bite is often obvious as a double puncture mark surrounded by ecchymosis. Hematemesis, melena, hemoptysis, and other manifestations of coagulopathy develop in severe cases. Respiratory difficulty and shock are the ultimate causes of death. Even in fatal rattlesnake bite, there is usually a period of 6–8 hours between the bite and death; there is, therefore, usually enough time to start effective treatment.

Coral snake envenomation causes little local pain, swelling, or necrosis, and systemic reactions are often delayed for 10 hours, although children may convulse within 1 hour after being bitten. The early signs of coral snake envenomation include bulbar paralysis, dysphagia, and dysphoria; these may appear in 5–10 hours and may be followed by total peripheral paralysis and death in 24 hours.

Snakebites are an important hazard in many parts of the world; in India there are thought to be over 30,000 deaths per year from cobra bites. The general principles outlined here apply to any bite, but specific therapy will naturally vary between species.

Treatment

The treatment of snakebite envenomation is controversial, but the following approach seems most useful.

A. Emergency (First Aid) Treatment: The most important first aid measure is reassurance. If possible, clean the wound with a germicidal preparation. Splint the affected extremity and minimize the patient's motion. Tourniquets are of questionable value, and ice packs are contraindicated.

Incision and suction are useful only if done soon after envenomation. Because most bites are into the deep subcutaneous layer or muscle, small skin incisions are not effective. In making an incision, consideration must be given to the danger of damaging underlying tendons, nerves, or vessels. Incision is not effective for coral snake bites.

B. Definitive Medical Management: Blood should be drawn for typing and cross-matching, hematocrit, clotting time and platelet function, and serum electrolyte determinations. Close monitoring of the hematocrit and electrolytes is indicated. The massive destruction of red cells may be associated with hyperkalemia. Establish 2 secure intravenous sites for the administration of antivenin, blood, and other medications.

Specific antivenin is indicated only when signs of severe envenomation are present. Polyvalent pit viper antivenin and coral snake antivenin (Wyeth Laboratories) are available from hospital pharmacies. Coral snake antivenin can also be obtained on an emergency basis from state epidemiologists and is stockpiled (mainly in the southeastern USA) at over 75 locations, including the Centers for Disease Control, Atlanta, GA 30333 (central telephone number: [404] 329–3311).

If horse serum sensitivity tests are negative, antivenin should be given intravenously (15–20 minutes per vial). Give 5–8 vials for minimal, 8–12 for moderate, and 13 or more for severe envenomation. Dilute each vial to 50–200 mL. (Antivenin should not be given intramuscularly or subcutaneously, because it is slow-acting, inefficient, and impossible to control if adverse reactions occur. Antivenin injected into the bite site has little effect and is dangerous.) If anaphylaxis occurs despite negative skin tests, it will occur at the onset of treatment. Epinephrine, 0.3 mL of 1:1000 solution, should be drawn up in a syringe before antivenin is administered. Horse serum sensitivity must be reevaluated if another course of antivenin is required over 36 hours after the first. The hemorrhagic tendency, pain, and shock are rapidly diminished by adequate amounts of antivenin.

Codeine, 1–1.5 mg/kg per dose orally, or meperidine, 0.6–1.5 mg/kg per dose orally or intramuscularly, is occasionally necessary to control pain during the first 24 hours. Cryotherapy is contraindicated because it commonly causes tissue damage severe enough to necessitate amputation. Early physiotherapy minimizes contractions. In rare cases, fasciotomy to relieve pressure within muscular compartments is required to save the function of a hand or foot. The evaluation of function as well as of pulses will better predict the need for fasciotomy. Corticosteroids (hydrocortisone, 1–2 g intravenously every 4–6 hours) are useful in the treatment of serum sickness or anaphylactic shock and may be useful treatment by themselves, especially if the patient is already sensitive to antivenin. Ampicillin (200 mg/kg/d orally) is given to treat gram-negative infections that are often associated with snakebite.

A fluid tetanus toxoid booster is adequate if the patient was previously immunized against tetanus.

Russell FE: *Snake Venom Poisoning.* Lippincott, 1980.

Russell FE et al: Snake venom poisoning in the United States: Experience with 550 cases. *JAMA* 1975; **233**:841.

SOAPS & DETERGENTS

1. SOAPS

Soap is made from salts of fatty acids. Some toilet soap bars contain both soap and detergent. Ingestion of soap bars may cause vomiting and diarrhea, but they have a low toxicity.

Dilute with milk or water. Induced emesis is unnecessary.

2. DETERGENTS

Detergents are nonsoap synthetic products used for cleaning purposes because of their surfactant properties. Commercial products include granules, powders, and liquids. Electric dishwasher detergents are very alkaline and can cause caustic burns. Low concentrations of bleaching and antibacterial agents as well as enzymes are found in many preparations. These pure compounds are moderately toxic, but the concentration used is too small to alter the product's toxicity significantly, although occasional primary or allergic irritative phenomena have been noted in housewives and in employees manufacturing these products.

There are 3 general types of detergents: cationic, anionic, and nonionic.

Cationic Detergents (Ceepryn, Diaperene, Phemerol, Zephiran)

Nausea, vomiting, collapse, coma, and convulsions may occur. Death may occur within an hour. As little as 2.25 g of some cationic agents have caused death in an adult. In 4 cases, 100–400 mg/kg of benzalkonium chloride caused death. Cationic detergents are rapidly inactivated by tissues and ordinary soap.

Because of the caustic potential and rapid onset of seizures, emesis is not recommended. Activated charcoal and a cathartic should be administered. Anticonvulsants may be needed.

Anionic Detergents

Most common household detergents are anionic. Laundry compounds have water softener (sodium phosphate) added, which is a strong irritant and may reduce ionized calcium. Anionic detergents irritate the skin by removing natural oils. Although ingestion causes diarrhea, intestinal distention, and vomiting, no fatalities have been reported. The LD50 in animals ranges from 1 to 5 g/kg.

The only treatment usually required is to discontinue use if skin irritation occurs and replace fluids and electrolytes. Induced vomiting is not indicated following ingestion of electric dishwasher detergent, because of its strong alkalinity. Dilute with water or milk.

Nonionic Detergents (Brij Products; Tritons X-45, X-100, X-102, & X-144)

These compounds include lauryl, stearyl, and oleyl alcohols and octyl phenol. They have a minimal irritating effect on the skin and are almost nontoxic when swallowed.

Deichmann WB, Gerarde HW: Hazards of alkaline laundry detergents. *JAMA* 1972;**220**:1014.

Enzyme detergents. (Editorial.) *Br Med J* 1970;**1**:518.

Jeven JE: Severe dermatitis and "biological" detergents. *Br Med J* 1970;**1**:299.

SPIDER BITES

At least 50 species of spiders have been implicated in human spider bites, but most toxic reactions in the USA are caused by the black widow spider (*Latrodectus mactans*) and the North American brown recluse (violin) spider (*Loxosceles reclusus*). Many spider venoms have common chemical and pharmacologic properties. It is helpful if positive identification of the spider can be made, since many spider bites may mimic those of the brown recluse spider.

Black Widow Spider

The black widow spider, which is endemic to nearly all areas of the USA, causes most of the deaths due to spider bites. The initial bite may be hemorrhagic and associated with a sharp fleeting pain. Local and systemic muscular cramping, abdominal pain, nausea and vomiting, and shock can occur. Convulsions are more commonly seen in small children. Systemic signs of black widow spider bite are often confused with other causes of acute abdomen. Although paresthesias, nervousness, and transient muscle spasms may persist for months in survivors, recovery from the acute phase is generally complete within 3 days.

Antivenin is no longer in general use, because of the self-limiting nature of the injury and the danger of serum sickness with its use. Antivenin is used in severe cases when other treatments fail. Give 50 mg/kg iv per dose, up to 250 mg/kg/24 hr of calcium gluconate intravenously to relieve muscle cramps. Methocarbamol (15 mg/kg orally) or diazepam may be useful. Morphine or barbiturates may occasionally be needed for control of pain or restlessness, but they increase the possibility of respiratory depression.

Local treatment of the bite is not helpful.

Brown Recluse Spider
(Violin Spider)

The North American brown recluse spider is most commonly seen in the central and midwestern areas of the USA. Its bite characteristically produces a localized reaction with progressively severe pain within 8 hours. The initial bleb on an erythematous ischemic base is replaced by a black eschar within a week. This eschar separates in 2–5 weeks, leaving a poorly healing ulcer that may result in keloid formation. Systemic signs include cyanosis, morbilliform rash, fever, chills, malaise, weakness, nausea and vomiting, joint pains, hemolytic reactions with hemoglobinuria, jaundice, and delirium. Fatalities are rare. Fatal disseminated intravascular coagulation due to the brown recluse spider has been reported.

Although of unproved efficacy, the following therapies have been used: dexamethasone (4 mg intravenously 4 times a day) during the acute phase; hydroxyzine 1 mg/kg/dose intramuscularly; polymorphonuclear leukocyte inhibitors, such as dapsone or colchicine, and oxygen applied to the bite site; and total excision of the lesion at the fascial level.

Arena JM & Drew RH: *Poisoning: Toxicology, Symptoms, Treatments*, 5th ed. Thomas, 1986.
Bolton M: The brown spider bite. *J Kans Med Soc* 1970; **71**:197.
Frazier CA: *Insect Allergy: Allergic and Toxic Reactions to Insects and Other Arthropods*. Warren Green, 1969.
Vorse H: Disseminated intravascular coagulopathy following fatal brown spider bite. *J Pediatr* 1971;**80**:1035.

THYROID PREPARATIONS
(Desiccated Thyroid, Sodium Levothyroxine)

Ingestion of the equivalent of 50–150 g of desiccated thyroid can cause signs of hyperthyroidism, including irritability, mydriasis, hyperpyrexia, tachycardia, and diarrhea. Maximal clinical effect occurs about 9 days after ingestion—several days after the protein-bound iodine level has fallen dramatically.

Induce vomiting. If the patient develops clinical signs of toxicity, propranolol is useful because of its anti-adrenergic activity.

Litovitz TL, White JD: Levothyroxine ingestions in children: An analysis of 78 cases. *Am J Emerg Med* 1985; **3**:297.

VITAMINS

Accidental ingestion of excessive amounts of vitamins rarely causes significant problems. Occasional cases of hypervitaminosis A and D do occur, however, particularly in patients with poor hepatic or renal function. The fluoride contained in many multivitamin preparations is not a realistic hazard, because a 2- or 3-year-old child could eat 100 tablets, containing 1 mg of sodium fluoride per tablet, without producing serious symptoms. Iron poisoning has been reported with multiple vitamin tablets containing iron.

Armstrong GD: Vitamin ingestions. *National Clearinghouse Poison Control Center Bull 1–6*, April–June, 1972.
Morrice G: Papilledema and hypervitaminosis A. *JAMA* 1970;**213**:1344.
Seelig MS: Vitamin D and cardiovascular, renal, and brain damage in infancy and childhood. *Ann NY Acad Sci* 1969;**147**:539.

WARFARIN

Warfarin is used as a pesticide. It causes hypoprothrombinemia and capillary injury. It is readily absorbed from the gastrointestinal tract but is absorbed poorly through the skin. A dose of 0.5 mg/kg of warfarin may be toxic in a child. A prothrombin time is helpful in establishing the severity of the poisoning.

Treatment consists of induced vomiting followed by a saline cathartic. If bleeding occurs or the prothrombin time is prolonged, give 1–5 mg of vitamin K_1 (phytonadione) intramuscularly or subcutaneously. For large ingestions with established toxicity, 0.6 mg/kg may be given.

Sellers EM: Potentiation of warfarin-induced hypoprothrombinemia by chloral hydrate. *N Engl J Med* 1970; **283**:827.

SELECTED REFERENCES

Arena JM, Drew RH: *Poisoning: Toxicology, Symptoms, Treatments,* 5th ed. Thomas Springfield, 1986.

Bayer MJ, Rumack BH (editors): *Poisonings and Overdose.* Aspen Systems, 1982.

Bayer MJ, Rumack BH, Wanke L: *Toxicologic Emergencies: A Manual of Diagnosis and Management.* Brady-Prentice Hall, 1983.

Billups NF: *American Drug Index,* 33th ed. Lippincott, 1989.

Browning E: *Toxicity of Industrial Metals,* 2nd ed. Butterworth, 1969.

Doull J, Klaassen C, Amdur M (editors): *Cassarett and Doull's Toxicology: The Basic Science of Poisons,* 3rd ed. Macmillan, 1985.

Ellenhorn MJ & Barceloux DG: Medical Toxicology: *Diagnosis and Treatment of Human Poisoning.* Elsever, New York, NY, 1988.

Gilman AG et al (editors): *Goodman and Gilman's The Pharmacological Basis of Therapeutics,* 7th ed. Macmillan, 1985.

Gosselin RE, Smith RP, Hodge HC: *Clinical Toxicology of Commercial Products,* 5th ed. Williams & Wilkins, 1984.

Finkel AJ (ed): Hamilton & Hardy's *Industrial Toxicology,* 4th ed. Publishing Sciences Group, Inc, 1983.

Handbook of Nonprescription Drugs, 7th ed. The American Pharmaceutical Association, 1982.

Lampe KF, McCann MA: *AMA Handbook of Poisonous and Injurious Plants.* American Medical Association, 1985.

Rumack BH, Spoerke DG (editors): *POISINDEX ® Information System.* [Published quarterly.] Micromedex, Inc, Denver, Colorado.

Rumack BH, Salzman E: *Mushroom Poisoning: Diagnosis and Treatment.* CRC Press, 1978.

Neoplastic Diseases

David G. Tubergen, MD

Cancer is the most common cause of death due to disease in children over the age of 1 year. Malignant diseases occur in about 10 per 100,000 children per year and account for about 4000 deaths annually. Leukemias and lymphomas constitute about 40% of pediatric malignant diseases, with the solid tumors, chiefly sarcomas, making up the remaining 60%. The signs and symptoms of pediatric cancer may be subtle. Any mass—solid, cystic, or mixed—should be considered malignant until a definitive histologic diagnosis is established or until specific therapy directed at another cause has resulted in its disappearance within the expected period.

The causes of cancer in children remain elusive. Genetic disorders play an important role in some cases, eg, retinoblastoma and the tumors associated with neurofibromatosis. Chromosomal excess, as in trisomy 21, or chromosomal instability, as in Fanconi's hypoplastic anemia, is associated with an increased incidence of cancer. Somatic growth disturbances, as seen in hemihypertrophy, may be associated with liver, kidney, or adrenal tumors.

A wide variety of immunologic deficiencies have been associated with an increased incidence of many types of cancer. This phenomenon may reflect a decrease in the host's surveillance mechanism against transformed cells or may result from prolonged exposure to oncogenic agents as a consequence of failure to mount an adequate immune response. Our lack of information regarding the causes of cancer makes prevention virtually impossible and emphasizes the importance of early detection and specific diagnosis followed by aggressive treatment.

Once cancer is suspected or diagnosed, there are several considerations that affect the ultimate outcome. The initial evaluation requires determination of the nature of the malignant tumor and the precise extent of disease. Because many pediatric tumors fit the broad description of "small cell neoplasm," the pathologic material should be examined by pathologists experienced in the special histologic techniques and molecular probes that can be of great value. Determination of the extent of disease requires a knowledge of potential metastatic sites and selected utilization of many imaging techniques, as well as biochemical and biopsy procedures. The surgeon must not only have sound judgment and expert technical skills but must also include with the operative notes an accurate description of the extent of tumor involvement and the location and extent of local metastases or extensions. These observations are critical to further therapeutic planning.

Therapy is multidisciplinary and ideally involves a surgeon, a radiation therapist, and a pediatric oncologist before therapy is started. Certainly once the diagnosis has been made, a comprehensive treatment plan must incorporate all 3 major modalities. The significant progress that has been made in the management of several pediatric cancers as a result of aggressive multimodal therapy emphasizes the importance of this approach and the advantage of beginning treatment in a medical center where personnel and facilities are available to implement this concept. The primary physician serves several roles as a member of this team: as the diagnostician best situated to facilitate early detection; as the person administering therapy in the home community; as the physician most likely to observe early complications or toxic reactions; and as counselor to the patients and their families.

The current goal of cancer chemotherapy is to cure the patient. This implies an aggressive approach, as will be evident in the following pages. Chemotherapeutic agents fall into several general classes based on mode of action, and almost all programs utilize combinations of agents of differing actions in an attempt to increase tumor kill. This goal can, of course, be reached only if each agent has some activity against the tumor in question. Ideally, the agents used together should have nonadditive toxicities. In other words, one attempts to use combinations with additive or synergistic antitumor effects and nonadditive toxic effects. In the treatment of solid tumors, the concept of adjunctive chemotherapy is important to achieve better results. In the case of many tumors, microscopic metastases are already present at the time of initial therapy, and local treatment alone will not be curative. Because of the growth characteristics of small tumor implants and probably because of their relatively better blood supply, these microscopic tumors appear more susceptible to drugs than are clinically obvious metastases. Thus, in beginning chemotherapy, one should reason that metastasis has already occurred, because the potential for cure is greater at this time than if one waits for clinical metastases to appear. In the management of some tumor types, the efficacy of drug therapy against microscopic residual disease lessens the need for extensive local tumor bed irradiation.

Specific drugs are mentioned in the following discussions of individual tumor types. Any of the general references will provide more specifics regarding doses, routes of administration, and toxicities.

LEUKEMIA

1. ACUTE LYMPHOBLASTIC LEUKEMIA

Essentials of Diagnosis

- Pallor, petechiae, purpura, fatigue, fever, bone pain.
- Hepatosplenomegaly, lymphadenopathy.
- Thrombocytopenia, normal or low hemoglobin.
- Diagnosis confirmed by bone marrow examination.

General Considerations

Acute lymphoblastic leukemia (ALL) comprises about 85% of leukemias in childhood. About 12% of cases are acute myeloblastic or monoblastic, and 3% are chronic granulocytic leukemia. ALL can be further classified on the basis of surface markers that identify the developmental line and stage of the leukemic cell.

The peak incidence of onset of acute lymphoblastic leukemia is at 4 years of age, but the disease may occur at any time during childhood. Before the advent of chemotherapy, this disease was usually fatal within 3–4 months, with virtually no survivors 1 year after diagnosis. Current estimates are that about 60% of children receiving aggressive combination chemotherapy and early central nervous system treatment may be expected to survive free of disease for 5 years or longer. Not all patients have the same likelihood of achieving long-term remission. Those with the best prognosis are 3–7 years of age with white counts at presentation of less than 10,000/μL. Patients who present with a white blood cell count over 50,000/μL or who are less than 1 year or more than 10 years of age have the poorest prognosis. Recent studies indicate that the DNA content of the leukemic cells and chromosomal abnormalities in the malignant line also have prognostic significance.

Clinical Findings

A. Symptoms and Signs: The variable presenting complaints of children with acute leukemia are referable to organ infiltration and marrow replacement with malignant cells that crowd out normal elements of the marrow. The absence of red cell precursors leads to anemia, which may make the child pale, listless, irritable, and chronically tired. The

lack of mature granulocytes makes the child more susceptible to infection, and a history of repeated infections prior to a definitive diagnosis of leukemia is not unusual. The thrombocytopenia predisposes the child to bleeding episodes: epistaxis, petechiae, hematomas, or life-threatening hemorrhage. Organs may be infiltrated by disease and not function properly; may cause discomfort because of their large size; or may cause symptoms due to pressure on other structures.

Organ infiltration, especially of the kidney, may cause significant dysfunction. This may result in serious uric acid toxicity when therapy is initiated and must be assessed prior to treatment.

B. Laboratory Findings: The white count at presentation is below normal in one-third of patients, normal in another third, and elevated in the remainder. Thrombocytopenia is present in about 85% of patients, and varying degrees of anemia are reported in almost that many. The peripheral blood smear may or may not demonstrate the malignant cells. The diagnosis is established by bone marrow examination, which shows a homogeneous infiltration of blast cells replacing the normal elements. Special stains may be useful in classification of the various types of leukemia, and T and B lymphocyte markers should be sought on the lymphoblasts. An elevated serum uric acid level requires careful monitoring and treatment (see below).

Diagnostic Workup

A. Complete History and Physical Examination: Important features of the history are a family history of cancer, drugs used, radiation exposure, immunizations, and infectious diseases.

B. Laboratory Studies:

1. Complete blood count, platelet count, reticulocyte count, prothrombin time, and bone marrow aspiration or biopsy (or both). (Bone marrow aspiration is discussed in Chapter 35.)

2. Lumbar puncture with study of a special Wright-stained smear of the sediment for blast cells.

3. Blood urea nitrogen and serum levels of creatinine, uric acid, bilirubin, AST (SGOT), alkaline phosphatase, proteins, sodium, potassium, lactate dehydrogenase, and immunoglobulins.

4. Urinalysis.

5. Cultures and smears of mouth, throat, blood, bone marrow, skin lesions, urine, cerebrospinal fluid, and stool should be taken immediately if infection is suspected. Fungal and viral cultures and serologic tests should also be done when needed.

6. PPD intermediate-strength skin test and endemic fungal skin tests.

C. Imaging: A chest x-ray should be obtained to look for mediastinal enlargement.

D. Psychosocial Evaluation: An inventory of the patient's and family's strengths, coping abilities, and economic status helps in anticipating problems.

Differential Diagnosis

Early in the course of the disease, leukemia may produce signs and symptoms similar to those of rheumatic fever, rheumatoid arthritis, viral diseases such as infectious mononucleosis or hepatitis, or other neoplastic diseases such as neuroblastoma or histiocytosis X. The peripheral blood picture may be indistinguishable from that of aplastic anemia.

Specific Treatment

The goal of therapy is to eradicate disease or, at a minimum, to produce a prolonged period free of disease. Therapy can be divided into (1) systemic therapy, consisting of induction and maintenance phases, and (2) treatment of the central nervous system.

A. Systemic Therapy: The theoretic objective of antileukemic therapy is elimination of lymphoblasts from the body. A child weighing 20–30 kg may present with a tumor weighing approximately 1 kg, which represents about 10^{12} cells. Current techniques do not permit detection of disease when cell numbers are 10^9 or fewer, so it is impossible to determine whether the objective is being approached.

Induction therapy is designed to achieve a complete remission, ie, absence of detectable tumor tissue and presence of normal bone marrow and peripheral blood counts. This generally requires 3–6 weeks of therapy and can be achieved in more than 98% of patients. Almost all programs use vincristine, a steroid such as prednisone, and asparaginase during induction. Some programs add a fourth drug such as doxorubicin or cyclophosphamide. Once remission has been obtained, patients may receive an additional several weeks of intensive treatment with a different group of drugs in a consolidation phase or may go on to maintenance therapy.

Maintenance therapy is designed to prevent reappearance of the disease while further reducing the number of leukemic cells. Current information indicates that therapy should be continued for at least 2 years, but the optimal duration has not yet been established. The most common maintenance programs consist of mercaptopurine daily plus methotrexate once a week. Other agents may be added at periodic intervals. Some programs add periodic (1–3 months) "mini-inductions" with vincristine and 5–14 days of a corticosteroid to attempt to eliminate cells that develop resistance to the other agents. The treatment programs for ALL vary in both duration and intensity, based upon the prognostic factors of the child and the disease.

In any treatment program, the dosages of drugs must be carefully adjusted to the patient's tolerance. The goals are to give the maximum tolerated amounts of drugs while preventing unacceptable toxicities or the hazards of severe marrow depression, particularly infections associated with profound neutropenia. This generally means maintaining the white count between 2000 and 3000/μL and the absolute neutrophil count above 1000/μL.

B. Therapy for Central Nervous System Leukemia: In the absence of specific therapy directed at leukemic cells within the central nervous system, as many as 50% of children with acute lymphoblastic leukemia may develop clinical central nervous system involvement. The symptoms are most commonly headache, stiff neck, vomiting, and lethargy and may include cranial nerve palsies, hyperphagia and rapid weight gain, polydipsia, and polyuria. Physical examination may show papilledema; in younger children, a skull x-ray film may reveal spread cranial sutures. The diagnosis is established by Wright-stained cytocentrifuge preparations of spinal fluid, which demonstrate the presence of lymphoblasts. Occasional patients will have definite symptoms of central nervous system leukemia without detectable lymphoblasts in the cerebrospinal fluid; in others, unequivocal lymphoblasts will be present in the absence of any associated symptoms.

Central nervous system leukemia appears to originate from leukemia cells that gain access to the central nervous system early in the course of the disease. Many of the antileukemic drugs do not penetrate the blood-brain barrier in adequate concentrations, and the cells can proliferate in the central nervous system while the disease is being controlled systemically.

Overt central nervous system leukemia can be prevented by "prophylactic" treatment. This can be accomplished by the use of cranial irradiation, 1800 rads, or by repeated injections of drugs such as methotrexate intrathecally. Cranial irradiation in young children is associated with neurologic toxicity as manifested by decreased cognitive functioning and learning disorders and is currently avoided for children with better prognostic features. Such prophylaxis will decrease the risk of central nervous system relapse to about 5%.

If overt central nervous system disease develops, the use of intrathecal methotrexate given twice weekly for 4–6 doses will usually relieve the symptoms and clear the spinal fluid of lymphoblasts. However, the disease tends to recur within a few months, and total eradication is rarely achieved. Cytarabine may also be used intrathecally, and a repeated course of irradiation may be used to control the debilitating symptoms. Oral corticosteroids may also offer some temporary relief. If central nervous system disease develops, a bone marrow examination is needed because systemic relapse may also be present.

The best means of achieving long-term survival is by prolongation of the first remission. If bone marrow relapse occurs, second and third remissions are obtainable in 40–70% of children using vincristine and corticosteroids. Maintenance programs may then employ combinations of drugs such as cytarabine, cyclophosphamide, daunorubicin, doxorubicin, asparaginase, epipodophyllotoxin, or newer experimental agents. Bone marrow transplantation is used after relapse to produce long-term remissions in some patients, although relapse recurs in a substantial percentage of transplanted patients.

Supportive & Adjunctive Treatment

A. Massive Tumor Tissue: Uric acid nephropathy, which can be fatal, can occur during initial therapy in the presence of leukemic leukocytosis, massive hepatosplenomegaly, mediastinal mass, or compromised renal function due to infiltrates. In some patients, hyperuricemia is present prior to therapy. Prevention of uric acid nephropathy depends upon decreasing uric acid production by the use of a xanthine oxidase inhibitor, increasing uric acid solubility in urine by keeping the urine pH above 6.5, and ensuring a large urine volume. These measures are important for the first 3–7 days of therapy.

Hyperphosphatemia and hypocalcemia may occur with rapid tumor destruction. On occasion, the patient will be symptomatic and require temporary calcium supplementation.

B. Hepatic Dysfunction: When there is evidence of hepatic dysfunction as manifested by elevated enzymes or bilirubin or prolonged prothrombin time, vincristine toxicity is likely, because vincristine is excreted by the liver. Subsequent doses of vincristine may need to be reduced if toxicity is moderate to severe.

C. Infection: Cultures of blood and bone marrow and smears and cultures of pharyngeal, nasopharyngeal (if no bleeding), rectal, and urine specimens should be taken on admission and repeated as necessary. Grain-stained smears of infected lesions and body orifices should be examined immediately. Full doses of appropriate bactericidal antibiotics should be used as soon as infection is suspected. If paronychia or other skin infections occur, 0.3 mL of saline solution should be injected and aspirated for smear and culture. Do not wait for "pointing." Urinary tract infections may exist without pyuria in the granulocytopenic child. Do not delay antibiotic chemotherapy. Suspect *Escherichia coli, Klebsiella-Enterobacter,* or staphylococcal infection if the child has been receiving penicillin. Therapy should be initiated with broad-spectrum combinations such as carbenicillin plus gentamicin or carbenicillin plus cephalothin. Tobramycin may also be useful. Therapy should be given intravenously. Prolonged antibiotic therapy should be avoided.

The organisms responsible for infections in leukemic children are almost always their own skin or enteric organisms. This has 2 important implications: "Reverse" precautions are unlikely to reduce the incidence of infections beyond that obtained by good hand washing (and this tends to make good medical and nursing care more difficult to provide), and prolonged use of antibiotics may modify the gut flora and select for increasingly resistant organisms.

Pneumocystis carinii pneumonia may be treated with trimethoprim-sulfamethoxazole (Bactrim, Septra) orally. Recent evidence indicates that *Pneumocystis* infection may be prevented in susceptible patients by daily low-dosage trimethoprim therapy. Fungal infections require prolonged treatment with amphotericin B given intravenously.

The classic symptoms of infection may be masked by immunosuppressive chemotherapy. Children may have life-threatening infections with rubeola and varicella. Parents, teachers, and school nurses need to be educated regarding notification of the physician when the child shows symptoms of infection or has been exposed to contagious diseases. Varicella-zoster immune globulin or convalescent plasma given within 48 hours of exposure may prevent or modify varicella. No live virus vaccines should be given to leukemic children or those receiving immunosuppressive therapy.

D. Thrombocytopenia and Anemia: The patient with thrombocytopenia is at risk of bleeding. Platelet transfusions should be given for episodes involving difficult to control epistaxis, gastrointestinal bleeding, or signs and symptoms of central nervous system hemorrhage (retinal hemorrhage is an important finding). Prophylactic platelet transfusion is usually not indicated in thrombocytopenic patients who are not bleeding, although some clinicians give platelets prior to lumbar puncture. Because patients with fever and infection tend to have more frequent serious bleeding episodes, prophylactic platelet transfusions may be indicated.

Anemia is present in more than two-thirds of patients at the time of diagnosis. Even with successful induction therapy, it takes 2–3 weeks before adequate numbers of erythrocytes can be produced, and red cell transfusion is often needed. An attempt is made to maintain the hemoglobin concentration at greater than 10 g/dL by the use of packed red blood cell transfusions. Each transfusion is limited to 8–10 mL/kg, and in thrombocytopenic patients the transfusions are given over 3–4 hours to prevent rapid expansion of the vascular space that might precipitate hemorrhage.

E. Additional Precautions:

1. A "no salt added" diet is prescribed when the patient is taking corticosteroids.

2. Avoid deep venipunctures, intramuscular injections, and instrumentation with catheters, laryngoscopes, etc, in children with bleeding tendencies. Avoid tight clothing.

3. Avoid administration of barium sulfate during vincristine therapy, and give the child fruit, fruit juice, and plenty of liquids to help prevent constipa-

tion due to vincristine. Stool softeners may be indicated.

4. For nausea and vomiting, give antiemetics orally (or as suppositories) and fluids if needed.

5. Good nutrition and well-balanced meals are essential. Providing extra fluids on the day before and the day of cyclophosphamide therapy helps decrease bladder toxicity.

F. Psychologic Support of Patient and Family: The emotional impact of the diagnosis of leukemia is usually overwhelming and affects the entire family. A thorough discussion with the parents regarding diagnosis, prognosis, therapy, toxic reactions to drugs, and their own role in the care of the child is mandatory initially and throughout the course of the disease. Psychologic problems are common in the patient's siblings, and anticipatory guidance is needed.

What to tell the patient depends upon the maturity of the child and the judgment of physicians and family about the problems at hand. The author recommends frank discussion of the disease with the adolescent patient. The discussion should be factual and honest, emphasizing the hopeful aspects and offering reassurance that progress is being made.

Psychologic guidance may be needed for siblings, parents, and patient, and appropriate professional consultation should be obtained.

Prognosis

Centers are now reporting greater than 60% projected 5-year survival rates with various programs that have in common aggressive combination chemotherapy, treatment for occult central nervous system disease, and the use of intensive supportive therapy as needed. We will now begin to see significant numbers of long-term survivors. The word "cure" as applied to leukemia is difficult to define but is undoubtedly a reality for some patients.

See references below.

2. ACUTE NONLYMPHOCYTIC LEUKEMIA

The acute nonlymphocytic leukemias include acute myeloblastic leukemia, acute monoblastic leukemia, and leukemias whose morphologic features suggest both cell lines, the myelomonocytic leukemias.

The clinical features are similar to those of acute lymphoblastic leukemia, and the supportive care is basically the same. Therapy is more difficult, with different drugs, and produces remission rates of about 70%. Bone marrow transplantation done after the patient is in remission offers a 40–50% opportunity for long-term remission and is the best treatment currently available.

See references below.

3. CHRONIC MYELOCYTIC LEUKEMIA

Chronic myelocytic leukemia (CML) of the adult form that demonstrates the Philadelphia (Ph) chromosome is treated with busulfan (Myleran).

The juvenile non-Philadelphia chromosome (Ph-negative) form of chronic myelocytic leukemia is seen in younger children. Bleeding secondary to thrombocytopenia, organomegaly, and repeated infections makes this form of disease difficult to control clinically. Attempts at various forms of chemotherapy have been only occasionally successful. Bone marrow transplantation has been used.

Kalvinsky DK, Mirco J, Dahl GV: Biology and therapy of childhood acute nonlymphoblastic leukemia. *Pediatr Ann* 1988;**17:**172.

Lampkin BC et al: Biologic characteristics and treatment of acute nonlymphoblastic leukemia in children. *Pediatr Clin North Am* 1988;**35:**743.

Poplack DG, Reaman G: Acute lymphoblastic leukemia in childhood. *Pediatr Clin North Am* 1988;**35:**903.

Rivera GK, Mauer AM: Controversies in the management of childhood acute lymphoblastic leukemia: Treatment intensification, CNS leukemia and prognostic factors. *Semin Hematol* 1987;**24:**12.

Sanders JE et al: Marrow transplantation for children with acute lymphoblastic leukemia in second remission. *Blood* 1987;**70:**324.

Steinberg PG: Acute lymphoblastic leukemia of childhood. *Hematol Oncol Clin North Am* 1987;**1:**549.

Trigg M: Bone marrow transplantation. *Pediatr Clin North Am* 1988;**35:**933.

LYMPHOMAS

1. HODGKIN'S DISEASE

Essentials of Diagnosis

- Lymphadenopathy.
- Hepatomegaly with or without splenomegaly.
- Fever, night sweats, fatigue, weight loss, generalized pruritus.

General Considerations

The clinical course of Hodgkin's disease has been favorably altered by advances in diagnostic techniques that have improved our understanding of the disease and by the application of combined modality therapy. Optimal results depend on precise definition of the extent of disease and selection of therapy based on these results.

The histologic classification currently used is shown in Table 31–1. Nodular sclerosing Hodgkin's disease is the type most commonly seen in the second decade. Hodgkin's disease is less frequent in the

Table 31–1. Histologic classification of Hodgkin's disease.

Designation	Distinctive Features	Relative Frequency
Lymphocyte predominance	Abundant stroma of mature lymphocytes, histiocytes, or both; no necrosis; Reed-Sternberg cells may be sparse.	10–15%
Nodular sclerosis	Nodules of lymphoid tissue partially or completely separated by bands of doubly refractile collagen of variable width; atypical Reed-Sternberg cells in clear spaces ("lacunae") in the lymphoid nodules.	20–50%
Mixed cellularity	Usually numerous Reed-Sternberg and atypical mononuclear cells with a pleomorphic admixture of plasma cells, eosinophils, lymphocytes, and fibroblasts; foci of necrosis commonly seen.	20–40%
Lymphocyte depletion	Reed-Sternberg and malignant mononuclear cells usually, though not always, numerous; marked paucity of lymphocytes; diffuse fibrosis and necrosis may be present.	5–15%

first decade but has occurred in children as young as 3 years. The mixed cellularity type is more common in younger children. The response to therapy is nearly equal in these 2 types. Lymphocyte-depleted Hodgkin's disease is less common and is much less responsive to therapy.

Clinical and pathologic staging of the disease is carried out according to the Ann Arbor classification (Table 31–2). The subclassification of (A) absence or (B) presence of systemic symptoms (fever, night sweats, or loss of over 10% of body weight) is also of prognostic value. For a given stage, treatment may be more aggressive in the presence of systemic symptoms.

Clinical Findings

A. Symptoms and Signs: The most common presentation of Hodgkin's disease is painless enlargement of lymph nodes. The most common sites of involvement are the cervical node areas. The involved nodes are firm or rubbery, often matted together and nontender to palpation. They may cause symptoms by compressing other structures, such as a chronic cough due to tracheal compression from a large mediastinal mass. Extranodal disease may occur in any organ. Symptoms may be absent but may include anorexia, fatigue, weight loss, night sweats,

and pain upon ingesting alcohol. Generalized pruritus may occur.

B. Laboratory Findings: Hematologic findings are often normal but may include anemia, elevated or depressed leukocytes and platelets, and, sometimes, modest eosinophilia. The sedimentation rate and the serum copper level may be elevated. With hepatic involvement, the serum alkaline phosphatase, AST (SGOT), and ALT (SGPT) may be elevated. Many patients have tumors that take up gallium, and in these patients the gallium scan may help identify areas of involvement. Gallium scanning does not differentiate between Hodgkin's disease and inflammatory tissue, and its usefulness is limited in the subdiaphragmatic area.

Immunologic abnormalities may occur, primarily in the cell-mediated system, with anergy to the common delayed hypersensitivity antigens. Coombs-positive hemolytic anemia and abnormal immunoglobulin levels have also been described.

The diagnosis is established by histologic examination of an excised lymph node or other involved tissue. After the diagnosis is made, bone marrow biopsy and imaging studies are done. This is followed in many cases by pathologic staging, involving laparotomy with multiple abdominal lymph node biopsies, liver biopsy, wedge bone marrow biopsy, and splenectomy and may include moving the ovaries laterally to remove them from the contemplated radiation field.

C. Imaging: Chest x-ray or CT scan may show parenchymal or mediastinal nodal disease. Skeletal survey may show bone involvement. CT scanning and ultrasonography may help identify abdominal and pelvic disease. Lymphangiography may reveal "foamy" filling defects in an enlarged node, which implies tumor involving the node. Allergy to iodides and severe pulmonary disease are contraindications to lymphangiography.

Table 31–2. Staging classification for Hodgkin's disease. (Ann Arbor classification.)

Stage I	Involvement of a single lymph node region (I) or a single extralymphatic organ or site (I$_E$).
Stage II	Involvement of 2 or more lymph node regions on the same side of the diaphragm (II) or localized involvement of an extralymphatic organ or site (II$_E$).
Stage III	Involvement of lymph node regions on both sides of the diaphragm (III) or localized involvement of an extralymphatic organ or site (III$_E$) or spleen (III$_{SE}$).
Stage IV	Diffuse or disseminated involvement of one or more extralymphatic organs with or without associated lymph node involvement. The organs involved should be identified by a symbol.
A = Asymptomatic. B = Fever, sweats, weight loss > 10% of body weight.	

Complications

Patients with Hodgkin's disease have an increased susceptibility to herpes zoster and fungal infections. Therapy may induce acute toxicities that include nausea, vomiting, anorexia, alopecia, bone marrow suppression, and radiation pneumonitis. The patient must be carefully monitored so that necessary adjustments can be made in treatment. Chronic toxic effects of therapy include retardation of bone growth and an increased incidence of second malignant tumors. The splenectomy that is done as part of pathologic staging is associated with an increased incidence of sepsis, most commonly pneumococcal, which can occur days to years after the splenectomy. These septic episodes have a high mortality rate. All such splenectomized patients should be given prophylactic antibiotics to prevent sepsis and should receive pneumococcal vaccine.

A fatal complication that may develop in up to 4% of Hodgkin's disease patients is acute myelogenous leukemia. It appears to be treatment-related in that it occurs with greater frequency in patients treated with both intensive radiation therapy and chemotherapy. This occurrence emphasizes the need to refine therapy to the minimum consistent with disease eradication, so as to minimize exposure to treatment that is itself carcinogenic.

The psychologic effects of this disease and its treatment in the adolescent age group require good rapport between the patient, the family, the school, and the physician.

Treatment

Following establishment of the patient's stage of disease, therapy is planned by the chemotherapist and radiation therapist. Optimum results will be obtained by a radiation therapist skilled in the treatment of growing children by means of megavoltage irradiation. Combination chemotherapy is vastly superior to single agent therapy. Several combinations have been used effectively, including mechlorethamine, vincristine (Oncovin), procarbazine, and prednisone (MOPP); cyclophosphamide, vincristine (Oncovin), procarbazine, and prednisone (COPP); and lomustine (CCNU), vinblastine, procarbazine, and prednisone. Programs using doxorubicin (Adriamycin), bleomycin, vinblastine, and dacarbazine (ABVD) also are effective. The dosage, frequency of administration, and duration of therapy depend upon the patient's tolerance to therapy and the stage of disease.

In general, for stage IA or IIA disease, treatment may consist of extended field irradiation alone or may employ irradiation only of clinically involved areas, with or without chemotherapy. When chemotherapy is used, doses of radiation therapy can be reduced. In stage IB or IIB, extended field irradiation is followed by 6 months of chemotherapy. In stage IIIA disease, therapy is initiated with 3 cycles

of chemotherapy and the patient then receives total nodal irradiation. Following hematologic recovery, chemotherapy is resumed for a total of 9 courses.

Stage IIIB or stage IV disease is treated with chemotherapy plus irradiation to areas of bulky disease. If the liver or lungs are involved, these organs are also irradiated as tolerated.

The goal of therapy is to eradicate malignant tissue. Recurrences in nonirradiated areas may require further irradiation. The various chemotherapy programs are not cross-resistant, and second prolonged remissions often can be obtained.

Prognosis

The 5-year survival rate of pathologically staged and aggressively treated patients with stage IA and IIA disease is about 90%. Most of these will be without relapse, and a high proportion are curable. In more advanced stage IIIA disease, the 5-year survival rate is about 70%, and even in stage IV disease, survival of more than 2 years with no evidence of disease can be achieved in a majority of cases.

Bonadonna G et al: Treatment strategies for Hodgkin's disease. *Semin Hematol* 1988;**25**:51.

Sullivan MP: Hodgkin's disease in children. *Hematol Oncol Clin North Am* 1987;**1**:603.

Windebank KP, Gilchrist GS: Hodgkin's disease. *Pediatr Ann* 1988;**17**:204.

2. NON-HODGKIN'S LYMPHOMA

The non-Hodgkin's lymphomas form a relatively diverse group of cancers of the lymphoid organs. Advances in our understanding of normal lymphocyte subpopulations have enabled investigators to clarify the origin of these cancers. Lymphoma cells may carry the membrane markers of T (thymus-dependent) lymphocytes, the surface markers of immunoglobulin-producing B lymphocytes, or no distinctive markers (null cells). Many classification systems have been used for the lymphomas, resulting in confusing terminology. For pediatric lymphomas, it appears sufficient to consider 2 major histologic categories: lymphoblastic lymphoma and nonlymphoblastic lymphoma. The latter category includes Burkitt's lymphoma and pleomorphic lymphoma. This simple classification system as applied by expert pathologists has been found to be very useful in planning therapy.

The lymphoblastic histologic type of lymphoma is often associated with T cell surface markers. Patients with this disease often have a mediastinal mass, and the disease tends to involve bone marrow and the central nervous system early. This disease appears very closely related to, if not identical with, T cell leukemia.

Burkitt's lymphoma is a lymphoma involving the

B lymphocyte line. It is responsible for over half the pediatric cancer deaths in Uganda and Central Africa, and in that area the Epstein-Barr virus appears to play an important role in tumor development. Its prevalence is much lower in the USA, where it tends to present with primary abdominal involvement and an extremely aggressive pattern of spread to viscera, marrow, and bones.

Clinical Findings

A. Symptoms and Signs: The non-Hodgkin's lymphomas in general are more common in boys than in girls, and the single most common site of origin is in the lymphoid structures of the intestinal tract, usually in the ileocecal area. The most common presentation in these children is with symptoms of an acute surgical abdomen. Disease originating elsewhere generally presents as nontender lymph node involvement, which may produce symptoms due to compression. Central nervous system involvement consists of symptoms due to cord compression or increased intracranial pressure.

B. Laboratory Findings: The evaluation is similar to that used in patients with Hodgkin's disease except that routine laparotomy and splenectomy are not done. Owing to the frequency of central nervous system involvement, lumbar puncture with careful cytologic examination of the fluid needs to be done on all patients. Clinical staging permits determination of whether disease is localized, involving a single or 2 contiguous nodal areas, or nonlocalized, with either widespread nodal involvement or extranodal involvement (eg, in bone marrow or the central nervous system).

Treatment

The lymphomas are sensitive to both chemotherapy and irradiation. A number of combination chemotherapy programs are effective in producing clinical remissions. The most commonly used agents are vincristine, prednisone, cyclophosphamide, asparaginase, methotrexate, and doxorubicin in varying doses, combinations, and sequences. Radiation therapy has generally been recommended for areas of bulky disease, although recent studies suggest that with the more effective chemotherapy programs, irradiation may not be necessary. Burkitt's lymphoma and lymphomas with a mediastinal primary site have a high incidence of involvement of the central nervous system, and presymptomatic treatment of the central nervous system with irradiation or intrathecal methotrexate (or both) is therefore recommended. Maintenance chemotherapy with multiple agents is continued for 6 months to 2 years, depending on the stage of disease and the particular program being followed. Relapses in early-stage disease are very uncommon after 1 year from diagnosis; in all stages, relapses are rare after 2 years of complete remission.

Prognosis

The prognosis for children with non-Hodgkin's lymphoma has improved dramatically in the past decade. Early-stage disease (isolated intestinal involvement or single lymph node involvement other than in the mediastinum) is curable in about 90% of patients. For all patients with non-Hodgkin's lymphoma, the 2-year survival rate is about 70%. Treatment failures are often related to relapses in the bone marrow or central nervous system. Because of rapid developments in treatment for children and the importance of careful histologic evaluation in determining optimum therapy, these patients must be treated at a major pediatric cancer center.

Magrath IT: Malignant non-Hodgkin's lymphomas in children. *Hematol Oncol Clin North Am* 1987;**1**:577

Murphy SB et al: Non-Hodgkin's lymphoma of childhood. *J Clin Oncol* 1989;**7**:186.

Wilson JF et al: The pathology of non-Hodgkin's lymphoma of childhood. *Hum Pathol* 1987;**18**:1008.

NEUROBLASTOMA

Essentials of Diagnosis

- Asymptomatic abdominal mass, subcutaneous nodules, posterior mediastinal mass, and organomegaly.
- Fever, anemia, weakness, "black eyes," proptosis, opsoclonus, diarrhea, and hypertension.
- Bone pain, paraplegia, and ataxia.

General Considerations

Neuroblastoma is a tumor arising from cells in the sympathetic ganglia and adrenal medulla. It is the third most frequent pediatric neoplasm. Clinically, the survival rates are much better in children under 2 years of age, in children with extra-adrenal tumor, and in those with localized disease. These tumors may spontaneously regress in 5–10% of cases. In routine autopsies of infants under 3 months of age dying of other causes, neuroblastoma in situ in the adrenal is seen 40 times more frequently than expected, suggesting a high rate of spontaneous regression or differentiation.

Clinical staging of extent of disease is the basis of therapeutic planning. The system developed by Evans is shown in Table 31–3.

Clinical Findings

A. Symptoms and Signs: The child most commonly presents at about age 2 with a palpable abdominal mass, although the tumor may present at any time from neonatal life to adolescence. Symptoms depend upon the extent of disease at the time of diagnosis. Bone pain, weight loss, and fever may be the presenting complaints. Newborn infants may present with subcutaneous nodules and adrenal

Table 31–3. Clinical staging of neuroblastoma (Evans).

Stage I	Tumors confined to the organ or structure of origin.
Stage II	Tumors extending in continuity beyond the organ or structure of origin but not crossing the midline. Regional lymph nodes on the ipsilateral side may be involved.
Stage III	Tumor extending in continuity beyond the midline. Regional lymph nodes bilaterally may be involved.
Stage IV	Remote disease involving skeleton, parenchymatous organs, soft tissues, or distant lymph node groups. (See IV-S.)
Stage IV-S	Tumors which would be stage I or II except for the presence of remote disease confined to one or more of the following sites: liver, skin, and bone marrow (without radiographic evidence of bone metastases on complete skeletal survey).

masses with marrow involvement. Early diagnosis depends on keeping the disease in mind so that obscure presentations will not be missed.

B. Laboratory Findings: Anemia and thrombocytopenia may be present secondary to marrow replacement by neuroblasts that may mimic leukemia.

The urinary excretion of catecholamines is elevated in the majority of patients. A 24-hour urine collection for vanilmandelic acid (VMA) and homovanillic acid (HVA) should be done preoperatively. This test is useful in following the patient if levels are elevated initially. If the vanilmandelic acid levels increase during follow-up, recurrence may be suspected and reevaluation is advised. Urinary cystathionine is increased in 50% of children with neuroblastoma; it is independent of vanilmandelic acid excretion and may offer additional diagnostic help if vanilmandelic acid levels are normal.

Measurement of other urinary catecholamines is sometimes useful.

C. Imaging: Chest x-ray, skeletal survey, and intravenous urography aid in preoperative staging of the disease. Angiography may aid the surgeon in identifying the extent of the tumor and its blood supply; the tumor may be extremely vascular. Bone scanning may detect skeletal metastases before gross lesions on x-rays can be observed.

Treatment & Prognosis

Therapy involves the combined use of surgery, irradiation, and chemotherapy. Initial surgical efforts are directed at removal of as much of the primary tumor as possible. The massive size of some tumors precludes a vigorous surgical approach, and only a biopsy may be advisable. Following irradiation and chemotherapy, a second surgical procedure may permit more definitive removal. Chemotherapy with drugs such as vincristine, cyclophosphamide, doxo-

rubicin, and dacarbazine produces remissions in about 80% of patients.

Infants under 1 year of age with stage IV-S disease have a generally good prognosis, with 80% or more 2-year disease-free survival. These infants may need little if any therapy of any kind to effect a cure.

Approximately two-thirds of children with neuroblastoma after age 2 years have widely disseminated disease at the time of diagnosis. Death due to the tumor occurs in over 80%, although chemotherapy may provide remissions. In children under age 2, the prognosis is significantly better.

Evans AE et al: Prognostic factors in neuroblastoma. *Cancer* 1987;**59**:1853.

Ferster A et al: Neuroblastoma today. *Biomed Pharmacother* 1988;**42**:247.

Kushner BH, Cheung NK: Neuroblastoma. *Pediatr Ann* 1988;**17**:269.

Oppedal BR et al: Prognostic factors in neuroblastoma: Clinical, histopathologic and immunochemical features and DNA ploidy in relation to prognosis. *Cancer* 1988;**62**:772.

WILMS' TUMOR

Essentials of Diagnosis

- Asymptomatic abdominal mass or abdominal pain.
- Hematuria, genitourinary anomalies, aniridia.
- Hypertension, fever.

General Considerations

Wilms' tumor follows neuroblastoma in frequency of occurrence of pediatric solid tumors. It is believed to be embryonal in origin, develops within the kidney parenchyma, and enlarges with distortion and invasion of the adjacent renal tissue. This tumor may be associated with congenital anomalies, and patients should be evaluated for Wilms' tumor if the following entities occur: hemihypertrophy, aniridia, ambiguous genitalia, hypospadias, undescended testes, duplications of the ureters or kidneys, horseshoe kidney, or Beckwith's syndrome.

Wilms' tumor more commonly presents as an abdominal mass—in contrast to renal tumors in adults, which usually present with hematuria. The incidence of bilateral Wilms' tumor is 5–10%. Metastatic disease in liver, lungs, bone, or (rarely) brain is present in about 11% of patients at the time of diagnosis.

The prognosis in Wilms' tumor is dependent upon 2 major criteria: the clinical grouping, which is a reflection of the extent of disease at the time of diagnosis; and the histologic features of the lesion. The clinical grouping as defined by the National Wilms' Tumor Studies extends from those lesions entirely confined to the kidney and totally resected through varying degrees of extension and finally hematogenous dissemination to such organs as lung, liver, bone, and brain. Beckwith and Palmer have identified 2 histologic variants of Wilms' tumor—the anaplastic and sarcomatous varieties—which in a large series comprised only 11.5% of the cases but accounted for over 50% of the deaths due to Wilms' tumor.

Clinical Findings

A. Symptoms and Signs: Children with Wilms' tumor may be asymptomatic, and a mass may be felt by the parent while dressing or washing the child, or less commonly, by a physician on a routine well-baby examination. Occasionally, a tumor may be ruptured by a fall or trauma to the abdomen, with symptoms of an acute surgical abdomen.

B. Laboratory Findings: Complete blood count, reticulocyte count, platelet count, and bone marrow examination are needed as baselines for staging and for following therapy. Wilms' tumor rarely metastasizes to bone marrow, whereas neuroblastoma does so frequently. Urinalysis and urine culture may reveal hematuria or infection. Blood urea nitrogen and serum creatinine, uric acid, bilirubin, alkaline phosphatase, lactate dehydrogenase, and AST (SGOT) are other baseline studies of importance for following treatment. Erythropoietin levels are followed in some centers and may aid in detecting tumor activity.

C. Imaging: Posteroanterior, lateral, and oblique views of the chest should be taken to search for pulmonary metastases. Ultrasonography, CT scans, or intravenous urograms to define the tumor mass and an inferior venacavogram to rule out vascular invasion are useful. A liver scan is helpful to rule out hepatic metastases.

Treatment & Prognosis

In 1956, a 47% cure rate with total excision of Wilms' tumor was reported. Radiation therapy to the renal fossa postoperatively increased the survival rate in some series to 60%. Therapy with megavoltage equipment is begun following surgery. Dosages of 2000–3500 rads are given, depending on the age of the patient and the stage of the tumor. If the tumor is ruptured, the entire abdomen should be treated using lead shields to protect the remaining kidney. The entire vertebral body is treated to prevent scoliosis if the spine is included in the radiation field. Radiation hepatitis may occur in the treatment of right-sided Wilms' tumor, and the early chemotherapy doses may need to be adjusted downward.

In 1966, survival rates of 89% were reported when chemotherapy with dactinomycin was added to surgery and radiation therapy in 53 patients with operable tumors; 53% survival rates were reported in 15 children presenting with metastases. Chemotherapy with vincristine and dactinomycin in courses of 6–12 weeks has been effective, with tolerable toxicity. Radiation therapy and chemotherapy are given

concurrently; wound healing and adequate nutrition are important factors in following patients postoperatively. Chest films, complete blood counts, and renal function studies should be monitored during therapy. The duration of therapy depends on the patient's age and the extent of the disease.

In patients with early-stage disease and favorable histologic features, there is now a tendency to decrease the amount and duration of therapy. Thus, in patients under 2 years of age who have grossly resectable tumors, no irradiation is given, and chemotherapy consists of several months of vincristine and dactinomycin. In the presence of more extensive local disease or metastases, irradiation is added, and chemotherapy is given for longer periods, with doxorubicin added.

Currently, the 2-year disease-free survival rate is about 80% in patients with tumor extending beyond the kidney by contiguity but without apparent hematogenous spread. It is about 90% in patients with tumor confined to the kidney, and in this group patients under 2 years of age do better than older patients. Even in patients with metastatic disease, an aggressive approach is rewarded with a significant number of cures.

Beckwith JB, Palmer NF: Histopathology and prognosis of Wilms' tumor: Results from the first National Wilms' Tumor Study. *Cancer* 1978;**41**:1937.

Breslow NE et al: Second malignant neoplasms in survivors of Wilms' tumor: A report from the National Wilms' Tumor Study. *J Natl Cancer Inst* 1988;**80**:592.

Ganick DJ: Wilms' tumor. *Hematol Oncol Clin North Am* 1987;**1**:695.

Wilimas JA et al: Reduced therapy for Wilms' tumor: Analysis of treatment results from a single institution. *J Clin Oncol* 1988;**6**:1630.

Zuppan CW, Beckwith JB, Luckey DW: Anaplasia in unilateral Wilms' tumor: A report from the National Wilms' Tumor Study Pathology Center. *Hum Pathol* 1988;**19**:1199.

HEPATIC TUMORS

Essentials of Diagnosis

- Abdominal mass.
- Weight loss, malaise, fever.
- Nausea, vomiting, diarrhea, rarely jaundice.
- Liver function studies usually normal; mild to moderate anorexia, hyperlipemia, osteoporosis, elevated alpha-fetoprotein, masculinization.

General Considerations

Hepatic carcinoma is the most commonly seen cancer in the newborn period, although hepatic cancer in general is a rare tumor. A survey of the Surgical Section of the American Academy of Pediatrics revealed data on 375 children with liver tumors over a period of 10 years: 252 (67%) were malignant; of these, 129 (51%) were hepatoblastoma and 98 (39%)

hepatocellular carcinoma. The leading benign tumors were hemangioma (38 cases), hamartoma (37 cases), and hemangioendothelioma (16 cases).

Hepatic tumors decline in incidence after a peak in the first year of life, although hepatocellular carcinoma shows a substantial increase in incidence during adolescence. Children with tyrosinemia are particularly susceptible to these tumors.

Norethandrolone and other androgenic hormones used in the treatment of aplastic anemias have been associated with benign and malignant tumors.

Clinical Findings

A. Symptoms and Signs: A painless, firm right upper quadrant mass is the most common finding; anorexia, weight loss, fever, or (rarely) jaundice may be the initial complaint.

B. Laboratory Findings: The workup should include specific inquiries about chemical or drug exposure or hepatitis in addition to bone marrow examination, reticulocyte count, and renal and liver function studies, including serum bilirubin, protein electrophoresis, serum alkaline phosphatase, serum lactate dehydrogenase, and tests for hepatitis-associated antigen titer and alpha-fetoprotein.

C. Imaging: Radiologic examination includes chest examination, skeletal and liver scans, and angiography in some cases.

D. Staging: The staging of primary hepatic tumors is based on resectability of the hepatic tumor and the extent of extrahepatic spread (Table 31–4). The value of differentiating stages II, III, and IV is questionable, because the outcome is virtually the same in these stages.

Treatment & Prognosis

The prognosis for children with primary hepatic tumors is grave. In the past, only 20–50% of patients with completely resectable lesions survived and very few with unresectable lesions. Data suggest improved survival with stage I tumors when multiagent chemotherapy is given. Chemotherapy often reduces or may completely destroy the tumor. A tumor that is initially unresectable may be reduced by chemotherapy so that resection is possible at a later time. When the liver is already compromised, multimodal

therapy is difficult and is associated with significant toxicity.

Chen WJ, Lee JC, Hung WT: Primary malignant tumor of liver in infants and children in Taiwan. *J Pediatr Surg* 1988;**23**:457.
DePotter CR et al: Hepatitis B related childhood hepatocellular carcinoma. *Cancer* 1987;**60**:414.

SOFT TISSUE TUMORS

Tumors arising in tissues of mesodermal origin may be malignant or benign. Histologically, they are of connective, fatty, or muscle tissue origin. The most common clinical complaint is of a painless lump that may arise at any site. These lumps should not be "watched" for long periods of time; surgical consultation with excisional biopsy is warranted. These tumors are too often diagnosed by means of incisional biopsy, which may disseminate the tumor and make a potentially curable lesion a widespread disease.

The malignant soft tissue tumors are rhabdomyosarcoma, malignant mesenchymoma, and fibrosarcoma.

1. RHABDOMYOSARCOMA

Rhabdomyosarcoma is the most common type of sarcoma among the somatic soft tissues of children. It is most commonly found in the first 2 decades of life and is an embryonal tumor. The 4 histologic types (with definite overlapping) are embryonal, alveolar, botryoid, and pleomorphic. Common sites of occurrence are the head and neck, extremities, orbits, and pelvic regions. The histologic pattern is variable and may be related to the site—ie, if arising in a luminal structure such as the bladder or nasopharynx where there is poor support, the tumor may assume a gelatinous or botryoid ("grapelike") appearance, in contrast to the fleshy sarcomatous tumor within the body of a muscle bundle in an extremity, where a more alveolar pattern with cross-striations may be noted. This tumor is often misdiagnosed as neuroblastoma; special electron microscopic studies may be needed for clarification and show primitive Z bands in the myofibrils.

Chest x-ray, intravenous urograms, and bone marrow examination should be done. Rhabdomyoblasts may appear in the marrow as primitive "tadpole" cells. Creatine phosphokinase and lactate dehydrogenase may be elevated. Renal and liver function studies should be obtained as baselines.

Staging is based on a scheme developed for a nationwide cooperative therapy trial (Table 31–5).

When single therapeutic modalities are used, cures are rare because of the tumor's microscopic local

Table 31–4. Staging of hepatic tumors.

Stage I	Tumor confined to liver and completely resected.
Stage II	Tumor confined to liver with microscopic residual tumor at the surgical margins.
Stage III	Tumor confined to liver but unresectable or with gross residual disease.
Stage IV	Extrahepatic tumor: A. Regional spread by contiguity. B. Hematogenous metastases.

Table 31–5. Staging of rhabdomyosarcoma.

Group I	Localized disease, completely resected: (a) Confined to muscle or organ of origin. (b) Infiltration outside the muscle or organ of origin, but regional nodes not involved.
Group II	(a) Grossly resected tumor with microscopic residual disease. (b) Regional disease completely resected. (c) Regional disease grossly resected but with evidence of microscopic residual.
Group III	Incomplete resection or biopsy with gross residual disease.
Group IV	Distant metastases present at diagnosis.

extensions and early infiltration of blood and lymphatic vessels. Surgical procedures should be designed to produce wide margins of normal tissue, but amputations or mutilating procedures need not be employed. Megavoltage therapy in the range of 4000–6000 rads is used locally for any residual disease or, in initially inoperable lesions, may precede surgical extirpation. Chemotherapeutic agents with demonstrated effectiveness include dactinomycin, cyclophosphamide, vincristine, doxorubicin, and dacarbazine.

Group I patients (Table 31–5) have a greater than 90% chance of long-term survival. With only microscopic residual disease and no regional spread, about 70% of children will survive for 3 years. With regional or distant metastases at the time of diagnosis, the long-term survival rate drops to about 30%. On a stage-for-stage basis, extremity lesions tend to do less well than more central ones. This reflects in part a poorer prognosis for alveolar as compared to embryonal histologic types and reflects in part the early spread of extremity tumors to regional nodes where microscopic disease may not be initially appreciated.

Malogolowkin MH, Ortega JA: Rhabdomyosarcoma of childhood. *Pediatr Ann* 1988;**17**:251.

Ruymann FB: Rhabdomyosarcoma in children and adolescents. *Hematol Oncol Clin North Am* 1987;**1**:621.

Treuner J et al: New aspects in the treatment of childhood rhabdomyosarcoma. *Prog Pediatr Surg* 1989;**22**:162.

2. MALIGNANT MESENCHYMOMA

Malignant mesenchymoma consists of 2 or more anaplastic mesenchymal elements. It is the second most frequent soft tissue cancer. It may be found in any superficial soft tissue as well as viscera.

Since the most common differentiated element is the rhabdomyosarcoma, treatment is as above.

3. FIBROSARCOMA

Fibrosarcoma may be found as a nodule of varying size that invades locally and may metastasize to the lung. It may be present at birth but more commonly is noted in the first year of life. A variant called neurilemoma, arising in the nerve sheath, may be seen in Recklinghausen's disease.

Surgical excision is the treatment of choice. The prognosis for the completely resected infantile variety of fibrosarcoma is good. In patients with incomplete resection, local recurrence is more common than metastases. Radiation therapy and drugs such as are used for rhabdomyosarcoma may be used to treat recurrences or metastases, although the responses are often poor.

BRAIN TUMORS

Brain tumors comprise about 20% of malignant disease in pediatrics. Two-thirds of these tumors arise in the infratentorial region. The most common histologic types are cerebellar **astrocytoma, medulloblastoma,** and **brain stem glioma.** Symptoms may be generalized as a result of increased intracranial pressure secondary to obstruction of normal cerebrospinal fluid flow or may be localized to the involved area of brain. In young children, the sutures may spread in response to increased pressure, and rapid head enlargement may occur. Headaches and vomiting—especially soon after rising in the morning—and lethargy are the most common symptoms of increased pressure. Papilledema is found in older children with increased pressure but may be absent in infants when the sutures spread to provide decompression.

In addition to a careful neurologic examination, brain scanning, CT scanning and magnetic resonance imaging are important noninvasive diagnostic procedures. Cerebral angiography may aid in precise tumor localization.

Therapy depends upon the tumor type. Cerebellar astrocytomas can often be totally excised, and no other therapy is indicated. With incomplete removal of more aggressive lesions, radiotherapy may be added. The 10-year survival rate is about 65%. Chemotherapy is not of proved effectiveness in primary management but may play a role in tumor recurrence.

Medulloblastoma is radiosensitive. Following surgery to reduce the tumor burden, radiation therapy is given to the primary and to the entire neuraxis because of the predilection of the tumor to metastasize to other areas of the brain and spinal cord via the cerebrospinal fluid. This therapy may produce 25% 10-year survival rates. Trials of various chemotherapeutic agents have now demonstrated an improved prognosis for some children receiving combined modality therapy.

Brain stem gliomas are usually not amenable to operation, and biopsy may not be feasible. Radiation therapy may produce survivals ranging from a few months in high-grade tumors to 3–5 years in low-grade ones. Chemotherapy with nitrosoureas and methotrexate, either intrathecally or in high doses by the intravenous route, has caused tumor regression, but the role of drugs is not established.

Finlay JL: Progress in the management of childhood brain tumors. *Hematol Oncol Clin North Am* 1987;**1**:753.

Finlay JL, Goins SC: Brain tumors in children. 3. Advances in chemotherapy. *Am J Pediatr Hematol Oncol* 1987;**9**:264.

Jenkins RDT et al: Brain stem tumors in childhood: A prospective randomized trial of irradiation with and without adjuvant CCNV, VCR and prednisone. *J Neurosurg* 1987;**66**:227.

Le Baron S et al: Assessment of quality of survival in children with medulloblastoma and cerebellar astrocytoma. *Cancer* 1988;**62**:1215.

BONE TUMORS

A variety of benign and malignant tumors may originate in bone. Bones are also common sites of metastatic disease. The principal symptoms of bone tumors, whether primary or metastatic, are pain and swelling. A fracture may first call attention to an area of cortical destruction due to cancer. The diagnosis must be based on careful and complete clinical evaluation and examination of an adequate biopsy specimen. (See Table 31–6.)

Ewing's sarcoma occurs most commonly in the long bones of the lower extremities and in the pelvis. Radiographically, it shows cortical bone destruction, often with periosteal elevation and an "onion skin" appearance beneath the periosteum. It must be differentiated from neuroblastoma, rhabdomyosarcoma, and non-Hodgkin's lymphoma. Metastasis occurs to other bones and to the lungs and may be present at diagnosis in one-third of patients. Ewing's sarcoma is treated with radiation doses of 6000–8000 rads over a 6- to 8-week period and with combination chemotherapy for 2 years employing vincristine, cyclophosphamide, doxorubicin, and dactinomycin. In patients without overt metastasis, 75% or more should live 3 years with no evidence of recurrent disease.

Surgical resection rather than irradiation should be considered for treatment of Ewing's sarcoma if resection can be done without an incapacitating loss of function. The high doses of radiation required may predispose adjacent normal tissues to the development of radiation-induced osteogenic sarcoma.

Osteogenic sarcoma is the most common malignant bone tumor in the pediatric age group. It is most frequently seen during adolescence and usually occurs in long bones, with the distal femur, proximal tibia, and proximal humerus being the most common sites. The diagnosis is made by biopsy, and the therapeutic approach is jointly planned after a careful

Table 31–6. Malignant neoplasms.

Disease	Clinical Features	X-Ray Features	Treatment	Prognosis
Osteosarcoma and chondrosarcoma	Pain the most common symptom. Mass, functional loss, limp occasionally present. Pathologic fracture common.	Destructive, expanding, invasive lesion. Minimal host reaction, but, if present, usually is a triangle between tumor, elevated periosteum, and cortex. Usually radiolucent, but lesional tissue may show ossification or calcification. Metaphyseal location common. Femur, tibia, humerus, and other long bones predominate.	Surgical excision or amputation. Radiation-resistant. Markedly improved prognosis (50–70%) results from use of surgery combined with doxorubicin and methotrexate in osteosarcoma.	Poor. Probably less than 5 or 10% cured. Metastases to lungs, occasionally to other bones. Life expectancy has been prolonged by use of chemotherapy.
Fibrosarcoma	Rare lesions in children.	Radiolucent, destructive, expanding, invasive lesion. Little or no host reaction. Long bones predominate.	Surgical excision or amputation.	Poor. Probably 10–15% cured. Metastases to lungs.
Ewing's tumor	Pain very common. Tenderness, fever, and leukocytosis also common. Frequent pathologic fracture. Frequently multicentric.	Radiolucent, destructive lesion, frequently in diaphyseal region of the bone. May be reactive bone formation about the lesion in successive layers—"onion skin" layering.	Radiation-sensitive but not curable. Surgical excision usually not desirable because of multiple areas of involvement. Chemotherapy by vincristine, doxorubicin, and cyclophosphamide.	Poor. Metastases to multiple organs.

review of the x-ray and histologic findings and the bone scan results.

Therapy for this tumor is undergoing rapid change. The traditional and still most widely used surgical approach is amputation above the joint proximal to the involved bone or, in the case of femoral lesions, amputation across the femur as high as possible to avoid the tumor while retaining enough femoral shaft to fit well into a prosthesis. This is followed by intensive chemotherapy with vincristine, high doses of methotrexate with folinic acid rescue, doxorubicin, and cisplatin. Chemotherapy extends over a period of 2 years. More recent approaches utilize aggressive preoperative chemotherapy, often with intra-arterial drugs. This approach may permit local tumor resection and limb sparing while improving the likelihood of cure.

Horowitz ME: Ewing's sarcoma: Current status of diagnosis and treatment. *Oncology* 1989;**3**:101.

Huth JF, Eilber FR: Patterns of recurrence after resection of osteosarcoma of the extremity: Strategies for treatment of metastases. *Arch Surg* 1989;**124**:122.

Jurgens H et al: Multidisciplinary treatment of primary Ewing's sarcoma of bone: A 6 year experience of a European cooperative trial. *Cancer* 1988;**61**:23.

Meyers PA: Malignant bone tumors in children: Ewing's sarcoma. *Hematol Oncol Clin North Am* 1987;**1**:667.

Springfield DS et al: Surgical treatment for osteosarcoma. *J Bone Joint Surg [Am]* 1988;**70**:1124.

Tebbi CK, Gaeta J: Osteosarcoma. *Pediatr Ann* 1988;**17**:285.

RETICULOENDOTHELIOSES

The diseases to be discussed under this heading comprise a heterogeneous group of proliferative disorders that involve the reticuloendothelial system and are of unknown cause. Eosinophilic granuloma of bone, Hand-Schüller-Christian disease, and Letterer-Siwe disease constitute a complex of diseases of unknown cause, of histiocytic proliferation, and of unpredictable prognosis. They are sometimes grouped under the term histiocytosis X. These disorders, frequently showing Langerhans' cells on ultrastructural study, should be differentiated from reactive histiocytosis seen in diseases caused by infection and immunodeficiency.

Certain patients present primarily with signs and symptoms of lytic lesions limited to the bones—especially the skull, ribs, clavicles, and vertebrae. These lesions are well demarcated and occasionally painful. Biopsy reveals eosinophilic granuloma, which may be the only lesion the patient will develop, although further bone and even visceral lesions may occur.

Another group of patients often present with otitis media, seborrheic skin rash, and evidence of bone lesions, usually in the mastoid or skull area. They frequently also have visceral involvement, which may be indicated by lymphadenopathy and hepatosplenomegaly. This chronic disseminated form is usually known as Hand-Schüller-Christian disease and is associated with "foamy histiocytes" on biopsy. The classic triad of Hand-Schüller-Christian disease (bony involvement, exophthalmos, and diabetes insipidus) is rarely seen; however, diabetes insipidus is a common complication.

A third group of patients present early in life primarily with visceral involvement. They often have a petechial or macular skin rash, generalized lymphadenopathy, enlarged liver and spleen, pulmonary involvement, and hematologic abnormalities such as anemia and thrombocytopenia. Bone lesions can occur. This acute visceral form—Letterer-Siwe disease—is often fatal.

The principal diseases to be differentiated from histiocytosis X are bone tumors (primary or metastatic), lymphomas or leukemias, granulomatous infections, storage diseases, reactive histiocytosis, sinus histiocytosis, and lymphohistiocytosis reticulosis. The diagnosis is established by biopsy of bone marrow, lymph node, liver, or mastoid or other bone. Tissue should be preserved for electron microscopy.

Almost any system or area can become involved during the course of the disease. Rarely, these will include the heart (subendocardial infiltrates), bowel, eye, mucous membranes such as vagina or vulva, and dura mater.

Isolated bony lesions are best treated by curettage and local radiotherapy. Multiple bony involvement and visceral involvement often respond well to prednisone, vinblastine (Velban), mechlorethamine (Mustargen), or methotrexate. The current treatment of choice at the author's institution is prednisone and vinblastine or etoposide, given in repeated courses or continuously until healing of lesions occurs.

If diabetes insipidus occurs, treatment with vasopressin (Pitressin) gives good control (see Chapter 26).

In idiopathic histiocytosis, the prognosis is often unpredictable. Many patients with considerable bony and visceral involvement have shown apparent complete recovery. In general, however, the younger the patient and the more extensive the visceral involvement, the worse the prognosis.

Berry DH et al: Natural history of histiocytosis X: A pediatric oncology group study. *Med Pediatr Oncol* 1986;**14**:1.

Broadbent V: Favorable prognostic features in histiocytosis X: Bone involvement and absence of skin disease. *Arch Dis Child* 1986;**61**:1219.

SELECTED REFERENCES

Chesler MA, Barbarin OA: *Childhood Cancer and the Family.* Brunner/Mazel, 1987.

McWhirter WR, Masel JP: *Paediatric Oncology: An Illustrated Introduction.* Williams & Wilkins, 1987.

Oakhill A (editor): *The Supportive Care of the Child with Cancer.* Butterworth, 1988.

Pizzo PA, Poplack DG (editors): *Principles and Practice of Pediatric Oncology.* Lippincott, 1989.

Riehm H (editor): *Malignant Neoplasms in Childhood and Adolescence.* Karger, 1986.

32   Allergic Disorders

David S. Pearlman, MD, & Carolyn R. Comer, MD

Allergic disorders include a variety of local and systemic manifestations that commonly are ultimate expressions of the union between antigen and antibody. Although this union triggers the chain of events that culminates in the clinical allergic reaction, nonimmunologic factors are important in modifying this chain of events. In some instances, nonimmunologic factors can be completely responsible for clinical reactions indistinguishable from immunologically induced reactions (eg, some forms of chronic urticaria).

Allergic reactivity is normal. The reaction that results from the transfusion of mismatched blood is an allergic reaction; the repeated injection of antitoxin in the form of foreign serum often leads to serum sickness; and contact with poison ivy frequently causes an allergic dermatitis. By definition, allergic reactions stem from an antigen-antibody interaction; identification of these participants is of prime importance both in the diagnosis and in the therapy of allergic disorders. It is often difficult to identify the antigens (allergens) responsible for a particular clinical disorder, but the most helpful procedure is a thorough and detailed history. Tests for the presence of a specific antibody that will implicate specific allergens are also helpful and may be necessary for diagnosis.

Some forms of allergic reactivity, however, occur only in certain members of the population. These disorders (allergic rhinitis, asthma, and atopic dermatitis) are called **atopic disorders,** a term signifying an unusual form of reactivity for which there is some unknown and probably genetic predisposition. An individual with such a disorder is sensitized to substances usually considered innocuous to other people. Animal danders, feathers, spores from indoor molds, and house dust mites are the most common perennial allergens. Animal danders and emanations of house dust mites (high in mattress flock) and of cockroaches (abundant in poor housing situations) are important factors contributing to the allergenicity of house dust. Many variants of tree, grass and weed pollens, and molds cause atopic disorders in a more or less seasonal incidence (trees in the spring; grasses in late spring and summer; weeds in late summer and fall; and outdoor molds in summer and fall). Foods and a number of other substances may contribute to perennial or seasonal problems.

Atopic individuals commonly become sensitized to one or more of these substances.

It is important to remember that many atopic disorders, including many cases of asthma and atopic dermatitis, are due to or are influenced by causes other than allergic sensitization.

PRINCIPLES OF DIAGNOSIS

The diagnosis of allergic disease is based primarily on the clinical findings. Laboratory procedures (including allergy testing) can be very helpful, but results should be interpreted in the light of the history and physical findings. Arriving at a diagnosis of any or all atopic diseases requires a detailed history and complete physical examination. More than one atopic disease may be present, and a history of familial atopic disorders or of other past or present atopic symptoms is especially useful. The following is a guideline for the overall history, physical examination, and supplementary diagnostic procedures.

History
A. Chief Complaint of Patient.

B. History of Present Illness: Details of development of first episode and circumstances of subsequent and most recent episodes. Areas of inquiry include infection, change in environment (family move, acquisitions of pets or toys, different household furnishings, improvement or worsening in symptoms with travel to different regions), season of year, ingestion of "new" food, special occasions, emotional and social upheavals.

C. Other Allergic Diseases: Associated atopic or other allergic diseases (past or present), especially allergic rhinitis, bronchial asthma, "allergic cough," atopic dermatitis, food intolerance (eg, colic, vomiting, abdominal pain, abnormal stools, skin rashes), eczema, hives, and angioedema.

D. Infections: History of pneumonia, bronchitis, bronchiolitis, croup, recurrent ear infections, sinusitis, removal of tonsils and adenoids.

E. Past Therapy and Response to It.

F. Emotional and Social Factors and Habits: Family structure; general attitudes and behavior; family, school, and social adjustments.

G. Family History.

H. Environmental History:
House pets; exposure to cigarette smoke; type of heating and air conditioning (including the presence of a central humidifier and other forms of heating such as a wood-burning stove); use of a portable vaporizer or humidifier; presence of mold or mildew in the home; details of patient's bedroom, including location in the home, composition and age of mattress and pillows, type of bedding and window dressing, and floor covering (age and type of carpet); details regarding day-care center or babysitter's home, including amount of time spent weekly, number of children, and presence of animals or cigarette smoke.

Physical Examination:

A complete physical examination is essential. The following signs deserve special emphasis:

A. General Appearance of Patient: State of nourishment and physical development, including weight and height; degree of activity; signs of fatigue; sneezing; cough and its character; dyspnea.

B. Attitudes: Responses and relationships of the patient to parents, physician, nurses, etc.

C. Vital Signs: Blood pressure, temperature, pulse rate, and character of respirations.

D. Skin: Rashes, pallor, cyanosis, temperature changes, sweating, degree of dryness.

E. Eyes: "Allergic shiners" (lower lid edema, eyeshadowing), conjunctival injection, blebs, itching, cataracts (in severe, long-standing atopic dermatitis), blepharitis (from chronic rubbing), tearing.

F. Nose: Itching ("allergic salute," "bunny nose," nasal crease), excoriation of nares, hyperemia, mucosal edema, polypoid changes, purplish pallor, excessive serous or mucoid discharge.

G. Ears: Auditory tube dysfunction, retraction of drums and decreased drum mobility; recurrent serous otitis media, hearing loss, changes in drum (immobility, distortion, retraction, fullness, opacity, narrow and "chalky" malleus), evidence of fluid in middle ear.

H. Mouth: Palatal malformations, character of speech, "canker sores," changes in tongue (geographism, grooving).

I. Throat: Presence and appearance of tonsils and pharyngeal lymphoid tissue, appearance of mucosal epithelium (anterior pillars, soft palate, pharyngeal wall), character of secretions.

J. Chest: Configuration ("barrel chest," "pigeon breast," prominent Harrison's grooves—all may be present in long-standing asthma), evidence of hyperinflation, pattern of breathing, development and use of accessory muscles for respiration (eg, hypertrophy of pectorals, trapezii, sternocleidomastoids), retractions.

K. Lungs: Relationship to inspiratory-expiratory cycle of gross or auscultatory wheezes (including wheezing brought on after exercise and forced expiration), rhonchi, or rales; degree and equality of air exchange; level and movement of diaphragm.

L. Heart: Tachycardia, size, accentuation of pulmonic second sound (for evidence of pulmonary hypertension in asthma), murmurs.

Supplementary Diagnostic Procedures

A. Allergy Tests: In all atopic disorders, reaginic or skin-sensitizing (IgE) antibody is important. Testing for the presence of IgE antibody is potentially useful in identifying allergens that may play a role in the disorder.

1. Skin tests—Scratch or prick testing should be done first, because it is less likely than intradermal testing to cause severe reactions in sensitive individuals. Intradermal testing is about 100 times more sensitive than scratch testing. The tests are read at the peak of the reaction, usually within 15–20 minutes. If these tests are negative, intradermal tests (on an extremity) may be performed. Skin testing is potentially dangerous in highly sensitive individuals; for this reason, epinephrine and a tourniquet should always be at hand.

A positive test reaction occurs when antigen combines with skin-sensitizing (IgE) antibody, thus producing erythema, wheal, and flare (triple response) from the liberation of histamine and other chemical mediators. In properly interpreting the skin tests and assessing their clinical significance, the following should be kept in mind: (1) Mild reactions are less likely to be clinically significant than more strongly positive reactions. (2) Strong (3–4 +) reactions to foods are likely to be of clinical significance (in contrast to mild reactions), but negative reactions do not rule out nonallergic (nor completely rule out allergic) clinical sensitivity. (3) A positive skin test suggests only that antibody is present in the skin. It may reflect past, present, or potential clinical hypersensitivity, but it is not necessarily clinically significant. The patient may or may not develop an atopic disease due to the specific allergen. The clinical importance of positive skin tests should be interpreted in correlation with the clinical history.

2. Serologic tests—The use of immunoassays to measure serum IgE antibody is increasing. The best known is the radioallergosorbent test (RAST), a radioimmunoassay, but enzyme-linked immunoassays that eliminate the need for radioactive material are also available.

Results of RAST and similar tests correlate well with those of skin tests, although the former are somewhat less sensitive. They are advantageous because they allow for testing of individuals in whom skin testing would be difficult (eg, patients with extensive dermatitis) and because there is no risk of provoking a hypersensitivity reaction. These tests would be especially useful in testing for severe hypersensitivity to drugs and stinging insects; however, these tests are less sensitive than skin tests. The usefulness of RAST and similar tests for this purpose is therefore somewhat limited. The number of antigens available for testing is also limited; furthermore, the greater expense of these tests and the delay in obtaining results make skin testing much preferable at this time.

B. Measurement of IgE Immunoglobulin Levels: The radioimmunosorbent test (RIST) measures the concentration of IgE immunoglobulin in the blood. Elevated IgE levels as measured by RIST or PRIST (paper RIST) suggest an atopic disorder, but the correlation is so imperfect that this is not a generally useful screening procedure. Greatly elevated IgE levels in infancy (> 2 SD above the mean) are highly predictive of an atopic diathesis, and elevated IgE levels in bronchiolitis suggest the diagnosis of asthma. However, a normal or low level of IgE does not rule out an atopic disorder or allergic sensitization.

C. Provocative Testing: The suspicion of the clinical importance of an allergen may be confirmed by the use of a "provocative test," ie, challenging a given individual with the suspected allergen and observing the response. Provocative testing may be employed but is not recommended as a routine procedure for any potentially severe disorder such as asthma and should not be performed with a substance suspected of causing a potentially life-threatening reaction. Provocative tests are most valuable in determining clinical sensitivity to foods. Elimination and subsequent challenge may be especially revealing if done properly but also can be misleading if an objective protocol for assessing the response is not followed. Direct provocative inhalant testing is potentially hazardous and is best performed in a hospital setting.

D. Eosinophilia: Increased numbers of eosinophils in the blood or bodily secretions (nasal, gastrointestinal) are frequently present in a variety of allergic conditions, especially in atopic disorders; the presence of eosinophilia may strengthen a suspicion of allergic diathesis. Nasal eosinophilia (> 15%) is highly suggestive of allergic rhinitis, but eosinophilia can occur in the absence of clinical allergies. Conversely, the absence of eosinophilia does not rule out allergy, particularly because a variety of factors (eg, concurrent infection) may suppress eosinophilia. The degree of eosinophilia correlates inversely with the degree of control of allergic and nonallergic asthma. Nasal eosinophilia in infants up to 3 months of age may be normal.

E. Controversial Techniques for Diagnosis And Treatment: Intracutaneous end point titration, sublingual and serial intracutaneous provocative titration tests, cytotoxic tests, and sublingual desensitization all have been claimed by some to be of value in diagnosing and treating allergic disorders. Their merit is yet to be validated scientifically, and they remain techniques of unproved value that are not recommended.

GENERAL PRINCIPLES OF TREATMENT

Environmental Control of Exposure

Because the clinical allergic reaction stems from the union of antigen with antibody, avoidance of the offending antigen is the most effective means of therapy of all allergic disorders. Moreover, there is reason to believe that continued exposure to an allergen can heighten sensitivity to other unrelated allergens and nonallergic irritants; thus, avoidance therapy has additional therapeutic implications, particularly in chronic allergic disorders. In many instances, complete avoidance of identified allergens is impossible, but it is frequently feasible to reduce the incidence and severity of reactions by minimizing the contact. Many nonimmune factors can precipitate or aggravate atopic disorders (eg, irritating smoke; cold air in asthma), and avoidance of such known or suspected irritants is also important.

The following are sample directions for environmental control of common allergens. They pertain mainly to the patient's bedroom, but the principles are applicable to the rest of the house as well.

1. House dust is a common offender as an irritant and allergen (especially from mites and insects, cats, and dogs). The accumulation of dust may be minimized by the avoidance of dust catchers and dust producers, such as wool (in rugs and blankets), flannel (in bedding and pajamas), upholstered furniture, toys stuffed with plant or animal products, chenille (bedspreads, drapes, and rugs), cotton quilts, stuffed cotton pads, and venetian blinds.

2. Rooms should be dusted daily with a damp or oiled cloth. The room should be cleaned thoroughly at least once a week—never with the patient present.

3. All forced air ducts, which frequently contain dust and molds and tend to stir up room dust, should be sealed off. An electric radiator may be substituted as a source of heat, if necessary. If pollinosis is a problem, windows should be kept closed during the pollen seasons. Air cleaners (central or room) and refrigerated air conditioners may be useful. Automatic humidifiers with provision for humidity not to exceed 40% can be helpful in dry climates and with heating systems. Humidifiers should be kept as free of mold as possible. In humid climates where dust mite, and mold sensitivity are more of a problem, dehumidification may be appropriate.

4. Plant products (kapok, cotton) and animal products sometimes used for pillows, stuffing of furniture, toys, bedding, and hair pads for rugs should be eliminated. Alternatively, all mattresses, box

springs, and pillows in the bedroom should be completely enclosed in impermeable plastic or rubber casings. Inexpensive casings may be obtained from department stores; better quality casings may be obtained from Environtrol P.O. Box 31313 St. Louis, MO 63131 Aller-Guard, Inc. Southgate Office Park 1645 S.W. 41st Street Topeka, Kansas 66609. Plastic casings especially should be checked periodically for tears or punctures. Furniture and bedding stuffed solely with synthetic products or rubber are permissible; rubber pillows, however, may harbor molds. Toys stuffed with old nylon stockings or synthetic foam and covered with plain, nonfuzzy cotton or synthetic materials are satisfactory.

5. Cleaning equipment, wool, and fur coats should not be kept in or near the child's room or closet.

6. Sensitization to animals develops so frequently in atopic individuals that close contact with animals of any sort should be avoided. Danders, saliva, and urine are the important sources of allergen. Depending on the degree of sensitivity, it may be important to rid the environment of animals altogether.

Hyposensitization (Immunotherapy)

If avoidance of offensive allergens is not possible, specific hyposensitization is sometimes attempted. The value of hyposensitization is limited mainly to atopic disorders and to severe insect allergy. There are a variety of hyposensitization procedures, but the same general principle applies to all: Extremely small amounts of allergen are injected subcutaneously at frequent intervals and in increasing amounts until a "top dose" is reached; this is usually the highest tolerated dose of a given allergen extract or that amount which induces a state of clinical hyporeactivity to the allergen as demonstrated after natural contact. When perennial therapy is adopted, the top tolerated dose is used as a maintenance dose, with carefully regulated lengthening of intervals (by not more than an additional week at a time) generally up to 4 weeks, as tolerated.

Most allergists agree that the majority of well-selected patients with pollen asthma or hay fever are significantly improved after 1–2 years of therapy on a "perennial" injection regimen of aqueous antigens, and there is evidence to substantiate the beneficial effects of hyposensitization even in perennial asthma. The effectiveness of therapy is dose-related. Repository therapy using alum-precipitated extracts (Allpyral, Center-Al) is useful mainly in increasing the antigen dosage in individuals who are extremely sensitive to small amounts of aqueous antigen. Theoretically, fewer injections of alum-precipitated material are required to reach a maintenance dose of antigen, and maintenance injections need to be given less frequently. Mold hyposensitization therapy is believed to offer significant protection, but adequate

documentation of this hypothesis is lacking. The value of hyposensitization against house dust mites is substantiated; it is beneficial but is no substitute for good environmental control. Venom therapy for sensitivity to stinging insects is efficacious. The use of bacterial extracts appears to be of little value and has been largely abandoned. Hyposensitization to foods is nonefficacious and may actually be dangerous.

Drug Therapy

Many drugs are effective in the treatment of allergic disorders (Table 32–1). The principal groups include adrenergic agents, antihistamines, methylxanthines, cromolyn sodium, anticholinergic agents, expectorants, oxygen, and adrenocorticosteroids. The selection of drugs depends upon the pathologic processes involved.

A. Adrenergic Agents: As a group, adrenergic agents exhibit many different pharmacologic effects. Their usefulness in allergic disorders depends mainly on their ability to constrict blood vessels and relax other smooth muscle. The manifestation of many allergic reactions is due, at least in part, to chemical mediators, such as histamine and leukotrienes, that produce varying degrees of vasodilatation, edema, and smooth muscle spasm. Adrenergic agents are the principal pharmacologic antagonists of these chemical mediators and at times may even reverse their effects completely. However, the pharmacologic properties of adrenergic drugs as a group are not shared uniformly by all members of the group, and these drugs cannot be used interchangeably to produce a given effect. In rhinitis, for example, phenylephrine, an effective vasoconstrictor but a poor smooth muscle dilator, is especially useful. Albuterol, on the other hand, although devoid of vasoconstrictor action, is an effective bronchodilator and is useful in asthma. In asthma and in anaphylaxis—in which vasodilatation, edema, and asthma may all be a problem—epinephrine, which is a potent antagonist of all of these effects, is the drug of choice.

Adrenergic drugs are not always effective in a given disorder and are not without undesirable effects. Epinephrine resistance may occur in severe asthma, for example, and the use of the drug in such cases may actually aggravate the disorder by increasing the patient's anxiety and contributing to venous congestion and mucus plugging. The injection of epinephrine when severe hypoxemia and acidosis are present may produce cardiac dysrhythmia or arrest. Adrenergic aerosols can be extremely effective in acute asthma, but some (eg, isoproterenol) have been shown to severely aggravate asthma if used excessively. Aerosols containing newer β_2-adrenergic drugs appear to be safer.

B. Antihistamines: The antihistamines act through competition with histamine for receptor sites, thereby preventing histamine from exerting its

Table 32–1. Preparations and dosages of drugs commonly used in allergic disorders.

Agent	Dosage
Adrenergic agents	
Epinephrine aqueous, 1:1000 (Adrenalin)	0.01 mL/kg SC or IM up to 0.3 mL. (May repeat at 20-minute intervals—total of 3 doses.)
Terbutaline[1] (Bricanyl), 1 mg/mL	0.01 mL/kg SC or IM up to 0.25 mL. (May repeat at 20-minute intervals—total of 2 doses.)
Epinephrine suspension, long-acting, 1:200 (Sus-Phrine)	0.1–0.2 mL SC every 8–12 hours. (Shake well before administering.)
Pseudoephedrine hydrochloride (Sudafed)	1 mg/kg/dose orally, 4–6 times a day.
Metaproterenol (Alupent, Metaprel)	10–20 mg orally, every 6–8 hours.
Terbutaline[1] (Brethine, Bricanyl)	2.5 mg orally, every 8 hours.
Albuterol[1] (salbutamol; Proventil, Ventolin), 2- to 4-mg tablets	2–4 mg orally, 3 times a day.
Adrenergic aerosols	
Albuterol[1] (Salbutamol; Proventil, Ventolin) Bitolterol[1] (Tornalate) Isoetharine mesylate (Bronkometer) Metaproterenol[1] (Alupent, Metaprel) Terbutaline[1] (Brethaire)	1–2 inhalations from pressurized aerosol. May use as often as every 4 hours. *Avoid excessive use.*
Isoetharine (Bronkosol) 1% solution	0.15–0.5 mL diluted with 1 mL water or saline and administered by hand or compressor-driven nebulizer.
Metaproterenol[1] (Alupent, Metaprel) 5% inhalant solution	0.1–0.3 mL diluted with 1 mL water or saline and administered by hand or compressor-driven nebulizer.
Albuterol[1] (Proventil, Ventolin) 0.5% inhalant solution	0.25–0.5 mL diluted with 2 mL water or saline and administered by hand or compressor-driven nebulizer.
Drugs with antihistaminic activity	
Diphenhydramine hydrochloride (Benadryl) Injectable	1 mg/kg/dose (up to 50 kg) orally, 4 times a day. 25–50 mg IV (slowly) or IM (ampules, 50 mg/mL; vials, 10 mg/mL).
Chlorpheniramine maleate (Chlor-Trimeton, Chlor-Trimeton Repetabs, Teldrin) Injectable	0.1 mg/kg/dose (up to 50 kg) orally, 4 times a day. 0.1–0.2 mg/kg/dose (up to 50 kg) orally, 2 times a day. 4–8 mg IV (slowly) or IM (10 mg/mL in 1-mL vials; 100 mg/mL in 2-mL vials).
Terfenadine[1] (Seldane) 60-mg tablets	1 tablet twice a day.
Clemastine fumarate[1] (Tavist) 2.68-mg tablets	1 tablet up to 3 times a day.
Hydroxyzine (Atarax, Vistaril)	0.2–0.5 mg/kg/dose (up to 50 kg) orally, 3 times a day.
Cyproheptadine (Periactin)	0.05 mg/kg/dose (up to 50 kg) orally, 3–4 times a day.
Combination drugs for allergic rhinitis and conjunctivitis	
Pseudoephedrine and triprolidine (Actifed)	Syrup: ½–2 tsp 3 times a day depending on age. Tablets: ½–1 tablet 3 times a day depending on age.
Pseudoephedrine and dexbrompheniramine[1] (Drixoral)	Tablets: 1 tablet 2 times a day (older children). Syrup: ½–1 tsp every 4–6 hours (younger children).
Pseudoephedrine and carbinoxamine (Rondec)	Drops: ¼–1 dropperful 4 times a day (infants). Syrup: ½–1 tsp 4 times a day (older children). Tablets: ½–1 tablet 4 times a day (older children).
Phenylpropanolamine, pyrilamine, and pheniramine (Triaminic)	Drops: 5–10 drops 3 times a day (infants). Syrup: ½–2 tsp 4 times a day depending on age. Juvulets: 1–2 tablets 4 times a day (older children).
Expectorants	
Guaifenesin (glyceryl guaiacolate; Robitussin)	1 tsp every 4–6 hours.
Methylxanthines	
Aminophylline, theophylline (Choledyl, Elixophyllin, Quibron, Respbid, Slo-Bid, Slo-Phyllin, Somophyllin, Sustaire, Theo-24, Theo-Dur, Theolair, Theophyl, Theospan, Theostat, Uniphyl)	IV: 4–6 mg^2/kg every 4–6 hours (infuse over 10- to 20-minute period or as 0.6–1 mg/kg/h at constant drip). Oral: 4–6 mg^2/kg every 6 hours. Longer-acting preparations can be used every 8–12 hours (eg, Slo-Bid, Theo-Dur) or every 24 hours (Theo-24, Uniphyl) in children over 12 years of age. Rectal: Enema (Somophyllin), 4–6 mg^2/kg every 6 hours.

Adrenal glucocorticoids
Most rapid therapeutic effect follows intravenous or oral administration, but there may be no perceptible effect for hours. In acute situations, high doses of corticosteroids (eg, 100–200 mg hydrocortisone or 40–80 mg methylprednisolone [Solu-Medrol] every 4–6 hours) are generally employed the first day and the dose tapered as rapidly as possible to maintenance levels or withdrawn completely.
Approximate equivalents of activity: 100 mg hydrocortisone = 4 mg dexamethasone = 25 mg prednisolone = 20 mg methylprednisolone.

Table 32–1 (cont'd.). Preparations and dosages of drugs commonly used in allergic disorders.

Agent	Dosage
Intravenous preparations	
Hydrocortisone sodium succinate (Solu-Cortef)	100 mg in 2-mL vials.
Methylprednisolone (Solu-Medrol)	40 mg in 1-mL vials.
Fluocinolone acetonide	0.025% cream or ointment and 0.01% cream.
Triamcinolone acetonide (Kenalog)	0.025% cream and 0.1% and 0.5% cream and ointment.
Hydrocortisone	0.5% and 1% hydrocortisone cream or ointment.
Topical corticosteroid preparations for severe asthma	
Beclomethasone dipropionate[3] (Beclovent, Vanceril)	Not to exceed 3 inhalations 4 times a day.
Flunisolide[3] (AeroBid)	2 inhalations 2 times a day.
Triamcinolone acetonide[3] (Azmacort)	1–2 inhalations 3 times a day.
Topical inhalant preparations for asthma prophylaxis	
Cromolyn sodium, 20-mg or vials or 1mg/spray in metered dose inhaler	1 capsule or vial or 2 puffs from the pressurized aerosol is inhaled 3–4 times a day or just prior to exercise or contact with asthma-precipitating agents.
Topical inhalant preparations for rhinitis	
Beclomethasone dipropionate[1] (Beconase, Vancenase)	1 inhalation in each nostril up to 3 times a day, or 2 inhalations in each nostril 2 times a day. Discontinue if there is any nasal bleeding.
Dexamethasone sodium phosphate[3] (Turbinaire Decadron Phosphate)	1–2 sprays in each nostril 2 times a day. (Should be used for short periods only.) Discontinue if there is any nasal bleeding.
Flunisolide 0.025% nasal solution[3] (Nasalide)	1 inhalation in each nostril 3 times a day, or 2 inhalations in each nostril 2 times a day. Discontinue if there is any nasal bleeding.
Cromolyn sodium[3] (Nasalcrom)	1–2 inhalations in each nostril every 3–4 hours.
Topical preparations for allergic conjunctivitis	
Decongestant-antihistamines	
Naphazoline 0.025% and pheniramine 0.3% solution (Muro's Opcon-A), 15-mL bottles	1–2 drops in each eye 3–4 times a day as needed.
Naphazoline 0.05% and antazoline 0.5% solution (Albalon-A Liquifilm), 15-mL bottles	1–2 drops in each eye 3–4 times a day as needed.
Phenylephrine 0.12%, pyrilamine 0.1% and antipyrine 0.1% solution (Prefrin-A), 15-mL bottles	1–2 drops in each eye 3–4 times a day as needed.
Corticosteroid preparations	
Dexamethasone phosphate 0.1% solution (Decadron phosphate), 2.5- and 5-mL bottles	1–2 drops up to every 1–2 hours initially until relief, then up to every 4 hours as needed.
Prednisolone phosphate 0.5% solution (Hydeltrasol, Metreton), 5-mL bottles	1–2 drops up to every 1–2 hours initially until relief, then up to every 4 hours as needed.
Medrysone 1% suspension (HMS Liquifilm), 5- and 10-mL bottles	1–2 drops every 4 hours as needed.
Preparations for prophylaxis	
Cromolyn sodium 4% solution[4] (Opticrom 4%), 10-mL bottles	1–2 drops in each eye 4–6 times a day.

[1]Not recommended by manufacturer for children under 12 years of age.
[2]Refers to theophylline dose. See text for further discussion of dosage.
[3]Not recommended by manufacturer for children under 6 years of age.
[4]Not recommended by manufacturer for children under 4 years of age.

activity. There are 3 classes of antihistamines: H_1 receptor inhibitors, the classic antihistamines used for many years in allergic disorders; H_2 receptor inhibitors, which are useful in inhibiting gastric acid secretion; and, finally, agents that affect a newly identified H_3 receptor. H_1 antihistamines are particularly useful in urticaria, anaphylaxis, and allergic rhinitis; however, their effectiveness is limited in many disorders because numerous mediators unrelated to histamine operate in most allergic conditions. In certain circumstances, such as chronic urticaria and anaphylaxis, the combination of H_1 and H_2 antihistamines is therapeutic when either alone is not sufficiently effective.

Although antihistamines may be useful in severe allergic disorders, they are not the drug of first choice in medical emergencies due to allergic reactions but may be administered after epinephrine has been given. Antihistamines have antipruritic properties and are useful in atopic dermatitis and in contact dermatitis, in which histamine may play a major role. The sedation that occurs as a side effect, although undesirable in many instances, may be an advantage in others. Some antihistamines possess atropinelike drying actions.

C. Methylxanthines: Theophylline and its ethylenediamine derivative, aminophylline, are effective bronchodilators that appear to act at a different point but in the same pathway through which epinephrine exerts its dilating effect on smooth muscle. The improper use of these agents has been associated with severe toxic reactions, in some cases resulting in death. Overdosage frequently occurs as a result of failure to appreciate the variability of rate and extent of absorption with different routes of administration. Toxic reactions include headache, palpitations, dizziness, stomachache, nausea and vomiting, excessive thirst, and hypotension. Nausea and stomachache may be related to local irritation but can also represent a central nervous system-mediated toxic effect of the drug when administered by any route. In recent years, more subtle but significant toxicity, including behavioral changes, has been recognized. When used properly, theophylline and aminophylline are valuable drugs with a potent bronchodilating effect. There is great individual variation in the metabolism of methylxanthines, and dosage must be highly individualized. Optimal therapeutic blood levels of theophylline are considered to be 10–20 μg/mL serum or plasma, with levels over 20 μg/mL more likely to be associated with drug toxicity. *However, side effects such as behavioral changes and effects on attention span and learning can occur, especially in young children, at significantly lower levels.* Also, levels below 10 μg/ml can be therapeutic. Average dosages likely to achieve blood levels of 10–20 μg/mL are 25 ± 5 mg/kg/d between ages 1 and 8, then 20 ± 5 mg/kg/d until about age 16; thereafter, average daily dose is closer to 12 ± 3 mg/kg/d. A single daily dose can be given, or the daily dosage can be divided into 2–4 doses (every 6–24 hours), depending on the preparation used. Safe peak blood levels appear to be those below 15 μg/mL. *In early to mid infancy, metabolism is markedly diminished, and theophylline should be employed with particular caution.*

Rectal administration of theophylline in fluid form usually results in prompt and efficient absorption of the drug that may be almost as efficient as intravenous administration. Absorption from rectal suppositories is unpredictable, and these preparations should not be used. For chronic administration of methylxanthines, long-acting preparations given orally are preferred. Theophylline levels should be monitored periodically in patients on chronic therapy.

D. Expectorants: Expectorants such as guaifenesin (glyceryl guaiacolate) are used mainly in bronchial asthma to liquefy thick, tenacious mucus, but it is not clear whether any therapeutic effectiveness of these agents is in fact due to their expectorant action. Iodides seem more effective than guaifenesin, but—especially with prolonged use—goiter, salivary gland inflammation, gastric irritation, skin eruptions, and acne may occur. *Note:* It is important to keep in mind that adequate hydration is essential to effective expectoration. In general, expectorant preparations containing narcotics should not be used in asthma.

E. Corticosteroids: Adrenal glucocorticoids have been used in the treatment of all of the allergic disorders. Their effectiveness is apparently due to their anti-inflammatory actions. The untoward side effects of prolonged systemic corticosteroid administration (eg, growth suppression, myopathy, Cushing's syndrome, hypertension, peptic ulcer [controversial], diabetes, and electrolyte imbalance) limit their use mainly to those conditions that are refractory to other measures or are life-threatening. Even then, however, their slow onset of action (even when given intravenously) precludes first-choice administration of these drugs in acute allergic emergencies. Most allergic syndromes are amenable to other forms of therapy, and the long-term systemic use of the corticosteroids usually is unnecessary. When chronic use is necessary, alternate-day corticosteroid therapy with a short-acting preparation (eg, prednisone) in the early morning every other day should be attempted. Alternatively, for asthma or rhinitis, use by inhalation can be considered. In fact, the recognition that chronic asthma is in large part an inflammatory disorder has prompted recent reconsideration with increased enthusiasm for chronic therapy with topical corticosteroids in even milder forms of chronic disease. There are virtually no advantages to the use of corticotropin over the glucocorticoids themselves when glucocorticoid action is deemed necessary.

The main indications for the use of systemic corticosteroids are acute severe asthma and control of chronic severe disorders, such as asthma, that are refractory to other appropriate therapy. In some instances, administration of a short course of corticosteroids for self-limiting allergic disorders (eg, serum sickness) may be warranted.

Topical corticosteroids are extremely effective anti-inflammatory agents in the control of allergic dermatitis (mainly contact dermatitis and atopic dermatitis) and allergic as well as nonallergic rhinitis and asthma. Topical application is the preferred route of administration in such disorders, keeping long-term use of the more potent preparations to a minimum.

F. Sedatives: Sedatives have been grossly misused in asthma and have been responsible for some deaths. Although the psyche undoubtedly exerts a significant influence on asthma and other allergic disorders, the anxiety associated with extreme asthma is more often a reflection of the severity of the respiratory distress than the main cause of it. Sedatives that suppress the respiratory center (as the barbiturates do) should not be used in the therapy of severe asthma.

G. Oxygen: Oxygen (4–6 L/min) is extremely important in the treatment of severe asthma. Hypoxemia usually occurs early in the course of moderately severe or severe asthma, much in advance of any detectable cyanosis. Oxygen is potentially very drying and should be humidified when administered. Excessively high concentrations of oxygen should be avoided because they can lead to atelectasis or the possible lessening of respiratory drive.

H. Antibiotics: There are no special indications for the use of antibiotics in allergic disorders. Antibiotics should of course be used when evidence of bacterial infection exists. However, their excessive use in children with allergic disorders should be avoided to reduce the risk of sensitization to these drugs.

Erythromycin seems to be one of the least sensitizing antibiotics and offers good coverage against many respiratory pathogens. It should be noted, however, that erythromycin interferes with theophylline metabolism and can elevate theophylline levels.

I. Cromolyn Sodium (Intal, Nasalcrom, Opticrom): This drug is used in the management of asthma and noninfectious rhinitis and conjunctivitis. It is believed to act in part by blocking the release of pharmacologic mediators such as histamine. In many children, cromolyn sodium is interchangeable with theophylline as a first-line drug for chronic asthma therapy and appears to be among the safest of antiallergic drugs. However, cromolyn sodium does not reverse tissue changes induced by chemical mediators and is therefore of no value in the treatment of acute asthmatic paroxysms. It is useful in blocking exercise-induced asthma and irritant- and allergen-provoked asthma if used prior to anticipated exposure to irritating agents.

J. Other Prospective Drugs: Major pharmacologic advances in the control of allergic diseases have occurred in recent years; currently, various drugs—many with novel pharmacologic properties—are under investigation. Some already are marketed in other countries. Some of the more interesting that may be available in the USA in the near future include nedocromil, and azelastine.

Prophylaxis of Atopic Disorders

There is suggestive evidence that the avoidance of cow products, eggs, wheat, and chicken during the first 9 months of life significantly lessens the child's likelihood of developing allergic rhinitis and asthma. There is also some evidence that a diet excluding cow products, fish, and eggs for the first 6 months of life, coupled with general environmental precautions to minimize contact with house dust and animal dander, is associated with a diminished likelihood of developing atopic dermatitis, at least in the first year. It seems prudent, therefore, to institute the dietary and environmental restrictions mentioned above in the first few months of life in children with a strong family history of atopy.

Bierman CW, Pearlman DS, Berman B: Injection therapy for allergic diseases. Chap 20, p 279, in: *Allergic Disease From Infancy to Adulthood,* 2nd ed. Bierman CW, Pearlman DS (editors). Saunders, 1988.

Buckley J, Pearlman DS: Controlling the environment for allergic diseases. Chap 2, p 239, in: *Allergic Disease from Infancy to Adulthood,* 2nd ed. Bierman CW, Pearlman DS (editors). Saunders, 1988.

Easton JG, Kaplan NS: Controversial concepts and practices in allergy. Chap 57, p 735, in: *Allergic Disease from Infancy to Adulthood,* 2nd ed. Bierman CW, Pearlman DS (editors). Saunders, 1988.

Johnstone, DE: The natural history of allergic disease in children and its intervention. *Pediatr. Asthma, Allergy and Immunol.* 1989;**3:**161.

Pollart SM, Chapman MD, Platts-Mills THE: House dust sensitivity and environmental control. *Prim Care* 1987; **14:**591.

Shapiro GG: Diagnostic methods for assessing the patient with possible allergic disease. Chap 17, p 224, in: *Allergic Disease from Infancy to Adulthood,* 2nd ed. Bierman CW, Pearlman DS (editors). Saunders, 1988.

Terr AI: *In vitro* tests for immediate hypersensitivity. *Ann Rev Med* 1988;**39:**135.

Weinberger M, Hendeles LH: Pharmacologic management of allergic diseases. Chap 19, p 253, in: *Allergic Disease from Infancy to Adulthood,* 2nd ed. Bierman CW, Pearlman DS (editors). Saunders, 1988.

MEDICAL EMERGENCIES DUE TO ALLERGIC REACTIONS

The most common causes of severe allergic reactions are skin testing, hyposensitization with allergen extracts, drugs, insect stings, and food sensitivity. Anaphylaxis related to strenuous exercise has been described. Anaphylactic shock, angioedema, and bronchial obstruction, alone or in combination, are the principal life-threatening manifestations of severe allergic reactions. Light-headedness, paresthesias, sweating, flushing, palpitations, and urticaria may precede or accompany severe reactions.

Prevention

Prevention consists mainly of avoiding allergens known or believed to be responsible for allergic reactions. A history suggestive of a reaction to a given drug is an indication that an alternative and unrelated drug should be selected for therapeutic use.

Treatment

A. Emergency Measures: Immediate treatment is essential for management of these reactions.

1. Epinephrine—Epinephrine, 1:1000, 0.2–0.4 mL, should be injected intramuscularly without delay. This may be repeated at intervals of 15–20 minutes as necessary. If the reaction is due to the recent injection of a drug, serum, or other substance, a tourniquet should be applied proximal to the injection. If the offending substance has been injected intradermally or subcutaneously, absorption of the material may be delayed further by injecting epinephrine, 0.1 mL subcutaneously, near the site of injection. Subsequent therapy depends partly upon the response.

2. Antihistamines—Antihistamines (Table 32–1) should be given intramuscularly or intravenously. When intravenous infusions are used, they should be given over a period of 5–10 minutes because untoward reactions, particularly hypotension, have been induced by too rapid administration. A combination of H_1 antihistamines (eg, chlorpheniramine) and H_2 antihistamines (eg, cimetidine) is recommended.

3. Theophylline—Theophylline is useful when bronchospasm occurs. (See also p 977.)

4. Tracheostomy—Tracheostomy may be lifesaving in cases of profound laryngeal edema.

5. Fluids—Because anaphylactic shock is in part produced by hypovolemia secondary to massive exudation of intravascular fluid, maintenance of a proper volume by intravenous fluids (isotonic saline, 5% dextrose in water, or 5% dextrose in saline) is particularly important.

B. Follow-Up Measures: Adrenocorticosteroids should be given only after epinephrine and antihistamines have been administered. The onset of action of these drugs is slow (hours, even by intravenous administration).

The patient should be watched for 24 hours because a recurrence (delayed anaphylaxis) has been noted in some cases many hours after initial treatment.

C. Hyposensitization for Insect Stings: Children who have experienced life-threatening reactions following an insect sting should be hyposensitized. A large local reaction or generalized urticaria *without* respiratory or cardiovascular compromise is probably *not* an indication for hyposensitization. The main allergens responsible for severe allergic reactions are found in the venoms of Hymenoptera (bees, wasps, hornets, and fire ants). Venom antigens for diagnosis and treatment are much more efficacious than whole body extracts, and the latter should no longer be employed. Hyposensitization with venom antigens, however, is associated with a high incidence of significant reactions in the course of treatment; testing and therapy are therefore best left to physicians experienced in dealing with insect allergy. Treatment kits for anaphylactic reactions should be available for immediate use in individuals with insect hypersensitivity and should be kept in the home or taken along by a responsible person when the sensitive person travels in an area likely to be infested with the offensive insects. The single most important item in such a kit is epinephrine. The pa-

tient and parents should be instructed in proper use of the kit and in ways to avoid insects. The kits should also be available for patients with severe recurrent allergic reactions from any cause.

Gershwin ME, Keslin MH (editors): Allergic emergencies. *Clin Rev Allergy* 1985;**3**:1 [Entire issue.]

Kniker WT: Anaphylaxis in children and adults. Chap 51, p 667, in: *Allergic Disease from Infancy to Adulthood*, 2nd ed. Bierman CW, Pearlman DS (editors). Saunders, 1988.

Yunginger JW: Insect allergy (adults and children). Chap 52, p 678, in: *Allergic Disease from Infancy to Adulthood*, 2nd ed. Bierman CW, Pearlman DS (editors). Saunders, 1988.

BRONCHIAL ASTHMA ("Reactive Airways Disorder")

Essentials of Diagnosis

- Paroxysmal or chronically exacerbating dyspnea characterized by bilateral wheezing, prolongation of expiration, hyperinflation of the lungs, and cough (overt wheezing may not occur).
- Reversal of abnormal pulmonary function to (or significantly toward) normal by injection of epinephrine, inhalation of adrenergic aerosols, or other therapeutic measures (can also reverse spontaneously).
- Eosinophilia of sputum and blood (common).
- Positive, immediate skin test reactions to provoking allergens (common but not necessary).

General Considerations

Bronchial asthma is a largely reversible obstructive process of the tracheobronchial tree caused by inflammation with epithelial denudation, mucosal edema, increased and unusually viscid secretions, and smooth muscle constriction. Especially in protracted asthmatic episodes, the obstructive pathologic changes may cause not only hypoxemia but also retention of CO_2 and respiratory acidosis.

The incidence of asthma is reportedly less than 5% of the total population, but in the authors' opinion, this figure is a gross underestimation. Before adolescence, boys are affected twice as frequently as girls. Onset in early childhood is common (but asthma frequently begins in adulthood). In the majority of cases in childhood, the onset occurs by the seventh year.

Evidence of sensitization to inhalant allergens is found in the majority of children with asthma. However, in many patients, offensive allergens cannot be identified by history or suggested by allergy testing, and, IgE-mediated allergy, at least, does not appear to be related to the pathogenesis of the disorder. One does *not* have to be allergic to have asthma. Nevertheless, allergic sensitization probably plays a major role in the pathogenesis of asthma in many if not *most* children and in many adults. When allergens contribute to or are major precipitants of asthma, ''allergy'' rarely is the sole significant factor involved (see below). The most common allergens causing asthma in children are inhalants: house dust mites, indoor molds, epidermals (especially the saliva and danders of cats and dogs), airborne pollens (trees, grasses, weeds), and out-of-doors seasonal molds. Foods occasionally provoke asthma, especially in infants, but do so less commonly in later childhood. The same allergens that cause asthma frequently cause allergic rhinitis in the same patient; many children who initially present with hay fever subsequently develop asthma.

An important pathogenic feature of asthma is an extraordinary ''nonspecific'' hyperreactivity of the tracheobronchial tree to various chemical mediators (eg, acetylcholine, histamine, leukotrienes) and, in turn, to various insulting agents or events that cause their activation or liberation. Because of this feature, asthma is sometimes called ''reactive airways disorder.'' (However, airway hyperreactivity is not always present in asthma.) In addition to allergic reactions, numerous factors trigger or aggravate asthma, principally upper and lower respiratory tract infections of *viral* origin. The role of bacterial organisms in the precipitation of asthma is a disputed question, although there is evidence indicating that acute and chronic sinusitis can exacerbate asthma. Other triggering factors are rapid changes in temperature or barometric pressure, the common air pollutants in cities, odors, smoke, paint fumes, cold air, and exercise. Psychologic factors appear to be important in some cases but are seldom the sole cause. Aspirin idiosyncrasy can be a cause of asthma in childhood as well as in adult life.

Clinical Findings

A. History: Onset may occur as early as the first few weeks of life. Particularly in infancy, the first attack usually is associated with a lower respiratory tract infection or bronchiolitis. As age increases, there is a progressively greater tendency for initial and subsequent episodes to be associated with inhalant allergens or irritants. The initial inciting event appears to render the tracheobronchial tree more susceptible to reactions to both similar and unrelated precipitants.

A history of atopic dermatitis or allergic rhinitis is often noted. A family history of atopic diseases (especially allergic rhinitis and bronchial asthma) is often present and may arouse suspicion of the diagnosis. Asthma can (and all too frequently does) occur in the *absence of overt wheezing,* and complaints may include ''chest congestion,'' chronic cough, exercise intolerance, dyspnea, and recurrent bronchitis/pneumonia. A careful physical examination, including chest auscultation on a forced expiratory maneuver rather than on simple tidal volume, can be revealing, especially when the patient is experiencing clinical discomfort.

Episodes of asthma associated with infections are frequently insidious in onset and prolonged; those due to specific, identifiable allergens tend to be acute in onset and relatively brief if the causative agent is removed.

Bronchial asthma in infants (under 2 years of age) deserves special comment. The first attack usually follows by a few days the onset of a respiratory infection; some degree of cough or wheezing may persist for prolonged periods and becomes worse with subsequent ''colds.'' In infants, the predominant symptoms may be dyspnea, excessive secretions, noisy and rattly breathing, cough, and, in many cases, some intercostal and suprasternal retractions—rather than the typical pronounced expiratory wheezes that occur in older children. Initial and repeated diagnoses of these episodes are apt to be croup, bronchiolitis, and pneumonia. Infection (viral) is often present.

A syndrome of paroxysmal cough, presumably tracheal in origin (''irritable trachea,'' ''allergic cough''), occurs and may be difficult to differentiate from true asthma, particularly because bronchodilator drugs are sometimes effective in this condition. In this condition, wheezing generally does not occur and signs of lower respiratory tract obstruction are absent. The condition frequently is provoked by a (viral) respiratory infection, and allergic factors may or may not play a role. This condition also may presage later asthma.

B. Physical Examination: The following may occur during an acute, severe attack or a prolonged attack:

1. Distressing cough, dyspnea, increasing prolongation of expirations, high-pitched rhonchi and wheezes throughout the chest (diminishing in intensity as the obstruction becomes more severe), secretions (variable), hyperinflation, retractions, use of accessory respiratory muscles, poor air exchange.

2. Restlessness, apprehension, fatigue, drowsiness, coma.

3. Increasing tachycardia; initially, perhaps mild hypertension; ultimately, hypotension; rarely, signs of cardiac failure; pulsus paradoxus.

4. Flushed, moist skin; pallid cyanosis; dry mucous membranes.

5. Initially good response to epinephrine or other adrenergic drugs or methylxanthines. If the attack is prolonged, the response to the above drugs may be poor.

C. Laboratory Findings: Eoisinophil accumulations (eg, clumps of eosinophils on sputum smear) and blood eosinophilia are commonly found but are often absent in infection or when corticosteroids are given. Their presence tends to reflect disease activity and does not necessarily mean that allergic factors are involved.

Hematocrit can be elevated with dehydration, as in prolonged attacks, or in severe chronic disease.

In severe asthma, the first sign is hypoxemia without CO_2 retention. Respiratory acidosis and increased CO_2 tension may ensue. (Moderately severe hypoxemia may occur with low CO_2 tension due to a combination of hyperventilation and ventilation-perfusion disturbances.)

D. Imaging: Bilateral hyperinflation, bronchial thickening, peribronchial infiltration, and areas of densities (patchy atelectasis or associated bronchopneumonia) may be present. (Patchy atelectasis is common and often misread as pneumonitis.) The pulmonary arteries may also appear prominent.

E. Pulmonary Function Studies: (See Chapter 15.) Increased airway resistance occurs with a decrease in flow rates, decreased vital capacity (VC), and increased functional residual capacity (FRC) and residual volume (RV). The first 3 may be normal in asymptomatic intervals, but residual hyperinflation is frequently chronic.

F. Allergy Tests: IgE antibodies to allergens may be present.

G. Provocative Tests:

1. Food and drugs—Clinical reactions occur within minutes to hours after ingestion.

2. Inhalants—A clinical reaction usually occurs immediately after inhalation and may occur again 4–8 hours after challenge (''late'' reaction). Asthma may occasionally be provoked by skin testing in unusually sensitive children.

Differential Diagnosis

Bronchial asthma may be confused with middle and lower respiratory tract infections (eg, laryngotracheobronchitis, acute bronchiolitis, bronchopneumonia, and pertussis), especially in the very young. Immunodeficiency (primarily defects in immunoglobulin production or function) may have associated cough and wheezing due to chronic lower respiratory tract infection.

Nasal ''wheezes'' may be transmitted to the chest (especially in infants) from upper airway edema, increased secretions, or other obstructing factors such as allergic rhinitis, upper respiratory tract infections, adenoidal hypertrophy, foreign body, choanal stenosis, and nasal polyps (eg, in cystic fibrosis).

Congenital laryngeal stridor is usually associated with other anomalies.

In cases of tracheal or bronchial foreign body, dyspnea or wheezing is usually of sudden onset; on auscultation, the wheezes are usually but not always unilateral. Characteristic x-ray findings are not always present.

The differentiation between bronchial asthma and cystic fibrosis is made on the basis of high sweat sodium and chloride, a history (often present) in cystic fibrosis of serious pulmonary infection since birth, a personal and family history of associated intestinal disturbances with profuse, bulky stools, and pancreatic enzyme deficiency. Chronic inflammatory changes seen on chest x-ray in cystic fibrosis also can be a helpful differential point. There is evidence, however, for a significant reactive airway (asthmatic) component with or without allergic precipitants in many children with cystic fibrosis, and it is clear that cystic fibrosis and asthma can coexist.

Tracheal or bronchial compression by extramural forces may resemble asthma and may be due to foreign body in the esophagus, aortic ring, anomalous vessels, or inflammatory or neoplastic lymphadenopathy.

Wheezing may be present in immotile cilia syndrome, but chronic upper respiratory tract infections (sinusitis and otitis media) and recurrent pneumonias are usually more common manifestations because of the lack of mucociliary clearance.

Treatment of Mild & Moderate Asthma

A. Specific Measures: The patient should avoid contact with proved or suspected irritants and allergens as much as possible. (See Environmental Control of Exposure.) Hyposensitization therapy is for allergens that cannot be avoided (eg, pollens, seasonal molds, and house dust mites) when such allergens play a substantial role in the disorder.

B. General Measures: Depending upon the frequency and severity of asthma, some or all of the measures listed below may be used, either with the onset of an asthmatic attack or as a constant regimen—especially during the times of year when asthma is most severe.

1. Education—The parents (and patient, if old enough) must understand the asthmatic process. Complete understanding of all recommendations is essential.

2. Liquefaction and expectoration of mucus—Maintain adequate hydration by encouraging oral fluid intake, or give intravenous fluids if necessary. The value of expectorants is dubious. Postural drainage, preceded by use of an adrenergic aerosol, up to every 4 hours *if tolerated,* may be useful.

3. Bronchodilation—The major bronchodilating drugs are theophylline (aminophylline) and adrenergic drugs used alone or in combination. Adrenergic aerosols are extremely useful but must not be abused. They can be as effective as injected drugs in reversing acute severe asthma and have fewer side effects.

4. Correction of metabolic acidosis—Correct metabolic acidosis, if present, by providing an adequate energy source to diminish ketosis (eg, 5% dextrose intravenously), food if tolerated, and bicarbonate (see p. 985).

5. Corticosteroids—In children with severe acute asthma or with chronic asthma unresponsive to other measures, adrenal glucocorticoids may be indicated (see p. 985). If chronic use of corticosteroids is necessary for adequate control of asthma, prednisone or other short-acting equivalent given before 8:00 AM on alternate days should be attempted. Topical aerosolized corticosteroids are a useful alternative. Before resorting to chronic systemic corticosteroid therapy, cromolyn sodium by inhalation 3–4 times daily, or topical aerosolized corticosteroids in maximum dose (or both) should be given a therapeutic trial for at least 4–6 weeks.

6. Antibiotics—If there is evidence of bacterial infection, give antibiotics. Leukocytosis up to 15,000/μL is common in severe asthma without any evidence of bacterial infection (even higher counts can be seen after epinephrine administration). Patchy atelectasis can be confused with pneumonitis on x-ray film.

7. Breathing and fitness exercise—In children with chronic or recurrent asthma, breathing and fitness exercises under the guidance of a properly trained physical therapist may assist the patient in aborting some attacks of asthma and improving muscular functions of the thoracic cage.

Exercise should be encouraged rather than restricted. Exercise-induced bronchospasm can be ameliorated, if necessary, by cromolyn sodium or adrenergic aerosol (albuterol is recommended), or both, just prior to exercise; by theophylline given 1–2 hours before exercise; or by a combination of these.

8. Airflow assessment—In instances when perception of the degree of airflow limitation may be poorly appreciated by the parents or patient, have the patient use a peak flow meter at home to assist in assessment of airflow.

9. Daily regimen for control of asthma—Children with frequent overt asthma attacks (eg, 1 or 2 per week) and evidence of more or less constant pulmonary obstruction should be on constant pharmacologic therapy. A daily regimen stimulating coughing and encouraging expectoration (eg, postural drainage at least twice a day) may be useful. Theophylline (taken orally) and cromolyn sodium (3–4 times daily by inhalation) may be considered first-line drugs for chronic symptomatic asthma in addition to adrenergic drugs. Topical corticosteroids may be added or used in place of cromolyn and/or theophylline. Anticholinergics may be useful for the patient with a strong cough or irritant component.

Treatment of Acute Severe Asthma (Status Asthmaticus, Intractable Asthma)

This is a medical emergency!

A. Emergency Care: Epinephrine (1:1000 solution; Sus-Phrine) or, if the child is cooperative, aerosolized adrenergic drugs given by a compressed air device, preferably with oxygen, are the drugs of first choice. Aerosolized adrenergic drugs have been found to be as effective as epinephrine, at least in

older children, and have the advantage of minimizing systemic side effects. These drugs can be used every ½–1 hour. The shorter-acting β_2 agonist isoetharine, metaproterenol sulfate, or the new β_2 agonist, albuterol (which has minimal systemic side effects) is recommended initially rather than isoproterenol. Dosages that do not induce jitteriness or tachycardia are used. The lack of therapeutic response to adrenergic drugs is sometimes used as the criterion for "status asthmaticus." Relative or apparently complete lack of responsiveness to these drugs may be due to hypoxemia and acidosis, bronchial obstruction with thick mucus plugs, pneumothorax, or simply severe asthma. Sensitivity to adrenergic drugs may improve after initiation of other therapy.

B. Hospital Care: If signs are relatively early, an overnight stay may suffice.

1. Give 5% dextrose solution with 0.2% saline intravenously at the first sign of resistance to epinephrine or when there is poor fluid intake, vomiting, or dehydration. (Use maintenance requirements; *do not overhydrate*.) Particularly if corticosteroids are used, remember to add potassium (10–20 meq/L of intravenous fluid) after urination is established.

2. Give moisturized oxygen (by mask or nasal prongs—not by tent) at a flow rate of approximately 4 L/min. All patients with acute severe asthma will be hypoxemic, largely as a result of the ventilation-perfusion imbalance that is integral to asthma.

3. Give aminophylline, 4–6 mg/kg in intravenous tubing over a 10- to 20-minute period (if not used in the previous 4 hours) and repeat every 4–6 hours, or give as a constant infusion beginning with a loading dose of 4–6 mg/kg over 15 minutes and then 0.6–1 mg/kg/h.*

Age	Average Total Daily Dose ± SD
12 months to 8 years	25 ± 5 mg/kg
8–16 years	20 ± 5 mg/kg
Over 16 years	12 ± 3 mg/kg

4. Take an arterial blood sample for pH, P_{CO_2}, and P_{O_2} determinations. Early in the course of an asthmatic paroxysm, the patient usually hyperventilates and blows off CO_2, with a resultant low Pa_{CO_2}. (A normal Pa_{CO_2} in acute severe asthma, in other words, is an indication of impending respiratory failure.)

---

*In patients receiving chronic theophylline therapy, use their usual total daily maintenance dose infused over a 24-hour period. Theophylline blood levels of 10–20 μg/mL serum are considered "optimally therapeutic" for hospitalized patients, but levels should be on the low side of this range when theophylline is used on a long-term basis. Average total daily dosages of theophylline to achieve therapeutic levels are listed below, but there is much individual variation in requirements. *Caution:* In the first few months of life, theophylline (aminophylline) is metabolized very slowly, and *this drug should be used with extreme caution in patients at this age.*

Continued close monitoring of blood gases and pH is essential to proper management of severe asthma. (Determination of gases or pH on capillary blood generally is unreliable.) An ear oximeter can be used to measure oxygen saturation of the blood; this is a useful substitute for measurement of arterial blood oxygen only.

5. Attempt to correct acidosis (pH 7.3 or below) with sodium bicarbonate. With the increased work of breathing and hypoxemia, there may be metabolic acidosis due to lactic acid production. This may be compensated by a respiratory alkalosis due to hyperventilation. The appropriate bicarbonate dose may be calculated with the following formula.

Bicarbonate needed (meq) = Negative base excess × 0.3 × Body weight (kg)

The bicarbonate can be given rapidly by the intravenous route. (Sodium bicarbonate for injection may be obtained in ampules or multidose vials that contain approximately 1 meq/mL.) Arterial or venous pH should be redetermined 5–10 minutes later, and further correction of acidosis, using bicarbonate, should be considered at that time if necessary. In respiratory failure, in the absence of a pH determination, 2 meq/kg may be infused initially.

6. Give albuterol, 0.5% by inhalation, (or other adrenergic aerosols) every 2–4 hours followed by postural drainage *as tolerated*. (The proper use of aerosolized adrenergic agents early in the course of acute severe asthma may obviate the need for injected epinephrine.)

7. If the patient is already receiving corticosteroids, do not withdraw the medication; rather, increase the dose temporarily. Patients requiring hospitalization should receive corticosteroids promptly, even though patients may not realize the full benefit from the medication for 48 hours. The use of corticosteroids in status asthmaticus reduces the morbidity and mortality and accelerates the recovery by reducing inflammation and by potentiating the effectiveness of adrenergic drugs. (For dosage schedule, see Table 32–1.) As the symptoms are relieved, the dose should be decreased as rapidly as possible and maintained at the lowest dose that controls symptoms. (If the patient has not been on prolonged corticosteroid therapy within the past year, the corticosteroids can be discontinued abruptly rather than tapered. It is frequently feasible to use high doses of corticosteroids for 48 hours or less.)

8. Give antibiotics as indicated.

9. Mist tents are not beneficial and may actually increase bronchospasm because of an irritant effect.

10. Respiratory failure that does not respond to the above therapy may require intravenous isoproterenol therapy or assisted ventilation by a mechanical respirator. Failure to respond to the above measures can be defined as 2 arterial PCO_2 determinations

above 45 mm Hg over a 15- to 30-minute period. This is the indication for the insertion of an indwelling arterial catheter, if the procedure has not already been done. If the steady-state arterial PCO_2 remains above 45 mm Hg in the blood drawn from the indwelling line, continuous isoproterenol infusions should be considered. This is *not* generally recommended for older adolescents or adults, however, because of the increased risk of inducing cardiac dysrhythmias. *Such an infusion should be undertaken only in an intensive care unit where continuous cardiac and blood pressure monitoring facilities are available and assisted ventilation is available.* An additional intravenous line for the isoproterenol should be started so that it is not infused into the only existing line. The infusion should be started at a rate of 0.1 μg/kg/min and increased by this amount every 10–15 minutes until there is clinical improvement or until the heart rate approaches 200 beats/min. The development of significant dysrhythmias is an indication for decreasing the rate of isoproterenol infusion. If a favorable response occurs, it is necessary to wean the patient from the isoproterenol very slowly, decreasing the rate of infusion over a period of 30–36 hours. Rebound bronchospasm may occur if the rate is decreased too rapidly.

If the arterial PCO_2 remains high or continues to increase despite the continuous isoproterenol infusion, endotracheal intubation should be performed and assisted ventilation initiated. A volume respirator capable of producing high inspiratory pressures should be used. Because these patients have prolonged expiratory times as a result of the marked airway resistance, it is necessary to set an adequate expiratory time on the ventilator to avoid further air trapping within the lung. The need for assisted ventilation for status asthmaticus in children has been reduced since the introduction of the continuous isoproterenol infusion. *Intubation and assisted ventilation should be performed only by medical personnel trained in such techniques.*

C. Precautions in Therapy: Note the following "don'ts":

1. Don't use narcotics or barbiturates. (They depress the respiratory center. Tranquilizers may do the same in the presence of severe hypoxemia.)

2. Don't use epinephrine excessively. (It tends to thicken secretions, deplete glycogen stores, and increase apprehension.)

D. Follow-Up Therapy:

1. Fluids—When the patient is improved and is able to take fluids or oral medications, give fluids orally in the form of fruit juices. Give no fluids that contain caffeine or chocolate. Give no milk or iced drinks.

2. Drugs—The following medications are of value at this stage:

a. Adrenergic aerosol every 4–6 hours, followed by postural drainage for 20 minutes as tolerated.

b. Theophylline orally (dosage according to weight).

c. If corticosteroids have been started, withdraw after 72 hours or taper gradually and discontinue as soon as possible.

Prognosis

In the past 25–30 years, the morbidity and mortality rates in asthma have increased. Mortality statistics indicate that a high percentage of deaths has been due to the indiscriminate use of sedatives, narcotics, and aminophylline. Many are also due to *undertreatment,* particularly in labile asthmatics and asthmatics whose perception of pulmonary obstruction is poor. "Continuity" symptoms of night cough, breathlessness, and wheezing provoked by exercise or stress usually indicate more serious disease than do occasional, spontaneous, and brief attacks due to recognizable allergens, with symptom-free periods in between. Prolonged exposure of asthmatic children to cigarette smoke ("passive smoking") is associated with increased risk of irreversible small airway obstruction in adulthood.

There is no evidence that bronchial asthma can be cured, and the old adage still holds: "Once an asthmatic, always an asthmatic." However, the prognosis for symptom-free control in childhood asthma is fairly good. The majority of asthmatic children have less symptomatic asthma in their teens, and some appear to lose any asthmatic symptomatology for life. Unfortunately, however, only a minority (probably < 30%) fall into this category, and it is usually the pediatrician rather than the disorder that the child outgrows. Many asthmatics have persistent, significant (though often unrecognized) chronic pulmonary obstruction, and others later redevelop symptomatic obstruction. Mild asthma is more likely to be outgrown than moderate or severe asthma.

Eggleston PA: Immunotherapy for asthma: Don't count it out. *J Respir Dis* 1988;**9:**13.

Haas A et al: Status asthmaticus: A housestaff manual. *Pediatr Asthma Allergy Immunol* 1987;**4:**231.

Konig P: Asthma: A pediatric pulmonary disease and a changing concept. *Pediatr Pulmonol* 1987;**3:**264.

Konig P: Inhaled corticosteroids: Their present and future role in the management of asthma. *J Allergy Clin Immunol* 1988;**82:**297.

Pearlman DS, Bierman CW: Asthma [bronchial asthma]. Chap 41, p 546, in: *Allergic Diseases from Infancy to Adulthood,* 2nd ed. Bierman CW, Pearlman DS (editors). Saunders, 1988.

Pearlman DS: Bronchial asthma: A perspective from childhood through adulthood. Update *Pediatr Asthma Allergy Immunol* 1989;**3:**191.

Phelan P: The natural history of childhood asthma into adult life. *Immunol Allergy Pract* 1988;**10:**334.

Sears MR: Fatal asthma: A perspective. *Immunol Allergy Pract* 1988;**10:**259.

Welliver RC: Pediatric asthma: The role of infection. *J Respir Dis* 1983;**4:**46.

Zieger RS: Special considerations in the approach to asthma in infancy and early childhood. *J Asthma* 1983; **20:**341.

ALLERGIC RHINITIS

Essentials of Diagnosis

- Chronic or recurrent nasal obstruction; itching and sneezing (frequently paroxysmal), with seromucoid discharge. There may be accompanying conjunctival injection and itching, with or without tearing.
- Mucosal hyperemia to purplish pallor and edema of nasal mucous membranes.
- Eosinophils of nasal secretions when symptomatic (frequent).
- Presence of IgE antibody to provoking allergens.

General Considerations

Allergic rhinitis is the most common atopic disease, perhaps because the nose is anatomically and physiologically vulnerable to inhalant allergens. The pathologic changes are chiefly hyperemia, edema, and increased serous and mucoid secretions due to mediator release, all of which lead to variable degrees of nasal obstruction, rhinorrhea, and pruritus. Inhalant allergens are principally responsible for symptoms, but food allergens on occasion may provoke rhinitis.

Classification

Allergic rhinitis may be classified as perennial, seasonal (hay fever), or episodic, but these entities frequently occur concomitantly. Children with allergic rhinitis seem to be more susceptible to upper respiratory infections, which in turn intensify the symptoms of existing allergic rhinitis.

A. Perennial Allergic Rhinitis: Perennial allergic rhinitis occurs to some degree all year long but may be more severe in winter. Nasal stuffiness, frequent sniffing, and constant rhinorrhea with evidence of mild to moderate itching (frequent nose rubbing) are often the dominant symptoms, although more severe symptoms, including paroxysmal sneezing, may occur. Sneezing is often most pronounced in the morning shortly after waking. Poor appetite, fatigue, and pharyngeal irritation from nasopharyngeal mucus drainage are not unusual accompanying symptoms. Greater exposure to house dust allergens during the winter months is due to increased indoor activities and heating systems that raise, disperse, and circulate dust. The increased dryness of heated air and greater exposure to pets housed indoors may also add to the problem.

This disease frequently begins before the second year of life. It often accompanies bronchial asthma and may be provoked by the same allergens. Dental abnormalities, including disturbances in dental arch growth and malocclusion, have been attributed to long-standing perennial allergic rhinitis with nasal obstruction.

B. Seasonal Allergic Rhinitis (Hay Fever):

Hay fever occurs seasonally as a result of exposure to specific wind-borne pollens. The major important pollen groups in the temperate zones are trees (late winter, early spring), grasses (spring to early summer), and weeds (late summer to early fall). Seasons may vary significantly in different parts of the country. Mold spores also cause seasonal allergic rhinitis, principally in the summer and fall.

The age of onset is generally later than that of perennial allergic rhinitis, usually after 2 years of age. Worsening or extension of pollen sensitivities over a period of several years after onset can be expected.

C. Vasomotor (Nonallergic, Noninfectious) Rhinitis:

This form of perennial rhinitis, which occurs in children and adults, masquerades as allergic rhinitis. Manifestations of the condition include variable degrees of serous or mucoid rhinorrhea and nasal stuffiness, often with pharyngeal drainage and with or without significant nasal itching. Diagnosis depends upon ruling out an allergic or infectious cause. Rarely, there may be nasal eosinophilia.

Clinical Findings

A. Symptoms and Signs: Nasal obstruction is manifested by mouth breathing, snoring, difficulty in nursing or eating, nasal speech, and inability to clear the nose with blowing. Nasal seromucoid secretions are increased, with anterior drainage, sniffling, "nasal stuffiness," postnasal drip, and loose cough. Nasal itching leads to nose rubbing ("allergic salute," "bunny nose"), nose picking, epistaxis, and sneezing. Eye manifestations consist of itching, tearing, conjunctival injection, lid and periorbital edema, and circumorbital cyanosis ("allergic shiners"). Palatal and pharyngeal irritation or frank fatigue often occurs. In perennial rhinitis, nasal obstruction tends to be a predominant symptom; in seasonal rhinitis, there tends to be more intense itching, coryza, and sneezing.

Examination shows decreased patency of nasal airways and increased seromucoid discharge (usually more serous in seasonal rhinitis). The mucous membranes range from reddened with little edema to pale blue, swollen, and boggy, with dimpling in the turbinates. Increased pharyngeal lymphoid tissue from chronic pharyngeal drainage or enlarged tonsillar and adenoid tissue may be present. Bleeding points or ulceration may be seen on the anterior nasal septum. There may be a horizontal crease extending across the lower third of the nose, owing to frequent upward rubbing of the nose. Malocclusion (overbite), presumably due to excess pressure of digit sucking to relieve palatal itching, may be seen in long-standing cases.

The florid conjunctival injection, coryza, intense itching of the eyes and nose, and violent sneezing experienced by older children and adults are not so commonly seen in young children. Paroxysmal sneezing, however, is frequent even in young children.

B. Laboratory Findings: Eosinophilia frequently can be demonstrated on smears of nasal secretions or blood. This is a frequent but not universal finding in allergic rhinitis and reflects mast cell or basophil mediator release. The presence of eosinophils, in addition to suggesting the probability of allergic mechanisms, indicates the likelihood that antiallergic medications will be helpful in therapy, whether or not allergic mechanisms are operative. Eosinophils in numbers consistently greater than 15% or in clusters on nasal smears are suggestive of this disorder.

C. Allergy Testing: Skin or serologic tests reveal IgE antibody to offending allergens.

D. Associated Conditions: Sinusitis may accompany allergic rhinitis and is frequently demonstrated on x-ray film (mucosal thickening, fluid levels, or complete opacification of sinuses). Vigorous treatment is indicated until there is complete resolution of x-ray as well as clinical findings.

Auditory tube dysfunction and chronic or recurrent serous or secretory otitis media can also be a complication of allergic rhinitis. The atopic young child seems particularly prone to the development of serous otitis media. The middle ear is probably only rarely a "shock organ" for allergy per se; rather, otitis media is related to auditory tube dysfunction that can be associated with allergic rhinitis. There is little evidence that allergy-associated serous otitis media exists in the absence of allergic rhinitis.

Nasal polyps are unusual in children and generally are not caused by allergy. When polyps are present, cystic fibrosis should be considered.

Differential Diagnosis

These disorders must be differentiated from the common cold, other infectious diseases (eg, purulent rhinitis and sinusitis), adenoidal hypertrophy, foreign bodies (usually unilateral), nasal polyposis associated with cystic fibrosis or aspirin idiosyncrasy (nasal polyposis is rarely due to allergy), choanal stenosis or atresia, nasopharyngeal neoplasms, palatal malformations (eg, congenitally high arch, cleft palate), and "vasomotor" rhinitis.

Treatment

A. Specific Measures:

1. Avoid exposure to proved allergens as much as reasonably possible.

2. Hyposensitization should be considered when symptoms are severe and other symptomatic measures have failed or when the disease is associated with complications such as chronic or recurrent sinusitis, recurrent serous otitis media, and hearing loss. There is controversial evidence that hyposensi-

tization for hay fever may prevent the onset of asthma.

B. General Measures:

1. Give antihistamines with or without vasoconstricting adrenergic drugs by mouth. (See Table 32–1).

2. Nasal cromolyn (Nasalcrom) may be used alone or in conjunction with the medications named in the first measure, above.

3. Treat associated infections.

4. Topical decongestants (eg, phenylephrine) can be used for no more than 5 days for severe episodes.

5. Topical corticosteroids can be used for nasal symptoms not controllable by other means or for months in severe cases, but care must be taken to prevent patient overuse or complications, including nasal bleeding and potential nasal septal perforation.

6. Surgical procedures (removal of nasal polyps, corrective surgery for maxillary sinusitis, insertion of ventilating tubes for chronic otitis media) should be considered only when medical therapy fails.

Prognosis

A. Perennial Allergic Rhinitis: Unless specific allergens can be identified and eliminated from the environment or diet (unusual cases), this atopic disease tends to be very protracted. However, nasal obstruction may become less troublesome as the child grows and the nasal airway increases in caliber.

B. Seasonal Allergic Rhinitis: Hay fever patients tend to suffer repeatedly from their seasonal symptoms if exposure to offending allergens is high. These symptoms are expected to be most severe from adolescence through early to mid adult life. On moving to a region devoid of problem allergens, patients may be free of seasonal allergic rhinitis for 1–3 years but frequently acquire new pollen hypersensitivities from airborne pollens in the areas to which they move.

Allansmith MR, Ross RN: Ocular allergy. *Clin Allergy* 1988;**18**:1.

International Symposium on Allergy and Associated Disorders in Otolaryngology. *J Allergy Clin Immunol* 1988; **81**(part 2):[Entire issue.]

Kaliner M, Eggleston PA, Matthews KP: Rhinitis and asthma. *JAMA* 1987;**258 (part 3):**2851.

Meltzer EO, Schatz M, Zieger RS: Allergic and nonallergic rhinitis. Chap 53, p 1253, in: *Allergy Principles and Practice,* 3rd ed. Middleton E Jr et al: (editors). Mosby, 1988.

ATOPIC DERMATITIS*
(Infantile Eczema)

Essentials of Diagnosis

- Lesions varying from erythematous and papular

---

*From the perspective of a pediatric allergist (see also Dermatitis, Chapter 11).

to scaling, vesicular, and oozing; lichenification in more chronic forms.

- Predilection in infants for cheeks and extensor areas and in older children and adolescents for flexural creases.
- Pruritus, frequently intense.

General Considerations

Atopic dermatitis is considered to be an atopic disorder because of its frequent association with allergic rhinitis and asthma and the high incidence of IgE antibodies in children with this disorder. However, the role of IgE antibody, particularly to inhalant allergens, in its pathogenesis has been controversial. Children with atopic dermatitis have many immune aberrations, but the role of these immune defects is also unclear. The common denominator in all individuals with atopic dermatitis appears to be a lowered threshold for itching; atopic dermatitis has been called "an itch that rashes."

In some infants and children, IgE antibody to one or more foods can be demonstrated; ingestion of a food(s) to which IgE antibody is present has been shown to be a major cause of the eczema in many cases. The presence of IgE antibody to a food also may be of no clinical importance, however; it appears to be a necessary but not sufficient condition for food-induced eczema. Foods implicated most frequently in atopic dermatitis include egg white, milk, legumes (including peanut butter), wheat, and corn. Certain foods, especially citrus fruits and tomatoes, may induce facial erythema in children with atopic dermatitis but generally do not induce more extensive dermatitis. Inhalant allergens also can play an important and even critical role in the pathogenesis of atopic dermatitis, in some instances probably by direct skin contact (eg, animal allergens, house dust mites).

Scratching plays a major role in the occurrence and progression of dermatitis, predisposing the skin to infection. Factors that aggravate itching include dryness, sweating, and contact with rough materials and detergents. Psychologic factors may intensify itching and complicate management at home and at school.

Clinical Findings

A. Symptoms and Signs: Although infantile eczema ordinarily begins in infancy, it can begin at almost any time in childhood. In infants, lesions typically appear after 2 months of age, beginning on the cheeks and forehead and spreading in a patchy or generalized distribution over the extremities and trunk. Initially, involvement of extremities is primarily on extensor surfaces, but after infancy, involvement of flexural creases (antecubital, popliteal, neck) predominates; frequently, the wrists, hands, feet, face, and eyelids are also involved. The lesions may vary from facial erythema and minimal scaling to frank oozing and "weeping." As the child grows older, the eczema tends to wax and wane, sometimes disappearing completely for months, and in many children abates altogether by age 3 years. The skin may be thickened and somewhat plaquelike (lichenified) because of long-standing irritation from scratching. Although scarring is unusual, hyperpigmentation and hypopigmentation may occur. Excessive skin dryness is a frequent concomitant finding in eczema, and a form of congenital ichthyosis often accompanies atopic dermatitis. Infection sometimes occurs; however, it is not usual, even though the concentration of staphylococci in and on the skin of children with atopic dermatitis tends to be much higher than normal.

B. Laboratory Findings: There are no practical tests for atopic dermatitis. IgE immunoglobulin levels are frequently elevated, and there may be specific IgE antibodies to various inhalant and food allergens. Evidence of IgE antibody to a food allergen may or may not be clinically relevant; in cases where such evidence is present, therefore, a trial elimination and challenge to that food is recommended. IgE antibody to inhalants also suggests only the possibility of clinical relevance to the disease. Eosinophilia may occur.

Differential Diagnosis

Seborrheic dermatitis may be distinguished by a lack of significant pruritus, its predilection for the scalp ("cradle cap"), and its coarse, yellowish "potato chip" scales. Seborrheic dermatitis may occur in association with atopic dermatitis. Candidiasis occurs predominantly in the diaper region and is characteristically intensely red, with satellite lesions. Contact dermatitis is distinguished chiefly by the distribution of lesions (usually on extensor and exposed areas), generally with a greater demarcation of dermatitis than in atopic dermatitis. Nummular eczema is characterized by coin-shaped plaques, with minimal to sometimes intense eczema. Scabies is more papulovesicular and relatively nonerythematous, occurring chiefly in the interdigital and waistline areas, with itching that may be intense, particularly at night; because of scratching, an eczematous dermatitis may develop.

Various other disorders have associated skin eruptions that may resemble atopic dermatitis. These include Wiskott-Aldrich syndrome, X-linked agammaglobulinemia, ataxia-telangiectasia, severe combined immunodeficiency disease, phenylketonuria, Hurler syndrome, Hartnup syndrome, and histidinemia.

In Buckley's syndrome, there is marked elevation of IgE, with a dermatitis associated with increased susceptibility to infectious agents, especially staphylococci. The skin eruption is easily distinguishable from atopic dermatitis.

Complications & Sequelae

Bacterial skin infections, particularly those produced by staphylococcal and streptococcal organisms, occur with some frequency. Viral infections, mainly with herpesvirus (Kaposi's varicelliform eruption), can occur from exposure to individuals with herpetic lesions, and varicella can be unusually severe in children with atopic dermatitis, although this generally is not a problem.

Nutritional disturbances may result from unwarranted and unnecessarily vigorous dietary restrictions imposed by physicians and parents. Cataracts in late childhood or adulthood occur in a small percentage of cases, even when corticosteroids are not used in treatment. Temporary or chronic emotional disturbances may occur as a result of feelings of disfigurement, imposed restrictions, and unhealthy attitudes of parents toward a child with this disease. Poor academic performance and behavioral disturbances may be a result of uncontrolled intense or frequent itching.

Treatment

Good general skin care and vigorous specific dermatologic treatment are the most important aspects of treatment of atopic dermatitis. Any foods that have been shown to aggravate eczema should be eliminated, provided that the diet remains nutritionally adequate. Minimizing direct contact with irritants (wood and other rough materials, irritating soaps and detergents) and allergens (eg, animal emanations, house dust mites, molds), avoiding excessive sweating, and maintaining good skin hydration are important. Hyposensitization is rarely of value.

A. General Skin Care: Provide good skin hydration and have the patient bathe at least once daily, using a bath oil (Alpha Keri or Lubath) added halfway through the bath; superfatted and nonirritating soaps (Basis, Dove, Lowila, or Neutrogena) should be used. The skin should be thoroughly rinsed. The skin may be patted partly dry, and areas that are ordinarily excessively dry can then be coated with a small amount of bland cream (eg, Eucerin) to help trap water in the skin.

B. Acute Weeping Stage: Apply Burow's solution (aluminum subacetate) soaks made up to 1:20 solution (Domeboro tablets or packets) for 20 minutes, using 3 layers of gauze or cloth thoroughly moistened with solution 4 times a day. Do not use for more than 3 days. Treat infection with a systemic antibiotic (eg, cephalexin, erythromycin). Antihistamines can be used as antipruritic agents but are of secondary importance to topical treatment in controlling pruritus. Hydroxyzine (Atarax) is of value.

C. Subacute and Chronic Stages: The liberal use of emollients along with the *cautious* use of corticosteroid topical agents to control inflammation is the mainstay of therapy. Encourage daily bathing followed by application of corticosteroid cream to allow for penetration of the corticosteroid through the skin barrier and to aid in trapping water in the skin. Although creams are generally preferred to ointments, ointments may be more effective in some situations, especially when the hands and feet are involved. Corticosteroids should be applied 2–3 times a day until inflammation is controlled. As active inflammation subsides, bland creams should be substituted. The choice of a corticosteroid preparation depends upon the degree of inflammation and, to some extent, the location of the lesions. Potent (fluorinated) topical agents are used for short periods of time to bring inflammation under control; with more chronic use, the weakest preparations compatible with control are used. (Hydrocortisone cream, 1%, is recommended.) Corticosteroid absorption from a potent agent used for a prolonged period and over large areas of inflamed skin (especially if used under occlusive dressing) can produce adrenal suppression and other complications of systemic corticosteroid therapy. Prolonged use of topical corticosteroids may also produce skin thinning. Potent topical corticosteroids should not be used with any frequency or duration on the face or periorbital areas.

An alternative approach to therapy (the Scholtz regimen) avoids bathing with water completely. A moist washcloth can be used to clean the groin and axillary areas. Cetaphil lotion, which consists primarily of propylene glycol, sodium lauryl sulfate, and acetyl alcohol in water, is applied liberally to other areas until it foams and is then gently wiped from the skin, so that a thin film of lotion is left on the skin. In the authors' experience, this regimen is of limited value in a dry climate. Topical ointments of any kind, with the exception of topical corticosteroid preparations in the form of creams or solutions, are avoided.

Prognosis

Most cases of atopic dermatitis resolve spontaneously by 3 years of age, but atopic dermatitis may persist through childhood and even into adult life. Emotional problems that stem from severe dermatitis may require special consideration. There is a high likelihood (up to 80% of children in some series) that a child with atopic dermatitis will develop allergic rhinitis, asthma, or both. Consequently, it seems wise to institute simple environmental control procedures in the homes of children with atopic dermatitis and to follow these children particularly closely for the development of these disorders.

Adinoff AD, Tellez P, Clark RAF: Atopic dermatitis and aeroallergen contact sensitivity. *J Allergy Clin Immunol* 1988;**81**:736.

Jacobs AH, Goldsobel AB: Atopic dermatitis. Chap 29, p 385, in: *Allergic Diseases from Infancy to Adulthood*, 2nd ed. Bierman CW, Pearlman DS (editors). Saunders, 1988.

Sampson HA: The role of food allergy and mediator release in atopic dermatitis. *J Allergy Clin Immunol* 1988; **81**:635.

ADVERSE REACTIONS TO FOODS

Adverse reactions to foods occur quite frequently and can be classified on the basis of the mechanism of the reaction. Although these reactions are often diagnosed as "allergic," the majority of adverse reactions to foods are, in fact, caused by many other factors that are nonimmune in origin, such as pharmacologic or metabolic mechanisms and food "idiosyncrasy" (mechanism unknown), or by food toxins. (See Table 32–2.) Reactions can occur in all body tissues. A wide variety of signs and symptoms can be encountered, many of which may appear extremely vague. Serious allergic reactions include anaphylaxis, acute angioedema of the upper airway, and severe bronchial asthma. Such reactions usually occur from within minutes to 2 hours. Other symptom complexes of lesser consequence, both allergic and nonallergic, can also occur in response to a variety of common foods. These are more likely to appear after several hours.

Several factors may influence a patient's potential to react to food. First, heredity influences the risk of developing food allergy. The incidence of food allergy increases if one or both parents are allergic. Also, early introduction of cow's milk or solid foods may induce a risk of food allergy. In general, those foods that cause an allergic reaction during early childhood are less likely to be a problem as the child grows than are those food sensitivities that are acquired later in life. For example, 60–90% of children who develop a milk allergy in infancy are able to tolerate milk in the diet by the age of 4 years (even though skin tests and RAST may remain positive to milk). Finally, the potential for an allergic reaction

Table 32–2. Adverse reactions to foods.

Food hypersensitivity (true allergic reactions)
Classic "allergic" reactions due to IgE antibody and release of mediators.
Nonanaphylactic reactions due to IgG or IgM or delayed-type hypersensitivity and release of mediators.
Food intolerance (mechanism unknown)
Idiosyncrasy
  Dyes
  Preservatives
  Exercise (may be allergic in part, in some cases)
Metabolic mechanisms
  Carbohydrate enzyme deficiencies
  Gluten sensitivity (celiac disease)
  G6PD deficiency
  Phenylketonuria
  Ceruloplasmin deficiency (Wilson's disease)
Pharmacologic mechanisms
  Histamine intoxication (ingestion of contaminated scombroid fish, (eg, tuna and mackerel)
  Vasoactive amines occurring naturally in foods (strawberries, melons, cheese, chocolate, some wines and beers)
  Methylxanthines (caffeine)

ALLERGIC DISORDERS / 991

to food is influenced by the rate and by the type of food particles that are absorbed across the intestinal mucosa. For example, infectious and toxic enteritis damages the mucosal lining, thereby permitting partially digested food allergens to be absorbed and increasing the potential for an allergic food reaction.

Syndromes Sometimes Associated with Food Sensitivity

A. Angioedema: Angioedema is often accompanied by urticaria. In mild cases, findings include periorbital and lip edema, a few hives, mild arthralgia, and malaise. In severe cases, there may be tongue, pharyngeal, and laryngotracheal edema and joint swelling. Death may occur from asphyxia. (See Medical Emergencies Due to Allergic Reactions.)

B. Anaphylaxis: Immediate reaction is characterized by light-headedness to syncope, flushing to pallor, paresthesias, generalized itching, palpitations, and tachycardia. There may be symptoms and signs of pulmonary edema, bronchial asthma, and vascular collapse. (See Medical Emergencies Due to Allergic Reactions.) Most often, food anaphylaxis results from the interaction of food allergen and IgE antibody with the release of histamine and other chemical mediators. There is, however, a reaction that is anaphylaxislike in clinical appearance, termed an **anaphylactoid reaction.** This reaction results from nonimmune release of chemical mediators.

C. Gastrointestinal Intolerance: In mild cases, findings may include nausea, diarrhea, flatulence, bloating, and abdominal discomfort. In severe cases, there may be forceful vomiting, severe colic, bloody and mucoid diarrhea, and dehydration. Prolonged episodes of gastrointestinal intolerance can result in malnutrition and growth retardation. In many instances, food-associated symptoms are attributed to "allergy," but the mechanism upon which the reaction is based is unclear.

D. Perennial Allergic Rhinitis, Bronchial Asthma, Atopic Dermatitis, Urticaria: See elsewhere in this chapter.

E. Tension-Fatigue Syndrome: A combination of the following symptoms has been reported: fatigue, lassitude, irritability, sleeplessness, disturbed behavior, apathy, pallor, "shadowy" eyes with "allergic pleats", "run-down feeling", and sometimes a generalized headache with vague abdominal complaints. This syndrome is claimed to be associated in particular with foods commonly and abundantly eaten, eg, cow's milk, cereal grains, chocolate, eggs, and pork. It is not clear that these symptoms (when they can be associated with the ingestion of a specific food) are mediated by an allergic mechanism.

F. Hyperactivity: Claims that salicylates, dyes, sugar, and other food ingredients may contribute to hyperactivity in children with minimal brain dysfunction are controversial. In the occasional case in which a child appears to benefit from restricted diets (eg, the "Feingold diet"), there is no evidence of an allergic reaction to the foodstuffs involved.

G. Migraine: In addition to other causes, foods may precipitate a migrainous episode either on an allergic or nonallergic basis. Certain foods in which significant amounts of vasoactive amines have been found, such as chocolate, cheese, liver, and some wines and beers, have been demonstrated to precipitate migraine.

Clinical Findings

A. History; Symptoms and Signs: (Refer to the section on history in the discussion of atopic disorders; see also individual disorders). Often, a symptom diary kept for 7 to 14 days is helpful in establishing a baseline pattern for symptoms.

B. Laboratory Findings:

1. Eosinophilia of stool mucus may be present in cases of gastrointestinal allergy but may be a normal finding in the first 3 months of life; blood eosinophilia may occur.

2. Large positive reactions in skin tests (use scratch or prick tests only) are likely to be clinically relevant; mild (1–2+) reactions correlate poorly with clinical sensitivity. Interpretations of skin tests in the child of less than 2 years may vary slightly because of decreased skin reactivity. Negative reactions do not rule out a nonimmune clinical reaction or even an allergic reaction to some elements of food (eg, partially hydrolyzed product). The most common food allergens in young children are cow's milk, eggs, peanuts, soy, and wheat. In older children and adults, fish, shellfish, and nuts are most often involved in allergic reactions. Keep in mind, however, that severe reactions can occur to almost any food.

3. Serologic tests are in principle the same as skin tests. RAST scores of less than 3 usually are not associated with clinical sensitivity.

4. Provocative food tests are important in the less serious entities. Elimination, challenge, and rechallenge must be relied upon for definitive diagnosis. In very serious reactions such as angioedema, anaphylaxis, and bronchial asthma, the causative food is usually known by the patient or parents or can be identified by the physician with the aid of a history. Food challenges and food skin testing would be hazardous in these situations. In the less serious and more obscure symptom entities, the likely food is a common one (eg, milk); the suspected food should be withdrawn for 1 week before challenge.

Differential Diagnosis of Important Symptoms

A. Gastrointestinal Intolerance: Differentiate from cystic fibrosis, pyloric stenosis, celiac disease, acute or chronic intestinal infections, gastrointestinal malformations, carbohydrate enzyme deficiencies (eg, lactase), and irritable bowel syndrome.

B. Angioedema of the Upper Airway: Differentiate from acute epiglottiditis and foreign body in the upper airway.

Treatment & Prognosis

Treatment consists of eliminating the offending food, but the physician must be careful to provide specific advice for ensuring the nutritional adequacy of the diet. If milk or a milk substitute is withdrawn from the diet for over 1 month, the daily maintenance requirement of calcium should be administered (see Chapter 5). *Note:* Especially in the growing child, the unnecessary and unjustified restriction of many foods over an indefinite period merely because they **might** be involved or because they happened to give a positive skin reaction is to be condemned. The majority of proved offending foods in young children can be tolerated as time passes and should be rechallenged at 6-month intervals (unless the symptoms have been life-threatening) until the food can be reintroduced without symptoms.

Treat specific signs or symptoms as indicated.

The prognosis is good if the offending food can be identified. In some of the vague chronic syndromes, identification may not be possible, in which case the patient will remain symptomatic. In the severe syndromes, the offending food is usually known and can be avoided.

Anderson JA, Sogn DD (editors): *Adverse Reactions to Foods: AAAI and NIAID Report.* US Department of Health and Human Services Publication No. (NIH) 84–2442, 1984.

Bahna SL: Diagnostic tests for food allergy. *Clin Rev Allergy* 1988;**6**:259.

Consensus Development Conference (NIH): Defined diets and childhood hyperactivity. *JAMA* 1982;**248**:290.

Heiner DC (editor): Food allergy. *Clin Rev Allergy* 1984; **2**:1. [Entire issue]

Metcalf DD (editor): Symposium proceedings on adverse reactions to foods and food additives. *J Allergy Clin Immunol* 1986;**78**:1. [Entire issue.]

Sampson HA: Food sensitivity in children. Page 52 in: *Current Therapy in Allergy, Immunology, and Rheumatology 3.* Lichtenstein LM, Fauci AS (editors). Decker, 1988.

CONTACT DERMATITIS

Essentials of Diagnosis

- Erythematous, papular eruption that may progress to include vesiculation, bullae formation, and denudation.
- Pruritus, often intense.
- Eruption confined more or less to areas of direct skin contact with allergen.

General Considerations

Contact dermatitis is a delayed hypersensitivity reaction in the skin. The allergen is believed to conjugate locally within skin tissue elements. Sensitization after initial contact requires at least a few days, but an already sensitized individual may react to allergen contact in as little as 24 hours. Fur, leather and fabric dyes, formalin, dichromates (used in leather), nickel, rubber compounds, ethylenediamine (used in topical medications), neomycin, poison ivy, poison oak, and poison sumac are the most common offenders in contact dermatitis. Although most contact is local, dermatitis can be induced systemically in an already sensitized individual by ingestion of the antigen.

Clinical Findings

A. History: A history of contact with possible allergens corresponding to the distribution of the lesions, in conjunction with the appearance of the lesions, may be sufficient for the diagnosis or may serve only as a starting point for further investigation. Itching, frequently intense, is the rule and may precede the onset of observable lesions.

B. Physical Examination: The appearance and distribution of the lesions are the main criteria for diagnosis. Eruptions may be confined to areas of contact with the offending allergen, and inflammations may be sharply demarcated from normal skin. With more severe and chronic eruptions, however, dissemination may occur as a result of scratching and repeated contact with the allergen. If the eruption is mild, only erythema with some papulation may be present; more intense reactions include vesiculation with denudation of skin and frank weeping. Exfoliative dermatitis and secondary infection can also occur. There may be evidence of excoriation reflecting the pruritic nature of these lesions. With chronic dermatitis, skin thickening may be present.

C. Patch Testing: Patch testing with suspected allergens can be used to identify the contactants involved. In general, patch testing should not be performed when the dermatitis is active because this procedure may exacerbate the dermatitis.

Prevention

Sensitizing substances should be avoided. Inflamed skin is more susceptible to sensitization than normal skin, and virtually any substance applied to the skin is potentially sensitizing; only those topical agents considered necessary for treatment should be used.

Parenteral or oral hyposensitization is not generally successful and can induce serious reactions. Moreover, the striking beneficial effects of a brief course of local or systemic corticosteroid treatment virtually nullify justification for hyposensitization at the present time.

Treatment

A. Early Treatment:

1. Terminate exposure to the contactant.

2. Soaks with Burow's solution (Domeboro powder or tablet, 1 package or tablet to 1–2 pints of water) or with 1:6000 solution of potassium permanganate (0.3-g tablet plus 2 quarts of water) may be used in the early stage of treatment, especially if oozing is present, to diminish itching.

B. Mild Dermatitis: A short period of treatment with a mild adrenocorticosteroid cream or ointment is recommended.

C. Severe Dermatitis: Creams or ointments containing potent corticosteroids are helpful. These should be applied liberally and frequently so that the inflamed areas are covered at all times. In unusual circumstances, eg, when the dermatitis is extremely severe and extensive, systemic corticosteroids should be considered. A short course of systemic corticosteroids followed by topical corticosteroid administration is frequently helpful in controlling acute severe contact dermatitis (eg, poison ivy dermatitis). Pastes, ointments, and creams should not be applied to weeping skin.

D. General Measures:

1. Avoid all secondary irritants to the skin, eg, wool and detergents.

2. Treat infection, if present. Early in the course of the dermatitis, potassium permanganate solution can be employed instead of Burow's solution. This topical treatment may be sufficient; however, when the lesions are extensive, systemic antibiotic therapy must be used. Topical antibiotics should not be used, because they have potential for sensitization.

3. Give antihistamines orally for pruritus (hydroxyzine is recommended). Colloidal soaks, such as starch baths, may be employed when the dermatitis is extensive.

Fisher AA: *Contact Dermatitis,* 3rd ed. Lea & Febiger, 1986.

Mallory SB: Allergic contact dermatitis. *Immunol Allergy Clin North Am* 1987;**7**:407.

Parker F: Contact dermatitis. Chap 30, p 405, in: *Allergic Disease from Infancy to Adulthood,* 2nd ed. Bierman CW, Pearlman DS (editors). Saunders, 1988.

DRUG HYPERSENSITIVITY

Drugs are so widely used that drug reactions of one type or another are commonplace. It is helpful to categorize drug reactions according to the mechanism of the reaction. **Toxic drug reactions** are due to the inherent pharmacologic properties of the drug and are most frequently encountered after drug overdosage. Some individuals exhibit inordinate sensitivity to the recognized pharmacologic effects of a drug, however, and may therefore develop toxicity after administration of amounts that are usually nontoxic. **Drug idiosyncrasy** is an unusual response to the pharmacologic action of the drug (eg, hyperactivity rather than sedation following the administration of phenobarbital). **Allergic reactions to drugs** are independent of the drug's pharmacologic action and are the result of antigen-antibody interaction. This interaction may cause the release of histamine and other chemical mediators from mast cells (as in anaphylaxis) or may cause the production and deposition of immune complexes (as in serum sickness). The allergen may not be the drug administered but a metabolic derivative of it produced in the body. Although the immune reaction is highly specific, cross-reactions with chemically related drugs are not infrequent, for example, among the various kinds of penicillins. **Anaphylactoid (pseudoallergic) reactions** mimic true allergic reactions but are caused by nonspecific release of histamine or other vasoactive mediators from mast cells (eg, some reactions to iodinated radiocontrast dyes).

The manifestations of drug allergy are extremely varied, and virtually all allergic syndromes can be produced by drugs. The most common manifestations are skin eruptions and fever. In serum sickness, symptoms may occur 7–10 days after the first encounter with the substance (particularly penicillins and sulfonamides). Reexposure to the antigen in an already sensitized individual may result in symptoms as early as 12–36 hours. This disorder usually begins with a low-grade fever and malaise, which are followed to a variable extent by skin rash (90% of cases), lymphadenopathy, polyarthritis, and neurologic symptoms.

In recent years, various syndromes related to reactivity to aspirin have been recognized, predominantly in adults but also in children. The reactions appear to be nonallergic, based rather on some peculiar biochemical idiosyncrasy. A syndrome of nasal polyposis, severe aspirin-induced bronchospasm, and rhinitis with sinusitis has been well publicized, but a more subtle bronchospastic influence also has been documented in many children with asthma. Urticaria or angioedema also occurs in association with rhinitis and nasal polyposis, generally without bronchospasm in the urticarial forms.

Although any drug is a potential sensitizer, some (particularly penicillin and the sulfonamides) are more often associated with allergic reactions by repeated exposure. It is also probable that parenteral administration is more sensitizing than oral administration. Topical administration of drugs, especially over inflamed skin, is particularly sensitizing.

Exposure to sunlight may activate skin reactions to photosensitizing drugs such as sulfonamides, tetracycline antibiotics, and topically applied coal tar products.

In questioning a patient about drug reactions, it should be remembered that certain drugs such as penicillin G benzathine remain in the body for a long time. Reactions to a single depot injection of penicillin have been known to last for months.

With the exception of patch testing in contact dermatitis, allergy testing has usually been a disappointing procedure in identifying or predicting drug allergy. The reasons are many, and—in some cases at least—the allergic reaction is due to a metabolically altered form of the drug. In the case of penicillin, some of the offensive metabolic derivatives have been identified. When these substances are used in testing, prediction of allergic reactions on the basis of a test reaction is more successful. However, these reagents are not readily available, and until the exact allergens in other drugs are identified and preparations containing the appropriate allergens become widely available, skin and serologic testing for drug allergy cannot be considered a reliable procedure. The basis for "hypersensitivity" reactions to urographic or other radiocontrast material is unknown, and skin testing and other tests, including use of a smaller "test dose" of the material, cannot reliably predict reactivity to these agents.

The history of previous reactions to drugs remains the best means of diagnosing drug sensitivity. This is often difficult, however. For this reason, an alternative drug should be used (if possible) in any instance where a reaction to a drug is questionable. Furthermore, the patient should be advised to avoid the drug even though a definite drug allergy has not been established.

Treatment & Prognosis

Regardless of the manifestation, the treatment of drug allergy includes discontinuance of the offending drug at the first sign of an adverse reaction, the use of antihistamines with or without adrenergic drugs, and, in more severe and prolonged cases, administration of adrenocorticosteroids. Further contact with the drug is avoided. Small amounts of drugs to which a patient may be sensitive may be found in vaccines, foods, and other substances. Individuals with extreme hypersensitivity to a given drug should be warned, therefore, of other hidden sources of contact with the drug. Although desensitization has been used successfully, it is not recommended; it is better to substitute a chemically unrelated drug for the offending drug.

Symptomatic treatment is usually effective. If the possibility of a reaction to a radiocontrast dye is suspected, the patient should be pretreated with corticosteroids and antihistamines if the use of the dye is considered necessary.

The prognosis is good, especially when drug allergies are identified early.

Goldstine RA, Patterson R (editors): Symposium proceedings on drug allergy: Prevention, diagnosis, and treatment. *J Allergy Clin Immunol* 1984;**74(Suppl)**:549. [Entire issue.]

Mathews KP: Clinical spectrum of allergic and pseudoallergic drug reactions. *J Allergy Clin Immunol* 1984;**74**:558.

Patterson R: Diagnosis and treatment of drug allergy. *J Allergy Clin Immunol* 1988;**81**:380.

Sullivan TJ: Drug allergy. Chap 65, p 1523, in: *Allergy Principles and Practice,* 3rd ed. Middleton E Jr et al: (editors). Mosby, 1988.

Van Arsdel PP Jr: Drug hypersensitivity. Chap 53, p 684, in: *Allergic Diseases from Infancy to Adulthood,* 2nd ed. Bierman CW, Pearlman DS (editors). Saunders, 1988.

URICARIA

Essentials of Diagnosis

- Multiple (occasionally single) macular lesions, consisting of localized edema (wheal) with surrounding erythema.
- Pruritus, frequently intense.

General Considerations

Urticaria is a vascular reaction of the upper dermis consisting mainly of vasodilation and perivascular transudation, resulting in the classic "hive" or wheal and flare. Lesions are characteristically pruritic. Ordinarily, this vascular reaction is due to the liberation of histamine, but other mediators may be involved.

Urticarial reactions are usually transient (hours) but can persist for months or more. They may be the sole allergic manifestation or may represent only a part of the clinical picture, as in serum sickness and erythema multiforme. They also may occur on a nonallergic basis. Emotional tension may be an aggravating factor. **Angioedema** is essentially an urticarial reaction of the lower parts of the dermis, resulting in the production of a more diffuse edema. **Hereditary angioedema** is a rare, nonallergic disorder characterized by periodic bouts of angioedema that are nonpruritic. It can be life-threatening. (See Chapter 18.)

There are various forms of urticaria and urticarial syndromes, with various classifications and etiologic origins (see Clinical Findings). Two deserve special attention because they can be life-threatening. **Cold-induced urticaria** is a syndrome in which exposure to cold air, cold water, or other cold objects induces localized urticaria or angioedema, sometimes in the rewarming phase. Death from sudden massive mediator release can occur, for example, from swimming in cold water. **Exercise-related urticaria** takes various forms. One form appears to be "cholinergic," relates to overheating, and is characterized by intense itching and small wheals with erythema. It rarely is life-threatening. However, urticaria and angioedema may occur as part of more generalized anaphylactic syndromes with or without pulmonary involvement and are potentially fatal.

Papular urticaria is a term given to a syndrome characterized by multiple papules from insect bites, found especially on the extremities. It is not true urticaria. Scabies also may present in papules secondary to infection and scratching.

Dermatographism is the appearance of a wheal and erythema on the skin when "written" on, ie, stroked with a fingernail, for example. Dermatographism can occur in allergic and nonallergic individuals. It generally is of no pathologic significance but may accompany chronic urticaria or urticaria pigmentosa (mastocytosis).

Clinical Findings

A. History: The history is of prime importance in ascertaining the possible cause. The most common causes of urticaria are categorized below. However, the cause most often is not identifiable, especially in chronic urticaria (urticaria lasting weeks to years).

1. Drugs, hyposensitization extracts, vaccines, toxoids, and hormone preparations.
2. Infections, including bacterial (especially staphylococcal and group A β-hemolytic streptococcal), parasitic, fungal, and viral, including viral hepatitis, herpesvirus, and various other common viral pathogens.
3. Foods (especially eggs, milk, soy, shellfish, fish, berries, peanuts, and nuts); food dyes and other food additives may be infrequent causes.
4. Inhalants, pollens, and molds (sometimes by direct contact as well as inhalation).
5. Psychologic factors (probably overrated).
6. Physical factors (cold, heat, vibration, delayed pressure), exercise, histamine liberators, and dermatographism.
7. Endocrine disorder (mainly thyroid and parathyroid disorders and diabetes). (uncommon).
8. Underlying systemic disease (eg, connective tissue disorders, cancer). (Rare in children.)

B. Symptoms and Signs: Urticarial lesions characteristically appear as erythematous areas with a pale center and usually occur in large numbers. Pruritus is the rule and is frequently intense; it may precede the appearance of the lesions. Pruritus is not, however, characteristic of angioneurotic edema, which occurs most often as a solitary lesion or together with multiple urticaria. When angioedema involves the laryngeal area, it may be a threat to life.

Dermatographism may be symptomatic and occurs in a small percentage of allergic and nonallergic patients.

C. Laboratory Findings: Diagnostic procedures may include drug elimination, dietary elimination and challenge of suspected foods, and a thorough search for infection elsewhere in the body. Allergy testing is occasionally of value.

Differential Diagnosis

Urticaria is a prominent feature of mastocytosis (urticaria pigmentosa) and may occur in systemic diseases such as lupus erythematosus, various liver diseases, lymphoma, leukemia, and carcinoma.

Treatment & Prognosis

Treatment consists mainly of the detection and elimination of the appropriate allergens, when possible. Aspirin should be avoided because it may secondarily aggravate the urticaria. Antihistamines are usually the most useful therapeutic agents in urticarial disorders, but adrenergic agents with vasoconstrictor properties can be a useful adjunct. Epinephrine is especially effective when rapid relief is needed. Hydroxyzine (Atarax, Vistaril) is among the most effective antihistamines, especially in treatment of chronic urticaria and dermatographism. In resistant cases, combining an H_1 antihistamine (eg, hydroxyzine) with an H_2 antihistamine (eg, cimetidine) may be helpful. Cyproheptadine hydrochloride (Periactin) is most effective in some patients with cold-induced urticaria. Mild sedation may also be indicated.

Adrenocorticosteroids are sometimes useful in the more chronic form of urticaria but are reserved for more refractory cases. Topical medications generally are not effective. Except for cases of life-threatening laryngeal edema, the prognosis is good. Identification of the offending agent is more important.

Kaplan AP: Urticaria and angioedema. Chap 59, p 1377, in: *Allergy: Principles and Practice*, 3rd ed. Middleton E Jr et al: (editors). Mosby, 1988.

Schocket A: Urticaria and angioedema. Chap 31, pp 415–424, in: *Allergic Diseases from Infancy to Adulthood*, 2nd ed. Bierman CW, Pearlman DS (editors). Saunders, 1988.

OTHER ALLERGIC PULMONARY DISORDERS

A syndrome thought to be related to **cow's milk hypersensitivity** has been described and consists of recurrent pulmonary infiltrates, wheezing, chronic cough, chronic or frequent otitis media and rhinorrhea, and iron deficiency anemia related to excessive gastrointestinal blood loss. Gastrointestinal symptoms (diarrhea, vomiting) and poor weight gain are also features of this disorder, which is seen in children chiefly in the first 2 years of life. Some of these children have evidence of pulmonary hemosiderosis, and blood eosinophilia is sometimes seen. Multiple precipitins to cow's milk can be demonstrated, but the significance of this finding is controversial. Dietary elimination of cow's milk is followed by improvement of the disorder, although symptoms also have been reported to subside spontaneously.

Hypersensitivity pneumonitis is an inflammatory reaction involving principally the alveoli and bronchioles and characterized clinically by malaise, fever, chills, cough, and dyspnea. Tissue damage stems from a hypersensitivity reaction to any of a variety of inhaled organic dusts or of fungi that may or may not also be infective. The disease is seen predominantly in adults as a result of occupational exposure to large concentrations of certain antigens (eg, thermophilic actinomycetes from hay, as in farmer's lung, or from contaminated air conditioners), but the disease can occur at any age. The onset may be insidious or acute. Symptoms of these disorders—particularly in the acute onset form— typically occur 4–8 hours after exposure to the offending antigen. In asthmatic individuals, wheezing also may be present, with involvement of IgE-mediated mechanisms.

Treatment consists mainly of avoiding the offensive inhalants. Glucocorticoids may be very helpful in minimizing the hypersensitivity reaction early in the disease.

Allergic bronchopulmonary aspergillosis, with or without tissue invasion by the organism, is seen with some frequency in Great Britain but is rare in the USA (especially in children). The syndrome occurs in allergic asthmatics and includes symptoms of asthma and recurrent pneumonitis. High levels of eosinophils in tissue and blood, high IgE levels, and the presence of IgE and precipitating antibody to

Aspergillus are characteristic laboratory findings. *Aspergillus* also may be found on sputum smear or culture. Treatment includes use of corticosteroids and antifungal agents.

An association between **tissue and blood eosinophilia** and **pulmonary infiltrates** has been observed in various disorders (eg, asthma, allergic bronchopulmonary aspergillosis, connective tissue diseases) and is thought to reflect an allergic mechanism in these disorders. A number of drugs (especially sulfonamides and nitrofurantoin), parasites (eg, *Ascaris*), and other antigens have been implicated at times in the production of this syndrome, but frequently no cause can be found.

Bierman CW, Pierson WE, Massie FS: Nonasthmatic allergic pulmonary disease. Chap 42, p 543, in: *Disorders of the Respiratory Tract in Children*, 4th ed. Kendig EL Jr, Cherniak V (editors). Saunders, 1983.

Greenberger PA: Allergic bronchopulmonary aspergillosis. Page 220 in: *Current Therapy in Allergy, Immunology and Rheumatology 3*. Lichtenstein LM, Fauci AS (editors). Dekker, 1988.

Stankus RP, Salvaggio JE (editors): Immunologically mediated lung disease. *Clin Rev Allergy* 1985;**3**:143. [Entire issue.]

SELECTED REFERENCES

References for Physicians

Bierman CW, Pearlman DS (editors): *Allergic Diseases from Infancy to Adulthood*, 2nd ed. Saunders, 1988.

Gershwin NE (editor): *Bronchial Asthma: Principles of Diagnosis and Treatment*. Grune & Stratton, 1981.

Middleton E Jr, Reed FE, Ellis EF (editors): *Allergy: Principles and Practice*, 2nd ed. Mosby, 1983.

Salvaggio JE (editor): Primer in allergic and immunologic diseases. *JAMA* 1982;**248**:2579.

References for Parents & Patients

Young SH, Shulman SA, Shulman MD: *The Asthma Handbook: A Complete Guide for Patients and Their Families*. Bantam Books, 1985.

Feldman ER with Carroll D: *The Complete Book of Children's Allergies: A Guide for Parents*. Times Books (Random House), 1986.

Plaut MF: *Children With Asthma: A Manual for Parents*, 2nd ed. Pediapress, 1988.

Useful Organizations for Parents, Patients, and Physicians

Asthma and Allergy Foundation of America, National Headquarters: 1302 18th Street N.W., Suite 303, Washington, D.C. [Chapters in various states.]

Mothers of Asthmatics, 10875 Main Street, Suite 210, Fairfax, VI 22030. Telephone (703) 285-4403. [These organizations provide information for understanding and treating allergic problems.]

Inborn Errors of Metabolism

33

Stephen I. Goodman, MD, & Carol L. Greene, MD

Disorders in which defects of single genes cause clinically significant blocks in metabolic pathways are called **inborn errors of metabolism.** For many years after Garrod first described them in 1908, these conditions were considered esoteric and rare. The number of known inborn errors has increased rapidly in recent years, however, and they are now recognized as important causes of disease in the pediatric age group. Many of them can now be treated effectively. Even when treatment is not available, correct diagnosis permits couples to make informed decisions about future offspring.

Pathogenesis is almost always due to accumulation of enzyme substrate behind the metabolic block or to deficiency of the reaction product. In some cases, the accumulated enzyme substrate is diffusible and has an adverse effect on distant organs; in others, as in lysosomal storage diseases, the substrate accumulates only locally.

The clinical manifestations of inborn errors vary significantly; there are mild and severe forms of virtually every disorder, and many patients do not match the classical phenotype. In many cases, this is because the mutations in different patients, even though they are in the same gene, are not identical.

Strategies used to treat inborn errors include avoiding enzyme substrate in the diet (eg, low-phenylalanine diet for phenylketonuria), removing accumulated substrate by pharmacologic means (eg, glycine therapy for isovaleric acidemia), supplementing an inadequately produced metabolite (eg, arginine administration for urea cycle disorders), providing additional coenzyme (eg, vitamin B_{12} therapy for methylmalonic acidemia), and providing normal enzyme (eg, liver transplantation for Wilson's disease). Gene replacement is a long-term goal, but problems of delivery and control of gene action make this an unrealistic option at the present.

Inborn errors can present at any time, affect virtually any organ system, and cause all but the most common pediatric problems. This chapter focuses first on when these conditions should be considered in the differential diagnosis of common pediatric problems and how to rule them out. Then a few of the more important disorders are discussed in detail.

DIAGNOSIS

Inborn errors must be considered in the differential diagnosis of the critically ill newborn and of the child with seizures, Reye-like syndromes, parenchymal liver disease, mental retardation or developmental delay, recurrent vomiting, unusual odor, unexplained acidosis, hyperammonemia, and hypoglycemia.

Inborn errors should be strongly suspected when (1) symptoms accompany changes in diet, (2) there is developmental slowing or regression, (3) there is a history of food preferences or aversions, or (4) there is a history of parental consanguinity or a similar disease in siblings or other family members. The last is especially important if the disease follows an X-linked pattern of inheritance.

Physical findings that should always raise the suspicion of an inborn error include alopecia or abnormal hair, retinal cherry-red spot or retinitis pigmentosa, cataracts or corneal opacity, hepatomegaly or splenomegaly, coarse features, skeletal changes (including gibbus), and ataxia. Features that are important, in combination with a suspicious history, include failure to thrive, microcephaly, jaundice, hypotonia, and hypertonia.

Finding a cause of symptoms is not enough to rule out an inborn error. Conditions such as renal tubular acidosis and cirrhosis are often due to an underlying inborn error. Some inborn errors predispose to infection, eg, gram-negative sepsis in patients with galactosemia. In other patients, acute crises may be brought on by intercurrent infections.

Table 33–1 lists common clinical and laboratory features of different groups of inborn errors. Table 33–2 lists laboratory tests used to diagnose these diseases and gives some comments on their use.

Laboratory studies are almost always needed for the diagnosis of inborn errors. Serum electrolytes and pH can be determined in a hospital laboratory

Table 33–1. Clinical and laboratory features of inborn errors.[1]

	Defects of Carbohydrate Metabolism	Defects of Amino Acid Metabolism[2]	Organic Acid Disorders[3]	Defects of Fatty Acid Oxidation	Defects of Purine Metabolism	Lysosomal Storage Diseases	Disorders of Peroxisomes
Neurodevelopmental							
Mental/developmental retardation	+++	+++	+++	−	++	+++	+++
Developmental regression	−	−	+	−	−	+++	+++
Acute encephalopathy	+++	+++	+++	+++	−	−	−
Seizures	++	+++	+++	+	−	+++	++
Ataxia/movement disorder	−	+	++	−	+++	−	−
Hypotonia	++	++	++	+++	−	+	+++
Hypertonia	−	++	+++	−	++	+	−
Abnormal behavior	−	++	++	−	++	+++	−
Growth							
Failure to thrive	+++	+++	+++	−	−	+	−
Short stature	++	−	+	−	−	++	−
Macrocephaly	−	−	+	−	−	+++	++
Microcephaly	+	++	+++	−	−	+	−
General							
Vomiting/anorexia	++	+++	+++	+++	−	−	++
Food aversion or craving	++	+++	+++	+++	−	−	−
Odor	−	++	++	−	−	−	−
Dysmorphic features	−	+	+	−	−	++	++
Congenital malformations	−	++	++	−	−	−	++
Organ specific							
Hepatomegaly	+++	−	++	+++	−	+++	+++
Liver disease/cirrhosis	++	+	−	−	−	−	+
Splenomegaly	−	−	−	−	−	++	+
Skeletal dysplasia	−	−	−	−	−	++	++
Cardiomyopathy	++	−	+	+++	−	++	−
Tachypnea/hyperpnea	++	++	++	++	−	−	−
Rash	−	++	++	−	−	−	−
Alopecia or abnormal hair	−	+	++	−	−	−	+
Cataracts or corneal opacity	++	−	−	−	−	++	−
retinal abnormality	−	+	+	−	−	++	++
...quent infections	++	−	++	−	++	−	−
...ness	−	−	+	−	−	++	−
...ory - general							
...cemia	+++	+	++	++	−	−	−
...monemia	−	++	++	++	−	−	−
...acidosis	++	++	+++	+++	−	−	−
El...alkalosis	−	++	−	−	−	−	−
Elev...te/pyruvate	++	−	+++	++	−	−	−
Neutro...nzymes	++	++	++	+++	−	+	+
Ketosis ...hrombocytopenia	+	−	+	−	++	+	−
Hypoketos...	+++	++	+++	−	−	−	−
	−	−	+	+++	−	−	−

[1] +++, mos...
[2] Includes disdions in group; ++, some; +, one or few; −, not found.
[3] Includes MSU... urea cycle but not maple syrup urine disease (MSUD).
...disorders of pyruvate oxidation.

Table 33–2. Obtaining and handling samples to diagnose inborn errors.

Test	Comments
Acid-base status	Accurate estimation of anion gap must be possible
	Samples for blood gases should be kept on ice and analyzed immediately
Blood ammonia	Sample should be collected without a tourniquet, kept on ice, and analyzed immediately
Blood lactic and pyruvic acids	Sample should be collected without a tourniquet, kept on ice, and analyzed immediately
	Reduction of pyruvic to lactic must be prevented
	Normal literature values are for the fasting state.
Amino acids	Blood *and* urine should be examined
	CSF glycine should be measured if nonketotic hyperglycinemia is to be ruled out
	Normal literature values are for the fasting state
	Growth of bacteria in urine should be prevented
	Autopsy: liver, kidney, or vitreous of eye may be analyzed if urine not available
Organic acids	Urine preferred for analysis
	Autopsy: liver, kidney, or vitreous of eye may be analyzed if urine not available
Urine mucopolysaccharides	Variations in urine concentration may cause errors in screening tests
	Diagnosis requires knowing which mucopolysaccharide(s) is increased
	Some Morquio patients do not have abnormal mucopolysacchariduria
Enzyme assays	Specific assay(s) must be requested
	Exposure to heat may cause loss of enzyme activity
	Enzyme activity in whole blood may become normal after transfusion or vitamin therapy
	Leukocyte or fibroblast pellets should be kept frozen prior to assays
	Fibroblasts may be grown from skin biopsies taken up to 72 hours after death
	Tissues such as liver and kidney should be taken as soon as possible after death, frozen immediately, and kept at −70° C until assayed

and should be used to estimate anion gap as well as acid-base status. Tests to determine serum lactate, pyruvate, and ammonia may be available only in large hospital laboratories. Amino and organic acid studies are almost always performed by more specialized facilities, to ensure adequate analysis and interpretation. Although it is becoming possible to diagnose an increasing number of inborn errors with DNA probes, this almost always requires an extensive genealogic chart or a knowledge of the precise mutation carried in the family. In most cases, these conditions cannot be satisfied.

The physician should know what conditions a test will detect and when it will detect them. For example, urine organic acids may be normal in patients with medium-chain acyl-CoA dehydrogenase deficiency or biotinidase deficiency, glycine may be elevated only in cerebrospinal fluid in patients with glycine encephalopathy, and a result that is normal in one physiologic state may be abnormal in another. For instance, the urine of a hypoglycemic child should not be negative for ketones; in such children, a ketone-negative urine test may suggest the presence of a defect in fatty acid oxidation.

Samples used to diagnose metabolic disease may be obtained at autopsy. They may be analyzed directly or stored frozen until a particular analysis is justified by the results of postmortem examination, new clinical information, or new developments in the field. Studies of other family members may also help to establish the diagnosis in a deceased patient; these include demonstrating that the parents are heterozygous carriers of a particular disorder or showing that another sibling has the condition.

ACUTE PRESENTATION IN NEONATE—THE CHILD WITH "RULE OUT SEPSIS"

Acute metabolic disease in the newborn may be clinically indistinguishable from sepsis and is most often caused by disorders of amino acid or carbohydrate metabolism. Initial symptoms may include poor feeding or vomiting, altered mental status or tone, jitteriness or seizures, and jaundice. Laboratory studies should include determination of electrolytes, ammonia, glucose, urine pH, urine-reducing substances, and urine ketones. Glycine in cerebrospinal fluid should be measured if glycine encephalopathy is suspected. Serum and urine to be used for amino and organic acid analysis should be collected before oral intake is stopped and sent for analysis if indicated by the results of initial studies.

VOMITING & ENCEPHALOPATHY IN THE INFANT OR OLDER CHILD

Even though vomiting and altered consciousness in the infant or child are more often due to infection and trauma than to an inborn error, the physician should order laboratory studies of electrolytes, ammonia, glucose, urine pH, urine-reducing substances, and urine ketones in all patients before the results are altered by treatment. Samples for amino and organic acid analysis should be obtained early and frozen pending the results of initial studies. An inborn error is even more likely when the presentation is typical of Reye syndrome (vomiting, encephalopathy, and hepatomegaly), and amino and organic acids should be studied immediately. If there is hypoglycemia with inappropriately low urine or serum ketones, studies of urine octanoylcarnitine and phenylpropionylglycine should be conducted.

MENTAL RETARDATION

Many inborn errors can cause mental retardation without other distinguishing characteristics. Laboratory studies of serum and urine amino acids should be obtained for every patient with nonspecific mental retardation. Because physical stigmas of certain mucopolysaccharidoses may be subtle, urine screens for mucopolysacchariduria may also be useful. Electrolytes should be examined because the presence of a high anion gap or renal tubular acidosis significantly increases the chance of finding an underlying inborn error. If developmental regression or specific neurologic findings are present, the evaluation should be expanded accordingly.

HYPOGLYCEMIA

Studies of electrolytes, ammonia, uric acid, urine-reducing substances, and urine ketones should be performed, and urine should be obtained to measure levels of organic acids. Ketone body production is usually not efficient in the neonate, and ketonuria in a hypoglycemic infant suggests an inborn error. In the older child, however, the absence of ketonuria suggests inborn error, particularly of fatty acid oxidation.

HYPERAMMONEMIA

Symptoms of hyperammonemia may appear rapidly or insidiously. Decreased appetite and irritability usually appear first, with vomiting, lethargy, seizures, and coma appearing as ammonia levels increase. Tachypnea is caused by a direct effect on respiratory drive. No single physical finding can exclude the presence of hyperammonemia, and serum ammonia should be measured whenever hyperammonemia is suspected.

Hyperammonemia may be due to urea cycle disorders, organic acidemias or, in infancy, to transient hyperammonemia of the newborn. The cause can usually be ascertained by measuring citrulline and electrolytes in serum and measuring amino acids, organic acids, and orotic acid in urine. Respiratory alkalosis is usually present in transient hyperammonemia of the newborn and hyperammonemia due to a urea cycle defect, whereas metabolic acidosis is usually associated with hyperammonemia due to organic acidemia. Urine organic acid analysis will demonstrate the cause if the condition is due to organic acidemia. Serum citrulline is usually low or undetectable in early urea cycle defects; normal or slightly high in transient hyperammonemia of the newborn; and very high in citrullinemia and argininosuccinic acidemia, and argininosuccinic acid is found in urine only in the latter. Of infants with early urea cycle defects, only those with hyperammonemia due to ornithine transcarbamoylase deficiency have increased urine orotic acid levels and (often) a family history of male newborn deaths due to defects that appear to be transmitted as an X-linked trait.

ACIDOSIS

Inborn errors may cause chronic or acute acidosis at any age, and with or without an increased anion gap. Certain clues should always increase suspicion of inborn error. Inborn errors should be considered when acidosis occurs with recurrent emesis or hyperammonemia, and when acidosis is out of proportion to the clinical state of the patient. Acidosis due to an inborn error is usually, but not always, difficult to correct. The presence of renal tubular acidosis does not exclude an underlying inborn error.

Serum glucose and ammonia, and urine pH and ketones should always be examined. Samples for amino and organic acids should be obtained at once and sent to the laboratory or saved in the freezer depending on how strongly an inborn error is suspected. It is useful to test blood lactate and pyruvate levels in the chronically acidotic patient if urine organic acid levels are normal. Lactic and pyruvate levels are difficult to interpret in the acutely ill patient, but in the absence of shock very high levels of lactic acid suggest primary lactic acidosis.

TREATMENT OF METABOLIC EMERGENCIES

Patients with severe acidosis, hypoglycemia, and hyperammonemia may be very ill; initially mild symptoms may worsen quickly, and coma and death may ensue within hours. With prompt and vigorous treatment, however, patients can recover completely, even from deep coma. All oral intake should be stopped. Glucose should be given intravenously in amounts sufficient to stop catabolic processes. Most conditions respond favorably to glucose administration, and few (eg, primary lactic acidosis due to pyruvate dehydrogenase deficiency) do not. Severe or increasing hyperammonemia should be treated pharmacologically or with dialysis, and severe acidosis should be treated with bicarbonate administration. Specific measures should be instituted when a diagnosis is established.

NEWBORN SCREENING

Criteria used to decide whether or not to screen newborns for a disorder include its frequency, the significance of consequences if it is not treated, the availability and cost of screening and diagnostic tests, and the availability and cost of treatment. All US states screen newborns for phenylketonuria, and many states also screen for hypothyroidism and galactosemia. Other disorders for which newborns are frequently screened include maple syrup urine disease, homocystinuria due to cystathionine synthase deficiency, and biotinidase deficiency.

Some screening tests measure a metabolite (eg, phenylalanine) that becomes abnormal only with time and exposure to diet, and in such instances the disease cannot be detected reliably until intake of the enzyme substrate has become established. Other tests (eg, for biotinidase deficiency) assay an enzyme and can be performed at any time; however, transfusions may cause false-negative results, and exposure of the sample to heat may cause false-positive results. Screening tests are not diagnostic, and diagnostic tests must be undertaken when an abnormal screening result is obtained. Also, because false-negative results are not unknown, a normal newborn screening test does not rule out a condition if symptoms develop.

The time of newborn screening recommended by the American Academy of Pediatrics is appropriate for the detection of phenylketonuria; hypothyroidism, for instance, can be missed when screening is carried out at this time.

Bickel, H: Early diagnosis and treatment of inborn errors of metabolism. *Enzyme* 1987;**38**:14.
Burton B: Inborn errors of metabolism: The clinical diagnosis in early infancy. *Pediatrics* 1987;**79**:359.
Childs B: Sir Archibald Garrod's conception of chemical individuality: A modern appreciation. *N Engl J Med* 1970; **282**:71.
Cohn RM, Roth KS: *Metabolic Disease: A Guide to Early Recognition*. Saunders, 1983.
Committee on Genetics, American Academy of Pediatrics: New issues in newborn screening for phenylketonuria and congenital hypothyroidism. *Pediatrics* 1982; **69**:104.
Emery JL et al: Investigation of inborn errors of metabolism in unexpected infant deaths. *Lancet* 1988;**2**:29.
Goodman SI: Inherited metabolic disease in the newborn: Approach to diagnosis and treatment. *Adv Pediatr* 1986; **33**:197.
Greene CL, Blitzer MG, Shapira E: Inborn errors of metabolism and Reye syndrome: Differential diagnosis. *J Pediatr* 1988;**113**:156.
Hirschhorn R: Therapy of genetic disorders. *N Engl J Med* 1987;**316:**623.
NEJM Case Records: Normal reference laboratory values. *N Engl J Med* 1986;**314:**39.
Nyhan WL, Sakati N: *Diagnostic Recognition of Genetic Disease*. Lea and Febiger, 1987.
Phillip M et al: An algorithmic approach to diagnosis of hypoglycemia. *J Pediatr* 1987;**110:**387.
Rivkees SA, Fine BP: The reliability of calculated bicarbonate in clinical practice. *Clini Pediatr* 1988;**27**:240.
Rosenn DW, Loeb LS, Jura MB: Differentiation of organic from non-organic failure to thrive in infancy. *Pediatrics* 1980;**66**:698.
Schweitzer LB, Desnick RJ: Inherited metabolic diseases: Advances in delineation, diagnosis and treatment. *Birth Defects* 1983;**19**:39.

DISORDERS OF CARBOHYDRATE METABOLISM

GLYCOGEN STORAGE DISEASES

Glycogen is a highly branched polymer of glucose that is stored in liver and muscle. Many different disorders of its biosynthesis and degradation have been described, and the enzyme defects responsible have been identified. The most common forms of glycogenosis are characterized by growth failure, hepatomegaly, and fasting hypoglycemia. Defects that cause these so-called hepatic forms of the disease include glucose-6-phosphatase (type I; von Gierke disease), debrancher enzyme (type III), hepatic phosphorylase (type VI), and phosphorylase kinase (type IX), which normally regulates hepatic phosphorylase activity. Further, there are 2 forms of glucose-6-phosphatase deficiency; in one the enzyme defect can be demonstrated in fresh or frozen liver; in the other, the defect can be demonstrated only in fresh tissue.

Forms of the disease affecting primarily muscle include acid maltase deficiency (type II; Pompe disease), which presents in infancy with cardiomegaly and macroglossia, and muscle phosphorylase (type V) and phosphofructokinase (type VII) deficiencies, in which the most striking features are easy fatigability and muscle weakness and stiffness.

Diagnosis

Precise diagnosis is by appropriate biochemical tests, such as responsiveness of blood glucose to glucagon and epinephrine, and enzyme assays on leukocytes, liver, or muscle. Disorders that can be diagnosed using red or white blood cells include deficiencies of debrancher enzyme (type III) and phosphorylase kinase (IX). Pompe disease can usually be diagnosed by assaying acid maltase in fibroblasts or peripheral leukocytes.

Treatment

In general, treatment is symptomatic. Treating hypoglycemia can lead to storage of even more glycogen in liver. In the most severe hepatic forms, some good results have been reported following continuous nighttime carbohydrate feeding.

Ambruso DR et al: Infectious and bleeding complications in patients with glycogenosis Ib. *Am J Dis Child* 1985; **139:**691.
Bashan N et al: Phosphorylase kinase in leukocytes and erythrocytes of a patient with glycogen storage disease type IX. *J Inherited Metab Dis* 1987;**10:**119.
Fernandes J et al: Glycogen storage disease: Recommendations for treatment. *Eur J Pediatr* 1988;**147:**226.
Greene HL et al: Type I glycogen storage disease: A metabolic basis for advances in treatment. *Adv Pediatr* 1979; **26:**63.

GALACTOSEMIA

Classical galactosemia is caused by almost total deficiency of galactose-1-phosphate uridyltransferase. Accumulation of galactose-1-phosphate in liver, brain, and renal tubules causes hepatic parenchymal disease, mental retardation, and renal Fanconi syndrome. Accumulation of galactitol (dulcitol) in the lens produces cataracts. With prompt institution of a galactose-free diet, the prognosis for life is excellent.

In the severe form of the disease, onset is marked by vomiting, jaundice, and hepatomegaly in the newborn period after milk feeding. Without treatment, death frequently occurs in the first month of life, often from *Escherichia coli* sepsis. Cataracts usually develop within 2 months in untreated cases, and hepatic cirrhosis is progressive. Some cases are not severe, however, as shown by the occasional recognition of undiagnosed patients in surveys of mental institutions. If untreated, galactosemia leads to seemingly irreversible mental retardation. Even when dietary restrictions are instituted early, patients with galactosemia are at increased risk for speech and language deficits and ovarian failure, and some patients develop progressive delay, tremor, and ataxia. Clinical and laboratory evidence of the disease abates gradually with effective treatment.

The disorder is inherited as an autosomal recessive trait with an incidence of approximately 1 in 40,000 live births. Because disease in infancy may be severe and difficult to diagnose, newborn screening is becoming increasingly common. Screening is accomplished either by demonstrating enzyme deficiency in red cells with the Beutler test or by demonstrating increased serum galactose. Prenatal diagnosis of fetal status can be made by enzyme assay of cultured amniotic cells or cells obtained by chorionic villus sampling.

Diagnosis

In infants receiving foods containing galactose, laboratory findings include galactosuria and hypergalactosemia together with proteinuria, aminoaciduria, and tyrosyluria. It is important not to exclude the diagnosis simply because the urine does not contain reducing substances. When the diagnosis is suspected, galactose-1-phosphate uridyltransferase should be assayed in erythrocytes; only blood transfusions will cause this test to be falsely negative, and only sample deterioration will cause it to be falsely positive.

Treatment

A galactose-free diet should be instituted as soon as the diagnosis is made, and compliance with the diet monitored. Avoidance of galactose should be lifelong in severe cases, although tolerance increases somewhat with age. Heterozygous and homozygous mothers are advised to follow a galactose-free diet during pregnancies.

Kaufman FR et al: Correlation of ovarian function with galactose-1-phosphate uridyl transferase levels in galactosemia. *J Pediatr* 1988;**112:**755.
Levy HL, Hammarsen G: Newborn screening for galactosemia and other galactose metabolic defects. *J Pediatr* 1978;**92:**871.
Levy HL et al: Sepsis due to *Escherichia coli* in neonates with galactosemia. *N Engl J Med* 1977;**297:**823.
Lo W et al: Neurologic sequelae in galactosemia. *Pediatrics* 1984;**73:**309.
Sardharwalla IB, Wraith JE: Galactosemia. *Nutr Health* 1987;**5:**175.

HEREDITARY FRUCTOSE INTOLERANCE

Hereditary fructose intolerance is an autosomal recessive disorder in which deficient activity of fructose-1-phosphate aldolase causes hypoglycemia and tissue accumulation of fructose-1-phosphate on fructose ingestion. Other abnormalities include failure to thrive, vomiting, jaundice, hepatomegaly, proteinuria, generalized aminoaciduria, and tyrosyluria. The untreated condition can progress to death as a result of liver failure.

Diagnosis

The diagnosis is supported by the demonstration of fructosuria following an oral fructose load. The appearance of hypoglycemia and hypophosphatemia after fructose loading (200 mg/kg) is diagnostic, as is reduced activity of fructose-1-phosphate aldolase in liver.

Treatment

Treatment consists of eliminating cane sugar from the diet and is complicated by the fact that many proprietary drugs and vitamins are in a sucrose base. If the diet is subsequently relaxed, there may be retardation of physical growth, but growth will resume when more stringent dietary restrictions are instituted. If the disorder is recognized early enough, the prospects for normal development are good. As less severely affected individuals grow up, they may recognize the association of nausea and vomiting with fructose-containing foods and selectively avoid them.

Melancon SB et al: Metabolic and biochemical studies in fructose-1,6-diphosphatase deficiency. *J Pediatr* 1973; **82**:650.

Mock DM et al: Chronic fructose intoxication after infancy in children with hereditary fructose intolerance: A cause of growth failure. *N Engl J Med* 1983;**309**:764.

Odierre M et al: Hereditary fructose intolerance in childhood: Diagnosis, management and course in 55 patients. *Am J Dis Child* 1978;**132**:605.

PRIMARY LACTIC ACIDOSIS

Lactic acidosis, ie, elevation of serum lactic acid levels over the normal 2 mmol/L (venous), is said to be primary when it is due to a defect in the metabolism of pyruvic acid and secondary when a change in cellular redox potential favors the reduction of pyruvate to lactate (as in shock). Some causes of primary lactic acidosis are shown in Table 33–3. In general, such disorders may present at any age with neurologic findings and, when the defect is in gluconeogenesis, with hypoglycemia. Patients with a defect in the E_1 component of the pyruvate dehydrogenase complex often show mild facial dysmorphism or CNS malformations.

Table 33–3. Causes of primary lactic acidosis in childhood.

Defects of the pyruvate dehydrogenase complex
1. E_1 (pyruvate decarboxylase) deficiency
2. E_2 (dihydrolipoyl transacetylase) deficiency
3. E_3 (lipoamide dehydrogenase) deficiency
4. Pyruvate decarboxylase phosphate phosphatase deficiency

Abnormalities of gluconeogenesis
1. Pyruvate carboxylase deficiency
   a) Isolated
   b) Biotinidase deficiency
   c) Holocarboxylase synthetase deficiency
2. Fructose-1,6-diphosphatase deficiency
3. Glucose-6-phosphatase deficiency (von Gierke disease;

Defects in mitochondrial respiratory chain
1. Disorders of respiratory chain complex I and III
2. Cytochrome oxidase deficiency (frequent cause of Leigh's disease)

Defects in the mitochondrial respiratory chain are also frequently associated with lactic acidosis; these conditions may present with hypotonia or eye findings such as ophthalmoplegia and optic atrophy. Ragged red fibers and mitochondrial abnormalities may be noted on histologic examination of muscle. These disorders may be progressive.

Diagnosis

Diagnosis of primary lactic acidosis is based on (1) demonstrating significant elevations of lactic and pyruvic acid and alanine in blood and (2) excluding disorders such as methylmalonic and propionic acidemia as the cause. Unless a specific diagnosis is suggested by fructose intolerance or by the typical physical findings of von Gierke disease or biotinidase deficiency, enzyme analysis of fibroblasts or skeletal muscle is often required. In many patients, the cause of the disorder cannot be defined.

Treatment

In some patients defects in gluconeogenesis can be treated with glucose administration, fructose avoidance, or administration of pharmacologic amounts of biotin. Thiamine or lipoic acid can be tried in patients with pyruvate dehydrogenase complex deficiencies, and coenzyme Q has been tried in patients with complex III deficiency states.

Brown GK et al: "Cerebral" lactic acidosis: Defects in pyruvate metabolism with profound brain damage and minimal systemic acidosis. *Eur J Pediatr* 1988;**147**:10.

DiMauro S et al: Mitochondrial myopathies. *Ann Neurol* 1985;**17**:521.

Robinson BH et al: Variable clinical presentation in patients with defective E_1 component of pyruvate dehydrogenase complex. *J Pediatr* 1987;**111**:525.

Trijbels JMF et al: Disorders of the mitochondrial respiratory chain: Clinical manifestations and diagnostic approach. *Eur J Pediatr* 1988;**148**:92.

DISORDERS OF AMINO ACID METABOLISM

DISORDERS OF THE UREA CYCLE

Ammonia is converted to an amino group in urea by enzymes of the urea cycle. Defects in early urea cycle enzymes, such as carbamoyl-phosphate synthetase (CPS) or ornithine transcarbamoylase (OTC), usually present in infancy with severe and rapidly fatal hyperammonemia, vomiting, and encephalopathy, but the course may also be milder, with vomiting and encephalopathy following protein ingestion or infections. Although defects in argininosuccinic acid synthetase (citrullinemia) and argininosuccinic acid lyase (argininosuccinic acidemia) may also present with severe hyperammonemia in infancy, a chronic course with mental retardation is more usual in these conditions.

Except for OTC deficiency, which is X-linked, urea cycle disorders are inherited as autosomal recessive traits. Citrullinemia and argininosuccinic acidemia can be diagnosed in utero by appropriate enzyme assays on cultured amniotic cells or material obtained from chorionic villus sampling, but CPS and OTC deficiency states can be diagnosed in utero only by using specific gene probes, and then only in certain families.

Diagnosis

Blood ammonia levels should be measured in any newborn who is acutely ill without obvious cause. A urea cycle defect should be suspected when severe hyperammonemia is associated with respiratory alkalosis. Serum citrulline is low or undetectable in CPS and OTC deficiency, high in argininosuccinic acidemia, and very high in citrullinemia. Large amounts of argininosuccinic acid are found in the urine of patients with argininosuccinic acidemia. Urine orotic acid is increased in infants with OTC deficiency, and there may also be a family history of male newborn deaths that appear to be transmitted as an X-linked trait.

Many female carriers of OTC deficiency show protein intolerance; some develop migrainelike symptoms after protein loads and others develop potentially fatal episodes of vomiting and encephalopathy after ingesting protein or contracting infections. Trichorrhexis nodosa is common in patients with the chronic form of argininosuccinic acidemia.

Treatment

In the newborn, measures to reduce serum ammonia by hemodialysis, peritoneal dialysis, or double-volume exchange transfusion should be instituted as soon as hyperammonemia is documented. Protein intake should be stopped, and glucose should be given to reduce endogenous protein breakdown. Arginine should be given intravenously, both because it is an essential amino acid for patients with urea cycle defects and because it increases the excretion of waste nitrogen in patients with citrullinemia and argininosuccinic acidemia. Sodium benzoate can also be given intravenously; after 2–3 days of therapy, blood ammonia levels usually fall and symptoms lessen.

Long-term treatment includes oral administration of arginine (or citrulline), adherence to a low-protein diet, and administration of sodium benzoate and sodium phenylacetate to increase excretion of nitrogen as hippuric acid and phenylacetylglutamine. Female OTC-deficient heterozygotes who develop hyperammonemia after protein loading should also receive such treatment.

The outcome of argininosuccinic acidemia and citrullinemia is better than that of OTC and CPS deficiency. Most patients with urea cycle defects, no matter what the enzyme defect, develop permanent neurologic and intellectual impairments, with cortical atrophy and ventricular dilatation seen on CT scan. The prognosis may be improved if the initial hyperammonemic episode is rapidly identified and treated.

Batshaw ML et al: Risk of serious illness in heterozygotes for ornithine transcarbamylase deficiency. *J Pediatr* 1986;**108**:236.

Brusilow SW: Arginine, an indispensable amino acid for patients with inborn errors of urea synthesis. *J Clin Invest* 1984;**74**:2144.

Brusilow SW et al: Treatment of episodic hyperammonemia in children with inborn errors of urea synthesis. *N Engl J Med* 1984;**310**:1630.

Hudak ML, Jones MD, Brusilow SW: Differentiation of transient hyperammonemia of the newborn and urea cycle enzyme defects by clinical presentation. *J Pediatr* 1985;**107**:712.

Msall M et al: Neurologic outcome in children with inborn errors of urea synthesis: Outcome of urea cycle enzymopathies. *N Engl J Med* 1984;**310**:1500.

Qureshi IA et al: Treatment of hyperargininemia with sodium benzoate and arginine-restricted diet. *J Pediatr* 1984;**104**:473.

PHENYLKETONURIA & THE HYPERPHENYLALANINEMIAS

Probably the best known disorder of amino acid metabolism is the classic form of phenylketonuria. It was first recognized in 1934 by Følling in several retarded children who excreted phenylpyruvic acid in the urine. The disorder is due to decreased activity of phenylalanine hydroxylase, the enzyme that converts phenylalanine to tyrosine. Phenylketonuria is inherited as an autosomal recessive trait, with a frequency in Caucasians of approximately 1 in 10,000 live births. On normal phenylalanine intake, affected patients develop hyperphenylalaninemia and produce and excrete phenylpyruvic, phenyllactic, phenylacetic, and 2-hydroxyphenylacetic acid. The untreated patient shows severe mental retardation, hyperactivity, seizures, a light complexion, and eczema. The patient's urine has a "mouselike" odor.

Clinicians had early success preventing severe mental retardation in phenylketonuric children by restricting phenylalanine from the diet starting in early infancy. This success led to the development of screening programs to detect the disease early. Since the outcome is best when treatment is begun in the first month of life, infants are usually screened during the first few days of life. A second test is necessary only when newborn screening is done before 24 hours of age, and in such cases the second test should be completed by the third week of life. Infants receiving hyperalimentation and premature infants should be screened at or near 7 days, and rescreened if they were transfused or not fed at the time of the initial test.

Enzymes involved with the interconversion of phenylalanine and tyrosine, and whose deficiencies can produce hyperphenylalaninemia, are shown in Fig 33–1. In classic phenylketonuria, there is little or no phenylalanine hydroxylase activity, but in the less severe hyperphenylalaninemias there is significant residual activity. Rare variants can be due to deficiency of dihydrobiopterin reductase or to defects in biopterin synthesis. All are inherited as autosomal recessive traits.

Prenatal diagnosis of PKU is often possible using DNA probes. Molecular approaches are replacing serum measurements of phenylalanine and tyrosine to determine carrier status. Prenatal diagnosis of defects in pterin metabolism can often be made by enzyme assay of amniocytes or by examination of pterin metabolites in amniotic fluid.

Diagnosis

The diagnosis of PKU in a severely retarded older child with typical biochemical and physical characteristics is straightforward, but in the newborn period, especially when there is no family history, the condition must be differentiated from other forms of hyperphenylalaninemia. This is done by determining serum phenylalanine and tyrosine levels on a normal diet, and by examining pterins and metabolites of phenylalanine in urine. Oral phenylalanine loads and liver biopsy are almost never necessary.

A. Classic Phenylketonuria: Findings include persistently elevated serum levels of phenylalanine (> 20 mg/dL on a regular diet), normal or low serum levels of tyrosine, urinary excretion of phenylpyruvic and 2-hydroxyphenylacetic acids, and normal pterins. Poor phenylalanine tolerance persists throughout life, and serum tyrosine levels do not rise after a phenylalanine load. Restriction of dietary phenylalanine intake is indicated to lower serum phenylalanine, and a favorable outcome is the rule.

B. Persistent Hyperphenylalaninemia: In infants receiving a normal protein intake, serum phenylalanine levels are usually 4–20 mg/dL. The serum tyrosine level rises after a phenylalanine load, urine pterins are normal, and phenylketones are either not excreted or excreted only transiently. Phenylalanine restriction may or may not be indicated, depending on the phenylalanine tolerance.

C. Transient Hyperphenylalaninemia: Serum phenylalanine levels are elevated early but progressively decline toward normal. If required at all, dietary restriction is only temporary.

D. Dihydropteridine Reductase Deficiency: Serum phenylalanine levels vary but may be in the range seen in hyperphenylalaninemia, and serum tyrosine is normal. Urine pterins are normal in amount, but the pattern of metabolites is abnormal. Seizures and psychomotor regression occur even with diet therapy, probably because the enzyme defect also causes neuronal deficiency of serotonin and dopamine. These deficiencies require treatment with levodopa, carbidopa, and 5-hydroxytryptophan, and possibly also with tetrahydrobiopterin.

E. Defects in Biopterin Biosynthesis: Serum phenylalanine levels vary but may be in the range seen in hyperphenylalaninemia, and serum tyrosine is normal. Total pterins in urine are low, and their pattern may suggest the specific defect, which can be at several steps in the biosynthetic pathway. Clinical findings include myoclonus, tetraplegia, and other movement disorders. Treatment is the same as for dihydropteridine reductase deficiency, but in general is not as effective.

F. Tyrosinemia of the Newborn: Serum phenylalanine levels are lower than those seen in PKU and

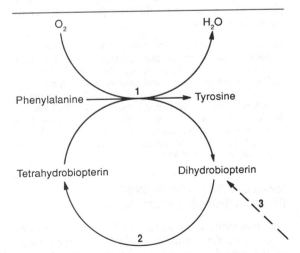

Figure 33–1. Oxidation of phenylalanine to tyrosine. 1. Phenylalanine hydroxylase. 2. Dihydropteridine reductase. 3. Enzymes of biopterin biosynthesis.

are accompanied by marked hypertyrosinemia. This usually occurs in premature infants and is due to immaturity of 4-hydroxyphenylpyruvic acid oxidase. The condition resolves spontaneously within 3 months, almost always without sequelae. If necessary, intramuscular injection of 100 mg ascorbic acid will normalize serum tyrosine (and phenylalanine) within 48 hours.

G. Maternal Phenylketonuria: Heterozygous offspring of phenylketonuric mothers have transient hyperphenylaninemia at birth; in such cases diagnosis is made by determining the serum phenylalanine level of the mother. Nearly all such offspring are mentally retarded, most are microcephalic, and many are small and have congenital heart disease or other malformations. The risk to the fetus is considerably lessened if phenylalanine restriction is begun before conception and maintained throughout pregnancy.

Treatment

Treatment of classic PKU is to limit dietary phenylalanine intake to amounts that permit normal growth and development without marked hyperphenylaninemia, and this can be done with several low-phenylalanine milk substitutes. Serum phenylalanine concentrations must be monitored frequently, while ensuring that growth, development, and nutrition are adequate. This monitoring is best done in clinics experienced in dealing with such problems. Although dietary treatment is most effective when initiated during the first months of life, it may also be of benefit in reversing behaviors such as hyperactivity, irritability, and distractibility when started later in life.

It is now generally accepted that phenylalanine restriction should continue throughout life. Females with phenylketonuria merit special attention during the childbearing years. Counseling should be given during adolescence, and the woman's diet should be closely monitored prior to conception and throughout pregnancy.

Children with classic PKU who are treated promptly after birth and achieve phenylalanine and tyrosine homeostasis will develop well physically and can be expected to have normal or nearly normal intellectual development.

Committee on Genetics, American Academy of Pediatrics: New issues in newborn screening for phenylketonuria and congenital hypothyroidism. *Pediatrics* 1982; **69**:104.

DiLella AG, Huang WM, Woo SLC: Screening for phenylketonuria mutations by DNA amplification with the polymerase chain reaction. *Lancet* 1988;**1**:497.

Niederwieser A, Ponzone A, Curtius H-Ch: Differential diagnosis of tetrahydrobiopterin deficiency. *J Inherited Metab Dis* 1985;**8(Suppl 1)**:34.

Niederwieser A et al: Prenatal diagnosis of "dihydrobiopterin synthetase" deficiency, a variant form of phenylketonuria. *Eur J Pediatr* 1986;**145**:176.

Soeters RP et al: Maternal phenylketonuria: Comparison of two treated full term pregnancies. *Eur J Pediatr* 1986;**145**:221.

Williamson ML et al: Correlates of intelligence test results in treated phenylketonuric children. *Pediatrics* 1981; **68**:161.

HEREDITARY TYROSINEMIA

Hereditary tyrosinemia is caused by deficiency of fumarylacetoacetase and is characterized by progressive hepatic parenchymal damage, renal tubular dystrophy with generalized aminoaciduria and hypophosphatemic rickets, hypermethioninemia, and tyrosine metabolites, succinylacetone, and δ-aminolevulinic acid in the urine. The course may be rapidly fatal in infancy or somewhat more chronic.

The condition is inherited as an autosomal recessive trait and is especially common in Scandinavia and in the Chicoutimi-Lac St Jean region of Quebec. Prenatal diagnosis can be established by demonstrating deficiency of fumarylacetoacetase in cultured amniocytes or increased concentrations of succinylacetone in amniotic fluid.

Diagnosis

Similar clinical and biochemical findings may occur in galactosemia and hereditary fructose intolerance, but increased succinylacetone occurs only in fumarylacetoacetase deficiency, and diagnosis is based on demonstrating this compound in urine. This may be done by gas chromatography-mass spectrometry or by demonstration that a urine extract can inhibit δ-aminolevulinic acid synthetase activity.

Treatment

A diet low in phenylalanine and tyrosine (50 mg each/kg/d) is indicated but not usually successful in preventing or reversing liver disease, and liver transplantation appears to be the only promising therapy for these children.

Berger R et al: Type I tyrosinemia: Lack of immunologically detectable fumarylacetoacetase enzyme protein in tissues and cell extracts. *Pediatr Res* 1987;**22**:394.

Kvittingen EA et al: Prenatal diagnosis of hereditary tyrosinemia by determination of fumarylacetoacetase in cultured amniotic fluid cells. *Pediatr Res* 1985;**19**:334.

Tuchman M et al: Contribution of extrahepatic tissues to biochemical abnormalities in hereditary tyrosinemia type 1: Study of three patients after liver transplantation. *J Pediatr* 1987;**110**:399.

MAPLE SYRUP URINE DISEASE
(Branched-Chain Ketoaciduria)

Maple syrup urine disease is due to deficiency of the enzyme that catalyzes oxidative decarboxylation of the branched-chain ketoacid derivatives of leucine, isoleucine, and valine. The accumulated ketoacids of leucine and isoleucine cause the characteristic odor, while only the ketoacid of leucine has been implicated in causing central nervous system dysfunction. Many variants of this disorder have been described, including mild, intermittent, and thiamine-dependent forms, and all are inherited as autosomal recessive traits. Fetal diagnosis of the disease is possible by demonstrating decreased branched-chain ketoacid dehydrogenase activity in cultured amniotic cells.

Patients with classical maple syrup urine disease are normal at birth but soon develop the characteristic odor, lethargy, feeding difficulties, coma, and seizures. Unless diagnosis is made and dietary restriction of branched-chain amino acids is begun, most will die in the first month of life, but normal growth and development can be achieved if treatment is begun before about 10 days of age. The requirement for early diagnosis has made this disorder one of those screened for in the newborn period.

Diagnosis

Marked elevations of branched-chain amino acids, including alloisoleucine, in serum and urine are characteristic. Alloisoleucine, a transamination product of the ketoacid of isoleucine, is almost pathognomonic. Branched-chain α-keto- and hydroxyacids are also present in the urine. The magnitude and consistency of amino and organic acid changes are altered in mild and intermittent forms of the disease.

Treatment

Products deficient in branched-chain amino acids but in other respects identical to milk are commercially available but must be supplemented with normal milk and other foods to supply enough branched-chain amino acids to permit normal growth and development. Serum levels of branched-chain amino acids must be monitored frequently, even at 1–2 day intervals in the first months of life, to cope with changing protein requirements.

Acosta PB et al: **Dietary Management of Inherited Metabolic Diseases.** Department of Pediatrics, Emory University School of Medicine, 1976.

Clow CL et al: Outcome of early and long-term management of classical maple syrup urine disease. *Pediatrics* 1981;**68:**856.

Hammersen G et al: Maple syrup urine disease: Treatment of the acutely ill newborn. *Eur J Pediatr* 1978;**129:**157.

HOMOCYSTINURIA

Homocystinuria is most often due to deficiency of cystathionine synthase, but it may also be due to deficiency of methylenetetrahydrofolate reductase or to defects in the biosynthesis of methyl-B_{12}, which is the coenzyme for N^5-methyltetrahydrofolate methyltransferase. All known inherited forms of homocystinuria are transmitted as autosomal recessive traits

and can be diagnosed in the fetus by assaying appropriate enzymes in cultured amniotic cells.

About half of untreated patients with cystathionine synthase deficiency are retarded, and most have arachnodactyly, osteoporosis, and a tendency to develop dislocated lenses and thromboembolic phenomena. Patients with remethylation defects usually show failure to thrive and a variety of neurologic symptoms, including microcephaly and seizures in infancy and early childhood.

Diagnosis

Diagnosis is made by demonstrating homocystinuria in a patient who is not severely deficient in vitamin B_{12}. Serum methionine levels are usually high in patients with cystathionine synthase deficiency and often low in patients with remethylation defects. When the remethylation defect is due to deficiency of methyl-B_{12}, megaloblastic anemia may be present, and an associated deficiency of adenosyl-B_{12} may cause methylmalonic aciduria. Studies of cultured fibroblasts may be necessary to make a specific diagnosis.

Treatment

About 50% of patients with cystathionine synthase deficiency respond to large doses, eg 250 mg/d, of pyridoxine administered orally. Early treatment of pyridoxine nonresponders by dietary methionine restriction may prevent mental retardation and delay lens dislocations, perhaps justifying screening of newborn infants for the condition. Oral administration of betaine (250 mg/kg/d) will increase methylation of homocystine to methionine in patients with remethylation defects and may also improve neurologic function. Large doses of cobalamin, eg 1 mg hydroxy-B_{12} administered intramuscularly every other day, are indicated in some patients.

Bartholomew DW et al: Therapeutic approaches to cobalamin-C methylmalonic acidemia and homocystinuria. *J Pediatr* 1988;**112:**32.

Mitchell GA et al: Clinical heterogeneity in cobalamin C variant of combined homocystinuria and methylmalonic aciduria. *J Pediatr* 1986;**108:**410.

Mudd SH et al: The natural history of homocystinuria due to cystathionine β-synthase deficiency. *Am J Hum Genet* 1985;**37:**1.

Rosenblatt DS et al: Vitamin B_{12} responsive homocystinuria and megaloblastic anemia: Heterogeneity in methylcobalamin deficiency. *Am J Med Genet* 1987;**26:**377.

NONKETOTIC HYPERGLYCINEMIA

Inherited deficiency of various subunits of the glycine cleavage enzyme causes nonketotic hyperglycinemia. In its most severe form, also termed **glycine encephalopathy,** the condition presents in the newborn period with unremitting seizures, hypotonia, hiccups, a burst suppression pattern on EEG, and (usually) death in infancy. Forms that present with seizures later in infancy or with developmental delay in childhood are less common. All forms of the condition are inherited as autosomal recessive traits.

Diagnosis

This deficiency should be suspected in any infant with intractable seizures, especially when hiccupping, and is confirmed by demonstrating a large increase in glycine in cerebrospinal fluid (CSF), with the CSF:serum glycine ratio being abnormally high. Demonstrating the specific enzyme defect by liver biopsy is necessary only if the couple is contemplating having more children, and prenatal diagnosis is possible only by assaying the enzyme in chorionic villus.

Treatment

Treatment is generally unsuccessful, although large doses of diazepam may be necessary to control seizures in some patients.

Hayasaka K et al: Nonketotic hyperglycinemia: Analyses of glycine cleavage system in typical and atypical cases. *J Pediatr* 1987;**110**:873.

Perry TL et al: Non-ketotic hyperglycinemia. *N Engl J Med* 1975;**292**:1269.

Tada K, Hayasaka K: Non-ketotic hyperglycinaemia: Clinical and biochemical aspects. *Eur J Pediatr* 1987;**146**:221.

ORGANIC ACIDEMIAS

Organic acidemias are disorders of amino (and fatty) acid metabolism in which nonamino organic acids accumulate in serum and urine. These conditions are usually diagnosed by examining organic acids in urine, a complex procedure that requires considerable interpretive expertise and is usually performed only in specialized laboratories. Clinical features of organic acidemias are given in Table 33–4, together with the urine organic acid patterns typical of each. Additional details about some of the more important organic acidemias are provided below.

KETOTIC HYPERGLYCINEMIAS (Propionic and Methylmalonic Acidemia)

Idiopathic hyperglycinemia was first reported in 1961 as a syndrome of mental retardation and episodic ketoacidosis, neutropenia, thrombocytopenia, osteoporosis, and hyperglycinemia induced by pro-

tein intake or infection. It was then renamed ketotic hyperglycinemia to distinguish it from nonketotic hyperglycinemia, described above. It is now known that the syndrome is almost always due to propionic or methylmalonic acidemia.

The oxidation of threonine, valine, isoleucine, and methionine through propionyl- and L-methylmalonyl-CoA is shown in Fig 33–2. Propionic acidemia is due to a defect in the biotin-containing enzyme propionyl-CoA carboxylase, and methylmalonic acidemia is due to a defect in methylmalonyl-CoA mutase. In most cases the latter is due to a defect in the mutase apoenzyme, but in others it is due to a defect in the biosynthesis of its adenosyl-B_{12} coenzyme. In some of these defects only the synthesis of adenosyl-B_{12} is blocked; in others, the synthesis of methyl-B_{12} is also blocked.

Clinical symptoms in propionic and methylmalonic acidemia vary according to the location and severity of the enzyme block. Those with severe blocks present with acute, life-threatening metabolic acidemia and hyperammonemia early in infancy or with metabolic acidemia, vomiting, and failure to thrive during the first few months of life. Children with less severe blocks may show only mild or moderate mental retardation.

All known forms of propionic and methylmalonic acidemia are transmitted as autosomal recessive traits and can be diagnosed in utero by performing appropriate enzyme assays of cultured amniotic fluid cells or by demonstrating characteristic abnormalities of organic acids in amniotic fluid.

Diagnosis

Laboratory findings include hyperglycinemia and hyperglycinuria, a positive methylmalonic aciduria screening test, the presence of diagnostic changes on urine organic acid chromatography (Table 33–4) and, in certain blocks of B_{12} metabolism, hypomethioninemic homocystinuria.

Treatment

Patients with enzyme blocks in B_{12} metabolism usually respond to massive (1 mg/d) doses of vitamin B_{12}, given orally or intramuscularly, whereas nonresponders require protein restriction and correction of their rather constant metabolic acidemia. Secondary carnitine deficiency has been reported, and blood carnitine should be measured and supplemented if required.

Matsui SM et al: The natural history of the inherited methylmalonic acidemias. *N Engl J Med* 1983;**308**:857.

Packman S et al: Severe hyperammonemia in a newborn infant with methylmalonyl-CoA-mutase deficiency. *J Pediatr* 1978;**92**:769.

Shinnar S, Singer HS: Cobalamin C mutation (methylmalonic aciduria and homocystinuria) in adolescence: A treatable cause of dementia and myelopathy. *N Engl J Med* 1984;**311**:451.

Table 33–4. Clinical and laboratory features of organic acidemias.

Disorder	Enzyme Defect	Clinical and Laboratory Features
Isovaleric acidemia	Isovaleryl-CoA dehydrogenase	Acidosis and "odor of sweaty feet" in infancy, or growth retardation and episodes of vomiting, lethargy, acidosis, and odor. Isovalerylglycine always present in urine, with 3-hydroxy-isovaleric acid during acute episodes.
3-methylcrotonyl-CoA carboxylase deficiency	3-methylcrotonyl-CoA carboxylase	Acidosis and feeding problems in infancy, or Reye-like episodes in older child. 3-Methylcrotonylglycine in urine, usually with 3-hydroxyisovaleric acid.
Combined carboxylase deficiency	Holocarboxylase synthetase	Hypotonia and lactic acidosis in infancy. 3-Hydroxyisovaleric acid in urine, often with small amounts of 3-hydroxypropionic and methylcitric acids. Often biotin responsive.
	Biotinidase	Alopecia, seborrheic rash, and ataxia in infancy or childhood. Urine organic acids as above. Usually biotin responsive.
3-hydroxy-3-methylglutaric acidemia	Hydroxymethylglutaryl-CoA lyase	Hypoglycemia and acidosis in infancy; Reye-like episodes with nonketotic hypoglycemia in older children. 3-Hydroxy-3-methyl-glutaric, 3-methylglutaconic, and 3-hydroxyisovaleric acids in urine.
3-ketothiolase deficiency	3-ketothiolase	Ketotic hyperglycinemia syndrome in infancy, or developmental and growth retardation with episodes of vomiting, acidosis, and encephalopathy. 2-Methyl-3-hydroxybutyric and 2-methylacetoacetic acids and tiglylglycine in urine, especially after isoleucine load.
Propionic acidemia	Propionyl-CoA carboxylase	Hyperammonemia and metabolic acidosis in infancy; ketotic hyperglycinemia syndrome later. 3-Hydroxypropionic and methylcitric acids in urine, with 3-hydroxy- and 3-ketovaleric during ketotic episodes.
Methylmalonic acidemia	Methylmalonyl-CoA mutase Defects in B_{12} biosynthesis	Clinical features same as propionic acidemia. Methylmalonic acid in urine, often with 3-hydroxypropionic and methylcitric acids. Clinical features same as above when only adenosyl-B_{12} synthesis is decreased; early neurological features prominent when accompanied by decreased synthesis of methyl-B_{12}. In latter instance, hypomethioninemia and homocystinuria accompany methylmalonic aciduria.
Pyroglutamic acidemia	Glutathione synthetase	Acidosis and hemolytic anemia in infancy; chronic acidosis later. Pyroglutamic acid in urine.
Glutaric acidemia type I	Glutaryl-CoA dehydrogenase	Progressive extrapyramidal movement disorder in childhood, with episodes of acidosis, vomiting and encephalopathy. Glutaric acid in urine, usually with 3-hydroxyglutaric acid.
Glutaric acidemia type II	Electron transfer flavoprotein (ETF) ETF:ubiquinone oxidoreductase (ETF dehydrogenase)	Hypoglycemia, acidosis, hyperammonemia and "smell of sweaty feet" in infancy, often with polycystic and dysplastic kidneys. Later onset may be with episodes of hypoketotic hypoglycemia, or slowly progressive skeletal myopathy. Glutaric, ethylmalonic, 3-hydroxy-isovaleric, isovalerylglycine, and 2-hydroxyglutaric acids in urine, often with sarcosine in serum and urine.
4-hydroxybutyric acidemia	Succinic semialdehyde dehydrogenase	Seizures and developmental retardation. 4-hydroxybutyric acid in urine.

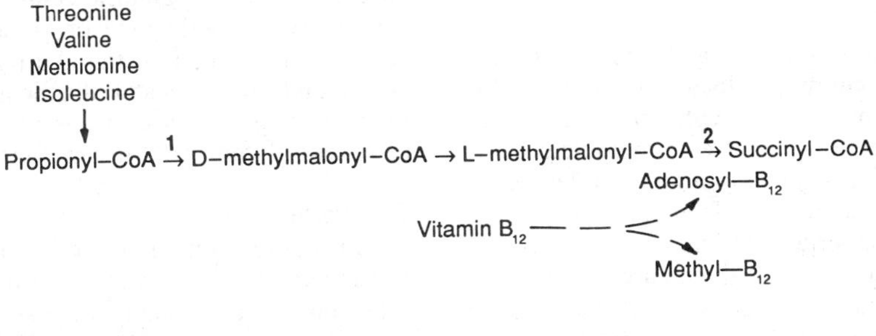

Threonine
Valine
Methionine
Isoleucine
↓
Propionyl–CoA $\xrightarrow{1}$ D–methylmalonyl–CoA → L–methylmalonyl–CoA $\xrightarrow{2}$ Succinyl–CoA

Adenosyl—B_{12}

Vitamin B_{12} — — $<$

Methyl—B_{12}

Figure 33–2. Oxidation of propionyl-CoA to succinyl-CoA. 1. Propionyl-CoA carboxylase. 2. Methylmalonyl-CoA mutase.

ISOVALERIC ACIDEMIA

This condition, due to deficiency of isovaleryl-CoA dehydrogenase in the leucine oxidative pathway, was the first organic acidemia to be described in humans. It usually presents with poor feeding, metabolic acidosis, seizures, and an odor of "sweaty feet" during the first few days of life, with coma and death occurring if the condition is not recognized and appropriate therapy quickly begun. Other patients show a more chronic course, with episodes of vomiting, lethargy, and urine (and body) odor precipitated by intercurrent infections or increased protein intake. Therapy by dietary means of by providing glycine is very effective. The condition is inherited as an autosomal recessive trait, and fetal disease can be diagnosed by demonstrating enzyme deficiency in cultured amniotic cells or the presence of isovalerylglycine in urine.

Diagnosis

Isovaleric acidemia and glutaric acidemia type II are the only conditions in which the characteristic odor of "sweaty feet" occurs. Isovalerylglycine is consistently detected in the urine by organic acid chromatography. During infections or following the intake of large amounts of protein, 3-hydroxy-isovaleric acid is also detected.

Treatment

Providing a low-protein diet or diets low in leucine or all three branched-chain amino acids is quite effective. Oral administration of glycine (250 mg/kg/d) appears to prevent complications during acute infections, but poses the risk of neurotoxicity due to severe hyperglycinemia. Oral administration of L-carnitine (40 mg/kg/d) may also be indicated.

Cohn RM et al: Isovaleric acidemia: Use of glycine therapy in neonates. *N Engl J Med* 1978;**299**:996.
de Sousa C et al: The response to L-carnitine and glycine therapy in isovaleric acidaemia. *Eur J Pediatr* 1986; **144**:451.

COMBINED CARBOXYLASE DEFICIENCY

Holocarboxylase synthetase and biotinidase are two enzymes of biotin metabolism in mammals. Holocarboxylase synthetase covalently binds biotin to the apocarboxylases for pyruvate, 3-methylcrotonyl-CoA and propionyl-CoA; and biotinidase releases biotin from these proteins and from proteins in the diet. Recessively inherited deficiency of either enzyme causes deficiency of all three carboxylases, ie, multiple carboxylase deficiency. Holocarboxylase synthetase deficiency usually presents in the neonatal period with hypotonia, and biotinidase deficiency more often presents somewhat later with a syndrome of ataxia, seborrhea, and alopecia. Because many patients with biotinidase deficiency do not show typical symptoms but do develop neurologic sequelae, newborn screening for the condition may be justified.

Diagnosis

This diagnosis should be excluded in patients with typical symptoms or in those with primary lactic acidosis. Urine organic acids are usually, but not always, abnormal (Table 33–4). Diagnosis is usually by enzyme assay. Biotinidase can be assayed in serum; holocarboxylase synthetase, in leukocytes or fibroblasts.

Treatment

Oral administration of biotin in large doses, 10–20 mg/d, often reverses the organic aciduria within days and the clinical symptoms within days to weeks. Incidence of hearing loss is high, even in treated patients.

Burri BJ, Sweetman L, Nyhan WL: Heterogeneity of holocarboxylase synthetase in patients with biotin-responsive multiple carboxylase deficiency. *Am J Hum Genet* 1985;**37**:326.
Wolf B et al: Clinical findings in four children with biotinidase deficiency detected through a statewide neonatal screening program. *N Engl J Med* 1985;**313**:16.

GLUTARIC ACIDEMIA TYPE I

Glutaric acidemia type I is due to deficiency of glutaryl-CoA dehydrogenase and causes a progressive extrapyramidal movement disorder in childhood, with dystonia and athetosis and neuronal degeneration in the caudate and putamen. Death usually occurs during the first decade of life. The condition is inherited as an autosomal recessive trait.

Diagnosis

Glutaric acidemia type I should be suspected in any patient with progressive dystonia or athetosis. The diagnosis is confirmed by demonstration of glutaric and 3-hydroxyglutaric acids in urine by organic acid analysis. Deficiency of glutaryl-CoA dehydrogenase can be demonstrated in fibroblasts, leukocytes, and, for prenatal diagnosis, amniotic cells. Prenatal diagnosis is also possible by demonstrating increased glutaric acid in amniotic fluid.

Treatment

Oral administration of riboflavin (100 mg/d) and restriction of dietary lysine and tryptophan are indicated but do not usually reverse or prevent neurologic deterioration. It is not yet known if valproic acid or lioresal have a place in treatment.

Amir N et al: Glutaric aciduria type I: Clinical heterogeneity and neuroradiologic features. *Neurology* 1987; **37**:1654.

Goodman SI, Frerman FE: Organic acidemias due to defects in lysine oxidation: 2-ketoadipic acidemia and glutaric acidemia. In: *The Metabolic Basis of Inherited Disease*, 6th ed. Scriver CR, Beaudet AL, Sly WS, Valle D (editors). McGraw-Hill, 1989.

Lipkin PH et al: A case of glutaric acidemia type I: Effect of riboflavin and carnitine. *J Pediatr* 1988;**112**:62.

DISORDERS OF FATTY ACID OXIDATION

LONG-CHAIN AND MEDIUM-CHAIN ACYL-CoA DEHYDROGENASE DEFICIENCIES

Deficiencies of long-chain and medium-chain acyl-CoA dehydrogenase (LCAD and MCAD), two enzymes of fatty acid β-oxidation, usually cause Reye-like episodes of hypoketotic hypoglycemia, mild hyperammonemia, hepatomegaly and encephalopathy, or less often, sudden death in infancy. The two conditions cannot be distinguished clinically, but MCAD deficiency is by far the more common, perhaps occurring in 1 of 5000 live births. Although Reye-like episodes may be fatal, they tend to become less frequent and severe with time, and prolonged survival is not unusual. Cardiomyopathy occurs in both conditions. In LCAD deficiency, cardiomyopathy is the result of the defect in the oxidation of long-chain fatty acids. In MCAD deficiency, cardiomyopathy occurs possibly because the loss of octanoylcarnitine in the urine causes carnitine deficiency, which restricts entry of long-chain fatty acids into mitochondria. Both conditions are inherited as autosomal recessive traits.

Diagnosis

Suspicion should be raised by the lack of an appropriate ketone response to fasting. Patients with MCAD deficiency excrete octanoylcarnitine and several unusual glycine esters in the urine; octanoylcarnitine is excreted only when the patient is not carnitine depleted. Elevated urinary phenylpropionylglycine levels may be a particularly accurate diagnostic indicator. Assays of MCAD (and LCAD) activity in fibroblasts are necessary only when the presence of octanoylcarnitine or phenylpropionylglycine cannot be demonstrated in urine. The finding of normal urine organic acids does not exclude these conditions, since excretion of dicarboxylic acids and other products of microsomal and peroxisomal oxidation of fatty acids can be intermittent.

Treatment

Acute management is directed to treating hypoglycemia, and long-term measures include providing carbohydrate snacks before bedtime and vigorous treatment of intercurrent infections. Because cardiomyopathy and muscle weakness in MCAD deficiency may be due to secondary carnitine deficiency, oral administration of carnitine may be indicated. Medium-chain triglycerides are contraindicated in MCAD deficiency, because they may raise serum octanoic acid to rise to neurotoxic concentrations, but they may be a useful energy source for patients with LCAD deficiency.

Duran M et al: Sudden child death and "healthy" affected family members with medium-chain acyl-coenzyme A dehydrogenase deficiency. *Pediatrics* 1986;**78**:1052.

Hale DE et al: Long-chain acyl coenzyme A dehydrogenase deficiency: An inherited cause of nonketotic hypoglycemia. *Pediatr Res* 1985;**19**:666.

Rinaldo P et al: Medium-chain acyl-CoA dehydrogenase deficiency; diagnosis by stable-isotope dilution measurement of urinary n-hexanoylglycine and 3-phenylpropionylglycine. *N Engl J Med* 1988;**319**:1308.

Roe CR, Coates PM: Acyl-CoA dehydrogenase deficiencies. In: *The Metabolic Basis of Inherited Disease*, 6th ed. Scriver CR, Beaudet AL, Sly WS, Valle D (editors). McGraw-Hill, 1989.

Taubman B, Hale DE, Kelley RI: Familial Reye-like syndrome: A presentation of medium-chain acyl-coenzyme A dehydrogenase deficiency. *Pediatrics* 1987;**79**:382.

GLUTARIC ACIDEMIA TYPE II

Glutaric acidemia type II (multiple acyl-CoA dehydrogenation deficiency) was first described in 1976 in a baby who died at 3 days of age with profound hypoglycemia, metabolic acidosis, and the "smell of sweaty feet." Since that time, many others have been diagnosed. Some have renal cysts and die in early infancy, and others have Reye-like episodes and skeletal muscle weakness beginning in childhood or adolescence. Some patients are deficient in electron transfer flavoprotein (ETF) and others in ETF:ubiquinone oxidoreductase, proteins that transfer electrons from many flavin-containing enzymes of fatty- and amino acid oxidation into the respiratory chain. Both enzyme deficiencies are inherited as autosomal recessive traits, and the infantile form of the disease can be diagnosed in utero by demonstrating increased glutaric acid in the amniotic fluid.

Diagnosis

Diagnosis can be made by demonstrating derivatives of the substrates of mitochondrial flavin-containing dehydrogenases on organic acid analysis of urine (Table 33–4). Tissue assays of ETF and ETF:ubiquinone oxidoreductase are not usually necessary.

Treatment

Dietary measures (carbohydrate feedings before bedtime, provision of bicarbonate, and restriction of fat) are usually not effective, but administration of riboflavin and carnitine has shown promise, usually in older patients.

Frerman FE, Goodman SI. Glutaric acidemia type II and defects of the mitochondrial respiratory chain. In: *The Metabolic Basis of Inherited Disease*, 6th ed. Scriver CR, Beaudet AL, Sly WS, Valle D (editors). McGraw-Hill, 1989.

Jacobs C et al: Prenatal diagnosis of glutaric aciduria type II by direct chemical analysis of dicarboxylic acids in amniotic fluid. *Eur J Pediat* 1984;**141**:153.

Mooy PD et al: Glutaric aciduria type II: Treatment with riboflavine, carnitine and insulin. *Eur J Pediatr* 1984; **143**:92.

DISORDERS OF PURINE METABOLISM

HYPOXANTHINE-GUANINE PHOSPHORIBOSYLTRANSFERASE DEFICIENCY (Lesch-Nyhan Syndrome)

Hypoxanthine-guanine phosphoribosyltransferase (HPRT) is the enzyme that converts the purine bases hypoxanthine and guanine to inosine monophosphate (IMP) and guanosine monophosphate (GMP), respectively. The X-linked recessive disorder due to its complete deficiency is characterized by central nervous system dysfunction and purine overproduction with hyperuricemia and hyperuricuria. Depending on the residual activity of the mutant enzyme, male hemizygotes may be severely retarded and show choreoathetosis, spasticity, and compulsive, mutilating lip and finger biting, or they may present with only gouty arthritis and urate ureterolithiasis. The enzyme deficiency can be demonstrated in erythrocytes, fibroblasts, and cultured amniotic cells; this disorder can thus be diagnosed with certainty in utero.

Although the cause of the central nervous system dysfunction in Lesch-Nyhan syndrome remains obscure, the absent or less severe central nervous system manifestations of purine nucleoside phosphorylase deficiency (in which HPRT is functionally inactive because of lack of substrate) suggest that the problem relates to accumulation of substrate behind the block.

Diagnosis

Diagnosis is made by demonstrating elevated uric acid:creatinine ratio in urine, followed by demonstration of enzyme deficiency in red blood cells.

Treatment

Allopurinol and probenecid may be given to reduce hyperuricemia but do not affect neurologic status. Insertions of the HPRT gene into cultured cells from affected patients and into experimental animals have been effective and offer promise as models for human gene therapy in the future.

Silverman LJ, Kelley WN, Palella TD: Genetic analysis of human hypoxanthine-guanine phosphoribosyltransferase deficiency. *Enzyme* 1987;**38**:36.

LYSOSOMAL DISEASES

Lysosomes are cellular organelles in which complex macromolecules are degraded by specific acid hydrolases. Deficiency of a lysosomal enzyme causes its substrate to accumulate in lysosomes of tissues that degrade it, creating a characteristic clinical picture. These so-called storage disorders are classified as mucopolysaccharidoses, lipidoses, or mucolipidoses, depending on the nature of the stored material. Two additional disorders, cystinosis and Salla disease, are caused by defects in lysosomal proteins that normally transport material from the lysosome to the cytoplasm.

Clinical and laboratory features of these conditions are shown in Table 33–5. Most are inherited as autosomal recessive traits, and all can be diagnosed in utero by enzyme assays of cultured amniotic cells.

The diagnosis of mucopolysaccharidosis is suggested by certain clinical and radiologic findings and confirmed by urine screening tests. Further tests are needed to determine which particular mucopolysaccharide(s) are present. Diagnosis should be confirmed by enzyme assays of cultured fibroblasts or leukocytes; this is especially important when the parents are contemplating having more children.

When a lipidosis or mucolipidosis is suspected, diagnosis is made by appropriate enzyme assays of biopsy specimens, cultured skin fibroblasts, and peripheral leukocytes.

Most of these conditions cannot be treated effectively, although there is increasing evidence that bone marrow transplantation may affect the course of some lysosomal diseases.

Beaudet A: Gaucher's disease. *N Engl J Med* 1987; **316**:619.

Muenzer J: Mucopolysaccharidoses. *Acta Pediatr* 1986; **33**:269.

Table 33–5. Clinical and laboratory features of lysosomal storage diseases.

Disorder	Enzyme Defect	Clinical and Laboratory Features
I. Mucopolysaccharidoses		
Hurler syndrome	α-iduronidase	Autosomal recessive. Mental retardation, hepatosplenomegaly, umbilical hernia, coarse facies, corneal clouding, dorsolumbar gibbus, severe heart disease. Heparan sulfate and dermatan sulfate in urine.
Scheie syndrome	α-iduronidase (incomplete)	Autosomal recessive. Corneal clouding, stiff joints, normal intellect. Clinical types intermediate between Hurler and Scheie common. Heparan sulfate and dermatan sulfate in urine.
Hunter syndrome	Sulfoiduronate sulfatase	X-linked recessive. Coarse facies, hepatosplenomegaly, mental retardation variable. Corneal clouding and gibbus not present. Heparan sulfate and dermatan sulfate in urine.

Sanfilippo syndrome:
  Type A
  Type B
 	
  Type C
 	
  Type D
	Sulfamidase
	α-N-acetylglucosaminidase
	Acetyl-CoA: α-glucosaminide-N-acetyltransferase
	α-N-acetylglucosamine-6-sulfatase
		Autosomal recessive. Severe mental retardation with comparatively mild skeletal changes, visceromegaly, and facial coarseness. Types cannot be differentiated clinically. Heparan sulfate in urine.

Morquio syndrome	N-Acetylgalactosamine-6-sulfatase	Autosomal recessive. Severe skeletal changes, platyspondylisis, corneal clouding. Keratan sulfate in urine.
Maroteaux-Lamy syndrome	N-acetylgalactosamine-4-sulfatase	Autosomal recessive. Coarse facies, growth retardation, dorsolumbar gibbus, corneal clouding, hepatosplenomegaly, normal intellect. Dermatan sulfate in urine.
β-Glucuronidase deficiency	β-glucuronidase	Autosomal recessive. Varies from mental retardation, dorsolumbar gibbus, corneal clouding, and hepatosplenomegaly to mild facial coarseness, retardation, and loose joints. Hearing loss common. Dermatan sulfate or heparan sulfate in urine.
II. Mucolipidoses		
Mannosidosis	α-mannosidase	Autosomal recessive. Varies from severe mental retardation, coarse facies, short stature, skeletal changes, and hepatosplenomegaly to mild facial coarseness and loose joints. Hearing loss common. Abnormal oligosaccharides in urine.
Fucosidosis	α-fucosidase	Autosomal recessive. Variable: coarse facies, skeletal changes, hepatosplenomegaly, occasional angiokeratoma corporis diffusum. Abnormal oligosaccharides in urine.
I-cell disease (mucolipidosis II)	N-Acetylglucosaminyl-phosphotransferase	Autosomal recessive; severe and mild forms known. Very short stature, mental retardation, early facial coarsening, clear cornea, stiffness of joints. Increased lysosomal enzymes in serum. Abnormal sialyl oligosaccharides in urine.
Sialidosis	N-acetylneuraminidase (sialidase)	Autosomal recessive. Mental retardation, coarse facies, skeletal dysplasia, myoclonic seizures, cherry-red macular spot. Abnormal sialyl oligosaccharides in urine.
III. Lipidoses		
Niemann-Pick disease	Sphingomyelinase	Autosomal recessive. Acute and chronic forms known. Acute neuronopathic form common in eastern European Jews. Accumulation of sphingomyelin in lysosomes of RE system and CNS. Hepatosplenomegaly, developmental retardation, macular cherry-red spot. Death by 1–4 years.
Metachromatic leukodystrophy	Arylsulfatase A	Autosomal recessive. Late infantile form, with onset at 1–4 years, most common. Accumulation of sulfatide in white matter. Gait disturbances (ataxia), motor incoordination, and dementia. Death usually in first decade.
Krabbe disease (globoid cell leukodystrophy)	Galactocerebroside β-galactosidase	Autosomal recessive. Globoid cells in white matter. Onset at 3–6 months with seizures, irritability, and retardation. Death by 1–2 years. Juvenile and adult forms are rare.
Fabry disease	α-galactosidase A	X-linked recessive. Storage of trihexosylceramide in endothelial cells. Pain in extremities, angiokeratoma corporis diffusum and (later) poor vision, hypertension, and renal failure.

Table 33–5 (cont'd.). Clinical and laboratory features of lysosomal storage diseases.

Farber disease	Ceramidase	Autosomal recessive. Storage of ceramide in tissues. Subcutaneous nodules, arthropathy with deformed and painful joints, and poor growth and development. Death within first year.
Gaucher disease	Glucocerebroside β-glucosidase	Autosomal recessive. Acute neuronopathic form: Accumulation of glucocerebroside in lysosomes of RE system and CNS. Retardation, hepatosplenomegaly, macular cherry-red spot, and Gaucher's cells in bone marrow. Death by 1–2 years. Chronic form common in eastern European Jews. Accumulation of spingomyelin in lysosomes of RE system. Hepatosplenomegaly and flask-shaped osteolytic bone lesions. Consistent with normal life expectancy.
GM₁ gangliosidosis	GM₁ ganglioside β-galactosidase	Autosomal recessive. Accumulation of GM₁ ganglioside in lysosomes of RE system and CNS. Infantile form: Abnormalities at birth with dysostosis multiplex, hepatosplenomegaly, macular cherry-red spot, and death by 2 years. Juvenile form: Normal development to 1 year of age, then ataxia, weakness, dementia, and death by 4–5 years. Occasional inferior beaking of vertebral bodies of L1 and L2.
GM₂ gangliosidoses; Tay-Sachs disease Sandhoff disease	β-N-acetylhexos-aminidase A β-N-acetylhexos-aminidases A & B	Autosomal recessive. Tay-Sachs disease common in eastern European Jews; Sandhoff disease is panethnic. Clinical phenotypes are identical, with accumulation of GM₂ ganglioside in lysosomes of CNS. Onset at age 3–6 months, with hypotonia, hyperacusis, retardation, and macular cherry-red spot. Death by 2–3 years. Juvenile and adult onset forms of Tay-Sachs disease are rare.
Wolman disease	Acid lipase	Autosomal recessive. Accumulation of cholesterol esters and triglycerides in lysosomes of reticuloendothelial system. Onset in infancy with gastrointestinal symptoms and hepatosplenomegaly, and death by 3–6 months. Adrenals commonly enlarged and calcified.

Spranger J: Inborn errors of complex carbohydrate metabolism. *Am J Med Genet* 1987;**28**:489.

von Figura K et al: Mutations affecting transport and stability of lysosomal enzymes. *Enzyme* 1987;**38**:144.

Whitley CB et al: Bone marrow transplantation for Hurler syndrome: Assessment of metabolic correction. *Birth Defects* 1986;**22**:7.

PEROXISOMAL DISEASES

Peroxisomes are intracellular organelles that contain a large number of enzymes, many of which are oxidases linked to catalase or peroxidase. Among the enzyme systems in peroxisomes is one for β-oxidation of very long chain fatty acids (which is analagous in many ways to the system for fatty acid oxidation in mitochondria) and another for plasmalogen biosynthesis. In addition, peroxisomes contain oxidases for D-and L-amino acids, pipecolic acid and phytanic acid, and an enzyme (alanine-glyoxylate aminotransferase) that effects transamination of glyoxylate to glycine.

In some peroxisomal diseases, many enzymes are deficient. Zellweger (cerebrohepatorenal) syndrome, the best known among these, is probably due to a defect in organelle assembly. Patients present in infancy with seizures, hypotonia, characteristic facies with a large forehead, and hepatomegaly, and at autopsy show renal cysts and absent peroxisomes. Neonatal adrenoleukodystrophy and hyperpipecolic acidemia are similar conditions, with similar clinical and laboratory findings and multiple enzyme deficiencies in cultured fibroblasts, but peroxisomes are usually detected in tissues.

In other perixosomal diseases, only a single enzyme is deficient. Primary hyperoxaluria (alanine-glyoxalate aminotransferase deficiency), X-linked adrenoleukodystrophy and adrenomyeloneuropathy (very long chain acyl-CoA ligase deficiency), and adult Refsum disease (phytanic acid oxidase deficiency) are disorders due to deficiency of single peroxisomal enzymes.

Except for childhood adrenoleukodystrophy, which is X-linked, all peroxisomal diseases are transmitted as autosomal recessive traits and can be diagnosed in utero by specific enzyme assays or by examining very long chain fatty acids in cultured amniotic cells. There is no treatment for most peroxisomal disorders but diet treatment is being studied in x-linked adrenomyelon europathy.

Diagnosis

The best screening test for Zellweger syndrome, hyperpipecolic acidemia, X-linked adrenoleukodystrophy, neonatal adrenoleukodystrophy, and infantile

Refsum disease is determination of very long chain fatty acids in serum or plasma; these acids are increased in all these conditions. Tissue biopsy may also be required to determine the presence and morphologic characteristics of peroxisomes.

Santos MJ et al: Peroxisomal membrane ghosts in Zellweger syndrome: Aberrant organelle assembly. *Science* 1988;**239**:1536.

Schutgens et al: Peroxisomal disorders: A newly recognized group of genetic diseases. *Eur J Pediatr* 1986; **144**:430.

Singh I, Johnson GH, Brown FR: Peroxisomal disorders: Biochemical and clinical diagnostic considerations. *Am J Dis Child* 1988;**142**:1297.

34

Genetics & Dysmorphology

David K. Manchester, MD, Janet Stewart, MD, & Eva Sujansky, MD

New techniques in molecular biology and biochemistry have changed the way clinicians think about and approach birth defects. Scientific reports appear almost daily that advance the understanding of human genetics and development. Molecular approaches to clinical problems now support "reverse genetics," the characterization of human disorders at the level of the gene before their clinical biochemistry and pathophysiology are described. Worldwide, scientists have united to map the human genome.

The clinical implications of these advances are far too numerous to discuss completely in this text. This chapter reviews human chromosomes and chromosome abnormalities, briefly describes diagnostic and therapeutic applications of recombinant DNA technology, and then outlines clinically important aspects of Mendelian genetics, dysmorphology, and teratology. The chapter concludes with a review of the scope and approach of genetic counseling. The reader is directed to the referenced publications for more comprehensive treatments of the rapidly expanding field of clinical genetics.

I. CHROMOSOMES & CELL DIVISIONS

Human chromosomes consist of deoxyribonucleic acid (DNA) and specific proteins. In a nondividing cell, chromosomes are tightly packaged in the nucleus. Chromosomes contain most of the genetic information necessary for growth and differentiation. Chromosome aberrations lead to physical and mental abnormalities. Documentation of chromosome abnormality is important for appropriate management of the affected child and for assessment of the risk of recurrence; sometimes this risk affects many family members.

Although the correct number of chromosomes was established in 1956, it was not until the early 1980s that newly developed cytogenetic techniques allowed the recognition of the more detailed characteristics of

chromosomes and the identification of a whole array of chromosome abnormalities.

The nuclei of all normal human cells, with the exception of gametes, contain 46 chromosomes, consisting of 23 pairs (Fig 34–1). Of these, 22 pairs are called **autosomes.** They are numbered according to their size; chromosome 1 is the largest, and chromosome 22 is the smallest. In addition, there are 2 **sex chromosomes:** 2 X chromosomes in females and one X and one Y chromosome in males. The 2 members of a chromosome pair are called **homologous chromosomes.** One homologue of each chromosome pair is maternal in origin (from the egg); the second is paternal (from the sperm). The egg and sperm each contain 23 chromosomes (**haploid cells**). During the formation of the zygote, they fuse into a cell with 46 chromosomes (**diploid cell**). The subsequent prenatal and postnatal growth of the human organism is through somatic cell divisions, called mitosis.

Mitosis (Fig 34–2) is a cell division of somatic cells. The process has different stages, during which the DNA replication takes place and 2 daughter cells genetically identical to the original parent cells are formed. During the **metaphase,** the phase after DNA replication but before cell division, individual chromosomes can be visualized. They consist of 2 arms, a short arm and a long arm separated by a centromere. Each arm consists of 2 identical parts, called **chromatids.** Chromatids of the same chromosome are called **sister chromatids.**

Meiosis (Fig 34–3), during which eggs and sperm are formed, is cell division limited to gametes. During meiosis, 3 unique processes take place.

(1) **Crossing over** of genetic material between 2 homologous chromosomes; this is preceded by the pairing of both members of each chromosome pair, thus facilitating the physical exchange of homologous genetic material between them.

(2) **Random assortment** of maternally and paternally derived homologous chromosomes into the daughter cells. The distribution of maternal or paternal chromosomes to a particular daughter cell is independent for each such cell.

(3) Two cell divisions, the first of which is a **reduction division,** ie, a parental cell with 46 chromosomes divides into 2 daughter cells with 23 chromosomes each.

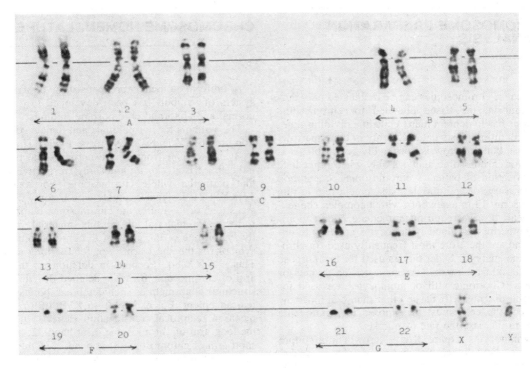

Figure 34–1. Normal male human chromosomes.

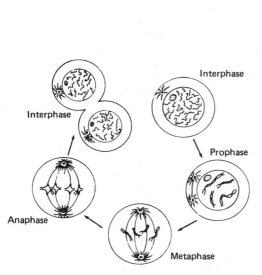

Figure 34–2. Diagram demonstrating the various stages of the mitotic cycle.

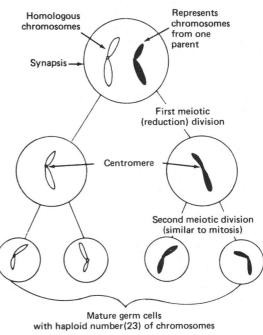

Figure 34–3. Diagram of meiosis, demonstrating the conversion from the diploid somatic cell to the haploid gamete.

CHROMOSOME PREPARATION & ANALYSIS

Because chromosomes can be delineated only during mitosis, the tissue obtained for chromosome analysis has to contain many cells in a dividing state. This condition exists naturally only in bone marrow. Because bone marrow is not readily accessible, it is used for chromosome analysis only when immediate identification of patient's chromosomal constitution is necessary for appropriate management (eg, to rule out trisomy 13 in a newborn with a complex congenital heart disease requiring immediate intervention).

The peripheral blood lymphocytes are easy to obtain and are therefore most frequently used for chromosome analysis. Other tissues used for this purpose include skin or internal organs, such as thymus or gonads. Chorionic villi or amniocytes are used for prenatal diagnosis. If tissue other than bone marrow is used, the cells must be exposed to a mitogenic agent to increase the rate of mitosis.

Lymphocytes require 3 days' growth in a culture medium, and other tissues require 1–2 weeks' growth before enough mitoses are present to allow complete analysis. The chromosome-preparation protocol calls for the processed cells to be placed on a glass slide and stained using new techniques that produce a light-and-dark band pattern across the arms of the chromosomes (see Fig 34–1). This band pattern is characteristic and reproducible for each chromosome, allowing the chromosomes to be arranged in homologous pairs and numeric and structural abnormalities to be identified. The layout of chromosomes on a sheet of paper in a predetermined order is called a **karyotype.**

In addition to the previously described routine chromosome analysis, these specific studies can be requested:

(1) **High-resolution** chromosome analysis of more elongated chromosomes, allowing visualization of more detailed chromosome bands and detection of abnormalities in a smaller segment of chromosome.
(2) **Fragile X** study (see the section on fragile X syndrome, later).
(3) **Assessment of chromosomal breaks and sister chromatid exchanges.** This study requires special techniques that may lead to enhancement of the breaks or special staining that allows visualization of the exchanged chromatids.

CHROMOSOME NOMENCLATURE

A uniform nomenclature consisting of a simple system of symbols has been developed to describe normal and abnormal chromosome findings.

The symbols for normal male and female constitution are 46,XY and 46,XX, respectively. The signs (+) and (−) in front of the chromosome number indicate a trisomy or a monosomy, respectively, for that particular whole chromosome. For example, 47,XY, + 21 designates a male with trisomy 21. The signs (+) or (−) after the chromosome number describe extra material or missing material, respectively, on one of the arms of the chromosome. The symbol for the short arm is p; for the long arm, q. Thus, 46,XX,8q − denotes a deletion on the long arm of chromosome 8. More detailed description of structural abnormalities includes break points in the rearrangement. For example, 46,XY,t(4:8)(q22;p21) means a reciprocal translocation (letter t) between the long arm of chromosome 4, at band 22, and the short arm of chromosome 8, at band 21. Other common symbols include *del* (deletion), *dup* (duplication), and *inv* (inversion).

CHROMOSOME ABNORMALITIES

Errors during cell division may result in numerical or structural abnormalities of chromosomes.

Numerical abnormalities are the result of unequal division, called **nondisjunction,** of chromosomes into the daughter cells. Any deviation from the normal diploid number of chromosomes is called **aneuploidy.** This most frequently involves the presence of an additional chromosome, called **trisomy** (eg, trisomy 21, Down syndrome) (Fig 34–4), or the presence of only a single copy of a chromosome, called **monosomy** (eg, monosomy X, Turner syndrome). Rarely, 3 copies (**triploidy**) of the whole set of 23 chromosomes are found. Four sets of chromosomes (**tetraploidy**) are not found in liveborns.

Structural abnormalities are the result of breaks in chromosomes, which join randomly to form new combinations. In contrast to the numerical abnormalities, which result in a trisomy or a monosomy of a whole chromosome, structural chromosome abnormalities result in a trisomy or a monosomy (or both) of only a part of a chromosome. The number of possible chromosome abnormalities is endless. The following types of chromosome rearrangements, ac-

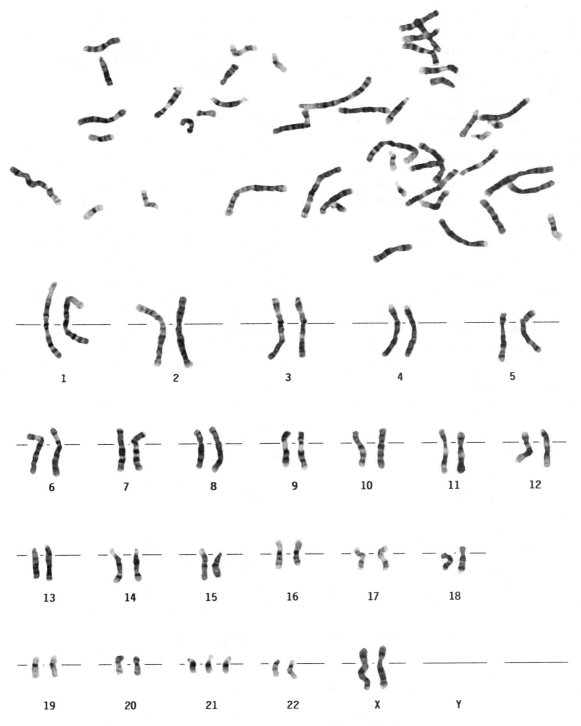

Figure 34–4. Karyotype of trisomy 21.

cording to the mechanism leading to the abnormality, are recognized (Fig 34–5):

(1) **Deletion** is the absence of a part of a chromosome. The deletion is called **terminal** if the distal end of a chromosomal arm is included and **interstitial** if it is not included in the deletion. A terminal deletion of both arms of a chromosome may result in reattachment of the remaining arms, leading to formation of a **ring** chromosome.

(2) **Translocation** is the detachment of a chromosome segment from its normal location and its attachment to another chromosome. The translocation is **balanced** if the cell contains 2 complete copies of all the chromosomal material, although in a different order. In an **unbalanced** translocation, the rearrangement results in partial trisomy or monosomy.

Translocations can be reciprocal or Robertsonian. A **reciprocal** translocation involves exchange of segments between two chromosomes; eg, part of the short arm of chromosome 4 trades place with a part of the long arm of chromosome 10. In **Robertsonian** translocations, 2 acrocentric chromosomes fuse at their centromeres. The most frequent Robertsonian translocation is formed between chromosomes 14 and 21.

(3) **Inversion** is the result of a double break in the same chromosome. The detached middle section turns upside down before reattaching. If both breaks are on the same side of the centromere, the inversion is **paracentric;** if the breaks are on the opposite arms of chromosomes, the inversion is **pericentric.**

MOSAICISM

Mosaicism is the presence of 2 or more different chromosomal constitutions in different cells of the same individual. For example, a patient may have some cells with 47 chromosomes and others with 46 chromosomes; 46,XX/47,XX, + 21 indicates mosaicism for trisomy 21; 45,X/46,XX/47,XXX indicates mosaicism for a monosomy and a trisomy X. Mosaicism should be suspected if clinical symptoms are milder than expected in a nonmosaic patient with the same chromosome abnormality. The prognosis is frequently better for a patient with mosaicism than one with a corresponding chromosome abnormality without mosaicism. In general, the smaller the proportion of the abnormal cell line, the better prognosis. In the same patient, however, the proportion of normal and abnormal cells in various tissues, such as in skin and peripheral blood, may be significantly different. A prognosis frequently cannot be made reliably and should be made with caution or deferred. Mosaicism for structural abnormalities is very rare.

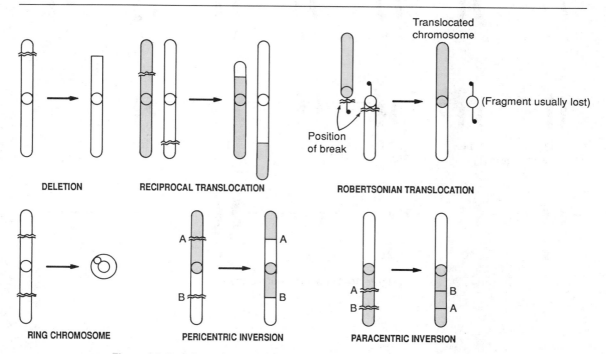

Figure 34–5. Schematic examples of structural chromosome abnormalities.

CLINICAL SIGNIFICANCE OF CHROMOSOME ABNORMALITIES

Chromosome abnormalities result in dysmorphic features, major malformations, developmental delays, or mental retardation. As a rule, abnormalities of autosomes have more severe consequences than abnormalities of sex chromosomes, some of which result only in behavioral problems. Numerical abnormalities resulting in a complete trisomy or monosomy are more deleterious than structural chromosome abnormalities resulting in a duplication or deletion of a chromosome segment. Frequently, the smaller the duplicated or deleted segment, the milder the clinical symptoms. However, comparison of patients with duplications or deletions of different sizes in a particular chromosome indicates that involvement of a small segment sometimes has a disproportionately great effect on mortality and morbidity.

ABNORMALITIES OF AUTOSOMES

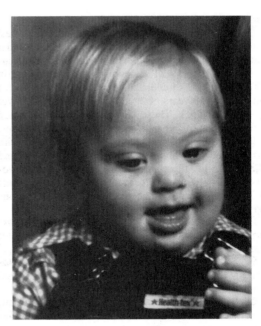

Figure 34–6. Child with Down syndrome.

DOWN SYNDROME

General Considerations

The term *Down syndrome* is preferred to *mongolism,* since the latter is descriptively inaccurate and offensive. The most constant characteristic of the disease is mental retardation. IQs vary between 20 and 80, with the great majority between 45 and 55. Down syndrome occurs in about 1 in 600 newborns; however, the incidence is greater among children of mothers over 35 years of age. The mother's age at the time of conception and the nature of the chromosome abnormality are important in genetic counseling.

Clinical Findings

A. Symptoms and Signs: The principal findings are a small, brachycephalic head; flat nasal bridge; ruddy cheeks; dry lips; large, protruding "scrotal" tongue; small ears; upslanted palpebral fissures that narrow laterally; epicanthic folds; occasionally Brushfield spots; and a short, fleshy neck (Fig 34–6). About one-third of children with Down syndrome have congenital heart disease, most often an endocardial cushion defect or other septal defect. Patients tend to have short, stubby, spadelike hands with transverse palmar simian lines and abnormal dermatoglyphics. Generalized hypotonia is often present, as well as umbilical hernia. The distance between the big toe and second toe is often greater than usual. Sexual development is retarded, especially in males. The affected newborn is prone to have a third fontanelle, prolonged physiologic jaun-

dice, polycythemia, and a transient leukemoid reaction. Cutis marmorata is often present. Later, there is an increased tendency for thyroid dysfunction, hearing loss, and atlanto-occipital instability. Leukemia is 20 times more common than in unaffected children. Susceptibility to intercurrent infections is increased. Patients with Down syndrome display an increased sensitivity to the mydriatic effects of atropine instilled into the conjunctiva.

B. Laboratory Findings: The chromosome abnormalities are pathognomonic. The great majority of cases (95%) have 47 chromosomes with trisomy of 21. However, about 4% of sporadic cases and about one-third of the familial cases have 46 chromosomes, including an abnormal translocated chromosome formed as the result of a centric fusion between 2 acrocentric chromosomes (Robertsonian translocation), one of which is chromosome 21. The translocation is found in 10% of patients whose mothers are younger, whereas in only 3% of those with older mothers.

Mosaicism of the 46/47 type can also occur in persons with Down syndrome. These patients may have milder symptoms, especially higher than expected IQ. Occasionally, normal parents of affected children have unapparent mosaicism.

Only band q22 on the long arm of chromosome 21 need be trisomic for Down syndrome to occur. Some genes located near this band, eg, those for superoxide dismutase, the interferon receptor, and several enzymes involved in the pathway of de novo purine biosynthesis, do not seem to be the cause of Down syndrome.

Prevention

Down syndrome is sporadic in most families; however, the recurrence risk may be increased under certain circumstances. The risk of having a child affected with trisomy 21 varies with maternal age (1 in 2000 for mothers under 25 years of age; 1 in 50 for mothers 35–39 years of age; 1 in 20 for mothers over 40 years of age). These figures are different when one of the parents is a balanced translocation carrier.

In counseling parents who have one child with Down syndrome about the risk of having a second affected child, the geneticist must study the karyotype of the affected child and sometimes the parents to achieve diagnostic accuracy. Several situations may occur.

A. Child with Trisomy 21, Parents with Normal Karyotypes: The risk is only slightly greater than for parents in the general population (1–2%).

B. Trisomic Child, One Parent with Mosaicism: The risk depends on the degree of gonadal mosaicism of the affected parent.

C. Child with 14/21 or 21/21 Translocation, Parents with Normal Karyotypes: The risks are unknown but should be considered only slightly increased.

D. Child with 14/21 Translocation, One Parent Is a Balanced Translocation Carrier:

1. When the mother is the carrier, there is a 10–15% chance that the child will be affected, a 33% chance that the child will be a balanced translocation carrier, and a 43–48% chance that the child will have a normal karyotype.

2. When the father is the carrier, there is a 3–5% chance of having another affected child, and 50% of the apparently unaffected children may be carriers.

E. Child with 21/21 Translocation and One Parent with the Translocation: The recurrence risk is 100%.

Treatment

There is not a convincing documentation of merit in any of the specific therapies, ranging from administration of megadoses of vitamins to specific exercise programs, proposed to eliminate physical and developmental abnormalities of Down syndrome. Therapy is thus directed toward specific problems, eg, cardiac surgery or digitalis administration for heart problems, antibiotic administration for infections, tests of thyroid function, infant stimulation programs, special education, and occupational training. The goal is to help affected children develop to their full potential. Parents' participation in support groups should be encouraged.

TRISOMY 18 SYNDROME

General Considerations

The incidence is about 1 in 4000 live births, and the ratio of affected males to females is approximately 1:3. The mean maternal age is advanced. Affected babies frequently die in early infancy, although patients occasionally survive into childhood.

Clinical Findings

A. Symptoms and Signs: Trisomy 18 is characterized by prenatal and postnatal growth retardation, hypertonicity, prominent occiput, lowset and malformed ears, micrognathia, abnormal flexion of the fingers (index over third and fifth over fourth), equinovarus or "rocker-bottom" feet, short sternum and narrow pelvis, congenital heart disease (often ventricular septal defect or patent ductus arteriosus), and inguinal or umbilical hernias (Fig 34–7). There is an increased occurrence of single umbilical artery.

Dermatoglyphics show simple arches on fingers, a single flexion crease on the fifth finger, and transverse palmar lines. Surviving children show significant developmental delay and mental retardation.

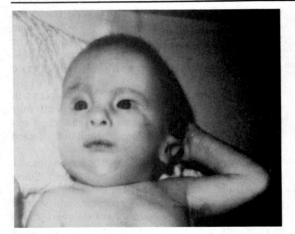
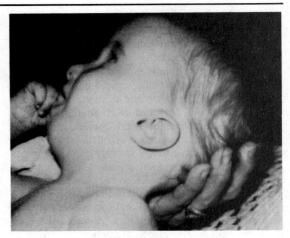

Figure 34–7. Child with trisomy 18.

B. Laboratory Findings: In place of uniform trisomy 18, chromosome analysis occasionally reveals mosaicism for trisomy 18 or an unbalanced translocation involving a third number 18 and other chromosome. Rarely, double trisomies have been found in which trisomy X or trisomy 21 is present in addition to trisomy 18.

Complications

Complications are related to associated lesions. Death is often due to heart failure or pneumonia.

Treatment & Prognosis

There is no treatment other than general supportive care. Death usually occurs in infancy or early childhood, although some patients have reached adulthood.

TRISOMY 13 SYNDROME

The incidence of trisomy 13 is about 1 in 12,000 live births, and 60% of the patients are female. The mean maternal age is increased. Death usually (but not always) occurs in infancy or by the second year of life, commonly as a result of heart failure or infection.

The symptoms and signs include prenatal and postnatal growth deficiency, arhinencephalia, sloping forehead, eye malformations (anophthalmia, colobomas), low-set ears, cleft lip and palate, capillary hemangiomas, polydactyly or syndactyly, and congenital heart disease (usually ventricular septal defect). The facies of an infant with trisomy 13 is shown in Fig 34–8. Other abnormal findings may

include hyperconvex, narrow fingernails; ''rocker-bottom'' feet; retroflexible tumbs; urinary tract anomalies; umbilical hernia; and cryptorchidism or bicornuate uterus. Surviving children demonstrate failure to thrive, developmental retardation, apneic spells, seizures, and deafness.

Treatment is supportive. Because it is sometimes necessary to decide immediately after birth how extensive therapy should be for a severely malformed infant, this diagnosis (as well as one of trisomy 18) can be immediately confirmed by direct examination of mitotic figures obtained from bone marrow. Prevention in the form of genetic counseling is indicated. Prenatal diagnosis is available. The recurrence risks are analogous to those of similar chromosomal situations in Down syndrome.

ABNORMALITIES OF SEX CHROMOSOMES

TURNER SYNDROME

General Considerations

The incidence is 1 in 10,000 among females. However, it is estimated that 95% of conceptuses with monosomy X are miscarried and only 5% are liveborn. Turner syndrome must be ruled out in all females with shortness of stature, webbing of the neck, coarctation of the aorta, or amenorrhea. The diagnosis is made by chromosome analysis. Patients with pseudohypoparathyroidism and Noonan syndrome have a similar phenotype with normal chromosomes.

Clinical Findings

A. Symptoms and Signs: In a newborn, Turner syndrome may be manifested by webbing of the neck, edema of hands and feet, coarctation of aorta, and a characteristic triangular face (Fig 34–9). Later symptoms include short stature, a shield chest with wide-set nipples, streak ovaries, amenorrhea, absence of secondary sex characteristics, and infertility. However, only short stature and amenorrhea and none of the other characteristics may be seen in some affected girls.

Complications relate primarily to the dangers of coarctation of the aorta, when present. Rarely, the dysgenetic gonads may become neoplastic (gonadoblastoma). Incidence of malformation of urinary tract is increased. Sexual infantilism and the perceptual motor difficulties to which these patients are prone may pose concomitant psychologic hazards.

B. Laboratory Findings: Monosomy X (45,X) is found in majority of patients with Turner syndrome. Mosaicism 45,X/46,XX or 45,X/46,XX/

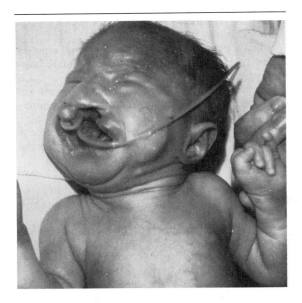

Figure 34–8. Child with trisomy 13.

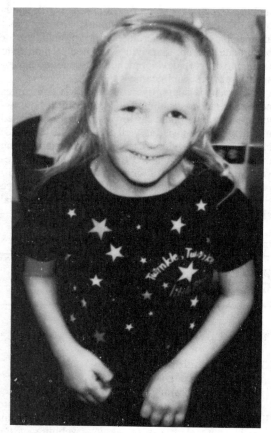

Figure 34–9. Child with Turner syndrome.

47,XXX may be present. Occasionally, the patient has 2 X chromosomes, one of which has a structural abnormality, eg, deletion or translocation of part of one X to one of autosomal chromosomes.

Treatment & Prognosis

Treatment consists of identifying and treating perceptual problems before they become established. Estrogen replacement therapy will cause development of secondary sex characteristics, permit normal menstruation, and prevent development of osteoporosis. Teenage patients need counseling to cope with the stigma of their condition and to understand the need for hormone therapy. In the recent years growth hormone therapy has been used successfully to increase the height of affected girls.

KLINEFELTER SYNDROME

General Considerations

The incidence in the newborn population is roughly 1 in 500, but it is about 1% among mentally retarded males and 3% among males seen at infertil-

ity clinics. The maternal age at birth is often advanced. The diagnosis is rarely made before puberty except as a result of prenatal diagnosis. Unlike gonadal dysgenesis, Klinefelter syndrome is rarely the cause of spontaneous abortions.

Clinical Findings

A. Symptoms and Signs: The characteristic findings do not usually appear until after puberty. Therefore, it is improper to diagnose a child with a 47,XXY karyotype as having Klinefelter syndrome. The most that can be said is that such a child is at increased risk of developing the clinical signs of the syndrome during adolescence. Micro-orchidism associated with otherwise normal external genitals, azoospermia, and sterility are almost invariable in diagnosed cases. Gynecomastia, normal to borderline IQ, diminished facial hair, lack of libido and potency, and a tall, eunuchoid build are frequent. In chromosomal variants with 3 and 4 X chromosomes (XXXY and XXXXY), mental retardation may be severe, and radioulnar synostosis may be present as well as anomalies of the external genitals and cryptorchidism. In the XXXXY cases, these findings are especially prominent, as well as microcephaly, hypertelorism, epicanthus, prognathism, short stature, and incurved fifth fingers.

The adult XXYY patient tends to be taller and more retarded than the average XXY patient.

In general, the physical and mental abnormalities associated with Klinefelter syndrome increase as the number of sex chromosomes increase.

B. Laboratory Findings: The majority of cases have a 47,XXY constitution. Rare variants are 48,XXXY, 49,XXXXY, and 48,XXYY. A variety of mosaicisms containing combinations of the above, as well as 46,XY/47,XXY mosaicism, have been reported. Some patients with 46,XY/47,XXY mosaicism are fertile.

Urinary excretion of gonadotropins is high in adults. Levels are comparable to those found in postmenopausal women.

Histologic analysis of the adult testis reveals hyalinization and atrophy of the majority of seminiferous tubules, with large clumps of abnormal Leydig's cells in between. A marked deficiency of germ cells (spermatogonia) has been found also in prepubertal patients (even in a 10-month-old child).

XYY SYNDROME

The incidence of the 47,XYY karyotype in the newborn population is as yet unknown, although current estimates are that it occurs in about 1 of 1000 male births. Affected newborns in general are perfectly normal and do not have the "XYY syndrome." This syndrome may be present in 10% of tall men (taller than 180 cm or 6 feet) who come into conflict with the law because of their grossly defective, aggressive personalities.

Affected individuals may on occasion exhibit an abnormal behavior pattern from early childhood and may be slightly retarded. Fertility may be normal.

There is no treatment. Many males with an XYY karyotype are normal. Long-term problems may relate to low IQ and environmental stress.

OTHER CHROMOSOME ABNORMALITIES

FRAGILE X SYNDROME

Fragile X syndrome, present in approximately 1 in 1000 males, accounts for 30–50% of X-linked mental retardation. It is associated in a high proportion of gene carriers with a fragile site (a chromatin gap) on the long arm of the X chromosome (Xq27.3) (Fig 34–10). This fragile site is visible only when the tissue culture medium used for chromosome analysis is deficient in folate or thymidine. Thus, the laboratory performing chromosome analysis must be informed in advance that a fragile X study is desired. Even under the optimal circumstances, the fragile site is not expressed in all cells. In affected males, 1 to 50% of cells are positive. In female carriers of the gene, the fragile site is usually expressed in a low percentage of cells, and 40% of carrier females do not express it at all. One percent of males who carry the gene do not express the fragile site.

In general, the percentage of cells expressing the fragile site is proportional to the degree of clinical difficulties. Because of the principles of X-linked inheritance (see the section "Single-Gene Defects"), it is not surprising that the clinical and cytogenetic abnormalities are more severe in males than females.

The majority of males with fragile X syndrome present with mental retardation, oblong face with large ears, and large testicles, especially after puberty. Other physical signs include evidence of connective tissue disorder, eg, hyperextensible joints and mitral valve prolapse. The majority are hyperactive and exhibit infantile autism or autisticlike behavior. However, a small percentage of males with the abnormal gene are of normal phenotype.

In contrast, only approximately one-third of females with fragile X syndrome show some degree of mental retardation. Typical physical features and behavioral problems are less common.

Genetic counseling in families with this disorder is difficult because incomplete penetrance of cytogenetic and clinical symptoms in both sexes precludes identification of all carriers of the gene. Identification of the gene using recombinant DNA technology will be very helpful in distinguishing nonpenetrant gene carriers from those without the gene.

SYNDROMES ASSOCIATED WITH CHROMOSOME FRAGILITY

It is well known that such environmental factors as exposure to radiation, certain chemicals, and viruses contribute to chromosome breaks and rearrangements. However, some well-defined autosomal recessive syndromes are associated with a greatly increased risk of chromosomal aberrations. These include **Bloom syndrome,** characterized by small stature and development of telangectasia upon exposure to sunlight; **Fanconi anemia,** frequently associated with a radial ray defect, pigmentary changes, hypogonadism, mild mental retardation, and development of panctyopenia; **ataxia-telangiectasia** (Louis-Bar syndrome), characterized by telangectasia of the skin and eyes, immunodeficiency, and progressive ataxia; **xeroderma pigmentosum,** resulting in the formation of skin lesions secondary to sun exposure; and **Werner syndrome,** which is associated with premature senility.

The knowledge that specific chromosome aberrations are associated with these syndromes is frequently the basis for cytogenetic confirmation of their diagnosis. For example, Bloom syndrome is associated with an increased tendency to exchange segments between homologous chromosomes during mitosis; this tendency is called sister chromatid exchange. In Fanconi anemia, translocations between nonhomologous chromosomes take place, resulting in formation of so-called quadriradii.

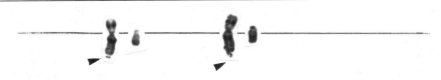

Figure 34–10. Partial karyotype showing fragile X and Y chromosomes. Arrow points to the fragile site.

CONTIGUOUS GENE SYNDROMES

Syndromes are disorders with recognizable patterns of malformations. Some syndromes are caused by chromosome abnormalities; others, by single-gene defects. Many syndromes of unknown etiology usually occur sporadically and are seldom familial. In some of these syndromes, high-resolution chromosome analysis can lead to the identification of small interstitial deletions. The deletion is visible under the microscope in the chromosomes of some, but not all, affected individuals. It is postulated that the syndrome is caused by the absence of a cluster of genes located in the deleted segment. It is believed that in the cases with normal chromosomes the deletion is submicroscopic, subject to detection by DNA analysis, or that other mechanisms interfere with the normal activity of the genes believed to be responsible for the syndrome. The group of genes causing the syndrome are related only through their linear placement on the same chromosome segments and do not influence each others' functions directly (thus the term *contiguous gene syndromes*). Table 34–1 lists the currently known contiguous gene syndromes and their associated chromosome abnormalities.

RECURRENCE RISKS

Most numerical chromosome abnormalities occur sporadically. However, occurrences in siblings or other relatives have been reported, suggesting a hereditary predisposition to nondisjunction in some kindreds. Attempts to identify a single cause have been unsuccessful. It is reasonable to assign parents of a child with aneuploidy an empirical recurrence risk of 1–2% and offer prenatal diagnosis for subsequent pregnancies. Determination of the recurrence risk in structural chromosome abnormalities requires chromosome analysis of the patient's parents to assess if the abnormality was a de novo event in the patient or if a balanced rearrangement of chromosomes exists in one of the parents. If a balanced rearrangement is found, chromosome analysis of other family members must be attempted until all family members with the rearrangement are identified. This analysis is important because, although members of kindreds with normal chromosomes are not at increased risk of recurrence, (except in a rare case of gonadal mosiacism), those with balanced structural rearrangements are. The specific risk varies according to the type of rearrangement and the chromosomes involved.

II. PRINCIPLES OF RECOMBINANT DNA

The revolutionary progress made in molecular biology during the past 2 decades have led to the development of recombinant DNA methods, which have greatly advanced our understanding of the structure and function of human genes. The recombinant DNA technology has major implication for all medical disciplines and especially for human genetics, since it allows location of genes on chromosomes, isolation and characterization of genes, and determination of DNA sequences and encoded protein sequences.

The development of recombinant DNA technology was based on the discovery of bacterial enzymes (**restriction enzymes**). These endonucleases cleave DNA at sites specific for each enzyme. Each restriction endonuclease recognizes a specific nucleotide sequence consisting of 4, 6, 8, or 10 nucleotides and cleaves DNA within that sequence, thus producing DNA fragments. A difference in DNA sequence caused by a normal variation of DNA or by a gene mutation either produces or eliminates an endonuclease recognition site, resulting in a DNA fragment of a different size. Thus, the number and arrangement of restriction sites (called a **restriction map**) are characteristic of a given DNA sequence. Mapping of DNA serves 3 purposes: (1) it is a signature, since each sequence has an unique map; (2) it is an aid to manipulation, such as subcloning and restriction fragment length polymorphism (RFLP) analysis; and (3) it is a prelude to nucleotide sequencing. Before a DNA fragment of interest can be analyzed, multiple copies of it must be produced. This can be achieved by incorporating the human DNA fragment into a **vector,** ie, a DNA segment containing the means of replication and selection in bacteria. The vector-containing human DNA insert is replicated,

Table 34–1. Currently recognized contiguous gene syndromes

Syndrome	Abnormal Chromosome Segment
Prader-Willi syndrome	del 15q11
DiGeorge syndrome	del 22q11
Langer-Gideon syndrome	del 8q24
Miller-Dicker syndrome	del 17p13
Retinoblastoma/mental retardation	del 13q14
Beckwith-Wiedemann syndrome	del 11p15
Wilms' tumor with aniridia, genitourinary malformations, and mental retardation	del 11p13

thus producing multiple copies of the segment of interest. Fig 34–11 shows a schematic representation of such cloning of human DNA. The source of inserts can be **genomic DNA,** obtained directly from the cleaving of the target organism, or **complementary DNA** (cDNA), obtained by copying messenger RNA (mRNA) into DNA by reverse transcription.

A **genomic library** can be constructed by randomly fragmenting human genomic DNA using restriction enzymes and then inserting the fragments into a vector. Such a library contains large numbers of different DNA sequences. Some of these specific DNA fragments are used to manufacture human proteins (eg insulin, growth hormone, interferon, and blood-clotting factors) for pharmacologic applications; others are used as **probes,** which may be thought of as DNA-segment specific, radioactively labeled reagents for mapping and diagnosis.

Molecular genetics is most commonly used to look for changes in genomic DNA detected by southern blot analysis, but a similar technique of northern blot analysis is being used increasingly to look for mRNA abnormalities. **Southern blot analysis** (Fig 34–12) relies on the use of restriction endo-

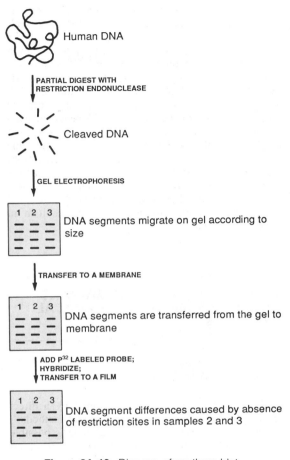

Figure 34–12. Diagram of southern blot.

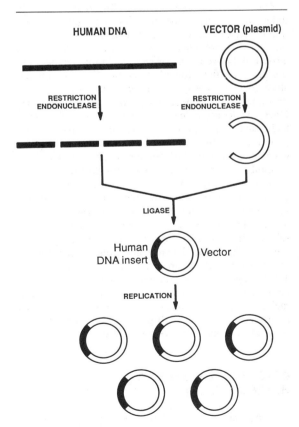

Figure 34–11. Cloning of human DNA segment in a vector.

nucleases to cleave human genomic DNA at specific nucleotide sequences and to produce DNA fragments of different lengths. These DNA fragments are then separated by agrose gel electrophoresis, transferred to a membrane, and overlaid with a radioactive probe, which hybridizes only with a fragment having complementary DNA. This fragment is identified by autoradiography, and its size is determined.

Recently a new gene-amplification technique, called **polymerase chain reaction** (PCR), has been developed. This technique will have a tremendous effect on the use of DNA probes in diagnosis, because it is simpler and less time-consuming than older methods. PCR substantially increases the amount of DNA sequence to be analyzed by easy enzymatic synthesis of 100,000 to 1,000,000 copies of the original DNA segment in a short time. Oligonucleotides, which usually consist of 120 bases and are complementary to the DNA flanking the target segment, are synthesized and used to prime DNA synthesis by DNA polymerase. Each cycle, consisting of denaturation of genomic DNA, primer annealing, and polymerase extension, produces new DNA strands complementary to the target DNA. During each cycle, the amount of amplified DNA doubles, accumulating rapidly in an exponential fashion. After 20 cycles, the DNA is amplified a millionfold.

The amplified DNA can be labeled with **synthetic oligonucleotide probes** (SOP). DNA sequence variation can be analyzed in a crude cell lysate of less than 100 cells in a dot blot format. Thus, this method eliminates the need for DNA purification, gel electrophoresis, and the use of radioactive probes. It can be performed on a small DNA sample in a short time. The disadvantage is that a small contamination with a foreign DNA can result in an incorrect diagnosis.

APPLICATION OF RECOMBINANT DNA TECHNOLOGIES IN CLINICAL GENETICS

GENETIC DIAGNOSIS

Genetic diagnosis can be performed by a direct detection of a mutant gene or by indirect methods.

Direct detection of an abnormal gene is possible only when the nature of the mutation is known. If the abnormal gene has a partial deletion, insertion, or rearrangement, restriction endonuclease analysis with southern blot is used. Cloned DNA fragments of the gene are used as molecular probes to label the gene, demonstrating the altered size of the gene in comparison with a normal control. Gene deletions have been found in α- and β-thalassemia, antithrombin III deficiency, congenital adrenal hyperplasia secondary to 21-hydroxylase deficiency, Duchenne muscular dystrophy, hemophilia A and B, Lesch-Nyhan syndrome, and ornithine transcarbamoylase deficiency.

An abnormal gene with a point mutation can be diagnosed by restriction analysis if the mutation either created or abolished a restriction recognition site, but a restriction recognition site is created or abolished in only 5 to 10% of point mutations. In the remainder of mutations, PCR can be used for DNA amplification, and the mutation can be documented by a mutant-specific oligonucleotide probe (MSO), which recognizes the mutant but not the normal alleles.

A diagnostic study employing the direct detection of the mutant gene can be performed on the affected individual only and does not require a study of many affected and unaffected family members.

Indirect detection of abnormal genes is used when (a) the gene is known, but there is extensive heterogeneity of the molecular defect between families, and (b) the gene responsible for a disease is unknown, but its chromosome location is known. In the former situation—the gene is known—it is not always necessary to know the exact molecular defect to determine the presence of the gene. It is, however, necessary to mark and trace the inheritance of the abnormal gene. This can be done on the basis of intragenic DNA polymorphism, which is characterized by the addition or removal of a restriction site and is thus identifiable by RFLP analysis. This DNA polymorphism, although intragenic, is not the mutation that causes the disorder; it simply marks and helps to differentiate the abnormal gene from the normal one. RFLP cannot be used, however, unless both parents of the tested individual are heterozygous. Thus, a family study is necessary to determine the haplotypes of the chromosomes with and without the mutant gene. However, crossover and recombination are not a problem, because the polymorhism is intragenic or in very close proximity to the gene. Examples of the disorders that can be screened by this method are phenylketonuria, hemophilia, β-thalasemia, and Fabry disease.

The latter situation—the abnormal gene is unknown—exists in the majority of single-gene disorders. In this case, linkage analysis using a large number of DNA polymorphic markers may reveal a close link between one or more such markers and the presence of the clinical disorder. Such a linkage study localizes the gene of interest to a specific chromosome or to a specific region of a chromosome. Once the location of the gene is known, the same technique (using probes known to be linked to the gene locus of interest) can be used to trace the presence or absence of the gene through the family. This method assumes that the two loci—the locus of the gene and the locus of the DNA polymorphism used to mark the gene—are so close that they will not segregate independently, but will be transmitted together. The presence of the marker, therefore, is a reliable indication of the presence of the gene of interest. Thus, the distance between the two loci is of utmost importance in determining the reliability of any linkage analysis, because crossing over and recombination between the gene and the marker during meiosis will result in an error in the diagnosis. To minimize the errors, multiple linked markers should be used in linkage analysis of any gene.

DETECTION OF GENETIC HETEROGENEITY

Sometimes genetic heterogeneity is suspected from clinical variability. In other instances, there is no clinical clue. For example, enzyme deficiencies may be caused by a number of different mutations, such as an abnormal active site in one case and abnormal coenzyme in another case. Alternatively, the phenotype may be caused in different families by different enzyme defects. Such heterogeneity cannot be suspected on a clinical basis; however, it can be detected using DNA technology.

TREATMENT

Recombinant DNA technology could facilitate treatment in following ways: (1) Production of large amounts of therapeutic agents, eg, growth hormone and interferon, which are present naturally in small quantities and are therefore very expensive. This is already being done.
(2) Gene therapy. The introduction of a normal gene into an individual affected with serious inherited disorder is predicted for the future. In principle, genes could be introduced either during embryonic life (germline therapy), in which case the gene could be transmitted to future generations, or the gene could be introduced only into somatic cells (somatic therapy), in which case it would be present only during the life of the recipient.

PREVENTION

Recombinant DNA technology has the potential to prevent genetic disease by facilitating the detection of carriers of defective genes and allowing prenatal diagnosis. Family studies can also clarify the mode of inheritance, thus allowing more accurate determination of recurrence risks and appropriate options. For example, differentiation of a gonadal mosaicism from decreased penetrance of a dominant gene or a new mutation has important implications for genetic counseling.

In the past, the diagnosis of a genetic disease characterized by a late onset of symptoms, eg, Huntington disease, could not be made prior to the appearance of clinical symptoms. In some inborn errors of metabolism, diagnostic tests (eg, measurement of enzyme activities) could be conducted only on inaccessible tissues. Gene identification techniques can enormously enhance our ability to diagnose symptomatic and presymptomatic individuals, conduct prenatal diagnosis, and detect heterozygous carriers.

Antonarakis SE: Diagnosis of genetic disorders at the DNA level. *N Engl J Med* 1989;**320**:153.

Caskey CT: Disease diagnosis by recombinant DNA methods. *Science* 1987;**236**:1223.

Childs B et al (editors): *Progress in Medical Genetics.* Vol 7. 1988.

Emanuel BS: Invited editorial: Molecular cytogenetics: toward dissection of the contiguous gene syndrome. *Am J Hum Genet* 1988;**43**:575.

Jones KL: *Smith's Recognizable Patterns of Human Malformation.* Saunders, 1988.

Opitz JM (editor): *X-linked Mental Retardation 2.* Liss, 1986.

Rooney DE, Czepulkowski BH (editors): *Human Cytogenetics: A Practical Approach.* IRL Press, 1986.

Schinzel A: *Catalogue of Unbalanced Chromosome Aberrations in Man.* Walter de Gruyter, 1984.

Smickel RD: Contiguous gene syndromes: A component of recognizable syndromes. *J Pediatr* 1986;**109**:231.

Smith AN, Scott JA (editors): *Genetic Applications: A Health Perspective.* Learner Managed Designs, 1988.

Therman E: *Human Chromosomes: Structure, Behavior, Effects.* Springer-Verlag, 1986.

III. MENDELIAN GENETICS

SINGLE-GENE DEFECTS

A **gene** is the unit of inheritance that determines the genetic makeup of an individual. Genes occur in pairs at a single locus or site on specific chromosomes. These paired genes, called **alleles,** determine the genotype of an individual at that locus. If the genes at a specific locus are identical, the individual is **homozygous;** if they are different, **heterozygous.** During normal meiosis, these alleles separate, one going to each of the 2 gametes. An understanding of this process is necessary for an understanding of single-gene inheritance.

Disorders due to an abnormality in a single gene are either autosomal or X-linked, depending upon the location of the gene on an autosome in the former and on the X chromosome in the latter. If the abnormality is present when the defective gene is in either the heterozygous or the homozygous state, it is dominantly inherited. If, however, it is present only when the gene involved is in the homozygous state, the disorder is recessively inherited.

AUTOSOMAL DOMINANT INHERITANCE

Autosomal dominant inheritance (AD) has these characteristics:

(1) Individuals in the same family may show very different manifestations of the same disorder. This

phenomenon is called **variable expressivity.** Typically, at least some persons who carry the gene are mildly affected, because an individual must be healthy enough and fertile enough to reproduce and pass on the trait. In some disorders, such as Huntington's disease, manifestations do not appear until after child bearing. In others, which tend to be more severe (eg, achondroplasia), there is a high mutation rate.

(2) Some persons who are obligatory carriers of the gene (ie, both a parent and a child are affected) may have no apparent manifestations. This phenomenon is called **nonpenetrance,** and the penetrance rate varies for each dominantly inherited condition.

(3) Males and females are equally affected, although the manifestations may vary according to sex. For example, baldness is a dominant trait but affects only males. In this case, the trait is said to be **sex-limited.** Both males and females can pass on the abnormality to children of either sex.

(4) Dominant inheritance is typically said to be "vertical," ie, the condition passes from one generation to the next in a vertical fashion (Fig 34–13).

(5) In some cases, the family history seems to be completely negative, and the affected individual appears to be the first abnormal case. This spontaneous appearance may be caused by a point mutation or a change in the structure of a specific gene. Such a change may be a deletion, a duplication, or an amino acid substitution. The mutation rate varies with each dominant condition, and in some cases the mutation rate increases with advancing paternal age. There are, however, several other possible explanations:

(a) Nonpaternity.

(b) Decreased penetrance or mild manifestations in one of the parents. For this reason, both parents must be carefully examined and a thorough family history taken.

(c) Germ cell mosaicism. In rare cases, there may be mosaicism in the germ cell line of either parent, in which case the risk of recurrence increases. This is a proposed explanation for cases in which 2 children of completely normal parents are affected with a dominant condition. Unfortunately, there is no way to predict or to confirm germ cell mosaicism.

(d) The possibility that the abnormality is not truly an autosomal dominant condition. It may be a phenocopy, ie, a nongenetic condition that mimics a certain genotype, or it may be a similar but genetically different abnormality with a different mode of inheritance.

(6) As a general rule, dominant conditions are not due to enzyme defects, since most biochemical defects are substrate rather than enzyme limited. Therefore, enzyme levels at 50% of the normal value are sufficient for normal function. There are exceptions, eg, acute intermittent porphyria. Dominant traits are more often related to structural abnormalities of protein, eg, as in Marfan syndrome.

(7) The risk of any offspring carrying an abnormal dominant gene is 50%, or 1 in 2 for each pregnancy. This is true whether the gene is penetrant or not, and the severity in the offspring is not related to the severity in the affected parent. If an abnormality represents a new mutation of a dominant trait, the parents of the affected individual run a low risk during subsequent pregnancies, but the risk for the offspring of the affected individual is 50%.

(8) Options available for future pregnancies include prenatal diagnosis in an increasing number of cases and artificial insemination if the father is the carrier of the abnormal gene.

NEUROFIBROMATOSIS

Essentials of Diagnosis

Two or more of the following:

- Six or more café-au-lait macules, greater than 15 mm in diameter in postpubertal and 5 mm in prepubertal individuals.
- Two or more neurofibromas of any type or one plexiform neuroma.
- Axillary or inguinal freckling.
- Two or more Lisch nodules (iris hamartomas).
- Distinctive bony lesions.
- An affected first-degree relative.

General Considerations

Neurofibromatosis (NFT) is one of the most common AD disorders, occurring in 1 in 3000 to 4000 births and seen in all races and ethnic groups. It has a wide range of variability and can present in many ways. In general, however, the disorder is progressive and new manifestations appear over time. There are at least 2 types of NFT: NFT I is characterized by multiple skin findings, and NFT II is character-

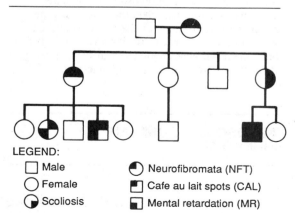

LEGEND:

☐ Male

○ Female

◑ Scoliosis

◐ Neurofibromata (NFT)

▨ Cafe au lait spots (CAL)

■ Mental retardation (MR)

Figure 34–13. Autosomal dominant inheritance: Neurofibromatosis, showing variable expressivity.

ized by bilateral acoustic neuromas, frequently unaccompanied by any skin manifestations. A third category includes all of the atypical forms. Because NFT II is less common and rarely presents before late adolescence, this discussion is limited to type I.

Clinical Findings

Café-au-lait macules may be present at birth or appear shortly thereafter, and most are apparent by 1 year of age. The typical skin lesion is 10 to 30 mm, ovoid, and smooth bordered, but there is great variation. There are 3 types of neurofibromas: cutaneous, subcutaneous, and plexiform. The last is a large, deep, interdigitating nerve tumor that may be a problem in early childhood, but other neurofibromas tend to occur later. The incidence of the Lisch nodules, which can be seen with a slit lamp, also increases with age. Common features of affected individuals include a large head (although only a small percentage have true hydrocephalus), bony abnormalities on x-ray studies, scoliosis, and a wide spectrum of developmental problems, ranging from learning disabilities to true mental retardation.

Differential Diagnosis

Areas of hyperpigmentation can be seen in other conditions, (eg, Albright's, Noonan's, and leopard syndromes), but the lesions are either single or different in character. Isolated neurofibromas and familial café-au-lait spots (fewer than 6 and with no other manifestations of NFT) have been described. The relationship of such cases to classical NFT I is uncertain.

Complications

It is difficult to differentiate a complication from a rare manifestation of the underlying disorder. Seen in less than 25% of persons with NFT are seizures, optic glioma, deafness, constipation, short stature, early puberty, and hypertension. The risk for malignancy is about 5% above baseline, and the most common malignant tumor is a neurofibrosarcoma. Other tumors may be benign but may cause significant morbidity and mortality because of their location in a vital and closed space. In childhood and adolescence, the major complications seen are scoliosis, developmental delay, and occasionally problems secondary to a plexiform neuroma.

Treatment

Appropriate therapy should be initiated as each new manifestation arises. Neurofibromas can be removed, but removal is of limited help if they are multiple or in a vital area. The most important part of therapy is close, ongoing follow-up. Because this disorder is progressive, affected individuals should be seen at regular intervals and have regular eye examinations, hearing tests, and developmental

screening, as well as other evaluations (eg, CT scans) as indicated.

Prognosis

Because there is such variability in NFT, it is difficult to make a prognosis. However, most affected persons have only skin lesions and few other problems. Severely affected individuals are rare, and close follow-up and early intervention may ameliorate complications.

Genetic Counseling

The gene for NFT has been localized to the long arm of chromosome 7 with several informative DNA probes flanking it. Between 30 and 50% of all cases are felt to be due to new mutations. The gene may be large, or there may be a fragile site or unstable locus within the gene itself. Before attributing an individual case to a new mutation, however, the geneticist must subject both parents to a careful evaluation, including a thorough examination of the skin and a slit lamp examination to look for Lisch nodules. Recent evidence would suggest that penetrance is quite high if individuals are carefully examined. The application of the new DNA probes not only makes prenatal diagnosis possible in many families but may also provide a more definitive way to identify affected persons. To date, however, DNA probes are of limited availability and very costly.

AUTOSOMAL RECESSIVE INHERITANCE

This type of inheritance also has some distinctive characteristics:

(1) There is less variability among affected persons. Parents are carriers and are clinically normal. (There are exceptions to this rule, however. For example, sickle cell disease is considered recessive. Under normal circumstances, carriers—those with sickle trait—are normal but may become symptomatic if they become hypoxic.)

(2) Both males and females are affected equally.

(3) Inheritance is horizontal; siblings may be affected, but both parents are normal (Fig 34–14).

(4) Recessive conditions are frequently rare; the rarer the condition, the more likely there is to be consanguinity. Conversely, if a child whose parents are related presents with an unrecognized abnormality, a recessive condition is likely.

(5) A negative family history is not unusual. In common conditions such as cystic fibrosis, there may be an affected second- or third-degree relative, but usually not. Because parents are clinically nor-

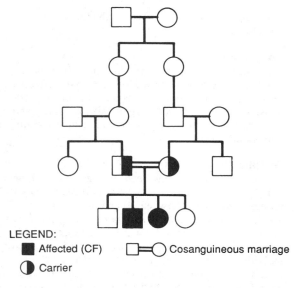

LEGEND:

■ Affected (CF)   □─○ Cosanguineous marriage

◐ Carrier

Figure 34–14. Autosomal recessive inheritance: Cystic fibrosis.

mal even though they are carriers, one must not be lulled into a false sense of security by the negative family history.

(6) Recessive conditions are frequently associated with enzyme defects. See Chapter 33.

(7) The recurrence risk is 25%, or 1 in 4 for each pregnancy. When there is a new partner, however, the risk drops and can be recalculated on the basis of the gene frequency in the population.

(8) Options available for future pregnancies include prenatal diagnosis in many cases and artificial insemination.

CYSTIC FIBROSIS

The gene for cystic fibrosis (CF) is one of the most common abnormal genes in the Caucasian population. Approximately 1 in 22 persons is a carrier. It appears to be a homogeneous condition, with most affected persons having an abnormality of the same gene. Before 1980, there was no reliable prenatal diagnostic technique, and the risk of having a second affected child (25%) could not be reduced. In 1983, however, the condition was found to be associated with decreased levels of certain enzymes in the amniotic fluid. These decreased enzyme levels seem to be secondary to decreased passage of meconium. The relatively high incidence of false-negative and false-positive results, however, limited the applicability and acceptability of this test. In 1985, the CF gene was located on the long arm of chromosome 7, and numerous DNA probes have been identified that detect restriction length polymorphisms (RLFP)

tightly linked to the gene. At the present, highly accurate prenatal diagnosis is available to a large number of families at risk. About 90% of families are informative or partially informative when the most closely linked markers are used to detect the gene. To be informative, one or both parents must be heterozygous for the marker in question, and blood must be available from both parents as well as an affected child. During a second pregnancy, enough tissue can be obtained by chorionic villous sampling for DNA studies on the fetus. In a proportion of cases, CF can be diagnosed or excluded with a high degree of probability, but in others, the results may be ambiguous. In the latter instance, amniotic fluid enzyme studies done at 16–18 weeks should increase the accuracy of the prediction. The most commonly used enzyme is alkaline phosphatase because its intestinal origin can be determined. Using the DNA technique, there is always a risk of crossover or recombination, but the risk seems to be small because the markers are very close to the gene. This mapping technique may also result in the isolation of the gene and, by reverse genetics, lead to an understanding of how it works and what mutations are involved.

X-LINKED INHERITANCE

When a gene for a specific disorder is on the X chromosome, the condition is said to be X-linked or sex-linked. Females may be either homogyzous or heterozygous, since they have 2 X chromosomes. Males, by contrast, have only one, and an affected male is said to be hemizygous. The severity of any disorder is more consistent in males than in females (within a specific family). According to the Lyon hypothesis, since one of the 2 X chromosomes is inactivated, and since this inactivation is random, the clinical picture in females depends on the percentage of mutant versus normal alleles inactivated. The X chromosome is not inactivated until about 14 days gestation, and parts of the short arm remain active throughout life.

X-LINKED RECESSIVE

The following are characteristic of X-linked recessive inheritance:

(1) Males are affected and carriers; heterozygous females are either normal or have mild manifestations.

(2) Inheritance is "diagonal" through the maternal side of the family (34–15).

(3) A female carrier has a 50% chance of having

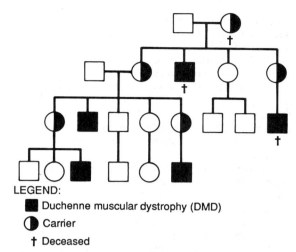

LEGEND:

■ Duchenne muscular dystrophy (DMD)

◐ Carrier

† Deceased

Figure 34–15. X-linked recessive inheritance: Duchenne type muscular dystrophy.

carrier daughters and a 50% chance of having affected sons.

(4) All of the daughters of an affected male are carriers, and none of his sons is affected. Since a father can give only his Y chromosome to his son, male-to-male transmission excludes X-linked inheritance.

(5) The mutation rate is high in some X-linked disorders, particularly when the affected male is infertile. In such instances, the mutation is felt to occur in the propositus in one-third of cases, in the mother in one-third of cases, and in earlier generations in one-third of cases. For this reason, genetic counseling is difficult in families with an isolated case.

(6) On rare occasions, a female may be fully affected. Several possible mechanisms may account for a fully affected female: (a) unfavorable lyonization, (b) 45,X karyotype, (c) homozygosity in the female, and (d) an X-autosome translocation in which the X chromosome of normal structure is preferentially inactivated.

DUCHENNE TYPE MUSCULAR DYSTROPHY

Duchenne type muscular dystrophy (DMD) has been recognized as an X-linked recessive condition for many years. There is also a milder type, Becker's muscular dystrophy (BMD), which is allelic. In the past, carrier detection has been unreliable because of nonspecific tests, such as serum creatine phosphokinase levels. The gene, now known to be in band Xp21, is one of the largest genes in the human genome. Its size may explain its high mutation rate. About 50% of families have a deletion (rather than a substitution) in the gene. In rare cases, this deletion visible on cytogenetic analysis, but most often DNA studies are required. Because of the length of the gene, there are many available informative RFLPs, both flanking the gene and within the gene. In addition, this gene has been shown to encode mRNA for a protein called dystrophin, which is localized to the muscle surface membrane, the sarcolemma. Males with low or undetectable levels of dystrophin have DMD, whereas those with nearly normal levels but dystrophin of an abnormal size have BMD. The levels of dystrophin seem to correlate well with clinical prognosis. All of these new advances have made accurate and predicitive counseling available to many families.

X-LINKED DOMINANT

This inheritance pattern is much less common than the X-linked recessive type. Examples include incontinentia pigmenti and hypophosphatemic or vitamin D–resistant rickets.

(1) The heterozygous female is symptomatic, and the disease is twice as common in females because they have 2 X chromosomes that can be affected.

(2) Clinical manifestations are more variable in females than in males.

(3) The risk for the offspring of heterozygous females is 50% regardless of sex.

(4) All of the daughters but none of the sons of affected males will have the disorder.

(5) Although a homogygous female is possible (particularly in an inbred population), she would be severely involved. All of her children would also be affected, but more mildly.

(6) Some disorders (eg, incontinentia pigmenti) are lethal in males (and in homozygous females). Affected women have twice as many daughters as sons and an increased incidence of miscarriages, because all affected males will be spontaneously aborted.

MITOCHONDRIAL INHERITANCE

Some unusual disorders seem to be transmitted only by the female members of a family and affect a high proportion of offspring. Examples include Leber's optic neuropathy and a variety of neurologic conditions in some described families. Since mitochondria are cytoplasmic and therefore inherited only from the mother, mitochondrial inheritance has been postulated. Mitochondrial DNA (mtDNA) codes for many enzymes, including enzymes of oxidative phosphorylation, which generate ATP. Those tissues most dependent on mitrochondrial energy, specifically central nervous system and skeletal muscle, seem to be most susceptible to mutations in mtDNA. New molecular approaches may help to identify more mitrochondrial abnormalities, and effective therapy may become available.

POLYGENIC DISEASE
(Multifactorial Inheritance)

The inheritance of many common traits and abnormalities does not seem to be due to a single gene. Multiple genes as well as a variety of environmental factors appear to be involved. The term *polygenic* refers to the effect of several genes, and the term *multifactorial* implies that environmental factors are important also. Inherited in a polygenic way are a variety of normal traits, eg, height, intelligence, and dermal ridge counts, as well as a variety of common abnormalities, eg, hypertension and allergies. In some conditions, there is an association with certain HLA types. For example, there is a high correlation between ankylosing spondilitis and B27. It is important to understand the difference between an association such as this and linkage of a certain disease with the HLA locus. In the latter instance, the gene for the disease is on chromosome 6, close to the HLA locus, but there is no association with a specific HLA type.

Many common congenital abnormalities, eg, cleft lip and palate, neural tube defects, and some kinds of congenital heart disease, are inherited in a polygenic manner. If the combination of predisposing genes from both parents and certain environmental factors (mostly unknown) exceed the "threshold," then the abnormality becomes manifest. Twin studies have been helpful in determining the relative importance of genetic versus environmental factors. If genetic factors are of little or no importance, then the concordance between monozygotic and dizygotic twins should be the same. (Dizygotic twins are no more genetically similar to each other than to other siblings.) If an abnormality is completely genetic, the concordance between identical twins should be 100%. Most polygenic conditions are associated with concordance rates somewhere in between.

Polygenic or multifactorial inheritance has some distinctive characteristics:

(1) The risk for relatives of affected persons is increased, and the risk is higher for first-degree relatives (those who have 50% of their genes in com-

mon) and lower for more distant relations, although the risk for the latter is higher than for the general population (Table 34–2).

(2) The recurrence risk varies with the number of affected family members. For example, after one child is born with a neural tube defect, the recurrence risk is 3 to 4%. If a second affected child is born, the risk increases to 10–12%. This is in contrast to single-gene disorders, where the risk is the same no matter how many family members are affected.

(3) The risk is higher if the defect is more severe. In Hirschsprung's disease, another polygenic condition, the longer the aganglionic segment, the higher the recurrence risk.

(4) Sex ratios may not be equal. If there is a marked discrepancy, the recurrence risk is higher if a child of the less commonly affected sex has the

Table 34–2. Empiric risks for some congenital disorders.

Mental deficiency of unknown cause: Incidence 3:1000
Risks for siblings
    Both parents normal: 5–13% retarded
    One parent retarded: 20% retarded
    Both parents retarded: 42% retarded
Anencephaly and spina bifida: Incidence (average) 1:1000
    One affected child: 2–3%
    Two affected children: 10–12%
    One affected parent: 2–3%
Hydrocephalus: Incidence 1:2000 newborns
    Occasional X-linked recessive
    Often associated with neural tube defect
    Some environmental etiologies, eg, toxoplasmosis
    Recurrence risk, one affected child
        Hydrocephalus: 1%
        Some CNS abnormality: 3%
Cleft Lip and/or palate: Incidence (average) 1:1000
    One affected child: 2–4%
    One affected parent: 2–4%
    Two affected children: 10%
    One affected parent, one affected child: 10–20%
Cleft palate: Incidence 1:2000
    One affected child: 2%
    Two affected children: 6–8%
    One affected parent: 4–6%
    One affected parent, one affected child: 15–20%
Congenital heart disease: Incidence 8:1000
    One affected child: 2–3%
    One affected parent, one affected child: 10%
Clubfoot: Incidence 1:1000 (male:female = 2:1)
    One affected child 2–3%
Congenital dislocated hip: Incidence 1:1000
    (female>male), with marked regional variation
    One child affected: 2–14%
Pyloric stenosis: Incidence, males: 1:200; females: 1:1000
    Male index patient

Brothers	3.2%
Sons	6.8%
Sisters	3.0%
Daughters	1.2%
Female index patient	
Brothers	13.2%
Sons	20.5%
Sisters	2.5%
Daughters	11.1%

disorder. This assumes that more genetic factors are required to raise the more resistant sex above the threshold than to raise the less resistant sex. For example, pyloric stenosis is more common in males. If the first affected child is a female, the recurrence risk is higher than if the child is a male.

(5) The risk for the offspring of an affected person is approximately the same as the risk for siblings, assuming that the spouse of the affected person has a negative family history.

Two common polygenic conditions are discussed in the following sections, which address genetic considerations as well as issues of management.

CLEFT LIP & CLEFT PALATE

General Considerations

From a genetic standpoint, cleft lip with or without cleft palate is distinct from isolated cleft palate. The former is more common in males; the latter, in females. Although both can occur in a single family, particularly in association with certain syndromes, this pattern is unusual. There is racial variation in the incidence of facial clefting. Among Asians, whites, and blacks, the incidence is 1.61, 0.9, and 0.31, respectively, per 1000 live births.

Clinical Findings

A cleft lip may be unilateral or bilateral and complete or incomplete. It may occur with a cleft of the entire palate or just the primary (anterior and gingival ridge) or secondary (posterior) palate. An isolated cleft palate can involve only the soft palate or both soft and hard palates. It can be a V-shaped or wide horseshoe cleft. A cleft associated with micrognathia and glossoptosis (a tongue that falls back) and causes respiratory or feeding problems is called the Pierre Robin syndrome. Among individuals with facial clefts, more commonly those with isolated cleft palate, there is an increased incidence of other congenital abnormalities. The incidence of congenital heart disease, for example, is between 1 and 2%, but among those with Pierre Robin syndrome, it can be as high as 15%. Associated abnormalities should be identified in the period immediately after birth, before surgery.

Differential Diagnosis

It is important to remember that a facial cleft may occur in many different circumstances. It may be an isolated abnormality or part of a more generalized syndrome. Prognosis, management, and accurate determination of recurrence risks all depend on an accurate diagnosis. The following etiologies must be considered in individuals with cleft lip and cleft palate or isolated cleft palate:

(1) Environmental factors, eg, a history of use of anticonvulsants (especially Dilantin) by the mother, fetal alcohol syndrome, and amniotic band syndrome.

(2) Chromosome abnormalities, particularly trisomies 13 and 18 and 4p−.

(3) Single-gene disorders, including Van der Woude syndrome (an autosomal dominant condition characterized by lip pits and either CL/CP or CP). Treacher Collins syndrome (CP), or Stickler syndrome (Pierre Robin with severe myopia, hearing loss, and arthropathies).

(4) Syndromes of unknown etiology, eg, Moebius syndrome (CP) or Cornelia de Lange syndrome (CP).

(5) Polygenic disorder.

Complications

The most immediate and potentially life-threatening complication in the newborn period is difficulty with feeding. This may be secondary to inadequate suction or to poorly coordinated sucking and swallowing. The Pierre Robin complex may also be associated with respiratory distress. Special bottles and nipples and occasionally a palatal prosthesis may be needed for feeding, and special positioning and supplemental O_2 may be necessary for children with Pierre Robin syndrome. Breast-feeding is not usually successful if the palate is involved. Rarely, gavage feedings and even a tracheostomy may be required. Later complications include recurrent serous otitis media and decreased or fluctuating hearing. The former is treated aggressively with medications and PE tubes, because evidence suggests that serous otitis contributes to delayed speech and language. Speech problems may also be the result of a short or poorly mobile palate or of multiple dental problems and malocclusion.

Treatment

The cleft lip is repaired surgically shortly after birth, within the first 3 months of life; the cleft palate, at about 12 months. The trend is toward earlier surgical repair as advances are made in pediatric anesthesia and nursing care. Additional surgery is usually needed to improve the appearance of the lip, correct nasal deformities, and provide adequate palatal length for normal speech. Hearing should be closely monitored and PE tubes replaced as needed. Most children with a cleft palate need speech therapy starting at age 2 to 3 years. They also need orthodontic intervention, sometimes as early as 8 or 9 years. Mid-face hypoplasia is commonly seen in children with facial clefts, and a mid-face advancement may be necessary at the end of the growth period. Because of the complexity of the management of these patients and the necessity for coordinated care, it is recommended that they be followed in a multidisciplinary cleft palate clinic.

Genetic Counseling

Accurate counseling depends on accurate diagnosis. A complete family history must be taken, and both parents must be examined. The choice of laboratory studies is guided by the presence of other abnormalities and clinical suspicions. They may include chromosomal analysis, eye examination, and x-ray studies. Clefts of both the lip and the palate have been detected on ultrasound prenatally, but intrauterine diagnosis is most likely in syndromes where other, more serious abnormalities can be identified.

NEURAL TUBE DEFECTS

General Considerations

The term **neural tube defect** (NTD) encompasses a variety of malformations including anencephaly, spina bifida (SB) or myelomeningocele, sacral agenesis, sacral lipomas, and other spinal dysraphisms. The pathogenesis is probably different for each defect. Anencephaly and high spina bifida are thought to be due to a primary neurulation defect or failure of the neural tube to close, whereas lower lesions may be caused by a problem with secondary neurulation or failure of the caudal neural rod to canalize. Hydrocephalus associated with the Arnold-Chiari malformation is commonly seen with spina bifida at all levels. Sacral agenesis, also called the caudal regression syndrome, is seen more frequently in infants of diabetic mothers than in other infants.

Clinical Findings

At birth, neural tube defects can present as rachischisis at any level, as a fluid-filled sac that may or may not be leaking, or as a variety of skin-covered lesions associated with a fatty mass, a hemangioma, a tuft of hair, or asymmetric buttock creases. In the latter cases, CT or MRI studies should be conducted to look for bony and neural involvement. The extent of associated abnormalities depends on the level of the lesion and may include a variety of foot deformities, flexion contractures, dislocated hips, or total flaccid paralysis below the level of the lesion. Hydrocephalus may be apparent at birth, but more often there is an increase in head circumference, irritability, and poor feeding, with vomiting beginning shortly after the back has been closed. Neurogenic bladder and bowel may present as constant urinary dribbling, frequent stooling, and occasionally rectal or even vaginal prolapse. There is also a higher incidence of unassociated abnormalities, particularly with higher lesions and anencephaly.

Differential Diagnosis

It is important to look for syndromes that may present as neural tube defects. Some chromosomal abnormalities, congenital rubella, and the fetal valproic acid syndrome have been associated with neural tube defects.

Complications & Management

If the spinal defect is leaking or open at birth, the major concerns are infection and drying of the nerve roots, leading to further loss of function. For this reason, surgical closure is recommended as soon as possible. The infant should be closely monitored, and a shunt, usually ventriculoperitoneal, should be inserted as soon as signs of hydrocephalus become apparent. The shunt may need to be replaced if it becomes obstructed, infected, or separated, or it may need to be lengthened as the child grows.

The child's ability to walk varies according to the level of the lesion. Children with low lumbar and sacral lesions walk with minimal support; those with high lumbar and thoracic lesions are rarely functional walkers; and those with midlumbar lesions vary. In any case, the child should receive physical therapy and assume the upright position at the appropriate developmental age. Orthopedic surgery may be necessary to get the child upright and ambulatory. Concerns about the bladder begin at birth. The bladder may be small and spastic or large and hypotonic, the sphincter may be flaccid or tight. The child may therefore be constantly wet because the bladder holds little urine, or there may be incomplete emptying of the bladder and ureteral reflux. In the latter case, there is a high risk for urinary tract infections. Management is guided by results of early studies to determine the type of bladder present. If the bladder is emptying, nothing need be done immediately, although crede is usually recommended to assist in complete emptying. If there is retention or reflux, clean intermittent catheterization should be started immediately. Continence can be achieved in a variety of ways. Usually medications are necessary to increase bladder capacity and tighten the sphincter. The mother and ultimately the child are taught the technique for clean intermittent catheterization. If the child still cannot achieve continence, an artificial urinary sphincter can be inserted at about 7 to 10 years of age. Diversionary procedures are rarely done unless there is damage to the upper tracts. Renal function should be monitored regularly by ultrasound studies. Cultures should also be obtained frequently, and symptomatic infections should be treated.

Bowel control can be more of a problem because a lax sphincter and poor peristalsis predispose to constipation and poor emptying. The principles of management include increasing the bulk of the stool to facilitate spontaneous and more complete evacuation and at the same time keep the child as free from accidents as possible. This is done with a combination of a high-fiber diet and suppositories. Enemas, digital stimulation or evacuation, and biofeedback have been used as well.

Areas of skin anesthesia or hypesthesia roughly correlate to motor level. Skin breakdown in the foot and perineal regions is always a threat, and skin care must be meticulous. Wheelchairs should have appropriate cushions, and new braces should be used very cautiously until it is certain that they fit. If skin breakdown does occur, all pressure must be relieved, the wound kept clean, and an artificial skin used to promote healing. Sometimes surgical closure is required. The advantages of prevention over treatment cannot be emphasized too strongly.

There is a wide range of intellectual capacity in children with neural tube defects, but most function in the low-normal to borderline area. Most children are now mainstreamed, but they have a higher incidence of fine motor and visual-perceptual problems. Because of early aggressive care, most children with neural tube defects are surviving into adolescence, when different problems are becoming apparent. Cord tethering may cause a loss of function and requires early surgical release, since lost function may not be regained. Scoliosis becomes apparent in adolescence, and surgery may be needed. A small percentage have progressive loss of renal function secondary to chronic infection and stones despite aggressive treatment, and some develop renal failure. Problems with bowel management and skin breakdown increase as individuals become obese and less ambulatory. The major problems, however, are psychosocial. The transition into independent adulthood is very difficult because of poor social skills, limited social contacts, inferior education, and poor preparation for the competitive work world. Society must do more for these disabled young adults.

Individuals with closed spinal cord abnormalities (eg, sacral lipomas) have similar problems, although hydrocephalus is rarely seen and intelligence is usually normal. Early surgical intervention is important to preserve function and prevent additional disability. Because needs are ongoing and management approaches change with time, all children with spinal defects of any type should be followed in a multidisciplinary clinic.

Genetic Counseling

Recurrence risks vary according to etiology, but most neural tube defects are polygenic. The risk for the offspring of an affected person is essentially the same. Prenatal diagnosis is available, and pregnancies can be monitored in a variety of ways. In fetuses with open neural tube defects, serum alpha fetoprotein levels, measured at 16–18 weeks' gestation, are elevated. In countries such as Great Britain, where the incidence is particularly high, in pregnant women are routinely screened. Routine screening has also been recommended by the American Academy of Obstetrics and Gynecology. Alpha fetoprotein levels in amniotic fluid are also elevated, and amniocentesis combined with experienced ultra-

sound studies will detect more than 90% of neural tube defects. There is no proved way to prevent neural tube defects, although some researchers are studying the effectiveness of vitamins taken prior to conception. Early data from Britain suggest that vitamin administration may lower the risk.

IV. DYSMORPHOLOGY

The term *birth defect* is conventionally used to describe dysmorphologies visible at birth; these may occur in 2 to 3% of infants. Various structural abnormalities can be found in up to 7% of the population at autopsy. The mortality rate among infants with congenital anomalies is high. Each year in the USA, about one-half million pregnancies end in miscarriage or in fetal or neonatal death as a direct result of congenital malformations. Survivors may have substantial defects, including incapacitating handicaps and severe impairment of organ function. Twenty to 30% of pediatric hospital admissions are for genetic conditions and birth defects.

Proper treatment of dysmorphic infants depends on an understanding of pathophysiology and an organized approach to diagnosis. This portion of the chapter describes mechanisms of teratogenesis and outlines a general and practical approach to the management of newborns with birth defects. Congenital abnormalities of specific organs are discussed in corresponding chapters as well.

INTERACTING MECHANISMS IN TERATOGENESIS

Congenital malformations can be caused by chromosomal aberrations, single-gene defects, mechanical stresses, and certain environmental agents (**teratogens**). Most birth defects are multifactorial, ie, they are the product of genetic, environmental, and developmental interactions. Single etiologic factors are recognized in only about 30% of cases.

GENETIC FACTORS

About 25% of birth defects can be directly attributed to single-gene defects and chromosomal aberrations. Although the phenotypes of several chromosome abnormalities are readily recognized, the mechanisms by which extra or missing chromosomes produce birth defects are not understood. Many single-gene disorders are also recognizable by the morphologic abnormalities they produce. In some of these disorders, abnormal morphogenesis is thought to be the result of alterations in structural proteins or enzymes have been identified. Genetic contributions to multifactorial disorders are more difficult to identify, but their presence is evident from studies in twins and from data documenting increased risk of recurrence in families of affected individuals.

ENVIRONMENTAL FACTORS

Epidemiologic studies consistently indicate that certain environmental factors (eg, season, residence, occupation, socioeconomic status, and exposures to drugs, chemicals, and environmental contaminants) increase the risk for congenital malformations. However, only a few specific teratogens have been identified. Animal studies of teratogenic mechanisms clearly indicate dose dependency. Therefore, it is important to consider levels of exposure to potential teratogens during pregnancy.

To be pharmacologically active, prescription drugs must be taken in high doses. Most drugs readily traverse the placenta and achieve pharmacologically active concentrations in the conceptus. However, extensive preclinical testing has led to the use of drugs that have a low potential for toxicity. Nonetheless, all drugs have a potential for adverse effects. Toxicity may be dose-related or idiosyncratic. Alcohol provides an example of dose-dependent toxicity. It is relatively safe at low doses in adults but is clearly toxic at higher levels. A similar spectrum is evident in the fetus. Idiosyncratic reactions occur at therapeutic concentrations but produce toxicity through unusual mechanisms. Idiosyncratic drug reactions in adults frequently result from genetically controlled differences in drug disposition or receptor interactions. Drugs that are frequently linked with idiosyncratic reactions in adults also appear to produce problems during fetal development.

Chemical contamination of the environment and exposures to natural toxins are also potentially teratogenic. Environmentally related cancer in adults suggests the potential for significant cytotoxicity during development. Most chemical carcinogens are also teratogens. Concentrations of these agents in the food and the environment are generally low but may be increased through inadvertent contamination of food or inadequate safety measures. An increase in exposure increases the risk for toxicity. Contamination of rice oil by polypropionated biphenyls produced dermatologic and central nervous system abnormalities in infants born to exposed Japanese and Taiwanese women. Contamination of food and the environment by methyl mercury has produced fetal neurotoxicity in Japan and Iran. Surveillance for adverse reproductive outcomes may be an important means of monitoring environmentally related toxicity in humans.

Not all teratogens are chemicals. Mechanical stresses, extremes of temperature, radiation exceeding usual diagnostic exposures, and infectious agents are also potential teratogens. The effects of congenital infections are discussed in Chapters 27–29.

DEVELOPMENTAL FACTORS

Each organ passes through a number of critical periods during its development (Fig 34–16). Interruption of normal development at any one of these stages is likely to produce a structural defect. The anlage for a single structure may be affected, but since critical periods overlap and there are important functional interactions between tissues. Genetic and environmental alterations may affect the development of several organs. At the cellular level, processes leading to cell death or to abnormal migration appear to contribute most significantly to structural defects.

Familiarity with human embryology is essential for an understanding of dysmorphology. Division of gestation into 5 stages allows a quick review of embryologically relevant events in individual cases. The first stage, preconception, includes the processes of gametogenesis and fertilization. New mutations occur during this stage.

The second stage, implantation, begins with fertilization and is complete by 13–14 days. During this period, the blastocyst invades the endometrium, and the placenta differentiates and begins to function. In humans, placentation precedes organogenesis. Although the trophoblastic tissues that separate maternal and embryonic circulation are readily permeable by most xenobiotics (compounds foreign to the biologic system), environmental exposures during this stage of development are not often associated with birth defects. The reason for this is unknown but could be explained by spontaneous abortion during implantation. Trophoblast failure may be a final common pathway for pregnancy loss from a variety of causes. Threatened miscarriage during this period may be an early manifestation of maldevelopment.

The third stage of prenatal development is organogenesis, extending from the second to the eighth week following conception. Most critical periods of organ formation occur during this stage; thus, most structural abnormalities can be traced to these or preceding weeks. While considerations of teratogenic mechanisms necessarily concentrate on this stage of development, it should not be assumed that adverse effects of environmental agents or genetic disorders are limited to this period.

The fourth stage, fetal development (weeks 9–38),

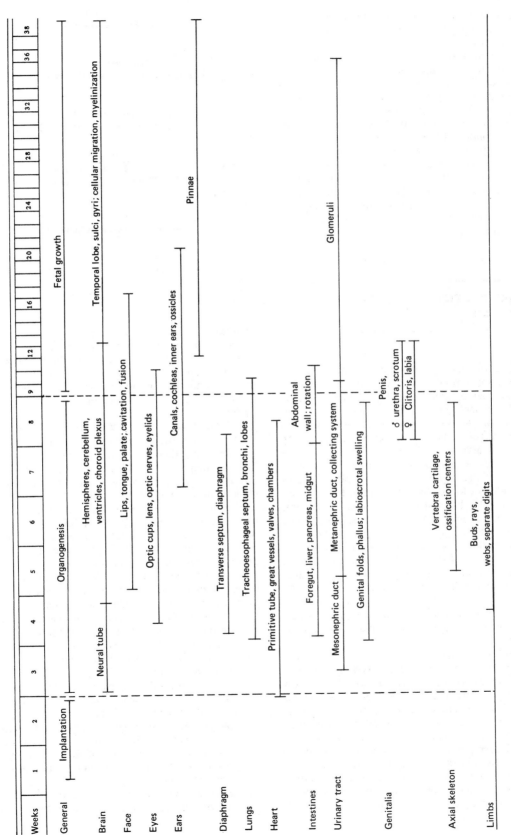

Figure 34–16. Critical periods in human gestation.

is the longest phase of human gestation. During this stage, cytotoxicity is less likely to be expressed as a structural defect but is not necessarily less likely to occur. Although organs are formed by this time, functional differentiation and growth occur during these weeks. This is an especially important period for the brain. Investigators in the field of behavioral teratology, which concentrates on this period, are just beginning to study relationships between events in fetal life and later brain function.

The final phase of intrauterine development is the intrapartum period. Fetal presentation at the time of delivery as well as route of delivery and any trauma sustained can affect morphologic features in the neonate. Many abnormal findings are related to molding of the head or the position of the extremities and are transient in nature.

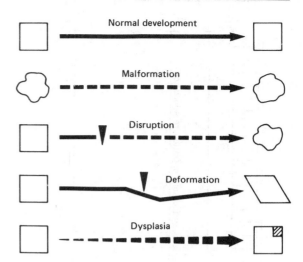

Figure 34–17. Etiologic classification of congenital anomalies.

CLASSIFICATION OF DYSMORPHIC FEATURES

Accurate diagnosis is the key to prognosis and management of birth defects. Recognition of specific syndromes and patterns of maldevelopment can be extremely valuable but is often difficult in the neonatal period. A dysmorphologist should be consulted, if possible, but classification of defects by etiology can also be useful and requires less firsthand experience than does recognition of specific syndromes. This approach to classification begins with an attempt to distinguish intrinsic from extrinsic causes on the basis of history and physical examination. Each anomaly found is then assigned to one of the etiologic categories listed in Fig 34–17.

Malformations are the result of intrinsically abnormal processes of development. The conceptus is abnormal from the outset of gestation, and malformations are generally attributed to genetic processes. The characteristic morphologic of Down's syndrome and the hypoplastic thumbs and pancytopenia associated with Fanconi's syndrome are classified as malformations.

Disruptions are the result of extrinsic processes. Development is perceived as proceeding normally when factors external to the conceptus interfere at a cellular level. Note that external factors need not be distributed in the general environment; they also include maternal factors. Drug-related embryopathies such as those associated with use of thalidomide are prototypic disruptions, but multifactorial processes such as neural tube defects are currently classified as disruptions despite their considerable genetic influence. The distinction between a disruption and a malformation may be difficult to discern on the basis

of form alone. Careful histories—especially family histories and cytogenic studies—are useful in this case. It is easier to establish the classification of malformation on the basis of a positive family history or abnormal karyotype than it is to rule out a disruption. Disruptions, however, are more common by far.

Deformations are the result of extrinsic mechanical forces. Deformations rarely involve internal organs but may range from minor malpositioning of limbs to major disturbances of the head and trunk. Intrauterine problems resulting in deformations include multiple pregnancies, abnormal uterine shape, fetal positioning, rupture of the amnion, and oligohydramnios caused by loss of or failure to produce fluid or by failure of the fetus to urinate. Deformations are characteristically asymmetric. Deforming processes may bend, cut, or fuse tissues.

Dysplasias occur as a result of abnormal tissue differentiation. In theory, extrinsic processes may be involved, but intrinsic, genetically determined factors are most often responsible. Dysplasias emphasize the link between cell function and morphogenesis. Examples include osteogenesis imperfecta (a disorder in which poorly ossified bone is easily fractured) and mucopolysaccharidoses (inborn errors of metabolism that result in growth deficiency, skeletal abnormalities, and unusual facies). Most dysplasias are the result of single gene mutations.

Etiologic categories imply prognoses. The presence of deformations, for instance, often means that the development and function of unaffected organs will be normal. When deformations are the result of neurologic abnormalities, however, the prognosis is poorer. Many dysplasias are not recognizable in the neonatal period. Those presenting at birth (eg, thanatophoric dwarfism) frequently have poor prognoses. Disruptions are probably the most common cause of birth defects and demonstrate the vulnerability of the developing human to extrinsic factors. Isolated disruptions, such as congenital heart defects, have excellent prognoses if repair is possible. Malformations are often multiple and, like dysplasias, often have poor prognoses.

Etiologic categorization also provides information about risks for recurrence. The highest risks are associated with single gene disorders, producing dysplasias and malformations. Most chromosomally mediated malformations occur sporadically, but careful cytogenetic analyses of family members may be required. Risks for recurrence are higher if parents carry balanced translocations. Disruptions also tend to occur sporadically, but many are the result of multifactorial processes with substantial genetic input. Empirical data indicate higher than normal risks for recurrence in relatives of infants affected with disruptions. Isolated deformations that do not occur as a result of uterine abnormalities have a low risk for recurrence.

MULTIPLE MALFORMATIONS

Many dysmorphic infants have more than one abnormality. Recognition of relationships between multiple malformations also provides important clues to etiology and prognosis.

A **developmental field** is a region or a group of cells in an embryo that responds as a coordinated unit to intrinsic or extrinsic stimuli. The pathogenesis of developmental field defects may involve functional disturbances in primordial cells, interactions among tissues, or processes common to multiple tissues. Disturbances of rostral mesoderm, for instance, may lead to multiple anomalies of the head and face. Genital and cardiac abnormalities may be related through disturbances in other organs such as the hypothalamus or vascular structures.

A **sequence** is a pattern of anomalies caused by a single event. Renal agenesis, for instance, results in decreased amniotic fluid, fetal compression, pulmonary hypoplasia, and limb deformation. This same sequence may occur as a result of loss of amniotic fluid or urethral obstruction. The sequence of micrognathia, glossoptosis, and cleft soft palate (Pierre Robin syndrome) may begin with mandibular hypoplasia, which pushes the developing tongue posteriorly so that it interferes with movements of the posterior palatal shelves.

The term **association,** when used to describe multiple anomalies, refers to their nonrandom occurrence outside any known developmental field. It denotes statistical but not necessarily causal relationships. The pathogenesis may involve both developmental field defects and sequences. Knowledge of associations is useful because it alerts the clinician to investigate other specific organs further if a defect is recognized in one.

The term **syndrome** is applied to patterns of multiple anomalies that recur with such regularity that they are considered to be pathogenetically related. Down syndrome and Turner's syndrome are disorders with morphologic features found in individuals with specific chromosomal abnormalities: trisomy 21 and 45,X karyotype, respectively.

DYSMORPHIC PATTERNS IN NEONATES

The following are examples of patterns of maldevelopment recognizable in the neonate. Numerous other patterns have been described in older children. Photographs of these entities are available in Jones K: *Smith's Recognizable Patterns of Human Malformation.* Saunders, 1988.

Chromosome Abnormalities

Several chromosome abnormalities are recognizable in neonates. These include trisomies 21, 13, and 18 and monosomy X (Turner syndrome). Chromosome abnormalities should be considered in the evaluation of all infants with multiple anomalies.

Cornelia de Lange Syndrome

Cornelia de Lange's syndrome, a sporadically occurring constellation of congenital anomalies, has typical features that can be recognized in the newborn. Intrauterine growth retardation and characteristic facial features, including prominent eyebrows with central fusion (synophrys) and thin, downturned lips are invariable. These infants are hirsute, and limb abnormalities occur in over 50%. Hypoplasia of the hand and feet is common, but major limb reductions occur in 30% and frequently involve the ulnar, rather than radial, ray. One infant in 4 has congenital heart disease. No specific chromosomal abnormalities have been found. The immediate prognosis depends largely on the presence of congenital heart disease or respiratory failure. Subsequent failure to thrive and severe mental deficiency are the rule.

Meckel Syndrome (Meckel-Gruber Syndrome)

Meckel's syndrome is rare and is inherited as an autosomal recessive trait. Infants with this syndrome have encephaloceles, polydactyly, renal cysts, and a characteristic pattern of hepatic fibrosis. The prognosis is generally poor, owing to central nervous system and renal dysfunction. Central nervous system anomalies are variably expressed and range from anencephaly and holoprosencephaly to small encephaloceles. Oligohydramnios due to renal hypoplasia may lead to a sequence including pulmonary hypoplasia and clubfeet. The renal cysts are bilateral and typically small and uniform. They must be distinguished from the more commonly occurring multicystic renal dysplasia, which may be associated with other anomalies. Meckel's syndrome is often recognized only at autopsy.

VATER (VACTERL) Association

Vertebral anomalies and abnormalities of the heart, trachea, esophagus, kidneys, and limbs are found in association with each other and in association with anal atresia more often than would be expected by chance alone. The acronym VATER (*ver*tebral defects, imperforate *a*nus, *t*racheo*e*sophageal fistula, and *r*adial and *r*enal dysplasia) is sometimes written as VACTERL to include *c*ardiac and *l*imb anomalies. The limb defects seen are usually preaxial (radial or fibular). The association occurs sporadically. Although the anomalies themselves may be immediately or ultimately life-threatening, neurologic abnormalities are absent and the prognosis for intellectual development is good if the VATER association is recognized early enough for proper treatment to be instituted.

CHARGE Association

The CHARGE association, *c*oloboma, *h*eart disease, choanal *a*tresia, *r*etarded growth, *g*enital anomalies, and *e*ar anomalies, was recognized through nonrandom association of facial anomalies. More recently, maldevelopment within a developmental field involving neural crest cells has been suggested. The importance of recognizing this condition is that the central nervous system is involved and that hypothalamic maldevelopment may affect secretion of pituitary trophic hormones.

Amnion Rupture Sequence

Rupture of the amniotic membrane in early gestation may lead to loss of fluid and entrapment of the developing conceptus. Early rupture is often associated with major structural abnormalities that are incompatible with life. Later rupture may lead to complex deformations of the head and limbs or to amputation of structures by constricting amniotic bands. It may be difficult to distinguish these deformations from malformations unless the placenta is carefully examined for the presence of amniotic bands. If the head has escaped significant deformation, neurologic development proceeds normally. The amniotic rupture sequence occurs sporadically, and its recognition allows counseling for low recurrence risks.

Twins

Multiple pregnancies are at high risk for abnormal development. Crowding may result in deformations in both identical and nonidentical twins. In one sense, monozygosity itself is a ''birth defect,'' since it occurs after conception. Depending on the timing of division, placental circulations and amniotic sacs may or may not be shared. Division after day 13 of gestation results in conjoined twins. Despite genetic concordance, congenital abnormalities in monozygotes are frequently discordant. This observation demonstrates the role of environmental factors in multifactorial birth defects. Monochorionic twins are particularly at risk for abnormalities resulting from vascular accidents, since emboli are more likely to form in shared circulations.

Skeletal Dysplasias

Several distinct dysplasias of bone and cartilage produce a phenotype with short, curved, or malformed limbs. The head and trunk may appear normal in a few of these disorders, but more frequently there is a protuberant abdomen with or without ascites. Many of these dysplasias result in death due to pulmonary hypoplasia associated with small or poorly compliant chest walls. The differential diagnosis includes achondroplasia, achondrogenesis, osteogenesis imperfecta, camptomelic syndrome, asphyxiating thoracic dystrophy, thanatophoric dwarfism, and several other rare syndromes. Many are the result of new dominant mutations, but recessive inheritance must always be considered. Accurate diagnosis is extremely important and is best made radiographically. Films should be taken of all extremities. A lateral view of the spine, which may be critical to the diagnosis, should be obtained as well. The immediate prognosis depends largely on the extent of pulmonary hypoplasia. Long-term prognoses are variable.

DRUG-RELATED DISORDERS

Thalidomide is the classic example of a human teratogen producing a specific syndrome. The compounds discussed below are also associated with specific abnormalities. Regional teratogen information services can provide additional information.

Warfarin

The use of warfarin derivatives as anticoagulants during pregnancy was initially felt to be safe, but closer examination of exposed fetuses has shown untoward effects, including nasal hypoplasia, optic nerve hypoplasia, extraosseous calcification, and abnormalities of brain development and function. Central nervous system abnormalities can occur in fetuses exposed to warfarin during the second or third trimester of pregnancy, demonstrating the potential susceptibility of the brain to drug-related disorders during this period. Approximately 1 in 3 exposed fetuses is affected. Mechanisms appear to involve transplacental anticoagulation and hemorrhage as well as direct effects on cartilage growth.

Anticonvulsants

The relationship between the use anticonvulsant drugs and congenital abnormalities seen in offspring of women with seizure disorders is controversial and complex. However, there is now general agreement that exposures to these agents increase risks for maldevelopment. Significant abnormalities may occur as frequently as once in every 10 pregnancies in this population. Growth of the brain and midface are consistently affected. A recognizable "fetal anticonvulsant syndrome," initially described in association with phenytoin use, has now also been recognized in children exposed in utero to carbamazepine and valproic acid. Additional structural anomalies are also associated with exposures to individual agents. Maternal use of phenytoin has been associated with cleft lip and palate, hypoplasia of distal phalanges and nails, and sacral teratomas. Maternal use of trimethadione has also been associated with growth retardation, decreased mentation, and unusual facies (fetal trimethadione syndrome). An increased risk for neural tube defects has recently been linked to maternal use of valproic acid.

13-*cis*-Retinoic Acid

Excessive doses of vitamin A have long been recognized as teratogenic in animals. The potent vitamin A analogue 13-*cis*-retinoic acid (isotretinoin, Accutane) was therefore considered a potential teratogen when it was introduced as a treatment for acne. Despite warnings, some women have taken this drug during pregnancy, and several infants with multiple anomalies have been born. A specific syndrome that includes abnormalities of the central nervous system, ears, and great vessels along with hypoplasia of the thymus and parathyroid gland has been described. This condition is a phenocopy of the DiGeorge sequence that occurs as a contiguous gene syndrome related to microdeletions of chromosome 22. It is now clear that both isotretinoin and the deletion produce the same developmental field defect. The mechanism involves failure of cells to migrate normally from the neural crest to form structures in the head and neck.

Ethyl Alcohol

Admonitions against heavy use of alcohol during pregnancy have been given since ancient times. More recently, a specific syndrome has been recognized in the offspring of heavy drinkers. The fetal alcohol syndrome consists of intrauterine and postnatal growth retardation, microcephaly, significant mental dysfunction, and craniofacial changes including short palpebral fissures, short nose, and a long, smooth philtrum. A variety of other structural abnormalities has also been reported.

Although it is clear that high concentrations of alcohol are cytotoxic, the mechanisms of alcohol toxicity are poorly understood. The dose-response relationship is not entirely clear, but maternal alcohol intake exceeding 2–3 oz daily is considered toxic. The timing of fetal exposure to alcohol is important. Structural abnormalities occur with increased frequency in offspring of chronic alcohol abusers, but neurologic abnormalities can be decreased if women stop drinking by 16–20 weeks of gestation. Approximately two-thirds of pregnancies in active alcoholics will have significant complications, including prematurity, growth retardation, and perinatal asphyxia. Fetal alcohol syndrome is seen in about one-third of offspring of active alcoholics. The relationship of episodic maternal use of alcohol or paternal alcoholism to congenital problems is less well defined.

Cocaine

As use of cocaine has increased, its effects on pregnancy have become more evident. Stimulation of central and peripheral sympathetic nervous systems by cocaine can produce intense uterine vasoconstriction, leading to placental ischemia and abruption. Cocaine readily crosses the placenta. Increasingly reports indicate that it is also vasoactive in the fetal circulation and may lead to ischemic injury of fetal limbs, intestines, and kidneys. The central nervous system appears to be particularly vulnerable. Intracranial hemorrhage and porencephalic cysts have been reported in as many as one-third of infants born to women abusing "crack" cocaine in combination with alcohol and other substances.

CLINICAL APPROACH TO THE DYSMORPHIC INFANT

Physicians caring for neonates with birth defects must frequently provide care and make accurate diagnoses under conditions of great stress. The extent of an infant's abnormalities may not be immediately apparent, and parents who feel grief and guilt are often desperate for information. As with any medical problem, however, the history and physical examination provide most of the clues to diagnosis. Special aspects of these procedures are outlined below.

HISTORY

Environmental, family, and pregnancy histories may contain important clues to the diagnosis. In the postpartum period, frightened parents are attempting to cope with their grief and fears. Feelings of guilt are likely to be heightened during a review of the pregnancy history. Thus, the interviewer must be prepared to answer as well as ask questions.

Parental recall after delivery of an infant with an anomaly is better than recall after a normal birth. An obstetric wheel can help document gestational age and events of the first trimester: the last menstrual period, the onset of symptoms of pregnancy, the date of diagnosis of the pregnancy, the date of the first prenatal visit, and the physician's impressions of fetal growth at that time.

Next, it is important to investigate fetal growth and development. Prenatal visits should be noted and, with the aid of the obstetric wheel, a record made of the patterns of fetal growth, the onset of fetal movement (usually at 16 weeks), and the mother's perceptions of fetal movements. Although the degree of movement is variable, normal fetal movement is usually strong enough to hurt the mother and be visible to the father. Abnormal fetal movement may indicate neuromuscular dysfunction or fetal constraint. These are particularly important when asphyxia accompanies the birth of a dysmorphic infant. A history of decreased fetal movement will distinguish neuromuscular abnormalities (which result in a low Apgar score) from intrapartum events (which depress the infant).

Abnormal patterns of uterine growth may also provide clues to fetal function. Increased uterine size may indicate accumulation of amniotic fluid (hydramnios). Fluid may accumulate if the fetus fails to swallow as a result of a neuromuscular disorder, obstruction of the fetal esophagus or proximal small bowel, or fetal heart failure. Hydramnios is also associated with diabetes and high output renal failure in the fetus. Lack or delay of uterine growth may reflect fetal growth directly or may indicate too little amniotic fluid (oligohydramnios). Amniotic fluid may be lost through premature rupture of membranes with or without formation of amniotic bands, or it may be the result of compromised function of fetal kidneys. The mother should be questioned about loss or leakage of amniotic fluid, which is often mistakenly perceived as a vaginal discharge. Information from prenatal ultrasound examination is often very helpful in distinguishing different entities associated with altered uterine growth.

The history should also include details about the onset and progression of labor. Breech presentation at term may indicate a uterine anomaly or abnormality of the fetal central nervous system.

Family histories, as described below, should always be included but may seem threatening to parents or relatives attempting to cope with strong feelings about birth defects. The interviewer should be prepared to respond to specific questions from family members.

Finally, an environmental history that includes parental habits and their work and home environments should be obtained. Maternal and paternal health, use of medications, and environmental exposures during the embryonic period should be reviewed.

Questions should be considered carefully because of their emotional impact. Society is currently preoccupied with the roles of drugs, radiation, and chemical exposures in birth defects.

PHYSICAL EXAMINATION

Meticulous physical examination is crucial to accurate diagnosis in dysmorphic infants. Delivery of an affected infant may necessitate immediate attention to potentially life-threatening problems, but it is precisely because intensive support may be required that a complete examination becomes urgent. The examination should be performed as soon as possible.

In addition to the routine procedures described in Chapter 3, special attention should be paid to the neonate's physical measurements (Fig 34–18). Photographs are very helpful and should include a scale of measurements for reference. The placenta should also be examined.

Since most syndromes occur infrequently in the general population and patterns of abnormalities are therefore difficult to recognize, an experienced dysmorphologist/geneticist should be consulted if possible.

LABORATORY STUDIES

Radiologic and ultrasonographic examinations can be extremely helpful in the evaluation of dysmorphic infants. In general, films of infants with apparent limb or skeletal anomalies should include views of the skull and all of the long bones in addition to frontal and lateral views of the axial skeleton. Chest and abdominal films should be obtained when indicated. The pediatrician should consult a radiologist for further workup. Nuclear scans and imaging by computed tomography, magnetic resonance, and ultrasound are all useful diagnostic tools, but their interpretation in the presence of birth defects may require considerable experience.

Cytogenetic analysis provides specific diagnoses in approximately 5% of dysmorphic infants who survive the newborn period. Chromosome abnormalities are recognized in 10–15% of infants who die. Karyotypes can be determined rapidly through analysis of cells in bone marrow. These allow limited interpretation and should always be accompanied by complete analysis of cultured cells. Any case requiring rapid diagnosis should be thoroughly discussed with an experienced cytogeneticist. The clinician should not base decisions about further workup and management on the results of only one test. A nor-

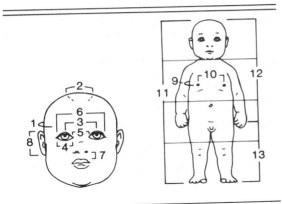

Measurement	Range (cm)	
	Term (38–40 weeks)	Preterm (32–33 weeks)
1 Head circumference	32–37	27–32
2 Anterior fontanelle $\left(\frac{L-W}{2}\right)$	0.7–3.7	. . .
3 Interpupillary distance	3.3–4.5	3.1–3.9
4 Palpebral fissure	1.5–2.1	1.3–1.6
5 Inner canthal distance	1.5–2.5	1.4–2.1
6 Outer canthal distance	5.3–7.3	3.9–5.1
7 Philtrum	0.6–1.2	0.5–0.9
8 Ear length	3–4.3	2.4–3.5
9 Chest circumference	28–38	23–29
10 Internipple distance*	6.5–10	5–6.5
11 Height	47–55	39–47
12 Ratio Upper body segment / 13 Lower body segment	1.7	. . .
14 Hand (palm to middle finger)	5.3–7.8	4.1–5.5
15 Ratio of middle finger to hand	0.38–0.48	0.38–0.5
16 Penis (pubic bone to tip of glans)	2.7–4.3	1.8–3.2

*Internipple distance should not exceed 25% of chest circumference.

Figure 34–18. Neonatal measurements.

mal karyotype does not rule out the presence of significant genetic disease.

PERINATAL AUTOPSY

When a dysmorphic infant dies, postmortem examination can provide important diagnostic information and should include sampling of tissue for cytogenetic analysis. The pediatrician and pathologist should consider whether samples of blood, urine, or tissue should be obtained for metabolic analyses. X-ray studies should be done whenever limb anomalies or disproportionate growth are present. Placental as well as from fetal tissue can be used for viral culture.

The pediatrician should discuss the case thoroughly with the pathologist, and photographs should always be taken.

IMMEDIATE MANAGEMENT OF THE DYSMORPHIC INFANT

Birth defects may be life-threatening. One physician should assume responsibility for overall care, but the skills of several other health professionals are usually required.

Vital functions should be supported until a thorough evaluation can be completed. When lethal or inoperable anomalies are recognized, humane and compassionate treatment directed at ensuring comfort should be provided. All neonates should be kept warm and given an opportunity to interact with their families.

DECISION MAKING

The birth of a dysmorphic infant is a highly emotional event and may raise difficult ethical and medical dilemmas. Modern medicine and technology now offer the potential to sustain life under extraordinary circumstances. Very often, the appropriate use of this capability is not immediately apparent. Society is currently agonizing over the dilemmas presented by infants with multiple anomalies, and it is clear that agreement on general principles does not always lead to agreement on what to do in individual cases. All decisions are best made in a supportive atmosphere by parents who are well informed and aware of the options open to them and who have been given clear medical recommendations. Most parents need both time and support from within their own community. A sense of the time available before a decision must be made should be given to the parents, and they should have an opportunity to discuss their feelings with supportive individuals. The infant's physician has an important role in this process but should not be the sole individual involved. Care of infants with birth defects requires access to medical, psychosocial, and ethical consultation.

Fabro S, Scialli A: *Drug and Chemical Action in Pregnancy.* Marcel Dekker, 1986.

Greenwood Genetic Center: *Growth References from Conception to Adulthood.* Proceedings of the Greenwood Genetic Center, suppl 1, 1988.

Jones K: *Smith's Recognizable Patterns of Human Malformation.* Saunders, 1988.

Niebyl J: *Drug Use in Pregnancy.* Lea and Febiger, 1988.

Wynne-Davies R, Hall C, Apley A: *Atlas of Skeletal Dysplasias.* Churchill Livingstone, 1987.

V. GENETIC COUNSELING

ISSUES

Genetic counseling is more than just a communication process about the risk for the recurrence of genetic disorders in a family. When families come for counseling, specific questions need to be addressed:

(1) What is it? An accurate *diagnosis* is the sine qua non of genetic counseling.

(2) What does it mean? For a family to make educated decisions concerning future pregnancies, they must understand the *prognosis* of the disorder. The birth of an infant with anencephaly is undoubtedly a traumatic experience, but caring for a child with a high myelomeningocele poses greater long-term stresses.

(3) What caused it? Determination of *etiology* is essential for correct counseling. The risk for recurrence of cleft lip and palate caused by amniotic bands is minimal, whereas the risk for recurrence of Van der Woude syndrome could be 50%.

(4) Is it curable or treatable? Possible *therapy*—its success, burden, and expense—need to be discussed.

(5) Will it happen again in future pregnancies? Only after the first 4 questions have been addressed can meaningful *recurrence risk figures* be given. At this time it is often necessary to review with the family some basic genetic information, showing pictures of chromosomes, explaining the difference between chromosomes and genes, and diagramming the more common mechanisms of inheritance.

(6) Can the abnormality be prevented or anticipated in future pregnancies? This question brings up the issue of *prenatal diagnosis* and other options available to the couple.

This may appear to be a formidable list of questions for the counselor to address, and answers may come from other members of the genetic counseling team and appropriate consultants. In addition, ongoing psychologic support is essential throughout the counseling process.

PROCESS

History

The cornerstone of a genetic evaluation is a thorough history, both of any pregnancy that resulted in an abnormal infant and of the family in general. Issues to be addressed in the pregnancy history include problems conceiving, bleeding, maternal illnesses or exposures, medications, smoking, the use of alcohol or any recreational drugs, possible exposures to teratogens, and lifetime histories of both parents' expo-

sure to x-rays. Information such as onset, intensity, and distribution of fetal activity may help to differentiate a prenatal from a postnatal problem. It is often helpful to ask if this pregnancy was "different" from others in any way. Information about the delivery should be obtained from birth records wherever possible. A family history should always be taken in a pedigree form. Parental ages, recurrent miscarriages, stillbirths, and infant deaths are all important. The possibility of consanguinity should be explored by asking for common family names and family origins. The general health and development of all first- and second-degree relatives should be ascertained. Information about ethnic background may be valuable. It is sometimes hard to know how extensive the family history should be. This depends to some extent on what may be suspected, but the major limiting factor is available information. Often, couples need to explore their family history in more depth and, in all cases, objective documentation should be sought when possible.

Physical Examination

The type of examination done as part of a genetic evaluation differs from others in that minor abnormalities are stressed as well as more obvious defects. It may also be necessary to examine parents, siblings, and even more distant relatives to make or confirm a diagnosis.

Laboratory Tests

The need for specific laboratory tests varies with the situation. Because these tests are expensive, they should be ordered with care but certainly done when important. Chromosomal analysis is indicated in any child with multiple major or minor anomalies, particularly if associated with mental retardation or development delay. High-resolution analysis or parental chromosomes may also be appropriate. Fragile X testing should be done in instances of mental retardation of unknown cause.

COUNSELING

Much has been written about directive versus nondirective genetic counseling, but in this country at least, the latter is recommended and more widely practiced. Although it is difficult to be totally objective, particularly if the geneticist is familiar with the long-term burden of a disorder, it is important to remember that the ultimate choice belongs to the parents. A geneticist may have concerns about society at large, but a counselor should be the advocate for the family and not for society. The timing of genetic counseling is also important. There is a fine line between counseling that is too early (because the family, still concerned about the welfare of the affected person, is emotionally unprepared) and counseling that is too late (because another at risk fetus has already been conceived). The possibility of a genetic etiology should be mentioned early, but ongoing contact is needed to delineate the diagnosis further and help the family understand the implications.

There are many ways to communicate information to the parents, but all explanations should be given in language that the family can understand and in a relaxed and unhurried atmosphere. The baseline risk for congenital abnormalities should be discussed and put into the perspective of the risk being quoted. The actual risk should be compared with the burden (or the parents' perception of the burden) of the abnormality in question. Examples can be helpful. The issues of guilt and blame must be addressed. This part of counseling can be difficult if one of the parents carries an abnormal gene or used a teratogenic substance, such as cocaine or alcohol. Ongoing psychologic counseling may be needed. It may be difficult for parents to understand how an isolated abnormality in a family can still be genetic and be associated with a significant recurrence risk; it may be necessary to review with them such concepts as phenocopy, new mutations, decreased penetrance, and variable expressivity.

All too often, no specific diagnosis can be made and no etiology can be determined. In these cases, recurrence risks can only be estimated. It may be helpful for families to explore possible mechanisms and for the geneticist to discuss with them the implications of each for subsequent pregnancies. In any case, parents should consider their own emotional response to the birth of a second affected child.

Genetic counseling is not a static process. Families often continue to have questions. A letter explaining clearly and concisely the information covered in the counseling session is helpful. Although a geneticist cannot assume responsibility for all problems that a family may have, appropriate referrals can be made. Ongoing contact is advisable to ensure adequate understanding and reopen counseling as new information and testing become available. A social worker, genetic nurse, or genetic associate who is a member of the counseling team is an ideal person to maintain contact.

A word should be said about responsibility to the extended family. As more genetic disorders become diagnosable by new molecular techniques, counseling needs to be expanded to the family at large. This requires both the cooperation of the consultand and collaboration between genetic units throughout the country. During counseling, it is necessary to educate families concerning this need and at the same time respect confidentiality.

OPTIONS

In situations of increased risk, families have a variety of options. They can have no further children or take the risk, but in many cases there are more and better choices. Some families for whom prenatal diagnosis is unacceptable or unavailable may prefer adoption. Artificial insemination is genetically appropriate if a disease is recessive or if the father is the carrier, and in vitro fertilization with donor ova may be possible if the mother is the carrier. Some families may consider sterilization, but they should realize that the risk for one of the parents may drop markedly if in the future that person takes another mate. For most families, however, some type of prenatal diagnosis is requested and often available. All of these options are expensive. Technology has outstripped society's responsiveness to the needs of these families. This problem must be addressed in the future.

PRENATAL DIAGNOSIS

It has been estimated that prenatal diagnosis is indicated in 7–8% of all pregnancies. As technology improves, the indications for and the accuracy of prenatal diagnosis can only increase. Today, a large proportion of pregnant women undergo at least one ultrasound study during pregnancy, and more congenital abnormalities are being detected prior to birth, even in low risk women. Prenatal diagnosis not only gives women the option to interrupt an abnormal pregnancy but also allows the physician to give optimal care during and immediately after delivery. As intrauterine therapy becomes feasible, prenatal diagnosis will become even more important.

METHODS

(1) Amniocentesis has been available for many years. Its accuracy and safety are well established. Fluid containing fetal cells is removed at 14 to 16 weeks' gestation. These cells are then cultured, and when adequate cell growth has occurred, cytogenetic and/or biochemical tests can be done. Studies such as alpha fetoprotein tests, predictive of neural tube defects, can also be done directly on the amniotic fluid. This is a safe procedure with a complication rate (primarily for miscarriage) of less than 1% in experienced hands. It is also readily available in many communities. There are two major disadvantage: (1) The test is not done until the second trimester, after fetal activity has been felt. The cells must be grown, which causes further delay before the results are available. This delay is emotionally difficult for the parents, particularly if they decide to abort the fetus. (2) It is difficult to get enough tissue for DNA studies.

(2) Chorionic villus sampling or biopsy (CVS) is now available in many centers. This test is done at 8 to 10 weeks of gestation. Since more tissue can be obtained, the cells can be examined or assayed directly, and results are available in a much shorter time. In addition, it is easier to obtain the required amount of tissue for DNA studies. To date, most CVS has been done transcervically, but the abdominal route may be preferred in the future. The complication rate in experienced hands is now under 5%, nearing 2%. This is the procedure of choice if DNA testing is indicated or if the risk for an abnormal fetus is high. If there is an abnormality, the parents have the option to terminate the pregnancy by a dilatation and curettage. At this time, however, the availability of CVS is limited, and it should be done only by experienced persons because of the potentially higher complication rate.

(3) The most commonly used prenatal test is ultrasound. At 18 weeks of gestation, it is now possible to view all major fetal organs, including the kidneys, heart, brain, spinal cord, bladder, and limbs. In addition, the finer structures of the eye, the vasculature, and digits are also visible. It is therefore possible to look for almost any genetic syndrome that is characterized by a structural defect. Although an abnormality could be missed and an unaffected child can never be guaranteed, many abnormalities are being detected by ultrasound in the second trimester. Routine ultrasound screening has demonstrated many unexpected abnormalities. Most of these are major defects, however, and minor anomalies are easily missed, especially if unexpected. In addition, procedures such as fetal blood sampling and skin biopsies can also be done under ultrasound guidance.

(4) X-ray studies of the fetus are rarely necessary because ultrasonography has improved so greatly. If a skeletal abnormality or bone dysplasia is suspected, however, x-ray films may be helpful.

(5) Fetoscopy has been done in the past to obtain fetal blood, biopsy fetal tissue, and visualize the fetus, but it has always been associated with significant morbidity. Fetoscopy has been replaced by ultrasonography in most cases.

INDICATIONS

Amniocentesis or chorionic villous sampling is indicated in the following instances:
(1) Maternal age over 35 years.
(2) Previous child with a chromosome abnormality.

(3) Either parent a translocation carrier. In this case, the risk for a fetus with an unbalanced chromosome abnormality is about 15% if the mother is a carrier and 5% if the father is a carrier.

(4) A history of any genetic disorder diagnosable by biochemical techniques or by DNA analysis. The list of such conditions changes daily, and a genetic center should be contacted for the most recent information.

(5) A request by the parents for fetal sexing because of a history of an X-linked disorder that is not diagnosable by current methods.

(6) Previous child or a parent with a neural tube defect. Unlike the indications listed above, for which either amniocentesis or chorionic villous sampling can be done, amniotic fluid is required in this case and therefore only an amniocentesis is appropriate.

(7) Either a high or a low value on alpha fetoprotein screening that has been confirmed on repeat testing. An elevated value is suggestive of a neural tube defect; a low one, of Down syndrome.

Fetal ultrasonography is indicated whenever an abnormality characterized by a structural defect is suspected.

FETAL SURGERY

Since fetal ultrasonography has become almost routine in many places, many unsuspected birth defects are being detected prior to delivery. In some cases, the diagnosis is made in the second trimester, and it is possible to terminate an abnormal pregnancy. Often, however, the defect is not suspected until 30 or 32 weeks. This has opened an entirely new field of fetal therapy for abnormalities such as hydrocephalus, but the results have been disappointing. Awareness of a fetal abnormality can be important for perinatal care. A mother may be transferred to a larger delivery center, where surgery for the newborn can be performed immediately. The timing of delivery may be influenced by the progression of hydrocephalus or bladder distention. This is a very difficult time for parents, however, and adequate psychologic support is essential. It is important for physicians and parents to realize that prenatal diagnosis has much to offer and that treatment of the newborn can be improved even if an abnormal pregnancy is continued.

SELECTED REFERENCES

General

Antonarakis, SE: Diagnosis of genetic disorders at the DNA level. *N Engl J Med* 1989;**320:**153.

Emery AEH, Rimoin DL: *Principles and Practice of Medical Genetics.* Churchill Livingstone, 1983.

Jones KL: *Smith's Recognizable Patterns of Human Malformation,* 4th ed. Saunders, 1988.

Kelly TE: *Clinical Genetics and Genetic Counseling,* 2nd ed. Year Book, 1986.

McKusick VA: *Mendelian Inheritance in Man,* 8th ed. Johns Hopkins University Press, 1988.

Specific

Collins FS, Ponder BAJ, Seizinger BR, Epstein CJ: The Von Recklinghausen neurofibromatosis region on chromosome 17: Genetic and physical maps come into focus. (Editorial.) *Am J Hum Genet* 1989;**44:**1.

Johnson JP: Genetic counseling using linked DNA probes: Cystic fibrosis as a phenotype. *J Pediatr* 1988;**113:**957.

Perruccello FW (editor): *Cleft Lip and Palate: Plastic Surgery, Genetics and the Team Approach.* Charles C. Thomas, 1987.

Riccardi VM, Eichner JE: *Neurofibromatosis: Phenotype, Natural History and Pathogenesis.* Johns Hopkins University Press, 1986.

Shurtleff DB (editor): *Myelodysplasias and Extrophies: Significance, Prevention and Treatment.* Harcourt-Brace-Jonanovich, 1986.

35

Diagnostic & Therapeutic Procedures

Ronald W. Gotlin, MD, & Anthony G. Durmowicz, MD

The optimal care of children requires that the physician be able to carry out a diagnostic and treatment plan in the most expedient manner. This objective is achieved only with an understanding of the specific procedures used in pediatrics as well as their adaptation according to the age of the child.

This chapter describes useful pediatric procedures that have proved effective. No claim of originality is made, and not all possible pediatric procedures are listed. It should be remembered that the need for a particular procedure needs to be weighed against the possible complications. An appropriate consent should be obtained prior to nonemergent, "invasive" procedures.

Finally, it should be added that this chapter is not a training manual and is not intended to substitute for personal instruction by those familiar with the techniques.

PREPARATION OF THE PATIENT & ORIENTATION OF THE PROCEDURE TEAM

It is essential in all diagnostic and treatment procedures, particularly in pediatrics, to orient the procedure team fully and to be certain prior to the procedure that all needed materials are readily available. This preparation includes the appropriate means of positioning and restraining the child. Unpreparedness and haste result in failure, increased apprehension in the child, and increased difficulty with subsequent attempts. Preparation should include providing a full explanation of the procedure to the parents or caretakers as well as an age-appropriate description to the child.

Patience and adequate preparation are also necessary when dealing with understandably anxious parents. A few words of explanation to concerned family members will be most reassuring. In general, procedures go more smoothly when parents are not in the procedure room. However, in the event that a parent wants to be present, forcible ejection from the scene may be associated with harmful effects both to the patient and to the procedure team, and it is usually advisable to allow the parent to remain under these circumstances. If parents are allowed to remain in the room, they should not be asked to become part of the procedure team or to play an active part in restraining the patient.

RESTRAINT & POSITIONING

The physician should be acquainted with various methods of properly restraining and positioning a patient. It is usually very difficult and sometimes dangerous to attempt any procedure on an unrestrained young patient. Before actually starting a procedure, the physician should be certain that all necessary items of equipment are available and arranged for immediate use.

Specially designed restraint devices (eg, "papoose boards") are commercially available. Following immobilization of any extremity, the fingers or toes should be examined for adequate circulation by noting the color and capillary filling of the nail bed.

When total body restraint is necessary, the physician must be certain before and during the procedure that cardiorespiratory function has not been impaired. A stethoscope may be taped to the anterior chest of the patient to permit frequent evaluation of cardiorespiratory function.

Local subcutaneous infiltration with procaine or lidocaine before performing a lumbar puncture, bone marrow aspiration, or thoracic, pericardial, or peritoneal aspiration is frequently necessary and advisable. Whenever drugs are employed, a history of previous reactions to the drugs should be ascertained, and equipment (suction apparatus, oral airway or endotracheal tube, laryngoscope, tourniquet, and epinephrine, 1:1000 solution) should be readily available to manage the rare but dangerous untoward reaction that may occur.

After any procedure is performed, the physician should personally observe the child long enough to be certain that no adverse reactions have developed.

DIAGNOSTIC PROCEDURES

COLLECTION & PROCESSING OF BLOOD SAMPLES

1. VENIPUNCTURE

The antecubital superficial veins of the hands, feet, and external jugular veins are used most frequently for venipuncture and withdrawal of blood. (See Fig 35–9). Venipuncture of the femoral and internal jugular veins may be associated with serious complications (see below), particularly in the newborn, and should be avoided if possible. In some instances, blood may be withdrawn from other peripheral veins. Large, accessible veins are best for purposes of injecting solutions and medications.

The skin should be cleansed thoroughly with an iodinated solution and alcohol. Gloves should be worn if there is a risk of blood-borne infections. Iodinated solutions should not be used when blood is to be tested for various iodinated compounds, and alcohol should be avoided when blood is drawn for alcohol levels. When blood is obtained for culture and for various tests, it should be put into media-containing tubes or bottles before being placed in vacutainer tubes, because the latter may not be sterile.

Antecubital Vein Puncture

If available, the antecubital vein should be used for venipuncture in children, infants, and newborns.

A soft elastic tourniquet is applied proximal (cephalad) to the vein and the venous pattern observed. Dilation of a vein may be facilitated by local warming in a wash basin or with warm, moist towels. Frequently, light palpation of the antecubital fossa reveals a distended vein not visible on the surface.

A short, sharp-beveled, 20- or 22-gauge needle (disposable syringes and needles are recommended) applied firmly to an appropriate-sized syringe is used.

The skin is entered with the needle at an approximately 10- to 30-degree angle with the bevel up. If gentle suction is applied to the syringe barrel, blood will be aspirated as the vessel is entered. Blood should be withdrawn gently and rapidly to avoid clotting and hemolysis. In a struggling patient, the use of a needle and catheter (eg, butterfly assembly) attached to the syringe will lessen leverage between the vein and needle. When the required quantity of blood has been obtained, the tourniquet is released and the needle withdrawn quickly. After the needle is removed, a dry sterile cotton ball is applied with pressure over the puncture site and held for approximately 3 minutes or until any evidence of bleeding has subsided. To avoid excessive hemolysis, the needle should be removed from the syringe and the stopper taken out of vacuum tubes prior to expelling the blood from the syringe into the specimen tube. Needles should be disposed of in appropriate containers to reduce the risk of injury or spread of contagious diseases.

Puncture of Superficial Dorsal Veins of the Hand & Wrist

The superficial dorsal veins of the hand and wrist are particularly readily accessible for diagnostic venipuncture in the newborn infant. After thorough preparation of the skin, a 22-gauge needle, preferably with a clear hub, can be inserted into the vein. Blood will be seen to flow into the hub and can be easily collected into capillary or specimen tubes.

External Jugular Vein Puncture (Fig 35–1)

Wrap the child firmly so that arms and legs are adequately restrained. The wraps should not extend higher than the shoulder girdle. Place the child on a flat, firm table so that both shoulders are touching the table; the head is rotated fully to one side and extended partly over the end of the table so as to stretch the vein. Adequate immobilization is essential.

Use a very sharp 20- or 22-gauge needle or a 21-gauge scalp vein needle with attached catheter (needle is shown in Fig 35–4) for withdrawing blood. The child should be crying and the vein distended when entered. First thrust the needle just under the skin; then enter the vein. Pull constantly on the barrel of the syringe and be certain that air is not drawn into the vein during aspiration.

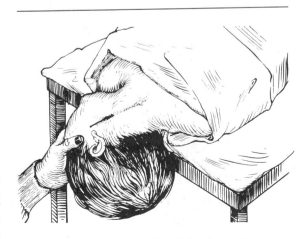

Figure 35–1. External jugular vein puncture.

After removing the needle, exert firm pressure over the vein for 3–5 minutes while the child is in a sitting position.

The next 2 procedures can result in significant complications, particularly in the newborn infant, and should be performed by someone skilled in their techniques.

Femoral Vein Puncture (Fig 35–2)

This is a hazardous procedure, particularly in the newborn, and should be employed only in emergencies.

Place the child on a flat, firm table. Abduct the leg so as to expose the inguinal region. Locate the femoral artery by its pulsation. The vein lies immediately medial to it. Be certain of the position of the femoral pulse at the time of puncture. Prepare the skin carefully with an antiseptic solution and carry out the procedure using strict sterile precautions. Insert a short-beveled, 21- or 22-gauge needle into the vein (perpendicularly to the skin) about 3 cm below the inguinal ligament; use the artery as a guide. If blood does not enter the syringe immediately, withdraw the needle slowly, gently drawing on the barrel of the syringe; the needle sometimes passes through both walls of the vein, and blood is obtained only when the needle is being withdrawn. Use a large enough syringe to produce adequate suction to assist in withdrawing the blood.

After removing the needle, exert firm, steady pressure over the vein for 3–5 minutes. If the artery has been entered, check the limb periodically for color, pulse, and perfusion for several hours.

Dangers: Septic arthritis of the hip may complicate femoral vein puncture secondary to accidental penetration of the joint capsule. Arteriospasm that has resulted in serious vascular compromise of the extremity, particularly in the debilitated and dehydrated infant, has been reported secondary to arterial puncture or venipuncture.

Internal Jugular Vein Puncture (Figure 35–3)

Prepare the child as for an external jugular vein puncture. Insert the needle beneath the sternocleidomastoid muscle at a point marking the junction of its lower and middle thirds. Aim at the suprasternal notch and advance the needle until the vein is entered. Avoid the trachea and the upper pleural space. Alternatively, the needle may be inserted at the apex of a triangle formed by the clavicle and the sternal and clavicular segments of the sternocleidomastoid muscle and advanced toward the ipsilateral nipple.

If no blood is obtained on inserting the needle, withdraw slowly and continue to pull gently on the barrel of the syringe. Not infrequently, the needle passes through both walls of the vein, and blood is obtained only when the needle is being withdrawn.

After completing the procedure, remove the needle and exert firm pressure over the area for 3–5 minutes with the child in a sitting position so as to reduce pressure in the vein.

Dangers: When the procedure is properly performed, complications are rare. However, deep, careless probing may lead to puncture of the internal carotid artery or injury to the trachea, vagus nerve, or pleura, resulting in pneumothorax or hemothorax.

Cote CJ et al: Two approaches to cannulation of a child's internal jugular vein. *Anesthesiology* 1979;**50**:371.

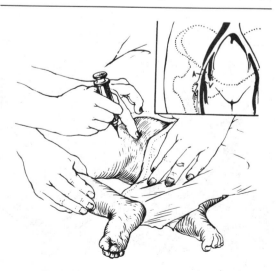

Figure 35–2. Femoral vein puncture.

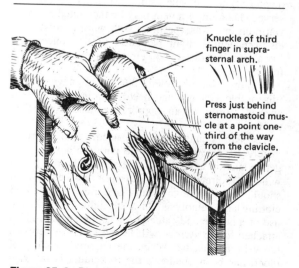

Knuckle of third finger in suprasternal arch.

Press just behind sternomastoid muscle at a point one-third of the way from the clavicle.

Figure 35–3. Direction of needle for internal jugular vein puncture.

2. COLLECTION OF CAPILLARY BLOOD

The majority of determinations may be made on blood obtained from a finger- or heelstick. An expertly performed heelstick is much less traumatic for a small infant than is a femoral puncture and has the additional advantage that it may be repeated frequently and does not have the same risk of complications. The earlobe is not a satisfactory site, because puncture here may be associated with excessive bleeding that may be relatively difficult to control.

After the skin is cleaned with alcohol, a stab is made with either a No. 11 Bard-Parker blade or a lancet. Free-flowing blood is collected in capillary tubes.

Frequent wiping of the puncture site with a dry swab may be necessary to prevent clotting and to ensure good blood flow. Collection of capillary blood may be difficult, and proficiency may be gained only after prolonged practice. Hemostasis can be obtained by applying pressure with a sterile cotton ball. The site of puncture should be examined several times during the next 1–2 hours for evidence of oozing or ecchymoses. A rare complication of this procedure is the development of osteomyelitis of the calcaneus as a result of puncture by the lancet. Because of the shallow depth of the calcaneus in small infants, premature newborns are at particular risk for this complication.

3. COLLECTION OF MULTIPLE SPECIMENS OF BLOOD

When a number of blood samples must be obtained over a short period of time (eg, when glucose and electrolyte determinations are needed for a diabetic patient with ketoacidosis), multiple venipunctures may be avoided by employing a pediatric scalp vein catheter (butterfly needle) or an indwelling 22-gauge or larger Teflon intravenous catheter. The catheter and stylet are inserted in an arm or hand vein in the usual manner. When the stylet is removed, the catheter hub is attached by means of a male Luer adapter to a reservoir filled with heparinized saline (10 units/mL) or, alternatively, to a 3-way stopcock. Blood may be withdrawn at intervals by applying a tourniquet to the extremity and inserting a needle attached to a syringe through the sterilely prepared rubber port or by opening the stopcock and drawing off and discarding the saline solution. A second needle and syringe are then used to collect the blood specimen. The tourniquet is removed, and the heparin lock and catheter are subsequently cleared by injecting heparinized saline through the rubber port.

4. ARTERIOPUNCTURE

Arteriopuncture is routinely employed in obtaining blood for blood gas determinations essential in monitoring many patients with cardiopulmonary disease. The radial, brachial, temporal, dorsalis pedis, and posterior tibial arteries are punctured most readily; the umbilical artery may be used in the newborn period. The femoral artery should be employed only in extreme emergencies.

Procedure

A. Radial and Brachial Arteries: The radial artery is the site of choice for obtaining arterial blood. It is relatively immobile in its position at the wrist, and because it does not course with an accompanying vein, erroneous sampling of venous blood will not easily occur. The right radial artery in the newborn has the advantage of providing preductal arterial blood samples. If the brachial artery is selected, it is entered either in the antecubital fossa or just proximal to the antecubital fossa along the anteromedial aspect of the arm. An effort should be made to maintain constant inspired oxygen delivery for the child or newborn receiving supplemental oxygen. A syringe fitted with a suitable needle (25-gauge for newborns and younger children to 22-gauge for adolescents) is flushed with heparin (200 units/mL), allowing a small amount to remain in the "dead space" of the syringe. A butterfly needle may be more useful in a struggling child. The wrist is supported slightly dorsiflexed and supine. The radial artery is located by palpation, and the overlying skin is cleaned first with an iodine-containing solution and then with alcohol. In the infant or edematous patient, a doppler probe may be useful for locating the course of the artery.

The needle is inserted into the artery at a 30- to 45-degree angle, and blood is withdrawn into the syringe. When a butterfly needle is used, pulsatile flow of blood can be observed in the tubing. After the pulsatile flow of bright red blood has cleared the tubing of solution, the syringe is connected and the sample collected. To avoid hematoma formation, firm pressure is applied for at least 5 minutes after specimen withdrawal.

B. Posterior Tibial Artery: The posterior tibial artery is relatively constant in its position between the medial malleolus and the Achilles tendon. Careful palpation will identify its course. Care should be taken to avoid the Achilles tendon.

C. Dorsalis Pedis Artery: The dorsalis pedis artery can be palpated along the dorsum of the foot and can be safely entered for sampling.

D. Branches of the Superficial Temporal Artery: These branches may be used for arterial sampling but not for indwelling catheters, which have been associated with cerebral thromboembolism and infarction. Either the frontal or parietal branch of the temporal artery is located by palpation. Overlying hair is shaved and the skin suitably cleansed. The palpating fingers partially immobilize the artery while the heparin-filled scalp vein needle is inserted with the bevel up (Fig 35–4). The needle is advanced until the artery is entered.

Dangers: Arterial punctures may be hazardous because of the risks of laceration, spasm, hematoma formation, and damage to adjacent structures. Septic arthritis may complicate inadvertent hip joint penetration deep in a femoral artery puncture. Damage to the median nerve may occur with repeated brachial artery blood sampling. Firm pressure should be applied for at least 10–15 minutes after withdrawal of the blood specimen to avoid hematoma formation. Temporary or persistent arteriospasm with serious vascular compromise may occur, leading to sloughing of the skin. Distal obstruction of an artery due to the inadvertent injection of clots into the vessel during arteriopuncture has been reported. Arteriospasm may be relieved by the application of heat or by the subcutaneous administration of 2% procaine proximal to the site of puncture.

Schlueter MA et al: Blood sampling from scalp arteries in infants. *Pediatrics* 1973;**51**:120.

UMBILICAL VESSEL CATHETERIZATION

The use of an indwelling catheter in an umbilical artery or vein has become a common procedure in hospital nurseries. Catheterization of the artery generally provides a more useful source of diagnostic information and is safer than catheterization of the umbilical vein. The umbilical vessels are employed to obtain reliable arterial access for sampling and pressure monitoring, to administer fluids and electrolytes, and to perform exchange transfusions. The risks of umbilical vessel catheterization are significant. Transcutaneous blood gas measurements, doppler ultrasound blood pressure measurements, and other noninvasive procedures should be substituted whenever possible.

Procedure

The catheter should be made of flexible, nontoxic radiopaque material that will not kink when advanced through a vessel and will not collapse during blood withdrawal. Nonwettable material and a single, smooth-surfaced end hole reduce clot formation. A 3.5-gauge catheter is used for infants weighing less than 1500 g and a 5-gauge for larger infants. Dead space of the catheter system should be determined prior to catheterization.

The infant is warmed (preferably under an overhead radiant heater) and loosely restrained. The procedure is carried out under sterile conditions.

A standard cut-down tray is opened, and the wide end of the umbilical artery catheter is cut off so that the blunt needle adapter fits snugly into the catheter. Discarding the wide end and utilizing the needle adapter reduces the catheter capacity. A sterile syringe is filled with flushing fluid (eg, heparinized saline) and attached to a 3-way stopcock and, in turn, to the umbilical catheter. The entire system is filled with flushing fluid.

An assistant may elevate the umbilical cord by the cord clamp while the operator prepares the cord and adjacent skin with 1% iodine solution, which should then be removed with alcohol to prevent an iodine burn of the skin. All areas of the skin should be inspected for the presence of iodine solution. The area is then draped. A loop of umbilical tape is placed at the base of the umbilical cord and tied loosely in order to control bleeding if necessary. The cord is then cut 1–1.5 cm above the skin with scissors or a scalpel blade.

The 2 thick-walled, round arteries and the single, thin-walled vein are identified. The rim of the cut vessel is grasped with a pointed forceps. The lumen of the vessel is then dilated with the tips of the forceps. Initially, the lumen may allow only one tip to enter. Both tips may then be inserted and allowed to spread, further dilating the vessel. The fluid-filled catheter is inserted into the lumen of the artery or vein and advanced. Any obstruction to advancement usually can be overcome by steady, gentle pressure. Forceful probing may lead to increased arteriospasm in the artery or perforation of the vein or artery. If the obstruction in one of the arteries cannot be over-

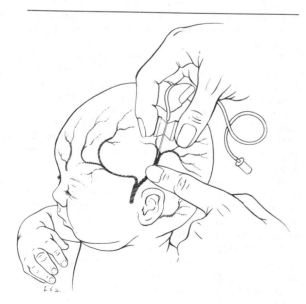

Figure 35–4. Scalp arteries suitable for blood sampling in infants. Note that the artery is palpated during cannulation to help immobilize the artery.

come, the catheter should be removed and an attempt made to catheterize the other umbilical artery. If a similar obstruction occurs, 0.1–0.2 mL of 1% or 2% lidocaine without epinephrine is instilled into the artery, and after 2–3 minutes the catheter can usually be advanced.

Frequent aspiration will demonstrate blood return. In arterial catheterization, the tip may be left at the level of the third to fifth lumbar vertebrae or the tenth to twelfth thoracic vertebrae (below and above the renal arteries, respectively). Position of the catheter is determined by both anteroposterior and lateral x-rays. The catheter is tied in place by a pursestring suture at the base of the umbilical cord, with the ends of the suture secured to the catheter and the catheter taped to the abdomen.

Complications

The principal complications of umbilical artery catheterization are thrombosis, embolism, and vasospasm. Portal vein thrombosis with subsequent development of presinusoidal portal hypertension may complicate umbilical vein catheterization. Infection and accidental disconnection of the catheter system may complicate either umbilical artery or vein catheterization. Thrombogenic complications of umbilical artery catheterization may result in paraplegia, infarction of the kidneys or bowel, gangrene of the buttocks or lower extremities, and renal hypertension in later childhood.

Adelman RD: Neonatal hypertension. *Pediatr Clin North Am* 1978;**25**:99.

Mokrohisky ST et al: Low positioning of umbilical-artery catheters increases associated complications in newborn infants. *N Engl J Med* 1978;**299**:561.

Moore TD (editor): *Iatrogenic Problems in Neonatal Care: Sixty-Ninth Ross Conference on Pediatric Research.* Ross Laboratories, 1976.

Wesström G: Umbilical artery catheterization in newborns: Clinical follow-up study. *Acta Paediatr Scand* 1980; **69**:371.

URINE COLLECTION

Attached Receptacle Method

A pediatric urine collector (a Sterilon product)—a plastic bag with a round opening surrounded by an adhesive surface that adheres to the skin—may be used. If a specimen is to be used for culture, the genitalia should be scrupulously cleansed with soap and water and benzalkonium chloride solution. In the male, the penis is placed in the plastic bag and the adhesive surface is applied to the surrounding skin. In the female, the opening of the bag is placed around the external genitalia. After voiding occurs, the bag is removed and emptied of urine. For collection of a 24-hour specimen, bags with a catheter outlet from which urine may be periodically removed are commercially available.

Clean-Catch Method

The "clean-catch" technique is a useful method for urine collection in toilet-trained children. The male prepuce and glans of the penis or the opening of the female urethra and external vaginal vestibule are cleansed with benzalkonium chloride-soaked cotton balls. (In uncircumcised males, the foreskin should first be retracted.) The benzalkonium chloride should be removed with sterile water. An uninterrupted midstream clean-catch specimen can then be obtained and sent to the laboratory.

Catheterization of the Urinary Bladder

Catheterization is necessary to obtain a sterile urine specimen from a child who cannot produce a clean catch sample or when continuous measurement of urine output is needed. When it is used, sterile technique, including the use of sterile gloves and towels and adequate antiseptic preparation with hexachlorophene and benzalkonium chloride, should be employed.

If catheterization is necessary, catheters measuring 3–6 mm in diameter are usually satisfactory for most patients. A No. 5 feeding tube may be used for all age groups beyond the newborn period. Catheters made of inert Silastic- or Teflon-coated materials are preferred. They may be either straight or indwelling. The latter are double lumen tubes with an inflatable balloon near the distal opening. When the balloon is inflated, removal is prevented until the bulb is deflated. This type of catheter is employed when continuous urine collection is necessary. If a retention catheter is employed, a closed drainage system should be used to reduce the risk of infection.

The patient is placed supine on a bed or table and immobilized and restrained when necessary. The skin is cleansed, and the catheter is inserted into the external urethra. In the male, the penis is held initially at a right angle to the body. In the female, the labia majora and minora are widely separated. The female urethra is somewhat C-shaped and is more easily traversed than the relatively acute-angled male urethra. Continue to thread the catheter gently until urine flow is obtained. Allow the first aliquot of urine to drain out of the catheter. Collect subsequent urine for culture. If a Foley catheter is used, inflate the balloon with the appropriate volume of normal saline solution (the volume is written on the catheter); inflation is through a one-way valve in the side-arm tubing. Pull back on the catheter to test that the balloon is in the bladder and that the catheter is secured. Tape the tubing to the thigh and attach the sterile collection unit and tubing. Trauma to the urethra or bladder can be minimized by using a catheter of the proper size and by gentle technique.

To prevent phimosis in male patients, remember to return the foreskin to its normal position after catheter insertion. Some authorities recommend use of a single dose of a urinary tract antibiotic (eg, nitrofurantoin, 2 mg/kg) following in-and-out catheterization in an attempt to prevent infection resulting from the possible introduction of bacteria into the bladder during the procedure.

Suprapubic Percutaneous Bladder Aspiration

This method is useful when a sterile urine sample is necessary—particularly in the newborn infant, in whom the bladder is high and easily accessible. This method is indicated in selected cases but does not lend itself to routine use.

The bladder *must* be full before the procedure is attempted and should be enlarged to palpation or percussion above the os pubis before an attempt is made to aspirate urine. Local anesthesia may be used but is generally not necessary.

A. Procedure:

1. Prepare the skin carefully with an antiseptic solution, using strict sterile precautions, while an assistant holds the child either in the frog-leg position or with thighs and hips together.

2. Firmly insert a sterile 22- or 25-gauge (for newborns) needle attached to a syringe through the skin and abdominal muscle in the midline 1–2 cm above the symphysis pubis, with the needle perpendicular to the skin. Slight negative pressure should be exerted as the needle is advanced into the bladder. The appearance of urine in the syringe will therefore indicate a successful tap. After the skin and anterior wall have been penetrated, the tip of the needle will be lying against the bladder.

3. After urine has been obtained, withdraw the needle with a single, swift motion and cover the area with a small dressing. Failure to obtain urine usually indicates either that the bladder was not full or that the needle did not enter the bladder but passed to one side. The procedure may be repeated.

B. Dangers: When the procedure is performed as outlined above, complications are uncommon but include transient hematuria, abdominal wall abscess, and penetration of the bowel.

COLLECTION OF NASOPHARYNGEAL FLUID

Nasopharyngeal secretions are frequently collected for culture in cases of upper respiratory infection and for use in rapid diagnosis techniques (eg, fluorescent antibody test for respiratory syncytial virus, chlamydia, pertussis, etc). In the newborn period, removal of fluid from the pharynx is frequently necessary after birth; passage of a nasopharyngeal tube, De Lee suction apparatus, or wall suction apparatus allows removal of and is helpful in excluding choanal atresia.

Collection of fluid is easily accomplished with the use of an ordinary polyvinyl feeding tube to which either a syringe or wall suction device with a trap is employed for suction. The tube is introduced into either nostril and directed downward as necessary while gentle suction is applied. A few drops of nonbacteriostatic saline may be instilled in the nares before the procedure to lubricate the nasopharynx and loosen secretions.

GASTRIC ASPIRATION

Gastric aspiration may be indicated to remove ingested drugs or toxins, to relieve intestinal distention, or to diagnose esophageal atresia in the newborn.

Infants and children unable to cooperate are restrained in the supine position. A cooperative older child is best intubated in the sitting position, with neck and chin held forward without flexion or extension of the neck. When restraint is necessary, the patient is placed on the left side after insertion of the nasogastric tube, allowing the stomach to assume a dependent position. When the danger of pulmonary aspiration is present (ie, toxic ingestions), the patient should be placed with the head in a dependent position while gastric aspiration is being carried out. In ingestions, use a large-bore orogastric tube (Ewald). If there is danger of aspiration, the patient should be intubated with an inflated cuffed orotracheal or endotracheal tube in place.

The desired tube length is determined by measuring the distance from the patient's nose to the xiphoid process and adding 10 cm. This point is marked on the tube, and another mark is made approximately 15 cm distal to that point for reference. The tube is lubricated and introduced into one nasal passage and directed posteriorly while the tip of the nose is held up (Fig 35–5). The tube is then ad-

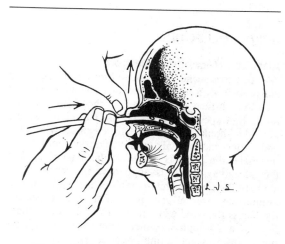

Figure 35–5. Inserting the nasogastric tube.

vanced for a distance of 5–7.5 cm as the patient swallows water. If the tube coils, it is best to remove it entirely and start over. To minimize coiling, the tube may be made stiff by prior cooling in ice. After passage of the tube, aspiration with a syringe is attempted. If gastric fluid is not obtained, a bolus of air is introduced while an assistant auscultates over the area of the stomach. A characteristic "gurgling" noise heard by the second observer will indicate that the stomach has been intubated properly; coughing indicates that the patient's respiratory tract has been intubated inadvertently.

The tube may have to be relocated by passing it farther or by withdrawing it 2.5–5 cm.

When prolonged intubation is necessary, the tube is secured to the cheekbone or forehead with nonirritating tape.

As an alternative, the oral route may be used and is preferable in the newborn.

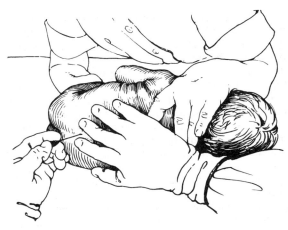

Figure 35–6. Restraining the infant for lumbar puncture with assistance of nurse. (Drapes omitted to show positioning.)

COLLECTION OF DUODENAL FLUID

Bile, duodenal, or pancreatic fluid may be needed for diagnostic analysis. The Miller-Abbott tube with weighted metal tip and double lumen is introduced as described above for gastric aspiration, and the gastric contents are aspirated with the patient placed on the right side. The tube is advanced approximately 15 cm and the patient asked to remain in that position for 30–60 minutes. In this position, the normal stomach will pass the tube beyond the gastric pylorus and into the duodenum. Alternatively, a standard feeding tube may be placed in the stomach and advanced 1–2 cm/h while the patient lies on the right side. The appearance of bile and change in pH of the aspirated duodenal fluid or roentgenographic visualization of the metal tip verifies proper positioning of the tube.

OBTAINING SPINAL FLUID

The 4 procedures for the collection of cerebrospinal fluid are lumbar, subdural, cisternal, and ventricular punctures. Lumbar puncture is most frequently used for obtaining cerebrospinal fluid for diagnostic purposes.

Lumbar Puncture

The patient should be restrained in either the sitting or lateral recumbent position according to the preference of the operator. (Fig 35–6). There is some evidence, however, that respiratory compromise is less in the sitting position than in the flexed lateral recumbent position.

The needle should be inserted through the L4–5 interspace into the subarachnoid space. This point is marked by the intersection of an imaginary line

drawn between the iliac crests and the spine. The interspace above and below this may also be used. Sterile gloves are worn, the skin around this area is cleansed with iodine and alcohol solutions, and the area is suitably draped. Local anesthetic may be used.

With the operator comfortably seated, the 22-gauge lumbar puncture needle with stylet in place is inserted into the chosen intervertebral space in the midline and perpendicular to the plane of the body. The needle is directed toward the umbilicus, with the bevel of the needle parallel to the spine. In older children, a distinct "give" is usually felt when the dura is pierced. However, this may not be appreciated in newborns or in young infants. If in doubt, remove the stylet and examine the needle hub for the appearance of fluid.

When fluid is obtained and with the child quiet, the 3-way stopcock and manometer are attached and the stopcock opened. Pressure measurements are made before collection (opening pressure) and at the completion of collection (closing pressure). In addition, the presence of pressure changes with compression of the neck veins (Queckenstedt's test) is indicative of patency between the intracranial system and cerebrospinal canal.

After the closing pressure is obtained, the needle is removed with a quick deliberate movement and pressure applied for several minutes with a sterile sponge over the puncture site. Pressure measurements are meaningless in the struggling, crying patient.

Note: When fluid is obtained in the infant or child for glucose determination, a concomitant blood sugar should be obtained for comparison. Without such a comparison, a low cerebrospinal fluid glucose may be difficult to interpret.

A "bloody tap" may occur without obvious cause and is most likely the result of penetration of the needle into the anterior venous plexus of the vertebral body. The counting of red blood cells in the first and third tubes of bloody spinal fluid will help distinguish a traumatic from a nontraumatic tap.

Dangers: Herniations of the cerebellar tonsils may occur when increased intracranial pressure is present in the posterior fossa at the time of lumbar puncture; preoperative ophthalmoscopic examination of the retina may be helpful in indicating increased pressure. Increased intracranial pressure is not necessarily an absolute contraindication to the procedure if provision is made for neurosurgical management of possible complications. Introduction of chemical irritants and infectious agents should be avoided by the use of proper technique. Postspinal headache is common when large amounts of cerebrospinal fluid are removed rapidly or when leakage from the spinal canal into the subarachnoid space occurs. An analgesic may be required. The use of needles without stylets for lumbar puncture has been associated with the development of intraspinal dermoids resulting from the introduction of islets of epidermis into the subarachnoid space.

Subdural Puncture
(Fig 35–7)

Subdural taps are performed to confirm the presence of and remove a postinfectious or posttraumatic subdural effusion. The anterior two-thirds of the scalp are shaved and cleaned with iodine and alcohol solutions. The patient is restrained as shown. Draw the scalp taut to one side and insert a short 19- or

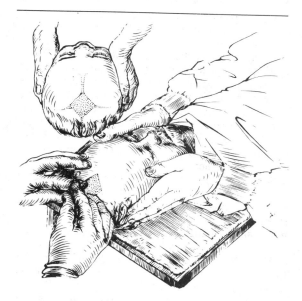

Figure 35–7. Subdural puncture.

20-gauge lumbar puncture needle with a very short bevel through the skin at the extreme lateral corner of the fontanelle or farther out through the suture line, depending on the size of the fontanelle. Release the tension and advance the needle for a distance of 0.2–0.5 cm. A hemostat clamped on the needle will prevent the operator from going too deep. Piercing the tough dura is easily recognized by a sudden "popping through" feeling. Normally, not more than a few drops (up to 1 mL) of clear fluid are obtained. If a subdural hematoma is present, the fluid will be grossly xanthochromic or bloody and more abundant. Repeat the procedure on the other side. Do not remove more than 15–20 mL of fluid at any one time and allow the fluid to drip from the needle without aspiration. Remove the needle, exert firm pressure for a few minutes, and apply a sterile collodion dressing.

If the fontanelle and sutures are closed, neurosurgical assistance should be sought.

Note: Hemorrhage may occur if the needle causes a laceration of a tiny vein communicating with the sagittal sinus. This may result in subsequent taps yielding xanthochromic fluid from the blood introduced during the preceding procedures. Fistulous drainage is prevented by covering the orifice with a sterile collodion dressing.

BONE MARROW ASPIRATION

Bone marrow puncture is indicated in the diagnosis of neuroblastomas, blood dyscrasias, metastatic disease, reticuloendothelioses, and "storage diseases" and is occasionally used for marrow culture.

Sites for Punctures

The sites that may be used at different ages are listed in Table 35–1.

The site of choice for children is the posterior iliac crest, because it is easy to locate and the child can easily be restrained in this position.

Procedure

For the performance of a posterior iliac crest aspiration, restrain the child on the abdomen with a rolled sheet placed under the hips. Sedation is often

Table 35–1. Sites for bone marrow puncture.[1]

Site	Age to Which Adaptable
Anterior iliac crest	Any age
Posterior iliac crest	Any age
Femur	Birth to 2 years
Spinous vertebral process	2 years and older
Sternum	6 years and older
Tibia	Birth to 2 years

[1]Reproduced, with permission, from Hughes WT: *Pediatric Procedures.* Saunders, 1964.

necessary for children. Prepare the skin surrounding the area as for a surgical procedure. Scrub and wear sterile gloves. Infiltrate with 1% procaine or lidocaine solution through the skin and subcutaneous tissues to the periosteum at a point 1 cm below the lip of the posterior crest.

Use an 18- or 19-gauge bone marrow needle in children and a 21-gauge needle in infants. Insert the needle with obturator in place perpendicular to the skin, through the skin and tissues, down to the periosteum. Push the needle through the cortex, using a screwing motion with firm, steady, well-controlled pressure. Some ''give'' is usually felt as the needle enters the marrow; the needle will then be firmly in place.

Fit a dry 20-mL syringe onto the needle and apply strong suction for a few seconds. A small amount of marrow will come up into the syringe. To prevent dilution of the marrow specimen by peripheral blood, no more than 0.5–1 mL of marrow should be aspirated. Marrow spicules should be smeared on glass coverslips or slides for subsequent staining and counting.

Remove the needle after replacing the obturator, and exert local pressure for 3–5 minutes or until all evidence of bleeding has ceased. Apply a dry dressing.

Bone marrow aspiration is a relatively safe procedure. Possible complications include infection and bleeding, e.g. in hemophiliacs.

COLLECTION OF FLUID FROM BODY CAVITIES

Thoracentesis

Thoracentesis is used in the removal of pleural fluid for diagnosis or treatment or in the emergency relief of a pneumothorax.

A. Site: Locate the fluid or air by physical examination and by x-ray or ultrasound when necessary.

B. Equipment: Use an 18- to 19-gauge needle with a very short bevel and a sharp point. The needle and a 10- or 20-mL syringe are attached to a 3-way stopcock (10-mL syringe is easier). If much fluid is to be removed, it can be pumped through a rubber tube attached to the sidearm of the stopcock, thereby avoiding leakage of air into the pleural space. A catheter with an external or internal needle can also be inserted; after the catheter has entered the pleural space, the needle is removed. This will lessen damage to the lung parenchyma.

C. Procedure: When possible, the patient should be in a flexed position and leaning forward against a chair back or bed stand. If too ill to sit, the patient can lie on the involved side on a firm, flat surface with an area of lateral chest wall extending over the edge of the procedure table.

Use strict sterile precautions, scrub, and wear sterile gloves. Prepare the skin surgically and use suitable drapes, preferably a large drape with a hole in the center. Infiltrate through the skin and down to the pleura with 1% procaine or lidocaine. A 3-way stopcock is attached to the aspiration needle, a section of rubber tubing is applied to the sidearm, and a 10-mL syringe is applied to the hub.

Insert the needle through an interspace, passing just above the edge of the rib. The intercostal vessels lie immediately below each rib. With gentle aspiration of the syringe, the needle is advanced a few millimeters at a time until the pleural space is reached. It is usually not difficult to know when the pleura is pierced: suction on the needle at any stage will show whether or not fluid has been reached. In long-standing infection, the pleura may be thick and the fluid may be loculated, necessitating more than one puncture site. To prevent accidental penetration of the lung after the needle is in place, apply a surgical hemostat to the needle adjacent to the skin. Pleural fluid is apt to coagulate unless it is frankly purulent, and an anticoagulant should be added after removal to facilitate examination. If a large amount of fluid is present, it should be removed slowly at intervals, 100–500 mL each time, depending on the size of the patient.

D. Dangers: Complications of this procedure include introduction of a new infection, pneumothorax or hemothorax from tearing of the lung, and hemoptysis. Careful sterile technique will decrease the risk of introducing infection. Insertion of the needle into a blood vessel, heart, liver, and spleen can be prevented by proper selection and positioning of the puncture site. Pneumothorax should not occur if care is taken to avoid advancing the needle beyond the point where fluid should be present.

If the patient starts to cough, the needle should be removed.

Pericardiocentesis (Fig 35–8)

Pericardiocentesis should be performed only by a practitioner experienced in the technique. The procedure is indicated for the diagnosis of purulent pericarditis or to relieve cardiac tamponade due to collection of large amounts of blood or other fluid.

A. Site: Several points for needle insertion are illustrated in Fig 35–8. The most common site used is at the chondroxiphoid angle. Echocardiography, fluoroscopy, and ultrasonography may aid in pericardial fluid location.

B. Procedure: The patient leans backward, restrained, at a 60-degree angle supported by bed or pillows. Using sterile technique, infiltrate the skin and subcutaneous tissues with 1% procaine. Connect a 50-mL syringe, 3-way stopcock, and 18-gauge needle. The V lead of an electrocardiograph machine attached with an alligator clip to the needle may be used to detect a current of injury tracing, should the myocardium be inadvertently entered. Insert the needle slowly at the lower border of the interspace just above the edge of the rib, directing it posteriorly and toward the spine. The needle is aimed posteriorly and upward when the chondroxiphoid approach is used. Aspirate slowly, and then turn the stopcock to discharge fluid via the rubber tubing. When fluid is being aspirated with ease, attach a surgical clamp to the needle next to the skin to prevent the needle from slipping farther.

The ECG should be continuously recorded and the needle pulled back if a current of injury pattern is observed. The blood pressure and pulse rate should be frequently recorded. The needle is removed in one quick movement at the completion of the procedure, and a dressing is applied.

C. Dangers: Cardiac dysrhythmias and penetration of the heart or coronary vessels have been reported.

Peritoneal Paracentesis

Peritoneal paracentesis can be used therapeutically to remove excessive fluid in cases of nephrotic syndrome or hepatic cirrhosis or diagnostically to seek evidence of blood or intestinal contents. In cases of known or suspected trauma, a puncture in each of the 4 quadrants of the abdomen may be made ("4-quadrant tap") in search of blood or intestinal contents. Infrequently, peritoneal paracentesis may be used as a diagnostic measure to obtain bacteriologic specimens in peritonitis, but this involves the danger of puncturing the distended bowel, which frequently is adherent to the abdominal wall. Electrolyte solutions, albumin, blood, and antibiotics may be administered by the peritoneal route. Peritoneal dialysis may be of value for renal insufficiency and in the treatment of certain poisonings.

A. Procedure: Use an 18- or 19-gauge needle with a short bevel and a sharp point. The skin is cleansed and surgical safeguards employed to avoid peritoneal infection. A local anesthetic is injected and a needle advanced along a zigzag course to prevent leakage. Enter at a level about halfway between the symphysis and the umbilicus in the lower quadrant or in the midline. The needle should enter obliquely to avoid leakage afterward. Ascitic fluid will flow out readily. Pus may require aspiration.

B. Dangers: Perforation of the intestine has resulted when the intestines are distended or adhesions are present. Perforation of the bladder has resulted when the bladder is not empty. The removal of excessive amounts or excessively rapid removal of fluid may result in circulatory embarrassment. Peritonitis from the introduction of infectious agents has been observed; "prophylactic" antibiotics are no substitute for proper surgical technique and are usually not indicated.

THERAPEUTIC PROCEDURES

ADMINISTRATION OF FLUIDS & MEDICATIONS

The administration of fluids and medications may be necessary in a number of clinical situations. The available routes of administration are as follows: (1) alimentary—oral, gastric (gavage or gastrostomy), duodenal, or rectal; (2) intravascular—intravenous or intra-arterial; (3) hypodermoclysis; (4) intraosseous; (5) intraperitoneal; and (6) intramuscular.

1. ALIMENTARY ROUTE

Oral, Gastric, or Duodenal

When available, the alimentary tract is the route of choice for the administration of all nutrients and fluids with the exception of blood. When the oral-gastric avenue is not competent, intubation of the stomach and duodenum is safe and easily accomplished.

Rectal

The rectal route may be used for diagnosis (cul-

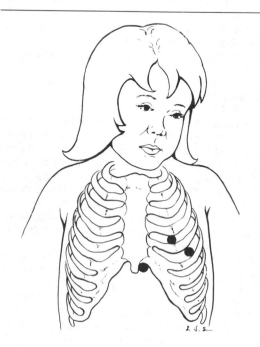

Figure 35–8. Sites of needle insertion for pericardiocentesis.

ture or roentgenologic examination with barium), for cleansing (fecal impaction), or for therapy (administration of fluids, electrolytes glucose, or medications).

Because the vascular drainage of the rectum does not enter the portal system, the liver is bypassed and administered fluids and drugs that are absorbed can enter the systemic circulation directly without hepatic conjugation or detoxification. The portal bypass may be avoided by administering fluids into the colon by high enema or colonic flush.

A. Procedure: The older patient is placed in either the left lateral recumbent or the knee-chest position. The small infant may be placed supine with legs flexed and elevated. A rectal examination should be performed initially to assume patency and to rule out the presence of a foreign body. A rectal catheter of appropriate size is lubricated and introduced beyond the anal sphincter. Fluids or medications (eg, anticonvulsants, aminophylline, ion exchange resins) are administered by the gravity method. The buttocks are held or taped together if necessary to prevent loss.

B. Dangers: Rectal perforation, particularly in the small infant, is not rare but can be avoided with the use of a soft rubber catheter.

2. INTRAVENOUS ROUTE

Intravenous fluid may be administered to infants and children by either a standard gravity apparatus or by a constant infusion pump. Fluids are best administered through a 21- or 23-gauge needle, however, the volume and required rate of infusion may dictate the use of other catheter sizes. In small babies, percutaneous insertion of very thin, flexible Silastic catheters may reduce the need for multiple attempts at insertion and complications of repeated skin and tissue trauma. *The rate of flow should be checked frequently.* An accurate record must be kept of the amount of fluid added. For small infants (particularly those who were prematurely born), never permit more than one-third of the daily fluid requirements to be in the container at any one time. It is advisable to remove the needle and change location each 48–72 hours to avoid phlebitis. If possible, avoid hypertonic solutions.

A. Site: (Fig 35–9.) For small infants, a scalp vein or one on the wrist, hand, foot, or arm will usually be most convenient. The superficial veins of the scalp do not have valves, and fluids may therefore be infused in either direction. In infants under the age of 2 years, these veins are easily visualized and can be distinguished from the superficial arteries of the scalp by palpation. Any accessible vein may be used in an older child. In infants and small children, a cool fiberoptic light source may be used for transillumination to demonstrate the course of the vein.

B. Procedure: The child should be positioned and the site for infusion immobilized. If an extremity is to be used, this should be taped to an adequately padded board. The skin is cleaned with iodine-containing solution and alcohol. When scalp veins are used, special care in cleansing the skin is mandatory, because they communicate with the dural sinuses. The dead space of a 21- to 25-gauge butterfly needle or similar gauge intravenous catheter needle (Medicut, Angiocath) should be filled with saline. A tourniquet is placed proximal to the site to enhance the distention of the vein. Warming in water or gentle percussion over the vein will increase its filling. The needle is introduced bevel up and parallel to the long axis of the vein at a point just beneath the skin. A characteristic ''give'' is perceptible, and blood usually flows back into the catheter. In the infant, venous pressure may be low and blood return not appreciated until negative pressure is applied with the syringe. The tourniquet is released and the flow tested by opening the intravenous clamp or by slowly injecting some saline. If there is no extravasation, the wing of the butterfly may be taped securely. Final restraints are applied when necessary and the flow rate adjusted. If a percutaneous needle catheter is used, the needle is inserted as described above. When blood is observed in the hub of the needle, the outer plastic catheter sleeve is gently ad-

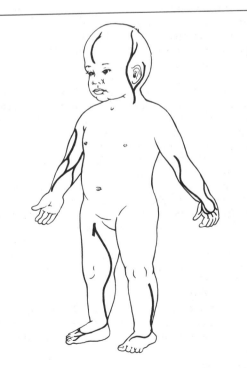

Figure 35–9. Superficial veins used most frequently for intravenous infusion.

vanced into the vein and the intravenous tubing connected. The plastic catheter is then securely taped in position.

Filston HC, Johnson DG: Percutaneous venous cannulation in neonates and infants: A method for catheter insertion without "cutdown." *Pediatrics* 1971;**48**:896.

Intravenous Cutdown

If fluids or intravenous medications are urgently needed by a seriously ill child and difficulty is encountered in entering a vein percutaneously, expose a vein surgically and tie a piece of polyethylene tubing in place or enter the vein subcutaneously with a plastic catheter equipped with an inner needle stylet.

A. Site: The internal saphenous vein has been found to be the most satisfactory site. Its position is constant, running anterior to the medial malleolus of the tibia to the groove between the upper medial end of the tibia and the calf muscle. It can be entered at any point along its course. The novice can easily identify it on his or her own leg first.

Other veins (external jugular, median, basilic, and cephalic) may also be used for cutdowns, but their courses are more variable and difficult to define.

B. Equipment:

1. Desired intravenous solutions.

2. A No. 4 or No. 5 French intravenous catheter or an 18- to 22-gauge needle within the catheter (eg, Medicut, Angiocath, or Jelco).

C. Procedure:

1. Preparation—Apply a tourniquet, cleanse the skin, and drape the leg as for a surgical procedure, using sterile precautions. The foot can be securely taped to a sandbag or board splint. Make a large wheal with 1% lidocaine solution in the skin over the vein.

2. Incision—With a scalpel, make an incision about 1 cm long just through the skin. The incision should be at a right angle to the direction of the vein. Using small, curved, sharp-pointed scissors or fine forceps, spread the incision widely.

3. Identifying the vein—The vein is usually seen lying on the fascia. Some dissection of subcutaneous fat may be necessary. Insert a curved clamp to the periosteum and bring the vein to the surface (Fig 35–10). Be certain it is a vein, not a nerve or tendon, by observing for the passage of blood. Using a small hook (eg, strabismus hook), dissect the vein free for a length of 1–2 cm. In small infants, the vein is small and fragile, and great care must be taken in handling it.

4. Placing ties—Using No. 000 or 4-0 black silk, tie the vein off at the extreme distal (lower) end of the exposed portion. Leave the ends of the suture long so that they may be used later for traction. At the proximal end of the vein, loop a piece of suture loosely around the vein.

5. Insertion and fixation of the catheter—Introduce the catheter with the stylet needle bevel

up. When the needle is in vessel lumen, hold the stylet stationary and gently advance the catheter. Withdraw the stylet and release tension on the proximal tie so that the catheter may be threaded and blood return ascertained. If there is no blood flow, remove the tourniquet and attempt to inject a small amount of intravenous solution into the vein. Watch for a wheal or extravasation of fluid, indicating that the catheter is not in the vessel. If the catheter flushes easily, remove the proximal ligatures and suture the plastic wings of the catheter hub to the skin. This can most easily be accomplished by placing a skin closure suture on either side of the catheter hub. Tie the suture, and then pass the free ends through holes provided in the wings of the plastic hub. Tie the suture again. This should hold the catheter securely in the vessel. Apply tape across the hub and tubing for further security.

When a needle or cannula is used, a pad of gauze under the hub will keep it in alignment with the vein. Cover the wound with gauze and roller bandage. Avoid restraint, which interferes with adequate circulation or causes pressure lesions.

3. INTRAOSSEOUS, INTRAPERITONEAL, & INTRAMUSCULAR THERAPY

The intraosseous route has again become a well-recognized, safe method of accessing the intravascular space. Intravenous fluids, cardiotonic agents, antibiotics, and even blood can be quickly infused in the critically ill child; availability to the systemic circulation occurs within seconds.

The most common sites for intraosseous infusion lines are the proximal and distal tibia. On the proximal tibia, the area just below and slightly medial to the tuberositas tibiae should be used; an area just proximal to the malleolus medialis is accessed when

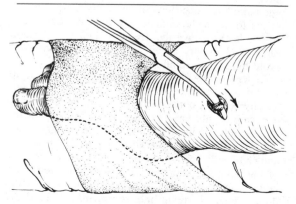

Figure 35–10. Isolation of vein for intravenous cutdown. (Drapes not shown.)

the distal tibia is used. The area should be prepared in a sterile fashion, with local anesthetic injected in the skin and periosteum if the child is conscious. Next, a needle with a stylet (18- to 20-gauge needle in an infant; 13- to 16-gauge bone marrow needle in an older child) should be firmly inserted perpendicular to the bone shaft, using a rotating motion. A characteristic "give" is felt when the bone cortex has been penetrated. Too great an applied pressure causes advancement of the needle through the opposite side of the bone, in which case an alternative site must be selected. If extravasation occurs, the needle should be withdrawn and another bone used as the infusion site. Aspiration of blood or bone marrow or the ability to inject sterile saline through the needle without evidence of extravasation confirms that the position of the needle is correct. There is usually slight resistance to fluid flow, and gentle pressure from an infusion pump or a syringe may be required to achieve adequate flow rates. Because of the risk of complications such as infection or extravasation, the intraosseous line should be used only until direct intravenous access is established.

Isotonic fluids and blood may be administered by the intraperitoneal route, but the intravenous route is generally preferred.

Intramuscular injections may be given into the upper outer quadrant of the gluteal area. With the child prone on a flat surface, locate the head of the greater trochanter of the femur and the posterior superior iliac spine. Direct the needle perpendicular to the table or bed in this space cephalad to the head of the trochanter. Other satisfactory sites include (1) the anterolateral aspect of the thigh (use a 2.5-cm needle), with the needle directed downward at an oblique angle toward the bone; and (2) the ventral gluteal muscles, to the center of an area outlined by locating the anterior iliac tubercle, placing the index finger on the tubercle, and extending the middle fingertip along the crest of the ileum as far as possible, forming a triangle. The needle is directed slightly toward the iliac crest. In infants and young children, the injected volume should be less than 2 mL; injecting larger amounts may lead to significant rhabdomyolysis.

EXCHANGE TRANSFUSION FOR NEONATAL JAUNDICE

After an adequate preparation of the infant (respirations and temperature stabilized and maintained, gastric contents removed, proper restraint), drape the umbilical area, employing sterile technique. Cut off the cord about 1.5 cm or less from the skin. Control any bleeding with umbilical tape. Identify the vein (the 2 arteries are white and cordlike; the single vein is larger and thin-walled). If the vein cannot be visualized in the cord stump, make a small transverse incision above the umbilicus, and cannulate the vein.

Selection & Amount of Blood

Employ sterile packaged equipment specifically prepared for this procedure (such as that supplied by Pharmaseal Laboratories).

Use freshly collected heparinized blood or blood preserved with anticoagulant acid-citrate-dextrose (ACD) or citrate-phosphate-dextrose (CPD). Blood should always be less than 3 days old and should be warmed before use. Give twice the blood volume (BV = 85 mL/kg) for a complete 2-volume exchange.

Remove blood in 5- to 20-mL amounts and save the first aliquot for laboratory studies. Replace with an equivalent amount of blood. The hydropic infant requires slow, carefully packed red cell exchanges with careful observation of signs of heart failure. The blood pressure and central venous pressure should also be frequently monitored in these patients. An assistant should accurately record each volume exchange as well as the total exchange volume.

The administration of calcium gluconate has been suggested by some when ACD blood is employed. If signs of hypocalcemia develop, administer calcium gluconate, 1 mL of 10% solution, slowly through the polyethylene tubing (rinsing tubing with saline solution before and after the drug is introduced). Do not give any further calcium if there is slowing of the pulse.

Give protamine sulfate, 0.5 mg intramuscularly, to terminate the heparin effect at the end of an exchange employing heparinized blood.

ARTERIAL ACCESS & MONITORING

Arterial access allows for accurate repeated blood gas determination, continuous pressure monitoring, and withdrawal of reliable blood specimens. An arterial line can eliminate the pain of repeated needle punctures for frequent tests; however, this should not be the sole indication for the procedure. Arterial access may be provided by percutaneous catheterization or by a cutdown procedure. The radial and posterior tibial arteries are most commonly used; each normally has an alternative arterial supply to distal tissue (eg, ulnar or dorsalis pedis arteries). This alternative supply prevents vascular compromise to the foot or hand in the event of occlusion of the catheterized artery. In the newborn, the umbilical artery is usually employed as described previously.

PERCUTANEOUS ARTERIAL CATHETERIZATION

Secure the forearm or leg to an armboard with the wrist in 30-degree extension or the foot dorsiflexed.

Determine patency of alternative arterial supply to distal parts of the extremity by doppler probe or palpation of the pulse. In the newborn, a cool fiberoptic bright light source carefully placed under or to the side of the area will, when pressed against the skin, allow visible pulsations to be seen. After locating the artery by palpation, prepare the area with an iodine-containing solution followed by alcohol. Anesthetize the area over the artery with 1% lidocaine. It is helpful to pierce the skin over the artery with an 18- to 20-gauge needle to help avoid shearing the catheter tip as it is being inserted. A 20- to 22-gauge catheter with a central needle is inserted through the pierced skin at a 45-degree angle; either the artery is entered directly, or both walls are pierced. If both walls have been pierced, remove the needle and very slowly withdraw the catheter until a gush of blood signifies that the catheter tip is in the artery. The catheter can then be advanced easily until only the hub is seen externally. Connect the catheter to the intravenous line containing heparinized normal saline (0.5–2 units/mL) and run under pressure at a rate of 2–3 mL/h. Connect to a pressure transducer and evaluate the wave form.

Although arterial punctures may be performed safely in the temporal artery, this artery should not be cannulated because there is a risk of secondary thrombosis and embolization resulting in ipsilateral cerebral infarcts and neurologic deficits.

Arterial catheterization can be complicated by bleeding, which is usually brief and can be controlled by direct pressure. More seriously, arterio-

spasm or thromboembolic events may severely impair distal blood flow and cause necrosis of areas of the extremity.

CUTDOWN ARTERIAL ACCESS

Secure the arm or leg to a board. After determining that alternative arterial supply is adequate, locate the artery by palpation and prepare the arm with an iodine-containing solution; anesthetize the area with 1% lidocaine. Drape the area with sterile towels. Make a 1-cm incision over the artery perpendicular to its course. Isolate the artery by blunt dissection. Pass one length of No. 000 or 4-0 silk suture around the artery at the distal end and a second length at the proximal end of the isolated vessel. Apply a hemostat to the ends of each suture for better control of the artery. Pierce the artery with a catheter with an interior needle-catheter and advance the catheter proximally while withdrawing the needle. A prompt flow of blood indicates correct placement. Attach the catheter to pressure intravenous solution with transducer, and observe the wave form. Remove the 2 sutures that were used to control the artery. No ligatures should be left around the artery. Close the skin wound and suture the catheter hub to the skin.

Complications include bleeding, which is generally brief and can be controlled by direct pressure, and loss of patency of the artery after discontinuation of the line. The latter is more common with this technique than with the percutaneous technique.

SELECTED REFERENCES

Block JA: *Pediatric Emergencies,* 2nd ed. Butterworths, 1987.

Dolcourt JL, Bose CL: Percutaneous insertion of Silastic central venous catheters in newborn infants. *Pediatrics* 1982;**70**:484.

Hodge D, Fleisher G: Pediatric catheter flow rates. *Am J Emerg Med* 1985;**3**:403.

Hughes WT Jr: *Pediatric Procedures,* 2nd ed. Saunders, 1980.

Millam DA: How to insert an IV. *Am J Nurs* 1979; **79**:1268.

Roberts JR, Hedges JR: *Clinical Procedures in Emergency Medicine.* Saunders, 1985.

Spivey WH: Intraosseous infusions. *J Pediatr* 1987; **111**:639.

Fluid & Electrolyte Therapy

36

James V. Lustig, MD

BODY FLUIDS

In term infants, the total body water (TBW) accounts for approximately 70–75% of the body weight. Following the normal postnatal fluid adjustment with its attendant weight loss, the TBW represents about 65% of the total body weight. This fraction remains constant until puberty, when the TBW decreases to 55–60% of the body weight. Approximately two-thirds of the TBW is intracellular water (ICW) and one-third is extracellular water (ECW). The ECW is further divided into plasma volume and interstitial fluid.

The intracellular and extracellular fluids are separated by the cell membranes of the body. For the purposes of addressing clinical disorders of hydration, these membranes may be conceptualized as one aggregate cell membrane that is water permeable. Further, the cell membrane facilitates the passage into and the maintenance of sodium (Na^+ in the ECW while potassium (K^+) is moved to and maintained in the intracellular environment via a membrane-associated "pump."

Because the cell membrane is water permeable and particles are dissolved in the water on each side of the cell membrane, shifts of water would occur if the number of particles dissolved on each side of the cell membrane were not the same. Normally the volumes of the ECW and ICW do not change because the concentration of dissolved particles is identical on each side of the membrane. The body maintains this ratio of water molecules to the number of dissolved particles on each side of the membrane. The actual number of dissolved particles per unit of water is seldom computed. In clinical situations the concept of osmolality is used. (Osmolality is usually expressed as mosm/L of water, which is equivalent to mmol/L times the number of particles formed when a molecule dissociates, eg, 2 particles for NaCl, and one particle for glucose.) Osmolality represents the osmolar concentration of a dissolved substance multiplied by the number of particles produced by dissociation of a molecule of the substance.

Osmolality is the same throughout the body water. Normally the osmolality of body water is approximately 285 mosm/L. Solutions with this osmolality are said to be "normal," because they are isosmolal or isotonic. Solutions of less than 285 mosm/L are hyposmolal or hypotonic, whereas those containing more than 285 mosm/L are hypertonic.

Conceptualizing osmotic shifts between the ECW and ICW is fundamental to understanding disorders of hydration. The "membrane" separating the extracellular and intracellular space must be freely permeable to water. Shifts occur only if there is an inequality on each side of the membrane in the concentration of solutes that cannot permeate the membrane. Normally Na^+, Cl^-, and HCO_3 are primarily excluded from most cellular environments, whereas K^+ is maintained within cells.

In addition to the isosmolality maintained between fluid compartments, electroneutrality is maintained within body fluids so that the concentration of cations equals the concentration of anions within a body fluid.

The clinician dealing with clinical disorders of hydration must remember that the extracellular fluid (ECF) is the only fluid compartment that can be readily monitored and that its composition reflects interactions between the ECF and intracellular fluid (ICF). Therapeutically it is generally desirable to maintain a normal osmolality (285 mosm/L).

FLUID COMPARTMENTS

Although the majority of body water is intracellular, direct measurement and characterization of ICF remains difficult. Clinically the status of ICF is inferred from analysis of plasma and the condition of the patient. This is obviously imprecise and frustrating because one cannot appreciate the early effects of hydration disorders upon the cell and its organelles.

The ECF is subdivided into the (1) plasma, (2) interstitial fluid (ISF), (3) transcellular fluid, and (4) bone fluid.

The connective tissue and bone fluid compartment has little role in the development of symptoms in disorders of hydration.

Transcellular fluids reside in a specific location as a result of a transport process through cells. These fluids include cerebrospinal fluid (CSF), bile, gastrointestinal fluid, and humors of the eye. These fluids normally account for a very small percentage of the TBW. It is important to remember that the volume of gastrointestinal fluid can expand vastly, creating a fluid pool of great size and clinical significance. The elimination of or redistribution of this fluid into another fluid compartment such as the ECF may pose a significant clinical problem.

The ISF represents a large compartment of body fluid. The size of the ISF allows it to withstand rapid change so that it "buffers" change occurring in the significantly smaller plasma compartment. ISF surrounds and bathes the cells.

The electrolyte composition of the ISF is similar to that of plasma. The concentrations of Na^+, K^+, Cl^-, and HCO_3^- in the ISF closely resemble the concentrations found in the plasma. Clinically, plasma electrolyte analysis can be said to reflect the composition of the ISF.

When the volume of the ISF is depleted, poor skin turgor, depressed fontanelles, and sunken eyes result, whereas an expanded ISF volume results in edema. Although it accounts for only about one-fifth of the ECF volume, plasma plays a critical role in the assessment of the status of the body's fluid compartments. Plasma is in contact with the gastrointestinal tract, kidney, and skin. The plasma is separated from the ISF by the endothelium lining blood vessels. The endothelium permits very rapid passage of water and ions but inhibits movement of protein molecules, confining most albumin and globulin to the intravascular compartment. The inhibition of

movement of protein molecules is presumably due to their size. Plasma proteins consist primarily of albumin, which has a molecular weight of about 60,000, and globulins, whose molecular weight ranges from 180,000 to over 1,000,000. Albumin molecules are more numerous than globulin molecules and exert three-fourths of the osmotic pressure exerted by plasma proteins. The protein osmotic pressure is referred to as colloid osmotic pressure. Although colloid osmotic pressure seems negligible compared to the osmotic pressure exerted by the low molecular weight electrolyte molecules, it is important in maintaining plasma volume.

As in other body fluids, electroneutrality is maintained in the plasma. As the previous discussion suggests, the majority of extracellular protein resides in the plasma. Alterations in plasma composition reflect the interaction of external forces on the internal environment. Fig 36–1 is a schematic depiction of the composition and distribution of the body fluids.

CONTROL OF THE ECF

Multiple mechanisms control the volume and content of the ECF. Among the more important control mechanisms are aldosterone, thirst, and antidiuretic hormone (ADH).

Aldosterone, from the adrenal cortex, enhances the tubular reabsorption of Na^+ in the kidney. As a

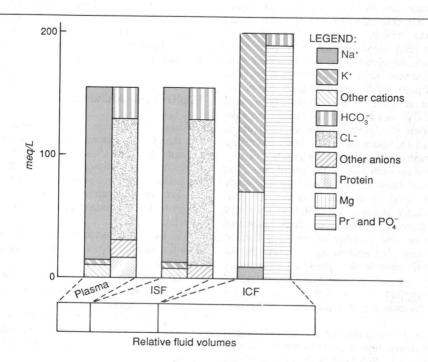

Figure 36–1. Composition of body fluids.

constant osmolality is maintained, retention of Na^+ leads to increased ECF volume.

Under normal physiologic conditions, plasma osmolality, as opposed to plasma volume, is the variable primarily regulated. Plasma osmolality and volume are maintained through the interaction of thirst and ADH. Thirst controls fluid intake, whereas ADH controls the volume of urine output.

Thirst controls the need to drink and reflects changes in the volume of ECF. Thirst provides precise control over a wide range of fluid volumes and can even be a response to an inhibition or absence of ADH with its attendant copious, dilute urine. However, thirst acts to maintain volume even at the expense of osmolality. An individual who cannot perceive thirst rapidly develops a significant problem with fluid balance. Neurologically impaired children or children who cannot respond to thirst pose serious management problems.

After being produced in the anterior hypothalamus, ADH is secreted from the posterior pituitary. ADH enhances the reabsorption of water in the kidney, and urine subsequently produced is low in volume and hypertonic relative to plasma. A small change in plasma osmolality precipitates a significant ADH response. ADH is secreted in response to a decrease in plasma ECF volume, an increase in osmolality, exercise, stress, and the ingestion of some drugs. Drugs that enhance ADH secretion include epinephrine, acetylcholine, histamine, morphine, barbiturates, and nicotine. Inhibition of ADH secretion results from decreased plasma osmolality, distention of the left atrium, and ethanol ingestion or administration.

Age also plays a role in regulating fluid volumes within the body, as the changes in the fluid compartments at birth and puberty demonstrate. In addition, growth necessitates a slight positive balance to accommodate the demands of the growing child.

ACID-BASE EQUILIBRIUM

The acidity of arterial blood is maintained within very narrow limits. The acidity is usually expressed in pH units, which represent $\log \frac{1}{H^+}$. Normally the pH is 7.40 ± 0.02 except in infants, in whom it ranges from 7.35 to 7.45. Acids dissociate into cations (C^+) and anions (A^-). The stronger the acid, the more complete the dissociation. The acidity of a lution is proportional to the concentration of hydrogen ions.

Buffers, which act to inhibit changes in the acidity of a solution, consist of a weak acid and its conjugate base. In the body, the primary role of buffers in maintaining pH is enhanced by physiologic mechanisms in the lung and kidney. The carbonic acid buffering system is perhaps the best known, but there are nonbicarbonate buffers, which include anion groups or plasma proteins and phosphates and

erythrocyte hemoglobin. Over 50% of the blood's buffering capacity is in the bicarbonate system. The action of buffers is strengthened by the lung's effect on carbonic acid and the alkalization or acidification of urine, which alters the concentration and amount of bicarbonate in the blood.

One can understand a buffer system's action by quantifying the system's reactions. Acid-base relationships are governed by the Henderson-Hasselbalch equation:

$$pH = pK' + \log \frac{[\text{conjugate base}]}{[\text{weak acid}]}$$

where pK' is a constant specific to the buffer system. In the carbonic acid system, whose pK' is 6.1, H_2CO_3 dissociates to H^+ and HCO_3^-. Knowing that the normal concentration of HCO_3^- is 24 meq/L and the normal concentration of H_2CO_3 is 1.2 mmol/L, one can rewrite the Henderson-Hasselbalch equation as follows:

$$pH = pK' + \log \frac{[HCO_3^-]}{[H_2CO_3]}$$

$$pH = 6.1 + \log \frac{[24 \text{ meq/L}]}{[1.2 \text{ mmol/L}]}$$

The equation can be rewritten in a number of equivalent forms. A clinically important form of the equation is based on the fact that blood in the pulmonary capillaries is in equilibrium with alveolar air. Therefore, the denominator of the log can be expressed as $P_{CO_2} \times S$ (solubility coefficient $= 0.03$ m-mol/L/mm Hg). Given a normal P_{CO_2} of 40 mm Hg, the denominator is again 1.2 mmol/L. The equation is then

$$pH = pK' + \log \frac{[HCO_3^-]}{S \times P_{CO_2}} = 6.1 + \log \frac{[HCO_3^-]}{1.2 \text{ mmol/L}}$$

To solve the equation, one must know 2 of the 3 variables (ie, pH, $[HCO_3^-]$, P_{CO_2}).

The bicarbonate system can interact with the nonbicarbonate system. Such interaction may be represented by the equation $H_2CO_3 + Hb^- \rightarrow HCO_3^- + H\ Prot$. The equation is shifted to the right by an increase of H_2CO_3 or P_{CO_2}. Although this shift would increase $[HCO_3^-]$ and decrease $[Hb^-]$, the sum of $[HCO_3^-] + [Hb^-]$ remains constant, and so the total buffer base remains the same. The total buffer base is normally 45–50 meq/L.

Both the lung and kidney can act to alter or stabilize pH. In respiratory alkalosis there is effective alveolar hyperventilation. Therefore, the denominator of the equation for pH

$$(pH = pK' + \log \frac{[HCO_3^-])}{S \times P_{CO_2}}$$

decreases, and the pH increases.

In metabolic acidosis, which results from an increase of a strong acid or loss of bicarbonate, the respiratory center increases respiratory drive, CO_2 is exhaled, and P_{CO_2} decreases so that the ratio of

$$\frac{[HCO_3^-]}{S \times P_{CO_2}}$$

tends to be maintained and there is a compensatory shift in pH toward normal.

Renal regulation of acid-base status primarily alters HCO_3^- concentration. Unwanted acid or base can be excreted in the urine, and subsequently the $[HCO_3^-]$ concentration can be altered throughout the entire ECF. Bicarbonate can be altered in 2 ways via the kidneys, since the urine may be either alkalized or acidified. When the urine is alkalized, HCO_3^- enters the kidney and is ultimately lost in the urine. This alkalinization of the urine can occur at any time that there is a relative or absolute excess of bicarbonate. This mechanism does not function if there is a deficiency of Na^+ or K^+, because the body could not maintain electroneutrality in this situation. A chloride deficiency also inhibits this mechanism.

If there is a relative or absolute decrease in HCO_3^-, the urine can be acidified. In this situation, water and CO_2 combine in the tubular cell to form carbonic acid, which then dissociates. H^+ is exchanged for Na^+, and the sodium bicarbonate gains access to the peritubular plasma and the ECF. This reaction facilitates the excretion of significant amounts of H^+. The reaction is limited by salt depletion or dehydration. Some of the processes controlling pH are illustrated schematically in Fig 36–2.

PRINCIPLES OF FLUID & ELECTROLYTE MANAGEMENT

The therapy for any disorder of fluids, and electrolytes is predicated on providing the patient with maintenance requirements of fluids and electrolytes, replacing any previous losses, and replenishing ongoing abnormal losses. In planning therapy, these 3 components should be addressed individually so that no basic needs are overlooked. In addition, therapy should be phased to meet these 3 needs: (1) maintaining adequate perfusion, (2) restoring fluid and electrolyte deficits while correcting acid-base defects, and (3) meeting nutritional needs.

The cornerstone of therapy is understanding maintenance requirements. The phrase "maintenance requirements" means enough water and electrolytes to prevent deterioration of body stores. When short-term (2–3 days) parenteral therapy is given, enough calories are given to blunt hunger and inhibit protein breakdown and ketosis. However, the amount given is usually little more than 20% of the patient's caloric needs.

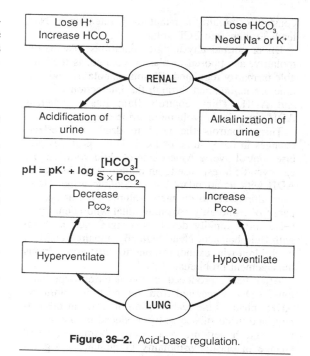

Figure 36–2. Acid-base regulation.

$$pH = pK' + \log \frac{[HCO_3]}{S \times P_{CO_2}}$$

Different schema have been devised to calculate maintenance fluid needs based on body weight, surface area, or caloric expenditures. A system based on caloric expenditures is helpful since we know that 1 ml of water every 24 hours is needed for each calorie expended and that metabolic needs, not size, determine the use of body stores.

Calories consumed per unit of body weight, or metabolic rate, decrease as size and age increase. The schema presented, which is based on caloric needs, is applicable to youngsters weighing over 3 kg (see Table 36–1).

As Table 36–1 shows, a child weighing 25 kg would need 1600 kcal daily and 1600 ml of water. If the child were admitted to the hospital for an elective procedure and received fluids intravenously for 2 days, the fluid would probably contain 5% glucose, which would provide 320 kcal per day, or about 20% of the maintenance needs. For short-term parenteral maintenance therapy in patients without

Table 36–1. Caloric and water needs per unit body weight.

Body weight in kg	Maintenance Needs	
	kcal/kg	ml Water/kg
3–10	100	100
11–20	50	50
> 20 kg	20	20

preexisting nutritional deficits, 5% glucose providing 20% of caloric needs is adequate. In general, all intravenous fluids should have at least 5% glucose. Maintenance fluid requirements take into account insensible water loss and water lost in sweat, urine, and stool. Patients are assumed to be relatively inactive or bed-ridden.

Electrolyte needs can be similarly approximated, although maintenance estimates vary considerably. Electrolyte losses vary significantly as the patient's output changes, and therefore no one figure reflects true needs. Reasonable initial approximations for maintenance needs are 3 meq Na^+/100 kcal and 2.5 meq K^+/100 kcal.

Altered metabolic states alter maintenance needs. Allowances must be made for such occurrences. Fever and hyperventilation are among the most commonly encountered of these conditions. For every degree (centigrade) of body temperature, fluid needs increase by 12%. Table 36–2 lists factors commonly altering fluid requirements.

Normally one need not measure individual components of output to ensure appropriate fluid balance. It is useful to monitor the patient's weight, output, input, and urine specific gravity. If there is an alteration of fluid or electrolyte balance, determination of electrolyte concentrations, urine osmolality, and pH may be necessary. Unless one is dealing with an osmotic diuresis, such as is seen in diabetic ketoacidosis, a urine osmolality between 200 and 600 mosm/L indicates adequate fluid intake. These measurements help the physician monitor the efficacy of therapy. In patients with significant burns, anuria, oliguria, or abnormal ongoing losses (eg, from a stoma), it is important to measure output and its fractions so that appropriate replacement can be instituted.

DEHYDRATION

Depletion of body fluids—dehydration—is one of the most commonly encountered problems in pediatrics. Dehydration, most often associated with gastroenteritis, remained a major cause of death in the

United States until well into this century and is still a major cause of morbidity and mortality in developing countries. The problems associated with dehydration remain common not only because of the frequency of gastroenteritis in young children but also because infants and young children often decrease their intake when ill. Furthermore, renal function in the first year of life does not maximally conserve water, the infant's high ratio of surface area to volume promotes evaporative fluid losses, and fever significantly increases fluid needs.

Dehydration results in protean changes in the body, leading to cellular dysfunction. The clinical effects of dehydration are proportional both to the degree of dehydration and to the relative ratio of salt to water lost. Briefly, dehydration decreases the extracellular volume, leading to decreased tissue perfusion. The decreased volume results in compensatory increases impulse rate as the heart attempts to increase output in the face of decreased stroke volume. The decreased tissue perfusion also impairs renal function, leading to acidosis and uremia. Decreased oxygen delivery due to dehydration may lead to lactic acidosis. If there is an associated decrease in caloric intake or an inability to metabolize ingested calories, ketoacidosis may ensue. These changes are illustrated in Fig 36–3.

The clinical sequelae of dehydration reflect the amount of fluid depletion. A number of clinical profiles have been suggested as a way to correlate the appearance of symptoms and physical signs with the degree of dehydration. Such a system is illustrated in Table 36–3. However, such schema are imprecise at best. The primary utility of such systems is to remind the physician to estimate the degree of dehydration (because treatment varies with the degree of dehydration) and to assess the adequacy of perfusion. They also serve as a reminder that the more physical signs present, the more likely it is that the dehydration is profound. Simple measures—eg, checking the patient's last recorded weight and comparing it to the present weight; carefully assessing blood pressure, capillary refill, and orthostatic blood pressure changes; and meticulously reviewing the history of fluids ingested and frequency of output—are often most helpful. Physicians dealing with growing children must remember the fluid shift that occurs around the time of puberty. Young children may not suffer shock until the degree of dehydration is approximately 15%. However, after the fluid shift at puberty, shock may occur when the degree of dehydration is 9–10%.

Dehydration is further characterized by the electrolyte composition of the plasma. When body salts are lost in proportion to water, the electrolyte readings yield normal values, and the dehydration is said to be isotonic. If relatively more solute than water is lost, the sodium concentration falls, and hyponatremic dehydration ($[Na^+] < 130$ meq/L) results.

Table 36–2. Alterations of maintenance fluid requirements.

Factor	Altered Requirement
Fever	12%/° C[1]
Hyperventilation	10–60 ml/100 kcal
Sweating	10–25 ml/100 kcal
Hyperthyroidism	Variable; 25–50%
Gastrointestinal loss and renal disease	Monitor and analyze output. Adjust therapy accordingly.

[1]Do not correct for 38 °C; correct 24% for 39 °C.

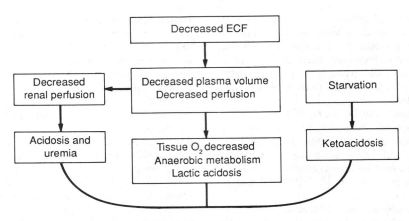

Figure 36–3. Sequelae of dehydration.

This finding is important because the hypotonicity of the plasma results in further volume loss from the ECF, and perfusion is therefore more significantly impaired for a given degree of hyponatremic dehydration than for the same degree of isotonic or hypertonic dehydration. Hypernatremic dehydration ([Na$^+$] > 150 meq/L) occurs when relatively less solute than body water is lost. Because plasma volume is protected, this might appear to be the least dangerous form of dehydration, but it poses the risk of an underestimation of the severity of dehydration. Further, if the hypertonicity is corrected too rapidly (a drop in [Na$^+$] of > 0.5–1 meq/L in 1 hour) cerebral edema, seizures, and severe central nervous system injury may occur. Typical electrolyte losses associated with each form of dehydration are listed in Table 36–4.

Table 36–3. Clinical manifestations of dehydration.[1]

	Degree of dehydration		
Clinical sign	**Mild**	**Moderate**	**Severe**
Decrease in body weight	3–5%	8–10%	12–15%
Skin			
Turgor	Normal (+/−)	Decreased	Markedly decreased
Color	Normal	Pale	Mottled or gray
Mucous membranes	Dry	—	Parched
Hemodynamics			
Pulse	Normal	—	Tachycardia
Blood pressure	Normal	—	Low
Perfusion	Normal	—	Circulatory collapse
Fluid loss			
Urinary output	Mild oliguria	—	Anuria
Tears	Decreased	—	Absent

[1]The manifestations of dehydration reflect the ECF in general, and the plasma in particular. Therefore hypotonic dehydration is clinically more apparent, and hypertonic dehydration is less apparent.

METABOLIC DERANGEMENTS

Metabolic acidosis results from either increased abnormal production of a strong acid or loss of a buffer base, such as bicarbonate. Acids produced include ketone bodies, lactic acid, or, in the presence of renal failure or azotemia, phosphoric or sulfuric acids. Ketone body production is increased in starvation, diabetic ketoacidosis, and salicylism. Lactic acidosis usually reflects poor tissue perfusion or hypoxia, although primary lactic acidosis may occur rarely.

Loss of bicarbonate is most often associated with loss of alkaline fluid from the small intestine. Such losses often accompany diarrheal disease, the use of suction to remove fluid from the intestine, or a small bowel fistula. Diarrheal stool is often acidic. The question arises as to how this occurs if the fluid from the small intestine is alkaline. The acidic pH reflects the bacterial fermentation of the intestinal fluid, which results in the production of organic acids. The stool has an anion gap. The stool of patients with cholera is as a result usually alkaline of the rapid transit time associated with this disorder. If a patient's stool is alkaline, the transit time should be assumed to be brief. Loss of bicarbonate is also seen in renal tubular acidosis.

Table 36–4. Estimated water and electrolyte deficits in dehydration (moderate to severe).[1]

Type of Dehydration	H$_2$O (mL/kg)	Na$^+$ (meq/kg)	K$^+$ (meq/kg)	Cl$^-$ and HCO$_3^-$ (meq/kg)
Isotonic	100–150	8–10	8–10	16–20
Hypotonic	50–100	10–14	10–14	20–28
Hypertonic	120–180	2–5	2–5	4–10

[1]Adapted from Winters RW: *Principles of Pediatric Fluid Therapy.* Little, Brown, 1982.

Metabolic acidosis is associated with a significant negative base excess and compensatory hyperventilation. Effective treatment depends on treating the underlying disorder. Bicarbonate may be used to ameliorate severe acidosis; however, it should be used carefully because overly rapid correction of pH may have deleterious sequelae. In general, one need not attempt to correct the pH if it is greater than 7.1, and one need not correct to values greater than 7.25 with bicarbonate. The dose of sodium bicarbonate used to correct pH is given by this formula:

$$\text{Dose (in meq)} = 0.3 \times \text{body weight (kg)} \times \text{base excess}$$

If sodium bicarbonate is given, the amount of sodium administered in maintenance should be adjusted.

Many physicians rely on determination of the anion gap (AG) to detect cases of metabolic acidosis due to the production of strong acid. The AG may be calculated from either formula below:

$$\text{Anion gap} = ([Na^+]) - ([Cl^-] + [HCO_3^-])$$

or

$$\text{Anion gap} = ([Na^+] + [K^+]) - ([Cl^-] + [HCO_3^-])$$

This calculation approximates the sum of the undetermined anions (proteanates, lactate, phosphate, sulfate beta-hydroxybutyrate). Normal values depend on the formula used and on laboratory protocol. Small variations are not significant, and the AG determinations should not be overinterpreted. The AG should be abnormal if a strong acid (not hydrochloric acid) is added, because the anion of the acid will appear in the undetermined fraction and increase the AG. The AG tends to be normal in diarrhea with its attendant hyperchloremic acidosis and bicarbonate loss. However, if azotemia ensues due to dehydration, the increase in phosphate and sulfate may increase the AG. It is of note that the AG should always be positive. An AG of zero or less indicates a laboratory error. Clinical situations in which an exaggerated AG is encountered include diabetic ketoacidosis uremia, salicylate intoxication, lactic acidosis, some other causes of metabolic acidosis. Therapy with various antibiotics, including carbenicillin and large doses of sodium penicillin, can also elevate the AG. A low AG is associated with hypoalbuminemia and dilution.

Emmett M, Narins RG: Clinical use of the anion gap. *Medicine* 1977;**56**:38.

Gabow PA, Kaehny WD, et al: Diagnostic importance of an increased serum anion gap. *N Engl J Med* 1980; **303**:854.

METABOLIC ALKALOSIS

Metabolic alkalosis is the result of gaining buffer base or losing strong acid, most commonly due to the loss of gastric juice from vomiting or nasogastric suctioning. Pyloric stenosis is the prototypical situation leading to the development of metabolic alkalosis. Other situations that may lead to metabolic alkalosis include chronic diarrhea, the administration of diuretics, and the use of silver nitrate in the treatment of burns. Metabolic anomalies in which sodium is conserved without chloride, such as 11β-hydroxylase deficiency, predispose patients to the development of metabolic alkalosis.

The laboratory profile of metabolic alkalosis includes, in addition to an elevated pH, a positive base excess and a normal or mildly elevated Pco_2.

The treatment of metabolic alkalosis includes, in addition to the treatment of the underlying disorder, the administration of chloride. Chloride may be supplied by a number of salts, including $NaCl$, NH_4Cl, or KCl. If a potassium deficiency is present, KCl becomes the drug of choice, and other chloride salts are of limited efficacy.

RESPIRATORY ACIDOSIS

Respiratory acidosis denotes a decrease in alveolar ventilation with an attendant increase in Pco_2 (both in the alveoli and in plasma). In acute respiratory acidosis, CO_2 is retained. In addition to a drop in pH and an increase in Pco_2, patients are likely to demonstrate an increased level of bicarbonate and a decreased level of chloride, which is lost as the urine is acidified. Clinically these patients are air hungry, and their respiration is characterized by retractions and the use of accessory muscles. Cyanosis may be present. This scenario may be seen in upper or lower airway obstruction, V/Q disturbances, inadequate perfusion, or respiratory failure. The goal of treatment is to provide adequate ventilation. HCO_3^- therapy is not efficacious because the elevated Pco_2 inhibits the shifting of the equation $H^+ + HCO_3^-$ H_2CO_3 to the right.

Chronic respiratory acidosis is characterized by gradual development of alveolar hypoventilation. A number of clinical entities, including primary lung problems, chest wall abnormalities, and neurologic problems, are associated with this disorder. Chronic respiratory acidosis is associated with kyphoscoliosis, chest wall deformities, osteogenesis imperfecta, rickets, polymyositis, cystic fibrosis, myasthenia gravis, muscular dystrophy, and poliomyelitis. Although respiratory acidosis has been seen in severe chronic asthma, such an occurrence should be very rare with present treatment modalities. Again, the goal of treatment is to control the underlying disorder and promote adequate ventilation.

RESPIRATORY ALKALOSIS

Respiratory alkalosis occurs when hyperventilation results in a decrease in P_{CO_2}. Patients describe tingling in the extremities paresthesia, dizziness, and palpitations. Syncope may occur, and very occasionally tetany associated with hypocalcemia or even seizures may be seen. The hyperventilation is the result of CNS stimulation. Causes of respiratory alkalosis include hysteria, CNS irritation from meningitis or encephalitis, and salicylism. Treatment varies from providing a paper bag to facilitate rebreathing by the hysterical patient to increasing the dead space in a patient with a CNS anomaly who requires ventilation.

Kassirer JP: Serious acid-base disorders. *N Engl J Med* 1974;**291**:773.

POTASSIUM DISORDERS

Potassium is the primary intracellular cation. Only about 2% of the body's K^+ is extracellular. The intracellular concentration of K^+ is over 40 times that found in the ECF. Skeletal muscle, which contains about 60% of the body's potassium, has an intracellular concentration of 150–160 meq/L, whereas the plasma concentration is only 4–5 meq/L. Over 90% of the potassium in the body is freely exchangeable. Maintenance of the appropriate potassium distribution and size of the body pool is maintained by the $Na^+ - K^+$ pump at the cell membrane and by the kidney. Potassium is filtered by the glomerulus, reabsorbed in the proximal tubule, and excreted in the distal tubule. The kidney can either excrete or conserve K^+ readily, but secretion of potassium occurs via the mechanism that results in acidification of the urine. Therefore, potassium secretion depends on the body's Na^+ level and pH. When Na^+ is reabsorbed in the tubular cell, it is exchanged for either H^+ or K^+. If an alkaline urine is to be excreted, K^+ is secreted preferentially. By contrast, acidification of the urine results in loss of H^+ and conservation of K^+. The kidney cannot conserve K^+ on short notice. In addition to the body's Na^+ load, the size of the body's potassium pool and steroids also affect K^+ balance. If K^+ is depleted, the urine is acidified, and systemic alkalosis ensues. Adrenal corticosteroids promote Na^+ retention, whereas Addison's disease results in Na^+ loss and K^+ retention. The concentration of K^+ in the ECF is increased by acidemia, whereas alkalosis, hypochloremia, and glycogen deposition result in decreased levels of K^+ in the ECF. Alkalosis promotes the entry of K^+ into cells, whereas acidemia results in K^+ leaving cells and entering the ECF. Treatment of a diabetic in ketoacidosis results in a decrease in the $[K^+]_s$ as the pH rises, and insulin administration results in glycogen deposition.

Potassium excretion continues for a significant period even if the intake of K^+ is decreased. By the time that a lowered urinary $[K^+]$ occurs, the body's K^+ pool has already been significantly depleted. A decreased urinary $[K^+]$ does exclude potassium-wasting states.

Diuretics, especially thiazides, acetazolamide, and mercurials, enhance the secretion of K^+. Aberrations in the concentration of potassium in the ECF alter myocardial contractility and can cause death from arrhythmia or cardiac standstill. When hypokalemia occurs with a loss of 10–20% of the body's potassium stores, apathy and muscle weakness occur. Occasionally paresthesias are reported, and tetany may be seen. Further, losses may result in flaccid paralysis and decreased respiration. Electrocardiographic changes associated with hypokalemia include T-wave depression, the appearance of U waves, ST segment depression and arrhythmia (see Fig 36–4). Arrhythmias associated with hypokalemia include premature ventricular contractions, atrial or nodal tachycardia, and ventricular tachycardia or fibrillation. Hypokalemia also heightens responsiveness to digitalis and may precipitate digitalis toxicity.

The first priority in the treatment of hypokalemia is maintaining an adequate concentration of K^+ in the serum. The magnitude of the total K^+ loss cannot be readily calculated because the vast majority of the body's K^+ is located intracellularly. Providing maintenance amounts of K^+ is usually sufficient to prevent problems. If hypochloremia is present, potassium should be given as KCl because other salts are not as effective in treating the potassium deficiency. In those situations in which $[K^+]_s$ is dangerously low and K^+ must be administered intravenously, it is imperative that the patient have a cardiac monitor, and the physician must be prepared to treat any arrhythmias. Potassium should not be administered at a rate exceeding 0.5 meq/kg per hour outside an intensive care unit. Once the $[K^+]_s$ is stabilized, the body's K^+ deficit may be replaced by providing foods rich in potassium.

Hyperkalemia is characterized by muscle weakness, occasional paresthesias and tetany, and ascending paralysis. Electrocardiographic changes associated with hyperkalemia include heightened T waves, widening of the QRS complex, and arrhythmias. The arrhythmias seen with hyperkalemia include sinus bradycardia or sinus arrest, AV block, nodal or idioventricular rhythms, and ventricular tachycardia or fibrillation. The severity of hyperkalemia depends on the electrocardiographic changes, the status of the other electrolytes, and the progression of the underlying disorder. If the $[K^+]_s$ is less than 6.5 meq/L, one seldom need do anything more than discontinue the administration of potassium. If potentiating factors (eg, hyponatremia, a brisk rise in $[K^+]_s$, alkalemia, digitalis toxicity, or renal failure) are present,

Hypokalemia

Apathy, Muscle weak-
ness, Paresthesia,
Tetany, Depressed
T wave, U wave, ST
depression

Arrhythmias.
Premature beats,
Atrial or nodal
tachycardia,
Ventricular
tachycardia or
fibrillation

Hyperkalemia

Ascending paralysis, Occasional
tetany and paresthesias, Muscle
weakness, Peaked T-wave, Prolonged PR interval, ST depression

Arrhythmias. Wide ORS comples,
Sinus bradycardia, AV block, Idio-
ventricular tachycardia or fibrillation,
Cardiac arrest

Figure 36–4. Clinical sequelae of abnormal potassium.

one needs to be more aggressive. Any suggestions of a dysrhythmia must be evaluated and treated aggressively. Because the most emergent effect of hyperkalemia is altered myocardial contractility, a rhythm strip should be obtained immediately whenever significant hyperkalemia is suspected. If electrocardiographic changes or arrhythmias are present, treatment must be promptly initiated to counteract the depolarization of cardiac muscle, shift potassium into cells, remove excess potassium from the body, and prevent tissue catabolism. Intravenous Ca^{++}, usually administered as 10% calcium gluconate (0.2–0.5 mL/kg over 2–10 minutes), will briefly ameliorate depolarization. The calcium should be administered with a cardiac monitor in place and should be discontinued immediately if bradycardia occurs. Administering Na^+ and increasing the pH with bicarbonate therapy will cause K^+ to move from the extracellular to intracellular environment. Insulin administration will result in glycogen deposition and a shift of K^+ to the intracellular environment. Insulin (0.1 unit/kg per hour) must be accompanied by glucose (approximately 3.5 g/unit of insulin) to prevent hypoglycemia. Potassium may be removed by ion exchange resins, such as sodium polystyrene sulfonate (Kayexalate), which may be given orally or as a retention enema (0.2 g/kg orally or 1 g/kg as an enema). Because ion exchange is not rapid, other measures must be employed simultaneously. Dialysis is efficacious, although it is costly and poses its own risks.

HYPERNATREMIA & HYPONATREMIA

The presence of hypernatremia indicates a loss of proportionately less solute than water. Because of the relative water deficit, hyperosmolality should be anticipated. Severe hypernatremia may precipitate CNS injury, seizures, intracerebral bleeding, retardation, and even death. Causes of hypernatremia include inadequate water intake, salt overloading, extrarenal water loss, defective osmoregulation, and water loss with simultaneous gain of solute.

Unconscious patients, patients who cannot swallow or drink, and retarded patients who cannot express thirst are at risk for the development of hypernatremic dehydration.

Salt overloading may occur if formula is mixed incorrectly or if a fluid with a high solute load is ingested. Salt overloading may be a form of child abuse.

Extrarenal water loss is seen in a variety of clinical situations, including prolonged fever, the presence of a tracheostomy, prolonged respiratory distress, heat stroke, and burns, or it may accompany the hyperpnea seen in metabolic disorders, such as diabetic ketoacidosis or salicylism. Anticipating such occurrences prevents the sequelae.

Defective osmoregulation is uncommonly seen in children. Tumors of the cerebral aqueduct, third ventricle, or anterior hypothalamus may lead to this disorder. Diabetes insipidus in its various forms may be associated with defective osmoregulation, which may be exacerbated by water deprivation or salt loading. Resistance to ADH may be present if there is chronic hypokalemia or hypercalciuria.

Water loss and simultaneous solute gain are associated with a variety of disorders. In straightforward infantile diarrhea, hypernatremia may ensue if the child's diet is high in sodium. Similarly the tube feeding of protein-rich foods to an unconscious patient or to an infant may precipitate an osmotic diuresis in which salt is conserved in greater proportion than water. A poorly controlled diabetic with chronic glycosuria may develop osmotic diuresis, attended by sodium conservation and the development of hypernatremia.

Patients with hypernatremia may be lethargic, confused, stuporous, or even comatose. Twitching, seizures, or irregular respirations may be present. The thirst reported in hypernatremic states is profound. Fever may occur due to an inability to sweat. Because there is a relative water deficit in the ECF, body fluids flow from the ICF to the ECF. This shift preserves the extracellular space, and occasionally patients with hypernatremic dehydration lose over 20% of body weight before experiencing vascular collapse. Blood pressure is maintained. Often the severity of hypernatremic dehydration is underestimated due to the maintenance of the vascular space. The skin of a patient with hypernatremic dehydration is doughy or yielding but inelastic.

Extreme care is required to treat hypernatremic dehydration successfully. The cellular space of the brain cannot equilibrate as rapidly as the ECF. If the $[Na^+]_s$ decreases too rapidly, the osmolality of the ECF drops more rapidly than that of the brain. As a result, water leaves the ECF and enters the brain to maintain osmotic neutrality. This shift can lead to cerebral edema, seizures, and death. To prevent this, the physician should ensure that the $[Na^+]_s$ does not drop more than 15 meq/L in 24 hours. Certainly, a drop in $[Na^+]_s$ greater than 1 meq/L per hour should be avoided. To affect this gradual decrease in $[Na^+]_s$, the physician should order isotonic solutions to restore deficits in ECW. Electrolyte concentrations and serum osmolality must be monitored frequently. If metabolic acidosis is present, it must be corrected gradually to avoid CNS irritability. If hypernatremia has developed gradually and the ECF and BUN are not significantly compromised, hypotonic solutions may be used for rehydration. However, the rate of fall of the serum sodium must not be greater than indicated above. This method involves very gradual administration of fluid and may not be of use if the degree of dehydration is significant. Alterations of blood glucose levels and BUN may contribute to the hyperosmolal state. Hyperglycemia is often seen in hypernatremic dehydration. Hyperglycemia should be monitored closely. Although it usually resolves as the dehydration is treated, it may contribute significantly to the osmolal disequilibrium.

Hyponatremia may occur with a decrease or increase in the ECF volume. Hyponatremia with a decrease in the volume of ECF is the more typical picture and may be present in association with gastroenteritis, diabetic ketoacidosis, vomiting, renal salt-losing disorders, or adrenal insufficiency. As expected, aldosterone conserves Na^+, which results in thirst, and increased glomerular filtration enhances the resorption of Na^+ and water. A decrease in ECF may inhibit the clearance of free water and lead to hyposmolality.

The typical symptoms and signs of dehydration are present in patients with hyponatremic dehydration. This form of dehydration brings the patient to medical attention rapidly because, in contrast to hypernatremic dehydration, the vascular space is selectively compromised as water leaves the vascular space to maintain osmotic neutrality.

The treatment of hyponatremic dehydration is straightforward. The magnitude of the sodium loss may be calculated by this formula:

$$Na^+ \text{ deficit (meq)} = ([\text{desired } Na^+] - [\text{observed } Na^+]) \times \text{body weight (kg)} \times \text{volume of distribution} \\ (0.6\text{--}0.7 \text{ for } Na^+)$$

Similar formulas exist for calculating chloride and bicarbonate deficits.

The presence of hyponatremia without a deficit in the ECF is troublesome because it implies a change in osmotic regulation. This picture is usually seen in conjunction with an underlying problem such as renal failure, liver disease, heart disease, or CNS damage. In these situations, water restriction and treatment of the underlying defect are the primary keys to therapy.

Whenever there is a rapid decrease in serum osmolality, the CNS is at risk. The risk of this situation was stressed in the discussion of hypernatremia, but similar fluid shifts out of the vascular space and into the CNS may occur with intravenous water overload, overly rapid dialysis, or in the treatment of diabetic ketoacidosis if glucose levels are allowed to drop precipitously. Nausea, vomiting, headaches, irritability, twitchiness, or neurologic changes should alert the physician to the possible presence of this disequilibrium syndrome, and steps should be taken to prevent CNS injury.

Although most patients tolerate a water load easily, patients with compromised renal function or an obstructive uropathy cannot. In response to a water load, such patients may develop hyponatremia, hyposmolality, and CNS insult. Such patients require fluid restriction in addition to treatment of the primary problem.

The syndrome of inappropriate secretion of ADH (SIADH) is also characterized by hyponatremia. SIADH is seen in wide variety of clinical settings, including meningitis, head injury, pneumonia, cystic fibrosis, intracranial tumors, stress, drugs (barbiturates and opiates), severe pain, and surgery. Patients with this syndrome pass small volumes of concentrated urine and experience thirst. For this reason, water is retained and $[Na^+]_s$ is decreased. Aldosterone secretion is eventually inhibited by the expansion of the ECF. The clinical manifestations of SIADH depend not only on the magnitude of the hyponatremia but also on the rapidity with which the syndrome evolved. The more rapid the change in $[Na^+]_s$, the more significant the clinical sequelae. If the hyponatremia develops gradually, patients do not usually experience symptoms unless the $[Na^+]_s$ is less than 120 meq/L. As in either form of hyponatremia and osmotic disequilibrium, CNS sequelae are often the most important complications. The effective treatment of SIADH depends on fluid restriction. Administration of isotonic or hypertonic saline elicits a brief, rapid response, but unfortunately this precipitates a saline diuresis and exacerbates the problem.

In cases of severe water intoxication a solution of 3% NaCl may be administered intravenously in the face of frank neurologic disturbances. This should be done to elevate the sodium only to a level at which seizures will not occur.

Finberg L: Hypernatremic (hypertonic) dehydration in infants. *N Engl J Med* 1973;**289**:196.

Kleisch RC, Oliver WJ: Hyponatremia in children. *Pediatr Rev* 1980;**2**:187.

Rahman O et al: Rapid intravenous hydration by means of a single polyelectroyte solution with or without dextrose. *J Pediatr* 1988;**113**:656.

REHYDRATION

Due to the high worldwide incidence of dehydration caused by infantile diarrhea, the development of effective, inexpensive, technologically independent rehydration fluids has been a major priority. The demonstration of effective oral rehydration in developing countries has led to the introduction of easily administered oral rehydration solutions in developed nations.

The first solutions endorsed by the World Health Organization contained 90 meq/L of Na^+. This concentration was reasonable in areas with a high incidence of cholera, but such solutions may cause hypernatremia in patients who lose less Na^+ or who live in cooler areas, where insensible losses are not as great. In the United States today, a typical effective solution for oral rehydration of patients with mild-to-moderate dehydration contains 50–60 meq/L of Na^+, 20–30 meq/L of K^+, 30 meq/L of HCO_3^-, and enough chloride to provide electroneutrality. Glucose in a concentration of 2–3% provides adequate calories for the short term and facilitates absorption of electrolytes. Some companies offer another oral rehydration formula with greater concentrations of sodium and chloride for more severe cases of dehydration.

In more severe cases of dehydration, especially in patients with intractable vomiting, parenteral (usually intravenous) therapy is necessary to correct dehydration. As mentioned previously, the initial goal of therapy is to provide adequate perfusion. Once perfusion is ensured, acid-base defects may be corrected and deficits of body electrolytes may be replaced. Finally, nutritional deficiencies should be corrected. Unless hypernatremia is present, deficits of water and electrolytes are typically replaced in 24 hours, although potassium replacement generally takes longer.

The physician's first job is to assess the magnitude of dehydration. If previous records are available, comparing the last recorded body weight with the present weight is very helpful. A reliable history enables the physician at least to estimate fluid losses and intake. The physician should be especially alert for any suggestion in the history or physical that anything other than isotonic dehydration exists. The physician must not only assess the degree of dehydration but also assess and treat factors that affect maintenance fluid requirement, such as respiratory distress or fever.

By separating fluid therapy into three components—previous losses, maintenance fluid needs, and ongoing loss—the physician can avoid many problems. Assessing previous losses allows the physician to anticipate the adequacy of perfusion and the type of dehydration that is likely to exist. If abnormal losses, eg, those associated with a stoma, nasogastric suction, or burns, have been present, the appropriate fluid can be analyzed and deficits replaced. The physician calculating maintenance needs must also take into account those metabolic factors that alter needs. Finally, in the vast majority of cases, abnormal losses stop once parenteral therapy is initiated. However, by addressing this issue directly, the physician will not overlook abnormal ongoing losses, eg, those associated with a fistula or tracheostomy.

Compromised perfusion (as evidenced by inadequate capillary refill, poor color, increased pulse, decreased urine output, or low blood pressure) constitutes an emergency that must be addressed at once. A 20 mL/kg bolus of fluid should be given intravenously as rapidly as possible. Either colloid or crystalloid may be used. The fluid may be administered intraosseously (the marrow space of the tibia is accessible) or even intraperitoneally if no IV site is available. If there is no response to the first bolus, a second may be given. It is important to document urine formation and output. Hypotonic solutions may create a problem unless it is known that hypernatremia is not present.

The magnitude of electrolyte deficit may be estimated from tables such as those previously presented or calculated from the formula (shown in the section on hyponatremic states):

$$\text{Deficit (meq)} = (\text{desired concentration} - \text{observed concentration}) \times \text{bodyweight (kg)} \times \text{volume of distribution}$$

Potassium defects must be estimated separately, because deficits cannot be calculated due to the primarily intracellular location of potassium.

Typically, one-half the previous deficits are administered in the first 8 hours of therapy, and the remainder are given over the next 16 hours. Maintenance needs are provided at a steady rate. Ongoing losses are analyzed as needed and replaced at a steady rate as well. If the patient is unable to eat for a prolonged period, nutritional needs must be anticipated and met either through enteral nutrition or hyperalimentation.

It is unfortunately fashionable simply to provide twice the maintenance fluids needed and to assume that time will cure the problem that precipitated the dehydration. This prevents early detection of secondary problems, such as fluid shifts or deficits caused by ongoing losses. By calculating deficits and needs, the physician can monitor the efficacy of therapy as the patient is being treated.

Finberg L et al: Oral rehydration for diarrhea. *J Pediatr* 1982;**101**:497.

Santosham M et al: Oral rehydration therapy for infantile diarrhea. *N Engl J Med* 1982;**306**:1070.

Santosham M et al: Oral rehydration therapy and dietary therapy for acute childhood diarrhea. *Pediatr Rev* 1987; **8**:273.

Winters RW: *Principles of Pediatric Fluid Therapy*, 2nd ed. Little, Brown, 1982.

Schrier RW (editor): *Renal and Electrolyte Disorders*, 3rd ed. Little, Brown, 1986.

Drug Therapy

37

Cynthia R. Gelman, BS Pharm, Barry H. Rumack, MD, & Robert G. Peterson, MD, PhD

INTRODUCTION

Precautions

Older children should never be given a dose greater than the adult dose. In the following pages, adult dosages are noted for the purpose of indicating the maximum dosage in older children when the dosage is calculated on the basis of weight. It must be recognized that on a milligram per kilogram basis, adult dosages are reached at 50 kilograms, not 70 kilograms. All drugs should be used with caution in children, and dosage should be individualized, based on age as well as weight. Once out of the neonatal period, children usually have more rapid hepatic metabolism than adults. Dosage may have to be adjusted downward for cases of kidney and liver disease, which may impair elimination of certain substances, and for individual metabolic capacities. The dosage recommendations on the following pages should be regarded only as estimates; careful clinical observations and the use of pertinent laboratory aids are necessary. Established drugs should be used in preference to newer and less familiar drugs, particularly because pediatric data are rarely submitted for new drugs.

Drugs should be used in early infancy only for significant disorders. In both full-term and premature infants, metabolizing enzymes may be deficient or absent; renal function relatively inefficient; and the blood-brain barrier and protein binding altered.

Dosages for newborn infants have not been determined as accurately as those for older children.

At any age, oliguria requires a reduction of dosage of drugs excreted via the urine.

Whenever possible, reference should also be made to the printed literature supplied by the manufacturer or to the recommendations of the American Academy of Pediatrics Committee on Drugs.

Determination of Drug Dosage

Dosage rules based on proportions of the adult dose are not satisfactory despite their wide use in the past. Dosage based on surface area is probably the most accurate method of estimating the dose for a child if extrapolated adult doses are ever used. Surface area in children can be estimated using Fig 37–1.

Administration of Drugs
A. Route of Administration:
1. Oral—Tablets may be crushed between spoons and given with chocolate, honey, jam, or maple or corn syrup. Many regularly prescribed drugs are commercially available in special pediatric preparations. The parent should be warned that the attractively flavored drug must be kept out of reach of children in the home. Avoid administering drugs with food. Attempt to administer the entire dose in one spoonful.

2. Parenteral—Parenteral administration of certain drugs is necessary, especially in the hospital. Its use as a matter of convenience should be evaluated in the light of the emotional trauma that may result.

3. Rectal—Rectal administration is often very useful, especially for home use. The physician must make certain, however, that rectal absorption is predictable before depending upon this route for a specific drug. Many drugs are prepared in suppository form, but pediatric dose forms are mandatory. It is not good practice to cut an adult suppository.

B. Flavoring Agents for Drugs:
Drugs for children should not be so flavorful that they are sought out as "candy." Syrups are more useful as flavoring agents than alcoholic elixirs, because the ethanol content of the latter may produce toxicity.

Refusal of Medications

The administration of a drug to a child requires tact and skill. The parent or nurse should proceed as if protest is not anticipated. Persuasion before it is necessary sets the stage for struggle. The child must understand that the drug will be given despite protest, but great care should be exercised to avoid aspiration in a struggling child.

SPECIAL CONSIDERATIONS IN PEDIATRIC DRUG DOSAGE

The pediatrician must not only be aware of the correct drug dosage and indication but must also take into account optimal frequency of administration as well as rates of absorption, metabolism, and elimination, which may vary widely at different ages and under different conditions. The following approach to rational drug administration in the pediatric age group takes into account various states of renal function, liver metabolism, and body size that affect drug dosage in children.

Therapeutic Range

Determination of plasma levels of drugs can be extremely useful in monitoring therapy. For some

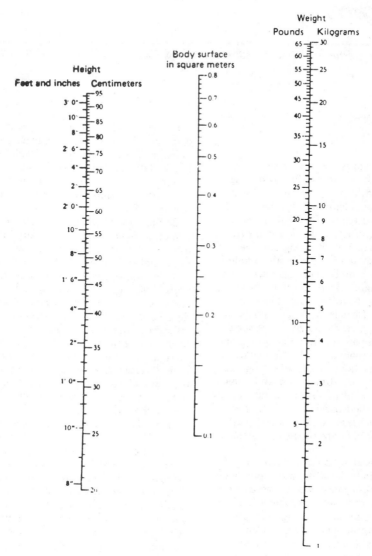

Figure 37–1. Nomogram for the determination of body surface area of children. (Reproduced, with permission, from DuBois EF: *Basal Metabolism in Health and Disease.* Lea & Febiger, 1936.)

drugs (eg, digoxin, theophylline, phenobarbital), the plasma level is well correlated with the drug's physiologic effect and is easier to quantify than the physiologic effect itself. For other classes of drugs (eg, antibiotics, anticoagulants, insulin), it is more important to measure the physiologic effect: serum bactericidal level, prothrombin time, blood glucose, etc.

The therapeutic range is defined as the range of plasma levels for any given drug at which the majority of a treated population will receive the drug's intended therapeutic benefit without experiencing serious toxic side effects. Table 37–1 lists the therapeutic ranges for some drugs commonly used in pediatric practice. Drug toxicity can be expected when plasma levels exceed the therapeutic range.

To obtain a therapeutic level for a particular drug, one must take into account the distribution of the drug throughout the body, whereas maintenance of a therapeutic level requires consideration of elimination processes.

Volume of Distribution

Following the intravenous administration of a drug, plasma levels will fall rapidly as the drug is distributed from the vascular compartment to the extracellular, cellular, central nervous system, and other "compartments" of the body. Its final concentration in the plasma will be dependent upon the dilution of the drug in the various body spaces. Mathematically, this is expressed as

$$\text{Plasma level} = \frac{\text{Dose}}{\text{Volume of distribution}}$$

Because different drugs have differing solubilities in the body fluids or bind to tissues to varying degrees, the volume of distribution (V_d) will vary from drug to drug. Table 37–2 gives the V_d values for a number of commonly used drugs. With the therapeu-

tic level (from Table 37–1) and the volume of distribution (from Table 37–2), one can calculate the appropriate loading dose for a number of drugs as follows:

$$\text{Dose (mg/kg)} = \text{Plasma level (mg/L)} \times V_d \text{ (L/kg)}$$

It should be emphasized that this calculation is appropriate for initial or loading doses only. Maintenance doses are discussed below.

Although the V_d is determined from data gathered after intravenous use, it is also a valuable constant for use with oral or intramuscular preparations. Pro-

Table 37–1. Therapeutic blood levels.[1]

Drug	Blood Levels	
	Expressed as Fraction of g/mL	Expressed as Fraction of mol/L (SI Units)
Acetaminophen	10–20 μg/mL[2]	65–130 μmol/L
Amikacin	15–30 μg/mL (peak) < 5 μg/mL (trough)	... ...
Amobarbital	< 5 μg/mL	< 20 μmol/L
Aprobarbital	< 5 μg/mL	< 20 μmol/L
Bromide	< 500 μg/mL	< 6 mmol/L
Bupivacaine	< 100 ng/mL	< 0.3 μmol/L
Butalbital	< 5 μg/mL	≤ 20 μmol/L
Carbamazepine	4–12 μg/mL	16–48 μmol/L
Chloramphenicol	15–30 μg/mL	45–90 μmol/L
Digoxin	0.9–2.4 ng/mL	1–2 nmol/L
Ethanol	1000 μg/mL ("under the influence")	20 mmol/L
Ethchlorvynol	10–20 μg/mL	70–140 μmol/L
Ethosuximide	40–100 μg/mL	280–700 μmol/L
Gentamicin	8–10 μg/mL (peak)	...
Glutethimide	< 4 μg/mL	< 20 μmol/L
Hexobarbital	< 5 μg/mL	< 20 μmol/L
Lidocaine	< 100 ng/mL (newborn) 1.5–2.5 μg/mL (adult)	< 0.4 μmol/L (newborn) 6–9 μmol/L (adult)
Meprobamate	5–20 μg/mL	20–80 μmol/L
Methsuximide as the metabolite N-des methsuximide	10–40 μg/mL	50–200 μmol/L
Methyprylon	< 5 μg/mL	< 25 μmol/L
Pentobarbital	< 5 μg/mL	< 20 μmol/L
Phenobarbital	15–40 μg/mL	60–160 μmol/L
Phensuximide	10–20 μg/mL	50–100 μmol/L
Phenytoin (diphenylhydantoin)	10–20 μg/mL	40–80 μmol/L
Primidone	4–12 μg/mL	20–55 μmol/L
Procainamide	4–6 μg/mL	15–20 μmol/L
Quinidine	3–5 μg/mL	10–15 μmol/L
Salicylate	< 350 μg/mL	< 2.5 mmol/L
Secobarbital	< 5 μg/mL	< 20 μmol/L
Sulfisoxazole	100 μg/mL	375 μmol/L
Theophylline	10–20 μg/mL	55–110 μmol/L
Tobramycin	8–10 μg/mL (peak)	17–21 μmol/L (peak)
Valproic acid	50–120 μg/mL	350–800 μmol/L

[1]Therapeutic level or range for drugs that can be routinely analyzed.
[2]Conversions: 1 μg/mL = 1 mg/L. 1 μg/mL = 0.1 mg/dL.

Table 37–2. Approximate volumes of distribution (V_d) in L/kg.

Acetaminophen	1.0
Amobarbital	1.1
Secobarbital	1.5
Phenobarbital	0.75 (1.0)[1]
Pentobarbital	1.0
Phenytoin	0.75 (1.0)
Amphetamine	0.6
Caffeine	0.9
Salicylate[2]	0.2 (therapeutic doses)
	0.6 (toxic doses)
Furosemide	0.2
Phenothiazines	> 30
Theophylline	0.46 (0.69)
Narcotics	> 5
Penicillins	0.2–0.3
Digoxin	7.5
Local anesthetics	1.0–1.5
Aminoglycosides	0.3–0.5
Benzodiazepines	> 10

[1] Values in parentheses are for newborns.
[2] The V_d of salicylate increases with increasing dose owing to saturation of plasma protein binding.

vided that the drug's absorption is complete, there is little difference between a slow intravenous infusion and an intramuscular injection. In an instance where an immediate effect is desired but intramuscular absorption is poor (eg, digoxin, phenytoin, diazepam), the slow intravenous route is preferred.

Renal Elimination

Maintenance of a therapeutic level requires that drugs be administered in amounts equivalent to their elimination. Charged or polar drugs (eg, penicillins, aminoglycosides) are directly excreted by the kidneys, and there is little danger of drug accumulation unless the drug is given more frequently than every half-life. Thus, the recommendation for dosage interval for this type of drug is approximately every 1–2 half-lives. When drugs are eliminated by renal processes alone, a steady state will be reached after approximately 5 half-lives, and the plasma level will depend upon the dose and volume of distribution of the drug (see above).

Recommendations for dose and frequency of administration of a large number of medications are given in Average Drug Dosages for Children (below).

Hepatic Elimination

Nonpolar drugs are first metabolized in the liver to make them polar and are then excreted by the kidneys. A steady-state plasma level will be achieved only when the dose given is equivalent to the amount of drug metabolized in the interval between doses.

In deciding on dosages of drugs metabolized in the liver, care must be exercised to make certain that an amount of drug given at a particular frequency does not overwhelm the liver's capacity to metabo-

lize it during the prescribed interval. Fig 37–2 demonstrates the effect of increasing dosage for a drug such as phenytoin upon the plasma level of the drug. As can be observed, one can determine a safe maximum dose (indicated by arrow) above which drug accumulation rapidly occurs. This dose approximates the maximum capacity of the liver for metabolism of this drug.

Drug toxicity can occur rapidly with drugs requiring hepatic elimination. When plasma levels in the upper portion of the therapeutic range are required, frequent plasma determinations should be utilized to avoid drug accumulation.

An example is as follows: A 20-kg child receiving phenytoin ($V_d = 0.75$ L/kg; see Table 37–2) has a plasma level of 18 μg/mL 4 hours following a daily oral dose. Just prior to the next dose (given at 24-hour intervals), a plasma level is 10 μg/mL. One can estimate the amount metabolized by this child and, therefore, the appropriate maintenance dose by means of the following equations:

$$\text{Fall in plasma level} = 8 \text{ mg/L}$$
$$V_d = 20 \text{ kg} \times 0.75 \text{ L/kg} = 15 \text{ L}$$
$$\text{Dose} = 15 \text{ L} \times 8 \text{ mg/L} = 120 \text{ mg}$$

In 20 hours, 120 mg was eliminated, or 144 mg would be eliminated in 24 hours. The appropriate dose of phenytoin for this child is 144 mg, or 7.2 mg/kg, given every 24 hours.

Table 37–3 outlines examples of drugs that are eliminated by the 2 routes discussed above.

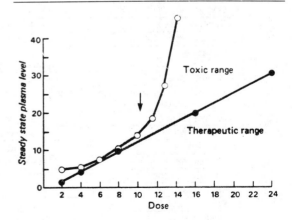

Figure 37–2. Plot (o—o) represents plasma level as a function of increasing dosage of any drug eliminated by hepatic metabolism. Arrow indicates dose at which rapid accumulation of drug occurs. This quantity of administered drug equals capacity of liver metabolism. Dosages above this level cause further rapid increase in plasma level. Plot (●—●) shows data observed with drugs eliminated directly by the kidney without metabolism; observe the difference.

Continuous intravenous infusions. Traditionally, several drugs have been administered by continuous intravenous infusion. Examples are theophylline, insulin, tolazoline, nitroprusside, lidocaine, and dopamine. Continuous intravenous infusion provides a constant amount of drug in the plasma and avoids the "peaks" and "troughs" in plasma levels. For several of the shorter-acting drugs such as dopamine or nitroprusside, it has not been important to measure an actual plasma level because the effect of the drug is readily apparent to the clinician and toxicity can be rapidly terminated by stopping the infusion. For other drugs such as theophylline or lidocaine, however, measurement of plasma levels during continuous infusion is essential, particularly if the drugs are used aggressively. For example, in the case of aminophylline (theophylline ethylenediamine), an infusion rate of 0.9 mg/kg/h is widely used, but this infusion rate is correct only in adults and will result in an average steady-state theophylline level of 10 μg/mL. Because this level is near the lower end of the therapeutic range (Table 37–1), many asthmatics in status asthmaticus will not be adequately treated with this infusion rate. A useful calculation in estimating the infusion rate required to obtain a higher steady-state continuous plasma level is as follows:

Infusion rate (mg/kg/h) = Plasma level (mg/L)
$$\times \text{ Plasma clearance (L/kg/h)}$$

The utility of this formula is that the clinician who has decided on the therapeutic plasma level that is appropriate for an asthmatic patient (low [10 μg/mL], middle [15 μg/mL], or high [20 μg/mL]) can then estimate an appropriate infusion rate. The plasma level in the formula is in mg/L for the sake of equality in the units, but 1 mg/L = 1 μg/mL. The additional value necessary for this estimation, the plasma clearance, is given in Table 37–4. Note that there are distinct differences in plasma clearance in different age groups; the greater theophylline clearance in younger children requires a larger rate of infusion than used in adults.

Table 37–3. Principal routes of drug elimination.

Renal	Liver
Aminoglycosides	Acetaminophen[1]
Digoxin	Alcohol
Furosemide	Caffeine
Penicillins	Digitoxin (75%)
Phenobarbital (25%)	Phenobarbital (75%)
	Phenytoin
	Salicylates
	Theophylline

[1]Liver metabolism is rapid, and kinetics appear to be similar to those of drugs excreted by primary renal elimination.

Table 37–4. Plasma theophylline clearance.

Age	Clearance (L/kg/h)
Newborn	0.018
Children (1–10 years)	0.10
Adults	0.07

If one wishes to estimate the theophylline infusion rate necessary to maintain a plasma level of 15 μg/mL in a 5-year-old child, the calculation would be:

$$\text{Rate (mg/kg/h)} = 15 \text{ (mg/L)} \times 0.1 \text{ (L/kg/h)}$$
$$= 1.5 \text{ (mg/kg/h)}$$

A continuous infusion should be initiated following a loading dose of theophylline based upon the V_d calculation to give an initial plasma level of 15 μg/mL.

These calculations do not take the place of laboratory monitoring of theophylline levels but provide a reference point to aid in dosage recommendations. In the case of theophylline, the use of a higher molecular weight dosage form, ie, aminophylline, will require an increment to be made in the dose administered. Also, theophylline elimination may not be linear at higher infusion rates. Drug accumulation should always be assessed by plasma levels.

DRUGS & BREAST FEEDING

Most drugs are excreted to some degree in breast milk, but this is not a pharmacologically important route for maternal drug elimination. Toxic quantities are rarely delivered to the infant by this route, and levels of drugs in breast milk rarely exceed levels in maternal plasma. In those cases where levels in milk have been reported to exceed the plasma level, the ratio is seldom beyond 1.5:1; ratios above 10:1 have not been reported for therapeutic agents. Quantitative drug overdose of the infant via breast milk is virtually never a problem.

Before administering a drug to a lactating woman, the following questions should be answered:

(1) Is the maternal drug therapy really necessary?

(2) Is this the least toxic drug that is effective?

(3) Can the dosing schedule be arranged to minimize delivery of the drug to the infant?

(4) Would this drug be given directly to the infant if the infant had an appropriate pediatric illness?

(5) In those instances where parenteral medications are given to the mother, is the drug absorbed by the oral route as it is delivered to the infant?

(6) Are idiosyncratic or allergic reactions a particular concern for this infant?

(7) Are there side effects? Will they be easily recognized (eg, drowsiness, rash, etc)?

(8) Does the infant have a known medical problem

(eg, hepatic disease or renal disease) that would diminish the drug's excretion and thereby allow it to accumulate in the infant?

(9) Does the infant have a suspected medical problem (eg, suspected infection masked by low-dose antibiotic delivery via milk) whose eventual diagnosis might be delayed by subtherapeutic doses of the maternal drug?

(10) Will the amount of drug delivered via breast milk come close to approaching a therapeutic dose in the infant?

The answers to these questions usually will give the health care provider the information needed to know whether a drug should be given to the mother.

Quantitative drug overdose of the infant via breast milk is virtually never an issue, but idiosyncratic or allergic reactions to drugs are often not dose-related, and this aspect of drug administration should be kept in mind.

Some drugs are relatively safe in the adult (eg, radioactive iodine) but are associated with higher toxicity rates in children. These drugs, as well as other radiolabeled compounds, many cancer chemotherapeutic agents, and organ-selective toxic substances, should not be given to the mother if breast feeding is to be continued.

SUMMARY

The therapeutic ranges for a number of drugs are presented in Table 37–1. The measurement of plasma levels during therapy will facilitate the regulation of dosage to produce therapeutic effects without toxicity. Drugs whose elimination is dependent chiefly upon hepatic metabolism require special surveillance. Average Drug Dosages for Children (below) lists a number of drugs used in pediatric patients along with the appropriate dose and frequency for each.

AVERAGE DRUG DOSAGES FOR CHILDREN*

Acetaminophen: Dose based on weight is 10–15 mg/kg orally. Dose based on age is generally as follows: 0–3 months, 40 mg; 4–11 months, 80 mg; 12–23 months, 120 mg; 2–3 years, 160 mg; 4–5 years,

180 mg; 6–8 years, 320 mg; 9–10 years, 400 mg; 11–12 years, 480 mg. May be repeated up to 5 times in 24 hours.

Acetazolamide: 5–30 mg/kg/d orally every 6–8 hours (Adult = 5 mg/kg/d.) For hydrocephalus, 20–55 mg/kg/d orally in 2 or 3 divided doses. For anticonvulsant use, see Table 24–3.

Acetylcysteine: For acetaminophen antidote, use 20% solution diluted 3:1 with juice, water, or carbonated beverage, 140 mg/kg orally (loading dose) followed by 17 doses of 70 mg/kg orally every 4 hours.

ACTH (adrenocorticotropic hormone, corticotropin): For infantile spasms, usually 20–40 units/d or (in gel form) 80 units every other day intramuscularly. For anticonvulsant use, see Seizure Disorders, Chapter 24.

Acyclovir: For herpes simplex infections and in neonates and children, 30 mg/kg/24 h intravenously every 8 hours for 10–14 days. For severe genital herpes, 15 mg/kg/24 h intravenously every 8 hours for 5 days.

Albumin, salt-poor: 0.5–1 g/kg intravenously as 25 g/dL solution. Maximum, up to 25 g per dose, as required.

Albuterol: For children 2–6 years, 0.1 mg/kg orally to a maximum of 2 mg/dose 3 times daily. For children 6–12 years, 2 mg orally 3–4 times daily.

Alprostadil (prostaglandin E_1): To maintain patency of ductus arteriosus in patients with congenital heart lesions, 0.05–0.1 μg/kg/min by continuous infusion.

Aluminum hydroxide gel: 5–15 mL orally with meals.

Amantadine hydrochloride: 4.4–8.8 mg/kg/d orally.

Aminocaproic acid: 200 mg/kg orally, then 100 mg/kg/dose orally every 6 hours for 3–7 days (adult maximum = 30 g/24 h).

Aminophylline: Intravenously, 4–6 mg/kg every 6 hours or by continuous infusion of 0.9 mg/kg/h. High infusion rates may be necessary in children (see Special Considerations in Pediatric Drug Dosage, above). Intramuscular or rectal administration not recommended.

Ammonium chloride: For urinary acidification, 75 mg/kg/d orally in 4 divided doses.

Amphetamine sulfate: 0.5 mg/kg/d orally in 3 divided doses. Maximum, 15 mg/d. (Adult = 5–15 mg/d.)

Apomorphine: Not indicated in pediatric practice.

Aspirin: Not recommended for routine analgesic or antipyretic use in children. For rheumatoid arthritis, 80–100 mg/kg/d to maintain a blood level of 20–30 mg/dL. (Adult maximum = 6–8 g/d.) Monitor plasma levels and liver function during therapy.

Atropine sulfate: 0.01–0.02 mg/kg subcutaneously, intravenously, or endotracheally. Maximum,

*For drugs discussed in other chapters, consult the index.

0.4 mg. (Adult = 0.3–1 mg.) For cardiac arrest, use intravenous or endotracheal route. For breath-holding spells, see Seizure Disorders, Chapter 24. *Caution.*

Azathioprine: 3–5 mg/kg/d orally.

Beclomethasone dipropionate: For reactive airway disease, 1–2 puffs every 6–8 hours. Metered aerosol delivers 42 µg per puff.

Benzoyl peroxide: Apply once daily after washing face. Begin with 2.5% gel, and increase gel concentration (5%, 10%) as tolerated and required.

Benztropine mesylate: Dose not established in younger children. For adolescents, 0.5–1.0 mg/dose every 12 hours or daily.

Bethanechol chloride: Orally, 0.6 mg/kg/d in 3 divided doses. (Adult = 10–30 mg 3 or 4 times daily.) Subcutaneously, 0.15–0.2 mg/kg/d. (Adult = 2.5–5 mg/d.)

Bisacodyl: 5 mg orally or rectally. Children over 2 years, up to 10 mg rectally.

Bretylium tosylate: For ventricular arrhythmias, 5 mg/kg/dose every 6 hours intramuscularly or diluted in 5% dextrose in water or in normal saline over 10–30 minutes.

Brompheniramine: For children under 6 years, 0.5 mg/kg/d orally. For children over 6 years, 4 mg 3 or 4 times daily. (Adult = 4–8 mg 3 or 4 times daily.)

Busulfan: 0.06 mg/kg/d orally. (Adult = 4–8 mg daily.)

Calcium chloride (27% calcium): For newborns and infants, 0.2 g/kg/d orally as a 2% solution. For children, 0.3 g/kg/d. (Adult = 2–4 g 3 times daily.) *Caution.*

Calcium glubionate (6% calcium): 600–2000 mg/kg/d given in 4 doses. (Adult = 6–18 g/d.)

Calcium gluconate (9% calcium): Intravenously, for cardiac arrest in children, give 10% solution, 1 mL/kg. Inject slowly and stop if bradycardia occurs. (Adult = 5–10 mL.) *Caution.*

Calcium lactate (13% calcium): 0.5 g/kg/d orally in divided doses as dilute solution. (Adult = 4–8 g 3 times daily.)

Captopril: For hypertension, 0.15 mg/kg/dose orally 1 hour prior to meals, 3 times daily. Double dose to achieve control of hypertension to maximum of 6 mg/kg/24 h.

Charcoal, activated: 1–2 g/kg mixed in water and given orally or by orogastric tube. 20–30 g should be diluted in 8 oz of water.

Chloral hydrate: As hypnotic, 12.5–50 mg/kg (up to 1 g) orally or rectally. (Adult = 0.5–2 g.) As sedative, 4–20 mg/kg (up to 1 g) orally or rectally. (Adult = 0.25–1 g.) May be repeated in 1 hour to obtain desired effect, and then may be repeated every 6–8 hours.

Chlorambucil: 0.1–0.2 mg/kg/d orally. (Adult = 0.2 mg/kg/d.)

Chlordiazepoxide: For children over 6 years, 0.5 mg/kg/d orally in 3 or 4 divided doses.

Chlorothiazide: For children under 6 months, 30 mg/kg/d orally in 2 divided doses. For older children, 20 mg/kg/d. (Adult = 0.5–1 g once or twice daily.)

Chlorpheniramine: 0.35 mg/kg/d orally in 4 divided doses or subcutaneously. (Adult = 2–4 mg 3 or 4 times daily; long-acting, 8–12 mg 2 or 3 times daily.)

Chlorpromazine: Orally, 0.5 mg/kg every 4–6 hours. (Adult maximum = 1–2 g/d.) Intramuscularly, for children up to 5 years, 0.5 mg/kg every 6–8 hours as necessary but not over 40 mg/d; for children 5–12 years, not over 75 mg/d. (Adult = 25–100 mg per dose.) Rectally, 1 mg/kg per dose. (Adult = 10–50 mg per dose.)

Cholestyramine: For children under 6 years, dose not yet established. For children over 6 years, 8 g/d in 2 divided doses increased to a maximum of 24 g for hyperlipidemias.

Cimetidine: 20–40 mg/kg/d orally or intravenously in 4 divided doses. (Adult = 300 mg 4 times daily.) Neonates, 10–20 mg/kg orally or intravenously in 4–6 doses.

Citrovorum factor (leucovorin calcium): 2–15 mg/d orally.

Clonazepam: 0.01 mg/kg/d orally in divided doses every 8 hours to start. Increase slowly to 0.1–0.2 mg/kg/d. See also Table 24–3.

Clonidine hydrochloride: For hypertension, 1–5 µg/kg/dose every 6 hours orally or as transdermal patch, 0.1–0.3 mg/24 hours. *Caution:* Rebound hypertension on discontinuation.

Cocaine: Topical, maximum dose = 1 mg/kg.

Codeine phosphate: Orally, 0.8–1.5 mg/kg as a single sedative or analgesic dose. (Adult = 8–60 mg every 4–6 hours.) Subcutaneously, 0.8 mg/kg. (Adult = 30 mg.) For cough, 0.2 mg/kg every 4–6 hours.

Corticotropin (adrenocorticotropic hormone, ACTH): For infantile spasms, usually 20–40 units/d or (in gel form) 80 units every other day intramuscularly. For anticonvulsant use, see Seizure Disorders, Chapter 24.

Cromolyn sodium: One 20-mg capsule inhaled with a Spinhaler 4 times daily or 2 inhalations from a metered dose dispenser. *Caution:* Should not be used during asthmatic attack.

Cyclizine: For children 6–10 years, 3 mg/kg/d orally in 3 divided doses. For adolescents, 50 mg every 4–6 hours as necessary (same as adult dose).

Cyclophosphamide: 2–8 mg/kg/d orally or intravenously for 7 or more days or 15–50 mg/kg once a week. See also Table 31–6.

Cyproheptadine hydrochloride: 0.25 mg/kg/d orally in 3 or 4 divided doses. (Adult = 12–16 mg/d.)

Cytarabine (cytosine arabinoside): 2 mg/kg/d by

direct injection or 2–6 mg/kg/d by infusion. See also Table 31–6.

Dactinomycin (actinomycin D): 0.015 mg/kg/d intravenously for 5 days (same as adult dose). See also Table 31–6.

Dantrolene sodium: For malignant hyperthermia prophylaxis, 1–2 mg/kg orally every 8 hours, starting 24–48 hours prior to anesthesia. For malignant hyperthermia treatment, 1 mg/kg intravenously as initial dose, and then increase by 0.5–1 mg/kg as required. Maximum dose, 10 mg/kg.

Deferoxamine mesylate: Intramuscularly, 90 mg/kg (up to 1 g) every 8 hours. Intravenously, 15 mg/kg/h by continuous infusion. *Caution:* Hypotension.

Dextroamphetamine: For children 3–5 years, 2.5 mg daily increased by 2.5 mg at weekly intervals; for children 6 years and older, 5–10 mg/d increased by 5 mg at weekly intervals. For anticonvulsant use, see Table 24–3.

Dextromethorphan hydrobromide: 1 mg/kg/d orally.

Diazepam: Orally, 0.12–0.8 mg/kg/d in 4 divided doses. (Adult = 5–10 mg per dose.) Intravenously, 0.04–0.2 mg/kg slowly as a single dose. (Adult = 5–10 mg per dose.) See also Table 24–3.

Diazoxide: For hypertensive crisis, 3–5 mg/kg intravenously as bolus into peripheral vein within 30 seconds (maximum dose 150 mg). May repeat in 5–15 minutes and then 4–24 hours. *Caution:* Monitor for sodium retention and hyperglycemia.

Dicyclomine hydrochloride: For infants, 5 mg orally (as syrup) 3 or 4 times daily. For children, 10 mg 3 or 4 times daily. (Adult = 10–20 mg 3 or 4 times daily.)

Digoxin: Digitalizing dose: 30 μg/kg over 24 hours as 15 μg/kg, then 7.5 μg/kg at 8- to 12-hour intervals orally or intravenously. Intramuscular administration not recommended. Maintenance: 10–15 μg/kg/24 h orally in 1 or 2 doses.

Dihydrotachysterol: Initially, 0.1–0.5 mg orally daily. (Adult = 0.5–1 mg/day.)

Dimenhydrinate: 1–1.5 mg/kg orally every 6 hours as needed. (Adult = 50–100 mg every 6 hours as needed.)

Dimercaprol (BAL): 2.5–3 mg/kg intramuscularly every 4 hours for 2 days, 4 times per day on day 3, then 2 times per day for 10 days.

Diphenhydramine hydrochloride: Orally, 4–6 mg/kg/d in 3 or 4 divided doses. (Adult = 100–200 mg/d.)

Diphenoxylate hydrochloride: Contraindicated in children under 2 years. Dose based on weight is 0.3–0.4 mg/kg administered in 4 divided doses. Dose based on age is generally as follows: 2 years, 1.5–3.0 mL 4 times per day; 3 years, 2–3 mL 4 times per day; 4 years, 2–4 mL 4 times per day; 5 years, 2.5–4.5 mL 4 times per day; 6–8 years, 2.5–5 mL 4 times per day; 9–12 years 3.5–5 mL 4 times per day.

Dobutamine: 2.5–15 μg/kg/min by continuous infusion. Incompatible with sodium bicarbonate in same line.

Docusate: Infants and children under 3 years, 10–40 mg/d orally; children 3–6 years, 20–60 mg/d orally; children 6–12 years, 40–120 mg/d orally. (Adults = 50–200 mg/day).

Dopamine: 5–20 μg/kg/min by continuous intravenous infusion.

Doxylamine succinate: 2 mg/kg/d orally.

Edrophonium chloride: As test dose for infant, 0.2 mg/kg intravenously. Give only one-fifth of dose slowly initially; if tolerated, give remainder. (Adult = 5–10 mg.) For myasthenia gravis, see Chapter 24. *Caution:* Atropine should be available as antidote.

EDTA (calcium disodium salt, calcium EDTA, edetate calcium disodium): 50–75 mg/kg/d intravenously or intramuscularly in solution containing procaine, 0.5–1.5%.

Ephedrine sulfate: Orally, 0.5–1 mg/kg. May repeat every 4–6 hours. (Adult = 25 mg per dose.) Intravenously, 50 mg/L, adjusting drip rate to patient's response (same as adult dose).

Epinephrine solution, 1:1000 aqueous: Subcutaneously, 0.01–0.025 mL/kg. Maximum, 0.5 mL. (Adult = 0.5–1 mL.) For cardiac arrest, 0.01 mL/kg intravenously or via endotracheal tube.

Epinephrine solution, 1:200 aqueous: 0.004–0.005 mL/kg subcutaneously, one dose only. Use smallest effective dose.

Ergocalciferol (vitamin D₂): For renal osteodystrophy, 25,000–200,000 units/d orally. For hypoparathyroidism, 2000 IU/d (50 μg/kg/d) orally.

Estradiol valerate: For teenage girls, 10 mg/month intramuscularly. (Adult = 10–20 mg every 2–3 weeks.)

Ethinyl estradiol: For teenage girls, 0.02–0.05 mg orally 1–3 times daily. (Adult = 0.05 mg 1–3 times daily.)

Ethosuximide: For children 3–6 years, 250 mg/d orally as starting dose. For children over 6 years, 250 mg twice daily as starting dose. See also Table 24–3.

Ferrous salts (medicinal iron): Elemental iron, 6–9 mg/kg/d orally in 3 divided doses. See also Table 5–1. For iron deficiency anemia, see Chapter 17.

Fluorouracil: 12 mg/kg intravenously (up to 800 mg/d) for 4 successive days. If no toxicity is observed, give 6 mg/kg on the sixth, eighth, tenth, and twelfth days. If toxicity has not been a problem, the course of therapy may be repeated beginning 30 days after the last day of the previous course. See also Table 31–6.

Flurazepam hydrochloride: Not recommended for children under 15 years. For adolescents and adults, 15–30 mg orally at bedtime for sleep.

Folic acid: 0.2–1 mg/d orally. (Adult = 1–3 mg/d.)

Furosemide: 1 mg/kg intravenously, intramuscularly, or 2 mg/kg orally. (Adult = 40–80 mg intravenously, intramuscularly, or orally in the morning for diuresis or 40 mg orally twice daily for hypertension.) For altered states of consciousness, see Chapter 24.

Glucagon: For newborns, 0.025–0.1 mg/kg intravenously as a single dose. Try smaller dose first. May repeat in 30 minutes. For older children, 0.25–1 mg subcutaneously, intramuscularly, or intravenously as a single dose. Maximum, 1 mg.

Gold sodium thiomalate: 1 mg/kg/wk intramuscularly.

Gonadotropin, chorionic: 500–1000 units intramuscularly 2 or 3 times a week for 5–8 weeks.

Guanethidine: 0.2 mg/kg/d orally as a single dose. Increase dose at weekly intervals by same amount. (Adult = 10 mg/d; larger doses possible for hospitalized adults.) *Caution.*

Haloperidol: Children 3–12 years, 0.05–0.15 mg/kg/d in 2–3 doses (maximum 6 mg/day). (Adult = 1–2 mg orally 2 or 3 times daily initially and then 1–2 mg 3 or 4 times daily for maintenance; maximum, 15 mg/d.)

Heparin: 50–100 units/kg intravenously as loading dose. May be followed by continuous infusion of 10–25 units/kg/h or by 40–100 units/kg subcutaneously every 4 hours. Control dosage with clotting times, and follow partial thromboplastin time. May prolong clotting for 24 hours.

Histamine: For provocative test, 0.0275 mg/kg subcutaneously. *Caution:* Phentolamine should be available.

Hydralazine hydrochloride: Orally, 0.15 mg/kg 4 times daily. Increase to tolerance. (Adult = 100 mg as single oral dose.) Intravenously or intramuscularly, 1.5–3.5 mg/kg/d in 4–6 divided doses. (Adult = 20–40 mg as initial parenteral dose.)

Hydrochlorothiazide: For children under 6 months, 2–3 mg/kg/d in 2 divided doses. For older children, 2 mg/kg/d as a single dose or in 2 divided doses. (Adult = 25–200 mg/d.)

Hydrocodone bitartrate: 0.6 mg/kg/d orally in 3 or 4 divided doses. (Adult = 5–10 mg/d.)

Hydroxyprogesterone caproate: For teenage girls, 375 mg intramuscularly.

Hydroxyzine: Orally, 1–2 mg/kg/d in 3 divided doses. (Adult = 25–50 mg 3 times daily.) Intramuscularly for preoperative use, 1 mg/kg/dose every 6 hours.

Ibuprofen: 20–70 mg/kg/d orally in 3 or 4 divided doses. (Adult = 1–3 g/d.)

Imipramine hydrochloride: Not generally recommended for children under 6 years. For older children, 25 mg/d orally as initial dose; may increase according to response and tolerance. For adolescents, generally not more than 75 mg/d. (Adult = 75 mg initially, increased to up to 150 mg/d.) *Caution.*

Indomethacin: For closure of patent ductus arteriosus, 0.1–0.25 mg/kg every 12–24 hours until 3 doses have been given. *Caution:* Monitor vital signs and urinary output.

Iodine solution, strong (Lugol's solution): 1–10 drops orally daily for 10–21 days.

Iodoquinol: 40 mg/kg/d orally in 2 or 3 divided doses.

Ipecac syrup: 15–20 mL orally initially. (Adult = 30 mL.) Give water. Ambulate. Repeat in 20 minutes if necessary. *Caution:* Never use fluid extract of ipecac as emetic.

Isoproterenol hydrochloride: For asthma in older children, 5–10 mg sublingually (never more often than every 3–4 hours or more than 3 times daily) or 5–15 breaths of 1:200 solution by oral inhalation (not more than 0.5 mL). (Adult = 5 mg sublingually 4 times daily.) For hypotension, 0.1–1 μg/kg/min by continuous intravenous infusion.

Isoproterenol sulfate: 1–2 inhalations of a 1:200 or 1:400 solution.

Kaolin with pectin: For children 3–6 years, 15–30 mL. For children 6–12 years, 30–60 mL.

Ketoconazole: For children older than 2 years, 3–6 mg/kg/d orally in single dose. Topically, 2% cream once daily for 2–4 weeks.

Leucovorin calcium (citrovorum factor): 2–15 mg/d orally.

Levothyroxine sodium (L-thyroxine): 0.1 mg of levothyroxine sodium = 65 mg of thyroid USP = 25–30 μg of triiodothyronine. For hypothyroidism, see Chapter 26.

Lidocaine: For ventricular ectopy, 0.5–1 mg/kg intravenously slowly. May repeat after 5–10 minutes for additional control. Give continuous intravenous infusion of 20–50 μg/kg/min following loading dose. Measure plasma levels during infusions. For seizures, 0.2–0.5 mg/kg as loading dose, followed by 5–15 μg/kg/min by continuous intravenous infusion. (Adult = 50–100 mg.) See also Table 24–3. Local infiltration, 7 mg/kg with epinephrine; 4.5 mg/kg without epinephrine. Topically, 3 mg/kg. *Caution:* Do not repeat within 2 hours.

Lindane: For scabies, 1% lotion, applied to entire body. Wash carefully after 6 hours. Not for use in infants. *Caution:* Toxic with long or repeated contact.

Lorazepam: For seizures, 0.03–0.05 mg/kg slowly intravenously. (Adult maximum = 2.5–10 mg.) Repeat once in 15 minutes if required.

Lypressin (8-lysine vasopressin): 1–2 sprays into each nostril 4 times a day.

Magnesium hydroxide (milk of magnesia): 0.5–1 mL/kg orally. (Adult = 30–60 mL.)

Magnesium sulfate: As cathartic, 250 mg/kg orally. As anticonvulsant for hypertension, use 20% solution, 20–40 mg/kg intramuscularly every 4–6 hours. *Caution:* Check blood pressure carefully, and have calcium gluconate available.

Mannitol: As test dose for oliguria, 0.75 g/kg

intravenously. For cerebral edema, 1–3 g/kg over a period of 30 minutes to 6 hours. For altered states of consciousness, see Chapter 24.

Mebendazole: For pinworm, 100 mg as a single oral dose; repeat after 2 weeks; for hookworm or roundworm, 100 mg twice a day for 3 days.

Mechlorethamine (nitrogen mustard): 0.1 mg/kg/d intravenously for 4 days (same as adult dose). Dilute and inject slowly.

Menadiol sodium diphosphate: For newborns, see Phytonadione. For older infants and children, 5–10 mg intramuscularly. (Adult = 5–15 mg.)

Meperidine hydrochloride (pethidine hydrochloride): 0.6–1.5 mg/kg intramuscularly, intravenously, or orally as a single analgesic dose. Maximum, 6 mg/kg/d. (Adult = 50–100 mg intramuscularly, intravenously, or orally every 4–6 hours.)

Mephenytoin: 3–15 mg/kg/d orally. Start with smaller dose and gradually increase. (Adult = 0.2–0.6 g daily.) See also Table 24–3.

Mercaptopurine (6-MP): 2.5 mg/kg/d orally (same as adult dose). See also Table 31–6. *Caution.*

Metaraminol: Subcutaneously or intramuscularly, 0.1 mg/kg. Intravenously, 0.01 mg/kg. Titrate by effect or by blood pressure readings. (Adult = 2–10 mg intramuscularly or 0.5–5 mg intravenously.)

Methadone hydrochloride: For analgesia, 0.7 mg/kg/d orally in 2 divided doses.

Methimazole: Initially, 0.5–0.7 mg/kg/d orally in 3 divided doses. Maximum, 30 mg/d. For maintenance, half of initial dose. (Adult = 30 mg/d.)

Methionine: 200–300 mg/d orally in 3 or 4 divided doses. (Adult dose to acidify urine = 12–15 g/d orally.)

Methocarbamol: For tetanus, 15 mg/kg intravenously every 6 hours.

Methoxamine hydrochloride: 0.25 mg/kg intramuscularly as a single dose. 0.08 mg/kg intravenously. (Adult = 15 mg.)

Methsuximide: 10 mg/kg/d orally in divided doses. (Adult = 300 mg 1–3 times daily.) See also Table 24–3.

Methyldopa: Intravenously, 5–10 mg/kg every 6–8 hours to a total of 65 mg/kg/d. Dilute in 50–100 mL of fluid and infuse over 30–60 minutes. Orally, 10 mg/kg/d in divided doses every 6 hours, increasing at 2-day or greater intervals to 65 mg/kg/d. (Adult = 250 mg orally 3 times daily initially, adjusted at 2- to 7-day intervals.) *Caution.*

Methylene blue: 1% solution, 0.1–0.2 mL/kg (1–2 mg/kg) slowly intravenously. (Adult = 100–150 mg per dose.)

Methylphenidate hydrochloride: Not recommended for children under 6 years. For children over 6 years, 0.2 mg/kg dose given orally with breakfast and lunch. (Adult = 10 mg 3 times daily.) For attention deficit disorder, see Chapter 24. *Caution.*

Methyltestosterone: 10–50 mg daily orally; 5–25 mg daily buccally.

Metoclopramide hydrochloride: 0.1 mg/kg orally intramuscularly, intravenously up to 4 times daily. Total daily dose not to exceed 0.5 mg/kg. For chemotherapy-induced emesis, 1–2 mg/kg intravenously.

Midazolam: For anesthesia induction, 0.15 mg/kg followed by 0.05 mg/kg every 2 minutes as required. For sedation, 0.08 mg/kg intramuscularly or 0.3 mg/kg rectally.

Mineral oil (liquid paraffin, liquid petrolatum): 10–20 mL twice daily. (Adult = 15–30 mL.)

Morphine sulfate: 0.1–0.2 mg/kg subcutaneously, intramuscularly, or intravenously every 4 hours as necessary. Single dose maximum, 10 mg. (Adult = 10–15 mg.)

Naloxone hydrochloride: Usual dose is 0.01 mg/kg intravenously. In patients who are significantly depressed, the first dose should be 0.4 mg for those under 5 years and 0.8 mg for those over 5 years. If patient is still unresponsive, 2–4 mg may be given once intravenously to rule out opiate overdose.

Neostigmine: Orally, 7.5–15 mg 3–4 times daily. (Adult = 15 mg 3 times a day.) For myasthenia test, 0.025–0.04 mg/kg intramuscularly (see also Chapter 24). *Caution:* Atropine should be available.

Nitroprusside: For hypertensive emergencies, 0.5–10 μg/kg/min as a continuous intravenous infusion. Start with lowest dose, and titrate blood pressure by increasing infusion by 0.3 μg/kg/min every 5 minutes.

Norepinephrine (levarterenol): Start at 0.1 μg/kg/min intravenously and titrate rate by blood pressure. For adrenal crisis, see Chapter 26.

Oxandrolone: 0.25–0.1 mg/kg/d orally.

Oxymetazoline hydrochloride: For children 2–5 years, 2–3 drops of a 0.025% solution in each nostril 2 times daily. For children greater than 6 years, 2–3 drops in each nostril 2 times daily. *Caution:* Do not use for more than 3 days.

Oxymetholone: 1–5 mg/kg/d orally.

Pancrelipase (pancreatic replacement): 3–12 capsules or 1–4 teaspoonsful of powder with each meal.

Paraldehyde: Orally, 0.1–0.15 mL/kg. (Adult = 4–16 mL.) Rectally, 0.15–0.3 mL/kg in 1 or 2 parts of vegetable oil. (Adult = 16–32 mL.) Do not use plastic equipment.

Paregoric (opium tincture, camphorated): Morphine content is 0.4 mg/mL. For newborns, 0.2–0.5 mL (0.08–0.2 mg morphine equivalents) every 3–4 hours until symptoms of withdrawal are controlled. For children, 0.25–0.5 mL/kg (not to exceed 10 mL) up to 4 times daily.

Penicillamine (D-isomer penicillamine): For arsenic poisoning, for infants over 6 months, 100 mg/kg/d orally in 4 divided doses. Maximum, 1 g/d. For Wilson's disease in infants, 250–500 mg daily.

Pentobarbital: 2–6 mg/kg orally. Intravenously, 3–5 mg/kg. (Adult = 100 mg.)

Phenobarbital: As sedative, 0.5–2 mg/kg orally every 4–6 hours. As anticonvulsant loading dose, 5–10 mg/kg intramuscularly (to receive 20 mg/kg in 24 hours). For maintenance, 5 mg/kg/d in 2 or 3 divided doses. See also Table 24–3.

Phentolamine: For hypertensive crisis, 0.05–0.1 mg/kg intravenously every 5 minutes until blood pressure is controlled. *Caution:* Avoid hypotension.

Phenytoin: For loading dose, 10–20 mg/kg intravenously slowly, not to exceed 1 mg/kg/min. (Adult = 500–1000 mg per dose.) For maintenance, 5–10 mg/kg/d orally as a single dose or in 2 divided doses. (Adult = 0.3–0.5 g/d.) See also Table 24–3.

Phytonadione (vitamin K_1): For prophylactic dose, 0.5–1 mg intramuscularly. For therapeutic dose, 1–2 mg intramuscularly, subcutaneously, or orally. (Mephyton for oral use; others for parenteral use.)

Pilocarpine: 0.25%, 0.5%, 1%, and 2% as eye drops.

Potassium iodide: Saturated solution, 0.1–0.3 mL/d in 2–3 doses orally in cold milk or fruit juice. (Adult = 0.3 mL.)

Pralidoxime: 5% solution, 25–50 mg/kg intravenously.

Primidone: 10–25 mg/kg/d orally. For children under 8 years, start with 125 mg daily; for those over 8 years, start with 250 mg daily. Increase dose slowly as necessary. (Adult = 250 mg as initial dose.) See also Table 24–3.

Probenecid: 25 mg/kg orally as initial dose and then 10 mg/kg every 6 hours. (Adult = 1–2 g as initial dose and then 0.5 g every 6 hours.)

Procainamide hydrochloride: Orally, 3–10 mg/kg every 4–6 hours. Intramuscularly, 6 mg/kg every 4–6 hours. Intravenously, for emergency use only, 2 mg/kg slowly over a 4- to 20-minute period. *Caution:* Monitor by continuous electrocardiography and blood pressure recording every minute.

Procarbazine hydrochloride: 50 mg/d orally as initial dose. See also Table 31–6. *Caution.*

Prochlorperazine: For children greater than 10 kg, 0.4 mg/kg/d in 3 or 4 divided doses orally or rectally. (Adult = 25 mg rectally twice daily or 5 mg orally 3 or 4 times daily.) Intramuscularly, 0.1–0.15 mg/kg/dose. *Caution:* Avoid overdosage; irritant to tissue.

Promethazine hydrochloride: As antihistaminic, 0.5 mg/kg orally at bedtime; 0.1 mg/kg orally 3 times daily. For nausea and vomiting, 0.25–0.5 mg/kg rectally or intramuscularly. For sedation, 0.5–1 mg/kg intramuscularly.

Propantheline bromide: 1–3 mg/kg/d orally in 4 divided doses after meals. (Adult = 15–30 mg 3 or 4 times daily.)

Propranolol: Intravenously, 0.01–0.15 mg/kg as slow push; tetralogy spells may require up to 0.25 mg/kg intravenously. Orally, 0.5–4 mg/kg/d given every 6–8 hours. For headaches, see Chapter 24.

Propylthiouracil: For children 6–10 years, 50–150 mg/d; for children older than 10 years, 150–300 mg/d.

Prostaglandin E_1 (alprostadil): To maintain patency of ductus arteriosus in patients with congenital heart lesions, 0.05–0.1 μg/kg/min by continuous infusion.

Protamine sulfate: 1 mg per 100 units of administered heparin.

Pseudoephedrine hydrochloride: 4 mg/kg/d orally in 4 divided doses. (Adult = 30–60 mg every 6–8 hours.)

Pyridostigmine bromide: 7 mg/kg/d orally in 4–6 divided doses. Increase as necessary. (Adult = 600 mg/d as average dose.) For myasthenia gravis, see Chapter 24.

Pyrimethamine: Children less than 10 kg, 6.25 mg/d for 3 days; children 10–20 kg, 12.5 mg/d for 3 days; children 20–40 kg, 25 mg/d for 3 days.

Quinidine: For test dose, 2 mg/kg orally. If tolerated, give 3–6 mg/kg every 2–3 hours. For therapeutic dose, 30 mg/kg/d orally in 4 or 5 divided doses.

Reserpine; Orally, 0.005–0.03 mg/kg/d in 4 divided doses. (Adult = 0.1–0.5 mg/d.)

Secobarbital sodium: Orally, 2–6 mg/kg as a single sedative or light hypnotic dose. (Adult = 100 mg.) Rectally, 6 mg/kg as a minimal hypnotic dose. (Adult = 200 mg.)

Sodium polystyrene sulfonate: 1 meq of potassium per gram of resin. Calculate dose on basis of desired exchange. Instill rectally in 10% glucose. May be administered every 6 hours. Usual dose is approximately 1 g/kg orally every 6 hours or rectally every 2–6 hours.

Spironolactone: For edema and ascites, 1.7–3.3 mg/kg/d orally in divided doses. Start with small dose. (Adult = 25 mg 3–6 times daily.) *Caution.*

Sulfasalazine: 4–60 mg/kg/d orally in 4–6 divided doses. (Adult = 1 g 4–6 times daily.)

Theophylline: 10–20 mg/kg/d orally in 4 divided doses. See discussion of aminophylline for intravenous use.

Thiopental sodium: For general anesthesia, 1–2 mg/kg intravenously, slowly.

Thioridazine hydrochloride: For children under 2 years, do not use. For behavior disorder in children 2–12 years, 0.5–3 mg/kg/d (maximum) orally; for older children 20–40 mg/d. (Adult = 200–800 mg/d for psychosis.)

Tolazoline hydrochloride: For newborns, 1–2 mg/kg intravenously, followed by 1–2 mg/kg/h by continuous intravenous infusion. *Caution:* potent vasodilator.

Trichlormethiazide: 0.03–0.1 mg/kg/d orally, (Adult = 2–8 mg/d.)

Triiodothyronine (liothyronine): 25–30 μg of triiodothyronine = 65 mg of thyroid USP = 0.1 mg of levothyroxine sodium.

Trimethaphan camsylate: 50–150 μg/kg/min intravenously. (Adult = begin at 0.5–1 mg/min and titrate rate by blood pressure.) *Caution:* Hypotension, including orthostatic hypotension.

Tripelennamine: 3–5 mg/kg/d orally in 3–6 divided doses. Maximum, 300 mg/d. (Adult = 50 mg 3 or 4 times daily.)

Tubocurarine (curare): Initially, 0.2–0.4 mg/kg intravenously. Subsequently, 0.04–0.2 mg/kg as needed to maintain paralysis. *Caution.*

Urea: Orally, 0.8 g/kg/d in 3 divided doses. Intravenously, 0.5–1 g/kg over a period of 30–60 minutes. (Adult = 1–1.5 g/kg/d intravenously.)

Valproic acid: 15 mg/kg/d as a single dose or in 2 or 3 divided doses. May increase by 5 mg/kg/d every 1–2 weeks. Maximum, 60 mg/kg/d. See also Table 24–3.

Vasopressin injection: 0.125–0.5 mL (20 units/mL) intramuscularly. Short duration. (Adult = 0.25–0.5 mL.)

Vasopressin tannate injection: 0.2–1 mL (5 units/mL in oil) intramuscularly every 2–4 days as necessary. Start with smaller dose and increase. Effective 1–3 days. (Adult = 0.3–1 mL per dose.)

Verapamil: For supraventricular tachycardia, 0.1 mg/kg intravenously over 30 seconds (repeat once if required) or 4–10 mg/kg/d orally in divided doses every 12 hours. *Caution:* Transient hypotension.

Vinblastine sulfate: 2.5 mg/m^2 intravenously as a single dose. (Adult = 3.7 mg/m^2 as a single dose.)

SELECTED REFERENCES

Benitz WE, Tatro DS: *Pediatric Drug Handbook,* 2nd ed. Yearbook Medical Publishers, 1988.

Gelman CR, Rumack BH: *DRUGDEX Information System,* Micromedex, 1988.

McEvoy G (editor): *American Hospital Formulary Service Drug Information 88.* American Society of Hospital Pharmacists, 1988.

Physicians' Desk Reference, 42nd ed. Medical Economics Company, 1988.

Roberts RJ (editor): *Drug Therapy in Infants: Pharmacologic Principles and Clinical Experience.* Saunders, 1984.

Antimicrobial Therapy of Pediatric Infections

38

James K. Todd, MD

Principles of Antimicrobial Treatment

The general process of decision making related to choosing appropriate antimicrobial treatment is summarized in Table 38–1. Accurate clinical diagnosis of the suspected site of infection—based on history, physical examination, and initial laboratory tests—leads to the appropriate consideration of common organisms usually associated with such infections, and their likely patterns of susceptibility to antimicrobial agents. After obtaining cultures to identify the precise cause of potentially serious infections, the physician initiates empiric antimicrobial therapy taking into account the above considerations as well as a knowledge (eg, personal or from the literature) of regimens that proved successful in the past. Therapy is modified according to patient response and culture results.

Important considerations include the age of the child, the presence of any host defense deficiencies, a thorough understanding of unusual exposures (eg, via travel or direct contact with others), and the severity of the child's illness. Those children who are severely ill (eg, with suspected meningitis) or who have infections known to progress rapidly to more severe illness (eg, bacteremia) should be evaluated quickly, hospitalized, and treated expeditiously with broad antimicrobial coverage until culture results allow a narrowing of therapy. Those patients with milder illness (eg, otitis media without severe systemic symptoms) may be treated empirically with a single agent administered orally. If that initial therapy fails, a more extensive workup is then done.

In those patients whose initial treatment is parenteral therapy, it is often desirable to change to oral therapy once symptoms are ameliorated and the causative agent is identified. As Table 38–2 shows, such a change in therapy cannot be made unless (1) an oral agent that allows sufficient blood levels is available; (2) the causative organism and its susceptibility patterns are known (or inferred by the response to single-agent parenteral therapy); (3) compliance with oral administration of antibiotic is likely; and (4) appropriate blood levels can be ensured by either the pharmacology of the drug or measurement of blood levels or serum killing powers.

It is important to recognize that these principles are merely guidelines. The only accurate measure of the success of antimicrobial therapy is the response

Table 38–1. Steps in decision making for use of antimicrobial agents.

Step	Action	Example
1	Determine diagnosis	Septic arthritis
2	Consider age and preexisting conditions	Normal 2-year-old
3	Consider common organisms	(*Staphylococcus aureus, Haemophilus influenzae*)
4	Consider organism susceptibility	(Penicillin/ampicillin-resistant)
5	Obtain proper cultures[1]	(Blood, joint fluid)
6	Initiate empiric therapy based on above considerations and past experience (eg, personal, literature)	(Nafcillin & cefotaxime)
7	Modify therapy based on culture results and patient response	(*S aureus* isolated; discontinue cefotaxime)
8	Follow clinical response	

[1]Indicated for serious or unusual infections or those with unpredictable clinical response to empiric therapy

Table 38–2. Steps in switching from parenteral to oral therapy for an initially serious infection.

Step	Action
1	Define infection
2	Determine causative organism and antimicrobial susceptibility
3	Achieve favorable response to parenteral therapy a. Systemic (eg, afebrile) b. Local (eg, decreased inflammation)
4	Determine if comparable blood levels can be achieved with an oral agent
5	Assess patient compliance potential
6	Initiate oral therapy
7	Measure blood levels (eg, serum killing powers)
8	Follow clinical response

of the patient. Tables 38–3 to 38–6 give general information about selecting and prescribing antimicrobial agents. Table 38–3 is a summary of common infecting organisms and their usual patterns of susceptibility to antimicrobial agents. Table 38–4 provides general information on various groups of antibacterial agents and their common or unique adverse reactions. Table 38–5 gives dosages for children 1 month of age or older, whereas Table 38–6 provides similar recommendations for use in the newborn. Of necessity, these tables are not comprehensive in that all possible information cannot be provided. For this reason, clinicians need to consult the specific chapter of this book related to the suspected disease and the more extensive dosage and side-effect information provided with the antibiotic or available from other sources (see Selected References). Clinicians must also learn to use a few drugs well rather than many different drugs infrequently. Using this strategy, the clinician can become familiar with various dosage forms of drugs, their palatability, their common as well as unusual side effects, and their cost. For the initial therapy for many infections, the physician may choose several different antibiotics, and it is reasonable to take cost into consideration if efficacy and side effects are comparable.

Antimicrobial Susceptibility Testing

It is critically important to obtain cultures and other diagnostic material from patients prior to initiating antimicrobial therapy. Obtaining cultures is especially important when the patient has a serious infection, initial attempts at therapy have failed, or the use of multiple antimicrobial agents is anticipated. If these cultures identify the causative agent, therapy can be narrowed or optimized according to susceptibility results. Antimicrobial susceptibility testing should be done in a laboratory using carefully defined procedures (National Committee for Clinical Laboratory Standards [NCCLS]). The use of non-

Table 38–3. Susceptibility of some common pathogenic microorganisms to various antimicrobial drugs.

Organism	Potentially Useful Antibiotics[1]
Bacteria	
Anaerobic bacteria[2]	Cefoxitin, chloramphenicol, clindamycin, metronidazole, penicillins
Bordetella pertussis	Erythromycin, tetracyclines
Branhamella (Moraxella catarrhalis)	Amoxicillin/clavulanate, ampicillins (if β-lactamase negative),[3] cephalosporins (III),[4] erythromycin, tetracycline, trimethoprim/sulfamethoxazole
Campylobacter spp	Erythromycin, furazolidone, tetracyclines
Clostridium spp	Clindamycin, penicillin, tetracyclines
Clostridium difficile	Bacitracin (PO), metronidazole, vancomycin (PO)
Corynebacterium diphtheria	Erythromycin, penicillins

Table 38–3 (cont'd.) Susceptibility of some common pathogenic microorganisms to various antimicrobial drugs.

Organism	Potentially Useful Antibiotics[1]
Enterobacteriaceae[5]	Aminoglycosides,[6] ampicillins, cephalosporins, trimethoprim/sulfamethoxazole, [quinolones][7]
Haemophilus influenzae	Amoxicillin/clavulanate, ampicillins (if β-lactamase negative), cephalosporins (II and III), chloramphenicol, rifampin, trimethoprim/sulfamethoxazole
Listeria monocytogenes	Ampicillin, trimethoprim/sulfamethoxazole
Neisseria gonorrhoeae	Ampicillins, cephalosporins (II and III), penicillins, spectinomycin, tetracyclines, trimethoprim/sulfamethoxazole
Neisseria meningitidis	Ampicillins, cephalosporins (II and III), chloramphenicol, penicillins, rifampin
Pasteurella multocida	Amoxicillin/clavulanate, ampicillins, chloramphenicol, penicillins, tetracyclines
Pseudomonas aeruginosa	Aminoglycosides, antipseudomonas penicillins,[8] ceftazidime, imipenem, [quinolones][7]
Salmonella spp	Ampicillin, cephalosporins (III), chloramphenicol, trimethoprim/sulfamethoxazole
Shigella spp	Ampicillin, cephalosporins (III), chloramphenicol, tetracyclines, trimethoprim/sulfamethoxazole
Staphylococcus aureus	Antistaphylococcal penicillins,[9] cephalosporins (I & II), clindamycin, erythromycin, rifampin, trimethoprim/sulfamethoxazole, vancomycin
Staphylococci (coagulase negative)	Cephalosporins (I & II), clindamycin, rifampin, vancomycin
Streptococci (most species)	Ampicillins, cephalosporins, clindamycin, erythromycin, penicillins, vancomycin
Streptococcus pneumoniae	Ampicillins, cephalosporins, erythromycin, penicillin, vancomycin
Enterococcus spp	Ampicillin (with/without aminoglycoside), vancomycin
Intermediate Organisms	
Chlamydia spp	Chloramphenicol, erythromycin, tetracyclines
Mycoplasma spp	Erythromycin, tetracyclines
Rickettsia spp	Chloramphenicol, tetracyclines
Fungi	
Candida spp	Amphotericin B, flucytosine, ketoconazole, miconazole, fluconazole
Fungi, systemic	Amphotericin B, ketoconazole, miconazole
Dermatophytes	Griseofulvin, topical antifungals
Viruses	
Herpes simplex	Acyclovir, vidarabine
Influenza A virus	Amantadine, ribavirin
Respiratory syncytial virus	Ribavirin
Varicella-zoster virus	Acyclovir
Cytomegalovirus	Ganciclovir

[1]In alphabetical order; selection dependent on age, diagnosis, site of infection, severity of illness, antimicrobial susceptibility of suspected organism, and drug hypersensitivity.
[2]Species dependent.
[3]Also applies to amoxicillin, bacampicillin, cyclacillin, hetacillin, and related compounds.
[4]Generation of cephalosporins: I—first, II—second, III—third.
[5]Includes: E coli, Klebsiella spp, Enterobacter spp, and others; antimicrobial susceptibilities should always be measured.
[6]Amikacin, gentamicin, kanamycin, netilmicin, tobramycin
[7]Not recommended for use in children.
[8]Carbenicillin, mezlocillin, piperacillin, ticarcillin
[9]Cloxacillin, dicloxacillin, methicillin, nafcillin, oxacillin

Table 38–4. Groups of common antibacterial agents.

Group	Examples	Some Common Susceptible Organisms (*Genus*)[1]	Common Resistant Organisms (*Genus*)	Common or Unique Adverse Reactions
Penicillins				Rash, anaphylaxis, drug fever, bone marrow suppression
Penicillins	Penicillin G, V	*Streptococcus, Neisseria*	*Staphylococcus, Haemophilus,* enterobacteriaceae	
Ampicillins	Ampicillin, amoxicillin cyclacillin, bacampicillin	(Same as penicillins), *Haemophilus* (β-lactamase negative), *Escherichia coli*	*Staphylococcus,* many enterobacteriaceae	Diarrhea, maculopapular rash
Antistaphylococcal penicillins	Methicillin, nafcillin, oxacillin, cloxacillin, dicloxacillin	*Streptococcus, Staphylococcus aureus*	Gram-negative, *Staphylococcus* (coagulase-negative) *Enterococcus*	Renal (interstitial nephritis)
Antipseudomonas penicillins	Carbenicillin, ticarcillin, mezlocillin, piperacillin, azlocillin	(Same as ampicillins), *Pseudomonas*	(Same as ampicillins)	Decreased platelet adhesiveness, hypokalemia, hypernatremia
Penicillin/beta-lactase inhibitor combination	Amoxicillin/clavulanate, ticarcillin/clavulanate ampicillin/sulbactam	Broad spectrum	Some enterobacteriaceae, *Pseudomonas*	Diarrhea
Other beta-lactams	Imipenem/cilastatin, aztreonam	Broad spectrum, gram-negative rods	Gram-positive	CNS, seizures
Cephalosporins				Rash; anaphylaxis, drug fever
First generation (I)	Cephalothin, cefazolin, cephalexin, cephradine, cephapirin	Gram-positive	Gram-negative, *Enterococcus,* some staphylococci (coagulase-negative)	
Second generation (II)	Cefamandole, cefaclor, cefuroxime, cefonicid	Gram-positive, some *Haemophilus,* some enterobacteriaceae	*Enterococcus, Pseudomonas,* some staphylococci (coagulase-negative)	Serum sickness (cefaclor)
	Cefoxitin, cefotetan	Anaerobes		
Third generation (III)	Cefotaxime, ceftizoxime, ceftriaxone, cefoperazone, cefixime, moxalactam	*Streptococcus, Haemophilus,* enterobacteriaceae, *Neisseria*	*Pseudomonas,* staphylococci	Increased prothrombin time (cefoperozone, moxalactam), biliary sludging (ceftriaxone)
	Ceftazidime	(Same as other third-generation cephalosporins), *Pseudomonas*		
Erythromycins		Gram-positive, *Mycoplasma, Chlamydia, Legionella*	Gram-negative, *Staphylococcus* (coagulase-negative)	Nausea, hepatic
Clindamycin	Clindamycin	Gram-positive, anaerobes	Gram-negative, *Enterococcus*	Nausea, diarrhea/colitis, rash
Vancomycins	Vancomycin, teicoplanin	Gram-positive	Gram-negative	Renal, hepatic, bone marrow suppression, rash (red man syndrome), shock
Quinolones[2]	Norfloxacin, ciprofloxacin	Broad spectrum	*Enterococcus*	Cartilage damage, GI, rash, CNS
Tetracyclines	Tetracycline, chlortetracycline, doxycycline	Anaerobes, *Mycoplasma, Chalmydia*	Many enterobacteriaceae, *Staphylococcus*	Teeth staining, rash, flora overgrowth, hepatic, pseudotumor cerebri
Chloramphenicol	Chloramphenicol	*S pneumoniae, H influenzae, Salmonella*	*Staphylococcus,* many enterobacteriaceae	Bone marrow, gray baby syndrome, neuritis
Sulfonamides	Many	Gram-negative (urine)	Gram-positive	Rash, renal, bone marrow suppression, Stevens-Johnson syndrome

Table 38–4 (cont'd.). Groups of common antibacterial agents.

Group	Examples	Some Common Susceptible Organisms (*Genus*)[1]	Common Resistant Organisms (*Genus*)	Common or Unique Adverse Reactions
Trimethoprim/ sulfamethoxazole		*S aureus*, gram-negative	*Streptococcus, Pseudomonas*	Rash, renal, bone marrow suppression, Stevens-Johnson syndrome
Rifampin		*Neisseria, Haemophilus, Staphylococcus*	Resistance develops rapidly if used as sole agent	Rash, GI, hepatic, CNS, bone marrow suppression
Aminoglycosides	Streptomycin, kanamycin, gentamicin, tobramycin, amikacin, netilmicin	Gram-negative	Gram-positive, anaerobes, some pseudomonads	Renal, ototoxicity, potentiates neuro-muscular blocking agent

[1]Not all strains susceptible; always obtain antimicrobial susceptibility tests on significant isolates.
[2]Not recommended for children.

standard media, inoculum size, or growth conditions may give markedly different and undependable results.

There are several different ways to test antimicrobial susceptibility. The identification of an antibiotic-destroying enzyme (eg, β-lactamase) implies resistance to that group of antimicrobial agents. Tube or microtiter broth dilution techniques can be used to determine the minimum inhibitory concentration (MIC) of antibiotic, which is the amount of antibiotic (μg/mL) necessary to inhibit the organism under specific laboratory conditions. The physician who also has a knowledge of the clinical pharmacology of the antimicrobial agent can infer antibiotic susceptibility if the MIC is less then the antibiotic concentration achievable in the patient using appropriate antibiotic dosages. Disk susceptibility testing (again, only under carefully controlled conditions) yields similar results.

It should be remembered that, for the most part, clinical laboratories report antimicrobial susceptibility (susceptible, intermediate, resistant) as it relates to levels of that antibiotic that can be achieved in the blood (or serum). In general, organisms are considered susceptible if their MIC is lower than levels of that antimicrobial agent that can be achieved in the blood using appropriate parenteral dosages. This assumption of susceptibility should be reconsidered if the patient has a focus of infection (eg, meningitis, osteomyelitis, abscess) where poor antibiotic penetration might occur; the levels of antibiotic might be lower than the MIC in such areas. Conversely, certain organisms may be reported as resistant to a certain antibiotic because sufficiently high blood concentrations cannot be achieved. However, urine, concentrations may be much higher. If so, a urinary tract infection would respond to that antibiotic, whereas septicemia would not.

Thus, antimicrobial susceptibility testing, although a very important part of therapeutic decision making, reflects assumptions that the clinician must understand before making therapeutic decisions, especially for patients with serious infections. Ultimately the true test of the efficacy of therapy is patient response. Those patients who do not seem to respond to appropriate therapy may require reassessment, including reculturing and repeat susceptibility testing, to determine whether resistant strains have evolved or a superinfection with another resistant organism is present. In addition, antimicrobial therapy cannot be expected to cure all infections unless additional supportive treatment is undertaken. Some antibiotics are only marginally effective against certain organisms, and many sequestered infections require surgical drainage procedures as an adjunct to antimicrobial therapy.

Alteration of Dose & Measurement of Blood Levels

Certain antimicrobial agents have not been approved (and often not tested) for use in newborns. For those that have, it is important to recognize that both dose and frequency of administration may need to be altered (see Table 38–6), especially in young (≤ 7 days) or low birth weight (< 2000 g) neonates.

Antimicrobial agents, like other drugs, are excreted through various physiologic mechanisms (eg, renal, hepatic). It is important to consider these routes of excretion and alter the antimicrobial dosage appropriately in any patient with some degree of organ failure. As indicated in Table 38–5, an assessment of renal or hepatic function may routinely be necessary for patients receiving certain drugs (eg, renal function for aminoglycosides, hepatic function for chloramphenicol); otherwise, harmful levels may accumulate. If some degree of organ failure is present, dosage modification may be necessary (see detailed description in individual drug information packet), and the measurement of drug levels may be indicated.

Table 38–5. Guidelines for use of common antimicrobial agents[1] in children ≥ 1 month of age.

Antimicrobial	Route	Dose[2] (mg/kg/day)	Maximum Daily Dose	Interval (hours)	Adjustment[3]	Blood Levels[4] (mμg/mL) Peak	Trough
Bacterial							
Amikacin	IM, IV	15–30	1.5 g	q8–12	R	15–30	5–10
Amoxicillin	PO	20–100	6 g	q8	R		
Amoxicillin/ clavulanate	PO	20–40	1.5 g	q8	R		
Ampicillin	PO, IM, IV	50–400	12 g	q4–6	R		
Azlocillin	IV	300–450	24 g	q4–6	R		
Bacampicillin	PO	25–50	1.6 g	q12			
Carbenicillin	IV	400–600	40 g	q4–6	R		
Cefaclor	PO	40	1.5 g	q8	R		
Cefamandole	IM, IV	50–150	6 g	q4–6	R		
Cefazolin	IM, IV	50–100	6 g	q8	R		
Cefixime	PO	8	400 mg	q12–24	R		
Cefotaxime	IM, IV	100–200	12 g	q6–8	R		
Cefoxitin	IM, IV	80–160	12 g	q6	R		
Ceftazidime	IM, IV	100–150	6 g	q8	R		
Ceftizoxime	IM, IV	150–200	12 g	q6–8	R		
Ceftriaxone	IM, IV	50–100	4 g	q12–24	R		
Cefuroxime	IM, IV, (PO)[5]	75–240(30)[5]	6 g	q6–8	R		
Cephalexin	PO	25–50	6 g	q6	R		
Cephalothin	IM, IV	75–125	12 g	q4–6	R		
Cephradine	IM, IV, (PO)[5]	50–150(25–50)[5]	8 g	q6	R		
Chloramphenicol	PO, IV	50–100	4 g	q6	R,H	15–25	5–10
Clindamycin	PO, IM, IV	10–40	4.8 g	q6–8	R,H		
Cloxacillin	PO	50–100	3 g	q6			
Cyclacillin	PO	50–100	2 g	q6	R		
Dicloxacillin	PO	12.5–100	6 g	q6			
Doxycycline[7]	PO	2–4	200 mg	q12			
Erythromycin	PO, (IV)[5]	20–50[6]	4 g	q6–8	H		
Erythromycin/ sulfasoxazole	PO	40 (erythro)	2 g (erythro)	q6–8	H,R		
Furazolidone	PO	5–8	8.8 mg/kg	q6			
Gentamicin	IM, IV	3–7.5	300 mg	q8	R	6–10	< 2
Isoniazid	PO	10–20	300 mg	q12–24			
Kanamycin	IM, IV	15–30	1.5 g	q8	R	15–30	5–10
Methicillin	IM, IV	100–200	12 g	q6	R		
Metronidazole	PO, IV	15–30	4 g	q6–8	H		
Mezlocillin	IV	200–350	24 g	q6			
Nafcillin	IM, IV	50–200	12 g	q6			
Netilmicin	IM, IV	3–8	300 mg	q8	R	6–12	0.5–2.0
Nitrofurantoin	PO	5–7	400 mg	q6			
Oxacillin	IM, IV	50–200	12 g				
Oxytetracycline[7]	PO	25–50	4 g	q6			
Penicillin G	IV	50,000–250,000 (units/kg)	20X10⁶units	q4–6	H,R		
Penicillin G (benzathine)	IM	50,000 (units/kg)	2.4X10⁶	1 dose			
Penicillin G (procaine)	IM	25,000–50,000 (units/kg)	4.8X10⁶	q12–24			
Penicillin V	PO	25–50	4 g	q6			
Rifampin	PO	10–20	600 mg	q12–24			
Sulfonamides	PO	See specific drug[5]			R		
Tetracycline[7]	PO, (IV)[5]	25–50(20–30)[5]	2 g	q6(12)	R		
Ticarcillin	IV	200–300	30 g	q4–6	R		
Tobramycin	IM, IV	3–7.5	300 mg	q8	R	6–10	< 2
Trimethoprim sulfa	PO, (IV)[5]	6–20(trimeth)	20(trimeth)	q6–12	R		
Vancomycin	IV	40	2 g	q6	R	20–40	5–10
Fungal							
Amphotericin B	IV	0.3–1.0	1 mg/kg	q24	R		
Flucytosine	PO	50–150	150 mg/kg	q6	R		
Griseofulvin	PO	15[5]	1 g[5]	q24			
Ketoconazole	PO	5–10	1 g	q12–24			
Miconazole	IV	20–40	3.6 g	q8			
Nystatin	PO	2–6 mL/dose	24 mL	q6			
Fluconazole	PO	1–8	400 mg	q24	R		

Table 38–5 (cont'd.). Guidelines for use of common antimicrobial agents[1] in children $\geq$ 1 month of age.

Antimicrobial	Route	Dose[2] (mg/kg/day)	Maximum Daily Dose	Interval (hours)	Adjustment[3]	Blood Levels[4] (mμg/mL) Peak	Trough
Viral							
Acyclovir	IV	15–30	1500 mg/m²	q8	R		
	(PO)[5]	Unknown	1 g	(5 doses)[5]	R		
Amantadine	PO	5–8	200 mg	q12	R		
Ribavirin	Aerosol	6 g vial	6 g	12–18 hr inhalation			
Vidarabine	IV	15–30	30 mg/kg	q24	R		

[1]Not including antiparasitic drugs, some newly released drugs, ones not recommended for use in children, or ones not widely used.
[2]Always consult package insert for complete prescribing information. Dosage may differ for alternate route, newborns (see Table 38–6), or patients with liver or renal failure (see Adjustment) and may not be recommended for use in pregnant women or newborns.
[3]Mode of excretion (R = renal, H = hepatic) of antimicrobial agent should be assessed at the onset of therapy and dosage modified or levels obtained as indicated in package insert.
[4]Suggested levels to reduce toxicity.
[5]Parentheses indicate less common route and dosage.
[6]Preparation dependent.
[7]Not recommended in children < 8 years of age.

Table 38–6. Guidelines for use of selected antimicrobial agents in newborns[1]

Antibiotics	Route	Body Weight (g)	Maximum Dosage (mg/kg/day) & Frequency < 7 days	8–30 days	Blood Levels (μg/ml) Peak	Trough
Amikacin[2]	IV, IM	< 2000	15 q12h	20 q8h	15–30	5–10
		> 2000	20 q12h	30 q8h		
Ampicillin	IV, IM	< 2000	100 q12h	150 q8h		
		> 2000	150 q8h	200 q6h		
Cefotaxime	IV, IM		100 q12h	150 q8h		
Ceftazidime	IV, IM		100 q12h	150 q8h		
Chloramphenicol[3]	IV, PO	< 2000	25 q24h	25 q24h	15–25	5–10
		> 2000	25 q24h	50 q12h		
Clindamycin	IV, IM, PO	< 2000	10 q12h	15 q8h		
		> 2000	15 q8h	20 q6h		
Erythromycin	PO		20 q12h	30 q8h		
Gentamicin[2]	IV, IM		5 q12h	7.5 q8h	6–10	< 2
Methicillin	IV, IM	< 2000	100 q12h	150 q8h		
		> 2000	150 q8h	200 q6h		
Mezlocillin	IV, IM		150 q12h	225 q8h		
Nafcillin	IV	< 2000	50 q12h	75 q8h		
		> 2000	50 q8h	75 q6h		
Netilmicin	IV, IM		5 q12h	7.5 q8h		
Oxacillin	IV, IM	< 2000	50 q12h	100 q8h		
		> 2000	75 q8h	150 q8h		
Penicillin G (units/kg/day)[4]	IV	< 2000	100,000 q12h	150,000 q8h		
		> 2000	150,000 q8h	200,000 q6h		
Ticarcillin	IV, IM	< 2000	150 q12h	225 q8h		
		> 2000	225 q8h	300 q6h		
Tobramycin[2]	IV, IM		4 q12h	6 q8h	6–10	< 2
Vancomycin[2]	IV	< 2000	20 q12h	30 q8h	20–40	5–10

[1]Adapted from Nelson JD: *Pocketbook of Pediatric Antimicrobial Therapy.* Williams & Wilkins, 1989.
[2]Neonates weighing < 1200 g may require even smaller doses. Antibiotic levels should be closely monitored.
[3]Chloramphenicol must be used with extreme caution. Levels should be measured in all patients to ensure proper dosing.
[4]Other preparations (eg, benzathine penicillin) may be given IM. See specific diseases for dosage.

Serum levels of those drugs posing a high risk of toxicity (eg, aminoglycosides, chloramphenicol, vancomycin) are ordinarily measured. For other drugs (eg, β-lactams) in certain circumstances it is useful to know the relative drug concentration as compared to the MIC of the organism (ie, the serum bactericidal assay, serum killing power). For certain infections, the target therapeutic levels are defined (eg, subacute bacterial endocarditis ≥ 1:64, osteomyelitis and septic arthritis ≥ 1:8). Appropriate levels for other infections are less well documented, but measurement of serum killing powers can also be used to assess compliance with an oral therapeutic regimen for serious infections.

The Use of New Antimicrobial Agents

New antibiotics are introduced frequently, and manufacturers often claim unique features that distinguish these usually more expensive products from their predecessors. The true role that new antimicrobials will play can be determined only over time, during which often new or previously unrecognized side effects are described and the true clinical efficacy of the agent is established in large numbers of patients. Because this process may take many years, a conservative approach to the implementation of new antibiotics seems appropriate, especially since the costs are often higher and appropriate antimicrobial choices for most common infections already exist. The development of new antibiotics is important to keep up with organism resistance patterns as they evolve and to identify new agents effective against some infections that are now currently difficult to treat (eg, viruses, fungi, and some resistant bacteria). Fortunately these infections are either rare or usually self limited in normal hosts, and for the most part we have reasonable initial therapies with which we are already experienced for treating most common infections.

New antimicrobial agents will continue to be developed, and some will ultimately have a significant impact on therapy. A conservative approach to the implementation of such therapies is to await objective clinical confirmation of initial marketing claims. In the end, it is appropriate to ask if this new antimicrobial therapy is proved to be clinically as effective (or more effective) then the current drug of choice, and, if so, whether its side effects are comparable or less and its cost reasonable.

SELECTED REFERENCES

McEvoy GK, McQuarrie GM (editors): *American Hospital Formulary Service: Drug Information.* American Society of Hospital Pharmacists, 1987.

Nelson JD: *Pocketbook of Pediatric Antimicrobial Therapy.* Williams & Wilkins, 1989.

Physicians Desk Reference, 42nd ed. Medical Economics Company, 1988.

Todd JK: Antimicrobial susceptibility testing in the office laboratory. *Pediatr Infect Dis* 1983;**2**:481.

39

Normal Biochemical & Hematologic Values

Keith B. Hammond, MS, FIMLS

Pediatricians and other health professionals caring for children have the responsibility to insist on accurate, rapid, and comprehensive laboratory testing. Collecting large blood samples for biochemical assay is not suitable for the proper care of children— especially for premature infants or older children in intensive care, where repetitive sampling may be essential. Technology for performing biochemical assays on blood samples of 100 μL or less has been available for 30 years or more. Most of the earlier automated systems for assay were better adapted to larger samples. However, the newest automated systems have the capacity to work with small volumes.

In infants and young children, blood samples attained by heel-prick are better collected by laboratory personnel than by physicians or nurses.

INTERPRETATION OF LABORATORY VALUES

Accreditation by the College of American Pathologists and by state or federal agencies has done much to ensure standardized laboratory working conditions. Methods employed in various laboratories differ, as do normal values for the methods. Normal range is, of course, a combination of biologic variation and of intrinsic laboratory variation; thus, an acceptable range of normal values should ideally be composed of data developed within the laboratory for the population it serves. Any laboratory should be able to provide information on the coefficient of variation and standard deviation applicable to each test performed in that laboratory. Each laboratory should maintain a rigorous procedure of checks with daily standards and control specimens. Errors may still occur but can usually be detected by retesting before a questionable result is reported. Fortunately, errors occur much less commonly today than in the past.

The clinical value of a test is related to its sensitivity and specificity. Sensitivity is an expression of the incidence of positive test results in those who have the disease. Specificity is an expression of the incidence of negative test results in those free of the disease. Sensitivity and specificity are calculated as follows:

$$\text{Sensitivity \%} = \frac{TP}{TP + FN} \times 100 \text{ (ie, how many TP are missed)}$$

$$\text{Specificity \%} = \frac{TN}{TN + FP} \times 100 \text{ (ie, how many TN are missed)}$$

where TP = true-positive result; FP = false-positive result; TN = true-negative result; and FN = false-negative result.

Screening tests must be interpreted with appreciation of sensitivity and specificity. These expressions are illustrated in Fig 39–1 in terms of a screening test for phenylketonuria in newborns. The figures are not strictly correct but serve the purpose of illustration. According to Fig 39–1, a blood phenylalanine level of 4 mg/dL is the discriminating point above which all infants are presumed to have the disease and below which they are presumed to be normal. However, no test is ever quite that exact. Some normal infants will have levels above 4 mg/dL; the test results in these will be false positive. Some abnormal infants will have levels below 4 mg/dL; the test results in these will be false negative. The discriminating point is a compromise between sensitivity and specificity. Moving the point to 2 mg/dL would effect 100% sensitivity, but there would be a large increase in the number of false-positive results. Moving it to 6 mg/dL would make it very specific, but this would increase the number of false-negative responses, which would result in failure to detect phenylketonuria in a much larger proportion of affected children.

These concepts can be viewed in yet another way. Suppose this test were set at a specificity of 99.9%. This would mean that in a sample of 10,000 tests, there would be 10 false-positive results. In a rare condition like phenylketonuria, however, the true incidence of the disease may be only 1 in 12,000. The ratio of true- to false-positive results is thus 1:12; this is a reflection of the low incidence of the disease and the relatively high incidence of false-positive results due to the nature of the assay. These considerations, of course, apply to the interpretation of all laboratory tests.

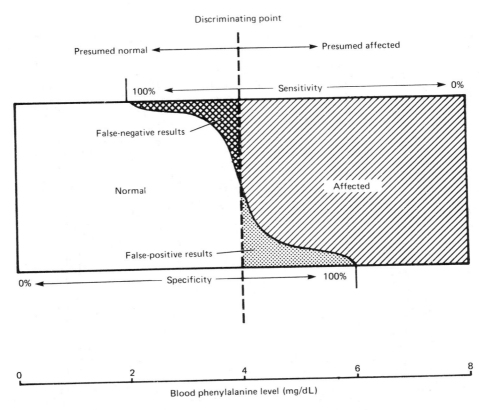

Figure 39–1. Screening test for phenylketonuria in newborns. Data have been simplified to illustrate the concepts of sensitivity and specificity (see text).

LABORATORY VALUES

Normal blood chemistry values and miscellaneous other laboratory values are shown in Tables 39–1 through 39–3.

Table 39–1. Normal values of amino acids and other Ninhydrin-positive substances in plasma[1] and urine.[2]

	Newborn	Premature		Full Term		Years 2–12		Adult		% Tubular Reabsorption		
	Plasma (Week 1)	Plasma (Week 6)	Urine (Week 6)	Plasma (Week 6)	Urine (Week 6)	Plasma	Urine	Plasma	Urine	Infancy	Childhood	Adult
Phosphoethanol-amine	tr	...	...	...	...	...	0.08–0.28	...	...	...	...	...
Taurine	0.01–0.20	0.05–0.08	0.03–0.08	0.02–0.11	0.01–0.18	0.06–0.11	0.76–1.9	0.05–0.08	0.4–1.3	96–98	93–95	72–95
Hydroxyproline	0–tr	tr–0.08	1.1–2.1	0–tr	0.7–2.6	0–tr	0	0–tr	0	See note 3.	...	...
Aspartic acid	tr–0.02	0.01–0.02	tr–0.04	0.008–0.02	tr–0.32	0.004–0.02	tr–0.07	0.004–0.01	0.03–0.09	See note 4.	92–99	85–98
Threonine	0.04–0.05	0.15–0.33	0.9–1.9	0.17–0.23	0.67–1.4	0.04–0.10	0.04–0.17	0.09–0.14	0.09–0.14	71–91	92–99.5	97–99
Serine	0.04–0.30	0.10–0.16	0.8–1.3	0.16–0.20	1.1–2.3	0.08–0.11	0.09–0.34	0.08–0.11	0.09–0.31	54–86	92–99	97–99
Asparagine Glutamine	0.3–2.1	0.40–0.44	0.5–1.5	0.36–0.57	1.1–2.0	0.06–0.47	0.04–0.75	0.4–0.5	0.17–0.48	90–96	98–9.99	99+
Proline	0.02–0.43	0.10–0.31	0.6–1.7	0.40–0.48	0.7–5.4	0.07–0.15	tr–0.04	0.15–0.25	0	53–94	99.5–100	99+
Glutamate	tr–0.26	0.08–0.14	0.02–0.13	0.06–0.21	0.04–0.62	0.02–0.25	0.01–0.13	0.05–0.20	0.008–0.16	95–99	98.5–99.8	99+
Citrulline	...	0.04–0.07	0.02–0.17	tr–0.04	tr–0.04	tr–0.03	tr–0.03	tr–0.03	0–tr	92–98	...	99+
Glycine	0.05–0.44	0.12–0.21	2.5–4.2	0.18–0.24	3.7–8.4	0.12–0.22	0.33–1.5	0.15–0.24	0.40–0.90	15–63	93–99	94–99
Alanine	0.04–0.44	0.20–0.39	0.5–0.7	0.46–0.52	1.2–2.1	0.14–0.30	0.04–0.35	0.35–0.37	0.09–0.27	87–92	99–99.9	99+
α – Amino adipic	...	0	0.1–0.23	0	0.17–0.23	...	...	0	0–0.02	See note 3.	...	See note 3.
α – Amino butyric	tr–0.07	0–tr	tr	tr–0.02	0	...	tr–0.06	0.01–0.03	0.01–0.04	...	...	99
Valine	0.03–0.32	0.12–0.22	tr–0.2	0.32–0.35	0.10–0.16	0.13–0.28	tr–0.06	0.05–0.08	tr–0.05	98–99+	99.6–99.9	99+
Homocitrulline	...	tr	0.13–0.37	0	0.12–0.24	...	tr–0.08	...	0.02–0.04	See note 3.	See note 3.	See note 3.
1/2 Cystine	0.02–0.07	tr–0.07	0.04–0.25	0	0.14–0.34	...	...	0	0.02–0.08	60–90	...	99+
Cystathionine	...	0.005–0.01	0.09–0.12	0–tr	0.11–0.17	...	...	0	0.01–0.02	0	...	See note 3.
Methionine	tr–0.08	0.02–0.04	0.08–0.14	0.03–0.05	0.12–0.14	0.01–0.02	0.01–0.04	0.01–0.04	0.02–0.04	85–97	98.3–99.7	98–99+
Isoleucine	0.01–0.09	0.04–0.08	0.03–0.07	0.08–0.12	0.10–0.16	0.03–0.08	0.01–0.07	0.05–0.08	0.01–0.04	96–99+	99.2–99.9	99+
Leucine	0.01–0.18	0.1–0.5	0.04–0.08	0.14–0.22	0.15–0.18	0.06–0.18	0.02–0.11	0.10–0.14	0.02–0.05	97–99+	99.6–99.9	99+
Tyrosine	0.05–0.30	0.1–0.4	0.17–0.60	0.11–0.21	0.22–0.38	0.03–0.07	0.03–0.12	0.04–0.07	0.06–0.10	93–99	98.2–99.3	99+
Phenylalanine	0.02–0.12	0.05–0.07	0.08–0.13	0.06–0.12	0.11–0.14	0.03–0.06	0.01–0.11	0.04–0.07	0.04–0.07	94–99	98.8–99.7	99+
β – Alanine	...	0	0	0	0	0.02–0.05	tr	0	0	...	...	...
BAIB	...	0	0.09–0.16	0	0.17–0.42	< 0.01	0–0.19	0	0.01–0.09	...	...	...
Methylglycine	...	...	...	...	...	...	< 0.05	0	...	...	...	...
Hydroxylysine	...	0	0.13–0.27	0	0.05–0.11	...	...	0	0–0.02	See note 3.	...	...
GABA	tr–0.1	0–tr	0–tr	0–tr	0–tr	...	...	0	tr	...	...	See note 3.
Ornithine	0.01–0.22	0.08–0.11	0–0.08	0.07–0.10	0.05–0.08	0.03–0.09	0.01–0.03	0.58–0.90	tr	96–99+	99.5–99.8	99+
Lysine	0.05–0.35	0.08–0.15	0.2–0.6	0.21–0.34	0.7–1.4	0.07–0.15	0.04–0.21	0.16–0.18	0.02–0.20	81–96	98.5–99.8	99+
1-Methylhistidine	0	0	0	0	0–0.03	...	...	0	0.58–0.90	...	...	...
Histidine	tr–0.13	0.05–0.13	0.34–0.83	0.05–0.08	0.8–1.8	0.02–0.08	0.11–1.0	0.06–0.07	0.15–0.53	30–80	90.3–98.4	92–98
3-Methylhistidine	0	0	0	0	0–0.07	...	...	0	0.08–0.28	...	...	...
Arginine	tr–0.12	tr–0.07	0.04–0.10	tr–0.1	tr–0.1	0.02–0.09	0.01–0.04	0.03–0.06	0.02–0.20	99+	99–99.9	99+

[1]Measured in μmol/mL (fasting).
[2]Measured in μmol/min/1.73 m².
[3]0—trace in plasma but significant amounts in urine.
[4]Detectable in plasma but not in urine except in traces.

Table 39–2. Normal blood chemistry values and miscellaneous other hematologic values.[1]
(Values may vary with the procedure employed.)

Determinations for:
(S) = Serum   (P) = Plasma
(B) = Whole blood   (RBC) = Red blood cells

Acid-Base Measurements (B)
pH: 7.38–7.42 from 14 minutes of age and older.
Pao_2: 65–76 mm Hg (8.66–10.13 kPa).
$Paco_2$: 36–38 mm Hg (4.8–5.07 kPa).
Base excess: −2 to +2 meq/L, except in newborns
(range, −4 to −0).

Acid Phosphatase (S, P)
Values using p-nitrophenyl phosphate buffered wth citrate
(end-point determination).
Newborns: 7.4–19.4 IU/L at 37 °C.
2–13 years: 6.4–15.2 IU/L at 37 °C.
Adult males: 0.5–11 IU/L at 37 °C.
Adult females: 0.2–9.5 IU/L at 37 °C.

ACTH: See Corticotropin.

Adenosine Triphosphate (RBC)
Premature infants: 5.66 μmol/g of hemoglobin.
Adults: 3.86 μmol/g of hemoglobin.

Alanine Aminotransferase (ALT, SGPT) (S)
Newborns (1–3 days): 1–25 IU/L at 37 °C.
Adult males: 7–46 IU/L at 37 °C.
Adult females: 4–35 IU/L at 37 °C.

Aldolase (S)
Newborns: 17.5–47.8 IU/L at 37 °C.
Children: 8.8–23.9 IU/L ay 37 °C.
Adults: 4.4–12 IU/L at 37 °C.

Aldosterone (P)
First year: 25–140 ng/dL.
Second year: 9–25 ng/dL.

Alkaline Phosphatase (S)
Values in IU/L at 37 °C using p-nitrophenol phosphate
buffered with AMP (kinetic).

Group	Males	Females
Newborns (1–3 days)	95–368	95–368
2–24 months	115–460	115–460
2–5 years	115–391	115–391
6–7 years	115–460	115–460
8–9 years	115–345	115–345
10–11 years	115–336	115–437
12–13 years	127–403	92–336
14–15 years	79–446	78–212
16–18 years	58–331	35–124
Adults	41–137	39–118

Amino Acids (P)
(See Table 39–1.)

Ammonia (P)
Newborns: 90–150 μg/dL (53–88 μmol/L); higher in premature and jaundiced infants.
Thereafter: 0–60 μg/dL (0–35 μmol/L) when blood is drawn with proper precautions.

Amylase (S)
Values using maltotetrose substrate (kinetic).
Neonates: Undetectable.
2–12 months: Levels increase slowly to adult levels.
Adults: 28–108 IU/L at 37 °C.

α_1-Antitrypsin (S)
1–3 months: 127–404 mg/dL.
3–12 months: 145–362 mg/dL.
1–2 years: 160–382 mg/dL.
2–15 years: 148–394 mg/dL.

Ascorbic Acid: See Vitamin C.

Aspartate Aminotransferase (AST, SGOT) (S)
Newborns (1–3 days): 16–74 IU/L at 37 °C.
Adult males: 8–46 IU/L at 37 °C.
Adult females: 7–34 IU/L at 37 °C.

Base Excess: See Acid-Base Measurements.

Bicarbonate, Actual (P)
Calculated from pH and Pa_{CO2}
Newborns: 17.2–23.6 mmol/L.
2 months–2 years: 19–24 mmo/L.
Children: 18–25 mmol/L.
Adult males: 20.1–28.9 mmol/L.
Adult females: 18.4–28.8 mmol/L.

Bilirubin (S)
Values in mg/dL (μmol/L)
Levels after 1 month are as follows:
Conjugated: 0–0.3 mg/dL (0–5 μmol/L).
Unconjugated: 0.1–0.7 mg/dL (2–12 μmol/L).

Peak Newborn Level	Percentage of Newborns (Birth Weight) Exceeding Peak Level		
	< 2001 g	2001–2500 g	> 2500 g
20 (342)	8.2%	2.6%	0.8%
18 (308)	13.5%	4.6%	1.5%
16 (274)	20.3%	7.6%	2.6%
14 (239)	33.0%	12.0%	4.4%
11 (188)	53.8%	23.0%	9.3%
8 (137)	77.0%	45.4%	26.1%

[1]Adapted from Meites S (editor): *Pediatric Clinical Chemistry,* 2nd ed. American Association for Clinical Chemistry, 1982, and many other sources.

Table 39–2 (cont'd.). Normal blood chemistry values and miscellaneous other hematologic values.[1]
(Values may vary with the procedure employed.)

Bleeding Time (Simplate)
2–9 minutes.

Blood Volume
Premature infants: 98 mL/kg.
At 1 year: 86 mL/kg (range, 69–112 mL/kg).
Older children: 70 mL/kg (range, 51–86 mL/kg).

BUN: See Urea Nitrogen.

C Peptide (S)
5–15 years (8:00 AM fasting): 1–4 ng/mL.
Adults (8:00 AM fasting): < 4 ng/mL.
Adults (nonfasting): < 8 ng/mL.

Calcium (S)
Premature infants (first week) 3.5–4.5 meq/L (1.7–2.3 mmol/L).
Full-term infants (first week): 4–5 meq/L (2–2.5 mmol/L).
Thereafter: 4.4–5.3 meq/L (2.2–2.7 mmol/L).

Carbon Dioxide, Total (S, P)
Cord blood: 15–20.2 mmol/L.
Children: 18–27 mmol/L.
Adults: 24–35 mmol/L.

Carboxyhemoglobin (B)
5% of total hemoglobin (0.05 mol/mol).

Carnitine (S)
Fasting levels: 20–45 μmol/L.

Carotene (S, P)
0–6 months: 0–40 μg/dL (0–0.75 μmol/L).
Children: 50–100 μg/dL (0.93–1.9 μmol/L).
Adults: 100–150 μg/dL (1.9–2.8 μmol/L).

Cation-Anion Gap (S, P)
5–15 mmol/L.

Ceruloplasmin (Copper Oxidase) (S, P)
21–43 mg/dL (1.3–2.7 μmol/L).

Chloride (S, P)
Premature infants: 95–110 mmol/L.
Full-term infants: 96–116 mmol/L.
Children: 98–105 mmol/L.
Adults: 98–108 mmol/L.

Cholesterol, Total (S, P)
Values in mg/dL (mmol/L)

Group	Males	Females
6–7 years	115–197 (2.97–5.09)	126–199 (3.25–5.14)
8–9 years	112–199 (2.89–5.14)	124–208 (3.20–5.37)
10–11 years	108–220 (2.79–5.68)	115–208 (2.97–5.37)
12–13 years	117–202 (3.02–5.21)	114–207 (2.94–5.34)
14–15 years	103–207 (2.66–5.34)	102–208 (2.63–5.37)
16–17 years	107–198 (2.76–5.11)	106–213 (2.73–5.50)

Cholinesterase (S, RBC)
2.5–5 μmol/min/mL of serum (pseudocholinesterase).
2.3–4 μmol/min/mL of red cells.

Christmas Factor (Factor IX) (P)
Children: 100 ± 22 units/dL.

Circulation Time, Decholin
3–6 years: 8–12 seconds.
6–12 years: 7.5–15 seconds.
12–15 years: 10–16 seconds.

Circulation Time, Fluorescein
Upper limit of normal, based on weight.
10 kg: 8 seconds.
20 kg: 8.4 seconds.
40 kg: 11.3 seconds.

Coagulation Time (Test Tube Method)
3–9 minutes.

Complement (S)
C3: 96–195 mg/dL.
C4: 15–20 mg/dL.

Copper (S)
Cord blood: 26–32 μg/dL (4.1–5.2 μmol/L).
Newborns: 26–32 μg/dL (4.1–5.2 μmol/L).
1 month: 73–93 μg/dL (11.5–14.6 μmol/L).
2 months: 59–69 μg/dL (9.3–10.9 μmol/L).
6 months–5 years: 27–153 μg/dL (4.2–24.1 μmol/L).
5–17 years: 94–234 μg/dL (14.8–36.8 μmol/L).
Adults: 70–118 μg/dL (11–18.6 μmol/L).

Copper Oxidase: See Ceruloplasmin.

Corticotropin (ACTH) (P)
Morning (8:00 AM): 20–100 pg/mL (4.4–22 pmol/L).

Cortisol (S, P)
Morning (8:00 AM): 5–25 μg/dL (0.14–0.68 μmol/L).
Evening: 5–15 μg/dL (0.14–0.41 μmol/L).

Creatine (S, P)
0.2–0.8 mg/dL (15.2–61 μmol/L).

Creatine Kinase (S, P)
Newborns (1–3 days): 40–474 IU/L at 37 °C.
Adult males: 30–210 IU/L at 37 °C.
Adult females: 20–128 IU/L at 37 °C.

Creatinine (S, P)
Values in mg/dL (μmol/L).

Group	Males	Females
Newborns (1–3 days)[1]	0.2–1.0 (17.7–88.4)	0.2–1.0 (17.7–88.4)
1 year	0.2–0.6 (17.7–53.0)	0.2–0.5 (17.7–44.2)
2–3 years	0.2–0.7 (17.7–61.9)	0.3–0.6 (26.5–53.0)
4–7 years	0.2–0.8 (17.7–70.7)	0.2–0.7 (17.7–61.9)
8–10 years	0.3–0.9 (26.5–79.6)	0.3–0.8 (26.5–70.7)
11–12 years	0.3–1.0 (26.5–88.4)	0.3–0.9 (26.5–79.6)
13–17 years	0.3–1.2 (26.5–106.1)	0.3–1.1 (26.5–97.2)
18–20 years	0.5–1.3 (44.2–115.0)	0.3–1.1 (26.5–97.2)

[1]Values may be higher in premature newborns.

Creatinine Clearance
Values show great variability and depend on specificity of analytical methods used.
Newborns (1 day): 5–50 mL/min/1.73 m (mean, 18 mL/min/1.73 m).
Newborns (6 days): 15–90 mL/min/1.73 m² (mean, 36 mL/min/1.73 m²).

Table 39–2 (cont'd). Normal blood chemistry values and miscellaneous other hematologic values.[1]
(Values may vary with the procedure employed.)

Adult males: 85–125 mL/min/1.73 m².
Adult females: 75–115 mL/min/1.73 m².

2,3-Diphosphoglycerate (B)
Values vary with method employed and with altitude.
4.5–6 mmol/L.

Factor: See Antihemophilic Globulin, Christmas Factor, Proaccelerin, and Prothrombin.

Fatty Acids, "Free" (P)
Newborns: 435–1375 μeq/L.
4 months–10 years (14-hour fast): 500–900 μeq/L.
4 months–10 years (19-hour fast): 730–1200 μeq/L.
Adults (14-hour fast): 310–590 μeq/L.
Adults (19-hour fast): 405–720 μeq/L.

Fatty Acids, Total Esterified (P, RBC)
Values in mg/dL.

Fatty Acid[1]	Plasma		Erythrocytes	
	mg/dL	% of Total	mg/dL	% of Total
16:0	29.4–55.8	20.7–28.3	24.8–49.0	18.5–28.3
16:1	1.4–6.8	1.1–2.5	0.0–9.4	0.0–4.9
18:0	11.2–28.6	6.9–16.1	13.7–47.3	13.1–26.5
18:1	21.9–51.1	16.9–24.5	11.6–46.8	12.7–23.3
18:2	24.5–78.5	19.5–39.1	0.7–47.9	6.1–22.1
20:3	0.0–8.0	0.0–4.9	0.8–7.6	0.8–4.4
20:4	5.5–26.9	3.2–15.6	14.2–46.2	12.5–26.3

[1]Ratio of number of carbons to number of unsaturated bonds.

Ferritin (S)
Newborns: 20–200 ng/ml (mean, 117 ng/mL).
1 month: 60–550 ng/mL (mean, 350 ng/mL).
1–15 years: 7–140 ng/mL (mean, 31 ng/mL).
Adult males: 50–225 ng/mL (mean, 140 ng/mL).
Adult females: 10–150 ng/mL (mean, 40 ng/mL).

Fibrinogen (P)
200–500 mg/dL (5.9–14.7 μmol/L).

Folate (S)
Prepubertal children: Mean folic acid values are reported to be slightly higher than mean adult values but remain within the normal range.
Adults: 3–21 ng/mL.

Galactose (S, P)
1.1–2.1 mg/dL (0.06–0.12 mmol/L).

Galactose 1-Phosphate (RBC)
Normal: 1 mg/dL of packed erythrocyte lysate; slightly higher in cord blood.
Infants with congenital galactosemia on a milk-free diet: < 2 mg/dL.
Infants with congenital galactosemia taking milk: 9–20 mg/dL.

Galactose-1-Phosphate Uridyl Transferase (RBC)
Normal: 308–475 mIU/g of hemoglobin.
Heterozygous for Duarte variant: 225–308 mIU/g of hemoglobin.
Homozygous for Duarte variant: 142–225 mIU/g of hemoglobin.
Heterozygous for congenital galactosemia: 142–225 mIU/g of hemoglobin.
Homozygous for congenital galactosemia: < 8 mIU/g of hemoglobin.

Gastrin (S)
Newborns (1–7 days): 20–300 pg/mL.
Children (8- to 12-hour overnight fast): < 10–125 pg/mL.
Adults (8- to 12-hour overnight fast): < 10–100 pg/mL.

GHL: See Growth Hormone.

Glomerular Filtration Rate
Newborns: About 50% of values for older children and adults.
Older children and adults: 75–165 mL/min/1.73 m² (levels reached by about 6 months).

Glucose (S, P)
Premature infants: 20–80 mg/dL (1.11–4.44 mmol/L).
Full-term infants: 30–100 mg/dL (1.67–5.56 mmol/L).
Children and adults (fasting): 60–105 mg/dL (3.33–5.88 mmol/L).

Glucose 6-Phosphate Dehydrogenase (RBC)
150–215 units/dL.

Glucose Tolerance Test (S)
(See Table, bottom of page.)

λ-Glutamyl Transpeptidase (S)
0–1 month: 12–271 IU/L at 37 °C (kinetic).
1–2 months: 9–159 IU/L at 37 °C (kinetic).

Glucose tolerance test results in serum.

Normal levels based on results in 13 normal children given glucose.
1.75 g/kg orally in one dose, after 2 weeks on a high-carbohydrate diet.

Time	Glucose		Insulin		Phosphorus	
	mg/dL	mmol/L	μU/mL	pmol/L	mg/dL	mmol/L
Fasting	59–96	3.11–5.33	5–40	36–287	3.2–4.9	1.03–1.58
30 minutes	91–185	5.05–10.27	36–110	258–789	2.0–4.4	0.64–1.42
60 minutes	66–164	3.66–9.10	22–124	158–890	1.8–3.6	0.58–1.16
90 minutes	68–148	3.77–8.22	17–105	122–753	1.8–3.6	0.58–1.16
2 hours	66–122	3.66–6.77	6–84	43–603	1.8–4.2	0.58–1.36
3 hours	47–99	2.61–5.49	2–46	14–330	2.0–4.6	0.64–1.48
4 hours	61–93	3.39–5.16	3–32	21–230	2.7–4.3	0.87–1.39
5 hours	63–86	3.50–4.77	5–37	36–265	2.9–4.4	0.94–1.42

Table 39–2 (cont'd). Normal blood chemistry values and miscellaneous other hematologic values.[1]
(Values may vary with the procedure employed.)

2–4 months: 7–98 IU/L at 37 °C (kinetic).
4–7 months: 5–45 IU/L at 37 °C (kinetic).
7–12 months: 4–27 IU/L at 37 °C (kinetic).
1–15 years: 3–30 IU/L at 37 °C (kinetic).
Adult males: 9–69 IU/L at 37 °C (kinetic).
Adult females: 3–33 IU/L at 37 °C (kinetic).

Glycogen (RBC)
Cord blood: 10–338 μg/g of hemoglobin.
4½–19 hours: 48–361 μg/g of hemoglobin.
2–12 months: 32–134 μg/g of hemoglobin.
1–12 years: 22–109 μg/g of hemoglobin.
Adults: 20–105 μg/g hemoglobin.

Glycohemoglobin (hemoglobin A$_{1c}$) (B)
Normal: 6.3–8.2% of total hemoglobin.
Diabetic patients in good control of their condition ordinarily have levels < 10%.
Values tend to be lower during pregnancy; they also vary with technique.

Growth Hormone (GH) (S)
After infancy (fasting specimen): 0–5 ng/mL.
In response to natural and artificial provocation (eg, sleep, arginine, insulin, hypoglycemia): > 8 ng/mL.
During the newborn period (fasting specimen); GH levels are high (15–40 ng/mL) and responses to provocation variable.

Haptoglobin (S)
50–150 mg/dL has hemoglobin-binding capacity.

Hematocrit (B)
At birth: 44–64%.
14–90 days: 35–49%.
6 months–1 year: 30–40%.
4–10 years: 31–43%.

Hemoglobin (P)
No more than 0.5 mg/dL (0.3 μmol/L).

Hemoglobin A$_{1c}$: See Glycohemoglobin.

Hemoglobin Electrophoresis (B)
A$_1$ hemoglobin: 96–98.5% of total hemoglobin.
A$_2$ hemoglobin: 1.5–4% of total hemoglobin.

Hemoglobin, Fetal (B)
At birth: 50–85% of total hemoglobin.
At 1 year: < 15% of total hemoglobin.
Up to 2 years: Up to 5% of total hemoglobin.
Thereafter: < 2% of total hemoglobin.

Immunoglobulins (S)
Values in mg/dL.

Group	IgG	IgA	IgM
Cord blood	766–1693	0.04–9	4–26
2 weeks–3 months	299–852	3–66	15–149
3–6 months	142–988	4–90	18–118
6–12 months	418–1142	14–95	43–223
1–2 years	356–1204	13–118	37–239
2–3 years	492–1269	23–137	49–204
3–6 years	564–1381	35–209	51–214
6–9 years	658–1535	29–384	50–228
9–12 years	625–1598	60–294	64–278
12–16 years	660–1548	81–252	45–256

Insulin: See Glucose Tolerance Test and Table (bottom of previous page).

Inulin Clearance
< 1 month: 29–88 mL/min/1.73 m².
1–6 months: 40–112 mL/min/1.73 m².
6–12 months: 62–121 mL/min/1.73 m².
< 1 year: 78–164 mL/min/1.73 m².

Iron (S, P)
Newborns: 20–157 μg/dL (3.6–28.1 μmol/L).
6 weeks–3 years: 20–115 μg/dL (3.6–20.6 μmol/L).
3–9 years: 20–141 μg/dL (3.6–25.2 μmol/L).
9–14 years: 21–151 μg/dL (3.8–27μmol/L).
14–16 years: 20–181 μg/dL (3.6–32.4 μmol/L).
Adults: 44–196 μg/dL (7.2–31.3 μmol/L).

Iron-Binding Capacity (S, P)
Newborns: 59–175 μg/dL (10.6–31.3 μmol/L).
Children and adults: 275–458 μg/dL (45–72 μmol/L).

Lactate (B)
Venous blood: 5–18 mg/dL (0.5–2 mmol/L).
Arterial blood: 3–7 mg/dL (0.3–0.8 mmol/L).

Lactate Dehydrogenase (LDH) (S, P)
Values using lactate substrate (kinetic).
Newborns (1–3 days): 40–348 IU/L at 37 °C.
1 month–5 years: 150–360 IU/L at 37 °C.
5–8 years: 150–300 IU/L at 37 °C.
8–12 years: 130–300 IU/L at 37 °C.
12–14 years: 130–280 IU/L at 37 °C.
14–16 years: 130–230 IU/L at 37 °C.
Adult males: 70–178 IU/L at 37 °C.
Adult females: 42–166 IU/L at 37 °C.

Lactate Dehydrogenase Isoenzymes (S)
LDH$_1$ (heart): 24–34%.
LDH$_2$ (heart, red cells): 35–45%.
LDH$_3$ (muscle): 15–25%.
LDH$_4$ (liver [trace], muscle): 4–10%.
LDH$_5$ (liver, muscle): 1–9%.

LDH: See Lactate Dehydrogenase.

Lead (B)
< 30 μg/dL (< 1.4 μmol/L).

Leucine Aminopeptidase (S, P)
Up to 1 month: 29–59 IU/L.
Thereafter: 15–50 IU/L.

Lipase (S, P)
20–136 IU/L based on 4-hour incubation.

Lipoprotein Cholesterol, High-Density (HDL) (S)
Values in mg/dL (mmol/L).

Group	Males	Females
6–7 years	35–77 (0.90–1.98)	24–76 (0.62–1.96)
8–9 years	31–80 (0.80–2.06)	34–77 (0.87–1.98)
10–11 years	34–81 (0.87–1.09)	30–74 (0.77–1.91)
12–13 years	30–82 (0.77–2.11)	33–73 (0.85–1.88)
14–15 years	26–72 (0.67–1.86)	29–73 (0.74–1.88)
16–17 years	25–66 (0.72–1.70)	27–78 (0.69–2.01)

Lipoprotein Cholesterol, Low-Density (LDL) (S)
Values in mg/dL (mmol/L).

Table 39–2 (cont'd). Normal blood chemistry values and miscellaneous other hematologic values.[1]
(Values may vary with the procedure employed.)

Group	Males	Females
6–7 years	56–134 (1.44–3.46)	52–149 (1.34–3.85)
8–9 years	52–129 (1.34–3.33)	57–143 (1.47–3.69)
10–11 years	45–149 (1.16–3.85)	56–140 (1.44–3.61)
12–13 years	55–135 (1.42–3.48)	58–138 (1.49–3.56)
14–15 years	48–143 (1.24–3.69)	47–140 (1.21–3.61)
16–17 years	53–134 (1.36–3.36)	44–147 (1.13–3.79)

Magnesium (RBC)
3.92–5.28 meq/L (1.96–2.64 mmol/L).

Magnesium (S, P)
Newborns: 1.5–2.3 meq/L (0.75–1.15 mmol/L).
Adults: 1.4–2 meq/L (0.7–1 mmol/L).

Manganese (S)
Newborns: 2.4–9.6 μg/dL (0.44–1.75 μmol/L).
2–18 years: 0.8–1.2 μg/dL (0.15–0.38 μmol/L).

Methemoglobin (B)
0–0.3 g/dL (0–186 μmol/L).

Osmolality (S, P)
270–290 mosm/kg.

Oxygen Capacity (B)
1.34 mL/g of hemoglobin.

Oxygen Saturation (B)
Newborns: 30–80% (0.3–0.8 mol/mol of venous blood).
Thereafter: 65–85% (0.65–0.85 mol/mol of venous blood).

Paco₂: See Acid-Base Measurements.

Pao₂: See Acid-Base Measurements.

Partial Thromboplastin Time (P)
Children: 42–54 seconds.

pH: See Acid-Base Measurements.

Phenylalanine (S, P)
0.7–3.5 mg/dL (0.04–0.21 mmol/L).

Phosphatase: See Acid Phosphatase and Alkaline Phosphatase.

Phospholipid (S)
Cord blood: 48–160 mg/dL (0.62–2.07 mmol/L).
2–13 years: 166–247 mg/dL (2.14–3.19 mmol/L).
13–20 years: 193–338 mg/dL (2.49–4.37 mmol/L).

Phosphorus, Inorganic (S, P)
Premature infants:
At birth: 5.6–8 mg/dL (1.81–2.58 mmol/L).

6–10 days: 6.1–11.7 mg/dL (1.97–3.78 mmol/L).
20–25 days: 6.6–9.4 mg/dL (2.13–3.04 mmol/L).
Full-term infants:
At birth: 5–7.8 mg/dL (1.61–2.52 mmol/L).
3 days: 5.8–9 mg/dL (1.87–2.91 mmol/L).
6–12 days: 4.9–8.9 mg/dL (1.58–2.87 mmol/L).
Children:
1 year: 3.8–6.2 mg/dL (1.23–2 mmol/L).
10 years: 3.6–5.6 mg/dL (1.16–1.81 mmol/L).
Adults: 3.1–5.1 mg/dL (1–1.65 mmol/L).
(See also Glucose Tolerance Test.)

Potassium (RBC)
87.2–97.6 mmol/L.

Potassium (S, P)
Premature infants: 4.5–7.2 mmol/L.
Full-term infants: 3.7–5.2 mmol/L.
Children: 3.5–5.8 mmol/L.
Adults: 3.5–5.5 mmol/L.

Prealbumin: See Transthyretin.

Proaccelerin (Factor V) (P)
Children: 61–127 units/dL.

Prostaglandin E (P)
Newborns: 1000–1730 pg/mL.
2–3 days: 60–150 pg/mL.
1–6 years: 125–200 pg/mL.
6–14 years: 160–340 pg/mL.
Adults: 450–550 pg/mL.

Proteins (S)
(See Table, bottom of page).

Prothrombin (Factor II) (P)
Children: 81–123 units/dL.

Prothrombin Time (P)
Children: 11–15 seconds.

Protoporphyrin, "Free" (FEP, ZPP) (B)
Values for free erythrocyte protoporphyrin (FEP) and zinc protoporphyrin (ZPP) are 1.2–2.7 μg/g of hemoglobin.

Pseudocholinesterase (S)
2.5–5 μmol/mL/min.

Pyruvate (B)
Resting adult males (arterial blood); 50.5–60.1 μmol/L.
Adults (venous blood): 34–102 μmol/L.

Pyruvate Kinase (RBC)
7.4–15.7 units/g of hemoglobin.

Proteins in serum.

Values are for cellulose acetate electrophoresis and are in g/dL. SI conversion factor: g/dL × 10 = g/L.

Group	Total Protein	Albumin	α₁-Globulin	α₂-Globulin	β-Globulin	γ-Globulin
At birth	4.6–7.0	3.2–4.8	0.1–0.3	0.2–0.3	0.3–0.6	0.6–1.2
3 months	4.5–6.5	3.2–4.8	0.1–0.3	0.3–0.7	0.3–0.7	0.2–0.7
1 year	5.4–7.5	3.7–5.7	0.1–0.3	0.5–1.1	0.4–1.0	0.2–0.9
> 4 years	5.9–8.0	3.8–5.4	0.1–0.3	0.4–0.8	0.5–1.0	0.4–1.3

Table 39–2 (cont'd.). Normal blood chemistry values and miscellaneous other hematologic values.[1]
(Values may vary with the procedure employed.)

Renin Activity (P)
3–6 days: 8–14 ng/mL/h.
0–3 years: 3–6 ng/mL/h.
Children: 1.3–2.6 ng/mL/h.

Sedimentation Rate (Micro) (B)
< 2 years: 1–5 mm/h.
> 2 years: 1–8 mm/h.

Serotonin (S, P)
Children: 127–187 ng/mL.
Adults: 119–171 ng/mL.

SGOT: See Aspartate Aminotransferase.

SGPT: See Alanine Aminotransferase.

Sodium (S, P)
Children and adults: 135–148 mmol/L.

Sugar: See Glucose.

T_3: See Triiodothyronine.

T_4: See Thyroxine.

TBG: See Thyroxine-Binding Globulin.

Thrombin Time (P)
Children: 12–16 seconds.

Thyroid-Stimulating Hormone (TSH) (S)
Levels increase shortly after birth to levels as high as 30–40 μIU/mL. Levels return to the adult normal range (1.6–10.9 μIU/mL) by about 10–14 days.

Thyroxine (T_4) (S)
1–2 days: 11.4–25.5 μg/dL (147–328 nmol/L).
3–4 days: 9.8–25.2 μg/dL (126–324 nmol/L).
1–6 years: 5–15.2 μg/dL (64–196 nmol/L).
11–13 years: 4–13 μg/dL (51–167 nmol/L).
> 18 years: 4.7–11 μg/dL (60–142 nmol/L).

Thyroxine, "Free" (Free T_4) (S)
1–2.3 ng/dL.

Thyroxine-Binding Globulin (TBG) (S)
1–7 months: 2.9–6 mg/dL.
7–12 months: 2.1–5.9 mg/dL.
Prepubertal children: 2–5.3 mg/dL.
Pubertal children and adults: 1.8–4.2 mg/dL.

α – Tocopherol: See Vitamin E.

Transaminase: See Alanine Aminotransferase and Asparate Aminotransferase.

Transthyretin (S, P)
2–5 months: 14–33 mg/dL
6–11 months: 12–27 mg/dL
12–17 months: 11–26 mg/dL
18–23 months: 14–24 mg/dL
24–36 months: 11–26 mg/dL

Triglyceride (S, P)
Fasting (> 12 hour) values in mg/mL (mmol/L)

Group	Males	Females
6–7 years	32–79 (0.36–0.89)	24–128 (0.27–1.44)
8–9 years	28–105 (0.31–1.18)	34–115 (0.38–1.29)
10–11 years	30–115 (0.33–1.29)	39–131 (0.44–1.48)
12–13 years	33–112 (0.37–1.26)	36–125 (0.40–1.41)
14–15 years	35–136 (0.39–1.53)	36–122 (0.40–1.37)
16–17 years	38–167 (0.42–1.88)	34–136 (0.38–1.53)

Note: Lower values represent 5th percentile, whereas upper values are calculated from mean + 2 SD.

Triiodothyronine (T_3) (S)
1–3 days: 89–405 ng/dL.
1 week: 91–300 ng/dL.
1–12 months: 85–250 ng/dL.
Prepubertal children: 119–218 ng/dL.
Pubertal children and adults: 55–170 ng/dL.

TSH: See Thyroid-Stimulating Hormone.

Tyrosine (S, P)
Premature infants: 3–30.2 mg/dL (0.17–1.67 mmol/L).
Full-term infants: 1.7–4.7 mg/dL (0.09–0.26 mmol/L).
1–12 years: 1.4–3.4 mg/dL (0.08–0.19 mmol/L).
Adults: 0.6–1.6 mg/dL (0.03–0.09 mmol/L).

Urea Clearance
Premature infants: 3.5–17.3 mL/min/1.73 m².
Newborns: 8.7–33 mL/min/1.73 m².
2–12 months: 40–95 mL/min/1.73 m².
≥ 2 years: > 52 mL/min/1.73 m².

Urea Nitrogen (S, P)
1–2 years: 5–15 mg/dL (1.8–5.4 mmol/L).
Thereafter: 10–20 mg/dL (3.5–7.1 mmol/L).

Uric Acid (S, P)
Males:
0–14 years: 2–7 mg/dL (119–416 μmol/L).
> 14 years: 3–8 mg/dL (178–476 μmol/L).
Females:
0–14 years: 2–7 mg/dL (119–416 μmol/L).
> 14 years: 2–7 mg/dL (119–416 μmol/L).

Vitamin A (S, P)
Total vitamin A: 19–81 μg/dL (0.66–2.82 μmol/L).
Retinol: 19–77 μg/dL (0.66–2.68 μmol/L).
Retinyl esters: 0.1–4.7 μg/dL (0.01–0.16 μmol/L).

Vitamin B_{12} (S, P)
330–1025 pg/ml (243–756 pmol/L).

Vitamin C (Ascorbic Acid) (S, P)
0.2–2 mg/dL (11–114 μmol/L).

Vitamin D (S)
1,25-Dihydroxycholecalciferol:
Normal: 37 ± 12 pg/mL.
X-linked vitamin D-resistant disease: 16 ± 8 pg/mL.
Vitamin D dependency: 9.5 ± 3 pg/mL in type I. Normal in type II.
Hypophosphatemic bone disease: 30 ± 6 pg/mL.
Lead poisoning: 20 ± 1 pg/mL.
25-Hydroxycholecalciferol:
Normal: 26–31 ng/mL.

Vitamin E (Tocopherol) (S, P)
Alpha-tocopherol:
< 12 y 3.8–15.5 μg/mL (9.1–37.2 μmol/L).
> 12 y 4.7–203 μg/mL (11.3–48.7 μmol/L).

Table 39–2 (cont'd). Normal blood chemistry values and miscellaneous other hematologic values.[1]
(Values may vary with the procedure employed.)

Gamma-tocopherol:
  The gamma isomer contributes 10–20% of the total tocopherols in plasma but is only 10% as active as the alpha form in vivo.
Vitamin E status is best assessed by performing chromatographic separation of the isomers and determining both alpha and gamma tocopherol levels. Levels should be expressed in terms of vitamin E/total lipid ratio:

  < 12 y > 0.6 mg/g (> 1.4 μmol/g)
  > 12 y > 0.8 mg/g (> 1.9 μmol/g)

Volume (B)
  Premature infants: 98 mL/kg (mean).
  Full-term infants: 75–100 mL/kg.
  1 year: 69–112 mL/kg (mean, 86 mL/kg).
  Older children: 51–86 mL/kg (mean, 70 mL/kg).

Volume (P)
  Full-term neonates: 39–77 mL/kg.
  Infants: 40–50 mL/kg.
  Older children: 30–54 mL/kg.

Water (B, S, RBC)
  Whole blood: 79–81 g/dL.
  Serum: 91–92 g/dL.
  Red blood cells: 64–65 g/dL.

Xylose Absorption Test (B)
  Following a 5-g loading dose, the laboratory will report the D-xylose concentration of the baseline and 60-minute samples in mg/dL. The difference between these 2 values should be corrected to a constant surface area of 1.73 m^2 according to the formula shown below.
  The actual surface area can be derived from a number of available nomograms using the patient's weight and height.
  Normal corrected blood values:[1] 9.8–20 mg/dL.
  Effect of age and sex: No significant differences between males and females. No significant differences in ages 14–92.

[1]Corrected blood value $= \dfrac{(\text{Value}_{60\ min} - \text{Value}_{baseline}) \times \text{Actual surface area}}{1.73}$

Zinc (S)
  Males: 83–88 μg/dL (12.7–13.5 μmol/L).
  Females: 85–91 μg/dL (13–13.9 μmol/L).
  Females taking oral contraceptives: 86–93 μg/dL (13.2–14.2 μmol/L).
  At 16 weeks of gestation: 66–70 μg/dL (10.1–10.7 μmol/L).
  At 38 weeks of gestation: 54–58 μg/dL (8.3–8.9 μmol/L).

Table 39–3. Normal values: Urine, bone marrow, duodenal fluid, feces, sweat, and miscellaneous.[1]

Urine

Acidity, Titratable
  20–50 meq/d.

Addis Count
  Red cells (12-hour specimen): < 1 million.
  White cells (12-hour specimen): < 2 million.
  Casts (12-hour specimen): < 10,000.
  Protein (12-hour specimen): < 55 mg.

Albumin
  First month: 1–100 mg/L.
  Second month: 0.2–34 mg/L.
  2–12 months: 0.5–19 mg/L.

Aldosterone
  Newborns: 0.5–5 μg/24 h (20–140 μg/g of creatinine).
  Prepubertal children: 1–8 μg/24 h (4–22 μg/g of creatinine).
  Adults: 3–19 μg/24 h (1.5–20 μg/g of creatinine).

Amino Acids
  (See Table 39–1.)

δ-Aminolevulinic Acid: See Porphyrins.

Ammonia
  2–12 months: 4–20 μeq/min/m^2.
  1–16 years: 6–16 μeq/min/m^2.

Calcium
  4–12 years: 4–8 meq/L (2–4 mmol/L).

Catecholamines (Norepinephrine, Epinephrine)
  Values in μg/24 in (nmol/24 h).
  (See Table, bottom of page.)

Chloride
  Infants: 1.7–8.5 mmol/24 h.
  Children: 17–34 mmol/24 h.
  Adults: 140–240 mmol/24 h.

Copper
  0–30 μg/24 h.

Coproporphyrin: See Porphyrins.

Corticosteroids (17-Hydroxycorticosteroids)
  0–2 years: 2–4 mg/24 h (5.5–11 μmol).
  2–6 years: 3–6 mg/24 h (8.3–16.6 μmol).
  6–10 years: 6–8 mg/24 h (16.6–22.1 μmol).
  10–14 years: 8–10 mg/24 h (22.1–27.6 μmol).

Creatine
  18–58 mg/L (1.37–4.42 mmol/L).

Creatinine
  Newborns: 7–10 mg/kg/24 h.
  Children: 20–30 mg/kg/24 h.
  Adult males: 21–26 mg/kg/24 h.
  Adult females: 16–22 mg/kg/24 h.

Epinephrine: See Catecholamines.

Homovanillic Acid
  Children: 3–16 μg/mg of creatinine.
  Adults: 2–4 μg/mg of creatinine.

[1]Adapted from Meites S (editor): *Pediatric Clinical Chemistry*, 2nd ed. American Association for Clinical Chemistry, 1982, and many other sources.

Table 39–3 (cont'd.). Normal values: Urine, duodenal fluid, feces, sweat, and miscellaneous.[1]

17-Hydroxycorticosteroids: See Corticosteroids.

5-Hydroxyindoleacetic Acid
0.11–0.61 µmol/kg/7 h, based on results in 15 well-nourished, apparently healthy, mentally defective children on a tryptophan load.

Hydroxyproline, Total
5–14 years: 38–126 mg/24 h (290–961 µmol/24 h).

Mercury
< 50 µg/24 h (249 nmol/24 h).

Metanephrine and Normetanephrine
< 2 years: < 4.6 µg/mg of creatinine (23.3 nmol).
2–10 years: < 3 µg/mg of creatinine (15.2 nmol).
10–15 years: < 2 µg/mg of creatinine (10.3 nmol).
> 15 years: < 1 µg/mg of creatinine (5.1 nmol).

Mucopolysaccharides
Acid mucopolysaccharide screen should yield negative results. Positive results after dialysis of the urine should be followed up with a thin-layer chromatogram for evaluation of the acid mucopolysaccharide excretion pattern.

Norepinephrine: See Catecholamines.

Normetanephrine: See Metanephrine and Normetanephrine.

Osmolality
Infants: 50–600 mosm/L.
Older children: 50–1400 mosm/L.

Phosphorus, Tubular Reabsorption
78–97%.

Porphobilinogen: See Porphyrins.

Porphyrins
δ-Aminolevulinic acid: 0–7 mg/24 h (0–53.4 µmol/24 h).
Porphobilinogen: 0–2 mg/24 h (0–8.8 µmol/24 h).
Coproporphyrin: 0–160 µg/24 h (0–244 nmol/24 h).
Uroporphyrin: 0–26 µg/24 h (0–31 nmol/24 h).

Potassium
26–123 mmol/L.

Pregnanetriol
2 weeks–2 years: 0–0.2 mg/24 h (0–0.59 µmol/24 h).
2–16 years: 0.3–1.1 mg/24 h (0.89–3.27 µmol/24 h).

Sodium
Infants: 0.3–3.5 mmol/24 h (6–10 mmol/m²).
Children and adults: 5.6–17 mmol/24 h.

Testosterone
Prepubertal children: 0.2–2.3 µg/24 h (0.3–5 µg/g of creatinine).

Adult males: 40–130 µg/24 h.
Adult females: 2–11 µg/24 h.

Urobilinogen
< 3 mg/24 h (< 5.1 µmol/24 h).

Uroporphyrin: See Porphyrins.

Vanilmandelic Acid (VMA)
Because of the difficulty in obtaining an accurately timed 24-hour collection, values based on microgram per milligram of creatinine are the most reliable indications of VMA excretion in young children.
1–12 months: 1–35 µg/mg of creatinine (31–135 µg/kg/24 h).
1–2 years: 1–30 µg/mg of creatinine.
2–5 years: 1–15 µg/mg of creatinine.
5–10 years: 1–14 µg/mg of creatinine.
10–15 years: 1–10 µg/mg of creatinine.
Adults: 1–7 µg/mg of creatinine (1–7 mg/24 h; 5–35 µmol/24 h).

VMA: See Vanilmandelic Acid.

Xylose Absorption Test
Mean 5-hour excretion expressed as percentage of ingested load.
< 6 months: 11–30%.
6–12 months: 20–32%.

Xylose Absorption (cont'd)
1–3 years: 20–42%.
3–10 years: 25–45%.
> 10 years: 25–50%.
Or: % excretion > (0.2 × age in months) + 12.

Duodenal Fluid Value

Enzymes
Amylase: (Anderson).
  0–2 months: 0–10 units/mL.
  2–6 months: 10–20 units/mL.
  6–12 months: 40–150 units/mL.
  1–2 years: 100–225 units/mL.
  2–5 years: 125–275 units/mL.
Carboxypeptidase:
  0.4–1 unit (Ravin).
Chymotrypsin:
  11–65 units (Ravin).
Protease:
  18–70 units (Free-Meyers).
Trypsin: (Anderson or as noted).
  0–2 months: 110–160 units/mL.
  2–6 months: 115–160 units/mL.
  6–12 months: 120–290 units/mL; 3–10 units (Nothman et al).
  1–2 years: 200–300 units/mL.
  2–5 years: 200–275 units/mL.

Catecholamines in urine.

Group	Total Catecholamines	Norepinephrine	Epinephrine
< 1 year	20	5.4–15.9 (32–94)	0.1–4.3 (0.5–23.5)
1–5 years	40	8.1–30.8 (48–182)	0.8–9.1 (4.4–49.7)
6–15 years	80	19.0–71.1 (112–421)	1.3–10.5 (7.1–57.3)
> 15 years	100	34.4–87.0 (203–514)	3.5–13.2 (19.1–72.1)

Table 39–3 (cont'd.). Normal values: Urine, duodenal fluid, feces, sweat, and miscellaneous.[1]

pH
 6–8.4.

Viscosity
 < 3 minutes (Shwachman).

Feces

Chymotrypsin
 3–14 mg/kg 72 h.

Fat, Percentage of Dry Weight
 2–6 months: 5–43%.
 6 months–6 years: 6–26%.

Fat, Total
 2–6 months: 0.3–1.3 g/d.
 6 months–1 year: < 4 g/d.
 Children: < 3 g/d.
 Adolescents: < 5 g/d.
 Adults: < 7 g/d.

Lipids, Split Fat
 Adults: > 40% of total lipids.

Lipids, Total
 Adults: Up to 7 g/d on normal diet, 10–27% of dry weight.

Nitrogen
 Infants: < 1 g/d.
 Children: < 1.2 g/d.
 Adults: < 3 g/d.

Urobilinogen
 2–12 months: 0.03–14 mg/d.
 5–10 years: 2.7–39 mg/d.
 10–14 years: 7.3–99 mg/d.

Sweat

Electrolytes
 Values for sodium or chloride or both. Elevated values in the presence of a family history or clinical findings of cystic fibrosis are diagnostic of cystic fibrosis.

Normal: < 55 mmol/L.
Borderline: 55–70 mmol/L.
Elevated: > 70 mmol/L.

Miscellaneous

Amylo-1,6-Glucosidase Debrancher (Liver)
 > 1 μmol/min/g of wet tissue.

Chloride
 Breast milk: 2.5–30 mmol/L.
 Cow's milk: 20–80 mmol/L.
 Muscle: 20–26 mmol/kg of wet-free tissue.
 Spinal fluid: 120–128 mmol/L.

Copper (Liver)
 < 20 μg/g of wet tissue.

Glucose 6-Phosphatase (Liver)
 > 5 μmol/min/g of wet tissue.

Lactate Dehydrogenase (LDH) (CSF)
 17–59 IU/L at 37 °C.

Potassium
 Breast milk: 12–17 mmol/L.
 Cow's milk: 20–45 mmol/L.
 Muscle: 160–180 mmol/kg of wet fat-free tissue.

Proteins (CSF)
 Total proteins:
  Newborn: 40–120 mg/dL (0.4–1.2 g/L).
  1 month: 20–70 mg/dL (0.2–0.7 g/L.
  Thereafter: 15–40 mg/dL (0.15–0.4 g/L).
 Gamma globulin:
  Children: Up to 9% of total.
  Adults: UP to 14% of total.

Sodium
 Breast milk: 4.7–8.3 mmol/L.
 Cow's milk: 22–26 mmol/L.
 Muscle: 33–43 mmol/kg of wet fat-free tissue.

Index